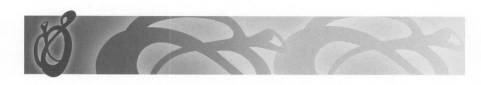

BRAUNWALD'S
HEART DISEASE

A Textbook of Cardiovascular Medicine

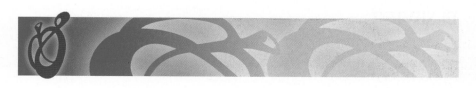

BRAUNWALD'S
HEART DISEASE
A Textbook of Cardiovascular Medicine
VOLUME II
NINTH EDITION

Edited by

Robert O. Bonow, MD
Max and Lilly Goldberg Distinguished Professor of Cardiology
Vice Chairman, Department of Medicine
Director, Center for Cardiac Innovation
Northwestern University Feinberg School of Medicine
Chicago, Illinois

Douglas L. Mann, MD
Lewin Chair and Professor of Medicine, Cell Biology, and Physiology
Chief, Division of Cardiology
Washington University School of Medicine in St. Louis
Cardiologist-in-Chief
Barnes-Jewish Hospital
Saint Louis, Missouri

Douglas P. Zipes, MD
Distinguished Professor
Professor Emeritus of Medicine, Pharmacology, and Toxicology
Director Emeritus, Division of Cardiology and the Krannert Institute of Cardiology
Indiana University School of Medicine
Indianapolis, Indiana

Peter Libby, MD
Mallinckrodt Professor of Medicine
Harvard Medical School
Chief, Cardiovascular Division
Brigham and Women's Hospital
Boston, Massachusetts

Founding Editor and Online Editor

Eugene Braunwald, MD, MD(Hon), ScD(Hon), FRCP
Distinguished Hersey Professor of Medicine
Harvard Medical School
Chairman, TIMI Study Group
Brigham and Women's Hospital
Boston, Massachusetts

ELSEVIER
SAUNDERS

ELSEVIER
SAUNDERS

1600 John F. Kennedy Blvd.
Ste. 1800
Philadelphia, PA 19103-2899

Notices

Knowledge and best practice in this field are constantly changing. As new research and experience
broaden our understanding, changes in research methods, professional practices, or medical
treatment may become necessary.

Practitioners and researchers must always rely on their own experience and knowledge in
evaluating and using any information, methods, compounds, or experiments described herein. In
using such information or methods they should be mindful of their own safety and the safety of
others, including parties for whom they have a professional responsibility.

With respect to any drug or pharmaceutical products identified, readers are advised to check the
most current information provided (i) on procedures featured or (ii) by the manufacturer of each
product to be administered, to verify the recommended dose or formula, the method and duration
of administration, and contraindications. It is the responsibility of practitioners, relying on their own
experience and knowledge of their patients, to make diagnoses, to determine dosages and the best
treatment for each individual patient, and to take all appropriate safety precautions.

To the fullest extent of the law, neither the Publisher nor the authors, contributors, or editors,
assume any liability for any injury and/or damage to persons or property as a matter of products
liability, negligence or otherwise, or from any use or operation of any methods, products, instructions,
or ideas contained in the material herein.

Library of Congress Cataloging-in-Publication Data
Robert O. Bonow … [et al.].—9th ed.
    p. ; cm.
    Heart disease
    Includes bibliographical references and index.
    ISBN 978-1-4377-0398-6 (single volume : hardcover : alk. paper)—ISBN 978-1-4377-2708-1 (two-volume
set : hardcover : alk. paper)—ISBN 978-0-8089-2436-4 (international ed. : hardcover : alk. paper)
    1. Heart—Diseases. 2. Cardiology. I. Braunwald, Eugene, 1929- II. Bonow, Robert O. III. Title: Heart
disease.
    [DNLM: 1. Heart Diseases. 2. Cardiovascular Diseases. WG 210]
    RC681.H36 2012
    616.1'2—dc22

                            2010044324

Executive Publisher: Natasha Andjelkovic
Developmental Editor: Anne Snyder
Publishing Services Manager: Patricia Tannian
Team Manager: Radhika Pallamparthy
Senior Project Manager: Sarah Wunderly
Project Manager: Joanna Dhanabalan
Design Direction: Steven Stave

Printed in China

Last digit is the print number: 9 8 7 6 5 4 3 2 1

BS

11/29/12

Dedication

We are proud to dedicate the ninth edition of *Braunwald's Heart Disease* to its founder, Eugene Braunwald, MD. The first edition of this work, published 30 years ago, established a standard of excellence that is rarely, if ever, achieved in publishing. Dr. Braunwald personally wrote half of the book and expertly edited the rest. He did the same for the next four editions, taking a 6-month sabbatical every 4 to 5 years to accomplish that. For the sixth edition, published in 2001, he invited two of us (PL, DPZ) to share the experience with him, increasing the editors by one (ROB) for the seventh edition. A new editor (DLM) joined for the eighth edition, and Dr. Braunwald no longer directly participated in the day-to-day editing of the print text, while still contributing some of the key chapters. However, he kept his finger on the pulse of the text and for that edition began *twice-weekly* electronic updates. Incorporating the most recent research, reviews, and opinions into the electronic text has continued through this ninth edition, making *Braunwald's Heart Disease* truly a living work and setting it apart from other texts. Dr. Braunwald, through his research, teaching, and mentorship, has shaped much of contemporary cardiovascular medicine, and it is with gratitude and admiration that we dedicate this edition of *his work* to him.

Robert O. Bonow

Douglas L. Mann

Douglas P. Zipes

Peter Libby

Acknowledgments

The editors gratefully acknowledge communication and correspondence from colleagues all over the world who have offered insightful suggestions to improve this text. We particularly wish to acknowledge the following individuals who have provided careful and studious commentary on numerous chapters: Shabnam Madadi, MD, Cardiac Imaging Center, Shahid Rajaei Heart Center, Tehran, Iran; Azin Alizadeh Asl, MD, Tabriz University of Medical Sciences and Madani Heart Hospital, Tabriz, Iran; Leili Pourafkari, MD, Razi Hospital, Tabriz, Iran; Banasiak Waldemar, MD, Centre for Heart Disease, Military Hospital, Wroclaw, Poland; Carlos Benjamín Alvarez, MD, PhD, Sacré Coeur Institute, Buenos Aires, Argentina; Elias B. Hanna, MD, Division of Cardiology, Louisiana State University, New Orleans, Louisiana.

We are also indebted to Dr. Jun-o Deguchi, Dr. Michael Markl, Dr. Vera Rigolin, and Dr. Carol Warnes for the images used on the cover.

Dr. Libby thanks Sara Karwacki for expert editorial assistance.

To:

Pat, Rob, and Sam

Laura, Stephanie, Jonathan, and Erica

Joan, Debra, Jeffrey, and David

Beryl, Oliver, and Brigitte

CONTRIBUTORS

William T. Abraham, MD
Professor of Internal Medicine, Physiology, and Cell Biology; Chair of Excellence in Cardiovascular Medicine; Director, Division of Cardiovascular Medicine; Deputy Director, The Davis Heart and Lung Research Institute, The Ohio State University, Columbus, Ohio
Devices for Monitoring and Managing Heart Failure

Michael A. Acker, MD
Professor of Surgery, University of Pennsylvania School of Medicine; Chief, Division of Cardiovascular Surgery, University of Pennsylvania Medical Center, Philadelphia, Pennsylvania
Surgical Management of Heart Failure

Michael J. Ackerman, MD, PhD
Professor of Medicine, Pediatrics, and Pharmacology; Consultant, Cardiovascular Diseases and Pediatric Cardiology; Director, Long QT Syndrome Clinic and the Windland Smith Rice Sudden Death Genomics Laboratory, Mayo Clinic, Rochester, Minnesota
Genetics of Cardiac Arrhythmias

Philip A. Ades, MD
Professor of Medicine, Division of Cardiology, Fletcher-Allen Health Care, University of Vermont College of Medicine, Burlington, Vermont
Exercise and Sports Cardiology

Elliott M. Antman, MD
Professor of Medicine, Harvard Medical School; Senior Investigator, TIMI Study Group, Brigham and Women's Hospital, Boston, Massachusetts
Design and Conduct of Clinical Trials; ST-Segment Elevation Myocardial Infarction: Pathology, Pathophysiology, and Clinical Features; ST-Segment Elevation Myocardial Infarction: Management; Guidelines: Management of Patients with ST-Segment Elevation Myocardial Infarction

Piero Anversa, MD
Professor of Anesthesia and Medicine; Director, Center for Regenerative Medicine, Brigham and Women's Hospital, Harvard Medical School, Boston, Massachusetts
Cardiovascular Regeneration and Tissue Engineering

Gary J. Balady, MD
Professor of Medicine, Boston University School of Medicine; Director, Non-Invasive Cardiovascular Laboratories, Section of Cardiology, Boston Medical Center, Boston, Massachusetts
Exercise and Sports Cardiology

Kenneth L. Baughman, MD (deceased)
Professor of Medicine, Harvard Medical School; Director, Advanced Heart Disease, Division of Cardiovascular Medicine, Brigham and Women's Hospital, Boston, Massachusetts
Myocarditis

Joshua Beckman, MD, MSc
Assistant Professor of Medicine, Harvard Medical School; Director, Cardiovascular Fellowship, Cardiovascular Division, Brigham and Women's Hospital, Boston, Massachusetts
Anesthesia and Noncardiac Surgery in Patients with Heart Disease; Guidelines: Reducing Cardiac Risk with Noncardiac Surgery

Michael A. Bettmann, MD
Professor and Vice Chair for Interventional Services, Department of Radiology, Wake Forest University Baptist Medical Center, Medical Center Boulevard, Winston-Salem, North Carolina
The Chest Radiograph in Cardiovascular Disease

Deepak L. Bhatt, MD, MPH
Associate Professor of Medicine, Harvard Medical School; Chief of Cardiology, VA Boston Healthcare System; Director, Integrated Interventional Cardiovascular Program, Brigham and Women's Hospital & VA Boston Healthcare System; Senior Investigator, TIMI Study Group, Brigham and Women's Hospital, Boston, Massachusetts
Percutaneous Coronary Intervention; Guidelines: Percutaneous Coronary Intervention; Endovascular Treatment of Noncoronary Obstructive Vascular Disease

William E. Boden, MD
Professor of Medicine and Preventive Medicine; Clinical Chief, Division of Cardiovascular Medicine, University at Buffalo Schools of Medicine & Public Health; Medical Director, Cardiovascular Services, Kaleida Health; Chief of Cardiology, Buffalo General and Millard Fillmore Hospitals, Buffalo, New York
Stable Ischemic Heart Disease; Guidelines: Chronic Stable Angina

Robert O. Bonow, MD
Max and Lilly Goldberg Distinguished Professor of Cardiology; Vice Chairman, Department of Medicine; Director, Center for Cardiovascular Innovation, Northwestern University Feinberg School of Medicine, Chicago, Illinois
Cardiac Catheterization; Nuclear Cardiology; Guidelines: Infective Endocarditis; Care of Patients with End-Stage Heart Disease; Valvular Heart Disease; Guidelines: Management of Valvular Heart Disease; Appropriate Use Criteria: Echocardiography

Eugene Braunwald, MD, MD(Hon), ScD(Hon), FRCP
Distinguished Hersey Professor of Medicine, Harvard Medical School; Founding Chairman, TIMI Study Group, Brigham and Women's Hospital, Boston, Massachusetts
Unstable Angina and Non–ST Elevation Myocardial Infarction; Guidelines: Unstable Angina and Non–ST Elevation Myocardial Infarction

Alan C. Braverman, MD
Alumni Endowed Professor in Cardiovascular Diseases; Professor of Medicine; Director, Marfan Syndrome Clinic; Director, Inpatient Cardiology Firm, Washington University School of Medicine, St. Louis, Missouri
Diseases of the Aorta

J. Douglas Bremner, MD
Professor of Psychiatry and Radiology, Department of Psychiatry and Behavioral Sciences, Emory University School of Medicine & Atlanta VAMC, Atlanta, Georgia
Psychiatric and Behavioral Aspects of Cardiovascular Disease

Hugh Calkins, MD
Nicholas J. Fortuin Professor of Cardiology; Professor of Medicine, The Johns Hopkins Medical University School of Medicine; Director of the Arrhythmia Service and Clinical Electrophysiology Laboratory, The Johns Hopkins Hospital, Baltimore, Maryland
Hypotension and Syncope

Christopher P. Cannon, MD
Associate Professor of Medicine, Harvard Medical School; Senior Investigator, TIMI Study Group, Cardiovascular Division, Brigham and Women's Hospital, Boston, Massachusetts
Approach to the Patient with Chest Pain; Unstable Angina and Non–ST Elevation Myocardial Infarction; Guidelines: Unstable Angina and Non–ST Elevation Myocardial Infarction

John M. Canty, Jr., MD
Albert and Elizabeth Rekate Professor of Medicine; Chief, Division of Cardiovascular Medicine, University at Buffalo, Buffalo, New York
Coronary Blood Flow and Myocardial Ischemia

Agustin Castellanos, MD
Professor of Medicine, University of Miami Miller School of Medicine; Director, Clinical Electrophysiology, University of Miami/Jackson Memorial Medical Center, Miami, Florida
Cardiac Arrest and Sudden Cardiac Death

Bernard R. Chaitman, MD
Professor of Medicine; Director, Cardiovascular Research, St. Louis University School of Medicine, Division of Cardiology, St. Louis, Missouri
Exercise Stress Testing; Guidelines: Exercise Stress Testing

Ming Hui Chen, MD, MMSc
Assistant Professor of Medicine, Harvard Medical School; Director, Cardiac Health for Hodgkin's Lymphoma Survivors; Associate in Cardiology, Department of Cardiology, Children's Hospital Boston, Boston, Massachusetts
The Cancer Patient and Cardiovascular Disease

Heidi M. Connolly, MD
Professor of Medicine, Mayo Clinic College of Medicine; Consultant, Division of Cardiovascular Diseases, Mayo Clinic, Rochester, Minnesota
Echocardiography

Mark A. Creager, MD
Professor of Medicine, Harvard Medical School; Director, Vascular Center, Brigham and Women's Hospital, Boston, Massachusetts
Peripheral Artery Diseases

Edécio Cunha-Neto, MD, PhD
Associate Professor of Immunology, University of São Paulo; Researcher of the Cardiac Immunology Laboratory, The Heart Institute (INCOR), University of São Paulo Medical School, São Paulo, Brazil
Chagas' Disease

Charles J. Davidson, MD
Professor of Medicine; Medical Director, Bluhm Cardiovascular Institute; Clinical Chief, Division of Cardiology, Northwestern University Feinberg School of Medicine, Chicago, Illinois
Cardiac Catheterization

Vasken Dilsizian, MD
Professor of Medicine and Diagnostic Radiology; Chief, Division of Nuclear Medicine; Director, Cardiovascular Nuclear Medicine and PET Imaging, University of Maryland School of Medicine, Baltimore, Maryland
Nuclear Cardiology

Stefanie Dimmeler, PhD
Professor and Director of the Institute of Cardiovascular Regeneration, Centre for Molecular Medicine, Goethe-University Frankfurt, Frankfurt, Germany
Emerging Therapies and Strategies in the Treatment of Heart Failure

Pamela S. Douglas, MD
Ursula Geller Professor of Research in Cardiovascular Diseases, Division of Cardiovascular Medicine, Duke University Medical Center, Durham, North Carolina
Cardiovascular Disease in Women

Andrew C. Eisenhauer, MD
Assistant Professor of Medicine, Harvard Medical School; Director, Interventional Cardiovascular Medicine Service; Associate Director, Cardiac Catheterization Laboratory, Brigham and Women's Hospital; Director, Cardiac Quality Assurance, Partners Health Care, Boston, Massachusetts
Endovascular Treatment of Noncoronary Obstructive Vascular Disease

Linda L. Emanuel, MD, PhD
Buehler Professor of Geriatric Medicine; Director, The Buehler Center on Aging, Northwestern University Feinberg School of Medicine, Chicago, Illinois
Care of Patients with End-Stage Heart Disease

Edzard Ernst, MD, PhD, FMed Sci, FRCP, FRCP(Edin)
Chair in Complementary Medicine, Peninsula Medical School, University of Exeter, Exeter, United Kingdom
Complementary and Alternative Approaches to Management of Patients with Heart Disease

James C. Fang, MD
Professor of Medicine, Division of Cardiovascular Medicine, Case Western Reserve University School of Medicine, Harrington-McLaughlin Heart and Vascular Institute, University Hospitals, Cleveland, Ohio
The History and Physical Examination: An Evidence-Based Approach

G. Michael Felker, MD, MHS
Associate Professor of Medicine, Division of Cardiology, Duke University School of Medicine, Durham, North Carolina
Diagnosis and Management of Acute Heart Failure Syndromes

Gerasimos S. Filippatos, MD
Head, Heart Failure Unit, Attikon University Hospital, Department of Cardiology, University of Athens, Athens, Greece
Diagnosis and Management of Acute Heart Failure Syndromes

Stacy D. Fisher, MD
Director of Women's and Complex Heart Disease, Department of Cardiology, University of Maryland Comprehensive Heart Center, Baltimore, Maryland
Cardiovascular Abnormalities in HIV-Infected Individuals

Lee A. Fleisher, MD
Roberts D. Dripps Professor and Chair of Anesthesiology and Critical Care; Professor of Medicine, University of Pennsylvania School of Medicine, Philadelphia, Pennsylvania
Anesthesia and Noncardiac Surgery in Patients with Heart Disease; Guidelines: Reducing Cardiac Risk with Noncardiac Surgery

Thomas Force, MD
Wilson Professor of Medicine, Thomas Jefferson University; Clinical Director, Center for Translational Medicine, Thomas Jefferson University Hospital, Philadelphia, Pennsylvania
The Cancer Patient and Cardiovascular Disease

J. Michael Gaziano, MD, MPH
Professor of Medicine, Harvard Medical School; Chief, Division of
Aging, Brigham and Women's Hospital; Director, Massachusetts
Veterans Epidemiology and Research Information Center
(MAVERIC), VA Boston Healthcare System, Boston, Massachusetts
*Global Burden of Cardiovascular Disease; Primary and Secondary
Prevention of Coronary Heart Disease*

Thomas A. Gaziano MD, MSc
Assistant Professor, Harvard Medical School; Associate Physician,
Cardiovascular Medicine, Brigham & Women's Hospital, Boston,
Massachusetts
Global Burden of Cardiovascular Disease

Jacques Genest, MD
Professor of Medicine; Scientific Director, Center for Innovative
Medicine, McGill University Health Center, McGill University,
Montreal, Quebec, Canada
Lipoprotein Disorders and Cardiovascular Disease

Mihai Gheorghiade, MD
Professor of Medicine and Surgery; Director, Experimental
Therapeutics/Center for Cardiovascular Innovation; Northwestern
University Feinberg School of Medicine, Chicago, Illinois;
Co-Director, Duke Cardiovascular Center for Drug Development,
Raleigh, North Carolina
Diagnosis and Management of Acute Heart Failure Syndromes

Ary L. Goldberger, MD
Professor of Medicine, Harvard Medical School & Wyss Institute for
Biologically Inspired Engineering at Harvard University; Director,
Margret and H.A. Rey Institute for Nonlinear Dynamics in
Medicine, Beth Israel Deaconess Medical Center, Boston,
Massachusetts
Electrocardiography; Guidelines: Electrocardiography

Samuel Z. Goldhaber, MD
Professor of Medicine, Harvard Medical School; Director, Venous
Thromboembolism Research Group; Staff Cardiologist,
Cardiovascular Medicine Division, Brigham and Women's Hospital,
Boston, Massachusetts
Pulmonary Embolism

Larry B. Goldstein, MD
Professor, Department of Medicine (Neurology), Duke Stroke Center;
Center for Clinical Health Policy Research, Duke University and
Durham VA Medical Center, Durham, North Carolina
Prevention and Management of Stroke

Richard J. Gray, MD
Medical Director, Sutter Pacific Heart Centers, California Pacific
Medical Center, San Francisco, California
Medical Management of the Patient Undergoing Cardiac Surgery

Barry Greenberg, MD
Professor of Medicine; Director, Advanced Heart Failure Treatment
Program, University of California, San Diego, California
Clinical Assessment of Heart Failure

Bartley P. Griffith, MD
The Thomas E. and Alice Marie Hales Distinguished Professor/
Professor of Surgery & Chief, Division of Cardiac Surgery,
Department of Surgery, Division of Cardiac Surgery, University of
Maryland School of Medicine, Baltimore, Maryland
Assisted Circulation in the Treatment of Heart Failure

William J. Groh, MD, MPH
Associate Professor of Medicine, Division of Cardiology, Indiana
University, Indianapolis, Indiana
Neurologic Disorders and Cardiovascular Disease

Joshua M. Hare, MD
Louis Lemberg Professor of Medicine; Professor of Biomedical
Engineering; Professor of Molecular and Cellular Pharmacology;
Director, Interdisciplinary Stem Cell Institute, University of Miami
Miller School of Medicine, Miami, Florida
The Dilated, Restrictive, and Infiltrative Cardiomyopathies

Gerd Hasenfuss, MD
Professor and Chair, Department of Cardiology and Pneumology,
Heart Center, University of Goettingen; Chair of Heart Research
Center, Goettingen, Germany
Mechanisms of Cardiac Contraction and Relaxation

David L. Hayes, MD
Professor of Medicine, College of Medicine; Consultant, Division of
Cardiovascular Diseases, Mayo Clinic, Rochester, Minnesota
*Pacemakers and Implantable Cardioverter-Defibrillators; Guidelines:
Cardiac Pacemakers and Cardioverter-Defibrillators*

Maria de Lourdes Higuchi, MD
Director of Laboratory of Research on Cardiac Inflammation and
Infection, Heart Institute (INCOR), University of São Paulo Medical
School, São Paulo, Brazil
Chagas' Disease

L. David Hillis, MD
Professor and Chair, Internal Medicine, University of Texas Health
Science Center, San Antonio, Texas
Toxins and the Heart

Farouc A. Jaffer, MD, PhD
Assistant Professor of Medicine, Cardiology Division and
Cardiovascular Research Center, Department of Medicine,
Massachusetts General Hospital, Harvard Medical School, Boston,
Massachusetts
Molecular Imaging in Cardiovascular Disease

Mariell Jessup, MD
Professor of Medicine; Associate Chief for Clinical Affairs,
Cardiovascular Division, University of Pennsylvania School of
Medicine; Medical Director, Penn Heart and Vascular Center,
University of Pennsylvania Health System, Philadelphia,
Pennsylvania
Surgical Management of Heart Failure

Andrew M. Kahn, MD, PhD
Assistant Professor of Medicine, University of California, San Diego,
California
Clinical Assessment of Heart Failure

Jan Kajstura, PhD
Associate Professor, Departments of Anesthesia and Medicine, and
Cardiovascular Division, Brigham and Women's Hospital, Harvard
Medical School, Boston, Massachusetts
Cardiovascular Regeneration and Tissue Engineering

Norman M. Kaplan, MD
Clinical Professor of Internal Medicine, University of Texas
Southwestern Medical Center at Dallas, Dallas, Texas
*Systemic Hypertension: Therapy; Guidelines: Treatment of
Hypertension*

Adolf W. Karchmer, MD
Professor of Medicine, Harvard Medical School; Division of Infectious Disease, Beth Israel Deaconess Medical Center, Boston, Massachusetts
Infective Endocarditis

Irwin Klein, MD
Professor of Medicine and Cell Biology; Associate Chairman, Department of Medicine, North Shore University Hospital, Manhasset, New York
Endocrine Disorders and Cardiovascular Disease

Harlan M. Krumholz, MD, SM
Harold H. Hines, Jr, Professor of Medicine and Epidemiology and Public Health; Section of Cardiovascular Medicine, Department of Medicine, Section of Health Policy and Administration, School of Public Health, Yale University School of Medicine; Center for Outcomes Research and Evaluation, Yale–New Haven Hospital, New Haven, Connecticut
Clinical Decision Making in Cardiology

Raymond Y. Kwong, MD, MPH
Assistant Professor of Medicine, Harvard Medical School; Director of Cardiac Magnetic Resonance Imaging, Cardiovascular Division, Brigham and Women's Hospital, Boston, Massachusetts
Cardiovascular Magnetic Resonance Imaging; Appropriate Use Criteria: Cardiovascular Magnetic Resonance

Philippe L. L'Allier, MD
Associate Professor of Medicine, Department of Medicine; Director, Interventional Cardiology; Desgroseillers-Bérard Chair in Interventional Cardiology, Montreal Heart Institute, University of Montreal, Montreal, Canada
Intravascular Ultrasound Imaging

Richard A. Lange, MD
Professor and Executive Vice Chairman, Medicine, University of Texas Health Science Center, San Antonio, Texas
Toxins and the Heart

Thomas H. Lee, MD
Professor of Medicine, Harvard Medical School; Network President, Partners Healthcare System, Boston, Massachusetts
Measurement and Improvement of Quality of Cardiovascular Care; Guidelines: Pregnancy and Heart Disease

Annarosa Leri, MD
Associate Professor, Departments of Anesthesia and Medicine and Cardiovascular Division, Brigham and Women's Hospital, Harvard Medical School, Boston, Massachusetts
Cardiovascular Regeneration and Tissue Engineering

Martin M. LeWinter, MD
Professor of Medicine and Molecular Physiology and Biophysics; Director, Heart Failure and Cardiomyopathy Program, University of Vermont College of Medicine; Attending Cardiologist, Fletcher Allen Health Care, Burlington, Vermont
Pericardial Diseases

Peter Libby, MD
Mallinckrodt Professor of Medicine, Harvard Medical School; Chief of Cardiovascular Medicine, Brigham and Women's Hospital, Boston, Massachusetts
Molecular Imaging in Cardiovascular Disease; The Vascular Biology of Atherosclerosis; Risk Markers for Atherothrombotic Disease; Lipoprotein Disorders and Cardiovascular Disease; Primary and Secondary Prevention of Coronary Heart Disease; Peripheral Artery Diseases

Steven E. Lipshultz, MD
George Batchelor Professor and Chairman, Department of Pediatrics; Batchelor Family Endowed Chair in Pediatric Cardiology; Professor of Epidemiology and Public Health; Professor of Medicine (Oncology); Associate Executive Dean for Child Health, Leonard M. Miller School of Medicine, University of Miami; Chief-of-Staff, Holtz Children's Hospital of the University of Miami–Jackson Memorial Medical Center; Director, Batchelor Children's Research Institute; Associate Director, Mailman Center for Child Development; Member, the Sylvester Comprehensive Cancer Center, Miami, Florida
Cardiovascular Abnormalities in HIV-Infected Individuals

Peter Liu, MD
Heart & Stroke/Polo Professor of Medicine and Physiology, Peter Munk Cardiac Centre, University Health Network, University of Toronto; Scientific Director, Institute of Circulatory and Respiratory Health, Canadian Institutes of Health Research, Toronto, Ontario, Canada
Myocarditis

Brian F. Mandell, MD, PHD
Professor and Chairman, Department of Medicine, Cleveland Clinic Foundation Lerner College of Medicine of Case Western Reserve University; Center for Vasculitis Care and Research, Department of Rheumatic and Immunologic Disease, The Cleveland Clinic, Cleveland, Ohio
Rheumatic Diseases and the Cardiovascular System

Douglas L. Mann, MD
Lewin Chair and Professor of Medicine, Cell Biology, and Physiology; Chief, Division of Cardiology, Washington University School of Medicine in St. Louis; Cardiologist-in-Chief, Barnes-Jewish Hospital, Saint Louis, Missouri
Pathophysiology of Heart Failure; Management of Heart Failure Patients with Reduced Ejection Fraction; Guidelines: Management of Heart Failure; Emerging Therapies and Strategies in the Treatment of Heart Failure

Barry J. Maron, MD
Director, Hypertrophic Cardiomyopathy Center, Minneapolis Heart Institute Foundation, Minneapolis, Minnesota
Hypertrophic Cardiomyopathy

Kenneth L. Mattox, MD
Professor and Vice Chairman, Distinguished Service Professor, Michael E. DeBakey Department of Surgery, Baylor College of Medicine, Houston, Texas
Traumatic Heart Disease

Peter A. McCullough, MD, MPH
Consultant Cardiologist, Chief Academic and Scientific Officer, St. John Providence Health System, Providence Park Heart Institute, Novi, Michigan
Interface Between Renal Disease and Cardiovascular Illness

Darren K. McGuire, MD, MHSc
Associate Professor, Internal Medicine, The University of Texas Southwestern Medical Center at Dallas, Dallas, Texas
Diabetes and the Cardiovascular System

Bruce McManus, MD, PhD
Professor of Pathology and Laboratory Medicine, Faculty of Medicine, University of British Columbia; Co-Director, Institute for Heart and Lung Health; Director, NCE CECR Centre of Excellence for Prevention of Organ Failure (PROOF Centre); Director, UBC James Hogg Research Centre, St. Paul's Hospital, University of British Columbia, Vancouver, British Columbia, Canada
Primary Tumors of the Heart

Mandeep R. Mehra, MBBS
Dr. Herbert Berger Professor of Medicine and Head of Cardiology; Assistant Dean for Clinical Services, University of Maryland School of Medicine, Baltimore, Maryland
Assisted Circulation in the Treatment of Heart Failure

John M. Miller, MD
Professor of Medicine, Krannert Institute of Cardiology, Indiana University School of Medicine; Director, Clinical Cardiac Electrophysiology, Clarian Health Partners, Indianapolis, Indiana
Diagnosis of Cardiac Arrhythmias; Guidelines: Ambulatory Electrocardiographic and Electrophysiologic Testing; Therapy for Cardiac Arrhythmias

David M. Mirvis, MD
Professor Emeritus, University of Tennessee Health Science Center, Memphis, Tennessee
Electrocardiography; Guidelines: Electrocardiography

Fred Morady, MD
McKay Professor of Cardiovascular Disease; Professor of Medicine, University of Michigan Health System, CVC Cardiovascular Medicine, Ann Arbor, Michigan
Atrial Fibrillation: Clinical Features, Mechanisms, and Management; Guidelines: Atrial Fibrillation

David A. Morrow, MD, MPH
Associate Professor of Medicine, Harvard Medical School; Senior Investigator, TIMI Study Group; Director, Samuel A. Levine Cardiac Unit, Brigham and Women's Hospital, Boston, Massachusetts
ST-Segment Elevation Myocardial Infarction: Management; Stable Ischemic Heart Disease; Guidelines: Chronic Stable Angina

Dariush Mozaffarian, MD, DrPH
Associate Professor, Division of Cardiovascular Medicine, Brigham and Women's Hospital and Harvard Medical School; Departments of Epidemiology and Nutrition, Harvard School of Public Health, Boston, Massachusetts
Nutrition and Cardiovascular Disease

Paul S. Mueller, MD, MPH
Associate Professor of Medicine, Mayo Clinic, Rochester, Minnesota
Ethics in Cardiovascular Medicine

Robert J. Myerburg, MD
Professor of Medicine and Physiology, University of Miami Miller School of Medicine, Miami, Florida
Cardiac Arrest and Sudden Cardiac Death

Elizabeth G. Nabel, MD
Professor of Medicine, Harvard Medical School; President, Brigham and Women's Hospital, Boston, Massachusetts
Principles of Cardiovascular Molecular Biology and Genetics

L. Kristin Newby, MD, MHS
Associate Professor of Medicine, Division of Cardiovascular Medicine, Duke University Medical Center, Durham, North Carolina
Cardiovascular Disease in Women

Patrick T. O'Gara, MD
Professor of Medicine, Harvard Medical School; Director, Clinical Cardiology, Cardiovascular Division, Brigham and Women's Hospital, Boston, Massachusetts
The History and Physical Examination: An Evidence-Based Approach

Jae K. Oh, MD
Professor of Medicine, Mayo Clinic College of Medicine, Consultant in Cardiovascular Diseases; Co-Director of the Echocardiography Laboratory, Mayo Clinic, Rochester, Minnesota
Echocardiography

Jeffrey Olgin, MD
Ernest Gallo-Kanu Chatterjee Distinguished Professor; Chief, Division of Cardiology; Chief, Cardiac Electrophysiology, University of California, San Francisco, California
Specific Arrhythmias: Diagnosis and Treatment

Lionel H. Opie, MD, DPhil, DSc
Professor of Medicine and Director Emeritus, Hatter Institute for Cardiovascular Research Institute, University of Cape Town, Cape Town, South Africa
Mechanisms of Cardiac Contraction and Relaxation

Catherine M. Otto, MD
Professor of Medicine, J. Ward Kennedy-Hamilton Endowed Chair in Cardiology; Director, Training Programs in Cardiovascular Disease, University of Washington School of Medicine; Associate Director, Echocardiography Laboratory; Co-Director, Adult Congenital Heart Disease Clinic, University of Washington Medical Center, Seattle, Washington
Valvular Heart Disease; Guidelines: Management of Valvular Heart Disease

Jeffrey J. Popma, MD
Associate Professor of Medicine, Harvard Medical School; Director, Interventional Cardiology Clinical Services, Beth Israel Deaconess Medical Center, Boston, Massachusetts
Coronary Arteriography; Guidelines: Coronary Arteriography; Percutaneous Coronary Intervention; Guidelines: Percutaneous Coronary Intervention

Reed E. Pyeritz, MD, PhD
Professor of Medicine and Genetics; Vice-chair for Academic Affairs, Department of Medicine, University of Pennsylvania School of Medicine, Philadelphia, Pennsylvania
Inherited Causes of Cardiovascular Disease

B. Soma Raju, MD
Professor & Head, Department of Cardiology, Hyderabad, Andhra Pradesh, India
Rheumatic Fever

José A.F. Ramires, MD, PhD
Head Professor of Cardiology and Director of Clinical Cardiology, Division of The Heart Institute (INCOR), University of São Paulo Medical School; Director of Health System and President of Professors Evaluation Committee, University of São Paulo, São Paulo, Brazil
Chagas' Disease

Margaret M. Redfield, MD
Professor of Medicine, Division of Cardiovascular Medicine, Mayo Clinic, Rochester, Minnesota
Heart Failure with Normal Ejection Fraction

Andrew N. Redington, MD
Professor and Head, Division of Cardiology, Paediatrics, Hospital for Sick Children, University of Toronto, Toronto, Canada
Congenital Heart Disease

Stuart Rich, MD
Professor of Medicine, Section of Cardiology, Center for Pulmonary Hypertension, University of Chicago, Chicago, Illinois
Pulmonary Hypertension

Paul M Ridker, MD, MPH
Eugene Braunwald Professor of Medicine, Harvard Medical School; Director, Center for Cardiovascular Disease Prevention, Brigham and Women's Hospital, Boston, Massachusetts
Risk Markers for Atherothrombotic Disease; Primary and Secondary Prevention of Coronary Heart Disease

Dan M. Roden, MD
Professor of Medicine and Pharmacology; Director, Oates Institute for Experimental Therapeutics; Assistant Vice-Chancellor for Personalized Medicine, Vanderbilt University School of Medicine, Nashville, Tennessee
Principles of Drug Therapy

Michael Rubart, MD
Assistant Professor of Pediatrics, Indiana University School of Medicine, Indianapolis, Indiana
Genesis of Cardiac Arrhythmias: Electrophysiologic Considerations

Marc S. Sabatine, MD, MPH
Associate Professor of Medicine, Harvard Medical School; Vice Chair, TIMI Study Group; Associate Physician, Division of Cardiovascular Medicine, Brigham and Women's Hospital, Boston, Massachusetts
Approach to the Patient with Chest Pain

Luis A. Sanchez, MD
Professor of Surgery and Radiology, Section of Vascular Surgery, Department of Surgery, Washington University School of Medicine, St. Louis, Missouri
Diseases of the Aorta

Janice B. Schwartz, MD
Clinical Professor of Medicine and Bioengineering and Therapeutic Sciences, University of California, San Francisco; Director, Research, Jewish Home of San Francisco, San Francisco, California
Cardiovascular Disease in the Elderly

Christine E. Seidman, MD
Thomas W. Smith Professor of Medicine and Genetics, Department of Medicine and Genetics, Brigham & Women's Hospital, Harvard Medical School, Howard Hughes Medical Institute, Boston, Massachusetts
Inherited Causes of Cardiovascular Disease

J. G. Seidman, PhD
Henrietta B. and Frederick H. Bugher Professor of Genetics, Department of Genetics, Harvard Medical School, Boston, Massachusetts
Inherited Causes of Cardiovascular Disease

Dhun H. Sethna, MD
Staff Cardiologist, Carilion Clinic, Christiansburg, Virginia
Medical Management of the Patient Undergoing Cardiac Surgery

Jeffrey F. Smallhorn, MBBS, FRACP, FRCP(C)
Professor of Pediatrics; Program Director, Pediatric Cardiology, Department of Pediatrics, University of Alberta, Edmonton, Alberta
Congenital Heart Disease

Virend K. Somers, MD, PhD
Professor of Medicine, Division of Cardiovascular Diseases, Mayo Clinic College of Medicine, Rochester, Minnesota
Sleep Apnea and Cardiovascular Disease; Cardiovascular Manifestations of Autonomic Disorders

Andrei C. Sposito
Associate Professor of Cardiology, University of Campinas; Past Director of The Heart Institute (INCOR), Brasilia, São Paulo, Brazil
Chagas' Disease

Charles D. Swerdlow, MD
Clinical Professor of Medicine, David Geffen School of Medicine at UCLA; Cedars-Sinai Heart Institute, Los Angeles, California
Pacemakers and Implantable Cardioverter-Defibrillators; Guidelines: Cardiac Pacemakers and Cardioverter-Defibrillators

Jean-Claude Tardif, MD
Professor of Medicine, University of Montreal; Director, Montreal Heart Institute Research Center; Endowed Research Chair in Atherosclerosis, Montreal Heart Institute, Université de Montréal, Montreal, Canada
Intravascular Ultrasound Imaging

Allen J. Taylor, MD
Professor of Medicine, Georgetown University; Director, Advanced Cardiovascular Imaging, Cardiology Section, Washington Hospital Center and Medstar Health Cardiovascular Research Institute, Washington, DC
Cardiac Computed Tomography; Appropriate Use Criteria: Cardiac Computed Tomography

David J. Tester, BS
Senior Research Technologist II-Supervisor, Mayo Clinic, Windland Smith Rice Sudden Death Genomics Laboratory, Rochester, Minnesota
Genetics of Cardiac Arrhythmias

Judith Therrien, MD
Associate Professor of Medicine, Department of Cardiology, McGill University, Montreal, Quebec, Canada
Congenital Heart Disease

Paul D. Thompson, MD
Professor of Medicine, University of Connecticut, Farmington, Connecticut; Director, Cardiology, Hartford Hospital, Hartford, Connecticut
Exercise-Based, Comprehensive Cardiac Rehabilitation

Robert W. Thompson, MD
Professor of Surgery, Division of General Surgery, Vascular Surgery Section, Radiology, and Cell Biology and Physiology, Washington University, St. Louis, Missouri
Diseases of the Aorta

Marc D. Tischler, MD
Associate Professor of Medicine, University of Vermont College of Medicine; Director, Cardiac Ultrasound Laboratory; Co-Director, Cardiac Magnetic Resonance Unit, Department of Internal Medicine, Burlington, Vermont
Pericardial Diseases

Peter I. Tsai, MD
Assistant Professor, Division of Cardiothoracic Surgery, Michael E. DeBakey Department of Surgery, Ben Taub General Hospital, Baylor College of Medicine, Houston, Texas
Traumatic Heart Disease

Zoltan G. Turi, MD
Professor of Medicine, Robert Wood Johnson Medical School; Director, Section of Vascular Medicine; Director, Cooper Structural Heart Disease Program, Cooper University Hospital, Camden, New Jersey
Rheumatic Fever

James E. Udelson, MD
Professor of Medicine, Department of Medicine; Chief, Division of Cardiology, The Cardiovascular Center, Tufts Medical Center and Tufts University School of Medicine, Boston, Massachusetts
Nuclear Cardiology; Appropriate Use Criteria: Nuclear Cardiology

Viola Vaccarino, MD, PhD
Professor and Chair, Department of Epidemiology, Emory University Rollins School of Public Health; Professor, Department of Medicine, Division of Cardiology, Emory University School of Medicine, Atlanta, Georgia
Psychiatric and Behavioral Aspects of Cardiovascular Disease

Ronald G. Victor, MD
Burns and Allen Professor of Medicine; Associate Director, Clinical Research; Director, Hypertension Center, The Heart Institute, Cedars-Sinai Medical Center, Los Angeles, California
Systemic Hypertension: Mechanisms and Diagnosis

Alexandra Villa-Forte, MD, MPH
Center for Vasculitis Care and Research, Department of Rheumatic and Immunologic Diseases, Cleveland Clinic, Cleveland, Ohio
Rheumatic Diseases and the Cardiovascular System

Matthew J. Wall, Jr., MD
Professor, Michael E. DeBakey Department of Surgery, Baylor College of Medicine; Deputy Chief of Surgery, Ben Taub General Hospital, Houston, Texas
Traumatic Heart Disease

Carole A. Warnes, MD, FRCP
Professor of Medicine, Mayo Clinic College of Medicine; Consultant, Division of Cardiovascular Diseases, Internal Medicine and Pediatric Cardiology, Mayo Clinic College of Medicine, Rochester, Minnesota
Pregnancy and Heart Disease; Guidelines: Pregnancy and Heart Disease

Gary D. Webb, MD
Professor, University of Cincinnati College of Medicine; Director, Cincinnati Adolescent and Adult Congenital Heart Center, Cincinnati Children's Hospital Heart Institute, Cincinnati, Ohio
Congenital Heart Disease

John G. Webb, MD
MacLeod Professor of Heart Valve Intervention, University of British Columbia; Director Cardiac Catheterization, St. Paul's Hospital, Vancouver, Canada
Percutaneous Therapies for Structural Heart Disease in Adults

Ralph Weissleder, MD, PhD
Professor, Harvard Medical School; Center for Systems Biology and Department of Radiology, Massachusetts General Hospital, Boston, Massachusetts
Molecular Imaging in Cardiovascular Disease

Jeffrey I. Weitz, MD, FRCP(C)
Professor of Medicine & Biochemistry, McMaster University; HSFO/J.F. Mustard Chair in Cardiovascular Research; Canada Research Chair (Tier 1) in Thrombosis; Executive Director, Thrombosis and Atherosclerosis Research Institute, Hamilton General Hospital Campus, Hamilton, Ontario, Canada
Hemostasis, Thrombosis, Fibrinolysis, and Cardiovascular Disease

Christopher J. White, MD
Professor of Medicine; Chairman, Department of Cardiology, Ochsner Clinic Foundation, New Orleans, Louisiana
Endovascular Treatment of Noncoronary Obstructive Vascular Disease

Stephen D. Wiviott, MD
Instructor of Medicine, Harvard Medical School; Investigator, TIMI Study Group; Associate Physician, Division of Cardiology, Brigham and Women's Hospital, Boston, Massachusetts
Guidelines: Management of Patients with ST-Segment Elevation Myocardial Infarction

Clyde W. Yancy, MD
Professor of Medicine; Chief, Division of Cardiology, Northwestern University Feinberg School of Medicine, Chicago, Illinois
Heart Disease in Varied Populations

Andreas M. Zeiher, MD
Professor of Cardiology; Chair, Department of Medicine, University of Frankfurt, Frankfurt, Germany
Emerging Therapies and Strategies in the Treatment of Heart Failure

Douglas P. Zipes, MD
Distinguished Professor; Professor Emeritus of Medicine, Pharmacology, and Toxicology; Director Emeritus, Division of Cardiology and the Krannert Institute of Cardiology, Indiana University School of Medicine, Indianapolis, Indiana
Genesis of Cardiac Arrhythmias: Electrophysiologic Considerations; Diagnosis of Cardiac Arrhythmias; Guidelines: Ambulatory Electrocardiographic and Electrophysiologic Testing; Therapy for Cardiac Arrhythmias; Pacemakers and Implantable Cardioverter-Defibrillators; Guidelines: Cardiac Pacemakers and Cardioverter-Defibrillators; Specific Arrhythmias: Diagnosis and Treatment; Atrial Fibrillation: Clinical Features, Mechanisms, and Management; Guidelines: Atrial Fibrillation; Hypotension and Syncope; Cardiovascular Disease in the Elderly; Neurologic Disorders and Cardiovascular Disease

Advances in cardiovascular science and practice continue at a breathtaking rate. As the knowledge base expands, it is important to adapt our learning systems to keep up with progress in our field. We are pleased to present the ninth edition of *Braunwald's Heart Disease: A Textbook of Cardiovascular Medicine* as the hub of an ongoing, advanced learning system designed to provide practitioners, physicians-in-training, and students at all levels with the tools needed to keep abreast of rapidly changing scientific foundations, clinical research results, and evidence-based medical practice.

In keeping with the tradition established by the previous editions of *Braunwald's Heart Disease*, the ninth edition covers the breadth of cardiovascular practice, highlighting new advances and their potential to transform the established paradigms of prevention, diagnosis, and treatment. We have thoroughly revised this edition to keep the content vibrant, stimulating, and up-to-date. Twenty-four of the 94 chapters are entirely new, including nine chapters that cover topics not addressed in earlier editions. We have added 46 new authors, all highly accomplished and recognized in their respective disciplines. All chapters carried over from the eighth edition have been thoroughly updated and extensively revised. This edition includes nearly 2500 figures, most of which are in full color, and 600 tables. We have continued to provide updated sections on current guidelines recommendations that complement each of the appropriate individual chapters.

A full accounting of these changes in the new edition cannot be addressed in the space of this Preface, but we are pleased to present a number of the highlights. The ninth edition includes two entirely new chapters—ethics in cardiovascular medicine by Paul Mueller and design and conduct of clinical trials by Elliot Antman—that supplement the initial section on the fundamentals of cardiovascular disease. Thomas Gaziano has joined J. Michael Gaziano in authoring the first chapter on the global burden of cardiovascular disease. With recognition of the increasing relevance of genetics, J.G. Seidman joins Reed Pyeritz and Christine Seidman in the updated chapter on inherited causes of cardiovascular disease, and David Tester and Michael Ackerman have contributed a new chapter on the genetics of cardiac arrhythmias.

Acknowledging the unremitting burden and societal impact of heart failure, the section on heart failure receives continued emphasis and has undergone extensive revision, including five new chapters. Barry Greenberg teams with Andrew Kahn in addressing the clinical approach to the patient with heart failure; Mihai Georghiade, Gerasimos Filippatos, and Michael Felker provide a fresh look at the evaluation and management of acute heart failure; Michael Acker and Mariell Jessup address advances in surgical treatment the failing heart; Mandeep Mehra and Bartley Griffith discuss the role of device therapy in assisted circulation; and William Abraham reviews the emerging role of devices for monitoring and managing heart failure.

The chapters that address cardiovascular imaging have kept abreast of all of the exciting advances in this field. Raymond Kwong and Allen Taylor have written excellent and comprehensive new chapters on cardiac magnetic resonance and cardiac computed tomography, respectively, with accompanying sections addressing the American College of Cardiology appropriate use criteria for the use of these advanced technologies. Updated ACC appropriate use criteria also follow the chapters on echocardiography and nuclear cardiology. In addition, the imaging section has been further enhanced by the inclusion of two new chapters focusing on the evolving applications of intravascular ultrasound, authored by Jean-Claude Tardif and Philippe

L'Allier, and cardiovascular molecular imaging, provided by Peter Libby, Farouc Jaffer, and Ralph Weissleder.

In recognition of the growing importance of atrial fibrillation in cardiovascular practice, a new chapter devoted to the evaluation and treatment of this rhythm disturbance, authored by Fred Morady and Douglas Zipes, has been added to the section on cardiac arrhythmias. The other updated chapters in the heart rhythm section continue to inform our readers on the current state-of-the-art in this important aspect of heart disease.

Dariush Mozaffarian and Edzard Ernst have added expertly authored new chapters on nutrition and complementary medicine, respectively, to the section on preventive cardiology. In the atherosclerotic disease section, Marc Sabatine joins Chris Cannon in the revised discussion of the approach to the patient with chest pain, and William Boden joins David Morrow in a new chapter on stable ischemic heart disease. Deepak Bhatt teams with Jeffrey Popma in creating a new chapter on percutaneous coronary intervention, and he joins Andrew Eisenhauer and Christopher White in updating the discussion on endovascular treatment of noncoronary vascular disease. We welcome John Webb to our authorship team with his new chapter on catheter-based interventions in structural heart disease that includes discussion of the exciting novel catheter-based techniques for repair and replacement of cardiac valves. Our other new chapters include a fresh commentary on diseases of the aorta by Alan Braverman, Robert Thompson, and Luis Sanchez; diabetes and cardiovascular disease by Darren McGuire; hemostasis, thrombosis, and fibrinolysis by Jeffrey Weitz; and psychiatric and behavioral aspects of cardiovascular disease by Viola Vaccarino and Douglas Bremner. Finally, we are delighted that José Ramires, Andrei Sposito, Edécio Cunha-Neto, and Maria de Lourdes Higuchi have expanded our discussion of the global nature of cardiovascular disease by contributing an excellent chapter on the pathophysiology, evaluation, and treatment of Chagas' disease.

We are indebted to all of our authors for their considerable time, effort, and commitment to maintaining the high standards of *Braunwald's Heart Disease*. As excited as we are about bringing this edition of the text to fruition, we are even more energized regarding the expanding *Braunwald's Heart Disease* website. The electronic version of this work on the companion Expert Consult website includes greater content in terms of figures and tables than the print version can accommodate. Figures and tables can be downloaded directly from the website for electronic slide presentations. In addition, we have a growing portfolio of video and audio content that supplements the print content of many of our chapters. Dr. Braunwald personally updates the chapter content on a weekly basis, thus creating a truly unique living textbook with expanding content that includes the latest research, clinical trials, and expert opinion.

Moreover, the family of *Braunwald's Heart Disease* companion texts continues to expand, providing detailed expert content for the subspecialist across the broad spectrum of cardiovascular conditions. These include: *Clinical Lipidology*, edited by Christie Ballantyne; *Clinical Arrhythmology and Electrophysiology*, authored by Ziad Issa, John Miller, and Douglas Zipes; *Heart Failure*, edited by Douglas Mann; *Valvular Heart Disease*, by Catherine Otto and Robert Bonow; *Acute Coronary Syndromes*, by Pierre Théroux; *Preventive Cardiology*, by Roger Blumenthal, JoAnne Foody, and Nathan Wong; *Cardiovascular Nursing*, by Debra Moser and Barbara Riegel; *Mechanical Circulatory Support*, by Robert Kormos and Leslie Miller; *Hypertension*, by Henry Black and William Elliott; *Cardiovascular Therapeutics*, by Elliott Antman and Marc Sabatine; *Vascular Medicine*, by Marc Creager, Joshua

Beckman, and Joseph Loscalzo; and recent atlases on cardiovascular imaging such as *Cardiovascular Magnetic Resonance*, by Christopher Kramer and Gregory Hundley; *Cardiovascular Computed Tomography*, by Allen Taylor; and *Nuclear Cardiology*, by Ami Iskandrian and Ernest Garcia.

The ninth edition of *Braunwald's Heart Disease* does indeed represent the central hub of a burgeoning cardiovascular learning system that can be tailored to meet the needs of all individuals engaged in cardiovascular medicine, from the accomplished subspecialist practitioner to the beginning student of cardiology. *Braunwald's Heart Disease* aims to provide the necessary tools to navigate the ever-increasing flow of complex information seamlessly.

Robert O. Bonow

Douglas L. Mann

Douglas P. Zipes

Peter Libby

Cardiovascular disease is the greatest scourge affecting the industrialized nations. As with previous scourges—bubonic plague, yellow fever, and smallpox—cardiovascular disease not only strikes down a significant fraction of the population without warning but also causes prolonged suffering and disability in an even larger number. In the United States alone, despite recent encouraging declines, cardiovascular disease is still responsible for almost 1 million fatalities each year and more than half of all deaths; almost 5 million persons afflicted with cardiovascular disease are hospitalized each year. The cost of these diseases in terms of human suffering and material resources is almost incalculable. Fortunately, research focusing on the causes, diagnosis, treatment, and prevention of heart disease is moving ahead rapidly.

In order to provide a comprehensive, authoritative text in a field that has become as broad and deep as cardiovascular medicine, I chose to enlist the aid of a number of able colleagues. However, I hoped that my personal involvement in the writing of about half of the book would make it possible to minimize the fragmentation, gaps, inconsistencies, organizational difficulties, and impersonal tone that sometimes plague multiauthored texts.

Since the early part of the 20th century, clinical cardiology has had a particularly strong foundation in the basic sciences of physiology and pharmacology. More recently, the disciplines of molecular biology, genetics, developmental biology, biophysics, biochemistry, experimental pathology, and bioengineering have also begun to provide critically important information about cardiac function and malfunction. Although *Heart Disease: A Textbook of Cardiovascular Medicine* is primarily a clinical treatise and not a textbook of fundamental cardiovascular science, an effort has been made to explain, in some detail, the scientific bases of cardiovascular diseases.

Eugene Braunwald
1980

CONTENTS

Look for these other titles in the Braunwald's Heart Disease Family

Braunwald's Heart Disease Companions

PIERRE THÉROUX
Acute Coronary Syndromes

ELLIOTT M. ANTMAN & MARC S. SABATINE
Cardiovascular Therapeutics

CHRISTIE M. BALLANTYNE
Clinical Lipidology

ZIAD ISSA, JOHN M. MILLER, & DOUGLAS P. ZIPES
Clinical Arrhythmology and Electrophysiology

DOUGLAS L. MANN
Heart Failure

HENRY R. BLACK & WILLIAM J. ELLIOTT
Hypertension

ROGER S. BLUMENTHAL, JOANNE M. FOODY, & NATHAN D. WONG
Preventive Cardiology

ROBERT L. KORMOS & LESLIE W. MILLER
Mechanical Circulatory Support

CATHERINE M. OTTO & ROBERT O. BONOW
Valvular Heart Disease

MARC A. CREAGER, JOSHUA A. BECKMAN, & JOSEPH LOSCALZO
Vascular Disease

Braunwald's Heart Disease Imaging Companions

ALLEN J. TAYLOR
Atlas of Cardiac Computed Tomography

CHRISTOPHER M. KRAMER & W. GREGORY HUNDLEY
Atlas of Cardiovascular Magnetic Resonance

AMI E. ISKANDRIAN & ERNEST V. GARCIA
Atlas of Nuclear Imaging

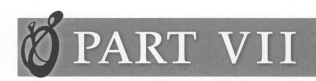

PART VII

ATHEROSCLEROTIC CARDIOVASCULAR DISEASE

CHAPTER **52**

Coronary Blood Flow and Myocardial Ischemia

John M. Canty, Jr.

The coronary circulation is unique in that it is responsible for generating the arterial pressure that is required to perfuse the systemic circulation and yet, at the same time, has its own perfusion impeded during the systolic portion of the cardiac cycle. Because myocardial contraction is closely connected to coronary flow and oxygen delivery, the balance between oxygen supply and demand is a critical determinant of the normal beat-to-beat function of the heart. When this relationship is acutely disrupted by diseases affecting coronary blood flow, the resulting imbalance can immediately precipitate a vicious cycle, whereby ischemia-induced contractile dysfunction precipitates hypotension and further myocardial ischemia. Thus, a knowledge of the regulation of coronary blood flow, determinants of myocardial oxygen consumption, and relationship between ischemia and contraction is essential for understanding the pathophysiologic basis and management of many cardiovascular disorders.[1]

Control of Coronary Blood Flow

There are pronounced systolic and diastolic coronary flow variations throughout the cardiac cycle, with coronary arterial inflow out of phase with venous outflow (**Fig. 52-1**).[2] Systolic contraction increases tissue pressure, redistributes perfusion from the subendocardial to the subepicardial layers of the heart, and impedes coronary arterial inflow, which reaches a nadir. At the same time, systolic compression reduces the diameter of intramyocardial microcirculatory vessels (arterioles, capillaries, and venules) and increases coronary venous outflow, which peaks during systole. During diastole, coronary arterial inflow increases with a transmural gradient that favors perfusion to the subendocardial vessels. At this time, coronary venous outflow falls.

Determinants of Myocardial Oxygen Consumption

In contrast to most other vascular beds, myocardial oxygen extraction is near-maximal at rest, averaging approximately 75% of arterial

oxygen content.[3] The ability to increase oxygen extraction as a means to increase oxygen delivery is limited to circumstances associated with sympathetic activation and acute subendocardial ischemia. Nevertheless, coronary venous oxygen tension (PvO_2) can only decrease from 25 to approximately 15 torr. Because of the high resting oxygen extraction, increases in myocardial oxygen consumption are primarily met by proportional increases in coronary flow and oxygen delivery (**Fig. 52-2**). In addition to coronary flow, oxygen delivery is directly determined by arterial oxygen content (PaO_2). This is equal to the product of hemoglobin concentration and arterial oxygen saturation plus a small amount of oxygen dissolved in plasma that is directly related to PaO_2. Thus, for any given flow level, anemia results in proportional reductions in oxygen delivery, whereas the nonlinear oxygen dissociation curve results in relatively small reductions in oxygen content until PaO_2 falls to the steep portion of the oxygen dissociation curve (below 50 torr).

The major determinants of myocardial oxygen consumption are heart rate, systolic pressure (or myocardial wall stress), and left ventricular (LV) contractility. A twofold increase in any of these individual determinants of oxygen consumption requires an approximately 50% increase in coronary flow. Experimentally, the systolic pressure-volume area is proportional to myocardial work and linearly related to myocardial oxygen consumption. The basal myocardial oxygen requirements needed to maintain critical membrane function are low (approximately 15% of resting oxygen consumption) and the cost of electrical activation is trivial when mechanical contraction ceases during diastolic arrest (as with cardioplegia) and diminishes during ischemia.

CORONARY AUTOREGULATION. Regional coronary blood flow remains constant as coronary artery pressure is reduced below aortic pressure over a wide range when the determinants of myocardial oxygen consumption are kept constant.[4] This phenomenon is termed *autoregulation* (**Fig. 52-3**). When pressure falls to the lower limit of autoregulation, coronary resistance arteries are maximally vasodilated to intrinsic stimuli and flow becomes pressure-dependent, resulting in the onset of subendocardial ischemia. Resting coronary blood flow under normal

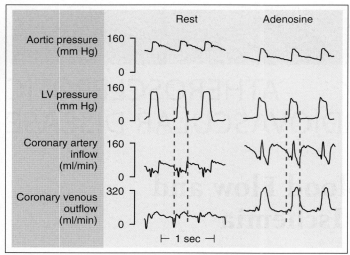

FIGURE 52-1 Phasic coronary arterial inflow and venous outflow at rest and adenosine vasodilation. Arterial inflow primarily occurs during diastole. During systole (dotted vertical lines), arterial inflow declines as venous outflow peaks, reflecting the compression of microcirculatory vessels during systole. After adenosine administration, the phasic variations in venous outflow are more pronounced. *(Modified from Canty JM Jr, Brooks A: Phasic volumetric coronary venous outflow patterns in conscious dogs. Am J Physiol 258:H1457, 1990.)*

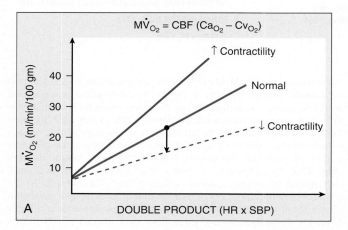

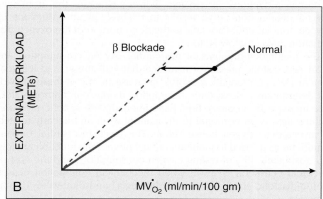

FIGURE 52-2 Fick equation and the relationship between heart rate (HR)–systolic pressure (SBP) double product and myocardial oxygen consumption ($M\dot{V}O_2$). **A,** Increases in $M\dot{V}O_2$ are primarily met by increases in coronary flow and linearly related to the double product. Twofold increases in HR, SBP, or contractility each result in approximately 50% increases in myocardial oxygen consumption. **B,** Beta blockade allows the same external workload to be accomplished at a lower cardiac workload ($M\dot{V}O_2$) by reducing the double product and myocardial contractility. CaO_2 = coronary arterial oxygen content; CBF = coronary blood flow; CvO_2 = coronary venous oxygen content.

hemodynamic conditions averages 0.7 to 1.0 mL/min/g and can increase between four- and fivefold during vasodilation.[5] The ability to increase flow above resting values in response to pharmacologic vasodilation is termed *coronary reserve*. Flow in the maximally vasodilated heart is dependent on coronary arterial pressure. Maximum perfusion and coronary reserve are reduced when the diastolic time available for subendocardial perfusion is decreased (tachycardia) or the compressive determinants of diastolic perfusion (preload) are increased. Coronary reserve is also diminished by anything that increases resting flow, including increases in the hemodynamic determinants of oxygen consumption (systolic pressure, heart rate, contractility) and reductions in arterial oxygen supply (anemia, hypoxia). Thus, circumstances can develop that precipitate subendocardial ischemia in the presence of normal coronary arteries.[1] Although initial studies have suggested that the lower pressure limit of autoregulation is 70 mm Hg, studies in conscious dogs in the basal state have shown that coronary flow can be autoregulated to mean coronary pressures as low as 40 mm Hg (diastolic pressures of 30 mm Hg).[4] These coronary pressure levels are similar to those recorded in humans without symptoms of ischemia, distal to chronic coronary occlusions, using pressure wire micromanometers. The lower autoregulatory pressure limit increases during tachycardia because of an increase in flow requirements, as well as a reduction in the time available for perfusion.[6]

Figure 52-4 illustrates important transmural variations in the lower autoregulatory pressure limit, which result in increased vulnerability of the subendocardium to ischemia.[1] Subendocardial flow primarily occurs in diastole and begins to decrease below a mean coronary pressure of 40 mm Hg.[4] In contrast, subepicardial flow occurs throughout the cardiac cycle and is maintained until coronary pressure falls below 25 mm Hg. This difference arises from increased oxygen consumption in the subendocardium, requiring a higher resting flow level, as well as the more pronounced effects of systolic contraction on subendocardial vasodilator reserve. The transmural difference in the lower autoregulatory pressure limit results in vulnerability of the subendocardium to ischemia in the presence of a coronary stenosis. Although there is no pharmacologically recruitable flow reserve during ischemia in the normal coronary circulation,[7] reductions in coronary flow below the lower limit of autoregulation can occur in the presence of pharmacologically recruitable coronary flow reserve under certain circumstances.[8]

ENDOTHELIUM-DEPENDENT MODULATION OF CORONARY TONE. Epicardial arteries do not normally contribute significantly to coronary vascular resistance, yet arterial diameter is modulated by a wide variety of paracrine factors that can be released from platelets, as well as circulating neurohormonal agonists, neural tone, and local control through vascular shear stress.[9] The most common factors related to cardiovascular disease are summarized in **Table 52-1** (see Fig. 52-e1 on website). The net effect of many of these agonists is critically dependent on whether a functional endothelium is present. Furchgott and Zawadzki[10] originally demonstrated that acetylcholine normally dilates arteries via an endothelium-dependent relaxing factor (EDRF) that was later identified to be nitric oxide (NO). This binds to guanylyl cyclase and increases cyclic guanosine monophosphate (cGMP), resulting in vascular smooth muscle relaxation. When the endothelium is removed, the dilation to acetylcholine is converted to vasoconstriction, reflecting the effect of muscarinic vascular smooth muscle contraction. Subsequent studies have demonstrated that coronary artery resistance arteries also exhibit endothelial modulation of diameter and that the response to physical forces such as shear stress, as well as paracrine mediators, vary with resistance vessel size.[11] The major endothelium-dependent biochemical pathways involved in regulating coronary epicardial and resistance artery diameter are as follows.

Nitric Oxide (Endothelium-Derived Relaxing Factor)

NO (EDRF) is produced in endothelial cells by the enzymatic conversion of L-arginine to citrulline via type III NO synthase (NOS). This reaction is controlled by calcium and calmodulin and is dependent on molecular oxygen, nicotinamide adenine dinucleotide phosphate, reduced form (NADPH), tetrahydrobiopterin, adenosine diphosphate (ADP), flavin adenine dinucleotide, and flavin mononucleotide. Endothelial NO diffuses abluminally into vascular smooth muscle, where it binds to guanylate cyclase, increasing cGMP production and causing relaxation through a reduction in intracellular calcium. NO-mediated vasodilation is enhanced by cyclical or pulsatile changes

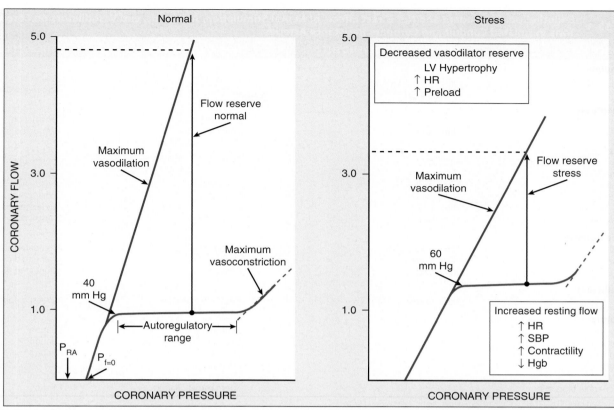

FIGURE 52-3 Autoregulatory relationship under basal conditions and following metabolic stress (e.g., tachycardia). The normal heart maintains coronary blood flow constant **(left panel)** as regional coronary pressure is varied over a wide range when the global determinants of oxygen consumption are kept constant (red lines). Below the lower autoregulatory pressure limit (approximately 40 mm Hg), subendocardial vessels are maximally vasodilated and myocardial ischemia develops. During vasodilation (blue lines), flow increases four to five times above resting values at a normal arterial pressure. Coronary flow ceases at a pressure higher than right atrial pressure (P_{RA}), called zero flow pressure ($P_{f=0}$), which is the effective backpressure to flow in the absence of coronary collaterals. Following stress **(right panel)**, tachycardia increases the compressive determinants of coronary resistance by decreasing the time available for diastolic perfusion and thus reduces maximum vasodilated flow. In addition, increases in myocardial oxygen demand or reductions in arterial oxygen content increase resting flow. These changes reduce coronary flow reserve, the ratio between dilated and resting coronary flow, and cause ischemia to develop at higher coronary pressures. Hgb = hemoglobin.

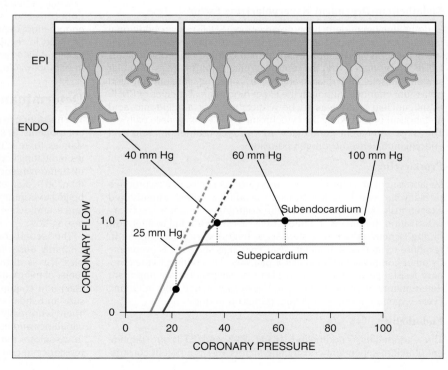

FIGURE 52-4 Transmural variations in coronary autoregulation and myocardial metabolism. Increased vulnerability of the subendocardium (ENDO; red) versus subepicardium (EPI; gold) to ischemia reflects the fact that autoregulation is exhausted at a higher coronary pressure (40 versus 25 mm Hg). This is the result of increased resting flow and oxygen consumption in the subendocardium and an increased sensitivity to systolic compressive effects, because subendocardial flow only occurs during diastole. Subendocardial vessels become maximally vasodilated before those in the subepicardium as coronary artery pressure is reduced. These transmural differences can be increased further during tachycardia or during conditions with elevated preload, which reduce maximum subendocardial perfusion.

TABLE 52-1	Endothelium-Dependent and Net Direct Effects of Neural Stimulation, Autacoids, and Vasodilators on Coronary Tone in Isolated Conduit and Coronary Resistance Arteries		
SUBSTANCE	**ENDOTHELIUM-DEPENDENT**	**NORMAL RESPONSE**	**ATHEROSCLEROSIS**
Acetylcholine			
Conduit	Nitric oxide	Net dilation	Constriction
Resistance	Nitric oxide, EDHF	Dilation	Attenuated dilation
Norepinephrine			
Alpha$_1$		Constriction	Constriction
Beta$_2$	Nitric oxide	Dilation	Attenuated dilation
Platelets			
Thrombin	Nitric oxide	Dilation	Constriction
Serotonin			
Conduit	Nitric oxide	Constriction	Constriction
Resistance	Nitric oxide	Dilation	Constriction
ADP	Nitric oxide	Dilation	Attenuated dilation
Thromboxane	Endothelin	Constriction	Constriction
Paracrine Agonists			
Bradykinin	Nitric oxide, EDHF	Dilation	Attenuated dilation
Histamine	Nitric oxide	Dilation	Attenuated dilation
Substance P	Nitric oxide	Dilation	Attenuated dilation
Endothelin (ET)			
ET-1	Nitric oxide	Net constriction	Increased constriction
Vasodilators			
Adenosine		Dilation	Dilation
Regadenoson		Dilation	Dilation
Dipyridamole		Dilation	Dilation
Papaverine		Dilation	Dilation
Nitroglycerin		Dilation	Dilation
Calcium channel blockers		Submaximal dilation	Dilation

ADP = adenosine diphosphate; EDHF = endothelium-dependent hyperpolarizing factor.

in coronary shear stress. Chronic upregulation of NO synthase occurs in response to episodic increases in coronary flow, such as during exercise training, which also potentiates the relaxation to various endothelium-dependent vasodilators. NO-mediated vasodilation is impaired in many disease states and in patients with one or more risk factors for coronary artery disease (CAD). This occurs via inactivation of NO by superoxide anion generated in response to oxidative stress. Such inactivation is the hallmark of impaired NO-mediated vasodilation in atherosclerosis, hypertension, and diabetes.

Endothelium-Dependent Hyperpolarizing Factor

Endothelium-dependent hyperpolarization (EDHF) is an additional mechanism for selected agonists (e.g., bradykinin), as well as shear stress–induced vasodilation, in the human coronary microcirculation. EDHF is produced by the endothelium, hyperpolarizes vascular smooth muscle, and dilates arteries by opening calcium-activated potassium channels. Although the exact biochemical species of EDHF is still unclear, it appears to be a metabolite of arachidonic acid metabolism produced by the cytochrome P-450 epoxygenase pathway. The most prominent candidates are epoxyeicosatrienoic acid and endothelium-derived hydrogen peroxide.

Prostacyclin

Metabolism of arachidonic acid via cyclooxygenase can also produce prostacyclin, which is a coronary vasodilator when administered exogenously. Although prostacyclin contributes to tonic coronary vasodilation in humans, inhibitors of cyclooxygenase fail to alter flow during ischemia distal to a stenosis or limit oxygen consumption in response to increases in metabolism. This suggests that it is overcome by other compensatory vasodilator pathways.[9] In contrast to the coronary resistance vasculature, vasodilator prostaglandins are important determinants of coronary collateral vessel resistance, and inhibiting cyclooxygenase reduces collateral perfusion in dogs.

Endothelin

The endothelins (endothelin-1 [ET-1], ET-2, and ET-3) are peptide endothelium-dependent constricting factors. ET-1 is a potent constric-

tor derived from the enzymatic cleavage of a larger precursor molecule (pre-proendothelin) via endothelin-converting enzyme. In contrast to the rapid vascular smooth muscle relaxation and recovery characteristic of endothelium-derived vasodilators (NO, EDHF, and prostacyclin), the constriction to ET is prolonged. Changes in ET levels are largely mediated through transcriptional control and produce longer term changes in coronary vasomotor tone. The effects of ET are mediated by binding to both ET-A and ET-B receptors. ET-A–mediated constriction is caused by the activation of protein kinase C in vascular smooth muscle. ET-B–mediated constriction is less pronounced and is counterbalanced by prominent ET-B–mediated endothelium-dependent NO production and vasodilation. ET is not involved in regulating coronary blood flow in the normal heart but can modulate vascular tone when circulating concentrations increase in pathophysiologic states, such as heart failure.

Determinants of Coronary Vascular Resistance

The resistance to coronary blood flow can be divided into three major components, as summarized in **Figure 52-5**.[5] Under normal circumstances, there is no measurable pressure drop in the epicardial arteries, indicating negligible conduit resistance (R_1). With the development of hemodynamically significant epicardial artery narrowing (more than 50% diameter reduction), the fixed conduit artery resistance begins to contribute an increasing component to total coronary resistance and, when severely narrowed (more than 90%), may reduce resting flow.

The second component of coronary resistance (R_2) is dynamic and primarily arises from microcirculatory resistance arteries and arterioles. This is distributed throughout the myocardium across a broad range of microcirculatory resistance vessel size (20 to 200 μm in diameter) and changes in response to physical forces (intraluminal pressure and shear stress), as well as the metabolic needs of the tissue. There is normally little resistance contributed by coronary venules and capillaries and their resistance remains fairly constant during changes in vasomotor tone. Even in the maximally vasodilated heart, capillary resistance accounts for no more than 20% of the microvascular resistance.[12] Thus, a twofold increase in capillary density would only increase maximal myocardial perfusion by approximately 10%. Minimal coronary vascular resistance of the microcirculation is primarily determined by the size and density of arterial resistance vessels and results in substantial coronary flow reserve in the normal heart.

The third component, or compressive resistance (R_3), varies with time throughout the cardiac cycle and is related to cardiac contraction and systolic pressure development within the left ventricle. In heart failure, compressive effects from elevated ventricular diastolic pressure also impede perfusion via passive compression of microcirculatory vessels by elevated extravascular tissue pressure during diastole. Increases in preload effectively raise the normal back pressure to coronary flow above coronary venous pressure levels.[8] Compressive effects are most prominent in the subendocardium and are discussed in greater detail later.

EXTRAVASCULAR COMPRESSIVE RESISTANCE (R_3).

During systole, cardiac contraction raises extravascular tissue pressure to values equal to LV pressure at the subendocardium. This declines to values near pleural pressure at the subepicardium.[3] The increased effective backpressure during systole produces a time-varying reduction in the driving pressure for coronary flow that impedes perfusion to the subendocardium. Although this paradigm can explain variations in systolic coronary inflow, it is not able to account for the increase in coronary venous systolic outflow. To explain both impaired inflow and accelerated venous outflow, some investigators have proposed the concept of the intramyocardial pump.[8] In this model, microcirculatory vessels are compressed during systole and produce a capacitive discharge of blood that accelerates flow from the microcirculation to the coronary venous system (**Fig. 52-6**). At the same time, the upstream capacitive discharge impedes systolic coronary arterial inflow. Although this explains the phasic variations in coronary arterial inflow and venous outflow, as well as its transmural distribution in systole, vascular capacitance cannot explain compressive effects related to elevated tissue pressure during diastole. Thus, components of intramyocardial capacitance, compressive changes in resistance, and time-varying driving pressure all contribute to the compressive determinants of phasic coronary blood flow.

TRANSMURAL VARIATIONS IN MINIMUM CORONARY RESISTANCE (R_2) AND DIASTOLIC DRIVING PRESSURE.

The subendocardial vulnerability to compressive determinants of vascular resistance[1] is partially compensated for by a reduced minimal resistance from an increased arteriolar and capillary density. Because of this vascular gradient, transmural flow during maximal pharmacologic vasodilation of the beating heart is uniform at rest. Coronary vascular resistance in the maximally vasodilated heart is also pressure-dependent, reflecting passive distention of arterial resistance vessels. Thus, the instantaneous vasodilated value of coronary resistance obtained at a normal coronary distending pressure will be lower than that at a reduced pressure.

The precise determinants of the effective driving pressure for diastolic perfusion continue to be controversial.[8] Most experimental studies have demonstrated that the effective backpressure to flow in the heart is higher than right atrial pressure. This has been termed *zero flow pressure* ($P_{f=0}$) and its minimum value is approximately 10 mm Hg

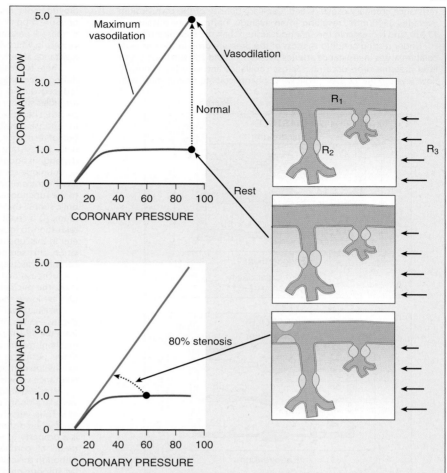

FIGURE 52-5 Schematic of components of coronary vascular resistance with and without a coronary stenosis. R_1 is epicardial conduit artery resistance, which is normally insignificant; R_2 is resistance secondary to metabolic and autoregulatory adjustments in flow and occurs in arterioles and resistance arteries; and R_3 is the time-varying compressive resistance that is higher in subendocardial than subepicardial layers. In the normal heart, $R_2 > R_3 \gg R_1$. The development of a proximal stenosis or pharmacologic vasodilation reduces arteriolar resistance (R_2). In the presence of a severe epicardial stenosis, $R_1 > R_3 > R_2$.

in the maximally vasodilated heart. This increases to values close to LV diastolic filling pressure when preload is elevated above 20 mm Hg. Elevated preload reduces coronary driving pressure and diminishes subendocardial perfusion. It is particularly important in determining flow when coronary pressure is reduced by a stenosis, as well as in the failing heart.

STRUCTURE AND FUNCTION OF THE CORONARY MICROCIRCULATION. The schematics in Figures 52-4 and 52-5 suggest a fairly localized site for the control of coronary vascular resistance that is useful for conceptualizing the major determinants of coronary vascular resistance. Individual coronary resistance arteries are a longitudinally distributed network and in vivo studies of the coronary microcirculation have demonstrated considerable spatial heterogeneity of specific resistance vessel control mechanisms (**Fig. 52-7**).[9,11] Each resistance vessel needs to dilate in an orchestrated fashion to meet the needs of the downstream vascular bed, which is frequently removed from the site of resistance artery control. This can be accomplished independently of metabolic signals by sensing physical forces such as intraluminal flow (shear stress–mediated control) or intraluminal pressure changes (myogenic control). Epicardial arteries (>400 μm in diameter) serve a conduit artery function, with diameter primarily regulated by shear stress, and contribute little pressure drop (<5%) over a wide range of coronary flow. Coronary resistance vessels can be divided into resistance arteries (100 to 400 μm), which regulate their tone in response to local shear stress and luminal pressure changes (myogenic response), and arterioles (>100 μm), which are sensitive to changes in local tissue metabolism and directly control perfusion of the low-resistance coronary capillary bed. Capillary density of the myocardium averages 3500/mm², resulting in an average intercapillary distance of 17 μm, and is greater in the subendocardium than the subepicardium.

Under resting conditions, most of the pressure drop in the microcirculation arises in resistance arteries between 50 and 200 μm in size, with little pressure drop occurring across capillaries and venules at normal flow levels (**Fig. 52-8A**).[12] Following pharmacologic vasodilation with

dipyridamole, resistance artery vasodilation minimizes the precapillary pressure drop in arterial resistance vessels. At the same time, there is an increased pressure drop and redistribution of resistance to venular vessels, in which smooth muscle relaxation is limited and the already low resistance is fairly fixed.

There is considerable heterogeneity in microcirculatory vasodilation during physiologic adjustments in flow. For example, as pressure is reduced during autoregulation, dilation is primarily accomplished by arterioles smaller than 100 μm, whereas larger resistance arteries tend to constrict because of the reduction in perfusion pressure (see Fig. 52-8B).[13] In contrast, metabolic vasodilation results from a more uniform vasodilation of resistance vessels of all sizes (see Fig. 52-8C).[14] Similar inhomogeneity in resistance vessel dilation occurs in response to endothelium-dependent agonists and pharmacologic vasodilators.

A unique component of subendocardial coronary resistance vessels are the transmural penetrating arteries that course from the epicardium to the subendocardial plexus.[9] These vessels are removed from the metabolic stimuli that develop when ischemia is confined to the subendocardium. As a result, local control from altered shear stress and myogenic relaxation to local pressure become very critical determinants of diameter in this "upstream" resistance segment. Even during maximal vasodilation, this segment creates an additional longitudinal component of coronary vascular resistance that must be traversed before the arteriolar microcirculation is reached. Because of this greater longitudinal pressure drop, the microcirculatory pressures in subendocardial coronary arterioles are lower than in the subepicardial arterioles.

INTRALUMINAL PHYSICAL FORCES REGULATING CORONARY RESISTANCE. Because much of the coronary resistance vasculature can be upstream from the effects of metabolic mediators of control, local vascular control mechanisms are critically important in orchestrating adequate regional tissue perfusion to the distal microcirculation. There is a differential expression of mechanisms among different sizes and classes of coronary resistance vessels, which coincides with their function.

MYOGENIC REGULATION. The myogenic response refers to the ability of vascular smooth muscle to oppose changes in coronary arteriolar diameter. Thus, vessels relax when distending pressure is decreased and constrict when distending pressure is elevated (**Fig. 52-9A**). Myogenic tone is a property of vascular smooth muscle and occurs across a large size range of coronary resistance arteries in animals and in humans.[15] Although the cellular mechanism is uncertain, it is dependent on vascular smooth muscle calcium entry, perhaps through stretch-activated L-type Ca²⁺ channels, eliciting cross-bridge activation. The resistance changes arising from the myogenic response tend to bring local coronary flow back to the original level. Myogenic regulation has been postulated to be one of the important mechanisms of the coronary autoregulatory response and, in vivo, appears to occur primarily in arterioles smaller than 100 μm (e.g., during autoregulation; see Fig. 52-8B).[13]

FLOW-MEDIATED RESISTANCE ARTERY CONTROL. Coronary resistance arteries and arterioles also regulate their diameter in response to changes in local shear stress (see Fig. 52-9B). Flow-induced dilation in isolated coronary arterioles was originally demonstrated by Kuo and colleagues.[11,16] They found this to be endothelium-dependent and mediated by NO, because it could be abolished with an L-arginine analogue. In contrast, isolated

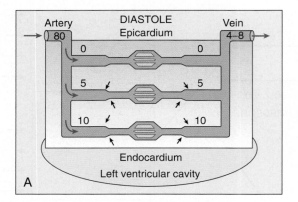

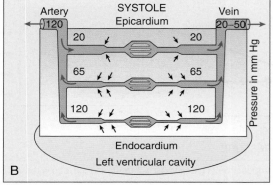

FIGURE 52-6 Effects of extravascular tissue pressure on transmural perfusion. **A,** Compressive effects during diastole are related to tissue pressures that decrease from the subendocardium to subepicardium. At diastolic LV pressures greater than 20 mm Hg, preload determines the effective backpressure to coronary diastolic perfusion. **B,** During systole, cardiac contraction increases intramyocardial tissue pressure surrounding compliant arterioles and venules. This produces a concealed arterial "backflow" that reduces systolic epicardial artery inflow, as depicted in Figure 52-1. Compression of venules accelerates venous outflow. (*Modified from Hoffman JIE, Baer RW, Hanley FL, et al: Regulation of transmural myocardial blood flow. J Biomech Eng 107:2, 1985.*)

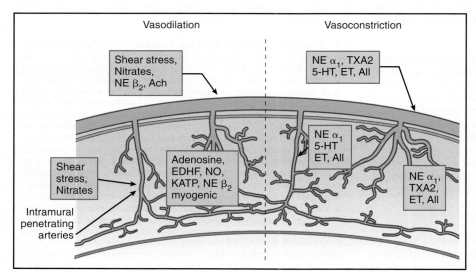

FIGURE 52-7 Transmural distribution of coronary resistance vessels—major vasodilatory and vasoconstrictor mechanisms in epicardial conduit arteries and different sites of the microcirculation. The epicardial conduit arteries arborize into subepicardial and subendocardial resistance arteries. Intramural penetrating resistance arteries are unique in that they are removed from subendocardial metabolic stimuli and theoretically are more dependent on regulating their tone in response to shear stress and luminal pressure as mechanisms to produce dilation in response to changes in metabolism of the distal subendocardial arteriolar plexus. See text for further discussion. Ach = acetylcholine; EDHF = endothelium-dependent hyperpolarizing factor; ET = endothelin; 5-HT = serotonin; KATP = ATP-dependent potassium channel; NE β₂ = norepinephrine beta₂ adrenergic; NE α₁ =norepinephrine alpha₁ adrenergic; TXA2 = thromboxane A₂. (*Modified from Duncker DJ, Bache RJ: Regulation of coronary vasomotor tone under normal conditions and during acute myocardial hypoperfusion. Pharmacol Ther 86:87, 2000.*)

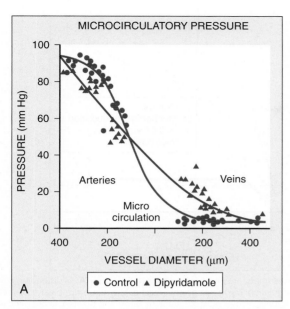

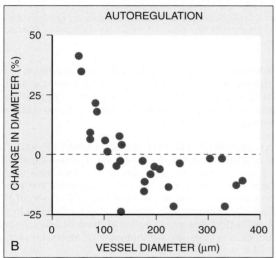

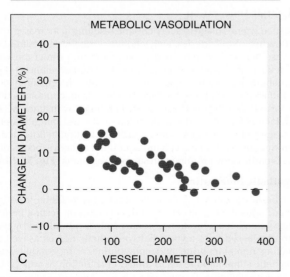

FIGURE 52-8 Microcirculatory pressure profile and local resistance changes to physiologic stimuli in subepicardial vessels. **A,** Under resting conditions, most of the pressure drop to flow arises from resistance arteries and arterioles. Following dipyridamole vasodilation, there is a redistribution of microcirculatory resistance. with a greater pressure drop occurring across postcapillary venules that do not alter their resistance. **B,** Heterogeneous arterial microvessel response during autoregulation. A reduction in pressure to 38 mm Hg elicited dilation in arterioles smaller than 100 μm, whereas larger arteries tended to constrict passively from the reduction in distending pressure. **C,** Homogeneous vasodilation of resistance arteries during increases in myocardial oxygen consumption. There is dilation in all microvascular resistance arteries that is greatest in vessels smaller than 100 μm. (**A** modified from Chilian WM, Layne SM, Klausner EC, et al: Redistribution of coronary microvascular resistance produced by dipyridamole. Am J Physiol 256:H383, 1989; **B** modified from Kanatsuka H, Lamping KG, Eastham CL, et al: Heterogeneous changes in epimyocardial microvascular size during graded coronary stenosis. Evidence of the microvascular site for autoregulation. Circ Res 66:389, 1990; **C** modified from Kanatsuka H, Lamping KG, Eastham CL, et al: Comparison of the effects of increased myocardial oxygen consumption and adenosine on the coronary microvascular resistance. Circ Res 65:1296, 1989.)

atrial vessels from patients undergoing cardiac surgery exhibit flow-mediated vasodilation that is mediated by EDHF.[17,18] The disparity with animal studies may reflect age or species variability in the relative importance of EDHF versus NO in the coronary circulation. The mechanisms also appear to vary as a function of vessel size, with studies in pigs demonstrating that hyperpolarization regulates epicardial conduit arteries[19] and NO predominates in the resistance vasculature.[16] Finally, EDHF may represent a compensatory pathway that is normally inhibited by NO and becomes upregulated in acquired disease states, in which NO-mediated vasodilation is impaired. Despite the variability in isolated vessels, blocking NO synthase with an L-arginine analogue in the coronary circulation of humans reduces vasodilation to pharmacologic endothelium-dependent agonists and attenuates flow increases during metabolic vasodilation, demonstrating that NO-mediated vasodilatation plays a role in determining physiologic vascular tone in some segments of the coronary resistance vasculature.[20]

METABOLIC MEDIATORS OF CORONARY RESISTANCE. Despite increasing knowledge regarding the distribution of coronary microvascular resistance, there is still no consensus regarding specific mediators of metabolic vasodilation. Coronary resistance in any segment of the microcirculation represents the integration of local physical factors (e.g., pressure and flow), vasodilator metabolites (e.g., adenosine, PO_2, pH), autacoids, and neural modulation. Each of these mechanisms contributes to net coronary vascular smooth muscle tone, which may ultimately be controlled by opening and closing vascular smooth muscle adenosine triphosphate (ATP)–sensitive K^+ (K^+-ATP) channels. There is considerable redundancy in the available local control mechanisms.[9] Because of this, blocking single mechanisms fails to alter coronary autoregulation or metabolic flow regulation at normal coronary pressures. This redundancy can, however, be unmasked by stressing the heart and evaluating flow regulation at reduced pressures distal to a coronary stenosis at rest or during exercise.[9] Some of the proposed candidates and their role in metabolic resistance control and ischemia-induced vasodilation are summarized here.[3]

Adenosine

There has been a longstanding interest in the role of adenosine as a metabolic mediator of resistance artery control. It is released from cardiac myocytes when the rate of ATP hydrolysis exceeds its synthesis during ischemia. Its production and release also increase with myocardial metabolism. Adenosine has an extremely short half-life (<10 seconds) caused by its rapid inactivation by adenosine deaminase. It binds to A2 receptors on vascular smooth muscle, increases cyclic adenosine monophosphate (cAMP), and opens intermediate calcium-activated potassium channels.[21] Adenosine has a differential effect on coronary resistance arteries, primarily dilating vessels smaller than 100 μm.[14] Although adenosine has no direct effect on larger resistance arteries and conduit arteries, these dilate through endothelium-dependent vasodilation from the concomitant increases

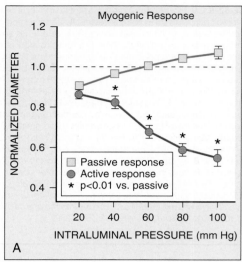

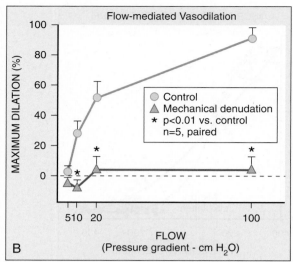

FIGURE 52-9 Effects of physical forces on coronary diameter in isolated human coronary resistance arteries (nominal diameter, 100 μm). **A,** As distending pressure is reduced from 100 mm Hg, there is progressive vasodilation consistent with myogenic regulation. Myogenic dilation reaches the maximum passive diameter of the vessel at 20 mm Hg. **B,** Flow-mediated vasodilation in cannulated human resistance arteries. As the pressure gradient across the isolated vessel is increased, intraluminal flow rises and causes progressive dilation that is abolished by removing the endothelium. Similar flow-mediated dilation occurs in most arterial vessels, including the coronary conduit arteries. (**A** modified from Miller FJ, Dellsperger KC, Gutterman DD: Myogenic constriction of human coronary arterioles. Am J Physiol 273:H257, 1997; **B** modified from Miura H, Wachtel RE, Liu Y, et al: Flow-induced dilation of human coronary arterioles: Important role of Ca²+-activated K+ channels. Circulation 103:1992, 2001.)

in local shear stress as arteriolar resistance falls.[22] Despite the attractiveness of adenosine as a local metabolic control mechanism, there is now substantial in vivo experimental data to demonstrate convincingly that it is not required for adjusting coronary flow to increases in metabolism or autoregulation.[23] It may, however, contribute to vasodilation during hypoxia and during acute exercise-induced myocardial ischemia distal to a stenosis.[9]

ATP-Sensitive K⁺ Channels

Coronary vascular smooth muscle K⁺-ATP channels are tonically active, contributing to coronary vascular tone under resting conditions. Preventing K⁺-ATP channel opening with glibenclamide causes constriction of arterioles smaller than 100 μm, reduces coronary flow, and accentuates myocardial ischemia distal to a coronary stenosis by overcoming intrinsic vasodilatory mechanisms.[9] The K⁺-ATP channels can modulate the coronary metabolic and autoregulatory responses. It is a potentially attractive mechanism, because many of the other candidates for metabolic flow regulation (e.g., adenosine, NO, beta₂ adrenoreceptors, and prostacyclin) are ultimately affected by blocking this pathway. It is likely that K⁺-ATP channel opening is a common effector rather than sensor of metabolic activity or of autoregulatory adjustments in flow. It is also possible that the reductions in coronary flow observed after blocking K⁺-ATP channel vasodilation are pharmacologic, caused by vasoconstriction of the microcirculation that overcomes intrinsic vasodilatory stimuli, as seen when other potent vasoconstrictors (e.g., endothelin or vasopressin) are administered at pharmacologic doses.

Hypoxia

Although a potent coronary vasodilatory stimulus, the role of local Po_2 in the regulation of arteriolar tone remains unresolved. Coronary flow increases in proportion to reductions in arterial oxygen content (reduced Po_2 or anemia) and there is a twofold increase in perfused capillary density in response to hypoxia.[3] Nevertheless, studies demonstrating a direct effect of oxygen on metabolic or autoregulatory adjustments are lacking and the vasodilatory response to reduced arterial oxygen delivery may simply reflect the close coupling between myocardial metabolism and flow.

Acidosis

Arterial hypercapnea and acidosis (Pco_2) are potent stimuli that have been demonstrated to produce coronary vasodilation independent of

hypoxia. Whereas their precise role in the local regulation of myocardial perfusion remains unclear, it seems reasonable that some of the vasodilation occurring with increased myocardial metabolism could arise from increased myocardial CO_2 production and tissue acidosis in the setting of acute ischemia.[3]

NEURAL CONTROL OF CORONARY CONDUIT AND RESISTANCE ARTERIES. Sympathetic and vagal nerves innervate coronary conduit arteries and segments of the resistance vasculature. Neural stimulation affects tone through mechanisms that alter vascular smooth muscle as well as by stimulating the release of NO from the endothelium. Diametrically opposite effects can occur in the presence of risk factors that impair endothelium-dependent vasodilation. Their actions in normal and pathophysiologic states are summarized in Table 52-1.

Cholinergic Innervation

Resistance arteries dilate to acetylcholine, resulting in increases in coronary flow. In conduit arteries, acetylcholine normally causes mild coronary vasodilation. This reflects the net action of a direct muscarinic constriction of vascular smooth muscle counterbalanced by an endothelium-dependent vasodilation caused by direct stimulation of NOS and an increased flow-mediated dilation from concomitant resistance vessel vasodilation. The response in humans with atherosclerosis or risk factors for CAD is distinctly different. The resistance vessel dilation to acetylcholine is attenuated and the reduction in flow-mediated NO production leads to net epicardial conduit artery vasoconstriction, which is particularly prominent in stenotic segments (**Fig. 52-10A**).

Sympathetic Innervation

Under basal conditions, there is no resting sympathetic tone in the heart and thus there is no effect of denervation on resting perfusion. During sympathetic activation, coronary tone is modulated by norepinephrine released from myocardial sympathetic nerves, as well as by circulating norepinephrine and epinephrine.[3,24] In conduit arteries, sympathetic stimulation leads to alpha₁ constriction as well as beta₂-mediated vasodilation. The net effect is to dilate epicardial coronary arteries. This dilation is potentiated by concomitant flow-mediated vasodilation from metabolic vasodilation of coronary resistance vessels. When NO-mediated vasodilation is impaired, alpha₁ constriction predominates and can dynamically increase stenosis severity in asymmetrical lesions in which the stenosis is compliant. This is one of the mechanisms that can provoke ischemia during cold pressor testing (see Fig. 52-10B).

The effects of sympathetic activation on myocardial perfusion and coronary resistance vessel tone are complex and dependent on the net actions of $beta_1$-mediated increases in myocardial oxygen consumption (resulting from increases in the determinants of myocardial oxygen consumption), direct $beta_2$-mediated coronary vasodilation, and $alpha_1$-mediated coronary constriction. Under normal conditions, exercise-induced $beta_2$-adrenergic feed-forward dilation predominates, resulting in a higher flow relative to the level of myocardial oxygen consumption.[23] This neural control mechanism produces transient vasodilation before the buildup of local metabolites during exercise and prevents the development of subendocardial ischemia during abrupt changes in demand. After nonselective beta blockade, sympathetic activation unmasks $alpha_1$-mediated coronary artery constriction. Although flow is mildly decreased, oxygen delivery is maintained by increased oxygen extraction and a reduction in coronary venous PO_2 at similar levels of cardiac workload. Intense $alpha_1$-adrenergic constriction can overcome intrinsic stimuli for metabolic vasodilation and result in ischemia in the presence of pharmacologic vasodilator reserve.[24] The role of pre- and postsynaptic $alpha_2$ responses is controversial. They appear to have a less significant role in controlling flow. This partly reflects the competing effects of presynaptic $alpha_2$ receptor stimulation, leading to reduced vasoconstriction by inhibiting norepinephrine release.

PARACRINE VASOACTIVE MEDIATORS AND CORONARY VASOSPASM. There are a large number of paracrine factors that can affect coronary tone in normal and pathophysiologic states that are unrelated to normal coronary circulatory control. The most important of these are summarized in Table 52-1 (see Fig. 52-e1 on website). Paracrine factors are released from epicardial artery thrombi after activation of the thrombotic cascade initiated by plaque rupture. They can modulate epicardial tone in regions near eccentric ulcerated plaques that are still responsive to stimuli that alter smooth muscle relaxation and constriction, leading to dynamic changes in the physiologic significance of a stenosis. Paracrine mediators can also have differential effects on downstream vessel vasomotion that are dependent on vessel size (conduit arteries versus resistance arteries) as well as on the presence of a functionally normal endothelium, because many also stimulate the release of NO and EDHF.

Serotonin released from activated platelets causes vasoconstriction in normal and atherosclerotic conduit arteries and can increase the functional severity of a dynamic coronary stenosis through superimposed vasospasm. In contrast, it dilates coronary resistance vessels (<100 μm) and increases coronary flow through the endothelium-dependent release of NO. In atherosclerosis or circumstances in which

NO production is impaired, the direct effects on smooth muscle predominate and the response of the microcirculation is converted to vasoconstriction. As a result, serotonin release generally exacerbates ischemia in CAD.

Thromboxane A_2 is a potent vasoconstrictor that is a product of endoperoxide metabolism and is released during platelet aggregation. It produces vasoconstriction of conduit arteries and isolated coronary resistance vessels and can accentuate acute myocardial ischemia.

ADP is another platelet-derived vasodilator that relaxes coronary microvessels and conduit arteries. It is mediated by NO and abolished by removing the endothelium.

Thrombin normally leads to vasodilation in vitro that is endothelium-dependent and mediated by the release of prostacyclin as well as NO. In vivo, it also releases thromboxane A_2, leading to vasoconstriction in epicardial stenoses in which endothelium-dependent vasodilation is

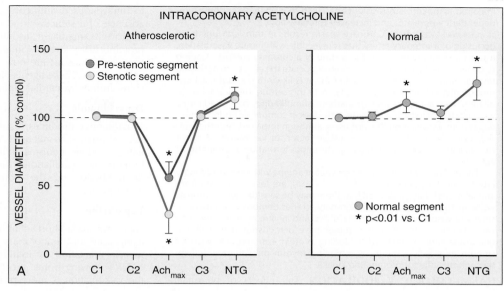

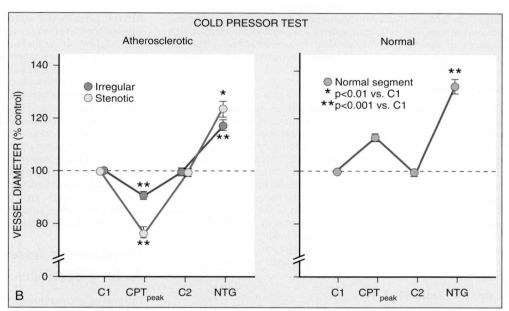

FIGURE 52-10 Differential conduit artery diameter responses in normal and atherosclerotic epicardial arteries. **A,** Acetylcholine. In normal arteries, acetylcholine elicits vasodilation but there is vasoconstriction in the atherosclerotic artery, which is particularly pronounced in the stenosis. **B,** Cold pressor testing. Activation of sympathetic tone normally leads to net epicardial dilation but there is vasoconstriction in irregular and stenotic coronary segments in patients with atherosclerosis. Ach = acetylcholine; C = control; CPT = cold pressor test; NTG = nitroglycerin. (**A** modified from Ludmer PL, Selwyn AP, Shook TL, et al: Paradoxical vasoconstriction induced by acetylcholine in atherosclerotic coronary arteries. N Engl J Med 315:1046, 1986; **B** modified from Nabel EG, Ganz P, Gordon JB, et al: Dilation of normal and constriction of atherosclerotic coronary arteries caused by the cold pressor test. Circulation 77:43, 1988.)

impaired. In the coronary resistance vasculature, it acts as an endothelium-dependent vasodilator and increases coronary flow.

CORONARY VASOSPASM. Coronary spasm results in transient functional occlusion of a coronary artery that is reversible with nitrate vasodilation. It most commonly occurs in the setting of a coronary stenosis, leading to dynamic stenosis behavior, and can dissociate the effects on perfusion from anatomic stenosis severity. In CAD, it is likely that endothelial disruption plays a role in focal vasospasm. In this setting, the normal vasodilation from autacoids and sympathetic stimulation is converted into a vasoconstrictor response because of the lack of competing endothelium-dependent vasodilation. Nevertheless, although impaired endothelium-dependent vasodilation is a permissive factor for vasospasm, it is not causal, and a trigger is required (e.g., thrombus formation or sympathetic activation).

The mechanisms responsible for variant angina with normal coronary arteries, or Prinzmetal angina (see Chap. 56), are less clear. Data from animal models have indicated that there may be sensitization of intrinsic vasoconstrictor mechanisms.[25] Coronary arteries demonstrate supersensitivity to vasoconstrictor agonists in vivo and in vitro as well as reduced vasodilatory responses. Some studies have demonstrated that Rho, a guanosine triphosphate (GTP)–binding protein, can sensitize vascular smooth muscle to calcium by inhibiting myosin phosphatase activity through the effector protein Rho kinase.

PHARMACOLOGIC VASODILATION. The effects of pharmacologic vasodilators on coronary flow reflect direct actions on vascular smooth muscle as well as secondary adjustments in resistance artery tone. Flow-mediated dilation can amplify the vasodilatory response, whereas autoregulatory adjustments can overcome vasodilation in a segment of the microcirculation and restore flow to normal. The potent resistance vessel vasodilators are specifically used in assessing coronary stenosis severity.[26]

Nitroglycerin

Nitroglycerin dilates epicardial conduit arteries and small coronary resistance arteries but does not increase coronary blood flow in the normal heart. This latter observation reflects the fact that transient arteriolar vasodilation is overcome by autoregulatory escape, which returns coronary resistance to control levels.[27] Although nitroglycerin does not increase coronary blood flow in the normal heart, it can produce vasodilation of large coronary resistance arteries, which improves the distribution of perfusion to the subendocardium when flow-mediated[9] NO-dependent vasodilation is impaired. It can also improve subendocardial perfusion by reducing LV end-diastolic pressure through systemic venodilation in heart failure. Similarly, coronary collateral vessels dilate in response to nitroglycerin, and the reduction in collateral resistance can improve regional perfusion in some settings.

Calcium Channel Blockers

All calcium channel blockers lead to vascular smooth muscle relaxation and are, to various degrees, pharmacologic coronary vasodilators. In epicardial arteries, the vasodilation is similar to that of nitroglycerin and is effective in preventing coronary vasospasm superimposed on a coronary stenosis as well as in normal arteries of patients with variant angina. They also submaximally vasodilate coronary resistance vessels. In this regard, dihydropyridine derivatives such as nifedipine are particularly potent and can sometimes precipitate subendocardial ischemia in the face of a critical stenosis. This arises from a transmural redistribution of blood flow as well and the tachycardia and hypotension that transiently occur with short half-life formulations of nifedipine.

Adenosine and A_2 Receptor Agonists

Adenosine dilates coronary arteries through activation of A2 receptors on vascular smooth muscle and is independent of the endothelium in coronary arterioles isolated from humans with heart disease.[21] Experimentally, there is a differential sensitivity of the microcirculation to adenosine, with the direct effects related to resistance vessel size and primarily restricted to vessels smaller than 100 µm.[14] Larger upstream resistance arteries dilate via an NO-dependent mechanism from the increase in shear stress. Thus, in states in which endothelium-dependent vasodilation is impaired, maximal coronary flow responses

to intravenous or intracoronary adenosine may be reduced in the absence of a stenosis[22] and can be increased by interventions that improve NO-mediated vasodilation, such as lowering low-density lipoprotein (LDL) levels.[28] Single-dose adenosine A_2 receptor agonists (e.g., regadenoson) are now clinically available and are as effective as adenosine. These agents circumvent the need for continuous infusions during myocardial perfusion imaging (see Chap. 17).[26]

Dipyridamole

Dipyridamole produces vasodilation by inhibiting the myocyte reuptake of adenosine released from cardiac myocytes. It therefore has actions and mechanisms similar to those of adenosine, with the exception that the vasodilation is more prolonged. It can be reversed via the administration of the nonspecific adenosine receptor blocker aminophylline.

Papaverine

Papaverine is a short-acting coronary vasodilator that was the first agent used for intracoronary vasodilation. It causes vascular smooth muscle relaxation by inhibiting phosphodiesterase and increasing cAMP. Following bolus injection, it has a rapid onset of action, but the vasodilation is more prolonged than after adenosine (approximately 2 minutes). Its actions are independent of the endothelium.

RIGHT CORONARY ARTERY FLOW. Although the general concepts of coronary flow regulation developed for the left ventricle apply to the right ventricle, there are differences related to the extent of the right coronary artery supply to the right ventricular free wall. This has been studied in dogs, in which the right coronary artery is a nondominant vessel.[29] In terms of coronary flow reserve, arterial pressure supplying the right coronary substantially exceeds right ventricular pressure, minimizing the compressive determinants of coronary reserve. Right ventricular oxygen consumption is lower than that in the left ventricle, and coronary venous oxygen saturations are higher than in the left coronary circulation. Because there is considerable oxygen extraction reserve, coronary flow decreases as pressure is reduced and oxygen delivery is maintained by increased extraction. These differences appear specific to the right ventricular free wall. In humans, in whom the right coronary artery is dominant (see Chap. 21) and supplies a large amount of the inferior left ventricle, factors affecting flow regulation to the LV myocardium are likely to predominate.

Physiologic Assessment of Coronary Artery Stenoses

The physiologic assessment of stenosis severity is a critical component of the management of patients with obstructive epicardial CAD.[30] Epicardial artery stenoses arising from atherosclerosis increase coronary resistance and reduce maximal myocardial perfusion. Abnormalities in coronary microcirculatory control can also contribute to causing myocardial ischemia in many patients. Separating the role of a stenosis from coronary resistance vessels can be accomplished by simultaneously assessing coronary flow and distal coronary pressure using intracoronary transducers that are currently available for clinical care.[31]

Stenosis Pressure-Flow Relationship

The angiographically visible epicardial coronary arteries are normally able to accommodate large increases in coronary flow without producing any significant pressure drop and thus serve a conduit function to the coronary resistance vasculature. This changes dramatically in CAD, in which the epicardial artery resistance becomes dominant. This fixed component of resistance increases with stenosis severity and limits maximal myocardial perfusion.

As a starting point, it is helpful to consider the idealized relationship between stenosis severity, pressure drop, and flow that has been validated in animals as well as humans studied in circumstances in which diffuse atherosclerosis and risk factors that can impair microcirculatory resistance vessel control are minimized. **Figure 52-11** summarizes the major determinants of stenosis energy losses. The relationship between pressure drop across a stenosis and coronary flow for stenoses between

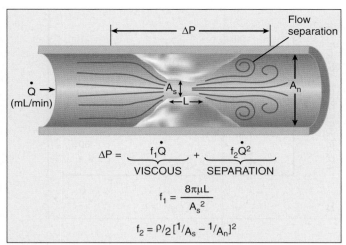

$$\Delta P = \underbrace{\frac{f_1 \dot{Q}}{}}_{\text{VISCOUS}} + \underbrace{\frac{f_2 \dot{Q}^2}{}}_{\text{SEPARATION}}$$

$$f_1 = \frac{8\pi\mu L}{A_s^2}$$

$$f_2 = \rho/2 \left[{}^1/A_s - {}^1/A_n \right]^2$$

FIGURE 52-11 Fluid mechanics of a stenosis. The pressure drop across a stenosis can be predicted by the Bernoulli equation. It is inversely related to the minimum stenosis cross-sectional area and varies with the square of the flow rate as stenosis severity increases. A_n = area of the normal segment; A_s = area of the stenosis; f_1 = viscous coefficient; f_2 = separation coefficient; L = stenosis length; ΔP = pressure drop; $\dot{Q}$ = flow; μ = viscosity of blood; ρ = density of blood.

30% and 90% diameter reduction can be described using the Bernoulli principle. The total pressure drop across a stenosis is governed by three hydrodynamic factors—viscous losses, separation losses, and turbulence, although the latter is usually a relatively minor component of pressure loss. The single most important determinant of stenosis resistance for any given level of flow is the minimum lesional cross-sectional area within the stenosis.[32] Because resistance is inversely proportional to the square of the cross-sectional area, small dynamic changes in luminal area caused by thrombi or vasomotion in asymmetric lesions (where vascular smooth muscle can relax or constrict in a portion of the stenosis) lead to major changes in the stenosis pressure-flow relationship and reduce maximal perfusion during vasodilation. Separation losses determine the curvilinearity or steepness of the stenosis pressure-flow relationship and become increasingly important as stenosis severity and/or flow rate increase(s). Stenosis length and changes in cross-sectional area distal to the stenosis are relatively minor determinants of resistance for most coronary lesions.

Diffuse abluminal outward remodeling with thickening of the arterial wall is common in coronary atherosclerosis but does not alter the pressure-flow characteristics of the stenosis for a given intraluminal geometry. In contrast, diffuse inward remodeling effectively reduces minimal lesion area along the length of the vessel and can underestimate stenosis severity using relative diameter measurements and contribute to a significant longitudinal pressure drop that can reduce maximum perfusion.[30]

Stenosis resistance increases exponentially as minimum lesional cross-sectional area decreases (**Fig. 52-12**). It is also flow dependent and varies with the square of the flow or flow velocity. As a result, the instantaneous stenosis resistance increases during vasodilation. This is particularly important in determining the stenosis pressure-flow behavior for severely narrowed arteries and leads to a situation in which small reductions in luminal area result in large reductions in poststenotic coronary pressure and maximum coronary perfusion as stenosis severity increases.

Interrelationship Among Distal Coronary Pressure, Flow, and Stenosis Severity

Because maximum myocardial perfusion is ultimately determined by the coronary pressure distal to a stenosis, it is helpful to place the epicardial stenosis pressure-flow relationship into the context of the coronary autoregulatory and vasodilated coronary pressure-flow relationships (**Fig. 52-13**). The effects of a stenosis on resting and vasodilated flow as a function of percentage diameter reduction when diffuse intraluminal narrowing is absent and coronary microcirculatory resistance is normal are summarized in Figure 52-13A. Because of coronary autoregulation, flow remains constant as stenosis severity increases. Thus, imaging resting perfusion cannot identify hemodynamically severe stenoses (see Chap. 17). In contrast, the maximally vasodilated pressure-flow relationship is

much more sensitive for detecting increases in stenosis severity. There is normally substantial coronary flow reserve and flow can increase approximately five times the resting flow values. Very little increase in epicardial conduit artery resistance (R_1) develops until stenosis severity reaches a 50% diameter reduction (see Fig. 52-13B). As a result, there is no significant pressure drop across a stenosis or stenosis-related alteration in maximal myocardial perfusion until stenosis severity exceeds a 50% diameter reduction (75% cross-sectional area). As stenosis severity increases further, the curvilinear coronary pressure-flow relationship steepens and increases in stenosis resistance are accompanied by concomitant increases in the pressure drop (ΔP) across the stenosis. This reduces distal coronary pressure, the major determinant of perfusion to the microcirculation, and maximum vasodilated flow decreases (see Fig. 52-13C). Above a value of 70% diameter reduction, small increases in stenosis severity are accompanied by further increases in stenosis pressure drop that reduce distal coronary pressure and result in progressive reductions in maximal vasodilated perfusion of the microcirculation. A critical stenosis, one in which subendocardial flow reserve is completely exhausted at rest, usually develops when stenosis severity exceeds 90%. Under these circumstances, pharmacologic vasodilation of subepicardial resistance vessels results in a reduction in distal coronary pressure that actually redistributes flow from the subendocardium, leading to a transmural steal phenomenon.

Concept of Maximal Perfusion and Coronary Reserve

Gould originally proposed the concept of coronary reserve.[30] With technologic advances, it has become possible to characterize this in humans using invasive catheter-based measurements of intracoronary pressure and flow (**Fig. 52-14**) and noninvasive imaging of myocardial perfusion with positron emission tomography (PET), single-photon emission tomography (SPECT; see Chap. 17) and, more recently, cardiac magnetic resonance imaging (CMR; see Chap. 18). With physiologically based approaches to quantify perfusion and coronary pressure, it has also become increasingly apparent that abnormalities in coronary microcirculatory control contribute to the functional significance of

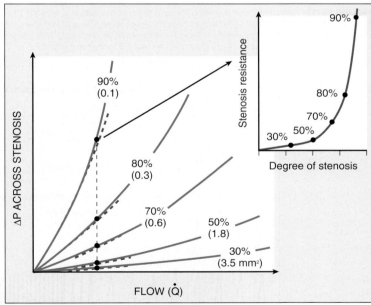

FIGURE 52-12 Curvilinearity of the pressure-flow relationship as stenosis severity increases. The relationship between pressure drop across the stenosis and flow for diameter narrowing of 30%, 50%, 70%, 80%, and 90% is calculated on the basis of a proximal reference internal diameter of 3 mm (area, 7.1 mm²). Measurements in parentheses are minimal lesional cross-sectional areas. Instantaneous resistance is the slope of the pressure-flow curve (dashed red line) and, for a given stenosis, increases as flow rate rises. At levels of resting flow (dashed vertical line), the stenosis resistance increases exponentially as stenosis severity rises (solid red line in inset). *(Modified from Klocke FJ: Measurements of coronary blood flow and degree of stenosis: Current clinical implications and continuing uncertainties. J Am Coll Cardiol 1:31, 1983.)*

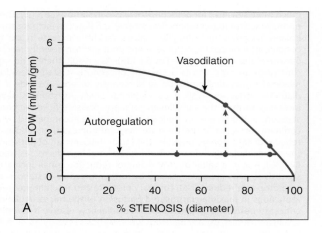

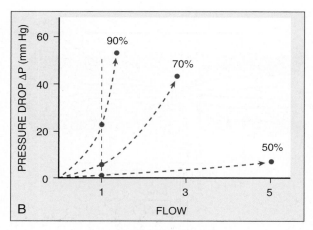

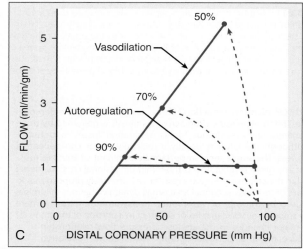

FIGURE 52-13 Interrelationship among stenosis flow reserve **(A),** the stenosis pressure-flow relationship **(B),** and autoregulation **(C).** Red circles depict resting flow and blue circles maximal vasodilation for stenoses of 50%, 70%, and 90% diameter reduction. There is very little pressure drop across a 50% stenosis, and distal coronary pressure and vasodilated flow remain near normal. In contrast, a 90% stenosis critically impairs flow, because the steep pressure flow relationship causes a marked reduction in distal coronary pressure. See text for further discussion.

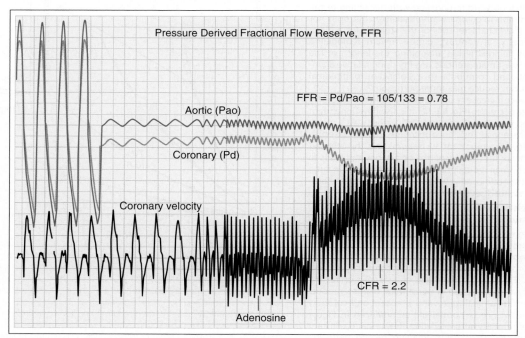

FIGURE 52-14 Coronary pressure and flow velocity tracings in a patient with an intermediate stenosis. Following intracoronary adenosine, flow velocity transiently increases and mean distal coronary pressure (Pd) falls. Absolute coronary flow reserve (CFR) is the ratio of peak flow to resting flow. Fractional flow reserve (FFR) is the ratio of Pd/Pao (distal coronary pressure divided by mean aortic pressure).

isolated epicardial artery stenoses in many patients with CAD. There are currently three major indices used to quantify coronary flow reserve—absolute, relative, and fractional. These are compared in **Figure 52-15**, and the relative advantages and limitations of each of the currently used indices are discussed here.

ABSOLUTE FLOW RESERVE. Initial approaches to assess functional stenosis severity focused on assessing the relative increase in flow following ischemic vasodilation (reactive hyperemic response following transient occlusion of the coronary artery) or pharmacologic vasodilation of the microcirculation with intracoronary papaverine, adenosine, or intravenous dipyridamole. Absolute flow reserve can be quantified using intracoronary Doppler velocity or thermodilution flow measurements, as well as by quantitative approaches to image absolute tissue perfusion based on PET. It is expressed as the ratio of maximally vasodilated flow to the corresponding resting flow value in a specific region of the heart and quantifies the ability of flow to increase above the resting value (see Fig. 52-15A). Clinically important reductions in maximum flow correlating with stress-induced ischemia on SPECT are generally associated with absolute flow reserve values below 2 (see Chap. 17).[31] Absolute flow reserve is altered not only by factors that affect maximal coronary flow (e.g., stenosis severity, impaired microcirculatory control, arterial pressure, heart rate) but also by the corresponding resting flow value. Resting flow can vary with hemoglobin content, baseline hemodynamics, and the resting oxygen extraction. As a result, reductions in absolute flow reserve can arise from inappropriate elevations in resting coronary flow and from reductions in maximal perfusion.

In the absence of diffuse atherosclerosis or LV hypertrophy, absolute flow reserve in conscious humans is similar to measurements in animals, with vasodilated flow increasing four to five times the value at rest. There is also fairly good reduplication of the idealized relationship between stenosis severity and absolute flow reserve in patients with isolated one- or two-vessel CAD (**Fig. 52-16A**) with intracoronary vasodilation. In contrast, in patients with risk factors such as hypercholesterolemia and no significant coronary luminal narrowing, values of absolute flow reserve using PET are lower than in normals, reflecting microcirculatory impairment in flow or attenuated vasodilator responsiveness.[33] Abnormalities in the coronary microcirculation and uncertainty in stenosis geometry or diffuse atherosclerosis lead to considerably more variability of the observed relationship between stenosis severity and absolute flow reserve in patients with more extensive disease (see Fig 52-16B). A significant limitation of absolute flow reserve measurements is that the importance of an epicardial stenosis cannot be dissociated from changes caused by functional abnormalities in the microcirculation that are common in patients (e.g., hypertrophy, impaired endothelium-dependent vasodilation).

RELATIVE FLOW RESERVE. Relative coronary flow reserve measurements are the cornerstone of noninvasive identification of hemodynamically important coronary stenoses using nuclear perfusion imaging (see Chap. 17). In this approach, relative differences in regional perfusion (per gram of tissue) are assessed during maximal pharmacologic vasodilation or exercise stress and expressed as a fraction of flow to normal regions of the heart (see Fig. 52-15B). This compares relative perfusion under the same hemodynamic conditions and thus is relatively insensitive to variations in mean arterial pressure and heart rate. An alternative invasive approach uses absolute flow reserve measurements and derives relative flow reserve by dividing measurements in a stenotic vessel by those in remote normally perfused territories.[31]

Although widely used to identify hemodynamically significant stenoses, there are significant limitations in using imaging to quantify relative flow reserve. First, conventional SPECT imaging requires a normal reference segment within the left ventricle for comparison. Because of this, relative flow reserve measurements cannot accurately quantify stenosis severity when diffuse abnormalities in flow reserve related to balanced multivessel CAD or impaired microcirculatory vasodilation are present. Large differences in relative vasodilated flow are required to detect SPECT perfusion differences because nuclear tracers become diffusion-limited and their myocardial uptake fails to

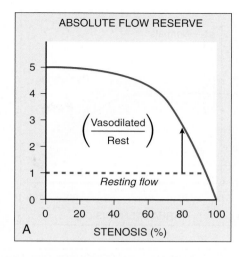

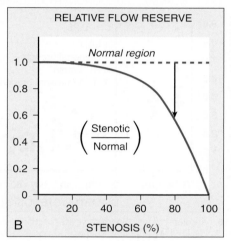

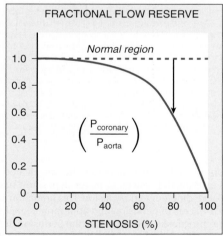

FIGURE 52-15 Absolute flow reserve, relative flow reserve, and fractional flow reserve. **A,** Absolute flow reserve is the ratio of coronary flow during vasodilation to the resting value. It can be obtained with invasive measurements of intracoronary flow velocity or quantitative kinetic perfusion measurements with PET. **B,** Relative flow reserve compares maximal vasodilated flow in a stenotic region with an assumed normal region in the same heart and is most commonly measured with perfusion imaging during stress. **C,** Fractional flow reserve is conceptually similar to relative flow reserve and assesses maximal flow indirectly from coronary pressure measurements distal to a stenosis during vasodilation. Neither relative flow reserve nor fractional flow reserve can identify the contribution of abnormalities in microcirculatory resistance control to the development of myocardial ischemia.

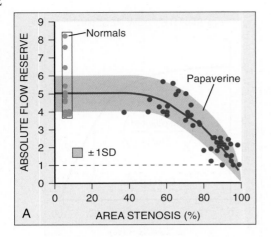

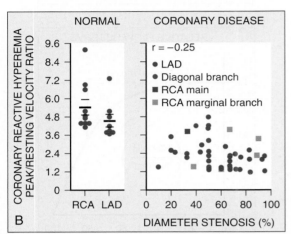

FIGURE 52-16 Absolute coronary flow reserve as a function of stenosis severity in patients. **A,** Idealized absolute flow reserve following intracoronary vasodilation in single-vessel disease without hypertrophy demonstrates a good correlation with values predicted theoretically. **B,** Absolute flow reserve assessed using intraoperative epicardial Doppler flow measurements following reactive hyperemia to a 20-second occlusion. Among all vessels, there is a poor relationship with stenosis severity. This reflects variability in stenosis severity with visual interpretation as well as abnormal microcirculatory responses to ischemia and multiple risk factors for impaired endothelial function. LAD = left anterior descending artery; RCA = right coronary artery. (*A modified from Wilson RF, Marcus ML, White CW: Prediction of the physiologic significance of coronary arterial lesions by quantitative lesion geometry in patients with limited coronary artery disease. Circulation 75:723, 1987; B modified from White CW, Wright CB, Doty DB, et al: Does visual interpretation of the coronary arteriogram predict the physiologic importance of a coronary stenosis? N Engl J Med 310:819, 1984.*)

increase proportionally with increases in vasodilated flow (see Chap. 17). As a result, differences in tracer deposition underestimate the actual relative difference in perfusion. This limitation can be overcome with PET tracers of perfusion and appropriate kinetic modeling. Finally, whereas prognostic data related to the perfusion deficit size are available, there are no imaging studies evaluating the quantitative severity of the stress or vasodilated flow reduction as a continuous outcome measure although, conceptually, this should be similar to fractional flow reserve.

FRACTIONAL FLOW RESERVE. Considerable focus has turned toward invasive point of care approaches that use pressure measurements distal to a coronary stenosis as an indirect index of stenosis severity (see Fig. 52-14).[31] This technique, pioneered by Pijls, is based on the principle that the distal coronary pressure measured during vasodilation is directly proportional to maximum vasodilated perfusion (see Fig. 52-15C). Fractional flow reserve (FFR) is an indirect index determined by measuring the driving pressure for microcirculatory flow distal to the stenosis (distal coronary pressure minus coronary venous pressure) relative to the coro-

nary driving pressure available in the absence of a stenosis (mean aortic pressure minus coronary venous pressure). The approach assumes linearity of the vasodilated pressure-flow relationship, which is known to be curvilinear at reduced coronary pressure,[34] and usually assumes that coronary venous pressure is zero. This results in the simplified clinical FFR index of mean distal coronary pressure/mean aortic pressure (Pd/Pao). Although derived, the measurements are conceptually similar to those of relative coronary flow reserve because they rely only on minimum mean coronary pressure measurements during intracoronary vasodilation and compare stenotic with normal regions (assumed to equal 1) under similar hemodynamic conditions. They are attractive in that they can immediately assess the physiologic significance of an intermediate stenosis to help guide decisions regarding coronary intervention and are unaffected by alterations in resting flow. Similarly, because they only require vasodilated coronary pressure measurements, FFR can be used to assess the functional effects of a residual lesion after percutaneous coronary intervention (PCI; see Chap. 58).

A significant advantage of FFR is that there is now considerable prognostic information, including recent data from a large prospective randomized study, indicating that FFR measurements more than 0.75 are associated with excellent outcomes with deferred rather than prophylactic intervention.[35] This study demonstrated that physiologically guided PCI using FFR versus angiographic criteria is safe and cost-effective and reduces the number of stents required to treat patients with multivessel CAD. Furthermore, the ischemia-driven strategy based on physiologic assessment of stenoses was accompanied by a significant reduction in major adverse cardiac events at one year (13.2% versus 18.3% in angiographically guided treatment (see Fig. 52-e2 on website). This provides further support for the role of ischemia in prognosis and a physiologically guided approach to percutaneous coronary intervention.

A limitation of FFR is that it can only assess the functional significance of epicardial artery stenoses and cannot assess physiologic contributions caused by abnormalities in microcirculatory flow reserve in resistance vessels. Although simple, the measurements are also critically dependent on achieving maximal pharmacologic vasodilation (underestimating stenosis severity if vasodilation is submaximal at the time of measurement). In addition, ignoring the backpressure to coronary flow by assuming that venous pressure is equal to zero and ignoring curvilinearity of the diastolic pressure-flow relationship will cause the FFR to underestimate the physiologic significance of a stenosis.[34] This is particularly problematic at low coronary pressures and when assessing the functional significance of coronary collaterals where venous pressure needs to be accounted for. Finally, inserting the guidewire across a stenosis can artifactually overestimate stenosis severity caused by the reduction in effective intralesional area when there is diffuse disease, when it is placed in small branch vessels, or in assessing a severe stenosis. Despite these limitations and its invasive nature, FFR is currently the most direct way to assess the physiologic significance of individual coronary lesions.

STENOSIS PRESSURE-FLOW RELATIONSHIP. The availability of high-fidelity pressure and flow measurements on a single wire has now facilitated the development of approaches to assess the stenosis pressure-flow relationship as well as abnormalities in microcirculatory reserve by determining the FFR and absolute coronary flow reserve simultaneously. When assessed together, these measurements have the potential to identify circumstances in which mixed abnormalities, stenosis and microcirculation, contribute to the net physiologic significance of a stenosis (**Fig. 52-17**). The instantaneous relationship between flow and pressure drop across the stenosis can also be obtained at the time of PCI. Although this has not yet been widely validated or used in clinical settings, it may afford a more accurate approach to assess contributions of a coronary stenosis versus those of the microcirculation.[31]

ADVANTAGES AND LIMITATIONS OF CORONARY FLOW RESERVE MEASUREMENTS. Assessing qualitative perfusion differences with noninvasive imaging is useful because relative perfusion deficit size is an important determinant of prognosis (see Chap. 17). Although the clinical role of invasive measurements that quantify functional stenosis severity continues to evolve, measurements of FFR, available at the point of interventional care, have been demonstrated to affect postprocedural outcomes favorably at reduced cost. The need to use these measurements in decision making may change in future clinical care guidelines.[31]

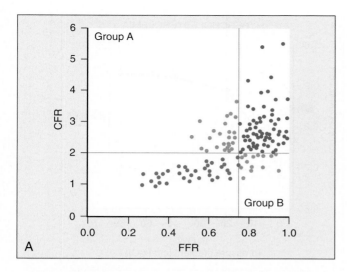

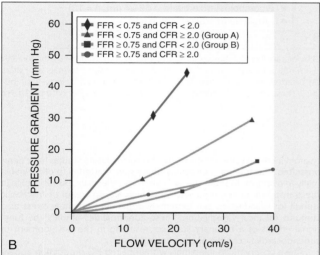

FIGURE 52-17 Characterization of coronary stenosis severity with simultaneous measurements of intracoronary pressure and flow. **A,** Vertical line represents a threshold fractional flow reserve (FFR) of 0.75 and the horizontal line predicts a threshold coronary flow reserve (CFR) of 2. Group A depicts patients with significant stenoses by FFR who have relatively preserved microvascular function and a CFR higher than 2. Group B depicts patients with microcirculatory impairment or submaximal vasodilation in whom CFR is limited but FFR is not reduced. **B,** Instantaneous stenosis pressure-flow relationships corresponding to the four groups depicted in **A**. *(Modified from Meuwissen M, Chamuleau S, Siebes M, et al: Role of variability in microvascular resistance on fractional flow reserve and coronary blood flow velocity reserve in intermediate coronary lesions. Circulation 103:184, 2001.)*

The major assumption common to all flow reserve measurements is that the pharmacologic vasodilator used consistently achieves maximal vasodilation of the resistance vasculature in normals as well as in patients with atherosclerotic disease and impaired endothelial function. The reductions in absolute flow reserve in people with angiographically insignificant stenoses (see Fig. 52-16B), as well as variability in quantitative perfusion measurements with normal epicardial arteries and coronary risk factors, indicate that this may not always be the case. The extent to which this is related to a structural abnormality in the microcirculation (e.g., caused by regional hypertrophy or vascular remodeling) versus a functional abnormality in the microcirculation (altered microcirculatory vasodilatory response versus impaired endothelium-dependent vasodilation) remains unclear. A second limitation is that currently available approaches can only measure coronary flow reserve averaged across the entire wall of the heart. This is because they are based on invasive epicardial coronary measurements or, in the case of imaging (SPECT and PET), have insufficient

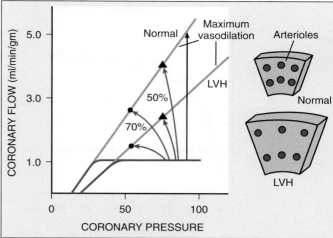

FIGURE 52-18 Effects of left ventricular hypertrophy (LVH) on maximal coronary flow. With acquired LVH, myocardial mass increases without proliferation of the microcirculatory resistance arteries (right side). Because the maximal absolute flow per minute during vasodilation remains unchanged, the maximum flow per gram of tissue falls inversely with the change in LV mass. In contrast, whereas the resting flow per gram of myocardium remains constant with hypertrophy, the increase in LV mass requires a higher absolute resting flow. The net effect of these opposing actions is to decrease coronary flow reserve at any coronary pressure. As a result of the reduction in microcirculatory reserve in the absence of a coronary stenosis, the functional significance of a 50% stenosis (triangles) in the hypertrophied heart could approach a more severe stenosis (in the example, 70%, circles) in normal myocardium. This can even result in ischemia with normal coronary arteries during stress.

spatial resolution to assess transmural variations in flow (see Chap. 17). An imaging technique that could assess the physiologic significance of a stenosis in the subendocardial layers would be a major advance, because this region is the most severely affected by an epicardial stenosis. This is feasible with CMR (see Chap. 18).[35a]

Pathophysiologic States Affecting Microcirculatory Coronary Flow Reserve

Various pathophysiologic states can accentuate the effects of a fixed-diameter coronary stenosis as well as precipitate subendocardial ischemia during stress in the presence of normal coronary arteries. Thus, it is important to incorporate measurements of stenosis severity with abnormalities of coronary resistance vessel control. In the former case, treatment will be directed at the epicardial stenosis, whereas in the latter, medical therapies designed to improve abnormalities in resistance vessel control will be required. The prognostic importance of abnormalities in coronary resistance vessel control is underscored by emerging data in women evaluated for chest pain thought to be of ischemic origin. Abnormalities in coronary flow reserve and endothelium-dependent vasodilation are common in women with insignificant coronary disease and can be accompanied by metabolic ischemia, assessed by magnetic resonance spectroscopy (see Chap. 18), and they negatively affect prognosis.[36] The two most common factors affecting microcirculatory resistance control independently of coronary stenosis severity in patients are LV hypertrophy and impaired NO-mediated resistance vessel vasodilation.

LEFT VENTRICULAR HYPERTROPHY. The effects of hypertrophy on coronary flow reserve are complex and need to be thought of in terms of the absolute flow level (e.g., measured with an intracoronary Doppler probe) as well as the flow per gram of myocardium. With acquired hypertrophy, resting flow per gram of myocardium remains constant, but the increase in LV mass necessitates an increase in the absolute level of resting flow (mL/min) through the coronary artery.[37] In terms of maximal perfusion, acquired hypertrophy does not result in vascular proliferation and coronary resistance vessels remain unchanged (**Fig. 52-18**). Because

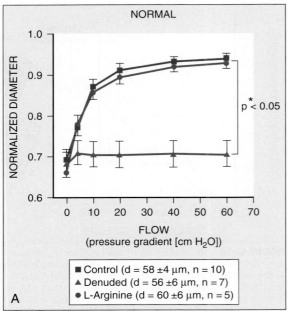
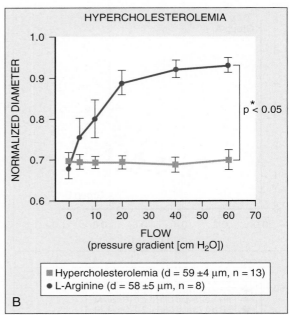

FIGURE 52-19 Flow-mediated vasodilation in coronary resistance arteries is abolished by dietary hypercholesterolemia in swine. **A,** In normal arterioles, increased flow (pressure gradient) elicits vasodilation that is abolished by removing the endothelium (denuded), similar to that in human vessels. **B,** In animals with dietary hypercholesterolemia but no significant epicardial stenosis, flow-mediated vasodilation of arterioles is abolished. It was restored by administering L-arginine to increase NO production. *(Modified from Kuo L, Davis MJ, Cannon MS, et al: Pathophysiological consequences of atherosclerosis extend into the coronary microcirculation: Restoration of endothelium-dependent responses by L-arginine. Circ Res 70:465, 1992.)*

maximum absolute flow (mL/min) remains unchanged, maximum perfusion per gram of myocardium falls. The net effect is that coronary flow reserve at any given coronary arterial pressure is reduced and inversely related to the change in LV mass. For example, in the absence of a change in mean aortic pressure, a twofold increase in LV mass, as is associated with severe LV hypertrophy, can reduce coronary flow reserve in a nonstenotic artery from 4 to 2 mL/min/g. This will increase the functional severity of any anatomic degree of coronary artery narrowing and can even precipitate subendocardial ischemia with normal coronary arteries.

Some degree of LV hypertrophy is common in patients with CAD and it likely contributes to reductions in coronary flow reserve that are independent of stenosis severity. The actual coronary flow reserve in hypertrophy will be critically dependent on the underlying cause of hypertrophy and its effects on coronary driving pressure. A similar degree of hypertrophy caused by untreated systemic hypertension will have a higher coronary flow reserve than in aortic stenosis, in which mean arterial pressure remains normal. Similarly, when hypertrophy is from systolic hypertension and increased pulse pressure caused by reduced aortic compliance, the accompanying reduction in diastolic pressure can lower coronary reserve.

IMPAIRED ENDOTHELIUM-DEPENDENT VASODILATION. Measurements of coronary flow reserve in humans with risk factors for atherosclerosis are systematically lower than normals without coronary risk factors and underscore the importance of abnormalities in microvascular control in determining coronary flow reserve. Much of this may reflect abnormal local resistance vessel control via impaired endothelial-dependent vasodilation arising from NO inactivation associated with risk factors for CAD. Kuo and colleagues have demonstrated that experimental hypercholesterolemia markedly attenuates the dilation of coronary arterioles in response to shear stress and pharmacologic agonists that stimulate NOS in the absence of epicardial stenoses (**Fig. 52-19**).[38] This was reversed with L-arginine, suggesting that it reflects impaired NO synthesis or availability.

Abnormalities in NO-mediated vasodilation in vivo are functionally significant and impair the ability of the heart to autoregulate coronary blood flow. **Figure 52-20** shows the effects of inhibiting NO on the coronary autoregulatory relationship in normal dogs.[39] Although resting blood flow is not altered, there is a marked increase in the coronary pressure at which intrinsic autoregulatory adjustments become exhausted, with flow beginning to decrease at a distal coronary pressure of 60 versus 45 mm Hg, approximately similar to the shift occurring in response to a

twofold increase in heart rate. In vivo microcirculatory studies have demonstrated that there is an inability of resistance arteries to dilate maximally in response to shear stress.[22] This likely reflects excess resistance in the transmural penetrating arteries, which are upstream of metabolic stimuli for vasodilation and extremely dependent on shear stress as a stimulus for local vasodilation. These abnormalities amplify the functional effects of a coronary stenosis, resulting in the development of subendocardial ischemia at a lower workload.[40]

These observations in animals with impaired NO production appear to be relevant to pathophysiologic states associated with impaired endothelium-dependent vasodilation in humans. For example, coronary flow reserve is markedly reduced in the absence of a coronary stenosis in familial hypercholesterolemia,[33] and improving endothelial function by lowering elevated LDL levels with statins produces a delayed improvement in coronary flow reserve in normal and stenotic arteries and also ameliorates clinical signs of myocardial ischemia.[28] Impaired NO-mediated vasodilation likely affects the regulation of myocardial perfusion in other disease states in which endothelium-dependent vasodilation is impaired.

Coronary Collateral Circulation

Following a total coronary occlusion, residual perfusion to the myocardium persists through native coronary collateral channels that open when an intercoronary pressure gradient between the source and recipient vessel develops. In animals, the native collateral flow during occlusion is less than 10% of the resting flow levels and is insufficient to maintain tissue viability for longer than 20 minutes. There is tremendous individual variability in the function of coronary collaterals among patients with chronic stenoses. In people without coronary collaterals, coronary pressure during balloon angioplasty occlusion falls to approximately 10 mm Hg. In other patients, collaterals proliferate to the point where they are sufficient not only to maintain normal resting perfusion but also to prevent stress-induced ischemia at submaximal cardiac workloads. Ischemia does not develop during PCI balloon occlusion when fractional flow reserve (based on coronary wedge pressure during occlusion minus venous pressure) is greater than 0.25.[31] A large observational cross-sectional study has demonstrated that patients with elevated distal coronary pressure arising

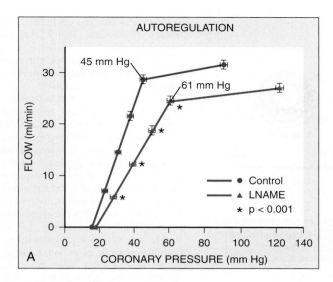

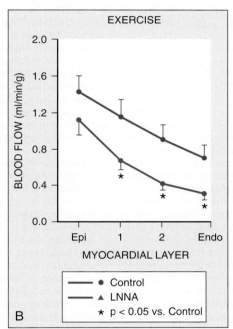

FIGURE 52-20 Impaired microcirculatory control with abnormal NO-mediated endothelium-dependent resistance artery dilation. **A,** Effects of blocking nitric oxide synthase (NOS) with the L-arginine analogue LNAME in chronically instrumented dogs. There is an increase in the lower autoregulatory pressure limit, resulting in the onset of ischemia at a coronary pressure of 61 mm Hg versus 45 mm Hg under normal conditions that occurred without a change in heart rate. **B,** Transmural perfusion before and after blocking NO-mediated dilation with LNNA in exercising dogs subjected to a coronary stenosis. Although coronary pressure and hemodynamics were similar, blood flow was lower in each layer of the heart after blocking NOS and not overcome by metabolic dilator mechanisms during ischemia. Collectively, these experimental data support the notion that abnormalities in endothelium-dependent vasodilation can amplify the functional effects of a coronary stenosis. Endo = endocardium; Epi = epicardium; LNAME = NG-nitro-L-arginine methyl ester; LNNA = NG-nitro-L-arginine. (**A** modified from Smith TP Jr, Canty JM Jr: Modulation of coronary autoregulatory responses by nitric oxide: Evidence for flow-dependent resistance adjustments in conscious dogs. Circ Res 73:232, 1993; **B** modified from Duncker DJ, Bache RJ: Inhibition of nitric oxide production aggravates myocardial hypoperfusion during exercise in the presence of a coronary artery stenosis. Circ Res 74:629, 1994.)

from recruitable collaterals during transient total balloon occlusion (fractional flow reserve > 0.25) have a lower cardiovascular event rate and improved survival (see Fig. 52-e3 on website).[41]

Arteriogenesis and Angiogenesis

Proliferation of coronary collaterals (see Chap. 21) occurs in response to repetitive stress-induced ischemia as well as the development of transient interarterial pressure gradients between the source and recipient vessel through a process termed *arteriogenesis*.[42] Resting distal coronary pressure consistently falls as stenosis severity exceeds 70% and the resultant interarterial pressure gradient increases endothelial shear stress in preexisting collaterals smaller than 200 µm in diameter. This causes progressive enlargement of collaterals through a process dependent on physical forces and growth factors, particularly vascular endothelial growth factor (VEGF) that is mediated via NO synthase. Thus, patients with impaired NO-mediated vasodilation resulting from coronary risk factors may have a limited ability to develop coronary collaterals in response to a chronic coronary stenosis.

Most functional collateral flow arises from arteriogenesis in existing epicardial anastomoses that enlarge into mature vessels that can reach 1 to 2 mm in diameter. Collateral perfusion can also originate from de novo vessel growth, or angiogenesis, which refers to the sprouting of smaller, capillary-like structures from preexisting blood vessels. These vessels may provide nutritive collateral flow when they develop in the border between ischemic and nonischemic regions. Capillary angiogenesis may also occur within the ischemic region and can reduce the intercapillary distance for oxygen exchange. Nevertheless, because capillary resistance is already a small component of microcirculatory resistance, increases in capillary density in the absence of changes in arteriolar resistance will not significantly increase myocardial perfusion.

There is currently great interest in experimental interventions to improve collateral flow (e.g., recombinant growth factors, in vivo gene transfer, and endothelial progenitor cells; see Chap. 11). Although many interventions have been shown to cause favorable angiogenesis of capillaries and improve myocardial function, few interventions have increased arteriogenesis in mature collaterals, and randomized human clinical trials have been disappointing.[43] Part of this may arise from the fact that no intervention has resulted in measurable increases in maximum vasodilated myocardial perfusion or coronary flow reserve indices, the sine qua non of functional collateral formation. Improvements in myocardial function have been used as an endpoint, but these may occur independently of increased perfusion and arise from mechanisms that alter cardiac myocyte growth and repair rather than angiogenesis.[44]

Regulation of Collateral Resistance

The control of blood flow to collateral-dependent myocardium is governed by a series resistance arising from interarterial collateral anastomoses, largely epicardial, as well as the native downstream microcirculation. Collateral resistance is therefore the major determinant of perfusion and coronary pressure distal to a chronic occlusion is already near the lower autoregulatory pressure limit. Because of this, subendocardial perfusion is critically dependent on mean aortic pressure and LV preload with ischemia easily provoked by systemic hypotension, increases in LV end-diastolic pressure, and tachycardia. Like the distal resistance vessels, collaterals constrict when NO synthesis is blocked, which aggravates myocardial ischemia and can be overcome by nitroglycerin.[9] In contrast to the native coronary circulation, experimental studies have shown that coronary collaterals are under tonic dilation from vasodilator prostaglandins, and blocking cyclooxygenase with aspirin exacerbates myocardial ischemia in dogs. The role of prostanoids in human coronary collateral resistance regulation is unknown.

The distal microcirculatory resistance vasculature in collateral-dependent myocardium appears to be regulated by mechanisms similar to those present in the normal circulation but is characterized by impaired endothelium-dependent vasodilation as compared with

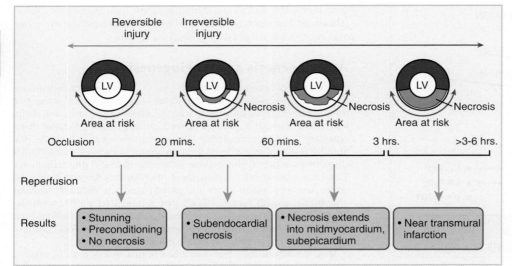

FIGURE 52-21 Wave front of necrosis in infarction in the absence of collaterals. Total occlusions shorter than 20 minutes do not cause irreversible injury but can cause myocardial stunning as well as precondition the heart and protect it against recurrent ischemic injury. Irreversible injury begins after 20 minutes and progresses as a wave front from endocardium to epicardium. After 60 minutes, the inner third of the LV wall is irreversibly injured. After 3 hours, there is a subepicardial rim of tissue remaining, with the transmural extent of infarction completed between 3 and 6 hours after occlusion. The most important factor delaying the progression of irreversible injury is the magnitude of collateral flow, which is primarily directed to the outer layers of the heart. *(Modified from Kloner RA, Jennings RB: Consequences of brief ischemia: Stunning, preconditioning, and their clinical implications: Part 1. Circulation 104:2981, 2001.)*

normal vessels. The extent to which these microcirculatory abnormalities alter the normal metabolic and coronary autoregulatory responses in collateral dependent myocardium is unknown.

Metabolic and Functional Consequences of Ischemia

Because oxygen delivery to the heart is closely coupled to coronary blood flow, a sudden cessation of regional perfusion following a thrombotic coronary occlusion quickly leads to the cessation of aerobic metabolism, depletion of creatine phosphate, and onset of anaerobic glycolysis. This is followed by the accumulation of tissue lactate, a progressive reduction in tissue ATP levels, and an accumulation of catabolites, including those of the adenine nucleotide pool. As ischemia continues, tissue acidosis develops and there is an efflux of potassium into the extracellular space. Subsequently, ATP levels fall below those required to maintain critical membrane function, resulting in the onset of myocyte death.

Irreversible Injury and Myocyte Death

The temporal evolution and extent of irreversible tissue injury after coronary occlusion are variable and dependent on transmural location, residual coronary flow, and the hemodynamic determinants of oxygen consumption. Irreversible myocardial injury begins after 20 minutes of coronary occlusion in the absence of significant collaterals.[45] Irreversible injury begins in the subendocardium and progresses as a wave front over time, from the subendocardial layers to the subepicardial layers (**Fig. 52-21**). This reflects the higher oxygen consumption in the subendocardium and the redistribution of collateral flow to the outer layers of the heart by the compressive determinants of flow at reduced coronary pressure. In experimental infarction, the entire subendocardium is irreversibly injured within 1 hour of occlusion and the transmural progression of infarction is largely completed within 4 to 6 hours after coronary occlusion. Factors that increase myocardial oxygen consumption (e.g., tachycardia) or reduce oxygen delivery (e.g., anemia, arterial hypotension) accelerate the progression of irreversible injury. In contrast, repetitive reversible ischemia or

angina prior to an occlusion can reduce irreversible injury through preconditioning.[46]

The magnitude of residual coronary flow through collaterals or through a subtotal coronary occlusion is the most important determinant of the actual time course of irreversible injury in patients with chronic CAD. The relationship between infarct size and the area at risk of ischemia during a total occlusion is inversely related to collateral flow and likely explains the important role of collateral vessel function in determining prognosis.[41] When subendocardial collateral flow is more than approximately 30% of resting flow values, it prevents infarction after periods of ischemia lasting longer than 1 hour. More moderate subendocardial ischemia from a subtotal occlusion (e.g., flow reduced by no more than 50%) can persist for at least 5 hours without producing significant irreversible injury.[47] This explains the fact that signs and symptoms of ischemia can be present for long periods without producing significant myocardial necrosis. It also explains the clinical observation that late coronary reperfusion with ongoing ischemia can salvage myocardium beyond the 6-hour time limit predicted from experimental models of infarction.

Cell death arises from multiple mechanisms in myocardial infarction (see Chap. 54).[48] Reperfusion immediately causes myocyte necrosis and sarcolemmal disruption, with the leakage of cell contents into the extracellular space. The injury is further amplified by the reentry of leukocytes into the area of injury. At later time points, myocytes initially salvaged can undergo programmed cell death or apoptosis, which can contribute to further delayed myocardial injury. Apoptosis is a coordinated involution of myocytes that circumvents the inflammation associated with necrotic cell death. Because apoptosis is an energy-dependent process, cells can be forced to switch to a necrotic pathway if energy levels are depleted below critical levels. In more chronic settings, autophagy can contribute to the mechanisms of myocyte death. Because of the temporal complexity of irreversible injury, the relative importance of each mechanism in myocardial infarction continues to be controversial. Nevertheless, modulating mechanisms contributing to late cell death could prevent deleterious LV remodeling.

Reversible Ischemia and Perfusion-Contraction Matching

Reversible ischemia is considerably more frequent than irreversible injury. Supply-induced ischemia can arise from transient coronary occlusion resulting from coronary vasospasm or transient thrombosis in a critically stenosed coronary artery, producing transmural ischemia similar to that present at the onset of infarction. Demand-induced ischemia arises from an inability to increase flow in response to increases in myocardial oxygen consumption in which ischemia predominantly affects the subendocardium. These have fundamentally different effects on myocardial diastolic relaxation, with supply-induced ischemia increasing LV compliance and demand-induced ischemia reducing it. There is a fairly stereotypical sequence of physiologic changes that develop during an episode of spontaneous transmural ischemia (**Fig. 52-22**). Coronary occlusion results in an immediate fall in coronary venous oxygen saturation, with a reduction in ATP production. This causes a decline in regional contraction within several beats, reaching dyskinesis within 1 minute. As regional contraction ceases, there is a reduction in global LV contractility (dP/dt), a progressive rise in LV end-diastolic pressure, and a fall in systolic pressure. The magnitude of the systemic hemodynamic changes varies with the severity of ischemia as well as the amount of the left ventricle subjected to ischemia. Significant electrocardiographic ST-segment changes develop within 2 minutes as efflux of potassium into the extra-

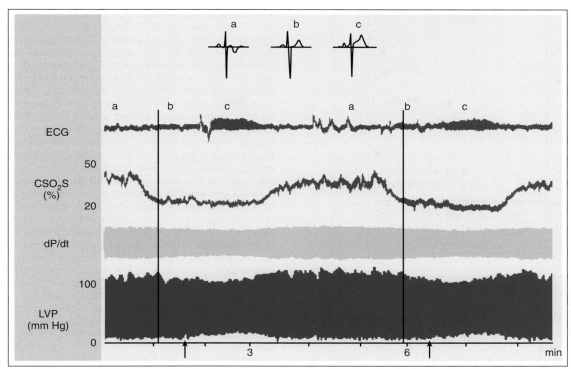

FIGURE 52-22 Physiologic changes during two episodes of spontaneous asymptomatic ischemia in a patient with acute coronary syndrome. High-speed electrocardiographic tracings depict the baseline ECG (a), pseudonormalization of T waves in early ischemia (b), and ST-segment elevation with late ischemia (c). A primary reduction in coronary flow is depicted by the sudden fall in coronary venous oxygen saturation (CSO₂S). Shortly thereafter, LV dP/dt falls, reflecting regional contractile dysfunction (solid vertical lines). Within 1 minute, LV end-diastolic pressure begins to rise (arrows) and is associated with a reduction in systolic pressure. Significant ST-segment elevation begins after the rise in LV end-diastolic pressure (c). On spontaneous resolution of ischemia (rise in CSO₂S), the changes resolve. Each episode lasted 2 minutes and was not associated with chest pain. LVP = left ventricular pressure. *(Modified from Chierchia S, Brunelli C, Simonetti I, et al: Sequence of events in angina at rest: Primary reduction in coronary flow. Circulation 61:759, 1980.)*

cellular space reaches a critical level. Symptoms of chest pain are variable and usually the last event to occur in the evolution of ischemia. On restoring perfusion, the sequence is reversed with resolution of chest pain occurring before hemodynamic changes resolve, but regional contraction can remain depressed, reflecting the development of stunned myocardium. A similar temporal sequence of events occurs during exercise-induced ischemia, although the time frame of evolution can be more protracted because ischemia primarily occurs in the subendocardium. Because of the temporal delay in the development of angina and other factors, many episodes of ST depression are symptomatically silent. It is also likely that very brief episodes of ischemia, as reflected by more sensitive indices, such as reduced regional contraction or elevations in end-diastolic pressure, can be electrocardiographically silent.

ACUTE PERFUSION-CONTRACTION MATCHING DURING SUBENDOCARDIAL ISCHEMIA. When coronary pressure distal to a stenosis falls below the lower limit of autoregulation, flow reserve is exhausted, resulting in the onset of subendocardial ischemia. In this case, reductions in subendocardial flow are closely coupled to reductions in regional contractile function of the heart as measured by sensitive approaches, such as regional wall thickening. There is an approximately linear relationship between relative reductions in subendocardial blood flow and relative reductions in regional wall thickening at rest,[4] during tachycardia,[6] and during exercise-induced dysfunction distal to a critical stenosis (**Fig. 52-23**).[49,50] This forms the basis for using regional myocardial function as an index of the severity of subendocardial ischemia during stress imaging (see Chap. 15).

SHORT-TERM HIBERNATION. In steady-state ischemia, the close matching between perfusion and contraction leads to reduced regional oxygen consumption and energy utilization, a phenomenon termed *short-term hibernation.*[47] This reestablishes a balance between supply and demand, as reflected by regeneration of creatine phosphate and ATP with the resolution of lactate production, despite persistent hypoperfusion. Short-term hibernation is an extremely tenuous state and small increases in the determinants of myocardial oxygen demand precipitate further ischemia and a rapid deterioration in function and metabolism. Thus, the ability of short-term hibernation to prevent necrosis is limited by the severity and duration of ischemia, with irreversible injury developing frequently after periods of more than 12 to 24 hours.[51]

Functional Consequences of Reversible Ischemia

There are various late consequences of ischemia after normal myocardial perfusion is reestablished (see Fig.17-28). These reflect acute and delayed effects on regional function, as well as protection of the heart from subsequent ischemic episodes. In the most chronic state, they result in hibernating myocardium, characterized by chronic contractile dysfunction and regional cellular mechanisms that downregulate contractile and metabolic function of the heart to protect it from irreversible injury. The complex interplay among these entities is summarized in **Figure 52-24**. Clinically, it is difficult to separate all the various mechanisms involved in contributing to ischemia-induced viable dysfunctional myocardium because they may all coexist to some extent in the same heart. They can, however, be separated experimentally, and the important features and mechanisms from basic studies are summarized here.

MYOCARDIAL PRECONDITIONING AND POSTCONDITIONING. Brief reversible ischemia preceding a prolonged coronary occlusion reduces myocyte necrosis, a phenomenon termed *acute preconditioning.*[46,52] Because acute infarction is frequently preceded by angina, preconditioning is an endogenous mechanism that can delay the evolution of irreversible myocardial injury. Acute preconditioning can be induced pharmacologically using adenosine A1 receptor stimulation as well as various pharmacologic agonists that stimulate protein kinase C or open K⁺-ATP channels. It has been demonstrated in humans during angioplasty with reduced subjective and objective ischemia during successive coronary occlusions as an endpoint. Preconditioning also develops on a chronic basis (termed *delayed preconditioning*) and, once induced, persists for up to 4 days.[53] It reduces myocardial infarct size and protects the heart from ischemia-induced stunning. The mechanisms of chronic preconditioning involve protein

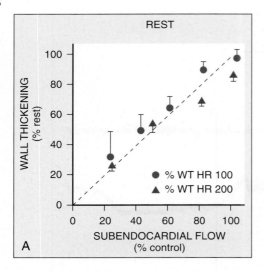

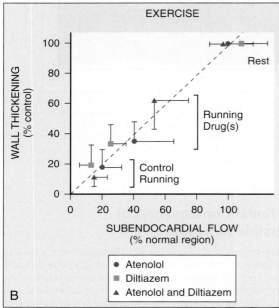

FIGURE 52-23 Perfusion contraction matching during acute ischemia. Relative reductions in function (regional wall thickening) are proportional to the relative reduction in subendocardial flow measured with microspheres in conscious dogs. This relationship is maintained over a wide range of heart rates during autoregulation **(A)** as well as during exercise with a fixed coronary stenosis **(B)**. In the latter case, medical interventions that ameliorate ischemia improve both subendocardial flow and wall thickening during exercise. HR = heart rate; WT = wall thickening. (**A** modified from Canty JM Jr: Coronary pressure-function and steady-state pressure-flow relations during autoregulation in the unanesthetized dog. Circ Res 63:821, 1988; and Canty JM Jr, Giglia J, Kandath D: Effect of tachycardia on regional function and transmural myocardial perfusion during graded coronary pressure reduction in conscious dogs. Circulation 82:1815, 1990; **B** modified from Matsuzaki M, Gallagher KB, Kemper WS, et al: Sustained regional dysfunction produced by prolonged coronary stenosis: Gradual recovery after reperfusion. Circulation 68:170, 1983.)

synthesis, with upregulation of the inducible form of NO synthase (iNOS), cyclooxygenase 2 (COX-2), and opening of the mitochondrial K+-ATP channel. A final protective mechanism, myocardial postconditioning,[54] refers to the ability to cause cardiac protection by producing intermittent ischemia or administering pharmacologic agonists at the time of reperfusion. It is a relatively new observation and, although less extensively studied, has a greater potential to affect irreversible injury because it can be induced after myocardial ischemia is established rather than requiring pretreatment.[46]

STUNNED MYOCARDIUM. Myocardial function normalizes rapidly after single episodes of ischemia lasting less than 2 minutes. As ischemia increases in duration and/or severity, there is a temporal delay in the recovery of function that occurs, despite the fact that blood flow has been restored. Kloner and Jennings[52] and Heyndrickx and associates[55] were the first to demonstrate that regional myocardial function remained depressed for up to 6 hours after resolution of ischemia following a 15-minute occlusion in the absence of tissue necrosis, a phenomenon termed *stunned myocardium* (**Fig. 52-25**). A defining feature of isolated myocardial stunning is that function remains depressed while resting myocardial perfusion is normal. Thus, there is a dissociation of the usual close relationship between subendocardial flow and function. Stunned myocardium also occurs after demand-induced ischemia. For example, exercise-induced ischemia can result in depressed regional function distal to a coronary stenosis for hours after perfusion is restored, and repetitive ischemia can lead to cumulative stunning. Prolonged sublethal ischemia, as in short-term hibernation, leads to stunning on restoration of perfusion that may take up to 1 week to resolve in the absence of necrosis and may be an important cause of reversibly dysfunctional myocardium in the setting of an acute reduction in flow, as in an acute coronary syndrome (ACS).[56] Stunned myocardium is also responsible for postoperative pump dysfunction following cardiopulmonary bypass. Finally, areas of stunned myocardium can coexist with irreversibly injured myocardium and contribute to time-dependent improvements in function following myocardial infarction.

Acutely stunned myocardium is clinically important to recognize because contractile function normalizes during stimulation with various inotropic agents, including beta-adrenergic agonists. In contrast to other dysfunctional states, function will spontaneously normalize within 1 week, provided that there is no recurrent ischemia. If repetitive episodes of reversible ischemia develop before function normalizes, they can cause a state of persistent dysfunction or chronic stunning. The cellular mechanism of stunning likely involves free radical–mediated myocardial injury and reduced myofilament calcium sensitivity.[57]

CHRONIC HIBERNATING MYOCARDIUM. Viable dysfunctional myocardium is defined as any myocardial region where contractile function improves after coronary revascularization.[58,59] This broad definition of reversible dyssynergy includes three distinct categories with fairly diverse pathophysiologic mechanisms, summarized in **Table 52-2**. Complete normalization of function is the rule after acute ischemia but the exception in chronically dysfunctional myocardium. Brief occlusions or prolonged moderate ischemia (short-term hibernation) result in postischemic stunning in the absence of infarction, with complete functional recovery occurring rapidly (within 1 week after reperfusion).[56,57] The time course of improvement is roughly dependent on the duration and severity of the ischemic episode. Reversible dyssynergy with delayed functional improvement can also arise from structural remodeling of the heart that is independent of ischemia or a coronary stenosis (e.g., remote myocardial remodeling in heart failure or the reduced infarct volume that occurs over the initial weeks following coronary reperfusion). The latter conditions can be readily identified when the clinical setting, coronary anatomy, and assessment of myocardial perfusion are taken into account. Many clinical studies have evaluated the presence of contractile reserve during dobutamine administration as a predictor of functional recovery. Although this identifies the likelihood of functional recovery (see Chap. 15), it cannot distinguish the diverse pathophysiologic states underlying reversible dyssynergy. Understanding the cause may be important to the extent that this affects the time course and magnitude of functional recovery after revascularization in patients undergoing revascularization to treat ischemic heart failure.[59]

Chronic segmental dysfunction arising from repetitive episodes of ischemia (frequently clinically silent) is common and present in at least one coronary distribution in over 60% of patients with ischemic cardiomyopathy (**Fig. 52-26**).[60] When resting flow relative to a remote

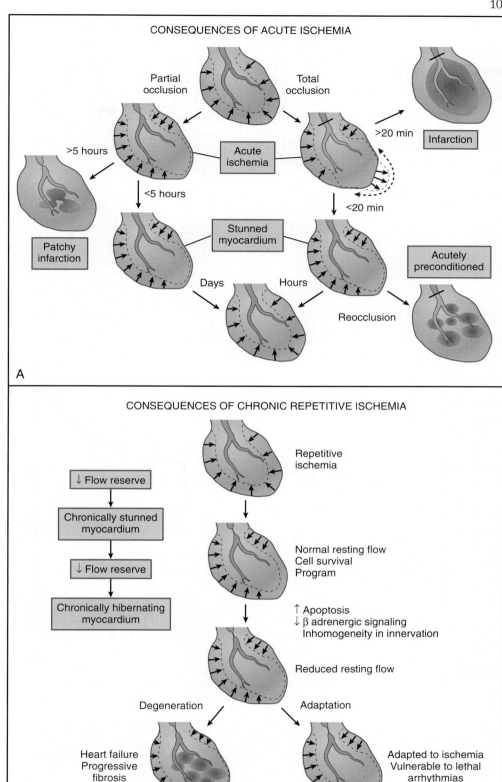

FIGURE 52-24 Effects of ischemia on LV function and irreversible injury. The ventriculograms illustrate contractile dysfunction (dashed lines and arrows). **A,** Consequences of acute ischemia. A brief total occlusion (right) or a prolonged partial occlusion (caused by an acute high-grade stenosis, left) leads to acute contractile dysfunction proportional to the reduction in blood flow. Irreversible injury begins after 20 minutes following a total occlusion but is delayed for up to 5 hours following a partial occlusion (or with significant collaterals) caused by short-term hibernation. When reperfusion is established before the onset of irreversible injury, stunned myocardium develops and the time required for recovery of function is proportional to the duration and severity of ischemia. With prolonged ischemia, stunning in viable myocardium coexists with subendocardial infarction and accounts for reversible dysfunction. Brief episodes of ischemia preceding prolonged ischemia elicit protection against infarction (acute preconditioning). **B,** Effects of chronic repetitive ischemia on function distal to a stenosis. As stenosis severity increases, coronary flow reserve decreases and the frequency of reversible ischemia increases. Reversible repetitive ischemia initially leads to chronic preconditioning against infarction and stunning (not shown). Subsequently, there is a gradual progression from contractile dysfunction with normal resting flow (chronically stunned myocardium) to contractile dysfunction with depressed resting flow (hibernating myocardium). This transition is related to the physiologic significance of a coronary stenosis and can occur in a time period as short as 1 week or develop chronically in the absence of severe angina. The cellular response during the progression to chronic hibernating myocardium is variable, with some patients exhibiting successful adaptation with little cell death and fibrosis and others developing degenerative changes difficult to distinguish from subendocardial infarction. See text for further discussion.

region is normal in dysfunctional myocardium distal to a stenosis, the region is chronically stunned. In contrast, when relative resting flow is reduced in the absence of symptoms or signs of ischemia, hibernating myocardium is present. Although there has previously been controversy over whether flow is normal or reduced at rest, both entities exist in patients and represent extremes in the spectrum of adaptive and maladaptive responses to chronic reversible ischemia. Viability studies are primarily required to distinguish infarction from hibernating myocardium because the myocardium is always viable when the resting flow is normal.[51]

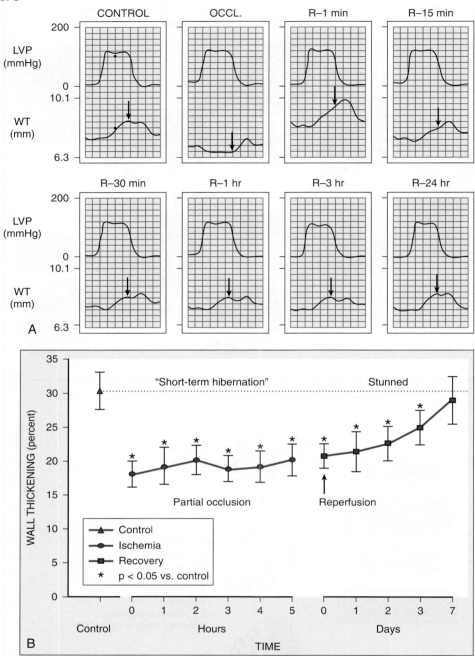

FIGURE 52-25 Stunned myocardium. **A,** Myocardial stunning following a brief total occlusion (OCCL.). Wall thickening (WT) measured by ultrasonic crystals is dyskinetic, with systolic thinning during occlusion. After reperfusion (R), function is completely normal after 24 hours. **B,** Myocardial stunning following a prolonged partial occlusion. During acute ischemia (red circles), there is short-term hibernation reflecting an acute match between reduced flow, wall thickening, and metabolism. With reperfusion (blue squares), wall thickening remains depressed and gradually returns to normal after 1 week. LVP = left ventricular pressure. (*A modified from Heyndrickx GR, Baig H, Nellens P, et al: Depression of regional blood flow and wall thickening after brief coronary occlusions. Am J Physiol 234:H653, 1978; B modified from Matsuzaki M, Gallagher KP, Kemper WS, et al: Sustained regional dysfunction produced by prolonged coronary stenosis: Gradual recovery after reperfusion. Circulation 68:170, 1983.*)

myocardium present with LV dysfunction rather than symptomatic ischemia. Serial studies in animals have now demonstrated that the reductions in relative resting flow are a consequence rather than a cause of the contractile dysfunction.[61,62] This paradigm, relevant to chronic coronary disease, was proposed after experimental studies with a slowly progressive left anterior descending artery (LAD) stenosis demonstrated that dysfunction with normal resting flow consistent with chronic stunning precedes the development of hibernating myocardium after 3 months (**Fig. 52-27**).[63] The progression from chronically stunned myocardium (with normal resting flow) to hibernating myocardium (with reduced flow) is related to the functional significance of the chronic stenosis supplying the region and is probably a reflection of its propensity to develop repetitive supply or demand-induced ischemia. This progression can develop in as little as 1 week after placement of a critical stenosis that exhausts coronary flow reserve.[64] As regional dysfunction progresses from chronically stunned to hibernating myocardium, the myocyte takes on regional characteristics similar to those from an explanted heart with advanced failure. Normally perfused remote zone cardiac myocytes can be normal or take on structural alterations similar to those in the dysfunctional region. Some of the major cellular responses are summarized here.

APOPTOSIS, MYOCYTE LOSS, AND MYOFIBRILLAR LOSS. The frequency of focal myocyte death from apoptosis varies during the development of viable dysfunctional myocardium and thus is probably responsible for the variability in the frequency of apoptosis when analyzing biopsies from patients.[65,66] Experimentally, apoptosis is particularly prominent during the transition from chronically stunned to hibernating myocardium, at which time there is a loss of approximately 30% of the regional myocytes (**Fig. 52-28**).[67] The myocyte loss results in compensatory regional myocyte hypertrophy to maintain approximately normal wall thickness. Vanoverschelde and coworkers[68] have previously described light microscopic and ultrastructural characteristics of hibernating myocardium from transmural biopsies, which are characterized by small increases in interstitial connective tissue, myofibrillar loss (myolysis), increased glycogen deposition, and minimitochondria. Experimental animal models of hibernating myocardium also develop these structural changes in as little as 2 weeks but they are also present in remote, normally perfused regions of the heart.[51,69] Global cellular changes have also been reported in patients in the absence of a stenosis, suggesting that the structural changes are probably the result of chronically elevated preload. Thus, although cellular dedifferentiation had been emphasized as a mechanism of adaptation, the global ultrastructural changes are probably not causally related to the regional responses to ischemia in hibernating myocardium.[59]

CELL SURVIVAL AND ANTIAPOPTOTIC PROGRAM IN RESPONSE TO REPETITIVE ISCHEMIA. There is variability in the regulation of cell survival pathways in response to repetitive ischemia. Some studies have demonstrated

It was originally thought that hibernating myocardium arises from a primary reduction in flow similar to experimental models of prolonged moderate ischemia and short-term hibernation. Whereas this is a plausible mechanism for the development of hibernating myocardium in association with an ACS, experimental studies have subsequently demonstrated that delayed subendocardial infarction is the rule rather than the exception when moderate flow reductions are maintained for more than 24 hours.[51] Many patients with hibernating

TABLE 52-2	Viable Dysfunctional Myocardium: Patterns of Contractile Reserve, Resting Perfusion, and Temporal Recovery of Function after Revascularization				
PARAMETER	**CONTRACTILE RESERVE**	**RESTING FLOW**	**EXTENT OF FUNCTIONAL RECOVERY**	**TIME COURSE OF RECOVERY**	
Transient Reversible Ischemia					
Postischemic stunning	Present	Normal	Normalizes	<24 hr	
Short-term hibernation	Present	Normal	Normalizes	<7 days	
Chronic Repetitive Ischemia					
Chronic hibernating myocardium	Variable	Reduced	Improves	Up to 12 mo	
Chronic stunning	Present	Normal	Improves	Days to weeks	
Structural Remodeling					
Subendocardial infarction	Variable	Reduced	Variable	Weeks	
Remodeled, tethered myocardium	Present	Normal	Improves	Months	

upregulation of cardioprotective mechanisms in response to repetitive reversible ischemia, which may be operative in minimizing myocyte cell death and fibrosis in the chronic setting.[70] An interesting mechanism potentially linking altered metabolism and protection is the regional downregulation of glycogen synthase kinase-3β, which can ameliorate cell death and also explains the increased tissue glycogen in hibernating myocardium.[71] In experimental studies in animals without heart failure, antiapoptotic and stress proteins such as HSP-70 have been found to be upregulated,[72] whereas increased proapoptotic proteins and a profile of progressive cell death and fibrosis have been reported in human biopsies of patients with hibernating myocardium and heart failure.[66] It is likely that the variability among studies reflects the frequency and severity of ischemia, modulation by neurohormonal activation in heart failure, and the complexity of the temporal expression of adaptive and maladaptive responses in myocardium subjected to chronic repetitive ischemia.

METABOLISM AND ENERGETICS IN HIBERNATING MYOCARDIUM. Once adapted, the metabolic and contractile response of hibernating myocardium appears to be dissociated from external determinants of workload. As a result, submaximal increases in oxygen consumption can occur without immediately leading to subendocardial ischemia.[73] Experimentally, the hibernating myocardial region appears to operate over a lower range of the normal myocardial supply-demand relationship in a fashion similar to that of the nonischemic failing heart. Although glycogen content is increased, maximum rates of glucose uptake during insulin stimulation are not altered. In addition, creatine phosphate and ATP levels are not regionally altered, contrasting with the depressed ATP levels in stunning. Recently, studies of isolated mitochondria from swine with hibernating myocardium have demonstrated a downregulation of energy uptake and oxygen consumption.[74] This slows ATP uptake and presumably maintains cell viability during superimposed acute ischemia. Proteomic analysis has demonstrated a reduction in multiple proteins involved in oxidative metabolism and electron transport.[72]

INHOMOGENEITY IN SYMPATHETIC INNERVATION, BETA-ADRENERGIC RESPONSES, AND SUDDEN DEATH. The contractile response of hibernating myocardium is blunted and partially related to a regional downregulation in beta-adrenergic adenylyl cyclase coupling, similar to that found globally in advanced heart failure.[75] This may be related to local norepinephrine overflow because the presynaptic uptake of norepinephrine is reduced when assessed using nuclear tracers such as ^{11}C-hydroxyephedrine.[76] The resultant inhomogeneity in myocardial sympathetic nerve function may be one of the reasons responsible for the vulnerability of experimental hibernating myocardium to develop lethal ventricular arrhythmias and ventricular fibrillation.[77] Thus, normalizing electrical instability and improving contractile dysfunction may account for the profound impact of revascularization on survival when hibernating myocardium is present.[59]

SUCCESSFUL ADAPTATION VERSUS DEGENERATION IN HIBERNATING MYOCARDIUM. There is considerable divergence among studies regarding the

Ventriculogram

FDG

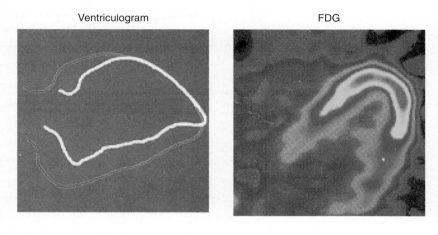

Resting flow

Vasodilated flow

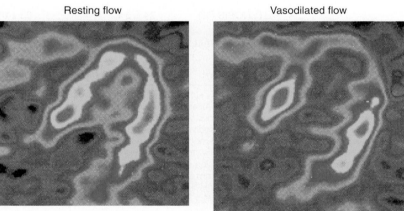

FIGURE 52-26 Hibernating myocardium in humans with a chronic LAD occlusion and collateral dependent myocardium. The RAO tracings of the left ventriculogram show anterior akinesis (upper left). Transaxial PET scans (see Chap. 17) illustrate [13]NH3 flow measurements at rest (lower left) and following pharmacologic vasodilation with dipyridamole (lower right). Quantitative perfusion measurements showed LAD flow to be critically impaired. Viability (following an oral glucose load) is identified by increased ^{18}F-fluorodeoxyglucose (FDG) uptake in the anterior wall (upper right). RAO = right anterior oblique. *(Modified from Vanoverschelde J-LJ, Wijns W, Depre C, et al: Mechanisms of chronic regional postischemic dysfunction in humans: New insights from the study of noninfarcted collateral-dependent myocardium. Circulation 87:1513, 1993.)*

pathology of reversibly dyssynergic hibernating myocardium. At one extreme, some investigators believe that it is destined to undergo irreversible myocyte death, which is supported by data showing large amounts of fibrosis (more than 30% of the tissue), markedly abnormal high-energy phosphate metabolism, and retrospective analysis suggesting that the degree of fibrosis is related to the duration of hibernating myocardium.[66] At the other extreme, there are circumstances in which fibrosis is not a prominent feature with normal myocardial energetics at

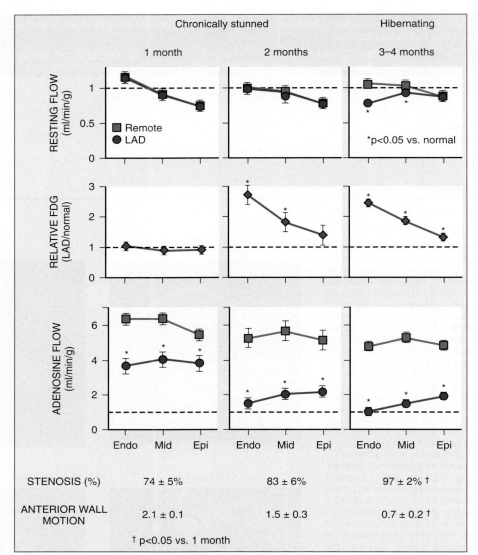

FIGURE 52-27 Progression from chronically stunned to hibernating myocardium as stenosis severity increases in swine with viable dysfunctional myocardium from a chronic LAD stenosis. Transmural flow measurements (microspheres) at rest and adenosine vasodilation are shown, along with regional FDG uptake (fasting conditions). Below are the angiographic stenosis severity and anterior wall motion score (3, normal; 2, mild hypokinesis; 1, severe hypokinesis). As stenosis severity increases over time, there is a reduction in vasodilated flow (adenosine) to the LAD region. Initially, there is anterior hypokinesis, with normal resting flow consistent with chronically stunned myocardium. After 3 months, the stenosis progresses to occlusion with collateral dependent myocardium. Subendocardial flow is critically reduced and there is a reduction in resting flow to the inner two thirds of the LAD myocardium. At this time, hibernating myocardium is present and there is no evidence of infarction. The temporal progression of abnormalities demonstrate that chronic stunning precedes the development of hibernating myocardium. In contrast to short-term hibernation resulting from acute ischemia, the reduction in resting flow is a consequence, rather than a cause, of the contractile dysfunction. Endo = endocardium; Epi = epicardium; FDG = ^{18}F-fluorodeoxyglucose. *(Modified from Fallavollita JA, Canty JM Jr: Differential ^{18}F-2-deoxyglucose uptake in viable dysfunctional myocardium with normal resting perfusion: Evidence for chronic stunning in pigs. Circulation 99:2798, 1999.)*

rest, suggesting that hibernating myocardium can be sustained for long periods without progressive degeneration.[77,78] The factors that determine the path to progressive structural degeneration versus adaptation are currently unknown but may be modulated by the superimposed neurohormonal activation, elevation in cytokine levels associated with advanced clinical heart failure, and structural degeneration that arises from small reductions in coronary flow reserve below the threshold required to maintain myocyte viability.

Future Perspectives

There has been considerable progress in advancing the mechanistic understanding of the coronary circulation and myocardial ischemia in health and disease, yet important gaps remain in basic knowledge and in its translation to clinical care. The major factors determining myocardial perfusion and oxygen delivery were established over 30 years ago,

have been incorporated into how angina is managed, and have stood the test of time. The basic understanding of the fluid mechanical behavior of coronary stenoses has only recently been translated to the cardiac catheterization laboratory, where it can facilitate routine clinical decision making. Here, measurements of coronary pressure distal to a stenosis and flow have been demonstrated to provide a physiologic approach to guiding interventional procedures (see Chap. 58). This ischemia-guided physiologic approach results in reduced major adverse cardiovascular events in comparison to an anatomically guided strategy based on the angiographic severity of potential lesions, and is likely to be increasingly used in future clinical decisions.

Basic research has led to the discovery of many new signaling pathways involved in the control of coronary blood flow, extended the understanding of flow regulation in microcirculatory vessels, and identified the importance of physical factors such as shear stress and local

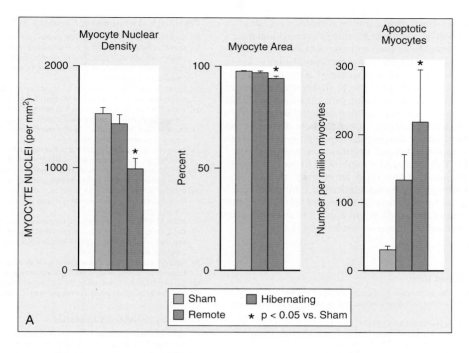

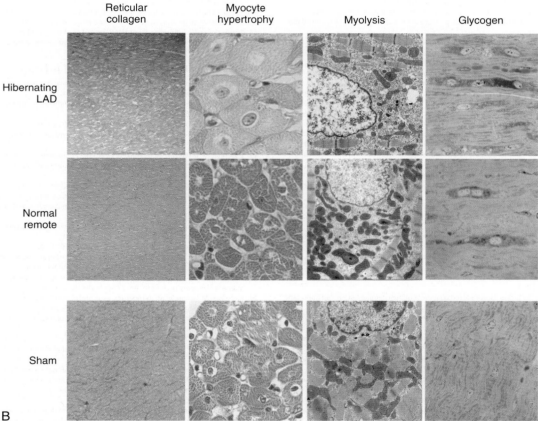

FIGURE 52-28 Apoptosis, hypertrophy, and myocyte cellular morphology in hibernating myocardium. Data in hibernating LAD regions are compared with remote regions as well as with LAD regions from normal animals. **A,** The progression from chronically stunned to hibernating myocardium is accompanied by regional apoptosis-induced myocyte loss. There is about a 30% reduction in myocyte nuclear number without significant fibrosis, because the myocyte area is almost normal. **B,** Myocyte cellular changes in hibernating myocardium. The increased myocyte loss results in compensatory myocyte cellular hypertrophy in hibernating myocardium. Whereas reticular collagen is regionally increased (about 2%), there is no evidence of infarction. The electron microscopic characteristics of hibernating myocardium demonstrate myofibrillar loss, an increased number of small mitochondria, and increased glycogen content. Although these are markedly different from normal myocardium (sham), biopsies of normal remote, nonischemic segments show similar morphologic changes, indicating that these structural abnormalities are not directly related to ischemia nor are they the cause of regional contractile dysfunction. (*A from Lim H, Fallavollita JA, Hard R, et al: Profound apoptosis-mediated regional myocyte loss and compensatory hypertrophy in pigs with hibernating myocardium. Circulation 100:2380, 1999; B from Canty JM, Fallavollita JA: Hibernating myocardium. J Nucl Cardiol 12:104, 2005.*)

coronary pressure in regulating local coronary resistance adjustments. Nevertheless, the question of how the mechanisms in individual microcirculatory vessels collectively interact to bring about the phenomenon of autoregulation and metabolic coronary vasodilation in the in vivo heart remains unanswered. At a myocardial level, the intrinsic mechanisms involved in patients with viable dysfunctional myocardium appear to be diverse, with some being protective and beneficial in maintaining myocyte viability in the setting of ischemia and others being detrimental. Understanding why some patients develop coronary collaterals and/or intrinsic adaptations to repetitive ischemia but others undergo progressive structural degeneration is an important gap in our knowledge. This information could lead to novel therapies and a better identification of the most appropriate patients and approach for high-risk myocardial revascularization. Continued bench to bedside translational investigation in these and other areas will allow us to expand our understanding and apply it to improving the management of patients with chronic ischemic heart disease.

REFERENCES

Control of Coronary Blood Flow

1. Hoffman JIE: Transmural myocardial perfusion. Prog Cardiovasc Dis 29:429, 1987.
2. Canty JM Jr, Brooks A: Phasic volumetric coronary venous outflow patterns in conscious dogs. Am J Physiol 258:H1457, 1990.
3. Feigl EO: Coronary physiology. Physiol Rev 63:1, 1983.
4. Canty JM Jr: Coronary pressure-function and steady-state pressure-flow relations during autoregulation in the unanesthetized dog. Circ Res 63:821, 1988.
5. Klocke FJ: Coronary blood flow in man. Prog Cardiovasc Dis XIX:117, 1976.
6. Canty JM Jr, Giglia J, Kandath D: Effect of tachycardia on regional function and transmural myocardial perfusion during graded coronary pressure reduction in conscious dogs. Circulation 82:1815, 1990.
7. Canty JM Jr, Smith TP Jr: Adenosine-recruitable flow reserve is absent during myocardial ischemia in unanesthetized dogs studied in the basal state. Circ Res 76:1079, 1995.
8. Hoffman JIE, Spaan JAE: Pressure-flow relations in coronary circulation. Physiol Rev 70:331, 1990.
9. Duncker DJ, Bache RJ: Regulation of coronary vasomotor tone under normal conditions and during acute myocardial hypoperfusion. Pharmacol Ther 86:87, 2000.

Coronary Microcirculation

10. Furchgott RF, Zawadzki JV: The obligatory role of endothelial cells in the relaxation of arterial smooth muscle by acetylcholine. Nature 288:373, 1980.
11. Kuo L, Davis MJ, Chilian WM: Longitudinal gradients for endothelium-dependent and -independent vascular responses in the coronary microcirculation. Circulation 92:518, 1995.
12. Chilian WM, Layne SM, Klausner EC, et al: Redistribution of coronary microvascular resistance produced by dipyridamole. Am J Physiol 256:H383, 1989.
13. Kanatsuka H, Lamping KG, Eastham CL, et al: Heterogeneous changes in epimyocardial microvascular size during graded coronary stenosis. Evidence of the microvascular site for autoregulation. Circ Res 66:389, 1990.
14. Kanatsuka H, Lamping KG, Eastham CL, et al: Comparison of the effects of increased myocardial oxygen consumption and adenosine on the coronary microvascular resistance. Circ Res 65:1296, 1989.
15. Miller FJ, Dellsperger KC, Gutterman DD: Myogenic constriction of human coronary arterioles. Am J Physiol Heart Circ Physiol 273:H257, 1997.
16. Kuo L, Davis MJ, Chilian WM: Endothelium-dependent, flow-induced dilation of isolated coronary arterioles. Am J Physiol 259:H1063, 1990.
17. Liu Y, Gutterman DD: Vascular control in humans: Focus on the coronary microcirculation. Basic Res Cardiol 104:211, 2009.
18. Miura H, Wachtel RE, Liu Y, et al: Flow-induced dilation of human coronary arterioles: Important role of Ca^{2+}-activated K^{+} channels. Circulation 103:1992, 2001.
19. Dube S, Canty JM Jr: Shear-stress induced vasodilation in porcine coronary conduit arteries is independent of nitric oxide release. Am J Physiol 280:H2581, 2001.
20. Quyyumi AA, Dakak N, Andrews NP, et al: Contribution of nitric oxide to metabolic coronary vasodilation in the human heart. Circulation 92:320, 1995.
21. Sato A, Terata K, Miura H, et al: Mechanism of vasodilation to adenosine in coronary arterioles from patients with heart disease. Am J Physiol Heart Circ Physiol 288:H1633, 2005.
22. Jones CJ, Kuo L, Davis MJ, et al: Role of nitric oxide in the coronary microvascular responses to adenosine and increased metabolic demand. Circulation 91:1807, 1995.
23. Duncker DJ, Bache RJ: Regulation of coronary blood flow during exercise. Physiol Rev 88:1009, 2008.

Coronary Vasoconstriction, Vasospasm, and Pharmacologic Vasodilation

24. Heusch G, Baumgart D, Camici P, et al: α-Adrenergic coronary vasoconstriction and myocardial ischemia in humans. Circulation 101:689, 2000.
25. Konidala S, Gutterman DD: Coronary vasospasm and the regulation of coronary blood flow. Prog Cardiovasc Dis 46:349, 2004.
26. Druz RS: Current advances in vasodilator pharmacological stress perfusion imaging. Semin Nucl Med 39:204, 2009.
27. Jones CJH, Kuo L, Davis MJ, et al: In vivo and in vitro vasoactive reactions of coronary arteriolar microvessels to nitroglycerin. Am J Physiol 271:H461, 1996.
28. Guethlin M, Kasel AM, Coppenrath K, et al: Delayed response of myocardial flow reserve to lipid-lowering therapy with fluvastatin. Circulation 99:475, 1999.
29. Zong P, Tune JD, Downey HF: Mechanisms of oxygen demand/supply balance in the right ventricle. Exp Biol Med (Maywood) 230:507, 2005.

Physiologic Assessment of Coronary Artery Stenosis

30. Gould KL: Does coronary flow trump coronary anatomy? J Am Coll Cardiol Img 2:1009, 2009.
31. Kern MJ, Lerman A, Bech JW, et al: Physiological assessment of coronary artery disease in the cardiac catheterization laboratory. A scientific statement from the American Heart Association Committee on Diagnostic and Interventional Cardiac Catheterization, Council on Clinical Cardiology. Circulation 114:1321, 2006.
32. Klocke FJ: Measurements of coronary blood flow and degree of stenosis: Current clinical implications and continuing uncertainties. J Am Coll Cardiol 1:31, 1983.
33. Yokoyama I, Ohtake T, Momomura S, et al: Reduced coronary flow reserve in hypercholesterolemic patients without overt coronary stenosis. Circulation 94:3232, 1996.
34. Spaan JA, Piek JJ, Hoffman JI, et al: Physiological basis of clinically used coronary hemodynamic indices. Circulation 113:446, 2006.
35. Tonino PA, De Bruyne B, Pijls NH, et al: Fractional flow reserve versus angiography for guiding percutaneous coronary intervention. N Engl J Med 360:213, 2009.
35a. Lee DC, Simonetti OP, Harris KR, et al: Magnetic resonance versus radionuclide pharmacologic stress perfusion imaging for flow-limiting stenoses of varying severity. Circulation 110:58, 2004.
36. Buchthal SD, den Hollander JA, Merz CN, et al: Abnormal myocardial phosphorus-31 nuclear magnetic resonance spectroscopy in women with chest pain but normal coronary angiograms. N Engl J Med 342:829, 2000.
37. Bache RJ: Effects of hypertrophy on the coronary circulation. Prog Cardiovasc Dis 31:403, 1988.
38. Kuo L, Davis MJ, Cannon MS, et al: Pathophysiological consequences of atherosclerosis extend into the coronary microcirculation: Restoration of endothelium-dependent responses by L-arginine. Circ Res 70:465, 1992.
39. Smith TP Jr, Canty JM Jr: Modulation of coronary autoregulatory responses by nitric oxide: Evidence for flow-dependent resistance adjustments in conscious dogs. Circ Res 73:232, 1993.
40. Duncker DJ, Bache RJ: Inhibition of nitric oxide production aggravates myocardial hypoperfusion during exercise in the presence of a coronary artery stenosis. Circ Res 74:629, 1994.

Coronary Collateral Circulation

41. Meier P, Gloekler S, Zbinden R, et al: Beneficial effect of recruitable collaterals: A 10-year follow-up study in patients with stable coronary artery disease undergoing quantitative collateral measurements. Circulation 116:975, 2007.
42. Schaper W: Collateral circulation: past and present. Basic Res Cardiol 104:5, 2009.
43. Simons M: Angiogenesis: Where do we stand now? Circulation 111:1556, 2005.
44. Suzuki G, Lee TC, Fallavollita JA, et al: Adenoviral gene transfer of FGF-5 to hibernating myocardium improves function and stimulates myocytes to hypertrophy and reenter the cell cycle. Circ Res 96:767, 2005.

Metabolic and Functional Consequence of Ischemia

45. Kloner RA, Jennings RB: Consequences of brief ischemia: Stunning, preconditioning, and their clinical implications: part 1. Circulation 104:2981, 2001.
46. Downey JM, Cohen MV: Reducing infarct size in the setting of acute myocardial infarction. Prog Cardiovasc Dis 48:363, 2006.
47. Heusch G: Hibernating myocardium. Physiol Rev 78:1055, 1998.
48. Dorn GW 2nd, Diwan A: The rationale for cardiomyocyte resuscitation in myocardial salvage. J Mol Med 86:1085, 2008.
49. Gallagher KP, Matsuzaki M, Osakada G, et al: Effect of exercise on the relationship between myocardial blood flow and systolic wall thickening in dogs with acute coronary stenosis. Circ Res 52:716, 1983.
50. Matsuzaki M, Guth B, Tajimi T, et al: Effect of the combination of diltiazem and atenolol on exercise-induced regional myocardial ischemia in conscious dogs. Circulation 72:233, 1985.
51. Heusch G, Schulz R, Rahimtoola SH: Myocardial hibernation: A delicate balance. Am J Physiol Heart Circ Physiol 288:H984, 2005.
52. Kloner RA, Jennings RB: Consequences of brief ischemia: Stunning, preconditioning, and their clinical implications: part 2. Circulation 104:3158, 2001.
53. Bolli R: The late phase of preconditioning. Circ Res 87:972, 2000.
54. Vinten-Johansen J, Zhao ZQ, Jiang R, et al: Preconditioning and postconditioning: Innate cardioprotection from ischemia-reperfusion injury. J Appl Physiol 103:1441, 2007.
55. Heyndrickx GR, Baig H, Nellens P, et al: Depression of regional blood flow and wall thickening after brief coronary occlusions. Am J Physiol 234:H653, 1978.
56. Matsuzaki M, Gallagher KP, Kemper WS, et al: Sustained regional dysfunction produced by prolonged coronary stenosis: Gradual recovery after reperfusion. Circulation 68:170, 1983.
57. Bolli R, Marban E: Molecular and cellular mechanisms of myocardial stunning. Physiol Rev 79:609, 1999.
58. Rahimtoola SH, Dilsizian V, Kramer CM, et al: Chronic ischemic left ventricular dysfunction: From pathophysiology to imaging and its integration into clinical practice. J Am Coll Cardiol Img 1:536, 2008.
59. Canty JM Jr, Fallavollita JA: Hibernating myocardium. J Nucl Cardiol 12:104, 2005.
60. Vanoverschelde J-LJ, Wijns W, Depre C, et al: Mechanisms of chronic regional postischemic dysfunction in humans: New insights from the study of noninfarcted collateral-dependent myocardium. Circulation 87:1513, 1993.
61. Fallavollita JA, Perry BJ, Canty JM Jr: ^{18}F-2-deoxyglucose deposition and regional flow in pigs with chronically dysfunctional myocardium: Evidence for transmural variations in chronic hibernating myocardium. Circulation 95:1900, 1997.
62. Fallavollita JA, Canty JM Jr: Differential ^{18}F-2-deoxyglucose uptake in viable dysfunctional myocardium with normal resting perfusion: Evidence for chronic stunning in pigs. Circulation 99:2798, 1999.
63. Canty JM Jr, Fallavollita JA: Chronic hibernation and chronic stunning: A continuum. J Nucl Cardiol 7:509, 2000.
64. Thomas SA, Fallavollita JA, Borgers M, et al: Dissociation of regional adaptations to ischemia and global myolysis in an accelerated swine model of chronic hibernating myocardium. Circ Res 91:970, 2002.
65. Dispersyn GD, Borgers M, Flameng W: Apoptosis in chronic hibernating myocardium: Sleeping to death? Cardiovasc Res 45:696, 2000.
66. Elsasser A, Vogt AM, Nef H, et al: Human hibernating myocardium is jeopardized by apoptotic and autophagic cell death. J Am Coll Cardiol 43:2191, 2004.

67. Lim H, Fallavollita JA, Hard R, et al: Profound apoptosis-mediated regional myocyte loss and compensatory hypertrophy in pigs with hibernating myocardium. Circulation 100:2380, 1999.

68. Vanoverschelde J-L, Wijns W, Borgers M, et al: Chronic myocardial hibernation in humans. From bedside to bench. Circulation 95:1961, 1997.

69. Thijssen VL, Borgers M, Lenders M-H, et al: Temporal and spatial variations in structural protein expression during the progression from stunned to hibernating myocardium. Circulation 110:3313, 2004.

70. Depre C, Vatner SF: Mechanisms of cell survival in myocardial hibernation. Trends Cardiovasc Med 15:101, 2005.

71. Kim SJ, Peppas A, Hong SK, et al: Persistent stunning induces myocardial hibernation and protection: Flow/function and metabolic mechanisms. Circ Res 92:1233, 2003.

72. Page B, Young R, Iyer V, et al: Persistent regional downregulation in mitochondrial enzymes and upregulation of stress proteins in swine with chronic hibernating myocardium. Circ Res 102:103, 2008.

73. Fallavollita JA, Malm BJ, Canty JM Jr: Hibernating myocardium retains metabolic and contractile reserve despite regional reductions in flow, function, and oxygen consumption at rest. Circ Res 92:48, 2003.

74. Hu Q, Suzuki G, Young RF, et al: Reductions in mitochondrial O_2 consumption and preservation of high-energy phosphate levels after simulated ischemia in chronic hibernating myocardium. Am J Physiol Heart Circ Physiol 297:H223, 2009.

75. Iyer V, Canty JM Jr: Regional desensitization of β-adrenergic receptor signaling in swine with chronic hibernating myocardium. Circ Res 97:789, 2005.

76. Luisi AJ Jr, Suzuki G, deKemp R, et al: Regional ^{11}C-hydroxyephedrine retention in hibernating myocardium: Chronic inhomogeneity of sympathetic innervation in the absence of infarction. J Nucl Med 46:1368, 2005.

77. Canty JM Jr, Suzuki G, Banas MD, et al: Hibernating myocardium: Chronically adapted to ischemia but vulnerable to sudden death. Circ Res 94:1142, 2004.

78. Dispersyn GD, Ramaekers FCS and Borgers M: Clinical pathophysiology of hibernating myocardium. Coron Artery Dis 12:381, 2001.

CH
52

CORONARY BLOOD FLOW AND MYOCARDIAL ISCHEMIA

CHAPTER **53** **Approach to the Patient with Chest Pain**

Marc S. Sabatine and Christopher P. Cannon

Acute chest pain is one of the most common reasons for presentation to the emergency department (ED), accounting for approximately 7 million ED visits annually in the United States. This presentation suggests acute coronary syndrome (ACS), but after diagnostic evaluation, only 15% to 25% of patients with acute chest pain actually have ACS.[1,2] The difficulty lies in discriminating patients with ACS or other life-threatening conditions from patients with noncardiovascular, non–life-threatening chest pain. The diagnosis of ACS is missed in approximately 2% of patients, leading to substantial consequences—for example, the short-term mortality for patients with acute myocardial infarction (MI) who are mistakenly discharged from the ED increases twofold over that expected for patients who are admitted to the hospital. For patients with a low risk of complications, however, these concerns must be balanced against the costs and inconvenience of admission and against the risk of complications from tests and procedures with a low probability of improving patient outcomes.

Several recent advances have enhanced the accuracy and efficiency of the evaluation of patients with acute chest pain, including better blood markers for myocardial injury,[3] decision aids to stratify patients according to their risk of complications, early and even immediate exercise testing[4] and radionuclide scanning for lower risk patient subsets (see Chap. 17),[5] multislice computed tomography for the anatomic evaluation of coronary artery disease, pulmonary embolism, and aortic dissection (see Chap. 19),[6] and the use of chest pain units[7] and critical pathways for efficient and rapid evaluation of lower-risk patients.[8]

Causes of Acute Chest Pain

In a typical population of patients presenting for the evaluation of acute chest pain in EDs, about 15% to 25% have acute MI or unstable angina.[2] A small percentage have other life-threatening problems, such as pulmonary embolism or acute aortic dissection, but most are discharged without a diagnosis or with a diagnosis of a noncardiac condition. These noncardiac conditions include musculoskeletal syndromes, disorders of the abdominal viscera (including gastroesophageal reflux disease), and psychological conditions (**Table 53-1**).

Myocardial Ischemia or Infarction

The most common serious cause of acute chest discomfort is myocardial ischemia or infarction (see Chaps. 54 to 56), which occurs when the supply of myocardial oxygen is inadequate compared with the demand. Myocardial ischemia usually occurs in the setting of coronary atherosclerosis, but it may also reflect dynamic components of coronary vascular resistance. Coronary spasm can occur in normal coronary arteries or, in patients with coronary disease, near atherosclerotic plaques and in smaller coronary arteries (see Chap. 52). Other less common causes of impaired coronary blood flow include syndromes that compromise the orifices or lumina of the coronary

arteries, such as coronary arteritis, proximal aortitis, spontaneous coronary dissection, proximal aortic dissection, coronary emboli from infectious or noninfectious endocarditis or thrombus in the left atrium or left ventricle, myocardial bridge, or a congenital abnormality of the coronary arteries (see Chap. 21).

The classic manifestation of ischemia is angina, which is usually described as a heavy chest pressure or squeezing, a burning feeling, or difficulty breathing (see Chap. 12). The discomfort often radiates to the left shoulder, neck, or arm. It typically builds in intensity over a period of a few minutes. The pain may begin with exercise or psychological stress, but ACS most commonly occurs without obvious precipitating factors.

Atypical descriptions of chest pain reduce the likelihood that the symptoms represent myocardial ischemia or injury. The American College of Cardiology (ACC) and American Heart Association (AHA) guidelines list the following as pain descriptions that are not characteristic of myocardial ischemia[8]:

- Pleuritic pain (i.e., sharp or knifelike pain brought on by respiratory movements or cough)
- Primary or sole location of discomfort in the middle or lower abdominal region
- Pain that may be localized at the tip of one finger, particularly over the left ventricular apex
- Pain reproduced with movement or palpation of the chest wall or arms
- Constant pain that persists for many hours
- Very brief episodes of pain that last a few seconds or less
- Pain that radiates into the lower extremities

Data from large populations of patients with acute chest pain indicate that ACS occurs in patients with atypical symptoms with sufficient frequency that no single factor should be used to exclude the diagnosis of acute ischemic heart disease. In particular, women, older persons, and individuals with diabetes may be more likely to report atypical symptoms of myocardial ischemia or infarction (see Chap. 81).

Pericardial Disease

The visceral surface of the pericardium is insensitive to pain, as is most of the parietal surface. Therefore, noninfectious causes of pericarditis (e.g., uremia; see Chap. 75) usually cause little or no pain. In contrast, infectious pericarditis almost always involves surrounding pleura, so that patients typically experience pleuritic pain with breathing, coughing, and changes in position. Swallowing may induce the pain because of the proximity of the esophagus to the posterior heart. Because the central diaphragm receives its sensory supply from the phrenic nerve, and the phrenic nerve arises from the third to fifth cervical segments of the spinal cord, pain from infectious pericarditis is frequently felt in the shoulders and neck. Involvement of the more lateral diaphragm can lead to symptoms in the upper abdomen and

TABLE 53-1 Common Causes of Acute Chest Pain

SYSTEM	SYNDROME	CLINICAL DESCRIPTION	KEY DISTINGUISHING FEATURES
Cardiac	Angina	Retrosternal chest pressure, burning, or heaviness; radiating occasionally to neck, jaw, epigastrium, shoulders, left arm	Precipitated by exercise, cold weather, or emotional stress; duration 2-10 min
	Rest or unstable angina	Same as angina, but may be more severe	Typically <20 min; lower tolerance for exertion; crescendo pattern
	Acute myocardial infarction	Same as angina, but may be more severe	Sudden onset, usually lasting ≥30 min; often associated with shortness of breath, weakness, nausea, vomiting
	Pericarditis	Sharp, pleuritic pain aggravated by changes in position; highly variable duration	Pericardial friction rub
Vascular	Aortic dissection	Excruciating, ripping pain of sudden onset in anterior of chest, often radiating to back	Marked severity of unrelenting pain; usually occurs in setting of hypertension or underlying connective tissue disorder such as Marfan syndrome
	Pulmonary embolism	Sudden onset of dyspnea and pain, usually pleuritic with pulmonary infarction	Dyspnea, tachypnea, tachycardia, signs of right heart failure
	Pulmonary hypertension	Substernal chest pressure, exacerbated by exertion	Pain associated with dyspnea and signs of pulmonary hypertension
Pulmonary	Pleuritis and/or pneumonia	Pleuritic pain, usually brief, over involved area	Pain pleuritic and lateral to midline, associated with dyspnea
	Tracheobronchitis	Burning discomfort in midline	Midline location, associated with coughing
	Spontaneous pneumothorax	Sudden onset of unilateral pleuritic pain, with dyspnea	Abrupt onset of dyspnea and pain
Gastrointestinal	Esophageal reflux	Burning substernal and epigastric discomfort, 10-60 min in duration	Aggravated by large meal and postprandial recumbency; relieved by antacid
	Peptic ulcer	Prolonged epigastric or substernal burning	Relieved by antacid or food
	Gallbladder disease	Prolonged epigastric or right upper quadrant pain	Unprovoked or following meal
	Pancreatitis	Prolonged, intense epigastric and substernal pain	Risk factors including alcohol, hypertriglyceridemia, medications
Musculoskeletal	Costochondritis	Sudden onset of intense fleeting pain	May be reproduced by pressure over affected joint; occasionally, swelling and inflammation over costochondral joint
	Cervical disc disease	Sudden onset of fleeting pain	May be reproduced with movement of neck
	Trauma or strain	Constant pain	Reproduced by palpation or movement of chest wall or arms
Infectious	Herpes zoster	Prolonged burning pain in dermatomal distribution	Vesicular rash, dermatomal distribution
Psychological	Panic disorder	Chest tightness or aching, often accompanied by dyspnea and lasting 30 minutes or more, unrelated to exertion or movement	Patient may have other evidence of emotional disorder

back, creating confusion with pancreatitis or cholecystitis. Pericarditis occasionally causes a steady, crushing substernal pain that resembles that of acute myocardial infarction.[9]

Vascular Disease

Acute aortic dissection (see Chap. 60) usually causes the sudden onset of excruciating ripping pain, the location of which reflects the site and progression of the dissection. Ascending aortic dissections tend to manifest with pain in the midline of the anterior chest, and posterior descending aortic dissections tend to manifest with pain in the back of the chest. Aortic dissections are rare, with an estimated annual incidence of 3/100,000, and usually occur in the presence of risk factors including Marfan and Ehlers-Danlos syndromes, bicuspid aortic valve, pregnancy (for proximal dissections), and hypertension (for distal dissections).

Pulmonary emboli (see Chap. 77) often cause the sudden onset of dyspnea and pleuritic chest pain, although they may be asymptomatic. The annual incidence is approximately 1 per 1000, though this number is likely an underestimate. Massive pulmonary emboli tend to cause severe and persistent substernal pain, attributed to distention of the pulmonary artery. Smaller emboli that lead to pulmonary infarction can cause lateral pleuritic chest pain. Hemodynamically significant pulmonary emboli may cause hypotension, syncope, and signs of right heart failure. Pulmonary hypertension (see Chap. 78) can cause chest pain similar to that of angina pectoris, presumably because of right heart hypertrophy and ischemia.

Pulmonary Conditions

Pulmonary conditions that cause chest pain usually produce dyspnea and pleuritic symptoms, the location of which reflects the site of pulmonary disease. Tracheobronchitis tends to be associated with a burning midline pain, whereas pneumonia can produce pain over the involved lung. The pain of a pneumothorax is sudden in onset and is usually accompanied by dyspnea. Primary pneumothorax typically occurs in tall, thin young men; secondary pneumothorax occurs in the setting of pulmonary disease such as chronic obstructive pulmonary disease, asthma, or cystic fibrosis. Asthma exacerbations can present with chest discomfort, typically characterized as tightness.

Gastrointestinal Conditions

Irritation of the esophagus by acid reflux can produce a burning discomfort that is exacerbated by alcohol, aspirin, and some foods. Symptoms often are worsened by a recumbent position and relieved by sitting upright and by acid-reducing therapies. Esophageal spasm can produce a squeezing chest discomfort similar to that of angina.[10] Mallory-Weiss tears of the esophagus can occur in patients who have had prolonged vomiting episodes. Severe vomiting can also cause esophageal rupture (Boerhaave syndrome) with mediastinitis. Chest pain caused by peptic ulcer disease usually occurs 60 to 90 minutes after meals and is typically relieved rapidly by acid-reducing therapies. This pain is usually epigastric in location but can radiate into the chest and shoulders. Cholecystitis produces a wide range of pain syndromes and usually causes right upper quadrant abdominal pain, but chest and back pain caused by this disorder is not unusual. The pain is often described as aching or colicky. Pancreatitis typically causes an intense, aching epigastric pain that may radiate to the back. Relief through acid-reducing therapies is limited.

Musculoskeletal and Other Causes

Chest pain can arise from musculoskeletal disorders involving the chest wall, such as costochondritis, by conditions affecting the nerves of the chest wall, such as cervical disc disease, by herpes zoster, or following heavy exercise. Musculoskeletal syndromes causing chest pain are often elicited by direct pressure over the affected area or by movement of the patient's neck. The pain itself can be fleeting, or can be a dull ache that lasts for hours. Panic syndrome is a major cause of chest discomfort in ED patients. The symptoms typically include chest tightness, often accompanied by shortness of breath and a sense of anxiety, and generally last 30 minutes or longer.

Diagnostic Considerations

Clinical Evaluation

When evaluating patients with acute chest pain, the clinician must address a series of issues related to prognosis and immediate management. Even before trying to arrive at a definite diagnosis, high-priority questions include the following:

- *Clinical stability:* Does the patient need immediate treatment for actual or impending circulatory collapse or respiratory insufficiency?
- *Immediate prognosis:* If the patient is currently clinically stable, what is the risk that he or she has a life-threatening condition such as an ACS, pulmonary embolism, or aortic dissection?
- *Safety of triage options:* If the risk of a life-threatening condition is low, is it safe to discharge the patient for outpatient management, or should he or she undergo further testing or observation to guide management?

Initial Assessment

Evaluation of the patient with acute chest pain can begin before the physician sees the patient, and thus effectiveness may depend on the actions of the office staff and other nonphysician personnel. Guidelines from the ACC and AHA[8] (see Chaps. 55 and 56, Guidelines sections) emphasize that patients with symptoms consistent with ACS should not be evaluated solely over the telephone but should be referred to facilities that allow evaluation by a physician and the recording of a 12-lead electrocardiogram (ECG).[11] These guidelines also recommend strong consideration of immediate referral to an ED or a specialized chest pain unit for patients with suspected ACS who experience chest discomfort at rest for longer than 20 minutes, hemodynamic instability, or recent syncope or near-syncope. Transport as a passenger in a private vehicle is considered an acceptable alternative to an emergency vehicle only if the wait would lead to a delay longer than 20 to 30 minutes.

The National Heart Attack Alert Program guidelines[12] recommend that patients with the following chief complaints should undergo immediate assessment by triage nurses and be referred for further evaluation:

- Chest pain, pressure, tightness, or heaviness; pain that radiates to neck, jaw, shoulders, back, or one or both arms
- Indigestion or heartburn; nausea and/or vomiting associated with chest discomfort
- Persistent shortness of breath
- Weakness, dizziness, lightheadedness, loss of consciousness

For such patients, the initial assessment involves taking a history, performing a physical examination, obtaining an ECG and chest radiograph, and measuring biomarkers of myocardial injury.

HISTORY. If the patient does not need immediate intervention because of impending or actual circulatory collapse or respiratory insufficiency, the physician's assessment should begin with a clinical history that captures the characteristics of the patient's pain, including its quality, location, and radiation, the time and tempo (abrupt or gradual) of onset, the duration of symptoms, provoking or palliating activities, and any associated symptoms, particularly those that are pulmonary or gastrointestinal. ACS is typically described as a diffuse substernal chest pressure that starts gradually, radiates to the jaw or arms, and is worsened by exertion and relieved by rest or nitroglycerin. Studies have suggested that response to nitroglycerin may not reliably discriminate cardiac chest pain from noncardiac chest pain.[13] In contrast to the tempo of the chest pain in ACS, pulmonary embolism, aortic dissection, and pneumothorax all present with chest pain that is sudden and severe in onset. Moreover, pain that is pleuritic or positional in nature suggests pulmonary embolism, pericarditis, pneumonia, or a musculoskeletal condition.

In addition to the characteristics of the acute episode, the presence of risk factors for atherosclerosis (e.g., advanced age, male sex, diabetes) increases the likelihood that the chest pain is caused by myocardial ischemia. A history of MI is associated not only with a high risk of obstructive coronary disease but also with an increased likelihood of multivessel disease. Younger patients have a lower risk of ACS but should be screened with greater care for histories of recent cocaine use (see Chap. 73).[14]

PHYSICAL EXAMINATION (see Chap. 12). The initial examination of patients with acute chest pain should aim to identify potential precipitating causes of myocardial ischemia (e.g., uncontrolled hypertension), important comorbid conditions (e.g., chronic obstructive pulmonary disease), and evidence of hemodynamic complications (e.g., congestive heart failure, new mitral regurgitation, hypotension).[8] In addition to vital signs, examination of the peripheral vessels should include assessment of the presence of bruits or absent pulses that suggest extracardiac vascular disease.

For patients whose clinical presentations do not suggest myocardial ischemia, the search for noncoronary causes of chest pain should focus first on potentially life-threatening issues (e.g., aortic dissection, pulmonary embolism), and then turn to the possibility of other cardiac diagnoses (e.g., pericarditis) and noncardiac diagnoses (e.g., esophageal discomfort). Aortic dissection is suggested by blood pressure or pulse disparities or by a new murmur of aortic regurgitation accompanied by back or midline anterior chest pain. Differences in breath sounds in the presence of acute dyspnea and pleuritic chest pain raise the possibility of pneumothorax. Tachycardia, tachypnea, and an accentuated pulmonic component of the second heart sound (P_2) may be the major manifestations of pulmonary embolism on physical examination.

ELECTROCARDIOGRAPHY (see Chap. 13). A critical source of data, the ECG, should be obtained within 10 minutes after presentation in patients with ongoing chest discomfort and as rapidly as possible in patients who have a history of chest discomfort consistent with ACS but whose discomfort has resolved by the time of evaluation, to identify patients who might benefit from immediate reperfusion therapy (mechanical or pharmacologic).[11]

The ECG provides critical information for both diagnosis and prognosis. New persistent or transient ST-segment abnormalities (≥ 0.05 mV) that develop during a symptomatic episode at rest and resolve when the symptoms resolve strongly suggest acute ischemia and severe coronary disease. Nonspecific ST-segment and T wave abnormalities are usually defined as lesser amounts of ST-segment deviation or T wave inversion of 0.2 mV or less, and are less helpful for risk stratification. A completely normal ECG does not exclude the possibility of ACS; the risk of acute MI is about 4% among patients with a history of coronary artery disease and 2% among patients with no such history.[15] However, patients with a normal or near-normal ECG have a better prognosis than patients with clearly abnormal ECGs at presentation. Moreover, a normal ECG has a negative predictive value of 80% to 90%, regardless of whether the patient was experiencing chest pain at the time the ECG was obtained.[16] Diffuse ST-segment elevation and PR-segment depression suggest pericarditis. Right axis deviation, right bundle branch block, T wave inversions in leads V_1 to V_4, and an S wave in lead I and Q wave and T wave inversion in lead III suggest pulmonary embolism.

The availability of a prior ECG improves diagnostic accuracy and reduces the rate of admission for patients with abnormal baseline tracings. Serial electrocardiographic tracings improve the clinician's ability to diagnose acute MI, particularly if combined with serial measurement of cardiac biomarkers. Continuous electrocardiographic monitoring to detect ST-segment shifts is technically feasible but makes an uncertain contribution to patient management. Posterior leads can be useful for identifying ischemia in the territory supplied by the left circumflex coronary artery, which is otherwise relatively silent electrocardiographically.

CHEST RADIOGRAPHY. A chest radiograph is typically obtained in all patients presenting with chest pain. It is usually nondiagnostic in patients with ACS, but can show pulmonary edema caused by ischemia-induced diastolic or systolic dysfunction. It is more useful for diagnosing or suggesting other disorders; for example, it may show a widened mediastinum or aortic knob in aortic dissection. The chest radiograph is usually normal in pulmonary embolism, but can show atelectasis, an elevated hemidiaphragm, a pleural effusion or, more rarely, Hampton's hump or Westermark's sign. The chest radiograph can reveal pneumonia or pneumothorax.

BIOMARKERS. Patients presenting with chest discomfort possibly consistent with ACS should have biomarkers of myocardial injury measured (see Chaps. 55 and 56). The preferred biomarker is a cardiac troponin (T or I; cTnT or cTnI); creatine kinase MB isoenzyme (CK-MB) is less sensitive.[8]

Diagnostic Performance

Studies of the diagnostic performance of cTnI, cTnT, or CK-MB indicate that when any of these test findings are abnormal, the patient has a high likelihood of having an ACS. It should be acknowledged, however, that it is inherently challenging to define the diagnostic performance of biomarkers for MI because part of the definition of MI includes the rise and fall of a cardiac biomarker of necrosis. Nevertheless, these assays are indispensible in the diagnosis of MI, and using the totality of clinical evidence as the reference standard for diagnosis, they have excellent sensitivity and specificity.

TROPONINS. Different genes encode troponins I and T in cardiac muscle, slow skeletal muscle, and fast skeletal muscle; hence, the assays for cardiac troponins are more specific than the assay for CK-MB for myocardial injury, and cardiac troponin is the preferred diagnostic biomarker.[17] The high specificity of cardiac troponins for myocardium make false-positive elevations (i.e., an elevated cardiac troponin in the absence of myocardial injury) exceedingly rare. Rather, elevations in the absence of other clinical data consistent with an ACS usually represent true myocardial damage from causes other than atherosclerotic coronary artery disease. Such damage may occur with other forms of myocardial injury, such as in the setting of myocarditis, myocardial contusion, or cardioversion or defibrillation, left ventricular strain from congestive heart failure,[18] hypertensive crisis, or extreme exercise, right ventricular strain from pulmonary embolus,[19] or other causes of acute pulmonary hypertension. Elevated levels of cardiac troponins have been reported in patients with renal disease.[20] The exact mechanism remains unclear, but in patients with a clinical history suggestive of ACS, an elevated cardiac troponin level conveys a similarly increased risk of ischemic complications in patients across a broad range of renal function.[21] Elevated cardiac troponin levels can also occur in patients with severe sepsis[22]; again, the mechanism remains unclear.

With serial sampling up to 12 hours after presentation, cardiac troponins offer a sensitivity higher than 95% and a specificity of 90%. When using only a single sample at presentation, performance has been substantially worse, with a sensitivity of only 70% to 75%. Recently, however, sensitive assays have been developed that offer a lower limit of detection, (approximately 0.001 to 0.01 ng/mL, depending on the specific assay) and acceptable imprecision at low levels that, importantly, are now below the 99th percentile in a normal reference population (typically 0.01 to 0.07 ng/mL), thereby improving the ability to detect myocardial injury. Using such assays, the sensitivity for detecting myocardial infarction using a single sample at presentation is approximately 90%, the specificity approximately 90%, and the negative predictive value approximately 97% to 99%.[3,23,24] Moreover, among patients presenting within 3 hours of the onset of chest pain, the superior performance of high-sensitivity assays is even more striking, a sensitivity of 80% to 85%, compared with approximately 55% for older assays. The area under the receiver operator characteristic curve is as high as 0.98 using serial samples for high-sensitivity assays.

Ultrasensitive assays with even lower limits of detection (e.g., <0.001 ng/mL or <1 pg/mL) are also being developed, allowing almost all individuals (including healthy persons) to have a quantifiable troponin result. Using such assays, in patients with non–ST-elevation MI, 72% had circulating troponin levels at baseline above the 99th percentile and another 28% had levels above the limit of detection. Moreover, in patients with unstable angina (defined as lack of elevation of troponin level using a current-generation commercial assay), 44% had circulating troponin levels above the 99th percentile and another 52% had levels above the limit of detection at baseline; 6 to 8 hours later, these values were 82% and 18%, respectively.[25] Similarly, ultrasensitive assays can detect increases in circulating troponin in proportion to the amount of ischemia experienced during exercise stress testing.[26] Thus, in the future, troponin may move from a semi-quantitative assay (negative in most individuals, quantified in a subset) to quantifiable in all. The clinical implications of very low level values reported from ultrasensitive assays will need to be defined.

CREATINE KINASE MB ISOENZYME. Until the advent of cardiac troponin assays, CK-MB was the biomarker of choice for the diagnosis of MI. The major limitation to CK-MB as a diagnostic biomarker is its relative lack of specificity, because it can be found in skeletal muscle, tongue, diaphragm, small intestine, uterus, and prostate. Use of the CK-MB relative index (the ratio of CK-MB to total CK) partially addresses this limitation for skeletal muscle as a source. However, the amount of CK-MB is increased in skeletal muscle in patients with conditions that cause chronic muscle destruction and regeneration, such as muscular dystrophy, high-performance athletics (e.g., marathon running), or rhabdomyolysis.[27] CK-MB elevations are particularly common in ED patients because they have higher rates of histories of alcohol abuse or trauma. One advantage of CK-MB is a shorter half-life in the circulation, which makes it useful for gauging the timing of an MI (a normal CK-MB with an elevated troponin level could represent a small MI or an MI that occurred several days ago) and for diagnosing reinfarction in a patient who has had an MI in the past week.

OTHER MARKERS. Serum myoglobin and heart-type fatty acid binding protein (H-FABP) are smaller molecules and diffuse through interstitial fluids more rapidly after cell death than the larger CK and troponin molecules; they become abnormal as early as 30 minutes after myocardial injury.[28] Because neither is specific to myocardial tissue, however, false-positive rates in ED populations are high.[29]

Many patients presenting with ACS, including those without evidence of myocyte necrosis, have elevated concentrations of inflammatory biomarkers such as C-reactive protein,[30] serum amyloid A, myeloperoxidase,[31] or interleukin-6 (IL-6). To date, no study has identified exact decision cut points or shown an incremental benefit on an admission or treatment strategy based on these new markers, so the clinical usefulness of these observations remains uncertain.

Ischemia-modified albumin (IMA) has been approved by the U.S. Food and Drug Administration for clinical use. The albumin cobalt binding test for the detection of IMA is based on the observation that the affinity of the N-terminus of human albumin for cobalt is reduced in patients with myocardial ischemia.[32] As with the other markers, however, the clinical specificity of IMA in the broad population of patients with chest pain and suspected ACS remains an area for further investigation.[33]

D-dimer testing is useful for patients with chest pain to help rule out pulmonary embolism, because a negative enzyme-linked immunosorbent assay (ELISA) test has a negative predictive value of more than 99% in patients with a low clinical probability (patients with a higher clinical probability should undergo an imaging study).[34]

B-type natriuretic peptides (BNP and N-terminal pro-BNP [NT-proBNP]) arise in the setting of increased ventricular wall stress. Natriuretic peptides are most commonly used to aid in the diagnosis of heart failure.[35] BNP levels can be elevated in the setting of transient myocardial ischemia,[36] and the magnitude of elevation in ACS is correlated with prognosis.[37] However, the lack of specificity of natriuretic peptide elevation for ACS limits its use as a diagnostic marker.

PROGNOSTIC IMPLICATIONS OF TEST RESULTS. Abnormal levels of CK-MB, cTnI, and cTnT predict an increased risk of complications.[8] Even if patients do not have CK-MB elevations, cTnI and cTnT are helpful for early risk stratification in patients with acute chest pain. The notion that a patient who has a slight elevation in troponin has an "infarctlet" of questionable prognostic significance should be abandoned.[38] The prognostic value of cTnI seems to be comparable to that of cTnT.

Testing Strategy

The 2007 National Academy of Clinical Biochemistry (NACB) practice guidelines recommend the measurement of biomarkers of cardiac injury in patients with symptoms that suggest ACS (**Table 53-2**). Furthermore, patients with a very low probability of ACS should not undergo measurement of biomarkers because false-positive results could lead to unnecessary hospitalizations, tests, procedures, and complications.

The ACC, AHA, and NACB guidelines recommend cTnI or cTnT as the preferred first-line markers, but CK-MB (by mass assay) is an acceptable alternative. The preference for cardiac troponins reflects the greater specificity of these markers compared with CK-MB and the prognostic value of troponin elevations in the presence of normal CK-MB levels. If the initial set of markers is negative in patients who have presented within the first 6 hours of the onset of pain, the guidelines recommend that another sample be drawn in the time frame of 8 to 12 hours after symptom onset.

Decision Aids

An algorithm for the diagnostic evaluation of chest pain is shown in **Figure 53-1**. The history, physical examination, ECG, and biomarkers of myocardial injury can be integrated to allow the clinician to assess the likelihood of ACS and the risk of complications (**Tables 53-3 and 53-4**). Furthermore, in terms of prognosis, multivariable algorithms have been developed and prospectively validated, with the goal of improving risk stratification in patients with acute chest pain. These algorithms can be used to estimate the probability of acute myocardial infarction, acute ischemic heart disease, or the risk of major cardiac complications in individual patients.[15] They serve mainly to identify patients who are at low risk for complications and who therefore do not require admission to the hospital or coronary care unit.

A prospectively validated algorithm for the prediction of the risk of complications requiring intensive care is presented as a flow chart in **Figure 53-2**.[39] In this algorithm, patients with suspected myocardial infarction on their ECGs are immediately classified as having a high risk (approximately 16%) of major complications within the next 72 hours. Patients whose ECGs are consistent with ischemia but not infarction are then classified as having an intermediate (approximately 8%) or high risk for complications, depending on the presence or absence of clinical risk factors, including systolic blood pressure below 110 mm Hg, bilateral rales heard above the bases, and known unstable ischemic heart disease (defined as worsening of previously stable angina, a new onset of angina after infarction or after a coronary revascularization procedure, or pain that was the same as that associated with a prior MI). These same risk factors help stratify patients without ischemic changes on their ECGs.

TABLE 53-2	**National Academy of Clinical Biochemistry Recommendations for Use of Biochemical Markers for Risk Stratification in Acute Coronary Syndrome**

Class I

1. Patients with suspected ACS should undergo early risk stratification based on an integrated assessment of symptoms, physical examination findings, electrocardiographic findings, and biomarkers (level of evidence: C).
2. A cardiac troponin is the preferred marker for risk stratification and, if available, should be measured in all patients with suspected ACS. In patients with a clinical syndrome consistent with ACS, a maximal (peak) concentration exceeding the 99th percentile of values for a reference control group should be considered indicative of increased risk of death and recurrent ischemic events (level of evidence: A).
3. Blood should be obtained for testing on hospital presentation followed by serial sampling, with timing of sampling based on the clinical circumstances. For most patients, blood should be obtained for testing at hospital presentation, and at 6 to 9 hours (level of evidence: B).

Class IIa

4. Measurement of hs-CRP may be useful, in addition to a cardiac troponin, for risk assessment in patients with a clinical syndrome consistent with ACS. The benefits of therapy based on this strategy remain uncertain (level of evidence: A).
5. Measurement of B-type natriuretic peptide (BNP) or N-terminal pro-BNP (NT-proBNP) may be useful, in addition to a cardiac troponin, for risk assessment in patients with a clinical syndrome consistent with ACS. The benefits of therapy based on this strategy remain uncertain (level of evidence: A).

Class IIb

6. Measurement of markers of myocardial ischemia, in addition to cardiac troponin and ECG, may aid in excluding ACS in patients with a low clinical probability of myocardial ischemia (level of evidence: C).
7. A multimarker strategy that includes measurement of two or more pathobiologically diverse biomarkers, in addition to a cardiac troponin, may aid in enhancing risk stratification in patients with a clinical syndrome consistent with ACS. BNP and high-sensitivity C-reactive protein (hsCRP) are the biomarkers best studied using this approach. The benefits of therapy based on this strategy remain uncertain (level of evidence: C).
8. Early repeat sampling of cardiac troponin (e.g., 2-4 hours after presentation) may be appropriate if tied to therapeutic strategies (level of evidence: C).

Class III

Biomarkers of necrosis should not be used for routine screening of patients with low clinical probability of ACS (level of evidence: C).

From Morrow DA, Cannon CP, Jesse RL, et al: National Academy of Clinical Biochemistry Laboratory medicine practice guidelines: Clinical characteristics and utilization of biochemical markers in acute coronary syndromes. Circulation 115:e356, 2007.

Immediate Management

The ACC and AHA guidelines suggest an approach to the immediate management of patients with possible ACS that integrates information from the history, physical examination, 12-lead ECG, and initial cardiac marker tests to assign patients to four categories—noncardiac diagnosis, chronic stable angina, possible ACS, and definite ACS (**Fig. 53-3**).[8] In this algorithm, patients with ST-segment elevations are triaged immediately for reperfusion therapy, in accordance with the ACC and AHA guidelines for acute MI. Patients with ACS who have ST wave or T wave changes, ongoing pain, positive cardiac markers, or hemodynamic abnormalities should be admitted to the hospital for the management of acute ischemia. Cost-effectiveness analyses support triage of such patients to the coronary care unit for their initial care. For patients with possible or definite ACS who do not have diagnostic ECGs and whose initial serum cardiac markers are within normal limits, observation in a chest pain unit or other nonintensive care facility is appropriate, with subsequent additional testing (see later).

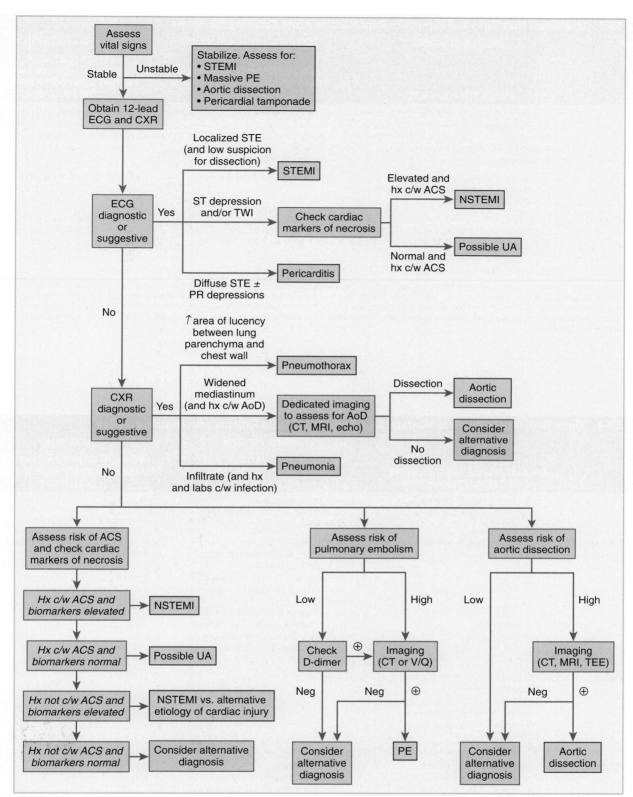

FIGURE 53-1 Algorithm for the initial diagnostic approach to a patient with chest pain. AoD = aortic dissection; c/w = consistent with; CXR = chest x-ray; hx = history; NSTEMI = non–ST-segment myocardial infarction; PE = pulmonary embolism; STE = ST elevation; STEMI = ST-segment myocardial infarction; TEE = transesophageal echocardiography; UA = unstable angina; V/Q = ventilation-perfusion scan.

CH
53

TABLE 53-3 Likelihood That Signs and Symptoms Represent an Acute Coronary Syndrome

FEATURE	HIGH LIKELIHOOD ANY OF THE FOLLOWING	INTERMEDIATE LIKELIHOOD ABSENCE OF HIGH-LIKELIHOOD FEATURES AND PRESENCE OF ANY OF THE FOLLOWING	LOW LIKELIHOOD ABSENCE OF HIGH- OR INTERMEDIATE-LIKELIHOOD FEATURES, BUT MAY HAVE ANY OF THE FOLLOWING
History	• Chest or left arm pain or discomfort as chief symptom reproducing documented angina prior • Known history of coronary artery disease, including MI	• Chest or left arm pain or discomfort as chief symptom • Age > 70 yr • Male sex • Diabetes mellitus	• Probable ischemic symptoms in absence of any of the intermediate-likelihood characteristics • Recent cocaine use
Examination	• Transient mitral regurgitation murmur, hypotension, diaphoresis, pulmonary edema, or rales	• Extracardiac vascular disease	• Chest discomfort reproduced by palpation
Electrocardiogram	• New, or presumably new, transient ST-segment deviation (≥0.1 mV) or T wave inversion (≥0.2 mV) in multiple precordial leads	• Fixed Q waves • ST-segment depression 0.05-0.1 mV or T wave inversion > 0.1 mV	• T wave flattening or inversion < 0.1 mV in leads with dominant R waves • Normal ECG
Cardiac markers	• Elevated cardiac TnI, TnT, or CK-MB	• Normal	• Normal

From Anderson JL, Adams CD, Antman EM, et al: ACC/AHA 2007 guidelines for the management of patients with unstable angina/non ST-elevation myocardial infarction: A report of the American College of Cardiology/American Heart Association Task Force on Practice Guidelines (Writing Committee to Revise the 2002 Guidelines for the Management of Patients With Unstable Angina/Non ST-Elevation Myocardial Infarction): Developed in collaboration with the American College of Emergency Physicians, the Society for Cardiovascular Angiography and Interventions, and the Society of Thoracic Surgeons: Endorsed by the American Association of Cardiovascular and Pulmonary Rehabilitation and the Society for Academic Emergency Medicine. Circulation 116:e148, 2007.

TABLE 53-4 Short-Term Risk of Death or Nonfatal Myocardial Ischemia in Patients with Unstable Angina

FEATURE	HIGH RISK AT LEAST ONE OF THE FOLLOWING FEATURES MUST BE PRESENT	INTERMEDIATE RISK NO HIGH-RISK FEATURES, BUT MUST HAVE ONE OF THE FOLLOWING	LOW RISK NO HIGH- OR INTERMEDIATE-RISK FEATURES, BUT MAY HAVE ANY OF THE FOLLOWING
History	• Accelerating tempo of ischemic symptoms in preceding 48 hours	• Prior MI, peripheral or cerebrovascular disease, or CABG; prior ASA use	
Character of pain	• Prolonged ongoing (>20 min) pain at rest	• Prolonged (>20 min) rest angina, now resolved, with intermediate or high likelihood of CAD • Rest angina (>20 min) or relieved with rest or sublingual nitroglycerin • Nocturnal angina • New-onset or progressive CCS class III or IV angina in past 2 wk without prolonged (20 min) rest pain, but with intermediate or high likelihood of CAD	• Increased angina frequency, severity, or duration • Angina provoked at a lower threshold • New-onset angina with onset 2 wk-2 mo prior to presentation
Clinical findings	• Pulmonary edema, most likely caused by ischemia • New or worsening MR murmur • S₃ or new or worsening rales • Hypotension, bradycardia, tachycardia • Age >75 yr	• Age > 70 yr	
Electrocardiogram	• Angina at rest with transient ST-segment changes > 0.05 mV • Bundle branch block, new or presumed new • Sustained ventricular tachycardia	• T wave changes • Pathologic Q waves or resting ST-segment depression < 0.1 mV in multiple lead groups (anterior, inferior, lateral)	• Normal or unchanged ECG
Cardiac markers	• Elevated cardiac TnI, TnT, or CK-MB	• Slightly elevated cardiac TnI, TnT, or CK-MB	• Normal

ASA = acetylsalicylic acid; CABG = coronary artery bypass grafting; CCS = *Canadian Cardiovascular Society;* MR = mitral regurgitation; NTG = nitroglycerin.
From Anderson JL, Adams CD, Antman EM, et al: ACC/AHA 2007 guidelines for the management of patients with unstable angina/non ST-elevation myocardial infarction: A report of the American College of Cardiology/American Heart Association Task Force on Practice Guidelines (Writing Committee to Revise the 2002 Guidelines for the Management of Patients With Unstable Angina/Non ST-Elevation Myocardial Infarction): Developed in collaboration with the American College of Emergency Physicians, the Society for Cardiovascular Angiography and Interventions, and the Society of Thoracic Surgeons: Endorsed by the American Association of Cardiovascular and Pulmonary Rehabilitation and the Society for Academic Emergency Medicine. Circulation 116:e148, 2007.

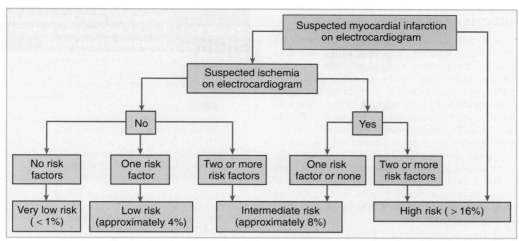

FIGURE 53-2 Derivation and validation of four groups into which patients can be categorized, according to the risk of major cardiac events within 72 hours after admission. Risk factors include: systolic blood pressure below 110 mm Hg, bilateral rales heard above the bases, and known unstable ischemic heart disease (see text for details). *(From Goldman L, Cook EF, Johnson PA, et al: Prediction of the need for intensive care in patients who come to emergency departments with acute chest pain. N Engl J Med 334:1498, 1996.)*

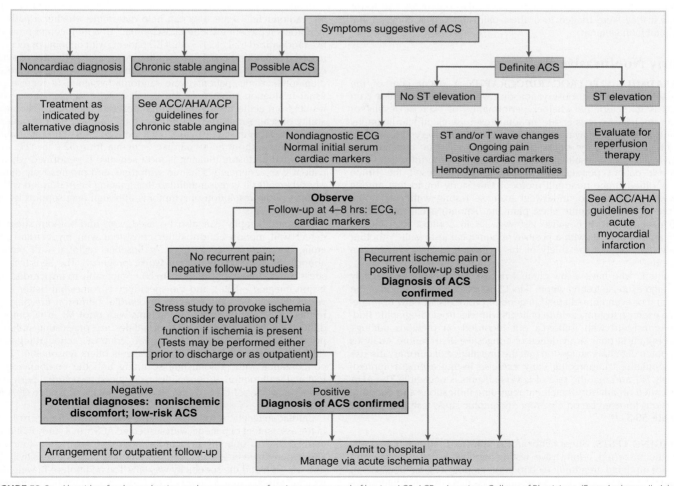

FIGURE 53-3 Algorithm for the evaluation and management of patients suspected of having ACS. ACP = American College of Physicians. *(From Anderson JL, Adams CD, Antman EM, et al: ACC/AHA 2007 guidelines for the management of patients with unstable angina/non ST-elevation myocardial infarction: A report of the American College of Cardiology/American Heart Association Task Force on Practice Guidelines [Writing Committee to Revise the 2002 Guidelines for the Management of Patients With Unstable Angina/Non ST-Elevation Myocardial Infarction]: Developed in collaboration with the American College of Emergency Physicians, the Society for Cardiovascular Angiography and Interventions, and the Society of Thoracic Surgeons: Endorsed by the American Association of Cardiovascular and Pulmonary Rehabilitation and the Society for Academic Emergency Medicine. Circulation 116:e148, 2007.)*

1084

Chest Pain Protocols and Units

The main elements of a typical chest pain critical pathway are included in Figure 53-3 (lower section). According to the ACC and AHA recommendations,[8] patients with a low risk of acute coronary syndrome or associated complications can be observed for 6 to 12 hours while undergoing electrocardiographic monitoring and serial measurement of cardiac markers. Patients who develop evidence of ischemia or other indicators of increased risk should be admitted to the coronary care unit for further management. Patients who do not develop recurrent pain or other predictors of increased risk can be triaged for early noninvasive testing (see later) before or after discharge. Outpatient stress testing is a reasonable option if the patient is at low risk for ACS and if the testing can be accomplished within 72 hours; such a strategy has been shown to be safe. In such patients, it is prudent to prescribe aspirin and possibly beta blockers, and to provide them with sublingual nitroglycerin.

To enhance the efficiency and reliability of implementation of such chest pain protocols, many hospitals triage low-risk patients with chest pain to special chest pain units.[40] These units often are located adjacent to or within EDs, but sometimes are located elsewhere in the hospital. In most of these units, the rate of MI has been about 1% to 2%, and they have proven to be safe and cost-saving sites of care for low-risk patients. Chest pain units are also sometimes used for intermediate-risk patients, such as those with a prior history of coronary disease but no other high-risk predictors. In one community-based randomized trial, patients with unstable angina and an overall intermediate risk of complications had similar outcomes and lower costs if they were triaged to a chest pain unit versus conventional hospital management.

Early Noninvasive Testing

TREADMILL ELECTROCARDIOGRAPHY. A major goal of the initial short period of observation of low-risk patients in chest pain units is to determine whether performance of exercise testing or other noninvasive tests is safe. Treadmill exercise electrocardiography is inexpensive and available at many hospitals every day, beyond traditional laboratory hours, and prospective data indicate that early exercise test results provide reliable prognostic information for low-risk patient populations. Most studies have used the Bruce or modified Bruce treadmill protocol. One study found that among low-risk patients who underwent exercise testing within 48 hours of presentation for acute chest pain, the 6-month event rate among 195 patients with a negative test was 2%, in contrast to a rate of 15% among patients with a positive or equivocal test result.[41] Another study documented the safety of this approach in 3000 consecutive patients.[4]

Patients who have a low clinical risk of complications can safely undergo exercise testing within 6 to 12 hours after presentation at the hospital or even immediately.[4] In general, protocols for early or immediate exercise testing exclude patients with electrocardiographic findings consistent with ischemia not recorded on previous tracings, ongoing chest pain, or evidence of congestive heart failure. Analyses of pooled data have suggested that the prevalence of coronary disease in populations undergoing early exercise testing averages approximately 5%, and that the rate of adverse events is negligible. The AHA has issued an advisory statement regarding indications and contraindications for exercise on electrocardiographic stress testing in the ED (**Table 53-5**).[4,42]

IMAGING TESTS. Stress echocardiography and radionuclide scans are the preferred noninvasive testing modalities for patients who cannot undergo treadmill electrocardiographic testing because of physical disability or who have resting ECGs that confound interpretation. Imaging studies are less readily available and more expensive than exercise electrocardiography, but have increased sensitivity for the detection of coronary disease and the ability to quantify the extent of, and localize, jeopardized myocardium. High-risk rest perfusion scans are associated with an increased risk of major cardiac

TABLE 53-5	Indications and Contraindications for Exercise Electrocardiographic Testing in the Emergency Department

Requirements before exercise electrocardiographic testing that should be considered in the Emergency Department setting:
- Two sets of cardiac enzymes at 4-hr intervals should be normal.
- ECG at the time of presentation and preexercise 12-lead ECG shows no significant abnormality.
- Absence of rest electrocardiographic abnormalities that would preclude accurate assessment of the exercise ECG
- From admission to time that results are available from the second set of cardiac enzymes: patient asymptomatic, lessening chest pain symptoms, or persistent atypical symptoms
- Absence of ischemic chest pain at the time of exercise testing

Contraindications to exercise electrocardiographic testing in the Emergency Department setting:
- New or evolving electrocardiographic abnormalities on the rest tracing
- Abnormal cardiac enzyme levels
- Inability to perform exercise
- Worsening or persistent ischemic chest pain symptoms from admission to the time of exercise testing
- Clinical risk profiling indicating that imminent coronary angiography is likely

complications, whereas patients with low-risk scans have low 30-day cardiac event rates (<2%).[43-45]

In addition to stress imaging studies to detect provocable ischemia, rest radionuclide scans also can help determine whether a patient's symptoms represent myocardial ischemia.[46] In a multicenter prospective randomized trial of 2475 adult ED patients with ongoing or recently resolved (<3 hours) chest pain or other symptoms suggestive of acute cardiac ischemia, and with normal or nondiagnostic initial electrocardiographic results, patients were randomly assigned to receive the usual evaluation strategy or the usual strategy supplemented with results from acute resting myocardial perfusion imaging.[47] The availability of scan results did not influence the management of patients with acute MI or unstable angina, but it reduced rates of hospitalization for patients without acute cardiac ischemia from 52% to 42%. Rest myocardial perfusion imaging is most sensitive if performed when a patient is experiencing ischemic symptoms, and progressively diminishes thereafter. It is recommended that imaging be performed within 2 hours of the resolution of symptoms, although data support its use for up to 4 hours.[48]

Echocardiography can also be used, with and without stress, to detect wall motion abnormalities consistent with myocardial ischemia. The presence of induced or baseline regional wall motion abnormalities correlates with a worse prognosis. The sensitivity of stress echocardiography appears to be comparable to myocardial perfusion imaging (~85%), and the specificity is somewhat better (95% versus 90%).[49] As is the case for myocardial perfusion imaging, the results are less interpretable in patients with prior MI, in whom it is difficult to exclude that the abnormalities are preexisting unless a prior study is available. Myocardial contrast echocardiography (MCE)[50] using microbubble imaging agents offers reasonable (77%) concordance with radionuclide scanning, and the combination of regional wall motion abnormalities or reduced myocardial perfusion has a sensitivity of 80% to 90% and a specificity of 60% to 90% for ACS.[51,52]

Cardiac magnetic resonance imaging (MRI) is also being explored in the assessment of patients with suspected ACS.[53] In a study that used cardiac MRI to quantify myocardial perfusion, ventricular function, and hyperenhancement in patients with chest pain, the sensitivity for ACS was 84% and the specificity was 85%. The addition of T2-weighted imaging, which can detect myocardial edema and thus help differentiate acute from chronic perfusion defects, improves the specificity to 96% without sacrificing sensitivity.[54] Integration of MRI coronary angiography is being studied.[55] Stress MRI using adenosine, although more labor intensive, has also been studied and shows excellent sensitivity and specificity.[56]

In contrast to the functional imaging data from stress testing, coronary computed tomography angiography (CTA) offers noninvasive anatomic data. Using multidetector computed tomography (MDCT), coronary CTA has a sensitivity of approximately 90% and a specificity of 65% to 90% for coronary stenosis greater than 50%. Coronary CTA has been evaluated in a single-center study of chest pain patients presenting to the ED.[6] Of 368 patients with a nondiagnostic ECG and negative initial biomarker of necrosis, 31 were ultimately diagnosed with ACS. Approximately half of the patients were free of coronary artery disease (CAD) on coronary CTA and 0% had an ACS, yielding a negative predictive value of 100%. The remaining 50% had evidence of atherosclerosis, with 32% having minor plaque and 18% having a stenosis greater than 50%. A final diagnosis of ACS was made in 6% of those with only minor plaque and in 35% with a significant stenosis. The negative predictive value of coronary stenosis by coronary CTA for ACS was 98%. Thus, given the anatomic rather than the functional data provided, coronary CTA may be best suited to rule out rather than rule in ACS. Of the patients who underwent CTA in a randomized comparison of myocardial perfusion imaging versus coronary CTA, 68% had a normal test and were discharged home. Another 24% had an intermediate or nondiagnostic test and underwent myocardial perfusion imaging; most of the results were negative. In total, 89% were discharged from the ED. Among patients who underwent myocardial perfusion imaging, 97% were discharged from the ED. The patients randomized to coronary CTA had a time to diagnosis that was 8 hours shorter, and consequently incurred lower hospital costs. Higher rates of cardiac catheterization and coronary revascularization occurred in the coronary CTA group (11% versus 3% and 5% versus 1%, respectively).[57] The most recent ACC and AHA guidelines acknowledge that coronary CTA is a reasonable alternative to stress testing in patients with low to intermediate probability of CAD.[8]

For both MRI and coronary CTA, additional multicenter studies and considerations related to radiation exposure are needed before such approaches are widely adopted clinically.

REFERENCES

Causes of Acute Chest Pain

1. Pope JH, Aufderheide TP, Ruthazer R, et al: Missed diagnoses of acute cardiac ischemia in the emergency department. N Engl J Med 342:1163, 2000.
2. Lindsell CJ, Anantharaman V, Diercks D, et al: The Internet Tracking Registry of Acute Coronary Syndromes (i*trACS): A multicenter registry of patients with suspicion of acute coronary syndromes reported using the standardized reporting guidelines for emergency department chest pain studies. Ann Emerg Med 48:666, 2006.
3. Morrow DA: Clinical application of sensitive troponin assays. N Engl J Med 361:913, 2009.
4. Amsterdam EA, Kirk JD, Diercks DB, et al: Exercise testing in chest pain units: Rationale, implementation, and results. Cardiol Clin 23:503, 2005.
5. Ekelund U, Forberg JL: New methods for improved evaluation of patients with suspected acute coronary syndrome in the emergency department. Emerg Med J 24:811, 2007.
6. Hoffmann U, Bamberg F, Chae CU, et al: Coronary computed tomography angiography for early triage of patients with acute chest pain: The ROMICAT (Rule Out Myocardial Infarction using Computer Assisted Tomography) trial. J Am Coll Cardiol 53:1642, 2009.
7. Blomkalns AL, Gibler WB: Chest pain unit concept: rationale and diagnostic strategies. Cardiol Clin 23:411, 2005.
8. Anderson JL, Adams CD, Antman EM, et al: ACC/AHA 2007 guidelines for the management of patients with unstable angina/non ST-elevation myocardial infarction: A report of the American College of Cardiology/American Heart Association Task Force on Practice Guidelines (Writing Committee to Revise the 2002 Guidelines for the Management of Patients With Unstable Angina/Non ST-Elevation Myocardial Infarction): Developed in collaboration with the American College of Emergency Physicians, the Society for Cardiovascular Angiography and Interventions, and the Society of Thoracic Surgeons: Endorsed by the American Association of Cardiovascular and Pulmonary Rehabilitation and the Society for Academic Emergency Medicine. Circulation 116:e148, 2007.
9. Lange RA, Hillis LD: Clinical practice. Acute pericarditis. N Engl J Med 351:2195, 2004.
10. Eslick GD: Noncardiac chest pain: Epidemiology, natural history, health care seeking, and quality of life. Gastroenterol Clin North Am 33:1, 2004.

Initial Assessment

11. Antman EM, Anbe DT, Armstrong PW, et al: ACC/AHA guidelines for the management of patients with ST-elevation myocardial infarction: A report of the American College of Cardiology/American Heart Association Task Force on Practice Guidelines (Committee to Revise the 1999 Guidelines for the Management of Patients with Acute Myocardial Infarction). Circulation 110:e82, 2004.
12. National Heart Attack Alert Program Coordinating Committee, 60 Minutes to Treatment Working Group: Emergency department: rapid identification and treatment of patients with acute myocardial infarction. Ann Emerg Med 23:311, 1994.
13. Diercks DB, Boghos E, Guzman H, et al: Changes in the numeric descriptive scale for pain after sublingual nitroglycerin do not predict cardiac etiology of chest pain. Ann Emerg Med 45:581, 2005.

14. McCord J, Jneid H, Hollander JE, et al: Management of cocaine-associated chest pain and myocardial infarction: A scientific statement from the American Heart Association Acute Cardiac Care Committee of the Council on Clinical Cardiology. Circulation 117:1897, 2008.
15. Lee TH, Goldman L: Evaluation of the patient with acute chest pain. N Engl J Med 342:1187, 2000.
16. Turnipseed SD, Trythall WS, Diercks DB, et al: Frequency of acute coronary syndrome in patients with normal electrocardiogram performed during presence or absence of chest pain. Acad Emerg Med 16:495, 2009.

Biomarkers

17. Thygesen K, Alpert JS, White HD: Universal definition of myocardial infarction. J Am Coll Cardiol 50:2173, 2007.
18. Peacock WF 4th, De Marco T, Fonarow GC, et al: Cardiac troponin and outcome in acute heart failure. N Engl J Med 358:2117, 2008.
19. Becattini C, Vedovati MC, Agnelli G: Prognostic value of troponins in acute pulmonary embolism: A meta-analysis. Circulation 116:427, 2007.
20. Khan NA, Hemmelgarn BR, Tonelli M, et al: Prognostic value of troponin T and I among asymptomatic patients with end-stage renal disease: A meta-analysis. Circulation 112:3088, 2005.
21. Wu AH, Jaffe AS, Apple FS, et al: National Academy of Clinical Biochemistry laboratory medicine practice guidelines: Use of cardiac troponin and B-type natriuretic peptide or N-terminal proB-type natriuretic peptide for etiologies other than acute coronary syndromes and heart failure. Clin Chem 53:2086, 2007.
22. Favory R, Neviere R: Significance and interpretation of elevated troponin in septic patients. Crit Care 10:224, 2006.
23. Reichlin T, Hochholzer W, Bassetti S, et al: Early diagnosis of myocardial infarction with sensitive cardiac troponin assays. N Engl J Med 361:858, 2009.
24. Keller T, Zeller T, Peetz D, et al: Sensitive troponin I assay in early diagnosis of acute myocardial infarction. N Engl J Med 61:868, 2009.
25. Wilson SR, Sabatine MS, Braunwald E, et al: Detection of myocardial injury in patients with unstable angina using a novel nanoparticle cardiac troponin I assay: Observations from the PROTECT-TIMI 30 Trial. Am Heart J 158:386, 2009.
26. Sabatine MS, Morrow DA, de Lemos JA, et al: Detection of acute changes in circulating troponin in the setting of transient stress test-induced myocardial ischaemia using an ultrasensitive assay: results from TIMI 35. Eur Heart J 30:162, 2009.
27. Leers MP, Schepers R, Baumgarten R: Effects of a long-distance run on cardiac markers in healthy athletes. Clin Chem Lab Med 44:999, 2006.
28. O'Donoghue M, de Lemos JA, Morrow DA, et al: Prognostic utility of heart-type fatty acid binding protein in patients with acute coronary syndromes. Circulation 2114:550, 2006.
29. Morrow DA, Cannon CP, Jesse RL, et al: National Academy of Clinical Biochemistry Laboratory Medicine Practice Guidelines: Clinical characteristics and utilization of biochemical markers in acute coronary syndromes. Circulation 115:e356, 2007.
30. Scirica BM, Morrow DA, Cannon CP, et al: Clinical application of C-reactive protein across the spectrum of acute coronary syndromes. Clin Chem 53:1800, 2007.
31. Schindhelm RK, van der Zwan LP, Teerlink T, Scheffer PG: Myeloperoxidase: A useful biomarker for cardiovascular disease risk stratification? Clin Chem 55:1462, 2009.
32. Peacock F, Morris DL, Anwaruddin S, et al: Meta-analysis of ischemia-modified albumin to rule out acute coronary syndromes in the emergency department. Am Heart J 152:253, 2006.
33. Sabatine MS: When prognosis precedes diagnosis: Putting the cart before the horse. CMAJ 172:1697, 2005.
34. van Belle A, Buller HR, Huisman MV, et al: Effectiveness of managing suspected pulmonary embolism using an algorithm combining clinical probability, D-dimer testing, and computed tomography. JAMA 295:172, 2006.
35. Braunwald E: Biomarkers in heart failure. N Engl J Med 358:2148, 2008.
36. Sabatine MS, Morrow DA, de Lemos JA, et al: Acute changes in circulating natriuretic peptide levels in relation to myocardial ischemia. J Am Coll Cardiol 44:1988, 2004.
37. Morrow DA, de Lemos JA, Blazing MA, et al: Prognostic value of serial B-type natriuretic peptide testing during follow-up of patients with unstable coronary artery disease. JAMA 294:2866, 2005.
38. Bonaca MP, Morrow DA: Defining a role for novel biomarkers in acute coronary syndromes. Clin Chem 54:1424, 2008.
39. Goldman L, Cook EF, Johnson PA, et al: Prediction of the need for intensive care in patients who come to the emergency departments with acute chest pain. N Engl J Med 334:1498, 1996.

Immediate Management

40. Farkouh ME, Smars PA, Reeder GS, et al: A clinical trial of a chest-pain observation unit for patients with unstable angina. N Engl J Med 339:1882, 1998.
41. Polanczyk CA, Johnson PA, Hartley LH, et al: Clinical correlates and prognostic significance of early negative exercise tolerance test in patients with acute chest pain seen in the hospital emergency department. Am J Cardiol 81:288, 1998.
42. Gibbons RJ, Balady GJ, Bricker JT, et al: ACC/AHA 2002 guideline update for exercise testing: summary article: A report of the American College of Cardiology/American Heart Association Task Force on Practice Guidelines (Committee to Update the 1997 Exercise Testing Guidelines). Circulation 106:1883, 2002.
43. Kontos MC, Tatum JL: Imaging in the evaluation of the patient with suspected acute coronary syndrome. Cardiol Clin 23:517, 2005.
44. Marcassa C, Bax JJ, Bengel F, et al: Clinical value, cost-effectiveness, and safety of myocardial perfusion scintigraphy: a position statement. Eur Heart J 29:557, 2008.
45. Wyrick JJ, Kalvaitis S, McConnell KJ, et al: Cost-efficiency of myocardial contrast echocardiography in patients presenting to the emergency department with chest pain of suspected cardiac origin and a nondiagnostic electrocardiogram. Am J Cardiol 102:649, 2008.
46. Klocke FJ, Baird MG, Lorell BH, et al: ACC/AHA/ASNC guidelines for the clinical use of cardiac radionuclide imaging—executive summary: A report of the American College of Cardiology/American Heart Association Task Force on Practice Guidelines (ACC/AHA/ASNC Committee to Revise the 1995 Guidelines for the Clinical Use of Cardiac Radionuclide Imaging). Circulation 108:1404, 2003.

APPROACH TO THE PATIENT WITH CHEST PAIN

47. Udelson JE, Beshansky JR, Ballin DS, et al: Myocardial perfusion imaging for evaluation and triage of patients with suspected acute cardiac ischemia: A randomized controlled trial. JAMA 288:2693, 2002.

48. Schaeffer MW, Brennan TD, Hughes JA, et al: Resting radionuclide myocardial perfusion imaging in a chest pain center including an overnight delayed image acquisition protocol. J Nucl Med Technol 35:242, 2007.

49. Conti A, Sammicheli L, Gallini C, et al: Assessment of patients with low-risk chest pain in the emergency department: Head-to-head comparison of exercise stress echocardiography and exercise myocardial SPECT. Am Heart J 149:894, 2005.

50. Kaul S: Myocardial contrast echocardiography: A 25-year retrospective. Circulation 118:291, 2008.

51. Kaul S, Senior R, Firschke C, et al: Incremental value of cardiac imaging in patients presenting to the emergency department with chest pain and without ST-segment elevation: A multicenter study. Am Heart J 148:129, 2004.

52. Korosoglou G, Labadze N, Hansen A, et al: Usefulness of real-time myocardial perfusion imaging in the evaluation of patients with first time chest pain. Am J Cardiol 94:1225, 2004.

53. Lockie T, Nagel E, Redwood S, Plein S: Use of cardiovascular magnetic resonance imaging in acute coronary syndromes. Circulation 119:1671, 2009.

54. Cury RC, Shash K, Nagurney JT, et al: Cardiac magnetic resonance with T2-weighted imaging improves detection of patients with acute coronary syndrome in the emergency department. Circulation 2118:837, 2008.

55. Yang Q, Li K, Liu X, et al: Contrast-enhanced whole-heart coronary magnetic resonance angiography at 3.0-T: A comparative study with X-ray angiography in a single center. J Am Coll Cardiol 54:69, 2009.

56. Ingkanisorn WP, Kwong RY, Bohme NS, et al: Prognosis of negative adenosine stress magnetic resonance in patients presenting to an emergency department with chest pain. J Am Coll Cardiol 47:1427, 2006.

57. Goldstein JA, Gallagher MJ, O'Neill WW, et al: A randomized controlled trial of multi-slice coronary computed tomography for evaluation of acute chest pain. J Am Coll Cardiol 49:863, 2007.

CHAPTER **54** # ST-Segment Elevation Myocardial Infarction: Pathology, Pathophysiology, and Clinical Features

Elliott M. Antman

The pathologic diagnosis of myocardial infarction (MI) requires evidence of myocyte cell death caused by prolonged ischemia. Characteristic findings include coagulation necrosis and contraction band necrosis, often with patchy areas of myocytolysis at the periphery of the infarct. During the acute phase of MI, most myocyte loss in the infarct zone occurs via coagulation necrosis and proceeds to inflammation, phagocytosis of necrotic myocytes, and repair eventuating in scar formation.

The clinical diagnosis of MI requires an integrated assessment of the history with some combination of indirect evidence of myocardial necrosis using biochemical, electrocardiographic, and imaging modalities (**Table 54-1**). The sensitivity and specificity of the clinical tools for diagnosing MI vary considerably, depending on the time after onset of the infarction (**Table 54-2**).

The World Heath Organization and American Heart Association previously required the presence of at least two of the following for the diagnosis of myocardial infarction: characteristic symptoms, electrocardiographic changes, and a typical rise and fall in biochemical markers. Advances in the techniques for diagnosing MI led to a consensus document published jointly by several prominent cardiac societies[1] (see Table 54-2). In addition to codifying the criteria for the diagnosis of MI, the revised definition classifies MI into five types, depending on the circumstances in which the MI occurs (**Table 54-3**). The revised definition of MI (see Table 54-2) has important implications not only for the clinical care of patients, but also for epidemiologic studies, public policy, and clinical trials.[2,3] The shift to cardiac-specific troponins as the markers of choice for the diagnosis of MI requires new cutoff values for cardiac injury. The term *normal range* has been replaced by the term *upper reference limit*, defined as the 99th percentile of a normal reference control group.[1]

The contemporary approach to patients presenting with ischemic discomfort is to consider them as experiencing an acute coronary syndrome. The 12-lead electrocardiogram (ECG) defines those presenting with ST-segment elevation, the subject of Chaps. 54 and 55, and those without ST-segment elevation, the subject of Chap. 56. Although the revised definition of MI has greater impact on the non–ST-segment elevation end of the acute coronary syndrome spectrum (i.e., distinction between unstable angina and non–ST-segment elevation MI), the issues also pertain to discussion of ST-segment elevation myocardial infarction (STEMI).

Changing Patterns in Clinical Care

Despite advances in diagnosis and management, STEMI continues to be a major public health problem in the industrialized world and is rising in developing countries (see Chap. 1).[4] In the United States, almost 1 million patients per year suffer from an acute MI, and more than 1 million patients with suspected acute MI yearly enter coronary care units in the United States.[5] The rate of MI rises for both men and women sharply with increasing age, and racial differences exist, with MI occurring more frequently in black men and women, regardless of age (**Fig. 54-1**). Of particular concern from a global perspective, the burden of MI in developing countries may approach those now afflicting developed countries. Limitations in available resources to treat STEMI in developing countries mandate major efforts on an international level to strengthen primary prevention programs.[6]

Improvements in Outcome

Mortality from STEMI has declined steadily.[7-9] This drop in mortality appears to result from a fall in the incidence of STEMI (replaced in part by an increase in the rate of unstable angina/non–ST-segment elevation MI [NSTEMI][10]) and a fall in the case fatality rate once STEMI has occurred.[5]

Several phases in the management of patients have contributed to the decline in mortality from STEMI.[11] The "clinical observation phase" of coronary care consumed the first half of the 20th century and focused on a detailed recording of physical and laboratory findings, with little active treatment for the infarction. The "coronary care unit phase" began in the mid-1960s and was notable for detailed analysis and vigorous management of cardiac arrhythmias. The "high-technology phase" heralded by the introduction of the pulmonary artery balloon flotation catheter set the stage for bedside hemodynamic monitoring and more precise hemodynamic management. The modern "reperfusion era" of coronary care was introduced by intracoronary and then intravenous fibrinolysis, increased use of aspirin, and the development of primary percutaneous coronary intervention (PCI; see Chap. 58).

Contemporary care of patients with STEMI has entered an evidence-based coronary care phase and is increasingly influenced by guidelines and performance measures for clinical practice.[12-14] Government websites now benchmark mortality rates for patients with MI who are treated at various hospitals (www.hospitalcompare.hhs.gov).

Limitations of Current Therapy

The short-term mortality rate of patients with STEMI who receive aggressive pharmacologic reperfusion therapy as part of a randomized trial is in the range of 6.5% to 7.5%,[15] whereas observational data bases suggest that the mortality rate in STEMI patients in the community is

TABLE 54-1	Aspects of Diagnosis of Myocardial Infarction by Different Techniques
TECHNIQUE	**FEATURES**
Pathology	Myocardial cell death
Biochemistry	Markers of myocardial cell death recovered from blood samples
Electrocardiography	Evidence of myocardial ischemia (ST and T wave abnormalities); evidence of loss of electrically functioning cardiac tissue (Q waves)
Imaging	Reduction or loss of tissue perfusion; cardiac wall motion abnormalities

Modified from Thygesen K, Alpert JS, White HD, et al: Universal definition of myocardial infarction. Circulation 116:2634, 2007.

TABLE 54-2 Revised Definition of Myocardial Infarction

Criteria for Acute, Evolving, or Recent MI

Either of the following criteria satisfies the diagnosis for acute, evolving, or recent MI:

1. Typical rise and/or fall of biochemical markers of myocardial necrosis with at least one of the following:
    a. Ischemic symptoms
    b. Development of pathologic Q waves in the ECG
    c. Electrocardiographic changes indicative of ischemia (ST-segment elevation or depression)
    d. Imaging evidence of new loss of viable myocardium or new regional wall motion abnormality
2. Pathologic findings of an acute myocardial infarction

Criteria for Healing or Healed Myocardial Infarction

Any one of the following criteria satisfies the diagnosis for healing or healed myocardial infarction:

1. Development of new pathologic Q waves in serial ECGs. The patient may or may not remember previous symptoms. Biochemical markers of myocardial necrosis may have normalized, depending on the length of time that has passed since the infarction developed.
2. Pathologic findings of a healed or healing infarction

From Thygesen K, Alpert JS, White HD, et al: Universal definition of myocardial infarction. Circulation 116:2634, 2007.

TABLE 54-3 Classification of Myocardial Infarction

TYPE	FEATURES
1	Spontaneous myocardial infarction related to ischemia caused by a primary coronary event such as plaque erosion and/or rupture, fissuring, or dissection
2	Myocardial infarction secondary to ischemia caused by increased oxygen demand or decreased supply (e.g., coronary artery spasm, coronary embolism, anemia, arrhythmias, hypertension, hypotension)
3	Sudden unexpected cardiac death, including cardiac arrest, often with symptoms suggestive of myocardial ischemia, accompanied by presumably new ST-segment elevation, or new LBBB, or presumably new major obstruction in a coronary artery by angiography and/or pathology, but death occurring before blood samples could be obtained, or before the appearance of cardiac biomarkers in the blood
4a	Myocardial infarction associated with PCI
4b	Myocardial infarction associated with stent thrombosis, as documented by angiography or autopsy
5	Myocardial infarction associated with CABG

CABG = coronary artery bypass grafting; LBBB = left bundle branch block.
From Thygesen K, Alpert JS, White HD, et al: Universal definition of myocardial infarction. Circulation 2007;116(22):2634-2653.

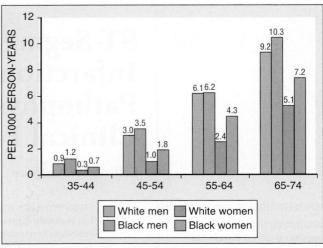

FIGURE 54-1 Annual rate of first heart attacks by age, sex, and race (data, Atherosclerosis Risk in Communities [ARIC] surveillance, 1987-2004). *(From Lloyd-Jones D, Adams R, Carnethon M, et al: Heart disease and stroke statistics—2009 update: A report from the American Heart Association Statistics Committee and Stroke Statistics Subcommittee. Circulation 119:e21, 2009.)*

15% to 20%.[16] About 30% of patients with STEMI who are eligible to receive reperfusion therapy do not receive that lifesaving treatment.[17] In part, this difference relates to the selection of patients without serious comorbidities for clinical trials.

Advanced age consistently emerges as one of the principal determinants of mortality in patients with STEMI.[18] Cardiac catheterization and other invasive procedures are being performed more commonly at some point during hospitalization in older patients with STEMI. Nevertheless, evidence suggests that the greatest reductions in mortality for older patients derive from those strategies used during the first 24 hours, a time frame during which prompt and appropriate use of lifesaving reperfusion therapy has paramount importance, emphasizing the need to extend advances in drug therapy for STEMI to older patients.[5]

Considerable variation exists in the management and outcomes of patients with STEMI.[19,20] Mortality rates for STEMI are lower in hospitals with a high clinical volume, a high rate of invasive procedures, and a top ranking in quality reports. Conversely, mortality rates are higher in STEMI patients not cared for by a cardiovascular specialist.[21] Variation also occurs in the treatment patterns of certain population subgroups with STEMI, notably women and blacks.[22] Evidence exists that much of the regional variation in outcomes derives from the characteristics of the patient and treatments received as opposed to the location where those treatments were delivered.

Pathology

Almost all MIs result from coronary atherosclerosis, generally with superimposed coronary thrombosis. Nonatherogenic forms of coronary artery disease are discussed later in this chapter, and causes of STEMI without coronary atherosclerosis are shown in **Table 54-4**.

Before the fibrinolytic era, clinicians typically divided patients with MI into those suffering a Q wave and those suffering a non–Q-wave infarction on the basis of evolution of the pattern on the ECG over several days. The term *Q-wave infarction* was frequently considered to be virtually synonymous with transmural infarction, whereas non–Q-wave infarctions were often referred to as subendocardial infarctions. Contemporary studies using cardiac magnetic resonance imaging indicate that the development of a Q wave on the ECG is determined more by the size of the infarct than the depth of mural involvement.[23,24] A more suitable framework that puts STEMI in perspective, along with unstable angina–NSTEMI (UA/NSTEMI) based on pathophysiology, is referred to as *acute coronary syndromes* (**Fig. 54-2**).

TABLE 54-4	Causes of Myocardial Infarction Without Coronary Atherosclerosis

Coronary Artery Disease Other Than Atherosclerosis
Arteritis
  Luetic
  Granulomatous (Takayasu disease)
  Polyarteritis nodosa
  Mucocutaneous lymph node (Kawasaki) syndrome
  Disseminated lupus erythematosus
  Rheumatoid spondylitis
  Ankylosing spondylitis
Trauma to coronary arteries
  Laceration
  Thrombosis
  Iatrogenic
  Radiation (radiation therapy for neoplasia)
Coronary mural thickening with metabolic disease or intimal proliferative disease
  Mucopolysaccharidoses (Hurler disease)
  Homocystinuria
  Fabry disease
  Amyloidosis
  Juvenile intimal sclerosis (idiopathic arterial calcification of infancy)
  Intimal hyperplasia associated with contraceptive steroids or with the postpartum period
  Pseudoxanthoma elasticum
  Coronary fibrosis caused by radiation therapy
Luminal narrowing by other mechanisms
  Spasm of coronary arteries (Prinzmetal angina with normal coronary arteries)
  Spasm after nitroglycerin withdrawal
  Dissection of the aorta
  Dissection of the coronary artery

Emboli to Coronary Arteries
Infective endocarditis
Nonbacterial thrombotic endocarditis
Prolapse of mitral valve
Mural thrombus from left atrium, left ventricle, or pulmonary veins
Prosthetic valve emboli
Cardiac myxoma
Associated with cardiopulmonary bypass surgery and coronary arteriography
Paradoxical emboli
Papillary fibroelastoma of the aortic valve (fixed embolus)
Thrombi from intracardiac catheters or guidewires

Congenital Coronary Artery Anomalies
Anomalous origin of left coronary from pulmonary artery
Left coronary artery from anterior sinus of Valsalva
Coronary arteriovenous and arteriocameral fistulas
Coronary artery aneurysms

Myocardial Oxygen Demand-Supply Disproportion
Aortic stenosis, all forms
Incomplete differentiation of the aortic valve
Aortic insufficiency
Carbon monoxide poisoning
Thyrotoxicosis
Prolonged hypotension
Takotsubo cardiomyopathy

Hematologic (In Situ Thrombosis)
Polycythemia vera
Thrombocytosis
Disseminated intravascular coagulation
Hypercoagulability, thrombosis, thrombocytopenic purpura

Miscellaneous
Cocaine abuse
Myocardial contusion
Myocardial infarction with normal coronary arteries
Complication of cardiac catheterization

Modified from Cheitlin MD, McAllister HA, de Castro CM: Myocardial infarction without atherosclerosis. JAMA 231:951, 1975.

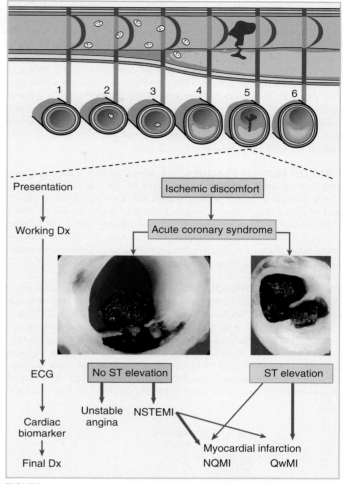

FIGURE 54-2 Acute coronary syndromes. The longitudinal section of an artery depicts the time line of atherogenesis from a normal artery (1), to lesion initiation and accumulation of extracellular lipid in the intima (2), to the evolution to the fibrofatty stage (3), and to lesion progression with procoagulant expression and weakening of the fibrous cap (4). An ACS develops when the vulnerable or high-risk plaque undergoes disruption of the fibrous cap (5); disruption of the plaque is the stimulus for thrombogenesis. Thrombus resorption may be followed by collagen accumulation and smooth muscle cell growth (6). Following disruption of a vulnerable or high-risk plaque, patients experience ischemic discomfort resulting from a reduction of flow through the affected epicardial coronary artery. The flow reduction may be caused by a completely occlusive thrombus (bottom half, right) or subtotally occlusive thrombus (bottom half, left). Patients with ischemic discomfort may present with or without ST-segment elevation on the ECG. Of patients with ST-segment elevation, most ultimately develop a Q-wave MI (QwMI), whereas a few develop a non–Q-wave MI (NQMI). Patients who present without ST-segment elevation are suffering from unstable angina or NSTEMI, a distinction that is ultimately made on the presence or absence of a serum cardiac marker such as CK-MB or a cardiac troponin detected in the blood. Most patients presenting with NSTEMI ultimately develop an NQMI on the ECG; a few may develop a QwMI. The spectrum of clinical presentations ranging from unstable angina through NSTEMI and STEMI are referred to as the acute coronary syndromes. Dx = diagnosis. (*Modified from Libby P: Circulation 104:365, 2001; Hamm CW, Bertrand M, Braunwald E: Lancet 358:1533, 2001; Davies MJ: Heart 83:361, 2000; and Antman EM, Anbe DT, Armstrong PW, et al: ACC/AHA guidelines for the management of patients with ST-elevation myocardial infarction: A report of the American College of Cardiology/American Heart Association Task Force on Practice Guidelines [Committee to Revise the 1999 Guidelines for the Management of Patients with Acute Myocardial Infarction]. Circulation 110:e82, 2004.*)

Plaque

During the natural evolution of atherosclerotic plaques, especially lipid-laden plaques, an abrupt and catastrophic transition can occur, characterized by plaque disruption (see Chap. 43).[25,26] Some patients have a systemic predisposition to plaque disruption that is independent of traditional risk factors.[27] Plaque disruption exposes substances that promote platelet activation and aggregation, thrombin generation, and ultimately thrombus formation. The resultant thrombus interrupts blood flow and leads to an imbalance between oxygen supply and demand and, if this imbalance is severe and persistent, to myocardial necrosis (**Fig. 54-3**).

COMPOSITION OF PLAQUES. The atherosclerotic plaques associated with a total thrombotic occlusion of an epicardial coronary artery, located in infarct-related vessels, are generally more complex and irregular than those in vessels not associated with STEMI. Histologic studies of these lesions often reveal plaque rupture or erosion (see Chap. 43). Thrombus composition may vary at different levels—white thrombi contain platelets, fibrin, or both, and red thrombi contain erythrocytes, fibrin, platelets, and leukocytes.

PLAQUE FISSURING AND DISRUPTION. Atherosclerotic plaques considered prone to disruption overexpress enzymes that degrade components of the plaque extracellular matrix (see Chap. 43).[28,29] Activated macrophages and mast cells abundant at the site of plaque disruption in patients who died of STEMI can elaborate these proteinases. In addition to these structural aspects of vulnerable or high-risk plaques, stresses induced by intraluminal pressure, coronary vasomotor tone, tachycardia (cyclic stretching and compression), and disruption of nutrient vessels combine to produce plaque disruption at the margin of the fibrous cap near an adjacent, less involved segment of the coronary artery wall (shoulder region of plaque).[30] A number of key physiologic variables such as systolic blood pressure, heart rate, blood viscosity, endogenous tissue plasminogen activator (t-PA) activity, plasminogen activator inhibitor type 1 (PAI-1) levels, plasma cortisol levels, and plasma epinephrine levels exhibit circadian and seasonal variations and increase at times of stress. These factors act in concert to heighten propensity to plaque disruption and coronary thrombosis, yielding the clustering of STEMI in the early morning hours, especially in the winter and after natural disasters.[31]

ACUTE CORONARY SYNDROMES. Plaque disruption exposes thrombogenic substances that may produce an extensive thrombus in the infarct-related artery (see Fig. 54-2). An adequate collateral network that prevents necrosis from occurring can result in clinically silent episodes of coronary occlusion. Characteristically, completely occlusive thrombi lead to transmural injury of the ventricular wall in the myocardial bed subtended by the affected coronary artery and typically produce ST-segment elevation on the ECG (see Figs. 54-2 to 54-4). Infarction alters the sequence of depolarization, ultimately reflected as changes in the QRS.[32] The most characteristic change in the QRS that develops in most patients initially presenting with ST-segment elevation is the evolution of Q waves in the leads overlying the infarct zone, leading to the term *Q-wave infarction* (see Fig. 54-2).[32] In the minority of patients presenting with ST-segment elevation, no Q waves develop, but other abnormalities of the QRS complex are frequently seen, such as diminution in R wave height and notching or splintering of the QRS. Patients presenting without ST-segment elevation are initially diagnosed as suffering from unstable angina or NSTEMI (see Fig. 54-2 and Chap. 56).

The acute coronary syndrome (ACS) spectrum concept, organized around a common pathophysiologic substrate, furnishes a useful framework for developing therapeutic strategies.[33] Patients presenting with persistent ST-segment elevation are candidates for reperfusion therapy (either pharmacologic or catheter-based) to restore flow in the occluded epicardial infarct-related artery. ACS patients presenting without ST-segment elevation are not candidates for pharmacologic reperfusion but should receive anti-ischemic therapy, followed by PCI. All patients with ACS should receive anticoagulant therapy and antiplatelet therapy, regardless of the presence or absence of ST-segment elevation. Thus, the 12-lead ECG remains at the center of the decision pathway for the management of patients with ACS to distinguish between presentations with ST-segment elevation and without ST-segment elevation (**Fig. 54-4**; see Fig. 54-2).[10] Prognostic considerations must take into account other important factors, such as whether the electrocardiographic abnormality is caused by a first infarct versus subsequent infarct, the location of infarction (anterior versus inferior [see Fig. 54-4]), infarct size, and demographic factors such as patient age.[32,33]

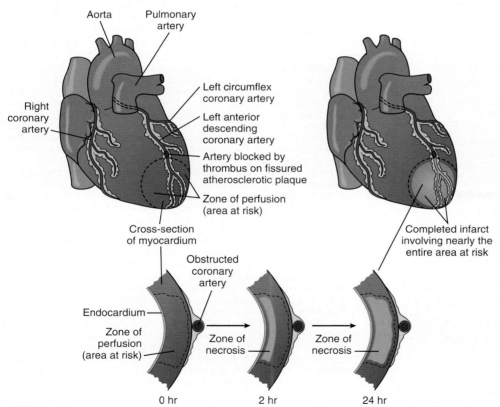

FIGURE 54-3 Schematic representation of the progression of myocardial necrosis after coronary artery occlusion. Necrosis begins in a small zone of the myocardium beneath the endocardial surface in the center of the ischemic zone. This entire region of myocardium (dashed outline) depends on the occluded vessel for perfusion and is the area at risk. A narrow zone of myocardium immediately beneath the endocardium is spared from necrosis because it can be oxygenated by diffusion from the ventricle. *(From Schoen FJ: The heart. In Kumar V, Abbas AK, Fausto N, Aster J [eds]: Robbins and Cotran Pathologic Basis of Disease. 8th ed. Philadelphia, WB Saunders, 2010, pp 529-587.)*

Heart Muscle

GROSS PATHOLOGY. On gross inspection, MI can be divided into two major types: transmural infarcts, in which myocardial necrosis involves the full thickness (or nearly full

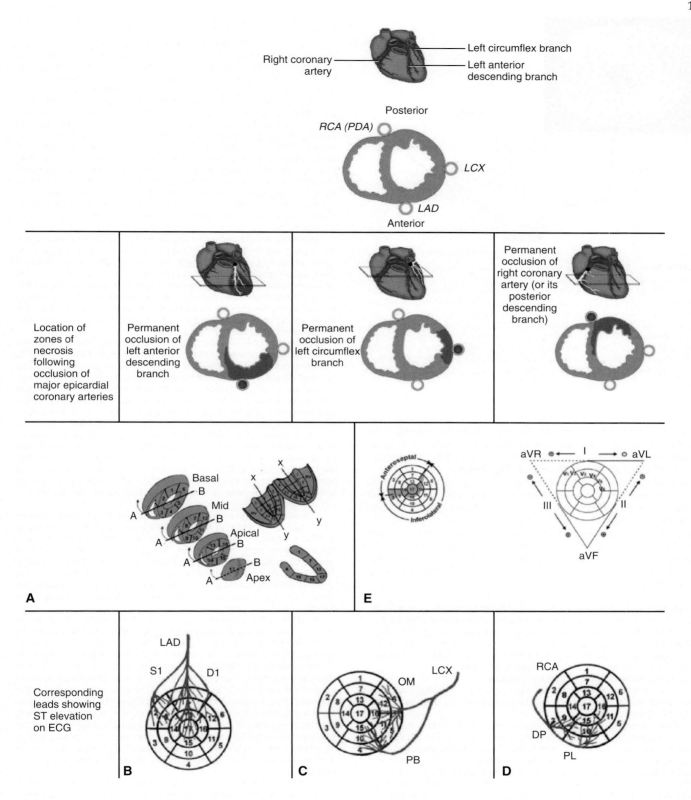

FIGURE 54-4 Correlation of sites of coronary occlusion, zones of necrosis, and electrocardiographic abnormalities. **Top,** Schematic diagram of the heart with the location of the major epicardial coronary arteries. Immediately below is another schematic diagram depicting a short-axis view of the left and right ventricles (LV, RV) and approximate location of the left anterior descending (LAD), left circumflex (LCX), and right coronary artery (RCA); the latter gives rise to the posterior descending artery (PDA) in most patients. **Middle,** Location of the zones of necrosis following occlusion of a major epicardial coronary artery. **Bottom,** Identification of the infarct artery from the 12-lead ECG. **A,** The 17 myocardial segments in a polar map format with superimposition of the arterial supply provided by the LAD **(B)**, LCX **(C)**, and RCA **(D)**. **E,** Position of the standard electrocardiographic leads relative to the polar map. The infarct artery can be deduced by identifying the leads that show ST-segment elevation and referencing that information to panels **A** through **D**. For example, ST-segment elevation seen most prominently in the leads overlying segments 1, 2, 7, 8, 13, 14, and 17 indicates that the LAD is the infarct artery. D_1 = first diagonal; DP = posterior descending; OM = obtuse marginal; PB = posterobasal; PL = posterolateral; S_1 = first septal. (From Bayes de Luna A, Wagner G, Birnbaum Y, et al: A new terminology for the left ventricular walls and location of myocardial infarcts that present Q wave based on the standard of cardiac magnetic resonance imaging. Circulation 114:1755, 2006.)

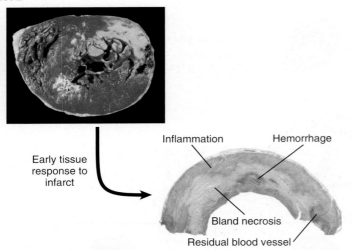

Early tissue response to infarct

Inflammation   Hemorrhage

Bland necrosis

Residual blood vessel

FIGURE 54-5 **Top,** Acute MI, predominantly of the posterolateral left ventricle, demonstrated histochemically by a lack of staining by the triphenyltetra-zolium chloride stain in areas of necrosis. The staining defect is caused by the enzyme leakage that follows cell death. The myocardial hemorrhage at one edge of the infarct was associated with cardiac rupture, and the anterior scar (lower left) was indicative of old infarct (specimen oriented with posterior wall at top). **Bottom,** The early tissue response to the infarction process involves a mixture of bland necrosis, inflammation, and hemorrhage. *(From Schoen FJ: The heart. In Kumar V, Abbas AK, Fausto N, Aster J [eds]: Robbins and Cotran Pathologic Basis of Disease. 8th ed. Philadelphia, WB Saunders, 2010, pp 529-587.)*

thickness) of the ventricular wall, and subendocardial (nontransmural) infarcts, in which the necrosis involves the subendocardium, the intramural myocardium, or both without extending all the way through the ventricular wall to the epicardium (**Fig. 54-5A**).

An occlusive coronary thrombosis appears to be far more common when the infarction is transmural and localized to the distribution of a single coronary artery (see Fig. 54-4). Nontransmural infarctions, however, frequently occur in the presence of severely narrowed but still patent coronary arteries. Patchy nontransmural infarction may arise from fibrinolysis or PCI of an originally occlusive thrombus with restoration of blood flow before the wave front of necrosis has extended from the subendocardium across the full thickness of the ventricular wall (see Fig. 54-3).

Gross alterations of the myocardium are difficult to identify until at least 6 to 12 hours have elapsed following the onset of necrosis (**Fig. 54-6**). However, a variety of histochemical stains can be used to identify zones of necrosis that can be discerned after only 2 to 3 hours (see Fig. 54-5A).[34] Subsequently, the infarcted myocardium undergoes a sequence of gross pathologic changes summarized in Figures 54-5 and 54-6.[35]

HISTOLOGIC AND ULTRASTRUCTURAL CHANGES

LIGHT MICROSCOPY: PATTERNS OF MYOCARDIAL NECROSIS. Histologic evaluation of MI reveals various stages of the healing process (**Fig. 54-7**; see Figs. 54-5B, and 54-6).

COAGULATION NECROSIS. Coagulation necrosis results from severe persistent ischemia and is usually present in the central region of infarcts, which results in the arrest of muscle cells in the relaxed state and the passive stretching of ischemic muscle cells. The myofibrils are stretched, many with nuclear pyknosis, vascular congestion, and healing by phagocytosis of necrotic muscle cells (see Fig. 54-6). Mitochondrial damage with prominent amorphous (flocculent) densities but no calcification is evident.

NECROSIS WITH CONTRACTION BANDS. This form of myocardial necrosis, also termed *contraction band necrosis* or *coagulative myocytolysis*, results primarily from severe ischemia followed by reflow.[35] It is characterized by hypercontracted myofibrils with contraction bands and mitochondrial damage, frequently with calcification, marked vascular congestion, and healing by lysis of muscle cells. Necrosis with contraction bands is caused by increased Ca^{2+} influx into dying cells, resulting in the arrest of cells in the contracted state, which occurs in the periphery of large infarcts and to a greater extent in nontransmural than in transmural infarcts. The

entire infarct may show this form of necrosis after reperfusion (see Fig. 54-7F).[36]

MYOCYTOLYSIS. Ischemia without necrosis generally causes no acute changes visible by light microscopy. However, severe prolonged ischemia can cause myocyte vacuolization, often termed *myocytolysis*. Prolonged severe ischemia, which is potentially reversible, causes cloudy swelling, as well as hydropic, vascular, and fatty degeneration.

ELECTRON MICROSCOPY. In experimental infarction, the earliest ultrastructural changes in cardiac muscle following ligation of a coronary artery, noted within 20 minutes, consist of reduction in the size and number of glycogen granules, intracellular edema, and swelling and distortion of the transverse tubular system, sarcoplasmic reticulum, and mitochondria (see Fig. 54-6).[37] These early changes are reversible. Changes after 60 minutes of occlusion include myocyte swelling, swelling and internal disruption of mitochondria, development of amorphous, flocculent aggregation and margination of nuclear chromatin, and relaxation of myofibrils. After 20 minutes to 2 hours of ischemia, changes in some cells become irreversible and there is progression of these alterations.[35]

APOPTOSIS. An additional pathway of myocyte death involves apoptosis, or programmed cell death. In contrast to coagulation necrosis, myocytes undergoing apoptosis exhibit shrinkage of cells, fragmentation of DNA, and phagocytosis, but without the usual cellular infiltrate indicative of inflammation (**Fig. 54-8**).[34] The role of apoptosis in the setting of MI is less well understood than that of classic coagulation necrosis. Apoptosis may occur shortly after the onset of myocardial ischemia. However, the major impact of apoptosis appears to be on late myocyte loss and ventricular remodeling after MI.[38]

MODIFICATION OF PATHOLOGIC CHANGES BY REPERFUSION. When reperfusion of myocardium undergoing the evolutionary changes from ischemia to infarction occurs sufficiently early (i.e., within 15 to 20 minutes), it can successfully prevent necrosis from developing. Beyond this early stage, the number of salvaged myocytes and therefore the amount of salvaged myocardial tissue (area of necrosis/area at risk) relates directly to the length of time of total coronary artery occlusion, level of myocardial oxygen consumption, and collateral blood flow (**Fig. 54-9**).[37] Typically, reperfused infarcts show a mixture of necrosis, hemorrhage within zones of irreversibly injured myocytes, coagulative necrosis with contraction bands, and distorted architecture of the cells in the reperfused zone (**Fig. 54-10**). Reperfusion of infarcted myocardium accelerates the washout of intracellular proteins, producing an exaggerated and early peak value of substances such as creatine kinase-MB (CK-MB) and cardiac-specific troponin T and I (see Fig. 54-6 and later).[39]

CORONARY ANATOMY AND LOCATION OF INFARCTION. Angiographic studies performed in the earliest hours of STEMI have revealed approximately a 90% incidence of total occlusion of the infarct-related vessel.[40] Recanalization from spontaneous fibrinolysis, as well as attrition caused by some mortality among those patients with total occlusion, diminishes angiographic total occlusion in the period following the onset of MI. Pharmacologic fibrinolysis and PCI markedly increase the proportion of patients with a patent infarct-related artery early after STEMI.

A STEMI with transmural necrosis typically occurs distal to an acutely totally occluded coronary artery, with thrombus superimposed on a ruptured plaque (see Fig. 54-4). The converse is not the case, however, in that chronic total occlusion of a coronary artery does not always cause MI. Collateral blood flow and other factors such as the level of myocardial metabolism, presence and location of stenoses in other coronary arteries, rate of development of the obstruction, and quantity of myocardium supplied by the obstructed vessel all influence the viability of myocardial cells distal to the occlusion. In many series of patients studied at necropsy or by coronary arteriography, a small number (5%) of patients with STEMI have normal coronary vessels. In these patients, an embolus that has lysed, a transiently occlusive platelet aggregate, or a prolonged episode of severe coronary spasm may have caused the infarct.

Studies of patients who ultimately develop STEMI after having undergone coronary angiography at some time before its occurrence have helped clarify coronary anatomy before infarction. Although high-grade stenoses, when present, more frequently lead to STEMI than less severe lesions, most occlusions actually occur in vessels with a previously identified stenosis of less than 50% on angiograms performed months to years earlier. This finding supports the concept that STEMI occurs as a result of sudden thrombotic occlusion at the site of rupture of previously nonobstructive but lipid-rich plaques. When collateral vessels perfuse an area of the ventricle, an infarct may occur at a distance from a coronary occlusion. For example, following the gradual obliteration of the lumen of the right coronary artery, the inferior wall of the left ventricle can be kept

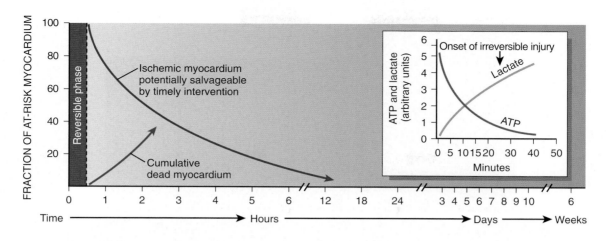

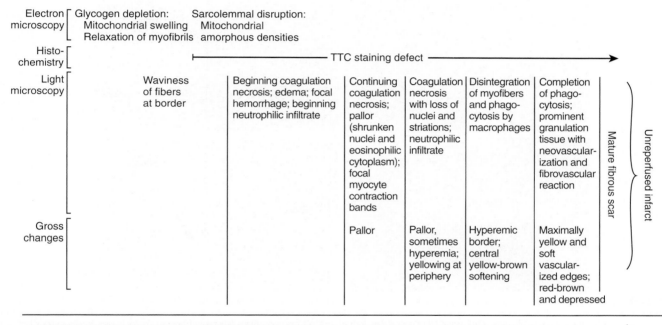

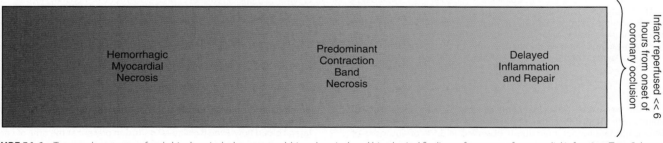

FIGURE 54-6 Temporal sequence of early biochemical, ultrastructural, histochemical, and histological findings after onset of myocardial infarction. **Top,** Schematics of the time frames for early and late reperfusion of the myocardium supplied by an occluded coronary artery. For approximately 30 minutes after the onset of even the most severe ischemia, myocardial injury is potentially reversible; after that, there is progressive loss of viability that is complete by 6 to 12 hours. The benefits of reperfusion (both early and late) are greatest when it is achieved early, with progressively smaller benefits occurring as reperfusion is delayed. Note the alterations in the temporal sequence in the reperfused infarct. The pattern of pathologic findings following reperfusion is variable, depending on the timing of reperfusion, prior infarction, and collateral flow. TTC = triphenyltetrazolium chloride. *(From Schoen FJ: The heart. In Kumar V, Abbas AK, Fausto N, Aster J [eds]: Robbins and Cotran Pathologic Basis of Disease. 8th ed. Philadelphia, WB Saunders, 2010, pp 529-587.)*

viable by collateral vessels arising from the left anterior descending coronary artery. Later, an occlusion of the left anterior descending artery may cause an infarct of the diaphragmatic wall.

RIGHT VENTRICULAR INFARCTION. Approximately 50% of patients with inferior infarction have some involvement of the right ventricle.[41] Among these patients, right ventricular infarction occurs exclusively in those with transmural infarction of the inferoposterior wall and posterior portion of the septum. Right ventricular infarction almost invariably develops in association with infarction of the adjacent septum and inferior left ventricular walls, but isolated infarction of the right ventricle is seen in 3% to 5% of autopsy-proven cases of MI (**Fig. 54-11**). Right ventricular infarction occurs less commonly than would be anticipated from the frequency of atherosclerotic lesions involving the right coronary artery. The right ventricle can sustain long periods of ischemia but still demonstrate excellent recovery of contractile function after reperfusion.[42]

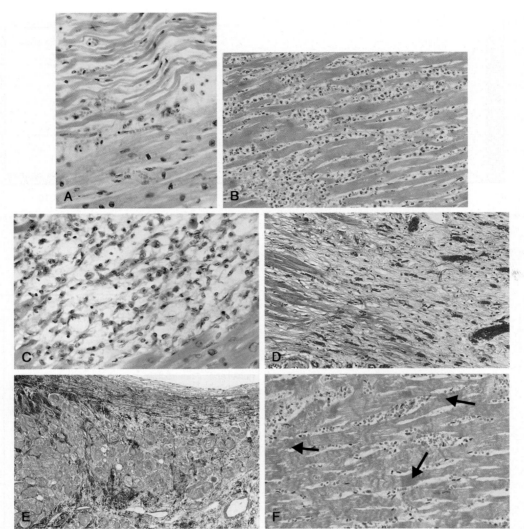

FIGURE 54-7 Microscopic features of myocardial infarction. **A,** 1-day-old infarct showing coagulative necrosis, wavy fibers with elongation, and narrowing compared with adjacent normal fibers (lower right). Widened spaces between the dead fibers contain edema fluid and scattered neutrophils. **B,** Dense polymorphonuclear leukocytic infiltrate in an area of acute myocardial MI of 3 to 4 days' duration. **C,** Almost complete removal of necrotic myocytes by phagocytosis (≈7 to 10 days). **D,** Granulation tissue with a rich vascular network and early collagen deposition, approximately 3 weeks after infarction. **E,** Well-healed myocardial infarct with replacement of the necrotic fibers by dense collagenous scar. A few residual cardiac muscle cells are present. (In **D** and **E**, collagen is highlighted as blue in this Masson trichrome stain.) **F,** Myocardial necrosis with hemorrhage and contraction bands, visible as dark bands spanning some myofibers (arrows). This is the characteristic appearance of markedly ischemic myocardium that has been reperfused. *(From Schoen FJ: The heart. In Kumar V, Abbas AK, Fausto N, Aster J [eds]: Robbins and Cotran Pathologic Basis of Disease. 8th ed. Philadelphia, WB Saunders, 2010, pp 529-587.)*

ATRIAL INFARCTION. Atrial infarction can be seen in up to 10% of patients with STEMI if PR-segment displacement is used as the criterion. Although isolated atrial infarction is observed in 3.5% of autopsies of patients with STEMI, it often occurs in conjunction with ventricular infarction and can cause rupture of the atrial wall.[43] This type of infarct is more common on the right side than on the left side, occurs more frequently in the atrial appendages than in the lateral or posterior walls of the atrium, and can result in thrombus formation. Atrial infarction is frequently accompanied by atrial arrhythmias.[44] It has also been linked to inadequate secretion of atrial natriuretic peptide and a low cardiac output syndrome when right ventricular infarction coexists.

COLLATERAL CIRCULATION IN ACUTE MYOCARDIAL INFARCTION. The coronary collateral circulation (see Chap. 52) is particularly well developed in patients with the following: (1) coronary occlusive disease, especially with reduction of the luminal cross-sectional area by more than 75% in one or more major vessels; (2) chronic hypoxia, as in cases of severe anemia, chronic obstructive pulmonary disease, and cyanotic congenital heart disease; and (3) left ventricular hypertrophy.

The magnitude of coronary collateral flow is one of the principal determinants of infarct size. Indeed, patients with abundant collaterals commonly can have totally occluded coronary arteries without evidence of infarction in the distribution of that artery; thus, the survival of the myocardium distal to such occlusions depends in large measure on collateral blood flow. Even if collateral perfusion present at the time of coronary occlusion does not prevent infarction, it may still exert a beneficial effect by preventing the formation of a left ventricular aneurysm. It is likely that the presence of a high-grade stenosis (90%), possibly with periods of intermittent total occlusion, permits the development of collaterals that remain only as potential conduits until a total occlusion occurs or recurs. Total occlusion then brings these channels into full operation.

NONATHEROSCLEROTIC CAUSES OF ACUTE MYOCARDIAL INFARCTION. Numerous pathologic processes other than atherosclerosis can involve the coronary arteries and result in STEMI (see Table 54-4). For example, coronary arterial occlusions can result from embolization of a coronary artery. The causes of coronary embolism are numerous and include infective endocarditis and nonbacterial thrombotic endocarditis (see Chap. 67), mural thrombi, prosthetic valves, neoplasms, air introduced at the time of cardiac surgery, and calcium deposits from manipulation of calcified valves at operation. In situ thrombosis of coronary arteries can occur secondary to chest wall trauma (see Chap. 76).

A variety of inflammatory processes can be responsible for coronary artery abnormalities, some of which mimic atherosclerotic disease and

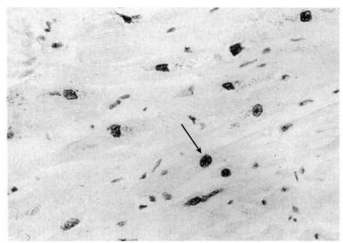

FIGURE 54-8 Apoptosis in STEMI. Myocytes at the infarct border in this specimen demonstrate nuclear staining by the nick-end labeling technique (arrow) suggesting that they have undergone apoptosis (×250). *(From Vargas SO, Sampson BA, Schoen FJ: Pathologic detection of early myocardial infarction: A critical review of the evolution and usefulness of modern techniques. Mod Pathol 12:635, 1999.)*

may predispose to true atherosclerosis. Epidemiologic evidence suggests that viral infections, particularly with Coxsackie B virus, may be an uncommon cause of MI. Viral illnesses precede MI occasionally in young persons who are later shown to have normal coronary arteries.

Syphilitic aortitis can produce marked narrowing or occlusion of one or both coronary ostia, whereas Takayasu arteritis can result in obstruction of the coronary arteries. Necrotizing arteritis, polyarteritis nodosa, mucocutaneous lymph node syndrome (Kawasaki disease), systemic lupus erythematosus (see Chap. 89), and giant cell arteritis can cause coronary occlusion. Therapeutic levels of mediastinal radiation can cause coronary arteriosclerosis, with subsequent infarction. MI can also result from coronary arterial involvement in patients with amyloidosis (see Chap. 68), Hurler syndrome, pseudoxanthoma elasticum, and homocystinuria.

As cocaine abuse has become more common, reports of MI after the use of cocaine have appeared with increasing frequency (see Chap. 73). Cocaine can cause MI in patients with normal coronary arteries, preexisting MI, documented coronary artery disease, or coronary artery spasm.

Myocardial Infarction with Angiographically Normal Coronary Vessels. Patients with STEMI and normal coronary arteries tend to be young, with relatively few coronary risk factors, except that they often have a history of cigarette smoking (see Table 54-4). Usually, they have no history of angina pectoris before the infarction. The infarction in these patients is usually not preceded by any prodrome, but the clinical, laboratory, and electrocardiographic features of STEMI are otherwise indistinguishable from those present in the overwhelming majority of patients with STEMI who have classic obstructive atherosclerotic coronary artery disease.

Patients who recover often have areas of localized dyskinesis and hypokinesis at left ventricular angiography. Many of these cases are caused by coronary artery spasm and/or thrombosis, perhaps with underlying endothelial dysfunction or small plaques inapparent on coronary angiography. The transient left ventricular apical ballooning syndrome (takotsubo cardiomyopathy) is characterized by transient wall motion abnormalities involving the left ventricular (LV) apex and midventricle.

This syndrome occurs in the absence of obstructive epicardial coronary disease and can mimic STEMI.[45] Typically, an episode of psychological stress precedes presentation with takotsubo cardiomyopathy. The etiology is not clear, but experts believe that catecholamine-mediated myocardial stunning and microvascular dysfunction play important roles.

Additional suggested causes include the following: (1) coronary emboli (perhaps from a small mural thrombus, a prolapsed mitral valve, or a myxoma); (2) coronary artery disease in vessels too small to be visualized by coronary arteriography or coronary arterial thrombosis with subsequent recanalization; (3) hematologic disorders causing in situ thrombosis in the presence of normal coronary arteries (e.g., polycythemia vera, cyanotic heart disease with polycythemia, sickle cell anemia, disseminated intravascular coagulation, thrombocytosis, thrombotic thrombocytopenic purpura); (4) augmented oxygen demand (e.g., thyrotoxicosis, amphetamine use); (5) hypotension secondary to sepsis, blood loss, or pharmacologic agents; and (6) anatomic variations such as anomalous origin of a coronary artery (see Chap. 21), coronary arteriovenous fistula, or myocardial bridge.

PROGNOSIS. The long-term outlook for patients who have survived a STEMI with angiographically normal coronary vessels on arteriography appears brighter than for patients with STEMI and obstructive coronary artery disease. After recovery from the initial infarct, recurrent infarction, heart failure, and death are unusual in patients with normal coronary arteries. Indeed, most of these patients have normal exercise ECGs, and only a minority develops angina pectoris.

Pathophysiology

Left Ventricular Function

SYSTOLIC FUNCTION. On interruption of antegrade flow in an epicardial coronary artery, the zone of myocardium supplied by that vessel immediately loses its ability to shorten and perform contractile work (see Fig. 54-10). Four abnormal contraction patterns develop in sequence: (1) dyssynchrony—that is, dissociation in the time course of contraction of adjacent segments; (2) hypokinesis, reduction in the extent of shortening; (3) akinesis, cessation of shortening; and (4) dyskinesis, paradoxical expansion, and systolic bulging. Hyperkinesis

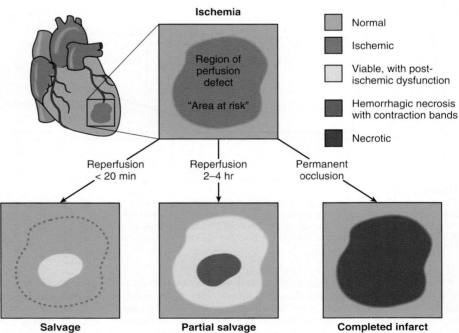

FIGURE 54-9 Consequences of reperfusion at various times after coronary adhesion. In this example, the midportion of the left anterior descending coronary artery is occluded and a large zone of ischemic myocardium develops—the "area at risk". Reperfusion in less than 20 minutes does not result in permanent tissue loss, but there may be a period of contractile dysfunction of the reperfused myocardium, a condition referred to as stunning. Later, reperfusion results in hemorrhagic necrosis, with contraction bands. Permanent occlusion results in necrosis of myocardium. *(From Schoen FJ: The heart. In Kumar V, Abbas AK, Fausto N, Aster J [eds]: Robbins and Cotran Pathologic Basis of Disease. 8th ed. Philadelphia, WB Saunders, 2010, pp 529-587.)*

CH
54

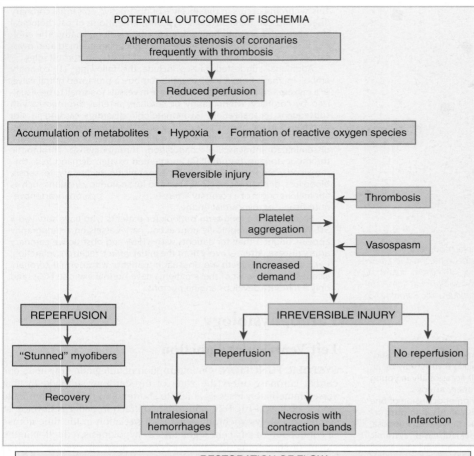

POTENTIAL OUTCOMES OF ISCHEMIA

Atheromatous stenosis of coronaries frequently with thrombosis

↓

Reduced perfusion

↓

Accumulation of metabolites • Hypoxia • Formation of reactive oxygen species

↓

Reversible injury

Thrombosis →
Platelet aggregation →
Vasospasm →
Increased demand →

REPERFUSION   IRREVERSIBLE INJURY

"Stunned" myofibers   Reperfusion   No reperfusion

Recovery

Intralesional hemorrhages   Necrosis with contraction bands   Infarction

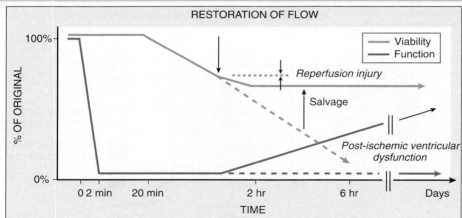

RESTORATION OF FLOW

Viability
Function

Reperfusion injury

Salvage

Post-ischemic ventricular dysfunction

% OF ORIGINAL

100%

0%

0 2 min   20 min   2 hr   6 hr   Days

TIME

FIGURE 54-10 Several potential outcomes of reversible and irreversible ischemic injury to the myocardium. The schematic diagram at the bottom depicts the timing of changes in function and viability. A key point is that although function drops dramatically after coronary occlusion, the tissue is still viable for a period of time. This is the basis for early aggressive efforts at reperfusion in STEMI. *(From Schoen FJ: The heart. In Kumar V, Abbas AK, Fausto N, Aster J [eds]: Robbins and Cotran Pathologic Basis of Disease. 8th ed. Philadelphia, WB Saunders, 2010, pp 529-587.)*

Patients with STEMI often also show reduced myocardial contractile function in noninfarcted zones. This finding may result from previous obstruction of the coronary artery supplying the noninfarcted region of the ventricle and loss of collaterals from the freshly occluded infarct-related vessel, a condition that has been termed *ischemia at a distance*.[46] Conversely, the presence of collaterals developing before STEMI may allow for greater preservation of regional systolic function in an area of distribution of the occluded artery and improvement in left ventricular ejection fraction (LVEF) early after infarction.

If a sufficient quantity of myocardium undergoes ischemic injury (see Fig. 54-10), left LV pump function becomes depressed; cardiac output, stroke volume, blood pressure, and peak dP/dt decline[47]; and end-systolic volume increases. The degree to which end-systolic volume increases is perhaps the most powerful hemodynamic predictor of mortality following STEMI.[48] Paradoxical systolic expansion of an area of ventricular myocardium further decreases LV stroke volume. As necrotic myocytes slip past each other, the infarct zone thins and elongates, especially in patients with large anterior infarcts, leading to infarct expansion. In some patients, a vicious circle of dilation ensues, causing further dilation. The degree of ventricular dilation, which depends closely on infarct size, patency of the infarct-related artery, and activation of the renin-angiotensin-aldosterone system (RAAS), can be favorably modified by inhibitors of this system, even in the absence of symptomatic LV dysfunction.[49]

With time, edema and cellular infiltration, and ultimately fibrosis, increase the stiffness of the infarcted myocardium back to and beyond control values. Increasing stiffness in the infarcted zone of myocardium improves LV function because it prevents paradoxical systolic wall motion (dyskinesia).

The likelihood of developing clinical symptoms such as dyspnea, and ultimately a shocklike state, correlates with specific parameters of LV function. The earliest abnormality is a ventricular stiffness in diastole (see later), which can be observed with infarcts that involve only a small portion of the left ventricle on angiographic examination. When the abnormally contracting segment exceeds 15%, the ejection fraction may decline, and elevations of LV end-diastolic pressure and volume occur. The risk of developing physical signs and symptoms of LV failure also increase proportionally to increasing areas of abnormal LV wall motion. Clinical heart failure accompanies areas of abnormal contraction exceeding 25%, and cardiogenic shock, often fatal, accompanies loss of more than 40% of the LV myocardium.

Unless infarct extension occurs, some improvement in wall motion takes place during the healing phase as recovery of function occurs in initially reversibly injured (stunned) myocardium

of the remaining normal myocardium initially accompanies dysfunction of the infarcting segment. The early hyperkinesis of the noninfarcted zones likely results from acute compensations, including increased activity of the sympathetic nervous system and the Frank-Starling mechanism. A portion of this compensatory hyperkinesis is ineffective work, because contraction of the noninfarcted segments of myocardium causes dyskinesis of the infarct zone. Increased motion of the noninfarcted region subsides within 2 weeks of infarction, during which time some degree of recovery often occurs in the infarct region as well, particularly if reperfusion of the infarcted area occurs and myocardial stunning diminishes.

DIASTOLIC FUNCTION. The diastolic properties of the left ventricle (see Chaps. 24, 25, and 30) change in infarcted and ischemic myocardium. These alterations are associated with a decrease in the peak rate of decline in LV pressure (peak −dP/dt), an increase in the time constant of the fall in LV pressure, and an initial rise in LV end-diastolic pressure. Over several weeks, end-diastolic volume increases and diastolic pressure begins to fall toward normal. As with impairment of systolic function, the magnitude of the diastolic abnormality appears to relate to the size of the infarct.

CIRCULATORY REGULATION. Patients with STEMI have an abnormality in circulatory regulation. The process begins with an anatomic or functional obstruction in the coronary vascular bed, which results in regional myocardial ischemia and, if the ischemia persists, in infarction (**Fig. 54-12**). If the infarct is of sufficient size, it depresses overall LV function so that LV stroke volume falls and filling pressures rise. A marked depression of LV stroke volume ultimately lowers aortic pressure and reduces coronary perfusion pressure; this condition may intensify myocardial ischemia and thereby initiate a vicious circle (see Fig. 54-12). Systemic inflammation secondary to the infarction process leads to the release of cytokines that contribute to vasodilation and a fall in systemic vascular resistance.[50]

The inability of the left ventricle to empty normally also increases preload; that is, it dilates the well-perfused, normally functioning portion of the left ventricle. This compensatory mechanism tends to restore stroke volume to normal levels, but at the expense of a reduced ejection fraction. The dilation of the left ventricle also elevates ventricular afterload, however, because Laplace's law dictates that at any given arterial pressure, the dilated ventricle must develop a higher wall tension. This increased afterload not only depresses LV stroke volume but also elevates myocardial oxygen consumption, which in turn intensifies myocardial ischemia. When regional myocardial dysfunction is limited and the function of the remainder of the left ventricle is normal, compensatory mechanisms—especially hyperkinesis of the nonaffected portion of the ventricle—sustain overall LV function. If a large portion of the left ventricle becomes necrotic, pump failure occurs.

Ventricular Remodeling

As a consequence of STEMI, the changes in LV size, shape, and thickness involving the infarcted and noninfarcted segments of the ventricle described earlier occur and are collectively termed *ventricular remodeling*, which can in turn influence ventricular function and prognosis. A combination of changes in LV dilation and hypertrophy of residual noninfarcted myocardium causes remodeling. After the size of infarction, the two most important factors driving the process of LV dilation are ventricular loading conditions and infarct artery patency (**Fig. 54-13**).[51] Elevated ventricular pressure contributes to increased wall stress and the risk of infarct expansion, and a patent infarct artery accelerates myocardial scar formation and increases tissue turgor in the infarct zone, reducing the risk of infarct expansion and ventricular dilation.

INFARCT EXPANSION. An increase in the size of the infarcted segment, known as infarct expansion, is defined as "acute dilation and thinning of the area of infarction not explained by additional myocardial necrosis."[52] Infarct expansion appears to be caused by the following: (1) a combination of slippage between muscle bundles, reducing the number of myocytes across the infarct wall; (2) disruption of the normal myocardial cells; and (3) tissue loss within the necrotic zone. It is characterized by disproportionate thinning and dilation of the infarct zone before formation of a firm fibrotic scar. The degree of infarct expansion appears to be related to the preinfarction wall thickness, with existing hypertrophy possibly protecting against infarct thinning. The apex is the thinnest region of the ventricle and an area of the heart that is particularly vulnerable to infarct expansion. Infarction of the apex secondary to occlusion of the left anterior descending coronary artery causes the radius of curvature at the apex to increase, exposing this normally thin region to a marked elevation in wall stress.

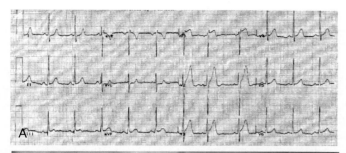
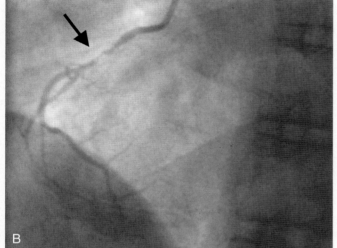
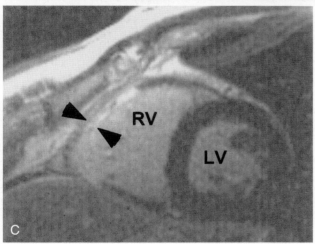

FIGURE 54-11 A 47-year-old man with no prior history of cardiac disease presented to an outside hospital describing "an awesome feeling that just sat in my chest," associated with bilateral arm weakness. **A,** The initial ECG revealed ST-segment elevation in the right precordial leads and, to a lesser extent, in the inferior leads. The patient was treated with fibrinolytic therapy and transferred for catheterization. **B,** Angiography revealed a tight stenosis of a proximal nondominant right coronary artery (arrow) without significant disease in the left coronary artery. **C,** Contrast-enhanced CMR demonstrated delayed hyperenhancement consistent with injury of the right ventricle (RV) with distinct involvement of the right ventricular free wall (arrowheads), sparing the left ventricle (LV) as well as the right ventricular apex. The patient remained hemodynamically stable throughout his hospital course and was discharged home. *(From Finn AV, Antman EM: Images in clinical medicine. Isolated right ventricular infarction. N Engl J Med 349:1636, 2003.)*

(see Figs. 54-9 and 54-10). Regardless of the age of the infarct, patients who continue to demonstrate abnormal wall motion of 20% to 25% of the left ventricle will likely manifest hemodynamic signs of LV failure, with its attendant poor prognosis for long-term survival.

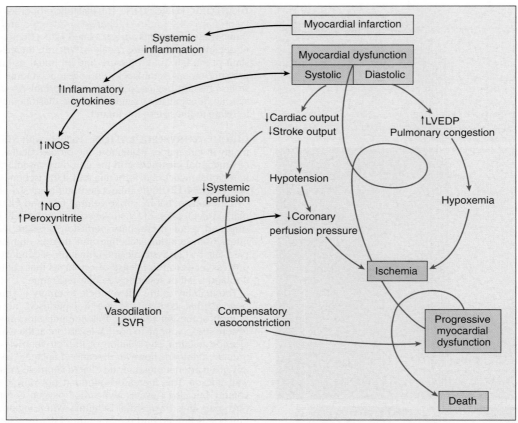

FIGURE 54-12 Classic shock paradigm is shown in black. The influence of the inflammatory response syndrome initiated by a large MI is illustrated in pink. iNOS = inducible nitric oxide synthase; LVEDP = LV end-diastolic pressure; NO = nitric oxide; SVR = systemic vascular resistance. *(From Hochman J: Cardiogenic shock complicating acute myocardial infarction: Expanding the paradigm. Circulation 107:2998, 2003.)*

Infarct expansion associates with both higher mortality and a higher incidence of nonfatal complications, such as heart failure and ventricular aneurysm. Infarct expansion is best recognized echocardiographically as elongation of the noncontractile region of the ventricle. When expansion is severe enough to cause symptoms, the most characteristic clinical finding is deterioration of systolic function associated with new or louder gallop sounds and new or worsening pulmonary congestion.

VENTRICULAR DILATION. Although infarct expansion plays an important role in the ventricular remodeling that occurs early following myocardial infarction, remodeling is also caused by dilation of the viable portion of the ventricle, commencing immediately after STEMI and progressing for months or years thereafter (see Fig. 54-13). Dilation may be accompanied by a shift of the pressure-volume curve of the left ventricle to the right, resulting in a larger LV volume at any given diastolic pressure. This dilation of the noninfarct zone can be viewed as a compensatory mechanism that maintains stroke volume in the face of a large infarction. STEMI places an extra load on the residual functioning myocardium, a burden that presumably is responsible for the compensatory hypertrophy of the uninfarcted myocardium. This hypertrophy could help compensate for the functional impairment caused by the infarct and may be responsible for some of the hemodynamic improvement seen in the months after infarction in some patients.

EFFECTS OF TREATMENT. Ventricular remodeling after STEMI can be affected by several factors, the first of which is infarct size (see Figs. 54-9, 54-10, and 54-13). Acute reperfusion and other measures to restrict the extent of myocardial necrosis limit the increase in ventricular volume after STEMI. The second factor is scar formation in the

infarct. Glucocorticosteroids and nonsteroidal anti-inflammatory drugs given early after MI can cause scar thinning and greater infarct expansion, whereas inhibitors of the RAAS attenuate ventricular enlargement (see Fig. 54-13). Additional beneficial consequences of inhibition of angiotensin II that may contribute to myocardial protection include attenuation of endothelial dysfunction and direct antiatherogenic effects. Inhibition of aldosterone action reduces collagen deposition and decreases the development of ventricular arrhythmias.[53]

Pathophysiology of Other Organ Systems

PULMONARY FUNCTION. An inverse relationship exists between arterial oxygen tension and pulmonary artery diastolic pressure. This suggests that increased pulmonary capillary hydrostatic pressure leads to interstitial edema, which results in arteriolar and bronchiolar compression that ultimately causes perfusion of poorly ventilated alveoli, with resultant hypoxemia (see Chap. 25). In addition to hypoxemia, diffusing capacity decreases. Hyperventilation often occurs in patients with STEMI and may cause hypocapnia and respiratory alkalosis, particularly in restless, anxious patients with pain. Pulmonary extravascular (interstitial) water content, LV filling pressure, and the clinical signs and symptoms of LV failure correlate. The increase in pulmonary extravascular water may be responsible for the alterations in pulmonary mechanics observed in patients with STEMI (i.e., reduction of airway conductance, pulmonary compliance, forced expiratory volume and midexpiratory flow rate, and an increase in closing volume, which is presumably related to the widespread closure of small dependent airways during the first 3 days after STEMI). Ultimately, severe increases in extravascular water may lead to pulmonary edema. Virtually all lung volume indices—total lung capacity, functional residual capacity, and residual volume, as well as vital capacity—fall during STEMI.

REDUCTION OF AFFINITY OF HEMOGLOBIN FOR OXYGEN. In patients with MI, particularly when complicated by LV failure or cardiogenic shock, the affinity of hemoglobin for oxygen falls (i.e., the P50 is increased).

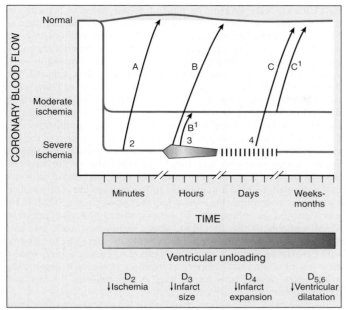

FIGURE 54-13 Therapeutic maneuvers in various stages of ischemia and infarction. Severely ischemic tissue (2) may be reperfused, thereby averting myocardial infarction (A). Infarcting tissue (3) may be reperfused, leading to sparing of myocardial tissue (B). If blood flow is restored only in part B, the myocardium may remain noncontractile, although viable (i.e., hibernating). After completion of the infarct (4), late reperfusion (C) may still be useful. Mechanical reperfusion of moderately ischemic myocardium (C^1) may restore contractility of hibernating myocardium to normal. Ventricular unloading may be useful throughout the preinfarct and postinfarct periods. Unloading may reduce ischemia (D_2), infarct size (D_3), infarct expansion (D_4), and ventricular dilatation ($D_{5,6}$). *(From Braunwald E, Pfeffer MA: Ventricular enlargement and remodeling following acute myocardial infarction: Mechanisms and management. Am J Cardiol 68:4D, 1991.)*

The increase in P50 results from increased levels of erythrocyte 2,3-diphosphoglycerate (2,3-DPG), which constitutes an important compensatory mechanism, responsible for an estimated 18% increase in oxygen release from oxyhemoglobin in patients with cardiogenic shock.

ENDOCRINE FUNCTION

PANCREAS. Although the absolute levels of blood insulin are often in the normal range, they are usually inappropriately low for the level of blood sugar, and there may be relative insulin resistance as well. Patients with cardiogenic shock often demonstrate marked hyperglycemia and depressed levels of circulating insulin. Abnormalities in insulin secretion and the resultant impaired glucose tolerance appear to be caused by a reduction in pancreatic blood flow as a consequence of splanchnic vasoconstriction accompanying severe LV failure. In addition, increased activity of the sympathetic nervous system with augmented circulating catecholamines inhibits insulin secretion and augments glycogenolysis, also contributing to the elevation of blood sugar.

Glucose appears to be a more favorable energy source than free fatty acids for the ischemic myocardium by permitting adenosine triphosphate (ATP) generation by anaerobic glycolysis.[54] Because hypoxic heart muscle derives a considerable portion of its energy from the metabolism of glucose (see Chap. 24) and because insulin is essential for the uptake of glucose by the myocardium, insulin deficiency has clear deleterious effects. These metabolic considerations, combined with epidemiologic observations that diabetic patients have a markedly worse prognosis, have served as the foundation for efforts to administer insulin-glucose infusions to diabetic patients with STEMI.[55]

ADRENAL MEDULLA. The plasma and urinary catecholamine levels peak during the first 24 hours after the onset of chest pain, with the greatest rise in plasma catecholamine secretion occurring during the first hour after the onset of STEMI. These high levels of circulating catecholamines in patients with STEMI correlate with the occurrence of serious arrhythmias and result in an increase in myocardial oxygen consumption, directly and indirectly, as a consequence of catecholamine-induced elevation of circulating free fatty acids. The concentration of circulating catecholamines correlates with the extent of myocardial damage and

incidence of cardiogenic shock, as well as with early and late mortality rates.

Circulating catecholamines enhance platelet aggregation; when this occurs in the coronary microcirculation, the release of the potent local vasoconstrictor thromboxane A_2 may further impair cardiac perfusion. The marked increase in sympathetic activity associated with STEMI serves as the foundation for beta-adrenergic receptor blocker regimens in the acute phase.

ACTIVATION OF THE RENIN-ANGIOTENSIN-ALDOSTERONE SYSTEM. Noninfarcted regions of the myocardium appear to exhibit activation of the tissue RAAS with increased angiotensin II production. Both locally generated and systemically generated angiotensin II can stimulate the production of various growth factors, such as platelet-derived growth factor and transforming growth factor-β, that promote compensatory hypertrophy in the noninfarcted myocardium, as well as control the structure and tone of the infarct-related coronary and other myocardial vessels. Additional potential actions of angiotensin II that have a more negative impact on the infarction process include the release of endothelin, PAI-1, and aldosterone, which may cause vasoconstriction, impaired fibrinolysis, and increased sodium retention, respectively.

NATRIURETIC PEPTIDES. The peptides atrial natriuretic factor (ANF) and N-terminal pro-ANF are released from cardiac atria in response to elevation of atrial pressure. B-type natriuretic peptide (BNP) and its precursor, N-terminal pro-BNP (NT-proBNP), are secreted by human atrial and ventricular myocardium. Given the larger mass of ventricular rather than atrial myocardium, the total amount of mRNA for BNP is higher in the ventricles than in the atria. Natriuretic peptides are released early after STEMI, peaking at about 16 hours. Evidence has shown that natriuretic peptides released from the left ventricle during STEMI originate from the infarcted myocardium and from viable noninfarcted myocardium. The rise in BNP and NT-proBNP levels after STEMI correlates with infarct size and regional wall motion abnormalities. Measurement of natriuretic peptides can provide useful information early and late in the course of STEMI.[56]

ADRENAL CORTEX. Levels of plasma and urinary 17-hydroxycorticosteroids and ketosteroids, as well as aldosterone, rise markedly in patients with STEMI. Their concentrations correlate directly with the peak level of serum CK, implying an association between the stress imposed by larger infarcts and greater secretion of adrenal steroids. The magnitude of the elevation of cortisol correlates with infarct size and mortality. Glucocorticosteroids also contribute to impaired glucose tolerance.

THYROID GLAND. Although patients with STEMI are generally clinically euthyroid, there is evidence of a transient decrease in serum triiodothyronine (T_3) levels, a fall that is most marked on approximately the third day after the infarct. This fall in T_3 is usually accompanied by a rise in reverse T_3, with variable changes or no change in thyroxine (T_4) and thyroid-stimulating hormone (TSH) levels. The alteration in peripheral T_4 metabolism appears to correlate with infarct size and may be mediated by the rise in endogenous levels of cortisol that accompanies STEMI.

RENAL FUNCTION.
Both prerenal azotemia and acute renal failure can complicate the marked reduction of cardiac output that occurs in cardiogenic shock. On the other hand, an increase in circulating atrial natriuretic peptide occurs following STEMI, which is correlated with the severity of LV failure. An increase in BNP is also found when right ventricular infarction accompanies inferior wall infarction, suggesting that this hormone may play a role in the hypotension that accompanies right ventricular infarction.

HEMATOLOGIC ALTERATIONS

PLATELETS. STEMI generally occurs in the presence of extensive coronary and systemic atherosclerotic plaques, which may serve as the site for the formation of platelet aggregates, a sequence that has been suggested as the initial step in the process of coronary thrombosis, coronary occlusion, and subsequent MI. Circulating platelets are hyperaggregable in patients with STEMI. Platelets from STEMI patients have an increased propensity for aggregation locally in the area of a disrupted plaque and also release vasoactive substances.[57]

HEMOSTATIC MARKERS. Elevated levels of serum fibrinogen degradation products, an end product of thrombosis, as well as the release of distinctive proteins when platelets are activated, such as platelet factor 4 and beta-thromboglobulin, have been reported in some patients with STEMI. Fibrinopeptide A (FPA), a protein released from fibrin by thrombin, is a marker of ongoing thrombosis and is increased during the early hours of STEMI. Marked elevations of hemostatic markers such as FPA, thrombin-antithrombin complex (TAT), and prothrombin fragment 1+2 (F1+2) are associated with an increased risk of mortality in STEMI patients. The interpretation of the coagulation tests in patients with STEMI may be complicated by elevated blood levels of catecholamines, concomitant shock, and/or pulmonary embolism—conditions that all may alter various tests of platelet and coagulation function. Additional factors that affect coagulation tests in STEMI include the type and dosage of antithrombotic agents and reperfusion of the infarct artery.

LEUKOCYTES. Leukocytosis usually accompanies STEMI in proportion to the magnitude of the necrotic process, elevated glucocorticoid levels, and possibly inflammation in the coronary arteries. The magnitude of elevation of the leukocyte count is associated with in-hospital mortality after STEMI.[58]

BLOOD VISCOSITY. Clinical and epidemiologic studies have suggested that several hemostatic and hemorheologic factors (e.g., fibrinogen, factor VII, plasma viscosity, hematocrit, red blood cell aggregation, total white blood cell count) participate in the pathophysiology of atherosclerosis and also play an integral role in acute thrombotic events. An increase in blood viscosity also occurs in patients with STEMI attributable to hemoconcentration during the first few days and later to elevated serum concentrations of alpha$_2$-globulin and fibrinogen, components of the acute-phase response to tissue necrosis, which is also responsible for the elevated sedimentation rate characteristic of STEMI.

Clinical Features

Predisposing Factors

In up to half of patients with STEMI, a precipitating factor or prodromal symptoms can be identified (see Chap. 44). Evidence suggests that unusually heavy exercise, particularly in fatigued or habitually inactive patients, and emotional stress can precipitate STEMI.[59] Such infarctions could result from marked increases in myocardial oxygen consumption in the presence of severe coronary arterial narrowing.

Accelerating angina and rest angina, two patterns of unstable angina, may culminate in STEMI (see Fig. 54-2). Noncardiac surgical procedures have also been noted as precursors of STEMI. Perioperative risk stratification may reduce the likelihood of STEMI and cardiac-related mortality (see Chap. 85).[60] Reduced myocardial perfusion secondary to hypotension (e.g., hemorrhagic or septic shock) and increased myocardial oxygen demands caused by aortic stenosis, fever, tachycardia, and agitation can also contribute to myocardial necrosis. Other factors reported as predisposing to STEMI include respiratory infections, hypoxemia of any cause, pulmonary embolism, hypoglycemia, administration of ergot preparations, use of cocaine, sympathomimetics, serum sickness, allergy, and on rare occasion, wasp stings. In patients with Prinzmetal angina (see Chap. 57), STEMI may develop in the territory of the coronary artery that repeatedly undergoes spasm. Rarely, munitions workers exposed to high concentrations of nitroglycerin develop MI when they are withdrawn from this exposure, suggesting that it is caused by vasospasm.

CIRCADIAN PERIODICITY. The time of onset of STEMI has a pronounced circadian periodicity, with a peak incidence of events between 6 AM and noon.[61] Circadian rhythms affect many physiologic and biochemical variables; the early morning hours are associated with rises in levels of plasma catecholamines and cortisol and increases in platelet aggregability. Interestingly, the characteristic circadian peak was absent in patients receiving a beta blocker or aspirin before their presentation with STEMI. The concept of triggering a STEMI is a complex one and likely involves the superimposition of multiple factors such as time of day, season, and the stress of natural disasters.[62]

History (see Chaps. 12 and 53)

PRODROMAL SYMPTOMS. The patient's history remains crucial to establishing a diagnosis. The prodrome is usually characterized by chest discomfort, resembling classic angina pectoris, but it occurs at rest or with less activity than usual and can therefore be classified as unstable angina. However, it is often not disturbing enough to induce patients to seek medical attention and, if they do, they may not be hospitalized. A feeling of general malaise or frank exhaustion often accompanies other symptoms preceding STEMI.

NATURE OF THE PAIN. The pain of STEMI varies in intensity; in most patients, it is severe and, in some cases, intolerable. The pain is prolonged, usually lasting for more than 30 minutes and frequently for a number of hours. The discomfort is described as constricting, crushing, oppressing, or compressing; often, the patient complains of a sensation of a heavy weight or squeezing in the chest. Although the discomfort is typically described as a choking, viselike, or heavy pain, it can also be characterized as a stabbing, knifelike, boring, or burning discomfort. The pain is usually retrosternal in location, spreading frequently to both sides of the anterior chest, with a predilection for the left side. Often, the pain radiates down the ulnar aspect of the left arm, producing a tingling sensation in the left wrist, hand, and fingers. Some patients note only a dull ache or numbness of the wrists in association with severe substernal or precordial discomfort. In some cases, the pain of STEMI may begin in the epigastrium and simulate a variety of abdominal disorders, a fact that often causes STEMI to be misdiagnosed as indigestion. In other patients, the discomfort of STEMI radiates to the shoulders, upper extremities, neck, jaw, and interscapular region, again usually favoring the left side. In patients with preexisting angina pectoris, the pain of infarction usually resembles that of angina with respect to location. However, it is generally much more severe, lasts longer, and is not relieved by rest and nitroglycerin.

The pain of STEMI may have subsided by the time the physician first encounters the patient (or the patient reaches the hospital), or it may persist for many hours. Opiates, in particular morphine, usually relieve the pain. Both angina pectoris and the pain of STEMI are thought to arise from nerve endings in ischemic or injured, but not necrotic, myocardium. Thus, in cases of STEMI, stimulation of nerve fibers in an ischemic zone of myocardium surrounding the necrotic central area of infarction probably gives rise to the pain.

The pain often disappears suddenly and completely when blood flow to the infarct territory is restored. In patients in whom reocclusion occurs after fibrinolysis, pain recurs if the initial reperfusion has left viable myocardium. Thus, what has previously been thought of as the pain of infarction, sometimes lasting for many hours, probably represents pain caused by ongoing ischemia. The recognition that pain implies ischemia and not infarction heightens the importance of seeking ways to relieve the ischemia, for which the pain is a marker. This finding suggests that the clinician should not be complacent about ongoing cardiac pain under any circumstances. In some patients, particularly older patients, diabetic patients, and heart transplantation recipients, STEMI manifests clinically not by chest pain, but rather by symptoms of acute LV failure and chest tightness or by marked weakness or frank syncope. Diaphoresis, nausea, and vomiting may accompany these symptoms.

OTHER SYMPTOMS. Nausea and vomiting may occur, presumably because of activation of the vagal reflex or stimulation of LV receptors as part of the Bezold-Jarisch reflex. These symptoms occur more commonly in patients with inferior STEMI than in those with anterior STEMI. Moreover, nausea and vomiting are common side effects of opiates. When the pain of STEMI is epigastric in location and is associated with nausea and vomiting, the clinical picture can easily be confused with that of acute cholecystitis, gastritis, or peptic ulcer. Occasionally, a patient complains of diarrhea or a violent urge to defecate during the acute phase of STEMI. Other symptoms include feelings of profound weakness, dizziness, palpitations, cold perspiration, and a sense of impending doom. On occasion, symptoms arising from an episode of cerebral embolism or other systemic arterial embolism herald a STEMI. Chest discomfort may not accompany these symptoms.

DIFFERENTIAL DIAGNOSIS. The pain of STEMI may simulate that of acute pericarditis (see Chap. 75), which usually associates with some pleuritic features. Pericardial discomfort is aggravated by respiratory movements and coughing and often involves the shoulder, the ridge of the trapezius, and the neck. An important feature that distinguishes pericardial pain from ischemic discomfort is that ischemic discomfort does not radiate to the trapezius ridge, a characteristic site of radiation of pericardial pain. Pleural pain is usually sharp, knifelike, and aggravated in a cyclical fashion by each breath, which distinguishes it from the deep, dull, steady pain of STEMI. Pulmonary embolism (see Chap. 77) generally produces pain laterally in the chest, is often pleuritic in nature, and may be associated with hemoptysis. The pain caused by acute aortic dissection (see Chap. 60) is usually localized to the center of the chest, is extremely severe and described by the patient as a "ripping" or "tearing" sensation, is at its maximal intensity shortly after onset, persists for many hours, and often radiates to the back or lower extremities. Often, one or more major arterial pulses are absent. Pain arising from the costochondral and chondrosternal articulations may be associated with localized swelling and redness; it is usually sharp and "darting" and is characterized by marked localized tenderness. Episodes of retrosternal discomfort induced by peristalsis in patients with increased esophageal stiffness and episodes of sustained esophageal contraction can mimic the pain of STEMI.

Silent STEMI and Atypical Presentation

Nonfatal STEMI can be unrecognized by the patient and discovered only on subsequent routine electrocardiographic or postmortem examinations. Of these unrecognized infarctions, approximately half are truly silent, with patients unable to recall any symptoms whatsoever. The other half of patients with so-called *silent infarction* can recall an event characterized by symptoms compatible with acute infarction when leading questions are posed after the electrocardiographic abnormalities are discovered. Unrecognized or silent infarction occurs more commonly in patients without antecedent angina pectoris and in patients with diabetes and hypertension.[63] Silent STEMI is often followed by silent ischemia (see Chap. 57). The prognoses of patients with silent and symptomatic presentations of STEMI appear to be similar.

Atypical presentations of STEMI include the following: (1) heart failure (i.e., dyspnea without pain beginning de novo or worsening of established failure); (2) classic angina pectoris without a particularly severe or prolonged episode; (3) atypical location of the pain; (4) central nervous system manifestations, resembling those of stroke, secondary to a sharp reduction in cardiac output in a patient with cerebral arteriosclerosis; (5) apprehension and nervousness; (6) sudden mania or psychosis; (7) syncope; (8) overwhelming weakness; (9) acute indigestion; and (10) peripheral embolization.

Physical Examination (see Chaps. 12 and 53)

GENERAL APPEARANCE. Patients suffering STEMI often appear anxious and in considerable distress. An anguished facial expression is common and—in contrast to patients with severe angina pectoris, who often lie, sit, or stand still, recognizing that all forms of activity increase the discomfort—some patients suffering STEMI may be restless and move about in an effort to find a comfortable position. They often massage or clutch their chests and frequently describe their pain with a clenched fist held against the sternum (the Levine sign). In patients with LV failure and sympathetic stimulation, cold perspiration and skin pallor may be evident; they typically sit or are propped up in bed, gasping for breath. Between breaths, they may complain of chest discomfort or a feeling of suffocation. Cough productive of frothy, pink, or blood-streaked sputum is common.

Patients in cardiogenic shock often lie listlessly, making few, if any, spontaneous movements. The skin is cool and clammy, with a bluish or mottled color over the extremities, with marked facial pallor and severe cyanosis of the lips and nail beds. Depending on the degree of cerebral perfusion, the patient in shock may converse normally or may evidence confusion and disorientation.

HEART RATE. The heart rate can vary from a marked bradycardia to a rapid regular or irregular tachycardia, depending on the underlying rhythm and degree of LV failure. Most commonly, the pulse is rapid

and regular initially (sinus tachycardia at 100 to 110 beats/min), slowing as the patient's pain and anxiety are relieved; premature ventricular beats are common.

BLOOD PRESSURE. Most patients with uncomplicated STEMI are normotensive, although the reduced stroke volume accompanying the tachycardia can cause declines in systolic and pulse pressures and elevation of diastolic pressure. Among previously normotensive patients, a hypertensive response is occasionally seen during the first few hours, with the arterial pressure exceeding 160/90 mm Hg, presumably as a consequence of adrenergic discharge secondary to pain, anxiety, and agitation. Previously hypertensive patients often become normotensive without treatment after STEMI, although many of these previously hypertensive patients eventually regain their elevated levels of blood pressure, generally 3 to 6 months after infarction. In patients with massive infarction, arterial pressure falls acutely because of LV dysfunction and venous pooling secondary to administration of morphine and/or nitrates. As recovery occurs, the arterial pressure tends to return to preinfarction levels.

Patients in cardiogenic shock by definition have systolic pressures below 90 mm Hg and evidence of end-organ hypoperfusion. Hypotension alone does not necessarily signify cardiogenic shock, however, because some patients with inferior infarction with Bezold-Jarisch reflex activation may also have a transient systolic blood pressure below 90 mm Hg. Their hypotension eventually resolves spontaneously, although the process can be accelerated by intravenous atropine (0.5 to 1 mg) and assumption of the Trendelenburg position. Other patients who are initially only slightly hypotensive may demonstrate gradually falling blood pressures with progressive reduction in cardiac output over several hours or days as they develop cardiogenic shock as a consequence of increasing ischemia and extension of infarction (see Fig. 54-12). Evidence of autonomic hyperactivity is common, varying in type with the location of the infarction. At some time during their initial presentation, more than half of patients with inferior STEMI have evidence of excess parasympathetic stimulation, with hypotension, bradycardia, or both, whereas about half of patients with anterior STEMI show signs of sympathetic excess, with hypertension, tachycardia, or both.

TEMPERATURE AND RESPIRATION. Most patients with extensive STEMI develop fever, a nonspecific response to tissue necrosis, within 24 to 48 hours of the onset of infarction. Body temperature often begins to rise within 4 to 8 hours after the onset of infarction, and rectal temperature may reach 38.3° to 38.9°C (101° to 102°F). Fever usually resolves by the fourth or fifth day after infarction.

The respiratory rate may be slightly elevated soon after the development of STEMI; in patients without heart failure, it results from anxiety and pain because it returns to normal with treatment of physical and psychological discomfort. In patients with LV failure, the respiratory rate correlates with the severity of failure; patients with pulmonary edema may have respiratory rates exceeding 40/min. But the respiratory rate is not necessarily elevated in patients with cardiogenic shock. Cheyne-Stokes (periodic) respiration may occur in older patients with cardiogenic shock or heart failure, particularly after opiate therapy or in the presence of cerebrovascular disease.

JUGULAR VENOUS PULSE. The jugular venous pulse usually fails to show any abnormalities. The *a* wave may be prominent in patients with pulmonary hypertension secondary to LV failure or reduced compliance. In contrast, right ventricular infarction (whether or not it accompanies LV infarction) often results in marked jugular venous distention and, when complicated by necrosis or ischemia of the right ventricular papillary muscles, tall *c-v* waves of tricuspid regurgitation are evident. Patients with STEMI and cardiogenic shock usually have elevated jugular venous pressure. In patients with STEMI, hypotension, and hypoperfusion (findings that may resemble those of patients with cardiogenic shock) but who have flat neck veins, it is likely that the depression of LV performance may relate, at least in part, to hypovolemia. The differentiation can be made only by assessing LV performance using echocardiography or by measuring LV filling pressure with a pulmonary artery flotation catheter.

CAROTID PULSE. Palpation of the carotid arterial pulse provides a clue to the LV stroke volume; a small pulse suggests a reduced stroke volume, whereas a sharp brief upstroke is often observed in patients with mitral regurgitation or ruptured ventricular septum with a left-to-right shunt. Pulsus alternans reflects severe LV dysfunction.

CHEST. Moist rales are audible in patients who develop LV failure and/or a reduction of LV compliance with STEMI. Diffuse wheezing can present in patients with severe LV failure. Cough with hemoptysis, suggesting pulmonary embolism with infarction, can also occur. In 1967, Killip and Kimball[64] proposed a prognostic classification scheme on the basis of the presence and severity of rales detected in patients presenting with STEMI. Class I patients are free of rales and a third heart sound. Class II patients have rales but only to a mild to moderate degree (<50% of lung fields), and they may or may not have an S_3. Patients in Class III have rales in more than half of each lung field and frequently have pulmonary edema. Finally, Class IV patients are in cardiogenic shock. Despite overall improvement in mortality rate in each class, compared with data observed during the original development of the classification scheme, the classification scheme remains useful today, as evidenced by data from large MI trials of STEMI patients.[65]

CARDIAC EXAMINATION

Palpation

Palpation of the precordium may yield normal findings, but in patients with transmural STEMI, it more commonly reveals a presystolic pulsation, synchronous with an audible fourth heart sound, which reflects a vigorous left atrial contraction filling a ventricle with reduced compliance. In the presence of LV systolic dysfunction, an outward movement of the left ventricle can be palpated in early diastole, coincident with a third heart sound.

Auscultation

HEART SOUNDS. The heart sounds, particularly the first sound, are frequently muffled and occasionally inaudible immediately after the infarct, and their intensity increases during convalescence. A soft first heart sound may also reflect prolongation of the P-R interval. Patients with marked ventricular dysfunction and/or left bundle branch block may have paradoxical splitting of the second heart sound.

A fourth heart sound is almost universally present in patients in sinus rhythm with STEMI. However, it has limited diagnostic value because it is commonly audible in most patients with chronic ischemic heart disease and is recordable, although not often audible, in many normal subjects older than 45 years of age.

A third heart sound in patients with STEMI usually reflects severe LV dysfunction with elevated ventricular filling pressure. It is caused by rapid deceleration of transmitral blood flow during protodiastolic filling of the left ventricle and is usually heard in patients with large infarctions. This sound is detected best at the apex, with the patient in the left lateral recumbent position. A third heart sound may be caused not only by LV failure but also by increased inflow into the left ventricle, as occurs when mitral regurgitation or ventricular septal defect complicates STEMI. Third and fourth heart sounds emanating from the left ventricle are heard best at the apex; in patients with right ventricular infarcts, these sounds can be heard along the left sternal border and increase on inspiration.

MURMURS. Transient or persistent systolic murmurs are commonly audible in patients with STEMI and generally result from mitral regurgitation secondary to dysfunction of the mitral valve apparatus (e.g., papillary muscle dysfunction, LV dilation). A new, prominent, apical holosystolic murmur, accompanied by a thrill, may represent rupture of a head of a papillary muscle (see Chap. 55). The findings in cases of rupture of the interventricular septum are similar, although the murmur and thrill are usually most prominent along the left sternal border and may be audible at the right sternal border as well. The systolic murmur of tricuspid regurgitation (caused by right ventricular

failure because of pulmonary hypertension and/or right ventricular infarction or by infarction of a right ventricular papillary muscle) is also heard along the left sternal border. It is characteristically intensified by inspiration and is accompanied by a prominent c-v wave in the jugular venous pulse and a right ventricular fourth sound.

FRICTION RUBS. Pericardial friction rubs may be heard in patients with STEMI, especially those sustaining large transmural infarctions.[66] Rubs are notorious for their evanescence and hence are probably even more common than reported. Although friction rubs can be heard within 24 hours or as late as 2 weeks after the onset of infarction, most commonly they are noted on the second or third day. Occasionally, in patients with extensive infarction, a loud rub can be heard for many days. Patients with STEMI and a pericardial friction rub may have a pericardial effusion on echocardiographic study, but only rarely does this cause the classic electrocardiographic changes of pericarditis. Delayed onset of the rub and the associated discomfort of pericarditis (as late as 3 months postinfarction) are characteristic of the now rare postmyocardial infarction syndrome (Dressler syndrome).

Pericardial rubs are most readily audible along the left sternal border or just inside the apical impulse. Loud rubs may be audible over the entire precordium and even over the back. Occasionally, only the systolic portion of a rub is heard; it can be confused with a systolic murmur, and the diagnosis of rupture of the ventricular septum or mitral regurgitation may be incorrectly considered.

OTHER FINDINGS

FUNDI. Hypertension, diabetes, and generalized atherosclerosis commonly accompany STEMI, and because these conditions can produce characteristic changes in the fundus, a funduscopic examination may provide information concerning the underlying vascular status. This is particularly useful for patients unable to provide a detailed history.

ABDOMEN. Pain in the abdomen associated with nausea, vomiting, restlessness, and even abdominal distention is often interpreted by patients as a sign of "indigestion," resulting in self-medication with antacids, and it can suggest an acute abdominal process to the physician. Right heart failure, characterized by hepatomegaly and a positive abdominojugular reflux, is unusual in patients with acute LV infarction, but does occur in patients with severe and prolonged LV failure or right ventricular infarction.

EXTREMITIES. Coronary atherosclerosis is often associated with systemic atherosclerosis, and therefore patients with STEMI may have a history of intermittent claudication and demonstrate physical findings of peripheral vascular disease (see Chap. 61). Thus, diminished peripheral arterial pulses, loss of hair, and atrophic skin in the lower extremities may be noted in patients with coronary artery disease. Peripheral edema is a manifestation of right ventricular failure and, like congestive hepatomegaly, is unusual in patients with acute LV infarction. Cyanosis of the nail beds is common in patients with severe LV failure and is particularly striking in patients with cardiogenic shock.

NEUROPSYCHIATRIC FINDINGS. Except for the altered mental status that occurs in patients with STEMI who have a markedly reduced cardiac output and cerebral hypoperfusion, neurologic findings are normal unless the patient has suffered cerebral embolism secondary to a mural thrombus. The coincidence between these two conditions can be explained by systemic hypotension caused by STEMI precipitating a cerebral infarction and the converse, as well as by mural emboli from the left ventricle causing cerebral emboli.

Patients with STEMI often exhibit alterations of the emotional state including intense anxiety, denial, and depression. Medical staff caring for STEMI patients must be sensitive to changes in the patient's emotional state; a calm, professional atmosphere, with thorough explanations of equipment and prognosis, can help alleviate the distress associated with STEMI.

Laboratory Findings

SERUM MARKERS OF CARDIAC DAMAGE. The availability of serum cardiac markers with markedly enhanced sensitivity for myocardial damage enables clinicians to diagnose MI in approximately an additional one third of patients who would not have fulfilled criteria for MI in the past.[67] The increased use of more sensitive biomarkers of MI, combined with more precise imaging techniques, has necessitated the establishment of new criteria for MI (see Table 54-2). As a consequence of the enhanced sensitivity for detection of smaller infarcts using cardiac-specific troponins, clinicians now face a new set of issues. More patients are discharged with a diagnosis of MI rather than UA, lifestyle and insurance implications need to be considered, and epidemiologic studies tracking the incidence of MI over time must account for the improved ability to diagnose MI in more contemporary patient cohorts.[1]

Although these considerations apply directly to patients on the UA/NSTEMI end of the ACS spectrum (see Chap. 56), a general discussion of cardiac biomarkers is presented here because the scientific aspects of the pathophysiologic concepts and assay methodology overlap when biomarkers are used to evaluate STEMI patients. It should be emphasized that clinicians should *not* wait for the results of biomarker assays to initiate treatment for the STEMI patient. Because there is a time urgency for reperfusion in STEMI, the 12-lead ECG should serve to initiate such strategies.

Necrosis compromises the integrity of the sarcolemmal membrane; intracellular macromolecules (serum cardiac markers) begin to diffuse into the cardiac interstitium, and ultimately into the microvasculature and lymphatics in the region of the infarct (**Fig. 54-14; Table 54-5**).[68,69] The rate of appearance of these macromolecules in the peripheral circulation depends on several factors, including intracellular location, molecular weight, local blood and lymphatic flow, and rate of elimination from the blood.[69,70]

Creatine Kinase

Serum CK activity exceeds the normal range within 4 to 8 hours after the onset of STEMI and declines to normal within 2 to 3 days (see Fig. 54-14). Although the peak CK level occurs on average at about 24 hours, peak levels occur earlier in patients who have had reperfusion as a result of the administration of fibrinolytic therapy or mechanical recanalization, as well as in patients with early spontaneous fibrinolysis (**Fig. 54-15**).

Although elevation of the serum CK concentration is a sensitive enzymatic detector of STEMI that is routinely available in most hospitals, important drawbacks include false-positive results in patients with muscle disease, alcohol intoxication, diabetes mellitus, skeletal muscle trauma, after vigorous exercise, convulsions, intramuscular injections, thoracic outlet syndrome, and pulmonary embolism.[71]

CREATINE KINASE ISOENZYMES. Three isoenzymes of CK exist (MM, BB, and MB). Extracts of brain and kidney contain predominantly the BB isoenzyme; skeletal muscle contains principally MM, but also contains some MB (1% to 3%), and cardiac muscle contains both MM and MB isoenzymes. The MB isoenzymes of CK can also be present in small quantities in the small intestine, tongue, diaphragm, uterus, and prostate. Strenuous exercise, particularly in trained long-distance runners or professional athletes, can cause elevation of both total CK and CK-MB.[72] Because CK-MB can be detected in the blood of healthy subjects, the cutoff value for abnormal elevation of CK-MB is usually set a few units above the upper reference limit for a given laboratory (see Fig. 54-14).[71] Although small quantities of CK-MB isoenzyme occur in tissues other than the heart, elevated levels of CK-MB may be considered, for practical purposes, to be the result of MI, except in the case of trauma or surgery on the organs noted.

Creatine kinase MB is analyzed in most laboratories by highly sensitive and specific enzyme immunoassays that use monoclonal antibodies directed against CK-MB.[71] It has been proposed that a ratio (relative index) of CK-MB mass to CK activity of approximately 2.5 indicates a myocardial rather than a skeletal source of the CK-MB elevation. Although this ratio may be satisfied by many patients with STEMI, it is inaccurate in several circumstances: (1) when high levels of total CK are present because of skeletal muscle injury (a large quantity of CK-MB must be released from the myocardium to satisfy criteria); (2) when chronic skeletal muscle injury releases large amounts of CK-MB; and (3) when total CK measurements are within the normal reference range for the laboratory and CK-MB is elevated, possibly indicating that a microinfarction has occurred. Clinicians should not rely on measurements of CK and CK-MB at a single time, but instead should evaluate the temporal rise and fall of serial values (see Fig. 54-14). Of note, because cardiac-specific troponins I and T (cTnI and cTnT; see Figs. 54-14 and 54-15 and Tables 54-2 and 54-5)

accurately distinguish skeletal from cardiac muscle damage, the troponins are now considered the preferred biomarker for diagnosing MI.[69]

In addition to STEMI secondary to coronary obstruction, other forms of injury to cardiac muscle, such as those resulting from myocarditis, trauma, cardiac catheterization, shock, and cardiac surgery, may also produce elevated serum CK-MB levels.[71] These latter causes of elevation of serum CK-MB values can usually be readily distinguished from STEMI by the clinical setting.

OTHER BIOMARKERS. Isoforms of the MM and MB isoenzymes have been identified,[73] but with the increased availability of assays for the cardiac-specific troponins, measurement of CK isoforms has little, if any, important clinical role (see Table 54-5 and Fig. 54-14).[69] Myoglobin has now given way to more cardiac-specific markers, such as cTnI or cTnT.[74]

Cardiac-Specific Troponins

The troponin complex consists of three subunits that regulate the calcium-mediated contractile process of striated muscle. These include troponin C, which binds Ca^{2+}, troponin I (TnI), which binds to actin and inhibits actin-myosin interactions, and troponin T (TnT), which binds to tropomyosin, thereby attaching the troponin complex to the thin filament. Although the majority of TnT is incorporated into the troponin complex, approximately 6% is dissolved in the cytosol; about 2% to 3% of TnI is found in a cytosolic pool. Following myocyte injury, the initial release of cTnT and cTnI is from the cytosolic pool, followed subsequently by release from the structural (myofilament-bound) pool (see Fig. 54-14).[1]

Different genes encode TnT and TnI in cardiac and skeletal muscle, thus permitting the production of specific antibodies for the cardiac form (cTnT and cTnI) that enable their quantitative assay (see Fig. 54-14 and Table 54-4).[68] The measurement of cTnT or cTnI is now at the center of the new diagnostic criteria for MI.[1]

When interpreting the results of assays for cTnT or cTnI, clinicians must be cognizant of several analytic issues.[75] The cTnT assays are produced by a single manufacturer, leading to relative uniformity of cutoffs, whereas several manufacturers produce cTnI assays. There is evidence that the release pattern of troponin complexes and degradation into various troponin fragments may affect the results of various commercial assays, especially for cTnI, and may be useful in the future to gain insight into pathophysiologic events (e.g., ischemia, reperfusion).[76]

CUTOFF VALUES. Variations in the cutoff concentration for abnormal levels of cTnI in the immunoassays clinically available may be caused in part by different specificities of the antibodies used for detecting free and complexed cTnI. Thus, when using the measurement of cTnI for diagnosing STEMI, clinicians should apply the cutoff values for the particular assay used in their laboratory.[74] For both cTnT and cTnI, the definition of an abnormally increased level is a value exceeding that of 99% of a reference control group.[1]

Furthermore, whereas CK-MB usually increases 10- to 20-fold above the upper limit of the reference range, cTnT and cTnI typically increase more than 20 times above the reference range (see Fig. 54-14). These features of the cardiac-specific troponin assays provide an improved signal-to-noise ratio, enabling the detection of even minor degrees of myocardial necrosis. In patients with MI, cTnT and cTnI levels first begin to rise above the upper reference limit by 3 hours from the onset of chest pain. Because of a continuous release from a degenerating contractile apparatus in necrotic myocytes, elevations of cTnI may persist for 7 to 10 days after MI; elevations of cTnT may persist for up to 10 to 14 days. The prolonged time course of elevation of cTnT and cTnI is advantageous for the late diagnosis of MI. Patients with STEMI who undergo successful recanalization of the infarct-related artery have a rapid release of cardiac troponins, which can indicate reperfusion (see Fig. 54-15).[33]

TROPONIN VERSUS CK-MB. When comparing the diagnostic efficiency of the cardiac troponins versus CK-MB for MI, it is important to remember that the troponin assays can probably detect episodes of myocardial necrosis that are below the detection limit of the current CK-MB assays. This can lead to false-positive cases of troponin elevations if CK-MB is used as the reference standard or, conversely, to false-negative cases of CK-MB elevation if troponin is used as the reference standard. From a clinical perspective, it is desirable to have diagnostic

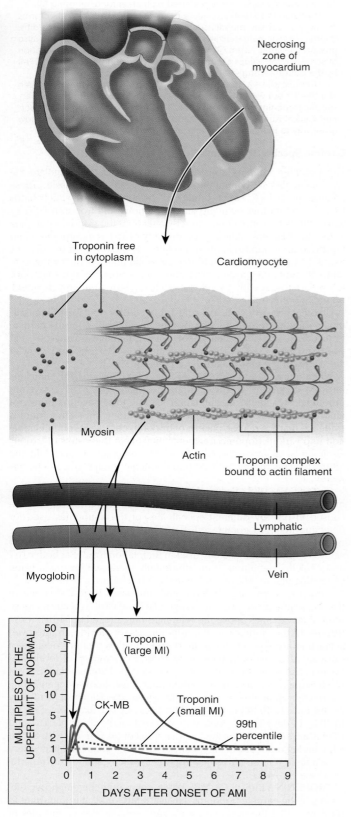

FIGURE 54-14 **Top,** Zone of necrosing myocardium, followed by a diagram of a cardiomyocyte that is in the process of releasing biomarkers **(middle)**. **Bottom,** After disruption of the sarcolemmal membrane of the cardiomyocyte, the cytoplasmic pool of biomarkers is released first (leftmost arrow). Markers such as myoglobin and CK isoforms are rapidly released, and blood levels rise quickly above the cutoff limit. This is then followed by a more protracted release of biomarkers from the disintegrating myofilaments that may continue for several days (three-headed arrow). Cardiac troponin levels rise to about 20 to 50 times the upper reference limit (the 99th percentile of values in a reference control group) in patients who have a classic acute MI and sustain sufficient myocardial necrosis to result in abnormally elevated levels of the MB fraction of creatine kinase (CK-MB). Clinicians can now diagnose episodes of microinfarction by sensitive assays that detect cardiac troponin elevations above the upper reference limit, even though CK-MB levels may still be in the normal reference range (not shown). CV = coefficient of variation. *(Modified from Antman EM: Decision making with cardiac troponin tests. N Engl J Med 346:2079, 2002; and Jaffe AS, Babiun L, Apple FS: Biomarkers in acute cardiac disease: The present and the future. J Am Coll Cardiol 48:1, 2006.)*

TABLE 54-5   Biomarkers for Evaluation of Patients with ST-Segment Elevation Myocardial Infarction

BIOMARKER	MOLECULAR WEIGHT (DA)	RANGE OF TIME TO INITIAL ELEVATION (HR)	MEAN TIME TO PEAK ELEVATIONS (NONREPERFUSED)	TIME TO RETURN TO NORMAL RANGE
Frequently Used in Clinical Practice				
MB-CK*	86,000	3-12	24 hr	48-72 hr
cTnI†	23,500	3-12	24 hr	5-10 days
cTnT	33,000	3-12	12 hr-2 days	5-14 days
Infrequently Used in Clinical Practice				
Myoglobin	17,800	1-4	6-7 hr	24 hr
MB-CK tissue isoform	86,000	2-6	18 hr	Unknown
MM-CK tissue isoform	86,000	1-6	12 hr	38 hr

*Increased sensitivity can be achieved with sampling every 6 or 8 hr.

†Multiple assays available for clinical use; clinicians should be familiar with the cutoff value used in their institution.

Modified from Antman EM, Anbe DT, Armstrong PW, et al: ACC/AHA guidelines for the management of patients with ST-elevation myocardial infarction: A report of the American College of Cardiology/American Heart Association Task Force on Practice Guidelines (Committee to Revise the 1999 Guidelines for the Management of Patients with Acute Myocardial Infarction). Circulation 110:e82, 2004.

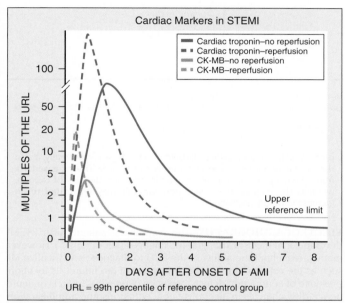

FIGURE 54-15 The kinetics of release of CK-MB and cardiac troponin in patients who do not undergo reperfusion are shown in the solid blue and pink curves as multiples of the upper reference limit (URL). When patients with STEMI undergo reperfusion (dashed blue and pink curves), the cardiac biomarkers are detected sooner and rise to a higher peak value, but decline more rapidly, resulting in a smaller area under the curve and limitation of infarct size. AMI = acute MI. (Modified from Antman EM, Anbe DT, Armstrong PW, et al: ACC/AHA guidelines for the management of patients with ST-elevation myocardial infarction: A report of the American College of Cardiology/American Heart Association Task Force on Practice Guidelines [Committee to Revise the 1999 Guidelines for the Management of Patients with Acute Myocardial Infarction]. Circulation 110:e82, 2004.)

tests for MI with increased sensitivity to increase the number of MI cases identified, and with increased specificity to reduce the number of cases incorrectly diagnosed and treated for MI. The prognostic value of the troponins is independent of other risk factors such as age and electrocardiographic abnormalities, as well as the measurement of older biomarkers such as CK-MB.[68]

Recommendations for Measurement of Serum Markers

It seems reasonable for clinicians to measure cTnT or cTnI in all patients with suspected MI. From a cost-effectiveness perspective, it is unnecessary to measure both a cardiac-specific troponin and CK-MB. Routine diagnosis of MI can be accomplished within 12 hours using CK-MB, cTnT, or cTnI by obtaining measurements approximately every 8 to 12 hours (see Tables 54-2 and 54-4). Retrospective diagnosis

or diagnosis of MI in the presence of skeletal muscle injury is more readily accomplished with cTnT or cTnI. Assays for the cardiac-specific troponins should supersede assays for CK-MB, not only for the diagnosis of MI but also for the assessment of reperfusion, reinfarction, and estimation of infarct size.[1]

The universal definition of MI not only recommends classifying infarctions into five types (see Table 54-3), but also recommends assessing the magnitude of the infarction by tabulating the fold elevation of cardiac biomarkers above the 99th percentile of a normal reference group. A suggested grid for reporting the results is shown in **Table 54-6**. An example from a clinical trial comparing prasugrel with clopidogrel as supportive antiplatelet therapy for moderate-high risk ACS patients undergoing PCI is shown in **Figure 54-16**.[3]

Clinicians should measure a cardiac biomarker reflective of muscle death in a patient with suspected MI. **Figure 54-17** illustrates the temporal rise and fall of such biomarkers of muscle death along the chronology of the disease process, which begins with the development of a vulnerable plaque and ends with the release of biomarkers of muscle overload.[29] Markers such as pregnancy-associated plasma protein (PAPP) and ischemia-modified albumin (IMA) are not routinely measured in patients with MI. Measurement of BNP and related compounds may be useful for the assessment of the hemodynamic impact of the MI, although no clear guidance is available as to how to structure specific therapeutic maneuvers in the setting of STEMI in response to BNP measurements.

OTHER LABORATORY MEASUREMENTS

SERUM LIPIDS. During the first 24 to 48 hours after admission, total cholesterol and high-density lipoprotein (HDL) cholesterol remain at or near baseline values but generally fall precipitously after that (see Chap. 47). The fall in HDL cholesterol after STEMI is greater than the fall in total cholesterol; thus, the ratio of total cholesterol to HDL cholesterol is no longer useful for risk assessment unless measured early after MI. A lipid profile should be obtained on all STEMI patients who are admitted within 24 to 48 hours of symptoms. The success of lipid-lowering therapy in primary and secondary prevention studies and evidence that hypolipidemic therapy improves endothelial function and inhibits thrombus formation[77] indicate that early management of serum lipids in patients hospitalized for STEMI is advisable.[78] For patients admitted beyond 24 to 48 hours, more accurate determinations of serum lipid levels are obtained approximately 8 weeks after the infarction has occurred.

HEMATOLOGIC FINDINGS. The elevation of the white blood cell count usually develops within 2 hours after the onset of chest pain, reaches a peak 2 to 4 days after infarction, and returns to normal in 1 week. The peak white blood cell count usually ranges from 12 to 15 × 10³/mL but occasionally rises to as high as 20 × 10³/mL in patients with large STEMI. Often, there is an increase in the percentage of polymorphonuclear leukocytes and a shift of the differential count to band forms. An epidemiologic association has been reported, indicating a worse angiographic appearance of culprit lesions and increased risk of adverse clinical outcomes the higher the white blood cell count is at presentation with an ACS.[79]

The erythrocyte sedimentation rate (ESR) is usually normal during the first day or two after infarction, even though fever and leukocytosis may

TABLE 54-6 Classification of Different Types of Myocardial Infarction: Suggested Grid for Reporting Results*

MULTIPLES X 99%	1 (SPONTANEOUS)	2 (SECONDARY)	MI Type 3† (SUDDEN DEATH)	4‡ (PCI)	5‡ (CABG)	TOTAL NO.
1-2×						
2-3×						
3-5×						
5-10×						
>10×						
Total no.						

TYPES OF MI	TREATMENT A NO. OF PATIENTS	TREATMENT B NO. OF PATIENTS
MI type 1		
MI type 2		
MI type 3		
MI type 4		
MI type 5		
Total no.		

*According to multiples of the 99th percentile of a control group of the applied cardiac biomarker.
†Biomarkers are not available for this type of myocardial infarction because the patients expired before biomarker determination could be performed.
‡For the sake of completeness, the total distribution of biomarker values should be reported. The shaded areas represent biomarker elevations below the decision limit used for these types of myocardial infarction.
From Thygesen K, Alpert JS, White HD, et al: Universal definition of myocardial infarction. Circulation 116:2634, 2007.

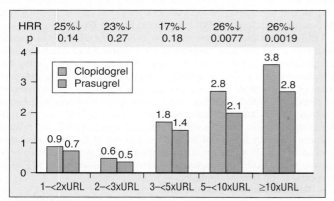

FIGURE 54-16 Effect of prasugrel compared with clopidogrel with respect to the total number of new or recurrent MIs classified using the biomarker categories recommended by the universal definition of MI (see Table 54-6). The biomarker categories are groupings of fold elevations above the upper reference limit (URL) of normal. The data shown for each bar are from Kaplan-Meier estimates for the incidence of MI; the percentage reductions represent the relative reductions in the hazard rate ratio (HRR) for the development of an MI in the prasugrel versus clopidogrel groups. *(From Morrow DA, Wiviott SD, White HD, et al: Effect of the novel thienopyridine prasugrel compared with clopidogrel on spontaneous and procedural myocardial infarction in the Trial to Assess Improvement in Therapeutic Outcomes by Optimizing Platelet Inhibition with Prasugrel-Thrombolysis in Myocardial Infarction 38: An application of the classification system from the universal definition of myocardial infarction. Circulation 119:2758, 2009.)*

be present. It then rises to a peak on the fourth or fifth day and may remain elevated for several weeks. The increase in the ESR does not correlate well with the size of the infarction or with the prognosis. The hematocrit often increases during the first few days after infarction as a consequence of hemoconcentration. An elevated C-reactive protein (CRP) level appears to identify patients presenting with STEMI, with worse angiographic appearance of the infarct artery and a greater likelihood of developing heart failure.[80]

The hemoglobin value at presentation with STEMI predicts major cardiovascular events powerfully and independently.[81] Of note is a J-shaped relationship between baseline hemoglobin values and clinical events. Cardiovascular mortality increases progressively as the presenting hemoglobin level falls below 14 to 15 g/dL; conversely, it also rises as the hemoglobin level increases above 17 g/dL. The increased risk from anemia probably relates to diminished tissue delivery of oxygen, whereas the increased risk with polycythemia may be related to an increase in blood viscosity.

ELECTROCARDIOGRAPHY. The majority of patients with STEMI develop serial electrocardiographic changes (see Chap. 13). However, many factors limit the ability of the ECG to diagnose and localize MI, such as the extent of myocardial injury, age of the infarct, its location, presence of conduction defects, presence of previous infarcts or acute pericarditis, changes in electrolyte concentrations, and administration of cardioactive drugs. Changes in the ST segment and T wave are nonspecific and may occur in a variety of conditions, including stable and unstable angina pectoris, ventricular hypertrophy, acute and chronic pericarditis, myocarditis, early repolarization, electrolyte imbalance, shock, and metabolic disorders, and following the administration of digitalis. Serial ECGs help differentiate these conditions from STEMI. Transient changes favor angina or electrolyte disturbances, whereas persistent changes argue for infarction if other causes such as shock, administration of digitalis, and persistent metabolic disorders can be eliminated. Nevertheless, serial standard 12-lead ECGs remain a potent and extremely useful method for the detection and localization of MI.[32] Analysis of the constellation of electrocardiographic leads showing ST-segment elevation may also be useful for identifying the site of occlusion in the infarct artery (see Fig. 54-4).[82] The extent of ST-segment deviation on the ECG, location of infarction, and QRS duration correlate with risk of adverse outcomes. Even when left bundle branch block is present on the ECG, MI can be diagnosed when striking ST-segment deviation is present beyond that which can be explained by the conduction defect. In addition to the diagnostic and prognostic information contained within the 12-lead ECG, it also provides valuable noninvasive information about the success of reperfusion for STEMI (see Chap. 55).[83]

Although general agreement exists on electrocardiographic and vectorcardiographic criteria for the recognition of infarction of the anterior and inferior myocardial walls, less agreement pertains to criteria for lateral and posterior infarcts; in this area, even the terminology can be confusing. A consensus group has recommended elimination of the term *posterior* and suggests using the term *lateral* to be consistent with current understanding of the segmental anatomy of the heart as it sits in the thorax.[84] Patients with an abnormal R wave in V_1 (0.04 second in duration and/or R/S ratio $\geq$ 1 in the absence of preexcitation or right ventricular hypertrophy), with inferior or lateral Q waves, have an increased incidence of isolated occlusion of a dominant left circumflex coronary artery without collateral circulation. These patients have a lower ejection fraction, increased end-systolic volume, and higher complication rate than patients with inferior infarction caused by isolated occlusion of the right coronary artery.

Although most patients bear the electrocardiographic changes from an infarction for the rest of their lives, particularly if they evolve Q waves, in a substantial minority the typical changes disappear, Q waves regress, and the ECG can even return to normal after a number of years. Under many circumstances, Q-wave patterns simulate MI. Conditions that may mimic the electrocardiographic features of MI by producing a pattern of "pseudoinfarction" include ventricular hypertrophy, conduction disturbances, preexcitation, primary myocardial disease, pneumothorax, pulmonary embolus, amyloid heart disease, primary and metastatic tumors of the heart, traumatic heart disease, intracranial hemorrhage, hyperkalemia, pericarditis, early repolarization, and cardiac sarcoidosis.

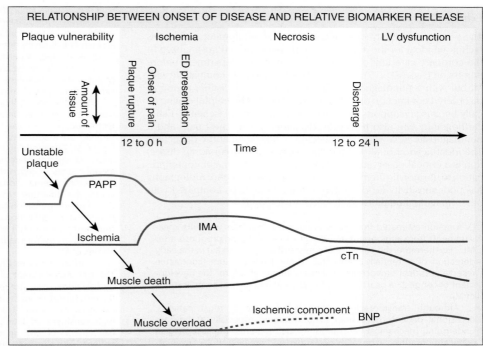

RELATIONSHIP BETWEEN ONSET OF DISEASE AND RELATIVE BIOMARKER RELEASE

FIGURE 54-17 Coronary artery plaques vulnerable to rupture are caused by infiltration of inflammatory elements that release cytokines and enzymes, resulting in degradation of the fibrous cap. PAPP-A is a metalloproteinase that is released into blood during the stage of plaque vulnerability. Once a plaque has ruptured, myocardial ischemia is the initial consequence. This can be detected by the IMA test. Prolonged ischemia leads to myocardial necrosis and the release of cTn. After 12 to 24 hours, there can be LV dysfunction and myocardial muscle overloading, causing the release of BNP. There may also be release of BNP because of myocardial ischemia (dotted line). IMA = ischemia-modified albumin. *(From Wu AHB: Early detection of acute coronary syndromes and risk stratification by multimarker analysis. Biomarkers Med 1:52, 2007.)*

Q-Wave and Non—Q-Wave Infarction

The presence or absence of Q waves on the surface ECG does not reliably distinguish between transmural and nontransmural (subendocardial) MI.[85] Q waves on the ECG signify abnormal electrical activity but are not synonymous with irreversible myocardial damage. Also, the absence of Q waves may simply reflect the insensitivity of the standard 12-lead ECG, especially in zones of the left ventricle supplied by the left circumflex artery (see Fig. 54-4). Angiographic studies in MI patients without ST-segment elevation show a higher incidence of subtotal occlusion of the culprit coronary vessel and greater collateral flow to the infarct zone. Observational data suggest that MI without ST-segment elevation occurs more commonly in older patients and in patients with a prior MI.

Ischemia at a Distance

Patients with new Q waves and ST-segment elevation diagnostic for STEMI in one territory often have ST-segment depression in other territories. These additional ST-segment changes, which imply a poor prognosis, are caused by ischemia in a territory other than the area of infarction, termed *ischemia at a distance*, or by reciprocal electrical phenomena. A good deal of attention has been directed to associated ST-segment depression in the anterior leads when it occurs in patients with acute inferior STEMI. However, despite the clinical importance of differentiation among causes of anterior ST-segment depression in such patients, including anterior ischemia, inferolateral wall infarction, and true reciprocal changes, such a differentiation cannot be made reliably by electrocardiographic or even vectorcardiographic techniques. Although precordial ST-segment depression is associated more commonly with extensive infarction of the lateral or inferior septal segments, rather than anterior wall subendocardial ischemia, imaging techniques such as echocardiography are necessary to ascertain whether an anterior wall motion abnormality is present.[86]

Right Ventricular Infarction

ST-segment elevation in the right precordial leads (V_1, V_3R to V_6R) is a relatively sensitive and specific sign of right ventricular infarction.[82,87] Occasionally, ST-segment elevation in leads V_2 and V_3 results from acute right ventricular infarction; this appears to occur only when the injury to the left inferior wall is minimal (see Fig. 54-11).[88] Usually, the concurrent inferior wall injury suppresses this anterior ST-segment elevation resulting from right ventricular injury. Similarly, right ventricular infarction appears to reduce the anterior ST-segment depression often observed with inferior wall myocardial infarction. A QS or QR pattern in leads V_3R and/or V_4R also suggests right ventricular myocardial necrosis but has less predictive accuracy than ST-segment elevation in these leads.

IMAGING

Roentgenography

The initial chest roentgenogram (see Chap. 16) in patients with STEMI is almost invariably a portable film obtained in the emergency department or coronary care unit. When present, prominent pulmonary vascular markings on the roentgenogram reflect elevated LV end-diastolic pressure, but significant temporal discrepancies can occur because of what have been termed *diagnostic lags* and *post-therapeutic lags*. Up to 12 hours can elapse before pulmonary edema accumulates after ventricular filling pressure has become elevated. The post-therapeutic phase lag represents a longer time interval; up to 2 days are required for pulmonary edema to resorb and the radiographic signs of pulmonary congestion to clear after ventricular filling pressure has returned toward normal. The degree of congestion and size of the left side of the heart on the chest film are useful for defining groups of patients with STEMI who are at increased risk of dying after the acute event.

Echocardiography

The relative portability of echocardiographic equipment makes this technique ideal for the assessment of patients with MI hospitalized in the coronary care unit or even in the emergency department before admission (see Chap. 15).[86] In patients with chest pain compatible with MI but with a nondiagnostic ECG, the finding of a distinct region of disordered contraction on echocardiography can be helpful diagnostically because it supports the diagnosis of myocardial ischemia. Echocardiography can also help evaluate patients with chest pain and a nondiagnostic ECG who are suspected of having an aortic dissection. The identification of an intimal flap consistent with an aortic dissection is a critical observation because it represents a major contraindication to fibrinolytic therapy (see Chap. 60). However, echocardiography has poor sensitivity for detection of the intimal flaps compared with other imaging modalities, such as CT angiography.

LV function estimated from echocardiograms correlates well with measurements from angiograms and is useful in establishing prognosis after MI.[86] Furthermore, the early use of echocardiography can aid in the early detection of potentially viable but stunned myocardium (contractile reserve), residual provocable ischemia, patients at risk for the development of congestive heart failure after MI, and mechanical complications of MI.

Although transthoracic imaging is adequate in most patients, occasional patients have poor echo windows, especially if they are undergoing mechanical ventilation. In such patients, transesophageal echocardiography can be safely performed and can be useful for evaluating ventricular septal defects and papillary muscle dysfunction.[33]

Doppler techniques allow the assessment of blood flow in the cardiac chambers and across cardiac valves. Used in conjunction with echocardiography, it can help detect and assess the severity of mitral or tricuspid regurgitation after STEMI. Identification of the site of acute ventricular septal rupture, quantification of shunt flow across the resulting defect, and assessment of acute cardiac tamponade are also possible.[33]

OTHER IMAGING MODALITIES

COMPUTED TOMOGRAPHY. This technique (see Chap. 19) can provide useful cross-sectional information in patients with MI. In addition to the assessment of cavity dimensions and wall thickness, LV aneurysms can be detected and, of particular importance in patients with STEMI, intracardiac thrombi can be identified. Although cardiac computed tomography is a less convenient technique, it probably is more sensitive than echocardiography for thrombus detection.

CARDIAC MAGNETIC RESONANCE IMAGING. In addition to localizing and sizing the area of infarction, cardiac magnetic resonance (CMR) techniques (see Chap. 18) permit early recognition of MI and can provide an assessment of the severity of the ischemic insult (see Fig. 56-5). This modality is attractive because it can assess perfusion of infarcted and noninfarcted tissue, as well as of reperfused myocardium; identify areas of jeopardized but not infarcted myocardium; identify myocardial edema, fibrosis, wall thinning, and hypertrophy; assess ventricular chamber size and segmental wall motion; and identify the temporal transition between ischemia and infarction (**Fig. 54-18**).[89] It has limited application during the acute phase because of the need to transport patients with MI to the MRI facility, but as discussed later, it is an extremely useful imaging technique during the subacute and chronic phases of MI.

Contrast-enhanced CMR can detect myocardial infarction accurately. The transmural extent of late gadolinium enhancement in regions of dysfunctional myocardium accurately predicts the likelihood of contractile recovery after successful restoration of coronary flow from mechanical revascularization.[90] Numerous clinical studies have also demonstrated high sensitivity of late gadolinium enhancement (delayed hyperenhancement) of CMR in detecting small amounts of myonecrosis. In patients with a prior MI, estimation of the size of the peri-infarct zone by CMR using the delayed enhancement technique provides incremental prognostic value beyond LV volumes and ejection fraction.[91] Beyond detecting infarction, this imaging technique can characterize the presence and size of microvascular obstruction from infarction, which portends an adverse clinical outcome postinfarction (see Fig. 18-4).[92] Clinically unrecognized myocardial scar detected by late gadolinium enhancement imaging is associated with a high risk of adverse cardiac events in patients with signs and symptoms of coronary artery disease but without a history of infarction.[93]

NUCLEAR IMAGING. Radionuclide angiography, perfusion imaging, infarct-avid scintigraphy, and positron emission tomography have been used to evaluate patients with STEMI (see Chap. 17).[94] Nuclear cardiac imaging techniques can be useful for detecting MI, assessing infarct size, collateral flow, and jeopardized myocardium, determining the effects of the infarct on ventricular function, and establishing a prognosis of patients with STEMI. However, the necessity of moving a critically ill patient from the coronary care unit to the nuclear medicine department limits practical application unless a portable gamma camera is available. Cardiac radionuclide imaging for the diagnosis of MI should be restricted to special limited situations in which the triad of clinical history, electrocardiographic findings, and serum marker measurements is unavailable or unreliable.

Estimation of Infarct Size

ELECTROCARDIOGRAPHY. Interest in limiting infarct size, in large part because of the recognition that the quantity of myocardium infarcted has important prognostic implications, has focused attention on the accurate determination of MI size. The sum of ST-segment elevations measured from multiple precordial leads correlates with the extent of myocardial injury in patients with anterior MI.[32] However,

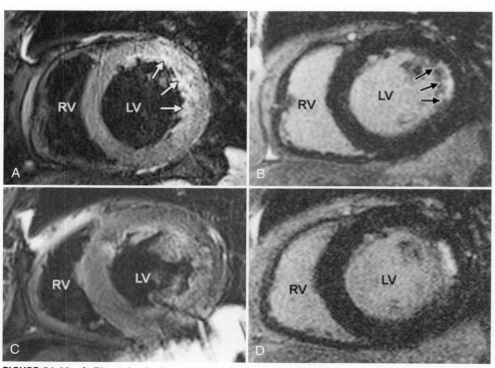

FIGURE 54-18 A, T2-weighted edema imaging showing acute transmural myocardial edema surrounding a subendocardial infarction *(arrows)* **(B)**. The patient suffered from an acute MI 2 days before the CMR, secondary to acute plaque rupture and thrombus formation in the proximal diagonal territory *(arrows)*. **C,** CMR was repeated 3 weeks after the initial presentation, showing marked resolution of the T2-weighted transmural myocardial edema. **D,** Infarct size is relatively unchanged compared with the first CMR study. *(Courtesy of Dr. Raymond Kwong, Brigham and Women's Hospital, Boston.)*

there is a relationship between the number of electrocardiographic leads showing ST-segment elevation and mortality rate. Patients with 8 or 9 of 12 leads with ST-segment elevation have 3 to 4 times the mortality of those with only 2 or 3 leads with ST-segment elevation. The duration of ischemia time, as estimated from continuous ST-segment monitoring, correlates with infarct size, ratio of infarct size to the area at risk, and extent of regional wall motion abnormality observed subsequently.[95]

SERUM CARDIAC MARKERS. Estimation of infarct size by the analysis of serum cardiac markers requires accounting for the quantity of the marker lost from the myocardium, its volume of distribution, and its release ratio. Serial measurements of proteins released by necrotic myocardium help determine MI size. Clinically, the peak CK or CK-MB value provides an approximate estimate of infarct size and is widely used prognostically. Coronary artery reperfusion dramatically changes the washout kinetics of CK and other markers from myocardium, resulting in early and exaggerated peak levels and limiting the usefulness of such curves as a measure of infarct size. Measuring a cardiac-specific troponin level several days after STEMI, even in cases of successful reperfusion, may provide a reliable estimate of infarct size, because such late troponin measurements reflect delayed release from the myofilament-bound pool in damaged myocytes.[96]

NONINVASIVE IMAGING TECHNIQUES. These imaging modalities can aid in the experimental and clinical assessment of infarct size.[94] Contrast-enhanced CMR can demonstrate regional heterogeneity of infarction patterns in patients with persistently occluded infarct arteries, compared with those with successfully reperfused vessels.[97]

REFERENCES

Changing Patterns in Clinical Care

1. Thygesen K, Alpert JS, White HD, et al: Universal definition of myocardial infarction. Circulation 116:2634, 2007.
2. Hochholzer W, Buettner HJ, Trenk D, et al: New definition of myocardial infarction: Impact on long-term mortality. Am J Med 121:399, 2008.
3. Morrow DA, Wiviott SD, White HD, et al: Effect of the novel thienopyridine prasugrel compared with clopidogrel on spontaneous and procedural myocardial infarction in the Trial to Assess Improvement in Therapeutic Outcomes by Optimizing Platelet Inhibition with Prasugrel-Thrombolysis in Myocardial Infarction 38: An application of the classification system from the universal definition of myocardial infarction. Circulation 119:2758, 2009.
4. Gaziano TA: Reducing the growing burden of cardiovascular disease in the developing world. Health Aff (Millwood) 26:13, 2007.
5. Lloyd-Jones D, Adams R, Carnethon M, et al: Heart disease and stroke statistics—2009 update: A report from the American Heart Association Statistics Committee and Stroke Statistics Subcommittee. Circulation 119:e21, 2009.
6. Napoli C, Cacciatore F: Novel pathogenic insights in the primary prevention of cardiovascular disease. Prog Cardiovasc Dis 51:503, 2009.
7. Goldberg RJ, Glatfelter K, Burbank-Schmidt E, et al: Trends in community mortality due to coronary heart disease. Am Heart J 151:501, 2006.
8. Kamalesh M, Subramanian U, Ariana A, et al: Similar decline in post-myocardial infarction mortality among subjects with and without diabetes. Am J Med Sci 329:228, 2005.
9. Myerson M, Coady S, Taylor H, et al: Declining severity of myocardial infarction from 1987 to 2002: The Atherosclerosis Risk in Communities (ARIC) Study. Circulation 119:503, 2009.
10. Anderson JL, Adams CD, Antman EM, et al: ACC/AHA 2007 guidelines for the management of patients with unstable angina/non-ST-elevation myocardial infarction: A report of the American College of Cardiology/American Heart Association Task Force on Practice Guidelines (Writing Committee to Revise the 2002 Guidelines for the Management of Patients With Unstable Angina/Non ST-Elevation Myocardial Infarction): Developed in collaboration with the American College of Emergency Physicians, the Society for Cardiovascular Angiography and Interventions, and the Society of Thoracic Surgeons: Endorsed by the American Association of Cardiovascular and Pulmonary Rehabilitation and the Society for Academic Emergency Medicine. Circulation 116:e148, 2007.
11. Braunwald E, Antman EM: Evidence-based coronary care. Ann Intern Med 126:551, 1997.
12. Antman EM, Peterson ED: Tools for guiding clinical practice from the American Heart Association and the American College of Cardiology: What are they and how should clinicians use them? Circulation 119:1180, 2009.
13. Krumholz HM, Anderson JL, Bachelder BL, et al: ACC/AHA 2008 performance measures for adults with ST-elevation and non-ST-elevation myocardial infarction: A report of the American College of Cardiology/American Heart Association Task Force on Performance Measures (Writing Committee to develop performance measures for ST-elevation and non-ST-elevation myocardial infarction): Developed in collaboration with the American Academy of Family Physicians and the American College of Emergency Physicians: Endorsed by the American Association of Cardiovascular and Pulmonary Rehabilitation, Society for Cardiovascular Angiography and Interventions, and Society of Hospital Medicine. Circulation 118:2596, 2008.
14. Kushner FG, Hand M, Smith SC Jr, et al: 2009 focused updates of the ACC/AHA guidelines for the management of patients with ST-elevation myocardial infarction (updating the 2004 guideline and 2007 focused update) and the ACC/AHA/SCAI guidelines on percutaneous coronary intervention (updating the 2005 guideline and 2007 focused update): A report of the American College of Cardiology Foundation/American Heart Association Task Force on Practice Guidelines. Circulation 120:2271, 2009.
15. Antman EM, Morrow DA, McCabe CH, et al: Enoxaparin versus unfractionated heparin with fibrinolysis for ST-elevation myocardial infarction. N Engl J Med 354:1477, 2006.
16. Canto JG, Rogers WJ, Chandra NC, et al: The association of sex and payer status on management and subsequent survival in acute myocardial infarction. Arch Intern Med 162:587, 2002.
17. Fox KA, Steg PG, Eagle KA, et al: Decline in rates of death and heart failure in acute coronary syndromes, 1999-2006. JAMA 297:1892, 2007.
18. Ahmed S, Antman EM, Murphy SA, et al: Poor outcomes after fibrinolytic therapy for ST-segment elevation myocardial infarction: Impact of age (a meta-analysis of a decade of trials). J Thromb Thrombolysis 21:119, 2006.
19. Orlandini A, Diaz R, Wojdyla D, et al: Outcomes of patients in clinical trials with ST-segment elevation myocardial infarction among countries with different gross national incomes. Eur Heart J 27:527, 2006.
20. Steinberg BA, Moghbeli N, Buros J, et al: Global outcomes of ST-elevation myocardial infarction: Comparisons of the Enoxaparin and Thrombolysis Reperfusion for Acute Myocardial Infarction Treatment-Thrombolysis In Myocardial Infarction study 25 (ExTRACT-TIMI 25) registry and trial. Am Heart J 154:54, 2007.
21. Birkhead JS, Weston C, Lowe D. Impact of specialty of admitting physician and type of hospital on care and outcome for myocardial infarction in England and Wales during 2004-5: Observational study. BMJ 332:1306, 2006.
22. Jani SM, Montoye C, Mehta R, et al: Sex differences in the application of evidence-based therapies for the treatment of acute myocardial infarction: The American College of Cardiology's Guidelines Applied in Practice projects in Michigan. Arch Intern Med 166:1164, 2006.

Pathology

23. Bayes de Luna A: Location of Q-wave myocardial infarction in the era of cardiac magnetic resonance imaging techniques: An update. J Electrocardiol 40:69, 2007.
24. Engblom H, Carlsson MB, Hedstrom E, et al: The endocardial extent of reperfused first-time myocardial infarction is more predictive of pathologic Q waves than is infarct transmurality: A magnetic resonance imaging study. Clin Physiol Funct Imaging 27:101, 2007.
25. Achenbach S: Can CT detect the vulnerable coronary plaque? Int J Cardiovasc Imaging 24:311, 2008.
26. Fox JJ, Strauss HW: One step closer to imaging vulnerable plaque in the coronary arteries. J Nucl Med 50:497, 2009.
27. Wasserman EJ, Shipley NM: Atherothrombosis in acute coronary syndromes: mechanisms, markers, and mediators of vulnerability. Mt Sinai J Med 73:431, 2006.
28. Katritsis DG, Pantos J, Efstathopoulos E: Hemodynamic factors and atheromatic plaque rupture in the coronary arteries: From vulnerable plaque to vulnerable coronary segment. Coron Artery Dis 18:229, 2007.
29. Wu AHB: Early detection of acute coronary syndromes and risk stratification by multimarker analysis. Biomarkers Med 1:45, 2007.
30. Barlis P, Serruys PW, Devries A, Regar E: Optical coherence tomography assessment of vulnerable plaque rupture: Predilection for the plaque 'shoulder'. Eur Heart J 29:2023, 2008.
31. Manfredini R, Boari B, Salmi R, et al: Circadian rhythms and reperfusion in patients with acute ST-segment elevation myocardial infarction. JAMA 294:2846, 2005.
32. Wagner GS, Macfarlane P, Wellens H, et al: AHA/ACCF/HRS recommendations for the standardization and interpretation of the electrocardiogram: Part VI: Acute ischemia/infarction: A scientific statement from the American Heart Association Electrocardiography and Arrhythmias Committee, Council on Clinical Cardiology; the American College of Cardiology Foundation; and the Heart Rhythm Society: Endorsed by the International Society for Computerized Electrocardiology. Circulation 119:e262, 2009.
33. Antman EM, Anbe DT, Armstrong PW, et al: ACC/AHA guidelines for the management of patients with ST-elevation myocardial infarction: A report of the American College of Cardiology/American Heart Association Task Force on Practice Guidelines (Committee to Revise the 1999 Guidelines for the Management of Patients with Acute Myocardial Infarction). Circulation 110:e82, 2004.
34. Chua S, Chang LT, Sun CK, et al: Time courses of subcellular signal transduction and cellular apoptosis in remote viable myocardium of rat left ventricles following acute myocardial infarction: Role of pharmacomodulation. J Cardiovasc Pharmacol Ther 14:104, 2009.
35. Schoen FJ: The heart. In Kumar V, Abbas AK, Fausto N (eds): Robbins & Cotran Pathologic Basis of Disease. 8th ed. Philadelphia, WB Saunders, 2010, pp 529-587.
36. Pasotti M, Prati F, Arbustini E: The pathology of myocardial infarction in the pre- and post-interventional era. Heart 92:1552, 2006.
37. Vargas SO, Sampson BA, Schoen FJ: Pathologic detection of early myocardial infarction: A critical review of the evolution and usefulness of modern techniques. Mod Pathol 12:635, 1999.
38. Abbate A, Bussani R, Sinagra G, et al: Right ventricular cardiomyocyte apoptosis in patients with acute myocardial infarction of the left ventricular wall. Am J Cardiol 102:658, 2008.
39. Noel TE, Kontos MC: Troponin and other markers of necrosis for risk stratification in patients with acute coronary syndromes. In de Lemos JA (ed): Biomarkers in Heart Disease. Oxford, Blackwell Publishing, 2008, pp 22-39.
40. DeWood MA, Spores J, Notske R, et al: Prevalence of total coronary occlusion during the early hours of transmural myocardial infarction. N Engl J Med 303:897, 1980.
41. Hamon M, Agostini D, Le Page O, Riddell JW: Prognostic impact of right ventricular involvement in patients with acute myocardial infarction: Meta-analysis. Crit Care Med 36:2023, 2008.
42. Popescu BA, Antonini-Canterin F, Temporelli PL, et al: Right ventricular functional recovery after acute myocardial infarction: Relation with left ventricular function and interventricular septum motion. GISSI-3 echo substudy. Heart 91:484, 2005.
43. Neven K, Crijns H, Gorgels A: Atrial infarction: A neglected electrocardiographic sign with important clinical implications. J Cardiovasc Electrophysiol 14:306, 2003.
44. Tjandrawidjaja MC, Fu Y, Kim DH, et al: Compromised atrial coronary anatomy is associated with atrial arrhythmias and atrioventricular block complicating acute myocardial infarction. J Electrocardiol 38:271, 2005.
45. Park SM, Prasad A, Rihal C, et al: Left ventricular systolic and diastolic function in patients with apical ballooning syndrome compared with patients with acute anterior ST-segment elevation myocardial infarction: A functional paradox. Mayo Clin Proc 84:514, 2009.

Pathophysiology

46. Schuster EH, Bulkley BH: Ischemia at a distance after acute myocardial infarction: A cause of early postinfarction angina. Circulation 62:509, 1980.

47. Forrester JS, Wyatt HL, Da Luz PL, et al: Functional significance of regional ischemic contraction abnormalities. Circulation 54:64, 1976.

48. Funaro S, La Torre G, Madonna M, et al: Incidence, determinants, and prognostic value of reverse left ventricular remodelling after primary percutaneous coronary intervention: results of the Acute Myocardial Infarction Contrast Imaging (AMICI) multicenter study. Eur Heart J 30:566, 2009.

49. McMurray J, Solomon S, Pieper K, et al: The effect of valsartan, captopril, or both on atherosclerotic events after acute myocardial infarction: An analysis of the Valsartan in Acute Myocardial Infarction Trial (VALIANT). J Am Coll Cardiol 47:726, 2006.

50. Hochman JS: Cardiogenic shock complicating acute myocardial infarction: Expanding the paradigm. Circulation 107:2998, 2003.

51. Ruan W, Lu L, Zhang Q, et al: Serial assessment of left ventricular remodeling and function by echo-tissue Doppler imaging after myocardial infarction in streptozotocin-induced diabetic swing. J Am Soc Echocardiogr 22:530, 2009.

52. Weisman HF, Bush DE, Mannisi JA, et al: Cellular mechanisms of myocardial infarct expansion. Circulation 78:186, 1988.

53. Konstam MA: Patterns of ventricular remodeling after myocardial infarction: Clues toward linkage between mechanism and morbidity. JACC Cardiovasc Imaging 1:592, 2008.

54. Kosiborod M, Inzucchi SE, Krumholz HM, et al: Glucose normalization and outcomes in patients with acute myocardial infarction. Arch Intern Med 169:438, 2009.

55. Hofsten DE, Logstrup BB, Moller JE, et al: Abnormal glucose metabolism in acute myocardial infarction: Influence on LV function and prognosis. JACC Cardiovasc Imaging 2:592, 2009.

56. Lorgis L, Zeller M, Dentan G, et al: Prognostic value of N-terminal pro-brain natriuretic peptide in elderly people with acute myocardial infarction: Prospective observational study. BMJ 338:b1605, 2009.

57. White HD, Chew DP: Acute myocardial infarction. Lancet 372:570, 2008.

58. Smit JJ, Ottervanger JP, Kolkman JJ, et al: Change of white blood cell count more prognostic important than baseline values after primary percutaneous coronary intervention for ST-segment elevation myocardial infarction. Thromb Res 122:185, 2008.

Clinical Features

59. Bodis J, Boncz I, Kriszbacher I: Permanent stress may be the trigger of an acute myocardial infarction on the first work-day of the week. Int J Cardiol 2009.

60. Fleischmann KE, Beckman JA, Buller CE, et al: ACCF/AHA 2009 focused update on perioperative beta blockade: A report of the American College of Cardiology Foundation/American Heart Association Task Force on Practice Guidelines. Circulation 120:2123, 2009.

61. Assali AR, Brosh D, Vaknin-Assa H, et al: The impact of circadian variation on outcomes in emergency acute anterior myocardial infarction percutaneous coronary intervention. Catheter Cardiovasc Interv 67:221, 2006.

62. Leiza JR, de Llano JM, Messa JB, et al: New insights into the circadian rhythm of acute myocardial infarction in subgroups. Chronobiol Int 24:129, 2007.

63. Feringa HH, Karagiannis SE, Vidakovic R, et al: The prevalence and prognosis of unrecognized myocardial infarction and silent myocardial ischemia in patients undergoing major vascular surgery. Coron Artery Dis 18:571, 2007.

64. Killip T 3rd, Kimball JT: Treatment of myocardial infarction in a coronary care unit. A two-year experience with 250 patients. Am J Cardiol 20:457, 1967.

65. Montalescot G, Wiviott SD, Braunwald E, et al: Prasugrel compared with clopidogrel in patients undergoing percutaneous coronary intervention for ST-elevation myocardial infarction (TRITON-TIMI 38): Double-blind, randomised controlled trial. Lancet 373:723, 2009.

66. Dorfman TA, Aqel R: Regional pericarditis: A review of the pericardial manifestations of acute myocardial infarction. Clin Cardiol 32:115, 2009.

67. Ravkilde J, Horder M, Gerhardt W, et al: Diagnostic performance and prognostic value of serum troponin T in suspected acute myocardial infarction. Scand J Clin Lab Invest 53:677, 1993.

68. Antman EM: Decision making with cardiac troponin tests. N Engl J Med 346:2079, 2002.

69. Jaffe AS, Babuin L, Apple FS: Biomarkers in acute cardiac disease: The present and the future. J Am Coll Cardiol 48:1, 2006.

70. Penttila K, Koukkunen H, Halinen M, et al: Myoglobin, creatine kinase MB isoforms and creatine kinase MB mass in early diagnosis of myocardial infarction in patients with acute chest pain. Clin Biochem 35:647, 2002.

71. Apple FS, Quist HE, Doyle PJ, et al: Plasma 99th percentile reference limits for cardiac troponin and creatine kinase MB mass for use with European Society of Cardiology/American College of Cardiology consensus recommendations. Clin Chem 49:1331, 2003.

72. Apple FS: Tissue specificity of cardiac troponin I, cardiac troponin T and creatine kinase-MB. Clin Chim Acta 284:151, 1999.

73. Roberts R, Kleiman NS: Earlier diagnosis and treatment of acute myocardial infarction necessitates the need for a 'new diagnostic mind-set.' Circulation 89:872, 1994.

74. Morrow DA, Cannon CP, Jesse RL, et al: National Academy of Clinical Biochemistry Laboratory Medicine Practice Guidelines: Clinical characteristics and utilization of biochemical markers in acute coronary syndromes. Circulation 115:e356, 2007.

75. Aviles RJ, Askari AT, Lindahl B, et al: Troponin T levels in patients with acute coronary syndromes, with or without renal dysfunction. N Engl J Med 346:2047, 2002.

76. Jaffe AS, Van Eyk JE: Degradation of cardiac troponins: implications for clinical practice. In Morrow DA (ed): Cardiovascular Biomarkers: Pathophysiology and Disease Management. Totowa, NJ, Humana Press, 2006, pp 161-174.

77. Wolfrum S, Jensen KS, Liao JK: Endothelium-dependent effects of statins. Arterioscler Thromb Vasc Biol 23:729, 2003.

78. Smith SC Jr, Allen J, Blair SN, et al: AHA/ACC guidelines for secondary prevention for patients with coronary and other atherosclerotic vascular disease: 2006 update: Endorsed by the National Heart, Lung and Blood Institute. Circulation 113:2363, 2006.

79. Barron HV, Cannon CP, Murphy SA, et al: Association between white blood cell count, epicardial blood flow, myocardial perfusion, and clinical outcomes in the setting of acute myocardial infarction: A thrombolysis in myocardial infarction 10 substudy. Circulation 102:2329, 2000.

80. Ziakas A, Gavrilidis S, Giannoglou G, et al: In-hospital and long-term prognostic value of fibrinogen, CRP, and IL-6 levels in patients with acute myocardial infarction treated with thrombolysis. Angiology 57:283, 2006.

81. Sabatine MS, Morrow DA, Giugliano RP, et al: Association of hemoglobin levels with clinical outcomes in acute coronary syndromes. Circulation 111:2042, 2005.

82. Zimetbaum PJ, Josephson ME: Use of the electrocardiogram in acute myocardial infarction. N Engl J Med 348:933, 2003.

83. Scirica BM, Morrow DA, Sadowski Z, et al: A strategy of using enoxaparin as adjunctive antithrombin therapy reduces death and recurrent myocardial infarction in patients who achieve early ST-segment resolution after fibrinolytic therapy: The ExTRACT-TIMI 25 ECG study. Eur Heart J 28:2070, 2007.

84. Bayes de Luna A, Wagner G, Birnbaum Y, et al: A new terminology for left ventricular walls and location of myocardial infarcts that present Q wave based on the standard of cardiac magnetic resonance imaging: A statement for health care professionals from a committee appointed by the International Society for Holter and Noninvasive Electrocardiography. Circulation 114:1755, 2006.

85. Moon JC, De Arenaza DP, Elkington AG, et al: The pathologic basis of Q-wave and non-Q-wave myocardial infarction: A cardiovascular magnetic resonance study. J Am Coll Cardiol 44:554, 2004.

86. Cheitlin MD, Armstrong WF, Aurigemma GP, et al: ACC/AHA/ASE 2003 Guideline Update for the Clinical Application of Echocardiography: Summary article. A report of the American College of Cardiology/American Heart Association Task Force on Practice Guidelines (ACC/AHA/ASE Committee to Update the 1997 Guidelines for the Clinical Application of Echocardiography). J Am Soc Echocardiogr 16:1091, 2003.

87. Lopez-Sendon J, Coma-Canella I, Alcasena S, et al: Electrocardiographic findings in acute right ventricular infarction: Sensitivity and specificity of electrocardiographic alterations in right precordial leads V4R, V3R, V1, V2, and V3. J Am Coll Cardiol 6:1273, 1985.

88. Finn AV, Antman EM: Images in clinical medicine. Isolated right ventricular infarction. N Engl J Med 349:1636, 2003.

89. Ibrahim T, Makowski MR, Jankauskas A, et al: Serial contrast-enhanced cardiac magnetic resonance imaging demonstrates regression of hyperenhancement within the coronary artery wall in patients after acute myocardial infarction. JACC Cardiovasc Imaging 2:580, 2009.

90. Silva C, Cacciavillani L, Corbetti F, et al: Natural time course of myocardial infarction at delayed enhancement magnetic resonance. Int J Cardiol 2009.

91. Yan AT, Shayne AJ, Brown KA, et al: Characterization of the peri-infarct zone by contrast-enhanced cardiac magnetic resonance imaging is a powerful predictor of post-myocardial infarction mortality. Circulation 114:32, 2006.

92. Habis M, Capderou A, Sigal-Cinqualbre A, et al: Comparison of delayed enhancement patterns on multislice computed tomography immediately after coronary angiography and cardiac magnetic resonance imaging in acute myocardial infarction. Heart 95:624, 2009.

93. Kwong RY, Chan AK, Brown KA, et al: Impact of unrecognized myocardial scar detected by cardiac magnetic resonance imaging on event-free survival in patients presenting with signs or symptoms of coronary artery disease. Circulation 113:2733, 2006.

94. Klocke FJ, Baird MG, Lorell BH, et al: ACC/AHA/ASNC guidelines for the clinical use of cardiac radionuclide imaging: A report of the American College of Cardiology/American Heart Association Task Force on Practice Guidelines (ACC/AHA/ASNC Committee to Revise the 1995 Guidelines for the Clinical Use of Radionuclide Imaging). Circulation 108:1404, 2003.

95. Krucoff MW, Johanson P, Baeza R, et al: Clinical utility of serial and continuous ST-segment recovery assessment in patients with acute ST-elevation myocardial infarction: assessing the dynamics of epicardial and myocardial reperfusion. Circulation 110:e533, 2004.

96. Giannitsis E, Katus HA: Biomarkers of necrosis for risk assessment and management of ST-elevation myocardial infarction. In Morrow DA (ed): Cardiovascular Biomarkers: Pathophysiology and Disease Management. Totowa, NJ, Humana Press, 2006, pp 119-128.

97. Baur LH: Magnetic resonance imaging of persistent myocardial obstruction after myocardial infarction. A tool becoming increasingly important in clinical cardiology? Int J Cardiovasc Imaging 25:549, 2009.

CHAPTER **55** # ST-Segment Elevation Myocardial Infarction: Management

Elliott M. Antman and David A. Morrow

Despite considerable advances in the care for patients with ST-segment elevation myocardial infarction (STEMI),[1-4] room for improvement exists, especially in special populations such as older adults, women, members of ethnic minority groups, and those with a low education level and low socioeconomic status.[5-7] A discussion of the phases of management of STEMI can follow the chronology of the interface of clinicians with the patient. Chap. 49 deals with the primary and secondary prevention of coronary artery disease. This chapter deals with the treatment at the time of onset of STEMI (prehospital issues, initial recognition and management in the emergency department, and reperfusion), hospital management (medications, arrhythmias, complications, and preparation for discharge), and secondary prevention after STEMI. Chap. 58 discusses percutaneous coronary intervention (PCI) in patients with STEMI.

Prehospital and Initial Management

Given the progressive loss of functioning myocytes with persistent occlusion of the infarct-related artery in STEMI (see Chap. 54), the initial management aims to restore blood flow to the infarct zone. Despite some deficiencies in the evidence base for selection of a reperfusion strategy, it is generally accepted that primary PCI is the preferred option, provided it can be delivered in a timely fashion by an experienced operator (>75 PCI procedures/year) and team (at least 200 PCI procedures/year, including at least 36 primary PCI procedures/year).[1,8] Missed opportunities for improvement of care for STEMI include failure to deliver any form of reperfusion therapy in about 30% of patients and failure to minimize delays in reperfusion because of perpetuation of inefficient systems of care.[2,9,10] The chain of survival for STEMI involves a highly integrated strategy, beginning with patient education about the symptoms of STEMI (see Chap. 54) and early contact with the medical system, coordination of destination protocols in emergency medical services (EMS) systems, efficient practices in emergency departments to shorten door-to-reperfusion time, and expeditious implementation of the reperfusion strategy by a trained team.[11-14] The next major breakthrough in the care of patients with STEMI will more likely come from the implementation of systems that shorten total ischemic time than from modifying adjunctive therapies that complement a reperfusion strategy or deal with the consequences of the infarction.[15-17] Much like the clinical research enterprise has been reorganized around translational steps, we must now follow a road map for the transformation of reperfusion therapy for STEMI (**Table 55-1**). The American Heart Association has launched a national initiative to engineer improved health care delivery for STEMI and

proposed the criteria for an ideal STEMI system (**Table 55-2**). When considering such initiatives to streamline timely delivery of reperfusion therapies, it is also important to focus on overall quality of care measures for STEMI.[18]

PREHOSPITAL CARE. The prehospital care of patients with suspected STEMI is a crucial element bearing directly on the likelihood of survival. Most deaths associated with STEMI occur within the first hour of its onset and are usually caused by ventricular fibrillation (see Chap. 41). Hence, the immediate implementation of definitive resuscitative efforts and of rapidly transporting the patient to a hospital is of prime importance. Major components of the delay from the onset of symptoms consistent with acute myocardial infarction (MI) to reperfusion include the following[1]: (1) the time for the patient to recognize the seriousness of the problem and seek medical attention; (2) prehospital evaluation, treatment, and transportation; (3) the time for diagnostic measures and initiation of treatment in the hospital (e.g., door-to-needle time for patients receiving a fibrinolytic agent and door-to-balloon time for patients undergoing a catheter-based reperfusion strategy); and (4) the time from initiation of treatment to restoration of flow (**Fig. 55-1**).

Patient-related factors that correlate with a longer time to the decision to seek medical attention include the following: older age; female sex; black race; low socioeconomic status; low emotional or somatic awareness; history of angina, diabetes, or both; consulting a spouse or other relative; and consulting a physician.[19,20] Health care professionals should heighten the level of awareness of patients at risk for STEMI (e.g., those with hypertension, diabetes, history of angina pectoris).[1,14] They should use each patient encounter as a teachable moment to review and reinforce with patients and their families the need to seek urgent medical attention for a pattern of symptoms, including chest discomfort, extreme fatigue, and dyspnea, especially if accompanied by diaphoresis, lightheadedness, palpitations, or a sense of impending doom. Although many patients shun such discussions and tend to minimize the likelihood of ever needing emergency cardiac treatment, emphasis should be placed on the prevention and treatment of potentially fatal arrhythmias, as well as salvage of the jeopardized myocardium by reperfusion, for which time is crucial.[21] Patients should also be instructed in the proper use of sublingual nitroglycerin and to call 911 emergency services if the ischemic-type discomfort persists for longer than 5 minutes.[22]

EMERGENCY MEDICAL SERVICES SYSTEMS. These systems have three major components—emergency medical dispatch, first

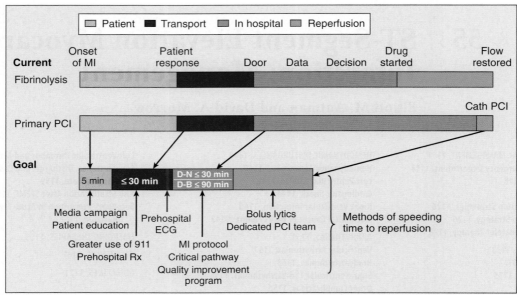

FIGURE 55-1 Major components of time delay between onset of infarction and restoration of flow in the infarct-related artery. Plotted sequentially from left to right are the time for patients to recognize symptoms and seek medical attention, transportation to the hospital, in-hospital decision making and implementing reperfusion strategy, and time for restoration of flow once the reperfusion strategy has been initiated. The time to initiate fibrinolytic therapy is the door-to-needle (D-N) time; this is followed by the period of time required for pharmacological restoration of flow. More time is required to move the patient to the catheterization laboratory for a PCI procedure, referred to as the door-to-balloon (D-B) time, but restoration of flow in the epicardial infarct-related artery occurs promptly after PCI. **Bottom,** Various methods for speeding the time to reperfusion are shown, along with the goals for the time intervals for the various components of the time delay. (*Modified from Antman EM, Anbe DT, Armstrong PW, et al: ACC/AHA guidelines for the management of patients with ST-elevation myocardial infarction: A report of the American College of Cardiology/American Heart Association Task Force on Practice Guidelines [Committee to Revise the 1999 Guidelines for the Management of Patients with Acute Myocardial Infarction]. Circulation 110:e82, 2004.*)

TABLE 55-1	Translational Approach to Systems of Care for STEMI	
TRANSLATIONAL STEP	**KEY ASPECTS OF TRANSLATIONAL STEP**	**REPERFUSION FOR STEMI**
1	Activity to test what care works: • Clinical efficacy research	Randomized clinical trials of fibrinolysis and catheter-based therapies
2	Activities to test who benefits from providing care: • Outcomes research • Comparative effectiveness research • Health services research	Registries such as the joint ACC/AHA ACTION-GWTG Registry
3	Activities to test how to deliver high-quality care reliably and in all settings: • Measurement and accountability of health care quality and cost • Implementation of interventions and health care system redesign • Scaling and spread of effective interventions • Research in above domains	ACC D2B Alliance; AHA Mission: Lifeline

ACC = American College of Cardiology; ACTION = Acute Coronary Treatment and Intervention Outcomes Network; AHA = American Heart Association; D2B = door-to-balloon; GWTG = Get With the Guidelines.
Modified from Dougherty D, Conway PH: The "3T's" road map to transform US health care: the "how" of high-quality care. JAMA 299:2319, 2008; and Antman EM: Time is muscle: translation into practice. J Am Coll Cardiol 52:1216, 2008.

TABLE 55-2	Criteria for a STEMI System of Care

1. The system should be registered with Mission: Lifeline.
2. There should be ongoing multidisciplinary team meetings that include EMS, non-PCI hospitals and STEMI referral centers, and PCI hospitals and STEMI receiving centers to evaluate outcomes and quality improvement data. Operational issues should be reviewed, problems identified, and solutions implemented.
3. Each STEMI system should include a process for prehospital identification and activation, destination protocols to STEMI receiving centers, and transfer for patients who arrive at STEMI referral centers and are primary PCI candidates and/or are fibrinolytic-ineligible and/or in cardiogenic shock.
4. Each system should have a recognized system coordinator, physician champion, and EMS medical director.
5. Each system component (EMS, STEMI referral centers and STEMI receiving centers) should meet the appropriate criteria.[13]

Modified from American Heart Association, Mission: Lifeline, 2010 (http://www.heart.org/HEARTORG/HealthcareProfessional/Mission-Lifeline-Home-Page_UCM_305495_SubHomePage.jsp).

arrival places EMS efforts at the center of the early response to STEMI.[24,25] Ongoing efforts to shorten the time to treatment of patients with STEMI include improvement in the medical dispatch component by expanding 911 coverage, providing automated external defibrillators to first responders, placing automated external defibrillators in critical public locations, and greater coordination of EMS ambulance response.[26,27] Well-equipped ambulances and helicopters staffed by personnel trained in the acute care of the STEMI patient allow definitive therapy to commence while the patient is being transported to the hospital (**Table 55-3**). To serve effectively, EMS units must be placed strategically within a community and have excellent radio communication systems. These units should be equipped with battery-operated monitoring equipment, a DC defibrillator, oxygen, endotracheal tubes and suction apparatus, and commonly used cardiovascular drugs. Radiotelemetry systems that allow transmission of the electrocardiographic signal to a medical control officer are highly desirable to facilitate triage of STEMI patients and are becoming increasingly

response, and EMS ambulance response. A major advance in the contribution of EMS systems is the expansion of the capability to record a prehospital 12-lead electrocardiogram (ECG).[23] The ability to transmit such ECGs and to activate the STEMI care team prior to hospital

TABLE 55-3   Reperfusion Checklist for Evaluation of the STEMI Patient

Step 1:

Has patient experienced chest discomfort for >15 min and <12 hr?

YES   NO

STOP

Step 2:

Are there contraindications to fibrinolysis?
If *ANY* of the following are checked, fibrinolysis *may* be contraindicated.

	YES	NO
Systolic blood pressure >180 mm Hg	☐ YES	☐ NO
Diastolic blood pressure >110 mm Hg	☐ YES	☐ NO
Right versus left arm systolic blood pressure difference >15 mm Hg	☐ YES	☐ NO
History of structural central nervous system disease	☐ YES	☐ NO
Significant closed head/facial trauma within the previous 3 mo	☐ YES	☐ NO
Recent (within 6 wk) major trauma, surgery (including laser eye surgery), gastrointestinal or genitourinary bleed	☐ YES	☐ NO
Bleeding or clotting problem on blood thinners	☐ YES	☐ NO
CPR more than 10 min	☐ YES	☐ NO
Pregnant female	☐ YES	☐ NO
Serious systemic disease (e.g., advanced/terminal cancer, severe liver or kidney disease)	☐ YES	☐ NO

Step 3:

Does the patient have severe heart failure or cardiogenic shock such that percutaneous coronary intervention is preferable?

	YES	NO
Pulmonary edema (rales more than halfway up)	☐ YES	☐ NO
Systemic hypoperfusion (cold, clammy)	☐ YES	☐ NO

CPR = cardiopulmonary resuscitation.
From Antman EM, Anbe DT, Armstrong PW, et al: ACC/AHA guidelines for the management of patients with ST-elevation myocardial infarction: A report of the American College of Cardiology/American Heart Association Task Force on Practice Guidelines (Committee to Revise the 1999 Guidelines for the Management of Patients with Acute Myocardial Infarction) Circulation 110:e82, 2004.

available in many communities (**Fig. 55-2**). Observations of simple variables such as age, heart rate, and blood pressure permit initial classification of patients into high- or low-risk subgroups.[28]

In addition to prompt defibrillation, the efficacy of prehospital care appears to depend on several factors, including early relief of pain with its deleterious physiologic sequelae, reduction of excessive activity of the autonomic nervous system, and abolition of prelethal arrhythmias such as ventricular tachycardia. Such efforts must not, however, impede rapid transfer to the hospital (see Fig. 55-2).

PREHOSPITAL FIBRINOLYSIS. Several randomized trials have evaluated the potential benefits of prehospital versus in-hospital fibrinolysis. Although none of the individual trials showed a significant reduction in mortality with prehospital-initiated fibrinolytic therapy, earlier treatment generally provides greater benefit; a meta-analysis of all the available trials demonstrated a 17% reduction in mortality. The CAPTIM trial reported a trend toward a lower rate of mortality among STEMI patients receiving prehospital fibrinolysis as compared with primary PCI, especially if patients were treated within 2 hours of the onset of symptoms.[1] Several registry reports have provided additional support for the benefit of prehospital lysis.[29-31]

Several factors enter consideration of whether ambulances and emergency transport vehicles should initiate fibrinolytic therapy. The greatest reduction in mortality is observed when reperfusion can be initiated within 60 to 90 minutes of the onset of symptoms.[1] Streamlining of emergency department triage practices so that treatment can be started within 30 minutes, when coupled with the 15- to

30-minute transport time that is common in most urban centers, may be more cost-effective than equipping all ambulances to administer prehospital fibrinolytic therapy (see Fig. 55-2).[19,20] The latter would require extensive training of personnel (see Table 55-3), installation of computer-assisted electrocardiography or systems for radio transmission of the electrocardiographic signal to a central station, and stocking of medicine kits with the necessary drug supplies. In some communities, in which transport delays may be 60 to 90 minutes or longer and experienced personnel are available on ambulances, prehospital fibrinolytic therapy is beneficial. Therefore, prehospital fibrinolysis is reasonable in settings in which physicians are present in the ambulance or there is a well-organized EMS system with full-time paramedics, capability for obtaining and transmitting 12-lead electrocardiographic readings from the field, and online medical command to authorize prehospital fibrinolysis.[32,33]

Management in the Emergency Department

When evaluating patients in the emergency department, physicians must confront the difficult task of rapidly identifying patients who require urgent reperfusion therapy, triaging lower-risk patients to the appropriate facility within the hospital, and not discharging patients inappropriately, while avoiding unnecessary admissions. A history of ischemic-type discomfort and the initial 12-lead ECG are the primary tools for screening patients with acute coronary syndromes in the emergency department.[34] More extensive use of prehospital 12-lead electrocardiographic recordings facilitate triage of STEMI patients in

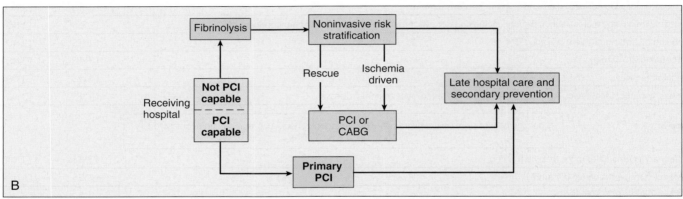

FIGURE 55-2 Options for transporting STEMI patients and initial reperfusion treatment. Reperfusion in patients with STEMI can be accomplished by the pharmacologic (fibrinolysis) or catheter-based (PCI) approach. Implementation of these strategies varies based on the mode of transportation of the patient and capabilities at the receiving hospital. **A,** Patient transported by EMS after calling 911. Transport time to the hospital varies from case to case, but the goal is to keep total ischemic time <120 minutes. There are three options: (1) If EMS has fibrinolytic capability and the patient qualifies for therapy, prehospital fibrinolysis should be started within 30 minutes of EMS arrival on scene. (2) If EMS is not capable of administering prehospital fibrinolysis and the patient is transported to a non–PCI-capable hospital, the hospital door-to-needle time should be ≤30 minutes for patients in whom fibrinolysis is indicated. (3) If EMS cannot administer prehospital fibrinolysis and the patient is transported to a PCI-capable hospital, the hospital door-to-balloon time should be ≤90 minutes. *Interhospital transfer:* It is also appropriate to consider emergency interhospital transfer of the patient to a PCI-capable hospital for mechanical revascularization if (1) there is a contraindication to fibrinolysis, (2) PCI can be initiated promptly (≤90 minutes after the patient presents to the initial receiving hospital or ≤60 minutes compared to when fibrinolysis could be initiated at the initial receiving hospital), or (3) fibrinolysis is administered and is unsuccessful (i.e., rescue PCI). Secondary nonemergency interhospital transfer can be considered for recurrent ischemia **(B).** *Patient self-transport:* Patient self-transportation is discouraged. If the patient arrives at a non–PCI-capable hospital, the door-to-needle time should be ≤30 minutes. If the patient arrives at a PCI-capable hospital, the door-to-balloon time should be ≤90 minutes. The treatment options and time recommendations after first hospital arrival are the same. **B,** For patients who receive fibrinolysis, noninvasive risk stratification is recommended to identify the need for rescue PCI (failed fibrinolysis) or ischemia-driven PCI. Regardless of the initial method of reperfusion treatment, all patients should receive late hospital care and secondary prevention of STEMI. †The medical system goal is to facilitate rapid recognition and treatment of patients with STEMI so that door-to-needle (or EMS-to-needle) for initiation of fibrinolytic therapy can be achieved within 30 minutes, or that door-to-balloon (or EMS-to-balloon) or PCI can be achieved within 90 minutes. These goals should not be understood as ideal times, but rather the longest times that should be considered acceptable for a given system. Systems that can achieve even more rapid times for treatment of patients with STEMI should be encouraged. *(Modified from Armstrong PW, Collen D, Antman E: Fibrinolysis for acute myocardial infarction: The future is here and now. Circulation 107:2533, 2003; and Antman EM, Anbe DT, Armstrong PW, et al: ACC/AHA guidelines for the management of patients with ST-elevation myocardial infarction: A report of the American College of Cardiology/American Heart Association Task Force on Practice Guidelines [Committee to Revise the 1999 Guidelines for the Management of Patients with Acute Myocardial Infarction]. Circulation 110:e82, 2004.)*

the emergency department.[23] ST-segment elevation on the ECG of a patient with ischemic discomfort highly suggests thrombotic occlusion of an epicardial coronary artery, and its presence should serve as the trigger for a well-rehearsed sequence of rapid assessment of the patient for contraindications to fibrinolysis and initiation of a reperfusion strategy (**Tables 55-4** and **55-5**).[1] Because the 12-lead ECG is at the center of the decision pathway for initiation of reperfusion therapy, it should be obtained promptly (≤10 minutes) in patients presenting with ischemic discomfort.

Because lethal arrhythmias can occur suddenly in patients with STEMI, all patients should be attached to a bedside electrocardiographic monitor and intravenous access should be obtained. If the initial reading shows ST-segment elevation of 1 mm or more in at least two contiguous leads or a new or presumably new left bundle branch block, the patient should be evaluated immediately for a reperfusion strategy. Critical factors that weigh into the selection of a reperfusion strategy include the following: (1) the time elapsed since the onset of symptoms; (2) the risk associated with STEMI; (3) the risk of

TABLE 55-4 Assessment of Reperfusion Options for STEMI Patients

Step 1: Assess time and risk.
- Time since onset of symptoms
- Risk of STEMI
- Risk of fibrinolysis
- Time required for transport to a skilled PCI laboratory

Step 2: Determine if fibrinolysis or invasive strategy is preferred.
- *If presentation is <3 hr and there is no delay to an invasive strategy, there is no preference for either strategy.*

Fibrinolysis is generally preferred if:
- Early presentation (≤3 hr from symptom onset and delay to invasive strategy; see below)
- Invasive strategy is not an option:
  - Catheterization laboratory occupied or not available
  - Vascular access difficulties
  - Lack of access to a skilled PCI laboratory*†
- Delay to invasive strategy:
  - Prolonged transport
  - (Door-to-balloon)–(door-to-needle) more than 1 hr‡§
  - Medical contact-to-balloon or door-to-balloon more than 90 min

An invasive strategy is generally preferred if:
- Skilled PCI laboratory is available with surgical backup
  - Skilled PCI laboratory is available, defined by†‡
  - Medical contact-to-balloon or door-to-balloon less than 90 min
  - (Door-to-balloon)–(door-to-needle) less than 1 hr‡
- High risk from STEMI
  - Cardiogenic shock
  - Killip class ≥ 3
- Contraindications to fibrinolysis, including increased risk of bleeding and ICH
- Late presentation
  - Symptom onset was more than 3 hr ago
- Diagnosis of STEMI is in doubt

*Operator experience > a total of 75 primary PCI cases/yr.
†Team experience > a total of 36 primary PCI cases/yr.
‡Applies to fibrin-specific agents.
§This calculation implies that the estimated delay to the implementation of the invasive strategy is >1 hr versus immediate initiation of fibrinolytic therapy.
ICH = intracranial hemorrhage.
From Antman EM, Anbe DT, Armstrong PW, et al: ACC/AHA guidelines for the management of patients with ST-elevation myocardial infarction: A report of the American College of Cardiology/American Heart Association Task Force on Practice Guidelines (Committee to Revise the 1999 Guidelines for the Management of Patients with Acute Myocardial Infarction) Circulation 110:e82, 2004.

TABLE 55-5 Contraindications and Cautions for Fibrinolytic Use in STEMI*

Absolute Contraindications
- Any prior intracranial hemorrhage
- Known structural cerebral vascular lesion (e.g., arteriovenous malformation)
- Known malignant intracranial neoplasm (primary or metastatic)
- Ischemic stroke within 3 mo *except* acute ischemic stroke within 3 hr
- Suspected aortic dissection
- Active bleeding or bleeding diathesis (excluding menses)
- Significant closed head or facial trauma within 3 mo

Relative Contraindications
- History of chronic severe poorly controlled hypertension
- Severe uncontrolled hypertension on presentation (SBP >180 mm Hg or DBP >110 mm Hg)†
- History of prior ischemic stroke > 3 mo, dementia, or known intracranial pathology not covered in contraindications
- Traumatic or prolonged (>10 min) CPR or major surgery (<3 wk)
- Recent (within 2-4 wk) internal bleeding
- Noncompressible vascular punctures
- For streptokinase, anistreplase: Prior exposure (>5 days ago) or prior allergic reaction to these agents
- Pregnancy
- Active peptic ulcer
- Current use of anticoagulants: the higher the INR, the higher the risk of bleeding

*Viewed as advisory for clinical decision-making and may not be all-inclusive or definitive.
†Could be an absolute contraindication in low-risk patients with myocardial infarction.
CPR = cardiopulmonary resuscitation; DBP = diastolic blood pressure; INR = international normalized ratio; SBP = systolic blood pressure.
From Antman EM, Anbe DT, Armstrong PW, et al: ACC/AHA guidelines for the management of patients with ST-elevation myocardial infarction: A report of the American College of Cardiology/American Heart Association Task Force on Practice Guidelines (Committee to Revise the 1999 Guidelines for the Management of Patients with Acute Myocardial Infarction). Circulation 110:e82, 2004.

administering a fibrinolytic; and (4) the time required to initiate an invasive strategy (see Table 55-4).

Given the importance of time to reperfusion,[8] the concept of medical system goals has arisen.[13] Benchmarks for medical systems to use when assessing the quality of their performance are a door-to-needle time of less than or equal to 30 minutes for initiation of fibrinolytic therapy and a door-to-balloon time of less than or equal to 90 minutes for percutaneous coronary perfusion (see Fig. 55-2).[35-37] Increasing sophistication of EMS systems facilitates initiating the process of evaluation and implementation of a reperfusion strategy even before the patient arrives in the emergency department.[23] For those patients transported by ambulance, the medical system goals can be restated as an EMS-to-needle time of less than or equal to 30 minutes for initiation of fibrinolysis and an EMS-to-balloon time of less than or equal to 90 minutes for initiation of PCI (see Fig. 55-2).[1,38]

Patients with an initial electrocardiographic reading that reveals new or presumably new ST-segment depression and/or T wave inversion, although not considered candidates for fibrinolytic therapy, should be treated as though they are suffering from MI without ST-segment elevation or unstable angina (a distinction to be made subsequently after scrutiny of serial ECGs and cardiac biomarker measurements; see Chap. 56).

In patients with a clinical history suggestive of STEMI (see Chap. 54) and an initial nondiagnostic electrocardiographic reading (i.e., no ST-segment deviation or T wave inversion), serial tracings should be obtained while the patients are being evaluated in the emergency department. Emergency department staff can be alerted to the sudden development of ST-segment elevation by periodic visual inspection of the bedside electrocardiographic monitor, by continuous ST-segment recording, or by auditory alarms when the ST-segment deviation exceeds programmed limits. Decision aids such as computer-based diagnostic algorithms, identification of high-risk clinical indicators, rapid determination of cardiac biomarkers, echocardiographic screening for regional wall motion abnormalities, and myocardial perfusion imaging have greatest clinical usefulness when the electrocardiographic reading is nondiagnostic. In an effort to improve the cost-effectiveness of care of patients with a chest pain syndrome, nondiagnostic electrocardiographic reading, and low suspicion of MI, but in whom the diagnosis has not been entirely excluded, many medical centers have developed critical pathways that involve a coronary observation unit with a goal of ruling out MI in less than 12 hours.[39,40]

GENERAL TREATMENT MEASURES

Aspirin

Aspirin is useful not only for the primary prevention of vascular events (see Chap. 49) but is also effective across the entire spectrum of acute coronary syndromes and forms part of the initial management strategy for patients with suspected STEMI (see Chap. 87). Because low doses (40 to 80 mg) take several days to achieve full antiplatelet effect, at least 162 to 325 mg should be administered acutely in the emergency department.[1] To achieve therapeutic blood levels rapidly, the patient should chew the tablet to promote buccal absorption rather than absorption through the gastric mucosa.[41]

Control of Cardiac Pain

Management of STEMI patients in the emergency department should aim to relieve pain. A tendency to underdose the patient for fear of obscuring response to antiischemic or reperfusion therapy should be avoided because pain heightens sympathetic activity during the early phase of STEMI. Control of cardiac pain typically uses a combination of nitrates, analgesics (e.g., morphine), oxygen, and in appropriately selected patients, beta-adrenergic blocking agents (referred to hereafter as beta blockers).[35] Similar pharmacologic principles apply in the coronary care unit, where many of the therapies discussed herein should continue after initial dosing in the emergency department. Because the pain associated with STEMI is related to ongoing ischemia, many interventions that improve the oxygen supply-demand relationship (by increasing supply or decreasing demand) can alleviate the cause of pain.

ANALGESICS. Although a wide variety of analgesic agents has been used to treat the pain associated with STEMI, including meperidine, pentazocine, and morphine, morphine remains the drug of choice, except in patients with well-documented morphine hypersensitivity. A dose of 4 to 8 mg should be administered intravenously, and doses of 2 to 8 mg should be repeated at intervals of 5 to 15 minutes until the pain is relieved or there is evident toxicity—hypotension, depression of respiration, or severe vomiting—which should preclude further administration of the drug.

The reduction of anxiety resulting from morphine diminishes the patient's restlessness and activity of the autonomic nervous system, with a consequent reduction of the heart's metabolic demands. Morphine has unequivocal beneficial effects in patients with pulmonary edema because of peripheral arterial and venous dilation (particularly among patients with excessive sympathoadrenal activity), reduction of the work of breathing, and slowing of heart rate secondary to combined withdrawal of sympathetic tone and augmentation of vagal tone.

Hypotension following the administration of nitroglycerin and morphine can be minimized by maintaining the patient in a supine position and elevating the lower extremities if systolic arterial pressure declines below 100 mm Hg. Such positioning is undesirable in the presence of pulmonary edema, but morphine rarely produces hypotension under these circumstances. The concomitant administration of atropine in doses of 0.5 to 1.5 mg intravenously may be helpful in treating eventual excessive vagomimetic effects of morphine, particularly when hypotension and bradycardia are present before it is administered.[1] Respiratory depression is an unusual complication of morphine in the presence of severe pain or pulmonary edema, but as the patient's cardiovascular status improves, impairment of ventilation may supervene. It can be treated with naloxone, in doses of 0.1 to 0.2 mg intravenous initially, repeated after 15 minutes if necessary. Nausea and vomiting may be troublesome side effects of large doses of morphine and can be treated with a phenothiazine.

NITRATES. Because of their ability to enhance coronary blood flow by coronary vasodilation and to decrease ventricular preload by increasing venous capacitance, sublingual nitrates are indicated for most patients with an acute coronary syndrome. At present, the only groups of patients with STEMI in whom sublingual nitroglycerin should *not* be given are those with inferior MI and suspected right ventricular infarction[42] or marked hypotension (systolic pressure <90 mm Hg), especially if accompanied by bradycardia.

Once hypotension is excluded, a sublingual nitroglycerin tablet should be administered and the patient observed for improvement in symptoms or change in hemodynamics. If an initial dose is well tolerated and appears to be of benefit, further nitrates should be administered, with monitoring of the vital signs. Even small doses can produce sudden hypotension and bradycardia, a reaction that can be life-threatening but is usually easily reversed with intravenous atropine if recognized quickly. Long-acting oral nitrate preparations should be avoided in the early course of STEMI because of the frequently changing hemodynamic status of the patient. In patients with a prolonged period of waxing and waning chest pain, intravenous nitroglycerin may help to control symptoms and correct ischemia, but requires frequent monitoring of blood pressure.

BETA BLOCKERS. Beta blockers relieve ischemic pain, reduce the need for analgesics in many patients, and reduce infarct size and life-threatening arrhythmias. Avoiding early intravenous beta blockade in patients presenting in Killip class II or higher is important, however,

because of the risk of precipitating cardiogenic shock.[1,43,44] A popular and relatively safe protocol for the use of a beta blocker in this situation is as follows:

1. Patients with heart failure (rales > 10 cm up from diaphragm), hypotension (blood pressure < 90 mm Hg), bradycardia (heart rate < 60 beats/min), or first-degree atrioventricular (AV) block (PR interval > 0.24 second) are first excluded.
2. Metoprolol is given in three 5-mg intravenous boluses.
3. Patients are observed for 2 to 5 minutes after each bolus and, if the heart rate falls below 60 beats/min or systolic blood pressure falls below 100 mm Hg, no further drug is given.
4. If hemodynamic stability continues 15 minutes after the last intravenous dose, the patient is begun on oral metoprolol, 50 mg every 6 hours for 2 days, and then switched to 100 mg twice daily.

An infusion of an extremely short-acting beta blocker, esmolol (50 to 250 μg/kg/min), may be useful for patients with relative contraindications to beta blocker administration in whom heart rate slowing is considered highly desirable.

OXYGEN. Hypoxemia can occur in patients with STEMI and usually results from ventilation-perfusion abnormalities that are sequelae of left ventricular failure; pneumonia and intrinsic pulmonary disease are additional causes of hypoxemia. Treating all patients hospitalized with STEMI with oxygen for at least 24 to 48 hours is common practice on the basis of the empiric assumption of hypoxia and evidence that increased oxygen in the inspired air may protect ischemic myocardium. But this practice may not be cost-effective. Augmentation of the fraction of oxygen in the inspired air does not elevate oxygen delivery significantly in patients who are not hypoxemic. Furthermore, it may increase systemic vascular resistance and arterial pressure and thereby lower cardiac output slightly.

In view of these considerations, arterial oxygen saturation can be estimated by pulse oximetry, and oxygen therapy can be omitted if it is normal. On the other hand, oxygen should be administered to patients with STEMI when arterial hypoxemia is clinically evident or can be documented by measurement (e.g., SaO_2 < 90%).[1] In these patients, serial arterial blood gas measurements can be employed to follow the efficacy of oxygen therapy. The delivery of 2 to 4 liters/min of 100% oxygen by mask or nasal prongs for 6 to 12 hours is satisfactory for most patients with mild hypoxemia. If arterial oxygenation is still depressed on this regimen, the flow rate may have to be increased, and other causes for hypoxemia should be sought. In patients with pulmonary edema, endotracheal intubation and positive-pressure controlled ventilation may be necessary.

LIMITATION OF INFARCT SIZE. Infarct size is an important determinant of prognosis in patients with STEMI. Patients who succumb from cardiogenic shock generally exhibit a single massive infarct or a small to moderate-sized infarct superimposed on multiple prior infarctions.[45] Survivors with large infarcts frequently exhibit late impairment of ventricular function, and the long-term mortality rate is higher than for survivors with small infarcts, who tend not to develop cardiac decompensation.[46]

In view of the prognostic importance of infarct size, the possibility of modification of infarct size has attracted a great deal of experimental and clinical attention (see Fig. 54-9).[8,12,47] Efforts to limit infarct size have been divided among several different (sometimes overlapping) approaches: (1) early reperfusion; (2) reduction of myocardial energy demands; (3) manipulation of sources of energy production in the myocardium; and (4) prevention of reperfusion injury. Despite the many advances in reperfusion therapy for STEMI, practical clinical decision making for individual patients is complex. Persistent uncertainties about the risk (bleeding)-benefit balance in older patients and those arriving late after the onset of symptoms appear to be the major factors explaining the underuse of reperfusion for STEMI in routine practice.[48]

Dynamic Nature of Infarction

STEMI is a dynamic process that does not occur instantaneously but evolves over hours. The fate of jeopardized ischemic tissue can be affected favorably by interventions that restore myocardial perfusion, reduce microvascular damage in the infarct zone, reduce myocardial oxygen requirements, inhibit accumulation of or facilitate washout of noxious metabolites, augment the availability of substrate for anaerobic metabolism, or blunt the effects of mediators of injury that compromise the structure and function of intracellular organelles and constituents of cell membranes. Strong evidence in experimental animals and suggestive evidence in patients have indicated that ischemic preconditioning, a form of endogenous protection against STEMI (see Chap. 24), before sustained coronary occlusion decreases infarct size and is associated with a more favorable outcome, with decreased risk of extension of infarction and recurrent ischemic events. Brief episodes of ischemia in one coronary vascular bed may precondition myocardium in a remote zone, attenuating the size of infarction in the latter when sustained coronary occlusion occurs.[49]

The perfusion of the myocardium in the infarct zone appears to be reduced maximally immediately following coronary occlusion. Up to one third of patients develop spontaneous recanalization of an occluded infarct-related artery beginning at 12 to 24 hours. This delayed spontaneous reperfusion may improve left ventricular function because it improves healing of infarcted tissue, prevents ventricular remodeling, and reperfuses hibernating myocardium. To maximize the amount of salvaged myocardium by accelerating the process of reperfusion and also implementing it in those patients who would otherwise have an occluded infarct-related artery, the strategies of pharmacologically induced and catheter-based reperfusion of the infarct vessel have been developed (**Fig. 55-3**; see Chap. 58). An overarching concept that applies to all methods of reperfusion is the critical importance of time. Mortality reduction from STEMI is highest the earlier the infarct artery is reperfused (**Fig. 55-4**).[47]

Additional factors that may contribute to limitation of infarct size in association with reperfusion include relief of coronary spasm, prevention of damage to the microvasculature, improved systemic hemodynamics (augmentation of coronary perfusion pressure and reduced left ventricular end-diastolic pressure), and development of collateral circulation. The prompt implementation of measures designed to protect ischemic myocardium and support myocardial perfusion may provide sufficient time for the development of anatomic and physiologic compensatory mechanisms that limit the ultimate extent of infarction (see Chap. 54). Interventions designed to protect ischemic myocardium during the initial event may also reduce the incidence of extension of infarction or early reinfarction.

Routine Measures for Infarct Size Limitation

Although timely reperfusion of ischemic myocardium is the most important technique for limiting infarct size, several routine measures to accomplish this goal apply to all patients with STEMI, whether or not they receive reperfusion therapy. The treatment strategies discussed in this section can be initiated in the emergency department and then continued in the coronary care unit.

It is important to maintain an optimal balance between myocardial oxygen supply and demand so that as much as possible of the jeopardized zone of the myocardium surrounding the most profoundly ischemic zones of the infarct can be salvaged. During the period before irreversible injury has occurred, myocardial oxygen consumption should be minimized by maintaining the patient at rest, physically and emotionally, and by using mild sedation and a quiet atmosphere that may lower heart rate, a major determinant of myocardial oxygen consumption. If the patient was receiving a beta blocker when the clinical manifestations of the infarction commenced, the drug should be continued unless a specific contraindication is noted, such as left ventricular systolic failure or bradyarrhythmia.[35] Marked sinus bradycardia (heart rate ≤ 50 beats/min) and the frequently coexisting hypotension should be treated with postural maneuvers (the Trendelenburg position) to increase central blood volume and with atropine and electrical pacing, but not with isoproterenol. On the other hand, the routine administration of atropine, with the resultant increase in heart rate, to patients without serious bradycardia is contraindicated. All forms of tachyarrhythmias require prompt treatment because they increase myocardial oxygen needs.[1]

Congestive heart failure should be treated promptly. Given their multiple beneficial actions in STEMI patients, inhibitors of the

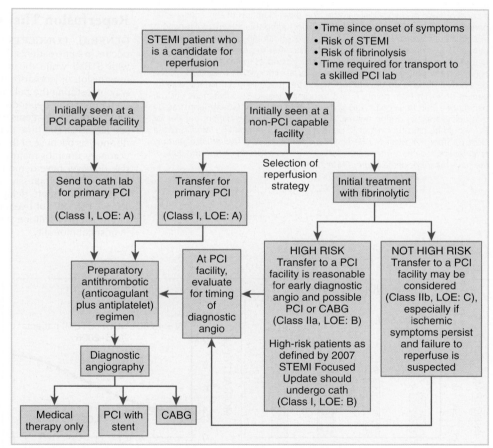

FIGURE 55-3 Each community, and each facility in that community, should have an agreed-on plan for how STEMI patients are to be treated. This plan should include which hospitals should do the following: (1) receive STEMI patients from EMS units capable of obtaining diagnostic ECGs, management at the initial receiving hospital, and written criteria and agreement for expeditious transfer of patients from non–PCI-capable to PCI-capable facilities; and (2) consider initiating a preparatory pharmacologic regimen as soon as possible in preparation for and during patient transfer to a catheterization laboratory. The optimal regimen is not yet established, although published studies (see text for details) have used various combinations of anticoagulants, oral antiplatelet agents, and IV antiplatelets. LOE = level of evidence. (*From Kushner FG, Hand M, Smith SC Jr, et al: 2009 Focused Updates: ACC/AHA Guidelines for the Management of Patients With ST-Elevation Myocardial Infarction (updating the 2004 Guideline and 2007 Focused Update) and ACC/AHA/SCAI Guidelines on Percutaneous Coronary Intervention [updating the 2005 Guideline and 2007 Focused Update]: A report of the American College of Cardiology Foundation/American Heart Association Task Force on Practice Guidelines. Circulation 120:2271, 2009.*)

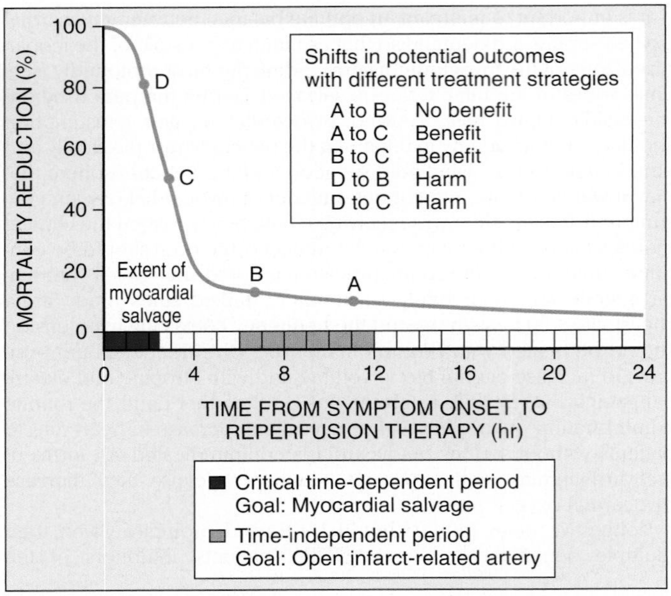

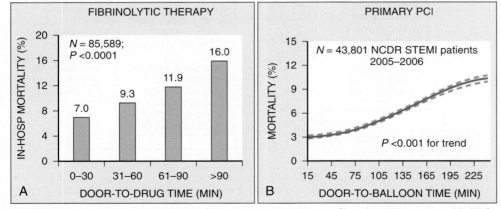

FIGURE 55-4 Mortality reduction as a benefit of reperfusion therapy is greatest in the first 2 to 3 hours after the onset of symptoms of acute MI, most likely a consequence of myocardial salvage. The exact duration of this critical early period may be modified by several factors, including the presence of functioning collateral coronary arteries, ischemic preconditioning, myocardial oxygen demands, and duration of sustained ischemia. After this early period, the magnitude of the mortality benefit is much reduced and, as the mortality reduction curve flattens, time to reperfusion therapy is less critical. The magnitude of the benefit will depend on how far up the curve the patient can be shifted. The benefit of a shift from points A or B to point C would be substantial, but the benefit of a shift from point A to point B would be small. A treatment strategy that delays therapy during the early critical period, such as patient transfer for PCI, would be harmful (shift from point D to point C or point B). *(Modified from Gersh BJ, Stone GW, White HD, Homes DR Jr: Pharmacological facilitation of primary percutaneous coronary intervention for acute myocardial infarction: Is the slope of the curve the shape of the future? JAMA 293:979, 2005.)*

renin-angiotensin-aldosterone system (RAAS) are indicated for the treatment of congestive heart failure associated with STEMI unless the patient is hypotensive. Inotropic agents that increase myocardial oxygen consumption (e.g., isoproterenol) should be avoided.

Arterial oxygenation should be restored to normal in patients with hypoxemia, such as occurs in patients with chronic pulmonary disease, pneumonia, or left ventricular failure. Oxygen-enriched air should be administered to patients with hypoxemia, and bronchodilators and expectorants should be used when indicated. Severe anemia, which also can extend the area of ischemic injury, should be corrected by the cautious administration of packed red blood cells, accompanied by a diuretic if there is any evidence of left ventricular failure. Associated conditions, particularly infections and the accompanying tachycardia, fever, and elevated myocardial oxygen needs, require immediate attention.

Systolic arterial pressure should not be allowed to deviate by more than approximately 25 to 30 mm Hg from the patient's usual level unless marked hypertension had been present before the onset of STEMI. It is likely that each patient has an optimal range of arterial pressure; as coronary perfusion pressure deviates from this level, the unfavorable balance that ensues between oxygen supply (which is related to coronary perfusion pressure) and myocardial oxygen demand (which is related to ventricular wall tension) increases the extent of ischemic injury.

Reperfusion Therapy

GENERAL CONCEPTS. Although late spontaneous reperfusion occurs in some patients, thrombotic occlusion persists in most patients with STEMI while the myocardium is undergoing necrosis. Timely reperfusion of jeopardized myocardium represents the most effective way of restoring the balance between myocardial oxygen supply and demand.[2,47] The dependence of myocardial salvage on time to treatment pertains to patients treated with fibrinolysis or PCI[1,12,50] (**Fig. 55-5**; see Fig. 55-4). The time dependence may be particularly critical with fibrinolysis because of the decreasing efficacy of fibrinolytic agents as coronary thrombi mature over time. Analyses adjusting for baseline risk, however, have demonstrated a statistically significant increase in mortality with progressive delays between the onset of symptoms and PCI. Each 30-minute delay from symptom onset to PCI increases the relative risk (RR) of 1-year mortality by 8%. Similarly, progressive delays in the door-to-balloon time have a significant adverse effect on in-hospital mortality.

FIGURE 55-5 Importance of time to reperfusion in patients undergoing fibrinolysis **(A)** or primary PCI **(B)** for STEMI. **A,** Graph based on data from 85,589 patients treated with fibrinolysis. For every 30-minute delay, there is a progressive increase in the in-hospital mortality rate. **B,** Based on data from 43,801 patients, this depicts the adjusted in-hospital mortality rate as a function of door-to-balloon time. Estimated mortality ranged from 3% with a door-to-balloon time of 30 minutes to 10.3% for patients with a door-to-balloon time of 240 minutes. NCDR = National Cardiovascular Data Registry. *(Data from Cannon CP, Gibson CM, Lambrew CT, et al: Relationship of symptom-onset-to-balloon time and door-to-balloon time with mortality in patients undergoing angioplasty for acute myocardial infarction. JAMA 283:2941, 2000; and Rathore SS, Curtis J, Chen J, et al: Association of door-to-balloon time and mortality in patients admitted to hospital with ST elevation myocardial infarction: National cohort study. BMJ 338:b1807, 2009.)*

In some patients, particularly those with cardiogenic shock, tissue damage occurs in a stuttering manner rather than abruptly, a condition that might more properly be termed *subacute infarction*. This concept of the nature of the infarction process, as well as the observation that the incidence of complications of STEMI in the early and late postinfarction periods is a function of infarct size, underscores the need for careful history taking to ascertain whether the patient appears to have had repetitive cycles of spontaneous reperfusion and reocclusion. Determining the time of onset of the infarction process in such patients can be difficult. In such patients, with waxing and waning ischemic discomfort, a rigid time interval from the first episode of pain should not be used when determining whether a patient is outside the window for benefit from acute reperfusion therapy.

PATHOPHYSIOLOGY OF MYOCARDIAL REPERFUSION. Prevention of cell death by the restoration of blood flow depends on the severity and duration of preexisting ischemia. Substantial experimental and clinical evidence has indicated that the earlier blood flow is restored, the more favorably influenced are recovery of left ventricular systolic function, improvement in diastolic function, and reduction in overall mortality.[12,51] Collateral coronary vessels also appear to influence left ventricular function following reperfusion.[52] They provide sufficient perfusion of myocardium to retard cell death and are probably of greater importance in patients having reperfusion later rather than 1 to 2 hours after coronary occlusion. Even after successful reperfusion and despite the absence of irreversible myocardial damage, a period of postischemic contractile dysfunction can occur, a phenomenon termed *myocardial stunning*.[53] Periods of myocardial stunning have been well described in experimental animals but also apply to STEMI patients who undergo PCI.

REPERFUSION INJURY. The process of reperfusion, although beneficial in terms of myocardial salvage, may come at a cost because of a process known as reperfusion injury.[54] Several types of reperfusion injury have been observed in experimental animals.[55] These consist of the following: (1) lethal reperfusion injury—reperfusion-induced death of cells that were still viable at the time of restoration of coronary blood flow; (2) vascular reperfusion injury—progressive damage to the microvasculature so that there is an expanding area of no reflow and loss of coronary vasodilatory reserve; (3) stunned myocardium—salvaged myocytes display a prolonged period of contractile dysfunction following restoration of blood flow because of abnormalities of intracellular metabolism leading to reduced energy production; and (4) reperfusion arrhythmias—bursts of ventricular tachycardia and, on occasion, ventricular fibrillation—that occur within seconds of reperfusion.[56] The available evidence suggests that vascular reperfusion injury, stunning, and reperfusion arrhythmias can all occur in patients with STEMI. The concept of lethal reperfusion injury of potentially salvageable myocardium remains controversial in experimental animals and in patients.[57]

Reperfusion increases the cell swelling that occurs with ischemia. Reperfusion of the myocardium in which the microvasculature is damaged leads to the creation of a hemorrhagic infarct (see Chap. 54). Fibrinolytic therapy appears more likely to produce hemorrhagic infarction than catheter-based reperfusion. Although concern has been raised that this hemorrhage may lead to extension of the infarct, this does not appear to be the case. Histologic study of patients not surviving in spite of successful reperfusion has revealed hemorrhagic infarcts, but this hemorrhage usually does not extend beyond the area of necrosis.

Protection Against Reperfusion Injury

A variety of adjunctive approaches may protect the myocardium against injury that occurs after reperfusion: (1) preservation of microvascular integrity by using antiplatelet agents and antithrombins to minimize embolization of atheroembolic debris; (2) prevention of inflammatory damage; and (3) metabolic support of the ischemic myocardium.[58] The effectiveness of agents directed against reperfusion injury rapidly declines the later they are administered after reperfusion[59]; eventually, no beneficial effect is detectable in animal models after 45 to 60 minutes of reperfusion has elapsed.

An alternative experimental approach to protection against reperfusion injury is called postconditioning, which involves introducing brief repetitive episodes of ischemia alternating with reperfusion.[60] This appears to activate a number of cellular protective mechanisms centering around prosurvival kinases.[61] Many of these protective kinases are also activated during ischemic preconditioning. Clinical studies in STEMI patients undergoing PCI have provided evidence that postconditioning protects the human heart and is associated with a reduction in infarct size and improvement in myocardial perfusion.[62]

REPERFUSION ARRHYTHMIAS. Transient sinus bradycardia occurs in many patients with inferior infarcts at the time of acute reperfusion; it is most often accompanied by some degree of hypotension. This combination of hypotension and bradycardia with a sudden increase in coronary flow may involve activation of the Bezold-Jarisch reflex.[63] Premature ventricular contractions, accelerated idioventricular rhythm, and nonsustained ventricular tachycardia also commonly follow successful reperfusion. Although some investigators have postulated that early afterdepolarizations participate in the genesis of reperfusion ventricular arrhythmias, early afterdepolarizations are present during ischemia and reperfusion and are therefore unlikely to be involved in the development of reperfusion ventricular tachycardia or fibrillation.

When present, rhythm disturbances may actually indicate successful restoration of coronary flow. While reperfusion arrhythmias have a high sensitivity for detecting successful reperfusion, the high incidence of identical rhythm disturbances in patients without successful coronary artery reperfusion limits their specificity for detection of restoration of coronary blood flow. In general, clinical features are poor markers of reperfusion, with no single clinical finding or constellation of findings being reliably predictive of angiographically demonstrated coronary artery patency.[1]

Although reperfusion arrhythmias may show a temporal clustering at the time of restoration of coronary blood flow in patients with successful fibrinolysis, the overall incidence of such arrhythmias appears to be similar in patients not receiving a fibrinolytic agent who may develop these arrhythmias as a consequence of spontaneous coronary artery reperfusion or the evolution of the infarct process itself. These considerations, as well as the fact that the brief electrical storm occurring at the time of reperfusion is generally innocuous, indicate that no prophylactic antiarrhythmic therapy is necessary when fibrinolytics are prescribed.

LATE ESTABLISHMENT OF PATENCY OF THE INFARCT VESSEL. Improved survival and ventricular function after successful reperfusion may not result entirely from limitation of infarct size.[64] Poorly contracting or noncontracting myocardium in a zone that is supplied by a stenosed infarct-related artery with slow antegrade perfusion may still contain viable myocytes. This situation is referred to as hibernating myocardium,[65] and its function can be improved by PCI to augment flow in the infarct-related artery.

SUMMARY OF EFFECTS OF MYOCARDIAL REPERFUSION. Plaque disruption in the culprit vessel produces complete occlusion of the infarct-related coronary artery. STEMI occurs with the ensuing development of left ventricular dilation and ultimate death through a combination of pump failure and electrical instability (**Fig. 55-6**; see Chap. 54). Early reperfusion shortens the duration of coronary occlusion, minimizes the degree of ultimate left ventricular dysfunction and dilation, and reduces the probability that the STEMI patient will develop pump failure or malignant ventricular tachyarrhythmias. Late reperfusion of stenosed infarct arteries may restore contractile function in hibernating myocardium.[65]

Fibrinolysis

Fibrinolysis recanalizes thrombotic occlusion associated with STEMI, and restoration of coronary flow reduces infarct size and improves myocardial function and survival over the short and the long term.[66,67] Most of the mortality benefit seen at 10-year follow-up in the GISSI trial

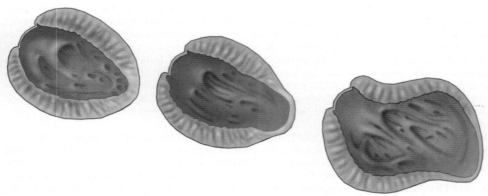

FIGURE 55-6 Remodeling of left ventricle after STEMI. **Left,** Apical STEMI (white zone of left ventricle). Over time, the infarct zone elongates and thins. Progressive remodeling of the left ventricle occurs **(center and right),** ultimately converting the left ventricle from an oval shape to a spherical shape. Pharmacologic and catheter-based reperfusion strategies for STEMI have a favorable impact on this process by minimizing the extent of myocardial necrosis **(left)** through prompt restoration of flow in the epicardial infarct vessel. *(Modified from McMurray JJV, Pfeffer MA [eds]: Heart Failure Updates. London, Martin Dunitz, 2003.)*

was obtained before hospital discharge because no survival difference was seen in fibrinolysed and control patients discharged alive except for those treated within the first hour after onset of symptoms.[1]

INTRACORONARY FIBRINOLYSIS. In current practice, patients are more likely to be treated by PCI. This has reopened the concept of delivering fibrinolytic agents via the intracoronary route, but such efforts at present are largely restricted to adjunctive use during complicated PCI procedures.[68]

INTRAVENOUS FIBRINOLYSIS

Thrombolysis in Myocardial Infarction Flow Grade

To provide a level of standardization for comparison of the various regimens, most investigators describe the flow in the infarct vessel according to the Thrombolysis in Myocardial Infarction (TIMI) trial grading system: grade 0, complete occlusion of the infarct-related artery; grade 1, some penetration of the contrast material beyond the point of obstruction but without perfusion of the distal coronary bed; grade 2, perfusion of the entire infarct vessel into the distal bed but with delayed flow compared with a normal artery; and grade 3, full perfusion of the infarct vessel with normal flow.[69] When evaluating reports of angiographic studies of fibrinolytic agents, it must be noted that only in studies in which a pretreatment coronary arteriogram documents occlusion of the culprit vessel can the term *recanalization* be applied if flow is restored. If the status of the culprit vessel is not known before treatment, one can only ascertain the patency rate of the vessel at the moment that the contrast material is injected. This snapshot in time does not reflect the fluctuating status of flow in the infarct vessel that characteristically undergoes repeated cycles of patency and reocclusion, as has been documented angiographically and by continuous ST-segment monitoring.

Issues of the fluctuating nature of patency of the infarct-related artery notwithstanding, most angiographic studies of reperfusion regimens for STEMI have used an assessment of the TIMI flow grade at 90 or preferably 60 minutes after the start of fibrinolytic therapy.[2,66] TIMI grade 3 flow is far superior to grade 2 in terms of infarct size reduction and short- and long-term mortality benefit. Therefore, TIMI grade 3 flow should be the goal when assessing flow in the epicardial infarct artery **(Fig. 55-7).**

TIMI Frame Count

To provide a more quantitative statement of the briskness of coronary blood flow in the infarct artery and to account for differences in the size and length of vessels (e.g., left anterior descending versus right

coronary artery) and interobserver variability, Gibson and colleagues[70] have developed the TIMI frame count, a simple count of the number of angiographic frames elapsed until the contrast material arrives in the distal bed of the vessel of interest. This objective and quantitative index of coronary blood flow independently predicts in-hospital mortality from STEMI and also discriminates patients with TIMI grade 3 flow into low-risk and high-risk groups. Using the TIMI frame count, they determined that the following are univariate predictors of delayed coronary blood flow after fibrinolytic administration: greater percentage diameter stenosis; decreased minimum lumen diameter; greater percentage of the culprit artery distal to stenosis; and presence of delayed achievement of patency, a culprit artery location in the left coronary circulation, pulsatile flow (i.e., reversible flow in systole), or intraluminal thrombus. The TIMI frame count can also be used to quantitate coronary blood flow (mL/second), as calculated by the following:

$$(21 \div \text{observed TIMI frame count}) \times 1.7$$

This is based on Doppler velocity wire data showing that normal flow equals 1.7 cm³/second, which is proportional to 21 frames. Calculated coronary perfusion relates to mortality for patients treated with

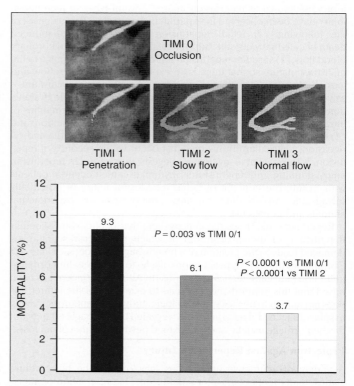

FIGURE 55-7 Correlation of TIMI flow grade and mortality. A pooled analysis of data from 5498 patients in several angiographic trials of reperfusion for STEMI showed a gradient of mortality when the angiographic findings were stratified by TIMI flow grade. Patients with TIMI 0 or TIMI 1 flow had the highest rate of mortality, TIMI 2 flow was associated with an intermediate rate of mortality, and the lowest rate of mortality was observed in patients with TIMI 3 flow. TIMI = Thrombolysis in Myocardial Infarction. *(Dr. Michael Gibson, personal communication, 2008.)*

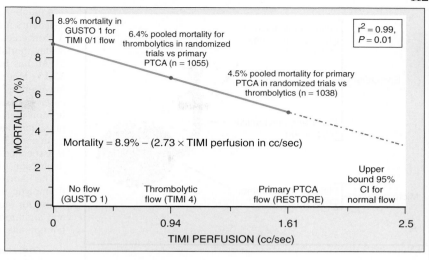

FIGURE 55-8 Relationship between coronary blood flow and mortality rate in patients with acute myocardial infarction. PTCA = percutaneous transluminal coronary angioplasty. *(From Gibson CM: Primary angioplasty, rescue angioplasty, and new devices. In Hennekens CH [ed]: Clinical Trials in Cardiovascular Disease: A Companion to Braunwald's Heart Disease. Philadelphia, WB Saunders, 1999, p 194.)*

fibrinolytics or primary PCI and serves to assess various modalities for reperfusion in STEMI (**Fig. 55-8**).

Myocardial Perfusion

Despite intense interest in the development of reperfusion regimens that normalize flow in the epicardial infarct-related artery, reperfusion in patients with STEMI aims to improve actual myocardial perfusion in the infarct zone. Myocardial perfusion cannot be improved adequately without restoration of flow in the occluded infarct-related artery. Yet, even patients with TIMI grade 3 flow may not achieve adequate myocardial perfusion, especially if there is a great delay between the onset of symptoms and restoration of epicardial flow.[71] The term *myocardial no-reflow* has been used to describe the state in which there is reduced myocardial perfusion after opening of an epicardial infarct artery.[72] The two major impediments to normalization of myocardial perfusion are microvascular damage (**Fig. 55-9**) and reperfusion injury. Obstruction of the distal microvasculature in the downstream bed of the infarct-related artery is caused by platelet microemboli and thrombi.[73] Fibrinolysis may actually exacerbate microembolization of platelet aggregates because of the exposure of clot-bound thrombin, an extremely potent platelet agonist. Spasm can also occur in the microvasculature because of the release of substances from activated platelets. Reperfusion injury results in cellular edema, formation of reactive oxygen species, and calcium overload. In addition, cytokine activation leads to neutrophil accumulation and inflammatory mediators that contribute to tissue injury.

Several techniques can evaluate the adequacy of myocardial perfusion. Electrocardiographic ST-segment resolution strongly predicts outcome in STEMI patients but is a better predictor of an occluded artery than of a patent infarct-related artery.[74,75] The absence of early ST-segment resolution after angiographically successful primary PCI identifies patients with a higher risk of left ventricular dysfunction and mortality, presumably because of microvascular damage in the infarct zone. Thus, the 12-lead ECG is a marker of the biologic integrity of myocytes in the infarct zone and can reflect inadequate myocardial perfusion, even in the presence of TIMI grade 3 flow.[71] ST-segment resolution in combination with cardiac biomarkers (e.g., troponins, natriuretic peptides) provides powerful prognostic information early in the management of STEMI patients.[76] Given the dynamic nature of coronary occlusion, continuous ST-segment monitoring may prove more informative than static 12-lead electrocardiographic recordings, but practical limitations have prevented continuous ST-segment monitoring in widespread clinical application.[77] Defects in perfusion patterns seen with myocardial contrast echocardiography correlate with regional wall motion abnormalities and lack of myocardial viability on dobutamine stress echocardiography. A practical

limitation to myocardial contrast echocardiography is the need for intracoronary injection of echo contrast, although this can be circumvented by the availability of new echo contrast agents that can be injected intravenously. Doppler flow wire studies, cardiac magnetic resonance (CMR), and nuclear imaging with positron emission tomography can also define abnormalities of myocardial perfusion.

An angiographic method for assessing myocardial perfusion has been developed by Gibson and coworkers,[71] the TIMI myocardial perfusion (TMP) grade (**Fig. 55-10**). Abnormalities of increasing myocardial perfusion as assessed by the TMP grade correlate with mortality risk even after adjusting for the presence of TIMI grade 3 flow or a normal TIMI frame count.

EFFECT OF FIBRINOLYTIC THERAPY ON MORTALITY. Early intravenous fibrinolysis undoubtedly improves survival in patients with STEMI.[1] Mortality varies considerably, depending on the patients included for study and the adjunctive therapies used. The benefit of fibrinolytic therapy appears to be greatest when agents are administered as early as possible, with the most dramatic results obtained when the drug is given less than 2 hours after symptoms begin.[2]

A comprehensive overview of nine trials of thrombolytic therapy has been performed, and each trial enrolled more than 1,000 patients; the absolute mortality rates for the control and fibrinolytic groups stratified by presenting features are shown in **Figure 55-11**. The overall results indicated an 18% reduction in short-term mortality, but as much as a 25% reduction in mortality for the subset of 45,000 patients with ST-segment elevation or bundle branch block. Two trials, LATE and EMERAS, viewed together have provided evidence that a mortality reduction may still be observed in patients treated with thrombolytic agents between 6 and 12 hours from the onset of ischemic symptoms. The data from LATE and EMERAS and the FTT overview form the basis for extending the window of treatment with fibrinolytics up to 12 hours from the onset of symptoms. Boersma and colleagues have pooled the trials in the FTT overview, two smaller studies with data on time to randomization, and 11 additional trials of more than 100 patients.[1] Patients were divided into six time categories from symptom onset to randomization. A nonlinear relationship of treatment benefit to time was observed, with the greatest benefit occurring in the first 1 to 2 hours from the onset of symptoms (**Fig. 55-12**).

The mortality effect of fibrinolytic therapy in older patients is of considerable interest and controversy. Although patients older than 75 years of age were initially excluded from randomized trials of fibrinolytic therapy, they now constitute about 15% of the patients studied in megatrials of fibrinolysis and about 35% of patients analyzed in

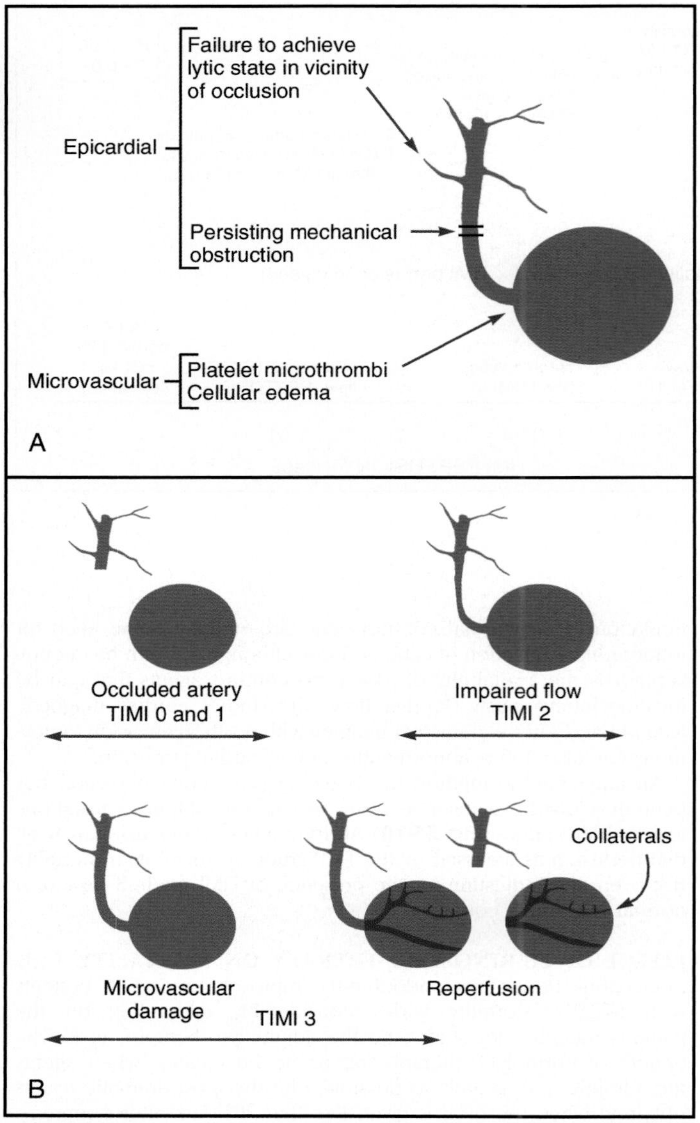

FIGURE 55-9 Patterns of response to fibrinolysis. **A,** Failure of epicardial reperfusion can occur because of failure to induce a lytic state or because of mechanical factors at the site of occlusion. Failure of microvascular reperfusion is caused by a combination of platelet microthrombi followed by endothelial swelling and myocardial edema (no reflow). **B,** Fibrinolysis may fail because of persistent occlusion of the epicardial infarct-related artery (TIMI grades 0 and 1), patency of an epicardial artery in the presence of impaired (TIMI grade 2) flow, or microvascular occlusion in the presence of angiographically normal (TIMI grade 3) flow. Successful reperfusion requires a patent artery with an intact microvascular network. Conversely, reperfusion may occur despite an occluded epicardial artery because of the presence of collateral arteries. *(From Davies CH, Ormerod OJ: Failed coronary thrombolysis. Lancet 351:1191, 1998.)*

A number of models integrate the many clinical variables that affect a patient's mortality risk before administration of fibrinolytic therapy. A convenient, simple, bedside risk-scoring system for predicting 30-day mortality at presentation for fibrinolytic-eligible patients with STEMI has been developed using the InTIME-II trial database (**Fig. 55-13**). Modeling of mortality risk cannot cover all clinical scenarios, however, and should not substitute for clinical judgment in individual cases. For example, patients with inferior STEMI who might otherwise be considered to have a low risk of mortality, and for whom many physicians have questioned the benefits of fibrinolytic therapy, might be in a much higher mortality risk subgroup if their inferior infarction is associated with right ventricular infarction, precordial ST-segment depression, or ST-segment elevation in the lateral precordial leads.

The short-term survival benefit enjoyed by patients who receive fibrinolytic therapy is maintained over the 1- to 10-year follow-up. Room for improvement remains. Advances in adjunctive antiplatelet and antithrombin therapies have led to reductions in the rate of reinfarction after fibrinolysis for STEMI.[2,66]

COMPARISON OF FIBRINOLYTIC AGENTS. Approved fibrinolytic agents for intravenous therapy have distinct features (**Table 55-6**; see Chap. 87). The tissue plasminogen activator (t-PA) molecule contains the following five domains: finger, epidermal growth factor, kringle 1 and kringle 2, and serine protease (**Fig. 55-14**).[66] In the absence of fibrin, t-PA is a weak plasminogen activator; fibrin provides a scaffold on which t-PA and plasminogen are held in such a way that the catalytic efficiency for plasminogen activation of t-PA is increased many-fold. Plasma clearance of t-PA is mediated to a varying degree by residues in each of the domains except the serine protease domain, which is responsible for the enzymatic activity of t-PA. The accelerated dose regimen of t-PA over 90 minutes produces more rapid thrombolysis than the standard 3-hour infusion of t-PA. The recommended dosage regimen for t-PA is a 15-mg intravenous bolus followed by an infusion of 0.75 mg/kg (maximum 50 mg) over 30 minutes, followed by an infusion of 0.5 mg/kg (maximum 35 mg) over 60 minutes.

Modifications of the native t-PA structure yielded a group of third-generation fibrinolytics (see Fig. 55-14 and Table 55-6). A common feature among these is prolonged plasma clearance, allowing them to be administered as a bolus rather than the bolus and double-infusion technique whereby an accelerated-dose t-PA is administered.[66]

RETEPLASE. Reteplase is a recombinant deletion mutant form of t-PA lacking the finger, epidermal growth factor, and kringle 1 domains, as well as the carbohydrate side chains (see Fig. 55-14 and Table 55-6).

The GUSTO III trial compared the 10 + 10 unit regimen of reteplase with accelerated t-PA in 15,059 patients.[1] The 30-day mortality rate was 7.47% in the reteplase group and 7.24% in the t-PA group, corresponding to an absolute difference of 0.23%, with a 95% confidence interval (CI) of −0.66 to +1.1%. The results of GUSTO III did not demonstrate superiority of reteplase over t-PA and, using a 1% absolute difference as a boundary for noninferiority, the mortality results also do not formally demonstrate noninferiority. The intracranial hemorrhage rate was 0.91% with reteplase and 0.87% with t-PA. The secondary composite endpoint of net clinical benefit (death or disabling stroke) was 7.89% with reteplase and 7.91% with accelerated t-PA. Although GUSTO III did not fulfill formal criteria for noninferiority of reteplase and t-PA, many clinicians consider the two agents to be therapeutically similar and consider the double-bolus method of administration of reteplase to be an advantage over t-PA.

TENECTEPLASE. Tenecteplase is a mutant form of t-PA with specific amino acid substitutions in the kringle 1 domain and protease domain introduced to decrease plasma clearance, increase fibrin specificity, and reduce sensitivity to plasminogen activator inhibitor-1 (see Fig. 55-14 and Table 55-6). ASSENT 2 was a randomized, double-blind, phase III equivalence trial comparing single-bolus tenecteplase with accelerated dose t-PA in 16,949 patients.[1] The 30-day mortality rate with tenecteplase was 6.179% and with t-PA it was 6.151% (*P* = 0.0059 for equivalence). The rate of intracranial hemorrhage was 0.93% with tenecteplase and 0.94% with t-PA. Major bleeding occurred in 4.66% of tenecteplase-treated patients compared with 5.94% of t-PA–treated patients (*P* = 0.0002). There was no specific subgroup of patients for whom tenecteplase or t-PA was significantly better, with the exception of patients treated after 4 hours from the onset of symptoms, among whom the mortality rate was 7.0% with tenecteplase and 9.2% with t-PA (*P* = 0.018).

OTHER FIBRINOLYTIC AGENTS. Urokinase is used on rare occasions as an intracoronary infusion (6000 IU/min) to an average cumulative dose of 5,000,000 IU to lyse intracoronary thrombi that are believed to be

registries of STEMI patients.[78] Barriers to the initiation of therapy in older patients with STEMI include a protracted period of delay in seeking medical care, a lower incidence of ischemic discomfort and greater incidence of atypical symptoms and concomitant illnesses, and an increased incidence of nondiagnostic electrocardiographic readings. Younger patients with STEMI achieve a slightly greater relative reduction in mortality compared with older patients, but the higher absolute mortality in older adults results in similar absolute mortality reductions.[79] Other important baseline characteristics that have an impact on the mortality effect of fibrinolytic therapy include the vital signs at presentation and presence of diabetes mellitus (see Fig. 55-11).

FIGURE 55-10 Relationship between TIMI myocardial perfusion (TMP) grade and mortality. TMP grade 0 or no perfusion of the myocardium is associated with the highest rate of mortality. If the stain of the myocardium is present (grade 1), mortality is also high. A reduction in mortality is seen if the contrast enters the microvasculature but is still persistent at the end of the washout phase (grade 2). The lowest mortality rate is observed in those patients with normal perfusion (grade 3) in whom the contrast is minimally persistent at the end of the washout phase. (*From Gibson CM, Cannon CP, Murphy SA, et al: Relationship of TIMI myocardial perfusion grade to mortality after administration of thrombolytic drugs. Circulation 101:125, 2000.*)

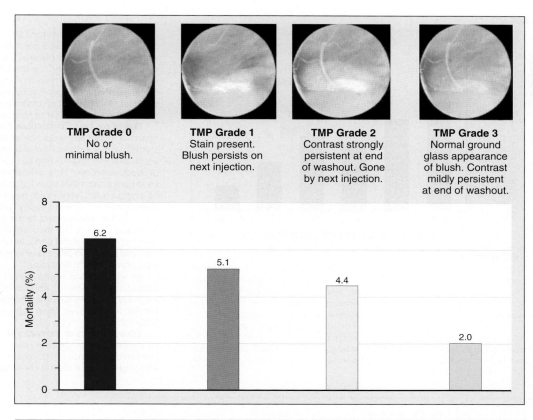

TMP Grade 0
No or minimal blush.

TMP Grade 1
Stain present. Blush persists on next injection.

TMP Grade 2
Contrast strongly persistent at end of washout. Gone by next injection.

TMP Grade 3
Normal ground glass appearance of blush. Contrast mildly persistent at end of washout.

FIGURE 55-11 Mortality differences during days 0 to 35 subdivided by presentation features in a collaborative overview of results from nine trials of thrombolytic therapy. The absolute mortality rates are shown for fibrinolytic and control groups in the center portion of the figure for each of the clinical features at presentation listed on the left side of the figure. The ratio of the odds of death in the fibrinolytic group to that in the control group is shown for each subdivision (magenta squares), along with its 99% confidence interval (horizontal line). The summary OR at the bottom of the figure corresponds to an 18% proportional reduction in 35-day mortality and is highly statistically significant. This translates to a reduction of 18 deaths/1000 patients treated with thrombolytic agents. BBB = bundle branch block; BP = blood pressure; SD = standard deviation. (*From Fibrinolytic Therapy Trialists' [FTT] Collaborative Group: Indications for fibrinolytic therapy in suspected acute myocardial infarction: Collaborative overview of mortality and major morbidity results from all randomized trials of more than 1000 patients. Lancet 343:311, 1994.*)

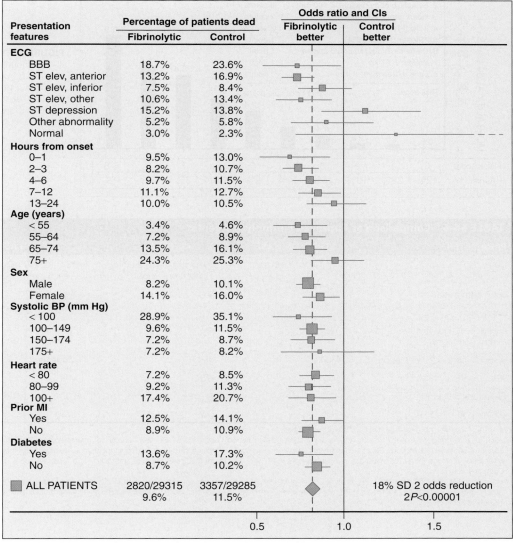

Presentation features	Percentage of patients dead		Odds ratio and CIs	
	Fibrinolytic	Control	Fibrinolytic better	Control better
ECG				
BBB	18.7%	23.6%		
ST elev, anterior	13.2%	16.9%		
ST elev, inferior	7.5%	8.4%		
ST elev, other	10.6%	13.4%		
ST depression	15.2%	13.8%		
Other abnormality	5.2%	5.8%		
Normal	3.0%	2.3%		
Hours from onset				
0–1	9.5%	13.0%		
2–3	8.2%	10.7%		
4–6	9.7%	11.5%		
7–12	11.1%	12.7%		
13–24	10.0%	10.5%		
Age (years)				
< 55	3.4%	4.6%		
55–64	7.2%	8.9%		
65–74	13.5%	16.1%		
75+	24.3%	25.3%		
Sex				
Male	8.2%	10.1%		
Female	14.1%	16.0%		
Systolic BP (mm Hg)				
< 100	28.9%	35.1%		
100–149	9.6%	11.5%		
150–174	7.2%	8.7%		
175+	7.2%	8.2%		
Heart rate				
< 80	7.2%	8.5%		
80–99	9.2%	11.3%		
100+	17.4%	20.7%		
Prior MI				
Yes	12.5%	14.1%		
No	8.9%	10.9%		
Diabetes				
Yes	13.6%	17.3%		
No	8.7%	10.2%		
ALL PATIENTS	2820/29315 9.6%	3357/29285 11.5%		18% SD 2 odds reduction 2P<0.00001

0.5   1.0   1.5

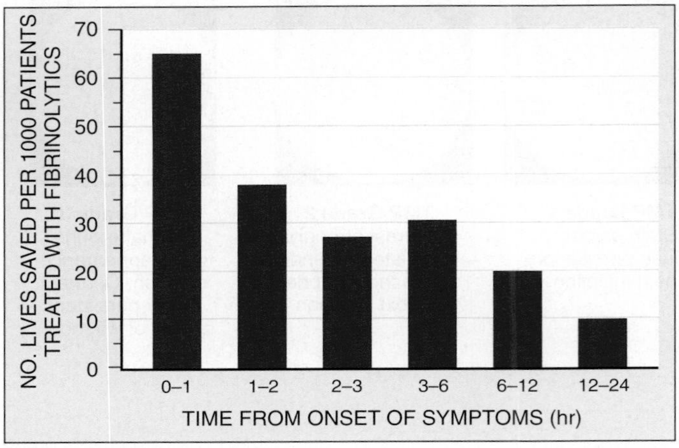

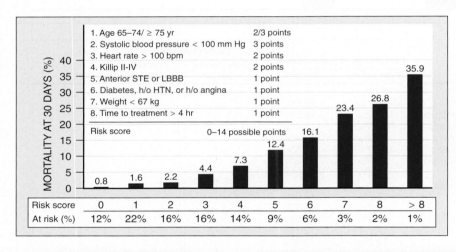

FIGURE 55-12 Importance of time to reperfusion in patients receiving fibrinolytic therapy for STEMI. The data from 22 trials of fibrinolytic therapy were pooled and the findings stratified by the six time categories shown in the figure. The number of lives saved/1000 patients treated with fibrinolytics compared with placebo is greatest the earlier treatment is initiated after the onset of symptoms, and this decreases in a nonlinear fashion with incremental time delays. Because the lifesaving effect of fibrinolysis is maximal in the first hour from onset of symptoms, this has been referred to as the "golden hour" for pharmacologic reperfusion. (From Boersma E, Maas AC, Deckers JW, et al: Early thrombolytic treatment in acute myocardial infarction: Reappraisal of the golden hour. Lancet 348:771, 1996.)

responsible for an evolving STEMI. Anistreplase, usually administered in a dose of 30 mg over 2 to 5 minutes intravenously, has a side effect profile similar to that of streptokinase, a patency profile similar to that of conventional dose t-PA, and a mortality benefit similar to that of streptokinase or t-PA (double-chain form, duteplase). Staphylokinase is a highly fibrin-specific plasminogen activator that requires priming on the surface of a clot. A pegylated recombinant form of staphylokinase yields TIMI grade 3 flow rates similar to those obtained with t-PA.[66]

EFFECT ON LEFT VENTRICULAR FUNCTION. Although precise measurements of infarct size would be an ideal endpoint for clinical reperfusion studies, such measures have proven impractical. Attempts to use the left ventricular ejection fraction as a surrogate for infarct size have not been productive because little difference is seen in ejection fraction between treatment groups that show a significant difference in mortality. Methods of assessing left ventricular function, such as end-systolic volume or quantitative echocardiography, are more revealing because patients with smaller volumes and better preserved ventricular shape have an improved survival. The myocardial salvage index, defined as the difference between an initial perfusion defect (e.g., by sestamibi scintigraphy) and final perfusion defect, is a useful means for comparing the effectiveness of reperfusion therapies.[80]

As with survival, improvement in global left ventricular function is related to the time of fibrinolytic treatment, with greatest improvement occurring with earliest therapy.[2] Greater improvement in left ventricular function has been reported with anterior than with inferior infarcts.[81]

COMPLICATIONS OF FIBRINOLYTIC THERAPY. Recent (<1 year) exposure to streptococci or streptokinase produces some degree of antibody-mediated resistance to streptokinase and anistreplase in most patients. Although this is of clinical consequence only rarely, it is recommended

FIGURE 55-13 TIMI risk score for STEMI predicting 30-day mortality. h/o = history of; HTN = hypertension; LBBB = left bundle branch block; STE = ST-segment elevation. (From Morrow DA, Antman EM, Charlesworth A, et al: The TIMI risk score for ST elevation myocardial infarction: A convenient, bedside, clinical score for risk assessment at presentation: An InTIME II substudy. Circulation 102:2031, 2000.)

Risk score	0	1	2	3	4	5	6	7	8	> 8
At risk (%)	12%	22%	16%	16%	14%	9%	6%	3%	2%	1%

Historical
1. Age 65–74/ ≥ 75 yr — 2/3 points
2. Systolic blood pressure < 100 mm Hg — 3 points
3. Heart rate > 100 bpm — 2 points
4. Killip II-IV — 2 points
5. Anterior STE or LBBB — 1 point
6. Diabetes, h/o HTN, or h/o angina — 1 point
7. Weight < 67 kg — 1 point
8. Time to treatment > 4 hr — 1 point

Risk score 0–14 possible points

TABLE 55-6 Comparison of Approved Fibrinolytic Agents*

PARAMETER	STREPTOKINASE	ALTEPLASE	RETEPLASE	TNK T-PA
Dose	1.5 MU in 30-60 min	Up to 100 mg in 90 min (based on weight)	10 U × 2 (30 min apart) each over 2 min	30-50 mg based on weight
Bolus administration	No	No	Yes	Yes
Antigenic				
Allergic reactions (hypotension most common)	Yes	No	No	No
Systemic fibrinogen depletion	Marked	Mild	Moderate	Minimal
90-min patency rates (%)	≈50	≈75	≈75	≈75[†]
TIMI grade 3 flow (%)	32	54	60	63
Cost per dose (U.S. $)[‡]	568	2750	2750	2750 for 50 mg

TIMI = Thrombolysis in Myocardial Infarction; TNK = tenecteplase.
*Data from Armstrong PW, Collen D: Fibrinolysis for acute myocardial infarction: Current status and new horizons for pharmacological reperfusion, part 1. Circulation 103:2862, 2001. [†]Data from Cannon CP, Gibson CM, McCabe CH, et al: TNK-tissue plasminogen activator compared with front-loaded alteplase in acute myocardial infarction: results of the TIMI 10B trial. Thrombolysis in Myocardial Infarction (TIMI) 10B Investigators. Circulation 98:2805, 1998. [‡]Data from Medical Economics Staff: 2001 Drug Topics Red Book. 105th ed. Montvale, NJ, Medical Economics Company, 2001.
From Antman EM, Anbe DT, Armstrong PW, et al: ACC/AHA guidelines for the management of patients with ST-elevation myocardial infarction: A report of the American College of Cardiology/American Heart Association Task Force on Practice Guidelines (Committee to Revise the 1999 Guidelines for the Management of Patients with Acute Myocardial Infarction). Circulation 110:e82, 2004.

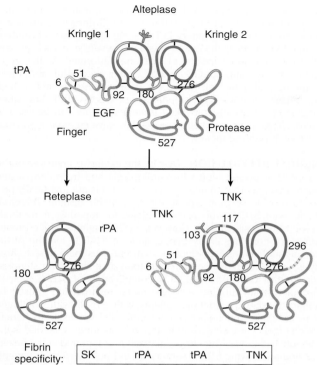

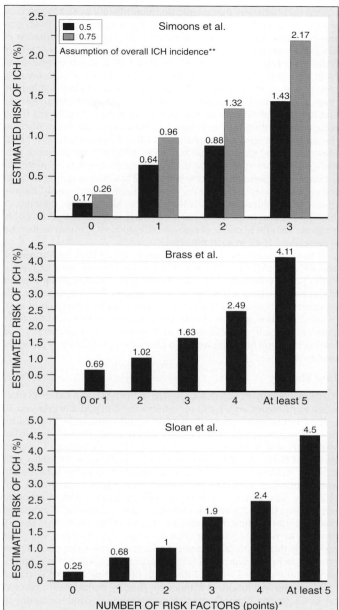

FIGURE 55-14 Molecular structure of alteplase (tPA), reteplase (rPA), and tenecteplase (TNK). Streptokinase (SK) is the least fibrin-specific thrombolytic agent in clinical use; the progressive increase in relative fibrin specificity for the various thrombolytics is shown at the bottom. *(Modified from Brener SJ, Topol EJ: Third-generation thrombolytic agents for acute myocardial infarction. In Topol EJ [ed]: Acute Coronary Syndromes. New York, Marcel Dekker, 1998, p 169.)*

FIGURE 55-15 Estimation of risk of intracranial hemorrhage (ICH) with fibrinolysis. The number of risk factors is the sum of the points based on criteria established in the studies shown. *Although the exact risk factors varied among the studies, common risk factors across all the studies included increased age, low body weight, and hypertension on admission. **If the overall incidence of ICH is assumed to be 0.75%, patients without risk factors who receive streptokinase have a 0.26% probability of ICH. The risk is 0.96%, 1.32%, and 2.17% in patients with one, two, or three risk factors, respectively. See references for further discussion. *(Data from Simoons ML, Maggioni AP, Knatterud G, et al: Individual risk assessment for intracranial haemorrhage during thrombolytic therapy. Lancet 342:1523, 1993; Brass LM, Lichtman JH, Wang Y, et al: Intracranial hemorrhage associated with thrombolytic therapy for elderly patients with acute myocardial infarction: results from the Cooperative Cardiovascular Project. Stroke 31:1802, 2000; Sloan et al: J Am Coll Cardiol 37(Suppl A):372A, 2001.)*

that patients not receive streptokinase for STEMI if they have been treated with a streptokinase product within the past year. Bleeding complications are most common and potentially the most serious. Most bleeding is relatively minor with all agents, with more serious episodes occurring in patients requiring invasive procedures.[82] Intracranial hemorrhage is the most serious complication of fibrinolytic therapy; its frequency varies with the clinical characteristics of the patient and the fibrinolytic agent prescribed (**Fig. 55-15**).[1]

There have been reports of an early hazard with fibrinolytic therapy—that is, an excess of deaths in the first 24 hours in fibrinolytic-treated patients compared with control subjects, especially in older patients treated more than 12 hours.[51] However, this excess early mortality is more than offset by the deaths prevented beyond the first day, culminating in an 18% (range, 13% to 23%) reduction in mortality by 35 days. The mechanisms responsible for this early hazard are not clear but are probably multiple, including an increased risk of myocardial rupture (particularly in older patients), fatal intracranial hemorrhage, inadequate myocardial reperfusion resulting in pump failure and cardiogenic shock, and possible reperfusion injury of reperfused myocardium. Reports of more unusual complications such as splenic rupture, aortic dissection, and cholesterol embolization have also appeared.

RECOMMENDATIONS FOR FIBRINOLYTIC THERAPY
Net Clinical Outcome with Fibrinolysis

Hesitancy in prescribing a fibrinolytic agent is often the result of uncertainty about the risk of bleeding. Patients with a higher baseline risk of mortality are more likely to benefit from fibrinolytic therapy. The mortality benefit associated with fibrinolytic therapy must be weighed against the excess risk of stroke. A useful concept that incorporates the benefits and risks of fibrinolytic therapy in a single composite endpoint is net clinical outcome. Thus, composite endpoints such as death or nonfatal stroke and death, nonfatal MI, or nonfatal major bleed may be used to compare various pharmacologic reperfusion regimens.[83]

Choice of Agent

Analysis of the net clinical outcome and cost-effectiveness of one agent versus another does not easily yield recommendations for treatment because clinicians must weigh the risk of mortality and the risk of intracranial hemorrhage when confronting a fibrinolytic-eligible patient with STEMI. Additional considerations may be the constraints placed on physicians' therapeutic decision making by the health care system in which they are practicing. In the subgroup of patients presenting within 4 hours of symptom onset, the speed of reperfusion of the infarct vessel is of paramount importance and a high-intensity fibrinolytic regimen such as accelerated t-PA is the preferred treatment, except in those for whom the risk of death is low (e.g., a young patient with a small inferior MI) and the risk of intracranial hemorrhage is increased (e.g., acute hypertension), in whom streptokinase and accelerated t-PA are approximately equivalent choices. For those patients presenting between 4 and 12 hours after the onset of chest discomfort, the speed of reperfusion of the infarct vessel is of lesser importance, and streptokinase and accelerated t-PA are therefore generally equivalent options, given the difference in costs. Of note, for those patients presenting between 4 and 12 hours from symptom onset with a low mortality risk but an increased risk of intracranial hemorrhage (e.g., older patients with inferior MI, systolic pressure > 100 mm Hg, and heart rate < 100 beats/min), streptokinase is probably preferable to t-PA because of cost considerations if fibrinolytic therapy is prescribed at all in such patients.

In those patients considered appropriate candidates for fibrinolysis and for whom t-PA would have been selected as the agent of choice in the past, we believe clinicians should now consider using a bolus fibrinolytic such as reteplase or tenecteplase. The rationale for this recommendation is that bolus fibrinolysis has the advantage of ease of administration, a lower chance of medication errors (and the associated increase in mortality when such medication errors occur), and less noncerebral bleeding, and also offers the potential for prehospital treatment.[66]

Late Therapy

No mortality benefit was demonstrated in the LATE and EMERAS trials when fibrinolytics were routinely administered to patients between 12 and 24 hours, although we believe it is still reasonable to consider fibrinolytic therapy in appropriately selected patients with persistent symptoms and ST-segment elevation on the ECG beyond 12 hours. Persistent chest pain late after the onset of symptoms correlates with a higher incidence of collateral or antegrade flow in the infarct zone and is therefore a marker for patients with viable myocardium that might be salvaged. Because older patients treated with fibrinolytic agents more than 12 hours after the onset of symptoms are at increased risk of cardiac rupture, it is preferable to restrict late fibrinolytic administration to patients younger than 65 years with ongoing ischemia, especially those with large anterior infarctions. The older patient with ongoing ischemic symptoms but presenting late (>12 hours) is probably better managed with PCI than with fibrinolytic therapy.

Before the institution of fibrinolytic therapy, consideration should be given to the patient's need for intravascular catheterization, as would be required for the placement of an arterial pressure monitoring line, pulmonary artery catheter for hemodynamic monitoring, or temporary transvenous pacemaker. If any of these are required, ideally they should be placed as expeditiously as possible before infusion of the fibrinolytic agent. If such procedures require an additional delay of more than 30 minutes, they should be deferred as long as possible after fibrinolytic therapy is begun. In the early hours after institution of fibrinolytic therapy, such catheterization should be performed only if crucial to the patient's survival, and then sites where excessive bleeding can be controlled should be chosen (e.g., subclavian vein catheterization should be avoided).

As noted, all patients with suspected STEMI should receive aspirin (160 to 325 mg) regardless of the fibrinolytic agent prescribed. Aspirin should be continued indefinitely. The issues surrounding antithrombin therapy as an adjunct to thrombolysis are complex and are discussed in detail later.

Catheter-Based Reperfusion Strategies

The infarct artery can also be reperfused by a catheter-based strategy (see Chap. 58). This approach has now evolved from passage of a balloon catheter over a guidewire to include potent antiplatelet therapy (intravenous glycoprotein [GP] IIb/IIIa inhibitors and P2Y12

adenosine diphosphate [ADP] antagonists), coronary stents, and thrombectomy.[35] When PCI is used in lieu of fibrinolytic therapy, it is referred to as direct or primary PCI (see Fig. 55-3). When fibrinolysis has failed to reperfuse the infarct vessel or a severe stenosis is present in the infarct vessel, a rescue PCI can be performed. A strategy of routine delayed angiography and PCI after successful fibrinolytic therapy may also be considered for patients who are not at high risk.[84,85] Lastly, a conservative approach of elective PCI only when spontaneous or exercise-provoked ischemia occurs can be used to manage STEMI patients, whether or not they have received a previous course of fibrinolytic therapy.

SURGICAL REPERFUSION. Despite the extensive improvement in intraoperative preservation with cardioplegia and hypothermia and numerous surgical techniques (see Chap. 84), it is not logistically possible to provide surgical reperfusion in a timely fashion. Therefore, patients with STEMI who are candidates for reperfusion routinely receive fibrinolysis or PCI. However, STEMI patients are currently referred for coronary artery bypass grafting (CABG) for one of the following indications: persistent or recurrent chest pain despite fibrinolysis or PCI, high-risk coronary anatomy (e.g., left main stenosis) discovered at catheterization, or a complication of STEMI such as ventricular septal rupture or severe mitral regurgitation caused by papillary muscle dysfunction. Patients with STEMI with continued severe ischemic and hemodynamic instability are likely to benefit from emergency revascularization. PCI with stenting as needed is the preferable technique when revascularization is required in the first 48 to 72 hours following STEMI; surgery should be reserved for patients in whom PCI has been unsuccessful or whose anatomy dictates the need for CABG, such as patients with left main or extensive multivessel coronary artery disease.

Patients undergoing successful fibrinolysis but with important residual stenoses, who on anatomic grounds are more suitable for surgical revascularization than for PCI, have undergone CABG with low rates of mortality (about 4%) and morbidity, provided that they are operated on more than 24 hours from STEMI. Those patients requiring urgent or emergency CABG within 24 to 48 hours of STEMI have mortality rates between 12% and 15%.[1] When surgery is performed under urgent conditions with active and ongoing ischemia or cardiogenic shock, the operative mortality rate rises steeply.

Selection of Reperfusion Strategy

Despite strong evidence in the literature that prompt use of reperfusion therapy improves survival of STEMI patients, reperfusion therapy remains underused and is too often tardy.[35] When performed rapidly after presentation in an experienced center, primary PCI is superior to pharmacologic reperfusion therapy.[86] Nevertheless, controversy exists about the optimum form of reperfusion therapy when there is an anticipated delay to PCI, such as in centers without 24-hour availability of primary PCI.[35] This controversy has been difficult to resolve in the context of a dynamic and rapidly changing evidence base regarding the best approach to reperfusion for patients with STEMI when immediate primary PCI is not an option. With respect to pharmacologic reperfusion, newer fibrinolytic agents and combinations of adjunctive treatments have improved medical measures to restore and maintain flow in the infarct artery (**Fig. 55-16**). From the perspective of PCI, improvements in catheterization laboratory facilities, new stents, evolution of adjunctive antithrombotic therapy, and thrombus aspiration devices have improved the efficacy and safety of PCI for patients with STEMI (see Chap. 58).[87] Importantly, the outcomes in patients treated with primary PCI also vary with the experience of the operator and the center. High-volume operators and centers can consistently achieve better outcomes in STEMI patients.[88] Selection of the optimal form of reperfusion therapy therefore involves judgment regarding system resources and individual patient characteristics.

Several issues should be considered in choosing the type of reperfusion therapy (see Fig. 55-3):
1. *Time from the onset of symptoms to initiation of reperfusion therapy.* This important variable predicts infarct size and patient outcome.

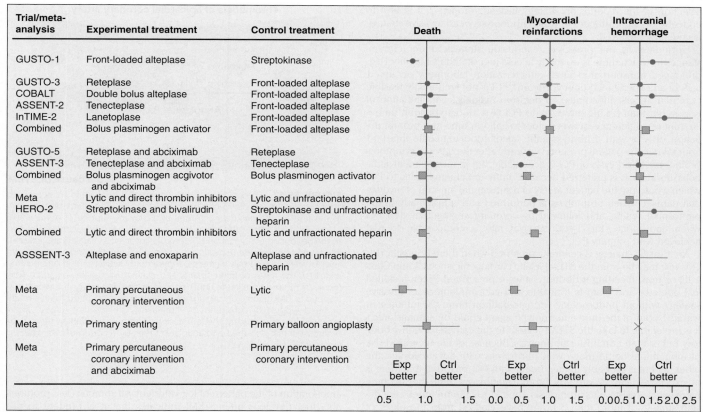

FIGURE 55-16 Relative treatment effect associated with several acute reperfusion modalities in patients presenting with STEMI. Data are odds ratios and 95% confidence intervals. Ctrl = control; Exp = experimental. *(Modified from Boersma E, Mercado N, Poldermans D, et al: Acute myocardial infarction. Lancet 361:851, 2003.)*

Although infarct size is one factor that affects patient outcomes, others include the coexistence of obstructions in non–infarct-related coronary arteries, level of electrical stability of the myocardium, extent of left ventricular remodeling, and appropriate use of evidence-based medical therapies following STEMI. Thus, for patients treated by fibrinolysis or PCI, time from the onset of symptoms predicts mortality, underscoring the need for prompt reperfusion, whichever strategy is selected (see Figs. 55-1 and 55-2).[35]

2. *Risk of death after STEMI.* Patients presenting with cardiogenic shock have an improved 1-year survival chance if they are treated with an early revascularization strategy (PCI and/or CABG, as indicated).[89] Patients at highest risk of mortality from STEMI account for the most deaths from STEMI (see Fig. 55-13). Accordingly, the mortality benefit associated with PCI is highest in patients who are at highest risk of mortality; the mortality benefit of PCI decreases progressively as the patient's risk of mortality from STEMI decreases, so that the mortality advantage of PCI is no longer evident among patients whose 30-day mortality rate is estimated to be between 2% and 3% if treated with fibrinolytic therapy.

3. *Risk of bleeding.* In patients with an increased risk of bleeding, particularly intracranial hemorrhage, therapeutic decision making strongly favors a PCI-based reperfusion strategy (see Fig. 55-15).[90] If PCI is unavailable, the benefit of pharmacologic reperfusion should be balanced against the risk of bleeding. A decision analysis has suggested that when PCI is not available, fibrinolytic therapy should still be favored over no reperfusion treatment until the risk of a life-threatening bleed exceeds 4%. For patients who are not candidates for acute reperfusion because of lack of availability of PCI and contraindications to fibrinolysis, aspirin and antithrombin therapy can be prescribed.

Thus, every effort should be made to provide reperfusion therapy, even in clinical circumstances in which there is a perceived increase in the risk of bleeding. Arrangements for urgent primary PCI should be made for patients with a constellation of advanced age, low body weight, and hypertension on presentation because of the substantially increased risk of intracranial hemorrhage with fibrinolytic therapy. When the estimated delay to implementation of primary PCI is substantial (>90 minutes), fibrinolysis (with a fibrin-specific agent) may be preferable to no reperfusion therapy in such patients when the risk from the STEMI is high (e.g., anterior infarction with hemodynamic compromise).[91] In the setting of absolute contraindications to fibrinolysis (see Table 55-5) and lack of access to PCI facilities, antithrombotic therapy should be prescribed because of the small but finite chance (10%) of restoration of TIMI grade 3 flow in the infarct vessel and decreasing the chance of thrombotic complications of STEMI.[1]

4. *Time required for transportation to a skilled PCI center.* The greatest operational impediment to routine implementation of a PCI reperfusion strategy is the delay required for transportation to a skilled PCI center (see Figs. 55-1 and 55-2).[92] Although several studies have reported that referral to a PCI center is superior to fibrinolysis administered in a local hospital, such studies were conducted in dedicated health care systems with extremely short transportation and door-to-balloon times at the PCI centers.[93] Some evidence has suggested that if the delay to implementation of primary PCI is longer than 1 hour, the mortality advantage compared with administration of a fibrin-specific agent is lost.[35]

Circumstances in which fibrinolysis or PCI is the preferred reperfusion strategy are summarized in Table 55-4. The assessment of reperfusion options for STEMI is a two-step process. Step 1 involves the integrated assessment of the time since onset of symptoms (see Figs. 55-1 to 55-4), risk of death after STEMI (see Fig. 55-13), risk of bleeding if fibrinolysis were to be administered (see Fig. 55-15), and time required for transportation to a skilled PCI center (see Fig. 55-5).[91] The complexities of clinical medicine do not permit decision making to be reduced to a simple equation or one-size-fits-all approach to selection of the reperfusion strategy. Instead, for step 2, it is best to conceive of circumstances in which fibrinolysis or an invasive strategy is generally preferred.

Fibrinolysis is the preferred reperfusion strategy under circumstances in which there is no ready access to a skilled PCI facility (e.g., prolonged transportation time, catheterization laboratory occupied, lack of an experienced operator/team), PCI is not technically feasible (vascular access difficulties), or decision making favors initiation of lysis rather than risking the delay to PCI (e.g., door-to-balloon time > 90 minutes; difference between door-to-balloon time and prompt initiation of lysis with a fibrin-specific agent [door-to-needle time] >1 hour). When the patient presents very early after the onset of symptoms (<3 hours), fibrinolysis or PCI is acceptable, but in most clinical situations, fibrinolysis is preferred because of the anticipated delay to PCI, which would put the patient at risk of a substantial amount of myocardial damage. When fibrinolysis is performed early, particularly in the prehospital setting, and followed by coronary angiography and PCI when appropriate, the 1-year survival rate is comparable to that achieved with primary PCI.[29]

An invasive strategy is generally preferred when there is greater risk. This risk may be from the STEMI itself (cardiogenic shock, Killip Class ≥ II) or from bleeding if fibrinolysis were prescribed. When a skilled PCI operator and team is available and can implement an invasive strategy without undue delay (door-to-balloon time <90 minutes, or within 1 hour of the time a fibrinolytic agent could be administered), it is preferable to take the STEMI patient to the catheterization laboratory rather than administer fibrinolysis. Because of the increased risk of intracranial hemorrhage with fibrinolysis with advanced age, the older patient is probably treated better with PCI, provided that there is no excessive delay. As coronary thrombi mature over time, they become increasingly resistant to fibrinolysis. Thus, PCI is the preferred reperfusion strategy if more than 3 hours have elapsed from the onset of symptoms, again assuming that there is no significant delay in the anticipated time to balloon inflation (see Fig. 55-2). Finally, when the diagnosis is in doubt, an invasive strategy is clearly the preferred strategy because it not only provides key diagnostic information regarding the patient's symptoms, but does so without the risk of intracranial hemorrhage associated with fibrinolysis.

Anticoagulant and Antiplatelet Therapy

ANTICOAGULANT THERAPY. The rationale for administering anticoagulant therapy acutely in STEMI patients includes prevention of deep venous thrombosis, pulmonary embolism, ventricular thrombus formation, and cerebral embolization. In addition, establishing and maintaining patency of the infarct-related artery, whether or not a patient receives fibrinolytic therapy, provides another rationale for anticoagulant therapy in cases of STEMI (**Fig. 55-17**).

EFFECT OF HEPARIN ON MORTALITY. Randomized trials in STEMI patients conducted in the prefibrinolytic era showed lower risks of pulmonary embolism, stroke, and reinfarction in patients who received intravenous heparin, supporting the administration of heparin to STEMI patients not treated with fibrinolytic therapy. With the introduction of the fibrinolytic era and, importantly, after the publication of the ISIS-2 trial, the situation became more complicated because of strong evidence of a substantial mortality reduction with aspirin alone and confusing and conflicting data regarding the risk-benefit ratio of heparin used as an adjunct to aspirin or in combination with aspirin and a fibrinolytic agent.[1] For every 1000 patients treated with heparin compared with aspirin alone, there are five fewer deaths ($P = 0.03$) and three fewer recurrent infarctions ($P = 0.04$), at the expense of three more major bleeds ($P = 0.001$).[94]

OTHER EFFECTS OF HEPARIN. A number of angiographic studies have examined the role of heparin therapy in establishing and maintaining patency of the infarct-related artery in patients with STEMI. The evidence favoring the use of heparin for enhancing patency of the infarct artery when a fibrin-specific fibrinolytic agent is prescribed is not conclusive. However, the suggestion of a mortality benefit and

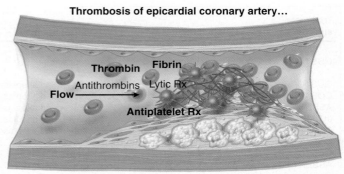

Thrombosis of epicardial coronary artery...

...the cause of STEMI

FIGURE 55-17 Pharmacologic dissolution of thrombus in infarct-related artery. This schematic view is of a longitudinal section of an infarct-related artery at the level of the obstructive thrombus. Following rupture of a vulnerable plaque (bottom center), the coagulation cascade is activated, ultimately leading to the deposition of fibrin strands (blue curvilinear arcs); platelets are activated and begin to aggregate (transition from flat discs, representing inactive platelets, to green spiked-ball elements, representing activated and aggregating platelets). The mesh of fibrin strands and platelet aggregates obstructs flow (normally moving from left to right) in the infarct-related artery; this would correspond to TIMI grade 0 on angiography. Pharmacologic reperfusion is a multipronged approach consisting of fibrinolytic agents that digest fibrin, antithrombins that prevent the formation of thrombin and inhibit the activity of thrombin that is formed, and antiplatelet therapy. (*Courtesy of Luke Wells, the Exeter Group, New York, NY.*)

amelioration of the pattern of left ventricular thrombus (less protuberant) that develops after STEMI indicates that it is prudent to use heparin for at least 48 hours after fibrinolysis and to maintain an activated partial thromboplastin time (aPTT) target of 1.5 to 2 times that of control.[35]

Although heparin may induce thrombocytopenia through an immunologic mechanism, this effect occurs only rarely, probably occurring in only 2% to 3% of patients (see Chap. 87).[95] The most serious complication of antithrombotic therapy is bleeding, especially intracranial hemorrhage, when fibrinolytic agents are prescribed.[96] Major hemorrhagic events occur more frequently in patients of low body weight, advanced age, and female sex, with marked prolongation of the aPTT (>90 to 100 seconds), and with the performance of invasive procedures. Frequent monitoring of the aPTT (facilitated by the use of a bedside testing device) reduces the risk of major hemorrhagic complications in patients treated with heparin. It should be noted, however, that during the first 12 hours following fibrinolytic therapy, the aPTT may be elevated from the fibrinolytic agent alone (particularly if streptokinase is administered), making it difficult to interpret accurately the effects of a heparin infusion on the patient's coagulation status.

NEWER ANTITHROMBOTIC AGENTS. Potential disadvantages of unfractionated heparin (UFH) include dependency on antithrombin III for inhibition of thrombin activity, sensitivity to platelet factor 4, inability to inhibit clot-bound thrombin, marked interpatient variability in therapeutic response, and the need for frequent aPTT monitoring. Even with standardized weight-based dosing nomograms, less than 35% of initial aPTT measurements are within the therapeutic range.[97] An effort to circumvent these disadvantages of UFH has stimulated interest in the development of alternative anticoagulants (see Chap. 87).

Hirudin and Bivalirudin

In patients undergoing fibrinolysis, direct thrombin inhibitors such as hirudin or bivalirudin reduce the incidence of recurrent MI by 25% to 30% compared with heparin but have not reduced mortality.[98] In addition, both hirudin and bivalirudin result in higher rates of major bleeding versus heparin when used with fibrinolytic agents. In contrast, when administered for a short period as an adjunct to primary PCI in an open-label trial, bivalirudin significantly reduced major bleeding by

40% compared with heparin and a GPIIb/IIIa receptor blocker and was associated with a significant reduction in mortality at 30 days and at 1 year (**Fig. 55-18**).[99] Bivalirudin was associated with an increased early risk of stent thrombosis, demonstrating an early trade-off of bleeding and antithrombotic efficacy.[100]

Low-Molecular-Weight Heparins

Advantages of low-molecular-weight heparins include a stable, reliable anticoagulant effect, high bioavailability, permitting administration via the subcutaneous route, and a high anti-Xa–to–anti-IIa ratio, producing blockade of the coagulation cascade in an upstream location, resulting in a marked decrement in thrombin generation. Compared with UFH, the rate of early (60 to 90 minutes) reperfusion of the infarct artery, either assessed angiographically or by noninvasive means, is not enhanced by the administration of a low-molecular-weight heparin.[94] However, the rates of reocclusion of the infarct artery, reinfarction, or recurrent ischemic events appear to be reduced by low-molecular-weight heparins.[101] This effect may underlie a significant reduction in recurrent MI with a strategy of extended anticoagulation with low-molecular-weight heparins or a factor Xa antagonist compared with standard therapy in patients with STEMI undergoing fibrinolysis.

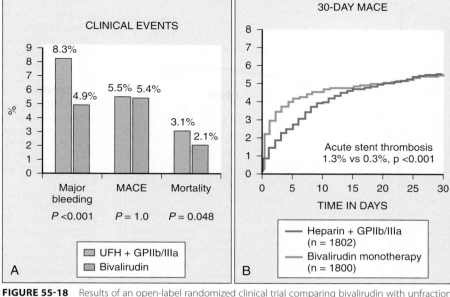

FIGURE 55-18 Results of an open-label randomized clinical trial comparing bivalirudin with unfractionated heparin (UFH) and a glycoprotein IIb/IIIa receptor antagonist (GPIIb/IIIa) as adjunctive medical therapy to support primary percutaneous coronary intervention in patients with ST-elevation STEMI. **A,** Treatment with bivalirudin was associated with a significantly lower rate of major bleeding and mortality at 30 days. **B,** Kaplan-Meier curves of the cumulative incidence of major adverse cardiac events (MACE), which did not differ between the two strategies at 30 days. Acute stent thrombosis during the first 24 hours was higher in patients treated with bivalirudin alone. *(From Stone GW, Witzenbichler B, Guagliumi G et al: Bivalirudin during primary PCI in acute myocardial infarction. N Eng J Med 358:2218, 2008.)*

The CREATE investigators have studied the effects of the low-molecular-weight heparin reviparin compared with placebo in 15,570 patients with STEMI, 73% of whom received a fibrinolytic (predominantly a non–fibrin-specific agent).[102] The primary composite outcome of death, recurrent MI, or stroke was reduced by 13% both at 7 days (*P* = 0.005) and at 30 days (*P* = 0.001) with reviparin. The AMI-SK investigators reported that ST-segment resolution at 90 and 180 minutes, as well as angiographic patency, was improved in streptokinase-treated STEMI patients who received enoxaparin compared with placebo. These observations support the hypotheses that antithrombin therapy is a useful adjunct to a pharmacologic reperfusion regimen and that low-molecular-weight heparins are clinically effective in STEMI.[94,95]

The ASSENT-3 trial compared UFH with enoxaparin (30 mg intravenous bolus followed by subcutaneous injections of 1 mg/kg every 12 hours until hospital discharge).[103] The composite endpoint of 30-day mortality, in-hospital reinfarction, or in-hospital refractory ischemia was reduced from 15.4% with UFH to 11.4% with enoxaparin (RR, 0.74; 95% CI, 0.63 to 0.87). The rate of intracranial hemorrhage was similar with UFH versus enoxaparin (0.93% versus 0.88%; *P* = 0.98). The ASSENT-3 PLUS study compared the same UFH and enoxaparin regimens but initiated therapy in the prehospital setting.[94,95] The composite endpoint of 30-day mortality, in-hospital reinfarction, or in-hospital refractory ischemia was reduced from 17.4% with UFH to 14.2% with enoxaparin (*P* = 0.08). Of concern, however, was the increased rate of intracranial hemorrhage observed in ASSENT-3 PLUS—1% with UFH versus 2.2% with enoxaparin (*P* = 0.05). The increase in intracranial hemorrhage in ASSENT-3 PLUS was seen predominantly in patients older than 75 years of age—0.8% with UFH versus 6.7% with enoxaparin (*P* = 0.01).

The ExTRACT-TIMI 25 trial, in a double-blind, double-dummy design, tested the hypothesis that a strategy of enoxaparin administered for the duration of the index hospitalization is superior to the conventional antithrombin strategy of UFH for 48 hours after fibrinolysis.[104] The enoxaparin dosing strategy was adjusted according to the patient's age and renal function. For patients younger than 75 years of age, enoxaparin (or matching placebo) was to be given as a fixed, 30-mg intravenous bolus followed 15 minutes later by a subcutaneous injection of 1 mg/kg, with injections administered every 12 hours. For patients 75 years of age and older, the intravenous bolus was eliminated and the subcutaneous dose was reduced to 0.75 mg/kg every 12 hours. The primary endpoint of death or recurrent nonfatal MI through

30 days occurred in 12% of patients in the UFH group and 9.9% of those in the enoxaparin group (17% reduction in RR; *P* = 0.001). Nonfatal reinfarction occurred in 4.5% of the patients receiving UFH and 3% of those receiving enoxaparin (33% reduction in RR; *P* = 0.001); 7.5% of patients given UFH died, as did 6.9% of those given enoxaparin (*P* = 0.11). The composite of death, nonfatal reinfarction, or urgent revascularization occurred in 14.5% of patients given UFH and 11.7% of those given enoxaparin (*P* = 0.001); major bleeding occurred in 1.4% and 2.1%, respectively (*P* = 0.001) (**Fig. 55-19**). The composite of death, nonfatal reinfarction, or nonfatal intracranial hemorrhage (a measure of net clinical benefit) occurred in 12.2% of patients given UFH and 10.1% of those given enoxaparin (*P* = 0.001).

FACTOR Xa ANTAGONISTS. The OASIS-6 trial evaluated the specific factor Xa antagonist fondaparinux (2.5 mg subcutaneously) in 12,092 patients with STEMI.[105] The trial design compared fondaparinux given for 8 days versus placebo in patients when the treating physician thought that UFH was not indicated (stratum I) and versus UFH for 48 hours when the treating physician thought that heparin was indicated (stratum II). The primary endpoint, death or reinfarction, occurred in 14% of placebo patients and 11.2% of fondaparinux patients in stratum I (HR 0.79; 95% CI, 0.68 to 0.92), and in 8.7% of UFH patients and 8.3% of fondaparinux patients in stratum II (HR 0.96; 95% CI, 0.81 to 1.13). Thus, fondaparinux was superior to placebo (stratum I) but yielded similar results to those achieved with UFH (stratum II). The outcome of patients in stratum II who underwent PCI tended to be worse when fondaparinux was used compared with UFH, probably because of an increased risk of catheter thrombosis when fondaparinux is administered without coadministration of another antithrombin that has anti-IIa activity. Severe hemorrhage occurred in 1.3% of control patients and 1% of fondaparinux patients through 9 days (*P* = 0.13).

Recommendations for Anticoagulant Therapy

ANTICOAGULATION WITH FIBRINOLYSIS. Given the pivotal role of thrombin in the pathogenesis of STEMI, antithrombotic therapy remains an important intervention (see Fig. 55-17). A regimen of intravenous unfractionated heparin bolus at 60 U/kg to a maximum of 4000 U, followed by an initial infusion of 12 U/kg/hr to a maximum of 1000 U/hr given for 48 hours, has established efficacy in patients receiving fibrinolytic therapy. However, infusions of unfractionated

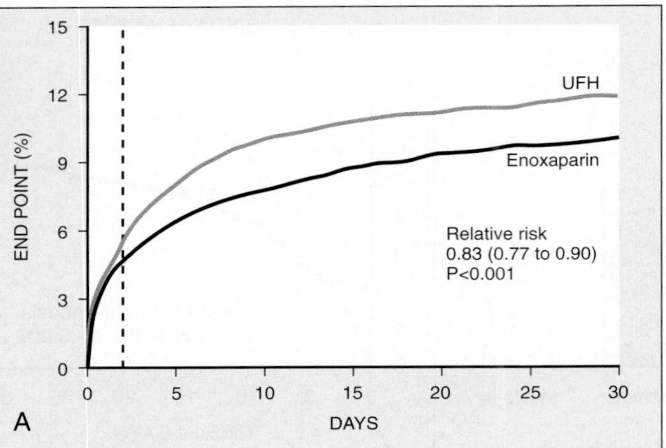

Number at risk:							
UFH	10223	9385	9188	9109	9064	9027	8994
Enox	10256	9595	9460	9362	9301	9263	9234

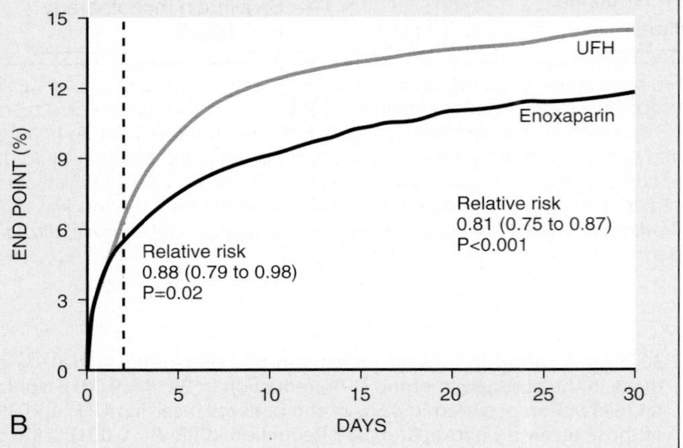

Number at risk:							
UFH	10223	9174	8955	8868	8818	8775	8738
Enox	10256	9479	9312	9200	9130	9084	9052

FIGURE 55-19 Comparison of enoxaparin with unfractionated heparin as adjunctive therapy in STEMI patients receiving fibrinolysis. **A,** The rate of the primary endpoint (death or nonfatal MI) at 30 days was significantly lower in the enoxaparin (Enox) group than in the unfractionated heparin (UFH) group (9.9% versus 12%; $P < 0.001$ by the log-rank test). The dashed vertical line indicates the comparison at day 2 (direct pharmacologic comparison), at which time a trend in favor of enoxaparin was seen. **B,** The rate of the main secondary endpoint (death, nonfatal MI, or urgent revascularization) at 30 days was significantly lower in the Enox group than in the UFH group (11.7% versus 14.5%; $P < 0.001$ by the log-rank test). The difference was already significant at 48 hours (6.1% in the UFH group versus 5.3% in the Emox group; $P = 0.02$ by the log-rank test). The interval shown is the time (in 24-hour intervals) from randomization to an event or the last follow-up visit. *(From Antman EM, Morrow DA, McCabe CH, et al: Enoxaparin versus unfractionated heparin with fibrinolysis for ST-elevation myocardial Infarction. N Engl J Med 354: 1477, 2006.)*

heparin are cumbersome to administer and provide unreliable levels of anticoagulation, requiring frequent measurements of aPTT to adjust the infusion rate.[106] In addition, because of the risk of heparin-induced thrombocytopenia with prolonged administration of unfractionated heparin, alternative anticoagulant regimens are preferred if administered for longer than 48 hours.[35]

Both ExTRACT-TIMI 25 and OASIS 6 have indicated that more prolonged administration of an antithrombin for the duration of hospitalization is beneficial compared with the prior practice of administering UFH only for 48 hours, unless clear-cut indications for continued anticoagulation were present. As such, patients managed with pharmacologic reperfusion therapy should receive anticoagulant therapy for a minimum of 48 hours and preferably for the duration of the hospitalization after STEMI, up to 8 days.[35]

Administration of enoxaparin or fondaparinux is preferred when administration of an anticoagulant for longer than 48 hours is planned for patients with STEMI treated with a fibrinolytic.[35] The benefits of enoxaparin over UFH are evident regardless of the type of fibrinolytic administered (streptokinase or fibrin-specific) and across a wide range of patient subgroups. An initial intravenous bolus of enoxaparin (30 mg) should be administered, followed by subcutaneous injections of 1 mg/kg every 12 hours for patients younger than 75 years of age; for patients 75 years of age and older, the initial intravenous bolus should be omitted and the maintenance dose should be 0.75 mg/kg every 12 hours. If the estimated creatinine clearance is less than 30 mL/min, the maintenance dose should be 1 mg/kg every 24 hours.

Fondaparinux was superior to placebo in OASIS 6. The convenience of once-daily subcutaneous injections of fondaparinux is also attractive compared with UFH, but its use is complicated by the need for coadministration of an additional antithrombin with anti-IIa activity if PCI is performed in a patient treated with fondaparinux. Further information regarding the appropriate dosing of additional antithrombins along with fondaparinux in the catheterization laboratory is needed.

In patients with a known history of heparin-induced thrombocytopenia, it is reasonable to consider bivalirudin as a useful alternative to heparin to be used in conjunction with streptokinase. Dosing according to the HERO 2 regimen (a bolus of 0.25 mg/kg followed by an intravenous infusion of 0.5 mg/kg/hr for the first 12 hours, and 0.25 mg/kg/hr for the subsequent 36 hours) is recommended but with a reduction in the infusion rate if the aPTT is longer than 75 seconds within the first 12 hours.[1]

For patients who are referred for CABG, the preferred antithrombin is UFH. When an alternative antithrombin has been used, it should be discontinued prior to surgery, with a sufficiently long interval to avoid double anticoagulation when the patient enters the operating room and receives UFH.

ADJUNCTIVE ANTICOAGULATION FOR PRIMARY PERCUTANEOUS INTERVENTION. Based on expert consensus, UFH is recommended for patients undergoing primary PCI (see Chap. 58). On the basis of the results of the HORIZONS-AMI trial,[99] bivalirudin is an alternative for adjunctive anticoagulation during primary PCI. Fondaparinux is not recommended as the sole anticoagulant in this setting.[35] A large randomized trial of fondaparinux in patients with STEMI, including 3789 patients undergoing primary PCI, revealed a possible hazard related to catheter thrombosis. Low-molecular-weight heparins have not had sufficient evaluation in primary PCI to formulate recommendations for treatment. Some investigators who have used enoxaparin to support primary PCI for STEMI administered 0.5 mg/kg intravenously at the time of the procedure.

PATIENTS TREATED WITHOUT REPERFUSION THERAPY. In STEMI patients not receiving reperfusion therapy, fondaparinux reduces the composite of death or recurrent MI without an increase in severe bleeding as compared with placebo or UFH.[107]

ANTIPLATELET THERAPY. Platelets play a major role in the response to disruption of a coronary artery plaque, especially in the early phase of thrombus formation (**Fig. 55-20**).[108] Platelets are also activated in response to fibrinolysis, and platelet-rich thrombi are more resistant to fibrinolysis than fibrin and erythrocyte-rich thrombi (see Fig. 55-17). Thus, there is a sound scientific basis for inhibiting platelet aggregation in all STEMI patients, regardless of the reperfusion management strategy. Comprehensive overviews of randomized trials of antiplatelet therapy have summarized the overwhelming evidence of benefit of antiplatelet therapy for a wide range of vascular disorders.[109] In patients at risk for STEMI, patients with a documented prior STEMI, and patients in the acute phase of STEMI, there is a 22% reduction in the odds of the composite endpoint of death, nonfatal recurrent infarction, and nonfatal stroke with antiplatelet therapy (**Fig. 55-21**). Not unexpectedly, the absolute benefits are greatest in those patients at highest baseline risk. Although several antiplatelet regimens have been evaluated, the agent most extensively tested has been aspirin.

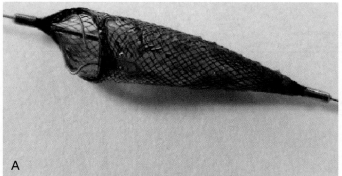

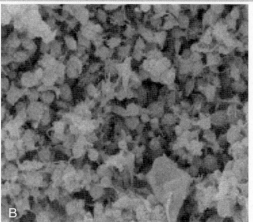

FIGURE 55-20 Importance of platelet aggregation early in STEMI. A 46-year-old man presented with STEMI resulting from occlusion of the right coronary artery. At the time of primary percutaneous PCI, which was performed within 90 minutes of the onset of symptoms, a nonocclusive distal protection filter was placed downstream from the obstruction in the infarct artery. **A,** Macroscopically, the obstructing thrombus was white. **B,** Scanning electron microscopy at high magnification (×2000) showed a platelet-rich thrombus without fibrin or erythrocytes. This case emphasizes the important role of platelet activation and aggregation early after the onset of disruption of a coronary artery plaque and underscores the necessity for antiplatelet therapy in STEMI patients. *(Modified from Beygui F, Collet JP, Nagaswami C, et al: Images in cardiovascular medicine. Architecture of intracoronary thrombi in ST-elevation acute myocardial infarction: Time makes the difference. Circulation 113:e21, 2006.)*

Antiplatelet Therapy with Fibrinolysis

The ISIS-2 study was the largest trial of aspirin in STEMI patients[1]; it provides the single strongest piece of evidence that aspirin reduces mortality in STEMI patients. In contrast to the observations of a time-dependent mortality effect of fibrinolytic therapy, the mortality reduction with aspirin was similar in patients treated within 4 hours (25% reduction in mortality), between 5 and 12 hours (21% reduction), and between 13 and 24 hours (21% reduction). There was an overall 23% reduction in mortality from aspirin in ISIS-2 that was largely additive to the 25% reduction in mortality from streptokinase, so patients receiving both therapies experienced a 42% reduction in mortality. The mortality reduction was as high as 53% in patients who received both aspirin and streptokinase within 6 hours of symptoms. Of particular interest was the finding that the combination of streptokinase and aspirin reduced mortality without increasing the risk of stroke or hemorrhage.

Obstructive platelet-rich arterial thrombi resist fibrinolysis and have an increased tendency to produce reocclusion after initial successful reperfusion in patients with STEMI. Despite the inhibition of cyclooxygenase by aspirin, platelet activation continues to occur through thromboxane A_2–independent pathways, leading to platelet aggregation and increased thrombin formation.[41] The addition of other antiplatelet agents to aspirin has been proven to benefit patients with STEMI. Inhibitors of the P2Y12 ADP receptor help prevent activation and aggregation of platelets. In the CLARITY-TIMI 28 trial, the addition of the P2Y12 inhibitor clopidogrel to background treatment with aspirin to STEMI patients younger than 75 years of age who received fibrinolytic therapy reduced the risk of clinical events (death, reinfarction, stroke) and reocclusion of a successfully reperfused infarct artery (**Fig. 55-22**).[110] An ST Resolution (STRes) electrocardiographic substudy from the CLARITY-TIMI 28 trial has provided insight into the mechanism of the benefit of clopidogrel in STEMI.[111] There was no difference in the rate of complete STRes between the clopidogrel and placebo groups at 90 minutes (38.4% versus 36.6% at 90 minutes). When patients were stratified by STRes category, treatment with clopidogrel resulted in greater benefit among those with evidence of early STRes, with greater odds of an open artery at late angiography in patients with partial (odds ratio [OR], 1.4; $P = 0.04$) or complete (OR, 2; $P = 0.001$) STRes, but no improvement in those with no STRes at 90 minutes (OR, 0.89; $P = 0.48$) (P for interaction, 0.003). Clopidogrel was also associated with a significant reduction in the odds of in-hospital death or MI in patients who achieved partial (OR, 0.30; $P = 0.003$) or complete STRes at 90 minutes (OR, 0.49; $P = 0.056$), whereas clinical benefit was not apparent in patients who had no STRes (OR, 0.98; $P = 0.95$) (P for interaction, 0.027). Thus it appears that clopidogrel did not increase the rate of complete opening of occluded infarct arteries when fibrinolysis was administered but was highly effective in preventing reocclusion of an initially reperfused infarct artery.

In the COMMIT trial, 45,852 patients with suspected MI were randomized to clopidogrel, 75 mg/day (without a loading dose), or placebo in addition to aspirin, 162 mg/day (see Fig. 55-22).[43] The patients in the clopidogrel group had a lower rate of the composite endpoint of death, reinfarction, or stroke (9.2% versus 10.1%; $P = 0.002$). They also had a significantly lower rate of death (7.5% versus 8.1%; $P = 0.03$). No excess of bleeding with clopidogrel occurred in this trial.

Combination Pharmacologic Reperfusion

Several studies have evaluated the combination of GP IIb/IIIa inhibitors and fibrinolytics.[1] The first series of trials combined full doses of thrombolytic agents with IIb/IIIa inhibitors. Although these initial trials provided proof of the hypothesis that the addition of an intravenous GP IIb/IIIa inhibitor enhanced the efficacy of a full dose of a fibrinolytic agent, unacceptably high rates of major bleeding were observed.

The combination of a reduced dose of a fibrinolytic agent and IIb/IIIa inhibitor was tested in a subsequent series of trials. The rates of TIMI grade 3 flow at 60 and 90 minutes were only slightly higher with combination reperfusion compared with full-dose fibrinolytic monotherapy. These trials generally showed improved myocardial perfusion, reflected in enhanced ST-segment resolution and faster angiographic frame counts.

The GUSTO V trial tested half-dose reteplase (5 U and 5 U) and full-dose abciximab compared with full-dose reteplase (10 U and 10 U) in 16,588 patients in the first 6 hours of STEMI. Thirty-day mortality rates were similar in the two treatment groups (5.9% versus 5.6%) but non-fatal reinfarction and other complications of MI were reduced in the group receiving combination reperfusion therapy. Although the rates of intracranial hemorrhage were the same in the two treatment groups (0.6%), moderate to severe bleeding was significantly increased from 2.3% to 4.6% with combination reperfusion therapy ($P = 0.001$). This excess bleeding risk appeared to be limited to patients older than 75 years of age. The greatest mortality benefit was observed in those patients who presented with anterior MI.

The ASSENT-3 trial randomized 6095 patients with STEMI to full-dose tenecteplase with UFH versus full-dose tenecteplase with enoxaparin or half-dose tenecteplase plus abciximab (with weight-adjusted reduced-dose UFH).[103] Similar to the GUSTO V trial, combination reperfusion therapy with half-dose tenecteplase and abciximab was not associated with a reduction in 30-day mortality; however, in-hospital reinfarction and refractory ischemia were reduced with combination reperfusion therapy. Of note, the major bleeding rate other than intracranial hemorrhage was increased from 2.2% to 4.3% with combination reperfusion therapy ($P = 0.0005$). Older patients were at greatest risk for excess bleeding, experiencing a threefold increase in the rate of that complication.

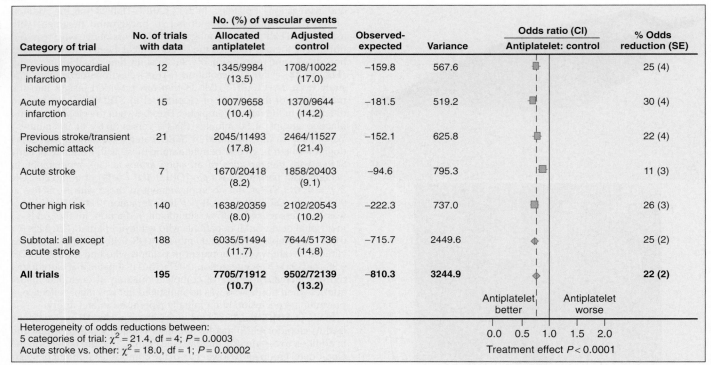

| Category of trial | No. of trials with data | No. (%) of vascular events | | Observed-expected | Variance | Odds ratio (CI) Antiplatelet: control | % Odds reduction (SE) |
		Allocated antiplatelet	Adjusted control				
Previous myocardial infarction	12	1345/9984 (13.5)	1708/10022 (17.0)	−159.8	567.6		25 (4)
Acute myocardial infarction	15	1007/9658 (10.4)	1370/9644 (14.2)	−181.5	519.2		30 (4)
Previous stroke/transient ischemic attack	21	2045/11493 (17.8)	2464/11527 (21.4)	−152.1	625.8		22 (4)
Acute stroke	7	1670/20418 (8.2)	1858/20403 (9.1)	−94.6	795.3		11 (3)
Other high risk	140	1638/20359 (8.0)	2102/20543 (10.2)	−222.3	737.0		26 (3)
Subtotal: all except acute stroke	188	6035/51494 (11.7)	7644/51736 (14.8)	−715.7	2449.6		25 (2)
All trials	**195**	**7705/71912 (10.7)**	**9502/72139 (13.2)**	**−810.3**	**3244.9**		**22 (2)**

Antiplatelet better | Antiplatelet worse

0.0 0.5 1.0 1.5 2.0

Treatment effect $P < 0.0001$

Heterogeneity of odds reductions between:
5 categories of trial: $\chi^2 = 21.4$, df = 4; $P = 0.0003$
Acute stroke vs. other: $\chi^2 = 18.0$, df = 1; $P = 0.00002$

FIGURE 55-21 Proportional effects of antiplatelet therapy on vascular events (MI, stroke, or vascular death) in the main high-risk categories. The stratified ratio of odds of an event in treatment groups to that in control groups is plotted for each group of trials (square) along with its 99% CI (horizontal line). Meta-analysis of results for all trials (95% CI) is represented by a diamond; SE = standard error. (*From Antithrombotic Trialists' Collaboration: Collaborative meta-analysis of randomised trials of antiplatelet therapy for prevention of death, myocardial infarction, and stroke in high-risk patients. BMJ 324:71, 2002.*)

Given the increased bleeding risk with combination reperfusion therapy, it cannot be recommended for routine clinical use. However, the combination of an intravenous GP IIb/IIIa inhibitor with a reduced dose of a fibrinolytic agent might be considered in high-risk patients (e.g., anterior STEMI) when long transfer delays for primary PCI are anticipated.[1]

Antiplatelet Therapy for Primary Percutaneous Intervention in STEMI

All patients with STEMI should receive aspirin as soon as possible after presentation, in the absence of contraindications. The addition of the P2Y12 inhibitor clopidogrel to aspirin appears to offer additional benefit in patients undergoing PCI after STEMI. An analysis of the subgroup of patients who underwent PCI in the CLARITY-TIMI 28 trial showed that pretreatment with clopidogrel significantly reduces the incidence of cardiovascular death, MI, or stroke following PCI (3.6% versus 6.2%; adjusted OR, 0.54 [95% CI, 0.35 to 0.85]; $P = 0.008$).[112] Pretreatment with clopidogrel also reduces the incidence of MI or stroke prior to PCI (4% versus 6.2%; OR, 0.62 [95% CI, 0.40 to 0.95]; $P = 0.03$). There was no significant excess in the rates of TIMI major or minor bleeding (2% versus 1.9%; $P = 0.99$).

Moreover, in patients undergoing primary or delayed PCI after initial therapy for STEMI, the more potent P2Y12 inhibitor prasugrel has been found to be superior to clopidogrel for reducing the risk of cardiovascular death, MI, or stroke.[113] In the subgroup of patients with STEMI enrolled in the TRITON-TIMI 38 trial ($N = 3534$), this endpoint was lowered by 32% at 30 days with prasugrel compared with aspirin (6.5% versus 9.5%; $P = 0.0017$) and by 21% at 15 months (10.0% versus 12.4%; $P = 0.022$) (**Fig. 55-23**).[114] Prasugrel reduced stent thrombosis by 42% compared with clopidogrel. This reduction in recurrent ischemic events with prasugrel was associated with a similar increase in major bleeding as seen in the overall trial population. Analogously, in the PLATO trial, compared with clopidogrel, treatment with the reversible P2Y12 inhibitor ticagrelor in patients with STEMI undergoing primary

PCI reduced the primary endpoint of cardiovascular death, recurrent MI, or stroke by 16%, a magnitude similar to that for the overall trial population.[114a] A discussion of the use of GP IIb/IIIa inhibitors as part of adjunctive therapy for patients with STEMI undergoing PCI is presented in Chap. 58.

Recommendations for Antiplatelet Therapy

Nonenteric-coated aspirin should be chewed by patients who have not taken aspirin prior to presentation with STEMI. The initial dose should be 162 to 325 mg. During the maintenance phase of antiplatelet therapy following STEMI, the dose of aspirin should be reduced to 75 to 162 mg to minimize bleeding risk.[115] If true aspirin allergy is present, other antiplatelet agents such as clopidogrel (loading dose, 300 to 600 mg; maintenance dose, 75 mg/day) or ticlopidine (loading dose, 500 mg; maintenance dose, 250 mg twice daily) can be substituted.

The addition of a P2Y12 inhibitor to aspirin is warranted for most patients with STEMI.[35] Based on the results of the COMMIT[116] and CLARITY-TIMI 28[110] trials, clopidogrel at 75 mg/day orally is an alternative for all patients with STEMI, regardless of whether they receive fibrinolytic therapy, undergo primary PCI, or do not receive reperfusion therapy.[35] The available data suggest that a loading dose of 300 mg of clopidogrel should be given to patients younger than 75 years of age who receive fibrinolytic therapy. There is insufficient data to recommend a loading dose in patients 75 years of age and older who receive a fibrinolytic. When primary PCI is the mode of reperfusion therapy, an oral loading dose of 300 to 600 mg of clopidogrel before stent implantation is an established alternative.[117] In addition, on the basis of the results of the TRITON-TIMI 38 trial, prasugrel administered with an oral loading dose of 60 mg and 10 mg orally daily thereafter is a superior alternative to clopidogrel, 300 mg, for patients not at particularly high risk of life-threatening bleeding, such as those with a history of cerebrovascular disease.[113,114] Similarly, ticagrelor administered with a loading dose of 180 mg and 90 mg twice daily thereafter is superior to clopidogrel.[114a]

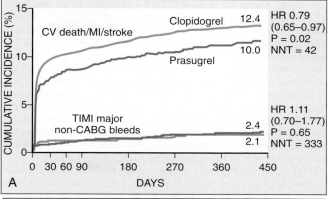

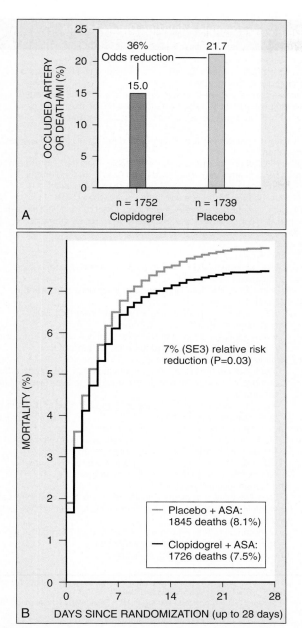

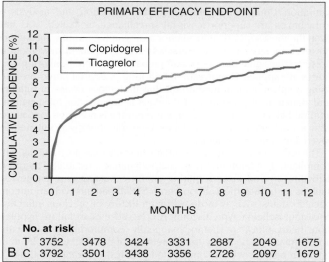

FIGURE 55-22 Impact of addition of clopidogrel to aspirin (ASA) in STEMI patients. **A,** Effects of the addition of clopidogrel in patients receiving fibrinolysis for STEMI. Patients in the clopidogrel group (n = 1752) had a 36% reduction in the odds of dying, sustaining a recurrent infarction, or having an occluded infarct artery compared with the placebo group (n = 1739) in the CLARITY-TIMI 28 trial. **B,** Effect of the addition of clopidogrel on in-hospital mortality after STEMI. These time-to-event curves show a 0.6% reduction in mortality in the group receiving clopidogrel plus aspirin (n = 22,961) compared with placebo plus aspirin (n = 22,891) in the COMMIT trial. (**A** modified from Sabatine MS, Cannon CP, Gibson, CM, et al: Addition of clopidogrel to aspirin and fibrinolytic therapy for myocardial infarction with ST-segment elevation. N Engl J Med 352:1179, 2005; **B** modified from Chen ZM, Jiang LX, Chen YP, et al: Addition of clopidogrel to aspirin in 45,852 patients with acute myocardial infarction: Randomised placebo-controlled trial. Lancet 366:1607, 2005.)

FIGURE 55-23 A, Efficacy and safety of prasugrel among the subgroup of patients with STEMI enrolled in a randomized clinical trial of prasugrel compared with clopidogrel in patients undergoing PCI after presentation with acute coronary syndrome. Treatment with prasugrel was associated with a 21% relative reduction in the risk cardiovascular death, myocardial infarction, or stroke during 15 months of follow-up. Major bleeding was increased with prasugrel in the trial overall, but not among patients with ST-elevation myocardial infarction. **B,** Efficacy results for ticagrelor (versus clopidogrel) in patients with STEMI enrolled in the PLATO trial. Ticagrelor reduced the primary endpoint (incidence of MI, stroke, or vascular death) versus clopidogrel, from 11.0% to 9.3% (hazard ratio [HR] 0.85; 95% CI, 0.74 to 0.97; P = 0.02). CV = cardiovascular; NNT = number needed to treat. (**A** from Montalescot G, Wiviott SD, Braunwald E, et al: Prasugrel compared with clopidogrel in patients undergoing percutaneous coronary intervention for ST-segment elevation myocardial infarction [TRITON-TIMI 38]: Double-blind, randomised controlled trial. Lancet 373:723, 2009; **B** from Steg G, et al: Circulation [in press].)

Hospital Management

Coronary Care Units

Deaths from primary ventricular fibrillation in patients with STEMI have been prevented because the coronary care unit (CCU) allows continuous monitoring of cardiac rhythm by highly trained nurses with the authority to initiate immediate treatment of arrhythmias in the absence of physicians, and because of the specialized equipment (e.g., defibrillators, pacemakers) and drugs available. Although all these benefits can be achieved for patients scattered throughout the hospital, the clustering of patients with STEMI in the CCU has greatly improved the efficient use of trained personnel, facilities, and equipment. With increasing emphasis on hemodynamic monitoring and treatment of the serious complications of STEMI with such modalities as pharmacologic or catheter-based reperfusion therapy, afterload reduction, and intra-aortic balloon counterpulsation, and other advanced hemodynamic support, the presence of a CCU and experienced teams of physicians has assumed even greater importance. As reperfusion strategies, including fibrinolytic therapy and PCI, are used more routinely for STEMI patients, facilities in which patients can undergo diagnostic and therapeutic angiographic procedures are being integrated into an expanded structure of a coronary care team.[11]

At the same time, the value of CCUs for patients with uncomplicated STEMI has undergone reevaluation. With increasing attention directed to the limitations of resources and to the economic impact of intensive care, efforts have been made to select patients likely to benefit from hospitalization in a CCU. The ECG, on presentation, particularly in conjunction with previous tracings and an immediate general clinical assessment, can be useful both for predicting which patients will have the diagnosis of STEMI confirmed and for identifying low-risk patients who may require less intensive care. Analysis of the quality of pain can help identify low-risk patients. Patients without a history of angina pectoris or MI who present with pain that is sharp or stabbing and pleuritic, positional, or reproduced by palpation of the chest wall are extremely unlikely to be experiencing STEMI (see Chap. 53).[118]

Today, CCUs typically have equipment available for the noninvasive monitoring of single or multiple electrocardiographic leads, cardiac rhythm, ST-segment deviation, arterial pressure, and arterial oxygen saturation. Computer algorithms for the detection and analysis of arrhythmias are superior to visual surveillance by skilled CCU staff. Even the most sophisticated electrocardiographic monitoring systems, however, are susceptible to artifacts because of patient movement or noise on the signal from poor skin preparation when monitoring electrodes are applied. Noninvasive monitoring of arterial blood pressure using a sphygmomanometric cuff that undergoes cycles of inflation and deflation at programmed intervals is suitable for most patients admitted to a CCU. Invasive arterial monitoring is preferred for patients with a low output syndrome when inotropic therapy is initiated for severe left ventricular failure.

The CCU remains the appropriate hospital unit for patients with complicated infarctions (e.g., hemodynamic instability, recurrent arrhythmias) and those requiring intensive nursing care for devices such as an intra-aortic balloon pump. STEMI patients with an uncomplicated status, such as those without a history of previous infarction, persistent ischemic-type discomfort, congestive heart failure, hypotension, heart block, or hemodynamically compromising ventricular arrhythmias, can be safely transferred out of the CCU within 24 to 36 hours. In patients with a complicated STEMI, the duration of the CCU stay should be dictated by the need for intensive care—that is, hemodynamic monitoring, close nursing supervision, intravenous vasoactive drugs, and frequent changes in the medical regimen.

For patients with a low risk of mortality from STEMI, the clinician should consider admission to an intermediate care facility (see later) equipped with simple electrocardiographic monitoring and resuscitation equipment.[1] This strategy has proven cost-effective and may reduce CCU use by one third, shorten hospital stays, and have no deleterious effect on a patient's recovery. Intermediate care units for low-risk STEMI patients can also be appealing to patients who stand to gain little benefit from the high staffing, intense activity, and elaborate technology available in current CCUs (but with their attendant high costs) and who may be disturbed by that activity and equipment.

GENERAL MEASURES. The CCU staff must be sensitive to patient concerns about mortality, prognosis, and future productivity. A calm, quiet atmosphere and the laying on of hands with a gentle but confident touch help allay anxiety and reduce sympathetic tone, ultimately leading to a reduction in hypertension, tachycardia, and arrhythmias.[1] To reduce the risk of nausea and vomiting early after infarction and to reduce the risk of aspiration, during the first 4 to 12 hours after admission patients should receive nothing by mouth or a clear liquid diet (**Table 55-7**). Subsequently, a diet with 50% to 55% of calories from complex carbohydrates and up to 30% from monounsaturated and unsaturated fats should be given. The diet should be enriched in foods that are high in potassium, magnesium, and fiber but low in sodium.

The results of laboratory tests obtained in the CCU should be scrutinized for any derangements potentially contributing to arrhythmias, such as hypoxemia, hypovolemia, disturbances of acid-base balance or of electrolytes, and drug toxicity. Oxazepam, 15 to 30 mg orally four times a day, is useful to allay the anxiety that is common in the first 24 to 48 hours (see Table 55-7). Delirium can be provoked by medications frequently used in the CCU, including antiarrhythmic drugs, H_2

TABLE 55-7	Sample Admitting Orders for the STEMI Patient

1. Condition: Serious
2. IV: NS on D_5W to keep vein open. Start a second IV if IV medication is being given. This may be saline lock.
3. Vital signs: Every 1.5 hr until stable, then every 4 hr and as needed. Notify physician if HR is <60 beats/min or >100 beats/min, BP is <100 mm Hg systolic or >150 mm Hg systolic, respiratory rate is <8 or >22.
4. Monitor: Continuous ECG monitoring for dysrhythmia and ST-segment deviation.
5. Diet: NPO except for sips of water until stable. Then start 2 g sodium/day, low saturated fat (<7% of total calories/day), low cholesterol (<200 mg/day) diet, such as total lifestyle change (TLC) diet.
6. Activity: Bedside commode and light activity when stable.
7. Oxygen: Continuous oximetry monitoring. Nasal cannula at 2 liters/min when stable for 6 hr, reassess for oxygen need (i.e., O_2 saturation of <90%) and consider discontinuing oxygen.
8. Medications:
   a. Nitroglycerin (NTG)
      1. Use sublingual NTG 0.4 mg every 5 min as needed for chest discomfort.
      2. Intravenous NTG for CHF, hypertension, or persistent ischemia.
   b. Aspirin (ASA; acetylsalicylic acid)
      1. If ASA not given in the emergency department (ED), chew nonenteric-coated ASA* 162-325 mg.
      2. If ASA has been given, start daily maintenance of 75-162 mg daily; may use enteric coated for gastrointestinal protection.
   c. Beta blocker
      1. If not given in the ED, assess for contraindication (i.e., bradycardia and hypotension); continue daily assessment to ascertain eligibility for beta blocker.
      2. If given in the ED, continue daily dose and optimize as dictated by heart rate and blood pressure.
   d. Angiotensin-converting enzyme (ACE) inhibitor
      1. Start ACE inhibitor orally in patients with pulmonary congestion or LVEF <40% if the following are absent: hypotension (SBP <100 mm Hg or <30 mm Hg below baseline) or known contraindications to this class of medications.
   e. Angiotensin receptor blocker (ARB)
      1. Start ARB orally in patients who are intolerant of ACE inhibitors and with either clinical or radiologic signs of heart failure or LVEF <40%.
   f. Pain medications
      1. IV morphine sulfate 2-4 mg with increments of 2-8 mg IV at 5- to 15-min intervals as needed to control pain.
   g. Anxiolytics (based on a nursing assessment)
   h. Daily stool softener

*Although some trials have used enteric-coated ASA for initial dosing, more rapid buccal absorption occurs with nonenteric-coated formulations.

BP = blood pressure; CHF = congestive heart failure; HR = heart rate; IV = intravenous; NS = normal saline; NPO = nothing by mouth.

Modified from Antman EM, Anbe DT, Armstrong PW, et al: ACC/AHA guidelines for the management of patients with ST-elevation myocardial infarction: A report of the American College of Cardiology/American Heart Association Task Force on Practice Guidelines (Committee to Revise the 1999 Guidelines for the Management of Patients with Acute Myocardial Infarction). Circulation 110:e82, 2004.

blockers, narcotics, and beta blockers. Potentially offending agents should be discontinued in patients with an abnormal mental status. Haloperidol, a butyrophenone, can be used safely in patients with STEMI, beginning with a dose of 2 mg intravenously for mildly agitated patients and 5 to 10 mg for progressively more agitated patients. Hypnotics, such as temazepam, 15 to 30 mg, or an equivalent, should be provided as needed for sleep. Docusate, 200 mg daily, or another stool softener should be used to prevent constipation and straining.

Coronary precautions that do not appear to be supported by evidence from clinical research include the avoidance of iced fluids, hot beverages, caffeinated beverages, rectal examinations, and back rubs.[1]

Physical Activity

In the absence of complications, patients with STEMI need not be confined to bed for more than 12 hours and, unless they are hemodynamically compromised, they may use a bedside commode shortly after admission (see Table 55-7). Progression of activity should be individualized depending on the patient's clinical status, age, and physical capacity.

In patients without hemodynamic compromise, early mobilization, including dangling the feet on the side of the bed, sitting in a chair, standing, and walking around the bed, does not cause important changes in heart rate, blood pressure, or pulmonary wedge pressure. Although heart rate increases slightly (usually by less than 10%), pulmonary wedge pressures fall slightly as the patient assumes the upright posture for activities. Early ambulatory activities are rarely associated with any symptoms, and when symptoms do occur, they generally are related to hypotension. Thus, when Levine and Lown proposed the armchair treatment of STEMI in the 1950s, they were undoubtedly correct that stress to the myocardium is less in the upright position. As long as blood pressure and heart rate are monitored, early mobilization offers considerable psychological and physical benefit, without any clear medical risk.

INTERMEDIATE CORONARY CARE UNIT. Patients with STEMI are at risk for late in-hospital mortality from recurrent ischemia or infarction, hemodynamically significant ventricular arrhythmias, and severe congestive heart failure after discharge from the CCU. Therefore, continued surveillance in intermediate CCUs (also called stepdown units) is justifiable. Risk factors for mortality in the hospital after discharge from the CCU include significant congestive heart failure evidenced by persistent sinus tachycardia for more than 2 days and rales in more than one third of the lung fields, recurrent ventricular tachycardia and ventricular fibrillation, atrial fibrillation or flutter while in the CCU, intraventricular conduction delays or heart block, anterior location of infarction, and recurrent episodes of angina with marked electrocardiographic ST-segment abnormalities at low activity levels.

The availability of intermediate care units may also be helpful for identifying those patients who remain free of complications and are suitable candidates for early discharge from the hospital. Aggressive reperfusion protocols with angioplasty or fibrinolytics can reduce the length of hospital stay without compromising mortality after discharge.[119] In patients who are thought to have undergone successful reperfusion, the absence of early sustained ventricular tachyarrhythmias, hypotension, or heart failure, coupled with a well-preserved left ventricular ejection fraction, predicts a low risk of in-hospital late complications. Such patients are suitable candidates for discharge from the hospital in less than 5 days from the onset of symptoms.

Following STEMI, patients are often eager for information, in need of reassurance, confused by misinformation and prior impressions, capable of counterproductive denial, and simply frightened. Intermediate care facilities provide ideal settings and ample opportunity to begin the rehabilitation process. The capacity for the early detection of problems following STEMI and the social and educational benefits of grouping such patients together strongly argue for continued use of intermediate CCUs. Furthermore, the economic advantage of grouping such patients together for the sharing of skilled personnel and resources outweighs any questions raised by the lack of a clear consensus regarding reduced mortality. An additional potential advantage is the facilitation of patient education in a group setting, with lectures and audiovisual programs.

Pharmacologic Therapy

BETA BLOCKERS. The effects of beta blockers for the treatment of patients with STEMI can be divided into those that are immediate (when the drug is given early in the course of infarction) and those that are long term (secondary prevention). The immediate intravenous administration of beta blockers reduces cardiac index, heart rate, and blood pressure.[120] The net effect is a reduction in myocardial oxygen consumption per minute and per beat. Favorable effects of acute intravenous administration of beta blockers on the balance of myocardial oxygen supply and demand are reflected in reductions in chest pain, in the proportion of patients with threatened infarction who actually evolve STEMI, and in the development of ventricular arrhythmias.[121]

Because beta-adrenergic blockade diminishes circulating levels of free fatty acids by antagonizing the lipolytic effects of catecholamines, and because elevated levels of fatty acids augment myocardial oxygen consumption and probably increase the incidence of arrhythmias, these metabolic actions of beta-blocking agents may also benefit the ischemic heart. Despite these favorable effects of early administration of intravenous beta blockers, there are potentially detrimental effects for some patients,[43] which have led to the modification of guidelines for early administration of intravenous beta blockers.[35]

More than 52,000 patients have been randomized in clinical trials studying beta-adrenergic blockade in acute MI. These trials cover a range of beta blockers and timing of administration and were largely conducted in the era before reperfusion strategies were developed for STEMI. The available data in the prereperfusion era have suggested there were favorable trends toward a reduction in mortality, reinfarction, and cardiac arrest. However, in the reperfusion era, the addition of an intravenous beta blocker to fibrinolytic therapy was not associated with a reduction in mortality but was helpful in reducing the rate of recurrent ischemic events.[122] Concern arose regarding the potential risk of provoking cardiogenic shock if early intravenous followed by oral beta-adrenergic blockade was routinely administered to all patients with STEMI.[121] The largest trial testing beta blockade in patients with acute MI was COMMIT, which randomized 45,852 patients within 24 hours of MI to metoprolol given as sequential intravenous boluses of 5 mg, up to 15 mg, followed by 200 mg/day orally or placebo.[43] There was no difference in the rate of the composite endpoint of death, reinfarction, or cardiac arrest in the metoprolol group (9.4%) compared with the placebo group (9.9%). But significant reductions occurred in reinfarction and episodes of ventricular fibrillation in the metoprolol group, translating into five fewer events for each of these endpoints per 1000 patients treated. However, there were 11 more episodes of cardiogenic shock in the metoprolol group per 1000 patients treated. The risk of developing cardiogenic shock, which was recorded as part of the COMMIT protocol in contrast to earlier studies, was greatest in those patients presenting with moderate to severe left ventricular dysfunction (Killip Class II or higher).

Combining the results of the low-risk patients from COMMIT with the data from earlier trials, an overview of the effects of early intravenous therapy followed by oral beta blocker therapy can be seen (**Fig. 55-24**). There is a 13% reduction in all-cause mortality (7 lives saved/1000 patients treated), 22% reduction in reinfarction (5 fewer events/1000 patients treated), and 15% reduction in ventricular fibrillation or cardiac arrest (5 fewer events/1000 patients treated).[43] To achieve these benefits safely, it is important to avoid the early administration of beta blockers to patients with relative contraindications, as outlined in **Table 55-8**.

Recommendations

Given the evidence of the benefits of early beta blocker administration in STEMI, patients without a contraindication (see Table 55-8), irrespective of administration of concomitant fibrinolytic therapy or performance of primary PCI, should promptly receive *oral* beta blockers. It is also reasonable to administer intravenously beta blockers promptly to STEMI patients, especially if a tachyarrhythmia or hypertension is present, in the absence of signs of heart failure or low output, increased risk of developing shock, indicators of high risk of developing shock, or other relative contraindications to beta blockers.[35] We use metoprolol 5 mg intravenously every 2 to 5 minutes for three doses, provided the heart rate does not fall below 60 beats/min and the systolic blood pressure does not drop below 100 mm Hg. Oral maintenance dosing

TABLE 55-8	Contraindications to Early Intravenous Beta Blocker Therapy in STEMI

Signs of heart failure
Evidence of a low-output state
Increased risk for cardiogenic shock*

*The more risk factors present, the higher the risk of developing cardiogenic shock: age older than 70 years, systolic blood pressure <120 mm Hg, sinus tachycardia >110 beats/min or heart rate <60 beats/min, and increased time since onset of symptom of STEMI.

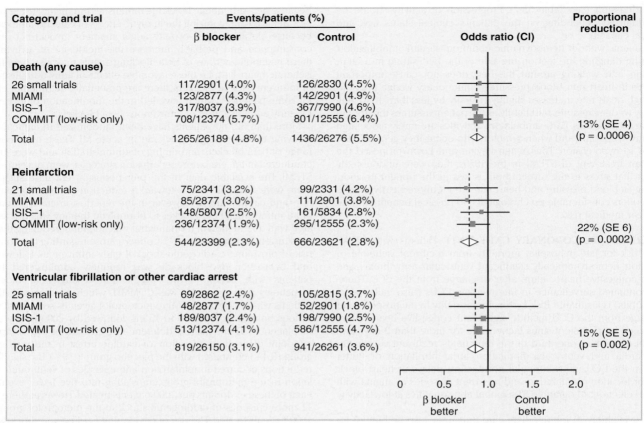

Category and trial	Events/patients (%)		Odds ratio (CI)	Proportional reduction
	β blocker	Control		
Death (any cause)				
26 small trials	117/2901 (4.0%)	126/2830 (4.5%)		
MIAMI	123/2877 (4.3%)	142/2901 (4.9%)		
ISIS–1	317/8037 (3.9%)	367/7990 (4.6%)		
COMMIT (low-risk only)	708/12374 (5.7%)	801/12555 (6.4%)		13% (SE 4)
Total	1265/26189 (4.8%)	1436/26276 (5.5%)		(p = 0.0006)
Reinfarction				
21 small trials	75/2341 (3.2%)	99/2331 (4.2%)		
MIAMI	85/2877 (3.0%)	111/2901 (3.8%)		
ISIS–1	148/5807 (2.5%)	161/5834 (2.8%)		
COMMIT (low-risk only)	236/12374 (1.9%)	295/12555 (2.3%)		22% (SE 6)
Total	544/23399 (2.3%)	666/23621 (2.8%)		(p = 0.0002)
Ventricular fibrillation or other cardiac arrest				
25 small trials	69/2862 (2.4%)	105/2815 (3.7%)		
MIAMI	48/2877 (1.7%)	52/2901 (1.8%)		
ISIS-1	189/8037 (2.4%)	198/7990 (2.5%)		
COMMIT (low-risk only)	513/12374 (4.1%)	586/12555 (4.7%)		15% (SE 5)
Total	819/26150 (3.1%)	941/26261 (3.6%)		(p = 0.002)

0   0.5   1.0   1.5   2.0

β blocker better   Control better

FIGURE 55-24 Meta-analysis of effects of intravenous and then oral beta blocker therapy on death, reinfarction, and cardiac arrest during the scheduled treatment periods in 26 small randomized trials, MIAMI, ISIS-1, and the low-risk subset of COMMIT. For COMMIT, data are included only for patients who presented with systolic blood pressure > 105 mm Hg, heart rate > 65 beats/min, and Killip Class I (as in MIAMI7). Five small trials included in the ISIS-1 report did not have any data on reinfarction. In the ISIS-1 trial, data on reinfarction in hospital were available for the last three quarters of the study, involving 11,641 patients. Odds ratios (ORs) in each (blue squares with area proportional to number of events) comparing outcome in patients allocated beta blockers to that in patients allocated controls, along with 99% CIs (horizontal line). Overall OR and 95% CI are indicated by diamonds. *(From Chen ZM, Pan HC, Chen YP, et al: Early intravenous then oral metoprolol in 45,852 patients with acute myocardial infarction: Randomised placebo-controlled trial. Lancet 366:1622, 2005.)*

is initiated with metoprolol, 50 mg every 6 hours for 2 days, and then 100 mg twice daily.

Beta blockers are especially helpful for patients in whom STEMI is complicated by persistent or recurrent ischemic pain, progressive or repetitive serum enzyme level elevations suggestive of infarct extension, or tachyarrhythmias early after the onset of infarction.[123] If adverse effects of beta blockers develop or if patients present with complications of infarction that are contraindications to beta blockade, such as heart failure or heart block, the beta blocker should be withheld. Unless there are contraindications (see Table 55-8), beta blockade probably should be continued in patients who develop STEMI.[35] Moreover, patients who initially have contraindications to a beta blocker, such as heart failure, should be reevaluated with respect to their candidacy for such therapy after 24 hours.

Selection of Beta Blocker

Favorable effects have been reported with metoprolol, atenolol, carvedilol, timolol, and alprenolol; these benefits probably occur with propranolol and with esmolol, an ultrashort-acting agent, as well. In the absence of any favorable evidence supporting the benefit of agents with intrinsic sympathomimetic activity, such as pindolol and oxprenolol, and with some unfavorable evidence for these agents in secondary prevention, beta blockers with intrinsic sympathomimetic activity probably should not be chosen for treatment of STEMI. The CAPRICORN trial randomized 1959 patients with MI and systolic dysfunction (ejection fraction < 40%) to carvedilol or placebo in addition to current pharmacotherapeutic agents, including angiotensin-converting enzyme (ACE) inhibitors in 98% of patients. All-cause mortality was

reduced over a mean follow-up of 1.3 years from 15.3% in the placebo group to 11.9% in the carvedilol group (23% RR reduction; $P = 0.031$), with a similar pattern during the first 30 days.[124] Thus, CAPRICORN confirms the benefit of beta blocker administration in addition to ACE inhibitor therapy for patients with transient or sustained left ventricular dysfunction after MI. An algorithm for the use of beta blockers in STEMI patients is shown in **Figure 55-25.**

Occasionally, the clinician may wish to proceed with beta blocker therapy even in the presence of relative contraindications, such as a history of mild asthma, mild bradycardia, mild heart failure, or first-degree heart block. In this situation, a trial of esmolol may help determine whether the patient can tolerate beta-adrenergic blockade. Because the hemodynamic effects of this drug, with a half-life of 9 minutes, disappear in less than 30 minutes, it offers considerable advantage over longer acting agents when the risk of a beta blocker complication is relatively high.

INHIBITORS OF THE RENIN-ANGIOTENSIN-ALDOSTERONE SYSTEM (RAAS). The rationale for inhibition of the RAAS includes experimental and clinical evidence of a favorable impact on ventricular remodeling, improvement in hemodynamics, and reductions in congestive heart failure. Unequivocal evidence from randomized, placebo-controlled trials has shown that ACE inhibitors reduce the rate of mortality from STEMI.[1] These trials can be grouped into two categories. The first group consisted of selected MI patients for randomization on the basis of features indicative of increased mortality, such as left ventricular ejection fraction less than 40%, clinical signs and symptoms of congestive heart failure, anterior location of infarction, and

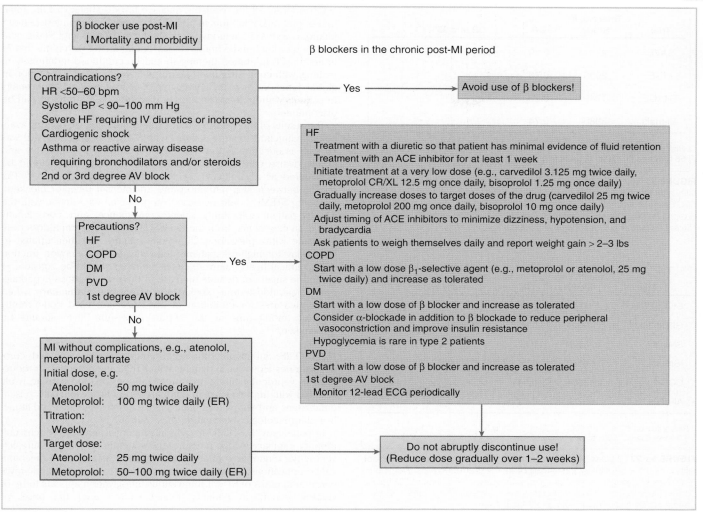

FIGURE 55-25 Algorithm for use of beta blockers in the treatment of patients with STEMI. COPD = chronic obstructive pulmonary disease; DM = diabetes mellitus; ER = extended release; HF = heart failure; PVD = peripheral vascular disease. *(From Gheorghiade M, Goldstein S: Beta-blockers in the post-myocardial infarction patient. Circulation 106:394, 2002.)*

abnormal wall motion score index (**Fig. 55-26**). Trials in the second group were unselective and randomized all patients with MI, provided they had a minimum systolic pressure of approximately 100 mm Hg (ISIS-4, GISSI-3, CONSENSUS II, and Chinese Captopril Study); (**Fig. 55-27**). With the exception of the SMILE trial, all the selective trials initiated ACE inhibitor therapy between 3 and 16 days after MI and maintained it for 1 to 4 years, whereas the unselective trials all initiated treatment within the first 24 to 36 hours and maintained it for only 4 to 6 weeks.

A consistent survival benefit was observed in all the trials already noted, except for CONSENSUS II, the one study that used an intravenous preparation early in the course of MI. An estimate of the mortality benefit of ACE inhibitors in the unselective, short duration trials was 5/1000 patients treated. Analysis of these unselective short-term trials indicates that approximately one third of lives was saved within the first 1 to 2 days. Certain subgroups, such as patients with anterior infarction, showed proportionately greater benefit from early administration (11 lives saved/1000) of ACE inhibitors. Not unexpectedly, greater survival benefits of 42 to 76 lives saved/1000 patients treated were obtained in the selective long-duration therapy trials. Of note, there was generally a 20% reduction in the risk of death attributable to ACE inhibitor treatment in the selective trials. The mortality reduction with ACE inhibitors is accompanied by significant reductions in the development of congestive heart failure, supporting the underlying pathophysiologic rationale for administering this class of drugs in patients with STEMI. In

addition, some data have suggested that chronic administration of ACE inhibitors after a STEMI reduces ischemic events, including recurrent infarction and the need for coronary revascularization.[125]

The mortality benefits of ACE inhibitors add to those achieved with aspirin and beta blockers. Thus, ACE inhibitors should not be considered a substitute for these other therapies with proven benefit in STEMI patients. The benefits of ACE inhibition appear to be a class effect, because mortality and morbidity have been reduced by several agents. To replicate these benefits in clinical practice, however, physicians should select a specific agent and prescribe the drug according to the protocols used in the successful clinical trials reported to date.[126]

The major contraindications to the use of ACE inhibitors in patients with STEMI include hypotension in the setting of adequate preload, known hypersensitivity, and pregnancy. Adverse reactions include hypotension, especially after the first dose, and intolerable cough with chronic dosing; much less commonly, angioedema can occur.

An alternative method of pharmacologic inhibition of the RAAS is by administration of angiotensin II receptor blockers (ARBs). The VALIANT trial compared the effects of the ARB valsartan versus captopril alone and in combination with captopril on mortality in patients with acute MI complicated by left ventricular systolic dysfunction and/or heart failure.[127] Patients were randomized within 10 days of MI to valsartan (20 mg initially, titrated to 160 mg twice daily), valsartan added to captopril (20 mg and 6.25 mg initially, titrated to 80 mg twice

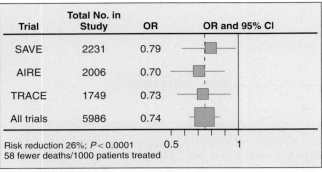

Trial	Total No. in Study	OR	OR and 95% CI
SAVE	2231	0.79	
AIRE	2006	0.70	
TRACE	1749	0.73	
All trials	5986	0.74	

Risk reduction 26%; *P* < 0.0001
58 fewer deaths/1000 patients treated

FIGURE 55-26 Effect of angiotensin-converting enzyme inhibitors on mortality after myocardial infarction—results from the long-term trials. *(From Gornik H, O'Gara PT: Adjunctive medical therapy. In Manson JE, Buring JE, Ridker PM, Gaziano JM [eds]: Clinical Trials in Heart Disease: A Companion to Braunwald's Heart Disease. Philadelphia, Elsevier Saunders, 2004, p 114.)*

Trial	Total No. in Study	OR	OR and 95% CI
CONSENSUS-II	6090	1.1	
GISSI-3	19394	0.88	
SMILE	1556	0.67	
ISIS-4	58050	0.94	
CCS-1	13634	0.94	
All trials	98724	0.93	

Risk reduction 6.7%; *P* < 0.006
4.9 fewer deaths/1000 patients treated

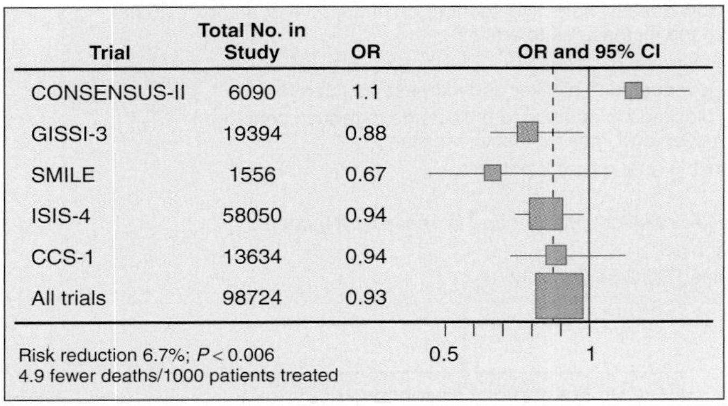

FIGURE 55-27 Effects of angiotensin-converting enzyme inhibitors on mortality after myocardial infarction—results from the short-term trials. *(From Gornik H, O'Gara PT: Adjunctive medical therapy. In Manson JE, Buring JE, Ridker PM, Gaziano JM [eds]: Clinical Trials in Heart Disease: A Companion to Braunwald's Heart Disease. Philadelphia, Elsevier Saunders, 2004, p 114.)*

daily and 50 mg three times daily), or captopril (6.25 mg initially, titrated to 50 mg three times daily) added to conventional therapy. Rates of mortality were similar in the three treatment groups—19.9% in the valsartan group, 19.3% in the valsartan plus captopril group, and 19.5% in the captopril alone group (**Fig. 55-28**).

Aldosterone blockade is another pharmacologic strategy for inhibition of the RAAS. The EPHESUS trial randomized 6642 patients with acute MI complicated by left ventricular dysfunction and heart failure to the selective aldosterone blocker eplerenone or placebo in conjunction with current postinfarction pharmacotherapy.[128] During a mean follow-up period of 16 months, there was a 15% reduction in the RR of mortality favoring eplerenone (**Fig. 55-29**). Cardiovascular mortality or hospitalization for cardiovascular events was also reduced by eplerenone. Serious hyperkalemia (serum potassium concentration ≥6 mmol/liter) occurred in 5.5% of patients in the eplerenone group compared with 3.9% of patients in the placebo group (*P* = 0.002).

Recommendations

After administration of aspirin and initiation of reperfusion strategies and, where appropriate, beta blockers, all STEMI patients should be considered for inhibition of the RAAS. Although there is little disagreement that high-risk STEMI patients (older, anterior infarction, prior infarction, Killip Class II or higher, and asymptomatic patients with evidence of depressed global ventricular function on an imaging study) should receive lifelong treatment with ACE inhibitors, short-term (4 to 6 weeks) therapy to a broader group of patients has also been proposed on the basis of the pooled results of the unselective mortality trials.[35,126]

Considering all the available data, we favor a strategy of an initial trial of oral ACE inhibitors in all STEMI patients with congestive heart failure, as well as in hemodynamically stable patients with ST-segment elevation or left bundle branch block, commencing within the first 24 hours.[129] ACE inhibition therapy should be continued indefinitely in patients with congestive heart failure, with evidence of a reduction in global function, or with a large regional wall motion abnormality. In patients without these findings at discharge, ACE inhibitors can be discontinued.

The results of the VALIANT trial expand the range of options available to clinicians treating patients with STEMI. Because the ARB was at least as effective as the ACE inhibitor in reducing mortality and other adverse cardiovascular outcomes following MI, it should be considered as a clinically effective alternative to captopril.[130] The choice between ACE inhibition and angiotensin receptor blockade following STEMI should be based on physician experience with the agents, patient tolerability, safety, convenience, and cost. Finally, based on experience from the EPHESUS study, long-term aldosterone blockade with eplerenone, 25 mg/day initially and then titrated to 50 mg/day for high-risk patients following STEMI (ejection fraction ≤40%, clinical heart failure, diabetes mellitus), should be considered. Given the small but definite increase in the risk of serious hyperkalemia when aldosterone blockade is prescribed, particularly when other measures for inhibition of the RAAS are used concurrently, periodic monitoring of the serum potassium level should be undertaken.[131]

NITRATES. Sublingual nitroglycerin rarely opens occluded coronary arteries. However, in patients with STEMI, the potential for reductions in ventricular filling pressures, wall tension, and cardiac work, coupled with improvement in coronary blood flow, especially in ischemic zones, and antiplatelet effects make nitrates a logical and attractive pharmacologic intervention (see Chap. 57).[35]

In patients with STEMI, the administration of nitrates reduces pulmonary capillary wedge pressure and systemic arterial pressure, left ventricular chamber volume, infarct size, and incidence of mechanical complications. As with other interventions to spare ischemic myocardium in cases of STEMI, intravenous nitroglycerin appears to be of greatest benefit in patients treated earliest after the onset of symptoms.

Clinical Trial Results

In the prefibrinolytic era, 10 randomized trials of acute administration of intravenous nitroglycerin (or nitroprusside, another nitric oxide donor) collectively enrolled 2042 patients. A meta-analysis of these trial results showed a reduction in mortality of 35% associated with nitrate therapy.[132]

In the fibrinolytic era, two megatrials of nitrate therapy have been conducted, GISSI-3 and ISIS-4.[1] In GISSI-3, there was no independent effect of nitrates on short-term mortality. Similarly, in ISIS-4, no effect of a mononitrate on 35-day mortality was observed. A pooled analysis of more than 80,000 patients treated with nitrate-like preparations intravenously or orally in 22 trials revealed a mortality rate of 7.7% in the control group, which was reduced to 7.4% in the nitrate group. These data suggest a small treatment effect of nitrates on mortality such that three to four fewer patients would die for every 1000 patients treated.

Nitrate Preparations and Mode of Administration

Intravenous nitroglycerin can be administered safely to patients with evolving STEMI as long as the dose is titrated to avoid induction of reflex tachycardia or systemic arterial hypotension. Patients with inferior wall infarction are particularly sensitive to an excessive fall in preload, particularly with concurrent right ventricular infarction.[35] In such cases, nitrate-induced venodilation could impair cardiac output and reduce coronary blood flow, thus worsening rather than improving myocardial oxygenation. A reasonable regimen begins with an initial infusion rate of 5 to 10 μg/min, with increases of 5 to 20 μg/min, until the mean arterial blood pressure is reduced by 10% of its baseline level in normotensive patients and by 30% for hypertensive patients, avoiding a systolic pressure lower than 90 mm Hg.

Adverse Effects

Clinically significant methemoglobinemia has been reported to occur during the administration of intravenous nitroglycerin. Although uncommon, this problem is seen when unusually large doses of nitrates are administered. It is important not only for its potential to cause symptoms of lethargy and headache, but also because elevated methemoglobin levels can impair the oxygen-carrying capacity of blood, potentially exacerbating ischemia. Dilation of the pulmonary vasculature supplying poorly ventilated lung segments may produce a ventilation-perfusion mismatch. Tolerance to intravenous nitroglycerin, as manifested by increasing nitrate requirements, develops in many patients, often as soon as 12 hours after the infusion is started. Despite the theoretical and demonstrated benefit of sulfhydryl agents in diminishing tolerance, their use has not become widespread.

Recommendations for Nitrates in Patients with STEMI

Nitroglycerin is indicated for the relief of persistent pain and as a vasodilator in patients with infarction associated with left ventricular failure. In the absence of recurrent angina or congestive heart failure, we do not routinely prescribe nitrates for STEMI patients. Higher-risk patients such as those with large infarctions, especially of the anterior wall, have the most to gain from nitrates in terms of reduction of ventricular remodeling, and therefore it is reasonable to consider using intravenous nitrates for 24 to 48 hours in such patients. There is no clear benefit to empirical long-term cutaneous or oral nitrates in the asymptomatic patient, and we therefore do not prescribe nitrates beyond the first 48 hours unless angina or ventricular failure is present.

CALCIUM CHANNEL ANTAGONISTS. Despite sound experimental and clinical evidence of an antiischemic effect, calcium antagonists have not been helpful in the acute phase of STEMI, and concern has been raised in several systematic overviews about an increased risk of mortality when they are prescribed on a routine basis. A distinction should be made between the dihydropyridine type of calcium channel antagonists (e.g., nifedipine) and the non-dihydropyridine agents (e.g., verapamil and diltiazem).

Nifedipine

In multiple trials involving more than 5000 patients, the immediate-release preparation of nifedipine has not resulted in any reduction in infarct size, prevention of progression to infarction, control of recurrent ischemia, or lowering of mortality rate. When trials of the immediate-release form of nifedipine are pooled in a meta-analysis, evidence suggests a dose-related increased risk of in-hospital mortality (especially at a dose of >80 mg of nifedipine), although posthospital mortality does not appear to be increased in nifedipine-treated patients. Nifedipine does not appear to be helpful in conjunction with fibrinolytic therapy or beta blockade. Thus, we do not recommend the use of immediate-release nifedipine early in the treatment of STEMI. No trials of the sustained-release preparations of nifedipine in patients with STEMI have been reported to date.

Verapamil and Diltiazem

When administered during the acute phase of STEMI, these drugs have not had any demonstrated favorable effect on infarct size or other important endpoints in patients with STEMI, with the exception of control of supraventricular arrhythmias.[1] The INTERCEPT trial compared 300 mg of diltiazem with placebo in patients who received fibrinolytic therapy for STEMI. Diltiazem did not reduce the cumulative

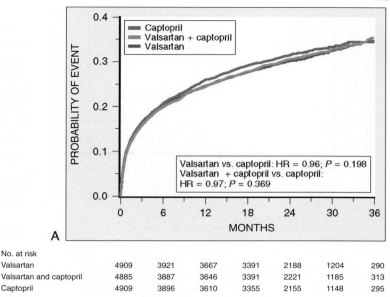

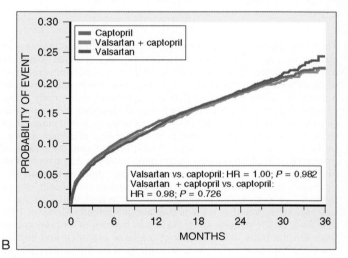

No. at risk

Valsartan	4909	3921	3667	3391	2188	1204	290
Valsartan and captopril	4885	3887	3646	3391	2221	1185	313
Captopril	4909	3896	3610	3355	2155	1148	295

No. at risk

Valsartan	4909	4464	4272	4007	2648	1437	357
Valsartan and captopril	4885	4414	4265	3994	2648	1435	382
Captopril	4909	4428	4241	4018	2635	1432	364

FIGURE 55-28 Effects of an ACE inhibitor (captopril), ARB (valsartan), or combination after myocardial infarction. The Kaplan-Meier estimates of **(A)** mortality and **(B)** cardiovascular death, reinfarction, or hospitalization for heart failure by treatment in the VALIANT trial are depicted. HR = hazard ratio. *(From Pfeffer M, McMurray JJ, Velasquez EJ, et al: Valsartan, captopril, or both in myocardial infarction complicated by heart failure, left ventricular dysfunction, or both. N Engl J Med 349:1893, 2003.)*

occurrence of cardiac death, nonfatal reinfarction, or refractory ischemia during a 6-month follow-up.

Based on the available data, we do not recommend the routine use of verapamil or diltiazem for patients with STEMI. Verapamil and diltiazem can be given for relief of ongoing ischemia or slowing of a rapid ventricular response in atrial fibrillation in patients for whom beta blockers are ineffective or contraindicated.[1] Their use should be avoided in patients with Killip Class II or greater hemodynamic findings.

OTHER THERAPIES

Magnesium

Patients with STEMI may have a total body deficit of magnesium because of a low dietary intake, advanced age, or prior diuretic use.

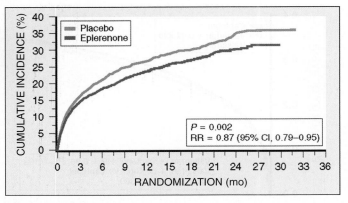

No. at risk
| Placebo | 3313 | 2754 | 2580 | 2388 | 2013 | 1494 | 995 | 558 | 247 | 77 | 2 | 0 | 0 |
| Eplerenone | 3319 | 2816 | 2680 | 2504 | 2096 | 1564 | 1061 | 594 | 273 | 91 | 0 | 0 | 0 |

FIGURE 55-29 Effect of a selective aldosterone receptor blocker (eplere-none) after myocardial infarction. The Kaplan-Meier estimates of the rate of death from cardiovascular causes or hospitalization for cardiovascular events in the EPHESUS trial are depicted. *(From Pitt B, Remme W, Zannad F, et al: Eplerenone, a selective aldosterone blocker, in patients with left ventricular dysfunction after myocardial infarction [abstract]. N Engl J Med 348:14, 2003.)*

They may also acquire a functional deficit of available magnesium caused by trapping of free magnesium in adipocytes, as soaps are formed when free fatty acids are released by catecholamine-induced lipolysis with the onset of infarction. Because of the risk of cardiac arrhythmias when electrolyte deficits are present in the early phase of infarction, all patients with STEMI should have their serum magnesium level measured on admission. We advocate repleting magnesium deficits to maintain a serum magnesium level of 2 mEq/liter or more. In the presence of hypokalemia (<4 mEq/liter) during the course of treatment of STEMI, the serum magnesium level should be rechecked and repleted if necessary because it is often difficult to correct a potassium deficit in the presence of a concurrent magnesium deficit. Episodes of torsades de pointes should be treated with 1 to 2 g of magnesium delivered as a bolus over about 5 minutes. Between 1980 and 2002, 68,684 patients were studied in a series of 14 randomized trials. On the basis of the totality of available evidence and current coronary care practice, there is no indication for the routine admin-istration of intravenous magnesium to patients with STEMI at any level of risk.[133]

Glucose Control During STEMI

During the acute phase of STEMI, there is an increase in catechol-amine levels in both the blood and ischemic myocardium. Insulin levels remain low, whereas cortisol, glucagon, and free fatty acid levels increase. These factors may contribute to an elevation of the blood glucose level, which should be measured routinely on admis-sion to the coronary care unit (see Chap. 64). An infusion of insulin is recommended to treat persistent hyperglycemia in STEMI patients with a complicated course.[134] Given the evidence supporting glucose control in critically ill patients, it is also reasonable to administer an insulin infusion to hyperglycemic STEMI patients, even if they have an uncomplicated course. However, intensive treatment of hyperglycemia to a target less than 110 mg/dL in the critical care setting is not recommended.

It was proposed that routine administration of infusions of glucose-insulin-potassium (GIK) to STEMI patients would reduce mortality. A series of small trials, most of which were performed in the prereperfu-sion era, along with some in the setting of fibrinolysis or PCI, has sug-gested that GIK infusions are of benefit. However, the CREATE-ECLA investigators randomized 20,201 STEMI patients (83% of whom received reperfusion therapy) to GIK or placebo and found no evi-dence of a mortality benefit (30-day mortality, 9.7% in control patients and 10% in GIK patients).[135] Thus, in the current era of STEMI manage-ment, in which other effective therapies (e.g., reperfusion, aspirin, ACE

inhibitors) are administered, there appears to be no benefit to the routine use of GIK infusions.

Other Agents

Several adjunctive pharmacotherapies have been investigated to prevent inflammatory damage in the infarct zone but have not been shown to provide a clinical benefit. For example, pexelizumab, a monoclonal antibody against the C5 component of complement, had no effect on infarct size in STEMI patients treated with fibrinolytics or PCI.[136,137] It also had no effect on mortality in STEMI patients treated with primary PCI.[138] The AMISTAD II trial was a dose-ranging study of adenosine in patients with anterior STEMI.[81] Although high-dose ade-nosine (70 μg/kg/min infusion for 3 hours) was associated with a reduction in infarct size, neither high- nor low-dose adenosine reduced the primary composite clinical endpoint of death or the development of heart failure at 6 months compared with placebo.[59]

Hemodynamic Disturbances

Hemodynamic Assessment

Patients with clinically uncomplicated STEMI do not require invasive hemodynamic monitoring because clinical evaluation can assess the status of the circulation. This approach ordinarily consists of monitor-ing of heart rate and rhythm, repeated measurement of systemic arte-rial pressure by cuff, obtaining chest radiographs to detect heart failure, repeated auscultation of the lung fields for pulmonary conges-tion, measurement of urine flow, examination of the skin and mucous membranes for evidence of the adequacy of perfusion, and arterial sampling for pO_2, pCO_2, and pH when hypoxemia or metabolic acido-sis is suspected.

In contrast, in patients with STEMI whose ventricular contractile performance is abnormal, as evidenced by clinical signs and symp-toms of heart failure, it is important to assess the degree of hemody-namic compromise to initiate therapy with drugs such as vasodilators and diuretics. In the past, central venous or right atrial pressure was used to gauge the degree of left ventricular failure in patients with STEMI. However, this technique is limited because central venous pressure reflects right rather than left ventricular function. Right ven-tricular function and therefore systemic venous pressure may be normal or almost normal in patients with significant left ventricular failure. Conversely, patients with right ventricular failure caused by right ventricular infarction or pulmonary embolism may exhibit elevated right atrial and central venous pressures, despite normal left ventricular function. Low values for right atrial and central venous pressures imply hypovolemia, whereas elevated right atrial pressures usually result from right ventricular failure secondary to left ventricular failure, pulmonary hypertension, or right ventricular infarc-tion or, less commonly, from tricuspid regurgitation or pericardial tamponade.

Major advances in the management of complicated STEMI have resulted from the hemodynamic monitoring that has become wide-spread in CCUs (**Table 55-9**). This approach often uses both an intra-arterial catheter and pulmonary artery catheter for the measurement of pulmonary artery, pulmonary artery occlusive (equivalent to pulmo-nary wedge), and right atrial pressures, and cardiac output by thermo-dilution. In patients with hypotension, a Foley catheter provides accurate and continuous measurement of urine output.

NEED FOR INVASIVE MONITORING. The use of invasive hemo-dynamic monitoring is based on the following needs and challenges:
1. Difficulty in interpreting clinical and radiographic findings of pul-monary congestion, even after a review of noninvasive studies such as an echocardiogram.
2. Need for identifying noncardiac causes of arterial hypotension, particularly hypovolemia.
3. Possible contribution of reduced ventricular compliance to impaired hemodynamics, requiring judicious adjustment of intra-vascular volume to optimize left ventricular filling pressure.

TABLE 55-9 Indications for Hemodynamic Monitoring in Patients with STEMI

Management of complicated acute myocardial infarction
   Hypovolemia versus cardiogenic shock
   Ventricular septal rupture versus acute mitral regurgitation
   Severe left ventricular failure
   Right ventricular failure
Refractory ventricular tachycardia
Differentiating severe pulmonary disease from left ventricular failure
Assessment of cardiac tamponade
Assessment of therapy in *selected* individuals
   Afterload reduction in patients with severe left ventricular failure
   Inotropic agent therapy
   Beta blocker therapy
   Temporary pacing (ventricular versus atrioventricular)
   Intra-aortic balloon counterpulsation
   Mechanical ventilation

From Gore JM, Zwernet PL: Hemodynamic monitoring of acute myocardial infarction. *In* Francis GS, Alpert JS (eds): Modern Coronary Care. Boston, Little, Brown, 1990, p 138.

TABLE 55-10 Hemodynamic Classifications of Patients with Acute Myocardial Infarction

Based on Clinical Examination*		Based on Invasive Monitoring†	
CLASS	DEFINITION	SUBSET	DEFINITION
I	Rales and S_3 absent	I	Normal hemodynamics; PCWP < 18 mm Hg, CI > 2.2
II	Crackles, S_3 gallop, elevated jugular venous pressure	II	Pulmonary congestion; PCWP > 18 mm Hg, CI > 2.2
III	Frank pulmonary edema	III	Peripheral hypoperfusion; PCWP < 18 mm Hg, CI < 2.2
IV	Shock	IV	Pulmonary congestion and peripheral hypoperfusion; PCWP > 18 mm Hg, CI < 2.2

CI = cardiac index; PCWP = pulmonary capillary wedge pressure.
*Modified from Killip T, Kimball J: Treatment of myocardial infarction in a coronary care unit. A two year experience with 250 patients. Am J Cardiol 20:457, 1967.
†Modified from Forrester J, Diamond G, Chatterjee K, et al: Medical therapy of acute myocardial infarction by the application of hemodynamic subsets. N Engl J Med 295:1356, 1976.

4. Difficulty in assessing the severity and sometimes the presence of complications such as mitral regurgitation and ventricular septal defect when the cardiac output or systemic pressures is (are) depressed.

5. Establishing a baseline of hemodynamic measurements and guiding therapy in patients with clinically apparent pulmonary edema or cardiogenic shock.

6. Underestimation of systemic arterial pressure by the cuff method in patients with intense vasoconstriction.

The prognosis and clinical status of patients with STEMI relate to the cardiac output and pulmonary artery wedge pressure. Patients with normal cardiac output after STEMI have a low expected mortality rate; prognosis worsens as cardiac output declines. Patients with intraventricular conduction defects, AV block, or both after anterior infarction have lower cardiac indices and higher pulmonary capillary wedge pressures than patients without these conduction disturbances. Conversely, patients with these conduction defects and inferior STEMI usually do not demonstrate such hemodynamic abnormalities.

PULMONARY ARTERY PRESSURE MONITORING. Patients most likely to benefit from pulmonary artery catheter monitoring include those whose STEMI is complicated by the following: (1) hypotension that is not easily corrected by fluid administration; (2) hypotension in the presence of congestive heart failure; (3) hemodynamic compromise severe enough to require intravenous vasopressors or vasodilators or intra-aortic balloon counterpulsation; (4) mechanical lesions (or suspected lesions) such as cardiac tamponade, severe mitral regurgitation, and a ruptured ventricular septum; and (5) right ventricular infarction.[139] Other indications for hemodynamic monitoring include assessment of the effects of mechanical ventilation, differentiating pulmonary disease from left ventricular failure as the cause of hypoxemia, and management of septic shock (see Table 55-9).[35] Before inserting a pulmonary artery catheter into a patient with STEMI, the physician must consider that the potential benefit of the information to be obtained outweighs any potential risks. Accumulating evidence from settings other than STEMI suggest that invasive hemodynamic monitoring does not improve outcomes.[140]

Major complications from pulmonary artery catheters are not common (about 3% to 5% of cases), but severe problems can occur, including sepsis, pulmonary infarction, and pulmonary artery rupture.[141] Minimized duration of catheterization and strict adherence to aseptic techniques can diminish risk. Catheter-related bloodstream infections can also be reduced by using antiseptic-impregnated dressings.[142] Noninvasive methods of determining cardiac output, such as pulse contour analysis and thoracic electrical bioimpedance, are under investigation.[143]

Accurate determination of hemodynamics by clinical assessment is difficult in critically ill patients. Consequently, the use of a pulmonary artery catheter often leads to important changes in therapy. Of note, it has been reported that rates of complications and mortality may be higher in patients who undergo pulmonary artery catheterization, although such patients are often at higher risk initially. These observations emphasize the importance of patient selection, meticulous technique, and correct interpretation of the data obtained.[141]

HEMODYNAMIC ABNORMALITIES. In 1976, Swan and coworkers measured the cardiac output and wedge pressure simultaneously in a large series of patients with acute MI and identified four major hemodynamic subsets of patients (**Table 55-10**): (1) patients with normal systemic perfusion and without pulmonary congestion (normal cardiac output and normal wedge pressure); (2) patients with normal perfusion and pulmonary congestion (normal cardiac output and elevated wedge pressure); (3) patients with decreased perfusion but without pulmonary congestion (reduced cardiac output and normal wedge pressure); and (4) patients with decreased perfusion and pulmonary congestion (reduced cardiac output and elevated wedge pressure). This classification, which overlaps with a crude clinical classification proposed earlier by Killip and Kimball (see Table 55-10), has proved to be useful, but it should be noted that patients frequently pass from one category to another with therapy and sometimes apparently even spontaneously.

Hemodynamic Subsets

The patient's clinical status generally reflects these subsets. Hypoperfusion usually becomes evident clinically when the cardiac index falls below approximately 2.2 liters/min/m², whereas pulmonary congestion is noted when the wedge pressure exceeds approximately 20 mm Hg. However, approximately 25% of patients with cardiac indices lower than 2.2 liters/min/m² and 15% of patients with elevated pulmonary capillary wedge pressures are not recognized clinically. Discrepancies in hemodynamic and clinical classification of patients with STEMI arise for a variety of reasons. Patients may exhibit phase lags as clinical pulmonary congestion develops or resolves, symptoms secondary to chronic obstructive pulmonary disease may be confused with those resulting from pulmonary congestion, or long-standing left ventricular dysfunction may mask signs of hypoperfusion because of compensatory vasoconstriction.

The hemodynamic findings shown in **Table 55-11** allow for rational approaches to therapy (see Table 55-10). The goals of hemodynamic therapy include maintenance of ventricular performance, blood pressure support, and protection of jeopardized myocardium. Because these goals occasionally may be at cross purposes, recognition of the

TABLE 55-11	Hemodynamic Patterns for Common Clinical Conditions				
	CHAMBER PRESSURE (MG HG)				
CARDIAC CONDITION	RA	RV	PA	PCW	CI
Normal	0-6	25/0-6	25/0-12	6-12	≥2.5
AMI without LVF	0-6	25/0-6	30/12-18	≤18	≥2.5
AMI with LVF	0-6	30-40/0-6	30-40/18-25	>18	>2.0
Biventricular failure	>6	50-60/>6	50-60/25	18-25	>2.0
RVMI	12-20	30/12-20	30/12	≤12	<2.0
Cardiac tamponade	12-16	25/12-16	25/12-16	12-16	<2.0
Pulmonary embolism	12-20	50-60/12-20	50-60/12	<12	<2.0

AMI = acute myocardial infarction; CI = cardiac index; LVF = left ventricular failure; PA = pulmonary artery; PCW = pulmonary capillary wedge; RA = right atrium; RV = right ventricle; RVMI = right ventricular myocardial infarction.

From Gore JM, Zwernet PL: Hemodynamic monitoring of acute myocardial infarction. In Francis GS, Alpert JS (eds): Modern Coronary Care. Boston, Little, Brown, 1990, pp 139-164.

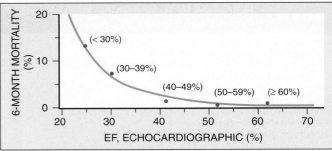

FIGURE 55-30 Impact of left ventricular function on survival following MI. The curvilinear relationship between left ventricular ejection fraction (EF) for patients treated in the fibrinolytic era is shown. Among patients with a left ventricular EF below 40%, the rate of mortality is markedly increased at 6 months. Thus, interventions such as thrombolysis, aspirin, and ACE inhibitors should be of considerable benefit in patients with acute MI to minimize the amount of left ventricular damage and interrupt the neurohumoral activation seen with congestive heart failure. (*Modified from Volpi A, De Vita C, Franzosi MG, et al: Determinants of 6-month mortality in survivors of myocardial infarction after thrombolysis. Results of the GISSI-2 data base. The Ad Hoc Working Group of the Gruppo Italiano per lo Studio della Sopravvivenza nell'Infarto Miocardico [GISSI]-2 Data Base. Circulation 88:416, 1993.*)

hemodynamic profile, as assessed clinically or as determined from hemodynamic monitoring, is required to design an optimal therapeutic management strategy.

Hypotension in the Prehospital Phase

During the prehospital phase of STEMI, invasive hemodynamic monitoring is not feasible and therapy should be guided by frequent clinical assessment and measurement of arterial pressure by cuff, recognizing that intense vasoconstriction can provide a falsely low pressure measured by this method. Hypotension associated with bradycardia often reflects excessive vagotonia. Relative or absolute hypovolemia is often present when hypotension occurs with a normal or rapid heart rate, particularly among patients receiving diuretics just before the infarction. Marked diaphoresis, reduction of fluid intake, or vomiting during the period preceding and accompanying the onset of STEMI may all contribute to the development of hypovolemia. Even if the effective vascular volume is normal, relative hypovolemia may be present because ventricular compliance is reduced in cases of STEMI, and a left ventricular filling pressure as high as 20 mm Hg may be necessary to provide an optimal preload.

MANAGEMENT. In the absence of rales involving more than one third of the lung fields, patients should be put in the reverse Trendelenburg position and, in patients with sinus bradycardia and hypotension, atropine should be administered (0.3 to 0.6 mg IV repeated at 3- to 10-minute intervals, up to 2 mg). If these measures do not correct the hypotension, normal saline should be administered intravenously, beginning with a bolus of 100 mL followed by 50-mL increments every 5 minutes. The patient should be observed and the infusion stopped when the systolic pressure returns to approximately 100 mm Hg, if the patient becomes dyspneic, or if pulmonary rales develop or increase. Because of the poor correlation between left ventricular filling pressure and mean right atrial pressure, assessment of systemic (even central) venous pressure is of limited value as a guide to fluid therapy. Administration of positive inotropic agents is indicated during the prehospital phase if systemic hypotension persists despite correction of hypovolemia and excessive vagotonia.

Hypovolemic Hypotension

Recognition of hypovolemia is of particular importance in hypotensive patients with STEMI because of the hazard it poses and because of the improvement in circulatory dynamics that can be achieved so readily and safely by augmentation of vascular volume. Because hypovolemia is often occult, it is frequently overlooked in the absence of invasive hemodynamic monitoring. Hypovolemia may be absolute, with low left ventricular filling pressure (8 mm Hg), or relative, with normal (8 to 12 mm Hg) or even modestly increased (13 to 18 mm Hg) left ventricular filling pressures.

Exclusion of hypovolemia as the cause of hypotension requires the documentation of a reduced cardiac output despite the left ventricular filling pressure exceeding 18 mm Hg. If, in a hypotensive patient, the pulmonary capillary wedge pressure (ordinarily measured as the pulmonary artery occlusive pressure) is below this level, fluid challenge should be carried out as noted. Hypotension caused by right ventricular infarction may be confused with that caused by hypovolemia because both are associated with a low, normal, or minimally elevated left ventricular filling pressure. The findings and management of right ventricular infarction are discussed elsewhere in this chapter.

Hyperdynamic State

When infarction is not complicated by hemodynamic impairment, no therapy other than general supportive measures and treatment of arrhythmias is necessary. However, if the hemodynamic profile is of the hyperdynamic state—that is, elevation of sinus rate, arterial pressure, and cardiac index, occurring singly or together in the presence of a normal or low left ventricular filling pressure—and if other causes of tachycardia such as fever, infection, and pericarditis can be excluded, treatment with beta blockers is indicated. Presumably, the increased heart rate and blood pressure result from inappropriate activation of the sympathetic nervous system, possibly because of the augmented release of catecholamines triggered by pain and/or anxiety.

Left Ventricular Failure

Left ventricular dysfunction is the single most important predictor of mortality following STEMI (**Fig. 55-30**).[144,145] In patients with STEMI, systolic dysfunction alone or both systolic and diastolic dysfunction can occur. Left ventricular diastolic dysfunction leads to pulmonary venous hypertension and pulmonary congestion. Clinical manifestations of left ventricular failure become more common as the extent of the injury to the left ventricle increases. In addition to infarct size, other important predictors of the development of symptomatic left ventricular dysfunction include advanced age and diabetes.[146,147] Mortality increases are related to the severity of the hemodynamic deficit.

THERAPEUTIC IMPLICATIONS. Classification of patients with STEMI by hemodynamic subsets has therapeutic relevance. As noted, patients with normal wedge pressures and hypoperfusion often benefit from the infusion of fluids because the peak value of stroke volume is usually not attained until left ventricular filling pressure reaches 18 to 24 mm Hg. However, a low level of left ventricular filling pressure does not necessarily imply that left ventricular damage is slight. Such patients may be relatively hypovolemic and/or may have suffered a right ventricular infarct, with or without severe left ventricular damage.

When preload is increased by fluid infusion, the relationship between ventricular filling pressure and cardiac index can provide valuable hemodynamic information in addition to that obtained from baseline measurements. For example, the ventricular function curve rises steeply (marked increase in cardiac index, small increase in filling pressure) in patients with normal left ventricular function and hypovolemia, whereas the curve rises gradually or remains flat in those patients with a combination of hypovolemia and depressed cardiac function. Invasive hemodynamic monitoring is essential to guide therapy of patients with severe left ventricular failure (pulmonary capillary wedge pressure > 18 mm Hg and cardiac index < 2.5 liters/min/m^2). Although positive inotropic agents can be useful, they do not represent the initial therapy of choice in patients with STEMI. Instead, heart failure is managed most effectively first by reduction of ventricular preload and then, if possible, by lowering of afterload. Arrhythmias can contribute to hemodynamic compromise and should be treated promptly in patients with left ventricular failure.

HYPOXEMIA. Patients with STEMI complicated by congestive heart failure characteristically develop hypoxemia caused by a combination of pulmonary vascular engorgement and, in some cases, pulmonary interstitial edema, diminished vital capacity, and respiratory depression from narcotic analgesics. Hypoxemia can impair the function of ischemic tissue at the margin of the infarct and thereby contribute to establishing or perpetuating the vicious cycle (see Chap. 54). The ventilation-perfusion mismatch that results in hypoxemia requires careful attention to ventilatory support. Increasing fractions of inspired oxygen (FiO$_2$) via face mask should be used initially, but if the oxygen saturation of the patient's blood cannot be maintained above 85% to 90% on 100% FiO$_2$, strong consideration should be given to endotracheal intubation with positive-pressure ventilation. The improvement of arterial oxygenation and hence myocardial oxygen supply may help restore ventricular performance. Positive end-expiratory pressure may diminish systemic venous return and reduce effective left ventricular filling pressure. This may require reduction in the amount of positive end-expiratory pressure, normal saline infusions to maintain left ventricular filling pressure, adjustment of the rate of infusion of vasodilators such as nitroglycerin, or some combination of these. Because myocardial ischemia frequently occurs during the return to unsupported spontaneous breathing, weaning should be accompanied by observation for signs of ischemia and is potentially facilitated by a period of intermittent mandatory ventilation or pressure support ventilation before extubation.

DIURETICS. Mild heart failure in patients with STEMI frequently responds well to diuretics such as furosemide, administered intravenously in doses of 10 to 40 mg and repeated at 3- to 4-hour intervals if necessary. The resultant reduction of pulmonary capillary pressure reduces dyspnea, and the lowering of left ventricular wall tension that accompanies the reduction of left ventricular diastolic volume diminishes myocardial oxygen requirements and may lead to improvement of contractility and augmentation of the ejection fraction, stroke volume, and cardiac output. The reduction of elevated left ventricular filling pressure may also enhance myocardial oxygen delivery by diminishing the impedance to coronary perfusion attributable to elevated ventricular wall tension. It may also improve arterial oxygenation by reducing pulmonary vascular congestion.

The intravenous administration of furosemide reduces pulmonary vascular congestion and pulmonary venous pressure within 15 minutes, before renal excretion of sodium and water has occurred; presumably, this action results from a direct dilating effect of this drug on the systemic arterial bed. It is important not to reduce left ventricular filling pressure much below 18 mm Hg, the lower range associated with optimal left ventricular performance in STEMI, because this could reduce cardiac output further and cause arterial hypotension. Excessive diuresis may also result in hypokalemia.

AFTERLOAD REDUCTION. Myocardial oxygen requirements depend on left ventricular wall stress, which in turn is proportional to the product of peak developed left ventricular pressure, volume, and wall thickness. Vasodilator therapy is recommended in patients with STEMI complicated by the following: (1) heart failure unresponsive to treatment with diuretics; (2) hypertension; (3) mitral regurgitation; or (4) ventricular septal defect. In these patients, treatment with vasodilator agents increases stroke volume and may reduce myocardial oxygen requirements and thereby lessen ischemia. Hemodynamic monitoring of systemic arterial and, in many cases, pulmonary capillary wedge (or at least pulmonary artery) pressure and cardiac output in patients treated with these agents is important. Improvement of cardiac performance and energetics requires three simultaneous effects: (1) reduction of left ventricular afterload; (2) avoidance of excessive systemic arterial hypotension to maintain effective coronary perfusion pressure; and (3) avoidance of excessive reduction of ventricular filling pressure with consequent diminution of cardiac output. In general, pulmonary capillary wedge pressure should be maintained at approximately 20 mm Hg and arterial pressure above 90/60 mm Hg in patients who were normotensive before developing STEMI.

Vasodilator therapy is particularly useful when STEMI is complicated by mitral regurgitation or rupture of the ventricular septum. In such patients, vasodilators alone or in combination with intra-aortic balloon counterpulsation can sometimes serve as a temporary measure and provide hemodynamic stabilization to permit definitive catheterization and angiographic studies and prepare the patient for early surgical intervention. Because of the precarious state of patients with complicated infarction and the need for meticulous adjustment of dosage, therapy is best initiated with agents that can be administered intravenously and that have a short duration of action (e.g., nitroprusside, nitroglycerin, isosorbide dinitrate). After initial stabilization, the medication of choice is generally an ACE inhibitor, but long-acting nitrates given by mouth, sublingually, or by ointment can also be useful.

Nitroglycerin

This drug has been shown in animal experiments to be less likely than nitroprusside to produce a coronary steal (i.e., to divert blood flow from the ischemic to the nonischemic zone). Therefore, apart from consideration of its routine use in STEMI patients discussed earlier, it may be a particularly useful vasodilator in patients with STEMI complicated by left ventricular failure. Ten to 15 mg/min is infused and the dose is increased by 10 mg/min every 5 minutes until the desired effect (improvement of hemodynamics or relief of ischemic chest pain) is achieved or a decline in systolic arterial pressure to 90 mm Hg, or by more than 15 mm Hg, has occurred. Although both nitroglycerin and nitroprusside lower systemic arterial pressure, systemic vascular resistance, and the heart rate–systolic blood pressure product, the reduction of left ventricular filling pressure is more prominent with nitroglycerin because of its relatively greater effect than nitroprusside on venous capacitance vessels. Nevertheless, in patients with severe left ventricular failure, cardiac output often increases, despite the reduction in left ventricular filling pressure produced by nitroglycerin.

Oral Vasodilators

The use of oral vasodilators in the treatment of chronic congestive heart failure is discussed in Chap. 28. Patients with STEMI and persistent heart failure should receive long-term inhibition of the RAAS.[35] Reduced ventricular load decreases the remodeling of the left ventricle that occurs commonly in the period after STEMI and thereby reduces the development of heart failure and risk of death.[148,149]

DIGITALIS. Although digitalis increases the contractility and oxygen consumption of normal hearts, when heart failure is present, the diminution of heart size and wall tension frequently results in a net reduction of myocardial oxygen requirements (see Chap. 28). In animal experiments, it fails to improve ventricular performance immediately following experimental coronary occlusion, but salutary effects are elicited when it is administered several days later. The absence of early beneficial effects may be caused by the inability of ischemic tissue to respond to digitalis or the already maximal stimulation of contractility of the normal heart by circulating and neuronally released catecholamines.

Although the issue is still controversial, arrhythmias can be increased by digitalis glycosides when they are given to patients in the first few hours after the onset of STEMI, particularly in the presence of hypokalemia. Also, undesirable peripheral systemic and coronary vasoconstriction can result from the rapid intravenous administration of rapidly acting glycosides such as ouabain.

Administration of digitalis to patients with STEMI in the hospital phase should generally be reserved for the management of supraventricular tachyarrhythmias, such as atrial flutter and fibrillation, and of heart failure that persists despite treatment with diuretics, vasodilators, and beta blockers. There is no indication for its use as an inotropic agent in patients without clinical evidence of left ventricular dysfunction, and it is too weak an inotropic agent to be relied on as the principal cardiac stimulant in patients with overt pulmonary edema or cardiogenic shock.

BETA-ADRENERGIC AGONISTS. When left ventricular failure is severe, as manifested by marked reduction of the cardiac index (<2 liters/min/m^2), and pulmonary capillary wedge pressure is at optimal (18 to 24 mm Hg) or excessive (>24 mm Hg) levels, despite therapy with diuretics, beta-adrenergic agonists are indicated.[150] Although isoproterenol is a potent cardiac stimulant and improves ventricular performance, it should be avoided in STEMI patients. It also causes tachycardia and augments myocardial oxygen consumption and lactate production; in addition, it reduces coronary perfusion pressure by causing systemic vasodilation, and in animal experiments it increases the extent of experimentally induced infarction. Norepinephrine also increases myocardial oxygen consumption because of its peripheral vasoconstrictor and positive inotropic actions. Nevertheless, in a randomized trial of norepinephrine as a first-line vasopressor in patients with shock, norepinephrine associated with similar survival to dopamine as the comparator, with fewer arrhythmias.[150a] Subgroup analysis suggested that use of norepinephrine associated with lower mortality in patients with cardiogenic shock.

Dopamine and dobutamine can be particularly useful for patients with STEMI and reduced cardiac output, increased left ventricular filling pressure, pulmonary vascular congestion, and hypotension. Fortunately, the potentially deleterious alpha-adrenergic vasoconstrictor effects exerted by dopamine occur only at higher doses than those required to increase contractility. The vasodilating actions of dopamine on renal and splanchnic vessels and its positive inotropic effects generally improve hemodynamics and renal function. In patients with STEMI and severe left ventricular failure, this drug should be administered at a dose of 3 µg/kg/min while pulmonary capillary wedge and systemic arterial pressures and cardiac output are monitored. The dose can be increased stepwise to 20 µg/kg/min to reduce pulmonary capillary wedge pressure to approximately 20 mm Hg and elevate the cardiac index to exceed 2 liters/min/m^2. Dopamine doses exceeding 5 µg/kg/min can, however, activate peripheral alpha receptors and cause vasoconstriction.

Dobutamine has a positive inotropic action comparable to that of dopamine but a slightly less positive chronotropic effect and less vasoconstrictor activity.[150] In patients with STEMI, dobutamine improves left ventricular performance without augmenting enzymatically estimated infarct size. It can be administered in a starting dose of 2.5 µg/kg/min and increased stepwise to a maximum of 30 µg/kg/min. Both dopamine and dobutamine must be given carefully and with constant monitoring of the ECG, systemic arterial pressure, pulmonary artery or pulmonary artery occlusive pressure and, if possible, frequent measurements of cardiac output. The dose must be reduced if the heart rate exceeds 100 to 110 beats/min, if supraventricular or ventricular tachyarrhythmias occur, or if ST-segment deviations increase.

OTHER POSITIVE INOTROPIC AGENTS. Milrinone is a noncatecholamine, nonglycoside, phosphodiesterase inhibitor with inotropic and vasodilating actions.[150] It is useful for selected patients whose heart failure persists despite treatment with diuretics, who are not hypotensive, and who are likely to benefit from both an enhancement in contractility and afterload reduction. Milrinone should be given as a loading dose of 0.5 µg/kg/min over 10 minutes, followed by a maintenance infusion of 0.375 to 0.75 µg/kg/min. The loading dose may be reduced or omitted if the patient has borderline hypotension.

Cardiogenic Shock

Cardiogenic shock is the most severe clinical expression of left ventricular failure and is associated with extensive damage to the left ventricular myocardium in more than 80% of STEMI patients in whom it occurs; the remainder have a mechanical defect such as ventricular septal or papillary muscle rupture or predominant right ventricular infarction. In the past, cardiogenic shock was reported to occur in up to 20% of patients with STEMI, but estimates from recent large trials and observational databases report an incidence in the range of 5% to 8%.[145] This low-output state is characterized by elevated ventricular filling pressures, low cardiac output, systemic hypotension, and evidence of vital organ hypoperfusion (e.g., clouded sensorium, cool extremities, oliguria, acidosis). Patients with cardiogenic shock caused by STEMI are more likely to be older, to have a history of diabetes mellitus, a prior MI or congestive heart failure, and to have sustained an anterior infarction at the time of development of shock. Mechanical complications should be strongly considered in patients with nonanterior MI who develop shock. Of note, although the incidence of cardiogenic shock in patients with STEMI has been relatively stable since the mid-1970s, the short-term mortality rate has decreased from 70% to 80% in the 1970s to 50% to 60% in the 1990s. Moreover, it is possible to stratify risk among patients with shock to identify those with a mortality rate lower than 50% with intensive therapy, including revascularization. Cardiogenic shock is the cause of death in about 60% of patients dying after fibrinolysis for STEMI.[89,151]

PATHOLOGIC FINDINGS. At autopsy, more than two thirds of patients with cardiogenic shock demonstrate stenosis of 75% or more of the luminal diameter of all three major coronary vessels, usually including the left anterior descending coronary artery. Almost all patients with cardiogenic shock are found to have thrombotic occlusion of the artery supplying the major region of recent infarction, with loss of about 40% of the left ventricular mass.[145] Patients who die as a consequence of cardiogenic shock often have piecemeal necrosis—that is, progressive myocardial necrosis from marginal extension of their infarct into an ischemic zone bordering on the infarction. This finding generally is associated with persistent elevation of cardiac biomarker levels. Such extensions and focal lesions are probably in part the result of the shock state itself. Early deterioration in left ventricular function secondary to apparent extension of infarction may, in some cases, result from expansion of the necrotic zone of myocardium without actual extension of the necrotic process. Hydrodynamic forces that develop during ventricular systole can disrupt necrotic myocardial muscle bundles, with resultant expansion and thinning of the akinetic zone of myocardium; this in turn results in the deterioration of overall left ventricular function.

Other causes of cardiogenic shock in patients with STEMI include mechanical defects such as rupture of the ventricular septum, a papillary muscle, or free wall with tamponade, right ventricular infarction, or a marked reduction of preload caused by conditions such as hypovolemia.[145]

PATHOPHYSIOLOGY. The shock state in patients with STEMI appears to be the result of a vicious cycle (see Chap. 54, Fig. 54-12).

DIAGNOSIS. Cardiogenic shock is characterized by marked and persistent (longer than 30 minutes) hypotension, with systolic arterial pressure lower than 80 mm Hg and a marked reduction of cardiac index (generally, <1.8 liters/min/m^2) in the face of elevated left ventricular filling pressure (pulmonary capillary wedge pressure

>18 mm Hg). Spurious estimates of left ventricular filling pressure based on measurements of the pulmonary artery wedge pressure can occur in the presence of marked mitral regurgitation, in which the tall v wave in the left atrial (and pulmonary artery wedge) pressure tracing elevates the mean pressure above the left ventricular end-diastolic pressure. Accordingly, mitral regurgitation and other mechanical lesions such as ventricular septal defect, ventricular aneurysm, and pseudoaneurysm must be excluded before the diagnosis of cardiogenic shock caused by impairment of left ventricular function can be established. Mechanical complications should be suspected in any patient with STEMI in whom circulatory collapse occurs. Immediate hemodynamic, angiographic, and echocardiographic evaluations are necessary in patients with cardiogenic shock. It is important to exclude mechanical complications because primary therapy of such lesions usually requires immediate operative treatment, with intervening support of the circulation by intra-aortic balloon counterpulsation.

MEDICAL MANAGEMENT. When the mechanical complications noted are absent, cardiogenic shock is caused by impairment of left ventricular function. Inotropic and vasopressor agents may be given as pharmacologic support and should be used in the lowest possible doses. Although dopamine or dobutamine usually improves the hemodynamics in these patients, unfortunately neither appears to improve hospital survival significantly. Similarly, vasodilators have been used to elevate cardiac output and reduce left ventricular filling pressure, but by lowering the already markedly reduced coronary perfusion pressure, myocardial perfusion can be compromised further, accelerating the vicious cycle illustrated in Figure 54-12. Vasodilators may nonetheless be used in conjunction with intra-aortic balloon counterpulsation and inotropic agents to increase cardiac output while sustaining or elevating coronary perfusion pressure.

The systemic vascular resistance is usually elevated in patients with cardiogenic shock, but occasionally resistance is normal and, in a few cases, vasodilation actually predominates.[152] When systemic vascular resistance is not elevated (i.e., <1800 dynes/sec/cm^5) in patients with cardiogenic shock, norepinephrine, which has both alpha- and beta-adrenergic agonist properties, can be used to increase diastolic arterial pressure, maintain coronary perfusion, and improve contractility, in doses ranging from 2 to 10 μg/min. The use of alpha-adrenergic agents such as phenylephrine and methoxamine is contraindicated in patients with cardiogenic shock unless systemic vascular resistance is inordinately low. Calcium sensitizing agents, such as levosimendan, have been studied but have shown little incremental value in randomized trials.[153]

MECHANICAL SUPPORT (see Chap. 32).

Intra-Aortic Balloon Counterpulsation

Intra-aortic balloon counterpulsation is used in the treatment of STEMI in three groups of patients: (1) those whose conditions are hemodynamically unstable and for whom support of the circulation is required for the performance of cardiac catheterization and angiography to assess lesions that are potentially correctable surgically or by angioplasty; (2) those with cardiogenic shock that is unresponsive to medical management; and (3) rarely, those with refractory ischemia that is unresponsive to other treatments. In experimental animals, intra-aortic balloon counterpulsation decreases preload, increases coronary blood flow, and improves cardiac performance. Unfortunately, among patients with cardiogenic shock, improvement is often only temporary. Although a response to intra-aortic balloon counterpulsation correlates with better outcomes, counterpulsation alone does not improve overall survival in patients with or without a surgically remediable mechanical lesion.

Percutaneous Left Ventricular Assist Devices

Temporary mechanical support with left ventricular assist devices may allow time for recovery of stunned or hibernating myocardium.[154] A percutaneous left ventricular assist device may be placed by cannulation of the left femoral vein and advancement to the left atrium via transseptal puncture.[155] Blood from the left atrium is then returned via a nonpulsatile motor into the femoral artery. This system may provide up to 5 liters/min of flow. Small randomized trials have not revealed any outcomes advantage compared with intraaortic balloon counterpulsation,[145] but hemodynamic improvement is greater with the percutaneous left ventricular assist device. Another percutaneous alternative is a motorized device that is placed across the aortic valve and provides continuous flow of blood from the left ventricle into the aorta; it has been shown to provide superior hemodynamic support to intra-aortic balloon pump in patients with MI.[156] External surgically placed left ventricular devices as a bridge to transplantation or as a destination therapy are discussed in Chap. 32.

Complications

Complications of intra-aortic balloon counterpulsation include damage to or perforation of the aortic wall, ischemia distal to the site of insertion of the balloon in the femoral artery, thrombocytopenia, hemolysis, atheroemboli, infection, and mechanical failure, such as rupture of the balloon. Patients at highest risk include those with peripheral vascular disease, older patients, and women, particularly if they are small. These risk indicators should be taken into consideration before the institution of intra-aortic balloon counterpulsation. Because of the potential for vascular bleeding complications, there has been a reluctance to use intra-aortic pumps in patients who have undergone fibrinolytic therapy. But despite the increased bleeding risk, because of the poor outcome among patients with shock following thrombolysis (usually ineffective thrombolysis), this modality should be considered for selected patients who are candidates for an aggressive approach to revascularization. In addition to vascular complications, and complications associated with transseptal puncture, percutaneous left ventricular assist devices are also associated with the development of a systemic inflammatory response syndrome (SIRS) in some cases.[154]

REVASCULARIZATION. Of the five therapeutic modalities frequently used to treat patients with cardiogenic shock (vasopressors, mechanical support, fibrinolysis, PCI, and CABG), the first two are useful temporizing maneuvers. Revascularization, however, is associated with an improvement in survival.

The SHOCK study evaluated early revascularization for the treatment of patients with MI complicated by cardiogenic shock. Patients with shock caused by left ventricular failure complicating STEMI were randomized to emergency revascularization ($n = 152$), accomplished by CABG or angioplasty, or initial medical stabilization ($n = 150$). In 86% of patients in both groups, intra-aortic balloon counterpulsation was performed. The primary endpoint was all-cause mortality at 30 days; a secondary endpoint was mortality at 6 months. At 30 days, the overall mortality rate was 46.7% in the revascularization group, not significantly different from the 56% mortality rate observed in the medical therapy group ($P = 0.11$). Subgroups of patients in the SHOCK trial that showed particular benefit from the early revascularization strategy (i.e., reduced 6-month mortality) were those who were younger than 75 years of age, had a prior MI, and were randomized less than 6 hours from onset of infarction. Long-term survival improved significantly in patients with cardiogenic shock who underwent early revascularization (**Fig. 55-31**).[89] A subsequent observational study of patients with MI complicated by shock indicated that well-selected older patients undergoing PCI had similar 1-year survival to younger patients undergoing early revascularization.[157]

RECOMMENDATIONS. We recommend assessment of patients on an individualized basis to determine their desire for aggressive care and overall candidacy for further treatment (e.g., age, mental status, comorbidities). Patients with shock who are potential candidates for revascularization receive intra-aortic balloon counterpulsation and undergo coronary arteriography as soon as possible. Those with suitable anatomy should be revascularized as completely as possible with PCI and/or CABG.[35,89,145] There appears to be a benefit of revascularization with respect to survival as long as 48 hours after MI and 18 hours after the onset of shock. Left ventricular assist devices

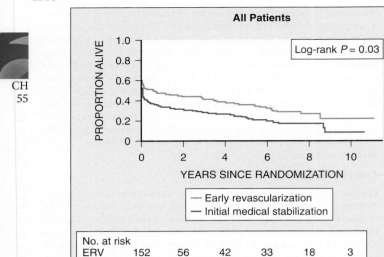

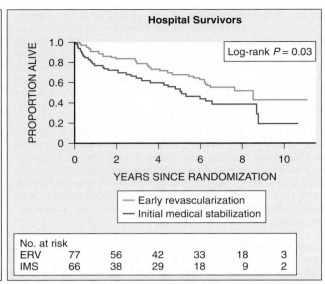

FIGURE 55-31 Impact of revascularization in patients in the SHOCK trial. Among all patients, the survival rates in the early revascularization (ERV) and initial medical stabilization (IMS) groups, respectively, were 41.4% versus 28.3% at 3 years and 32.8% versus 19.6% at 6 years. With the exclusion of eight patients with aortic dissection, tamponade, or severe mitral regurgitation identified shortly after randomization, the survival curves remained significantly different (P = 0.02), with a 14% absolute difference at 6 years. Among hospital survivors, the survival rates in the ERV and IMS groups, respectively, were 78.8% versus 64.3% at 3 years and 62.4% versus 44.4% at 6 years. *(From Hochman JS, Sleeper LA, Webb JG, Dzavik V, et al: Early revascularization and long-term survival in cardiogenic shock complicating acute myocardial infarction. JAMA 295:2511, 2006.)*

may be considered for patients with refractory shock after revascularization.

Right Ventricular Infarction

Right ventricular infarction can have a range of clinical presentations, from mild right ventricular dysfunction through cardiogenic shock. A characteristic hemodynamic pattern (**Fig. 55-32**) has been observed in patients with clinically significant right ventricular infarction, which frequently accompanies inferior left ventricular infarction or rarely occurs in isolated form. Right heart filling pressures (central venous, right atrial, and right ventricular end-diastolic pressures) are elevated, whereas left ventricular filling pressure is normal or only slightly raised, right ventricular systolic and pulse pressures are decreased, and cardiac output is often markedly depressed. Rarely, this disproportionate elevation of right-sided filling pressure causes right-to-left shunting through a patent foramen ovale. This possibility should be considered in patients with right ventricular infarction who have unexplained systemic hypoxemia. The finding of an elevation in the atrial natriuretic factor level in patients with this condition has led to the suggestion that abnormally high levels of this peptide might be partly responsible for the hypotension seen in patients with right ventricular infarction.

DIAGNOSIS. Many patients with the combination of normal left ventricular filling pressure and depressed cardiac index have right ventricular infarcts, with accompanying inferior left ventricular infarcts. The hemodynamic picture may superficially resemble that seen in patients with pericardial disease (see Chap. 75). It includes elevated right ventricular filling pressure, steep, right atrial *y* descent, and an early diastolic drop and plateau (resembling the square root sign) in the right ventricular pressure tracing. Moreover, patients with right ventricular infarction may display the Kussmaul sign (an increase in jugular venous pressure with inspiration) and pulsus paradoxus (a fall in systolic pressure of more than 10 mm Hg with inspiration; see Fig. 55-32).[158] The Kussmaul sign in the setting of inferior STEMI strongly predicts right ventricular involvement.

The ECG can provide the first clue that right ventricular involvement is present in the patient with inferior STEMI (see Fig. 55-32). Most patients with right ventricular infarction have ST-segment elevation in lead V_4R (right precordial lead in the V_4 position).[159] Transient

elevation of the ST segment in any of the right precordial leads can occur with right ventricular MI, and the presence of ST-segment elevation of 0.1 mV or more in any one or a combination of leads V_4R, V_5R, and V_6R in patients with the clinical picture of acute MI indicates the diagnosis of right ventricular MI. Wellens[160] has emphasized that in addition to noting the presence or absence of convex upward ST-segment elevation in V_4R, clinicians should determine whether the T wave is positive or negative; such distinctions help distinguish proximal versus distal occlusion of the right coronary artery versus occlusion of the left circumflex artery (see Fig. 55-32). Elevation of the ST segments in leads V_1 through V_4 caused by right ventricular infarction can be confused with elevation caused by anteroseptal infarction. Although the elevated ST segments are oriented anteriorly in both cases, the frontal plane can provide important clues; the ST segments are oriented to the right in right ventricular infarction (e.g., +120 degrees), whereas they are oriented to the left in anteroseptal infarction (e.g., −30 degrees).

Noninvasive Assessment

Echocardiography is helpful in the differential diagnosis because in right ventricular infarction, in contrast to pericardial tamponade, little or no pericardial fluid accumulates. The echocardiogram shows abnormal wall motion of the right ventricle, as well as right ventricular dilation and depression of right ventricular ejection fraction.[161] CMR can also aid in the recognition of right ventricular infarction.[162] Serial studies have shown that some degree of recovery of an initially depressed right ventricular ejection fraction is the rule with right ventricular infarction, to a greater degree than with the left ventricular ejection fraction.[158]

Hemodynamics

Impaired left atrial filling in patients with right ventricular infarction can result in marked reductions in stroke volume and arterial blood pressure. Disproportionate elevation of the right-sided filling pressure is the hemodynamic hallmark of right ventricular infarction. Therefore, ventricular pacing may fail to increase cardiac output and atrioventricular sequential pacing may be required.

TREATMENT. Because of their ability to reduce preload, medications routinely prescribed for left ventricular infarction may produce profound hypotension in patients with right ventricular infarction. In

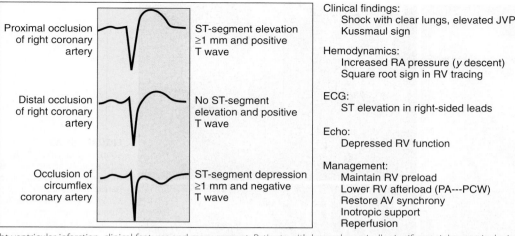

Clinical findings:
    Shock with clear lungs, elevated JVP
    Kussmaul sign

Hemodynamics:
    Increased RA pressure (*y* descent)
    Square root sign in RV tracing

ECG:
    ST elevation in right-sided leads

Echo:
    Depressed RV function

Management:
    Maintain RV preload
    Lower RV afterload (PA---PCW)
    Restore AV synchrony
    Inotropic support
    Reperfusion

FIGURE 55-32 Right ventricular infarction, clinical features and management. Patients with hemodynamically significant right ventricular infarction present with shock but clear lungs and elevated JVP. ST-segment elevation exists in right-sided electrocardiographic leads with variation in the repolarization pattern depending on the infarct artery and the location of the occlusion. Management recommendations are shown at the bottom, right. Echo = echocardiogram; JVP = jugular venous pressure; PA = pulmonary artery; PCW = pulmonary capillary wedge; RA = right atrial; RV = right ventricular. *(Modified from Wellens HJ: The value of the right precordial leads of the electrocardiogram. N Engl J Med 340:381, 1999; and Antman EM, Anbe DT, Armstrong PW, et al: ACC/AHA guidelines for the management of patients with ST-elevation myocardial infarction: A report of the American College of Cardiology/American Heart Association Task Force on Practice Guidelines [Committee to Revise the 1999 Guidelines for the Management of Patients with Acute Myocardial Infarction]. Circulation 110:e82, 2004.)*

patients with hypotension caused by right ventricular MI, hemodynamics can be improved by a combination of expanding plasma volume to augment right ventricular preload and cardiac output and, when left ventricular failure is present, arterial vasodilators.[1] The initial therapy for hypotension in patients with right ventricular infarction should almost always be volume expansion. If hypotension has not been corrected after brisk administration of 1 liter or more of fluid, however, consideration should be given to hemodynamic monitoring with a pulmonary artery catheter, because further volume infusion may be of little use and may produce pulmonary congestion. Vasodilators reduce the impedance to left ventricular outflow and in turn left ventricular diastolic, left atrial, and pulmonary (arterial) pressures, thereby lowering the impedance to right ventricular outflow and enhancing right ventricular output.

Right ventricular infarction is common among patients with inferior left ventricular infarction. Therefore, otherwise unexplained systemic arterial hypotension or diminished cardiac output, or marked hypotension in response to small doses of nitroglycerin in patients with inferior infarction, should lead to the prompt consideration of this diagnosis. Patients requiring pacing should have atrial or atrioventricular sequential pacing. Successful reperfusion of the right coronary artery significantly improves right ventricular mechanical function and lowers in-hospital mortality in patients with right ventricular infarction. Replacement of the tricuspid valve and repair of the valve with annuloplasty rings have been carried out in the treatment of severe tricuspid regurgitation caused by right ventricular infarction.

Mechanical Causes of Heart Failure

FREE WALL RUPTURE. The most dramatic complications of STEMI are those that involve tearing or rupture of acutely infarcted tissue (**Fig. 55-33**). The clinical characteristics of these lesions vary considerably and depend on the site of rupture, which may involve the papillary muscles, interventricular septum, or free wall of either ventricle. The overall incidence of these complications is hard to assess because clinical and autopsy series differ considerably, but the incidence appears to be decreasing with the increasing use of reperfusion therapy.[163,164] **Table 55-12** shows the comparative clinical profile of these complications, as gathered from different studies. Rupture of the free wall of the infarcted ventricle (see Fig. 55-33) occurs in up to 10% of patients dying in the hospital of STEMI. Thinness of the apical wall,

marked intensity of necrosis at the terminal end of the blood supply, poor collateral flow, the shearing effect of muscular contraction against an inert and stiffened necrotic area, and aging of the myocardium with laceration of the myocardial microstructure may all promote rupture.

Clinical Characteristics

The following are some features that characterize this serious complication of STEMI[164]:

1. Occurs more frequently in older patients, and possibly more frequently in women than in men with infarction.
2. Appears to be more common in hypertensive than in normotensive patients.
3. Occurs more frequently in the left than in the right ventricle and seldom occurs in the atria.
4. Usually involves the anterior or lateral walls of the ventricle in the area of the terminal distribution of the left anterior descending coronary artery.
5. Is usually associated with a relatively large transmural infarction involving at least 20% of the left ventricle.
6. Occurs between 1 day and 3 weeks, but most commonly 1 to 4 days, after infarction.
7. Is usually preceded by infarct expansion—that is, thinning and a disproportionate dilation within the softened necrotic zone.
8. Most commonly results from a distinct tear in the myocardial wall or a dissecting hematoma that perforates a necrotic area of myocardium (see Fig. 55-33).
9. Usually occurs near the junction of the infarct and the normal muscle.
10. Occurs less frequently in the center of the infarct, but when rupture occurs here, is usually during the second rather than the first week after the infarct.
11. Rarely occurs in a greatly thickened ventricle or in an area of extensive collateral vessels.
12. Most often occurs in patients without previous infarction.
13. No evidence that the intensity of anticoagulation influences the occurrence of rupture.
14. Occurs more commonly in patients who have received reperfusion therapy with a fibrinolytic versus PCI.[1]

Rupture of the free wall of the left ventricle usually leads to hemopericardium and death from cardiac tamponade. Occasionally, rupture

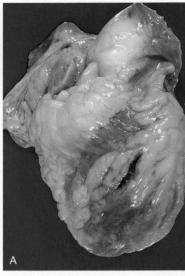
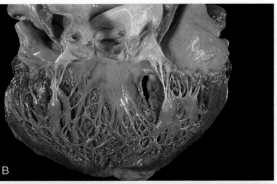
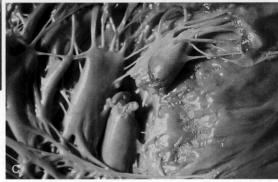

FIGURE 55-33 Cardiac rupture syndromes complicating STEMI. **A,** Anterior myocardial rupture in an acute infarct. **B,** Rupture of the ventricular septum. **C,** Complete rupture of a necrotic papillary muscle. *(From Schoen FJ: The heart. In Kumar V, Abbas AK, Fausto N [eds]: Robbins & Cotran Pathologic Basis of Disease. 8th ed. Philadelphia, Saunders, 2010, pp 529-587.)*

TABLE 55-12 Features of Ventricular Septal Rupture (VSR), Rupture of Ventricular Free Wall, and Papillary Muscle Rupture

FEATURE	VSR	RUPTURE OF VENTRICULAR FREE WALL	PAPILLARY MUSCLE RUPTURE
Incidence	1%-3% without reperfusion therapy, 0.2%-0.34% with fibrinolytic therapy, 3.9% among patients with cardiogenic shock	0.8%-6.2%; fibrinolytic therapy does not reduce risk; primary PTCA seems to reduce risk	About 1% (posteromedial more frequent than anterolateral papillary muscle)
Time course	Bimodal peak; within 24 hr and 3-5 days; range, 1-14 days	Bimodal peak; within 24 hr and 3-5 days; range, 1-14 days	Bimodal peak; within 24 hr and 3-5 days; range, 1-14 days
Clinical manifestations	Chest pain, shortness of breath, hypotension	Anginal, pleuritic, or pericardial chest pain, syncope, hypotension, arrhythmia, nausea, restlessness, sudden death	Abrupt onset of shortness of breath and pulmonary edema; hypotension
Physical findings	Harsh holosystolic murmur, thrill (+), S_3, accentuated second heart sound, pulmonary edema, RV and LV failure, cardiogenic shock	Jugular venous distention (29% of patients), pulsus paradoxus (47%), electromechanical dissociation, cardiogenic shock	A soft murmur in some cases, no thrill, variable signs of RV overload, severe pulmonary edema, cardiogenic shock
Echocardiographic findings	VSR, left-to-right shunt on color flow Doppler echocardiography through the ventricular septum, pattern of RV overload	>5 mm pericardial effusion not visualized in all cases; layered, high-acoustic echoes within the pericardium (blood clot); direct visualization of tear; signs of tamponade	Hypercontractile LV, torn papillary muscle or chordae tendineae, flail leaflet, severe MR on color flow Doppler echocardiography
Right-heart catheterization	Increase in oxygen saturation from the RA to RV, large v waves	Ventriculography insensitive, classic signs of tamponade not always present (equalization of diastolic pressures among the cardiac chambers)	No increase in oxygen saturation from the RA to RV, large v waves,* very high pulmonary-capillary wedge pressures

*Large v waves are from the pulmonary capillary wedge pressure.
LV = left ventricle or left ventricular; MR = mitral regurgitation; PTCA = percutaneous transluminal coronary angioplasty; RA = right atrium; RV = right ventricle or right ventricular.
From Antman EM, Anbe DT, Armstrong PW et al: ACC/AHA guidelines for the management of patients with ST-elevation myocardial infarction: A report of the American College of Cardiology/American Heart Association Task Force on Practice Guidelines (Committee to Revise the 1999 Guidelines for the Management of Patients with Acute Myocardial Infarction). Circulation 110:e82, 2004.

of the free wall of the ventricle occurs as the first clinical manifestation in patients with undetected or silent MI, and then it may be considered a form of sudden cardiac death (see Chap. 41).

The course of rupture varies from catastrophic, with an acute tear leading to immediate death, to subacute, with nausea, hypotension, and pericardial type of discomfort being the major clinical clues to its presence. Survival depends on the recognition of this complication, on hemodynamic stabilization of the patient—usually with inotropic agents and/or intra-aortic balloon pump—and, most importantly, on prompt surgical repair.[1] Initial percutaneous treatment of small or medium-sized ventricular septal defects with an occluder device offers a promising alternative to surgical closure or as an approach to initial medical stabilization facilitating delayed, definitive, surgical correction.[154,165]

Pseudoaneurysm

Incomplete rupture of the heart may occur when organizing thrombus and hematoma, together with pericardium, seal a rupture of the left ventricle and thus prevent the development of hemopericardium (**Fig. 55-34**). With time, this area of organized thrombus and pericardium can become a pseudoaneurysm (false aneurysm) that maintains communication with the cavity of the left ventricle. In contrast to true aneurysms, which always contain some myocardial elements in their walls, the walls of pseudoaneurysms are composed of organized hematoma and pericardium and lack any elements of the original myocardial wall. Pseudoaneurysms can become large, even equaling the true ventricular cavity in size, and communicate with the left ventricular cavity through a narrow neck. Frequently, pseudoaneurysms contain significant quantities of old and recent thrombi, superficial portions of which can cause arterial emboli. Pseudoaneurysms can drain off a portion of each ventricular stroke volume in the same manner as true aneurysms. The diagnosis of pseudoaneurysm can usually be made by echocardiography and contrast angiography, although at times, differentiation between true aneurysm and pseudoaneurysm can be difficult by any imaging technique.[166]

Diagnosis

The rupture usually presents with sudden profound shock, often rapidly leading to pulseless electrical activity caused by pericardial tamponade. Immediate pericardiocentesis confirms the diagnosis and relieves the pericardial tamponade, at least momentarily. If the patient's condition is relatively stable, echocardiography may help in establishing the diagnosis of tamponade.[1] Under the most favorable conditions, cardiac catheterization can be carried out, not necessarily to confirm the diagnosis of rupture but to delineate the coronary anatomy. This information helps guide CABG in patients with high-grade obstructive lesions during ventricular repair. In patients with critically compromised hemodynamics, establishment of the diagnosis should be followed immediately by surgical resection of the necrotic and ruptured myocardium with primary reconstruction. When rupture is subacute and a pseudoaneurysm is suspected or present, prompt elective surgery is indicated because rupture of the pseudoaneurysm occurs relatively frequently.[167]

RUPTURE OF THE INTERVENTRICULAR SEPTUM. Clinical features associated with an increased risk of rupture of the interventricular septum (see Table 55-12) include lack of development of a collateral network, advanced age, hypertension, anterior location of infarction, and possibly fibrinolysis.[168] Rupture of the interventricular septum after STEMI confers a high 30-day mortality.[164] The perforation can range in length from 1 cm to several centimeters (see Fig. 55-33). It can be a direct through-and-through opening or more irregular and serpiginous. The size of the defect determines the magnitude of the left-to-right shunt and the extent of hemodynamic deterioration, which in turn affects the likelihood of survival. As in rupture of the free wall of the ventricle, transmural infarction underlies rupture of the ventricular septum. Rupture of the septum with an anterior infarction tends to be apical in location, whereas inferior infarctions are associated with perforation of the basal septum and have a worse prognosis than those in an anterior location. In contrast with rupture of the free wall, rupture of the ventricular septum is more often associated with complete heart block, right bundle branch block, or atrial fibrillation. Almost all patients have multivessel coronary artery disease, with most exhibiting lesions in all the major vessels. The likelihood of survival depends on the degree of impairment of ventricular function and the size of the defect.

A ruptured interventricular septum is characterized by the appearance of a new harsh, loud holosystolic murmur that is heard best at the lower left sternal border and that is usually accompanied by a thrill.[1] Biventricular failure generally ensues within hours to days. The defect can also be recognized by echocardiography with color flow Doppler imaging (**Fig. 55-35**; see Fig. 15-31) or insertion of a pulmonary artery balloon catheter to document the left-to-right shunt. Catheter placement of an umbrella-shaped device within the ruptured septum may stabilize the condition of critically ill patients with acute septal rupture after STEMI.

RUPTURE OF A PAPILLARY MUSCLE. Partial or total rupture of a papillary muscle is a rare but often fatal complication of transmural MI (see Fig. 55-33).[169,170] Inferior wall infarction can lead to rupture of

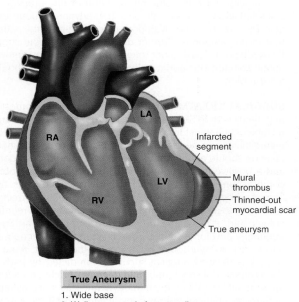

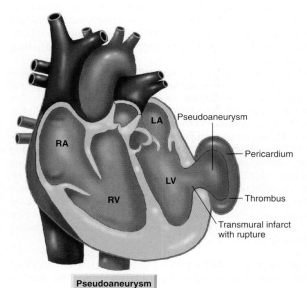

FIGURE 55-34 Differences between a pseudoaneurysm and a true aneurysm. LA = left atrium; LV = left ventricle; RA = right atrium; RV = right ventricle. *(From Shah PK: Complications of acute myocardial infarction.* In *Parmley W, Chatterjee K [eds]: Cardiology. Philadelphia, JB Lippincott, 1987.)*

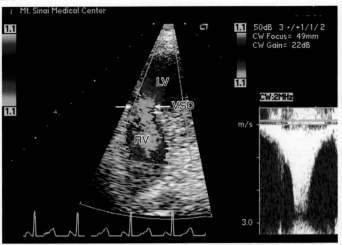

FIGURE 55-35 Two-dimensional echocardiography in an older female patient with a ventricular septal defect (VSD) that developed after a STEMI caused by occlusion of the left anterior descending coronary artery. Close-up of ventricular septum in apical four-chamber view **(left)** demonstrates turbulent systolic color flow Doppler across large VSD. Continuous wave Doppler **(right)** demonstrates systolic flow across VSD. LV = left ventricle; RV = right ventricle. *(From Kamran M, Attari M, Webber G: Images in cardiovascular medicine. Ventricular septal defect complicating an acute myocardial infarction. Circulation 112:e337, 2005.)*

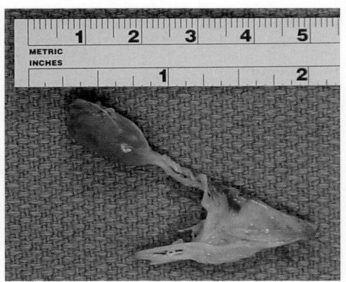

FIGURE 55-36 Surgical specimen showing papillary muscle **(top left),** chordae, and anterior mitral leaflet **(bottom right)** from a patient who had partial rupture of the papillary muscle and underwent mitral valve replacement for severe mitral regurgitation after STEMI. *(Courtesy of Dr. John Byrne.)*

the posteromedial papillary muscle, which occurs more commonly than rupture of the anterolateral muscle, a consequence of anterolateral MI. Rupture of a right ventricular papillary muscle is unusual but can cause massive tricuspid regurgitation and right ventricular failure. Complete transection of a left ventricular papillary muscle is incompatible with life because the sudden massive mitral regurgitation that develops cannot be tolerated. Rupture of a portion of a papillary muscle, usually the tip or head of the muscle, resulting in severe, although not necessarily overwhelming, mitral regurgitation, is much more frequent and is not immediately fatal (**Fig. 55-36**). Unlike rupture of the ventricular septum, which occurs with large infarcts, papillary muscle rupture occurs with a relatively small infarction in approximately half of the cases seen. The extent of coronary artery disease in these patients sometimes is modest as well. In a small number of patients, rupture of more than one cardiac structure is noted clinically or at postmortem examination; all possible combinations of rupture of the free left ventricular wall, interventricular septum, and papillary muscles can occur.[171]

As with patients who have a ruptured ventricular septal defect, those with papillary muscle rupture manifest a new holosystolic murmur and develop increasingly severe heart failure.[170] In both conditions, the murmur may become softer or disappear as arterial pressure falls. Mitral regurgitation caused by partial or complete rupture of a papillary muscle can be promptly recognized echocardiographically. Color flow Doppler imaging is particularly helpful in distinguishing acute mitral regurgitation from a ventricular septal defect in the setting of STEMI (see Table 55-12).[1] Therefore, an echocardiogram should be obtained immediately on any patient in whom the diagnosis is suspected because hemodynamic deterioration can ensue rapidly. Echocardiography also often permits differentiation of papillary muscle rupture from other, generally less severe forms of mitral regurgitation that occur with STEMI.

DIFFERENTIATION BETWEEN VENTRICULAR SEPTAL RUPTURE AND MITRAL REGURGITATION. It may be difficult, on clinical grounds, to distinguish between acute mitral regurgitation and rupture of the ventricular septum in patients with STEMI who suddenly develop a loud systolic murmur.[170] This differentiation can be made most readily by color flow Doppler echocardiography. In addition, a right-heart catheterization with a balloon-tipped catheter can readily distinguish between these two complications. Patients with

ventricular septal rupture demonstrate a "step-up" in oxygen saturation in blood samples from the right ventricle and pulmonary artery compared with those from the right atrium. Patients with acute mitral regurgitation lack this step-up. They also may demonstrate tall *c-v* waves in both the pulmonary capillary and pulmonary arterial pressure tracings.

Invasive monitoring, which is essential in these patients, also allows for the critically important assessment of ventricular function.[1] Right and left ventricular filling pressures (right atrial and pulmonary capillary wedge pressures) guide fluid administration or the use of diuretics, whereas measurements of cardiac output and mean arterial pressure permit the calculation of systemic vascular resistance to direct vasodilator therapy. Unless systolic pressure is below 90 mm Hg, this therapy, generally using nitroglycerin or nitroprusside, should be instituted as soon as possible once hemodynamic monitoring is available. This may be critically important for stabilizing the patient's condition in preparation for further diagnostic studies and surgical repair. If vasodilator therapy is not tolerated or if it fails to achieve hemodynamic stability, intra-aortic balloon counterpulsation should be instituted rapidly.

SURGICAL TREATMENT. Operative intervention is most successful in patients with STEMI and circulatory collapse when a surgically correctable mechanical lesion such as ventricular septal defect or mitral regurgitation can be identified and repaired. In such patients, the circulation should at first be supported by intra-aortic balloon pulsation and a positive inotropic agent such as dopamine or dobutamine in combination with a vasodilator, unless the patient is hypotensive. Surgery should not be delayed in patients with a correctable lesion who agree to an aggressive management strategy and require pharmacologic and/or mechanical (counterpulsation) support. Such patients frequently develop a serious complication (e.g., infection, adult respiratory distress syndrome, extension of the infarct, renal failure) if surgery is delayed. Surgical survival is predicted by early operation, short duration of shock, and mild degrees of right and left ventricular impairment.[164,172] When the hemodynamic status of a patient with one of these mechanical lesions complicating STEMI remains stable after the patient has been weaned from pharmacologic and/or mechanical support, it may be possible to postpone the operation for 2 to 4 weeks to allow some healing of the infarct to occur).[1] Surgical repair involves correction of mitral regurgitation, insertion of a prosthetic mitral valve

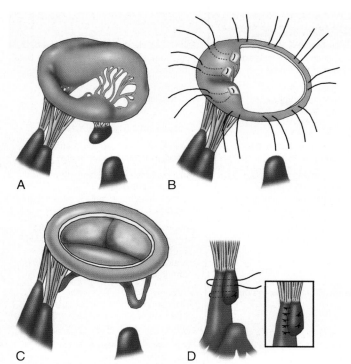

FIGURE 55-37 Surgical management of mitral regurgitation caused by ruptured papillary muscle. **A,** Acute papillary muscle rupture results in severe mitral regurgitation caused by leaflet and commissural prolapse. Mitral valve replacement is usually necessary. **B,** Mitral débridement with retention of the unruptured commissural and leaflet segment is performed to preserve partial annular papillary continuity. **C,** Mitral valve replacement is then performed. **D,** Occasionally, mitral valve repair can be performed by transfer of a papillary head to a nonruptured segment. *(Courtesy of Dr. David Adams, Division of Cardiac Surgery, Mount Sinai Hospital, New York.)*

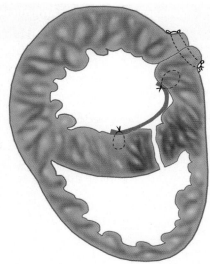

FIGURE 55-38 Repair of ischemic ventricular septal defect. The infarct typically involves a free wall and septum. Repair of the defect is performed through an incision in the ventricular wall infarct. The septal defect is closed with a prosthetic patch and a second patch is used to close the incision in the free wall. *(Courtesy of Dr. David Adams, Division of Cardiac Surgery, Mount Sinai Hospital, New York.)*

repair, or closure of a ventricular septal defect, usually accompanied by coronary revascularization (**Figs. 55-37** and **55-38**).

Arrhythmias

Arrhythmias that can complicate the course of patients with STEMI and their prevention and treatment in this setting are discussed here and summarized in **Table 55-13**.

The incidence of arrhythmias is higher in patients the earlier they are seen after the onset of symptoms. Many serious arrhythmias develop before hospitalization, even before the patient is monitored. Some abnormality of cardiac rhythm also occurs in most patients with STEMI treated in CCUs. Patients seen very early during the course of STEMI almost invariably exhibit evidence of increased activity of the autonomic nervous system. Thus, sinus bradycardia, sometimes associated with AV block, and hypotension reflect augmented vagal activity.

MECHANISM OF ARRHYTHMIAS. A leading hypothesis for a major mechanism of arrhythmias in the acute phase of coronary occlusion is reentry caused by inhomogeneity of the electrical characteristics of ischemic myocardium.[173,174] The cellular electrophysiologic mechanisms for reperfusion arrhythmias appear to include washout of various ions, such as lactate and potassium, and toxic metabolic substances that have accumulated in the ischemic zone.

HEMODYNAMIC CONSEQUENCES. Patients with significant left ventricular dysfunction have a relatively fixed stroke volume and depend on changes in heart rate to alter cardiac output. However, there is a narrow range of heart rate over which the cardiac output is maximal, with significant reductions occurring at faster and slower rates. Thus, all forms of bradycardia and tachycardia can depress cardiac output in patients with STEMI. Although the optimal rate insofar as cardiac output is concerned may exceed 100 beats/min, it is important to consider that heart rate is one of the major determinants of myocardial oxygen consumption and that at more rapid heart rates, myocardial energy needs can be elevated to levels that adversely affect the ischemic myocardium. Therefore, in patients with STEMI, the optimal rate is usually lower, in the range of 60 to 80 beats/min.

A second factor to consider in assessing the hemodynamic consequences of a particular arrhythmia is the loss of the atrial contribution to ventricular preload. In patients without STEMI, loss of atrial transport decreases left ventricular output by 15% to 20%. In patients with reduced diastolic left ventricular compliance of any cause (including STEMI), however, atrial systole is of greater importance for left ventricular filling. In patients with STEMI, atrial systole boosts end-diastolic volume by 15%, end-diastolic pressure by 29%, and stroke volume by 35%.

Ventricular Arrhythmias (see Chap. 39)

VENTRICULAR PREMATURE DEPOLARIZATIONS. Before the widespread use of reperfusion therapy, aspirin, beta blockers, and intravenous nitrates in the management of STEMI, it was believed that frequent ventricular premature complexes (VPCs; more than five/min), VPCs with multiform configuration, early coupling (the R-on-T phenomenon), and repetitive patterns in the form of couplets or salvos presaged ventricular fibrillation. It is now clear, however, that such warning arrhythmias are present in as many patients who do not develop fibrillation as in those who do. Several reports have shown that primary ventricular fibrillation (see later) occurs without antecedent warning arrhythmias and may even develop in spite of suppression of warning arrhythmias.[1] Both primary ventricular fibrillation and VPCs, especially R-on-T beats, occur during the early phase of STEMI, when considerable heterogeneity of electrical activity is present. Although R-on-T beats expose this heterogeneity and can precipitate ventricular fibrillation in a small minority of patients, the ubiquitous nature of VPCs in patients with STEMI and the extremely infrequent nature of ventricular fibrillation in the current era of STEMI management produce unacceptably low sensitivity and specificity of electrocardiographic patterns observed on monitoring systems for identifying patients at risk of ventricular fibrillation.

CH
55

TABLE 55-13 Management of Cardiac Arrhythmias During Acute Myocardial Infarction

CATEGORY	ARRHYTHMIA	OBJECTIVE OF TREATMENT	THERAPEUTIC OPTIONS
Electrical instability	Ventricular premature beats	Correction of electrolyte deficits and increased sympathetic tone	Potassium and magnesium solutions, beta blocker
	Ventricular tachycardia	Prophylaxis against ventricular fibrillation, restoration of hemodynamic stability	Antiarrhythmic agents; cardioversion/defibrillation
	Ventricular fibrillation	Urgent reversion to sinus rhythm	Defibrillation; bretylium tosylate
	Accelerated idioventricular rhythm	Observation unless hemodynamic function is compromised	Increase sinus rate (atropine, atrial pacing); antiarrhythmic agents
	Nonparoxysmal atrioventricular junctional tachycardia	Search for precipitating causes (e.g., digitalis intoxication); suppress arrhythmia only if hemodynamic function is compromised	Atrial overdrive pacing; antiarrhythmic agents; cardioversion relatively contraindicated if digitalis intoxication present
Pump failure, excessive sympathetic stimulation	Sinus tachycardia	Reduce heart rate to diminish myocardial oxygen demands	Antipyretics; analgesics; consider beta blocker unless congestive heart failure present; treat latter if present with anticongestive measures (diuretics, afterload reduction)
	Atrial fibrillation and/or atrial flutter	Reduce ventricular rate; restore sinus rhythm	Verapamil, digitalis glycosides; anticongestive measures (diuretics, afterload reduction); cardioversion; rapid atrial pacing (for atrial flutter)
	Paroxysmal supraventricular tachycardia	Reduce ventricular rate; restore sinus rhythm	Vagal maneuvers; verapamil, cardiac glycosides, beta-adrenergic blockers; cardioversion; rapid atrial pacing
Bradyarrhythmias and conduction disturbances	Sinus bradycardia	Acceleration of heart rate only if hemodynamic function is compromised	Atropine; atrial pacing
	Junctional escape rhythm	Acceleration of sinus rate only if loss of atrial "kick" causes hemodynamic compromise	Atropine; atrial pacing
	Atrioventricular block and intraventricular block		Insertion of pacemaker

Modified from Antman EM, Rutherford JD (eds): Coronary Care Medicine: A Practical Approach. Boston, Martinus Nijhoff, 1986, p 78.

Management

Because the incidence of ventricular fibrillation in patients with STEMI seen in CCUs over the past three or four decades appears to be declining, the prior practice of prophylactic suppression of ventricular premature beats with antiarrhythmic drugs no longer is necessary, and its use may actually increase the risk of fatal bradycardic and asystolic events.[175] Therefore, we pursue a conservative course when VPCs are observed in STEMI patients and do not routinely prescribe antiarrhythmic drugs, but instead determine whether recurrent ischemia or electrolyte or metabolic disturbances are present.[1] When, at the inception of an infarction, VPCs accompany sinus tachycardia, augmented sympathoadrenal stimulation is often a contributing factor and can be treated by beta-adrenergic blockade. In fact, the early administration of an intravenous beta blocker is effective in reducing the incidence of ventricular fibrillation in cases of evolving MI.

ACCELERATED IDIOVENTRICULAR RHYTHM. This arrhythmia is seen in up to 20% of patients with STEMI. It occurs frequently during the first 2 days, with about equal frequency in anterior and inferior infarctions. Most episodes are of short duration. Accelerated idioventricular rhythm is often observed shortly after successful reperfusion has been established. However, the frequent occurrence of this rhythm in patients without reperfusion limits their reliability as markers of restoration of patency of the infarct-related coronary artery.[1] In contrast to rapid ventricular tachycardia, accelerated idioventricular rhythm is thought not to affect prognosis, and we do not routinely treat accelerated idioventricular rhythms.

VENTRICULAR TACHYCARDIA. Nonsustained runs of ventricular tachycardia early after presentation do not appear to be associated with an increased mortality risk, either during hospitalization or over the first year. Ventricular tachycardia occurring late in the course of STEMI is more common in patients with transmural infarction and left ventricular dysfunction, is likely to be sustained, usually induces marked hemodynamic deterioration, and is associated with increased rates of hospital and long-term mortality.

Management

Because hypokalemia can increase the risk of developing ventricular tachycardia, low serum potassium levels should be identified quickly after a patient's admission for STEMI and should be treated promptly. We strive to maintain the serum potassium level above 4.5 mEq/liter and serum magnesium level above 2 mEq/liter. Rapid abolition of sustained ventricular tachycardia in patients with STEMI is mandatory because of its deleterious effect on pump function and because it frequently deteriorates into ventricular fibrillation. After reversion to sinus rhythm, every effort should be made to correct underlying abnormalities, such as hypoxia, hypotension, acid-base or electrolyte disturbances, and digitalis excess. Although no definitive data are available, it is a common clinical practice to continue maintenance infusions of antiarrhythmic drugs for several days after an index episode of ventricular tachycardia, discontinue the drug, and either observe the patient for recurrence or perform a diagnostic electrophysiology study. Patients with recurrent or refractory ventricular tachycardia should be considered for specialized procedures, such as implantation of antitachycardia devices or surgery. Occasionally, urgent attempts at revascularization with angioplasty or CABG can help control refractory ventricular tachycardia.

VENTRICULAR FIBRILLATION. Ventricular fibrillation can occur in three settings in hospitalized patients with STEMI. (Its occurrence as a mechanism of sudden death is discussed in Chap. 41.) Primary ventricular fibrillation occurs suddenly and unexpectedly in patients with no or few signs or symptoms of left ventricular failure. Although primary ventricular fibrillation occurred in up to 10% of patients hospitalized with STEMI several decades ago, analyses have suggested that its incidence has declined. Secondary ventricular fibrillation is often the final event of a progressive downhill course with left ventricular failure and cardiogenic shock. So-called late ventricular fibrillation develops more than 48 hours after STEMI and frequently but not exclusively occurs in patients with large infarcts and ventricular dysfunction. Patients with intraventricular conduction defects and anterior wall infarction, with persistent sinus tachycardia, atrial flutter, or fibrillation early in the clinical course, and with right ventricular infarction who require ventricular pacing are at higher risk for suffering late in-hospital ventricular fibrillation than are patients without these features.

Prognosis

Debate continues on the effect of primary ventricular fibrillation on prognosis.[176] Now, with the availability of amiodarone and implantable cardioverter-defibrillators (ICDs), the prognosis of late ventricular fibrillation is improving and is probably driven more by residual ventricular function and recurrent ischemia than by the arrhythmic risk per se.

Prophylaxis

Lidocaine prophylaxis to prevent primary ventricular fibrillation is no longer advised. Hypokalemia is associated with the risk of ventricular fibrillation in the CCU.[1] Although it has not been conclusively shown that correction of hypokalemia to a level of 4.5 mEq/liter actually reduces the incidence of ventricular fibrillation, our experience suggests that this probably is protective and of little risk. Despite the lack of a consistent relationship between hypomagnesemia and ventricular fibrillation, magnesium deficits may still be linked to the risk of ventricular fibrillation because intracellular magnesium levels are reduced in patients with STEMI and are not adequately reflected by serum measurements. For these reasons, and because it is often difficult to repair a potassium deficit without administering supplemental magnesium, we routinely replete magnesium to a level of 2 mEq/liter. The only situation in which we might consider prophylactic lidocaine (bolus of 1.5 mg/kg, followed by 20 to 50 μg/kg/min) would be the unusual circumstance in which a patient within the first 12 hours of a STEMI must be managed in a facility in which cardiac monitoring is not available and equipment for prompt defibrillation is not readily accessible.

Management

Treatment for ventricular fibrillation (see Chaps. 37 and 39) consists of an unsynchronized electrical countershock with at least 200 to 300 J, implemented as rapidly as possible.[1] When ventricular fibrillation occurs outside an intensive care unit, resuscitative efforts are much less likely to be successful, primarily because the time interval between the onset of the episode and institution of definitive therapy tends to be prolonged. Failure of electrical countershock to restore an effective cardiac rhythm is almost always caused by rapidly recurrent ventricular tachycardia or ventricular fibrillation, electromechanical dissociation, or, rarely, electrical asystole.

Successful interruption of ventricular fibrillation or prevention of refractory recurrent episodes can also be facilitated by administration of intravenous amiodarone. When synchronous cardiac electrical activity is restored by countershock but contraction is ineffective (i.e., pulseless electrical activity), the usual underlying cause is extensive myocardial ischemia or necrosis or rupture of the ventricular free wall or septum. If rupture has not occurred, intracardiac administration of calcium gluconate or epinephrine may promote restoration of an effective heartbeat. We do not usually administer bicarbonate injections to correct acidosis because of the high osmotic load they impose and the fact that hyperventilation of the patient is probably a more suitable means of clearing the acidosis.

Bradyarrhythmias (see Chap. 39)

SINUS BRADYCARDIA. Sinus bradycardia occurs commonly during the early phases of STEMI, particularly in patients with inferior and posterior infarction.[1] On the basis of data obtained in experimental infarction studies and from some clinical observations, the increased vagal tone that produces sinus bradycardia during the early phase of STEMI may actually be protective, perhaps because it reduces myocardial oxygen demands. Thus, the acute mortality rate appears similar in patients with sinus bradycardia to the rate in those without this arrhythmia.

Management

Isolated sinus bradycardia, unaccompanied by hypotension or ventricular ectopy, should be observed rather than treated initially. In the first 4 to 6 hours after infarction, if the sinus rate is extremely slow (<40 to 50 beats/min) and associated with hypotension, intravenous atropine in doses of 0.3 to 0.6 mg every 3 to 10 minutes (with a total dose not exceeding 2 mg) can be administered to bring the heart rate up to approximately 60 beats/min.

ATRIOVENTRICULAR AND INTRAVENTRICULAR BLOCK. Ischemic injury can produce conduction block at any level of the AV or intraventricular conduction system. Such blocks can occur in the AV node and the bundle of His, producing various grades of AV block, in either main bundle branch, producing right or left bundle branch block, and in the anterior and posterior divisions of the left bundle, producing left anterior or left posterior (fascicular) divisional blocks. Disturbances of conduction can occur in various combinations. Clinical features of proximal and distal AV conduction disturbances in patients with STEMI are summarized in **Table 55-14.**

First-Degree Atrioventricular Block

First-degree AV block generally does not require specific treatment. Beta blockers and calcium antagonists (other than nifedipine) prolong AV conduction and may be responsible for first-degree AV block as well. However, discontinuation of these drugs in the setting of STEMI has the potential of increasing ischemia and ischemic injury. Therefore, it is our practice not to decrease the dosage of these drugs unless the PR interval is longer than 0.24 second. Only if higher degree block or hemodynamic impairment occurs should these agents be stopped. If the block is a manifestation of excessive vagotonia and is associated with sinus bradycardia and hypotension, administration of atropine, as already outlined, may be helpful. Continued electrocardiographic monitoring is important in such patients in view of the possibility of progression to higher degrees of block.

Second-Degree Atrioventricular Block

First-degree and type I second-degree AV blocks do not appear to affect survival, are most commonly associated with occlusion of the right coronary artery, and are caused by ischemia of the AV node (see Table 55-14). Specific therapy is not required in patients with second-degree type I AV block when the ventricular rate exceeds 50 beats/min and premature ventricular contractions, heart failure, and bundle branch block are absent. However, if these complications develop or if the heart rate falls below approximately 50 beats/min and the patient is symptomatic, immediate treatment with atropine (0.3 to 0.6 mg) is indicated; temporary pacing systems are almost never needed in the management of this arrhythmia.

Type II second-degree block usually originates from a lesion in the conduction system below the His bundle (see Table 55-14). Because of its potential for progression to complete heart block, type II second-degree AV block should be treated with a temporary external or transvenous demand pacemaker, with the rate set at approximately 60 beats/min.[1]

CH
55

TABLE 55-14 **Atrioventricular Conduction Disturbances in Acute Myocardial Infarction**

PARAMETER	Location of Disturbance	
	PROXIMAL	DISTAL
Site of block	Intranodal	Infranodal
Site of infarction	Inferoposterior	Anteroseptal
Compromised arterial supply	RCA (90%), LCX (10%)	Septal perforators of LAD
Pathogenesis	Ischemia, necrosis, hydropic cell swelling, excess parasympathetic activity	Ischemia, necrosis, hydropic cell swelling
Predominant type of AV nodal block	(a) First-degree (PR > 200 msec) Mobitz type I, second-degree	(a) Mobitz type II, second-degree Third-degree
Common premonitory features of third-degree AV block	(a) First- or second-degree AV block (b) Mobitz I pattern	(a) Intraventricular conduction block (b) Mobitz II pattern
Features of escape rhythm following third-degree block (a) Location (b) QRS width (c) Rate (d) Stability of escape rhythm	(a) Proximal conduction system (His bundle) (b) <0.12/sec* (c) 45-60/min but may be as low as 30/min (d) Rate usually stable; asystole uncommon	(a) Distal conduction system (bundle branches) (b) >0.12/sec (c) Often <30/min (d) Rate often unstable with moderate to high risk of ventricular asystole
Duration of high-grade AV block	Usually transient (2-3 days)	Usually transient, but some form of AV conduction disturbance and/or intraventricular defect may persist
Associated mortality rate	Low unless associated with hypotension and/ or congestive heart failure	High because of extensive infarction associated with power failure or ventricular arrhythmias
Pacemaker therapy (a) Temporary (b) Permanent	(a) Rarely required; may be considered for bradycardia associated with left ventricular power failure, syncope, or angina (b) Almost never indicated because conduction defect is usually transient	(a) Should be considered in patients with anteroseptal infarction and acute bifascicular block (b) Indicated for patients with high-grade AV block with block in His-Purkinje system and those with transient advanced AV block and associated bundle branch block

*Some studies have suggested that a wide QRS escape rhythm (>0.12 second) following high-grade AV block in inferior infarction is associated with a worse prognosis.
LAD = left anterior descending coronary artery; LCX = left circumflex coronary artery; RCA = right coronary artery.
Modified from Antman EM, Rutherford JD: Coronary Care Medicine: A Practical Approach. Boston, Martinus Nijhoff, 1986; and Dreifus LS, Fisch C, Griffin JC, et al: Guidelines for implantation of cardiac pacemakers and antiarrhythmia devices. J Am Coll Cardiol 18:1, 1991.

Complete (Third-Degree) Atrioventricular Block

Complete AV block can occur in patients with anterior or inferior infarction. Complete heart block in patients with inferior infarction usually results from an intranodal or supranodal lesion and develops gradually, often progressing from first-degree or type I second-degree block.[177] The escape rhythm is usually stable, without asystole and often junctional, with a rate exceeding 40 beats/min and a narrow QRS complex in 70% of cases and a slower rate and wide QRS in the others. This form of complete AV block is often transient, may be responsive to pharmacologic antagonism of adenosine with methylxanthines,[178] and resolves in most patients within a few days (see Table 55-14).

In patients with anterior infarction, third-degree AV block often occurs suddenly, 12 to 24 hours after the onset of infarction, although it is usually preceded by intraventricular block and often type II (not first-degree or type I) AV block. Such patients have unstable escape rhythms with wide QRS complexes and rates less than 40 beats/min; ventricular asystole may occur suddenly. In patients with anterior infarction, AV block usually develops as a result of extensive septal necrosis that involves the bundle branches. The high rate of mortality in this group of patients with slow idioventricular rhythm and wide QRS complexes is the consequence of extensive myocardial necrosis, which results in severe left ventricular failure and often shock (see Table 55-14).

Patients with inferior infarction often have concomitant ischemia or infarction of the AV node secondary to hypoperfusion of the AV node artery. However, the His-Purkinje system usually escapes injury in such individuals. Patients with inferior STEMI who develop AV block generally have lesions in both right and left anterior descending coronary arteries. Similarly, patients with inferior STEMI and AV block have larger infarcts and more depressed right ventricular and left ventricular function than patients with inferior infarct and no AV block. As noted, junctional escape rhythms with narrow QRS complexes occur commonly in this setting.

Although data suggest that complete AV block is not an independent risk factor for mortality, whether temporary transvenous pacing per se improves survival of patients with anterior STEMI remains controversial. Some investigators have contended that ventricular pacing is of no value when used to correct complete AV block in patients with anterior infarction in view of the poor prognosis in this group, regardless of therapy. However, pacing may protect against transient hypotension, with its attendant risks of extending infarction and precipitating malignant ventricular tachyarrhythmias. Also, pacing protects against asystole, a particular hazard in patients with anterior infarction and infranodal block. Improved survival with pacing probably occurs in only a small fraction of patients with complete AV block and anterior wall infarcts, because the extensive destruction of the myocardium that almost invariably accompanies this condition results in a high mortality rate, even in paced patients. Given these considerations, an extremely large series of patients would be required to demonstrate the small reduction of mortality that might be achieved by pacing. The absence of data supporting such an effect, however, by no means excludes the possibility that it may be present.

Pacing is not usually necessary in patients with inferior wall infarction and complete AV block that is often transient in nature, but it is indicated if the ventricular rate is slow (<40 to 50 beats/min), if ventricular arrhythmias or hypotension is present, or if pump failure develops; atropine is only rarely of value in these patients. Only when complete heart block develops in less than 6 hours after the onset of symptoms is atropine likely to abolish the AV block or cause acceleration of the escape rhythm. In such cases, the AV block is more likely to be transient and related to increases in vagal tone, rather than the more persistent block seen later in the course of STEMI, which generally requires cardiac pacing.

INTRAVENTRICULAR BLOCK. The right bundle branch and left posterior division have a dual blood supply from the left anterior descending and right coronary arteries, whereas the left anterior division is supplied by septal perforators originating from the left anterior descending coronary artery. Not all conduction blocks observed in patients with STEMI can be considered to be complications of infarcts because almost half are already present when the first ECG is recorded, and they may represent antecedent disease of the conduction system.[179] Compared with patients without conduction defects, STEMI patients with bundle branch blocks have more comorbid conditions, are less likely to receive therapies such as thrombolytics, aspirin, and beta blockers, and have an increased in-hospital mortality rate.[180] In the prefibrinolytic era, studies of intraventricular conduction disturbances (i.e., block within one or more of the three subdivisions [fascicles] of the His-Purkinje system [the anterior and posterior divisions of the left bundle and the right bundle]) had been reported to occur in 5% to 10% of patients with STEMI. More recent series in the reperfusion era have suggested that intraventricular blocks occur in about 2% to 5% of patients with MI.[181] Investigators performing primary PCI for STEMI have reported an association between new-onset bundle branch block and abnormal myocardial perfusion, even if flow through epicardial arteries is restored.[182]

Isolated Fascicular Block

Isolated left anterior divisional block is unlikely to progress to complete AV block. Mortality is increased in these patients, although not as much as in patients with other forms of conduction block. The posterior fascicle is larger than the anterior fascicle and, in general, a larger infarct is required to block it. As a consequence, mortality is markedly increased. Complete AV block is not a frequent complication of either form of isolated divisional block.

Right Bundle Branch Block

This conduction defect alone can lead to AV block because it is often a new lesion, associated with anteroseptal infarction. Isolated right bundle branch block is associated with an increased mortality risk in patients with anterior STEMI, even if complete AV block does not occur, but this appears to be the case only if it is accompanied by congestive heart failure.

Bifascicular Block

The combination of right bundle branch block with left anterior or posterior divisional block, or the combination of left anterior and posterior divisional blocks (i.e., left bundle branch block), is known as bidivisional or bifascicular block. If new block occurs in two of the three divisions of the conduction system, the risk of developing complete AV block is high. Mortality is also high because of the occurrence of severe pump failure secondary to the extensive myocardial necrosis required to produce such an extensive intraventricular block.[183] Patients with intraventricular conduction defects, particularly right bundle branch block, account for the majority of patients who develop ventricular fibrillation late in their hospital stay. However, the high rate of mortality in these patients occurs even in the absence of high-grade AV block and appears to be related to cardiac failure and massive infarction, rather than to the conduction disturbance.

Preexisting bundle branch block or divisional block is less often associated with the development of complete heart block in patients with STEMI than are conduction defects acquired during the course of the infarct. Bidivisional block in the presence of prolongation of the P-R interval (first-degree AV block) may indicate disease of the third subdivision rather than of the AV node; it is associated with a greater risk of complete heart block than if first-degree AV block is absent.

Complete bundle branch block (left or right), the combination of right bundle branch block and left anterior divisional (fascicular) block, and any of the various forms of trifascicular block are all more often associated with anterior than with inferoposterior infarction. All these forms are more frequent with large infarcts and in older patients, and have a higher incidence of other accompanying arrhythmias than that seen in patients without bundle branch block.

USE OF PACEMAKERS IN PATIENTS WITH ACUTE MYOCARDIAL INFARCTION (see Chap. 38)

Temporary Pacing

Just as is the case for complete AV block, transvenous ventricular pacing has not resulted in a statistically demonstrable improvement in prognosis in patients with STEMI who develop intraventricular conduction defects. However, temporary pacing is advisable in some of these patients because of the high risk of developing complete AV block. This includes patients with new bilateral (bifascicular) bundle branch block (i.e., right bundle branch block with left anterior or posterior divisional block and alternating right and left bundle branch block); first-degree AV block adds to this risk. Isolated new block in only one of the three fascicles, even with P-R prolongation and preexisting bifascicular block and a normal P-R interval, poses somewhat less risk; these patients should be monitored closely, with insertion of a temporary pacemaker deferred unless higher degree AV block occurs.

Noninvasive external temporary cardiac pacing is possible routinely in conscious patients and is acceptable to many patients, despite the discomfort. Used in a standby mode, it is almost free of complications and contraindications and provides an important alternative to transvenous endocardial pacing.[1] Once it is clinically evident that continuous pacing is required, external pacing, which is generally not well tolerated for more than minutes to hours, should be replaced by a temporary transvenous pacemaker.

Asystole

The presence of apparent ventricular asystole on monitor displays of continuously recorded ECGs may be misleading because the rhythm may actually be fine ventricular fibrillation. Because of the predominance of ventricular fibrillation as the cause of cardiac arrest in this setting, initial therapy should include electrical countershock, even if definitive electrocardiographic documentation of this arrhythmia is not available. In the rare case in which asystole can be documented as the responsible electrophysiologic disturbance, immediate transcutaneous pacing, or stimulation with a transvenous pacemaker if one is already in place, is indicated.[1]

Permanent Pacing

The question of the advisability of permanent pacemaker insertion is complicated because not all sudden deaths in STEMI patients with conduction defects are caused by high-grade AV block. A high incidence of late ventricular fibrillation occurs in CCU survivors with anterior STEMI complicated by right or left bundle branch block. Therefore, ventricular fibrillation, rather than asystole caused by failure of AV conduction and infranodal pacemakers, could be responsible for late sudden death.

Long-term pacing is often helpful when complete heart block persists throughout the hospital phase in a patient with STEMI, when sinus node function is markedly impaired, or when type II second- or third-degree block occurs intermittently.[1] When high-grade AV block is associated with newly acquired bundle branch block or other criteria of impairment of conduction system function, prophylactic long-term pacing may also be justified. Additional considerations that drive a decision to insert a permanent pacemaker include whether the patient is a candidate for an ICD or has severe heart failure that might be improved with biventricular pacing (see Chap. 28).

Supraventricular Tachyarrhythmias (see Chaps. 39 and 40)

SINUS TACHYCARDIA. This arrhythmia is typically associated with augmented sympathetic activity and may provoke transient hypertension or hypotension. Common causes are anxiety, persistent pain, left ventricular failure, fever, pericarditis, hypovolemia, pulmonary embolism, and the administration of cardioaccelerator drugs such as atropine, epinephrine, or dopamine; rarely, it occurs in patients with atrial infarction. Sinus tachycardia is particularly common in patients with anterior infarction, especially if there is significant accompanying left ventricular dysfunction. It is an undesirable rhythm in patients with STEMI because it results in an augmentation of myocardial oxygen consumption, as well as a reduction in the time available for coronary perfusion, thereby intensifying myocardial ischemia and/or external myocardial necrosis. Persistent sinus tachycardia can signify persistent heart failure and, under these circumstances, connotes poor prognosis and excess mortality. An underlying cause should be sought and appropriate treatment instituted, such as analgesics for pain, diuretics for heart failure, oxygen, beta blockers, and nitroglycerin for ischemia, and aspirin for fever or pericarditis.

Administration of beta blockers, in the dosage and manner described elsewhere in this chapter, may be helpful in the treatment of sinus tachycardia, particularly when this arrhythmia is a manifestation of a hyperdynamic circulation, which is seen particularly in young patients with an initial STEMI without extensive cardiac damage. Beta blocker administration is contraindicated, however, in patients in whom the sinus tachycardia is a manifestation of hypovolemia or of pump failure; the latter is indicated by a systolic arterial pressure below 100 mm Hg, rales involving more than one third of the lung fields, a pulmonary capillary wedge pressure exceeding 20 to 25 mm Hg, or a cardiac index below approximately 2.2 liters/min/m². A possible exception to this is a patient in whom persistent ischemia is believed to be the cause or the result of tachycardia—cautious administration of an ultrashort-acting beta blocker such as esmolol (25 to 200 µg/kg/min) can evaluate the patient's response to slowing of the heart rate.

ATRIAL FLUTTER AND FIBRILLATION. Atrial flutter is usually transient and, in patients with STEMI, is typically a consequence of augmented sympathetic stimulation of the atria, often occurring in patients with left ventricular failure, pulmonary emboli in whom the arrhythmia intensifies hemodynamic deterioration, or atrial infarction (see Table 55-13).

As with atrial premature complexes and atrial flutter, fibrillation is usually transient and tends to occur in patients with left ventricular failure but also occurs in those with pericarditis and ischemic injury to the atria and right ventricular infarction.[184] The increased ventricular rate and loss of the atrial contribution to left ventricular filling result in a significant reduction in cardiac output. Atrial fibrillation during STEMI is associated with increased mortality and stroke, particularly in patients with anterior wall infarction.[185] However, because it is more common in patients with clinical and hemodynamic manifestations of extensive infarction and a poor prognosis, atrial fibrillation is probably a marker of poor prognosis, with only a small independent contribution to increased mortality.

Management

Atrial flutter and fibrillation in patients with STEMI are treated in a manner similar to that in other settings (see Chap. 40). Patients with recurrent episodes of atrial fibrillation should be treated with oral anticoagulants to reduce the risk of stroke, even if sinus rhythm is present at the time of hospital discharge, because no antiarrhythmic regimen can be relied on to be completely effective in suppressing atrial fibrillation. In the absence of contraindications, patients should receive a beta blocker after STEMI; in addition to their several other beneficial effects, these agents are helpful in slowing the ventricular rate if atrial fibrillation recurs. Digitalis may also be helpful in slowing the ventricular rate and managing ventricular dysfunction when atrial fibrillation develops after STEMI.[186]

Other Complications

RECURRENT CHEST DISCOMFORT. Evaluation of postinfarction chest discomfort is sometimes complicated by previous abnormalities on the ECG and a vague description of the discomfort by the patient,

who may be exquisitely sensitive to fleeting discomfort or may deny a potential recrudescence of symptoms. The critical task for clinicians is to distinguish recurrent angina or infarction from nonischemic causes of discomfort that might be caused by infarct expansion, pericarditis, pulmonary embolism, and noncardiac conditions. Important diagnostic maneuvers include a repeat physical examination, repeat reading of the ECG, and assessment of the response to sublingual nitroglycerin, 0.4 mg. (The use of noninvasive diagnostic evaluation for recurrent ischemia in patients whose symptoms appear only with moderate levels of exertion is discussed elsewhere in this chapter.)

Recurrent Ischemia and Infarction

The incidence of postinfarction angina without reinfarction is reduced in patients undergoing primary PCI for STEMI compared with fibrinolysis.[187] More effective antiplatelet and antithrombin therapies significantly reduce the rate of recurrent ischemic events after fibrinolysis to a range similar to that reported for primary PCI.[104,110,113] When accompanied by ST and T wave changes in the same leads where Q waves have appeared, it may be caused by occlusion of an initially patent vessel, reocclusion of an initially recanalized or stented vessel, or coronary spasm.

Diagnosis

Extension of the original zone of necrosis or reinfarction in a separate myocardial zone can be a difficult diagnosis, especially within the first 24 hours after the index event. It is more convenient to refer to extension and reinfarction collectively under the more general term *recurrent infarction*. Serum cardiac marker levels may remain elevated from the initial infarction, and it may not be possible to distinguish the electrocardiographic changes that are part of the normal evolution after the index infarction from those caused by recurrent infarction. Within the first 18 to 24 hours following the initial infarction, when serum cardiac marker levels may not have returned to the normal range, recurrent infarction should be strongly considered when there is repeat ST-segment elevation on the ECG. Although pericarditis remains a possibility in such patients, the two can usually be distinguished by the presence of a rub and lack of responsiveness to nitroglycerin in patients with pericardial discomfort. Beyond the first 24 hours, recurrent infarction can be diagnosed either by re-elevation of the cardiac markers or the appearance of new Q waves on the ECG.[1] Reinfarction is more common in patients with diabetes mellitus and those with a previous MI. The predominant angiographic predictors of reinfarction in patients undergoing primary PCI include a final coronary stenosis larger than 30%, post-PCI coronary dissection, and post-PCI intracoronary thrombus. Diabetic patients and those with advanced Killip class are more likely to experience reinfarction.[188]

Prognosis

Regardless of whether postinfarction angina is persistent or limited, its presence is important because the short-term morbidity rate is higher among such patients; mortality is increased if the recurrent ischemia is accompanied by electrocardiographic changes and hemodynamic compromise.[1] Recurrent infarction, often caused by reocclusion of the infarct-related coronary artery, carries serious adverse prognostic information because it is associated with higher rates of in-hospital complications (e.g., congestive heart failure, heart block) and early and long-term mortality.[189] Presumably, the higher mortality rate is related to the larger mass of myocardium whose function becomes compromised.

Management

As with the acute phase of treatment of STEMI, algorithms for the management of patients with recurrent ischemic discomfort at rest center on the 12-lead ECG (**Fig. 55-39**). Patients with ST-segment re-elevation should be referred for urgent catheterization and PCI; repeat fibrinolysis can be considered if PCI is not available. Insertion of an intra-aortic balloon pump may help stabilize the patient while other procedures are being arranged. For patients who are thought to have recurrent ischemia but no evidence of hemodynamic compromise, an attempt should be made to control symptoms

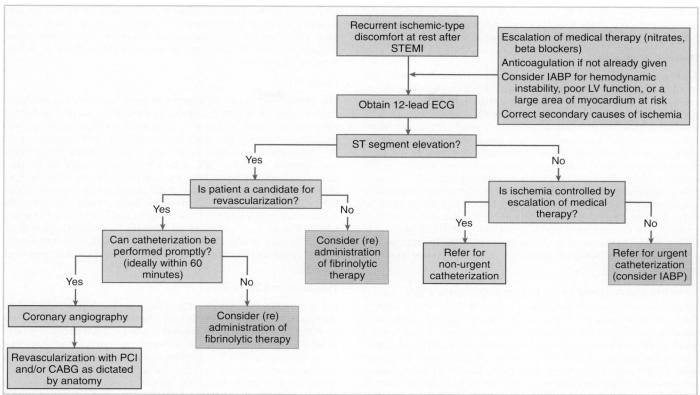

FIGURE 55-39 Algorithm for management of ischemia/infarction after STEMI. IABP = intra-aortic balloon pump; LV = left ventricular. *(Modified from Antman EM, Anbe DT, Armstrong PW, et al: ACC/AHA guidelines for the management of patients with ST-elevation myocardial infarction: A report of the American College of Cardiology/ American Heart Association Task Force on Practice Guidelines [Committee to Revise the 1999 Guidelines for the Management of Patients with Acute Myocardial Infarction]. Circulation 110:e82, 2004.)*

with sublingual or intravenous nitroglycerin and intravenous beta blockade to slow the heart rate to 60 beats/min. When hypotension, congestive heart failure, or ventricular arrhythmias develop during recurrent ischemia, urgent catheterization and revascularization are indicated.

High-risk patients with STEMI who receive fibrinolysis benefit from a strategy of routine referral for catheterization and revascularization (<24 hours).[85] However, current trials that compared primary PCI with PCI performed as soon as possible after a preparatory pharmacologic regimen had been administered have not shown such a facilitated PCI approach to be more effective than primary PCI; there are even suggestions of increased mortality because of excess bleeding in the facilitated PCI group.[35]

Finally, with increasing use of PCI in the management of patients with STEMI, clinicians should be alert to the problem of stent thrombosis as a cause of recurrent ischemia. Stent thrombosis can occur acutely (hours to days after deployment of a stent) or in a more sub-acute fashion (many months after deployment of a stent; see Chap. 58).

PERICARDIAL EFFUSION AND PERICARDITIS (see Chap. 75)

Pericardial Effusion

Effusions are generally detected echocardiographically and their incidence varies with technique, criteria, and laboratory expertise.[190] Effusions are more common in patients with anterior STEMI and with larger infarcts and when congestive failure is present. Most pericardial effusions that occur following STEMI do not cause hemodynamic compromise; when tamponade occurs, it is usually caused by ventricular rupture or hemorrhagic pericarditis. The reabsorption rate of a postinfarction pericardial effusion is slow, with resolution often taking several months. The presence of an effusion does not indicate that pericarditis is present; although they may occur together, most effusions occur without other evidence of pericarditis.

Pericarditis

Pericarditis can produce pain as early as the first day and as late as 6 weeks after STEMI. The pain of pericarditis may be confused with that resulting from postinfarction angina, recurrent infarction, or both. An important distinguishing feature is the radiation of the pain to either trapezius ridge, a finding that is almost pathognomonic of pericarditis and is rarely seen with ischemic discomfort. Transmural MI, by definition, extends to the epicardial surface and is responsible for local pericardial inflammation. An acute fibrinous pericarditis (pericarditis epistenocardiaca) occurs commonly after transmural infarction, but most patients do not report any symptoms from this process. Although transient pericardial friction rubs are relatively common in patients with transmural infarction within the first 48 hours, pain or electrocardiographic changes occur much less often. However, the development of a pericardial rub appears to be correlated with a larger infarct and greater hemodynamic compromise. The discomfort of pericarditis usually becomes worse during a deep inspiration, but it can be relieved or diminished when the patient sits up and leans forward.

Although anticoagulation clearly increases the risk for hemorrhagic pericarditis early after STEMI, this complication does not occur with sufficient frequency during heparinization or following fibrinolytic therapy to warrant absolute prohibition of such agents when a rub is present. Nevertheless, the detection of a pericardial effusion on echo is usually an indication for discontinuation of anticoagulation. In patients for whom continuation or initiation of anticoagulant therapy is strongly indicated (e.g., during cardiac catheterization or following coronary angioplasty), heightened monitoring of clotting parameters and observation for clinical signs of possible tamponade are necessary. Late pericardial constriction caused by anticoagulant-induced hemopericardium has been reported.

Treatment of pericardial discomfort consists of aspirin, but usually in higher doses than prescribed routinely following infarction; doses of 650 mg orally every 4 to 6 hours may be necessary. Nonsteroidal anti-inflammatory drugs (NSAIDs) and steroids should be avoided because they may interfere with myocardial scar formation.[1,191]

Dressler Syndrome

Also known as the postmyocardial infarction syndrome, Dressler syndrome usually occurs 1 to 8 weeks after infarction. Dressler cited an incidence of 3% to 4% of all MI patients in 1957, but the incidence has decreased dramatically since then. Clinically, patients with Dressler syndrome present with malaise, fever, pericardial discomfort, leukocytosis, an elevated sedimentation rate, and a pericardial effusion. At autopsy, patients with this syndrome usually demonstrate localized fibrinous pericarditis containing polymorphonuclear leukocytes. The cause of this syndrome is not clearly established, although the detection of antibodies to cardiac tissue has raised the notion of an immunopathologic process. Treatment is with aspirin, 650 mg, as often as every 4 hours. Glucocorticosteroids and NSAIDs are best avoided in patients with Dressler syndrome within 4 weeks of STEMI because of their potential to impair infarct healing, cause ventricular rupture, and increase coronary vascular resistance. Aspirin in large doses is effective.[192]

VENOUS THROMBOSIS AND PULMONARY EMBOLISM. Almost all peri-MI pulmonary emboli originate from thrombi in the veins of the lower extremities; much less commonly, they originate from mural thrombi overlying an area of right ventricular infarction. Bed rest and heart failure predispose to venous thrombosis and subsequent pulmonary embolism, and both these factors occur commonly in patients with STEMI, particularly those with large infarcts. At a time when patients with STEMI were routinely subjected to prolonged periods of bed rest, significant pulmonary embolism was found in more than 20% of patients with STEMI coming to autopsy, and massive pulmonary embolism accounted for 10% of deaths from MI. In current practice, with early mobilization and the widespread use of low-dose anticoagulant prophylaxis, especially using low-molecular-weight heparins, pulmonary embolism has become an uncommon cause of death in patients with STEMI. When pulmonary embolism does occur in patients with STEMI, management is generally similar to that described for noninfarction patients (see Chap. 77).

LEFT VENTRICULAR ANEURYSM. The term *left ventricular aneurysm* (often termed *true aneurysm*) is generally reserved for a discrete dyskinetic area of the left ventricular wall with a broad neck to differentiate it from pseudoaneurysm caused by a contained myocardial rupture. Dyskinetic or akinetic areas of the left ventricle are far more common than true aneurysms after STEMI; such poorly contracting segments are termed *regional wall motion abnormalities*. True left ventricular aneurysms probably develop in less than 5% of all patients with STEMI and perhaps somewhat more frequently in patients with transmural infarction (especially anterior).[193] The wall of the true aneurysm is thinner than the wall of the rest of the left ventricle (see Fig. 55-34); it is usually composed of fibrous tissue and necrotic muscle, occasionally mixed with viable myocardium.

Pathogenesis

Aneurysm formation presumably occurs when intraventricular tension stretches the noncontracting infarcted heart muscle, thus producing infarct expansion, a relatively weak thin layer of necrotic muscle, and fibrous tissue that bulges with each cardiac contraction. With the passage of time, the wall of the aneurysm becomes more densely fibrotic, but it continues to bulge with systole, causing some of the left ventricular stroke volume during each systole to be ineffective.

When an aneurysm is present after anterior STEMI, there is generally a total occlusion of a poorly collateralized left anterior descending coronary artery. An aneurysm rarely occurs with multivessel disease when there are extensive collaterals or a nonoccluded left anterior descending artery. Aneurysms usually range from 1 to 8 cm in diameter. They occur approximately four times more often at the apex and in the anterior wall than in the inferoposterior wall. The overlying pericardium is usually densely adherent to the wall of the aneurysm, which

may even become partially calcified after several years. True left ventricular aneurysms, in contrast to pseudoaneurysms, rarely rupture soon after development. Late rupture, when the true aneurysm has become stabilized by the formation of dense fibrous tissue in its wall, almost never occurs.

Diagnosis

The presence of persistent ST-segment elevation in an electrocardiographic area of infarction, classically thought to suggest aneurysm formation, actually indicates a large infarct with a regional wall motion abnormality but does not necessarily imply an aneurysm. The diagnosis of aneurysm is best made noninvasively by an echocardiographic study, by CMR, or by left ventriculography at the time of cardiac catheterization. With the loss of shortening from the area of the aneurysm, the remainder of the ventricle may become hyperkinetic to compensate. With relatively large aneurysms, complete compensation is impossible. The stroke volume falls or, if it is maintained, it is at the expense of an increase in end-diastolic volume, which in turn leads to increased wall tension and myocardial oxygen demand. Heart failure may ensue, and angina may appear or worsen.

Prognosis and Treatment

Left ventricular aneurysm increases the risk of a mortality, even when compared with that in patients with comparable left ventricular ejection fraction. Death in these patients is often sudden and presumably related to the high incidence of ventricular tachyarrhythmias that occur with aneurysms.[194] Aggressive management of STEMI, including prompt reperfusion, may diminish the incidence of ventricular aneurysms. Surgical aneurysmectomy generally only succeeds if there is relative preservation of contractile performance in the nonaneurysmal portion of the left ventricle. In such a case, when the operation is performed for worsening heart failure or angina, operative mortality is relatively low and clinical improvement can be expected. Because of the importance of maintaining as normal a left ventricular shape as possible, several surgical techniques for ventricular reconstruction have been developed; these may be combined with the general approach shown in **Figure 55-40**.[195] Because of the risk of mural thrombosis and systemic embolization, we favor long-term oral anticoagulation with warfarin in patients with a left ventricular aneurysm after STEMI.

Left Ventricular Thrombus and Arterial Embolism

Endocardial inflammation during the acute phase of infarction probably provides a thrombogenic surface for clots to form in the left ventricle. With extensive transmural infarction of the septum, however, mural thrombi may overlie infarcted myocardium in both ventricles. The incidence of left ventricular thrombus formation after STEMI appears to have dropped from about 20% to 5% with more aggressive use of antithrombotic strategies.[196] Prospective studies have suggested that patients who develop a mural thrombus early, within 48 to 72 hours of infarction, have an extremely poor early prognosis, with a high rate of mortality from the complications of a large infarction (e.g., shock, reinfarction, rupture, ventricular tachyarrhythmia), rather than emboli from the left ventricular thrombus.

Although a mural thrombus adheres to the endocardium overlying the infarcted myocardium, superficial portions of it can become detached and produce systemic arterial emboli. Although estimates vary on the basis of patient selection, about 10% of mural thrombi result in systemic embolization. Echocardiographically detectable features that suggest a given thrombus is more likely to embolize include increased mobility and protrusion into the ventricular chamber, visualization in multiple views, and contiguous zones of akinesis and hyperkinesis.

MANAGEMENT. Data from previous trials with limited sample size have suggested that anticoagulation (intravenous heparin or high-dose

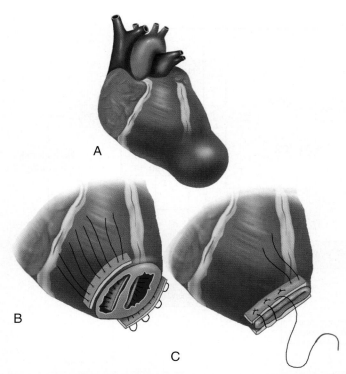

FIGURE 55-40 Surgical management of ventricular aneurysm. **A,** In this case, the aneurysm is located at the apex. **B,** The aneurysmal segment is resected and felt pledget strips are used to reinforce interrupted suture closure of the apex. **C,** Completed repair partially restores apical geometry. *(Courtesy of Dr. David Adams, Division of Cardiac Surgery, Mount Sinai Hospital, New York.)*

subcutaneous heparin) reduce the development of left ventricular thrombi by 50% but, because of the low event rate, it is not possible to demonstrate a reduction in the incidence of systemic embolism. Fibrinolysis reduces the rate of thrombus formation and the character of the thrombi so that they are less protuberant. However, the data from fibrinolytic trials are difficult to interpret because of the confounding effect of antithrombotic therapy with heparin. Recommendations for anticoagulation vary considerably, and fibrinolysis has precipitated fatal embolization. Nevertheless, anticoagulation for 3 to 6 months with warfarin is advocated for many patients with demonstrable mural thrombi.[1,197]

On the basis of the available data, it is our practice to recommend anticoagulation (intravenous heparin to elevate the aPTT to 1.5 to 2 times that of control, followed by a minimum of 3 to 6 months of warfarin) in the following clinical situations: (1) an embolic event has already occurred or (2) the patient has a large anterior infarction whether or not a thrombus is visualized echocardiographically. We are also inclined to follow the same anticoagulation practice in patients with infarctions other than in the anterior distribution if a thrombus or large wall motion abnormality is detected. Aspirin, although probably not able to affect thrombus size in most patients, may prevent further platelet deposition on existing thrombi and also protects against recurrent ischemic events. Aspirin should be prescribed in conjunction with warfarin to patients who are candidates for long-term anticoagulation therapy on the basis of the indications discussed earlier.

Convalescence, Discharge, and Post–Myocardial Infarction Care

TIMING OF HOSPITAL DISCHARGE. The timing of discharge from the hospital is variable. As noted, patients who have undergone aggressive reperfusion protocols and have no significant ventricular arrhythmias, recurrent ischemia, or congestive heart failure have been safely discharged in less than 5 days. More commonly, discharge occurs 5 or 6 days after admission for patients who experience no complications, who can be followed readily at home, and whose family setting is conducive to convalescence. Most complications that would preclude early discharge occur within the first day or two of admission; therefore, patients suitable for early discharge can be identified early during their hospitalization.[1] Several controlled trials and many uncontrolled trials of early discharge after STEMI have failed to show any increase in risk in patients appropriately selected for early discharge. The decision regarding timing of discharge in the patients with uncomplicated STEMI should take into account the patient's psychological state after STEMI, the adequacy of the dose titration for essential drugs such as beta blockers and inhibitors of the RAAS, and the availability and timing of follow-up with visiting nurses and the patient's primary care physician. For patients who have experienced a complication, discharge is deferred until their condition has been stable for several days and it is clear that they are responding appropriately to necessary medications such as antiarrhythmic agents, vasodilators, or positive inotropic agents or that they have undergone the appropriate workup for recurrent ischemia.

COUNSELING. Before discharge from the hospital, all patients should receive detailed instruction concerning physical activity. Initially, this should consist of walking at home with avoidance of isometric exercise such as lifting; several rest periods should be taken daily. In addition, the patient should be given fresh nitroglycerin tablets and instructed in their use (see Chap. 57) and should receive careful instructions about the use of any other medications prescribed. As convalescence progresses, graded resumption of activity should be encouraged (see Chaps. 50 and 83). Many approaches have been used, ranging from formal rigid guidelines to general advice advocating moderation and avoidance of any activity that evokes symptoms. Sexual counseling is often overlooked during recovery from STEMI and should be included as part of the educational process. Such counseling should begin early after STEMI and include the recommendation that sexual activity be resumed after successful completion of early submaximal or later symptom-limited exercise stress testing.[1]

Some evidence indicates that behavioral alteration is possible after recovery from STEMI and that this may improve prognosis. A cardiac rehabilitation program with supervised physical exercise and an educational component has been recommended for most STEMI patients after discharge. Although the overall clinical benefit of such programs continues to be debated, there is little question that most people derive considerable information and psychological security from such interventions, and they continue to be endorsed by experienced clinicians.[1] Meta-analyses of randomized trials of medically supervised rehabilitation programs versus usual care that were conducted in an era before widespread use of beta blockers and aggressive reperfusion strategies have shown a reduction in cardiovascular death but no change in the incidence of nonfatal reinfarction. Given the relationship between depression and STEMI, interest has arisen in psychosocial intervention programs during the convalescent phase of STEMI (see Chaps. 50 and 91).[198,199] Psychosocial intervention programs can decrease symptoms of depression and are a useful adjunct to standard cardiac rehabilitation programs after STEMI; however, they do not have a significant impact on the risk of mortality or recurrent MI after STEMI.[200]

Risk Stratification After STEMI

The process of risk stratification following STEMI occurs in several stages—initial presentation, in-hospital course (CCU, intermediate care unit), and at the time of hospital discharge. The tools used to form an integrated and dynamic assessment of the patient consist of baseline demographic information, serial ECGs and serum and plasma cardiac biomarker measurements, hemodynamic monitoring data, noninvasive tests and, if performed, the findings at cardiac catheterization (**Fig. 55-41**).[1] These are integrated with the occurrence of in-hospital complications to provide information regarding survival.

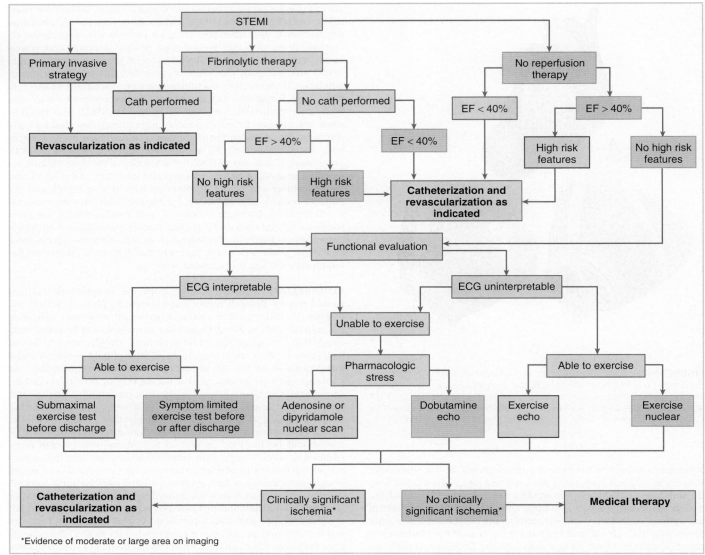

FIGURE 55-41 Algorithm for catheterization and revascularization after STEMI. The algorithm shows the treatment paths for patients who initially undergo a primary invasive strategy, receive fibrinolytic therapy, or do not undergo reperfusion therapy for STEMI. Patients who have not undergone a primary invasive strategy and have no high-risk features should undergo functional evaluation using one of the noninvasive tests shown. When clinically significant ischemia (evidence of moderate or large area of ischemia by imaging) is detected, patients should undergo catheterization and revascularization as indicated; if no clinically significant ischemia is detected, medical therapy is prescribed post-STEMI. cath = catheterization; echo = echocardiography; EF = ejection fraction. *(From Antman EM, Anbe DT, Armstrong PW, et al: ACC/AHA guidelines for the management of patients with ST-elevation myocardial infarction: A report of the American College of Cardiology/American Heart Association Task Force on Practice Guidelines [Committee to Revise the 1999 Guidelines for the Management of Patients with Acute Myocardial Infarction]. Circulation 110:e82, 2004.)*

INITIAL PRESENTATION. Certain demographic and historical factors portend a worse prognosis in patients with STEMI, including female gender, age older than 65 years, a history of diabetes mellitus, prior angina pectoris, and previous MI (see Fig. 55-13). Diabetes mellitus, in particular, appears to confer a more than 40% increase in adjusted risk of death by 30 days (see Chap. 64).[201] Surviving diabetic patients also experience a more complicated post-MI course, including a greater incidence of postinfarction angina, infarct extension, and heart failure.[1] These higher rates of complications likely relate to the extensive accelerated atherosclerosis and higher risk of thrombosis and heart failure associated with diabetes mellitus.

In addition to playing a central role in the decision pathway for the management of patients with STEMI based on the presence or absence of ST-segment elevation, the 12-lead ECG carries important prognostic information.[202] Mortality is higher in patients experiencing anterior wall STEMI than after inferior STEMI, even when corrected for infarct size. Patients with right ventricular infarction complicating inferior

infarction, as suggested by ST-segment elevation in V_4R, have a higher mortality rate than patients sustaining an inferior infarction without right ventricular involvement.[158] Patients with multiple leads showing ST-segment elevation and a high sum of ST-segment elevation have an increased mortality rate, especially if their infarct is anterior in location. Patients whose ECG demonstrates persistent advanced heart block (e.g., type II, second-degree, or third-degree AV block) or new intraventricular conduction abnormalities (bifascicular or trifascicular) in the course of STEMI have a worse prognosis than patients without these abnormalities. The influence of a high degree of heart block is particularly important in patients with right ventricular infarction because such patients have a markedly increased mortality risk. Other electrocardiographic findings that augur poorly are persistent horizontal or downsloping ST-segment depression, Q waves in multiple leads,[203] evidence of right ventricular infarction accompanying inferior infarction, ST-segment depressions in anterior leads in patients with inferior infarction, and atrial arrhythmias, especially atrial fibrillation.

Several validated clinical risk stratification tools may be used at presentation to assess the short- and long-term risk of death after MI.[204] In addition to the patient's age and historical factors such as diabetes and prior MI, clinical signs of heart failure, including tachycardia and hypotension, are common to many of these clinical scores for risk assessment.

HOSPITAL COURSE. Soon after CCUs were instituted, it became apparent that left ventricular function is an important early determinant of survival. Hospital mortality from STEMI depends directly on the severity of left ventricular dysfunction. Risk stratification via physical findings, estimation of infarct size and, in appropriate patients, invasive hemodynamic monitoring in the CCU, provide an assessment of the likelihood of a complicated hospital course and may also identify important abnormalities, such as hemodynamically significant mitral regurgitation, that convey an adverse long-term prognosis (see Table 55-10). In particular, the development of heart failure after MI entails a higher risk of sudden cardiac death.[205]

Recurrent ischemia and infarction following STEMI, in the same location as the index infarction or at a distance, influence prognosis adversely.[206] Poor prognosis comes from the loss of viable myocardium, with the resulting larger area of infarction creating a greater compromise in ventricular function. Postinfarction angina generally connotes a less favorable prognosis because it indicates the presence of jeopardized myocardium. In the current era of aggressive revascularization, early postinfarction angina often leads to early interventions that tend to improve outcome, diminishing the long-term impact and significance of angina soon after STEMI.[205,207]

ASSESSMENT AT HOSPITAL DISCHARGE. Both short- and long-term survival after STEMI depend on three factors—resting left ventricular function, residual potentially ischemic myocardium, and susceptibility to serious ventricular arrhythmias. The most important of these factors is the state of left ventricular function (see Fig. 55-30).[1] The second most important factor is how the severity and extent of the obstructive lesions in the coronary vascular bed perfusing residual viable myocardium affect the risk of recurrent infarction, additional myocardial damage, and serious ventricular arrhythmias. Thus, survival relates to the quantity of myocardium that has become necrotic and the quantity at risk of becoming necrotic. At one end of the spectrum, the prognosis is best for the patient with normal intrinsic coronary vessels whose completed infarction constitutes a small fraction (5%) of the left ventricle as a consequence of a coronary embolus and who has no jeopardized myocardium. At the other extreme is the patient with a massive infarct with left ventricular failure whose residual viable myocardium is perfused by markedly obstructed vessels. Progression of atherosclerosis or lowering of perfusion pressure in these vessels impairs the function and viability of the residual myocardium on which left ventricular function depends. Revascularization may reduce the threat to the jeopardized myocardium, even in such a patient. The third risk factor, the susceptibility to serious arrhythmias, is reflected in ventricular ectopic activity and other indicators of electrical instability, such as reduced heart rate variability or baroreflex sensitivity and an abnormal signal-averaged ECG.[204] All these identify patients at increased risk of death.

Left Ventricular Function

Left ventricular ejection fraction may be the most easily assessed measurement of left ventricular function and is extremely useful for risk stratification (see Fig. 55-30). However, imaging of the left ventricle at rest may not distinguish adequately among infarcted, irreversibly damaged, and stunned or hibernating myocardium. To circumvent this difficulty, various techniques have been investigated to assess the extent of residual viable myocardium including exercise and pharmacologic stress echocardiography, stress radionuclide ventricular angiography, perfusion imaging in conjunction with pharmacological stress, positron emission tomography, and gadolinium-enhanced CMR.[208,209] All these techniques can be performed safely in postinfarction patients. Because no study has clearly shown one imaging modality to be superior to others, clinicians should be guided in their selection of ventricular imaging technique by the availability and level of expertise with a given modality at their institution.[210] Because of the dynamic nature of LV function recovery after STEMI, clinicians should consider the timing of the imaging study relative to the index event when assessing LV function.[1]

In patients with low left ventricular ejection fraction, the measurement of exercise capacity is useful for further identifying those patients at particularly high risk and also for establishing safe exercise limits after discharge.[1] Patients with a good exercise capacity despite a reduced ejection fraction have a better long-term outcome than those with exercise impairment (see Chaps. 50 and 83).

Myocardial Ischemia

Because of the potent adverse consequences of recurrent MI after STEMI, it is important to assess a patient's risk for future ischemia and infarction. Given the increasing array of pharmacologic, interventional, and surgical options available to modify the likelihood of developing recurrent episodes of myocardial ischemia, most clinicians find it helpful to identify patients at risk for provocable myocardial ischemia before discharge. A predischarge evaluation for ischemia allows clinicians to select patients who might benefit from catheterization and revascularization following fibrinolysis for STEMI and to assess the adequacy of medical therapy for those patients who are suitable for a more conservative management strategy (see Fig. 55-41).

EXERCISE TESTING. An exercise test also offers the clinician an opportunity to formulate a more precise exercise prescription and is helpful for boosting patients' confidence in their ability to conduct their daily activities after discharge. Patients who are unable to exercise can be evaluated by the use of a pharmacologic stress protocol, such as an infusion of dobutamine or dipyridamole with echocardiography or perfusion imaging (see Fig. 55-41).

Treadmill exercise testing after STEMI has traditionally used a submaximal protocol that requires the patient to exercise until symptoms of angina appear, electrocardiographic evidence of ischemia is seen, or a target workload (≈5 metabolic equivalents) has been reached (see Chap. 50). Symptom-limited exercise tests can be performed safely before discharge in patients with an uncomplicated in-hospital postinfarction course. Variables derived from exercise tests after STEMI that have been evaluated for their ability to predict the occurrence of death or recurrent nonfatal infarction include the development and magnitude of ST-segment depression, development of angina, exercise capacity, and systolic blood pressure response during exercise.[204]

Electrical Instability

After STEMI, patients are at greatest risk for the development of sudden cardiac death caused by malignant ventricular arrhythmias over the course of the first 1 to 2 years.[1,211] Several techniques have been proposed to stratify patients into those who are at increased risk of sudden death following STEMI, including the following: measurement of Q-T dispersion (variability of Q-T intervals between electrocardiographic leads); ambulatory electrocardiographic recordings for detection of ventricular arrhythmias (Holter monitoring); invasive electrophysiologic testing; recording a signal-averaged ECG (a measure of delayed, fragmented conduction in the infarct zone); and measuring heart rate variability (beat to beat variability in R-R intervals) or baroreflex sensitivity (slope of a line relating beat to beat change in sinus rate in response to alteration of blood pressure). However, these have not proved sufficiently useful to recommend their use in routine practice.[204]

Despite the increased risk of arrhythmic events following STEMI in patients who are found to have abnormal results on one or more of the noninvasive tests described earlier, several points should be emphasized. The low positive predictive value (<30%) for the noninvasive screening tests limits their usefulness when viewed in isolation. Although the predictive value of screening tests can be improved by combining several of them together, the therapeutic implications of an increased risk profile for arrhythmic events have not been established. The mortality reductions achievable with the general use of beta blockers, ACE inhibitors, aspirin, and revascularization when appropriate after infarction, coupled with concerns about the efficacy and safety of antiarrhythmic drugs and the cost of implanted defibrillators, leave considerable uncertainty about the therapeutic implications of an abnormal noninvasive test for electrical instability in an asymptomatic patient. Additional data on patient outcomes when clinicians act on the results of an abnormal finding are required before definitive recommendations can be made for asymptomatic patients.[1] The management of patients with sustained, hemodynamically compromising arrhythmias is discussed in Chaps. 37 to 39.

PROPHYLACTIC ANTIARRHYTHMIC THERAPY. Although it has been recognized for decades that antiarrhythmic therapy can control atrial and ventricular arrhythmias effectively in many patients, reviews of clinical trials following STEMI have reported an increased risk of mortality with type I drugs. The most notable postinfarction trial in this area was the Cardiac Arrhythmia Suppression Trial (CAST), which tested whether encainide, flecainide, or moricizine for suppression of ventricular arrhythmias detected on ambulatory electrocardiographic monitoring would reduce the risk of cardiac arrest and death over the long term. Both the first phase of the trial (encainide or flecainide versus placebo) and the second phase of the trial (moricizine versus placebo) were stopped prematurely because of increased mortality in the active treatment groups. The mechanism of the increased risk after STEMI remains a subject of investigation. One hypothesis that has been proposed is an adverse interaction between recurrent ischemia and the presence of an antiarrhythmic drug because the risk of death or cardiac arrest was greater in patients with a non–Q-wave acute MI than with Q-wave MI. Sodium channel blockade by antiarrhythmics may exacerbate electrophysiologic differences between subepicardial and subendocardial zones of myocardium, rendering the latter more susceptible to ischemic injury.

Subsequent to CAST, another postinfarction, prophylactic, antiarrhythmic drug trial was undertaken with oral D-sotalol (Survival With ORal D-sotalol, or SWORD). SWORD also was stopped prematurely after enrollment of only 3121 of a planned 6400 patients because statistical evidence of increased mortality emerged in the active treatment group. The Canadian Amiodarone Myocardial Infarction Trial (CAMIAT) showed that amiodarone reduces the frequency of ventricular premature depolarization in patients with recent MI; this is correlated with a reduction in arrhythmic death or resuscitation from ventricular fibrillation. However, 42% of patients discontinued amiodarone during maintenance therapy in CAMIAT because of intolerable side effects. The European Amiodarone Myocardial Infarction Trial (EMIAT) showed a reduction in arrhythmic death after MI in patients with depressed left ventricular function, but there was no reduction in total mortality or other cardiovascular-related mortality.

The routine use of antiarrhythmic agents (including amiodarone) cannot be recommended. Given the data cited earlier on the protective effects of beta blockers against sudden death and the ability of aspirin to reduce the risk of reinfarction, it is unclear that additional mortality reductions would be achieved by the empirical addition of amiodarone in the patient who is convalescing from a STEMI and is free of symptomatic sustained ventricular arrhythmias.

Several trials that included post-STEMI patients in the study population have shown significant mortality reductions in patients randomized to ICD implantation versus conventional medical therapy (see Chap. 38). However, early implantation of an ICD in the first few weeks after MI has not been shown to be beneficial; at present, there is insufficient evidence to support routine risk stratification to guide ICD placement soon after STEMI.[212] At present, the selection of STEMI patients who are candidates for ICD implantation is based on the algorithm in **Figure 55-42**.

Secondary Prevention of Acute Myocardial Infarction

Patients who survive the initial course of STEMI still have considerable risk of recurrent events rendering imperative efforts to reduce this risk (see Chap. 49).

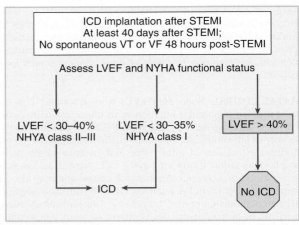

FIGURE 55-42 Algorithm for implantation of an ICD in STEMI patients without ventricular fibrillation (VF) or sustained ventricular tachycardia (VT) more than 48 hours after STEMI. The appropriate management path is based on measurement of the left ventricular ejection fraction (LVEF); measurements obtained 3 days or less after STEMI should be repeated before proceeding with the algorithm. Patients with an LVEF < 30% to 40% at least 40 days post-STEMI are referred for insertion of an ICD if they are in New York Heart Association (NYHA) Class II or III. Patients with a more depressed LVEF < 30% to 35% are referred for ICD implantation even if they are NYHA Class I because of their increased risk of sudden cardiac death. Patients with preserved left ventricular function (LVEF > 40%) do not receive an ICD and are treated with medical therapy post-STEMI. (Modified from Zipes DP, Camm AJ, Borggrefe M, et al: ACC/AHA/ESC 2006 guidelines for management of patients with ventricular arrhythmias and the prevention of sudden cardiac death: A report of the American College of Cardiology/American Heart Association Task Force and the European Society of Cardiology Committee for Practice Guidelines [Writing Committee to Develop Guidelines for Management of Patients with Ventricular Arrhythmias and the Prevention of Sudden Cardiac Death]. Developed in collaboration with the European Rhythm Association and the Heart Rhythm Society. Circulation 114:e385, 2006.)

LIFESTYLE MODIFICATION. Efforts to improve survival and quality of life after MI that relate to lifestyle modification of known risk factors are considered in Chap. 49. Of these, cessation of smoking and control of hypertension are probably most important. Within 2 years of quitting smoking, the risk of a nonfatal MI in former smokers falls to a level similar to that in patients who never smoked. Being hospitalized for STEMI is a powerful motivation for patients to cease cigarette smoking, and this is an ideal time to encourage that clearly beneficial and highly cost-effective lifestyle change. Use of hospital-based smoking cessation programs and referral to cardiac rehabilitation programs have been associated with successful smoking cessation.[213] Smoking cessation intervention should therefore be a routine part of the discharge planning post-STEMI for all smokers. It is also an ideal time to begin to treat hypertension, counsel patients to achieve optimal body weight, and consider various strategies to improve the patient's lipid profile.[1]

TREATING DEPRESSION. Physicians caring for patients following a STEMI need to be sensitive to the prevalence of major depression after infarction (see Chap. 91).[214] This problem is associated independently with a higher risk of death. In addition, lack of an emotionally supportive network in the patient's environment after discharge is associated with an increased risk of recurrent cardiac events.[1] The precise mechanisms relating depression and lack of social support to a worse prognosis after STEMI are not clear, but one possibility is lack of adherence to prescribed treatments, a behavior that has been shown to be associated with increased risk of mortality after infarction. Evidence exists that a comprehensive rehabilitation program using primary health care personnel who counsel patients and make home visits favorably affects the clinical course of patients after infarction and reduces the rate of rehospitalization for recurrent ischemia and infarction.[215] A supportive physician attitude can also have a positive impact on the rate of return to work after STEMI.

MODIFICATION OF LIPID PROFILE. Increased cholesterol level, and most importantly an increased low-density lipoprotein (LDL) cholesterol level, is associated with an increased risk of coronary heart disease and is a modifiable risk factor for recurrent events (see Chaps. 47 and 49). A target LDL cholesterol level lower than 100 mg/dL with an optimal target lower than 70 mg/dL has been recommended for patients with clinically evident coronary heart disease.[216] This recommendation clearly applies to patients with STEMI, and it is therefore important to obtain a lipid profile on admission in all patients admitted with acute infarction. (It should be recalled that cholesterol levels may fall 24 to 48 hours after infarction.) In addition to lowering LDL cholesterol, therapy with statins reduces levels of C-reactive protein, suggesting an anti-inflammatory effect.[217] Surveys of physician practice in the past have revealed a disappointingly low rate of treatment of hypercholesterolemia to recommended targets in patients with proven coronary artery disease, indicating considerable room for improvement in this aspect of secondary prevention.[218]

Recommendations

The dietary prescription after STEMI should be low saturated fat (<7% of total calories) and low cholesterol (<200 mg/day).[219] Patients with an LDL cholesterol level higher than 100 mg/dL should be discharged on statin therapy with the goal of reducing the LDL level to less than 70 mg/dL (see Chaps. 47 and 49). It is also reasonable to prescribe statin therapy to patients recovering from STEMI whose LDL cholesterol level is unknown or is lower than 100 mg/dL.[1] For many patients recovering from an acute MI, a low high-density lipoprotein cholesterol level is their primary lipid abnormality.

ANTIPLATELET AGENTS. On the basis of the compelling data from the Antiplatelet Trialists' Collaboration of a 22% reduction in the risk of recurrent infarction, stroke, or vascular death in high-risk vascular patients receiving prolonged antiplatelet therapy (see Chap. 87) in the absence of a true aspirin allergy, all STEMI patients should receive 75 to 162 mg of aspirin daily indefinitely.[109,216] Additional benefits of long-term aspirin that can accrue in the STEMI patient are an increased likelihood of patency of the infarct artery and smaller infarcts if recurrent MI does take place. Patients with true aspirin allergy can be treated with clopidogrel (75 mg once daily) on the basis of experience from patients with unstable angina/non–ST-segment elevation MI (UA/NSTEMI). Given the results of the CLARITY-TIMI 28[110] and COMMIT[116] trials, as well as experience with clopidogrel in UA/NSTEMI, clopidogrel (75 mg/day) should be added to aspirin in patients discharged after a STEMI.[35] Prasugrel (10 mg/day) may be considered for patients with STEMI who have undergone PCI for STEMI.[113] The optimum duration of treatment with dual antiplatelet therapy needs further study, but benefit has been shown to continue after 30 days and it seems reasonable to continue a thienopyridine for at least 1 year after STEMI and maintain aspirin treatment indefinitely.[220,221] In addition, there is accumulating evidence that more potent antiplatelet therapy than aspirin and clopidogrel is beneficial for the patient treated for an acute coronary syndrome with a drug-eluting stent, at least for a period of 30 days.[222]

INHIBITION OF THE RENIN-ANGIOTENSIN-ALDOSTERONE SYSTEM. The rationale for inhibition of this neurohormonal axis after STEMI was discussed earlier. To prevent late remodeling of the left ventricle and also to decrease the likelihood of recurrent ischemic events, we advocate indefinite therapy with an ACE inhibitor to all patients with clinically evident congestive heart failure, a moderate decrease in global ejection fraction, or a large regional wall-motion abnormality, even in the presence of a normal global ejection fraction. Once the STEMI patient is discharged from the hospital, the evidence based on long-term management of patients with chronic coronary artery disease is the most relevant for long-term decision making. Based on the results of the HOPE and EUROPA trials, we advocate indefinite treatment with an ACE inhibitor for all STEMI patients with an ejection fraction less than 40%, renal dysfunction, or diabetes regardless of ejection fraction, provided no contraindications exist.[216] As discussed earlier, the VALIANT trial results suggest that valsartan

may be used as an alternative to an ACE inhibitor for the long-term management of patients with left ventricular dysfunction after STEMI.

BETA BLOCKERS. Meta-analyses of trials from the prethrombolytic era involving more than 24,000 patients who received beta blockers in the convalescent phase of STEMI have shown a 23% reduction in long-term mortality.[1] When beta blockers are administered early (6 hours) in the acute phase of infarction and continued in the chronic phase of treatment, some of the benefit may result from a reduction in infarct size. In most patients who have beta blockade initiated during the convalescent phase of STEMI, however, reduction in long-term mortality is probably the result of a combination of an antiarrhythmic effect (prevention of sudden death) and prevention of reinfarction.

Given the well-documented benefits of beta blocker therapy, it is disturbing that this form of therapy continues to be underused, especially in high-risk groups such as older adults.[1] Patients with a relative contraindication to beta blockers (moderate heart failure, bradyarrhythmias) should undergo a monitored trial of therapy in the hospital. The dosage should be sufficient to blunt the heart rate response to stress or exercise. Much of the impact of beta blockers in preventing mortality occurs in the first weeks; treatment should commence as soon as possible. Evidence exists that programs providing physician feedback improve adherence to guidelines such as those noted earlier for prescription of beta adrenoceptor blockers after acute MI.[223]

Some controversy exists as to how long patients should be treated. The collective data from five trials providing information on long-term follow-up of beta blockers after infarction have suggested that therapy be continued for at least 2 to 3 years.[1] At that time, if the beta blocker is well tolerated and if there is no reason to discontinue therapy, such therapy probably should be continued in most patients.

Not all patients derive the same benefit from beta blocker therapy. The cost-effectiveness of treatment in medium- or high-risk persons compares favorably with that of many other accepted interventions, such as CABG, angioplasty, and lipid-lowering therapy. In patients with an extremely good prognosis (first acute MI, good ventricular function, no angina, negative stress test result, and no complex ventricular ectopy) among whom a mortality rate of approximately 1%/year can be anticipated, beta blockers would have a smaller impact on survival. However, it is our preference to prescribe beta blockers to such patients for whatever postinfarction benefit is achieved and also to include them as part of the patient's usual regimen should MI recur at an unpredictable time in the future.

NITRATES. Although nitrates are suitable for the management of specific conditions after STEMI, such as recurrent angina or as part of a treatment regimen for congestive heart failure, little evidence indicates that they reduce mortality over the long term when prescribed on a routine basis to all patients with infarction.[1]

ANTICOAGULANTS. After several decades of evaluation, the weight of evidence now suggests that anticoagulants have a favorable effect on late mortality, stroke, and reinfarction in patients hospitalized with STEMI (**Table 55-15**). Given the complexities of combining long-term therapy with warfarin alone with antiplatelet therapy, clinicians must weigh the need for warfarin based on established indications for anticoagulation and the risk of bleeding.[96] An algorithm to guide decision making with respect to warfarin is shown in **Figure 55-43**.

There are at least three hypothetical reasons for anticipating that anticoagulants might be beneficial in the long-term management of patients after STEMI:

1. Because the coronary occlusion responsible for the STEMI is often caused by a thrombus, anticoagulants might be expected to halt progression, slow progression, or prevent the development of new thrombi elsewhere in the coronary arterial tree.
2. Anticoagulants might be expected to diminish the formation of mural thrombi and resultant systemic embolization.
3. Anticoagulants might be expected to reduce the incidence of venous thrombosis and pulmonary embolization.

TABLE 55-15 Aspirin Versus Warfarin Therapy after ST-Elevation Myocardial Infarction (STEMI)

STUDY	STUDY DESIGN	DRUGS USED	ASA	SECOND ARM	THIRD ARM	PATIENTS	ENDPOINTS	Results (%) ASA ALONE	WARFARIN ALONE	ASA + WARFARIN
STEMI-Specific Trials										
WARIS II*	Randomized Open label, N = 3630, FU = 4 yr (mean)	ASA monotherapy vs. warfarin monotherapy vs. warfarin + ASA	160 mg daily	Dosed to target INR 2.8-4.2	Dosed to target INR 2.0-2.5 + ASA 75 mg daily	Age <75 yr Hospitalized for acute MI, % STEMI = 71.8	Death, nonfatal reinfarction, or thromboembolic stroke; Major, nonfatal bleeding (P <0.001)	20; 0.17	16.7 (P = 0.03 vs. ASA); 0.68	15 (P = 0.001 vs. ASA); 0.57
APRICOT II†	Randomized Open label, N = 308, FU = 3 mo	ASA monotherapy vs. warfarin + ASA	If TIMI grade 3, post-48 hr UFH, then 160 mg initially and then 80 mg daily	Dosed to target INR 2-3 if TIMI 3 post-48 hr, UFH + 160 mg initially and then 80 mg daily	N/A	Age ≤76 yr Acute STEMI ≤6 yr prior to thrombolytic Tx, % STEMI = 100	Reocclusion (TIMI ≤ 2) (P <0.02); Total occlusion (TIMI 0-1) (P <0.02); Revascularization (P < 0.01); Reinfarction (P <0.05); Event-free survival rate* (P <0.01); Bleeding (TIMI major and minor (P = NS)	28; 20; 31; 8; 66; 3	N/A	15; 9; 13; 2; 86; 5
Trials Not Specific to STEMI										
ASPECT II‡	Randomized Open label, N = 999, FU = 26 mo	ASA monotherapy vs. warfarin monotherapy vs. warfarin + ASA	80 mg daily	Dosed to target INR 3-4	Dosed to target INR 2-2.5 + ASA 80 mg daily	Acute MI or UA within preceding 8 wk	Death, MI, or stroke (P = 0.02479); Major bleeding; Minor bleeding (P <0.0001); Almost 20% of warfarin and combined group discontinued therapy; 40% in therapeutic range	9; 1; 5	5; 1; 8	5; 2; 15
CHAMP§	Randomized Open label, N = 5059, FU = median 2.7 yr	ASA monotherapy vs. warfarin + ASA	162 mg daily	Dosed to target INR 1.5-2.5 + 81 mg ASA daily	N/A	Acute MI within preceding 14 days prior to enrollment	Death (P = 0.76); Recurrent MI (P = 0.78); Stroke (P = 0.52); Major bleeding (P = 0.001)	17.3; 13.1; 3.5; 0.72**	N/A	17.6; 13.3; 3.1; 1.2**
CARS¶	Randomized Blinded, N = 8803, FU = 33 mo, Median = 14 mo	ASA monotherapy vs. warfarin 1 mg + ASA	160 mg daily (avg INR @ wk 4 = 1.02)	1 mg + 80 mg ASA (avg INR @ wk 4 = 1.05)	N/A	Age 21-85 yr (82% <70 yr) MI 3-21 days (mean, 9.6 days) prior to enrollment	Ischemic stroke (P = 0.0534)	0.6	N/A	1.1

*Hurlen M, Abdelnoor M, Smith P, et al: Warfarin, aspirin, or both after myocardial infarction. N Engl J Med 347:969, 2002.

†Brouwer MA, van den Bergh PJ, Aengevaeren WR, et al: Aspirin plus coumarin versus aspirin alone in the prevention of reocclusion after fibrinolysis for acute myocardial infarction: Results of the Antithrombotics in the Prevention of Reocclusion In Coronary Thrombolysis (APRICOT)-2 Trial. Circulation 106:659, 2002.

‡Van Es RF, Jonker JJ, Verheugt FW, et al: Aspirin and coumadin after acute coronary syndromes (the ASPECT-2 study): A randomised controlled trial. Lancet 360:109, 2002.

§Fiore LD, Ezekowitz MD, Brophy MT, et al: Department of Veterans Affairs Cooperative Studies Program Clinical Trial comparing combined warfarin and aspirin with aspirin alone in survivors of acute myocardial infarction: Primary results of the CHAMP study. Circulation 105:557, 2002.

¶O'Connor CM, Gattis WA, Hellkamp AS, et al: Comparison of two aspirin doses on ischemic stroke in post-myocardial infarction patients in the warfarin (Coumadin) Aspirin Reinfarction Study (CARS). Am J Cardiol 88:541, 2001.

** Reported as number of events per 100 person-years of follow-up.

ASA = acetylsalicylic acid (aspirin); FU = follow-up; INR = international normalized ratio; MI = myocardial infarction; N/A = not applicable; STEMI = ST-segment myocardial infarction ; TIMI = Thrombosis In Myocardial Infarction; Tx = treatment; UA = unstable angina; UFH = unfractionated heparin; vs. = versus.

Modified from Antman EM, Anbe DT, Armstrong PW, et al: ACC/AHA Guidelines for the Management of Patients with ST-Elevation Myocardial Infarction: A report of the American College of Cardiology/American Heart Association Task Force on Practice Guidelines (Committee to Revise the 1999 Guidelines for the Management of Patients with Acute Myocardial Infarction). Circulation 110:e82, 2004.

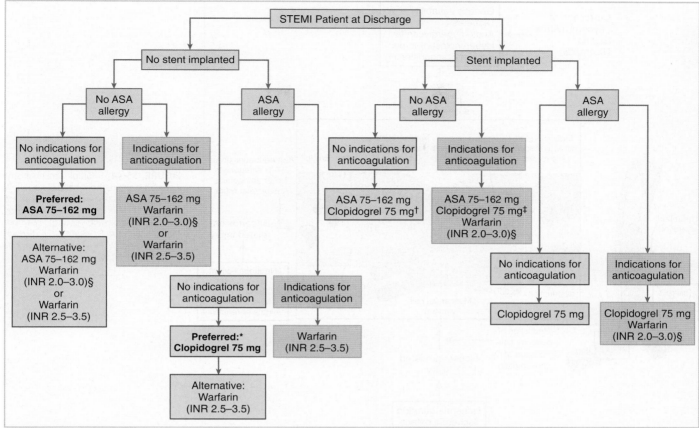

FIGURE 55-43 Algorithm for antithrombotic therapy at hospital discharge after STEMI. *Clopidogrel is preferred over warfarin because of an increased risk of bleeding and low patient compliance in warfarin trials. †For 12 months. ‡Discontinue clopidogrel 1 month after implantation of a bare metal stent or several months after implantation of a drug-eluting stent (3 months after sirolimus and 6 months after paclitaxel) because of the potential increased risk of bleeding with warfarin and two antiplatelet agents. Continue ASA and warfarin long term if warfarin is indicated for other reasons such as atrial fibrillation, LV thrombus, cerebral emboli, or extensive regional wall motion abnormality. §An INR of 2 to 3 is acceptable with tight control, but the lower end of this range (2.0-2.5) is preferable. The combination of antiplatelet therapy and warfarin may be considered in patients younger than 75 years, with low bleeding risk, who can be monitored reliably. ASA = acetylsalicylic acid; INR = international normalized ratio; LV = left ventricular. *(Modified from Antman EM, Anbe DT, Armstrong PW, et al: ACC/AHA guidelines for the management of patients with ST-elevation myocardial infarction: A report of the American College of Cardiology/American Heart Association Task Force on Practice Guidelines [Committee to Revise the 1999 Guidelines for the Management of Patients with Acute Myocardial Infarction]). Circulation 110:e82, 2004.)*

Alternative oral anticoagulants, such as the oral factor Xa inhibitors, that have the advantage of more predictable anticoagulation without stable oral dosing, have undergone initial evaluation in patients with acute coronary syndrome, including STEMI, and are being evaluated in larger trials.[224,225]

CALCIUM CHANNEL ANTAGONISTS. At present, we do not recommend the routine use of calcium antagonists for secondary prevention of infarction. A possible exception is a patient who cannot tolerate a beta blocker because of adverse effects on bronchospastic lung disease but who has well-preserved left ventricular function; such patients may be candidates for a rate-slowing calcium antagonist such as diltiazem or verapamil.

HORMONE THERAPY. The decision to prescribe hormone therapy (see Chap. 81) is often a complex one that involves the desire to suppress postmenopausal symptoms versus the risks of breast and endometrial cancer and vascular events. Despite improvement in lipid profiles, hormone therapy with estrogen plus progestin in postmenopausal women with established coronary heart disease does not prevent recurrent coronary events and is associated with a significantly increased risk of coronary and venous thromboembolic events.[1] At present, we recommend not starting hormone therapy with estrogen plus progestin after STEMI and discontinuing it in postmenopausal women after STEMI.

ANTIOXIDANTS. Dietary supplementation with omega-3 polyunsaturated fatty acids has been associated with a reduction in coronary heart disease death and nonfatal reinfarction in patients within 3 months of a MI (see Chap. 48). Vitamin E (300 mg/day) does not confer any significant clinical benefit, however.[1]

NONSTEROIDAL ANTI-INFLAMMATORY DRUGS. Evidence has emerged that cyclooxygenase-2 (COX-2) selective drugs and NSAIDs that have varying COX-1:COX-2 inhibitory ratios promote a prothrombotic state, and their use is associated with an increased risk of atherothrombotic events.[226,227] Given the increased risk of atherothrombosis related to the index STEMI event, the desire not to interfere with the beneficial pharmacologic actions of low-dose aspirin post-STEMI, and reports of increased mortality and reinfarction when they are used after MI, clinicians should avoid prescribing NSAIDs to patients recovering from STEMI.[35] If NSAIDs must be prescribed for pain relief, the lowest dose required to control symptoms should be administered for the shortest period of time required.[228]

Emerging Therapies

Although there has been a substantial increase in the number of patients with STEMI who receive primary PCI, there remains considerable room for improvement. Although PCI usually restores flow through epicardial arteries, many patients do not achieve adequate nutrient

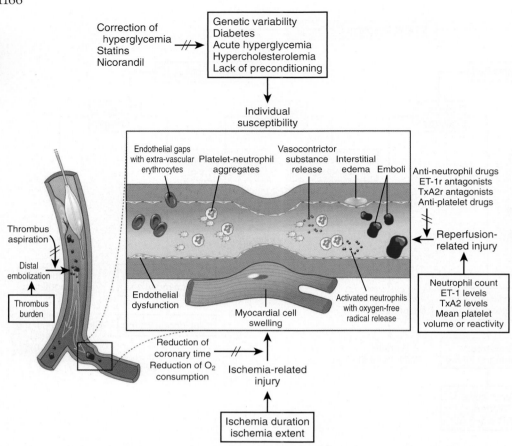

Correction of
hyperglycemia
Statins
Nicorandil

Genetic variability
Diabetes
Acute hyperglycemia
Hypercholesterolemia
Lack of preconditioning

Individual
susceptibility

Endothelial gaps
with extra-vascular
erythrocytes

Platelet-neutrophil
aggregates

Vasocontrictor
substance
release

Interstitial
edema

Emboli

Anti-neutrophil drugs
ET-1r antagonists
TxA2r antagonists
Anti-platelet drugs

Reperfusion-
related injury

Endothelial
dysfunction

Myocardial cell
swelling

Activated neutrophils
with oxygen-free
radical release

Neutrophil count
ET-1 levels
TxA2 levels
Mean platelet
volume or reactivity

Thrombus
aspiration

Distal
embolization

Thrombus
burden

Reduction of
coronary time
Reduction of O₂
consumption

Ischemia-related
injury

Ischemia duration
ischemia extent

FIGURE 55-44 Multiple mechanisms involved in the pathogenesis of no-reflow that might be targeted by appropriate therapy. ET = endothelin; r = receptor; TxA2 = thromboxane A2. *(Modified from Niccoli G, Burzotta F, Galiuto L, Crea F: Myocardial no-reflow in humans. J Am Coll Cardiol 54:281, 2009.)*

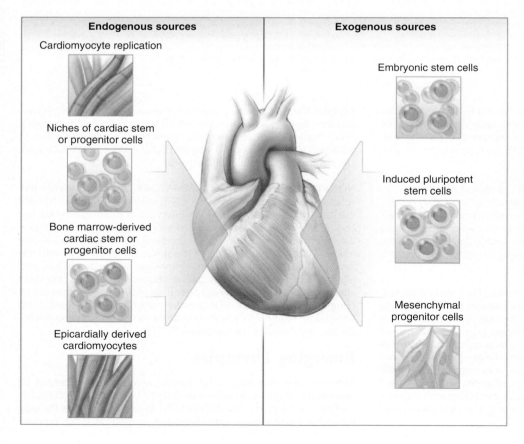

Endogenous sources

Exogenous sources

Cardiomyocyte replication

Embryonic stem cells

Niches of cardiac stem
or progenitor cells

Induced pluripotent
stem cells

Bone marrow-derived
cardiac stem or
progenitor cells

Mesenchymal
progenitor cells

Epicardially derived
cardiomyocytes

FIGURE 55-45 The demonstration that some cardiomyocytes are regenerated after birth highlights the promise and challenges of future regenerative cardiac therapies. Autologous and allogeneic sources of cells that may give rise to cardiomyocytes are under investigation. See Chap. 11. *(From Parmacek MS, Epstein JA: Cardiomyocyte renewal. N Engl J Med 361:86, 2009.)*

flow at the myocardial level in the infarct zone because of a process referred to as no-reflow.[72] The no-reflow phenomenon occurs more frequently when there is a large thrombus burden, high platelet count, increased platelet reactivity, presence of hyperglycemia, and lack of preconditioning. The duration and extent of myocardial ischemia also bear directly on the likelihood of the occurrence of the no-reflow phenomenon. Potential therapies designed to address the pathogenetic mechanisms underlying the no-reflow phenomenon are summarized in **Figure 55-44**.

Even if reperfusion is achieved in a timely fashion and no-reflow is minimized, there is an inevitable loss of a finite number of myocytes in a patient with STEMI. The secondary damage to the left ventricle after STEMI occurs through a process of postinfarction ventricular remodeling. Treatments to minimize ventricular remodeling include the standard approaches to disruption of the RAAS and potential new therapies, such as renin inhibition, reducing the amount of central nervous system generation of aldosterone, enhancing the synthesis of endothelial nitric oxide synthase, modulating beta-adrenergic signaling, and minimizing the processes that lead to cardiac apoptosis.[229]

Finally, in contradistinction to the traditional teaching that the heart is a terminally differentiated organ, it is now clear that myocytes are capable of entering the cell cycle and dividing (see Chaps. 11 and 33).[230] The burgeoning field of cardiac regenerative medicine is now focusing on several approaches using endogenous and exogenous sources of cells that may give rise to myocytes (**Fig. 55-45**).[231]

REFERENCES

General

1. Antman EM, Anbe DT, Armstrong PW, et al: ACC/AHA guidelines for the management of patients with ST-elevation myocardial infarction: A report of the American College of Cardiology/American Heart Association Task Force on Practice Guidelines (Committee to Revise the 1999 Guidelines for the Management of Patients with Acute Myocardial Infarction). Circulation 110:e82, 2004.
2. White HD, Chew DP: Acute myocardial infarction. Lancet 372:570, 2008.
3. Kuch B, von Scheidt W, Ehmann A, et al: Extent of the decrease of 28-day case fatality of hospitalized patients with acute myocardial infarction over 22 years: Epidemiological versus clinical view: The MONICA/KORA Augsburg Infarction Registry. Circ Cardiovasc Qual Outcomes 2:313, 2009.
4. Krumholz HM, Wang Y, Chen J, et al: Reduction in acute myocardial infarction mortality in the United States: Risk-standardized mortality rates from 1995-2006. JAMA 302:767, 2009.
5. Lloyd-Jones D, Adams R, Carnethon M, et al: Heart disease and stroke statistics—2009 update: A report from the American Heart Association Statistics Committee and Stroke Statistics Subcommittee. Circulation 119:e21, 2009.
6. Ting HH, Bradley EH, Wang Y, et al: Factors associated with longer time from symptom onset to hospital presentation for patients with ST-elevation myocardial infarction. Arch Intern Med 168:959, 2008.
7. Floyd KC, Yarzebski J, Spencer FA, et al: A 30-year perspective (1975-2005) into the changing landscape of patients hospitalized with initial acute myocardial infarction: Worcester Heart Attack Study. Circ Cardiovasc Qual Outcomes 2:88, 2009.
8. Antman EM: Time is muscle: translation into practice. J Am Coll Cardiol 52:1216, 2008.
9. Fox KA, Steg PG, Eagle KA, et al: Decline in rates of death and heart failure in acute coronary syndromes, 1999-2006. JAMA 297:1892, 2007.

Emergency Department Management

10. Tricomi AJ, Magid DJ, Rumsfeld JS, et al: Missed opportunities for reperfusion therapy for ST-segment elevation myocardial infarction: Results of the Emergency Department Quality in Myocardial Infarction (EDQMI) study. Am Heart J 155:471, 2008.
11. Jacobs AK, Antman EM, Faxon DP, et al: Development of systems of care for ST-elevation myocardial infarction patients: Executive summary. Circulation 116:217, 2007.
12. Rathore SS, Curtis JP, Chen J, et al: Association of door-to-balloon time and mortality in patients admitted to hospital with ST elevation myocardial infarction: National cohort study. BMJ 338:b1807, 2009.
13. American Heart Associaton, Mission: Lifeline, 2010 (http://www.heart.org/HEARTORG/HealthcareProfessional/Mission-Lifeline-Home-Page_UCM_305495_SubHomePage.jsp).
14. Jones DW, Peterson ED, Bonow RO, et al: Partnering to reduce risks and improve cardiovascular outcomes: American Heart Association initiatives in action for consumers and patients. Circulation 119:340, 2009.
15. Le May MR, So DY, Dionne R, et al: A citywide protocol for primary PCI in ST-segment elevation myocardial infarction. N Engl J Med 358:231, 2008.
16. Peterson ED, Roe MT, Mulgund J, et al: Association between hospital process performance and outcomes among patients with acute coronary syndromes. JAMA 295:1912, 2006.
17. Frendl DM, Palmeri ST, Clapp JR Jr, et al: Overcoming barriers to developing seamless ST-segment elevation myocardial infarction care systems in the United States: Recommendations from a comprehensive Prehospital 12-lead Electrocardiogram Working Group. J Electrocardiol 42:426, 2009.

18. Wang TY, Fonarow GC, Hernandez AF, et al: The dissociation between door-to-balloon time improvement and improvements in other acute myocardial infarction care processes and patient outcomes. Arch Intern Med 169:1411, 2009.
19. Mensah GA, Hand MM, Antman EM, et al: Development of systems of care for ST-elevation myocardial infarction patients: the patient and public perspective. Circulation 116:e33, 2007.
20. Moser DK, Kimble LP, Alberts MJ, et al: Reducing delay in seeking treatment by patients with acute coronary syndrome and stroke: A scientific statement from the American Heart Association Council on cardiovascular nursing and stroke council. Circulation 114:168, 2006.
21. Ting HH, Bradley EH, Wang Y, et al: Delay in presentation and reperfusion therapy in ST-elevation myocardial infarction. Am J Med 121:316, 2008.
22. National Heart Lung and Blood Institute: Act in Time to Heart Attack Signs (http://www.nhlbi.nih.gov/actintime).
23. Rokos IC, French WJ, Koenig WJ, et al: Integration of pre-hospital electrocardiograms and ST-elevation myocardial infarction receiving center (SRC) networks: Impact on door-to-balloon times across 10 independent regions. JACC Cardiovasc Interv 2:339, 2009.
24. Granger CB: Accelerating ST-segment elevation myocardial infarction care: Emergency medical services take center stage. JACC Cardiovasc Interv 2:347, 2009.
25. Sivagangabalan G, Ong AT, Narayan A, et al: Effect of prehospital triage on revascularization times, left ventricular function, and survival in patients with ST-elevation myocardial infarction. Am J Cardiol 103:907, 2009.
26. Jacobs AK, Antman EM, Ellrodt G, et al: Recommendation to develop strategies to increase the number of ST-segment-elevation myocardial infarction patients with timely access to primary percutaneous coronary intervention. Circulation 113:2152, 2006.
27. Millin MG, Brooks SC, Travers A, et al: Emergency medical services management of ST-elevation myocardial infarction. Prehosp Emerg Care 12:395, 2008.
28. Wiviott SD, Morrow DA, Frederick PD, et al: Performance of the thrombolysis in myocardial infarction risk index in the National Registry of Myocardial Infarction-3 and -4: A simple index that predicts mortality in ST-segment elevation myocardial infarction. J Am Coll Cardiol 44:783, 2004.
29. Danchin N, Coste P, Ferrieres J, et al: Comparison of thrombolysis followed by broad use of percutaneous coronary intervention with primary percutaneous coronary intervention for ST-segment-elevation acute myocardial infarction: Data from the French registry on acute ST-elevation myocardial infarction (FAST-MI). Circulation 118:268, 2008.
30. Bjorklund E, Stenestrand U, Lindback J, et al: Pre-hospital thrombolysis delivered by paramedics is associated with reduced time delay and mortality in ambulance-transported real-life patients with ST-elevation myocardial infarction. Eur Heart J 27:1146, 2006.
31. Zeymer U, Arntz HR, Dirks B, et al: Reperfusion rate and inhospital mortality of patients with ST-segment elevation myocardial infarction diagnosed already in the prehospital phase: Results of the German Prehospital Myocardial Infarction Registry (PREMIR). Resuscitation 80:402, 2009.
32. Morrison LJ, Brooks S, Sawadsky B, et al: Prehospital 12-lead electrocardiography impact on acute myocardial infarction treatment times and mortality: A systematic review. Acad Emerg Med 13:84, 2006.
33. Goldstein P, Lapostolle F, Steg G, et al: Lowering mortality in ST-elevation myocardial infarction and non-ST-elevation myocardial infarction: Key prehospital and emergency room treatment strategies. Eur J Emerg Med 16:244, 2009.
34. Atzema CL, Austin PC, Tu JV, Schull MJ: Emergency department triage of acute myocardial infarction patients and the effect on outcomes. Ann Emerg Med 53:736, 2009.
35. Antman EM, Hand M, Armstrong PW, et al: 2007 focused update of the ACC/AHA 2004 guidelines for the management of patients with ST-elevation myocardial infarction: A report of the American College of Cardiology/American Heart Association Task Force on Practice Guidelines: Developed in collaboration With the Canadian Cardiovascular Society: Endorsed by the American Academy of Family Physicians: 2007 Writing Group to Review New Evidence and Update the ACC/AHA 2004 Guidelines for the Management of Patients With ST-Elevation Myocardial Infarction, Writing on Behalf of the 2004 Writing Committee. Circulation 117:296, 2008.
36. Bradley EH, Herrin J, Wang Y, et al: Strategies for reducing the door-to-balloon time in acute myocardial infarction. N Engl J Med 355:2308, 2006.
37. Wang OJ, Wang Y, Lichtman JH, et al: "America's Best Hospitals" in the treatment of acute myocardial infarction. Arch Intern Med 167:1345, 2007.
38. Van de Werf F, Bax J, Betriu A, et al: Management of acute myocardial infarction in patients presenting with persistent ST-segment elevation: The Task Force on the Management of ST-Segment Elevation Acute Myocardial Infarction of the European Society of Cardiology. Eur Heart J 29:2909, 2008.
39. Cannon CP: Updated Strategies and Therapies for Reducing Ischemic and Vascular Events (STRIVE) unstable angina/non-ST elevation myocardial infarction critical pathway toolkit. Crit Pathw Cardiol 7:43, 2008.
40. Ross MA, Amsterdam E, Peacock WF, et al: Chest pain center accreditation is associated with better performance of centers for Medicare and Medicaid services core measures for acute myocardial infarction. Am J Cardiol 102:120, 2008.
41. Sweeny JM, Gorog DA, Fuster V: Antiplatelet drug 'resistance'. Part 1: Mechanisms and clinical measurements. Nat Rev Cardiol 6:273, 2009.
42. Hamon M, Agostini D, Le Page O, Riddell JW: Prognostic impact of right ventricular involvement in patients with acute myocardial infarction: meta-analysis. Crit Care Med 36:2023, 2008.
43. Chen ZM, Pan HC, Chen YP, et al: Early intravenous then oral metoprolol in 45,852 patients with acute myocardial infarction: randomised placebo-controlled trial. Lancet 366:1622, 2005.
44. Sabatine MS: Something old, something new: Beta blockers and clopidogrel in acute myocardial infarction. Lancet 366:1587, 2005.
45. Goldberg RJ, Spencer FA, Gore JM, et al: Thirty-year trends (1975 to 2005) in the magnitude of, management of, and hospital death rates associated with cardiogenic shock in patients with acute myocardial infarction: a population-based perspective. Circulation 119:1211, 2009.
46. Roik M, Opolski G: Long-term outcome among patients with ST-segment elevation myocardial infarction complicated by shock. J Am Coll Cardiol 52:315, 2008.

Reperfusion Therapy

47. Gersh BJ, Stone GW, White HD, Holmes DR Jr: Pharmacological facilitation of primary percutaneous coronary intervention for acute myocardial infarction: Is the slope of the curve the shape of the future? JAMA 293:979, 2005.

48. Alter DA, Ko DT, Newman A, Tu JV: Factors explaining the under-use of reperfusion therapy among ideal patients with ST-segment elevation myocardial infarction. Eur Heart J 27:1539, 2006.

49. Gross ER, Gross GJ: Ischemic preconditioning and myocardial infarction: An update and perspective. Drug Discov Today Dis Mech 4:165, 2007.

50. De Luca G, Suryapranata H, Ottervanger JP, Antman EM: Time delay to treatment and mortality in primary angioplasty for acute myocardial infarction: Every minute of delay counts. Circulation 109:1223, 2004.

51. Fibrinolytic Therapy Trialists' (FTT) Collaborative Group: Indications for fibrinolytic therapy in suspected acute myocardial infarction: Collaborative overview of early mortality and major morbidity results from all randomised trials of more than 1000 patients. Lancet 343:311, 1994.

52. Park HJ, Chang K, Park CS, et al: Coronary collaterals: The role of MCP-1 during the early phase of acute myocardial infarction. Int J Cardiol 130:409, 2008.

53. Depre C, Vatner SF: Cardioprotection in stunned and hibernating myocardium. Heart Fail Rev 12:307, 2007.

54. Wu KC: Fighting the "fire" of myocardial reperfusion injury: How to define success? J Am Coll Cardiol 53:730, 2009.

55. Piper HM, Garcia-Dorado D: Cardiac protection takes off. Cardiovasc Res 83:163, 2009.

56. Majidi M, Kosinski AS, Al-Khatib SM, et al: Reperfusion ventricular arrhythmia 'bursts' in TIMI 3 flow restoration with primary angioplasty for anterior ST-elevation myocardial infarction: A more precise definition of reperfusion arrhythmias. Europace 10:988, 2008.

57. Garcia-Dorado D, Ruiz-Meana M, Piper HM: Lethal reperfusion injury in acute myocardial infarction: facts and unresolved issues. Cardiovasc Res 83:165, 2009.

58. Cannon RO 3rd: Mechanisms, management and future directions for reperfusion injury after acute myocardial infarction. Nat Clin Pract Cardiovasc Med 2:88, 2005.

59. Kloner RA, Forman MB, Gibbons RJ, et al: Impact of time to therapy and reperfusion modality on the efficacy of adenosine in acute myocardial infarction: The AMISTAD-2 trial. Eur Heart J 27:2400, 2006.

60. Laskey WK, Yoon S, Calzada N, Ricciardi MJ: Concordant improvements in coronary flow reserve and ST-segment resolution during percutaneous coronary intervention for acute myocardial infarction: A benefit of postconditioning. Catheter Cardiovasc Interv 72:212, 2008.

61. Granfeldt A, Lefer DJ, Vinten-Johansen J: Protective ischaemia in patients: Preconditioning and postconditioning. Cardiovasc Res 83:234, 2009.

62. Thibault H, Piot C, Staat P, et al: Long-term benefit of postconditioning. Circulation 117:1037, 2008.

63. Kawasaki T, Akakabe Y, Yamano M, et al: Vagal enhancement as evidence of residual ischemia after inferior myocardial infarction. Pacing Clin Electrophysiol 32:52, 2009.

64. Takemura G, Nakagawa M, Kanamori H, et al: Benefits of reperfusion beyond infarct size limitation. Cardiovasc Res 83:269, 2009.

65. Kelly RF, Sluiter W, McFalls EO: Hibernating myocardium: Is the program to survive a pathway to failure? Circ Res 102:3, 2008.

66. Van de Werf FJ, Topol EJ, Sobel BE: The impact of fibrinolytic therapy for ST-segment-elevation acute myocardial infarction. J Thromb Haemost 7:14, 2009.

67. Kiernan TJ, Gersh BJ: Thrombolysis in acute myocardial infarction: Current status. Med Clin North Am. 91:617, 2007.

68. Kelly RV, Crouch E, Krumnacher H, et al: Safety of adjunctive intracoronary thrombolytic therapy during complex percutaneous coronary intervention: Initial experience with intracoronary tenecteplase. Catheter Cardiovasc Interv. 66:327, 2005.

69. TIMI Study Group: The Thrombolysis in Myocardial Infarction (TIMI) trial. Phase I findings. N Engl J Med 312:932, 1985.

70. Gibson CM, Murphy S, Menown IB, et al: Determinants of coronary blood flow after thrombolytic administration. TIMI Study Group. Thrombolysis in Myocardial Infarction. J Am Coll Cardiol 34:1403, 1999.

71. Appelbaum E, Kirtane AJ, Clark A, et al: Association of TIMI myocardial perfusion grade and ST-segment resolution with cardiovascular magnetic resonance measures of microvascular obstruction and infarct size following ST-segment elevation myocardial infarction. J Thromb Thrombolysis 27:123, 2009.

72. Niccoli G, Burzotta F, Galiuto L, Crea F: Myocardial no-reflow in humans. J Am Coll Cardiol 54:281, 2009.

73. Kirtane AJ, Vafai JJ, Murphy SA, et al: Angiographically evident thrombus following fibrinolytic therapy is associated with impaired myocardial perfusion in STEMI: A CLARITY-TIMI 28 substudy. Eur Heart J 27:2040, 2006.

74. Rakowski T, Dziewierz A, Siudak Z, et al: ST-segment resolution assessed immediately after primary percutaneous coronary intervention correlates with infarct size and left ventricular function in cardiac magnetic resonance at 1-year follow-up. J Electrocardiol 42:152, 2009.

75. Rekik S, Mnif S, Sahnoun M, et al: Total absence of ST-segment resolution after failed thrombolysis is correlated with unfavorable short- and long-term outcomes despite successful rescue angioplasty. J Electrocardiol 42:73, 2009.

76. Bjorklund E, Jernberg T, Johanson P, et al: Admission N-terminal pro-brain natriuretic peptide and its interaction with admission troponin T and ST-segment resolution for early risk stratification in ST elevation myocardial infarction. Heart 92:735, 2006.

77. Terkelsen CJ, Norgaard BL, Lassen JF, et al: Potential significance of spontaneous and interventional ST-changes in patients transferred for primary percutaneous coronary intervention: Observations from the ST-MONitoring in Acute Myocardial Infarction study (the MONAMI study). Eur Heart J 27:267, 2006.

78. Gershlick AH: Managing myocardial infarction in the elderly: Time to bury inappropriate concerns instead. Eur Heart J 30:887, 2009.

79. Schiele F, Meneveau N, Seronde MF, et al: Changes in management of elderly patients with myocardial infarction. Eur Heart J 30:987, 2009.

80. Acikel S, Akdemir R, Cagirci G, et al: The treatment of clopidogrel resistance: Triple antiplatelet therapy and future directions. Int J Cardiol 144:79, 2009.

81. Ross AM, Gibbons RJ, Stone GW, et al: A randomized, double-blinded, placebo-controlled multicenter trial of adenosine as an adjunct to reperfusion in the treatment of acute myocardial infarction (AMISTAD-II). J Am Coll Cardiol 45:1775, 2005.

82. Assessment of the Safety and Efficacy of a New Treatment Strategy with Percutaneous Coronary Intervention (ASSENT-4 PCI) investigators: Primary versus tenecteplase-facilitated percutaneous coronary intervention in patients with ST-segment elevation acute myocardial infarction (ASSENT-4 PCI): Randomised trial. Lancet 367:569, 2006.

83. Carter NJ, McCormack PL, Plosker GL: Enoxaparin: A review of its use in ST-segment elevation myocardial infarction. Drugs 68:691, 2008.

84. Fernandez-Aviles F, Alonso JJ, Castro-Beiras A, et al: Routine invasive strategy within 24 hours of thrombolysis versus ischaemia-guided conservative approach for acute myocardial infarction with ST-segment elevation (GRACIA-1): a randomised controlled trial. Lancet 364:1045, 2004.

85. Cantor WJ, Fitchett D, Borgundvaag B, et al: Routine early angioplasty after fibrinolysis for acute myocardial infarction. N Engl J Med 360:2705, 2009.

86. Huynh T, Perron S, O'Loughlin J, et al: Comparison of primary percutaneous coronary intervention and fibrinolytic therapy in ST-segment-elevation myocardial infarction: bayesian hierarchical meta-analyses of randomized controlled trials and observational studies. Circulation 119:3101, 2009.

87. Stone GW: Angioplasty strategies in ST-segment-elevation myocardial infarction: part I: primary percutaneous coronary intervention. Circulation 118:538, 2008.

88. Srinivas VS, Hailpern SM, Koss E, et al: Effect of physician volume on the relationship between hospital volume and mortality during primary angioplasty. J Am Coll Cardiol 53:574, 2009.

89. Hochman JS, Sleeper LA, Webb JG, et al: Early revascularization and long-term survival in cardiogenic shock complicating acute myocardial infarction. JAMA 295:2511, 2006.

90. Grzybowski M, Clements EA, Parsons L, et al: Mortality benefit of immediate revascularization of acute ST-segment elevation myocardial infarction in patients with contraindications to thrombolytic therapy: A propensity analysis. JAMA 290:1891, 2003.

91. Pinto DS, Kirtane AJ, Nallamothu BK, et al: Hospital delays in reperfusion for ST-elevation myocardial infarction: Implications when selecting a reperfusion strategy. Circulation 114:2019, 2006.

92. Chakrabarti A, Krumholz HM, Wang Y, et al: Time to reperfusion in patients undergoing interhospital transfer for primary percutaneous coronary intervention in the U.S: An analysis of 2005 and 2006 data from the National Cardiovascular Data Registry. J Am Coll Cardiol 51:2442, 2008.

93. Busk M, Maeng M, Rasmussen K, et al: The Danish multicentre randomized study of fibrinolytic therapy vs. primary angioplasty in acute myocardial infarction (the DANAMI-2 trial): Outcome after 3 years follow-up. Eur Heart J 29:1259, 2008.

94. Morrow DA: Heparin and low-molecular-weight heparin. In Manson JE, Buring JE, Ridker PM, Gaziano JM (eds): Clinical Trials in Heart Disease: A Companion to Braunwald's Heart Disease. 2nd ed. Philadelphia, Elsevier Saunders, 2004, pp 45-65.

95. Crespo EM, Oliveira GB, Honeycutt EF, et al: Evaluation and management of thrombocytopenia and suspected heparin-induced thrombocytopenia in hospitalized patients: The Complications After Thrombocytopenia Caused by Heparin (CATCH) registry. Am Heart J 157:651, 2009.

96. Holmes DR Jr, Kereiakes DJ, Kleiman NS, et al: Combining antiplatelet and anticoagulant therapies. J Am Coll Cardiol 54:95, 2009.

97. Cheng S, Morrow DA, Sloan S, et al: Predictors of initial nontherapeutic anticoagulation with unfractionated heparin in ST-segment elevation myocardial infarction. Circulation 119:1195, 2009.

98. Bittl JA, White HD, Antman EM: Direct thrombin inhibitors. In Manson JE, Buring JE, Ridker PM, Gaziano JM (eds): Clinical Trials in Heart Disease: A Companion to Braunwald's Heart Disease. 2d ed. Philadelphia, Elsevier Saunders; 2004, pp 83-96.

99. Stone GW, Witzenbichler B, Guagliumi G, et al: Bivalirudin during primary PCI in acute myocardial infarction. N Engl J Med 358:2218, 2008.

100. Morrow DA: Antithrombotic therapy to support primary PCI. N Engl J Med 358:2280, 2008.

101. Singh S, Bahekar A, Molnar J, et al: Adjunctive low molecular weight heparin during fibrinolytic therapy in acute ST-segment elevation myocardial infarction: A meta-analysis of randomized control trials. Clin Cardiol 32:358, 2009.

102. Yusuf S, Mehta SR, Xie C, et al: Effects of reviparin, a low-molecular-weight heparin, on mortality, reinfarction, and strokes in patients with acute myocardial infarction presenting with ST-segment elevation. JAMA 293:427, 2005.

103. Assessment of the Safety and Efficacy of a New Thrombolytic Regimen (ASSENT)-3 Investigators: Efficacy and safety of tenecteplase in combination with enoxaparin, abciximab, or unfractionated heparin: the ASSENT-3 randomised trial in acute myocardial infarction. Lancet 358:605, 2001.

104. Antman EM, Morrow DA, McCabe CH, et al: Enoxaparin versus unfractionated heparin with fibrinolysis for ST-elevation myocardial infarction. N Engl J Med 354:1477, 2006.

105. Yusuf S, Mehta SR, Chrolavicius S, et al: Effects of fondaparinux on mortality and reinfarction in patients with acute ST-segment elevation myocardial infarction: The OASIS-6 randomized trial. JAMA 295:1519, 2009.

106. Eikelboom JW, Weitz JI: Anticoagulation for ST-segment elevation myocardial infarction. Circulation 119:1186, 2009.

107. Oldgren J, Wallentin L, Afzal R, et al: Effects of fondaparinux in patients with ST-segment elevation acute myocardial infarction not receiving reperfusion treatment. Eur Heart J 29:315, 2008.

108. Beygui F, Collet JP, Nagaswami C, et al: Images in cardiovascular medicine. Architecture of intracoronary thrombi in ST-elevation acute myocardial infarction: Time makes the difference. Circulation 113:e21, 2006.

109. Antithrombotic Trialists' Collaboration: Collaborative meta-analysis of randomised trials of antiplatelet therapy for prevention of death, myocardial infarction, and stroke in high risk patients. BMJ 324:71, 2002.

110. Sabatine MS, Cannon CP, Gibson CM, et al: Addition of clopidogrel to aspirin and fibrinolytic therapy for myocardial infarction with ST-segment elevation. N Engl J Med 352:1179, 2005.

111. Scirica BM, Sabatine MS, Morrow DA, et al: The role of clopidogrel in early and sustained arterial patency after fibrinolysis for ST-segment elevation myocardial infarction: The ECG CLARITY-TIMI 28 Study. J Am Coll Cardiol 48:37, 2006.

112. Sabatine MS, Cannon CP, Gibson CM, et al: Effect of clopidogrel pretreatment before percutaneous coronary intervention in patients with ST-elevation myocardial infarction treated with fibrinolytics: The PCI-CLARITY study. JAMA 294:1224, 2005.

Hospital Management

113. Wiviott SD, Braunwald E, McCabe CH, et al: Prasugrel versus clopidogrel in patients with acute coronary syndromes. N Engl J Med 357:2001, 2007.

114. Montalescot G, Wiviott SD, Braunwald E, et al: Prasugrel compared with clopidogrel in patients undergoing percutaneous coronary intervention for ST-elevation myocardial infarction (TRITON-TIMI 38): Double-blind, randomised controlled trial. Lancet 373:723, 2009.

114a. Wallentin L, Becker RC, Budaj A, et al: Ticagrelor versus clopidogrel in patients with acute coronary syndromes. N Engl J Med 361:1045, 2009.

115. Peters RJ, Mehta SR, Fox KA, et al: Effects of aspirin dose when used alone or in combination with clopidogrel in patients with acute coronary syndromes: Observations from the Clopidogrel in Unstable angina to prevent Recurrent Events (CURE) study. Circulation 108:1682, 2003.

116. Chen ZM, Jiang LX, Chen YP, et al: Addition of clopidogrel to aspirin in 45,852 patients with acute myocardial infarction: Randomised placebo-controlled trial. Lancet 366:1607, 2005.

117. King SB 3rd, Smith SC Jr, Hirshfeld JW Jr, et al: 2007 focused update of the ACC/AHA/SCAI 2005 guideline update for percutaneous coronary intervention: A report of the American College of Cardiology/American Heart Association Task Force on Practice Guidelines: 2007 Writing Group to Review New Evidence and Update the ACC/AHA/SCAI 2005 Guideline Update for Percutaneous Coronary Intervention, Writing on Behalf of the 2005 Writing Committee. Circulation 117:261, 2008.

118. Anderson JL, Adams CD, Antman EM, et al: ACC/AHA 2007 guidelines for the management of patients with unstable angina/non ST-elevation myocardial infarction: A report of the American College of Cardiology/American Heart Association Task Force on Practice Guidelines (Writing Committee to Revise the 2002 Guidelines for the Management of Patients With Unstable Angina/Non ST-Elevation Myocardial Infarction): Developed in collaboration with the American College of Emergency Physicians, the Society for Cardiovascular Angiography and Interventions, and the Society of Thoracic Surgeons: Endorsed by the American Association of Cardiovascular and Pulmonary Rehabilitation and the Society for Academic Emergency Medicine. Circulation 116:e148, 2007.

119. Berger AK, Duval S, Jacobs DR Jr, et al: Relation of length of hospital stay in acute myocardial infarction to postdischarge mortality. Am J Cardiol 101:428, 2008.

120. Bates ER: Role of intravenous beta-blockers in the treatment of ST-elevation myocardial infarction: Of mice (dogs, pigs) and men. Circulation 115:2904, 2007.

121. Freemantle N, Cleland J, Young P, et al: Beta blockade after myocardial infarction: Systematic review and meta regression analysis. BMJ 318:1730, 1999.

122. The TIMI Study Group: Comparison of invasive and conservative strategies after treatment with intravenous tissue plasminogen activator in acute myocardial infarction. Results of the thrombolysis in myocardial infarction (TIMI) phase II trial. N Engl J Med 320:618, 1989.

123. Piccini JP, Hranitzky PM, Kilaru R, et al: Relation of mortality to failure to prescribe beta blockers acutely in patients with sustained ventricular tachycardia and ventricular fibrillation following acute myocardial infarction (from the VALsartan In Acute myocardial iNfarcTion trial [VALIANT] Registry). Am J Cardiol 102:1427, 2008.

124. Fonarow GC, Lukas MA, Robertson M, et al: Effects of carvedilol early after myocardial infarction: Analysis of the first 30 days in Carvedilol Post-Infarct Survival Control in Left Ventricular Dysfunction (CAPRICORN). Am Heart J 154:637, 2007.

125. Rutherford JD, Pfeffer MA, Moye LA, et al: Effects of captopril on ischemic events after myocardial infarction. Results of the Survival and Ventricular Enlargement trial. SAVE Investigators. Circulation 90:1731, 1994.

126. Schocken DD, Benjamin EJ, Fonarow GC, et al: Prevention of heart failure: A scientific statement from the American Heart Association Councils on Epidemiology and Prevention, Clinical Cardiology, Cardiovascular Nursing, and High Blood Pressure Research; Quality of Care and Outcomes Research Interdisciplinary Working Group; and Functional Genomics and Translational Biology Interdisciplinary Working Group. Circulation 117:2544, 2008.

127. Pfeffer MA, McMurray JJ, Velazquez EJ, et al: Valsartan, captopril, or both in myocardial infarction complicated by heart failure, left ventricular dysfunction, or both. N Engl J Med 349:1893, 2003.

128. Pitt B, Remme W, Zannad F, et al: Eplerenone, a selective aldosterone blocker, in patients with left ventricular dysfunction after myocardial infarction. N Engl J Med 348:1309, 2003.

129. Pedrazzini G, Santoro E, Latini R, et al: Causes of death in patients with acute myocardial infarction treated with angiotensin-converting enzyme inhibitors: Findings from the Gruppo Italiano per lo Studio della Sopravvivenza nell'Infarto (GISSI)-3 trial. Am Heart J 155:388, 2008.

130. Tokmakova M, Solomon SD: Inhibiting the renin-angiotensin system in myocardial infarction and heart failure: lessons from SAVE, VALIANT and CHARM, and other clinical trials. Curr Opin Cardiol 21:268, 2006.

131. Phillips CO, Kashani A, Ko DK, et al: Adverse effects of combination angiotensin II receptor blockers plus angiotensin-converting enzyme inhibitors for left ventricular dysfunction: A quantitative review of data from randomized clinical trials. Arch Intern Med 167:1930, 2007.

132. Gornik H, O'Gara PT: Adjunctive medical therapy. In Manson JE, Buring JE, Ridker PM, Gaziano JM (eds): Clinical Trials in Heart Disease: A Companion to Braunwald's Heart Disease. Philadelphia, Elsevier Saunders, 2004, pp 109-128.

133. MAGIC Investigators: Early administration of intravenous magnesium to high-risk patients with acute myocardial infarction in the Magnesium in Coronaries (MAGIC) Trial: A randomised controlled trial. Lancet 360:1189, 2002.

134. Moghissi ES, Korytkowski MT, DiNardo M, et al: American Association of Clinical Endocrinologists and American Diabetes Association consensus statement on inpatient glycemic control. Endocr Pract 15:353, 2009.

135. Mehta SR, Yusuf S, Diaz R, et al: Effect of glucose-insulin-potassium infusion on mortality in patients with acute ST-segment elevation myocardial infarction: The CREATE-ECLA randomized controlled trial. JAMA 293:437, 2005.

136. Granger CB, Mahaffey KW, Weaver WD, et al: Pexelizumab, an anti-C5 complement antibody, as adjunctive therapy to primary percutaneous coronary intervention in acute myocardial infarction: The COMPlement inhibition in Myocardial infarction treated with Angioplasty (COMMA) trial. Circulation 108:1184, 2003.

137. Mahaffey KW, Granger CB, Nicolau JC, et al: Effect of pexelizumab, an anti-C5 complement antibody, as adjunctive therapy to fibrinolysis in acute myocardial infarction: The COMPlement inhibition in myocardial infarction treated with thromboLYtics (COMPLY) trial. Circulation 108:1176, 2003.

138. Armstrong PW, Granger CB, Adams PX, et al: Pexelizumab for acute ST-elevation myocardial infarction in patients undergoing primary percutaneous coronary intervention: A randomized controlled trial. JAMA 297:43, 2007.

Hemodynamic Disturbances

139. Chatterjee K: The Swan-Ganz catheters: Past, present, and future. A viewpoint. Circulation 119:147, 2009.

140. Stewart RM, Park PK, Hunt JP, et al: Less is more: Improved outcomes in surgical patients with conservative fluid administration and central venous catheter monitoring. J Am Coll Surg. 208:725, 2009.

141. Finfer S, Delaney A: Pulmonary artery catheters. BMJ 333:930, 2006.

142. Timsit JF, Schwebel C, Bouadma L, et al: Chlorhexidine-impregnated sponges and less frequent dressing changes for prevention of catheter-related infections in critically ill adults: A randomized controlled trial. JAMA 301:1231, 2009.

143. Funk DJ, Moretti EW, Gan TJ: Minimally invasive cardiac output monitoring in the perioperative setting. Anesth Analg 108:887, 2009.

144. Frisch DR, Giedrimas E, Mohanavelu S, et al: Predicting irreversible left ventricular dysfunction after acute myocardial infarction. Am J Cardiol 103:1206, 2009.

145. Reynolds HR, Hochman JS: Cardiogenic shock: Current concepts and improving outcomes. Circulation 117:686, 2008.

146. Harinstein ME, Flaherty JD, Fonarow GC, Gheorghiade M: Directions for research in the post-myocardial infarction patient with left ventricular dysfunction. Am J Cardiol 102:57G, 2008.

147. Lewis EF, Velazquez EJ, Solomon SD, et al: Predictors of the first heart failure hospitalization in patients who are stable survivors of myocardial infarction complicated by pulmonary congestion and/or left ventricular dysfunction: A VALIANT study. Eur Heart J 29:748, 2008.

148. Flaherty JD, Udelson JE, Gheorghiade M, et al: Assessment and key targets for therapy in the post-myocardial infarction patient with left ventricular dysfunction. Am J Cardiol 102:5G, 2008.

149. Ishii H, Amano T, Matsubara T, Murohara T: Pharmacological intervention for prevention of left ventricular remodeling and improving prognosis in myocardial infarction. Circulation 118:2710, 2008.

150. Overgaard CB, Dzavik V: Inotropes and vasopressors: Review of physiology and clinical use in cardiovascular disease. Circulation 118:1047, 2008.

150a. De Backer D, Biston P, Devriendt J, et al: Comparison of dopamine and norepinephrine in the treatment of shock. N Engl J Med 362:779, 2010.

151. Babaev A, Frederick PD, Pasta DJ, et al: Trends in management and outcomes of patients with acute myocardial infarction complicated by cardiogenic shock. JAMA 294:448, 2005.

152. Hochman JS: Cardiogenic shock complicating acute myocardial infarction: Expanding the paradigm. Circulation 107:2998, 2003.

153. Mebazaa A, Nieminen MS, Packer M, et al: Levosimendan vs dobutamine for patients with acute decompensated heart failure: The SURVIVE Randomized Trial. JAMA 297:1883, 2007.

154. Thiele H, Smalling RW, Schuler GC: Percutaneous left ventricular assist devices in acute myocardial infarction complicated by cardiogenic shock. Eur Heart J 28:2057, 2007.

155. Al-Husami W, Yturralde F, Mohanty G, et al: Single-center experience with the TandemHeart percutaneous ventricular assist device to support patients undergoing high-risk percutaneous coronary intervention. J Invasive Cardiol 20:319, 2008.

156. Seyfarth M, Sibbing D, Bauer I, et al: A randomized clinical trial to evaluate the safety and efficacy of a percutaneous left ventricular assist device versus intra-aortic balloon pumping for treatment of cardiogenic shock caused by myocardial infarction. J Am Coll Cardiol 52:1584, 2008.

157. Lim HS, Farouque O, Andrianopoulos N, et al: Survival of elderly patients undergoing percutaneous coronary intervention for acute myocardial infarction complicated by cardiogenic shock. JACC Cardiovasc Interv 2:146, 2009.

158. Pfisterer M: Right ventricular involvement in myocardial infarction and cardiogenic shock. Lancet 362:392, 2003.

159. Zimetbaum PJ, Josephson ME: Use of the electrocardiogram in acute myocardial infarction. N Engl J Med 348:933, 2003.

160. Wellens HJ: The value of the right precordial leads of the electrocardiogram. N Engl J Med 340:381, 1999.

161. Anavekar NS, Skali H, Bourgoun M, et al: Usefulness of right ventricular fractional area change to predict death, heart failure, and stroke following myocardial infarction (from the VALIANT ECHO Study). Am J Cardiol 101:607, 2008.

162. Larose E, Ganz P, Reynolds HG, et al: Right ventricular dysfunction assessed by cardiovascular magnetic resonance imaging predicts poor prognosis late after myocardial infarction. J Am Coll Cardiol 49:855, 2007.

163. Figueras J, Alcalde O, Barrabes JA, et al: Changes in hospital mortality rates in 425 patients with acute ST-elevation myocardial infarction and cardiac rupture over a 30-year period. Circulation 118:2783, 2008.

164. Poulsen SH, Praestholm M, Munk K, et al: Ventricular septal rupture complicating acute myocardial infarction: Clinical characteristics and contemporary outcome. Ann Thorac Surg. 85:1591, 2008.

165. Maltais S, Ibrahim R, Basmadjian AJ, et al: Postinfarction ventricular septal defects: Towards a new treatment algorithm? Ann Thorac Surg 87:687, 2009.

166. Freixa X, Sitges M, Pare C: Images in cardiology. Left ventricular pseudoaneurysm complicating acute myocardial infarction: Improved diagnosis by real-time three-dimensional echocardiography. Heart 92:154, 2006.

167. Atik FA, Navia JL, Vega PR, et al: Surgical treatment of postinfarction left ventricular pseudoaneurysm. Ann Thorac Surg 83:526, 2007.

168. Birnbaum Y, Fishbein MC, Blanche C, Siegel RJ: Ventricular septal rupture after acute myocardial infarction. N Engl J Med 347:1426, 2002.

169. Bursi F, Enriquez-Sarano M, Jacobsen SJ, Roger VL: Mitral regurgitation after myocardial infarction: A review. Am J Med 119:103, 2006.

170. Stout KK, Verrier ED: Acute valvular regurgitation. Circulation 119:3232, 2009.

171. Liuzzo JP, Shin YT, Choi C, et al: Simultaneous papillary muscle avulsion and free wall rupture during acute myocardial infarction. Intra-aortic balloon pump: A bridge to survival. J Invasive Cardiol 18:135, 2006.

172. Russo A, Suri RM, Grigioni F, et al: Clinical outcome after surgical correction of mitral regurgitation due to papillary muscle rupture. Circulation 118:1528, 2008.

173. Carmeliet E: Cardiac ionic currents and acute ischemia: From channels to arrhythmias. Physiol Rev 79:917, 1999.

174. Tang L, Deng C, Long M, et al: Thrombin receptor and ventricular arrhythmias after acute myocardial infarction. Mol Med. 14:131, 2008.

175. Yadav AV, Zipes DP: Prophylactic lidocaine in acute myocardial infarction: Resurface or reburial? Am J Cardiol 94:606, 2004.

176. Piccini JP, Berger JS, Brown DL: Early sustained ventricular arrhythmias complicating acute myocardial infarction. Am J Med 121:797, 2008.

177. Hreybe H, Saba S: Location of acute myocardial infarction and associated arrhythmias and outcome. Clin Cardiol 32:274, 2009.

178. Altun A, Kirdar C, Ozbay G: Effect of aminophylline in patients with atropine-resistant late advanced atrioventricular block during acute inferior myocardial infarction. Clin Cardiol 21:759, 1998.

179. Di Chiara A: Right bundle branch block during the acute phase of myocardial infarction: Modern redefinitions of old concepts. Eur Heart J 27:1, 2006.

180. Wong CK, Stewart RA, Gao W, et al: Prognostic differences between different types of bundle branch block during the early phase of acute myocardial infarction: insights from the Hirulog and Early Reperfusion or Occlusion (HERO)-2 trial. Eur Heart J 27:21, 2006.

181. Kleemann T, Juenger C, Gitt AK, et al: Incidence and clinical impact of right bundle branch block in patients with acute myocardial infarction: ST elevation myocardial infarction versus non-ST elevation myocardial infarction. Am Heart J 156:256, 2008.

182. Suzuki M, Sakaue T, Tanaka M, et al: Association between right bundle branch block and impaired myocardial tissue-level reperfusion in patients with acute myocardial infarction. J Am Coll Cardiol 47:2122, 2006.

183. Bogale N, Orn S, James M, et al: Usefulness of either or both left and right bundle branch block at baseline or during follow-up for predicting death in patients following acute myocardial infarction. Am J Cardiol 99:647, 2007.

184. Køber L, Swedberg K, McMurray JJ, et al: Previously known and newly diagnosed atrial fibrillation: A major risk indicator after a myocardial infarction complicated by heart failure or left ventricular dysfunction. Eur J Heart Fail 8:591, 2006.

185. Saczynski JS, McManus D, Zhou Z, et al: Trends in atrial fibrillation complicating acute myocardial infarction. Am J Cardiol 104:169, 2009.

186. Berton G, Cordiano R, Cucchini F, et al: Atrial fibrillation during acute myocardial infarction: Association with all-cause mortality and sudden death after 7-year of follow-up. Int J Clin Pract. 63:712, 2009.

187. Keeley EC, Boura JA, Grines CL: Primary angioplasty versus intravenous thrombolytic therapy for acute myocardial infarction: A quantitative review of 23 randomised trials. Lancet 361:13, 2003.

188. Kruk M, Kadziela J, Reynolds HR, et al: Predictors of outcome and the lack of effect of percutaneous coronary intervention across the risk strata in patients with persistent total occlusion after myocardial infarction: Results from the OAT (Occluded Artery Trial) study. JACC Cardiovasc Interv 1:511, 2008.

189. Fokkema ML, van der Vleuten PA, Vlaar PJ, et al: Incidence, predictors, and outcome of reinfarction and stent thrombosis within one year after primary percutaneous coronary intervention for ST-elevation myocardial infarction. Catheter Cardiovasc Interv 73:627, 2009.

190. Gueret P, Khalife K, Jobic Y, et al: Echocardiographic assessment of the incidence of mechanical complications during the early phase of myocardial infarction in the reperfusion era: A French multicentre prospective registry. Arch Cardiovasc Dis 101:41, 2008.

191. Jugdutt BI: Cyclooxygenase inhibition and adverse remodeling during healing after myocardial infarction. Circulation 115:288, 2007.

192. Imazio M, Negro A, Belli R, et al: Frequency and prognostic significance of pericarditis following acute myocardial infarction treated by primary percutaneous coronary intervention. Am J Cardiol 103:1525, 2009.

193. Napodano M, Tarantini G, Ramondo A, et al: Myocardial abnormalities underlying persistent ST-segment elevation after anterior myocardial infarction. J Cardiovasc Med (Hagerstown) 10:44, 2009.

194. Abildstrom SZ, Ottesen MM, Rask-Madsen C, et al: Sudden cardiovascular death following myocardial infarction: The importance of left ventricular systolic dysfunction and congestive heart failure. Int J Cardiol 104:184, 2005.

195. Marchenko AV, Cherniavsky AM, Volokitina TL, et al: Left ventricular dimension and shape after postinfarction aneurysm repair. Eur J Cardiothorac Surg 27:475, 2005.

196. Rehan A, Kanwar M, Rosman H, et al: Incidence of post myocardial infarction left ventricular thrombus formation in the era of primary percutaneous intervention and glycoprotein IIb/IIIa inhibitors. A prospective observational study. Cardiovasc Ultrasound 4:20, 2006.

197. Hirsh J, Fuster V, Ansell J, Halperin JL: American Heart Association/American College of Cardiology Foundation guide to warfarin therapy. Circulation 107:1692, 2003.

198. Jaffe AS, Krumholz HM, Catellier DJ, et al: Prediction of medical morbidity and mortality after acute myocardial infarction in patients at increased psychosocial risk in the Enhancing Recovery in Coronary Heart Disease Patients (ENRICHD) study. Am Heart J 152:126, 2006.

199. Alter DA, Chong A, Austin PC, et al: Socioeconomic status and mortality after acute myocardial infarction. Ann Intern Med 144:82, 2006.

200. Mendes de Leon CF, Czajkowski SM, Freedland KE, et al: The effect of a psychosocial intervention and quality of life after acute myocardial infarction: The Enhancing Recovery in Coronary Heart Disease (ENRICHD) clinical trial. J Cardiopulm Rehabil 26:9, 2006.

201. Donahoe SM, Stewart GC, McCabe CH, et al: Diabetes and mortality following acute coronary syndromes. JAMA 298:765, 2007.

202. Petrina M, Goodman SG, Eagle KA: The 12-lead electrocardiogram as a predictive tool of mortality after acute myocardial infarction: current status in an era of revascularization and reperfusion. Am Heart J 152:11, 2006.

203. Wong CK, Gao W, Raffel OC, et al: Initial Q waves accompanying ST-segment elevation at presentation of acute myocardial infarction and 30-day mortality in patients given streptokinase therapy: An analysis from HERO-2. Lancet 367:2061, 2006.

204. Morrow DA: Cardiovascular risk prediction in patients with stable and unstable coronary heart disease. Circulation 121:2681, 2010.

205. Adabag AS, Therneau TM, Gersh BJ, et al: Sudden death after myocardial infarction. JAMA 300:2022, 2008.

206. Gibson CM, Karha J, Murphy SA, et al: Early and long-term clinical outcomes associated with reinfarction following fibrinolytic administration in the Thrombolysis in Myocardial Infarction trials. J Am Coll Cardiol 42:7, 2003.

207. De Luca G, Ernst N, van 't Hof AW, et al: Predictors and clinical implications of early reinfarction after primary angioplasty for ST-segment elevation myocardial infarction. Am Heart J 151:1256, 2006.

208. Bodi V, Sanchis J, Nunez J, et al: Prognostic value of a comprehensive cardiac magnetic resonance assessment soon after a first ST-segment elevation myocardial infarction. JACC Cardiovasc Imaging 2:835, 2009.

209. Wright J, Adriaenssens T, Dymarkowski S, et al: Quantification of myocardial area at risk with T2-weighted CMR: Comparison with contrast-enhanced CMR and coronary angiography. JACC Cardiovasc Imaging 2:825, 2009.

210. Di Carli MF, Hachamovitch R: New technology for noninvasive evaluation of coronary artery disease. Circulation 115:1464, 2007.

Arrhythmias

211. Zipes DP, Camm AJ, Borggrefe M, et al: ACC/AHA/ESC 2006 Guidelines for Management of Patients With Ventricular Arrhythmias and the Prevention of Sudden Cardiac Death: A report of the American College of Cardiology/American Heart Association Task Force and the European Society of Cardiology Committee for Practice Guidelines (writing committee to develop Guidelines for Management of Patients With Ventricular Arrhythmias and the Prevention of Sudden Cardiac Death): Developed in collaboration with the European Heart Rhythm Association and the Heart Rhythm Society. Circulation 114:e385, 2006.

212. Estes NA 3rd: The challenge of predicting and preventing sudden cardiac death immediately after myocardial infarction. Circulation 120:185, 2009.

Other Complications

213. Dawood N, Vaccarino V, Reid KJ, et al: Predictors of smoking cessation after a myocardial infarction: The role of institutional smoking cessation programs in improving success. Arch Intern Med 168:1961, 2008.

214. Thombs BD, de Jonge P, Coyne JC, et al: Depression screening and patient outcomes in cardiovascular care: A systematic review. JAMA 300:2161, 2008.

215. Milani RV, Lavie CJ: Impact of cardiac rehabilitation on depression and its associated mortality. Am J Med 120:799, 2007.

216. Smith SC Jr, Allen J, Blair SN, et al: AHA/ACC guidelines for secondary prevention for patients with coronary and other atherosclerotic vascular disease: 2006 update: Endorsed by the National Heart, Lung, and Blood Institute. Circulation 113:2363, 2006.

217. Morrow DA, de Lemos JA, Sabatine MS, et al: Clinical relevance of C-reactive protein during follow-up of patients with acute coronary syndromes in the Aggrastat-to-Zocor Trial. Circulation 114:281, 2006.

218. Waters DD, Brotons C, Chiang CW, et al: Lipid treatment assessment project 2: A multinational survey to evaluate the proportion of patients achieving low-density lipoprotein cholesterol goals. Circulation 120:28, 2009.

219. Lichtenstein AH, Appel LJ, Brands M, et al: Diet and lifestyle recommendations revision 2006: A scientific statement from the American Heart Association Nutrition Committee. Circulation 114:82, 2006.

220. Morrow DA, Wiviott SD, White HD, et al: Effect of the novel thienopyridine prasugrel compared with clopidogrel on spontaneous and procedural myocardial infarction in the Trial to Assess Improvement in Therapeutic Outcomes by Optimizing Platelet Inhibition with Prasugrel-Thrombolysis in Myocardial Infarction 38: An application of the classification system from the universal definition of myocardial infarction. Circulation 119:2758, 2009.

221. Antman EM, Wiviott SD, Murphy SA, et al: Early and late benefits of prasugrel in patients with acute coronary syndromes undergoing percutaneous coronary intervention: A TRITON-TIMI 38 (TRial to Assess Improvement in Therapeutic Outcomes by Optimizing Platelet InhibitioN with Prasugrel-Thrombolysis In Myocardial Infarction) analysis. J Am Coll Cardiol 51:2028, 2008.

222. Abdel-Latif A, Moliterno DJ: Antiplatelet polypharmacy in primary percutaneous coronary intervention: Trying to understand when more is better. Circulation 119:3168, 2009.

223. Fonarow GC: Beta-blockers for the post-myocardial infarction patient: Current clinical evidence and practical considerations. Rev Cardiovasc Med 7:1, 2006.

224. Mega JL, Braunwald E, Mohanavelu S, et al: Rivaroxaban versus placebo in patients with acute coronary syndromes (ATLAS ACS-TIMI 46): A randomised, double-blind, phase II trial. Lancet 374:29, 2009.

225. Alexander JH, Becker RC, Bhatt DL, et al: Apixaban, an oral, direct, selective factor Xa inhibitor, in combination with antiplatelet therapy after acute coronary syndrome: Results of the Apixaban for Prevention of Acute Ischemic and Safety Events (APPRAISE) trial. Circulation 119:2877, 2009.

226. Antman EM, Bennett JS, Daugherty A, et al: Use of nonsteroidal antiinflammatory drugs: An update for clinicians: A scientific statement from the American Heart Association. Circulation 115:1634, 2007.

227. Gibson CM, Pride YB, Aylward PE, et al: Association of non-steroidal anti-inflammatory drugs with outcomes in patients with ST-segment elevation myocardial infarction treated with fibrinolytic therapy: An ExTRACT-TIMI 25 analysis. J Thromb Thrombolysis 27:11, 2009.

228. Garcia Rodriguez LA, Tacconelli S, Patrignani P: Role of dose potency in the prediction of risk of myocardial infarction associated with nonsteroidal anti-inflammatory drugs in the general population. J Am Coll Cardiol 52:1628, 2008.

229. Dorn GW 2nd: Novel pharmacotherapies to abrogate postinfarction ventricular remodeling. Nat Rev Cardiol 6:283, 2009.

230. Bergmann O, Bhardwaj RD, Bernard S, et al: Evidence for cardiomyocyte renewal in humans. Science 324:98, 2009.

231. Parmacek MS, Epstein JA: Cardiomyocyte renewal. N Engl J Med 361:86, 2009.

GUIDELINES STEPHEN D. WIVIOTT AND ELLIOTT M. ANTMAN

Management of Patients with ST-Segment Elevation Myocardial Infarction

The American College of Cardiology and American Heart Association (ACC/AHA) comprehensive recommendations for the management of ST-segment elevation myocardial infarction (STEMI) were initially published in 2004,[1] followed by focused updates.[2,3]

PRE-STEMI GOALS, EARLY RISK STRATIFICATION, AND MANAGEMENT

The ACC/AHA guidelines on pre-STEMI management aim to identify patients at risk for STEMI and to provide therapies to prevent STEMI and promote patient education to identify symptoms and signs of STEMI to allow for early activation of emergency medical systems (EMS) rather than self-transport. The early risk stratification and management guidelines for STEMI aim to provide early access to known therapies that improve outcomes.

Prehospital, EMS providers should administer aspirin (162 to 325 mg) to all patients not already taking aspirin (Class I; level of evidence [LOE], C), obtain a 12-lead electrocardiogram (ECG) in patients suspected of having STEMI (Class IIa; LOE, B), review a reperfusion checklist, and relay this information to a medical facility (Class IIa; LOE, C; see Fig. 55-2). Patients with STEMI who have cardiogenic shock, those with contraindications to lytics (Class I; LOE, A), and those at high-risk of dying because of heart failure (Class IIa; LOE, B) should be channeled immediately to a facility capable of cardiac catheterization.

INITIAL RECOGNITION AND EVALUATION IN THE EMERGENCY DEPARTMENT

Initial evaluation in the emergency department focuses on identification of STEMI, early therapy, and reperfusion strategy. Selection of reperfusion strategy depends on hospital and patient characteristics (**Fig. 55G-1;** see Table 55-4). Time to reperfusion therapy strongly influences outcomes in STEMI. Patients presenting to a hospital with percutaneous coronary intervention (PCI) capability should undergo PCI within 90 minutes of first medical contact as a systems goal. Patients with STEMI presenting to a non-PCI–capable hospital should be considered for transfer to a PCI-capable hospital based on patient characteristics, time from symptom onset, and time to available PCI therapy. STEMI patients presenting to a hospital without PCI capability and who cannot be transferred to a PCI center and undergo PCI within 90 minutes of first medical contact should receive fibrinolytic therapy within 30 minutes of hospital presentation as a systems goal in the absence of contraindications (Class I; LOE, B). Communities should have well-developed plans for transfer of patients with STEMI to PCI-capable hospitals (Class I; LOE, C).

Achieving these goals requires rapid and focused evaluation (Class I; LOE, C), including the following:

■ History of coronary artery disease (CAD), cerebrovascular disease (CVD),

and risk factors associated with fibrinolytic therapy, including prior stroke, bleeding risk, or signs and symptoms of stroke
■ Physical examination to assess the extent and complications of STEMI and to identify evidence of prior stroke or cognitive deficits
■ 12-lead ECG interpreted by an experienced physician within 10 minutes of hospital arrival at the emergency department in patients with suggestive symptoms
■ Laboratory examinations, including cardiac-specific troponin levels should be performed—but not delay reperfusion
■ Patients with STEMI should have portable chest X-ray, when possible, without delaying reperfusion (unless a potential contraindication, such as aortic dissection, is suspected)—if the distinction between STEMI and aortic dissection remains unclear, imaging should be used.

Initial medical therapies in the emergency department should include the following:

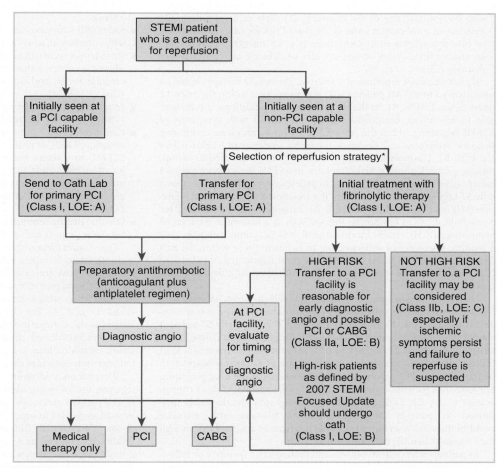

FIGURE 55G-1 Each community and each facility in that community should have an agreed-on plan for how STEMI patients are to be treated. It should include which hospitals should receive STEMI patients from emergency medical services units capable of obtaining diagnostic ECGs, management at the initial receiving hospital, and written criteria and agreements for expeditious transfer of patients from non-PCI–capable to PCI-capable facilities. Consideration should be given to initiating a preparatory pharmacologic regimen as soon as possible in preparation for and during patient transfer to the catheterization laboratory. The optimal regimen has not yet been established, although published studies have used various combinations for the following: anticoagulant, oral antiplatelet agents, intravenous antiplatelet. *Time since onset of symptoms, risk of STEMI, risks associated with fibrinolytic therapy; time required for transport to a skilled PCI laboratory. Angio, angiography; Cath Lab, catheterization laboratory. (*Modified from Kushner FG, Hand M, Smith SC Jr, et al: 2009 Focused Updates: ACC/AHA Guidelines for the Management of Patients With ST-Elevation Myocardial Infarction (updating the 2004 Guideline and 2007 Focused Update) and ACC/AHA/SCAI Guidelines on Percutaneous Coronary Intervention (updating the 2005 Guideline and 2007 Focused Update): a report of the American College of Cardiology Foundation/American Heart Association Task Force on Practice Guidelines. Circulation 120:2271, 2009.*)

- *Supplemental oxygen:* Supplemental oxygen should be administered to patients with arterial oxygen desaturation (i.e., $SaO_2 < 90\%$) (Class I; LOE, B), but it is reasonable to administer supplemental oxygen to all patients with uncomplicated STEMI during the first 6 hours (Class IIa; LOE, C).
- *Nitroglycerin:* Sublingual nitroglycerin should be given to patients with ongoing ischemic discomfort, 0.4 mg every 5 minutes, for a total of three doses. Intravenous (IV) nitroglycerin is then indicated for relief of ongoing ischemic discomfort, control of hypertension, or management of pulmonary congestion (Class I; LOE, C). Nitrates should not be administered to patients with systolic blood pressure (SBP) < 90 mm Hg or SBP ≥ 30 mm Hg below baseline, severe bradycardia (<50 beats/min), tachycardia (>100 beats/min), or suspected right ventricular (RV) infarction (Class III; LOE, C).
- *Analgesia:* Morphine sulfate (2 to 4 mg IV, with increments of 2 to 8 mg IV repeated at 5- to 15-minute intervals) is the analgesic of choice for management of pain associated with STEMI (Class I; LOE, C).
- *Aspirin:* Aspirin should be chewed by patients who have not taken aspirin before presentation with STEMI (Class I). The initial dose should be 162 mg (LOE, A) to 325 mg (LOE, C). Nonenteric-coated aspirin provides more rapid buccal absorption.
- *Beta blockers:* Oral beta blocker therapy should be initiated for patients who do not have any of the following: (1) signs of heart failure; (2) evidence of a low output state; (3) increased risk for cardiogenic shock; or (4) other relative contraindications (e.g., PR interval > 0.24 second, second- or third-degree atrioventricular (AV) block, or reactive airway disease) (Class I; LOE, B).

If pharmacologic reperfusion is selected, fibrinolytic therapy should be administered to STEMI patients with symptom onset within the prior 12 hours (Class I; LOE, A). In the absence of contraindications, it is reasonable to administer fibrinolytic therapy to patients with symptoms of STEMI beginning within the prior 12 to 24 hours who have continuing ischemic symptoms and electrocardiographic evidence of STEMI (Class IIa; LOE, C). Fibrinolytic therapy should not be administered to asymptomatic patients whose initial symptoms of STEMI began more than 24 hours earlier (Class III; LOE, C) nor to patients whose 12-lead ECG shows only ST-segment depression, except if a true posterior myocardial infarction (MI) is suspected (Class III; LOE, A). Patients should be evaluated for contraindications to fibrinolytic therapy such as a history of intracranial hemorrhage (ICH), significant closed head or facial trauma within the past 3 months, uncontrolled hypertension, or ischemic stroke within the past 3 months (Class I; LOE, A). STEMI patients at substantial (≥4%) risk of ICH should be treated with PCI rather than with fibrinolytic therapy (Class I; LOE, A).

Diagnostic angiography should be available to most patients with STEMI, even when the initial strategy is fibrinolytic therapy. It is reasonable (Class IIa; LOE, B) for high-risk patients (e.g., extensive ST-segment elevation, left bundle branch block [LBBB], congestive heart failure, hypotension, Killip Class 2 or higher, inferior MI with ejection fraction ≤ 35%) initially treated with reperfusion therapy at non-PCI—capable hospitals to be transferred to PCI-capable hospitals for consideration of angiography. For lower risk patients, transfer to a PCI-capable hospital is also a consideration (Class IIb; LOE, B). Coronary angiography should not be performed in patients following fibrinolytic therapy with extensive comorbidities in whom the risks of revascularization are likely to outweigh the benefits (Class III; LOE, C).

In patients with indications who can undergo PCI (primary or following fibrinolytics), the procedure should be performed by skilled personnel. PCI should not be performed in a noninfarct artery at the time of primary PCI in patients without hemodynamic compromise (Class III; LOE, C). Primary PCI should not be performed in asymptomatic patients more than 12 hours after the onset of STEMI if they are hemodynamically and electrically stable (Class III; LOE, C).

A strategy of coronary angiography with intent to perform PCI (or emergency coronary artery bypass grafting [CABG]) is recommended for patients who have received fibrinolytic therapy and have any of the following: (1) cardiogenic shock, younger than 75 years, and are suitable candidates for revascularization; (2) severe congestive heart failure and/or pulmonary edema (Killip Class III); or (3) hemodynamically compromising ventricular arrhythmias (Class I; LOE, C). It is reasonable to perform rescue PCI for patients with one or more of the following: hemodynamic or electrical instability, persistent ischemic symptoms or fibrinolytic therapy has failed (ST-segment elevation < 50%, resolved after 90 minutes following initiation of fibrinolytic therapy in the lead showing the worst initial elevation), and a moderate or large area of myocardium at risk (Class II; LOE, B).

Indications for PCI following STEMI depend on clinical considerations and coronary anatomy. In patients whose anatomy is suitable, PCI should be performed in the following situations: (1) when there is objective evidence of recurrent MI (Class I; LOE, C); (2) for moderate or severe spontaneous or provocable myocardial ischemia during recovery from STEMI (Class I; LOE, B); or (3) for cardiogenic shock or hemodynamic instability (Class I; LOE, B).

Emergency CABG can be useful as the primary reperfusion strategy in patients who have suitable anatomy, are not candidates for fibrinolysis or PCI, and are within 6 to 12 hours of an evolving STEMI, especially with severe multivessel or left main disease (Class IIa; LOE, B). Emergency CABG should not be performed in patients with persistent angina and a small area of myocardium at risk if they are hemodynamically stable or after successful reperfusion with PCI but persistent ischemia on the basis of microvascular obstruction (Class III; LOE, C). Additionally, emergency or urgent CABG in patients with STEMI should be considered for the following:

- Failed PCI with persistent pain or hemodynamic instability in patients with coronary anatomy suitable for surgery (Class I; LOE, B)
- Persistent or recurrent ischemia refractory to medical therapy in patients who have coronary anatomy suitable for surgery, have substantial myocardium at risk, and are not candidates for PCI or fibrinolytic therapy (Class I; LOE, B)
- At the time of surgical repair of postinfarction ventricular septal rupture (VSR) or mitral valve insufficiency (Class I; LOE, B)
- Cardiogenic shock in patients younger than 75 years with ST-segment elevation, LBBB, or posterior MI who develop shock within 36 hours of STEMI, have severe multivessel or left main disease, and are suitable for revascularization that can be performed within 18 hours of shock, unless further support is futile because of the patient's wishes or there are contraindications or unsuitability for further invasive care (Class I; LOE, A)
- Life-threatening ventricular arrhythmias in the presence of 50% or more left main stenosis and/or triple-vessel disease (Class I; LOE, B)

Reperfusion therapy should be supported with ancillary anticoagulants and antiplatelet therapies. Patients undergoing reperfusion with fibrinolytics should receive anticoagulant therapy for a minimum of 48 hours (Class IIa; LOE, C) and preferably for the duration of the index hospitalization, up to 8 days when using regimens other than unfractionated heparin (UFH) (Class IIa; LOE, A). For UFH, therapy is generally limited to 48 hours to lessen the risk of heparin-induced thrombocytopenia. Anticoagulant regimens with established efficacy include UFH, enoxaparin (provided the serum creatinine level < 2.5 mg/dL in men and 2.0 mg/dL in women), fondaparinux (provided the creatinine level < 3.0 mg/dL).

For patients undergoing PCI after having received an anticoagulant regimen, the following additional therapies should be considered (Class I). For patients previously receiving UFH additional boluses of UFH can be used as needed to support the procedure, taking into account whether glycoprotein (GP) IIb/IIIa antagonists have been administered (LOE, C). Bivalirudin is useful as a supportive measure for primary PCI, with or without prior treatment with UFH (Class I; LOE, B), and is a reasonable consideration in patients at high risk for bleeding. For patients with prior treatment with enoxaparin, if the last subcutaneous dose was administered at least 8 to 12 hours earlier, an additional intravenous dose should be given (Class I; LOE, B). Because of the risk of catheter thrombosis, fondaparinux should not be used as the sole anticoagulant to support PCI. An additional anticoagulant with anti-IIa activity should be administered (Class III; LOE, C).

Adjunctive antiplatelet therapies play a key role in the management of STEMI. A daily dose of aspirin (initial dose, 162 to 325 mg orally; maintenance dose, 75 to 162 mg) should be given indefinitely after STEMI to all patients without a true aspirin allergy (Class I; LOE, A). Clopidogrel, 75 mg/day orally, should be added to aspirin in patients with STEMI if fibrinolytic therapy or no reperfusion therapy is administered (Class I;

LOE, A). Treatment with clopidogrel in these settings should continue for at least 14 days (Class I; LOE, B).

A loading dose of a thienopyridine is recommended for STEMI patients for whom PCI is planned. The regimen should be one of the following:

- At least 300 to 600 mg of clopidogrel should be given as early as possible before or at the time of primary or nonprimary PCI (Class I; LOE, C).
- Prasugrel, 60 mg, should be given as soon as possible for primary PCI (Class I; LOE, B)

For STEMI patients undergoing nonprimary PCI, the following regimens are recommended:

- If the patient has received fibrinolytic therapy and has been given clopidogrel, clopidogrel should be continued as the thienopyridine of choice (Class I; LOE, C).
- If the patient has received fibrinolytic therapy without a thienopyridine, a loading dose of 300 to 600 mg of clopidogrel should be given as the thienopyridine of choice (Class I; LOE, C).
- If the patient did not receive fibrinolytic therapy, either a loading dose of 300 to 600 mg of clopidogrel should be given (Class I; LOE, C) or, once the coronary anatomy is known and PCI is planned, a loading dose of 60 mg of prasugrel should be given promptly, no later than 1 hour after the PCI (Class I; LOE, B).
- In STEMI patients with a history of prior stroke or transient ischemic attack for whom primary PCI is planned, prasugrel is not recommended (Class III; LOE, C).

The duration of thienopyridine therapy should be as follows:

- In patients receiving a stent (bare metal stent [BMS] or drug-eluting stent [DES]) during PCI for acute coronary syndrome (ACS), clopidogrel, 75 mg daily, or prasugrel, 10 mg daily, should be given for at least 12 months (Class I; LOE, B).
- If the risk of morbidity because of bleeding outweighs the anticipated benefit afforded by thienopyridine therapy, earlier discontinuation should be considered (Class I; LOE, C).
- In patients with DES, consideration of continuation of clopidogrel or prasugrel beyond 15 months may be considered (Class IIb; LOE, C).

Beyond these recommendations, consideration of long-term maintenance therapy (e.g., 1 year) with clopidogrel (75 mg/day, orally) is reasonable in STEMI patients whether they undergo reperfusion with fibrinolytic therapy or do not receive reperfusion therapy (Class IIa; LOE, C). In patients taking a thienopyridine for whom CABG is planned and can be delayed, it is recommended that the drug be discontinued to allow dissipation of the antiplatelet effect. The period of withdrawal should be at least 5 days in patients receiving clopidogrel and at least 7 days in patients receiving prasugrel, unless the need for revascularization and/or the net benefit of the thienopyridine outweighs the potential risks of excess bleeding (Class I; LOE, C) .

It is reasonable to start treatment with GP IIb/IIIa antagonists at the time of primary PCI (with or without stenting) in selected patients with STEMI (Class IIa; LOE, A, abciximab; LOE, B, tirofiban or eptifibatide). GP IIb/IIIa antagonists, as part of a preparatory pharmacologic strategy for patients with STEMI before their arrival in the cardiac catheterization laboratory for angiography and PCI, have uncertain usefulness (Class IIb; LOE, B).

HOSPITAL MANAGEMENT

After initial patient evaluation and management in the emergency department and selection of reperfusion therapy, STEMI guidelines focus on the in-hospital management on monitoring for and treating secondary complications of STEMI, initiation of secondary preventive measures and transition to long-term management of STEMI. Care should be structured around protocols that promote guideline-based management. Critical pathways, protocols, and other quality improvement tools (e.g., ACC, "Guidelines Applied in Practice,"[4] and AHA, "Mission: Lifeline"[5]) can aid in the application of evidence-based treatments for patients with STEMI by caregivers and institutions (Class I; LOE, C). A standard set of admitting orders summarizes the key features of care (see Table 55-7).

STEMI patients should be admitted to a coronary care unit (CCU) or step-down unit (for low-risk patients) (Class I; LOE, C). Nursing care should be provided by individuals certified in critical care (Class I; LOE,

C). STEMI patients originally admitted to the CCU who are stable after 12 to 24 hours should be transferred to the step-down unit (Class I; LOE, C). Additional general measures include limiting bed rest to less than 12 to 24 hours for stable patients.

A medical assessment to determine the appropriateness of adjunctive medical therapies should include the following:

1. Beta-adrenergic blocking agents (beta blockers)
   - Patients receiving beta-blockers within the first 24 hours of STEMI without adverse effects should continue their use during the early convalescent phase of STEMI (Class I; LOE, A).
   - Patients without contraindications to beta blockers who did not receive them within the first 24 hours after STEMI should have them started in the early convalescent phase (Class I; LOE, A).
   - Patients with early contraindications within the first 24 hours of STEMI should be reevaluated for candidacy for beta blocker therapy (Class I; LOE, X).
2. Nitroglycerin
   - Intravenous nitroglycerin is indicated in the first 48 hours after STEMI for the treatment of persistent ischemia, congestive heart failure (CHF), or hypertension. The decision to administer intravenous nitroglycerin and the dose used should not preclude therapy with other proven mortality-reducing interventions, such as beta blockers or angiotensin-converting enzyme (ACE) inhibitors (Class I; LOE, B).
   - Intravenous, oral, or topical nitrates are useful beyond the first 48 hours after STEMI for treatment of recurrent angina or persistent CHF if their use does not preclude therapy with beta blockers or ACE inhibitors (Class I; LOE, B).
   - Nitrates should not be administered to patients with systolic pressure lower than 90 mm Hg or 30 mm Hg or more below baseline, severe bradycardia (less than 50 beats/min), tachycardia (more than 100 beats/min), or RV infarction (Class III; LOE, C).
3. Inhibition of the renin-angiotensin-aldosterone system
   - An ACE inhibitor should be administered orally during convalescence from STEMI in patients who tolerate this class of medication (Class I; LOE, A).
   - An angiotensin receptor blocker (ARB) should be administered to STEMI patients who cannot tolerate ACE inhibitors and have clinical or radiologic signs of heart failure or left ventricular ejection fraction (LVEF) less than 0.40 (Class I; LOE, B).
   - Long-term aldosterone blockade should be prescribed for post-STEMI patients without significant renal dysfunction (creatinine level ≤2.5 mg/dL in men and ≤ 2.0 mg/dL in women) or without hyperkalemia (potassium level ≤ 5.0 mEq/L) who are already receiving therapeutic doses of an ACE inhibitor, have an LVEF ≤0.40, and have either symptomatic heart failure or diabetes (Class I; LOE, A).
   - In STEMI patients who tolerate ACE inhibitors, an ARB can be useful as an alternative to ACE inhibitors provided there are clinical or radiologic signs of heart failure or LVEF <0.40 (Class IIa; LOE, B).

COMPLICATIONS FOLLOWING STEMI

The management of patients with hypotension, pulmonary edema, arrhythmias, or shock depends on the most likely underlying disorder (Fig. 55G-2). For most conditions, LV function and the presence of a mechanical complication should be assessed by echocardiography if not previously evaluated invasively. Recommended treatments for low-output states include inotropic support, intra-aortic counterpulsation (IABP), mechanical reperfusion with PCI or CABG, and surgical correction of mechanical complications (Class I; LOE, B). Beta blockers or calcium channel antagonists should not be administered to patients in a low-output state because of pump failure (Class III; LOE, B).

For patients with cardiogenic shock not quickly reversed with pharmacologic therapy, the IABP is a stabilizing measure for angiography and prompt revascularization (Class I; LOE, B). Early revascularization, either PCI or CABG, is recommended for patients younger than 75 years with ST-segment elevation or LBBB who develop shock within 36 hours of MI and are suitable for revascularization that can be performed within 18 hours of shock, unless further support is futile because of the patient's

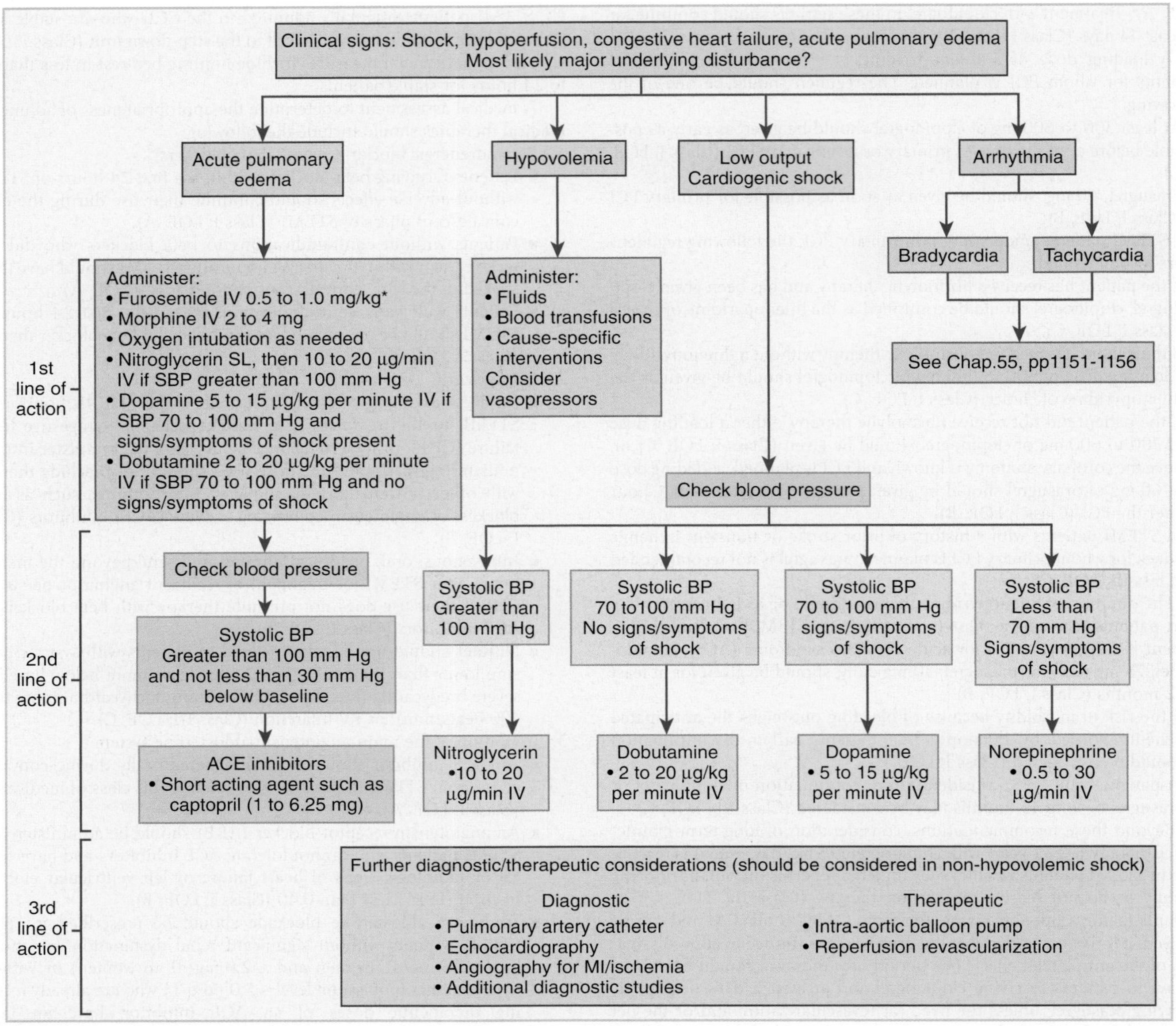

CH
55

FIGURE 55G-2 Emergency management of complicated STEMI. The emergency management of patients with cardiogenic shock, acute pulmonary edema, or both is outlined. *Furosemide < 0.5 mg/kg for new-onset acute pulmonary edema without hypovolemia, 1 mg/kg for acute or chronic volume overload, renal insufficiency. Nesiritide has not been studied adequately in patients with STEMI. Combinations of medications (e.g., dobutamine and dopamine) may be used. BP = blood pressure; SL = sublingual; SBP = systolic BP. *(Modified from the American Heart Association in collaboration with the International Liaison Committee on Resuscitation: Guidelines 2000 for Cardiopulmonary Resuscitation and Emergency Cardiovascular Care. Part 7: The era of reperfusion: Section 1: Acute coronary syndromes [acute myocardial infarction]. Circulation 102:1172, 2000.)*

wishes or contraindications or unsuitability for further invasive care (Class I; LOE, A).

RV infarction should be considered for patients with inferior STEMI and hemodynamic compromise and should be assessed with a right precordial V$_4$R lead to detect ST-segment elevation and an echocardiogram to screen for RV infarction (Class I; LOE, B). For such patients, early reperfusion should be achieved, if possible, AV synchrony should be achieved, and bradycardia should be corrected. RV preload should be optimized (intravenous volume challenge), RV afterload should be optimized (therapy of concomitant LV dysfunction), and inotropic support should be used for hemodynamic instability not responsive to volume challenge (Class I; LOE, C).

Mechanical causes of heart failure or low-output syndrome, including mitral valve regurgitation, ventricular septal rupture, and left-ventricular free wall rupture, should prompt consideration for urgent cardiac surgical repair unless further support is considered futile because of the patient's

wishes or contraindications or unsuitability for further invasive care (Class I; LOE, B or C). CABG should generally be undertaken at the same time as repair of these defects when coronary anatomy is appropriate (Class I; LOE, C).

Tachyarrhythmias after STEMI include ventricular fibrillation, ventricular tachycardia, and atrial fibrillation or flutter. In general, ventricular and atrial arrhythmias in the setting of STEMI are treated according to advanced cardiac life support (ACLS) guidelines that include electrical and pharmacologic therapies. Beyond standard measures, it is reasonable to manage refractory arrhythmias in the setting of recent STEMI, particularly polymorphic ventricular tachycardia (VT), by aggressive attempts to reduce myocardial ischemia and adrenergic stimulation, including therapies such as beta-adrenergic blockade, IABP use, consideration of emergency PCI-CABG surgery (Class IIa; LOE, B), and normalization of serum potassium and magnesium levels (Class IIa; LOE, B). The routine use of prophylactic antiarrhythmic drugs is not indicated for suppression of isolated ventricular premature beats, couplets, runs of accelerated idioventricular rhythm, or nonsustained VT (Class III). The use of implantable cardioverter-defibrillator (ICD) implantation post-STEMI is summarized in Figure 55-42. For episodes of sustained atrial fibrillation or flutter without hemodynamic compromise or ischemia, rate control is indicated (Class I; LOE, C). In addition, patients with sustained atrial fibrillation or flutter should be given anticoagulant therapy unless contraindications exist (Class I; LOE, C). Consideration should be given to cardioversion to sinus rhythm for patients with a history of atrial fibrillation or flutter prior to STEMI (Class I; LOE, C).

The guidelines provide an approach to the management of bradyarrhythmias and AV block (**Table 55G-1**). There are four possible actions for bradycardias: observation, medical therapy with atropine, transcutaneous pads with standby pacing, or temporary venous pacing. Actions depend on the severity of bradycardia, type of STEMI, and likely anatomic site of block. Permanent ventricular pacing is indicated for persistent second-degree AV block in the His-Purkinje system with bilateral bundle branch block or third-degree AV block within or below the His-Purkinje system after STEMI, transient advanced second- or third-degree infranodal AV block, and associated bundle-branch block. Uncertainty regarding the site of the block may warrant an electrophysiologic study for persistent and symptomatic second- or third-degree AV block. Permanent ventricular pacing may be considered for persistent second- or third-degree AV block at the AV node level. Permanent ventricular pacing is not recommended for transient AV block in the absence of intraventricular conduction defects, in the presence of isolated left anterior fascicular block, for acquired left anterior fascicular block in the absence of AV block, or first-degree AV block in the presence of bundle branch block that predated STEMI or is of indeterminate age.

Recurrent chest pain after STEMI may indicate pericarditis or recurrent ischemia. Aspirin is recommended for treatment of pericarditis after STEMI. Doses as high as 650 mg orally (enteric) every 4 to 6 hours may be needed, and anticoagulation should be immediately discontinued if pericardial effusion develops or increases (Class I; LOE, B). Nonsteroidal anti-inflammatory drugs (NSAIDs) may be considered for pain relief; however, they should not be used for extended periods because of their continuous effect on platelet function, an increased risk of myocardial scar thinning, and infarct expansion (Class IIb; LOE, B). Corticosteroids might be considered only as a last resort in patients with pericarditis refractory to aspirin or NSAIDs (Class IIb; LOE, C).

The guidelines recommend an approach to management of recurrent ischemic discomfort (**Fig. 55G-3**). Initial assessment is based on the presence or absence of recurrent ST-elevation. Patients with recurrent ischemic chest discomfort after initial reperfusion therapy for STEMI should undergo escalation of medical therapy with nitrates and beta blockers. Intravenous anticoagulation should be initiated if not already started (Class I; LOE, B). In addition to intensified medical therapy, patients with recurrent ischemic chest discomfort with recurrent ST-segment elevation, hemodynamic instability, poor LV function, or a large area of myocardium at risk should be referred urgently for cardiac catheterization and revascularization as needed. Insertion of an IABP should also be considered (Class I; LOE, C). Patients with recurrent ischemic-type chest discomfort who are considered candidates for revascularization should undergo coronary arteriography and PCI or CABG, as dictated by coronary anatomy (Class I; LOE, B).

CONVALESCENCE, DISCHARGE, AND POST–MYOCARDIAL INFARCTION CARE

After the acute phase of STEMI management, assessment of ventricular function, exercise testing, and further invasive assessment merit consideration. Echocardiography should be used for patients with STEMI not undergoing LV angiography to assess baseline LV function, especially if the patient is hemodynamically unstable (Class I; LOE, C). Echocardiography should also be used to evaluate suspected mechanical complications, shock, intracardiac thrombus, and pericardial effusion (Class I; LOE, B).

The guidelines offer an approach to exercise testing and repeat catheterization (see Fig. 55-41). Exercise testing is not recommended routinely for patients who have undergone successful revascularization. Functional

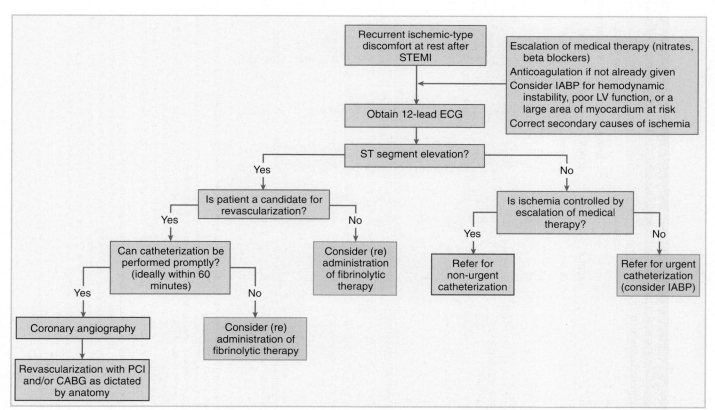

FIGURE 55G-3 Algorithm for the management of ischemia or infarction after STEMI. *(Modified from Antman EM, Anbe DT, Armstrong PW, et al: ACC/AHA guidelines for the management of patients with ST-elevation myocardial infarction: A report of the American College of Cardiology/American Heart Association Task Force on Practice Guidelines [Committee to Revise the 1999 Guidelines for the Management of Patients with Acute Myocardial Infarction]. Circulation 110:e82, 2004.)*

TABLE 55G-1 Recommendations for Treatment of Atrioventricular and Intraventricular Conduction Disturbances during STEMI

Intraventricular Conduction	Action	Atrioventricular Conduction						
		NORMAL Class	FIRST-DEGREE AV BLOCK Anterior MI Class	FIRST-DEGREE AV BLOCK Nonanterior MI Class	MOBITZ I SECOND-DEGREE AV BLOCK Anterior MI Class	MOBITZ I SECOND-DEGREE AV BLOCK Nonanterior MI Class	MOBITZ II SECOND-DEGREE AV BLOCK Anterior MI Class	MOBITZ II SECOND-DEGREE AV BLOCK Nonanterior MI Class
(Normal)	Observe	I	I	I	IIb	IIa	III	III
	A / A*	III	III	III	III	III	III	III
	TC	III	IIb	IIb	I	I	I	I
	TV	III	III	III	III	III	IIa	IIa
Old or new fascicular block (left anterior or left posterior or fascicular block)	Observe	I	IIb	IIb	IIb	IIb	III	III
	A / A*	III	III	III	III	III	III	III
	TC	IIb	I	IIa	I	I	I	I
	TV	III	III	III	III	III	IIa	IIb
Old bundle branch block (BBB)	Observe	I	III	III	III	III	III	III
	A / A*	III	III	III	III	III	III	III
	TC	IIb	I	I	I	I	I	I
	TV	III	IIb	IIb	IIb	IIb	IIa	IIa
New bundle branch block	Observe	III	III	III	III	III	III	III
	A / A*	III	III	III	III	III	III	III
	TC	I	I	I	I	I	IIb	IIb
	TV	IIb	IIa	IIa	IIa	IIa	I	I
Fascicular block + right bundle branch block	Observe	III	III	III	III	III	III	III
	A / A*	III	III	III	III	III	III	III
	TC	I	I	I	I	I	IIb	IIb
	TV	IIb	IIb	IIa	IIa	IIa	I	I
Alternating left and right bundle branch block	Observe	III	III	III	III	III	III	III
	A / A*	III	III	III	III	III	III	III
	TC	IIb	IIb	IIb	IIb	IIb	IIb	IIb
	TV	I	I	I	I	I	I	I

Explanation of table: This table is designed to summarize the atrioventricular (column headings) and intraventricular (row headings) conduction disturbances that may occur during acute anterior or nonanterior STEMI, the possible treatment options, and the indications for each possible therapeutic option.

Actions: There are four possible actions, or therapeutic options, listed and classified for each bradyarrhythmia or conduction problem:

1. Observe: Continued electrocardiographic monitoring, no further action planned.
2. A, A*: Atropine administered at 0.6 to 1.0 mg intravenously every 5 minutes, up to 0.04 mg/kg. In general, because the increase in sinus rate with atropine is unpredictable, this is to be avoided unless there is symptomatic bradycardia that will likely respond to a vagolytic agent (e.g., sinus bradycardia or Mobitz I), as denoted by the asterisk, above.
3. TC: Application of transcutaneous pads and standby transcutaneous pacing, with no further progression to transvenous pacing imminently planned.
4. TV: Temporary transvenous pacing. It is assumed, but not specified in the table, at the discretion of the clinician, that transcutaneous pads will be applied and standby transcutaneous pacing will be in effect as the patient is transferred to the fluoroscopy unit for temporary transvenous pacing.

Class: Each possible therapeutic option is further classified according to ACC/AHA criteria as I, IIa, IIb, and III. There are no randomized trials available that address or compare specific treatment options. Moreover, the data for this table and recommendations are largely derived from observational data of prefibrinolytic era databases. Thus, the recommendations above must be taken as recommendations and tempered by the clinical circumstances.

Level of evidence: This table was developed from the following: (1) published observational case reports and case series; (2) published summaries, not meta-analyses, of these data; and (3) expert opinion, largely from the prereperfusion era. There are no published randomized trials comparing different strategies of managing conduction disturbances post-STEMI. Thus, the level of evidence for the recommendations in the table is C.

How to use the table: For example, a 54-year-old man is admitted with an anterior STEMI and a narrow QRS on admission. On day 1, he develops a right bundle branch block (RBBB), with a PR interval of 0.28 second. RBBB is an intraventricular conduction disturbance, so look at row "New BBB." Find the column for "First-Degree AV Block." Find the "Action" and "Class" cells at the convergence. Note that "Observe" and "Atropine" are Class III, not indicated; transcutaneous pacing (TC) is Class I. Temporary transvenous pacing (TV) is Class IIb.

testing should be performed in the hospital or early after discharge in STEMI patients not selected for cardiac catheterization, and without high-risk features, to assess the presence and extent of inducible ischemia (Class I; LOE, B). In patients judged to be unable to exercise, pharmacologic stress nuclear scintigraphy or dobutamine echocardiography before or early after discharge should be used for patients with STEMI who are not undergoing cardiac catheterization to assess for inducible ischemia (Class I; LOE, B).

Coronary arteriography should be performed in patients with spontaneous episodes of myocardial ischemia or episodes of myocardial ischemia provoked by minimal exertion during recovery from STEMI (Class I; LOE, A). Coronary arteriography should be performed for intermediate- or high-risk findings on noninvasive testing after STEMI or in survivors of STEMI who had clinical heart failure during the acute episode but subsequently demonstrated well-preserved LV function (Class I; LOE, B or C). It is reasonable to perform coronary arteriography when STEMI is suspected to have occurred by a mechanism other than thrombotic occlusion (Class IIa; LOE, C). These circumstances would include coronary embolism, certain metabolic or hematologic diseases, or coronary artery spasm. Coronary arteriography is also considered reasonable for STEMI patients with any of the following: diabetes mellitus, LVEF < 0.40, CHF, prior revascularization, or life-threatening ventricular arrhythmias, without the above features (Class I; LOE, C).

SECONDARY PREVENTION AND LONG-TERM MANAGEMENT

Patients who survive the acute phase of STEMI should have plans initiated for secondary prevention therapies (Class I; LOE, A). Contemporary recommendations for secondary prevention after STEMI include the following:

- Complete smoking cessation
- Blood pressure at goal < 140/90 mm Hg unless diabetes or chronic kidney disease is present (blood pressure < 130/90 mm Hg)
- Physical activity 30 minutes, 3 to 4 days/week, optimally daily
- Hemoglobin A1c (HbA1c) < 7%
- Body mass index (BMI), 18.5 to 24.9

In addition, cardiac rehabilitation and secondary prevention programs are recommended for patients with STEMI, particularly those with a number of modifiable risk factors and/or those moderate- to high-risk patients for whom supervised exercise training is warranted. Before discharge, follow-up therapy with a medical provider should be arranged to evaluate functional recovery, assess medication use and titrate doses as needed, and address physical activity, return to work, sexual activity, and travel in detail (Class I; LOE, C).

REFERENCES

1. Antman EM, Anbe DT, Armstrong PW, et al: ACC/AHA guidelines for the management of patients with ST-elevation myocardial infarction: A report of the American College of Cardiology/American Heart Association Task Force on Practice Guidelines (Committee to Revise the 1999 Guidelines for the Management of Patients with Acute Myocardial Infarction). Circulation 110:e82, 2004.
2. Antman EM, Hand M, Armstrong PW, et al: 2007 Focused Update of the ACC/AHA 2004 Guidelines for the Management of Patients with ST-Elevation Myocardial Infarction: A report of the American College of Cardiology/American Heart Association Task Force on Practice Guidelines: Developed in collaboration with the Canadian Cardiovascular Society endorsed by the American Academy of Family Physicians: 2007 Writing Group to Review New Evidence and Update the ACC/AHA 2004 Guidelines for the Management of Patients With ST-Elevation Myocardial Infarction, Writing on Behalf of the 2004 Writing Committee. Circulation 117:296, 2008.
3. Kushner FG, Hand M, Smith SC Jr, et al: 2009 Focused Updates: ACC/AHA Guidelines for the Management of Patients With ST-Elevation Myocardial Infarction (updating the 2004 Guideline and 2007 Focused Update) and ACC/AHA/SCAI Guidelines on Percutaneous Coronary Intervention (updating the 2005 Guideline and 2007 Focused Update): A report of the American College of Cardiology Foundation/American Heart Association Task Force on Practice Guidelines. Circulation 120:2271, 2009.
4. Montoye CK, Eagle KA; Michigan ACC-GAP Investigators; ACC-GAP Steering Committee; American College of Cardiology: An Organizational Framework for the AMI ACC-GAP Project. J Am Coll Cardiol 46 (10 Suppl):1, 2005.
5. American Heart Associaton, Mission: Lifeline, 2010 (http://www.heart.org/HEARTORG/HealthcareProfessional/Mission-Lifeline-Home-Page_UCM_305495_SubHomePage.jsp).

CHAPTER 56

Unstable Angina and Non– ST Elevation Myocardial Infarction

Christopher P. Cannon and Eugene Braunwald

Each year, approximately one million patients in the United States are hospitalized for unstable angina or non–ST elevation myocardial infarction (UA/NSTEMI), a condition also referred to as non–ST elevation acute coronary syndrome (NSTE-ACS).[1,2] Acute total occlusion of a coronary artery usually causes STEMI (see Chap. 54), whereas UA/NSTEMI most commonly results from severe obstruction, but not total occlusion, of the culprit coronary artery. The incidence of NSTE-ACS, both absolute and relative to STEMI, is increasing, probably as a result of demographic changes in the population, including progressively increasing numbers of older persons and higher rates of diabetes.[3]

Definition

Stable angina pectoris typically manifests as a deep, poorly localized chest or arm discomfort (rarely described as pain), reproducibly precipitated by physical exertion or emotional stress, and relieved within 5 to 10 minutes by rest or sublingual nitroglycerin (see Chaps. 53 and 54). In contrast, *unstable* angina is defined as angina pectoris (or equivalent type of ischemic discomfort) with at least one of three features: (1) occurring at rest (or minimal exertion) and usually lasting >20 minutes (if not interrupted by the administration of a nitrate or an analgesic); (2) being severe and usually described as frank pain; or (3) occurring with a crescendo pattern (i.e., pain that awakens the patient from sleep or that is more severe, prolonged, or frequent than previously). Approximately two thirds of patients with unstable angina have evidence of myocardial necrosis on the basis of elevated cardiac serum markers, such as cardiac-specific troponin T or I and creatine kinase isoenzyme (CK)–MB, and thus have a diagnosis of NSTEMI. As troponin measurements become progressively more sensitive, an increasing fraction of patients with NSTE-ACS exhibit some release of troponin, and therefore these should be considered cases of NSTEMI with a reciprocal reduction in the fraction with unstable angina.

Pathophysiology

Five pathophysiologic processes may contribute to the development of UA/NSTEMI (**Fig. 56-1A**)[4]:
1. plaque rupture or erosion with superimposed nonocclusive thrombus (this causes by far the most UA/NSTEMI);
2. dynamic obstruction due to
   a. spasm of an epicardial coronary artery, as in Prinzmetal variant angina;
   b. constriction of the small, intramural muscular coronary arteries, that is, the coronary resistance vessels[5];
   c. local vasoconstrictors, such as thromboxane A_2, released from platelets;
   d. dysfunction of the coronary endothelium; and
   e. adrenergic stimuli including cold and cocaine;
3. severe coronary luminal narrowing caused by progressive coronary atherosclerosis or post–percutaneous coronary intervention restenosis;
4. inflammation; and
5. secondary unstable angina, that is, severe myocardial ischemia related to increased myocardial oxygen demand or decreased oxygen supply (e.g., tachycardia, fever, hypotension, or anemia).

Individual patients may have several of these processes coexisting as the cause of UA/NSTEMI. Several serum markers can serve as effective tools in identifying these pathophysiologic processes. As noted later, these serum markers form the foundation of a "multimarker strategy" for evaluation and risk stratification (**Fig. 56-1B**).

Thrombosis

Six sets of observations support the central role of coronary artery thrombosis in the pathogenesis of UA/NSTEMI: (1) the findings, at autopsy, of thrombi in the coronary arteries, usually localized to the site of a ruptured or eroded coronary plaque[6]; (2) the demonstration in coronary atherectomy specimens from patients with UA/NSTEMI of a high incidence of thrombotic lesions compared with those obtained from patients with stable angina; (3) the frequent finding of thrombus at coronary angioscopy; (4) the demonstration at coronary angiography (**Fig. 56-2**), intravascular ultrasound, optical coherence tomography, and computed tomography angiography of plaque ulceration or irregularities suggesting a ruptured plaque or thrombus; (5) the elevation of several serum markers of platelet activity and fibrin formation; and (6) the improvement in clinical outcome by antiplatelet and antithrombotic therapy.

Platelet Activation and Aggregation

Platelets play a key role in the transformation of a stable atherosclerotic plaque to an unstable lesion (**Fig. 56-3**). Rupture or ulceration of an atherosclerotic plaque often exposes the subendothelial matrix (e.g., collagen and tissue factor) to circulating blood. The first step in

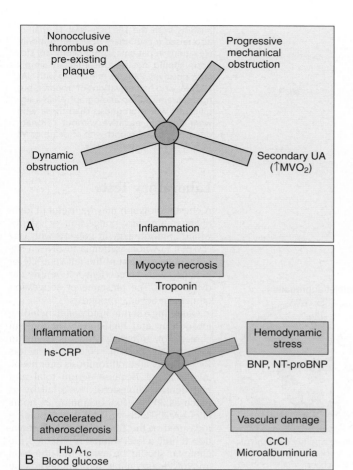

FIGURE 56-1 **A,** Schematic representation of the causes of unstable angina (UA). MVO_2 = myocardial O_2 consumption. *(Reproduced from Braunwald E: Unstable angina: An etiologic approach to management. Circulation 98:2219, 1998.)* **B,** A multimarker strategy for evaluation of the etiology and prognosis of UA/NSTEMI. In addition, these now have been seen to be independent markers of an adverse prognosis. BNP = B-type natriuretic peptide; CrCl = creatinine clearance; Hb A_{1c} = hemoglobin A_{1c}; hs-CRP = high-sensitivity C-reactive protein; NT-proBNP = N-terminal–pro-BNP; UA/NSTEMI = unstable angina or non–ST elevation myocardial infarction. *(Modified with permission from Morrow DA, Braunwald E: Future of biomarkers in acute coronary syndromes: Moving toward a multimarker strategy. Circulation 108:250, 2003.)*

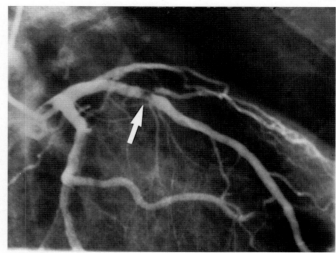

FIGURE 56-2 Coronary artery thrombus in a 60-year-old patient with unstable angina. Coronary angiography shows an irregular hazy filling defect in the left anterior descending artery at the level of the second diagonal branch (arrow). Contrast medium surrounds the globular thrombus, which extends into the diagonal branch.

Thrombin molecules are incorporated into coronary thrombi and can form the nidus of rethrombosis.

Clinical Presentation

Among patients with ACS, women present more often with unstable angina, representing 30% to 45% of patients with this condition, compared with 25% to 30% of patients with NSTEMI and only 20% of patients with STEMI.[7] In comparison to the latter, patients with UA/NSTEMI are older and have higher rates of prior MI, stable angina, diabetes, previous coronary revascularization, and extracardiac vascular disease than do patients with STEMI.[7] Indeed, approximately 80% of patients with UA/NSTEMI have a history of coronary artery disease (CAD) before the acute event.[8]

Clinical Examination

The physical examination may be unremarkable or may support the diagnosis of cardiac ischemia. Signs suggesting that ischemia involves a large fraction of the left ventricle include diaphoresis, pale cool skin, sinus tachycardia, a third or fourth heart sound, and basilar rales on lung examination. In some patients, ischemia of a large area of myocardium reduces left ventricular dysfunction and causes hypotension.

Electrocardiography

ST depression (or transient ST elevation) and T wave changes occur in up to 50% of patients with UA/NSTEMI[9] (see Chap. 13). New (or presumably new) ST-segment deviation (≥0.1 mV) is a useful measure of ischemia and prognosis. When electrocardiograms preceding the acute event are available, further ST depression of only 0.05 mV is a sensitive although nonspecific finding of UA/NSTEMI.[9] Transient (i.e., <20 minutes) ST elevation, which occurs in approximately 10% of patients with UA/NSTEMI, portends a high risk of future cardiac events. T wave changes are sensitive but not specific for acute ischemia unless they are marked (>0.3 mV) (**Fig. 56-4**).

CONTINUOUS ELECTROCARDIOGRAPHIC MONITORING. Continuous electrocardiographic monitoring serves two purposes in UA/NSTEMI: (1) to identify arrhythmias and (2) to identify recurrent ST-segment deviation indicative of ischemia. Recurrent ST-segment deviation is a strong *independent* marker of adverse outcome,[10] even in the presence of troponin release.

thrombus formation is platelet *adhesion* via platelet glycoprotein (GP) Ib binding to von Willebrand factor and GP VI binding to collagen. The ensuing platelet *activation* leads to (1) a shape change in the platelet (from a smooth discoid shape to a spiculated form, which increases the surface area on which thrombin generation can occur); (2) degranulation of the platelet alpha and dense granules, releasing thromboxane A_2, serotonin, and other platelet aggregatory and chemoattractant agents; (3) increased expression of the GP IIb/IIIa receptor on the platelet surface followed by a conformational change of the receptor that enhances its affinity for fibrinogen; and (4) platelet *aggregation,* in which fibrinogen binds to the activated platelet fibrinogen inhibitor GP IIb/IIIa, causing a growing platelet plug.

SECONDARY HEMOSTASIS. Simultaneous with the formation of the platelet plug, the plasma coagulation system is activated. Tissue factor triggers most coronary artery thrombosis (see Chaps. 43 and 87). Ultimately, factor X is activated (to factor Xa), which leads to the generation of thrombin (factor IIa, which plays a central role in arterial thrombosis). Thrombin, which converts fibrinogen to fibrin, is also a powerful stimulant of platelet aggregation and activates factor XIII, which leads to cross-linking of fibrin and stabilization of the clot.

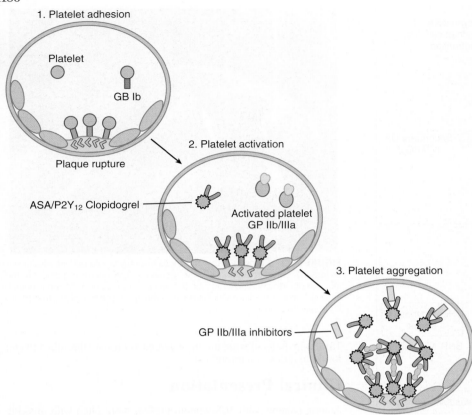

1. Platelet adhesion

Platelet

GB Ib

Plaque rupture

2. Platelet activation

ASA/P2Y$_{12}$ Clopidogrel

Activated platelet
GP IIb/IIIa

3. Platelet aggregation

GP IIb/IIIa inhibitors

FIGURE 56-3 Platelet adhesion (1), activation (2), and aggregation (3). Platelets initiate thrombosis at the site of a ruptured or eroded plaque: the first step is platelet adhesion (1) via the GP Ib receptor in conjunction with von Willebrand factor. This is followed by platelet activation (2), which leads to a shape change in the platelet, degranulation of the alpha and dense granules, and expression of GP IIb/IIIa receptors on the platelet surface with activation of the receptor, such that it can bind fibrinogen. The final step is platelet aggregation (3), in which fibrinogen (yellow) binds to the activated GP IIb/IIIa receptors of two platelets. Aspirin (ASA) and clopidogrel act to decrease platelet activation (see text for details), whereas the GP IIb/IIIa inhibitors inhibit the final step of platelet aggregation. GP = glycoprotein. (See Fig. 87-3.)

Markers of Cardiac Necrosis

Among patients presenting with symptoms consistent with UA/NSTEMI, elevations of markers of myocardial necrosis (i.e., CK-MB, troponin T or I) identify patients with the diagnosis of NSTEMI. With the use of troponins, which are more sensitive than CK-MB, a greater percentage of patients are classified as having NSTEMI, which is associated with a worse prognosis.[11] Persistent elevation of troponin after an acute event also associates with worse clinical outcomes.[12]

Although the appropriate cut point to define an elevation of troponin I has engendered controversy, growing consensus has focused on use of the 99th percentile of a normal population (approximately 0.10 ng/mL) with a coefficient of variation (a measure of reproducibility of the assay) not greater than 10% and a sensitivity (lower level of detection) of as low as 0.02 ng/mL. As more sensitive assays for troponin are being developed, revision of these characteristics will be required. Even slight elevations of cardiac troponin presage a higher risk of death or recurrent ischemic events.[11,12]

Because assays differ, each hospital needs to review the specific cut points defined by the assay used. Most point-of-care tests for troponins provide a binary (positive or negative) result, whereas some provide a quantitative result, although the sensitivity and diagnostic accuracy of some of these tests have only recently matched the accuracy of current-generation laboratory-based assays.

Despite increasingly accurate assays, apparent false-positive troponin elevations have been found in patients later found at coronary angiography not to have epicardial stenoses.[13] These elevations result from an alternative diagnosis, such as congestive heart failure, in which troponin elevations in the absence of CAD portend an adverse prognosis. An

analysis from the TACTICS–TIMI 18 trial[14,15] also raised a cautionary note that troponin elevations in patients without coronary stenosis should not be discarded as simply false-positives. Patients presenting with UA/NSTEMI who had elevations of troponin but no apparent CAD on angiography had a significantly worse prognosis than those who were troponin negative without coronary disease, with a 6-month rate of death or MI of 5.3% and 0%, respectively.[14]

Laboratory Tests

A chest radiograph may be useful in identifying pulmonary congestion or edema, which is more likely in patients with UA/NSTEMI in whom ischemia involves a significant proportion of the left ventricle or in those with antecedent left ventricular dysfunction. The presence of congestion confers an adverse prognosis.

Obtaining a serum lipid panel including low-density and high-density lipoprotein cholesterol and triglyceride is useful in identifying important, treatable risk factors for coronary atherothrombosis after hospital discharge. Because serum total and high-density cholesterol levels fall by as much as 30% to 40% beginning 24 hours after UA/NSTEMI or STEMI, they should be measured at the time of initial presentation. If only a later sample is obtained, the clinician should be aware that the total and low-density cholesterol values may be as much as 30% to 40% lower than the patient's actual baseline concentration (see Chap. 47). Other circulating markers of increased risk are discussed subsequently. Evaluation for other secondary causes of UA/NSTEMI[16] may also be appropriate in selected patients (e.g., assessing thyroid function in patients who present with UA/NSTEMI and persistent tachycardia).

Noninvasive Testing

In the management of UA/NSTEMI, noninvasive testing is employed for several purposes: (1) at presentation, usually in the emergency department, to diagnose the presence or absence of CAD (see Chap. 53); (2) to evaluate the extent of residual ischemia after medical therapy has been initiated and to guide further therapy as part of an "early conservative" strategy; (3) to evaluate left ventricular function; and (4) in risk stratification. The markers of high risk include evidence of severe ischemia or ventricular tachyarrhythmia on continuous electrocardiography or stress testing and the development of left ventricular dysfunction, either at rest or stress induced.

The safety of early stress testing in patients with UA/NSTEMI has been debated, but observations made in several trials have suggested that pharmacologic or symptom-limited stress testing is safe after a period of at least 24 hours of stabilization.[17] Contraindications to stress testing are a recent (less than 24 hours) occurrence of rest pain, especially if it is associated with electrocardiographic changes or other signs of hemodynamic instability or arrhythmia.

The merits of various modalities of stress testing have been compared. Stress myocardial perfusion imaging with sestamibi or stress echocardiography is slightly more sensitive than electrocardiographic stress testing alone and has greater prognostic value, but myocardial perfusion has been proven cost-effective only in higher-risk patients. A useful approach is to individualize the choice on the basis of patient characteristics, local availability, and expertise in interpretation. For most patients, electrocardiographic stress testing is recommended if the

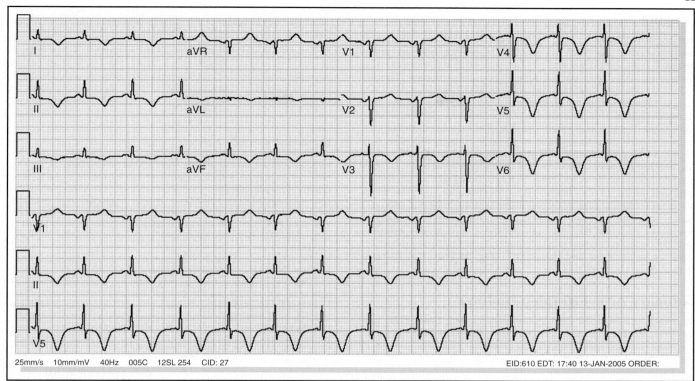

FIGURE 56-4 Electrocardiogram showing deep symmetric inferolateral T wave inversion with 1-mm ST-segment deviation. Such electrocardiographic findings are frequently associated with critical stenosis of a coronary artery (although localization of which artery is often difficult). These findings are also a useful marker of patients at high risk of subsequent death or myocardial infarction.

TABLE 56-1 Braunwald Clinical Classification of UA/NSTEMI

CLASS	DEFINITION	DEATH OR MI TO ONE YEAR* (%)
Severity		
Class I	New onset of severe angina or accelerated angina; no rest pain	7.3
Class II	Angina at rest within past month but not within preceding 48 hr (angina at rest, subacute)	10.3
Class III	Angina at rest within 48 hr (angina at rest)	10.8[†]
Clinical Circumstances		
A. Secondary angina	Develops in the presence of extracardiac condition that intensifies myocardial ischemia	14.1
B. Primary angina	Develops in the absence of extracardiac condition	8.5
C. Postinfarction angina	Develops within 2 wk after acute myocardial infarction	18.5[‡]
Intensity of treatment	Patients with unstable angina may also be divided into three groups according to whether unstable angina occurs: (1) in the absence of treatment for chronic stable angina, (2) during treatment for chronic stable angina, or (3) despite maximal anti-ischemic drug therapy. The three groups may be designated by subscripts 1, 2, and 3, respectively.	
Electrocardiographic changes	Patients with unstable angina may be further divided into those with or without transient ST-T wave changes during pain.	

*Data from TIMI III Registry: Scirica BM, Cannon CP, McCabe CH, et al: Prognosis in the thrombolysis in myocardial ischemia III registry according to the Braunwald unstable angina pectoris classification. Am J Cardiol 90:821, 2002.
[†]$P = 0.057$.
[‡]$P = 0.001$.
UA/NSTEMI = unstable angina/non–ST elevation myocardial infarction.
From Braunwald E: Unstable angina: A classification. Circulation 80:410, 1989.

electrocardiogram at rest lacks significant ST-segment abnormalities. If ST abnormalities at rest exist, then perfusion or echocardiographic imaging is recommended. Exercise testing is generally recommended unless the patient cannot walk sufficiently to achieve a significant workload, in which case pharmacologic stress testing provides an alternative (see Chaps. 14 and 50).

Clinical Classification

Because UA/NSTEMI comprises such a heterogeneous group of patients, classification schemes based on clinical features are useful.

A clinical classification of UA/NSTEMI (**Table 56-1**)[16] provides a useful means to stratify risk. Patients fall into three groups according to the clinical circumstances of the acute ischemic episode: (1) primary unstable angina caused by reductions of myocardial perfusion; (2) secondary unstable angina (e.g., with ischemia related to precipitating factors such as anemia or an acute MI); and (3) post-MI unstable angina. Patients are classified simultaneously according to the severity of the ischemia. This classification provides valuable prognostic information (with postinfarction angina at rest having the worst prognosis).

Imaging

Intravascular ultrasound (IVUS) was the first imaging technique to demonstrate that patients who had recently had an acute coronary event had disrupted plaques that exhibited more positive remodeling (i.e., less encroachment on the coronary lumen) and larger plaque areas than did patients with chronic stable CAD. Computed tomography angiography (CTA) has also shown that ruptured plaques were characterized by positive vascular remodeling, low plaque density, and spotty calcification. Patients presenting to the emergency department without these features could have ACS ruled out with great reliability.[18,19] Motoyama and colleagues[20] showed that contrast-enhanced CTA could also identify vulnerable plaques that had not yet ruptured but were at risk of doing so. This interesting approach might, in the future, allow identification of patients in whom prevention of rupture by invasive means might be considered.[21] Cardiac magnetic resonance (CMR) imaging with T2-weighted imaging, assessment of left ventricular wall thickness, myocardial perfusion, and detection of delayed enhancement permits accurate detection of ACS as well as acute and chronic MI[22] (**Fig. 56-5**; see Figs. 18-4 and 54-18).

Coronary Arteriographic Findings

The extent of epicardial CAD among patients with UA/NSTEMI randomized to the invasive arm of the TACTICS–TIMI 18 trial, who systematically underwent angiography, was as follows: 34% had significant obstruction (>50% luminal diameter stenosis) of three vessels; 28% had two-vessel disease; 26% had single-vessel disease; and 13% had no coronary stenosis >50%. Approximately 10% had left main stem stenosis >50%.[16] Registries of unselected UA/NSTEMI patients have reported similar findings. Women and nonwhites with UA/NSTEMI have less extensive coronary disease than their counterparts do,[7] whereas patients with NSTEMI have more extensive disease on coronary angiography than do those who present with unstable angina alone.

Women and nonwhites represent a larger proportion of patients with symptoms of UA/NSTEMI without epicardial CAD, suggesting a different pathophysiologic mechanism for their clinical presentation, leading to difficulty in making a firm diagnosis of UA/NSTEMI in these patient groups.[7] Approximately one third of patients with UA/NSTEMI without a critical epicardial obstruction have impaired coronary flow assessed angiographically, suggesting a pathophysiologic role for coronary microvascular dysfunction. The short-term prognosis in this group of patients with UA/NSTEMI without angiographic evidence of epicardial disease is excellent.[23]

The culprit lesion in UA/NSTEMI typically exhibits an eccentric stenosis with scalloped or overhanging edges and a narrow neck (see Chap. 21). These angiographic findings may represent disrupted atherosclerotic plaque, thrombus, or a combination. Features suggesting thrombus include globular intraluminal masses with a rounded or polypoid shape (see Fig. 56-2). "Haziness" of a lesion suggests the presence of thrombus, but this finding is not specific. Patients with angiographically visualized thrombus have impaired coronary blood flow and worse clinical outcomes compared with those without thrombus.

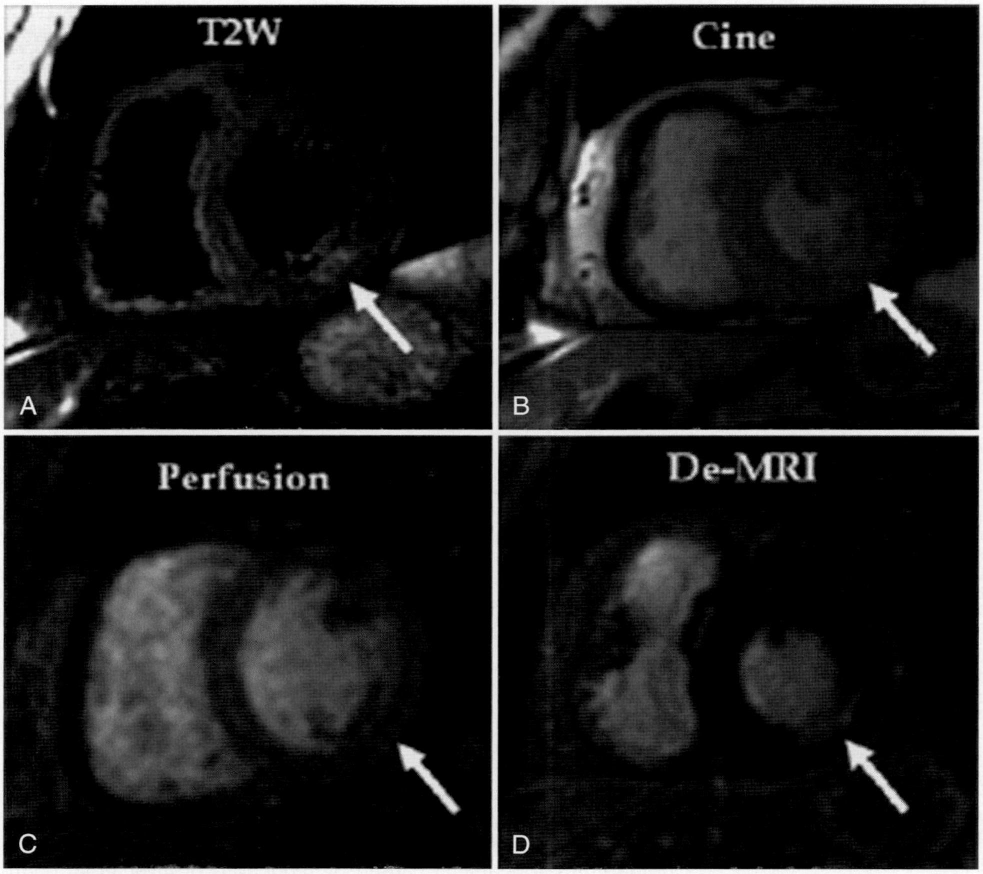

RISK STRATIFICATION

RISK AFTER ACUTE CORONARY SYNDROME. An important emerging concept is that the risk of recurrent ischemic events is more dependent on the presence of multifocal lesions other than the culprit lesion responsible for the ACS event. Studies of coronary anatomy by angiography, IVUS, or angioscopy have shown multiple active plaques in addition to the culprit lesion. Thus, as aggressive interventional approaches are used increasingly successfully to treat the culprit lesion, the remaining plaques often provoke recurrent events. The percentage of patients with more than one active plaque on angiography relates to an increasing baseline level of C-reactive protein (CRP),[23] a marker of inflammation. These findings provide an important pathophysiologic link between inflammation, more diffuse active CAD, and recurrent cardiac events in the months to years after a clinical ACS event.

NATURAL HISTORY. Patients with unstable angina have lower *short-term* mortality (1.5% to 2.0% from first presentation to 30 days) than do those with NSTEMI or STEMI; the early mortality risk of the two types of MI is similar and between 3% and 5%. The *early* mortality risk in UA/NSTEMI relates to the extent of myocardial damage and resulting hemodynamic compromise and is less than in patients with STEMI. In contrast, *long-term* outcome—for both mortality and nonfatal events—is actually *worse* for patients with UA/NSTEMI compared with STEMI. This finding probably results from the greater likelihood of recurrence of ACS in patients with UA/NSTEMI as well as their older age, greater extent of coronary disease, prior MI, and comorbidities such as diabetes and impaired renal function.

FIGURE 56-5 Example of a patient with NSTEMI. CMR imaging was performed in a 63-year-old man 1 hour after his arrival at the emergency department with initially normal cardiac enzymes; it revealed a small area of T2 hyperintensity **(A)** in the inferolateral wall (myocardial edema) with associated subtle hypokinesis **(B)**, a resting perfusion defect **(C)**, and delayed hyperenhancement **(D)**; (myocardial necrosis) in the same area (arrows). Troponin level was elevated 7 hours after CMR imaging. Invasive angiography revealed triple-vessel disease with a 95% stenosis in the posterolateral branch. *(From Cury RC, Shash K, Nagurney JT, et al: Cardiac magnetic resonance with T2-weighted imaging improves detection of patients with acute coronary syndrome in the emergency department. Circulation 118:837, 2008.)*

Methods of Risk Stratification

CLINICAL VARIABLES

High-Risk Clinical Subgroups

The aforementioned classification of unstable angina (see Table 56-1) has proved clinically useful in several studies for the identification of high-risk patients, notably those with ongoing or recurrent rest pain, post-MI unstable angina, or secondary unstable angina.[15] Increasing age associates with a significant increase in adverse outcomes.[24] Patients with UA/NSTEMI and diabetes mellitus or extracardiac vascular disease (i.e., cerebrovascular disease or peripheral arterial vascular disease) are at approximately 50% higher risk than those without these comorbidities even after controlling for other differences in baseline characteristics (**Table 56-2**). As with STEMI, patients with UA/NSTEMI who present with evidence of congestive heart failure (Killip class ≥II) also have an increased risk of death.

RISK ASSESSMENT BY ELECTROCARDIOGRAPHY. In the TIMI III registry of patients with UA/NSTEMI, independent predictors of 1-year death or MI included left bundle branch block (risk ratio, 2.8); and ST-segment deviation >0.05 mV (risk ratio, 2.45); both $P < 0.001$.[9] There appears to be a gradient of risk based on the degree of ST-segment deviation.[25]

RISK ASSESSMENT BY CARDIAC MARKERS (Table 56-3)

Markers of Myocyte Necrosis

Patients with NSTEMI, defined as associated with an elevated biomarker of necrosis (CK-MB or troponin), have a worse long-term prognosis than do those with unstable angina.[26] Beyond just a positive versus negative test result, there is a linear relation between the level of circulating troponin T or I and subsequent risk of death.[27] However, in several studies, a higher risk of MI (or recurrent MI) was observed even with small elevations of positive troponins.[11,28]

C-Reactive Protein and Other Markers of Inflammation (see Chaps. 44 and 49)

Elevated levels of CRP relate to increased risk of death, MI, and the need for urgent revascularization. Because CRP is an acute-phase reactant, it is elevated by MI, with or without ST-segment elevation. Thus, the level of CRP in patients with very recent ACS is approximately five times that of stable patients.[25] Among patients with negative troponin I, CRP can discriminate between high- and low-risk groups. When both CRP and troponin T are used, mortality can be stratified from 0.4% for patients with both markers negative, to 4.7% if either CRP or troponin is positive, to 9.1% if both are positive.[29] CRP measured after stabilization post-ACS strongly predicts outcome after 3 to 12 months.[30]

Study of other inflammatory markers has offered consistent evidence of an association between systemic inflammation and recurrent adverse events, including serum amyloid A, monocyte chemoattractant protein

TABLE 56-2	Clinical Indicators of Increased Risk in UA/NSTEMI

History
Advanced age (>70 yr)
Diabetes mellitus
Post–myocardial infarction angina
Prior peripheral vascular disease
Prior cerebrovascular disease

Clinical Presentation
Braunwald class II or III (acute or subacute rest pain)
Braunwald class B (secondary unstable angina)
Heart failure or hypotension
Multiple episodes of pain within 24 hr

Electrocardiogram
ST-segment deviation ≥0.05 mV
T wave inversion ≥0.3 mV
Left bundle branch block

Cardiac Markers
Increased troponin T or I or creatine kinase–MB
Increased C-reactive protein or white blood cell count
Increased B-type natriuretic peptide
Elevated creatinine
Elevated glucose or hemoglobin A_{1c}

Angiogram
Thrombus
Multivessel disease
Left ventricular dysfunction

UA/NSTEMI = unstable angina/non–ST elevation myocardial infarction.

TABLE 56-3 Emerging Biomarkers in Acute Coronary Syndrome

	POSSIBLE MECHANISM	MAJOR FINDINGS
Markers Predicting the Development of ACS		
von Willebrand factor[1]	Mediates platelet adhesion, aggregation (at high shear stress), and stabilizes factor VIIIc	OR = 3.0 for the 4th quartile compared with 1st quartile in patients developing ACS
Erythrocyte membrane–bound interleukin-8[2]	Increases inflammatory response on release from erythrocyte membrane during intraplaque hemorrhage	1 SD increase was associated with 5.1-fold higher odds of having ACS (compared with chronic stable angina), adjusted for baseline characteristics and other markers
Platelet collagen receptor glycoprotein (GP) VI[3]	Enhances platelet aggregability	Mean fluorescence intensity above the cutoff of >18.6 (i.e., an elevated level of surface expression of GP VI) had a 1.4-fold relative risk for ACS
Platelet-bound stromal cell–derived factor 1[4]	May play a role in vascular and myocardial remodeling or regeneration	1.4-fold higher level in patients with ACS compared with stable angina
Linoleic acid[5]	Varies inversely with low-density lipoprotein Other undefined mechanism	1 SD decrease was associated with a >3-fold increase in the odds of being a case (ACS) compared with controls
Trans isomer of oleic acid[6]	Unfavorable effects on lipid profile, endothelial function, and inflammatory markers	1 SD increase was associated with an OR of 1.2 of being a case (ACS) compared with controls
Markers Predicting Prognosis in Patients with ACS		
Thrombus precursor protein[7]	Reflects enhanced systemic activation of the coagulation system	Elevated levels independently associated with increased risk of death, reMI, or recurrent ischemia (HR, 1.5) and death or MI (HR, 1.6), adjusted for baseline characteristics and other biomarkers
Chromogranin A[8]	Negative inotropy, induction of apoptosis, inhibition of catecholamine secretion, vasodilation	1 SD increase associated with increases in mortality (1.3-fold), CHF hospitalizations (1.2-fold) after adjustment for conventional cardiovascular risk markers
Free plasma homocysteine[9]	Causes endothelial damage and dysfunction	Level >4.11 μmol/liter (highest quintile) was independently associated with increased risk of cardiovascular death, MI, or stroke (HR, 2.3) after a median follow-up of 2.7 years

ACS = acute coronary syndrome; CHF = congestive heart failure; HR = hazard ratio; OR = odds ratio; reMI = recurrent infarction; SD = standard deviation.
From Giugliano RP, Braunwald E: The year in non–ST-segment elevation acute coronary syndrome. J Am Coll Cardiol 54:1544, 2009. See this paper for references in the table.

1,[30a] and interleukin-6. Neopterin, a marker of monocyte activation, has been reported to be an independent predictor of long-term adverse outcomes.[31] Elevated levels of this inflammatory biomarker (as well as of CRP) can be reduced by high doses of potent statins (e.g., 80 mg/daily of atorvastatin or 40 mg/daily of rosuvastatin). These studies, taken together, indicate that inflammation relates to patient instability and to an increased risk of recurrent cardiac events.

WHITE BLOOD CELL COUNT. This is an even simpler, universally available but nonspecific marker of inflammation. Several studies of patients with UA/NSTEMI[32] have reported that patients with elevated white cell counts have a higher risk of mortality and recurrent MI. This association was independent of CRP, suggesting that no one marker, such as CRP, captures all of the information about the influence of inflammation on outcomes.

MYELOPEROXIDASE. Myeloperoxidase (MPO) is a heme protein released during degranulation of neutrophils and some monocytes that generates hypochlorous acid, a potent pro-oxidant. Elevated concentrations in patients presenting with a significantly higher risk of recurrent ACS have associated with increased short-term risk of recurrent ischemic events.[33] Elevations of MPO occur even in coronary arteries remote from the culprit lesion of a UA/NSTEMI episode.[33,34] Thus, leukocyte activation appears to extend beyond a single coronary artery lesion in patients with ACS.

NATRIURETIC PEPTIDES (BNP AND NT-proBNP). B-type natriuretic peptide (BNP) is a neurohormone that is synthesized in ventricular myocardium and is released in response to increased wall stress (see Chap. 25). Its actions include natriuresis, vasodilation, inhibition of sympathetic nerve activity, and inhibition of the renin-angiotensin-aldosterone system. BNP is a useful diagnostic and prognostic marker among patients with heart failure. BNP has prognostic value across the full spectrum of patients with ACS, including those with UA/NSTEMI. In OPUS–TIMI 16, patients with elevated levels of BNP (>80 pg/mL) or NT-proBNP had a twofold to threefold higher risk of death by 10 months,[35] a finding that has been confirmed.[36,37] Together, these data suggest that measurement of natriuretic peptides in patients presenting with UA/NSTEMI adds importantly to current tools for risk stratification.

CREATININE. Another simple tool for risk stratification is the use of creatinine or calculation of creatinine clearance.[38] The risk of impaired renal function appears to be independent of other standard risk factors, such as troponin elevation. Reduced renal function may also play a role in reduced drug clearance, indicating the need for downward adjustment of doses of medications frequently used in the treatment of ACS, such as low-molecular-weight heparin (LMWH) or the small molecule GP IIb/IIIa blockers eptifibatide and tirofiban.

GLUCOSE. Elevated admission values of glucose or hemoglobin A1c predict adverse outcomes among diabetic and nondiabetic patients with acute UA/NSTEMI compared with those without hyperglycemia (see Chap. 64).[39] A synergistic relationship between hyperglycemia and inflammation has also been described.[40] The risk associated with hyperglycemia was amplified in patients with an elevated CRP level compared with a normal one.

THROMBUS PRECURSOR PROTEIN. This soluble fibrin polymer is a precursor to the formation of insoluble fibrin that may be increased in patients with acute MI. A significant correlation between thrombus precursor protein levels and the incidence of adverse clinical outcomes in ACS has been reported.[41]

Combined Risk Assessment Scores

Integrating all of these factors, several groups have developed comprehensive risk scores that use clinical variables and findings from the electrocardiogram or from serum cardiac markers.[42,43] The TIMI risk score identified seven independent risk factors: age >65 years, >3 risk factors for CAD, documented CAD at catheterization, ST deviation >0.5 mm, >2 episodes of angina in last 24 hours, ASA within prior week, and elevated cardiac markers. Use of this scoring system allowed risk stratification of patients across an almost 10-fold gradient of risk, from 4.7% to 40.9% (P < 0.001) (**Fig. 56-6A**). More important, this risk score predicts the response to several of the therapies in UA/NSTEMI. Patients with higher TIMI risk scores had significant reductions in events when treated with enoxaparin compared with unfractionated heparin,[43] with a GP IIb/IIIa inhibitor compared with placebo, and with an invasive versus conservative strategy (Fig. 56-6B).

The Global Registry of Acute Coronary Events (GRACE) has also identified factors that were associated independently with increased mortality; the most important baseline determinants of higher mortality were increased age, Killip class, increased heart rate, ST-segment depression, signs of heart failure, lower systolic pressure, cardiac arrest at presentation, and elevated serum creatinine or cardiac marker enzymes.[44]

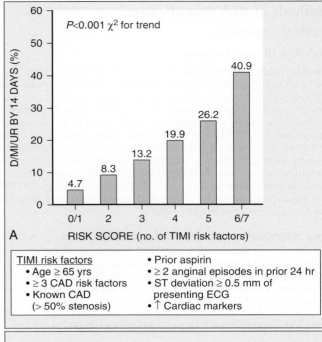

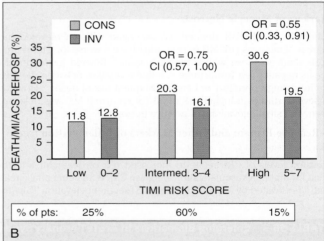

FIGURE 56-6 A, Thrombolysis In Myocardial Ischemia (TIMI) risk score for unstable angina or non–ST elevation myocardial infarction (UA/NSTEMI). The risk factors are shown at the bottom, and the risk of death (D), myocardial infarction (MI), or urgent revascularization (UR) is shown along the vertical axis. **B,** Use of the TIMI risk score for UA/NSTEMI to predict the benefit of an early invasive strategy. In a prospectively defined analysis, the TIMI risk score was applied in the Treat Angina with Aggrastat and determine Cost of Therapy with an Invasive or Conservative Strategy (TACTICS)–TIMI 18 trial. As shown, 75% of patients had a risk score of 3 or higher, and a significant benefit of an invasive strategy was observed in these patients. ACS = acute coronary syndrome; CAD = coronary artery disease; CI = confidence interval; CONS = conservative; ECG = electrocardiogram; INV = invasive; OR = odds ratio. (**A,** modified from Antman EM, Cohen M, Bernink PJLM, et al: The TIMI risk score for unstable angina/non–ST elevation MI: A method for prognostication and therapeutic decision-making. JAMA 284:835, 2000. **B,** data from Cannon CP, Weintraub WS, Demopoulos LA, et al: Comparison of early invasive and conservative strategies in patients with unstable coronary syndromes treated with the glycoprotein IIb/IIIa inhibitor tirofiban. N Engl J Med 344:1879, 2001.)

With the ever-growing number of new cardiac markers, comprehensive risk scores will likely include these new markers as they become more widely available in clinical practice, as shown in several studies using three markers in a "multimarker strategy" evaluation for prediction of mortality[45] or of nonfatal events.[46]

A risk score to predict major bleeding has also been developed from the CRUSADE registry. Patients with worsening creatinine clearance, women, diabetics, patients with lower blood pressure, and patients with higher heart rates had higher rates of bleeding.[47] In addition, when antithrombotic agents were not dose-adjusted for renal function or weight, rates of bleeding were two to three times higher.[48]

Medical Therapy

General Measures

Patients with UA/NSTEMI at medium or high risk should be admitted to an intensive (cardiac) or intermediate care unit; patients at low risk should be admitted to a monitored bed, preferably in a cardiac step-down unit.[2] In these settings, continuous electrocardiographic monitoring (i.e., telemetry) is used to detect tachyarrhythmias, alterations in atrioventricular and intraventricular conduction, and changes in ST-segment deviation. Bed rest should be prescribed initially. Ambulation, as tolerated, is permitted if the patient has been stable without recurrent chest discomfort for at least 12 to 24 hours. It is advisable to provide supplemental oxygen to patients with cyanosis or extensive rales and when arterial oxygen saturation, measured by oximetry, declines below 90%.

Relief of chest pain is an initial goal of treatment. In patients with persistent pain despite therapy with nitrates and beta blockers (see later), morphine sulfate by intravenous bolus in doses of 2 to 5 mg may be administered. Contraindications to morphine include allergy for this drug, for which meperidine can be substituted, and hypotension. With careful blood pressure monitoring, repeated doses can be administered every 5 to 30 minutes. Morphine may act as both an analgesic and an anxiolytic, but its venodilatory effects may produce beneficial hemodynamic effects by reducing ventricular preload, which is especially useful in the presence of pulmonary congestion. However, morphine may also cause hypotension, and if that occurs, supine positioning and intravenous saline should restore blood pressure; pressors are rarely needed. If respiratory depression develops, naloxone (0.4 to 2.0 mg) may be given.

NITRATES. Nitrates are endothelium-independent vasodilators that both increase myocardial blood flow by coronary vasodilation and reduce myocardial oxygen demand. The latter effect results from arteriolar and venous dilation leading to reduced myocardial afterload, preload, and ventricular wall stress. If the patient is experiencing ischemic pain, nitrates should initially be given sublingually or by buccal spray (0.3 to 0.6 mg). If pain persists after three sublingual tablets (or buccal sprays) administered at 5-minute intervals, intravenous nitroglycerin by use of nonabsorbing tubing (5 to 10 μg/min) is recommended. The rate of the nitroglycerin infusion may be increased by 10 μg/min every 3 to 5 minutes until relief of symptoms occurs or systolic blood pressure falls to below 100 mm Hg.[2] Although there is no absolute maximum dose, a dose of 200 μg/min is generally used as a ceiling.

Contraindications to the use of nitrates are hypotension and the use of sildenafil or related phosphodiesterase type 5 inhibitors within the previous 24 to 48 hours. Topical or long-acting oral nitrates can be used if the patient has been pain free for 12 to 24 hours. Dosing of nitrates depends on the formulation, but an attempt should be made to have an 8- to 10-hour nitrate-free interval to avoid the development of tolerance. Chronic nitrate therapy can frequently be tapered in the long-term management of patients unless they develop chronic, stable angina (see Chap. 57).

The effect of nitrates on mortality was evaluated in ISIS-4, a large randomized trial for patients with suspected MI (both STEMI and NSTEMI).[49] No effect on mortality was observed in the overall population or in the subgroup of patients with NSTEMI.

BETA BLOCKERS. Early placebo-controlled trials in UA/NSTEMI demonstrated the benefit of beta blockers in reducing subsequent MI or recurrent ischemia.[46] In patients with acute MI (both STEMI and NSTEMI), beta blockers have also been shown to reduce reinfarction and ventricular fibrillation (see Chap. 57).[50] A reduction in mortality achieved by beta blockers in more recent times (i.e., the 21st century) is less clear.[51]

Oral beta blockers in doses used in chronic stable angina (see Chap. 57) should be begun 24 hours after presentation and should be continued at discharge in patients with UA/NSTEMI who do not have contraindications. Oral beta blocker therapy should be initiated within the first 24 hours for patients who do not have one or more of the following: (1) signs of heart failure, (2) evidence of a low-output state, (3) increased risk for cardiogenic shock, or (4) other relative contraindications to beta blockade (PR interval >0.24 second, second- or third-degree heart block, active asthma, or reactive airway disease). Beta blockers can be administered at low doses to patients with heart failure once they are stabilized. If ischemia and chest pain are ongoing despite intravenous nitrate therapy, intravenous beta blockers may be used cautiously, followed by oral administration. The choice of beta blocker can be individualized on the basis of the drug's pharmacokinetics, cost, and physician familiarity. However, those with intrinsic sympathomimetic activity, such as pindolol, should not be selected.

CALCIUM CHANNEL BLOCKERS. Calcium channel blockers have vasodilatory effects and reduce blood pressure. Some, such as verapamil and diltiazem, also slow heart rate and reduce myocardial contractility. Early studies suggested that they reduce recurrent MI.[52] Calcium antagonists may be used in patients with persistent ischemia despite treatment with full-dose nitrates and beta blockers, in patients with contraindications to beta blockers (see earlier), and in those with hypertension. Such patients should be treated with heart rate–slowing calcium channel blockers (e.g., diltiazem or verapamil). Oral doses of diltiazem and verapamil range from 30 to 90 mg four times daily to 360 mg once daily of the long-acting preparation. Nifedipine (short acting), which accelerates heart rate, has been shown to be harmful in patients with acute MI when it is not coadministered with a beta blocker. No harm with long-term treatment with the long-acting drugs (amlodipine and felodipine) was observed in patients with documented left ventricular dysfunction and CAD,[53] indicating that these agents may be safely used in patients with UA/NSTEMI with left ventricular dysfunction. In addition, two recent trials documented the benefit of amlodipine in patients with hypertension and stable CAD.[54,55]

Antithrombotic Therapy (see Chap. 87)

ANTIPLATELET AGENTS. The importance of platelets in the pathogenesis of UA/NSTEMI was discussed earlier. Accordingly, antiplatelet therapy plays a central role in management.

Aspirin (ASA)

This drug acetylates platelet cyclooxygenase 1 (COX-1), thereby blocking the synthesis and release of thromboxane A_2, a platelet activator (**Fig. 56-7**). ASA thereby decreases overall platelet aggregation and arterial thrombus formation. Because this inhibition of COX-1 is irreversible, the antiplatelet effects last for the lifetime of the platelets, approximately 7 to 10 days. Several trials have demonstrated clear beneficial effects of ASA in patients with UA/NSTEMI[56] (**Fig. 56-8**). In addition to reducing adverse clinical events early in the course of treatment of UA/NSTEMI, ASA also prevents recurrence of ischemic events in secondary prevention.

In the randomized trials of ASA versus placebo, the dose of aspirin ranged from 75 mg/day to 1300 mg/day, and each trial showed an approximately 25% reduction in death or MI.[56] Thus, there does not appear to be a dose-response in the efficacy of aspirin.[57] In the case of patients with UA/NSTEMI, after an initial loading dose of 162 to 325 mg, doses of 75 or 81 mg daily appear to be efficacious and cause less gastrointestinal irritation or bleeding than higher doses. The OASIS-7 trial randomized 25,087 ACS patients (UA/NSTEMI, 70.8%; STEMI, 29.2%) to receive high-dose (300 to 325 mg/day) versus low-dose (75 to 100 mg/day) aspirin for 30 days (and to high-dose versus regular-dose clopidogrel; see later). Preliminary results found no difference in the risk of cardiovascular death, MI, or stroke, and no difference in the overall rate of major bleeding—2.3% in each group. More complete analysis of this short-term comparison of aspirin dosing will be needed.

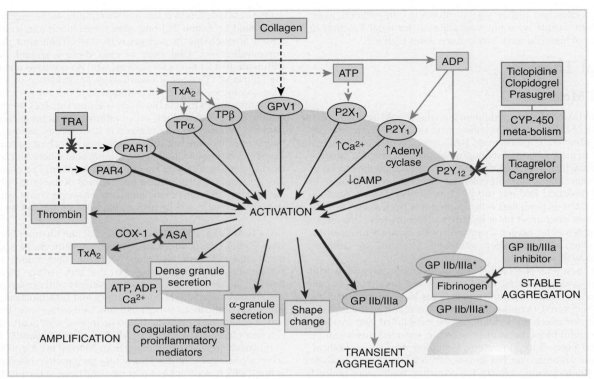

FIGURE 56-7 Platelet activation mechanisms and sites of blockade of antiplatelet therapies. Platelet activation is initiated by soluble agonists, such as thrombin, thromboxane A$_2$, 5HT, ADP (via P2Y$_1$), and ATP, and by adhesive ligands, such as collagen and von Willebrand factor. Consequently, dense granule secretion of platelet agonists and secretion of thromboxane A$_2$ (as a result of phospholipase A$_2$ activation) lead to amplification of platelet activation and the associated responses. The P2Y$_{12}$ receptor plays a major role in the amplification of platelet activation, supported also by outside-in signaling via the $\alpha_{IIb}\beta_3$ (GP IIb/IIIa) receptor. Combined P2Y$_{12}$ and $\alpha_{IIb}\beta_3$ blockade, therefore, has additive effects on platelet activation and the associated platelet responses. See text for details. ADP = adenosine; cAMP = cyclic adenosine monophosphate; COX = cyclooxygenase diphosphate; GP = glycoprotein; TxA$_2$ = thromboxane A$_2$. (*Modified after Storey RF: Biology and pharmacology of the platelet P2Y$_{12}$ receptor. Curr Pharm Des 12:1255, 2006. From Wallentin L: P2Y$_{12}$ inhibitors: Differences in properties and mechanisms of action and potential consequences for clinical use. Eur Heart J 30:1964, 2009, with permission.*)

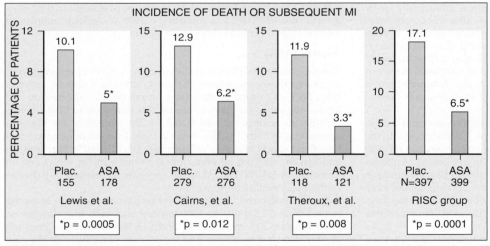

FIGURE 56-8 Four randomized trials showing the benefit of aspirin in UA/NSTEMI, in which the incidence of death or MI was reduced by more than 50% in each of the four trials. The doses of aspirin in the four trials were 325 mg, 1300 mg, 650 mg, and 75 mg daily, indicating no difference in efficacy for aspirin across these doses. ASA = aspirin; Plac. = placebo. (*Data from Lewis HD, et al: N Engl J Med 309:396, 1983; Cairns JA, et al: N Engl J Med 313:1369, 1985; Theroux P, et al: N Engl J Med 319:1105, 1988; RISC Group: Lancet 349:827, 1990.*)

In patients who have an allergy or who cannot tolerate aspirin, clopidogrel is recommended.[2]

"Aspirin resistance" may occur during chronic therapy.[58,59] Small studies have identified 2% to 8% of patients in whom treatment with ASA appears to have a limited antiplatelet effect (i.e., minimal change in the degree of platelet aggregation). These patients tend to have a greater risk of recurrent cardiac events.[60] There is increasing evidence that so-called aspirin resistance is often related to poor compliance. Other causes include poor absorption, interaction with ibuprofen, and overexpression of COX-2 mRNA. Whether routine monitoring of antiplatelet effects by light transmission aggregometry or point-of-care devices with adjustment of dose is an effective strategy has not been evaluated in large trials or registries, but such monitoring would seem to be a potentially useful approach.

Contraindications to ASA therapy include documented allergy (e.g., asthma), active bleeding, and a known platelet disorder. Dyspepsia and other gastrointestinal symptoms with long-term ASA therapy (i.e., aspirin intolerance) do not usually preclude therapy in the short term.

ADP ANTAGONISTS

Thienopyridines

These agents (ticlopidine, clopidogrel, and prasugrel) are prodrugs that are converted to active metabolites through oxidation by the

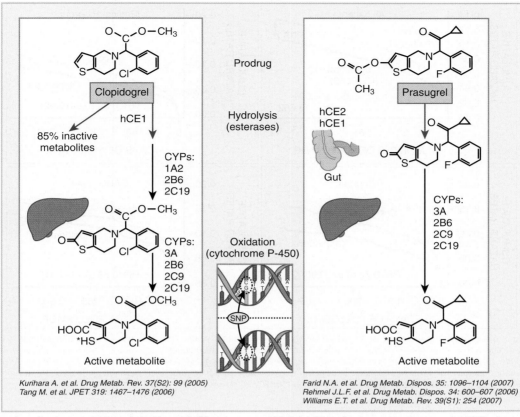

FIGURE 56-9   Formation of active metabolites of clopidogrel **(left)** and prasugrel **(right)**. hCE 1 = human carboxylesterase 1; hCE 2 = human carboxylesterase 2; CYP = cytochrome P-450 enzyme. *(Courtesy of Dr. E. Antman.)*

hepatic cytochrome P-450 system[61] (**Fig. 56-9**). The active metabolites inhibit platelet aggregation by inhibiting irreversibly the binding of adenosine diphosphate (ADP) to platelet $P2Y_{12}$ receptors and increase bleeding time (see Fig. 56-7).

CLOPIDOGREL.   This drug largely avoids the hematologic complications associated with ticlopidine, the first thienopyridine agent that was widely used. Ticlopidine is now rarely prescribed because of the occasional development of neutropenia or, even less commonly, thrombotic thrombocytopenic purpura. The combination of clopidogrel and aspirin appears to be as effective as ticlopidine and aspirin in preventing stent thrombosis.[57] When clopidogrel is absorbed, approximately 85% is hydrolyzed by esterases in the bloodstream and is rendered inactive. The remaining clopidogrel must be oxidized by the hepatic cytochrome P-450 system to generate the active metabolites that block the $P2Y_{12}$ receptor (see Fig. 56-9).

The addition of clopidogrel to aspirin was studied in the CURE trial of 12,562 patients with UA/NSTEMI, in which patients were treated with ASA (75 to 325 mg), unfractionated or low-molecular weight heparin, and other standard therapies and were randomized to receive a 300-mg loading dose of clopidogrel followed by 75 mg daily or placebo.[62] The combination of clopidogrel and ASA, referred to as dual antiplatelet therapy, conferred a 20% reduction in cardiovascular death, MI, or stroke compared with aspirin alone, in both low- and high-risk patients with UA/NSTEMI and whether patients were managed with medical therapy, percutaneous coronary intervention (PCI), or coronary bypass grafting (CABG) (**Fig. 56-10**).[62] Benefit was seen as early as 24 hours, with the Kaplan-Meier curves beginning to diverge after just 2 hours.[63] Moreover, the benefit continued throughout the trial's 1-year treatment period. Benefit of treatment *before* PCI was also seen, with a 31% reduction in cardiac events at 30 days and 1 year in UA/NSTEMI patients randomized to dual antiplatelet therapy, compared with ASA alone. [64]

In a meta-analysis of three trials, pretreatment with clopidogrel was associated with a significant 29% reduction in cardiovascular death or MI after PCI compared with no pretreatment. These benefits of clopidogrel

accrued with or without the concomitant use of GP IIb/IIIa inhibitors.[65] This led to a Class IA recommendation in the ACC/AHA Guidelines for clopidogrel treatment before PCI.[66] This recommendation supports the benefit of initiating clopidogrel as soon as possible after presentation.

For patients undergoing CABG, those who had received clopidogrel within 5 days of surgery had an increased risk of major bleeding and the need for reoperation secondary to bleeding and longer length of stay in the hospital,[67] leading to the recommendation that clopidogrel be discontinued at least 5 days before surgery, if possible.[2]

Two prevailing strategies for initiation of clopidogrel therapy in patients with UA/NSTEMI have evolved: (1) to start clopidogrel at the time of presentation or of hospital admission and (2) to delay treatment with clopidogrel until after coronary angiography and then to administer the drug on the catheterization table if PCI is carried out. The early treatment strategy affords the benefits of reducing early ischemic events and providing the benefit from pretreatment before PCI, but at the cost of an increase in bleeding in the patients who undergo CABG instead of or immediately after PCI. Thus, although a bleeding risk exists if early CABG cannot be deferred, the overall benefit-to-risk ratio still favors the strategy of early initiation of clopidogrel.[68]

In UA/NSTEMI, the initial loading dose of 300 to 600 mg clopidogrel is followed by a maintenance dose of 75 mg/day. Initiation with only 75 mg daily will achieve the target level of platelet inhibition after 3 to 5 days, whereas the loading dose of 300 mg will achieve effective platelet inhibition within 4 to 6 hours.[69] Use of a 600-mg loading dose achieves a steady-state level of platelet inhibition after just 2 hours. Several PCI trials have used this dose, including one direct comparison of 300 mg versus 600 mg. In this study of 254 patients undergoing PCI, pretreated 4 to 8 hours before the procedure, the 600-mg loading dose was associated with a significantly lower rate of major cardiovascular events.[70]

The OASIS-7 trial randomized 25,087 ACS patients with an intent for an invasive strategy to high-dose versus low-dose aspirin (see earlier)

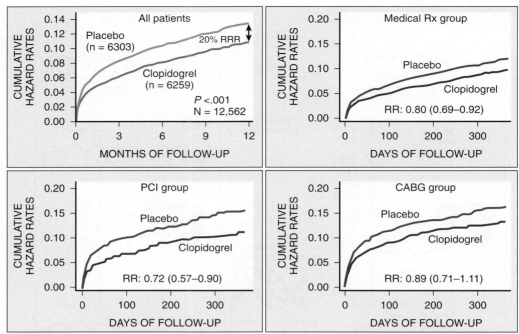

FIGURE 56-10 Benefit of clopidogrel in reducing cardiovascular death, MI, or stroke to 1 year in the CURE trial conducted in patients with UA/NSTEMI and in patients managed medically, with PCI or CABG. RR = risk ratio; RRR = relative risk reduction. *(Reproduced from Yusuf S, Zhao F, Mehta SR, et al: Effects of clopidogrel in addition to aspirin in patients with acute coronary syndromes without ST-segment elevation. N Engl J Med 345:494, 2001; and Fox KA, Mehta SR, Peters R, et al: Benefits and risks of the combination of clopidogrel and aspirin in patients undergoing surgical revascularization for non–ST-elevation acute coronary syndrome: The Clopidogrel in Unstable angina to prevent Recurrent ischemic Events [CURE] Trial. Circulation 110:1202, 2004.)*

and to two doses of clopidogrel for 1 week: high dose (600 mg loading dose and 150 mg/day for 1 week) versus standard dose (300 mg loading dose and 75 mg/day) followed by 75 mg/day for 30 days. Preliminary results found no difference in the trial as a whole in the risk of cardiovascular death, MI, or stroke (4.2% for high-dose and 4.4% for standard-dose clopidogrel). But there was a statistical interaction noted between the aspirin and clopidogrel randomization strata (*P* = 0.043), meaning that one should evaluate the four groups separately. In the high-dose aspirin group, the primary efficacy event rate was lower in the high-dose clopidogrel group than in the standard-dose clopidogrel group (4.6% versus 3.8%; RR, 0.83; 95% CI, 0.70-0.99; *P* = 0.036). But there was no difference between the high-dose clopidogrel group and the standard-dose group in the low-dose aspirin cohort. Overall, there was a higher risk of major bleeding according to the trial definition in the high-dose versus standard-dose clopidogrel group (2.0% versus 2.5%; *P* = 0.01). These data can be judged in two ways—supportive of the use of higher doses of clopidogrel for 1 week and of aspirin for 1 month, but more complete analysis of the trial data will be needed.[71]

Nonresponders or hyporesponders to clopidogrel have been identified in several studies.[72-74] Hyporesponsiveness to clopidogrel is more common among diabetics as well as in patients with obesity, advanced age, and a genetic polymorphism of the cytochrome P-450 system (see later).[75] Clopidogrel hyporesponders have lower concentrations of the active metabolite, indicating a failure of this necessary conversion. However, when the active metabolite of clopidogrel was added to platelets ex vivo, the platelet response was similar in normal and hyporesponsive subjects, indicating that the defect in hyporesponders is related to the lower concentration of the clopidogrel active metabolite in vivo.[73]

Hyporesponders have higher rates of recurrent cardiac events, including stent thrombosis and acute MI.[76-78] Some investigators are testing a strategy of checking platelet response by platelet aggregometry or bedside testing and increasing the dose of clopidogrel in nonresponders or hyporesponders, an approach that was suggested in the 2005 ACC/AHA Guidelines for high-risk PCI procedures.[66] However, the

outcomes in patients managed with this strategy are not yet available.

Patients with hyporesponsiveness to clopidogrel may be managed by increasing the maintenance dose of clopidogrel to 150 mg/daily, switching to prasugrel 10 mg/day (see later),[79] or potentially by adding cilostazol, a selective phosphodiesterase inhibitor.[80]

As already pointed out, thienopyridines must undergo biotransformation into active metabolites by cytochrome P-450 enzymes, and it is these active metabolites that exert their antiplatelet effect.[61] Alleles of genes that interfere with this biotransformation can interfere with P2Y$_{12}$ blockade. The enzyme CYP2C19 is important in this biotransformation. Polymorphisms in CYP2C19 occur in approximately one third of whites and appear to be more frequent in Asians. These polymorphisms, especially the *C2 allele, a "reduced-function allele," interfere with clopidogrel-induced inhibition of platelet aggregation and are associated with an increase in adverse clinical outcomes in patients treated with clopidogrel in the TRITON–TIMI 38 trial[81] (**Fig. 56-11**). In other studies, this polymorphism was associated with an increase in stent thrombosis.[82-85] The presence of this reduced-function allele in approximately 30% of whites and 50% of Asians explains, at least in part, the hyporesponsiveness to clopidogrel discussed before. It reduces the concentration of the active metabolite and therefore impairs the inhibition of platelet aggregation.

Testing for these polymorphisms in patients who are candidates for thienopyridine treatment can identify patients who are likely to be unresponsive or hyporesponsive to clopidogrel and are candidates for the replacement by prasugrel or ticagrelor when the latter becomes available (see following). Common functional CYP genetic variants do not affect active drug metabolite levels, inhibition of platelet aggregation, or clinical cardiovascular event rates in patients treated with prasugrel.[86]

PRASUGREL. This thienopyridine, like ticlopidine or clopidogrel, is a prodrug whose active metabolite is an irreversible inhibitor of the platelet P2Y$_{12}$ receptor, and thereby of platelet aggregation. Although the biologic efficacies of the active metabolites of clopidogrel and

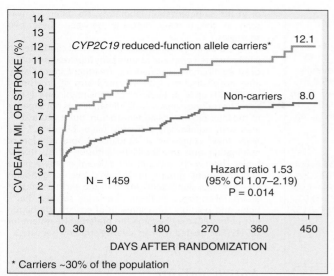

FIGURE 56-11 Association between status as a carrier of a CYP2C19 reduced-function allele and the primary efficacy outcome or stent thrombosis in subjects receiving clopidogrel. Among 1459 subjects who were treated with clopidogrel and could be classified as CYP2C19 carriers or noncarriers, the rate of the primary efficacy outcome (a composite of death from cardiovascular [CV] causes, myocardial infarction [MI], or stroke) was significantly higher among carriers compared with noncarriers.

prasugrel studied in vitro exert equal antiplatelet effects, the generation of the prasugrel metabolite is approximately 10 times as great as with clopidogrel administration, resulting in a roughly 10 times greater potency.

The TRITON–TIMI 38 trial randomized 13,608 patients with ACS (10,074 with UA/NSTEMI) in whom PCI was planned.[79] The loading dose of prasugrel was 60 mg, followed by a 10-mg daily maintenance dose. The loading dose of clopidogrel was 300 mg, followed by a maintenance dose of 75 mg daily with a follow-up of 15 months. The primary efficacy endpoint (cardiovascular death, MI, and stroke) was reduced significantly by 19% (**Fig. 56-12**); 12,844 patients received coronary stents at the time of the PCI. In the prasugrel group, the incidence of stent thromboses was reduced in half compared with clopidogrel[79] (see Fig. 56-12). This relative reduction of stent thrombosis was similar with bare metal and drug-eluting stents.[87]

These findings of the superiority of prasugrel to clopidogrel are consistent with the aforementioned concept that the limited efficacy of clopidogrel compared with prasugrel is relative to the slower and less effective generation of the active metabolite of clopidogrel[81] (see Fig. 56-9). Indeed, in a crossover study in patients undergoing PCI for stable angina, Wiviott and colleagues[74] reported that loading with 60 mg of prasugrel resulted in greater platelet inhibition than with a 600-mg clopidogrel loading dose. The same was observed during maintenance therapy, in which the comparison was made between 10 mg and 150 mg daily, respectively.

Not surprisingly, the greater platelet inhibitory effect of prasugrel was associated with more common serious bleeding. In TRITON–TIMI 38, there was a 32% higher relative incidence of serious, including fatal, bleeding. The risk of bleeding was especially higher in the elderly (≥75 years), in whom the use of prasugrel should be limited to those at high risk, and in those with reduced body weight (<60 kg, 132 pounds). It is advisable to avoid treating the latter with prasugrel unless they are at high risk of thrombosis. Consider treating them with a 5-mg instead of a 10-mg maintenance dose. Prasugrel is contraindicated in patients with a history of stroke or a transient ischemic attack.[79] Prasugrel should be discontinued at least a week before surgery whenever possible.

Ticagrelor

In contrast to the thienopyridines (ticlopidine, clopidogrel, and prasugrel), whose active metabolites are irreversible platelet inhibitors,

ticagrelor* is a *reversible* blocker of the P2Y$_{12}$ platelet receptor that acts directly on the platelet.[88,89] Although it has an active metabolite, its potency is similar to that of the parent drug; both are excreted into the bile. Like prasugrel, ticagrelor can inhibit P2Y$_{12}$-mediated platelet aggregation almost completely. The DISPERSE-2 trial was a phase II dose-ranging trial[90] and led to the phase III pivotal trial (PLATO) that compared the combination of ticagrelor (90 mg twice daily) and clopidogrel (300 or 600 mg loading dose and 75 mg daily maintenance dose); both groups also received ASA. PLATO enrolled 18,624 patients, 15,381 (62%) of whom had UA/NSTEMI.[91] The primary endpoint, a composite of cardiovascular death, MI, and stroke, was reduced significantly by 16% (**Fig. 56-13**). There were also significant 16% reductions in MI, 21% in cardiovascular death, and 22% relative (1.4% absolute) reduction in total mortality. The greater clinical efficacy of ticagrelor was observed across a broad array of subgroups, including patients who had previously received clopidogrel, patients treated with a noninvasive strategy, and patients with STEMI.

There was no difference with ticagrelor in total *major* bleeding, but a significantly higher 19% occurrence of non-CABG major bleeding (*P* = 0.03) and an 11% significant increase in major plus minor bleeding. Episodes of dyspnea and ventricular pauses exceeding 5 seconds occurred more frequently in the ticagrelor-treated patients than in the clopidogrel-treated patients.

The PLATO investigators calculated that if 1000 hospitalized patients with ACS treated with ticagrelor and ASA were compared with a similar group treated with clopidogrel and ASA, there would be 14 fewer deaths, 11 fewer MIs, and 6 to 8 fewer cases of stent thrombosis, with 9 patients switching to a thienopyridine because of dyspnea. Because ticagrelor is a reversible agent, this agent could be started at the time of presentation to the emergency department and continued for medically managed patients or those undergoing PCI; but if necessary, it could be stopped and CABG could be carried out 48 to 72 hours later.

GLYCOPROTEIN IIb/IIIa INHIBITORS. These drugs block the final common pathway of platelet aggregation, the fibrinogen-mediated cross-linkage of platelets (see Fig. 56-7). GP IIb/IIIa blockers interfere with platelet aggregation caused by all types of stimuli (e.g., thrombin, ADP, collagen, serotonin). Three agents of this class are currently available—abciximab, a monoclonal antibody, approved only in patients undergoing PCI, and eptifibatide and tirofiban (small molecule inhibitors). Each of these three agents is administered by intravenous bolus followed by continuous infusion. The receptor-blocking activity of the small molecule receptor blockers and the accompanying bleeding risk subside promptly after discontinuation of the infusion.

Several trials have shown benefit of GP IIb/IIIa inhibition in the management of patients with UA/NSTEMI.[92] Tirofiban plus heparin and ASA significantly reduced the rate of death, MI, or refractory ischemia at 7 days compared with heparin plus ASA. In a trial involving 10,948 patients, eptifibatide also reduced significantly the rate of death or MI at 30 days. However, no benefit and a higher early mortality were found with the use of abciximab in UA/NSTEMI patients for whom an early conservative strategy was planned. Overall, in the meta-analysis, the benefit of GP IIb/IIIa inhibition was a significant 9% relative reduction in death or MI at 30 days.[92]

Risk Stratification to Target GP IIb/IIIa Inhibitors

The benefit of GP IIb/IIIa inhibition appears greater in high-risk patients with UA/NSTEMI, such as those with ST-segment changes, those with elevated troponin concentrations, and diabetics.[93,94] These subgroups have more thrombus at coronary angiography and thus are at higher risk for microvascular embolization. The benefit of GP IIb/IIIa inhibition has been confirmed even on a background of clopidogrel pretreatment[93] and was seen in high-risk patients with or without revascularization.

---

*Not marketed in the United States at the time of writing.

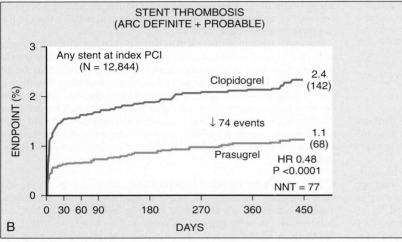

FIGURE 56-12 A, Comparison of efficacy (top) and safety (bottom) in the TRITON–TIMI 38 trial, which compared prasugrel with clopidogrel in patients with ACS undergoing PCI. HR = hazard ratio; NNH = number of patients needed to be treated to cause harm (TIMI major bleed); NNT = number of patients needed to prevent one primary endpoint event. *(From Wiviott SD, Braunwald E, McCabe CH, et al: Prasugrel versus clopidogrel in patients with acute coronary syndromes. N Engl J Med 357:2001, 2007.)* **B,** Comparison of prasugrel and clopidogrel on the development of stent thrombosis. ARC = Academic Research Consortium. *(Modified from Wiviott SD, Braunwald E, McCabe CH, et al: Intensive oral antiplatelet therapy for reduction of ischaemic events including stent thrombosis in patients with acute coronary syndromes treated with percutaneous coronary intervention and stenting in the TRITON–TIMI 38 trial: A subanalysis of a randomised trial. Lancet 371:1356, 2008.)*

Safety

In a meta-analysis of placebo-controlled trials, the rates of major hemorrhage were significantly higher for patients treated with GP IIb/IIIa inhibitors, occurring in 2.4% compared with 1.4% for placebo.[92] The rate of severe thrombocytopenia (<50,000/mm³) was approximately 0.5% in patients treated with a GP IIb/IIIa inhibitor and heparin, versus 0.3% in those receiving heparin alone. Thrombocytopenia was associated with both increased bleeding and recurrent thrombotic events and indicates a need to monitor platelet count daily during the GP IIb/IIIa infusion.

TIMING OF GP IIb/IIIa INHIBITION. Opinion is divided on the optimal timing of the administration of GP IIb/IIIa inhibitors. Some advocate starting these drugs at the time of presentation, whereas others reserve it for use during PCI. The ACC/AHA Guidelines have indicated that either strategy is acceptable.[2]

Three trials have examined the timing of GP IIb/IIIa inhibitors. The Acute Catheterization and Urgent Intervention Triage Strategy (ACUITY) trial randomized patients to treatment with a GP IIb/IIIa inhibitor (eptifibatide or tirofiban) either in the emergency department

or in the catheterization laboratory. No difference was seen in the primary outcome between these two strategies.[95]

The EARLY ACS trial, a double-blind trial conducted in 9492 patients, compared routine early (upstream) double-dose eptifibatide, commencing treatment immediately after hospitalization, with a control arm of provisional eptifibatide given just before PCI at the physician's discretion. The routine early use of eptifibatide was not superior to the later provisional administration, but it was associated with significantly increased major bleeding.[94] The BRIEF trial[96] compared a standard 18-hour infusion of eptifibatide with an abbreviated infusion of less than 2 hours. There were no significant differences between the two treatment groups in ischemic events, although bleeding was significantly lower in the shorter infusion group. Taken together, these three trials suggest that a bolus and possibly short infusion of eptifibatide begun just before PCI may become the preferred treatment for UA/NSTEMI treated with an invasive strategy (see later).

Anticoagulants

In addition to antiplatelet therapy, as described earlier, an anticoagulant should be added in patients with UA/NSTEMI as soon as possible after presentation.

HEPARIN. Anticoagulation, traditionally with unfractionated heparin (UFH), has been a cornerstone of therapy for patients with UA/NSTEMI.[97] A meta-analysis showed a 33% reduction in death or MI comparing UFH plus aspirin to aspirin alone.[98] Variability in the anticoagulant effects of UFH, which is common, is thought to result from the heterogeneity of UFH and the neutralization of heparin by circulating plasma factors and by proteins released by activated platelets.[99] Monitoring of the anticoagulant response by activated partial thromboplastin time (APTT) is recommended with titrations made according to a standardized nomogram, aiming for an APTT of 50 to 70 seconds or 1.5 to 2.5 times control (**Table 56-4**). On the basis of available data, the ACC/AHA Guidelines[2] recommend a weight-adjusted dose of UFH (60 units/kg bolus and 12 units/kg/hr infusion) as well as frequent monitoring of APTT (every 6 hours until the target range is reached and every 12 to 24 hours thereafter) and adjustment of dose if necessary. Adverse effects include bleeding, especially when APTT is elevated, and heparin-induced thrombocytopenia, which is more common with longer durations of treatment (see Chap. 87).[100]

Low-Molecular-Weight Heparin

These forms of heparin have been tested widely as a means of improving anticoagulation with UFH. LMWHs combine inhibition of factors IIa and Xa and have several potential advantages over UFH: (1) their greater anti–factor Xa activity inhibits thrombin generation more effectively; (2) LMWH also induces a greater release of tissue factor pathway inhibitor than does UFH, and it is not neutralized by platelet factor 4[101]; (3) LMWH causes thrombocytopenia at a lower rate than does UFH[100]; (4) the high bioavailability of LMWH allows subcutaneous administration; and (5) LMWH binds less avidly than UFH to plasma proteins and therefore has a more consistent anticoagulant effect. Monitoring of the level of anticoagulation is not necessary. However, in the event of bleeding, the anticoagulant effect of LMWH can be reversed less effectively with protamine than that of UFH. Also, LMWHs are more affected by renal dysfunction than UFH is, and the dose should be reduced in patients with a creatinine clearance <30 mL/min. The standard dose of enoxaparin is 1 mg/kg subcutaneously every 12 hours, with dosing only once daily for patients with a creatinine clearance <30 mL/min.

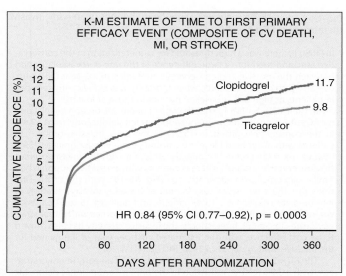

FIGURE 56-13 The primary endpoint of the PLATO trial—a composite of death from cardiovascular (CV) causes, myocardial infarction (MI), or stroke—occurred significantly less often in the ticagrelor group than in the clopidogrel group (9.8% versus 11.7% at 12 months; HR, 0.84; 95% CI, 0.77 to 0.92; P < 0.001). K-M = Kaplan-Meier; HR = hazard ratio; CI = confidence interval. (From Wallentin L, Becker R, Budaj A, et al: Ticagrelor versus clopidogrel in patients with acute coronary syndromes. N Engl J Med 361:1045, 2009.)

TABLE 56-4	**Standardized Nomogram for Titration of Heparin***	
APTT (SEC)†	**CHANGE**	**IV INFUSION (UNITS/KG/HR)**
<35	70 units/kg bolus	+3
35-49	35 units/kg bolus	+2
50-70	0	0
71-90	0	−2
>100	Hold infusion for 30 min	−3

*Initial dose: 60 units/kg bolus and 12 units/kg/hr infusion.
†Activated partial thromboplastin time (APTT) should be checked and infusion adjusted at 6, 12, and 24 hours after initiation of heparin, daily thereafter, and 4 to 6 hours after any adjustment in dose.
From Becker RC, Ball SP, Eisenberg P, et al: A randomized, multicenter trial of weight-adjusted intravenous heparin dose titration and point-of-care coagulation monitoring in hospitalized patients with active thromboembolic disease. Am Heart J 137:59, 1999.

LMWH, when added to ASA, has proved to be effective compared with ASA alone, leading to a 66% reduction in the odds of death or MI.[98] Early trials with enoxaparin showed a 20% reduction in death, MI, or recurrent ischemia compared with UFH.[102] In two more recent trials, enoxaparin was found to be noninferior to UFH.[103,104] In a meta-analysis of all trials in ACS, enoxaparin yielded a statistically significant 16% reduction in the odds of death or MI at 30 days.[102] Enoxaparin provides significant benefit over UFH in patients with UA/NSTEMI who are managed conservatively and who typically receive UFH or LMWH for at least 48 hours, but not in patients managed invasively who are taken to the catheterization laboratory within 24 hours.[105] Treatment with enoxaparin was associated with an excess of major bleeding compared with UFH.[102] Although several LMWHs have been approved, the weight of evidence supports the choice of enoxaparin.[2]

FONDAPARINUX. Fondaparinux, a synthetic pentasaccharide, is an *indirect* factor Xa inhibitor and requires the presence of antithrombin for its action. The OASIS-5 trial compared fondaparinux, administered at a relatively low dose (2.5 mg subcutaneously once daily) with standard-dose enoxaparin in 20,078 patients with high-risk UA/NSTEMI.

The rates of death, MI, or refractory ischemia throughout the first 9 days were similar.[106] Of importance, however, the rate of major bleeding was reduced significantly—almost by half—in the fondaparinux arm (2.2% versus 4.1%). By 30 days, mortality was significantly lower in the fondaparinux arm (2.9% versus 3.5%). However, in patients undergoing PCI, fondaparinux has associated with more than a three-fold increased risk of catheter-related thrombi, a complication also observed in STEMI patients treated with fondaparinux.[107] Supplemental UFH at the time of catheterization appeared to minimize the risk of this problem with fondaparinux. Thus, fondaparinux is an alternative for patients with UA/NSTEMI. It is associated with a lower risk of bleeding and is recommended, in particular, in patients at a higher risk of bleeding.[2]

DIRECT THROMBIN INHIBITORS. Direct thrombin inhibitors have a potential advantage over indirect thrombin inhibitors, such as UFH, LMWH, and fondaparinux, in that they do not require antithrombin and can inhibit clot-bound thrombin. They do not interact with plasma proteins, provide a stable level of anticoagulation, and do not cause thrombocytopenia. A meta-analysis of all direct thrombin inhibitors, including hirudin, bivalirudin, argatroban, efegatran, or inogatran, showed a modest 9% reduction in death or MI at 30 days, favoring the direct thrombin inhibitor over unfractionated heparin.[108] The only current indication approved by the Food and Drug Administration for lepirudin and argatroban is for anticoagulation in patients with heparin-induced thrombocytopenia and associated thromboembolic disease.

Bivalirudin binds reversibly to thrombin. The open-label ACUITY trial randomized 13,819 patients with UA/NSTEMI managed with an early invasive strategy to one of three treatments: (1) UFH or enoxaparin with or without a GP IIb/IIIa inhibitor, (2) bivalirudin with a GP IIb/IIIa inhibitor, and (3) bivalirudin alone. The primary endpoint was the composite of death, MI, unplanned revascularization for ischemia, and major bleeding at 30 days.[109] No differences were observed for efficacy or major bleeding in the direct comparison of the anticoagulants, that is, between UFH or enoxaparin plus a GP IIb/IIIa inhibitor and bivalirudin plus a GP IIb/IIIa inhibitor. For the bivalirudin-alone group, compared with the group receiving UFH or enoxaparin plus a GP IIb/IIIa inhibitor, there were no differences in efficacy but a significantly lower rate of bleeding (3.0% versus 5.7%).[109] Thus, the substitution of bivalirudin for UFH or enoxaparin as the anticoagulant among patients receiving supplemental GP IIb/IIIa inhibitors did not change efficacy or safety outcomes, but the strategy of bivalirudin alone (i.e., without a GP IIb/IIIa inhibitor) was associated with less bleeding than the combination of a GP IIb/IIIa inhibitor with either UFH or enoxaparin. The ISAR–REACT 3[110] trial compared UFH and bivalirudin in patients who had received 600 mg of clopidogrel. The reduced rate of major bleeding with bivalirudin was largely offset by an increase in ischemic events.

ORAL ANTICOAGULATION. Several trials have examined oral anticoagulation with warfarin after ACS, with the rationale that prolonged treatment might extend the benefit of early anticoagulation with a parenteral antithrombin agent. They have suggested that if a sufficient degree of anticoagulation were achieved, a benefit accrued from the combination of ASA plus warfarin.[111,112] In the WARIS trial, patients with ACS within the prior 8 weeks were randomized to warfarin alone (target international normalized ratio [INR] of 2.8 to 4.2), ASA alone (160 mg daily), or aspirin (80 mg daily) combined with warfarin (target INR of 2.0).[111] During a follow-up of 4 years, the rate of death, MI, or thromboembolic stroke occurred in 20% of patients receiving ASA alone, 16.7% of patients receiving warfarin alone (P = 0.03), and 15% of patients receiving warfarin and ASA (P = 0.001). Rates of major bleeding were 0.62% per treatment-year in both groups receiving warfarin and 0.17% in patients receiving ASA (P < 0.001). Thus, the combination of ASA plus warfarin was more effective than aspirin alone for long-term secondary prevention but was associated with increased serious bleeding.

However, given the similar benefits seen with clopidogrel and warfarin added to ASA, the lack of need for monitoring of the INR, and the frequent use of PCI and stenting in the patient population in whom the need for clopidogrel is well established, the clinical use of ASA and warfarin has been limited. Among patients *without a coronary stent* but with another indication for warfarin, such as chronic atrial fibrillation or severe left ventricular dysfunction, who are at high risk of systemic embolization, the combination of ASA and warfarin would be preferable as the long-term antithrombotic strategy. The combination of all three agents (ASA, clopidogrel, and warfarin) has not been tested prospectively to date, but it may be associated with a high bleeding risk during long-term therapy. Use of this combination is sometimes required in UA/NSTEMI patients after stenting with atrial fibrillation or other strong indications for warfarin. In such patients, it is recommended to use low-dose aspirin (75 to 81 mg daily), warfarin (titrated meticulously to an INR of 2.0 to 2.5), and clopidogrel for as short a time as recommended for the type of stent placed.[2]

FACTOR XA INHIBITORS. Two potent oral direct factor Xa inhibitors with a high bioavailability are undergoing phase III testing. In the ATLAS ACS–TIMI 46 trial, a phase II dose-finding study with rivaroxaban, the addition of this drug to ASA in patients with recent ACS[113] was associated with a significant 31% reduction of the hard endpoints of death, MI, and stroke, but a significant increase in bleeding. In the APPRAISE trial, carried out with apixaban (a factor Xa inhibitor with properties similar to those of rivaroxaban), a dose-related increase in bleeding and a trend to a reduction in ischemic events were observed.[114] In both trials, the reduction of ischemic events trended to be greater with the ASA plus a factor Xa inhibitor combination, whereas bleeding was higher in the group receiving triple therapy (ASA, clopidogrel, and factor Xa inhibitor).

Ongoing phase III trials will help in the elucidation of the clinical role of this therapeutic class.

PROTEASE-ACTIVATED RECEPTOR (PAR-1) ANTAGONISTS. Thrombin potently stimulates platelets by activating PAR-1. The thrombin receptor blocker Vorapaxar blocks this interaction.[115-117] This thrombin receptor antagonist was tested in a phase II trial of patients undergoing PCI, in whom it was associated with a trend toward a lower incidence of death or MI but without an increase in bleeding.[118] It is now undergoing testing in two large phase III trials. One trial, Thrombin Receptor Antagonist for Clinical Events Reduction (TRACER), is in patients who recently experienced an ACS; the other trial is in patients with chronic CAD.[119]

Treatment Strategies and Interventions

There are two general approaches to the use of cardiac catheterization and revascularization in UA/NSTEMI: (1) an early *invasive* strategy, involving routine early cardiac catheterization followed by PCI, CABG, or continuing medical therapy, depending on the coronary anatomy; and (2) a more *conservative* approach, with initial medical management and catheterization reserved for patients with recurrent ischemia either at rest or on a noninvasive stress test and, if the anatomy is suitable, revascularization. To date, the relative merits of these two strategies have been studied in 10 randomized trials. The first three and the most recent trial did not demonstrate a significant difference;

however, six trials have shown a significant benefit of an early invasive therapy (**Fig. 56-14**).[119-121]

In FRISC II, there was a high threshold for catheterization in the conservative arm, and therefore a large difference in the rate of revascularization between the invasive and conservative strategies. In a 5-year follow-up, overall death or MI was lower, while mortality was significantly reduced in patients at high risk at baseline but not in those at low risk.[122]

In the TACTICS–TIMI 18 trial, the rate of death, MI, or rehospitalization for ACS at 6 months (the primary endpoint) fell significantly, from 19.4% in the conservative group to 15.9% in the early invasive group.[15] In patients with a troponin I level >0.1 ng/mL, there was a significant 39% relative risk reduction in the primary endpoint with the invasive versus the conservative strategy, whereas patients with a negative troponin had similar outcomes with either strategy (**Fig. 56-15**). With use of the TIMI risk score, there was significant benefit of the early invasive strategy in intermediate-risk (score, 3 to 4) patients and high-risk (5 to 7) patients, whereas low-risk (0 to 2) patients had similar outcomes with either strategy[15] (see Fig. 56-6B). Interestingly, the invasive strategy has also proved to be cost-effective, with the estimated cost per year of life gained for the invasive strategy of $12,739 in TACTICS–TIMI 18.[123]

The RITA-3 trial also demonstrated a benefit of an early invasive strategy, with a 34% relative reduction in the primary endpoint of death, MI, or refractory angina at 4 months; this benefit was driven primarily by a reduction in refractory angina. By 5 years, there was a significantly lower cardiovascular mortality rate in the early invasive arm.[124] In the most recent trial (ICTUS) that examined an invasive versus a conservative approach, all patients received ASA, enoxaparin, and abciximab for PCI, followed by intensive statin therapy. At 1 year, there was no significant difference in the rate of the primary endpoint—death, MI, or rehospitalization for angina.[125] In this trial, a very low threshold was used in the definition of periprocedural MI, and thus there was a much higher periprocedural MI rate compared with earlier trials, explaining, at least in part, the disparate results of this trial. However, even in ICTUS, the risk of rehospitalization was significantly lower in the invasive arm.

A meta-analysis of the more recent trials has confirmed an overall significant reduction in death, MI, or rehospitalization and of mortality during follow-up (see Fig. 56-14).[121] A sex-specific collaborative meta-analysis demonstrated benefit of an invasive strategy in all men and in high-risk women, but not in low-risk women, consistent with the 2007 Guidelines[120] (**Fig. 56-16**; see Fig. 81-6). Subgroup analyses of registries and clinical trials have shown a benefit of an early invasive strategy among women,[120] the elderly,[126] and patients with chronic

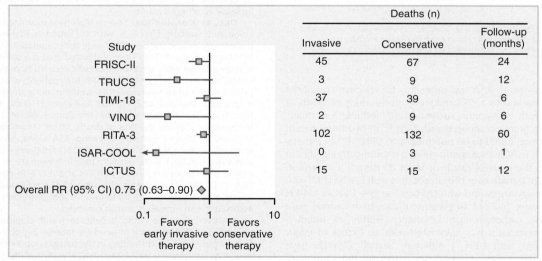

		Deaths (n)		
Study		Invasive	Conservative	Follow-up (months)
FRISC-II		45	67	24
TRUCS		3	9	12
TIMI-18		37	39	6
VINO		2	9	6
RITA-3		102	132	60
ISAR-COOL		0	3	1
ICTUS		15	15	12
Overall RR (95% CI) 0.75 (0.63–0.90)				

FIGURE 56-14 Meta-analysis of the benefit of a routine invasive versus "selective" invasive (i.e., conservative) strategy for patients with unstable angina or NSTEMI on the rate of death, myocardial infarction, or rehospitalization through follow-up. FRISC-II = Fragmin and Fast Revascularization During Instability in Coronary Artery Disease; ICTUS = Invasive Versus Conservative Treatment in Unstable Coronary Syndromes; ISAR-COOL = Intracoronary Stenting With Antithrombotic Regimen Cooling-Off; RITA-3 = Randomized Intervention Trial of Unstable Angina; RR = risk ratio; TACTICS–TIMI 18 = Treat Angina With Aggrastat and Determine the Cost of Therapy With an Invasive or Conservative Strategy–Thrombolysis in Myocardial Infarction; TRUCS = Treatment of Refractory Unstable Angina in Geographically Isolated Areas Without Cardiac Surgery; VINO = Value of First Day Coronary Angiography/Angioplasty in Evolving Non–ST-Segment Elevation Myocardial Infarction. (*Reproduced with permission from Bavry AA, Kumbhani DJ, Rassi AN, et al: Benefit of early invasive therapy in acute coronary syndromes: A meta-analysis of contemporary randomized clinical trials. J Am Coll Cardiol 48:1319, 2006.*)

kidney disease[127]—groups that are less likely to undergo early coronary arteriography.

Indications for Invasive Versus Conservative Management Strategies

On the basis of several recent randomized trials and meta-analyses, an early invasive strategy is now recommended in patients with UA/NSTEMI who have ST-segment changes or positive troponin on admission or who evolve these high-risk features during the subsequent 24 hours. Other high-risk indicators, such as recurrent ischemia and evidence of congestive heart failure, are also indications for an early invasive strategy. An early invasive strategy is also advised in patients who present with UA/NSTEMI within 6 months of a prior PCI and in whom restenosis may be the cause. An early invasive approach is also indicated in patients with UA/NSTEMI with prior CABG.[2]

The Intracoronary Stenting with Antithrombotic Regimen Cooling-Off (ISAR-COOL) trial found a benefit of an immediate invasive strategy with an average time of only 2 hours from randomization to catheterization, compared with a delayed invasive strategy, in which the average time to catheterization was 4 days.[128] The TIMACS trial compared early (median = 14 hours after randomization) with later (median = 50 hours) angiography.[129] It showed a trend for reduction of the primary endpoint (death, MI, and stroke) in the group as a whole but a significant reduction in the primary endpoint in patients with a high GRACE risk score. There was also a significant 28% reduction of the secondary endpoint of death, MI, and refractory ischemia with earlier angiography. Both of these trials lend support to a very early invasive strategy, especially in high-risk patients.

PERCUTANEOUS CORONARY INTERVENTION. (See Chap. 58.) Current angiographic success rates of PCI are high, generally >95%, although the presence of UA/NSTEMI or visualized thrombus can increase the risk of acute complications, such as abrupt closure and MI. Thus, use of GP IIb/IIIa inhibitors or a thienopyridine (clopidogrel or prasugrel) in such patients improves both acute and long-term outcomes after PCI. Implantation of drug-eluting stents reduces the risk of restenosis. There is a risk of late stent thrombosis after drug-eluting stent implantation, especially when clopidogrel is stopped. This serious complication can be reduced by long-term (at least 1 year or perhaps longer) dual antiplatelet therapy (i.e., ASA and a thienopyridine) in patients treated in this manner.

PERCUTANEOUS CORONARY INTERVENTION VERSUS CORONARY ARTERY BYPASS GRAFTING. Several trials have compared PCI and CABG in patients with ischemic heart disease, many of whom had UA/NSTEMI (see Chap. 58). On the basis of the results, CABG is recommended for patients with disease of the left main coronary artery as well as for those with multivessel disease and impaired left ventricular function or diabetes mellitus. For other patients treated invasively, PCI is ordinarily employed if the coronary anatomy is suitable. If it is not, CABG is the treatment of choice. PCI associates with a slightly lower initial morbidity and mortality than CABG, but there is a higher need of repeated PCI.

Other Therapies

ANGIOTENSIN-CONVERTING ENZYME INHIBITORS AND ANGIOTENSIN RECEPTOR BLOCKERS. Large trials have shown a

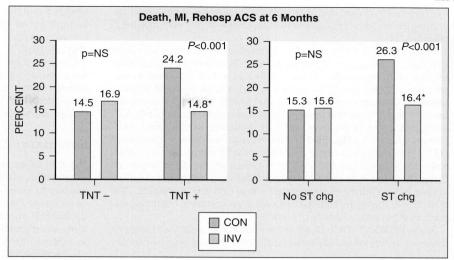

FIGURE 56-15 Risk stratification with troponin T (TnT) or ST-segment changes to determine the benefit of an early invasive (INV) versus conservative (CON) strategy in the TACTICS–TIMI 18 trial. *(Data from Cannon CP, Weintraub WS, Demopoulos LA, et al: Comparison of early invasive and conservative strategies in patients with unstable coronary syndromes treated with the glycoprotein IIb/IIIa inhibitor tirofiban. N Engl J Med 344:1879, 2001.)*

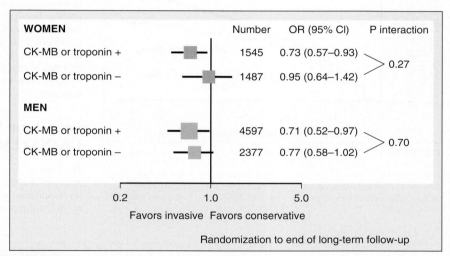

FIGURE 56-16 Meta-analysis, by sex, of the benefit of a routine invasive versus "selective" invasive (i.e., conservative) strategy for patients with unstable angina or NSTEMI on the rate of death, myocardial infarction, or rehospitalization through follow-up. *(From O'Donoghue M, Boden WE, Braunwald E, et al: Early invasive vs. conservative treatment strategies in women and men with unstable angina and non–ST-segment elevation myocardial infarction. A meta-analysis. JAMA 300:71, 2008.)*

0.5% absolute mortality benefit of early (initiated within 24 hours) angiotensin-converting enzyme (ACE) inhibitor therapy in patients with acute MI. However, the ISIS-4 trial did not show a benefit in patients without ST elevation.[49] Long-term use of ACE inhibition prevents recurrent ischemic events and mortality (see Chap. 55). Angiotensin receptor blockers (ARBs) may be substituted for ACE inhibitors on the basis of the Valsartan in Acute Myocardial Infarction Trial (VALIANT), which showed equivalent outcomes in post-MI patients treated with the ACE inhibitors captopril and the ARB valsartan.[130] ARBs are certainly indicated in patients who cannot tolerate ACE inhibitors.

LIPID-LOWERING THERAPY. Long-term treatment with lipid-lowering therapy, especially with statins, has shown benefit in patients after acute MI and UA/NSTEMI (see Chaps. 47 and 55).[131] In a prespecified subgroup of more than 3200 patients with unstable angina, in the Long-Term Intervention with Pravastatin in Ischemic Disease (LIPID) trial, pravastatin therapy led to a significant 26% reduction in total mortality.[132] When statins are initiated in-hospital at the time of an ACS, long-term benefits in outcome compared with placebo have been reported.[133]

In the PROVE IT–TIMI 22 trial, conducted in 4162 patients who were enrolled an average of 10 days after an ACS, intensive lipid-lowering therapy with atorvastatin 80 mg resulted in a 16% reduction in the primary endpoint and a 25% reduction in death, MI, or urgent revascularization, compared with moderate lipid-lowering therapy with pravastatin (40 mg).[134] A benefit emerged only 30 days after randomization,[135] highlighting the importance of early initiation of intensive statin therapy after ACS (**Fig. 56-17**). The average low-density lipoprotein (LDL) levels achieved in the two arms were 62 mg/dL and 95 mg/dL, respectively. In part on the basis of these results, the Adult Treatment Panel III of the National Cholesterol Education Program issued an update in which they recommended a new optional therapeutic LDL goal of <70 mg/dL in high-risk patients with coronary heart disease, such as those with a history of an ACS.[136]

Since PROVE IT–TIMI 22, there have been four additional trials of intensive versus moderate (standard) statin therapy, one in patients

after ACS and three in patients with stable CAD. A meta-analysis of the four published trials showed a highly significant 16% reduction in coronary death or MI with intensive versus standard statin therapy (**Fig. 56-18**).[137]

Intensive statin therapy should start at least at the time of hospital discharge, according to the ACC/AHA guidelines. However, benefit of intensive statin therapy before PCI has been seen in five small- to moderately-sized randomized trials,[138] suggesting that high-dose statin therapy should be started at the time of admission.

Summary: Acute Management of UA/NSTEMI

The evaluation of patients with UA/NSTEMI begins with the clinical examination, electrocardiography, and measurement of cardiac biomarkers to assess (1) the likelihood of CAD and (2) the risk of death or recurrent cardiac events. Patients with a low likelihood of having UA/NSTEMI should undergo a "diagnostic pathway" evaluation via serial electrocardiograms, cardiac biomarkers, and early stress testing to evaluate for CAD. This can be accomplished frequently in an observation/chest pain unit or in association with a hospital emergency department. Patients with a clinical history strongly consistent with UA/NSTEMI should undergo risk stratification by a clinical scoring system, such as the TIMI or GRACE risk scores,[43,44] as well as troponin measurement. Those at low risk should be treated with antiplatelet therapy with aspirin and clopidogrel as well as an anticoagulant, nitrates, and beta blockers. An early conservative strategy is adequate in low-risk patients. For moderate- to high-risk patients (e.g., those with positive troponin, ST-segment changes, TIMI risk score >3), the aforementioned medications should be used, and an early invasive strategy is preferred. GP IIb/IIIa inhibition should be added for patients who are unstable or at the time of PCI. Clopidogrel should be begun on admission. For patients in whom prasugrel is intended, omitting a loading dose of clopidogrel at the time of presentation would be warranted.

Long-Term Secondary Prevention After UA/NSTEMI (see Chap. 49)

The time of hospital discharge after UA/NSTEMI affords a "teachable moment" for the patient,[139] when the physician and staff can review and optimize the medical regimen for long-term treatment. Risk factor modification is critical and includes discussions with the patient (as appropriate to the risk factors) on the importance of smoking cessation, achieving optimal weight, exercise, following appropriate diet, good blood pressure control, control of hyperglycemia in diabetic patients, and intensive statin therapy (**Table 56-5**).

Six classes of therapies that have improved outcomes after UA/NSTEMI in large randomized trials should be instituted for long-term treatment. Each may contribute to long-term clinical stability in different ways:

1. Intensive LDL-C reduction with high-dose statins.[134,137,140]
2. ACE inhibitors or ARBs are recommended for long-term treatment that may facilitate plaque stabilization or retard progression of atherosclerosis.
3. Beta blockers are indicated for antiischemic therapy and may help decrease triggers for MI during follow-up.
4. For antiplatelet therapy, the combination of low-dose aspirin and a P2Y$_{12}$ inhibitor for at least a year confers clinical benefit

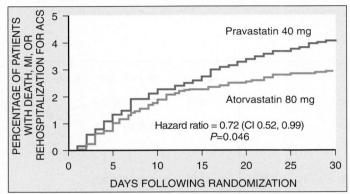

FIGURE 56-17 The benefit of intensive statin therapy initiated early after acute coronary syndrome (ACS) in the PROVE IT–TIMI 22 trial. A significant reduction in events is seen in the first 30 days. *(Modified from Ray KK, Cannon CP, McCabe C, et al: Early and late benefits of high-dose atorvastatin in patients with acute coronary syndromes: Results from the PROVE IT–TIMI 22 Trial. J Am Coll Cardiol 46:1405, 2005.)*

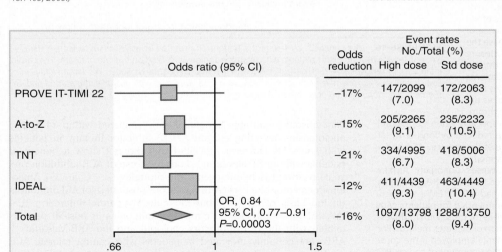

FIGURE 56-18 Meta-analysis of trials of intensive versus standard statin therapy, showing a highly significant 16% reduction in the risk of coronary death or myocardial infarction (P < 0.0001). A-to-Z = Aggrastat-to-Zocor trial; IDEAL = Incremental Decrease in End Points Through Aggressive Lipid-Lowering trial; PROVE IT–TIMI 22 = Pravastatin or Atorvastatin Evaluation and Infection Therapy–Thrombolysis In Myocardial Infarction 22 trial; TNT = Treating to New Targets trial. *(Reproduced from Cannon CP, Steinberg BA, Murphy SA, et al: Meta-analysis of cardiovascular outcomes trials comparing intensive versus moderate statin therapy. J Am Coll Cardiol 48:438, 2006.)*

TABLE 56-5   Cardiac Checklist for UA/NSTEMI*

CARDIAC CHECKLIST—ADMISSION	CARDIAC CHECKLIST—DISCHARGE
Admit Date: _____	Admit Date: _____
Patient Name:_____ (First Name) (Middle Initial) (Last Name)	Patient Name:_____ (First Name) (Middle Initial) (Last Name)
Brief History:_____	Brief History:_____
Medications: 1. Aspirin.. ☐ 2. Clopidogrel or ticagrelor.......................... ☐ 3. Heparin, LMWH, or other anticoagulant.......... ☐ 4. GP IIb/IIIa inhibitor................................. ☐ 5. Beta blocker... ☐ 6. Nitrate.. ☐ 7. ACE inhibitor.. ☐	**Medications:** 1. Aspirin (low dose)................................. ☐ 2. Clopidogrel/prasugrel/ticagrelor.............. ☐ 3. Statin (high dose)................................ ☐ 4. ACE inhibitor...................................... ☐ 5. Beta blocker....................................... ☐
Interventions: 8. Cath/revascularization for recurrent ischemia or in intermediate- and high-risk patients.......... ☐	**Interventions:** 6. LDL controlled to goal........................... ☐ 7. Blood pressure controlled...................... ☐ 8. Diabetes controlled.............................. ☐ 9. Smoking cessation counseling (if applicable) ☐ 10. Cardiac rehabilitation/lifestyle change........ ☐
Risk Factor Modification: 9. Cholesterol—check and treat as needed.......... ☐ 10. Treat other risk factors (e.g., smoking)......... ☐	

*These simple lists serve as reminders of guideline-recommended therapies, such as aspirin, clopidogrel, heparin, or LMWH. This "cardiac checklist" could be used in two ways: the physician could keep a copy on a small index card in a pocket or in a personal digital assistant (PDA) and run down the list when writing admission orders for patients, or it could be used in developing standard orders for UA/NSTEMI—either printed order sheets or computerized orders. See text for details of specific indications and contraindications for medications.
ACE = angiotensin-converting enzyme; cath = catheterization; GP = glycoprotein; LDL = low-density lipoprotein; LMWH = low-molecular-weight heparin.

by preventing or decreasing the severity of any thrombosis that occurs if a plaque ruptures and reducing thrombosis if a stent has been implanted. Longer duration of dual antiplatelet therapy may be appropriate in patients at high risk of recurrent ischemic events and is generally recommended in patients with drug-eluting stents.
5. Smoking cessation programs involving counseling, the use of nicotine patches or gum, the anxiolytic agent bupropion, or the acetylcholine partial agonist varenicline should be strongly encouraged.[141]
6. Exercise-based cardiac rehabilitation programs coupled with education on weight control, diet, and drug adherence are also advisable.

Thus, a multifactorial approach to long-term medical therapy can address the various components of atherothrombosis.

REGISTRY EXPERIENCE. A major problem identified in clinical practice is that a large proportion of patients fail to receive guideline-recommended therapies after UA/NSTEMI. Many large registries, in the United States and worldwide, have documented that 10% to 15% of patients do not receive any antithrombotic therapy and 40% to 50% of medically managed patients do not receive clopidogrel, despite Class I recommendations for their use.[142,143] These data suggest that in addition to guideline development and education, there is a need for specific tools to improve implementation of guideline recommendations on a patient-by-patient basis. Most important, lack of adherence to the guidelines has associated with adverse outcomes.[144] Paradoxically, patients at high risk for recurrent events (the elderly and patients with diabetes mellitus, renal dysfunction, and heart failure) were less likely than lower-risk patients to receive guideline-recommended therapies.[145]

CRITICAL PATHWAYS AND QUALITY IMPROVEMENT. Critical pathways and the process of Continuous Quality Improvement (CQI) are means of trying to improve care[146,147] (see Chap. 5). Critical pathways are standardized protocols for the management of specific diseases (e.g., ACS) that aim to optimize and streamline patient care.[148] In general, these pathways involve standardized or computerized order sets or simple pocket cards, reminders, or checklists of the appropriate therapies. The process of pathway

implementation generally involves physician and nursing education, including presentations at grand rounds, "in-services," and other educational meetings throughout the institution to the relevant caregivers. Another key part of an overall CQI effort is to monitor performance—that is, actual use of guideline-recommended therapies.[148]

CRITICAL PATHWAYS IMPROVE OUTCOMES. There are now several well-conducted studies showing that the use of critical pathways can improve the quality of care. The American Heart Association's Get With The Guidelines (GWTG) program aims to support and facilitate improvement in the quality of care of patients with cardiovascular disease. The GWTG-CAD program includes learning sessions, didactic sessions, best-practice sharing, interactive workshops, postmeeting follow-up, and a web-based Patient Management Tool, which provides the opportunity for concurrent data collection, ongoing real-time feedback of hospital data, and clinical decision support to enable rapid cycle improvement. GWTG-CAD also has a performance recognition program.[147] Participation in GWTG-CAD improves the use of therapies such as ASA, beta blockers, ACE inhibitors, and statins at the time of hospital discharge.

The American College of Cardiology–sponsored Guidelines Applied in Practice (GAP) program has also provided important multicenter data supporting the efficacy of critical pathways.[149] Better compliance with the use of guideline-recommended therapies is associated with lower mortality (**Fig. 56-19**). In the GAP program, patients in whom the clinical records showed that the pathways and tools had been used had the highest rates of treatment with the recommended therapies and better outcomes.[149]

Prinzmetal Variant Angina

In 1959, Prinzmetal and colleagues described a syndrome of ischemic pain that occurred at rest, accompanied by ST-segment elevation.[150] This syndrome, known as Prinzmetal variant angina (PVA), may be associated with acute MI, ventricular tachycardia or fibrillation, and sudden cardiac death. The incidence of PVA has always been greater in Japan than in Western countries, but across the world, the incidence appears to have fallen markedly during the past three decades; this

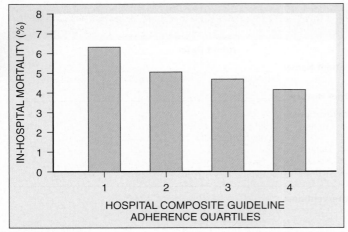

FIGURE 56-19 Association between hospital guideline adherence and in-hospital mortality. Hospitals in quartile 1 had the poorest adherence. *(Modified with permission from Peterson ED, Roe MT, Mulgund J, et al: Association between hospital process performance and outcomes among patients with acute coronary syndromes. JAMA 295:1912, 2006.)*

decline may be related, in part, to the more aggressive use of calcium antagonists for hypertension.[151]

Mechanisms

The original hypothesis of Prinzmetal and colleagues was that variant angina results from transient increases in coronary vasomotor tone or vasospasm. The focal vasospasm in PVA should not be confused with the generalized vasoconstriction of both the large and small coronary vessels, a normal response to stimuli such as cold exposure; the latter response, although widespread in the coronary vascular bed, is much less intense.

The precise mechanisms responsible for PVA have not been established, but a reduction in nitric oxide production by the coronary arterial endothelium or an imbalance between endothelium-derived relaxing and contracting factors may prevail.[152] Enhanced phospholipase C (PLC) activity has also been documented. Because PLC (through activation of the inositol triphosphate pathway) mobilizes Ca^{2+} from intracellular stores, it may enhance contraction of smooth muscle cells.[153] An inflammatory cause is supported by the finding of elevated levels of serum hs-CRP in many patients.[154] Polymorphisms of the alpha$_2$ presynaptic and the postsynaptic beta$_2$ receptor may also associate with PVA.[155]

Histologic findings in patients with PVA who underwent coronary atherectomy suggest that repetitive coronary vasospasm may provoke vascular injury and lead to the formation of neointimal hyperplasia at the initial site of spasm, which in turn caused rapid progression of coronary stenosis in some patients. Imaging with iodine-123–labeled metaiodobenzylguanidine (^{123}I-MIBG) has demonstrated regional myocardial sympathetic denervation in the area of distribution of the vessel in which vasospasm developed.[156]

Clinical and Laboratory Findings

Patients with PVA tend to be younger than patients with chronic stable angina or unstable angina secondary to coronary atherosclerosis, and many do not exhibit classic coronary risk factors, except that they are often heavy cigarette smokers. The anginal pain is often extremely severe and may be accompanied by syncope related to atrioventricular block, asystole, or ventricular tachyarrhythmias.[156]

Attacks of PVA tend to cluster between midnight and 8 AM,[157] and they sometimes occur in clusters of two or three within 30 to 60 minutes. Although exercise capacity is generally well preserved in patients with PVA, some patients experience typical pain and ST-segment elevations not only at rest but also during or after exertion. Patients with the combination of PVA and severe fixed coronary obstruction may have a combination of exertion-induced angina with ST-segment depression and episodes of angina at rest with ST-segment elevation. Some patients appear to have a distinct relation between

emotional distress and episodes of coronary vasospasm, in agreement with studies suggesting that sympathovagal imbalance may precipitate spasm in patients with PVA. In rare cases, PVA develops after coronary artery bypass surgery and may occur adjacent to a drug-eluting stent[158]; on occasion, PVA appears to be a manifestation of a generalized vasospastic disorder associated with migraine or Raynaud phenomenon. PVA can also occur in association with ASA-induced asthma and administration of 5-fluorouracil and cyclophosphamide.

ELECTROCARDIOGRAPHY. The key to the diagnosis of PVA lies in the detection of episodic ST-segment elevation often accompanied by severe chest pain, usually occurring at rest (**Fig. 56-20**). Many patients also exhibit multiple episodes of asymptomatic (silent) ST-segment elevation. ST-segment deviations may be present in any leads, depending on the artery involved. Serious arrhythmias can sometimes be precipitated by the cold pressor test. Transient conduction disturbances may occur during episodes of ischemia. Myocardial cell damage may occur in the absence of persistent electrocardiographic changes in patients with prolonged attacks of PVA. STEMI caused by coronary artery spasm in the absence of angiographically demonstrable obstructive CAD has been well documented.[159]

Exercise testing in patients with PVA can yield variable responses. Approximately equal numbers of patients show ST-segment depression, no change, or ST-segment elevation. These changes reflect the presence of underlying fixed CAD in some patients, the absence of significant lesions in others, and the provocation of spasm by exercise in the remainder. Ambulatory electrocardiographic monitoring or the use of a telephone transmitter may be helpful in capturing ST-segment elevations during symptomatic episodes.

Serious arrhythmias including sinus node dysfunction causing asystole and syncope, complete atrioventricular block, ventricular tachycardia, ventricular fibrillation, and sudden cardiac death have been reported.[160,161] Implantation of a pacemaker or an implanted automatic defibrillator may be required.[162]

CORONARY ARTERIOGRAPHY. (see Chap. 21) Spasm of a proximal coronary artery with resultant transmural ischemia and abnormalities in left ventricular function are the diagnostic hallmarks of PVA (see Fig. 56-20). Patients with no or mild fixed coronary obstruction tend to experience a more benign course than patients with PVA and associated severe obstructive lesions.[163] The vasospastic process almost always involves large segments of the epicardial vessels at a single site, but other sites may be involved at different times. The right coronary artery is the most frequent site, followed by the left anterior descending coronary artery. Simultaneous spasm of all three major coronary arteries may mimic three-vessel atherosclerotic disease.[164]

PROVOCATIVE TESTS

ERGONOVINE. Several provocative tests for coronary spasm have been developed. Of these, the ergonovine test is the most sensitive. Ergonovine maleate, an ergot alkaloid, stimulates both alpha-adrenergic and serotonergic receptors, and therefore exerts a direct constrictor effect on vascular smooth muscle and can induce coronary artery spasm.

When it is administered intravenously in bolus doses rising from 0.05 to 0.20 mg, ergonovine provides a sensitive and specific test for provocation of coronary artery spasm. The majority of patients who have a response to ergonovine do so at a dose of less than 0.20 mg. In low doses, and in carefully controlled clinical situations, ergonovine is a relatively safe drug, but prolonged coronary artery spasm precipitated by ergonovine may cause MI. On occasion, conduction disturbances (heart block) or severe tachyarrhythmias develop. Because of these hazards, it is recommended that ergonovine be administered only to patients in whom coronary arteriography has demonstrated normal or nearly normal coronary arteries and in gradually increasing doses, beginning with a very low dose. Intracoronary nitrates and calcium antagonists are usually effective in providing prompt relief from drug-induced spasm. Absolute contraindications to ergonovine testing include pregnancy, severe hypertension, severe left ventricular dysfunction, moderate to severe aortic stenosis, and high-grade left main coronary artery stenosis.

ACETYLCHOLINE. Stimulation of acetylcholine receptors produces a uniform endothelium-dependent dilation of normal coronary arteries but leads to vasoconstriction when endothelial function is impaired. In patients with PVA, intracoronary injections of acetylcholine can induce severe coronary spasm and reproduce the clinical syndrome.[165] This focal spasm should not be confused with the mild diffuse constriction that acetylcholine induces in patients with abnormal coronary endothelium. Acetylcholine is infused during a 1-minute period into a coronary artery in incremental doses of 10, 25, 50, and 100 µg, and doses should be separated by 5-minute intervals.

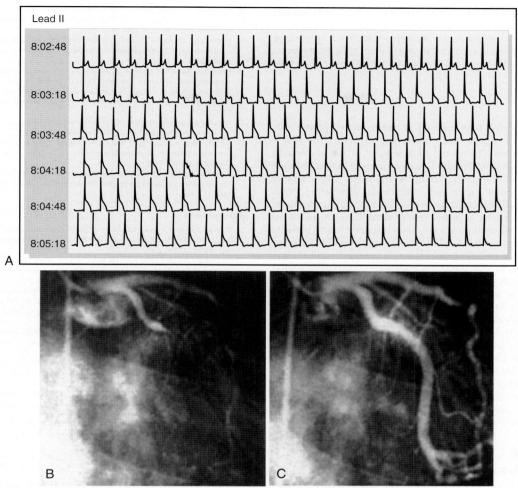

FIGURE 56-20 Continuous electrocardiography in a 39-year-old man with Prinzmetal angina. **A,** During an episode of angina, transient ST-segment elevation (in lead II) was noted on continuous telemetry. **B,** Hyperventilation-induced total occlusion of the proximal left circumflex artery (visible on angiography from the right anterior oblique caudal view). **C,** Spasm that resolved with the administration of intracoronary nitroglycerin and diltiazem. The patient's symptoms were controlled with oral nitrates and calcium channel blockade during a follow-up of 2 years. *(From Chen HSV, Pinto DS: Prinzmetal angina. N Engl J Med 349:e1, 2003.)*

Histamine, dopamine, and serotonin can also induce coronary artery spasm. Exercise, the cold pressor test, and alkalosis induced by hyperventilation[166] can all cause coronary spasm in patients with PVA, but none of these tests is as sensitive as ergonovine or acetylcholine.

Management

Patients with PVA should be urged strongly to discontinue smoking. The mainstay of therapy is a calcium antagonist alone or in combination with a long-acting nitrate. There are several similarities and differences between the optimal management of PVA and that of classic (stable and unstable) angina.

1. Patients with both PVA and classic angina usually respond well to nitrates; sublingual or intravenous nitroglycerin often abolishes attacks of PVA promptly, and long-acting nitrates are useful in preventing attacks. Calcium antagonists have proved extremely effective in preventing the coronary artery spasm of PVA,[167] and they should ordinarily be prescribed in maximally tolerated doses on a long-term basis. Because calcium antagonists act through a mechanism different from that of nitrates, these two classes of drugs may exert additive vasodilatory effects. All first- and second-generation calcium antagonists have similar (approximately 90%) efficacy in producing relief of symptoms, and they also suppress asymptomatic ischemia.

2. Response to beta blockade in patients with PVA is variable.[168,169] Some, particularly those with associated fixed lesions, exhibit a reduction in the frequency of exertion-induced angina caused primarily by augmentation of myocardial oxygen requirements. In others, however, nonselective beta blockers may actually be detrimental because blockade of beta$_2$ receptors, which mediate coronary dilation, allows unopposed alpha receptor–mediated coronary vasoconstriction to occur; in these patients, the duration of episodes of vasospastic angina may be prolonged by beta blockers.

3. Prazosin, a selective alpha-adrenergic receptor blocker, may also have value in the treatment of patients with PVA.[170] Nicorandil, a coronary vasodilator that acts by activating the potassium channel, also appears to be effective.[171] This agent has been approved in Europe but not in the United States.

4. ASA, helpful in unstable angina, may theoretically increase the severity of ischemic episodes in patients with PVA because it inhibits biosynthesis of the naturally occurring coronary vasodilator prostacyclin.

5. PCI and occasionally CABG may be helpful in patients with PVA and discrete, proximal fixed obstructive lesions. However, spasm may develop at a site different from the initial stenosis; therefore, calcium antagonists should be continued for at least 6 months after successful revascularization in patients with PVA. PCI and CABG

are contraindicated in patients with isolated coronary artery spasm without accompanying fixed obstructive disease.

6. Patients who have experienced ischemia-associated ventricular fibrillation who continue to manifest ischemia despite maximal medical treatment should receive an implantable cardioverter-defibrillator.[162,172]

Prognosis

Many patients with PVA pass through an acute, active phase, with frequent episodes of angina and cardiac events during the first 6 months after diagnosis. The extent and severity of the underlying CAD and the tempo of the syndrome have a major effect on the incidence of late mortality and MI. Patients with PVA in whom serious arrhythmias (ventricular tachycardia, ventricular fibrillation, high-degree atrioventricular block, or asystole) develop during spontaneous episodes of pain have a higher risk of sudden death unless an implanted cardioverter-defibrillator has been inserted. In most patients who survive an infarction or the initial 3- to 6-month period of frequent ischemic episodes, the condition stabilizes, and symptoms and cardiac events tend to diminish with time.[173] In patients who experience such remissions, cautious tapering of calcium antagonists may be attempted. In one series, 16% of patients had spontaneous remission 3 months after withdrawal of therapy, 44% continued to have symptoms despite treatment with calcium antagonists and nitrates, and the other 40% were free of angina but receiving treatment. Remission occurred more frequently in patients without significant coronary artery stenoses and in those who stopped smoking.[174]

For reasons that are not clear, some patients, after a relatively quiescent period of months or even years, experience a recrudescence of vasospastic activity with frequent and severe episodes of ischemia. Fortunately, these patients usually respond to re-treatment with calcium antagonists and nitrates.

REFERENCES

Epidemiology and Pathophysiology

1. Lloyd-Jones D, Adams R, Carnethon M, et al: Heart disease and stroke statistics—2009 update: A report from the American Heart Association Statistics Committee and Stroke Statistics Subcommittee. Circulation 119:480, 2009.
2. Anderson JL, Adams CD, Antman EM, et al: ACC/AHA 2007 guidelines for the management of patients with unstable angina/non–ST-elevation myocardial infarction: Executive summary. A report of the American College of Cardiology/American Heart Association Task Force on Practice Guidelines. Circulation 116:803, 2007.
3. Giugliano RP, Braunwald E: The year in non–ST-segment elevation acute coronary syndrome. J Am Coll Cardiol 54:1544, 2009.
4. Braunwald E: Unstable angina: An etiologic approach to management. Circulation 98:2219, 1998.
5. Ong P, Athanasiadis A, Hill S, et al: Coronary artery spasm as a frequent cause of acute coronary syndrome: The CASPAR (Coronary Artery Spasm in Patients with Acute Coronary Syndrome) study. J Am Coll Cardiol 52:523, 2008.
6. Davies MJ: The composition of coronary-artery plaques. N Engl J Med 336:1312, 1997.
7. Hochman JS, Tamis JE, Thompson TD, et al: Sex, clinical presentation, and outcome in patients with acute coronary syndromes. N Engl J Med 341:226, 1999.
8. Khot UN, Khot MB, Bajzer CT, et al: Prevalence of conventional risk factors in patients with coronary heart disease. JAMA 290:898, 2003.
9. Cannon CP, McCabe CH, Stone PH, et al: The electrocardiogram predicts one-year outcome of patients with unstable angina and non–Q wave myocardial infarction: Results of the TIMI III Registry ECG Ancillary Study. J Am Coll Cardiol 30:133, 1997.
10. Scirica BM, Morrow DA, Budaj A, et al: Ischemia detected on continuous electrocardiography following acute coronary syndrome: Observations from the MERLIN-TIMI 36 trial. J Am Coll Cardiol 53:1411, 2009.

Biomarkers

11. Morrow DA, Cannon CP, Rifai N, et al: Ability of minor elevations of troponin I and T to predict benefit from an early invasive strategy in patients with unstable angina and non–ST elevation myocardial infarction: Results from a randomized trial. JAMA 286:2405, 2001.
12. Eggers KM, Lagerqvist B, Venge P, et al: Persistent cardiac troponin I elevation in stabilized patients after an episode of ACS predicts long-term mortality. Circulation 116:1907, 2007.
13. Fleming SM, O'Byrne L, Finn J, et al: False-positive cardiac troponin I in a routine clinical population. Am J Cardiol 89:1212, 2002.
14. Dokainish H, Pillai M, Murphy S, et al: Prognostic implications of elevated troponin in patients with suspected acute coronary syndromes but no epicardial coronary disease. J Am Coll Cardiol 45:19, 2005.
15. Cannon CP, Weintraub WS, Demopoulos LA, et al: Comparison of early invasive and conservative strategies in patients with unstable coronary syndromes treated with the glycoprotein IIb/IIIa inhibitor tirofiban. N Engl J Med 344:1879, 2001.

16. Braunwald E: Unstable angina: A classification. Circulation 80:410, 1989.
17. Karha J, Cannon CP, Murphy S, et al: Safety of stress testing following an acute coronary syndrome. Am J Cardiol 94:1534, 2004.
18. Hollander JE, Chang AM, Shofer F, et al: Coronary computed tomographic angiography for rapid discharge of low-risk patients with potential acute coronary syndromes. Ann Emerg Med 53:295, 2009.
19. Hoffmann U, Bamberg F, Chae CU, et al: Coronary computed tomography angiography for early triage of patients with acute chest pain. J Am Coll Cardiol 53:1642, 2009.
20. Motoyama S, Sarai M, Harigaya H, et al: Computed tomographic angiography characteristics of atherosclerotic plaques subsequently resulting in acute coronary syndrome. J Am Coll Cardiol 54:49, 2009.
21. Braunwald E: Noninvasive detection of vulnerable coronary plaques: Locking the barn door before the horse is stolen. J Am Coll Cardiol 54:58, 2009.
22. Cury RC, Shash K, Nagurney JT, et al: Cardiac magnetic resonance with T2-weighted imaging improves detection of patients with acute coronary syndrome in the emergency department. Circulation 118:837, 2008.
23. Zairis MN, Papadaki OA, Manousakis SJ, et al: C-reactive protein and multiple complex coronary artery plaques in patients with primary unstable angina. Atherosclerosis 164:355, 2002.

Management

24. Bach RG, Cannon CP, Weintraub WS, et al: The effect of routine, early invasive management on outcome for elderly patients with non–ST segment elevation acute coronary syndromes. Ann Intern Med 141:186, 2004.
25. Westerhout CM, Fu Y, Lauer MS, et al: Short- and long-term risk stratification in acute coronary syndromes: The added value of quantitative ST-segment depression and multiple biomarkers. J Am Coll Cardiol 48:939, 2006.
26. Kleiman N, Lakkis N, Cannon C, et al: Prospective analysis of creatine kinase muscle-brain fraction and comparison with troponin T to predict cardiac risk and benefit of an invasive strategy in patients with non–ST elevation acute coronary syndromes. J Am Coll Cardiol 40:1044, 2002.
27. Antman EM, Tanasijevic MJ, Thompson B, et al: Cardiac-specific troponin I levels to predict the risk of mortality in patients with acute coronary syndromes. N Engl J Med 335:1342, 1996.
28. Kastrati A, Mehilli J, Neumann FJ, et al: Abciximab in patients with acute coronary syndromes undergoing percutaneous coronary intervention after clopidogrel pretreatment: The ISAR-REACT 2 randomized trial. JAMA 295:1531, 2006.
29. Morrow DA, Rifai N, Antman EM, et al: C-reactive protein is a potent predictor of mortality independently and in combination with troponin T in acute coronary syndromes: A TIMI 11A substudy. J Am Coll Cardiol 31:1460, 1998.
30. Morrow DA, de Lemos JA, Sabatine MS, et al: Clinical relevance of C-reactive protein during follow-up of patients with acute coronary syndromes in the Aggrastat-to-Zocor Trial. Circulation 114:281, 2006.
30a de Lemos JA, Morrow DA, Sabatine MS, et al: Association between plasma levels of monocyte chemoattractant protein-1 and long-term clinical outcomes in patients with acute coronary syndromes. Circulation 107:690, 2003.
31. Ray KK, Morrow DA, Sabatine MS, et al: Long-term prognostic value of neopterin: A novel marker of monocyte activation in patients with acute coronary syndrome. Circulation 115:3071, 2007.
32. Sabatine MS, Morrow DA, Cannon CP, et al: Relationship between baseline white blood cell count and degree of coronary artery disease and mortality in patients with acute coronary syndromes: A TACTICS-TIMI 18 substudy. J Am Coll Cardiol 40:1761, 2002.
33. Baldus S, Heeschen C, Meinertz T, et al: Myeloperoxidase serum levels predict risk in patients with acute coronary syndromes. Circulation 108:1440, 2003.
34. Buffon A, Biasucci LM, Liuzzo G, et al: Widespread coronary inflammation in unstable angina. N Engl J Med 347:5, 2002.
35. de Lemos JA, Morrow DA, Bentley JH, et al: The prognostic value of B-type natriuretic peptide in patients with acute coronary syndromes. N Engl J Med 345:1014, 2001.
36. Omland T, de Lemos JA, Morrow DA, et al: Prognostic value of N-terminal pro-atrial and pro-brain natriuretic peptide in patients with acute coronary syndromes. Am J Cardiol 89:463, 2002.
37. Morrow DA, de Lemos JA, Sabatine MS, et al: Evaluation of B-type natriuretic peptide for risk assessment in unstable angina/non–ST-elevation myocardial infarction: B-type natriuretic peptide and prognosis in TACTICS-TIMI 18. J Am Coll Cardiol 41:1264, 2003.
38. Gibson CM, Pinto DS, Murphy SA, et al: Association of creatinine and creatinine clearance on presentation in acute myocardial infarction with subsequent mortality. J Am Coll Cardiol 42:1535, 2003.
39. Bhadriraju S, Ray KK, DeFranco AC, et al: Association between blood glucose and long-term mortality in patients with acute coronary syndromes in the OPUS-TIMI 16 trial. Am J Cardiol 97:1573, 2006.
40. Ray KK, Cannon CP, Morrow DA, et al: Synergistic relationship between hyperglycemia and inflammation with respect to clinical outcomes in non–ST elevation acute coronary syndromes: Analyses from OPUS-TIMI 16 and TACTICS-TIMI 18. Eur Heart J 28:806, 2007.
41. Mega JL, Morrow DA, de Lemos JA, et al: Thrombus precursor protein and clinical outcomes in patients with acute coronary syndromes. J Am Coll Cardiol 51:2422, 2008.
42. Boersma E, Pieper KS, Steyerberg EW, et al: Predictors of outcome in patients with acute coronary syndromes without persistent ST-segment elevation. Results from an international trial of 9461 patients. Circulation 101:2557, 2000.
43. Antman EM, Cohen M, Bernink PJ, et al: The TIMI risk score for unstable angina/non–ST elevation MI: A method for prognostication and therapeutic decision making. JAMA 284:835, 2000.
44. Granger CB, Goldberg RJ, Dabbous O, et al: Predictors of hospital mortality in the global registry of acute coronary events. Arch Intern Med 163:2345, 2003.
45. Sabatine MS, Morrow DA, de Lemos J, et al: Multimarker approach to risk stratification in non–ST elevation acute coronary syndromes: Simultaneous assessment of troponin I, C-reactive protein, and B-type natriuretic peptide. Circulation 105:1760, 2002.

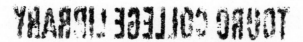

46. Gottlieb SO, Weisfeldt ML, Ouyang P, et al: Effect of the addition of propranolol to therapy with nifedipine for unstable angina: A randomized, double-blind, placebo-controlled trial. Circulation 73:331, 1986.
47. Subherwal S, Bach RG, Chen AY, et al: Baseline risk of major bleeding in non–ST-segment elevation myocardial infarction: The CRUSADE bleeding score. Circulation 119:1873, 2009.
48. Alexander KP, Chen AY, Roe MT, et al: Excess dosing of antiplatelet and antithrombin agents in the treatment of non–ST-segment elevation acute coronary syndromes. JAMA 294:3108, 2009.
49. ISIS-4 (Fourth International Study of Infarct Survival) Collaborative Group): Randomized factorial trial assessing early oral captopril, oral mononitrate, and intravenous magnesium sulphate in 58,050 patients with suspected acute myocardial infarction. Lancet 345:669, 1995.
50. Yusuf S, Peto R, Lewis J, et al: Beta-blockade during and after myocardial infarction: An overview of the randomized trials. Prog Cardiovasc Dis 27:335, 1985.
51. Chen ZM, Pan HC, Chen YP, et al: Early intravenous then oral metoprolol in 45,852 patients with acute myocardial infarction: Randomised placebo-controlled trial. Lancet 366:1622, 2005.
52. The Multicenter Diltiazem Postinfarction Trial Research Group: The effect of diltiazem on mortality and reinfarction after myocardial infarction. N Engl J Med 319:385, 1998.
53. Cohn JN, Ziesche S, Smith R, et al: Effect of the calcium antagonist felodipine as supplementary vasodilator therapy in patients with chronic heart failure treated with enalapril: V-HeFT III. Circulation 96:856, 1997.
54. Jamerson K, Weber MA, Bakris GL, et al: Benazepril plus amlodipine or hydrochlorothiazide for hypertension in high-risk patients. N Engl J Med 359:2417, 2008.
55. Nissen SE, Tuzcu EM, Libby P, et al: Effect of antihypertensive agents on cardiovascular events in patients with coronary disease and normal blood pressure: The CAMELOT study: A randomized controlled trial. JAMA 292:2217, 2004.
56. Antithrombotic Trialists' Collaboration: Collaborative meta-analysis of randomised trials of antiplatelet therapy for prevention of death, myocardial infarction, and stroke in high risk patients. BMJ 324:71, 2002.
57. Bhatt DL, Bertrand ME, Berger PB, et al: Meta-analysis of randomized and registry comparisons of ticlopidine with clopidogrel after stenting. J Am Coll Cardiol 39:9, 2002.
58. Patrono C, Rocca B: Aspirin, 110 years later. J Thromb Haemost 7(Suppl 1):258, 2009.
59. Frelinger AL 3rd, Furman MI, Linden MD, et al: Residual arachidonic acid–induced platelet activation via an adenosine diphosphate–dependent but cyclooxygenase-1– and cyclooxygenase-2–independent pathway: A 700-patient study of aspirin resistance. Circulation 113:2888, 2006.
60. Eikelboom JW, Hirsh J, Weitz JI, et al: Aspirin-resistant thromboxane biosynthesis and the risk of myocardial infarction, stroke, or cardiovascular death in patients at high risk for cardiovascular events. Circulation 105:1650, 2002.
61. Cattaneo M: New $P2Y_{12}$ blockers. J Thromb Haemost 7(Suppl 1):262, 2009.
62. Clopidogrel in Unstable Angina to Prevent Recurrent Events Trial Investigators: Effects of clopidogrel in addition to aspirin in patients with acute coronary syndromes without ST-segment elevation. N Engl J Med 345:494, 2001.
63. Yusuf S, Mehta SR, Zhao F, et al: Early and late effects of clopidogrel in patients with acute coronary syndromes. Circulation 107:966, 2003.
64. Mehta SR, Yusuf S, Peters RJ, et al: Effects of pretreatment with clopidogrel and aspirin followed by long-term therapy in patients undergoing percutaneous coronary intervention: The PCI-CURE study. Lancet 358:527, 2001.
65. Sabatine MS, Cannon CP, Gibson CM, et al: Effect of clopidogrel pretreatment before percutaneous coronary intervention in patients with ST-elevation myocardial infarction treated with fibrinolytics: The PCI-CLARITY study. JAMA 294:1224, 2005.
66. Smith SC Jr, Feldman TE, Hirshfeld JW Jr, et al: ACC/AHA/SCAI 2005 Guideline Update for Percutaneous Coronary Intervention—Summary Article: A Report of the American College of Cardiology/American Heart Association Task Force on Practice Guidelines (ACC/AHA/SCAI Writing Committee to Update the 2001 Guidelines for Percutaneous Coronary Intervention). J Am Coll Cardiol 47:216, 2006.
67. Fox KAA, Mehta SR, Peters R, et al: Benefits and risks of the combination of clopidogrel and aspirin in patients undergoing surgical revascularization for non–ST-elevation acute coronary syndrome: The Clopidogrel in Unstable angina to prevent Recurrent ischemic Events (CURE) trial. Circulation 110:1202, 2004.
68. Berger JS, Frye CB, Harshaw Q, et al: Impact of clopidogrel in patients with acute coronary syndromes requiring coronary artery bypass surgery: A multicenter analysis. J Am Coll Cardiol 52:1693, 2008.
69. Montalescot G, Sideris G, Meuleman C, et al: A randomized comparison of high clopidogrel loading doses in patients with non–ST-segment elevation acute coronary syndromes: The ALBION (Assessment of the Best Loading Dose of Clopidogrel to Blunt Platelet Activation, Inflammation, and Ongoing Necrosis) trial. J Am Coll Cardiol 48:931, 2006.
70. Patti G, Colonna G, Pasceri V, et al: Randomized trial of high loading dose of clopidogrel for reduction of periprocedural myocardial infarction in patients undergoing coronary intervention: Results from the ARMYDA-2 (Antiplatelet therapy for Reduction of MYocardial Damage during Angioplasty) study. Circulation 111:2099, 2005.
71. OASIS 7. Mehta S, presented at the European Society of Cardiology, Barcelona, 2009.
72. Gurbel PA, Bliden KP, Hayes KM, et al: The relation of dosing to clopidogrel responsiveness and the incidence of high post-treatment platelet aggregation in patients undergoing coronary stenting. J Am Coll Cardiol 45:1392, 2005.
73. Erlinge D, Varenhorst C, Braun OO, et al: Patients with poor responsiveness to thienopyridine treatment or with diabetes have lower levels of circulating active metabolite, but their platelets respond normally to active metabolite added ex vivo. J Am Coll Cardiol 52:1968, 2008.
74. Wiviott SD, Trenk D, Frelinger AL, et al: Prasugrel compared with high loading- and maintenance-dose clopidogrel in patients with planned percutaneous coronary intervention. The Prasugrel in Comparison to Clopidogrel for Inhibition of Platelet Activation and Aggregation–Thrombolysis in Myocardial Infarction 44 trial. Circulation 116:2923, 2007.
75. Cuisset T, Frere C, Quilici J, et al: Relationship between aspirin and clopidogrel responses in acute coronary syndrome and clinical predictors of non response. Thromb Res 123:597, 2009.
76. Matetzky S, Shenkman B, Guetta V, et al: Clopidogrel resistance is associated with increased risk of recurrent atherothrombotic events in patients with acute myocardial infarction. Circulation 109:3171, 2004.
77. Marcucci R, Gori AM, Paniccia R, et al: Cardiovascular death and nonfatal myocardial infarction in acute coronary syndrome patients receiving coronary stenting are predicted by residual platelet reactivity to ADP detected by a point-of-care assay: A 12-month follow-up. Circulation 119:237, 2009.
78. van Werkum JW, Heestermans AA, Zomer AC, et al: Predictors of coronary stent thrombosis: The Dutch Stent Thrombosis Registry. J Am Coll Cardiol 53:1399, 2009.
79. Wiviott SD, Braunwald E, McCabe CH, et al: Prasugrel versus clopidogrel in patients with acute coronary syndromes. N Engl J Med 357:2001, 2007.
80. Han Y, Li Y, Wang S, et al: Cilostazol in addition to aspirin and clopidogrel improves long-term outcomes after percutaneous coronary intervention in patients with acute coronary syndromes: A randomized, controlled study. Am Heart J 157:733, 2009.
81. Mega JL, Close SL, Wiviott SD, et al: Cytochrome p-450 polymorphisms and response to clopidogrel. N Engl J Med 360:354, 2009.
82. Simon T, Verstuyft C, Mary-Krause M et al: Genetic determinants of response to clopidogrel and cardiovascular events. N Engl J Med 360:363, 2009.
83. Collet J-P, Hulot J-S, Pena A, et al: Cytochrome P450 2C19 polymorphism in young patients treated with clopidogrel after myocardial infarction: A cohort study. Lancet 373:309, 2009.
84. Sibbing D, Stegherr J, Latz W, et al: Cytochrome P450 2C19 loss-of-function polymorphism and stent thrombosis following percutaneous coronary intervention. Eur Heart J 30:916, 2009.
85. Trenk D, Hochholzer W, Fromm MF, et al: Cytochrome P450 2C19 681G>A polymorphism and high on-clopidogrel platelet reactivity associated with adverse 1-year clinical outcome of elective percutaneous coronary intervention with drug-eluting or bare-metal stents. J Am Coll Cardiol 51:1925, 2008.
86. Mega JL, Close SL, Wiviott SD, et al: Cytochrome P450 genetic polymorphisms and the response to prasugrel. Relationship to pharmacokinetic, pharmacodynamic, and clinical outcomes. Circulation 119:2553, 2009.
87. Montalescot MM, Wiviott SD, Braunwald E, et al: Prasugrel compared with clopidogrel in patients undergoing percutaneous coronary intervention for ST-elevation myocardial infarction (TRITON-TIMI 38): Double-blind, randomized controlled trial. Lancet 373:723, 2009.
88. Husted S, Emanuelsson H, Heptinstall S, et al: Pharmacodynamics, pharmacokinetics, and safety of the oral reversible $P2Y_{12}$ antagonist AZD6140 with aspirin in patients with atherosclerosis: A double-blind comparison to clopidogrel with aspirin. Eur Heart J 27:1038, 2006.
89. Wallentin L: $P2Y_{12}$ inhibitors: Differences in properties and mechanisms of action and potential consequences for clinical use. Eur Heart J 30:1964, 2009.
90. Storey RF, Husted S, Harrington RA, et al: Inhibition of platelet aggregation by AZD6140, a reversible oral $P2Y_{12}$ receptor antagonist, compared with clopidogrel in patients with acute coronary syndromes. J Am Coll Cardiol 50:1852, 2007.
91. Wallentin L, Becker R, Budaj A, et al: Ticagrelor versus clopidogrel in patients with acute coronary syndromes. N Engl J Med 361:1045, 2009.
92. Boersma E, Harrington RA, Moliterno DJ, et al: Platelet glycoprotein IIb/IIIa inhibitors in acute coronary syndromes: A meta-analysis of all major randomised clinical trials. Lancet 359:189, 2002.
93. Kastrati A, Mehilli J, Neumann FJ, et al: Abciximab in patients with acute coronary syndromes undergoing percutaneous coronary intervention after clopidogrel pretreatment: The ISAR-REACT 2 randomized trial. JAMA 295:1531, 2006.
94. Giugliano RP, White JA, Bode C, et al: Early versus delayed, provisional eptifibatide in acute coronary syndromes. N Engl J Med 360:2176, 2009.
95. Stone GW, Bertrand ME, Moses JW, et al: Routine upstream initiation vs deferred selective use of glycoprotein IIb/IIIa inhibitors in acute coronary syndromes: The ACUITY Timing trial. JAMA 297:591, 2007.
96. Fung AY, Saw J, Starovoytov A, et al: Abbreviated infusion of eptifibatide after successful coronary intervention: The BRIEF-PCI (Brief Infusion of Eptifibatide Following Percutaneous Coronary Intervention) randomized trial. J Am Coll Cardiol 53:837, 2009.
97. Theroux P, Ouimet H, McCans J, et al: Aspirin, heparin or both to treat unstable angina. N Engl J Med 319:1105, 1988.
98. Eikelboom JW, Anand SS, Malmberg K, et al: Unfractionated heparin and low-molecular-weight heparin in acute coronary syndrome without ST elevation: A meta-analysis. Lancet 355:1936, 2000.
99. Rich JD, Maraganore JM, Young E, et al: Heparin resistance in acute coronary syndromes. J Thromb Thrombolysis 23:93, 2007.
100. Warkentin TE, Kelton JG: Temporal aspects of heparin-induced thrombocytopenia. N Engl J Med 344:1286, 2001.
101. Hirsh J, Warkentin TE, Shaughnessy SG, et al: Heparin and low-molecular-weight heparin: Mechanisms of action, pharmacokinetics, dosing, monitoring, efficacy, and safety. Chest 119:64S, 2001.
102. Murphy SA, Gibson CM, Morrow DA, et al: Efficacy and safety of the low-molecular weight heparin enoxaparin compared with unfractionated heparin across the acute coronary syndrome spectrum: A meta-analysis. Eur Heart J 28:2077, 2007.
103. Blazing MA, de Lemos JA, White HD, et al: Safety and efficacy of enoxaparin vs unfractionated heparin in patients with non–ST-segment elevation acute coronary syndromes who receive tirofiban and aspirin: A randomized controlled trial. JAMA 292:55, 2004.
104. Ferguson JJ, Califf RM, Antman EM, et al: Enoxaparin vs unfractionated heparin in high-risk patients with non–ST-segment elevation acute coronary syndromes managed with an intended early invasive strategy: Primary results of the SYNERGY randomized trial. JAMA 292:45, 2004.
105. de Lemos JA, Blazing MA, Wiviott SD, et al: Enoxaparin versus unfractionated heparin in patients treated with tirofiban, aspirin and an early conservative initial management strategy: Results from the A phase of the A-to-Z trial. Eur Heart J 25:1688, 2004.

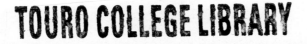

106. Yusuf S, Mehta SR, Chrolavicius S, et al: Comparison of fondaparinux and enoxaparin in acute coronary syndromes. N Engl J Med 354:1464, 2006.

107. Yusuf S, Mehta SR, Chrolavicius S, et al: Effects of fondaparinux on mortality and reinfarction in patients with acute ST-segment elevation myocardial infarction: The OASIS-6 randomized trial. JAMA 295:1519, 2006.

108. Direct Thrombin Inhibitor Trialists' Collaborative Group: Direct thrombin inhibitors in acute coronary syndromes: Principal results of a meta-analysis based on individual patients' data. Lancet 359:294, 2002.

109. Stone GW, McLaurin BT, Cox DA, et al: Bivalirudin for patients with acute coronary syndromes. N Engl J Med 355:2203, 2006.

110. Kastrati A, Neumann F-J, Mehilli J, et al: Bivalirudin versus unfractionated heparin during percutaneous coronary intervention. N Engl J Med 359:688, 2008.

111. Hurlen M, Abdelnoor M, Smith P, et al: Warfarin, aspirin, or both after myocardial infarction. N Engl J Med 347:969, 2002.

112. van Es RF, Jonker JJC, Verheugt FWA, et al: Aspirin and coumadin after acute coronary syndromes (the ASPECT-2 study): A randomised controlled trial. Lancet 360:109, 2002.

113. Mega J, Braunwald E, Mohanavelu S, et al: Rivaroxaban versus placebo in patients with acute coronary syndromes (ATLAS ACS–TIMI 46): A randomized, double blind, phase II trial. Lancet 374:29, 2009.

114. APPRAISE Steering Committee and Investigators: Apixaban, an oral, direct, selective factor Xa inhibitor, in combination with antiplatelet therapy after acute coronary syndrome: Results of the Apixaban for Prevention of Acute Ischemic and Safety Events (APPRAISE) trial. Circulation 119:2877, 2009.

115. Becker RC, Smyth S: The evolution of platelet-directed pharmacotherapy. J Thromb Haemost 7:266, 2009.

116. Chakalamannil S, Wang Y, Greenlee WJ, et al: Discovery of a novel, orally active himbacine-based thrombin receptor antagonist (SCH 530348) with potent antiplatelet activity. J Med Chem 51:3061, 2008.

117. Smuth SS, Woulfe DS, Weitz CG, et al: G-protein coupled receptors as signaling targets for antiplatelet therapy. Arterioscler Thromb Vasc Biol 29:449, 2009.

118. Becker RC, Moliterno DJ, Jennings LK, et al: Safety and tolerability of SCH 530348 in patients undergoing non-urgent percutaneous coronary intervention: A randomised, double-blind, placebo-controlled phase II study. Lancet 373:919, 2009.

119. Morrow DA, Scirica BM, Fox KA, et al: Evaluation of a novel antiplatelet agent for secondary prevention in patients with a history of atherosclerotic disease: Design and rationale for the Thrombin-Receptor Antagonist in Secondary Prevention of Atherothrombotic Ischemic Events (TRA 2 P)–TIMI 50 trial. Am Heart J 158:335, 2009.

120. O'Donoghue M, Boden WE, Braunwald E, et al: Early invasive vs. conservative treatment strategies in women and men with unstable angina and non–ST-segment elevation myocardial infarction. A meta-analysis. JAMA 300:71, 2008.

121. Bavry AA, Kumbhani DJ, Rassi AN, et al: Benefit of early invasive therapy in acute coronary syndromes: A meta-analysis of contemporary randomized clinical trials. J Am Coll Cardiol 48:1319, 2006.

122. Lagerqvist B, Husted S, Kontny F, et al: 5-Year outcomes in the FRISC-II randomised trial of an invasive versus a non-invasive strategy in non–ST-elevation acute coronary syndrome: A follow-up study. Lancet 368:998, 2006.

123. Mahoney EM, Jurkovitz CT, Chu H, et al: Cost and cost-effectiveness of an early invasive versus conservative strategy for the treatment of unstable angina and non–ST elevation myocardial infarction. JAMA 288:1851, 2002.

124. Fox KA, Poole-Wilson P, Clayton TC, et al: 5-Year outcome of an interventional strategy in non–ST-elevation acute coronary syndrome: The British Heart Foundation RITA 3 randomised trial. Lancet 366:914, 2005.

125. de Winter RJ, Windhausen F, Cornel JH, et al: Early invasive versus selectively invasive management for acute coronary syndromes. N Engl J Med 353:1095, 2005.

126. Bauer T, Koeth O, Junger C, et al: Effect of an invasive strategy on in-hospital outcome in elderly patients with non–ST-elevation myocardial infarction. Eur Heart J 28:2873, 2007.

127. Charytan DM, Wallentin L, Lagerqvist B, et al: Early angiography in patients with chronic kidney disease: A collaborative systematic review. Clin J Am Soc Nephrol 4:1032, 2009.

128. Neumann FJ, Kastrati A, Pogatsa-Murray G, et al: Evaluation of prolonged antithrombotic pretreatment ("cooling-off" strategy) before intervention in patients with unstable coronary syndromes: A randomized controlled trial. JAMA 290:1593, 2003.

129. Mehta SR, Granger CB, Boden WE, et al: Early versus delayed invasive intervention in acute coronary syndromes. N Engl J Med 360:2165, 2009.

130. Pfeffer MA, McMurray JJ, Velazquez EJ, et al: Valsartan, captopril, or both in myocardial infarction complicated by heart failure, left ventricular dysfunction, or both. N Engl J Med 349:1893, 2003.

131. Heart Protection Study Collaborative Group: MRC/BHF Heart Protection Study of cholesterol lowering with simvastatin in 20,536 high-risk individuals: A randomised placebo controlled trial. Lancet 360:7, 2002.

132. Tonkin AM, Colquhoun D, Emberson J, et al: Effects of pravastatin in 3260 patients with unstable angina: Results from the LIPID study. Lancet 356:1871, 2000.

133. Hulten E, Jackson JL, Douglas K, et al: The effect of early, intensive statin therapy on acute coronary syndrome: A meta-analysis of randomized controlled trials. Arch Intern Med 166:1814, 2006.

134. Cannon CP, Braunwald E, McCabe CH, et al: Intensive versus moderate lipid lowering with statins after acute coronary syndromes. N Engl J Med 350:1495, 2004.

135. Ray KK, Cannon CP, McCabe C, et al: Early and late benefits of high-dose atorvastatin in patients with acute coronary syndromes: Results from the PROVE IT–TIMI 22 Trial. J Am Coll Cardiol 46:1405, 2005.

136. Grundy SM, Cleeman JI, Merz CNB, et al: Implications of recent clinical trials for the National Cholesterol Education Program Adult Treatment Panel III Guidelines. Circulation 110:227, 2004.

137. Cannon CP, Steinberg BA, Murphy SA, et al: Meta-analysis of cardiovascular outcomes trials comparing intensive versus moderate statin therapy. J Am Coll Cardiol 48:438, 2006.

138. Di Sciascio G, Patti G, Pasceri V, et al: Efficacy of atorvastatin reload in patients on chronic statin therapy undergoing percutaneous coronary intervention: Results of the ARMYDA-RECAPTURE (Atorvastatin for Reduction of Myocardial Damage During Angioplasty) randomized trial. J Am Coll Cardiol 54:558, 2009.

139. Fonarow GC: In-hospital initiation of statins: Taking advantage of the "teachable moment." Cleve Clin J Med 70:502, 504, 2003.

140. Baigent C, Keech A, Kearney PM, et al: Efficacy and safety of cholesterol-lowering treatment: Prospective meta-analysis of data from 90,056 participants in 14 randomised trials of statins. Lancet 366:1267, 2005.

141. Tonstad S, Tonnesen P, Hajek P, et al: Effect of maintenance therapy with varenicline on smoking cessation: A randomized controlled trial. JAMA 296:64, 2006.

142. Fox KA, Steg PG, Eagle KA, et al: Decline in rates of death and heart failure in acute coronary syndromes, 1999-2006. JAMA 297:1892, 2007.

143. Tricoci P, Roe MT, Mulgund J, et al: Clopidogrel to treat patients with non–ST-segment elevation acute coronary syndromes after hospital discharge. Arch Intern Med 166:806, 2006.

144. Peterson ED, Roe MT, Mulgund J, et al: Association between hospital process performance and outcomes among patients with acute coronary syndromes. JAMA 295:1912, 2006.

145. Roe MT, Peterson ED, Newby LK, et al: The influence of risk status on guideline adherence for patients with non–ST-segment elevation acute coronary syndromes. Am Heart J 151:1205, 2006.

146. Cannon CP, O'Gara PT: Goals, design and implementation of critical pathways in cardiology. In Cannon CP, O'Gara PT (eds): Critical Pathways in Cardiology. Philadelphia, Lippincott Williams & Wilkins, 2001, pp 3-6.

147. Califf RM, Peterson ED, Gibbons RJ, et al: Integrating quality into the cycle of therapeutic development. J Am Coll Cardiol 40:1895, 2002.

148. Cannon CP, Hand MH, Bahr R, et al: Critical pathways for management of patients with acute coronary syndromes: An assessment by the National Heart Attack Alert Program. Am Heart J 143:777, 2002.

149. Eagle KA, Montoye CK, Riba AL, et al: Guideline-based standardized care is associated with substantially lower mortality in Medicare patients with acute myocardial infarction: The American College of Cardiology's Guidelines Applied in Practice (GAP) Projects in Michigan. J Am Coll Cardiol 46:1242, 2005.

Prinzmetal Variant Angina

150. Prinzmetal M, Kennamer R, Merliss R, et al: A variant form of angina pectoris. Am J Med 27:375, 1959.

151. Sueda S, Kohno H, Fukuda H, Uraoka T: Did the widespread use of long-acting calcium antagonists decrease the occurrence of variant angina? Chest 124:2074, 2003.

152. Mayer S, Hillis LD: Prinzmetal's variant angina. Clin Cardiol 21:243, 1998.

153. Okumura K, Osanai T, Kosugi T, et al: Enhanced phospholipase C activity in the cultured skin fibroblast obtained from patients with coronary spastic angina: Possible role for enhanced vasoconstrictor response. J Am Coll Cardiol 36:1847, 2000.

154. Hung MJ, Cherng WJ, Yang NI, et al: Relation of high-sensitivity C-reactive protein level with coronary vasospastic angina pectoris in patients without hemodynamically significant coronary artery disease. Am J Cardiol 96:1484, 2005.

155. Park JS, Zhang SY, Jo SH, et al: Common adrenergic receptor polymorphisms as novel risk factors for vasospastic angina. Am Heart J 151:864, 2006.

156. Sakata K, Miura F, Sugino H, et al: Assessment of regional sympathetic nerve activity in vasospastic angina: Analysis of iodine 123–labeled metaiodobenzylguanidine scintigraphy. Am Heart J 133:484, 1997.

157. Kawano H, Motoyama T, Yasue H, et al: Endothelial function fluctuates with diurnal variation in the frequency of ischemic episodes in patients with variant angina. J Am Coll Cardiol 40:266, 2002.

158. Abe M, Yoshida A, Otsuka Y: Intractable Prinzmetal's angina three months after implantation of sirolimus-eluting stent. J Invasive Cardiol 20:E306, 2008.

159. Lip GY, Gupta J, Khan MM, Singh SP: Recurrent myocardial infarction with angina and normal coronary arteries. Int J Cardiol 51:65, 1995.

160. Ledakowicz-Polak A, Ptaszynski P, Polak L, Zielinska M: Prinzmetal's variant angina associated with severe heart rhythm disturbances and syncope: A therapeutic dilemma. Cardiol J 16:269, 2009.

161. Hung M-J, Cheng CW, Yang NI, et al: Coronary vasospasm–induced acute coronary syndrome complicated by life-threatening cardia arrhythmias in patients without hemodynamically significant coronary artery disease. Int J Cardiol 117:37, 2007.

162. Meisel SR, Mazur A, Chetboun I, et al: Usefulness of implantable cardioverter-defibrillators in refractory variant angina pectoris complicated by ventricular fibrillation in patients with angiographically normal coronary arteries. Am J Cardiol 89:1114, 2002.

163. Crea F: Variant angina in patients without obstructive coronary atherosclerosis: A benign form of spasm. Eur Heart J 17:980, 1996.

164. Ahooja V, Thetai D: Multivessel coronary vasospasm mimicking triple-vessel obstructive coronary artery disease. J Invasive Cardiol 19:E178, 2007.

165. Hirano Y, Uehara H, Nakamura H, et al: Diagnosis of vasospastic angina: Comparison of hyperventilation and cold-pressor stress echocardiography, hyperventilation and cold-pressor stress coronary angiography, and coronary angiography with intracoronary injection of acetylcholine. Int J Cardiol 116:331, 2007.

166. Nakao K, Ohgushi M, Yoshimura M, et al: Hyperventilation as a specific test for diagnosis of coronary artery spasm. Am J Cardiol 80:545, 1997.

167. Antman E, Muller J, Goldberg S, et al: Nifedipine therapy for coronary artery spasm. Experience in 127 patients. N Engl J Med 302:1269, 1980.

168. De Cesare N, Cozzi S, Apostolo A, et al: Facilitation of coronary spasm by propranolol in Prinzmetal's angina: Fact or unproven extrapolation? Coron Artery Dis 5:323, 1994.

169. Petrov D, Sardowski S, Gesheva M: "Silent" Prinzmetal's ST elevation related to atenolol overdose. J Emerg Med 33:123, 2007.

170. Tzivoni D, Keren A, Benhorin J, et al: Prazosin therapy for refractory variant angina. Am Heart J 105:262, 1983.

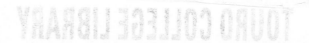

171. Kaski JC: Management of vasospastic angina—role of nicorandil. Cardiovasc Drugs Ther 9(Suppl 2):221, 1995.
172. Al-Sayegh A, Shukkur AM, Akbar M: Automatic implantable cardioverter defibrillator for the treatment of ventricular fibrillation following coronary artery spasm: A case report. Angiology 58:122, 2007.
173. Tashiro H, Shimokawa H, Koyanagi S, Takeshita A: Clinical characteristics of patients with spontaneous remission of variant angina. Jpn Circ J 57:117, 1993.
174. Bory M, Pierron F, Panagides D, et al: Coronary artery spasm in patients with normal or near normal coronary arteries. Long-term follow-up of 277 patients. Eur Heart J 17:1015, 1996.

 # GUIDELINES CHRISTOPHER P. CANNON AND EUGENE BRAUNWALD

Unstable Angina and Non–ST Elevation Myocardial Infarction

American College of Cardiology/American Heart Association (ACC/AHA) guidelines for the management of unstable angina and non–ST elevation myocardial infarction (UA/NSTEMI) were published in 2007,[1] presenting updates from prior versions.

Recommendations made in these guidelines pertaining to the initial evaluation of the patient with acute chest pain are included in the text of Chap. 53. For other recommendations relevant to this topic in guidelines for the use of percutaneous coronary interventions (PCI), see Chap. 58.

Like other ACC/AHA guidelines, these use the standard ACC/AHA classification system for indications:

Class I: conditions for which there is evidence and/or general agreement that the treatment is useful and effective.

Class II: conditions for which there is conflicting evidence and/or a divergence of opinion about the usefulness or efficacy of performing the treatment.

Class IIa: weight of evidence or opinion is in favor of usefulness or efficacy.

Class IIb: usefulness or efficacy is less well established by evidence or opinion.

Class III: conditions for which there is evidence and/or general agreement that the treatment is not useful or effective, and in some cases may be harmful.

Three levels are used to rate the evidence on which recommendations have been based. Level A recommendations are derived from data from multiple randomized clinical trials; level B recommendations are derived from a single randomized trial or nonrandomized studies; and level C recommendations are based on the consensus opinion of experts.

EARLY RISK STRATIFICATION AND MANAGEMENT

The initial evaluation of patients with UA/NSTEMI involves risk stratification, which the guidelines term an "integral prerequisite to decision making." This process involves two related but actually separate decision trees. The first, a diagnostic evaluation, estimates the likelihood that obstructive coronary artery disease is the cause of the presenting symptoms and asks, Does this patient have symptoms due to acute ischemia from obstructive coronary artery disease? For this process, the guidelines offer a table of characteristics that portend a high, intermediate, or low likelihood that the patient's presentation is due to ischemia (**Table 56G-1**). For patients of low and sometimes intermediate probability, a diagnostic pathway is provided to determine rapidly if the patient does or does not have an acute coronary syndrome (**Fig. 56G-1**).

The second part of stratification assesses the risk that a patient with UA/NSTEMI has for myocardial infarction or death during the next few weeks. Factors associated with an increased risk are listed in **Table 56G-2**. The guideline notes that risk stratification is useful in (1) selection of the site of care (coronary care unit, monitored step-down unit, or outpatient setting) and (2) selection of therapy, including platelet glycoprotein (GP) IIb/IIIa inhibitors and an invasive versus conservative management strategy.

HOSPITAL CARE

The guidelines recommend that patients admitted for acute coronary syndromes with continuing discomfort or hemodynamic instability, or both, be hospitalized for at least 24 hours in a coronary care unit characterized by a nurse-to-patient ratio sufficient to provide continuous rhythm monitoring and rapid resuscitation and defibrillation should it be necessary. Patients who do not have continuing discomfort or hemodynamic instability can be admitted to a step-down unit.

The 2007 guidelines recommend that the second step after risk stratification is to choose a management strategy (**Table 56G-3**), and then to proceed to the choice of antithrombotic therapy, because choices differ slightly on the basis of which strategy is followed.

TABLE 56G-1	Likelihood That Signs and Symptoms Represent an Acute Coronary Syndrome Secondary to Coronary Artery Disease		
FEATURE	**HIGH LIKELIHOOD**	**INTERMEDIATE LIKELIHOOD**	**LOW LIKELIHOOD**
	Any of the Following:	*Absence of High-Likelihood Features and Presence of Any of the Following:*	*Absence of High- or Intermediate-Likelihood Features But May Have:*
History	Chest or left arm pain or discomfort as chief symptom reproducing prior documented angina Known history of CAD, including MI	Chest or left arm pain or discomfort as chief symptom Age >70 years Male sex Diabetes mellitus	Probable ischemic symptoms in absence of any of the intermediate-likelihood characteristics Recent cocaine use
Examination	Transient MR murmur, hypotension, diaphoresis, pulmonary edema, or rales	Extracardiac vascular disease	Chest discomfort reproduced by palpation
ECG	New, or presumably new, transient ST-segment deviation (1 mm or greater) or T wave inversion in multiple precordial leads	Fixed Q waves ST depression 0.5 to 1 mm or T wave inversion greater than 1 mm	T wave flattening or inversion less than 1 mm in leads with dominant R waves Normal ECG
Cardiac markers	Elevated cardiac TnI, TnT, or CK-MB	Normal	Normal

CAD = coronary artery disease; CK-MB = MB fraction of creatine kinase; ECG = electrocardiogram; MI = myocardial infarction; MR = mitral regurgitation; TnI = troponin I; TnT = troponin T.
From Anderson JL, Adams CD, Antman EM, et al: ACC/AHA 2007 guidelines for the management of patients with unstable angina/non–ST-elevation myocardial infarction: A report of the American College of Cardiology/American Heart Association Task Force on Practice Guidelines (Writing Committee to Revise the 2002 Guidelines for the Management of Patients With Unstable Angina/Non–ST-Elevation Myocardial Infarction) developed in collaboration with the American College of Emergency Physicians, the Society for Cardiovascular Angiography and Interventions, and the Society of Thoracic Surgeons endorsed by the American Association of Cardiovascular and Pulmonary Rehabilitation and the Society for Academic Emergency Medicine. J Am Coll Cardiol 50:e1, 2007.

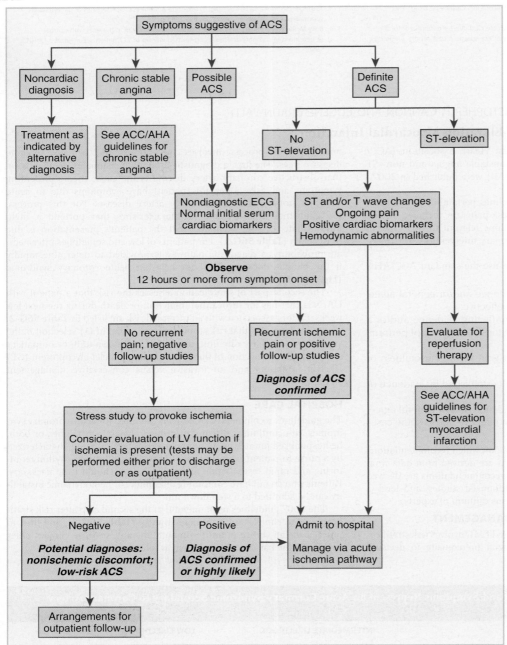

FIGURE 56G-1 ACC/AHA guideline algorithm for acute coronary syndrome (ACS).

beta blocker therapy should be initiated within the first 24 hours in patients who do not have one or more of the following: signs of heart failure, evidence of a low-output state, increased risk for cardiogenic shock, or other relative contraindications to beta blockade (PR interval greater than 0.24 second, second- or third-degree heart block, active asthma, or reactive airway disease). If a contraindication to beta blocker therapy exists, patients with recurrent ischemia can be treated with a nondihydropyridine calcium antagonist (e.g., verapamil or diltiazem). Morphine sulfate should be used for patients whose condition is not controlled with nitrates or for patients who have pulmonary congestion, severe agitation, or both. An angiotensin-converting enzyme (ACE) inhibitor should be started if hypertension persists despite anti-ischemic therapy or if patients have left ventricular systolic dysfunction or diabetes. A new recommendation in the 2007 guidelines is that because of the increased risks of mortality, reinfarction, hypertension, heart failure, and myocardial rupture associated with their use, nonsteroidal anti-inflammatory drugs, except for aspirin, whether nonselective or cyclooxygenase 2—selective agents, should be discontinued at the time a patient presents with UA/NSTEMI.

For both treatment strategies, aspirin is indicated, at an initial dose of 160 to 325 mg daily. In addition, the guidelines note that all patients should receive anticoagulants. In the invasive approach, there are four choices: unfractionated heparin (UFH), enoxaparin (Lovenox), bivalirudin (Angiomax), or fondaparinux (Arixtra). Regarding additional antiplatelet therapy, the 2007 guidelines recommend that before diagnostic angiography, at least one of clopidogrel (Plavix) or an intravenous GP IIb/IIIa inhibitor should be initiated. Use of both agents is listed as reasonable; factors favoring administration of both include a delay to the time of angiography, high-risk features, and early recurrent ischemic discomfort.

For patients managed with an initial conservative strategy (see Fig. 56G-3), in addition to aspirin, the ACC/AHA guidelines recommend anticoagulant therapy but have only three options—enoxaparin, fondaparinux, or UFH—with the subcutaneously administered drugs enoxaparin and fondaparinux preferred to UFH as a Class IIa recommendation. In patients with an increased risk of bleeding, fondaparinux is preferable on the basis of lower bleeding risk. Clopidogrel should be started at the time of presentation in conservatively managed patients.

The 2007 ACC/AHA guidelines emphasize reevaluation of medications after angiography (**Fig. 56G-4**). If a patient is selected for coronary artery bypass grafting (CABG), aspirin and UFH should be continued; clopidogrel, GP IIb/IIIa inhibitors, and anticoagulants other than UFH should be stopped. For medically managed patients, reevaluation for the need of clopidogrel is encouraged—so that if it had not been given before angiography (if the physician wished to define the coronary anatomy

An early invasive strategy involves prompt coronary angiography (within approximately 48 hours) followed by revascularization if the anatomy is appropriate. This strategy is recommended for patients with high-risk features as outlined in Tables 56G-2 and 56G-3 and **Figure 56G-2**. In contrast, an early conservative strategy, in which patients are stabilized with medical therapy and angiography is performed only if patients have recurrent symptoms or ischemia, heart failure, or serious arrhythmias, is generally recommended for low-risk patients. As noted in **Figure 56G-3**, patients managed according to the early conservative strategy should undergo an assessment of left ventricular function and a stress test; they should also undergo angiography if they have an ejection fraction below 40% or if they have an intermediate- or high-risk exercise test result. For low-risk women, the 2007 guidelines give a Class I recommendation for an early conservative approach.

Anti-ischemic medical therapy should include nitrates and, in the absence of contraindications, beta blockers (**Table 56G-4**). The 2007 ACC/AHA guidelines emphasize, however, that oral (not intravenous)

TABLE 56G-2 ACC/AHA System for Risk Stratification of Patients with Unstable Angina

FEATURE	HIGH RISK	INTERMEDIATE RISK	LOW RISK
	At Least One of the Following Features:	*No High-Risk Feature But Must Have One of the Following:*	*No High- or Intermediate-Risk Feature But May Have Any of the Following Features:*
History	Accelerating tempo of ischemic symptoms in preceding 48 hr	Prior MI, peripheral or cerebrovascular disease, or CABG; prior aspirin use	
Character of pain	Prolonged ongoing (>20 min) rest pain	Prolonged rest angina, now resolved, with moderate or high likelihood of CAD Rest angina <20 min or relieved with rest or sublingual NTG	New-onset or progressive CCS class III or IV angina the past 2 wk without prolonged rest pain but with moderate or high likelihood of CAD
Clinical findings	Pulmonary edema, most likely caused by ischemia New or worsening MR murmur S_3 or new worsening rales Hypotension, bradycardia, tachycardia Age >75 yr	Age >70 yr	
ECG	Angina at rest with transient ST-segment changes >0.05 mV Bundle branch block, new or presumed new Sustained ventricular tachycardia	T wave inversions >0.2 mV Pathologic Q waves	Normal or unchanged ECG during an episode of chest discomfort
Cardiac markers	Elevated	Slightly elevated	Normal

CABG = coronary artery bypass graft; CAD = coronary artery disease; CCS = Canadian Cardiovascular Society; ECG = electrocardiogram; MI = myocardial infarction; MR = mitral regurgitation; NTG = nitroglycerin.
From Anderson JL, Adams CD, Antman EM, et al: ACC/AHA 2007 guidelines for the management of patients with unstable angina/non–ST-elevation myocardial infarction: A report of the American College of Cardiology/American Heart Association Task Force on Practice Guidelines (Writing Committee to Revise the 2002 Guidelines for the Management of Patients With Unstable Angina/Non–ST-Elevation Myocardial Infarction) developed in collaboration with the American College of Emergency Physicians, the Society for Cardiovascular Angiography and Interventions, and the Society of Thoracic Surgeons endorsed by the American Association of Cardiovascular and Pulmonary Rehabilitation and the Society for Academic Emergency Medicine. J Am Coll Cardiol 50:e1, 2007.

TABLE 56G-3 ACC/AHA Guideline Recommendations for Selection of Initial Treatment Strategy: Invasive Versus Conservative Strategy

PREFERRED STRATEGY	PATIENT CHARACTERISTICS
Invasive	Recurrent angina or ischemia at rest or with low-level activities, despite intensive medical therapy Elevated cardiac biomarkers (TnT or TnI) New or presumably new ST-segment depression Signs or symptoms of HF or new or worsening mitral regurgitation High-risk findings from noninvasive testing Hemodynamic instability Sustained ventricular tachycardia PCI within 6 months Prior CABG High-risk score (e.g., TIMI, GRACE) Reduced left ventricular function (LVEF <40%)
Conservative	Low-risk score (e.g., TIMI, GRACE) Patient or physician preference in the absence of high-risk features

CABG = coronary artery bypass graft surgery; GRACE = Global Registry of Acute Coronary Events; HF = heart failure; LVEF = left ventricular ejection fraction; PCI = percutaneous coronary intervention; TIMI = Thrombolysis In Myocardial Infarction; TnI = troponin I; TnT = troponin T.
From Anderson JL, Adams CD, Antman EM, et al: ACC/AHA 2007 guidelines for the management of patients with unstable angina/non–ST-elevation myocardial infarction: A report of the American College of Cardiology/American Heart Association Task Force on Practice Guidelines (Writing Committee to Revise the 2002 Guidelines for the Management of Patients With Unstable Angina/Non–ST-Elevation Myocardial Infarction) developed in collaboration with the American College of Emergency Physicians, the Society for Cardiovascular Angiography and Interventions, and the Society of Thoracic Surgeons endorsed by the American Association of Cardiovascular and Pulmonary Rehabilitation and the Society for Academic Emergency Medicine. J Am Coll Cardiol 50:e1, 2007.

before starting this agent), it should be given if coronary artery disease is confirmed at angiography. Indeed, use of clopidogrel in medically managed patients is listed as a "test" performance measure in the 2008 ACC/AHA myocardial infarction performance measures.[2]

LATER RISK STRATIFICATION AND MANAGEMENT

Table 56G-5 lists the ACC/AHA guidelines recommendations for risk stratification before discharge. As shown in Figure 56G-1, early stress testing is performed in low-risk patients (see Table 56G-2 for risk category definition); for intermediate-risk patients managed with an early conservative strategy, stress testing can be performed after they have been free of ischemia and heart failure for a minimum of 2 to 3 days. The first choice in noninvasive tests is exercise electrocardiography; imaging technologies and pharmacologic stress tests should be used for subsets of patients for whom exercise electrocardiography would be expected to have a high likelihood of providing inadequate data. Data from noninvasive tests can restratify patients into high-, intermediate-, and low-risk groups (**Table 56G-6**).

For patients who require coronary revascularization, the principles for choosing between CABG and PCI are similar to those used for patients with chronic stable angina (see Chap. 57). The guidelines recommend CABG over PCI for patients with significant left main coronary artery disease and for patients with multivessel disease and diminished ejection fraction or diabetes (**Fig. 56G-5**). Either CABG or PCI is considered appropriate for patients with two-vessel disease (**Table 56G-7**).[3] The UA/NSTEMI guidelines and the 2009 ACC/AHA appropriate use criteria provide some support for revascularization with CABG or PCI for patients with proximal left anterior descending coronary artery disease alone.

HOSPITAL DISCHARGE AND POSTHOSPITAL DISCHARGE CARE

The ACC/AHA guidelines emphasize the importance of aggressive risk factor modification and of teaching patients about management of ischemic episodes (**Table 56G-8**). Five classes of drugs are indicated: aspirin,

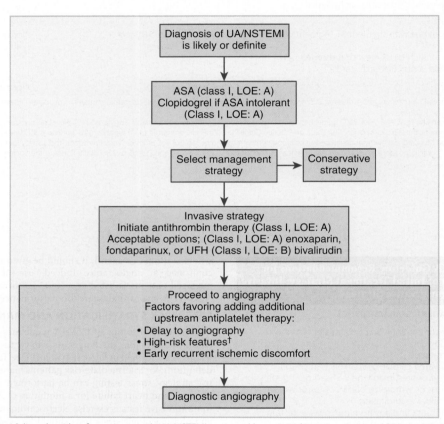

FIGURE 56G-2 ACC/AHA guideline algorithm for patients with UA/NSTEMI managed by an initial invasive strategy. ASA = aspirin; LOE = level of evidence; UFH = unfractionated heparin.

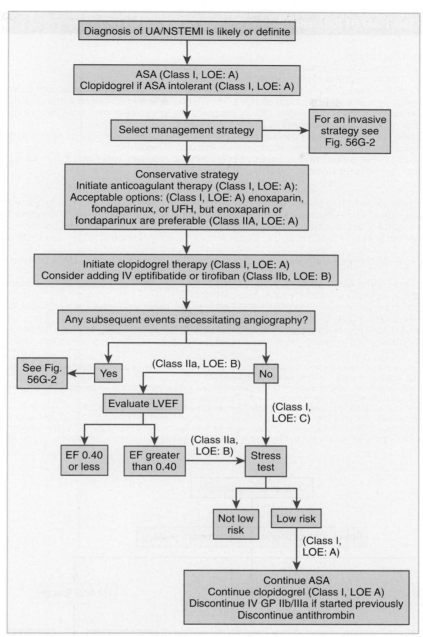

FIGURE 56G-3 ACC/AHA guideline algorithm for patients with UA/NSTEMI managed by an initial conservative strategy. ASA = aspirin; EF = ejection fraction; GP = glycoprotein; IV = intravenous; LOE = level of evidence; LVEF = left ventricular ejection fraction; UFH = unfractionated heparin.

UNSTABLE ANGINA AND NON–ST ELEVATION MYOCARDIAL INFARCTION

CH 56

TABLE 56G-4   ACC/AHA Class I and III Recommendations for Anti-Ischemic Therapy

Class I

1. Bed/chair rest with continuous ECG monitoring
2. NTG 0.4 mg sublingually every 5 min for a total of 3 doses; afterward, assess need for IV NTG
3. NTG IV for first 48 hr after UA/NSTEMI for treatment of persistent ischemia, HF, or hypertension
4. Decision to administer NTG IV and dose should not preclude therapy with other mortality-reducing interventions such as beta blockers or ACE inhibitors
5. Beta blockers (via oral route) within 24 hr without a contraindication (e.g., HF) irrespective of concomitant performance of PCI
6. When beta blockers are contraindicated, a nondihydropyridine calcium antagonist (e.g., verapamil or diltiazem) should be given as initial therapy in the absence of severe LV dysfunction or other contraindications
7. ACE inhibitor (via oral route) within first 24 hr with pulmonary congestion, or LVEF ≤0.40, in the absence of hypotension (systolic blood pressure <100 mm Hg or <30 mm Hg below baseline) or known contraindications to that class of medications
8. ARB should be administered to UA/NSTEMI patients who are intolerant of ACE inhibitors and have either clinical or radiologic signs of heart failure or LVEF ≤0.40. Valsartan and candesartan have demonstrated efficacy for this indication.

Class III

1. Nitrates should not be administered to UA/NSTEMI patients with systolic blood pressure <90 mm Hg or ≥30 mm Hg below baseline, severe bradycardia (<50 beats/min), tachycardia (>100 beats/min) in the absence of symptomatic HF, or right ventricular infarction. *(Level of Evidence: C)*
2. Nitroglycerin or other nitrates should not be administered to patients with UA/NSTEMI who have received a phosphodiesterase inhibitor for erectile dysfunction within 24 hr of sildenafil or 48 hr of tadalafil use. The suitable time for the administration of nitrates after vardenafil has not been determined. *(Level of Evidence: C)*
3. Immediate-release dihydropyridine calcium antagonists should not be administered to patients with UA/NSTEMI in the absence of a beta blocker. *(Level of Evidence: A)*
4. An intravenous ACE inhibitor should not be given to patients within the first 24 hours of UA/NSTEMI because of the increased risk of hypotension. (A possible exception may be patients with refractory hypertension.) *(Level of Evidence: B)*
5. It may be harmful to administer intravenous beta blockers to UA/NSTEMI patients who have contraindications to beta blockade, signs of HF or low-output state, or other risk factors* for cardiogenic shock. *(Level of Evidence: A)*
6. Nonsteroidal anti-inflammatory drugs (except for aspirin), whether nonselective or COX-2–selective agents, should not be administered during hospitalization for UA/NSTEMI because of the increased risks of mortality, reinfarction, hypertension, HF, and myocardial rupture associated with their use. *(Level of Evidence: C)*

*Risk factors for cardiogenic shock (the greater the number of risk factors present, the higher the risk of developing cardiogenic shock): age >70 years, systolic blood pressure <120 mm Hg, sinus tachycardia >110 or heart rate <60, increased time since onset of symptoms of UA/NSTEMI.

ACE = angiotensin-converting enzyme; ARB = angiotensin receptor blocker; COX-2 = cyclooxygenase 2; HF = heart failure; IV = intravenous; LV = left ventricular; LVEF = left ventricular ejection fraction; MI = myocardial infarction; NTG = nitroglycerin; PCI = percutaneous coronary intervention.

From Anderson JL, Adams CD, Antman EM, et al: ACC/AHA 2007 guidelines for the management of patients with unstable angina/non–ST-elevation myocardial infarction: A report of the American College of Cardiology/American Heart Association Task Force on Practice Guidelines (Writing Committee to Revise the 2002 Guidelines for the Management of Patients With Unstable Angina/Non–ST-Elevation Myocardial Infarction) developed in collaboration with the American College of Emergency Physicians, the Society for Cardiovascular Angiography and Interventions, and the Society of Thoracic Surgeons endorsed by the American Association of Cardiovascular and Pulmonary Rehabilitation and the Society for Academic Emergency Medicine. J Am Coll Cardiol 50:e1, 2007.

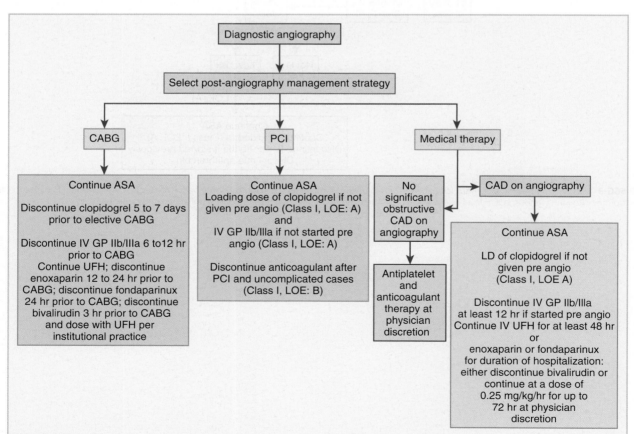

FIGURE 56G-4   ACC/AHA guideline for management after diagnostic angiography in patients with UA/NSTEMI. ASA = aspirin; CABG = coronary artery bypass graft; CAD = coronary artery disease; GP = glycoprotein; IV = intravenous; LD = loading dose; LOE = level of evidence; PCI = percutaneous coronary intervention; pre angio = before angiography; UFH = unfractionated heparin.

TABLE 56G-5 ACC/AHA Guidelines for Risk Stratification Before Discharge in Patients with Acute Coronary Syndromes

Class I

1. Noninvasive stress testing is recommended in low-risk patients who have been free of ischemia at rest or with low-level activity and of HF for a minimum of 12 to 24 hr. *(Level of Evidence: C)*
2. Noninvasive stress testing is recommended in patients at intermediate risk who have been free of ischemia at rest or with low-level activity and of HF for a minimum of 12 to 24 hr. *(Level of Evidence: C)*
3. Choice of stress test is based on the resting ECG, ability to perform exercise, local expertise, and technologies available. Treadmill exercise is useful in patients able to exercise whose ECG lacks baseline ST-segment abnormalities, bundle branch block, LV hypertrophy, intraventricular conduction defect, paced rhythm, preexcitation, or digoxin effect. *(Level of Evidence: C)*
4. An imaging modality should be added in patients with resting ST-segment depression (≥0.1 mV), LV hypertrophy, bundle branch block, intraventricular conduction defect, preexcitation, or digoxin. In patients undergoing a low-level exercise test, an imaging modality can add sensitivity. *(Level of Evidence: B)*
5. Pharmacologic stress testing with imaging is recommended when physical limitations (e.g., arthritis, amputation, severe peripheral vascular disease, severe chronic obstructive pulmonary disease, or general debility) preclude adequate exercise stress. *(Level of Evidence: B)*
6. Prompt angiography without noninvasive risk stratification should be performed for failure of stabilization with intensive medical treatment. *(Level of Evidence: B)*
7. A noninvasive test (echocardiogram or radionuclide angiogram) is recommended to evaluate LV function in patients with definite ACS who are not scheduled for coronary angiography and left ventriculography. *(Level of Evidence: B)*

ACS = acute coronary syndrome; ECG = electrocardiogram; HF = heart failure; LV = left ventricular.
From Anderson JL, Adams CD, Antman EM, et al: ACC/AHA 2007 guidelines for the management of patients with unstable angina/non–ST-elevation myocardial infarction: A report of the American College of Cardiology/American Heart Association Task Force on Practice Guidelines (Writing Committee to Revise the 2002 Guidelines for the Management of Patients With Unstable Angina/Non–ST-Elevation Myocardial Infarction) developed in collaboration with the American College of Emergency Physicians, the Society for Cardiovascular Angiography and Interventions, and the Society of Thoracic Surgeons endorsed by the American Association of Cardiovascular and Pulmonary Rehabilitation and the Society for Academic Emergency Medicine. J Am Coll Cardiol 50:e1, 2007.

TABLE 56G-6 ACC/AHA Noninvasive Risk Stratification

High Risk (>3% Annual Mortality Rate)

1. Severe resting LV dysfunction (LVEF <0.35)
2. High-risk treadmill score (score ≤ −11)
3. Severe exercise LV dysfunction (exercise LVEF <0.35)
4. Stress-induced large perfusion defect (particularly if anterior)
5. Stress-induced multiple perfusion defects of moderate size
6. Large, fixed perfusion defect with LV dilation or increased lung uptake (thallium-201)
7. Stress-induced moderate perfusion defect with LV dilation or increased lung uptake (thallium-201)
8. Echocardiographic wall motion abnormality (involving > two segments) developing at a low dose of dobutamine (≤10 mg/kg/min) or at a low heart rate (<120 beats/min)
9. Stress echocardiographic evidence of extensive ischemia

Intermediate Risk (1%-3% Annual Mortality Rate)

1. Mild/moderate resting LV dysfunction (LVEF 0.35-0.49)
2. Intermediate-risk treadmill score (−11 < score < 5)
3. Stress-induced moderate perfusion defect without LV dilation or increased lung intake (thallium-201)
4. Limited stress echocardiographic ischemia with a wall motion abnormality only at higher doses of dobutamine involving two segments or less

Low Risk (<1% Annual Mortality Rate)

1. Low-risk treadmill score (score ≥5)
2. Normal or small myocardial perfusion defect at rest or with stress
3. Normal stress echocardiographic wall motion or no change of limited resting wall motion abnormalities during stress

LV = left ventricular; LVEF = left ventricular ejection fraction.
From Gibbons RJ, Chatterjee K, Daley J, et al: ACC/AHA/ACP-ASIM guidelines for the management of patients with chronic stable angina. J Am Coll Cardiol 33:2092, 1999.

FIGURE 56G-5 ACC/AHA guideline for revascularization strategy in UA/NSTEMI. CABG = coronary artery bypass graft; LAD = left anterior descending coronary artery; PCI = percutaneous coronary intervention.

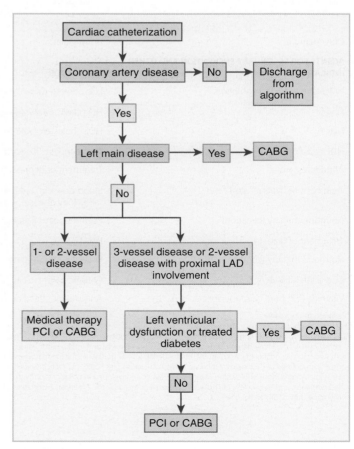

CH
56

TABLE 56G-7 ACC/AHA Appropriateness Ratings for Type of Revascularization

	CABG			PCI		
	NO DIABETES AND NORMAL LVEF	DIABETES	DEPRESSED LVEF	NO DIABETES AND NORMAL LVEF	DIABETES	DEPRESSED LVEF
Two-vessel coronary artery disease with proximal LAD stenosis	A	A	A	A	A	A
Three-vessel coronary artery disease	A	A	A	U	U	U
Isolated left main stenosis	A	A	A	I	I	I
Left main stenosis and additional coronary artery disease	A	A	A	I	I	I

A = appropriate; I = inappropriate; U = uncertain; CABG = coronary artery bypass graft; LAD = left anterior descending coronary artery; LVEF = left ventricular ejection fraction; PCI = percutaneous coronary intervention.
From Patel MR, Dehmer GJ, Hirshfeld JW, et al: ACCF/SCAI/STS/AATS/AHA/ASNC 2009 Appropriateness Criteria for Coronary Revascularization: A report by the American College of Cardiology Foundation Appropriateness Criteria Task Force, Society for Cardiovascular Angiography and Interventions, Society of Thoracic Surgeons, American Association for Thoracic Surgery, American Heart Association, and the American Society of Nuclear Cardiology Endorsed by the American Society of Echocardiography, the Heart Failure Society of America, and the Society of Cardiovascular Computed Tomography. J Am Coll Cardiol 53:530, 2009.

TABLE 56G-8 Medications Used for Stabilized UA/NSTEMI Patients

ANTI-ISCHEMIC AND ANTITHROMBOTIC/ ANTIPLATELET AGENTS	DRUG ACTION	CLASS/LEVEL OF EVIDENCE
Aspirin	Antiplatelet	I/A
Clopidogrel* or ticlopidine	Antiplatelet when aspirin is contraindicated	I/A
Beta blockers	Anti-ischemic	I/B
ACEI	EF <0.40 or HF EF >0.40	I/A, IIa/A
Nitrates	Antianginal	I/C for ischemic symptoms
Calcium channel blockers (short-acting dihydropyridine antagonists should be avoided)	Antianginal	I for ischemic symptoms; when beta blockers are not successful (B) or contraindicated, or cause unacceptable side effects (C)
Dipyridamole	Antiplatelet	III/A

AGENTS FOR SECONDARY PREVENTION AND OTHER INDICATIONS	RISK FACTOR	CLASS/LEVEL OF EVIDENCE
HMG-CoA reductase inhibitors	LDL cholesterol >70 mg/dL	Ia
Fibrates	HDL cholesterol <40 mg/dL	IIa/B
Niacin	HDL cholesterol <40 mg/dL	IIa/B
Niacin or fibrate	Triglycerides 200 mg/dL	IIa/B
Antidepressant	Treatment of depression	IIb/B
Treatment of hypertension	Blood pressure >140/90 mm Hg or >130/80 mm Hg if kidney disease or diabetes present	I/A
Hormone therapy (initiation)[†]	Postmenopausal state	III/A
Treatment of diabetes	HbA1c >7%	I/B
Hormone therapy (continuation)[†]	Postmenopausal state	III/B
COX-2 inhibitor or NSAID	Chronic pain	IIa/C, IIb/C, or III/C
Vitamins C, E, beta-carotene; folic acid, B_6, B_{12}	Antioxidant effect; homocysteine lowering	III/A

*Preferred to ticlopidine.
[†]For risk reduction of coronary artery disease.
ACEI = angiotensin-converting enzyme inhibitor; COX-2 = cyclooxygenase 2; EF = ejection fraction; HDL = high-density lipoprotein; HF = heart failure; HMG-CoA = hydroxymethylglutaryl coenzyme A; LDL = low-density lipoprotein; NSAID = nonsteroidal anti-inflammatory drug.
From Anderson JL, Adams CD, Antman EM, et al: ACC/AHA 2007 guidelines for the management of patients with unstable angina/non–ST-elevation myocardial infarction: a report of the American College of Cardiology/American Heart Association Task Force on Practice Guidelines (Writing Committee to Revise the 2002 Guidelines for the Management of Patients With Unstable Angina/Non–ST-Elevation Myocardial Infarction) developed in collaboration with the American College of Emergency Physicians, the Society for Cardiovascular Angiography and Interventions, and the Society of Thoracic Surgeons endorsed by the American Association of Cardiovascular and Pulmonary Rehabilitation and the Society for Academic Emergency Medicine. J Am Coll Cardiol 50:e1, 2007.

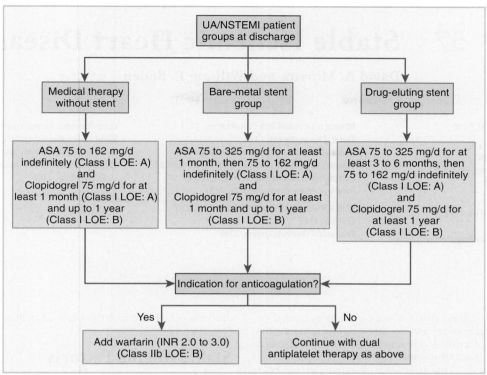

FIGURE 56G-6 ACC/AHA guideline for long-term antithrombotic therapy at hospital discharge after UA/NSTEMI. ASA = aspirin; INR = international normalized ratio; LOE = level of evidence.

clopidogrel, beta blockers, ACE inhibitors, and statins. The 2007 guidelines recommend that statins be given at the time of discharge, regardless of low-density lipoprotein level. Recommendations for antithrombotic therapy are given in **Figure 56G-6**. The dose of aspirin is recommended to be 81 to 162 mg for medically managed patients; after PCI, a slightly higher dose is recommended (162 to 325 mg) for a period of 1, 3, or 6 months, depending on the type of stent, followed by the lower dose. If a patient has an indication for warfarin, it should be added but titrated to an international normalized ratio of 2.0 to 2.5, and aspirin 81 mg daily is recommended.

REFERENCES

1. Anderson JL, Adams CD, Antman EM, et al: ACC/AHA 2007 guidelines for the management of patients with unstable angina/non—ST-elevation myocardial infarction: A report of the American College of Cardiology/ American Heart Association Task Force on Practice Guidelines (Writing Committee to Revise the 2002 Guidelines for the Management of Patients With Unstable Angina/Non—ST-Elevation Myocardial Infarction) developed in collaboration with the American College of Emergency Physicians, the Society for Cardiovascular Angiography and Interventions, and the Society of Thoracic Surgeons endorsed by the American Association of Cardiovascular and Pulmonary Rehabilitation and the Society for Academic Emergency Medicine. J Am Coll Cardiol 50:e1, 2007.

2. Masoudi FA, Bonow RO, Brindis RG, et al: ACC/AHA 2008 statement on Performance Measurement and Reperfusion Therapy: A report of the ACC/ AHA Task Force on Performance Measures (Work Group to address the challenges of Performance Measurement and Reperfusion Therapy). J Am Coll Cardiol 52:2100, 2008.

3. Patel MR, Dehmer GJ, Hirshfeld JW, et al: ACCF/SCAI/STS/AATS/AHA/ ASNC 2009 Appropriateness Criteria for Coronary Revascularization: A report by the American College of Cardiology Foundation Appropriateness Criteria Task Force, Society for Cardiovascular Angiography and Interventions, Society of Thoracic Surgeons, American Association for Thoracic Surgery, American Heart Association, and the American Society of Nuclear Cardiology Endorsed by the American Society of Echocardiography, the Heart Failure Society of America, and the Society of Cardiovascular Computed Tomography. J Am Coll Cardiol 53:530, 2009.

CHAPTER **57** # Stable Ischemic Heart Disease

David A. Morrow and William E. Boden

Stable ischemic heart disease (IHD) is most commonly caused by obstruction of the coronary arteries by atheromatous plaque (the pathogenesis of atherosclerosis is described in Chap. 43). Factors that predispose to this condition are discussed in Chap. 44, control of coronary blood flow in Chap. 52, acute myocardial infarction (MI) in Chaps. 54 and 55, and unstable angina in Chap. 56; sudden cardiac death, another significant consequence of coronary artery disease (CAD), is presented in Chap. 41.

The clinical presentations of IHD are highly variable. Chest discomfort is usually the predominant symptom in chronic (stable) angina, unstable angina, Prinzmetal (variant) angina, microvascular angina, and acute myocardial infarction (MI). However, presentations of IHD also occur in which chest discomfort is absent or not prominent, such as asymptomatic (silent) myocardial ischemia, heart failure, cardiac arrhythmias, and sudden death. Obstructive CAD also has nonatherosclerotic causes, including congenital abnormalities of the coronary vessels, myocardial bridging, coronary arteritis in association with the systemic vasculitides, and radiation-induced coronary disease. Myocardial ischemia and angina pectoris may also occur in the absence of obstructive CAD, as in the case of aortic valve disease (see Chap. 66), hypertrophic cardiomyopathy (see Chap. 69), and idiopathic dilated cardiomyopathy (see Chap. 68). Moreover, CAD may coexist with these other forms of heart disease.

Magnitude of the Problem

The importance of IHD in contemporary society is attested to by the almost epidemic number of persons afflicted (see Chap. 1). It is estimated that 17,600,000 Americans have IHD, of whom 10,200,00 have angina pectoris and 8,500,000 have had an MI.[1] Based on data from the Framingham Heart Study, the lifetime risk of developing symptomatic CAD after age 40 is 49% for men and 32% for women. In 2006, IHD accounted for 52% of all deaths caused by cardiovascular disease and was the single most frequent cause of death in American men and women, resulting in more than one in six deaths in the United States. The economic cost of IHD in the United States in 2010 has been estimated at $177.1 billion. Despite a steady decline in age-specific mortality from CAD over the past several decades,[2] ischemic heart disease is now the leading cause of death worldwide, and it is expected that the rate of CAD will only accelerate in the next decade with the burden shifting progressively to lower socioeconomic groups. Contributory factors include aging of the population, alarming increases in the worldwide prevalence of obesity, type 2 diabetes, and a rise in cardiovascular risk factors in younger people. The World Health Organization has estimated that by 2020, the global number of

deaths from CAD will have risen from 7.6 million in 2005 to 11.1 million (see Chap. 1).[3]

Stable Angina Pectoris

Clinical Manifestations

CHARACTERISTICS OF ANGINA. Angina pectoris (see Chap. 12) is a discomfort in the chest or adjacent areas caused by myocardial ischemia. It is usually brought on by exertion and is associated with a disturbance in myocardial function. Acute MI, which is usually associated with prolonged severe pain occurring at rest (see Chap. 54), and unstable angina, which is characterized by an accelerated pattern and/ or occurrence at rest (see Chap. 56), are discussed separately. Heberden's initial description of angina as conveying a sense of "strangling and anxiety" is still remarkably pertinent. Other adjectives frequently used to describe this distress include tight, constricting, suffocating, crushing, heavy, and squeezing. In other patients, the quality of the sensation is more vague and described as a mild pressure-like discomfort, an uncomfortable numb sensation, or a burning sensation. The site of the discomfort is usually retrosternal, but radiation is common and usually occurs down the ulnar surface of the left arm; the right arm and the outer surfaces of both arms may also be involved (**Fig. 57-1**). Epigastric discomfort alone or in association with chest pressure may occur. Anginal discomfort above the mandible or below the epigastrium is rare. Anginal equivalents (i.e., symptoms of myocardial ischemia other than angina), such as dyspnea, faintness, fatigue, and eructations, are common, particularly in older patients. A history of abnormal exertional dyspnea may be an early indicator of IHD, even when angina is absent or no evidence of CAD can be found on the electrocardiogram (ECG). Dyspnea at rest or with exertion may be a manifestation of severe ischemia, leading to increases in left ventricular (LV) filling pressure.[4] Nocturnal angina should raise the suspicion of sleep apnea (see Chap. 79). Postprandial angina, presumably caused by redistribution of coronary blood flow away from the territory supplied by severely stenosed vessels, may be a marker of severe CAD.

The typical episode of angina pectoris usually begins gradually and reaches its maximum intensity over a period of minutes before dissipating. It is unusual for angina pectoris to reach its maximum severity within seconds, and it is characteristic that patients with angina usually prefer to rest, sit, or stop walking during episodes. Chest discomfort while walking in the cold or uphill is suggestive of angina. Features suggesting the absence of angina pectoris include pleuritic pain, pain localized to the tip of one finger, pain reproduced by movement or palpation of the chest wall or arms, and constant pain lasting

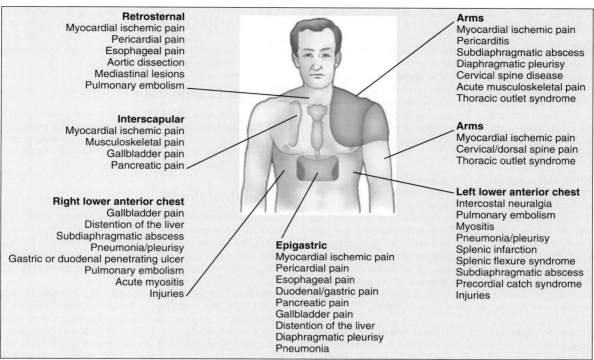

FIGURE 57-1 Location of discomfort and cause of chest symptoms. The location of angina is usually retrosternal but radiation is common. An epigastric location of angina may also occur. *(Modified from Braunwald E: The history. In Zipes D, Libby P, Bonow RO, Braunwald E [eds]: Braunwald's Heart Disease. 7th ed. Philadelphia, WB Saunders, 2005, p 68.)*

many hours or, alternatively, very brief episodes of pain lasting seconds. Pain radiating into the lower extremities is also a highly unusual manifestation of angina pectoris.

Typical angina pectoris is relieved within minutes by rest or the use of nitroglycerin. The response to the latter is often a useful diagnostic tool, although it should be remembered that esophageal pain and other syndromes may also respond to nitroglycerin. A delay of more than 5 to 10 minutes before relief is obtained by rest and nitroglycerin suggests that the symptoms are either not caused by ischemia or are caused by severe ischemia, as with acute MI or unstable angina. The phenomenon of first-effort or warm-up angina is used to describe the ability of some patients in whom angina develops with exertion to continue subsequently at the same or even greater level of exertion without symptoms after an intervening period of rest. This attenuation of myocardial ischemia observed with repeated exertion has been postulated to be caused by ischemic preconditioning and appears to require preceding ischemia of at least moderate intensity to induce the warm-up phenomenon.

GRADING OF ANGINA PECTORIS. A system of grading the severity of angina pectoris proposed by the Canadian Cardiovascular Society (CCS) has gained widespread acceptance (see Table 12-1).[5] The system is a modification of the New York Heart Association (NYHA) functional classification but allows patients to be categorized in more specific terms. Other grading systems[6] include a specific activity scale developed by Goldman and associates and an anginal score developed by Califf and colleagues. The Goldman scale is based on the metabolic cost of specific activities and appears to be valid when used by physicians and nonphysicians. The anginal score of Califf and coworkers integrates the clinical features and tempo of angina together with ST and T wave changes on the ECG and offers independent prognostic information beyond that provided by age, gender, LV function, and coronary angiographic anatomy. A limitation of all these grading systems is their dependence on accurate patient observation and patients' widely varying tolerance for symptoms. Functional estimates based on the CCS criteria have shown a reproducibility of only 73% and do not correlate well with objective measures of exercise performance.

MECHANISMS. The mechanisms of cardiac pain and the neural pathways involved are poorly understood. It is presumed that angina pectoris results from ischemic episodes that excite chemosensitive and mechanosensitive receptors in the heart.[7] Stimulation of these receptors results in the release of adenosine, bradykinin, and other substances that excite the sensory ends of the sympathetic and vagal afferent fibers.[8] The afferent fibers traverse the nerves that connect to the upper five thoracic sympathetic ganglia and upper five distal thoracic roots of the spinal cord. Impulses are transmitted by the spinal cord to the thalamus and hence to the neocortex. Data from animal studies have identified the vanilloid receptor-1 (VR_1), an important sensor for somatic nociception, as present on the sensory nerve endings of the heart and have suggested that VR_1 functions as a transducer of myocardial tissue ischemia.[9] In a murine VR_1 gene knockout model, ischemia-induced activation of VR_1 appeared to play a role in ischemic preconditioning.[10]

Within the spinal cord, cardiac sympathetic afferent impulses may converge with impulses from somatic thoracic structures, which may be the basis for referred cardiac pain—for example, to the chest. In comparison, cardiac vagal afferent fibers synapse in the nucleus tractus solitarius of the medulla and then descend to excite the upper cervical spinothalamic tract cells, which may contribute to the anginal pain experienced in the neck and jaw. Positron emission tomography (PET) imaging of the brain in subjects with silent ischemia has suggested that failed transmission of signals from the thalamus to the frontal cortex may contribute to this phenomenon, along with impaired afferent signaling, such as that caused by autonomic neuropathy. Silent ischemia in diabetic patients, for example, has been proposed to relate to failed development of the cardiac sensory system due to reduced nerve growth factor.[11]

Differential Diagnosis of Chest Pain

ESOPHAGEAL DISORDERS. Common disorders that may simulate or coexist with angina pectoris are gastroesophageal reflux and disorders of esophageal motility, including diffuse spasm and nutcracker esophagus. To compound the difficulty in distinguishing between angina and esophageal pain, both may be relieved by nitroglycerin.

However, esophageal pain is often relieved by milk, antacids, foods or, occasionally, warm liquids.

ESOPHAGEAL MOTILITY DISORDERS. Esophageal motility disorders are not uncommon in patients with retrosternal chest pain of unclear cause and should be specifically excluded or confirmed, if possible. In addition to chest pain, most such patients have dysphagia. Both IHD and esophageal disease are common clinical entities that may coexist. Diagnostic evaluation for an esophageal disorder may be indicated for patients with IHD who have a poor symptomatic response to antianginal therapy in the absence of documentation of severe ischemia.

BILIARY COLIC. Although visceral symptoms are commonly associated with myocardial ischemia (particularly acute inferior MI; see Chap. 54), cholecystitis and related hepatobiliary disorders may also mimic ischemia and should always be considered in patients with atypical chest discomfort, particularly those with diabetes. The pain is steady, usually lasts 2 to 4 hours, and subsides spontaneously, without any symptoms between attacks. It is generally most intense in the right upper abdominal area but may also be felt in the epigastrium or precordium. This discomfort is often referred to the scapula, may radiate around the costal margin to the back, or may in rare cases be felt in the shoulder and suggest diaphragmatic irritation.

COSTOSTERNAL SYNDROME. In 1921, Tietze first described a syndrome of local pain and tenderness, usually limited to the anterior chest wall and associated with swelling of costal cartilage. The full-blown Tietze syndrome—pain associated with tender swelling of the costochondral junctions—is uncommon, whereas costochondritis causing tenderness of the costochondral junctions (without swelling) is relatively common. Pain on palpation of these joints is usually well localized and is a useful clinical sign. Local pressure should be applied routinely to the anterior chest wall during examination of a patient with suspected angina pectoris. Although palpation of the chest wall often reproduces pain in patients with various musculoskeletal conditions, it should be appreciated that chest wall tenderness may also be associated with and does not exclude symptomatic CAD.

OTHER MUSCULOSKELETAL DISORDERS. Cervical radiculitis may be confused with angina. This condition may occur as a constant ache, sometimes resulting in a sensory deficit. The pain may be related to motion of the neck, just as motion of the shoulder triggers attacks of pain from bursitis. Occasionally, pain mimicking angina can be caused by compression of the brachial plexus by the cervical ribs, and tendinitis or bursitis involving the left shoulder may also cause angina-like pain. Physical examination may also detect pain brought about by movement of an arthritic shoulder or a calcified shoulder tendon.

OTHER CAUSES OF ANGINA-LIKE PAIN. Severe pulmonary hypertension may be associated with exertional chest pain with the characteristics of angina pectoris and, indeed, this pain is thought to be caused by right ventricular ischemia that develops during exertion (see Chap. 78). Other associated symptoms include exertional dyspnea, dizziness, and syncope. Associated findings on physical examination, such as parasternal lift, a palpable and loud pulmonary component of the second sound, and right ventricular hypertrophy on the ECG, are usually readily recognized.

Pulmonary embolism is initially characterized by dyspnea as the cardinal symptom, but chest pain may also be present (see Chap. 77). Pleuritic pain suggests pulmonary infarction and a history of exacerbation of the pain with inspiration, along with a pleural friction rub, usually helps distinguish it from angina pectoris. Pleuritic discomfort also may be caused by pneumonia or other causes of pleuritis.

The pain of acute pericarditis (see Chap. 75) may at times be difficult to distinguish from angina pectoris. However, pericarditis tends to occur in younger patients and the diagnosis depends on the combination of chest pain not relieved by rest or nitroglycerin,

exacerbation by movement, deep breathing, and lying flat, a pericardial friction rub, which may be evanescent, and electrocardiographic changes.

The classic symptom of aortic dissection is a severe, often sharp pain that radiates to the back (see Chap. 60).

Physical Examination

Many patients with stable IHD present with normal physical findings and thus the single best clue to the diagnosis of angina is the clinical history. Nonetheless, careful examination may reveal the presence or evidence of risk factors for coronary atherosclerosis or the consequences of myocardial ischemia (see Chap. 12).

Pathophysiology

Angina pectoris results from myocardial ischemia, caused by an imbalance between myocardial O_2 requirements and myocardial O_2 supply. The former may be elevated by increases in heart rate, LV wall stress, and contractility (see Chap. 52); the latter is determined by coronary blood flow and coronary arterial O_2 content (**Fig. 57-2**).

ANGINA CAUSED BY INCREASED MYOCARDIAL O_2 REQUIREMENTS. In this condition, sometimes termed *demand angina*, the myocardial O_2 requirement increases in the face of a constant and usually restricted O_2 supply. The increased requirement commonly stems from norepinephrine release by adrenergic nerve endings in the heart and vascular bed, a physiologic response to exertion, emotion, or mental stress. Of great importance to the myocardial O_2 requirement is the rate at which any task is carried out. Hurrying is particularly likely to precipitate angina, as are efforts involving motion of the hands over the head. Mental and emotional stress may also precipitate angina, presumably by increased hemodynamic and catecholamine responses to stress, increased adrenergic tone, and reduced vagal activity. The combination of physical exertion and emotion in association with sexual activity may precipitate angina pectoris. Anger may produce constriction of coronary arteries with pre-existing narrowing, without necessarily affecting O_2 demand. Other precipitants of angina include physical exertion after a heavy meal and the excessive metabolic demands imposed by fever, thyrotoxicosis, tachycardia from any cause, and hypoglycemia.

ANGINA CAUSED BY TRANSIENTLY DECREASED O_2 SUPPLY. Evidence has suggested that not only unstable angina but also chronic stable angina may be caused by transient reductions in O_2 supply, a condition sometimes termed *supply angina*, as a consequence of coronary vasoconstriction that results in dynamic stenosis. In the presence of organic stenoses, platelet thrombi and leukocytes may elaborate vasoconstrictor substances, such as serotonin and thromboxane A_2. Also, endothelial damage in atherosclerotic coronary arteries decreases production of vasodilator substances and may result in an abnormal vasoconstrictor response to exercise and other stimuli. A variable threshold of myocardial ischemia in patients with chronic stable angina may be caused by dynamic changes in peristenotic smooth muscle tone and also by constriction of arteries distal to the stenosis.

In rare patients without organic obstructing lesions, severe dynamic obstruction alone can cause myocardial ischemia and result in angina at rest (see Prinzmetal [variant] angina and Chaps. 52 and 56). On the other hand, in patients with severe fixed obstruction to coronary blood flow, only a minor increase in dynamic obstruction is necessary for blood flow to fall below a critical level and cause myocardial ischemia.

FIXED-THRESHOLD COMPARED WITH VARIABLE-THRESHOLD ANGINA. In patients with fixed-threshold angina precipitated by increased O_2 demands with few if any dynamic (vasoconstrictor) components, the level of physical activity required to precipitate angina is relatively constant. Characteristically, these patients can predict the amount of physical activity that will precipitate angina—for example, walking up exactly two flights of stairs at a customary pace. When tested on a treadmill or

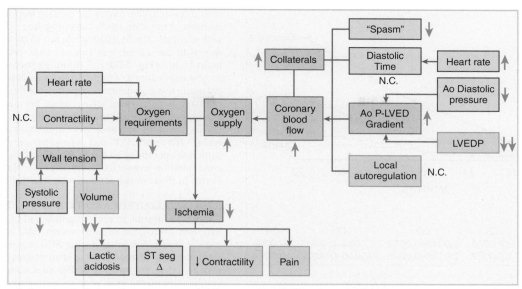

FIGURE 57-2 Factors influencing the balance between myocardial O_2 requirement **(left)** and supply **(right)**. Purple arrows indicate effects of nitrates. In relieving angina pectoris, nitrates exert favorable effects by reducing O_2 requirements and increasing supply. Although a reflex increase in heart rate would tend to reduce the time for coronary flow, dilation of collaterals and enhancement of the pressure gradient for flow to occur as the left ventricular end-diastolic pressure (LVEDP) decreases tend to increase coronary flow. Ao P-LVED = aortic pressure–left ventricular end-diastolic; N.C. = no change. *(From Frishman WH: Pharmacology of the nitrates in angina pectoris. Am J Cardiol 56:8I, 1985.)*

bicycle, the pressure-rate product (the so-called double product, a correlate of the myocardial O_2 requirement) that elicits angina and/or electrocardiographic evidence of ischemia is relatively constant.

Most patients with variable-threshold angina have atherosclerotic coronary arterial narrowing, but dynamic obstruction caused by vasoconstriction plays an important role in causing myocardial ischemia. These patients typically have good days, when they are capable of substantial physical activity, as well as bad days, when even minimal activity can cause clinical and/or electrocardiographic evidence of myocardial ischemia or angina at rest. They often complain of a circadian variation in angina that is more common in the morning. Angina on exertion and sometimes even at rest may be precipitated by cold temperature, emotion, and mental stress.

MIXED ANGINA. The term *mixed angina* has been proposed by Maseri and colleagues to describe the many patients who fall between the two extremes of fixed-threshold and variable-threshold angina.

The pathophysiologic and clinical correlations of ischemia in patients with stable IHD may have important implications for the selection of anti-ischemic agents, as well as for their timing. The greater the contribution from increased myocardial O_2 requirements to the imbalance between supply and demand, the greater the likelihood that beta-blocking agents will be effective, whereas nitrates and calcium channel blocking agents, at least hypothetically, are likely to be especially effective in episodes caused primarily by coronary vasoconstriction. The finding that in most patients with chronic stable angina, an increase in myocardial O_2 requirement precedes episodes of ischemia—that is, that they have demand angina—argues in favor of controlling heart rate and blood pressure as a primary therapeutic approach.

Evaluation and Management

Testing modalities include noninvasive and invasive procedures.

Noninvasive Testing

BIOCHEMICAL TESTS. In patients with stable IHD, including those with chronic angina, metabolic abnormalities that are risk factors for the development of CAD are frequently detected. These abnormalities include hypercholesterolemia and other dyslipidemias (see Chap. 47), carbohydrate intolerance, and insulin resistance. Moreover, chronic kidney disease is strongly associated with the risk of atherosclerotic

vascular disease (see Chap. 93).[12] All patients with established or suspected CAD warrant biochemical evaluation of total cholesterol, low-density lipoprotein (LDL) cholesterol, high-density lipoprotein (HDL) cholesterol, triglyceride, serum creatinine (estimated glomerular filtration), and fasting blood glucose levels.

Other biochemical markers have also been shown to be associated with higher risk of future cardiovascular events (see Chap. 44). Measurement of lipoprotein(a) and other lipid elements that are particularly atherogenic, such as apoprotein B and small dense LDLs, appears to add prognostic information to the measurement of total cholesterol and LDL, and may be considered as a secondary target for therapy in patients who have achieved therapeutic targets for LDL.[13] However, no consensus has been reached regarding routine measurement and a simple approach based on calculation of non-HDL cholesterol may capture the information available from measurement of specific apolipoproteins.[14] Similarly, lipoprotein-associated phospholipase A_2 (Lp-PLA2) is associated with the risk of coronary heart disease as well as recurrent events independent of traditional risk factors.[15] An assay for Lp-PLA2 is available for clinical use but has not been incorporated into guidelines for routine risk assessment.[16] Inhibitors of Lp-PLA2 are under investigation for treatment of IHD and, if proven useful for clinical practice, may stimulate new applications for Lp-PLA2 as a biomarker.[17] Homocysteine has also been linked to atherogenesis and correlates with the risk of CAD; however, in aggregate, prospective studies have supported, at most, a modest increase in risk associated with elevated homocysteine levels and have not consistently demonstrated a relationship independent of traditional risk factors or other biochemical markers. Therefore, general screening for elevated homocysteine levels is not recommended.[18]

Advances in understanding regarding the pathobiology of atherothrombosis (see Chap. 43) have generated interest in inflammatory biomarkers as noninvasive indicators of underlying atherosclerosis and cardiovascular risk. The serum concentration of high-sensitivity C-reactive protein (hsCRP) has shown a consistent relationship to the risk of incident cardiovascular events. The prognostic value of hsCRP is additive to traditional risk factors, including lipids[19]; however, the incremental clinical value for screening continues to be debated.[20] Measurement of hsCRP in patients judged at intermediate risk by global risk assessment (10% to 20% risk of coronary heart disease [CHD]/10 years) may help direct further evaluation and therapy in the primary prevention of CHD (see Chap. 44) and may be useful as an

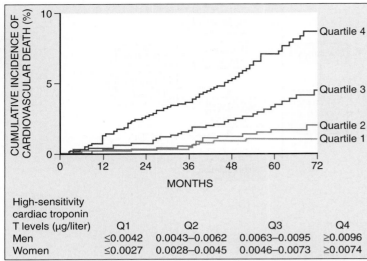

High-sensitivity
cardiac troponin

T levels (µg/liter)	Q1	Q2	Q3	Q4
Men	≤0.0042	0.0043–0.0062	0.0063–0.0095	≥0.0096
Women	≤0.0027	0.0028–0.0045	0.0046–0.0073	≥0.0074

FIGURE 57-3 Incidence of cardiovascular death according to the concentration of high-sensitivity troponin T (hs-TnT) in patients with stable CAD, subgrouped by quartiles of hs-TnT concentration. In a cohort of patients with stable CAD, 97.7% of individuals had detectable circulating cardiac troponin using a sensitive assay, with 11.1% having a concentration that exceeded the 99th percentile reference limit. During a median follow-up of 5.2 years, the incidence of cardiovascular death was associated with the baseline concentration of hs-TnT. This relationship was apparent at concentrations of hs-TnT below the 99th percentile reference limit (0.013 µg/L). *(From Omland T, de Lemos JA, Sabatine MS, et al: A sensitive cardiac troponin T assay in stable coronary artery disease. N Engl J Med 361:2538, 2009.)*

TABLE 57-1	Pretest Likelihood of Coronary Artery Disease in Symptomatic Patients According to Age and Gender*					
	Nonanginal Chest Pain		Atypical Angina		Typical Angina	
AGE (YR)	MEN	WOMEN	MEN	WOMEN	MEN	WOMEN
30-39	4	2	34	12	76	26
40-49	13	3	51	22	87	55
50-59	20	7	65	31	93	73
60-69	27	14	72	51	94	86

*Each value represents the percentage with significant coronary artery disease at coronary angiography.
From Gibbons RJ, Abrams J, Chatterjee K, et al: ACC/AHA 2002 guideline update for the management of patients with chronic stable angina: A report of the American College of Cardiology/American Heart Association Task Force on Practice Guidelines (Committee to update the 1999 guidelines for the management of patients with chronic stable angina) (http://www.acc.org/clinical/guidelines/stable/stable.pdf).

independent marker of prognosis in patients with established CAD. In a randomized double-blind trial in patients free of known atherosclerosis with LDL lower than 130 mg/dL who were identified at higher vascular risk by an elevated hsCRP level (>2 mg/L), treatment with a 3-hydroxy-3-methylglutaryl coenzyme A (HMG-CoA) reductase inhibitor (rosuvastatin) compared with placebo significantly reduced the risk of cardiovascular death and incident atherosclerotic vascular events.[21] On the basis of this finding, some professional society guidelines recommend the use of hsCRP as a risk indicator to support statin therapy in candidates for prevention who are at moderate global risk.[22] Other biomarkers of inflammation, such as myeloperoxidase, growth factors, and metalloproteinases, remain under study as markers of underlying atherosclerosis.[23]

Blood levels of cardiac markers of necrosis are typically used to differentiate patients with acute MI from those with stable IHD. However,

with more sensitive assays for cardiac troponin, circulating biomarkers of myocyte injury have now been detected in patients with clinically stable IHD and shown to have a graded relationship with the subsequent risk of cardiovascular mortality and heart failure (**Fig. 57-3**).[24,25] Although such evidence may lead to new applications of troponin in patients with stable IHD, clinical use in this population is currently not recommended.[26] Novel biomarkers of myocardial ischemia are also under study. For example, the plasma concentration of brain natriuretic peptide (BNP) increases in response to spontaneous or provoked ischemia.[27] Although BNP and N-terminal pro-BNP may not have sufficient specificity to aid in the diagnosis of stable IHD, their concentration is associated with the risk of future cardiovascular events in those at risk for and with established CAD.[28]

RESTING ELECTROCARDIOGRAPHY. The resting ECG (see Chap. 13) is normal in approximately half of patients with stable IHD, and even patients with severe CAD may have a normal tracing at rest. A normal resting ECG suggests the presence of normal resting LV function and is an unusual finding in a patient with an extensive previous MI. The most common electrocardiographic abnormalities in patients with chronic CAD are nonspecific ST-T wave changes, with or without abnormal Q waves. In addition to myocardial ischemia, other conditions that can produce ST-T wave abnormalities include LV hypertrophy and dilation, electrolyte abnormalities, neurogenic effects, and antiarrhythmic drugs. In patients with known CAD, however, the occurrence of ST-T wave abnormalities on the resting ECG can correlate with the severity of the underlying heart disease. In contrast, a normal resting ECG is a favorable long-term prognostic sign in patients with suspected or definite CAD.

Interval ECGs may reveal the development of Q wave MIs that have gone unrecognized clinically. Various conduction disturbances, most frequently left bundle branch block and left anterior fascicular block, may occur in patients with stable IHD and are often associated with impairment of LV function and reflect multivessel CAD and previous myocardial damage. Hence, such conduction disturbances are an indicator of a relatively poor prognosis. Abnormal Q waves are relatively specific but insensitive indicators of previous MI. Various arrhythmias, especially ventricular premature beats, may be present on the ECG, but they too have low sensitivity and specificity for CAD. LV hypertrophy on the ECG is an indicator of worse prognosis in patients with chronic stable angina. This finding suggests the presence of underlying hypertension, aortic stenosis, hypertrophic cardiomyopathy, or prior MI with remodeling and warrants further evaluation, such as echocardiography to assess LV size, wall thickness, and function.

During an episode of angina pectoris, the ECG becomes abnormal in 50% or more of patients with normal resting ECGs. The most common finding is ST-segment depression, although ST-segment elevation and normalization of resting ST-T wave depression or inversion (pseudonormalization) may develop. Ambulatory electrocardiographic monitoring has shown that many patients with symptomatic myocardial ischemia also have episodes of silent ischemia that would otherwise go unrecognized during normal daily activities. Although this form of electrocardiographic testing provides a quantitative estimate of the frequency and duration of ischemic episodes during routine activities, its sensitivity for detecting CAD is less than that of exercise electrocardiography.

NONINVASIVE STRESS TESTING. Noninvasive stress testing (see Chaps. 14, 15, and 17) can provide useful and often indispensable information to establish the diagnosis and estimate the prognosis in patients with chronic stable angina. However, the indiscriminate use of such tests provides limited incremental information beyond that provided by the physician's detailed and thoughtful clinical assessment. Appropriate application of noninvasive tests requires consideration of Bayesian principles, which state that the reliability and predictive accuracy of any test are defined not only by its sensitivity and specificity but also by the prevalence of disease (or pretest probability) in the population under study. A reasonable estimate of the pretest probability of CAD may be made on clinical grounds (**Table 57-1**).

Noninvasive testing should be performed only if the incremental information provided by a test is likely to alter the planned management strategy. The value of noninvasive stress testing is greatest when the pretest likelihood is intermediate because the test result is likely to have the greatest effect on the post-test probability of CAD and, hence, on clinical decision making.

EXERCISE ELECTROCARDIOGRAPHY

DIAGNOSIS OF CORONARY ARTERY DISEASE. The exercise ECG (see Chap. 14) is particularly helpful for patients with chest pain syndromes who are considered to have a moderate probability of CAD and in whom the resting ECG is normal, provided that they are capable of achieving an adequate workload. Although the incremental diagnostic value of exercise testing is limited in patients in whom the estimated prevalence of CAD is high or low, the test provides useful additional information about the degree of functional limitation in both groups of patients and about the severity of ischemia and prognosis in patients with a high pretest probability of CAD.[29] Interpretation of the exercise test should include consideration of the exercise capacity (duration and metabolic equivalents) and clinical, hemodynamic, and electrocardiographic responses.

INFLUENCE OF ANTIANGINAL THERAPY. Antianginal pharmacologic therapy reduces the sensitivity of exercise testing as a screening tool. Therefore, if the purpose of the exercise test is to diagnose ischemia, it should be performed, if possible, in the absence of antianginal medications. Two or 3 days of interruption is required for patients receiving long-acting beta blockers. For long-acting nitrates, calcium antagonists, and short-acting beta blockers, discontinuing use of the medications the day before testing usually suffices if the purpose of the exercise test is to identify safe levels of daily activity or the extent of functional disability.

NUCLEAR CARDIOLOGY TECHNIQUES (See Chap. 17.)

STRESS MYOCARDIAL PERFUSION IMAGING. Exercise perfusion imaging with simultaneous electrocardiographic testing is superior to exercise electrocardiography alone in detecting CAD, identifying multivessel CAD, localizing diseased vessels, and determining the magnitude of ischemic and infarcted myocardium. Exercise single-photon emission computed tomography (SPECT) yields an average sensitivity and specificity of 88% and 72%, respectively (ranges, 71% to 98% and 36% to 92%, respectively) compared with 68% sensitivity and 77% specificity for exercise electrocardiography alone (**Table 57-2**).[30] Referral bias may account, in part, for the low specificity of many studies, and the few studies that have adjusted for referral bias report a specificity higher than 90%. Perfusion imaging is also valuable for detecting myocardial viability in patients with regional or global LV dysfunction, with or without Q waves, and provides important information in regard to prognosis in all patients.

Stress myocardial scintigraphy is particularly helpful in the diagnosis of CAD in patients with abnormal resting ECGs and in those in whom ST-segment responses cannot be interpreted accurately, such as patients with repolarization abnormalities caused by LV hypertrophy, those with left bundle branch block, and those receiving digitalis. Because stress myocardial perfusion imaging is a relatively expensive test (three to four times the cost of an exercise ECG), stress myocardial perfusion scintigraphy should not be used as a screening test in patients in whom the prevalence of CAD is low, because most abnormal tests will yield false-positive results, and a regular exercise ECG should always be considered first in patients with chest pain and a normal resting ECG for screening and detection of CAD.[30]

PHARMACOLOGIC NUCLEAR STRESS TESTING. For patients unable to exercise adequately, especially older patients and patients with peripheral vascular disease, pulmonary disease, arthritis, other orthopedic limitations, obesity, or a previous stroke, pharmacologic vasodilator stress with dipyridamole or adenosine derivatives may be used.[31] In most nuclear cardiology laboratories, such patients account for approximately 40% of those referred for perfusion imaging. Although the diagnostic accuracy of pharmacologic vasodilator stress perfusion imaging is comparable to that achieved with exercise perfusion imaging (see Table 57-2), treadmill testing is preferred for patients who are capable of exercising because the exercise component of the test provides additional diagnostic and prognostic information, including ST-segment changes, effort tolerance and symptomatic response, and heart rate and blood pressure response. Vasodilator stress agents are also used with PET to diagnose CAD and determine its severity (see Chap. 17).

STRESS ECHOCARDIOGRAPHY. Two-dimensional echocardiography is useful for the evaluation of patients with chronic CAD because it can assess global and regional LV function under basal conditions and during ischemia, as well as detect LV hypertrophy and associated valve disease.[32] Stress echocardiography (see Chap. 15) may be performed using exercise or pharmacologic stress and allows for the detection of regional ischemia by identifying new areas of wall motion disorders. Adequate images can be obtained in more than 85% of patients, and the test is highly reproducible. Numerous studies have shown that exercise echocardiography can detect the presence of CAD with an accuracy similar to that of stress myocardial perfusion imaging and superior to exercise electrocardiography alone (see Table 57-2). Stress echocardiography is also valuable in localizing and quantifying ischemic myocardium (see Fig. 15-25). As with perfusion imaging, stress echocardiography also provides important prognostic information about patients with known or suspected CAD. Pharmacologic stress, such as with dobutamine, should be used for patients unable to exercise, those unable to achieve adequate heart rates with exercise, and those in whom the quality of the echocardiographic images during or immediately after exercise is poor.

Stress echocardiography is an excellent alternative to nuclear cardiology procedures. Limitations imposed by poor visualization of endocardial borders in a sizable subset of patients have been reduced by newer contrast-assisted and imaging technologic modalities (see Chap. 15).[32] Although less expensive than nuclear perfusion imaging, stress echocardiography is more expensive than and not as widely available as exercise electrocardiography.

STRESS CARDIAC MAGNETIC RESONANCE IMAGING. Pharmacologic stress perfusion imaging with cardiac magnetic resonance (CMR) imaging also compares favorably with other methods and is being used clinically in some centers, particularly in individuals who present limitations for the use of other imaging modalities (see Chap. 18).[33,34]

CLINICAL APPLICATIONS OF NONINVASIVE TESTING

GENDER DIFFERENCES IN THE DIAGNOSIS OF CAD. On the basis of earlier studies that indicated a much higher frequency of false-positive stress test results in women than in men, it is generally accepted that electrocardiographic stress testing is not as reliable in women (see Chap. 81). However, the prevalence of CAD in women in the patient populations under study was low, and the lower positive predictive value of exercise electrocardiography in women can be accounted for, in large part, on the basis of Bayesian principles (see Table 57-1).[35] Once men and women are stratified appropriately according to the pretest prevalence of disease, the results of stress testing are similar, although the specificity is probably slightly less in women. Exercise imaging modalities have greater diagnostic accuracy than exercise electrocardiography in men and women.

IDENTIFICATION OF PATIENTS AT HIGH RISK. When applying noninvasive tests to the diagnosis and management of CAD, it is useful to grade the results as negative, indeterminate, positive, not high risk, and positive,

TABLE 57-2	**Sensitivity and Specificity of Stress Testing***		
MODALITY	TOTAL NO. OF PATIENTS	SENSITIVITY†	SPECIFICITY†
Exercise ECG	24,047	0.68	0.77
Exercise SPECT	5,272	0.88	0.72
Adenosine SPECT	2,137	0.90	0.82
Exercise echocardiography	2,788	0.85	0.81
Dobutamine echocardiography	2,582	0.81	0.79

*Without correction for referral bias.
†Weighted average pooled across individual trials.
Data from Gibbons RJ, Abrams J, Chatterjee K, et al: ACC/AHA 2002 guideline update for the management of patients with chronic stable angina: A report of the American College of Cardiology/American Heart Association Task Force on Practice Guidelines (Committee to update the 1999 guidelines for the management of patients with chronic stable angina) (http://www.acc.org/clinical/guidelines/stable/stable.pdf).

high risk. The criteria for high-risk findings on stress electrocardiography, myocardial perfusion imaging, and stress echocardiography are listed in **Table 57-3**.

Regardless of the severity of symptoms, patients with high-risk non-invasive test results have a high likelihood of CAD and, if they have no obvious contraindications to revascularization, should undergo coronary arteriography. Such patients, even if asymptomatic, are at risk for left main or triple-vessel CAD, and many have impaired LV function. In contrast, patients with clearly negative exercise test results, regardless of symptoms, have an excellent prognosis that cannot usually be improved by revascularization. If they do not have other high risk features or refractory symptoms, coronary arteriography is generally not indicated.

ASYMPTOMATIC PERSONS. Exercise testing in asymptomatic individuals without known CAD is generally not recommended.[36] Exercise testing may be appropriate for asymptomatic individuals with diabetes mellitus who plan to begin vigorous exercise,[37] for those with evidence of myocardial ischemia on ambulatory ECG monitoring, or for those with severe coronary calcifications on cardiac computed tomography (CT; see Chap. 19).

CHEST ROENTGENOGRAPHY. The chest roentgenogram (see Chap. 16) is usually within normal limits in patients with stable IHD, particularly if they have a normal resting ECG and have not experienced an MI. If cardiomegaly is present, it is indicative of severe CAD with previous MI, preexisting hypertension, or an associated nonischemic condition, such as concomitant valvular heart disease, pericardial effusion, or cardiomyopathy.

COMPUTED TOMOGRAPHY. Cardiac multidetector CT (MDCT) has made substantial advances as a noninvasive approach to imaging atherosclerosis (see Chap. 19).[38] In addition to providing a highly sensitive method for detecting coronary calcification which is diagnostic of coronary atherosclerosis, MDCT can also provide an angiogram of the coronary arterial tree.[39]

TABLE 57-3	Risk Stratification Based on Noninvasive Testing

High Risk (>3% Annual Mortality Rate)
1. Severe resting left ventricular dysfunction (LVEF < 0.35)
2. High-risk treadmill score (score ≤ −11)
3. Severe exercise left ventricular dysfunction (exercise LVEF < 0.35)
4. Stress-induced large perfusion defect (particularly if anterior)
5. Stress-induced multiple perfusion defects of moderate size
6. Large, fixed perfusion defect with LV dilation or increased lung uptake (thallium-201)
7. Stress-induced moderate perfusion defect with LV dilation or increased lung uptake (thallium-201)
8. Echocardiographic wall motion abnormality (involving more than two segments) developing at low dose of dobutamine (≤10 μg/kg/min) or at low heart rate (<120 beats/min)
9. Stress echocardiographic evidence of extensive ischemia

Intermediate Risk (1%-3% Annual Mortality Rate)
1. Mild or moderate resting LV dysfunction (LVEF = 0.35-0.49)
2. Intermediate-risk treadmill score (−11 < score < 5)
3. Stress-induced moderate perfusion defect without LV dilation or increased lung intake (thallium-201)
4. Limited stress echocardiographic ischemia with a wall motion abnormality only at higher doses of dobutamine involving two segments or less

Low Risk (<1% Annual Mortality Rate)
1. Low-risk treadmill score (score ≥ 5)
2. Normal or small myocardial perfusion defect at rest or with stress*
3. Normal stress echocardiographic wall motion or no change of limited resting wall motion abnormalities during stress*

*Although the published data are limited, patients with these findings will probably not be at low risk in the presence of a high-risk treadmill score or severe resting LV dysfunction (LVEF < 0.35).

From Gibbons RJ, Abrams J, Chatterjee K, et al: ACC/AHA 2002 guideline update for the management of patients with chronic stable angina: A report of the American College of Cardiology/American Heart Association Task Force on Practice Guidelines (Committee to update the 1999 guidelines for the management of patients with chronic stable angina). (http://www.acc.org/clinical/guidelines/stable/stable.pdf).

The calcium score is a quantitative index of total coronary artery calcium detected by CT, and this score has been shown to be a good marker of the total coronary atherosclerotic burden.[40] Although coronary calcification is a highly sensitive (approximately 90%) finding in patients who have CAD, the specificity for identifying patients with obstructive CAD is low (approximately 50%).[41] In view of this limitation and the potential consequences of unnecessary testing as the result of false-positive results, CT is currently not recommended as a routine approach for screening for obstructive CAD in individuals at low risk for IHD (<10% 10-year estimated risk of coronary events). Moreover, in patients with known or suspected CAD, functional testing is preferable to CT imaging for determining the extent of CAD, the presence of ischemia, and indications for coronary angiography. However, selective screening of individuals at intermediate risk of CAD events may be reasonable to consider because a high calcium score may reclassify an individual at higher risk and thereby lead to more intense risk factor modification. This information should be weighed against the risk of exposure to ionizing radiation.[41a]

CT technology has progressed such that in selected individuals, high-quality images of the coronary arteries may be obtained. As such, CT angiography may be reasonable for symptomatic patients at intermediate risk for coronary disease after initial evaluation—in particular, those with indeterminate results of stress testing.[39] In experienced centers with advanced technology, CT has also been used to characterize plaque composition and, when paired with imaging with PET in a hybrid PET-CT scanner, can offer an assessment of coronary anatomy concurrent with information regarding myocardial blood flow and metabolism.[38] Nevertheless, despite these advances, at present, in most individuals, the temporal resolution of coronary CT angiography is lower than optimal for accurate, complete coronary artery depiction because of nonevaluable segments and limited accuracy in estimating the degree of luminal stenosis. The ability of CT for determination of plaque composition is also currently not sufficient for routine application. The results of ongoing investigation and new technologic innovations will guide evolution of the role of cardiac CT in the assessment and management of IHD.

CARDIAC MAGNETIC RESONANCE IMAGING. Cardiac magnetic resonance imaging (CMR; see Chap. 18) is established as a valuable clinical tool for imaging the aorta and cerebral and peripheral arterial vasculature and is evolving as a versatile noninvasive cardiac imaging modality that has multiple applications for patients with IHD.[39] The clinical use of CMR for myocardial viability assessment has grown based on evidence demonstrating its ability to predict functional recovery after percutaneous or surgical revascularization and its excellent correlation with PET. Pharmacologic stress perfusion imaging with CMR compares favorably with SPECT imaging and also offers accurate characterization of LV function, as well as delineating patterns of myocardial disease that are often useful in discriminating ischemic from nonischemic myocardial dysfunction.

Because of its ability to visualize arteries in three dimensions and differentiate tissue constituents, CMR has received interest as a method to characterize arterial atheroma and assess vulnerability to rupture on the basis of compositional analysis.[42] Arterial plaque has been characterized in the aorta and carotid arteries in humans and has been shown to be predictive of subsequent vascular events.[39] Moreover, CMR coronary angiography in humans is established as a modality to characterize congenital coronary anomalies (see Chaps. 21 and 65), and has shown promise as a method to detect stenoses in the proximal and middle segments of major epicardial vessels or surgical bypass grafts. As such, CMR is continuing to develop as a single approach to assessment of cardiac function, structure, blood flow, and viability without exposing the patient to ionizing radiation.

Catheterization and Coronary Arteriography

The clinical examination and noninvasive techniques described are extremely valuable for establishing the diagnosis of CAD and are indispensable to an overall assessment of patients with this condition.

Currently, however, definitive diagnosis of CAD and precise assessment of its anatomic severity still require cardiac catheterization and coronary arteriography (see Chaps. 20 and 21). In patients with chronic stable angina referred for coronary arteriography, approximately 25% each have single-, double-, or triple-vessel CAD (i.e., more than 70% luminal diameter narrowing); 5% to 10% have obstruction of the left main coronary artery and, in approximately 15%, no flow-limiting obstruction is detectable. Advanced invasive imaging techniques such as intravascular ultrasonography (IVUS) provide a cross-sectional view of the coronary artery and have substantially enhanced the detection and quantification of coronary atherosclerosis, as well as the potential to characterize the vulnerability of coronary atheroma (see Chap. 22).[43] Studies incorporating both coronary angiography and IVUS have demonstrated that the severity of CAD may be underestimated by angiography alone. Intravascular optical coherence tomography, angioscopy, and thermography are evolving as additional tools for more complete characterization of coronary atheroma.[44,45]

Coronary angiographic findings differ between patients presenting with acute MI and those with chronic stable angina. Patients with unheralded MI have fewer diseased vessels, fewer stenoses and chronic occlusions, and less diffuse disease than patients with chronic stable angina, suggesting that the pathophysiologic substrate and propensity for thrombosis differ between these two groups. In patients with chronic angina who have a history of prior MI, total occlusion of at least one major coronary artery is more common than in those without such a history.

CORONARY ARTERY ECTASIA AND ANEURYSMS. Patulous aneurysmal dilation involving most of the length of a major epicardial coronary artery is present in approximately 1% to 3% of patients with obstructive CAD at autopsy or angiography. This angiographic lesion does not appear to affect symptoms, survival, or incidence of MI. Most coronary artery ectasia and/or aneurysms are caused by coronary atherosclerosis (50%), and the rest are caused by congenital anomalies and inflammatory diseases, such as Kawasaki disease.[46] Despite the absence of overt obstruction, 70% of patients with multivessel fusiform coronary artery ectasia or aneurysms have demonstrated evidence of cardiac ischemia based on cardiac lactate levels during ergometry and atrial pacing.

Coronary ectasia should be distinguished from discrete coronary artery aneurysms, which are almost never found in arteries without severe stenosis, are most common in the left anterior descending (LAD) coronary artery, and are usually associated with extensive CAD. These discrete atherosclerotic coronary artery aneurysms do not appear to rupture and their resection is not warranted.

CORONARY COLLATERAL VESSELS. Provided that they are of adequate size, collaterals (see Chap. 21) may protect against MI when total occlusion occurs. In patients with abundant collateral vessels, myocardial infarct size is smaller than in patients without collaterals, and total occlusion of a major epicardial artery may not lead to LV dysfunction. In patients with chronic occlusion of a major coronary artery but without MI, collateral-dependent myocardial segments show almost normal baseline blood flow and O_2 consumption, but severely limited flow reserve. This finding helps explain the ability of collaterals to protect against resting ischemia but not against exercise-induced angina.

MYOCARDIAL BRIDGING. Bridging of coronary arteries (see Chap. 21) is observed by coronary angiography at a rate of less than 5% in otherwise angiographically normal coronary arteries and ordinarily does not constitute a hazard. Occasionally, compression of a portion of a coronary artery by a myocardial bridge can be associated with clinical manifestations of myocardial ischemia during strenuous physical activity and may even result in MI or initiate malignant ventricular arrhythmias. In an autopsy study, increased myocardial bridge thickness and length, as well as proximal vessel location, correlated with an increased risk of MI, proposed to be caused by promotion of proximal atherosclerosis.[47] The functional consequences of myocardial bridging may be characterized with intracoronary Doppler measurements.

LEFT VENTRICULAR FUNCTION. LV function can be assessed by biplane contrast ventriculography (see Chaps. 20 and 21). Global abnormalities of LV systolic function are reflected by elevations in LV end-diastolic and end-systolic volumes and depression of the ejection fraction. These changes are, however, nonspecific and can occur in many forms of heart disease. Abnormalities of regional wall motion (e.g., hypokinesis, akinesia, dyskinesia) are more characteristic of CAD. LV relaxation, as reflected in the early diastolic ventricular filling rate, may be impaired at rest in patients with stable IHD. Diastolic filling becomes even more abnormal (slowed) during exercise, when ischemia intensifies. In patients with stable IHD, the frequency of elevated LV end-diastolic pressure and reduced cardiac output at rest, generally attributed to abnormal LV dynamics, increases with the number of vessels exhibiting critical narrowing and with the number of prior MIs. LV end-diastolic pressure may be elevated secondary to reduced LV compliance, LV systolic failure, or a combination of these two processes.

CORONARY BLOOD FLOW AND MYOCARDIAL METABOLISM. Cardiac catheterization can also document abnormal myocardial metabolism in patients with stable IHD. With a catheter in the coronary sinus, arterial and coronary venous lactate measurements are obtained at rest and after suitable stress, such as the infusion of isoproterenol or pacing-induced tachycardia. Because lactate is a byproduct of anaerobic glycolysis, its production by the heart and subsequent appearance in coronary sinus blood is a reliable sign of myocardial ischemia.

Studies of coronary flow reserve (maximum flow divided by resting flow) and endothelial function are frequently abnormal in patients with CAD and may play an important role in determining the functional significance of a stenosis[48] or detecting microvascular dysfunction in those without obstructive epicardial disease. These techniques are discussed in Chap. 52.

Natural History and Risk Stratification

In a registry of patients with a history of stable angina followed in general practices, 29% of patients experienced angina one or more times per week, with associated greater physical limitation and worse quality of life. The frequency of reported angina varied substantially between clinics, suggesting significant heterogeneity in the success of identifying and managing angina.[49] Women have a similar incidence of stable angina to men, and angina in both genders is associated with a higher risk of mortality compared with the general population.[50] Data from the Framingham Study, obtained before the widespread use of aspirin, beta blockers, and aggressive modification of risk factors, revealed an average annual mortality rate of patients with stable IHD of 4%. The combination of these treatments has improved prognosis with an annual mortality rate of 1% to 3% and a rate of major ischemic events of 1% to 2%. For example, among 38,602 outpatients with stable IHD enrolled in 2003 to 2004, the 1-year rate of cardiovascular death was 1.9% (95% confidence interval [CI], 1.7 to 2.1), all-cause mortality was 2.9% (95% CI 2.6 to 3.2), and cardiovascular death, MI, or stroke was 4.5% (95% CI, 4.2 to 4.8).[51] Clinical, noninvasive, and invasive tools are useful for refining the estimate of risk for the individual patient with stable IHD. Moreover, noninvasively acquired information is valuable in identifying patients who are candidates for invasive evaluation with cardiac catheterization.

CLINICAL CRITERIA. Clinical characteristics that include age, male gender, diabetes mellitus, previous MI, and the presence of symptoms typical of angina are predictive of the presence of CAD.[6] A number of studies have attested to the adverse prognostic implications of heart failure in patients with stable IHD. The severity of angina, especially the tempo of intensification, and the presence of dyspnea are also important predictors of outcome.[6]

NONINVASIVE TESTS (see Chaps. 14, 15, and 17)

Exercise Electrocardiography

The prognostic importance of the treadmill exercise test was determined by observational studies in the 1980s and early 1990s. One of the most important and consistent predictors is the maximal exercise capacity, regardless of whether it is measured by exercise duration or workload achieved or whether the test was terminated because of dyspnea, fatigue, or angina.[4] After adjustment for age, the peak exercise capacity measured in metabolic equivalents (METs) is among the strongest predictors of mortality in men with cardiovascular disease.[29] Other factors associated with a poor prognosis identified in patients with chronic stable angina are delineated in Table 57-3.[52]

Stress Nuclear Myocardial Perfusion Imaging

The prognostic value of myocardial perfusion imaging is now well established (see Chap. 17). In particular, the ability of myocardial perfusion SPECT to identify patients at low (less than 1%), intermediate (1% to 5%), or high (more than 5%) risk for future cardiac events is valuable for patient management decisions. The prognostic data obtained from myocardial perfusion SPECT are incremental over clinical and treadmill exercise data for predicting future cardiac events.[38] In patients with normal SPECT imaging findings, the annual risk of death or MI is less than 1%.

Echocardiography

Echocardiographic assessment of LV function is one of the most valuable aspects of noninvasive imaging. Such testing is not necessary for all patients with angina pectoris and, in patients with a normal ECG and no previous history of MI, the likelihood of preserved LV systolic function is high. In contrast, in patients with a history of MI, ST-T wave changes, or conduction defects or Q waves on the ECG, LV function should be measured with echocardiography or an equivalent technique. The presence or absence of inducible regional wall motion abnormalities and the response of the ejection fraction to exercise or pharmacologic stress appear to provide incremental prognostic information to the data provided by the resting echocardiogram. Moreover, a negative stress test portends a low risk for future events (less than 1%/person-year).

ANGIOGRAPHIC CRITERIA. The independent impact of multivessel CAD and LV dysfunction and their interaction with the prognosis of patients with CAD are well established (**Fig. 57-4**). The adverse effects of impaired LV function on prognosis are more pronounced as the number of stenotic vessels increases. Although several indices have been used to quantify the extent of severity of CAD, the simple classification of disease into single-, double-, or triple-vessel or left main CAD is the most widely used and is effective. Additional prognostic information is provided by the severity of obstruction and its location, whether proximal or distal. The concept of the gradient of risk is illustrated in **Figure 57-5**. The importance to survival of the quantity of myocardium that is jeopardized is reflected in the observation that an obstructive lesion proximal to the first septal perforating branch of the LAD coronary artery is associated with a 5-year survival rate of 90% in comparison with 98% for patients with more distal lesions.

High-grade lesions of the left main coronary artery or its equivalent, as defined by severe proximal LAD artery and proximal left circumflex CAD, are particularly life-threatening. Mortality in medically treated patients has been reported to be 29% at 18 months and 43% at 5 years. Survival is better for patients with 50% to 70% stenosis (1- and 3-year survival rates of 91% and 66%, respectively) than for patients with a left main coronary artery stenosis more than 70% (1- and 3-year survival rates of 72% and 41%, respectively).

LIMITATIONS OF ANGIOGRAPHY. The pathophysiologic significance of coronary stenoses lies in their impact on resting and exercise-induced blood flow and in their potential for plaque rupture, with superimposed thrombotic occlusion. It is generally accepted that a stenosis of more than 60% of the luminal diameter is hemodynamically significant in that it may be responsible for a reduction in exercise-induced myocardial blood flow that causes ischemia. The immediate functional significance of obstruction of intermediate severity (approximately 50% diameter stenosis) is less well established. Coronary angiography is not a reliable indicator of the functional significance of stenosis. Moreover, the coronary angiographic determinants of the severity of stenosis are based on a decrease in the caliber of the lumen at the site of the lesion relative to adjacent reference segments, which are considered, often erroneously, to be relatively free of disease. This approach may lead to significant underestimation of the severity and extent of atherosclerosis.

The most serious limitation to the routine use of coronary angiography for prognosis in patients with stable IHD is its inability to identify which coronary lesions can be considered to be at high risk, or vulnerable, for future events, such as MI or sudden death. Although it is widely accepted that MI is the result of thrombotic occlusion at the site of

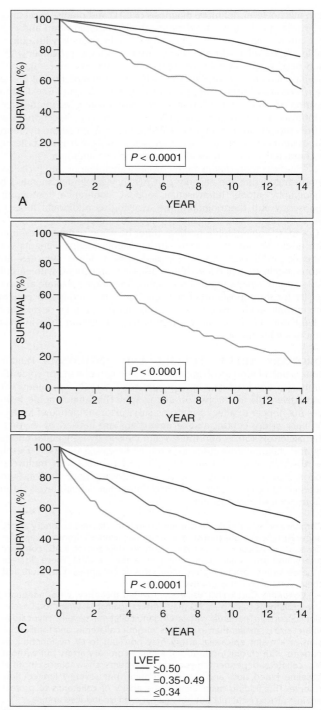

FIGURE 57-4 A, Patients with single-vessel coronary disease stratified by normal, moderately, or severely reduced left ventricular ejection fraction (LVEF). **B,** Patients with double-vessel coronary disease stratified by normal, moderately, or severely reduced LVEF. **C,** Patients with triple-vessel coronary disease stratified by normal, moderately, or severely reduced left ventricular LVEF. *(Modified from Emond M, Mock MB, Davis KB, et al: Long-term survival of medically treated patients in the Coronary Artery Surgery Study [CASS] Registry. Circulation 90:2651, 1994.)*

plaque rupture or erosion (see Chaps. 43 and 54), it is clear that it is not necessarily the plaque causing the most severe stenosis that subsequently ruptures. Lesions causing mild obstructions can rupture, thrombose, and occlude, thereby leading to MI and sudden death. Approaches to quantifying the extent of coronary disease, inclusive of nonobstructive lesions, appear to offer additional prognostic information. In contrast, arteries with severe pre-existing stenoses may proceed to clinically silent complete occlusion, often without MI, presumably because of the formation of collaterals as the ischemia gradually becomes more severe.

In summary, angiographic documentation of the extent of CAD provides useful information toward assessment of the patient's risk of death and future ischemic events and is an indispensable step in the selection of patients for coronary revascularization, particularly if the interaction between the anatomic extent of disease, LV function, and the severity of ischemia is taken into account. However, angiography is not helpful for predicting the site of subsequent plaque rupture or erosion that can precipitate MI or sudden cardiac death. Additional tools that improve the imaging of coronary atheroma (e.g., IVUS; see Chap. 22) or the functional assessment of a stenosis (e.g., Doppler determination of coronary flow reserve; see Chap. 52) may be helpful in deciding on the flow-limiting significance of a specific lesion and the need for coronary revascularization.[48] Characterization of the atheroma using CT or CMR remains under evaluation but is not yet a routine clinical tool.

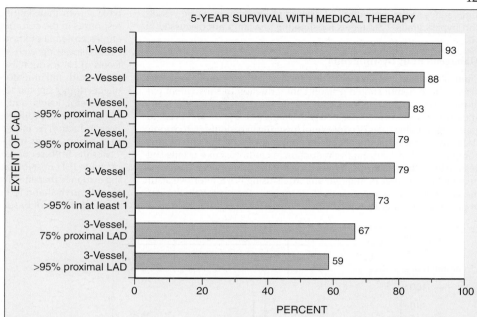

FIGURE 57-5 Angiographic extent of CAD and subsequent survival with medical therapy. A gradient of mortality risk is established based on the number of diseased vessels and the presence and severity of disease of the proximal LAD artery. *(Data from Califf RM, Armstrong PW, Carver JR, et al: Task Force 5: Stratification of patients into high-, medium-, and low-risk subgroups for purposes of risk factor management. J Am Coll Cardiol 27:964, 1996.)*

Medical Management

Comprehensive management of stable IHD has five aspects: (1) identification and treatment of associated diseases that can precipitate or worsen angina and ischemia; (2) reduction of coronary risk factors; (3) application of pharmacologic and nonpharmacologic interventions for secondary prevention, with particular attention to adjustments in lifestyle; (4) pharmacologic management of angina; and (5) revascularization by catheter-based percutaneous coronary intervention (PCI) or by coronary artery bypass grafting (CABG), when indicated. Although discussed individually in this chapter, all five of these approaches must be considered, often simultaneously, in each patient. Of the medical therapies, three (aspirin, angiotensin-converting enzyme [ACE] inhibition, and effective lipid lowering) have been shown to reduce mortality and morbidity in patients with stable IHD and preserved LV function. Other therapies such as nitrates, beta blockers, calcium antagonists, and ranolazine have been shown to improve symptomatology and exercise performance but their effect, if any, on survival in patients with stable IHD has not been demonstrated.

In stable patients with LV dysfunction following MI, evidence has consistently indicated that ACE inhibitors and beta blockers reduce both mortality and the risk of repeat MI, and these agents are recommended for such patients, with or without chronic angina, along with aspirin and lipid-lowering drugs.

TREATMENT OF ASSOCIATED DISEASES. Several common medical conditions that can increase myocardial O_2 demand or reduce O_2 delivery may contribute to the onset of new angina pectoris or the exacerbation of previously stable angina. These conditions include anemia, marked weight gain, occult thyrotoxicosis, fever, infections, and tachycardia. Cocaine, which can cause acute coronary spasm and MI, is discussed in Chap. 73. In patients with CAD, heart failure, by causing cardiac dilation, mitral regurgitation, or tachyarrhythmias (including sinus tachycardia), can increase myocardial O_2 need, along with an increase in the frequency and severity of angina. Identification and treatment of these conditions are critical to the management of stable IHD.

REDUCTION OF CORONARY RISK FACTORS

Hypertension

Epidemiologic links between increased blood pressure (see Chaps. 45, 46, and 49) and CAD severity and mortality are well established. For individuals aged 40 to 70 years, the risk of IHD doubles for each 20-mm Hg increment in systolic blood pressure across the entire range of 115 to 185 mm Hg.[53] Hypertension predisposes to vascular injury, accelerates the development of atherosclerosis, increases myocardial O_2 demand, and intensifies ischemia in patients with preexisting obstructive coronary vascular disease. Although the relationship between hypertension and CAD is linear, LV hypertrophy is a stronger predictor of MI and CAD death than the actual degree of increase in blood pressure.[53] A meta-analysis of clinical trials of treatment of mild to moderate hypertension has shown a statistically significant 16% reduction in CAD events and mortality in patients receiving antihypertensive therapy.[54] This treatment effect is almost twice as great in older compared with younger persons. It is logical to extend these observations about the benefits of antihypertensive therapy to patients with established CAD. Moreover, the number of individuals treated to avoid one death is lower in subjects with established cardiovascular disease. Therefore, blood pressure control is an essential aspect of the management of patients with stable IHD. Although professional society recommendations have advocated a goal of less than 130/80 mm Hg,[53] the results of the Action to Control Cardiovascular Risk in Diabetes (ACCORD) trial, in which 34% of the study population had established cardiovascular disease, did not reveal a significant benefit of targeting a systolic blood pressure below 120 mm Hg versus a level below 140 mm Hg; however, serious adverse events were more frequent in the intensive-therapy group.[54a]

Cigarette Smoking

This remains one of the most powerful risk factors for the development of CAD in all age groups (see Chap. 44). In patients with angiographically documented CAD, cigarette smokers have a higher 5-year risk of sudden death, MI, and all-cause mortality than those who have stopped smoking. Moreover, smoking cessation lessens the risk of adverse coronary events in patients with established CAD. Cigarette smoking may be responsible for aggravating angina other than through the progression of atherosclerosis. It may increase myocardial O_2 demand and reduce coronary blood flow by an alpha-adrenergically mediated increase in coronary artery tone and thereby cause acute ischemia. Moreover, passive exposure to smoke has adverse cardiovascular effects that are almost as great as those of active smoking.[55] Smoking cessation is one of the most effective and cost-effective approaches to the prevention of disease progression in native vessels and bypass grafts.[56] Strategies for smoking cessation are discussed in Chap. 50.

Management of Dyslipidemia

Clinical trials in patients with established atherosclerotic vascular disease have demonstrated a significant reduction in subsequent cardiovascular events in patients with a wide range of serum cholesterol and LDL cholesterol levels treated with statins (see Chap. 47).[57] In aggregate, angiographic trials of cholesterol lowering in patients with chronic CAD have shown that the effects on coronary obstruction are modest compared with the substantive reduction in cardiovascular events, suggesting that atherosclerosis regression is not the primary mechanism of benefit. Nonetheless, in angiographic trials using IVUS, intensive statin therapy has led to regression of coronary atherosclerotic burden in patients with angiographic CAD.[58,59] Also, several, but not all, studies

have shown that statins significantly improve endothelium-mediated responses in the coronary and systemic arteries of patients with hypercholesterolemia or known atherosclerosis.

Lipid-lowering with statins has been shown to reduce circulating levels of hsCRP, decrease thrombogenicity, and favorably alter the collagen and inflammatory components of arterial atheroma; these effects do not appear to correlate well with the change in serum LDL cholesterol levels and suggest antiatherothrombotic properties of statins.[60] These properties may contribute to improvement in blood flow, reduction in inducible myocardial ischemia, and the reduction in coronary events in patients treated with statins.

Results from secondary prevention trials of patients with a history of stable IHD, unstable angina, or previous MI have provided convincing evidence that effective lipid-lowering therapy significantly improves overall survival and reduces cardiovascular mortality in patients with CAD, regardless of baseline cholesterol. The National Cholesterol Education Program Guidelines (see Chaps. 47 and 49) advocate cholesterol-lowering therapy for all patients with CAD or extracardiac atherosclerosis to LDL levels below 100 mg/dL, and these guidelines have been adopted in recommendations from the American College of Cardiology/American Heart Association (ACC/AHA).[57] Moreover, results from trials of intensive versus moderate dose statin therapy in patients with recent acute coronary syndrome (ACS) and in patients with stable IHD have provided evidence for a reduction in major cardiovascular events with more aggressive lipid lowering therapy to an LDL concentration lower than 100 mg/dL (**Fig. 57-6**).[61-63] These findings have led to the recommendation that it is reasonable to treat all patients with CAD to an achieved LDL concentration of less than 70 mg/dL (see Chap. 49).

LOW LEVEL OF HDL CHOLESTEROL. Patients with established CAD and low levels of HDL cholesterol represent a subgroup at considerable risk for future coronary events, even when LDL cholesterol is low.[64,65] Low HDL levels are often associated with obesity, hypertriglyceridemia, and insulin resistance and often signify the presence of small lipoprotein remnants and small, dense, LDL particles that are thought to be particularly atherogenic (see Chap. 47). Therapy has focused on diet and exercise, as well as on LDL cholesterol reduction, in patients with a concomitant increase in HDL cholesterol levels. The Veterans Affairs High-Density Lipoprotein Cholesterol Intervention Trial (VA-HIT) Study Group has demonstrated the efficacy of gemfibrozil treatment in men with low HDL cholesterol (40 mg/dL or lower) without elevations in LDL cholesterol (140 mg/dL or lower) or triglyceride levels (mean, 160 mg/dL). Gemfibrozil resulted in a 6% increase in HDL cholesterol and a 31% decrease in triglyceride levels, and these changes were associated with a 24% reduction in death, nonfatal MI, and stroke. Emerging therapies aimed at promoting reverse cholesterol transport and/or interfering

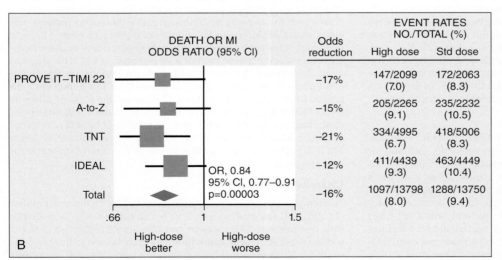

FIGURE 57-6 Pooled evaluation of intensive versus standard statin therapy for patients with established coronary artery disease in the Pravastatin or Atorvastatin Evaluation and Infection Therapy Trial (PROVE-IT-TIMI 22; atorvastatin, 80 mg daily, versus pravastatin, 40 mg daily), Aggrastat-to-Zocor Trial (A-to-Z; simvastatin, 40 mg daily, for 30 days followed by 80 mg daily, versus placebo for 4 months, followed by simvastatin, 20 mg daily), Treat to New Targets Trial (TNT; atorvastatin, 80 mg daily, versus atorvastatin, 10 mg daily), and Incremental Decrease in Endpoints Through Aggressive Lipid-Lowering Trial (IDEAL; atorvastatin, 80 mg daily versus simvastatin, 20 mg daily). Intensive statin therapy was associated with significantly lower achieved levels of low-density lipoprotein cholesterol, LDL-C (**A**) and a 16% lowering of the risk of death or myocardial infarction, MI (**B**). OR = odds ratio. *(From Cannon CP, Steinberg BA, Murphy SA, et al: Meta-analysis of cardiovascular outcomes trials comparing intensive versus moderate statin therapy. J Am Coll Cardiol 48:438, 2006.)*

with HDL metabolism to raise the concentration of HDL or the related apolipoprotein A-I (the main protein in HDL) are under investigation.[66] In two large randomized trials, torcetrapib, a cholesteryl ester transfer protein (CETP) inhibitor, increased HDL cholesterol by 61% and reduced LDL cholesterol by 20%, but did not decrease progression of atherosclerosis[67] and was associated with an increase in ischemic events, which may be explained by an increase in blood pressure with torcetrapib.[68] It is not known whether there are other unexpected adverse effects specific to this molecule or its drug class.

MANAGEMENT OF DIABETES MELLITUS. Patients with diabetes mellitus (see Chaps. 49 and 64) are at significantly higher risk of atherosclerotic vascular disease. Although a favorable impact of control of glycemia on microvascular complications of diabetes is established, the effect on macrovascular complications (including CAD) is unclear. During a mean follow-up of 17 years in participants in the Diabetes Control and Complications Trial, patients with type 1 diabetes assigned to intensive glycemic therapy were at lower risk of cardiovascular complications.[69] In an analysis of a secondary endpoint of the Prospective Pioglitazone Clinical Trial in Macrovascular Events Trial (PROACTIVE), treatment of patients with type 2 diabetes with the oral hypoglycemic agent pioglitazone reduced the risk of death, nonfatal MI, or stroke.[70] Caution is raised regarding interpretation of this finding from PROACTIVE on controlling hyperglycemia given the neutral result of the trial with respect to its primary endpoint and effects of pioglitazone on metabolic elements other than blood glucose level. Several large trials evaluating the effects of oral hypoglycemic agents on cardiovascular outcomes are ongoing. Management of hypercholesterolemia and hypertension are particularly important in patients with type 2 diabetes.[57,69]

ESTROGEN REPLACEMENT. In view of the collective data from randomized clinical trials, it is not advised that hormone replacement therapy be initiated or continued for secondary cardiovascular prevention in women with CAD (see Chap. 81).[57]

Exercise

The conditioning effect of exercise (see Chap. 50) on skeletal muscles allows a greater workload at any level of total body O_2 consumption. By decreasing the heart rate at any level of exertion, a higher cardiac output can be achieved at any level of myocardial O_2 consumption. The combination of these two effects of exercise conditioning permits patients with chronic stable angina to increase physical performance substantially following the institution of a continuing exercise program.[71,72]

Most information about the physiologic effects of exercise and their effect on prognosis in patients with CAD has come from studies on patients entered into cardiac rehabilitation programs, many of whom previously sustained a MI. Less information is available on the benefits of exercise in patients with stable IHD without a prior MI., Collectively, small randomized trials evaluating exercise training in patients with stable IHD have indicated improved effort tolerance, O_2 consumption, quality of life, and reduced evidence of ischemia with myocardial perfusion imaging.[71] One randomized trial of exercise training compared with angioplasty in 101 patients with stable angina showed fewer hospitalizations and revascularization procedures in those allocated to regular exercise.[73] Others have demonstrated a striking and direct relationship between the intensity of exercise and favorable changes in inflammatory and hemostatic mediators of cardiovascular risk,[74] the morphology of obstructive lesions on angiography, and vascular endothelial function, thought to be mediated through the expression and phosphorylation of endothelial nitric oxide synthase. Whether exercise accelerates the development of collateral vessels in patients with chronic CAD is unclear.

Exercise is safe if begun under supervision and increased gradually[75] and, if survivors of MI can be used as a yardstick, is probably cost-effective. The psychological benefits of exercise are difficult to evaluate. However, a single nonrandomized study has demonstrated significant improvement in well-being scores and positive affect scores, as well as a reduction in disability scores, in patients in a structured exercise program. Patients who are involved in exercise programs are also more likely to be health conscious, pay attention to diet and weight, and discontinue cigarette smoking. For all these reasons, patients should be urged to participate in regular exercise programs, usually walking, in conjunction with their drug therapy.[72]

Inflammation

Atherothrombosis has been recognized as an inflammatory disease (see Chaps. 43, 44, and 49).[76] Moreover, markers of systemic inflammation, of which hsCRP is the most extensively studied, identify patients with established vascular disease who are at higher risk for death and future ischemic events. Therefore, inflammation has been identified as a potential target for therapeutic intervention in patients with IHD. For example, in a number of studies, treatment with statins has lowered the serum concentration of hsCRP. In addition, lower levels of hsCRP achieved with statin therapy in patients 1 month after an ACS are associated with better long-term prognosis.[77,78] Also, in a large randomized, placebo-controlled trial in individuals with average LDL levels and no known atherosclerosis but an increased risk of atherothrombosis identified with elevated hsCRP, statin therapy reduced the risk of first major cardiovascular events.[21] Although it is challenging to dissect the potential benefit of anti-inflammatory effects of statins from those derived from lowering LDL cholesterol, these findings lend support to the hypothesis that statins are effective in modifying the risk associated with evidence of systemic inflammation and that inflammatory markers may complement LDL measurement in guiding statin therapy.[22] Other established preventive interventions, as well as novel therapeutic strategies, may also have anti-inflammatory effects that could target inflammation. Aspirin, ACE inhibitors, thiazolidinediones, thienopyridines, and fibric acid derivatives are among those agents that have been shown to exert anti-inflammatory or immunoregulatory actions.[76] Additional research is needed to clarify whether inflammation should be a target for routine strategies for risk reduction or novel therapeutic agents in patients with stable IHD.

Obesity

Obesity (see Chaps. 44 and 64) is an independent contributor to the risk for IHD and is associated with a constellation of other risk factors, including hypertension, dyslipidemia, and abnormal glucose metabolism. Weight loss can improve or prevent many of the cardiovascular consequences of obesity.[79]

ADDITIONAL DISEASE-MODIFYING PHARMACOTHERAPY FOR SECONDARY PREVENTION

ASPIRIN. A meta-analysis of 140,000 patients in 300 studies has confirmed the prophylactic benefit of aspirin (see Chaps. 49 and 87) in men and women with angina pectoris, previous MI, or stroke and after CABG. In a Swedish trial of men and women with chronic stable angina, 75 mg of aspirin in conjunction with the beta blocker sotalol conferred a 34% reduction in acute MI and sudden death. In a smaller study confined to men with chronic stable angina but without a history of MI, 325 mg of aspirin on alternate days reduced the risk of MI by 87% during 5 years of follow-up. Therefore, administration of aspirin daily is advisable for patients with stable IHD without contraindications to this drug.[57,80] Dosing at 75 to 162 mg daily appears to have comparable effects for secondary prevention with dosing at 160 to 325 mg daily and appears to be associated with lower bleeding risk. Aspirin 75 to 162 mg daily is thus preferred for secondary prevention in the absence of recent intracoronary stenting. Although warfarin has proved beneficial in patients after MI, no evidence supports the use of chronic anticoagulation in patients with stable angina.

CLOPIDOGREL. Other orally acting antiplatelet agents have been studied in patients with stable IHD. Clopidogrel, a thienopyridine derivative, may be substituted for aspirin in patients with aspirin hypersensitivity or those who cannot tolerate aspirin (see Chap. 87).[57] In a randomized comparison between clopidogrel and aspirin in patients with established atherosclerotic vascular disease (the Clopidogrel versus Aspirin in Patients at Risk of Ischaemic Events [CAPRIE] trial), treatment with clopidogrel resulted in a modest 8.7% relative reduction in the risk of vascular death, ischemic stroke, or MI ($P = 0.043$) over 2 years. Studies evaluating the addition of clopidogrel to aspirin in patients with non–ST-segment elevation ACS or after PCI have demonstrated robust risk reductions. However, the Clopidogrel for High Atherothrombotic Risk and Ischemic Stabilization Management and Avoidance (CHARISMA) trial showed no overall benefit of the addition of clopidogrel to aspirin with respect to the primary endpoint of cardiovascular death, MI, or stroke over a median of 28 months (6.8%% versus 7.3%; $P = 0.22$) in patients with clinically evident cardiovascular disease ($N = 12,153$) or multiple risk factors ($N = 3,284$).[81] In the subgroup of those with established vascular disease, the addition of clopidogrel was associated with a 1% lower risk of these events (6.9 versus

7.9%; $P = 0.046$), supporting a hypothesis of a potential modest benefit from clopidogrel in patients with stable IHD taking aspirin.[82] Ongoing studies are testing the hypothesis that more potent antiplatelet therapy than aspirin alone is useful for patients with stable IHD.[83]

BETA BLOCKERS. The value of beta blockers in reducing death and recurrent MI in patients who have experienced a MI is well established (see Chaps. 49 and 55), as is their usefulness in the treatment of angina. Moreover, patients receiving beta blockers for hypertension are more likely to present with stable angina rather than MI as their first manifestation of CAD.[84] Whether these drugs are also of value in preventing MI and sudden death in patients with stable IHD without previous MI is uncertain and, despite at least one observational study suggesting lower mortality in the patients who were taking beta blockers,[85] there have been no controlled trials against placebo. However, there is no reason to assume that the favorable effects of beta blockers on ischemia and perhaps on arrhythmias should not apply to patients with stable IHD. In addition, observational data have raised the possibility that beta blockers may reduce the progression of coronary atherosclerosis, in part through reduced turbulence and reduced intramural arterial wall stress.[86] Therefore, although the use of beta blockers as first-line agents for uncomplicated hypertension has been questioned, it is sensible to use these drugs when angina, hypertension, or both are present in patients with stable IHD and when these drugs are well tolerated.[87] Emerging evidence also has identified genetic polymorphisms of the beta$_2$-adrenergic receptor gene (ADRB1 and ADRB2) that may influence beta blocker responsiveness.[88]

ANGIOTENSIN-CONVERTING ENZYME INHIBITORS AND ANGIOTENSIN RECEPTOR BLOCKERS. Although inhibitors of the renin-angiotensin-aldosterone system are not indicated for the treatment of angina, these drugs appear to have important benefits in reducing the risk of future ischemic events in some patients with cardiovascular disease.[89] An unexpected finding from randomized trials of ACE inhibitors in postinfarction and other patients with ischemic and nonischemic causes of LV dysfunction was a significant reduction in the incidence of subsequent coronary ischemic events. The potentially beneficial effects of ACE inhibitors include reductions in LV hypertrophy, vascular hypertrophy, progression of atherosclerosis, plaque rupture, and thrombosis, in addition to a potentially favorable influence on myocardial O$_2$ supply and demand relationships, cardiac hemodynamics, sympathetic activity, and coronary endothelial vasomotor function. In addition, in vitro experiments have shown that angiotensin II induces inflammatory changes in human vascular smooth muscle cells, and treatment with ACE inhibitors can reduce signs of inflammation in animal models of atherosclerosis.

Two trials have provided strong evidence supporting the therapeutic benefit of ACE inhibitors in patients with normal LV function and absence of heart failure (**Fig. 57-7**). In the Heart Outcomes Protection Evaluation (HOPE) study, ramipril significantly decreased the risk of the primary

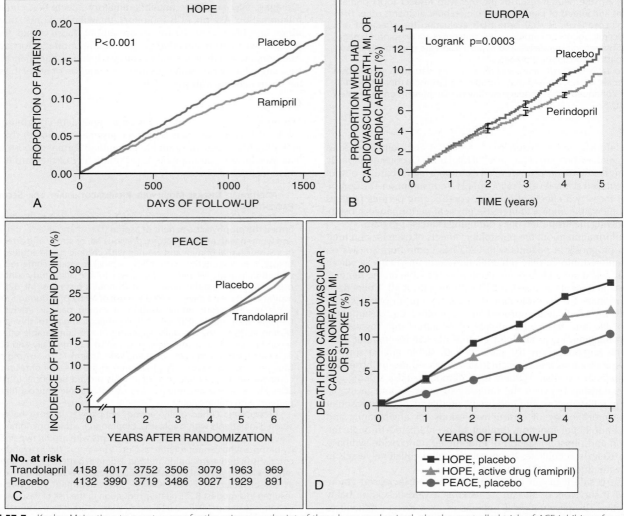

FIGURE 57-7 Kaplan-Meier time to event curves for the primary endpoint of three large randomized, placebo-controlled trials of ACE inhibitors for patients at high risk for or with established cardiovascular disease without heart failure. **A,** Cumulative incidence of cardiovascular death, MI, or stroke with ramipril versus placebo among patients in the HOPE trial. **B,** Cumulative incidence of cardiovascular death, MI, or cardiac arrest with perindopril or placebo in the European Trial on the EUROPA trial. **C,** Cumulative incidence of cardiovascular death, MI, or coronary revascularization in the PEACE trial. **D,** Comparison of cardiovascular death, MI, or stroke in the HOPE and PEACE trials. The cumulative incidence of major cardiovascular events was lower in patients treated with placebo in PEACE than in the patients treated with ramipril in HOPE. (**A,** from HOPE Study Investigators: Effects of an angiotensin-converting enzyme inhibitor, ramipril, on cardiovascular events in high risk patients. N Engl J Med 342:145, 2000; **B,** from EUROPA Investigators: Efficacy of perindopril in reduction of cardiovascular events among patients with stable coronary artery disease: Randomized double-blind, placebo-controlled, multicenter trial [the EUROPA study]. Lancet 363:782, 2003; **C,** from PEACE Trial Investigators: Angiotensin-converting enzyme inhibition in stable coronary artery disease. N Engl J Med 351:2058, 2004.)

composite endpoint of cardiovascular death, MI, and stroke from 17.7% to 14.1% (relative risk reduction of 22%; $P < 0.001$) compared with placebo in 9297 patients with atherosclerotic vascular disease or diabetes mellitus. In addition, the European Trial on Reduction of Cardiac Events with Perindopril in stable CAD (EUROPA) provided additional convincing support for the benefit of ACE inhibitors, with a 20% relative reduction in the risk of cardiovascular death, MI or cardiac arrest in 13,655 patients with stable CAD in the absence of heart failure.[57] In contrast, in the Prevention of Events with Angiotensin Converting Enzyme Inhibition (PEACE) trial, trandolapril administered to a target dose of 4 mg daily showed no effect on the risk of cardiovascular death, MI, or coronary revascularization (21.9% versus 22.5%; $P = 0.43$) in 8,290 patients with stable CAD and preserved LV function receiving intensive preventive therapy, usually including revascularization and lipid-lowering agents (see Fig. 57-7).[90] Notably, in patients with evidence of renal dysfunction (estimated glomerular filtration rate < 60 mL/min/1.73 m^2), trandolapril was associated with lower all-cause mortality.[91] Hence, ACE inhibitors are recommended for all patients with CAD with LV dysfunction and for those with hypertension, diabetes, or chronic kidney disease.[57] ACE inhibitors may be considered for optional use in all other patients with stable IHD with normal LV ejection fraction and cardiovascular risk factors that are well controlled in whom revascularization has been performed.

In patients with established vascular disease or high risk diabetes, telmisartan, an angiotensin receptor blocker (ARB), was equivalent to ramipril with respect to secondary prevention of major cardiovascular events in patients tolerant of ACE inhibitors[92] but was not superior to placebo in patients intolerant of ACE inhibitors.[93] The combination of telmisartan and ramipril provided no additional benefit compared with ramipril alone and resulted in an increased rate of complications.

ANTIOXIDANTS. Oxidized LDL particles are strongly linked to the pathophysiology of atherogenesis, and descriptive, prospective cohort, and case-control studies have suggested that a high dietary intake of antioxidant vitamins (A, C, and beta-carotene) and flavonoids (polyphenolic antioxidants), naturally present in vegetables, fruits, tea, and wine, is associated with a decrease in CAD events (see Chap. 49). However, large randomized trials of antioxidant supplements, including vitamin E, vitamin C, beta-carotene, folic acid, and vitamins B_6 and B_{12}, indicated that they did not reduce the risk of major cardiovascular events.[94,95] Thus, based on current evidence, there is no basis for recommending that individuals take supplemental folate, vitamin E, vitamin C, or beta-carotene for the purpose of treating CAD.[57] Additional investigation of other approaches to antioxidant therapy is ongoing.[96]

COUNSELING AND CHANGES IN LIFESTYLE. The psychosocial issues faced by a patient who develops stable angina are similar to, although usually less intense than, those experienced by a patient with an acute MI. Depressive symptoms are strongly associated with health status as reported by the patient, including the burden of symptoms and overall quality of life, independently of LV function and the presence of provokable ischemia.[97] In addition, the association between depressive symptoms and IHD may reflect a causal relationship between the former and atherothrombosis. Depressive symptoms are associated with higher levels of circulating biomarkers of inflammation.[98] In conjunction with counseling, treatment with a selective serotonin reuptake inhibitor appears to be safe and effective for managing depression in patients with IHD.[99] Thus, efforts to evaluate and treat depression in patients with CAD is an important element of their overall management. Moreover, psychosocial stress at work, home, or both is associated with an increased risk of MI and may be a target for preventive interventions.[100]

An important aspect of the physician's role is to counsel patients with respect to dietary habits, goals for physical activity,[101,102] the types of work they can do, and their leisure activities. Certain changes in lifestyle may be helpful, such as modifying strenuous activities if they constantly and repeatedly produce angina. A history of CAD and stable angina is not inconsistent with the patients' ability to continue to exert themselves, which is important not only in regard to recreational activities and lifestyle but also for patients in whom some physical exertion is required in their employment. However, isometric activities such as weightlifting and other activities such as shoveling snow, which involves an energy expenditure between 60% and 65% of peak oxygen consumption, and cross-country or downhill skiing are undesirable. In addition, these latter activities expose the individual to the detrimental effects of cold on the O_2 demand and supply

relationship, and these activities should also be avoided whenever possible.

Eliminating or reducing the factors that precipitate anginal episodes is of obvious importance. Patients learn their usual threshold by trial and error. Patients should avoid sudden bursts of activity, particularly after long periods of rest, after meals, and in cold weather. Both chronic and unstable angina exhibit a circadian rhythm characterized by a lower angina threshold shortly after arising. Therefore, morning activities such as showering, shaving, and dressing should be done at a slower pace and, if necessary, with the use of prophylactic nitroglycerin. The stress of sexual intercourse is approximately equal to that of climbing one flight of stairs at a normal pace or any activity that induces a heart rate of approximately 120 beats/min. With proper precautions (i.e., commencing more than 2 hours postprandially and taking an additional dose of a short-acting beta blocker 1 hour before and nitroglycerin 15 minutes before), most patients with stable angina are able to continue satisfactory sexual activity. Although it is desirable to minimize the number of bouts of angina, an occasional episode is not to be feared. Indeed, unless patients occasionally reach their angina threshold, they may not appreciate the extent of their exercise capacity. Patients with stable IHD may use a phosphodiesterase type 5 (PDE5) inhibitor, such as sildenafil, tadalafil, or vardenafil, but not in conjunction with nitrates.[103]

Pharmacologic Management of Angina

NITRATES

Mechanism of Action

Even though the clinical effectiveness of amyl nitrite in angina pectoris was first described in 1867 by Brunton, organic nitrates are still the drugs most commonly used for the treatment of patients with this condition. The action of these agents is to relax vascular smooth muscle. The vasodilator effects of nitrates are evident in systemic (including coronary) arteries and veins, but they appear to be predominant in the venous circulation. The venodilator effect reduces ventricular preload, which in turn reduces myocardial wall tension and O_2 requirements. The action of nitrates in reducing preload and afterload makes them useful in the treatment of heart failure (see Fig. 57-2) as well as angina. By reducing the heart's mechanical activity, volume, and O_2 consumption, nitrates increase exercise capacity in patients with IHD, thereby allowing a greater total body workload to be achieved before the angina threshold is reached. Thus, in patients with stable angina, nitrates improve exercise tolerance and time to ST-segment depression during treadmill exercise tests. When used in combination with calcium channel blockers and/or beta blockers, the antianginal effects appear greater.[80]

Effects on the Coronary Circulation

Nitroglycerin causes dilation of epicardial stenoses (**Table 57-4**). These stenoses are often eccentric lesions, and nitroglycerin causes relaxation of the smooth muscle in the wall of the coronary artery that is not encompassed by plaque. Even a small increase in a narrowed arterial lumen can produce a significant reduction in resistance to blood flow across obstructed regions. Nitrates may also exert a beneficial effect in patients with impaired coronary flow reserve by alleviating the vasoconstriction caused by endothelial dysfunction.

REDISTRIBUTION OF BLOOD FLOW. Nitroglycerin causes redistribution of blood flow from normally perfused to ischemic areas, particularly in the subendocardium. This redistribution may be mediated in part by an increase in collateral blood flow and in part by lowering of LV diastolic pressure, thereby reducing subendocardial compression. Nitroglycerin appears to reduce coronary vascular resistance preferentially in viable myocardium with ischemia, as detected by SPECT imaging.[104] In patients with chronic stable angina responsive to nitroglycerin, topical nitroglycerin under resting conditions alters myocardial perfusion by preferentially increasing flow to areas of reduced perfusion, with little or no change in global myocardial perfusion.

ANTITHROMBOTIC EFFECTS. Stimulation of guanylate cyclase by nitric oxide (NO) results in an inhibitory action on platelets in addition to vasodilation. Although the antithrombotic effects of intravenous

TABLE 57-4 Effects of Antianginal Agents on Indices of Myocardial Oxygen Supply and Demand

INDEX	NITRATES	Beta-Adrenoceptor Blockers ISA NO	ISA YES	CARDIOSELECTIVE NO	CARDIOSELECTIVE YES	Calcium Antagonists NIFEDIPINE	VERAPAMIL	DILTIAZEM
Supply								
Coronary resistance								
Vascular tone	↓↓	↑	0	↑	0↑	↓↓↓	↓↓↓	↓↓↓
Intramyocardial diastolic tension	↓↓↓	↑	0	↑	↑	↓↓	0	0
Coronary collateral circulation	↑	0	0	0	0	↑	0	↑
Duration of diastole	0 (↓)	↑↑↑	0↓	↑↑↑	↑↑↑	0↑ (↓↓)	↑↑↑(↓)	↑↑(↓)
Demand								
Intramyocardial systolic tension								
Preload	↓↓↓	↑	0	↑	↑	↓0	↑0↓	0↓
Afterload (peripheral vascular resistance)	↓	↑	↑	↑↑	↑	↓↓	↓	↓
Contractility	0 (↑)	↓↓↓	↓	↓↓↓	↓↓↓	↓ (↑↑)†	↓↓(↑)†	↓(↑)†
Heart rate	0 (↑)	↓↓↓	0↓	↓↓↓	↓↓↓	0 (↑↑)	↓↓ (↑)	↓↓ (↑)

↑ = Increase; ↓ = decrease; 0 = little or no definite effect. The number of arrows represents the relative intensity of effect. Symbols in parentheses indicate reflex-mediated effects.
†Effect of calcium entry on left ventricular contractility, as assessed in the intact animal model. The net effect on left ventricular performance is variable because it is influenced by alterations in afterload, reflex cardiac stimulation, and underlying state of the myocardium.
From Shub C, Vlietstra RE, McGoon MD: Selection of optimal drug therapy for the patient with angina pectoris. Mayo Clin Proc 60:539, 1985.

nitroglycerin have been demonstrated in patients with unstable angina and in those with stable IHD, the clinical significance of these actions is not clear.

CELLULAR MECHANISM OF ACTION. Nitrates have the ability to cause vasodilation, regardless of whether the endothelium is intact. After entering the vascular smooth muscle cell, nitrates are converted to reactive NO or S-nitrosothiols, which activate intracellular guanylate cyclase to produce cyclic guanosine monophosphate (cGMP), which in turn triggers smooth muscle relaxation and antiplatelet aggregator effects (see Fig. 57-e1 on the website). Evidence now indicates that the biotransformation of nitroglycerin occurs via mitochondrial aldehyde dehydrogenase and that inhibition of this enzyme may contribute to the development of tolerance.[105] Although the aggregate evidence supports the release of NO as the major cellular mechanism of action of oral nitrates, experimental data have raised challenges to this conclusion. In particular, the arterial vasodilatory effects of nitroglycerin in vitro depend at least in part on endothelial calcium-activated potassium channels.

POTENTIAL FOR ADVERSE EFFECTS OF LONG-TERM ADMINISTRATION. Experimental studies have raised questions regarding potentially competing long-term effects of oral nitrates.[106] A number of animal experiments and at least one human study have demonstrated that extended exposure to nitrates can impair endothelial-dependent vasodilation through the generation of free radical species. This effect appears to be reversed by antioxidant therapy.[107] In contrast, in an animal model of hypercholesterolemia, large doses of a nitrate had endothelial protective effects and attenuated the increase in intima-media thickness. Long-term studies in humans are necessary to determine the clinical relevance of these findings.[108]

Types of Preparations and Routes of Administration

Nitroglycerin administered sublingually remains the drug of choice for the treatment of acute angina episodes and for the prevention of angina (**Table 57-5**). Because sublingual administration avoids first-pass hepatic metabolism, a transient but effective concentration of the drug rapidly appears in the circulation. The half-life of nitroglycerin itself is brief and it is rapidly converted to two inactive metabolites, both of which are found in the urine. Within 30 to 60 minutes, hepatic breakdown has abolished the hemodynamic and clinical effects. The usual sublingual dose is 0.3 to 0.6 mg, and most patients respond within 5 minutes to one or two 0.3-mg tablets. If symptoms are not relieved by a single dose, additional doses of 0.3 mg may be taken at 5-minute intervals, but no more than 1.2 mg should be used within a 15-minute period. The development of tolerance (see later) is rarely a problem with intermittent use. Sublingual nitroglycerin is especially useful when taken prophylactically shortly before undertaking physical activities that are likely to cause angina. When used for this purpose, it may prevent angina for up to 40 minutes.

ADVERSE REACTIONS. Adverse reactions are common and include headache, flushing, and hypotension. The last is rarely severe

TABLE 57-5 Recommended Dosing Regimens for Long-Term Nitrate Therapy

PREPARATION OF AGENT	DOSE	SCHEDULE
Nitroglycerin*		
Ointment	0.5-2 inches	Two or three times daily
Transdermal patch	0.2-0.8 mg/hr	q 24 hr; remove at bedtime for 12-14 hr
Sublingual tablet	0.3-0.6 mg	As needed, up to three doses 5 min apart
Spray	One or two sprays	As needed, up to three doses 5 min apart
Isosorbide dinitrate*		
Oral	10-40 mg	Two or three times daily
Oral sustained release	80-120 mg	Once or twice daily (eccentric schedule)
Isosorbide 5-mononitrate		
Oral	20 mg	Twice daily (given 7-8 hr apart)
Oral sustained release	30-240 mg	Once daily

*A 10- to 12-hour nitrate-free interval is recommended.

but, in some patients with volume depletion and in an upright posture, nitrate-induced hypotension is accompanied by a paradoxical bradycardia, consistent with a vasovagal or vasodepressor response. This reaction is more common in older patients, who are less able to tolerate hypovolemia. Administration of nitrates before or soon after a meal, particularly in patients with a tendency toward postprandial hypotension, may augment venous pooling, preload reduction, and extent of the fall in blood pressure after the meal. In addition, the partial pressure of O_2 in arterial blood may fall after large doses of nitroglycerin because of a ventilation-perfusion imbalance caused by inability of the pulmonary vascular bed to constrict in areas of alveolar hypoxia, thereby leading to perfusion of less hypoxic tissues. Methemoglobinemia is a rare complication of very large doses of nitrates; commonly used doses of nitrates cause small elevations of methemoglobin levels that are probably not of clinical significance.

PREPARATIONS

Nitroglycerin Tablets

Nitroglycerin tablets tend to lose their potency, especially if exposed to light, and should thus be kept in dark containers. Other nitrate preparations are available in sublingual, buccal, oral, spray, and ointment forms (see Table 57-5). An oral nitroglycerin spray that dispenses metered, aerosolized doses of 0.4 mg may be better absorbed than the sublingual form by patients with dry mucosal membranes. It can also be quickly sprayed onto or under the tongue. For prophylaxis, the spray should be used 5 to 10 minutes before angina-provoking activities.

Isosorbide Dinitrate

This drug is an effective antianginal agent but has low bioavailability after oral administration. It undergoes hepatic metabolism rapidly, and marked variation in plasma concentrations may be seen after oral administration. It has two metabolites, one with potent vasodilator action, which are cleared less rapidly than the parent drug and excreted unchanged in the urine. It is available in tablets for sublingual use, in chewable form, in tablets for oral use, and in sustained-release capsules.

Partial or complete nitrate tolerance (see later) develops with regimens of isosorbide dinitrate when administered as 30 mg three or four times daily. A dosage schedule should be adopted that allows a 10- to 12-hour nitrate-free interval. If the drug is administered on a three times daily schedule (e.g., at 8 AM, 1 PM, and 6 PM), the antianginal benefit lasts for approximately 6 hours, and the magnitude of the antianginal benefit decreases with each successive dose.

Isosorbide 5-Mononitrate

This active metabolite of the dinitrate is completely bioavailable with oral administration because it does not undergo first-pass hepatic metabolism; it is efficacious in the treatment of chronic stable angina. Plasma levels of isosorbide 5-mononitrate reach their peak between 30 minutes and 2 hours after ingestion, and the drug has a plasma half-life of 4 to 6 hours. A single 20-mg tablet still exhibits activity 8 hours after administration. Tolerance has not been demonstrated with once-daily or eccentric dosing intervals but does occur with a twice-daily dosing regimen at 12-hour intervals. The sustained-release preparation of isosorbide 5-mononitrate may be given once daily in a dosage of 30 to 240 mg. Presumably, this preparation avoids tolerance by providing a sufficiently low nitrate level or a duration of action of 12 hours or less. Once-daily dosing of oral nitrates improves compliance and may offer better efficacy in reducing angina.[109,110]

Topical Nitroglycerin

1. *Ointment.* Nitroglycerin ointment (15 mg/inch) is efficacious when applied (most commonly to the chest) in strips of 0.5 to 2.0 inches. The delay in onset of action is approximately 30 minutes. Because this form of the drug is effective for 4 to 6 hours, it is particularly useful for patients with severe angina or unstable angina who are confined to bed and chair. Nitroglycerin ointment may also be used prophylactically after retiring by patients with nocturnal angina. Skin permeability increases with increased hydration, and absorption is also enhanced if the paste is covered with plastic, with the edges taped to the skin.

2. *Transdermal Patches.* Application of silicone gel or polymer matrix impregnated with nitroglycerin results in absorption for 24 to 48 hours at a rate determined by various methods of preparation of the patch, including a semipermeable membrane placed between the drug reservoir and the skin. The release rate of the patches varies from 0.1 to 0.8 mg/hr. Relatively low doses (0.1 to 0.2 mg/hr) may not produce sufficient plasma and tissue concentrations to sustain consistent, effective antianginal effects. Transdermal nitroglycerin therapy has been shown to increase exercise duration and maintain anti-ischemic effects for 12 hours after patch application throughout 30 days of therapy, without significant evidence of nitrate tolerance or rebound phenomena, provided that the patch is not applied for more than 12 out of 24 hours.

NITRATE TOLERANCE. A major problem with the use of nitrates is the development of nitrate tolerance, which has been demonstrated with all forms of nitrate administration delivering continuous, relatively stable blood levels of the drug. Although nitrate tolerance is rapid in onset, renewed responsiveness is easily established after a short nitrate-free interval. The problem of tolerance applies to all nitrate preparations; it is particularly important in patients with chronic angina, as opposed to those receiving short-acting courses of nitrates (e.g., with unstable angina and MI). Nitrate tolerance appears to be limited to the capacitance and resistance vessels and has not been noted in the large conductance vessels, including the epicardial coronary arteries and radial arteries, despite continuous administration of nitroglycerin for 48 hours.

MECHANISMS. Several mechanisms of nitrate tolerance have been proposed. Evidence has supported the hypothesis that increased generation of vascular superoxide anion ($\cdot O_2^-$) is central to the process.[111] There are various possible contributors to generation of oxygen free radicals, including the effects of nitroglycerin on endothelial nitric oxide synthase (NOS) uncoupling and counterregulatory neurohormonal activation. There are a number of consequences of increased superoxide anion formation; these include plausible links to many of the proposed mechanisms of nitrate tolerance: (1) plasma volume expansion and neurohormonal activation; (2) impaired biotransformation of nitrates to NO; and (3) decreased end-organ responsiveness to NO.

MANAGEMENT. The primary strategy to manage nitrate tolerance is to prevent it by providing a nitrate-free interval. The optimal interval is unknown, but with patches or ointment of nitroglycerin or preparations of isosorbide dinitrate or isosorbide 5-mononitrate, a 12-hour off-period is recommended.

NITRATE WITHDRAWAL. A common form of nitrate withdrawal (rebound) is observed in patients whose angina is intensified after discontinuation of large doses of long-acting nitrates. In this situation, patients may also have heightened sensitivity to constrictor stimuli. The potential for rebound can be modified by adjusting the dose and timing of administration in addition to the use of other antianginal drugs.

INTERACTION WITH PDE5 INHIBITORS. The combination of nitrates and PDE5 inhibitors, such as sildenafil, may cause serious, prolonged, and potentially life-threatening hypotension.[112] Nitrate therapy is an absolute contraindication to the use of PDE5 inhibitors, and vice versa. Patients who wish to take this class of medications should be aware of the serious nature of this adverse drug interaction and be warned about taking a PDE5 inhibitor within 24 hours of any nitrate preparation, including short-acting sublingual nitroglycerin tablets.

BETA-ADRENERGIC BLOCKING AGENTS. Beta-adrenergic blocking drugs (beta blockers) constitute a cornerstone of therapy for angina.[113] In addition to their antiischemic properties, beta blockers are effective antihypertensives (see Chap. 46) and antiarrhythmics (see Chap. 37). They have also been shown to reduce mortality and reinfarction in patients after MI (see Chap. 55) and to reduce mortality in patients with heart failure (see Chap. 28). This combination of actions makes them extremely useful in the management of stable IHD. A number of studies have shown that beta blockers, in doses that are generally well tolerated, reduce the frequency of anginal episodes and raise the anginal threshold when given alone and when added to other antianginal agents.

The beneficial actions of these drugs depend on their ability to cause competitive inhibition of the effects of neuronally released and circulating catecholamines on beta adrenoceptors (**Table 57-6**). Beta blockade reduces myocardial O_2 requirements, primarily by slowing the heart rate; the slower heart rate in turn increases the fraction of the cardiac cycle occupied by diastole, with a corresponding increase in the time available for coronary perfusion (**Fig. 57-8**; see Table 57-4). These drugs also reduce exercise-induced increases in blood pressure and limit exercise-induced increases in contractility. Thus, beta blockers reduce myocardial O_2 demand primarily during activity or excitement, when surges of increased sympathetic activity occur. In the face of impaired myocardial perfusion, the effects of beta blockers on myocardial O_2 demand may critically and favorably alter the imbalance between supply and demand, thereby resulting in the elimination of ischemia.

Beta blockers may reduce blood flow to most organs by means of the combination of beta$_2$ receptor blockade and unopposed alpha-adrenergic vasoconstriction and (**Table 57-7**). Complications are relatively minor but, in patients with peripheral vascular disease, the reduction in blood flow to skeletal muscles with the use of nonselective beta blockers may reduce maximal exercise capacity. In patients with preexisting LV dysfunction, beta blockade may increase LV volume and thereby increase O_2 demand.

TABLE 57-6	Physiologic Actions of Beta-Adrenergic Receptors	
ORGAN	RECEPTOR TYPE	RESPONSE TO STIMULUS
Heart		
SA node	Beta$_1$	Increased heart rate
Atria	Beta$_1$	Increased contractility and conduction velocity
AV node	Beta$_1$	Increased automaticity and conduction velocity
His-Purkinje system	Beta$_1$	Increased automaticity and system conduction velocity
Ventricles	Beta$_1$	Increased automaticity, contractility, and conduction velocity
Arteries		
Peripheral	Beta$_2$	Dilation
Coronary	Beta$_2$	Dilation
Carotid	Beta$_2$	Dilation
Other	Beta$_2$	Increased insulin release; increased liver and muscle glycogenolysis
Lungs	Beta$_2$	Dilation of bronchi
Uterus	Beta$_2$	Smooth muscle relaxation

AV = atrioventricular; SA = sinoatrial.

From Abrams J: Medical therapy of stable angina pectoris. In Beller G, Braunwald E (eds): Chronic Ischemic Heart Disease. Atlas of Heart Disease. Vol 5. Philadelphia, WB Saunders 1995, p 7.19.

BETA BLOCKADE EFFECTS ON ISCHEMIC HEART

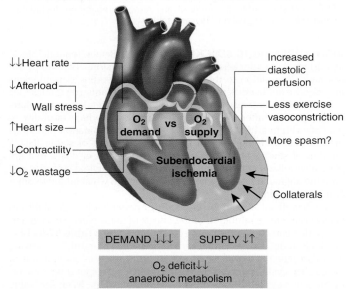

FIGURE 57-8 Effects of beta blockade on the ischemic heart. Beta blockade has a beneficial effect on ischemic myocardium unless (1) the preload rises substantially, as in left-sided heart failure, or (2) vasospastic angina is present, in which case spasm may be promoted in some patients. Note the suggestion that beta blockade diminishes exercise-induced vasoconstriction. *(Modified from Opie LH: Drugs for the Heart. 4th ed. Philadelphia, WB Saunders, 1995, p 6.)*

CHARACTERISTICS OF DIFFERENT BETA BLOCKERS

SELECTIVITY. Two major subtypes of beta receptors, designated beta$_1$ and beta$_2$, are present in different proportions in different tissues. Beta$_1$ receptors predominate in the heart, and stimulation of these receptors leads to an increase in heart rate, atrioventricular (AV) conduction, and contractility, release of renin from juxtaglomerular cells in the kidneys, and lipolysis in adipocytes. Beta$_2$ stimulation causes bronchodilation, vasodilation, and glycogenolysis. Nonselective beta-receptor-blocking drugs (e.g., propranolol, nadolol, penbutolol, pindolol, sotalol, timolol, carteolol) block both beta$_1$ and beta$_2$ receptors, whereas cardioselective beta blockers (e.g., acebutolol, atenolol, betaxolol, bisoprolol, esmolol,

metoprolol, nebivolol) block beta$_1$ receptors while having less effect on beta$_2$ receptors. Thus, cardioselective beta blockers reduce myocardial O$_2$ requirements while tending not to block bronchodilation, vasodilation, or glycogenolysis. However, as the doses of these drugs are increased, this cardioselectivity diminishes. Because cardioselectivity is only relative, the use of cardioselective beta blockers in doses sufficient to control angina may still cause bronchoconstriction in some susceptible patients. Nevertheless, beta blockers are relatively well tolerated in most patients with obstructive pulmonary disease.[114]

Some beta blockers also cause vasodilation. Such drugs include labetalol (an alpha-adrenergic blocking agent and beta$_2$ agonist; see Chap. 46), carvedilol (with alpha- and beta$_1$-blocking activity), bucindolol (a nonselective beta blocker that causes direct [non–alpha-adrenergic mediated] vasodilation), and nebivolol (a cardioselective beta blocker with a direct stimulatory effect on endothelial nitric oxide synthase, eNOS).[115]

ANTIARRHYTHMIC ACTIONS. Beta blockers have antiarrhythmic properties as a direct effect of their ability to block sympathoadrenal myocardial stimulation, which in certain situations may be arrhythmogenic (see Chap. 37).

INTRINSIC SYMPATHOMIMETIC ACTIVITY. Beta blockers with intrinsic sympathomimetic activity (ISA), such as acebutolol, bucindolol, carteolol, celiprolol, penbutolol, and pindolol, are partial beta agonists that also produce blockade by shielding beta receptors from more potent beta agonists. Pindolol and acebutolol produce low-grade beta stimulation when sympathetic activity is low (at rest), whereas these partial agonists behave more like conventional beta blockers when sympathetic activity is high. Agents with ISA may not be as effective as those without this property in reducing the heart rate or frequency, duration, and magnitude of ambulatory ST-segment changes or increasing the duration of exercise in patients with severe angina.

POTENCY. Potency can be measured by the ability of beta blockers to inhibit the tachycardia produced by isoproterenol. All drugs are considered in reference to propranolol, which is given a value of 1.0 (see Table 57-7). Timolol and pindolol are the most potent agents, and acebutolol and labetalol are the least potent.

LIPID SOLUBILITY. The hydrophilicity or lipid solubility of beta blockers is a major determinant of their absorption and metabolism. The lipid-soluble (lipophilic) beta blockers propranolol, metoprolol, and pindolol are readily absorbed from the gastrointestinal tract, are metabolized predominantly by the liver, have a relatively short half-life, and usually require administration twice or more daily to achieve continuing pharmacologic effects. If metoprolol or propranolol is administered intravenously, a much higher concentration reaches the bloodstream, and therefore intravenous dosing has much greater potency than oral dosing. The water-soluble (hydrophilic) beta blockers (e.g., atenolol, sotalol, nadolol) are not as readily absorbed from the gastrointestinal tract, are not as extensively metabolized, have relatively long plasma half-lives, and can be administered once daily. Water-soluble beta blockers are usually eliminated unchanged by the kidneys. Lipid-soluble agents are often preferable for patients with significant renal dysfunction for whom clearance of water-soluble agents is reduced. Greater lipid solubility is associated with greater penetration to the central nervous system and may contribute to side effects (e.g., lethargy, depression, hallucinations) that are not clearly related to beta-blocking activity.

ALPHA-ADRENERGIC BLOCKING ACTIVITY. The alpha-blocking potency of labetalol (approximately 10% that of phentolamine) is approximately 20% of its beta-blocking potency (see Table 57-7). Labetalol's combined alpha- and beta-blocking effects make it a particularly useful antihypertensive agent (see Chap. 46), especially in patients with hypertension and angina. The major side effects of labetalol are postural hypotension and retrograde ejaculation. Carvedilol also possesses alpha-adrenergic blocking activity with an alpha$_1$-to–beta-blocking ratio of approximately 1:10.

GENETIC POLYMORPHISMS. The metabolism of metoprolol, carvedilol, and propranolol may be influenced by genetic polymorphisms or other medications that influence hepatic metabolism.[116] The oxidative metabolism of metoprolol occurs primarily through the cytochrome P-450 enzyme CYP2D6 and exhibits the debrisoquin type of genetic polymorphism; poor hydroxylators or metabolizers (10% of whites or less) have significant prolongation of the elimination half-life of the drug in comparison to extensive hydroxylators or metabolizers. Thus, angina might be controlled by a single daily dose of metoprolol in poor metabolizers, whereas extensive metabolizers require the same dose two or three times daily. If a patient exhibits an exaggerated clinical response (e.g., extreme bradycardia) following the administration of metoprolol, propranolol, or other lipid-soluble beta blockers, it may be the result of prolongation of the elimination half-life because of slow oxidative metabolism. Metabolism of metoprolol may also be altered by drugs that interact with CYP2D6. Preliminary evidence has raised the possibility of differences in survival in patients with unstable IHD and provoked ischemia in stable IHD treated with beta blockers based on polymorphisms of the beta$_2$-adrenergic receptor (*ADRB1* and *ADRB2*).[117,118] Moreover, polymorphisms of the beta-adrenergic receptor may lead to variability in response to beta blockers in patients with heart failure.[119]

EFFECTS ON SERUM LIPID LEVELS. Beta blocker therapy (with agents lacking ISA) usually causes no significant changes in total or LDL cholesterol levels but increases triglyceride and reduces HDL cholesterol levels. The most commonly studied drug has been propranolol, which can increase plasma triglyceride concentrations by 20% to 50% and reduce HDL cholesterol levels by 10% to 20%. Increasing beta$_1$ selectivity is associated with lesser effects on lipid levels. Adverse effects on the lipid profile may be more frequent with nonselective than with beta$_1$-selective blockers. The effects of these changes in serum lipid levels by long-term administration of beta blockers must be considered when this therapy is begun or maintained for hypertension or angina.

Dosage

For optimal results, the dosage of a beta blocker should be carefully adjusted. In the case of atenolol, it is useful to start with a dosage of 50 mg once daily. The usual effective dosage is 50 to 100 mg daily; however, some patients benefit from up to 200 mg daily. In the case of metoprolol, it is often preferable from a perspective of the patient's compliance to use an extended-release formulation, which may be started at a dose of 100 mg once daily. Other beta blockers should be started at comparable doses.

Efficacy is determined by the effect on heart rate and symptoms and, when these are unclear, the effect on exercise performance can be evaluated by treadmill exercise testing. The resting heart rate should be reduced to between 50 and 60 beats/min, and an increase of less than 20 beats/min should occur with modest exercise (e.g., climbing one flight of stairs). Therapy with beta blockers needs to be individualized and requires repeated clinical evaluation during the initial period of drug administration.

Adverse Effects and Contraindications

Most of the adverse effects of beta blockers occur as a consequence of the known properties of these drugs and include cardiac effects (e.g., severe sinus bradycardia, sinus arrest, AV block, reduced LV contractility), bronchoconstriction, fatigue, mental depression, nightmares, gastrointestinal upset, sexual dysfunction, intensification of insulin-induced hypoglycemia, and cutaneous reactions (**Table 57-8**; see Table 57-6). Lethargy, weakness, and fatigue may be caused by reduced cardiac output or may arise from a direct effect on the central nervous system. Bronchoconstriction results from blockade of beta$_2$ receptors in the tracheobronchial tree. As a consequence, asthma and chronic obstructive lung disease may be considered as relative contraindications to beta blockers, even to beta$_1$-selective agents.[114]

In patients who already have impaired LV function, heart failure may be intensified, an effect that can be counteracted in part by the use of digitalis or diuretics. Beginning therapy with a very low dose (e.g., metoprolol succinate extended release, 25 mg daily, for 2 weeks in patients with NYHA functional Class II) and then gradually increasing the dose over the course of several weeks has been shown to be well tolerated and beneficial in patients with idiopathic dilated cardiomyopathy and those with heart failure caused by IHD (see Chap. 28). This approach is recommended when using beta blockers for patients with angina and heart failure.[120,121]

Beta blockers should be prescribed with caution for patients with cardiac conduction disease involving the sinus node or AV conduction system. In patients with symptomatic conduction disease, beta blockers are contraindicated unless a pacemaker is in place. In patients with asymptomatic sinus node dysfunction or first-degree AV block, beta blockers may be tolerated, but their administration requires careful observation. Pindolol, because of its ISA activity, may be preferable in this situation. Blockade of noncardiac beta$_2$ receptors inhibits catecholamine-induced glycogenolysis, so noncardioselective beta blockers can mask the premonitory signs of insulin-induced

hypoglycemia. Nevertheless, beta blockers are generally well tolerated by patients with diabetes mellitus. Moreover, carvedilol has been shown to exhibit modest insulin-sensitizing properties and can relieve some manifestations of the metabolic syndrome.[122,123] Blockade of beta$_2$ receptors also inhibits the vasodilating effects of catecholamines in peripheral blood vessels and leaves the constrictor (alpha-adrenergic) receptors unopposed, thereby enhancing vasoconstriction. Noncardioselective beta blockers may precipitate episodes of Raynaud phenomenon in patients with this condition and may cause uncomfortable coldness in the distal extremities. Reduced flow to the limbs may occur in patients with peripheral vascular disease.

Abrupt withdrawal of beta-adrenergic blocking agents after prolonged administration can result in increased total ischemic activity in patients with chronic stable angina. This increased ischemia may be caused by a return to the previously high levels of myocardial O$_2$ demand while the underlying atherosclerotic process has progressed, but a rebound phenomenon resulting in increased beta-adrenergic sensitivity probably occurs in some patients. Occasionally, such withdrawal can precipitate unstable angina and may, in rare cases, even provoke MI. Chronic beta blocker therapy can be safely discontinued by slowly withdrawing the drug in a stepwise manner over the course of 2 to 3 weeks. If abrupt withdrawal of beta blockers is required, patients should be instructed to reduce exertion and manage angina episodes with sublingual nitroglycerin and/or substitute a calcium antagonist.

CALCIUM ANTAGONISTS. The critical role of calcium ions in the normal contraction of cardiac and vascular smooth muscle is discussed in Chaps. 24 and 52. The calcium antagonists (see Chap. 46) are a heterogeneous group of compounds that inhibit calcium ion movement through slow channels in cardiac and smooth muscle membranes by noncompetitive blockade of voltage-sensitive L-type calcium channels.[124] The three major classes of calcium antagonists are the dihydropyridines (nifedipine is the prototype), the phenylalkylamines (verapamil is the prototype), and the modified benzothiazepines (diltiazem is the prototype). Amlodipine and felodipine are additional dihydropyridines that are among the most commonly used calcium antagonists in the United States. The two predominant effects of calcium antagonists result from blocking the entry of calcium ions and slowing recovery of the channel. Phenylalkylamines have a marked effect on recovery of the channel and thereby exert depressant effects on cardiac pacemakers and conduction, whereas dihydropyridines, which do not impair channel recovery, have little effect on the conduction system.

MECHANISM OF ACTION. The efficacy of calcium antagonists in patients with angina pectoris is related to the reduction in myocardial O$_2$ demand and the increase in O$_2$ supply that they induce (see Table 57-4). The latter effect is particularly important in patients with conditions in which a prominent vasospastic or vasoconstrictor component may be present, such as Prinzmetal (variant) angina (see Chaps. 52 and 56), variable-threshold angina, and angina related to impaired vasodilator reserve of small coronary arteries. Calcium antagonists may be effective on their own or in combination with beta-adrenergic blockers and nitrates in patients with chronic stable angina. Several calcium antagonists are effective for the treatment of angina pectoris (**Table 57-9**). Each relaxes vascular smooth muscle in the systemic arterial and coronary arterial beds. In addition, blockade of the entry of calcium into myocytes results in a negative inotropic effect, which is counteracted to some extent by peripheral vascular dilation and by activation of the sympathetic nervous system in response to drug-induced hypotension.[124] However, the negative inotropic effect must be taken into consideration in patients with significant LV dysfunction.

With a rapid onset of action and metabolism by the liver, calcium antagonists have a limited bioavailability of between 13% and 52% and a half-life of between 3 and 12 hours. Amlodipine and felodipine are exceptions in that both drugs have long half-lives and may be administered once daily. In the case of some of the other calcium antagonists (e.g., nifedipine and diltiazem), sustained-release preparations have been shown to be effective.

ANTIATHEROGENIC ACTION. Hyperlipidemia-induced changes in the permeability of smooth muscle cells to calcium may play a role in atherogenesis; thus, the hypothesis that calcium antagonists might inhibit

CH
57

TABLE 57-7 Pharmacokinetics and Pharmacology of Some Beta-Adrenoceptor Blockers

CHARACTERISTIC	ATENOLOL	METOPROLOL/ METOPROLOL XL	NADOLOL	PINDOLOL	PROPRANOLOL/ PROPRANOLOL LA	TIMOLOL	ACEBUTOLOL
Extent of absorption (%)	~50	>95	~30	>90	>90	>90	~70
Extent of bioavailability (% of dose)	~40	~50/77	~30	~90	~30/20	75	~50
Beta-blocking plasma concentration	0.2-0.5 µg/mL	50-100 ng/mL	50-100 ng/mL	50-100 ng/mL	50-100 ng/mL	50-100 ng/mL	0.2-2.0 µg/mL
Protein binding (%)	<5	12	~30	57	93	~10	30-40
Lipophilicity*	Low	Moderate	Low	Moderate	High	Low	Low
Elimination half-life (hr)	6-9	3-7	14-25	3-4	3.5-6/8-11	3-4	3-4†
Drug accumulation in renal disease	Yes	No	Yes	No	No	No	Yes‡
Route of elimination	RE (mostly unchanged)	HM	RE	RE (40% unchanged and HM)	HM	RE (20% unchanged and HM)	HM‡
Beta blocker potency ratio (propranolol = 1)	1.0	1	1.0	6.0	1	6.0	0.3
Adrenergic-receptor blocking activity	β_1¶	β_1¶	β_1/β_2	β_1/β_2	β_1/β_2	β_1/β_2	β_1¶
Intrinsic sympathetic activity	0	0	0	+	0	0	+
Membrane-stabilizing activity	0	0	0	+	++	0	+
Usual maintenance dose	50-100 mg/day	50-100 mg bid-qid/50-400 mg/day	40-80 mg/day	10-40 mg/day (bid-tid)	80-320 mg/day (bid-tid)/ 80-160 mg/day	10-30 mg bid	200-600 mg bid
FDA-approved indications:							
Hypertension	Yes	Yes/yes	Yes	Yes	Yes/yes	Yes	Yes
Angina	Yes	Yes/yes	Yes	No	Yes/yes	No	No
Post-MI	Yes	Yes/no	No	No	Yes/no	Yes	No
Heart failure	No	Yes/yes	No	No	No/no	No	No

*Determined by the distribution ratio between octanol and water.
†Half-life of the active metabolite, diacetolol, is 12 to 15 hours.
‡Acebutolol is mainly eliminated by the liver, but its major metabolite, diacetolol, is excreted by the kidney.

TABLE 57-8 Candidates for Use of Beta-Blocking Agents for Angina

Ideal Candidates
Prominent relationship of physical activity to attacks of angina
Coexistent hypertension
History of supraventricular or ventricular arrhythmias
Previous myocardial infarction
Left ventricular systolic dysfunction
Mild to moderate heart failure symptoms (NYHA functional Classes II, III)
Prominent anxiety state

Poor Candidates
Asthma or reversible airway component in chronic lung disease patients
Severe left ventricular dysfunction with severe heart failure symptoms
  (NYHA functional Class IV)
History of severe depression
Raynaud phenomenon
Symptomatic peripheral vascular disease
Severe bradycardia or heart block
Brittle diabetes

Modified from Abrams JA: Medical therapy of stable angina pectoris. In Beller G, Braunwald E (eds): Chronic Ischemic Heart Disease. Atlas of Heart Disease. Vol. 5. Philadelphia, WB Saunders, 1995. p 7.22.

atherogenesis has been explored since the 1970s but has not yet achieved consensus. Experimental work with calcium channel blockers, in particular with more lipophilic second-generation agents such as amlodipine, have demonstrated improved endothelial function, inhibition of smooth muscle cell proliferation, migration, and ameliorated unfavorable membrane alterations.[125] In a randomized trial in patients with established CAD without hypertension, treatment with amlodipine, compared with placebo, reduced coronary atherosclerosis progression.[126] In a similar trial, nifedipine, compared with placebo, improved coronary endothelial function but did not reduce plaque volume.[125] In summary, although the evidence remains mixed, calcium antagonists may have some role in atheroprotection.

First-Generation Calcium Antagonists

NIFEDIPINE. Nifedipine, a dihydropyridine, is a particularly effective dilator of vascular smooth muscle and is a more potent vasodilator than diltiazem or verapamil. Although its in vitro actions on myocardium and specialized cardiac tissue are similar to those of other agents, the concentration required to reproduce effects on these tissues is not reached in vivo because of the early appearance of its powerful vasodilating effects. Thus, in clinical practice, the potential negative chronotropic, inotropic, and dromotropic (on AV conduction) effects of nifedipine are seldom a problem, with the exception that nifedipine has been reported to worsen heart failure in patients with pre-existing chronic heart failure.

The beneficial effects of nifedipine in the treatment of angina result from its ability to reduce myocardial O_2 requirements because of its afterload-reducing effect and to increase myocardial O_2 delivery as a result of its dilating action on the coronary vascular bed (see Table 57-4). Oral nifedipine in capsule form exerts hypotensive effects within 20 minutes of administration. This immediate-release formulation is no longer recommended because of concerns regarding adverse

	LABETALOL	BISOPROLOL	BETAXOLOL	CARTEOLOL	PENBUTOLOL	CARVEDILOL/ CARVEDILOL CR	ESMOLOL (IV)	SOTALOL
	>90	>90	>90	>90	100	ND	ND	ND
	~25	80	90	85	100	~30/~25	100	>90
	0.7-3.0 µg/mL	0.01-0.1 µg/mL	20-50 ng/mL	40-160 ng/mL	ND	ND	0.15-2.0 µg/mL	ND
	~50	30	50-60	23-30	80-98	95-98	55	0
	Low	Moderate	Moderate	Low	High	High	Low	Low
	~6	7-15	12-22	5-7	17-26	6-10/11	4.5 min	12
	No	Yes	Yes	Yes	Yes	No	No	Yes
	HM	HM 50%; RE 50%	HM	RE	HM	HM	§	RE
	0.3	10	4	10	1	10	0.02	0.3
	$\beta_1/\beta_2/\alpha_1$	β_1¶	β_1ᵃ	β_1/β_2	β_1/β_2	$\beta_1/\beta_2/\alpha_1$	β_1¶	β_1/β_2
	0	0	0	+	+	0	0	0
	0	0	0	0	0	+	0	0
	100-400 mg bid	5-20 mg/day	5-20 mg/day	2.5-10 mg/day	10-40 mg/day	3.125-50 mg bid 10-18 mg/day	Bolus of 500 µg/kg; infusion at 50-200 µg/kg/min	80-160 mg
	Yes	Yes	Yes	Yes	Yes	Yes/Yes	Yes	No
	No	No	No	No	No	No/No	No	No
	No	No	No	No	No	No/No	Yes	No
	No	No	No	No	No	Yes/Yes	No	No

§Rapid metabolism by esterases in the cytosol of red blood cells.
¶Beta₁ selectivity is maintained at lower doses, but beta₂ receptors are inhibited at higher doses.
FDA = U.S. Food and Drug Administration; HM = hepatic metabolism; MI = myocardial infarction; ND = no data; RE = renal excretion.

events. An extended-release formulation using the gastrointestinal therapeutic system of drug delivery (see Table 57-9) is designed to deliver 30, 60, or 90 mg of nifedipine in a single daily dose at a relatively constant rate over a 24-hour period and is useful for the treatment of chronic stable angina, Prinzmetal angina, and hypertension. Steady-state plasma levels are typically achieved within 48 hours of initiation. The efficacy of the extended-release preparation, either alone or in conjunction with beta blockers, in reducing episodes of angina and ischemia on ambulatory monitoring has been documented.

Adverse Effects

These occur in 15% to 20% of patients and require discontinuation of medication in about 5%. Most adverse effects are related to systemic vasodilation and include headache, dizziness, palpitations, flushing, hypotension, and leg edema (unrelated to heart failure). Gastrointestinal side effects, including nausea, epigastric pressure, and vomiting, are noted in approximately 5% of patients. In rare cases, in patients with extremely severe fixed coronary obstructions, nifedipine aggravates angina, presumably by lowering arterial pressure excessively, with subsequent reflex tachycardia. For this reason, combined treatment of angina with nifedipine and a beta blocker is particularly effective and superior to nifedipine alone. Most adverse effects are reduced by the use of extended-release preparations.

Several clinical case-control studies of hypertension and associated reviews have suggested that short-acting nifedipine may cause an increase in mortality. However, a meta-analysis of 15 studies of long-acting calcium channel antagonists, including nifedipine, in patients with CAD demonstrated a significant reduction in angina, stroke, and heart failure with similar rates of other cardiovascular outcomes.[127] Long-acting nifedipine should be considered as an effective and safe antianginal drug for the treatment of symptomatic patients with chronic CAD who are already receiving beta blockers, with or without nitrates. Short-acting nifedipine should ordinarily be avoided.

Because of its potent vasodilator effects, nifedipine is contraindicated for patients who are hypotensive or have severe aortic valve stenosis and for patients with unstable angina who are not simultaneously receiving a beta blocker in whom reflex-mediated increases in the heart rate may be harmful. Nifedipine (or a second-generation dihydropyridine) is the calcium antagonist of choice in patients with sinus bradycardia, sick sinus syndrome, or AV block, particularly if a beta-adrenergic blocking agent is administered concurrently and additional drug therapy for angina is indicated. This recommendation is based on the observation that in doses used clinically, nifedipine has fewer negative effects on myocardial contractility, heart rate, and AV conduction than verapamil or diltiazem.

Nifedipine interacts significantly with cimetidine and phenytoin (resulting in increased bioavailability of nifedipine). In patients with Prinzmetal angina, abrupt cessation of nifedipine therapy may result in a rebound increase in the frequency and duration of attacks.

VERAPAMIL. Verapamil dilates systemic and coronary resistance vessels and large coronary conductance vessels. It slows the heart rate

TABLE 57-9 Pharmacokinetics of Some Calcium Antagonists Used for Angina Pectoris

CHARACTERISTIC	DILTIAZEM/ DILTIAZEM SR	NICARDIPINE	NIFEDIPINE/ NIFEDIPINE SR	VERAPAMIL/ VERAPAMIL SR	AMLODIPINE	FELODIPINE	ISRADIPINE	NISOLDIPINE
Usual adult dose	IV: 0.25 mg/kg bolus, then 5-15 mg/hr Oral: 30-90 mg tid-qid SR: 60-180 mg bid CD: 120-480 mg/day	IV: 3-15 mg/hr Oral: 20-40 mg tid SR: 30-60 mg bid	Oral: 10-30 mg tid SR: 90 mg/d	IV: 0.075-0.15 mg/kg Oral: 80-120 mg tid-qid SR: 180-480 mg/day	Oral: 2.5-10 mg/ day	Oral SR: 2.5-10 mg/day	Oral CR: 2.5-10 mg bid	Oral SR: 10-40 mg/day
Extent of absorption (%)	80-90	100	90	90	>90	>90	>90	ND
Extent of bioavailability (%)	40-70	30	65-75/86	20-35	60-90	20	25	5
Onset of action	IV: 3 min Oral: 30-60 min	IV: 1 min Oral: 20 min	20 min	IV: 2-5 min Oral: 30 min	0.5-1.0 hr	2 hr	20 min	1-3 hr
Time to peak serum concentration (hr)	2-3/6-11	0.5-2.0	0.5/6	IV: 3-5 min Oral: 1-2; SR: 7-9	6-12	2-5	1.5	6-12
Therapeutic serum levels (ng/mL)	50-200	30-50	25-100	80-300	5-20	1-5	2-10	ND
Elimination half-life (hr)	3.5/5-7	2.0-4.0	2.0-5.0	3.0-7.0*	30-50	11-16	8	7-12
Elimination	60% metabolized by liver; remainder excreted by kidneys	High first-pass hepatic metabolism	High first-pass hepatic metabolism	85% eliminated by first-pass hepatic metabolism	Hepatic	High first-pass hepatic metabolism	High first-pass hepatic metabolism	Hepatic
Heart rate	↓	↑	↑↑	↓	0	↑	0	0
Peripheral vascular resistance	↓	↓↓↓	↓↓↓	↓↓	↓↓↓	↓↓↓	↓↓↓	↓↓↓
FDA-approved indications	IR / SR		IR / SR	IR / SR				
Hypertension	No	Yes†	No	Yes	Yes	Yes	Yes	Yes
Angina	Yes	Yes	Yes	Yes	Yes	No	No	Yes
Coronary spasm	Yes	No	Yes	Yes	Yes	No	No	No

*Half-life of 4.5 to 12 hr with multiple dosing; may be prolonged in older patients.
†The sustained-release formulation may be preferred for hypertension.
CD = combination drug; CR = controlled release; IR = immediate release; ND = no data; SR = sustained release.

and reduces myocardial contractility. This combination of actions results in a reduction in myocardial O_2 requirement, which is the basis for the drug's efficacy in the management of chronic stable angina.

Verapamil reduces the frequency of angina and prolongs exercise tolerance in patients with symptomatic chronic CAD, and the combination of verapamil and a beta blocker provides clinical benefit that is additive. When evaluated in the International Verapamil-Trandolapril Study (INVEST), a strategy combining sustained-release verapamil and trandolapril compared with atenolol and a diuretic for the treatment of patients with hypertension and CAD showed equivalent outcomes with respect to death, MI, or stroke, including patients with prior MI.[128] Despite the marked negative inotropic effects of verapamil in isolated cardiac muscle preparations, changes in contractility are modest in patients with normal cardiac function. However, in patients with cardiac dysfunction, verapamil may reduce cardiac output, increase LV filling pressure, and cause clinical heart failure. In clinically useful doses, verapamil inhibits calcium influx into specialized cardiac cells, sometimes causing slowing of the heart rate and AV conduction. Therefore, it is contraindicated for patients with pre-existing AV nodal disease or sick sinus syndrome, heart failure, and suspected digitalis or quinidine toxicity.

The usual starting dose of verapamil for oral administration is 40 to 80 mg three times daily to a maximal dose of 480 mg daily (see Table 57-9). Sustained-release preparations of verapamil are available, and starting doses are 120 to 240 mg twice daily, with a usual optimal dosage range of 240 to 360 mg daily.

Verapamil interacts significantly with several other drugs. Intravenous verapamil should generally not be used together with a beta blocker (given intravenously or orally), nor should a beta blocker be administered intravenously in patients receiving oral verapamil. Both drugs can be administered orally but with caution in view of the potential for the development of bradyarrhythmias and negative inotropic effects. The bioavailability of verapamil is increased by cimetidine and carbamazepine, whereas verapamil may increase plasma levels of cyclosporine and digoxin and may be associated with excessive hypotension in patients receiving quinidine or prazosin. Hepatic enzyme inducers such as phenobarbital may reduce the effects of verapamil. Verapamil should not be administered in conjunction with the antiarrhythmic drug dofetilide.

Adverse effects of verapamil are noted in approximately 10% of patients and relate to systemic vasodilation (hypotension and facial flushing), gastrointestinal symptoms (constipation and nausea), and central nervous system reactions, such as headache and dizziness. A rare side effect is gingival hyperplasia, which appears after 1 to 9 months of therapy.

DILTIAZEM. Diltiazem's actions are intermediate between those of nifedipine and verapamil. In clinically useful doses, its vasodilator effects are less profound than those of nifedipine, and its cardiac depressant action, on the sinoatrial and AV nodes and myocardium, is less than that of verapamil. This profile may explain the remarkably low incidence of adverse effects of diltiazem. Diltiazem is a systemic vasodilator that lowers arterial pressure at rest and during exertion and increases the workload required to produce myocardial ischemia, but it may also increase myocardial O_2 delivery. Although this drug causes little vasodilation of epicardial coronary arteries under basal conditions, it may enhance perfusion of the subendocardium distal to a flow-limiting coronary stenosis; it also blocks exercise-induced coronary vasoconstriction. In patients with chronic stable angina receiving maximally tolerated doses of diltiazem, the heart rate is significantly reduced at rest, but no effect on peak blood pressure is achieved during exercise, and the duration of symptom-limited treadmill exercise is prolonged.

Several sustained-release formulations of diltiazem are available for once-daily treatment of systemic hypertension and angina pectoris. The usual starting dosage of sustained-release formulations is 120 mg once daily up to a typical maintenance dosage of 180 to 360 mg once daily. The maximum effect on blood pressure may not be observed until 14 days after starting therapy.

Diltiazem is a highly effective antianginal agent. Atenolol and diltiazem have similar efficacy in increasing nonischemic exercise duration

in patients with variable-threshold angina and act primarily by slowing the resting heart rate. High doses (mean dose, 340 mg) have been shown to be a relatively safe addition to maximally tolerated doses of isosorbide dinitrate and a beta blocker and cause increases in exercise tolerance and resting and exercise LV ejection fractions. Major side effects are similar to those of the other calcium channel blockers and are related to vasodilation, but they are relatively infrequent, particularly if the dosage does not exceed 240 mg daily. As is the case with verapamil, diltiazem should be prescribed with caution for patients with sick sinus syndrome or AV block. In patients with pre-existing LV dysfunction, diltiazem may exacerbate or precipitate heart failure.

Diltiazem interacts with other drugs, including beta-adrenergic blocking agents (causing enhanced negative inotropic, chronotropic, and dromotropic effects), flecainide, and cimetidine (which increases the bioavailability of diltiazem). It has been associated with increased plasma levels of cyclosporine, carbamazepine, and lithium carbonate. Diltiazem may cause excessive sinus node depression if administered with disopyramide and may reduce digoxin clearance, especially in patients with renal failure.

Second-Generation Calcium Antagonists

The second-generation calcium antagonists (e.g., nicardipine, isradipine, amlodipine, felodipine) are mainly dihydropyridine derivatives, with nifedipine being the prototypical agent. Considerable experience has also accumulated with nimodipine, nisoldipine, and nitrendipine. These agents differ in potency, tissue specificity, and pharmacokinetics and, in general, are potent vasodilators because of greater vascular selectivity than that seen with the first-generation antagonists (e.g., verapamil, nifedipine, diltiazem).

AMLODIPINE. This agent, which is less lipid-soluble than nifedipine, has a slow smooth onset and ultralong duration of action (plasma half-life of 36 hours). It causes marked coronary and peripheral dilation and may be useful in the treatment of patients with angina accompanied by hypertension. It may be used as a once-daily hypotensive or antianginal agent. In a series of randomized placebo-controlled studies in patients with stable exercise-induced angina pectoris, amlodipine was shown to be effective and well tolerated. In two trials in patients with established CAD, amlodipine reduced the risk of major cardiovascular events. Amlodipine has little, if any, negative inotropic action and may be especially useful for patients with chronic angina and LV dysfunction.

The usual dosage of amlodipine is 5 to 10 mg once daily. Downward adjustment of the starting dose is appropriate for patients with liver disease and older patients. Significant changes in blood pressure are typically not evident until 24 to 48 hours after initiation. Steady-state serum levels are achieved at 7 to 8 days.

NICARDIPINE. This drug has a half-life similar to that of nifedipine (2 to 4 hours), but appears to have greater vascular selectivity. Nicardipine may be used as an antianginal and antihypertensive agent and requires administration three times daily, although a sustained-release formulation is available for twice-daily dosing in hypertension. For chronic stable angina pectoris, it appears to be as effective as verapamil or diltiazem, and its efficacy is enhanced when combined with a beta blocker.

FELODIPINE AND ISRADIPINE. In the United States, both drugs are approved by the U.S. Food and Drug Administration for the treatment of hypertension but not for angina pectoris. One study has documented similar efficacy between felodipine and nifedipine in patients with chronic stable angina. Felodipine has also been reported to be more vascular-selective than nifedipine and to have a mild positive inotropic effect as a result of calcium channel agonist properties. Isradipine has a longer half-life than nifedipine and demonstrates greater vascular sensitivity.

OTHER PHARMACOLOGIC AGENTS
RANOLAZINE. Ranolazine is a piperazine derivative that was approved in 2006 in the United States for use in patients with chronic stable angina.[129] Ranolazine is unique among currently approved antianginals in that its anti-ischemic effects are achieved without a clinically meaningful change in heart rate or blood pressure.[130] The mechanism of action of this agent remains under investigation. When studied at high

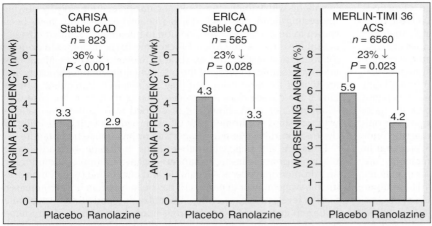

FIGURE 57-9 Reduction in the frequency of angina in three randomized, double-blind, placebo-controlled trials of ranolazine in patients with established CAD. Patients with stable CAD with early positive stress testing treated with standard doses of atenolol, amlodipine, or diltiazem were studied in the Combination Assessment of Ranolazine In Stable Angina (CARISA) trial. Patients with stable CAD and at least three episodes of angina weekly, despite amlodipine, 10 mg daily, were studied in the Efficacy of Ranolazine in Chronic Angina (ERICA) trial. Patients after presentation with non–ST-segment elevation ACS were studied for an average of 12 months in the Metabolic Efficiency With Ranolazine for Less Ischemia in Non-ST-Elevation Acute Coronary Syndromes (MERLIN) trial. In each trial, ranolazine reduced the frequency of angina. *(Data from Chaitman BR, Pepine CJ, Parker JO, et al: Effects of ranolazine with atenolol, amlodipine, or diltiazem on exercise tolerance and angina frequency in patients with severe chronic angina: A randomized controlled trial. JAMA 291:309, 2004; Stone PS, Gratsiansky NA, Blokhin A, et al: Antianginal efficacy of ranolazine when added to treatment with amlodipine. J Am Coll Cardiol 48:566, 2006; and Morrow DA, Scirica BM, Karwatowska-Prokopczuk E, et al: Effects of ranolazine on recurrent cardiovascular events in patients with non-ST-elevation acute coronary syndromes: The MERLIN-TIMI 36 Randomized Trial. JAMA 297:1775, 2007.)*

concentrations in in vitro experiments, ranolazine was shown to shift myocardial substrate utilization from fatty acid to glucose and thus was considered to be a potential metabolic agent. However, subsequent studies at concentrations of ranolazine consistent with doses tested in clinical trials have suggested that ranolazine exerts favorable effects on ischemia through a reduction in calcium overload in the ischemic myocyte via inhibition of the late sodium current (I_{Na}). In animal models of ischemia and reperfusion, ranolazine preserves tissue levels of adenosine triphosphate, improves myocardial contractile function, and reduces the extent of irreversible myocardial injury measured by biomarkers of necrosis and by electron microscopy.

A sustained-release formulation of ranolazine has been studied in three randomized, placebo-controlled clinical trials in patients with stable IHD and has improved exercise performance and increased the time to ischemia during exercise treadmill testing when used as monotherapy or when used in combination with the most frequently used doses of atenolol, amlodipine, or diltiazem.[131] Ranolazine also decreases angina frequency and nitroglycerin use when used in combination with a beta blocker or calcium channel blocker.

When studied in a randomized, blinded, placebo-controlled trial of 6560 patients with non–ST-segment elevation ACS, ranolazine, administered for an average of approximately 1 year, did not add to standard therapy for the secondary prevention of major cardiovascular events.[132] However, ranolazine reduced the incidence of recurrent ischemia, in particular worsening angina, in a significantly more diverse population with established CAD than studied previously with ranolazine (**Fig. 57-9**).[132] Consistent with prior studies, the reduction in angina and improvement in exercise performance were evident only in patients with a history of chronic angina.[133]

The half-life of the sustained-release formulation of ranolazine is approximately 7 hours. A steady state is generally achieved within 3 days of dosing twice daily. Ranolazine is metabolized primarily through the cytochrome P-450 (CYP3A4) pathway and thus the plasma concentration is increased if administered in combination with moderate (e.g., diltiazem) or strong (e.g., ketoconazole and macrolide antibiotic) inhibitors of this system. Verapamil increases the absorption of ranolazine by inhibition of P-glycoprotein. Plasma concentrations of simvastatin are increased approximately twofold after administration of ranolazine.

Ranolazine should be started as 500 mg twice daily and may be increased to a maximum of 1000 mg twice daily in patients with persistent angina. The most commonly reported adverse effects in clinical studies are nausea, generalized weakness, and constipation. Dizziness has also been reported, as has a small dose-related increase in the corrected QT interval, an average of 2 to 5 milliseconds in the dosage range of 500 to 1000 mg twice daily.[129] The electrophysiologic effects of ranolazine include inhibition of the delayed rectifier current and inhibition of I_{Na}; the net effect is to shorten action potential duration and suppress early afterdepolarizations.[134] Thus, ranolazine does not have the electrophysiologic profile that has been observed with QT-prolonging drugs associated with torsades de pointes. Ranolazine should be used with caution in patients receiving other QT-prolonging medications and is contraindicated in patients with clinically significant hepatic impairment, which has been associated with a steeper relationship between ranolazine and the QTc.

There was no adverse trend in the incidence of symptomatic documented arrhythmias, all-cause mortality, or sudden cardiac death with ranolazine in a randomized trial of 6560 patients with recent ACS. A significant reduction in the incidence of arrhythmias detected by 7 days of Holter monitoring with ranolazine compared with placebo in this study suggests possible antiarrhythmic actions of the agent that may warrant additional investigation.[135] In addition to these electrophysiologic effects, ranolazine also appears to have glycometabolic effects, including a reduction in hemoglobin A1c.[136]

IVABRADINE*. Ivabradine is a specific and selective inhibitor of the I_f ion channel, the principal determinant of the sinoatrial node pacemaker current.[137] Ivabradine reduces the spontaneous firing rate of sinoatrial pacemaker cells and thus slows heart rate through a mechanism that is not associated with negative inotropic effects. Ivabradine reduces peak heart rate during exercise, increases the time to limiting angina compared with placebo, and is equivalent to atenolol with respect to exercise performance and time to ischemia (ST-segment depression) in patients with stable angina undergoing exercise treadmill testing.[138] In a randomized trial of 10,917 patients with CAD and reduced LV function, ivabradine did not reduce the primary endpoint of cardiovascular death, hospitalization for MI, or hospitalization for heart failure.[139] Fewer hospitalizations for MI were observed in the subgroup of patients with a baseline heart rate higher than 70 beats/min who were randomized to ivabradine compared with placebo and in patients with a history of limiting angina.[140]

INVESTIGATIONAL AGENTS

NICORANDIL*. Nicorandil is a nicotinamide ester that dilates peripheral and coronary resistance vessels via action on ATP-sensitive potassium channels and possesses a nitrate moiety that promotes systemic venous and coronary vasodilation.[141] As a result of these dual actions, nicorandil reduces preload and afterload and results in an increase in coronary blood flow. In addition to these effects, nicorandil may have cardioprotective actions mediated through the activation of potassium channels. Nicorandil has been associated with ulcerations of the gastrointestinal tract.[142]

Nicorandil has antianginal efficacy similar to those of beta blockers, nitrates, and calcium channel blockers. In a recent randomized clinical trial ($N = 5126$), nicorandil reduced the risk of cardiac death, MI, or hospital admission for angina (hazard ratio, 0.83; $P = 0.014$) compared with placebo when added to standard antianginal therapy.[143]

FASUDIL*. Fasudil is an orally available inhibitor of rho kinase, an intracellular signaling molecule that participates in vascular smooth muscle contraction. Fasudil was shown to increase the time to ischemia in a study of 84 patients with CAD undergoing exercise treadmill testing.[144]

METABOLIC AGENTS*. Agents aimed at increasing the metabolic efficiency of cardiac myocytes have also been studied in patients with chronic stable angina. Partial inhibitors of fatty acid oxidation appear to shift myocardial metabolism to more oxygen-efficient pathways. Trimetazidine and perhexiline are agents that have been shown to inhibit fatty acid metabolism and to reduce the frequency of angina without hemodynamic effects in patients with chronic stable angina.[145]

---

*Has not been approved by the U.S. Food and Drug Administration at the time of this writing.

OTHER CONSIDERATIONS OF MEDICAL MANAGEMENT OF ANGINA PECTORIS

Relative Advantages of Beta Blockers and Calcium Antagonists

The choice between a beta blocker and calcium channel antagonist as initial therapy in patients with chronic stable angina is controversial because both classes of agents are effective in relieving symptoms and reducing ischemia (**Table 57-10**).[80] Trials comparing beta blockers and calcium antagonists have not shown any difference in the rate of death or MI, although in some studies beta blockers appeared to have greater clinical efficacy and less frequent discontinuation because of side effects. Because long-term administration of beta blockers has been demonstrated to prolong life in patients after acute MI, it is reasonable to consider beta blockers over calcium antagonists as the agents of choice in treating patients with stable IHD. However, it must be recognized that beta blockers (without ISA) increase serum triglyceride levels and decrease HDL cholesterol levels, with uncertain long-term consequences. In addition, these drugs may produce fatigue, depression, and sexual dysfunction. In contrast, although calcium antagonists do not show these adverse effects, their long-term administration has not been shown to improve long-term survival after acute MI. However, diltiazem is apparently effective in preventing severe angina and early reinfarction after non–Q-wave MI. Verapamil reduces reinfarction rates in patients post-MI and, when combined with trandolapril, achieves similar outcomes to atenolol together with a diuretic for the treatment of patients with hypertension and CAD.

The choice of drug with which to initiate therapy is influenced by a number of clinical factors (see Table 57-10)[80]:

1. Calcium antagonists are the preferred agents in patients with a history of asthma or chronic obstructive lung disease with wheezing on clinical examination, in whom beta blockers, even relatively selective agents, are contraindicated. Consideration to a trial of beta blockers should be given if the patient has a history of prior MI.

2. Nifedipine (long-acting), amlodipine, and nicardipine are the calcium antagonists of choice in patients with chronic stable angina and sick sinus syndrome, sinus bradycardia, or significant AV conduction disturbances, whereas beta blockers and verapamil should be used only with great caution in such patients. In patients with symptomatic conduction disease, neither a beta blocker nor a calcium channel blocker should be used unless a pacemaker is in place. If a beta blocker is required in patients with asymptomatic evidence of conduction disease, pindolol, which has the greatest ISA, is useful. In the case of calcium channel blockers in patients with conduction system disease a dihydropyridine is preferable to verapamil and diltiazem, but careful observation for deterioration of conduction is mandatory.

3. Calcium antagonists are clearly preferred for patients with suspected Prinzmetal (variant) angina (see Chap. 56); beta blockers may even aggravate angina under these circumstances.

4. Calcium antagonists may be preferred over beta blockers in patients with significant, symptomatic peripheral arterial disease because the latter may cause peripheral vasoconstriction.

5. Beta blockers should usually be avoided in patients with a history of significant depressive illness and should be prescribed cautiously for patients with sexual dysfunction, sleep disturbance, nightmares, fatigue, or lethargy.

6. The presence of moderate to severe LV dysfunction in patients with angina limits the therapeutic options. The beneficial effects of beta blockers on survival in patients with LV dysfunction after MI, coupled with their beneficial effects on survival and LV performance in patients with heart failure,[121] have established beta blockers as the drug class of choice for the treatment of angina in patients with LV dysfunction, with or without symptoms of heart failure, together with ACE inhibitors, diuretics, and digitalis. If a beta blocker is not tolerated or angina persists despite beta blockade and nitrates, amlodipine can be administered. Ranolazine is also an option for such patients. Verapamil, nifedipine, and diltiazem should be avoided.

7. Short-acting nifedipine should not be used because the reflex-mediated tachycardia may aggravate ischemia.

8. Hypertensive patients with angina pectoris do well with beta blockers or calcium antagonists because both agents have antihypertensive effects. However, beta blockers are the preferred initial agent for treating angina in such patients, as noted earlier, and an ACE inhibitor should be strongly considered for all patients with CAD with hypertension.

Combination Therapy

The combination of multiple agents is widely used in the management of chronic stable angina with options that include a beta blocker, calcium antagonist, long-acting nitrate, or newer agents such as ranolazine, which may be particularly useful when heart rate, blood pressure, or LV dysfunction limit escalation or initiation of other therapy. When adrenergic blockers and calcium antagonists are used together in the treatment of angina pectoris, several issues should be considered:

1. The addition of a beta blocker enhances the clinical effect of nifedipine and other dihydropyridines.

2. In patients with moderate or severe LV dysfunction, sinus bradycardia, or AV conduction disturbances, combination therapy with calcium antagonists and beta blockers should be avoided or initiated with caution. In patients with AV conduction system disease, the preferred combination is a long-acting dihydropyridine and a beta blocker. The negative inotropic effects of calcium antagonists are not usually a problem in combined therapy with low doses of beta blockers but can become significant with higher doses. With such doses, amlodipine is the calcium antagonist of choice, but it should be used cautiously. Ranolazine may be useful for patients who do not tolerate the combination of a beta blocker and calcium channel antagonist.

3. The combination of a dihydropyridine and a long-acting nitrate (without a beta blocker) is not an optimal combination because both are vasodilators.

APPROACH TO PATIENTS WITH CHRONIC STABLE ANGINA.
This approach is as follows:

1. Identify and treat precipitating factors such as anemia, uncontrolled hypertension, thyrotoxicosis, tachyarrhythmias, uncontrolled heart failure, and concomitant valvular heart disease.

TABLE 57-10	Recommended Use of Beta Blockers or Calcium Antagonists for Patients Who Have Angina in Conjunction with Other Medical Conditions
CLINICAL CONDITION	**RECOMMENDED DRUG***
Cardiac Arrhythmia or Conduction Disturbance	
Sinus bradycardia	Nifedipine, amlodipine
Sinus tachycardia (not caused by cardiac failure)	Beta blocker
Supraventricular tachycardia	Beta blocker (verapamil)
Atrioventricular block	Nifedipine or amlodipine
Rapid atrial fibrillation	Verapamil or beta blocker
Ventricular arrhythmia	Beta blocker
Left Ventricular Dysfunction	
Heart failure	Beta blocker
Miscellaneous Medical Conditions	
Systemic hypertension	Beta blocker (calcium antagonist)
Severe preexisting headaches	Beta blocker (verapamil or diltiazem)
COPD with bronchospasm or asthma	Nifedipine, amlodipine, verapamil, or diltiazem
Hyperthyroidism	Beta blocker
Raynaud syndrome	Nifedipine or amlodipine
Claudication	Calcium antagonist
Severe depression	Calcium antagonist

*Alternatives in parentheses.
COPD = chronic obstructive pulmonary disease.

2. Initiate risk factor modification, physical exercise, diet, and lifestyle counseling. Initiate therapy with a statin, as needed, to reduce the LDL cholesterol level to at least below 100 mg/dL.

3. Initiate pharmacotherapy with aspirin and a beta blocker. Initiate an ACE inhibitor in all patients with an LV ejection fraction of 40% or lower and in those with hypertension, diabetes, or chronic kidney disease. In addition, an ACE inhibitor should be considered for all other patients.

4. Use sublingual nitroglycerin for alleviation of symptoms and for prophylaxis.

5. If angina persists, the next step is usually the addition of a calcium antagonist or long-acting nitrate via dosing schedules to prevent nitrate tolerance. The decision to add a calcium antagonist or long-acting nitrate is not based entirely on the frequency and severity of symptoms. The need to treat concomitant hypertension or the presence of LV dysfunction and symptoms of heart failure may be an indication for the use of one of these agents, even in patients in whom episodes of symptomatic angina are infrequent.

6. If angina persists despite two antianginal agents (a beta blocker with a long-acting nitrate preparation or calcium antagonist), add a third antianginal agent. The selection of the agent will be guided by potential side effects and the presence or absence of concomitant hypertension, relative hypotension, conduction system disease, tachyarrhythmias, or LV dysfunction.

7. Coronary angiography, with a view to considering coronary revascularization, is indicated for patients with refractory symptoms or ischemia despite optimal medical therapy. It should also be carried out in patients with high-risk noninvasive test results (see Table 57-3) and in those with occupations or lifestyles that require a more aggressive approach.

OTHER THERAPIES

SPINAL CORD STIMULATION. An option for patients with refractory angina who are not candidates for coronary revascularization is spinal cord stimulation using a specially designed electrode inserted into the epidural space.[146] The beneficial effects of neuromodulation on pain via this technique are based on the gate theory, in which stimulation of axons in the spinal cord that do not transmit pain to the brain will reduce input to the brain from axons that do transmit pain. Irrespective of the mechanism, several observational studies have reported success rates of up to 80% in terms of reducing the frequency and severity of angina. One small, randomized, sham-controlled study has demonstrated an improvement in symptoms and functional status.[147] What is less easily explained is an apparent anti-ischemic effect of this technique. In a small randomized trial in patients with angina and CAD not amenable to PCI, spinal cord stimulation was associated with similar symptom relief and long-term quality of life compared with CABG. This approach should be reserved for patients in whom all other treatment options have been exhausted.

ENHANCED EXTERNAL COUNTERPULSATION. The use of enhanced external counterpulsation (EECP) is another alternative treatment of refractory angina.[148] EECP is generally administered as 35 1-hour treatments over 7 weeks. Observational data have suggested that EECP reduces the frequency of angina and the use of nitroglycerin and improves exercise tolerance and quality of life, and that the responses can last for up to 2 years.[149] In a randomized, double-blind, sham-controlled study of EECP for patients with chronic stable angina, active counterpulsation was associated with an increase in time to ST-segment depression during exercise testing and a reduction in angina, as well as an improvement in health-related quality of life that extended to at least 1 year. There are no definitive data that EECP reduces the extent of ischemia determined by myocardial perfusion imaging.

The mechanisms underlying the effects of EECP are poorly understood. Possible mechanisms include the following: (1) durable hemodynamic changes that reduce myocardial O_2 demand; (2) improvement in myocardial perfusion caused by the ability of increased transmyocardial pressure to open collaterals; and (3) the elaboration of various substances that improve endothelial function and vascular remodeling caused by augmented flow through the arterial vascular bed.[148,150] Finally, the possibility of placebo effects should be recognized; most of the evidence demonstrating favorable effects of EECP is from uncontrolled studies, and data from sham-controlled studies are few.

CHELATION. Randomized trials have shown no benefit, and these agents may be harmful.

Revascularization of Coronary Artery Disease
(see Chap. 58)

APPROACH TO DECISIONS REGARDING REVASCULARIZATION. IHD manifests as a continuum of disease with a variable natural history that may, over decades, encompass many phases of clinical expression, ranging from asymptomatic periods, the development of chronic exertional angina, subsequent quiescent periods, progression to accelerating angina, and culmination in unstable angina or acute MI (see Chaps. 54 and 56). Therefore, the approach to treatment should be tailored to the individual's clinical status. Moreover, atherosclerosis is typically a diffuse or multifocal process in which non–flow-limiting coronary stenoses are the principal progenitors of most "hard" clinical events[76] and require a comprehensive systemic approach to management. In general, the principles guiding patient management are predicated on addressing two simultaneous goals, if possible: (1) use of disease-modifying therapies or approaches to prolong life and reduce major cardiovascular events such as acute MI, hospitalization for ACS, or heart failure; (2) optimization of the patient's health status, quality of life, and functional capacity such that angina or ischemia do not adversely affect the activities of daily living.[80]

It is widely accepted that the benefits of revascularization are proportional to the patient's underlying risk, which makes it essential to quantify the patient's prognosis as accurately as possible (see Table 57-3). In addition to the patient's risk for major cardiovascular events, sociodemographic factors, such as age, physical capacity, and ability to adhere to prescribed treatments and lifestyle interventions, overall quality of life, other medical conditions, and patient preferences should be considered. Each of these aspects should be integrated in considering how best to achieve these two fundamental goals of therapy for patients with stable IHD. Revascularization approaches are an integral component of an overall management strategy to improve outcomes and are used when needed in addition to optimal medical therapy. The success of catheter-based or surgical treatment is predicated on the overall success of guideline-directed secondary prevention and lifestyle intervention as a platform for management of all patients with stable IHD.

PATIENT SELECTION. Each of the following considerations may be used to guide decisions regarding the indications for and approach to revascularization: (1) presence and severity of symptoms; (2) physiologic significance of coronary lesions and other anatomic considerations; (3) extent of myocardial ischemia and the presence of LV dysfunction; and (4) other medical conditions that influence the risks of percutaneous or surgical revascularization.

Presence and Severity of Symptoms

A goal of therapy is the complete elimination of angina and resumption of full physical function to the greatest extent possible.[80] Mechanical revascularization (surgical or catheter-based) should be considered if ischemic symptoms persist after intensification of medical therapy, including stringent risk factor modification, or if unacceptable side effects limit antianginal therapy.

Significance of Coronary Lesions and Other Anatomic Considerations

The presence of a 70% or greater stenosis of an epicardial coronary artery is considered to be significant (50% or greater for left main coronary stenosis). Thus, professional guidelines that have informed clinical practice regarding revascularization have been framed principally around these anatomic criteria (number of diseased vessels, extent and severity of anatomic disease), integrating functional considerations (magnitude and distribution of ischemia, and amount of threatened myocardium subtending coronary stenosis).[80,151] However, clinicians also quite often face clinical uncertainty regarding the potential significance of borderline visual coronary stenoses, nominally defined as those lesions in the 50% to 70% range.[152] It is widely acknowledged that angiographic stenosis severity (as a percentage) is often an inaccurate measure of a lesion's functional significance.[45] Whereas cardiac surgeons have used a 50% or greater stenosis as the criterion for significant,[153] many factors other than visual stenosis severity (e.g., lesion eccentricity, tortuousity, presence of plaque rupture or asymmetric luminal filling defects, presence of additional serial lesions) can potentially render a 50% to 70% stenosis functionally or hemodynamically significant. In a study of 325 patients with intermediate stenosis scheduled for PCI, patients with a fractional flow reserve (FFR) more than 0.75 (56%) were randomized to PCI or medical therapy. Patients managed medically had a risk of cardiac death or MI of less than 1%/year that was not increased compared with the group that was stented.[154] Optimally stress testing can be used to determine whether a borderline visual coronary stenosis subtends a segment (or segments) of ischemic myocardium. However, an invasive physiologic tool such as FFR (see Chap. 52) can be used to guide appropriate decisions regarding revascularization of the intermediate stenosis. Judgments regarding the need for revascularization should incorporate angiographic (anatomic) and physiologic (functional) data, including that obtained by intravascular ultrasonography (see Chap. 22).

Other anatomic features, in addition to lesion severity, influence the approach to revascularization for a given patient. These features include vessel size, extent of calcification, tortuosity, and relationships to side branches (see Chap. 58). Each of these characteristics may influence the likelihood of successful catheter-based or, in some cases, surgical revascularization. For example, a patient with single-vessel CAD with a long, complex, and calcified bifurcation lesion of the proximal LAD artery and first diagonal branch may in some cases be a candidate for surgical revascularization. Patients with diffuse severe disease of the distal coronary arteries may be poor candidates for any revascularization procedure.

Extent of Ischemia and Presence of Left Ventricular Dysfunction

The four major determinants of risk in CAD are the extent of ischemia, number of vessels diseased, LV function, and electrical substrate. The extent of ischemia on noninvasive testing is an important predictor for subsequent adverse outcomes and identifies patients for whom revascularization may provide clinical benefit compared with medical therapy beyond the relief of symptoms (**Fig. 57-10**).[155,156] The major effect of coronary revascularization is on ischemia, and the magnitude of the benefit compared with that of medical therapy is enhanced with LV dysfunction, particularly in the presence of reversibly ischemic jeopardized myocardium. Moreover, the greatest survival benefits of CABG, as well as symptomatic and functional improvements, are evident in patients with impaired LV function (generally defined as an ejection fraction of less than 40%; **Tables 57-11** and **57-12**).

Risks of the Procedure

Patients with stable IHD more often than not have other medical conditions, such as renal dysfunction, peripheral atherosclerosis, or pulmonary disease, which may influence the patient's suitability for surgical or percutaneous revascularization. For example, in a patient with peptic ulcer disease and history of GI bleeding, the potential need for long-term dual antiplatelet therapy after a procedure should be

considered. Moreover, a patient with three-vessel CAD and impaired LV function who might derive a more durable survival benefit from CABG may be too high risk clinically to undergo surgery and might be a better candidate for multivessel PCI.

In addition, some general principles regarding the choice of treatment in patients with stable IHD should be considered:

1. For most patients with chronic angina, revascularization should not constitute the initial management strategy before evidence-based medical therapy (e.g., pharmacologic antianginal therapy, disease-modifying treatments, therapeutic lifestyle intervention) is initiated and optimized.
2. When improvement in survival is not a relevant consideration, the severity of angina or impairment in health status should play a significant role in determining whether revascularization is appropriate (i.e., limiting angina on optimal medical therapy is a more compelling indication than episodic exertional angina on minimal medical therapy).
3. The patient's treatment preferences and sociodemographic and/or clinical circumstances should always be a consideration in choosing which treatment strategy to use.

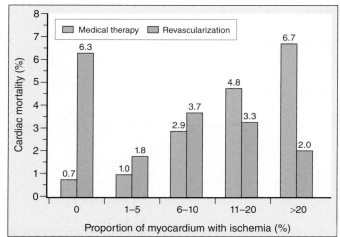

FIGURE 57-10 Rate of cardiac death in patients treated with medical therapy versus revascularization, stratified by the proportion of ischemic myocardium on stress nuclear imaging. A total of 10,627 consecutive patients without prior MI or revascularization were followed for a mean of 1.6 years after exercise or adenosine myocardial perfusion imaging. Patients with moderate to severe ischemia who underwent percutaneous or surgical coronary revascularization within 60 days of stress imaging had lower mortality than those treated with medical therapy (P < 0.0001). However, those patients with no or mild ischemia had no survival advantage with revascularization. *(From Hachamovitch R, Hayes SW, Friedman JD, et al: Comparison of the short-term survival benefit associated with revascularization compared with medical therapy in patients with no prior coronary artery disease undergoing stress myocardial perfusion single photon emission computed tomography. Circulation 107:2900, 2003.)*

TABLE 57-11	Impact of Coronary Bypass Surgery on Survival*			
CATEGORY OF RISK	**NUMBER OF DISEASED VESSELS**	**SEVERITY OF ISCHEMIA**	**EJECTION FRACTION**	**RESULTS OF SURGERY ON SURVIVAL**
Mild	2	Mild	>0.50	Unchanged[†]
	3	Mild	>0.50	Unchanged[†]
Moderate	2	Moderate to severe	>0.50	Unchanged[†]
	3	Moderate to severe	>0.50	Improved[†]
	2	Mild	<0.50	Unchanged[†]
	3	Mild	<0.50	Improved[‡]
Severe	2	Moderate to severe	<0.50	Improved[‡]
	3	Moderate to severe	<0.50	Improved[‡]

*In subsets of patients studied in the CASS randomized trial and registry studies.
†Randomized trial.
‡Survival improved with surgery versus medicine. In the European Coronary Surgery Trial, patients with double-vessel disease and involvement of the proximal left anterior descending coronary artery had improved survival with surgery, irrespective of left ventricular function.

TABLE 57-12	Effects of Coronary Artery Bypass Grafting on Survival*	
SUBGROUP	**MEDICAL TREATMENT MORTALITY RATE (%)**	**P VALUE FOR CABG VERSUS MEDICAL TREATMENT**
Vessel Disease		
One vessel	9.9	0.18
Two vessels	11.7	0.45
Three vessels	17.6	<0.001
Left main artery	36.5	0.004
No LAD Disease		
One or two vessels	8.3	0.88
Three vessels	14.5	0.02
Left main artery	45.8	0.03
Overall	12.3	0.05
LAD Disease Present		
One or two vessels	14.6	0.05
Three vessels	19.1	0.009
Left main artery	32.7	0.02
Overall	18.3	0.001
LV Function		
Normal	13.3	<0.001
Abnormal	25.2	0.02
Exercise Test Status		
Missing	17.4	0.10
Normal	11.6	0.38
Abnormal	16.8	<0.001
Severity of Angina		
Class 0, I, II	12.5	0.005
Class III, IV	22.4	0.001

*Systematic overview of the effect of CABG versus medical therapy on survival based on data from seven randomized trials comparing a strategy of initial CABG with one of initial medical therapy. Subgroup results at 5 years are shown.
From Yusuf S, Zucker D, Peduzzi P, et al: Effect of coronary artery bypass surgery on survival: Overview of 10-year results from randomized trials by the Coronary Artery Bypass Surgery Trialists Collaboration. Lancet 344:563, 1994.

4. In certain clinical circumstances, it may be difficult to ascertain reliably whether anginal symptoms or anginal equivalents such as exertional dyspnea or fatigue are a direct manifestation of underlying CAD, especially in patients with significant obesity, those who are sedentary, or those who may have coexisting chronic obstructive pulmonary disease. In such settings, symptoms that are atypical or nondiagnostic for obstructive CAD may not necessarily improve with revascularization, even when such symptoms coexist with physiologically significant coronary disease.

5. The decision to proceed with myocardial revascularization must be individualized according to the specific clinical features and personal preferences of a given patient, often in collaboration with family members and the patient's referring physician, with informed discussion about the potential risks and benefits of all three therapeutic options.

Percutaneous Coronary Intervention

PCI, which includes percutaneous transluminal coronary angioplasty (PTCA), stenting, and related techniques, has continued to evolve significantly over the past three decades (see Chap. 58).[157] PTCA has been largely replaced since the advent of bare metal stents (BMS) in the mid-1990s, with continued evolution over the past 15 years, particularly with the introduction of drug-eluting stents (DES) in 2003. First-generation DES have subsequently been modified through evolutionary design to include thinner struts and improved drug-eluting platforms and delivery systems to minimize restenosis and acute and subacute stent thrombosis. Moreover, the practice of interventional cardiology has changed radically with increased operator experience, improved adjunctive pharmacotherapy, and advances in technology other than stenting, such as distal protection devices and devices directed at specific technical issues (e.g., thrombectomy and atherectomy catheters). As such, PCI is an important treatment modality for patients with stable IHD, particularly those patients with chronic angina who remain symptomatic despite medial therapy.

OUTCOMES

Early Outcome

Continued improvement in the technical aspects of PCI (predominantly coronary stenting), as well as increasing operator experience, has had a favorable impact on the rate of primary success and the rate of reductions in complications.[158] Among the many desirable features of PCI is the fact that it can be performed during the same clinical encounter as the diagnostic angiography. Stable patients can often be discharged on the same or next day and clinical recovery is usually complete within a week or less. In many cases, symptomatic relief can be immediate and dramatic. Such attributes may motivate some patients to elect to undergo PCI, even when optimal medical therapy alone may lower overall risk with equivalent long-term outcomes. A recent examination of data on over 2.6 million patients undergoing PCI between 2005 and 2007 at 968 U.S. sites in the American College of Cardiology National Cardiovascular Data Registry (ACC-NCDR) revealed that among elective PCIs, 58% were performed in patients with stable IHD, of whom 35% had diabetes mellitus.[159] The ACC-NCDR reported an angiographic success rate of 96% and a procedural success rate (angiographic success without death, heart attack, or emergency revascularization) of 93% in patients undergoing PCI. The incidence of death prior to hospital discharge was less than 1% and emergency CABG was required in 0.3% of patients. The ACC-NCDR reported a periprocedural MI rate of 1%, but studies using routine assessments of cardiac biomarkers reported higher rates, although the significance of these periprocedural biomarker increases has been debated.[160,161] Finally, the rate of restenosis with DES is reported to be less than 10%, with a corresponding approximately 20% decrease in the need for repeat revascularization procedures compared with the era of BMS.[162] Outcomes in specific challenging subgroups of patients, such as those with chronic total occlusions or left main coronary stenosis, are discussed in Chap. 58.

Long-Term Outcome

Long-term outcome after PCI is well characterized, with LV function, extent of coronary disease, diabetes, renal function, and the patient's age being the major determinants of mortality risk, and restenosis at the site of intervention being a major contributor to recurrent ischemia and the need for subsequent procedures. The introduction of BMS and DES has dramatically reduced the incidence of restenosis compared with balloon angioplasty. The evolution of stent technology, comparisons of long-term outcomes, and decision-making regarding device selection are discussed in Chap. 58.

Restenosis and Late Stent Thrombosis

(See Chap. 58.)

COMPARISONS BETWEEN PERCUTANEOUS CORONARY INTERVENTION AND MEDICAL THERAPY. Studies comparing balloon angioplasty with medical therapy are of uncertain clinical relevance today because both PCI and medical treatments have undergone profound changes over the last one or two decades. Moreover, randomized clinical trials comparing PCI with medical therapy are few in number and have involved less than 5000 patients (in total). Most have enrolled patients with predominantly single-vessel disease and were completed prior to the routine use of coronary stenting and enhanced adjunctive pharmacotherapy. In aggregate, the results of these 11 trials have supported superior control of angina, improved exercise capacity, and improved quality of life in patients treated with angioplasty compared with medical therapy (**Fig. 57-11**).[163] In 1997, the second Randomized Intervention Treatment of Angina (RITA-2) investigators reported that balloon angioplasty improved angina compared with medical therapy, although this was followed by a higher incidence of ischemic events (combined death and MI) as compared

1237

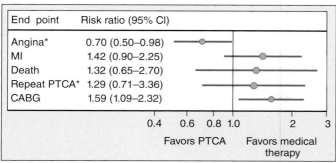

FIGURE 57-11 Relative risk of recurrent cardiac events with PTCA versus medical therapy from a meta-analysis of six randomized trials (*N* = 1904). Compared with medical therapy, angioplasty reduced the relative risk of recurrent angina by 30%. Randomized trials have not included sufficient numbers of patients for informative estimates of the effect of angioplasty on MI, death, or subsequent revascularization; however, trends in the available data do not favor angioplasty. These trials do not reflect the widespread use of coronary stenting. *Test for heterogeneity, *P* < 0.0001. (*From Bucher HC, Hengstler P, Schindler C, et al: Percutaneous transluminal coronary angioplasty versus medical therapy for treatment of non-acute coronary heart disease: A meta-analysis of randomised controlled trials. BMJ 321:73, 2000.*)

with medical therapy, which consisted principally of aspirin, beta blockers, and anti-ischemic therapy. The authors observed an excess of death and periprocedural MI with angioplasty compared with medical therapy (6.3 versus 3.3%; *P* < 0.02). After 7 years, there was no difference in the composite of death or MI, whereas the initial improvement in angina and exercise times with balloon angioplasty versus medical therapy narrowed, mainly because one third of medical patients eventually required PCI because of severe angina.

Meta-analyses of trials of routine stenting compared with balloon angioplasty have not demonstrated differences in the incidence of death, MI, or emergency CABG. In an analysis of 23 trials of 10,347 patients, bare metal stenting compared with balloon angioplasty produced similar rates of mortality (odds ratio, 0.92; *P* = 0.60), and similar rates of a combined endpoint of death or MI (odds ratio, 0.86; *P* = 0.2).[164] However, stenting led to significantly fewer major adverse cardiac events (odds ratio, 0.59; *P* < 0.001), driven exclusively by reduced revascularization. Brophy and coworkers[164a] have analyzed 27 trials with 9918 patients and found that stenting compared with balloon angioplasty produces similar mortality (odds ratio, 0.65; *P* = NS), death or MI (odds ratio, 0.90; P = not significant [NS]), and need for subsequent CABG surgery (odds ratio, 1.01; *P* = NS), but less frequent restenosis (odds ratio, 0.52; 95% CI, 0.37 to 0.69). The Medicine, Angioplasty, or Surgery Study (MASS) II study enrolled 651 patients between 1995 and 2000 who were randomized to PCI, CABG, or medical therapy. After 5 years, patients who had undergone PCI were more likely to be free of angina than were medical therapy patients (77% versus 55%; *P* < 0.001), but equally likely to have experienced death, MI, or revascularization for refractory angina and to have undergone subsequent elective revascularization procedures.[165] Currently, no randomized trial or meta-analysis to date has demonstrated a reduction in death or MI with PCI compared with medical therapy for patients with chronic stable angina, although all these comparative studies, by design, assessed PCI in apposition to, not in combination with, medical therapy; no study incorporated guideline-driven disease-modifying medical therapies such as statins or inhibitors of the renin-angiotensin system.

Between 1999 and 2004, the Clinical Outcomes Utilization Revascularization and Aggressive DruG Evaluation (COURAGE) Trial Research Group randomized 2287 patients with objective evidence of ischemia and proximal angiographic CAD (70% visual stenosis) to optimal medical therapy (OMT) with or without PCI.[166] Importantly, the aim and design of COURAGE was to test a strategy of routine, anatomically driven PCI plus OMT versus a strategy of selective, ischemia-driven PCI, if needed, for a failure of initial OMT. Follow-up from 2.5 to 7 years (median, 4.6 years) demonstrated that the combination of death or MI occurred with similar frequency in both arms. The 4.6-year cumulative

primary event rates were 19.0% and 18.5% in the PCI + OMT and OMT groups, respectively (hazard ratio [HR] in the PCI + OMT group compared with the OMT group, 1.05; 95% CI, 0.87 to 1.27; *P* = 0.62; **Fig. 57-12**). Comparing PCI and medical therapy groups, there were no differences in death, MI, or stroke (20.0% versus 19.5%; HR, 1.05; 95% CI, 0.87 to 1.27; *P* = 0.62); hospitalization for ACS (12.4% versus 11.8%; HR, 1.07; 95% CI, 0.84 to 1.37; *P* = 0.56); or MI (13.2% versus 12.3%; HR, 1.13; 95% CI, 0.89 to 1.43; *P* = 0.33). Thus, the main study findings indicated that as an initial management strategy in patients with stable CAD, PCI does not reduce death, MI, or other major cardiovascular events when added to OMT. Patients initially treated with PCI had less angina at 1 and 3 years, but not at 5 years, compared with patients initially treated without PCI. As expected, patients who received initial OMT had more frequent subsequent PCIs compared with patients initially treated with PCI, although only 16.5% of OMT patients required revascularization during the first year of follow-up; the remaining 16.5% of patients crossed over to revascularization between year 1 and 7. Subgroup analyses of COURAGE have suggested that there is no difference in the combined endpoint of death and MI in patients with multivessel CAD (compared with those who had single-vessel disease), low ejection fraction (compared with those with ejection fraction > 50%), Class II or III angina (compared with those with Class 0 or I angina), or diabetes (compared with no diabetes; see Fig. 57-12).[166]

Review of the baseline characteristics from COURAGE[167] has revealed that the population was not low risk—34% were diabetic, 71% were dyslipidemic, 67% were hypertensive, 29% were current smokers, 39% had prior MI, and 26% had undergone previous revascularization. Most patients (58%) were in CCS Class II or III and 30% were in Class I (12% had asymptomatic myocardial ischemia); the average number of anginal episodes was six/week, whereas the median was three/week. A total of 95% of patients had ischemia testing and, of those who underwent myocardial perfusion scintigraphy, two thirds had multiple reversible perfusion defects and the remaining third had a single reversible perfusion defect. Almost 70% of patients had multivessel CAD (70% diameter stenosis estimated visually), and LAD coronary disease was common (68%), being significantly more prevalent in the OMT group (37%) than in the PCI group (31%). In the aggregate, these findings indicate that the enrolled patients were highly symptomatic at baseline, had appreciable clinical comorbidity, high prevalence of objective evidence of myocardial ischemia, and extensive angiographic CAD, and thus fall into the population in which a clinical benefit of PCI is expected.[166]

A separately published substudy from COURAGE has demonstrated that patients randomized to receive PCI in addition to OMT had greater reduction in high-grade ischemia on stress nuclear imaging compared with patients who received OMT alone, although such findings were observed in only 20% of the 314 patients in this subgroup.[168] Thus, data support the premise that severe ischemia may identify an important subset of patients with stable IHD who might derive clinical benefit from PCI, but prospective studies in a larger cohort of such patients will be required to evaluate this possibility.

In summary, based on the best available data from randomized trials, it appears reasonable to pursue a strategy of initial medical therapy for most patients with stable IHD and CCS class I or II symptoms and to reserve revascularization for those with persistent and/or more severe symptoms, despite optimal medical therapy, or those with high-risk criteria on noninvasive testing, such as inducible ischemia involving a moderate or large territory of myocardium.[80] The results from the COURAGE trial also underscore the favorable impact that intensive medical therapy and lifestyle interventions have on mitigating clinical events in patients treated with and without PCI. OMT as an initial management strategy in patients with stable IHD is safe and effective.

PATIENT SELECTION. In addition to general considerations regarding the indications and approach to revascularization (see "Approach to Decisions Regarding Revascularization"), additional factors that need to be weighed in patient selection for PCI include the following:

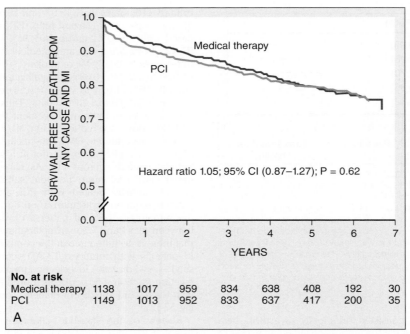

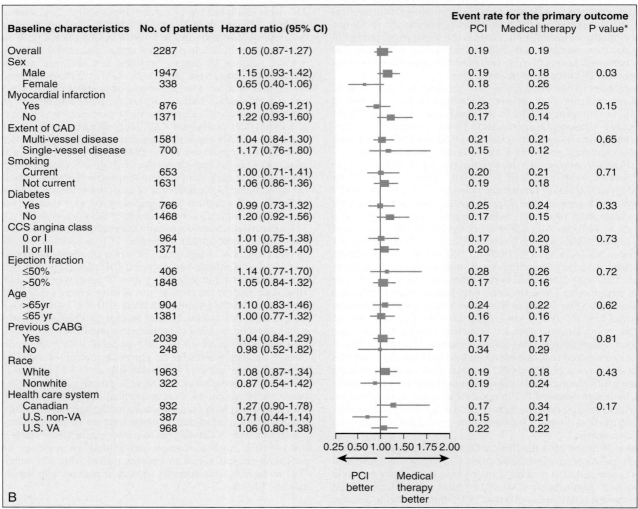

FIGURE 57-12 Outcome in 2287 patients with objective evidence of myocardial ischemia and significant coronary artery disease enrolled in the COURAGE trial and randomized to PCI and optimal medical therapy or optimal medical therapy alone (Medical therapy). **A,** No difference in the primary endpoint of death from any cause or MI was observed between the two treatment groups. **B,** The finding of no difference between the two treatment groups was consistent across multiple subgroups, including patients with multivessel disease, diabetes, severe angina, and prior revascularization. *Interaction p-value. *(From Boden WE, O'Rourke RA, Teo KK, et al: Optimal medical therapy with or without PCI for stable coronary disease. N Engl J Med 356:1503, 2007.)*

1. The likelihood of successful catheter-based revascularization based on the angiographic characteristics of the lesion
2. The risk and potential consequences of acute failure of PCI, which are a function, in part, of the coronary artery anatomy (multivessel and/or diffuse disease), percentage of viable myocardium at risk, presence of heart failure, and underlying LV function
3. The likelihood of restenosis, which has been associated with clinical (e.g., diabetes, prior restenosis) and angiographic factors (e.g., small vessel diameter, long lesion length, total occlusion, saphenous vein graft disease; see Chap. 58)
4. The need for complete revascularization based on the extent of CAD, volume of myocardium, and severity of ischemia in the distribution of the artery(ies) amenable to PCI

PERCUTANEOUS CORONARY INTERVENTION IN SUBGROUPS OF PATIENTS WITH STABLE ISCHEMIC HEART DISEASE

DIABETES MELLITUS. Patients with diabetes are at substantially higher risk for complications after PCI (see Chap. 64). Possible explanations for the higher rate of adverse outcomes include an altered vascular biologic response in diabetic patients to balloon injury and rapid progression of disease in nondilated segments. The diabetic atherosclerotic milieu is characterized by a procoagulant state, decreased fibrinolytic activity, increased proliferation, and inflammation. Restenosis is more frequent in diabetic patients, as is disease progression. For this reason, CABG, which bypasses most of the vessel instead of a specific lesion, may offer a better intermediate- to long-term outcome.[169] The optimal strategy for revascularization in patients with diabetes is discussed later in this chapter. A strategy of initial optimal medical therapy appears reasonable for most patients with diabetes with stable IHD.[170]

LEFT VENTRICULAR DYSFUNCTION. Despite advances in interventional cardiology, LV dysfunction remains independently associated with higher in-hospital and long-term mortality after PCI. Specifically, in patients with stable CAD and estimated ejection fractions of 40% or less, 41 to 49, and 50% or higher in the National Heart, Lung, and Blood Institute (NHLBI) Dynamic Registry, mortality at 1 year after PCI was 11.0, 4.5, and 1.9%, respectively. Contemporary trials of PCI versus medical therapy have included too few patients with impaired LV function to guide therapeutic decision-making in this important subset of patients.

WOMEN AND OLDER PATIENTS. Specific issues related to PCI in women and older adults are discussed in Chaps. 80 and 81.

PREVIOUS CORONARY BYPASS GRAFTING. CABG and PCI are often considered competitive procedures, but it is more appropriate to view them as complementary. An increasing number of patients who have had CABG and later have recurrent ischemia undergo revascularization with PCI. Technical aspects and procedural outcomes of PCI in venous bypass grafts are discussed in Chap. 58.

Coronary Artery Bypass Grafting

In 1964, Garrett and colleagues first used CABG as a "bailout" procedure. Widespread use of the technique by Favoloro and Johnson and their respective collaborators followed in the late 1960s. Use of the internal mammary artery (IMA) graft was pioneered by Kolessov in 1967 and by Green and associates in 1970. Since then, CABG has evolved progressively over the past four decades, and today remains an important treatment modality for many patients with stable IHD. Most bypass operations continue to be performed through a median sternotomy, using cardiopulmonary bypass (CPB) and cardioplegic myocardial arrest or without bypass on a beating heart. Less invasive approaches have become increasingly commonplace in select patients who may be appropriate candidates for more limited coronary revascularization, and include anterior and lateral thoracotomies, partial sternotomies, and epigastric incisions.[171] The technical goal of bypass surgery is to obtain, whenever possible, complete revascularization by grafting all coronary arteries of sufficient caliber that have physiologically significant proximal stenoses. CABG has been documented to prolong survival, relieve angina, and improve quality of life in specific subgroups of patients with CAD.[172]

The annual number of CABG operations in the United States rose steadily over its first three decades, peaking in the late 1990s. Since then, however, rates of CABG have steadily declined, which likely relates to the sustained growth of the use of PCI, particularly in patients with multivessel CAD.[1] CABG provides excellent short- and intermediate-term results in the management of stable IHD; its long-term results are affected by failure of venous grafts. Long-term data with totally arterial surgical revascularization (i.e., using bilateral internal mammary artery [IMA] grafts) are few.

MINIMALLY INVASIVE CORONARY ARTERY BYPASS GRAFTING. Less invasive or minimally invasive approaches may be divided into four major categories based on the approach and use of CPB (see Chap. 84). Port access CABG is performed using limited incisions with femoral-femoral CPB and cardioplegic arrest. Port access technology has also now enabled totally endoscopic robotically assisted CABG (TECAB) to be performed on the arrested heart.[173] Off-pump CABG is performed using a standard median sternotomy, with generally small skin incisions, and stabilization devices to reduce motion of the target vessels while anastomoses are performed without CPB. Finally, minimally invasive direct coronary artery bypass (MIDCAB) is performed through a left anterior thoracotomy without CPB. Thus, off-pump approaches to CABG include off-pump CAB (OPCAB) and MIDCAB techniques (see Fig. 57-e2 on website).

The potential advantages of the minimally invasive approaches include reduced postoperative patient discomfort, minimized risk of wound infection, and shorter recovery times.[174] The avoidance of CPB may mitigate the risk of bleeding, systemic thromboembolism, renal insufficiency, myocardial stunning, stroke, and the damaging neurologic effects of CABG that could result in cognitive impairment, particularly in older patients and patients with heavily calcified aortas.[175] Amelioration of the systemic inflammatory response that occurs after CABG using CPB is viewed as an additional advantage that might affect these clinical outcomes. The learning curve of minimally invasive CABG has led to some reports of early graft failure. It should be emphasized that with conventional surgical techniques, the early patency rates of an IMA graft are excellent (98.7% in one large series).

Short-term clinical and angiographic outcomes have suggested that the less invasive techniques can be used to achieve results comparable to those of traditional CABG. However, in 2009, a comparative trial of OPCAB versus CABG using CPB in 2203 patients revealed that there was no difference in death or complications at 30 days (7.0% versus 5.6%, respectively; $P = 0.19$) but a significantly worse 1-year composite outcome of all-cause mortality, nonfatal MI, need for repeat revascularization in off-pump versus on-pump procedures (9.9% versus 7.4%, respectively; $P = 0.04$).[176] Additionally, in those patients undergoing follow-up angiography, there was a significantly lower graft patency rate in OPCAB recipients, and no treatment-based differences in neuropsychological outcomes or short-term resource use. Additional data regarding long-term graft patency and more prospective randomized trials of these two approaches will permit the comparative effectiveness of these two approaches on clinical outcomes to be assessed critically.

Novel approaches to coronary revascularization may also include CABG with PCI by combining a minimally invasive surgical CABG procedure on the LAD coronary artery (i.e., a left IMA implant to the proximal LAD artery using OPCAB) with PCI on the remaining vessels. Further experience with these so-called hybrid revascularization procedures is needed to clarify appropriate selection criteria further and to determine whether this strategy offers important advantages over multivessel CABG alone.[177]

OUTCOMES IN MINIMALLY INVASIVE CORONARY ARTERY BYPASS GRAFTING. Meta-analyses of observational and randomized trials of OPCAB versus CPB[178] have failed to demonstrate clear superiority of OPCAB over CPB with respect to mortality or major morbidity. Intraoperative conversion from OPCAB to CPB appears to be approximately 8%.[179] Early postoperative complications appear to be reduced with OPCAB, along with nonsignificant trends toward lower rates of death, MI, or stroke (see Chap. 84). Generally consistent findings across randomized and observational data sets have revealed comparable completeness of revascularization, reductions in blood loss and/or transfusion requirements, fewer wound infections, less postoperative atrial fibrillation, lower indices of myocardial injury, shorter duration of mechanical ventilation, and earlier hospital discharge with OPCAB. However, the largest randomized trial raises concern regarding possible long-term worse outcomes than with traditional CABG with CPB.[176]

ARTERIAL AND VENOUS CONDUITS. The current standard for bypass grafting advocates routine use of the left IMA for grafting the LAD artery, with supplemental saphenous vein grafts to other vessels. Although the benefits of a single IMA graft over a saphenous vein graft alone are not in dispute, the superiority of bilateral IMA grafts over a single IMA graft and one saphenous vein graft is less well accepted.[180] Initial enthusiasm for the use of bilateral IMA grafts was tempered by a higher rate of postoperative complications, including bleeding, wound infection, and prolonged ventilatory support.[181] Wound infection, most notably, deep sternal wound infection, has been of particular concern, but remains modest in frequency, <3%, except in patients who are obese or diabetic or those who require prolonged ventilatory support. Subsequent series have shown that bilateral versus single IMA grafting is associated with lower rates of recurrent angina pectoris, reoperation, and MI, improved survival in nonrandomized studies and, in some series, the risk of wound infection does not differ substantially from that with single IMA grafts. The increased technical demands and longer operative times of bilateral IMA grafting have also been a barrier to more widespread adoption but may be overcome if evidence supporting a survival advantage continues to accumulate.[182]

Patency of Venous and Arterial Grafts

Early occlusion (before hospital discharge) occurs in 8% to 12% of venous grafts and, by 1 year, 15% to 30% of vein grafts have become occluded. After the first year, the annual occlusion rate is 2% and rises to approximately 4% annually between years 6 and 10. Patency rates with IMA grafts are superior.

DISTAL VASCULATURE. The state of the distal coronary vasculature is important for the fate of bypass grafts. Late patency of grafts is related to coronary arterial runoff as determined by the diameter of the coronary artery into which the graft is inserted, size of the distal vascular bed, and severity of coronary atherosclerosis distal to the site of insertion of the graft. The highest graft patency rates are found when the lumina of the vessels distal to the graft insertion are larger than 1.5 mm in diameter, perfuse a large vascular bed, and are free of atheroma obstructing more than 25% of the vessel lumen. For saphenous veins, optimal patency rates are achieved with a lumen of 2.0 mm or larger.

PROGRESSION OF DISEASE IN NATIVE ARTERIES. The rate of disease progression appears highest in arterial segments already showing evidence of disease, and is between three and six times higher in grafted native coronary arteries than in nongrafted native vessels. These data have suggested that bypassing an artery with minimal disease, even if initially successful, may ultimately be harmful to patients, who incur both the risk of graft closure and the increased risk of accelerated obstruction of native vessels. Lesions in the native vessel that are long (more than 10 mm) and more than 70% in diameter are at increased risk of progressing to total occlusion.

EFFECTS OF THERAPY ON VEIN GRAFT OCCLUSION AND NATIVE VESSEL PROGRESSION. Measures aimed at enhancing long-term patency are generally directed at delaying the overall process of atherosclerosis, and thus may have several additional benefits. Secondary preventive therapy, in particular lipid-lowering treatment, is important to reducing the risk of failure of venous grafts. Chronic anticoagulant therapy has not been shown to alter outcomes convincingly. Other novel approaches, such as pretreatment of venous grafts to increase resistance to atherothrombosis, have not been definitively evaluated.

ANTIPLATELET THERAPY. Several trials have demonstrated the efficacy of aspirin therapy when started 1, 7, or 24 hours preoperatively, but the benefit is lost when aspirin is started more than 48 hours postoperatively. Aspirin, 80 to 325 mg daily, should be continued indefinitely. The addition of dipyridamole or warfarin in conventional doses has not been shown definitively to provide added benefit.[183] Although the effects of clopidogrel on graft patency have not been studied specifically, it is likely to be at least as effective as aspirin and is recommended for those who have an allergy to aspirin or who have had a recent ACS.[184]

LIPID-LOWERING THERAPY. Three randomized trials of lipid-lowering therapy have shown a favorable impact on the development of graft disease.[57] The rationale for lowering LDL cholesterol concentration to less than 100 mg/dL in patients with CAD was extended to postoperative patients in the Post-Coronary Artery Bypass Graft Trial.

PATIENT SELECTION. Indications for CABG are centered on the need for improvement in the quality and/or duration of life.[153] The

decision to perform revascularization with PCI or CABG is based largely on coronary anatomy, LV function, other medical comorbidities that may affect the patient's risk for either revascularization procedure, and patient preference (see "Approach to Decisions Regarding Revascularization" and "Choosing Among Percutaneous Coronary Intervention, Coronary Artery Bypass Grafting, and Medical Therapy").[169] CABG is indicated, regardless of symptoms, for patients with CAD in whom survival is likely to be prolonged and for patients with multivessel CAD in whom noninvasive testing suggests high risk (see Table 57-11). Patients with more extensive and severe CAD have an increasing magnitude of benefit from CABG over medical therapy (**Fig. 57-13**; see Fig. 57-10 and Table 57-12). Other factors that must

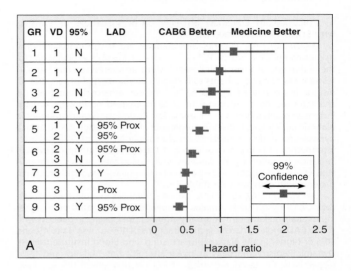

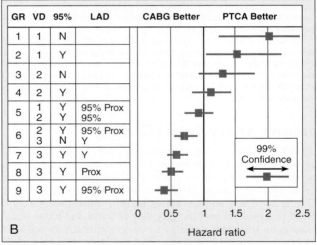

FIGURE 57-13 **A,** Adjusted hazard (mortality) ratios comparing CABG and medical therapy for nine coronary anatomy severity groups (GR) according to the number of vessels diseased (VD), presence or absence of a 95% proximal stenosis (95%), and involvement of the LAD artery. **B,** Adjusted hazard (mortality) ratios comparing CABG and PTCA for nine coronary anatomy groups according to the number of vessels diseased, presence or absence of a 95% proximal stenosis, and LAD artery involvement. In patients with the least severe categories of disease, 5-year survival appears to be better with PTCA (single-vessel disease without proximal stenosis and without LAD artery involvement), whereas for patients with triple-vessel disease and higher grade, more complex, double-vessel disease, a survival benefit is noted with surgery. For other subsets of patients with double-vessel disease, no difference in survival was seen in those treated with CABG or PTCA, and many of these patients are probably similar to those included in the randomized trials. *(Data from the Duke University data base; A and B, from Jones RH, Kesler K, Phillips HR III, et al: Long-term survival benefits of coronary artery bypass grafting and percutaneous transluminal angioplasty in patients with coronary artery disease. J Thorac Cardiovasc Surg 111:1013, 1996.)*

always be considered in the decision are general health and noncoronary comorbid conditions.

SURGICAL OUTCOMES AND LONG-TERM RESULTS. The patient population undergoing CABG has been changing over time, particularly with the wider use of PCI. In comparison with the 1970s, patients undergoing CABG today are older, include a higher percentage of women, and are sicker, in that a greater proportion have unstable angina, triple-vessel CAD, previous coronary revascularization with CABG or PCI, LV dysfunction, and comorbid conditions, including hypertension, diabetes, and peripheral vascular disease. Despite the increasing risk profile of this population, outcomes with CABG have generally remained stable or have improved.

Operative Mortality

Risk factors for death following CABG may be separated into five categories: (1) preoperative factors related to CAD, including recent acute MI, hemodynamic instability, LV dysfunction, extensive CAD, presence of left main CAD, and severe or unstable angina; (2) preoperative factors related to the aggressiveness of the arteriosclerotic process, as reflected in associated carotid or peripheral vascular disease; (3) preoperative biologic factors (older age at surgery, diabetes mellitus, other comorbidities, including pulmonary and renal disease, and perhaps female gender); (4) intraoperative factors (intraoperative ischemic damage, failure to use IMA grafts); and (5) environmental or institutional factors, including the specific surgeon and treatment protocols used.[185] Of these factors, several variables have consistently emerged as the most potent predictors of mortality after CABG: (1) age; (2) urgency of operation; (3) prior cardiac surgery; (4) LV function; (5) percentage stenosis of the left main coronary artery; and (6) number of epicardial vessels with significant disease.

In-hospital mortality after isolated CABG has continued to decline over the last several decades. Despite a shift toward higher risk demographics, increasing age, and clinical comorbidity, early mortality continued to decline in the 1990s. The cumulative mortality for CABG-only operations among more than 1.4 million CABG-only operations recorded in the Society of Thoracic Surgeons (STS) data base declined from 3.05% between 1997 and 1999 to approximately 2% in 2009.[186] Operative mortality rates for isolated CABG surgery now range from approximately 1.5% to 2.0%. Several models have been developed and refined, with the objective of predicting perioperative mortality.[187] Application of such models have demonstrated even greater declines in CABG mortality over the past decade when adjusted for changes in clinical risk profile.

PERIOPERATIVE COMPLICATIONS. Perioperative morbidity (see Chap. 84) has increased because of a larger fraction of higher risk patients. Major morbidity (e.g., death, stroke, renal failure, reoperation, prolonged ventilation, sternal infection) occurred in 13.4% through 30 days among the 503,478 CABG-only operations recorded in the STS data base between 1997 and 1999.[186]

MYOCARDIAL INFARCTION. Perioperative MI, particularly if associated with hemodynamic or arrhythmic complications or pre-existing LV dysfunction, has a major adverse effect on early and late prognosis. The reported incidence varies widely (0% to more than 10%), in large part because of heterogeneous diagnostic criteria, with an average of 3.9% (median, 2.9%). Elevation of the myocardial creatine kinase-MB (CK-MB) isoenzyme level more than five times the upper limit of normal is commonly considered diagnostic of MI in this setting. Data from a prospectively performed study of routine monitoring of CK-MB postoperatively has shown CK-MB to be independently associated with mortality.[188] Predictors of perioperative MI in the Coronary Artery Surgery Study (CASS) were female gender, severe perioperative angina pectoris, severe stenosis of the left main coronary artery, and triple-vessel CAD. It is possible that mortality associated with perioperative MI may be reduced with acadesine, an experimental agent that increases the concentration of adenosine in ischemic tissue.[189]

CEREBROVASCULAR COMPLICATIONS. Neurologic abnormalities following cardiac surgery are dreaded complications and are associated with higher long-term mortality (see Chap. 84).[190] Postulated mechanisms include emboli from atherosclerosis of the aorta or other large arteries, emboli possibly from the CPB machine circuit and its tubing, and intraoperative hypotension, particularly in patients with pre-existing

hypertension.[191] Type I injury is associated with major neurologic deficits, stupor, and coma, and type II injury is characterized by a deterioration in intellectual function and memory. The incidence of neurologic abnormalities is variably estimated, depending on how the deficits are defined. The incidence of stroke reported in the Northern New England Cardiovascular Disease Study Group data base between 1992 to 2001 was 1.6% and has been documented as higher in prospective studies (1.5% to 5%).[190] Studies aimed at careful evaluation of neurologic deficits report more frequent neurologic sequelae; type I deficits have been documented in 6% of patients early after CABG, with short-term cognitive decline in 33% to 83%. A prospective long-term study using sophisticated neurocognitive testing revealed cognitive decline in 53% of patients at the time of hospital discharge, 36% at 6 weeks, and 24% at 6 months.[175] In regard to the neurologic sequelae of CPB (including stroke, delirium, and neurocognitive dysfunction), older age, in addition to other comorbid conditions (particularly diabetes), and intraoperative manipulation of the aorta are the more powerful predictors. In most, but not all, studies, atherosclerosis of the proximal aorta has also been a strong predictor of stroke, as has the use of an intra-aortic balloon pump.[192] Mild hypothermia in the intra- and perioperative periods may improve neurocognitive function after CABG.

ATRIAL FIBRILLATION. This arrhythmia is one of the most frequent complications of CABG.[193] It occurs in up to 40% of patients, primarily within 2 to 3 days. In the early postoperative period, rapid ventricular rates and loss of atrial transport may compromise systemic hemodynamics, increase the risk of embolization, and lead to a significant increase in the duration and cost of the hospital stay; it is associated with a twofold to threefold increase in postoperative stroke. Older age, hypertension, prior atrial fibrillation, and heart failure are associated with higher risk of developing atrial fibrillation after cardiac surgery.[194] Prior statin therapy may be associated with less frequent postoperative atrial fibrillation.[195]

Prophylactic use of beta blockers reduces the frequency of postoperative atrial fibrillation; these should be administered routinely before and after CABG to patients without contraindications. Amiodarone is also effective in prophylaxis against postoperative atrial fibrillation and may be considered for patients at high risk for developing this dysrhythmia (see Chap. 84). Off-pump techniques may be associated with less frequent postoperative atrial fibrillation.[175,179] Up to 80% of patients spontaneously revert to sinus rhythm within 24 hours without treatment other than digoxin or other agents used for controlling the ventricular rate. In a randomized trial of patients with postoperative atrial fibrillation that had resolved prior to discharge, there was no detectable benefit of extended antiarrhythmic therapy beyond a short course of 1 week.[193] Most patients return to sinus rhythm by 6 weeks after surgery.

RENAL DYSFUNCTION. The incidence of renal failure requiring dialysis after CABG remains low (0.5% to 1.0%) but is associated with significantly greater morbidity and mortality (see Chap. 84). A decline in renal function defined by a postoperative serum creatinine level higher than 2.0 mg/dL or an increase of more than 0.7 mg/dL is more frequent (7% to 8%). Predictors of postoperative renal dysfunction include advanced age, diabetes, pre-existing renal dysfunction, and heart failure. Patients with preoperative renal dysfunction and a serum creatinine level higher than 2.5 mg/dL appear to be at increased risk of the need for hemodialysis and may be candidates for alternative approaches to revascularization or prophylactic dialysis. A randomized trial of *N*-acetylcysteine for the prevention of development of renal dysfunction in 295 patients undergoing CABG showed no difference compared with placebo.[196]

Relief of Angina

Trials in which the contemporary practice of using one or more arterial grafts was prevalent have demonstrated similar or superior rates of freedom from angina during short- and mid-term follow-up. The major randomized trials all have demonstrated greater relief of angina, better exercise performance, and a lower requirement for antianginal medications for surgically compared with medically treated patients 5 years postoperatively. Independent predictors of recurrence of angina are female gender, obesity, preoperative hypertension, and lack of use of the IMA as a conduit. In patients with triple-vessel CAD undergoing CABG surgery, the completeness of revascularization is a significant determinant of the relief of symptoms at 1 year and over a 5-year period.

In summary, after 5 years, approximately 75% of surgically treated patients can be predicted to be free of an ischemic event, sudden death, occurrence of MI, or recurrence of angina; about 50% remain free for approximately 10 years and about 15% for 15 years or

CH
57

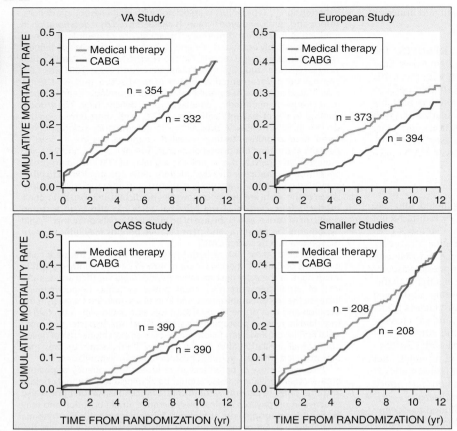

FIGURE 57-14 Survival curves of three large randomized trials and four smaller studies combined. *(From Eagle KA, Guyton RA, Davidoff R, et al: ACC/AHA guidelines for coronary artery bypass graft surgery: A report of the American College of Cardiology/American Heart Association Task Force on Practice Guidelines [Committee to Revise the 1991 Guidelines for Coronary Artery Bypass Graft Surgery]. American College of Cardiology/American Heart Association. J Am Coll Cardiol 34:1262, 1999.)*

main CAD; (2) single- or double-vessel CAD with proximal LAD artery disease; (3) LV systolic dysfunction; and (4) a composite evaluation that indicates high risk, including severity of symptoms, high-risk exercise tolerance test, history of prior MI, and the presence of ST-segment depression on the resting ECG.

Taken together, the results of all the trials and registries indicate that the sicker the patient—based on the severity of symptoms or ischemia, age, number of diseased vessels, and presence of LV dysfunction—the greater the benefit of surgical over medical therapy on survival (see Figs. 57-10 and 57-13 and Table 57-12). CABG prolongs survival in patients with significant left main CAD irrespective of symptoms, in those with multivessel CAD and impaired LV function, and in patients with triple-vessel CAD that includes the proximal LAD artery, irrespective of LV function. Surgical therapy has also been demonstrated to prolong life in patients with double-vessel CAD and LV dysfunction, particularly those with proximal narrowing of one or more coronary arteries and in the presence of severe angina. Although no study has documented a survival benefit with surgical treatment in patients with single-vessel disease, some evidence has indicated that such patients, who have impaired LV function, have a poor long-term survival with medical therapy.

PATIENTS WITH DEPRESSED LEFT VENTRICULAR FUNCTION. Depressed LV function (see Chap. 52) is one of the most powerful predictors of perioperative and late mortality. In the New York State CABG registry, an ejection fraction of 25% or less was associated with 6.5% in-hospital mortality compared with 1.4% in those with an ejection fraction greater than 40%.[197] In the STS data base, the mean ejection fraction in approximately 136,330 patients undergoing initial CABG in 1999 was 0.51, and approximately 25% had an ejection fraction of less than 0.45. Moreover, as the population ages and the proportion undergoing reoperation increases, the number of patients with preoperative LV dysfunction and clinical heart failure will increase. In the CABG Patch trial confined to patients with an ejection fraction of 0.35 or less, perioperative mortality was 3.5% for patients without clinical signs of heart failure versus 7.7% for those with NYHA Classes I to IV heart failure.

Although the effect of a reduced ejection fraction on operative mortality cannot be eliminated, careful attention to intraoperative metabolic, inotropic, and mechanical support, including preoperative intra-aortic balloon counterpulsation in some patients, may decrease perioperative mortality in comparison with the mortality rates expected from prediction models. In addition to advances in myocardial protection for those undergoing CABG with CPB, off-pump approaches to CABG may also lead to improved surgical outcomes in this high-risk population. Thus, in experienced centers, the in-hospital mortality for patients with severe LV dysfunction is less than 4%.

The powerful effect of the preoperative ejection fraction on late survival currently emphasizes that the presence of LV dysfunction, in association with viable myocardium, has changed from a relative contraindication to CABG to a strong indication. This shift in focus has been caused by the realization that viable dysfunctional myocardium may improve after coronary revascularization.[198] The most striking survival benefits of CABG, as well as symptomatic and functional improvements, are shown by patients with seriously impaired LV function in whom the prognosis of medical therapy is poor. In patients with a history of heart failure and multivessel (particularly triple-vessel) disease, CABG may also reduce the incidence of sudden cardiac death. Although preoperative LV dysfunction creates the potential for significant benefit, the perioperative risk should not be underestimated, particularly in the setting of clinical congestive heart failure.[199] Selection of patients with viable myocardium supplied by a reasonable target vessel(s) for grafting appears critical when considering CABG for patients with severe LV dysfunction.

more. Symptomatic improvement is best maintained in patients with the most complete revascularization.

Effects on Survival

Current clinical practice has been shaped by three major randomized trials of CABG compared with medical therapy that enrolled patients between 1972 and 1984—the Veterans Affairs (VA) Trial, the European Cardiac Society Study (ECSS), and the National Institutes of Health–supported CASS (**Fig. 57-14**).[153] The evidence base comprises data from 2649 patients participating in these and several smaller trials and has several important limitations with respect to application to current practice because the risk profile of patients referred for surgery, as well as the available surgical and medical interventions, have evolved substantially since these trials were conducted. In particular, these trials antedated the widespread use of one or two IMAs and the disease-modifying therapies (e.g., aspirin, statins, inhibitors of the renin-angiotensin system) that are currently used as guideline-driven intensive medical therapy.

The results of the trials of surgical versus medical therapy have generally been highly consistent, and thus the major points guiding clinical practice may still be drawn from a meta-analysis of the results. In each of the trials, a survival benefit of CABG emerged during mid-term follow-up (2 to 6 years), but this advantage eroded during long-term follow-up and remained statistically significant only in the ECSS. Considered together, the results of these trials support a 4.1% absolute reduction in long-term mortality (10 years) with CABG (*P* = 0.03). Subgroup analyses have revealed several high-risk criteria that identify patients likely to sustain a more substantial survival benefit: (1) left

TABLE 57-13	Markers of Viable Myocardium	
CLINICAL INDICATOR	**DIAGNOSTIC TEST**	**ALTERNATIVE TEST**
Diastolic wall thickness	Echo	CT, CMR
Systolic wall thickening	Echo	CT, CMR, gated SPECT
Regional wall motion	Echo	CT, CMR, gated SPECT
Regional blood flow	SPECT	PET, CMR
Myocardial metabolism	PET	SPECT
Cell membrane integrity	SPECT	PET
Contractile reserve	Dobutamine echocardiography	Angiography, CT, CMR
Myocardial fibrosis	CMR	CT

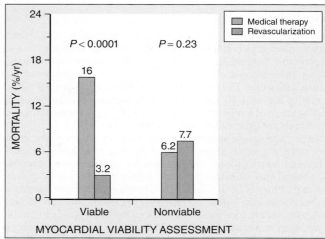

FIGURE 57-15 Meta-analysis of observational studies examining late survival with revascularization versus medical therapy for patients with CAD and LV dysfunction. Analysis of results from 24 studies (*N* = 3088) demonstrated that revascularization is associated with a significant reduction in annual mortality compared with medical therapy in patients with myocardial viability. No advantage of revascularization was detected in patients without myocardial viability. *(Modified from Allman KC, Shaw LJ, Hachamovitch R, et al: Myocardial viability testing and impact of revascularization on prognosis in patients with coronary artery disease and left-ventricular dysfunction: A meta-analysis. J Am Coll Cardiol 39:1151, 2002.)*

MYOCARDIAL HIBERNATION. Improvement in survival and LV function following CABG depends on the successful reperfusion of viable but noncontractile or poorly contracting myocardium (see Chap. 52). Two related pathophysiologic conditions have been described to explain reversible ischemic contractile dysfunction: (1) myocardial stunning (prolonged but temporary postischemic LV dysfunction without myocardial necrosis); and (2) myocardial hibernation (persistent LV dysfunction when myocardial perfusion is chronically reduced or repetitively stunned but sufficient to maintain the viability of tissue).[200] The reduction in myocardial contractility in hibernating myocardium conserves metabolic demands and may be protective, but more prolonged and severe hibernation may lead to severe ultrastructural abnormalities, irreversible loss of contractile units, and apoptosis.

Hibernating myocardium can cause abnormal systolic or diastolic LV function, or both. The predominant clinical feature of myocardial ischemia in these patients may not be angina but dyspnea secondary to increased LV diastolic pressure. Symptoms of heart failure resulting from chronic LV dysfunction may be inappropriately ascribed to myocardial necrosis and scarring when the symptoms may, in fact, be reversed after the chronic ischemia is relieved by coronary revascularization.

DETECTION OF HIBERNATING MYOCARDIUM. Several clinical markers may be used to determine the likelihood that a dysfunctional myocardial segment is viable or nonviable (**Table 57-13**). The presence of angina and the absence of Q waves on the ECG or a history of prior MI are useful clues. A severe reduction in the diastolic wall thickness of dysfunctional LV segments is indicative of scarring. On the other hand, akinetic or dyskinetic segments with preserved diastolic wall thickness may represent a mixture of scarred and viable myocardium. Although a number of imaging tools may be used for this assessment, the most readily available in most settings is low-dose dobutamine echocardiography[201] (see Chap. 15). PET (see Chap. 17) has emerged as an excellent method for demonstrating viable myocardium in patients with impaired LV function.[156] In comparative studies, PET has yielded the highest predictive accuracy of all imaging modalities for detecting dysfunctional myocardium that will improve after revascularization. However, the high cost, technical difficulty, and need for a cyclotron continue to limit this technique's widespread applicability. Contrast-enhanced CMR is emerging as a valuable alternative technique for the assessment of myocardial viability (see Chap. 18)[202] and thallium-201 rest-redistribution imaging continues to be an alternative (see Chap. 17).

PROGNOSTIC IMPLICATIONS OF IDENTIFYING VIABLE MYOCARDIUM. A growing body of evidence has indicated that the detection of viable myocardium in patients with CAD and LV dysfunction not only identifies those for whom improvement in cardiac function is likely after revascularization, but also identifies a group of high-risk patients for whom revascularization improves survival (**Fig. 57-15**).[156] Studies with PET, thallium-201, and dobutamine echocardiography have uniformly demonstrated that patients with LV dysfunction and evidence of hibernating myocardium have a high mortality rate during medical therapy and appear to have a better outcome with revascularization.[203] All these studies have limitations, including a small number of patients, the retrospective nature of the analysis, and lack of a randomized control group.[198] However, the consistency of the findings has been striking. Viability assessment is also helpful in the selection of patients for revascularization because patients selected for revascularization on the basis of an imaging study demonstrating myocardial viability have lower operative mortality and a higher long-term survival rate than those with no evidence of important myocardial viability, or those in whom a viability assessment is not performed.

The mechanisms for improved survival after revascularization in patients with hibernating myocardium in these retrospective studies may be related to improvement in LV function. However, it is likely that other factors are also operative, including reductions in LV remodeling, propensity for serious arrhythmias, and likelihood of a future fatal acute ischemic event. Prospective trials are needed to provide definitive evidence about whether myocardial viability testing identifies patients with LV dysfunction for whom revascularization improves survival and quality of life. The ongoing follow-up of the revascularization hypothesis treatment groups in the Surgical Treatment of Ischemic Heart Failure (STICH) trial is designed to address this issue.[204]

SURGICAL TREATMENT IN SPECIAL GROUPS

Women

Women are less likely than men to be referred for coronary angiography and subsequent revascularization (see Chap. 81). In some studies, gender-based differences in referral for revascularization are fully explained by clinical factors. Moreover, it has not been established whether gender-based differences represent systematically less consideration of referrals for women, inappropriately more consideration of referrals for men, or both. In comparison with men, women who undergo CABG are sicker, as defined by age, comorbid conditions, severity of angina, and history of heart failure.[205] In-hospital mortality and perioperative morbidity after CABG have remained, on average, two times higher in women compared with men.[206] However, when adjusted for the greater risk profile of women referred for CABG, short-term mortality rates and long-term outcomes are similar to those for men in most, but not all, studies. The independent predictors of long-term prognosis in women are similar to those in men and include older age, previous CABG surgery, previous MI, and diabetes.

With generally similar long-term outcomes after surgical revascularization, gender should not be a significant factor in decisions regarding whether to offer CABG.[205]

Older Patients

An evolving change in demographics, in combination with marked improvement in perioperative care and in the outcomes of CABG, has resulted in a burgeoning population of older patients with extensive disease undergoing such surgery (see Chap. 80). The number of individuals older than 75 years in the United States is expected to quadruple in the next 50 years, with cardiovascular disease being the leading cause of morbidity and mortality in this population. Many such individuals are likely to become candidates for CABG.

Older patients are sicker than their younger counterparts in that they have a greater frequency of comorbid conditions, including peripheral vascular and cerebrovascular disease, more extensive triple-vessel and left main CAD, and a higher frequency of LV dysfunction and history of heart failure.[153] Not unexpectedly, these differences are translated into higher perioperative mortality and complication rates, with a sharp increase in the slope of the curve relating mortality to age seen in patients older than 70 years. Despite these differences, in-hospital mortality for older patients has declined over time to 7% to 9% in those undergoing CABG only and has been reported to be as low as 3% to 4% in the subgroup of octogenarians without significant medical comorbidities.[153] Given marked variation in the outcomes in older patients undergoing revascularization, decisions should be based on individual risk and needs assessment.[207]

Renal Disease

Cardiovascular disease is the major cause of mortality in patients with end-stage renal disease (ESRD) and accounts for 54% of deaths (see Chap. 93). Patients with ESRD, as well as those with less severe renal insufficiency, have numerous risk factors that not only accelerate the development of CAD but also complicate its medical management. These risk factors include diabetes, hypertension with LV hypertrophy, systolic and diastolic dysfunction, abnormal lipid metabolism, anemia, and increased homocysteine levels. Therefore, mild or more severe renal dysfunction is prevalent in as many as 50% of patients presenting for CABG.[208] Coronary revascularization with PCI or CABG is feasible and well documented in patients with ESRD, but mortality and complication rates are increased. Patients with milder degrees of renal insufficiency who are not dependent on dialysis are also at higher risk of major perioperative complications, longer recovery times, and lower rates of short- and mid-term survival.[209] Observational data have suggested that in patients on chronic dialysis, CABG is the preferred strategy for revascularization over PCI. However, randomized data are few, and 30-day mortality in patients with ESRD undergoing CABG ranges from 9% to as high as 20%.

Patients with Diabetes

In comparison with age-matched nondiabetic patients, diabetic patients (see Chap. 64) with angiographically proven CAD are more likely to be women with evidence of peripheral vascular disease and a higher number of coronary occlusions. Diabetes is an important independent predictor of mortality among patients undergoing surgical revascularization.[210] Patients with diabetes have smaller distal vessels, which are judged to be poorer targets for bypass grafting. Nevertheless, the patency of arterial and venous grafts appears similar in diabetics and nondiabetic patients. Despite these higher risks with operative intervention, because of the potential long-term benefits of CABG in patients with diabetes and severe CAD, such patients should be considered as candidates for CABG (see "Comparisons Between Percutaneous Coronary Intervention and Coronary Artery Bypass Grafting" and "Choosing Among Percutaneous Coronary Intervention, Coronary Artery Bypass Grafting, and Medical Therapy").

CORONARY BYPASS SURGERY IN PATIENTS WITH ASSOCIATED VASCULAR DISEASE. Management of patients with combined CAD and peripheral vascular disease involving the carotid arteries, the abdominal aorta, or the vessels of the lower extremities presents many challenges (see Chaps. 60 and 61). Polyvascular disease is becoming increasingly frequent as the population of patients under consideration for CABG ages and as technical improvements allow the application of coronary revascularization to ever more complex cases.

IMPACT OF COMBINED CORONARY ARTERY DISEASE AND PERIPHERAL VASCULAR DISEASE. Clinically apparent CAD occurs frequently in patients with peripheral vascular disease. In patients undergoing peripheral vascular surgery, late outcomes are dominated by cardiac causes of morbidity and mortality. Conversely, in patients with CAD, the presence of peripheral vascular disease, even if asymptomatic, is associated with an adverse prognosis, presumably because of the greater total atherosclerotic burden borne by these patients.

Because patients with CAD and peripheral atherosclerosis tend to be older and have more widespread vascular disease and end-organ damage than patients without peripheral atherosclerosis, the perioperative mortality and morbidity consequent to CABG are high and the late outcome is not as favorable.[211] In the Northern New England Cardiovascular data base, in-hospital mortality after CABG was 2.4-fold greater in patients with peripheral vascular disease than in those without it, particularly for patients with lower extremity disease. Diffuse atheroembolism is a particularly serious complication of CABG in patients with peripheral vascular disease and aortic atherosclerosis. It is a major cause of perioperative death, stroke, neurocognitive dysfunction, and multiorgan dysfunction after CABG.

Peripheral vascular disease is also a strong marker of an adverse long-term outcome. For example, in the Northern New England Cardiovascular data base, the 5-year mortality was approximately twofold greater in patients with peripheral vascular disease than in those without it, even after adjusting for other comorbid conditions, which are more frequent in patients with peripheral vascular disease. Nevertheless, given the diffuse nature of coronary disease in patients with peripheral vascular disease, there may be advantages to surgical coronary revascularization rather than PCI in many of these patients.[212]

CAROTID ARTERY DISEASE. In patients with stable CAD and carotid artery disease for whom carotid endarterectomy is planned, exercise stress testing and consideration of coronary revascularization can ordinarily be performed after the carotid surgery. The prevalence of significant carotid disease in an increasingly older population being considered for CABG is high; approximately 20% have a stenosis of 50% or greater, 6% to 12% have a stenosis of 80% or greater, and the percentage is higher in patients with left main CAD. In patients for whom surgical treatment is considered for both carotid artery disease and CAD, the merits of a combined versus a staged approach have been debated. Neither strategy has been demonstrated to be unequivocally superior to the other, and an individualized approach, depending on the patient's initial condition, severity of symptoms, anatomy of the coronary and carotid vessels, and individual institutional experience, is most appropriate. Preoperative or simultaneous carotid stenting is under investigation as an alternative approach to combined carotid endarterectomy and CABG.

MANAGEMENT OF PATIENTS WITH ASSOCIATED VASCULAR DISEASE. Patients with severe or unstable CAD requiring revascularization can be categorized into two groups according to the severity and instability of the accompanying vascular disease (see Chap. 61). When the noncoronary vascular procedures are elective, they can generally be postponed until the cardiac symptoms have stabilized, either by intensive medical therapy or by revascularization. A combined procedure is necessary in patients with unstable CAD and an unstable vascular condition, such as frequent recurrent transient ischemic attacks or a rapidly expanding abdominal aortic aneurysm. In some patients in this category, PCI offers the potential for stabilizing the patient's cardiac condition before proceeding with a definitive vascular repair. A problem is posed by the use of a thienopyridine after stenting; this will increase bleeding unless surgery is performed at least 5 days after discontinuation of the thienopyridine.

PATIENTS REQUIRING REOPERATION. Currently, approximately 12% of coronary artery procedures are reoperations and, in some centers, particularly tertiary care centers, the proportion is increasing rapidly and accounts for 20% of all CABG operations. The major indication for reoperation is late disease of saphenous vein grafts. An additional factor underlying recurrent symptoms is progression of disease in native vessels between the first and second operations. Several series have emphasized the sicker preoperative status of patients undergoing reoperation, including older age, more serious comorbidity, associated valvular heart disease, and a greater prevalence of LV dysfunction and greater extent of ischemic jeopardized myocardium.[213]

Not unexpectedly, the mortality associated with reoperation is significantly higher than that of initial CABG procedures. For patients undergoing first operations, mortality was 2.6% for urgent and 6% for emergency procedures in comparison with 7.4% and 13.5%, respectively, in patients undergoing repeat CABG.

COMPARISONS BETWEEN PERCUTANEOUS CORONARY INTERVENTION AND CORONARY ARTERY BYPASS GRAFTING

Observational Studies

Catheter-based revascularizations in most comparative studies have been limited mainly to PTCA, and the findings were largely consistent.[153] Over a period of 1 to 5 years, the rates of mortality and nonfatal MI were not significantly different between patients revascularized with CABG versus PTCA, but recurrent events, including angina pectoris and the need for repeat revascularization procedures, were significantly more frequent in the PTCA than the CABG group, largely as a consequence of incomplete revascularization and restenosis. However, several subgroups of patients who may derive a survival benefit from CABG compared with PTCA have been identified. These include patients with LV dysfunction, probably because of the ability to achieve more complete revascularization with CABG. In addition, CABG provides a survival benefit compared with PTCA when proximal LAD artery stenosis (>70%) is present.

More recent studies have included patients undergoing stenting. In an analysis of approximately 60,000 patients with multivessel CAD treated with coronary stenting or CABG and recorded in the New York State Registry between 1997 and 2000, CABG was found to be associated with higher survival after adjustment for medical comorbidities in patients with two or more diseased vessels, with or without involvement of the LAD artery.[214] Nevertheless, the similarity of the unadjusted rates of survival highlights the role of clinical judgment in selecting the optimal therapy for the individual patient and the ability to achieve good outcomes for appropriately selected patients with two-vessel CAD, particularly without involvement of the proximal LAD artery.[169]

Randomized Trials

Overall, the findings from randomized trials indicate that in selected patients with multivessel CAD and preserved ejection fraction, compared with multivessel PCI, CABG results in fewer repeat revascularizations and fewer symptoms, without a significant difference in survival.

PERCUTANEOUS CORONARY INTERVENTION VERSUS CORONARY ARTERY BYPASS GRAFTING IN PATIENTS WITH SINGLE-VESSEL DISEASE. Both the Lausanne and the MASS trials were limited to patients with isolated disease of the proximal LAD coronary artery.[153] The results of these small trials were consistent in that over 2 to 3 years, the rates of mortality and MI were similar in the two treatment arms, as was improvement in symptoms, but at the cost of more frequent reintervention in patients treated with PCI. In a trial comparing minimally invasive direct CABG to stenting for patients with isolated stenosis in the proximal LAD artery (N = 220), patients treated with CABG were less likely to have recurrent symptoms or undergo repeat revascularization, but showed no detectable difference in the risk of death or MI with PCI.

MULTIVESSEL DISEASE. At least 10 published studies have compared PCI with CABG in patients with multivessel CAD. Despite the heterogeneity of the trials in regard to design, methods, and patient population enrolled, the results are generally comparable and provide a consistent perspective of CABG and PCI in selected patients with multivessel CAD. Nevertheless, there are limitations that should be recognized. Conducted over several decades, the trials evolved substantially with respect to the technology used for both procedures and disease-modifying preventive therapy. Moreover, most patients entered into the trials had well-preserved LV function. Therefore, patients enrolled in these trials were at relatively low risk, with predominantly double-vessel CAD and normal LV ejection fraction—that is, a high proportion of patients in whom CABG surgery had not been previously shown to be superior to medical therapy in regard to survival. Thus, one would not expect a significant mortality difference between PCI and CABG.[80]

As an example, between 1988 and 1991, the Bypass Angioplasty Revascularization Investigation (BARI) trial enrolled 1829 patients with multivessel CAD in the United States and Canada. At 5 years, overall survival rates were not different between the two groups (89.3% with CABG and 86.3% with PTCA; P = 0.19), nor was any difference noted in the incidence of MI. CABG was initially associated with greater improvement in angina. Moreover, as anticipated from the observational data, repeat revascularization procedures were more frequent after PCI. This absolute difference was less in subsequent trials in which progressive improvements in stent technology were made. In the Synergy between PCI with Taxus and Cardiac Surgery (SYNTAX) trial, between 2005 and 2007, 1800 patients with three-vessel or left main CAD were randomly assigned to undergo CABG or PCI, for which a multidisciplinary team consisting of a local cardiac surgeon and interventional cardiologist determined that equivalent anatomic revascularization could be achieved with either treatment.[215] The primary outcome measure was the noninferiority comparison of the two groups for major adverse cardiac or cerebrovascular events (i.e., death from any cause, stroke, MI, or repeat revascularization) during the 12-month period after randomization. Rates of major adverse cardiac or cerebrovascular events at 12 months were significantly higher in the PCI group (17.8% versus 12.4% for CABG; P = 0.002; **Fig. 57-16**), in large part because of an increased rate of repeat revascularization (13.5% versus 5.9%; P < 0.001); thus, the criterion for noninferiority was not met. At 12 months, the rates of death and MI were similar between the two groups. However, stroke was significantly more likely to occur with CABG (2.2% versus 0.6% with PCI; P = 0.003).

In-hospital costs are lower for patients undergoing PCI. However, the need for recurrent hospitalization and repeat revascularization procedures over the long term contribute to an increase in postdischarge cost in patients treated with PCI, resulting in similar overall cost over 3 to 5 years.

PATIENTS WITH DIABETES. An initially unexpected finding in the BARI trial was that patients with previously treated diabetes who underwent PTCA had a 5-year mortality of 34.5% versus 19.4% for those who underwent CABG (P = 0.003; see Chap. 64). This advantage of CABG over PTCA for patients with diabetes became more robust by 10 years of follow-up in BARI and was supported in other studies.[216] More rapid progression of atherosclerosis and high rates of restenosis in patients undergoing PCI were plausibly major contributors to this difference. However, subsequent analyses of smaller randomized trials and large clinical registries with mixed results and the introduction of BMS and DES have led to the reevaluation of the relevance of the findings from BARI.[217] Nevertheless, in a collaborative meta-analysis of individual patient data from 7812 patients in ten trials of PCI versus CABG, there was a significant 30% reduction in total mortality with CABG in the subset of 1233 diabetic patients, findings that persisted even after exclusion of the BARI trial (**Fig. 57-17**).[218]

The findings of the Bypass Angioplasty Revascularization Investigation 2 Diabetes (BARI 2D) trial did not directly compare PCI and CABG but provide additional information with respect to revascularization in patients with diabetes mellitus.[170] In the BARI 2D trial, 2368 patients with established diabetes and CAD were randomized to prompt revascularization (PCI or CABG) versus delayed or no revascularization and optimal medical therapy. A notable feature of the prompt revascularization strategy was prespecification to PCI or CABG before randomization, with patients with more severe CAD being allocated to CABG. At 5 years, all-cause mortality did not differ between these two treatment groups (**Fig. 57-18**), However, two prespecified analyses of a secondary composite endpoint (death, MI, or stroke) provide important scientific and clinical insights: (1) compared with optimal medical therapy without revascularization, the CABG cohort had a significantly lower rate of death, MI, or stroke driven mainly by a reduction in nonfatal MI, but accompanied also by a nonsignificant 16% relative decrease in mortality; (2) in contrast to CABG, there was absolutely no difference in the primary survival or secondary composite endpoints in PCI patients versus optimal medical therapy.

In BARI 2D, only 35% of patients received DES; the ongoing Future REvascularization Evaluation in patients with Diabetes mellitus: Optimal management of Multivessel disease (FREEDOM) trial of patients with multivessel CAD who are randomized to either DES or CABG will provide additional information to guide clinical practice.[219]

CHOOSING AMONG PERCUTANEOUS CORONARY INTERVENTION, CORONARY ARTERY BYPASS GRAFTING, AND MEDICAL THERAPY. Optimal medical therapy of stable IHD involves a reduction in reversible risk factors, counseling in lifestyle alteration, treatment of conditions that intensify angina, and pharmacologic management of ischemia. Unlike in ACS patients,[220] revascularization has not been shown to reduce death or MI when used

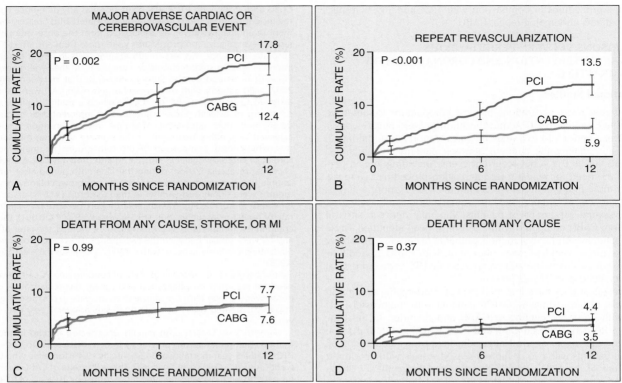

FIGURE 57-16 Outcomes in 1800 patients with stable ischemic heart disease and multivessel coronary artery disease randomized to CABG or PCI. **A,** CABG was superior to PCI at 1 year with respect to the primary outcome measure of death from any cause, MI, stroke, or repeat revascularization. **B,** This result was driven by the need for repeat revascularization, which was reduced significantly in the CABG group. **C, D,** There was no difference in the rate of death, MI, or stroke or death from any cause in the two treatment groups. *(Modified from Serruys PW, Morice MC, Kappetein AP, et al: Percutaneous coronary intervention versus coronary-artery bypass grafting for severe coronary artery disease. N Engl J Med 360:961, 2009.)*

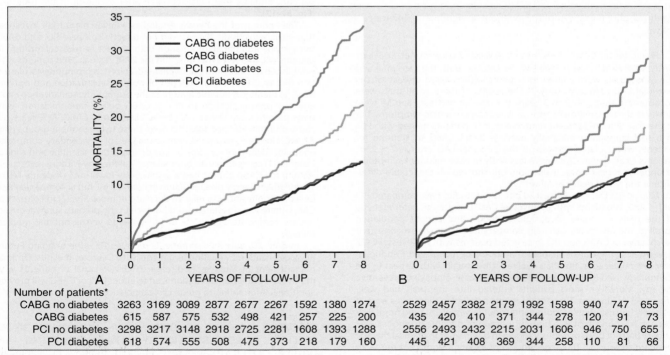

FIGURE 57-17 Kaplan-Meier estimates of death from any cause in a collaborative analysis of individual patient data from 10 randomized trials in patients with stable CAD with and without diabetes mellitus assigned to multivessel PCI or CABG. Patients with diabetes had a significant reduction in mortality with CABG compared with PCI. **A,** Cumulative incidence among patients from all 10 trials. **B,** Cumulative incidence among all trials, excluding the BARI trial. *(Modified from Hlatky MA, Boothroyd DB, Bravata DM, et al: Coronary artery bypass surgery compared with percutaneous coronary interventions for multivessel disease: A collaborative analysis of individual patient data from ten randomised trials. Lancet 373:1190, 2009.)*

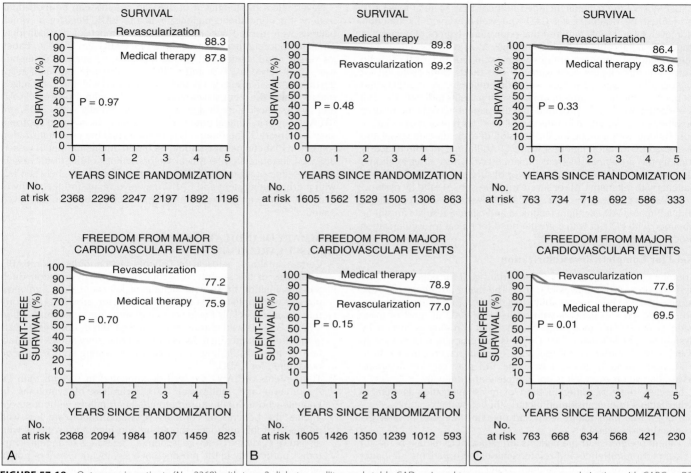

FIGURE 57-18 Outcomes in patients (*N* = 2368) with type 2 diabetes mellitus and stable CAD assigned to prompt coronary revascularization with CABG or PCI versus intensive medical therapy alone in the BARI-2D trial. Intent to revascularize with PCI or CABG was recorded at the time of randomization. **A,** There was no significant difference in the rates of survival (top) or major cardiovascular events (death, myocardial infarction, or stroke; bottom) by treatment group in the overall cohort. **B,** In the PCI stratum, there was no difference between treatment groups with respect to either endpoint. **C,** In patients selected by the investigator to undergo CABG, the rate of major cardiovascular events was significantly lower in patients who underwent prompt revascularization compared with medical therapy alone. (*Modified from Frye RL, August P, Brooks MM, et al: A randomized trial of therapies for type 2 diabetes and coronary artery disease. N Engl J Med 360:2503, 2009.*)

in patients with stable IHD (with the exception of surgery in patients meeting specific anatomic criteria). Recommendations for PCI or CABG should be based both on the extent and severity of ischemia by noninvasive stress testing or invasive assessment of the hemodynamic significance of anatomic stenosis and the severity of anginal symptoms or functional impairment. When an unacceptable level of angina persists despite medical management, the patient has troubling side effects from the anti-ischemic drugs, and/or exhibits a high-risk result on noninvasive testing, the coronary anatomy should be defined to allow selection of the appropriate technique for revascularization.[153] Accordingly, based on these data, and after elucidation of the coronary anatomy, selection of the technique of revascularization should be made as described here (**Table 57-14**; see Figs. 57-16 and 57-18).

Single-Vessel Disease

In patients with single-vessel disease in whom revascularization is deemed necessary and the lesion is anatomically suitable, PCI is almost always preferred over CABG.

Multivessel Disease

The first step is to decide whether a patient falls into the category of those who were included in randomized trials comparing PCI and

TABLE 57-14	Comparison of Revascularization Strategies in Multivessel Disease	
ADVANTAGES	**DISADVANTAGES**
Percutaneous Coronary Intervention	
Less invasive	Restenosis
Shorter hospital stay	High incidence of incomplete revascularization
Lower initial cost	
Easily repeated	Relative inefficacy in patients with severe left ventricular dysfunction
Effective in relieving symptoms	
	Less favorable outcome in diabetics
	Limited to specific anatomic subsets
Coronary Artery Bypass Grafting	
Effective in relieving symptoms	Cost
Improved survival in certain subsets	Morbidity
Ability to achieve complete revascularization	
Wider applicability (anatomic subsets)	

Modified from Faxon DP: Coronary angioplasty for stable angina pectoris. *In* Beller G, Braunwald E (eds): Chronic Ischemic Heart Disease. Atlas of Heart Disease. Vol 5. Philadelphia, WB Saunders, 1995, p 9.15.

CABG. Most of the patients included in these trials were at lower risk, as defined by double-vessel CAD and well-preserved LV function. Moreover, several trials required that equivalent degrees of revascularization be achievable by both techniques. Most patients with chronically occluded coronary arteries were excluded and, of those who were clinically eligible, approximately two thirds were excluded for angiographic reasons. The lack of any difference in late mortality and MI between the two treatment arms in such patients indicates that PCI is a reasonable strategy, provided that the patient accepts the distinct possibility of symptom recurrence and need for repeat revascularization. Patients with a single localized lesion in each affected vessel and preserved LV function fare best with PCI. Additional anatomic factors, such as the presence of severe proximal LAD artery disease, should also be considered and weigh in favor of surgery (see Fig. 57-13). For patients with left main CAD or severe triple-vessel CAD and LV dysfunction, CABG is generally the best approach. However, in selected patients with left main CAD, excellent technical and clinical results can still be obtained with PCI but with a greater need for repeat revascularization procedures than with CABG.[215,220]

Need for Complete Revascularization

Complete revascularization is an important goal for patients with LV dysfunction and/or multivessel CAD.[221] The major advantage of CABG surgery over PCI is its greater ability to achieve complete revascularization, particularly in patients with triple-vessel CAD. In most of these patients, particularly those with chronic total coronary occlusion, LV dysfunction, or left main CAD, CABG is the procedure of choice. In patients with borderline LV function (ejection fraction from 0.40 to 0.50) and milder degrees of ischemia, PCI may provide adequate revascularization, even if it is not complete anatomically.

In many patients, either method of revascularization is suitable. Other factors to be considered include the following:

1. Access to a high-quality team and operator (surgeon or interventional cardiologist).
2. Patient preference. Some patients are reluctant to remain at risk for symptom recurrence and reintervention; these patients are better candidates for surgical treatment. Other patients are attracted by the less invasive nature and more rapid recovery from PCI; they prefer to have PCI as their initial revascularization, with the possibility of undergoing CABG if symptoms persist and/or an excellent revascularization has not been achieved.
3. Advanced patient age and comorbidity. Much older patients and those with comorbid conditions are often better candidates for PCI.
4. Younger patient age. PCI is also often preferable for younger patients (<50 years), with the expectation that they may require CABG at some time in the future and that PCI will postpone the need for surgery; this sequence may be preferable to two operations. Patient preference is a pivotal aspect of the decision to perform PCI or CABG in these patient groups.

Patients with Diabetes

The poorer outcomes after PCI than after CABG in treated diabetic patients in the BARI trial, together with similar findings in the ARTS trial, had raised concern whether all diabetic patients with multivessel CAD should be treated surgically (see Chap. 64). The BARI-2D trial results reinforce the principal finding of the COURAGE trial[166] that an initial strategy of PCI provides no incremental clinical benefit over optimal medical therapy, even in patients with diabetes. However, in those patients who remain symptomatic despite medical therapy, or where there is demonstration of significant ischemia or extensive CAD, then a revascularization strategy is warranted. Either PCI or CABG may be reasonable choices, depending on the anatomic complexity of disease. In patients with severe disease, as selected for CABG in the BARI 2D, current evidence supports CABG as the preferred revascularization strategy. A potential advantage is that bypass grafts to the midcoronary vessel both treat the culprit lesion (regardless of anatomic complexity) and may afford prophylaxis against new proximal disease progression, whereas stents only treat suitable stenotic segment(s), with no benefit against the development of new disease.[172]

Nevertheless, the treatment of diabetic patients can be individualized, as for nondiabetic patients.[210] In the BARI Registry, in which patients were treated according to the preference of the individual physician, poorer outcomes were noted for CABG and PTCA in diabetics versus nondiabetics but, among diabetics, no survival difference was noted between PTCA and CABG.[169] A plausible explanation for the differences in results in the registry compared with the randomized trials is that in the latter, sicker diabetic patients with triple-vessel CAD and LV dysfunction, by design, were treated equally with CABG and PTCA, whereas in clinical practice, such patients are referred appropriately for surgery.[169] Therefore, it is reasonable that the revascularization strategy in diabetic patients should be based on the number of vessels diseased, lesion-related technical factors, caliber of the distal vessels, and presence or absence of LV dysfunction. The choice between PCI with a drug-eluting stent and CABG may revolve around the ability of each procedure to achieve complete revascularization in any given patient.[210,219,222]

SUMMARY OF INDICATIONS FOR CORONARY REVASCULARIZATION

1. Certain anatomic subsets of patients are candidates for CABG, regardless of the severity of symptoms or LV dysfunction. Such patients include those with significant left main CAD and most patients with triple-vessel CAD that includes the proximal LAD coronary artery, especially those with LV dysfunction (ejection fraction < 50%). Patients with chronic stable angina and double-vessel CAD with significant proximal disease of the LAD artery and LV dysfunction or high-risk findings on noninvasive testing should also be considered for CABG.[80]

2. The benefits of CABG are well documented in patients with LV dysfunction and multivessel CAD, regardless of symptoms. In patients whose dominant symptom is heart failure without severe angina, the benefits of coronary revascularization are less well defined, but this approach should be considered for patients who also have evidence of severe ischemia (regardless of angina symptoms), particularly in the presence of a significant extent of potentially viable dysfunctional (hibernating) myocardium.[153]

3. The primary objective of coronary revascularization in patients with single-vessel disease is relief of significant symptoms or objective evidence of severe ischemia. For most of these patients, PCI is the revascularization modality of choice.

4. In patients with angina who are not considered to be at high risk, survival is similar for surgery, PCI, and medical management.

5. All the indications discussed earlier relate to the potential benefits of surgery over medical therapy on survival. Coronary revascularization with PCI or CABG is highly efficacious in relieving symptoms and may be considered for patients with moderate to severe ischemic symptoms who are not controlled by and/or who are dissatisfied with medical therapy, even if they are not in a high-risk subset. For such patients, the optimal method of revascularization is selected on the basis of LV function and arteriographic findings and the likelihood of technical success.

OTHER SURGICAL PROCEDURES FOR ISCHEMIC HEART DISEASE. CABG may be combined with surgical procedures aimed at correction of atherosclerotic disease elsewhere in the cardiovascular system, correction of mechanical complications of MI (mitral regurgitation or ventricular septal defect), LV aneurysms, and concomitant valvular heart disease. Not unexpectedly, morbidity and mortality are correspondingly increased because of the added complexity of the procedure and, in many patients who require these other procedures, the presence of underlying LV dysfunction (see later).

Transmyocardial Laser Revascularization

Transmyocardial laser revascularization (TMLR) is performed by placing a laser on the epicardial surface of the left ventricle, exposed through a lateral thoracotomy, and creating small channels from the epicardial to endocardial surfaces. TMLR has been reported to improve symptoms in patients with refractory angina; however, the mechanism and magnitude of benefit remain uncertain. The initial assumption was that laser-mediated channels would provide a network of functional connections between the LV cavity and ischemic myocardium. Subsequent observations demonstrating closure of the channels within hours or days, despite apparent relief of symptoms, have led to other explanations for the apparent clinical success of the procedure. These explanations include improved perfusion by stimulation of angiogenesis, a placebo effect, and an anesthetic effect mediated by the destruction of sympathetic nerves carrying pain-sensitive afferent fibers or periprocedural MI. The failure of two sham-controlled trials of percutaneous laser myocardial revascularization to show any benefit has highlighted the impact of the placebo effect in response to laser myocardial revascularization. On the basis of data from the randomized trials, it would appear that the widespread use of TMLR as a stand-alone method cannot be justified. Because of the perioperative morbidity associated with surgical TMLR, careful selection of patients is necessary.[223]

Other Manifestations of Coronary Artery Disease

Prinzmetal (Variant) Angina

(See Chaps. 52 and 56.)

Chest Pain with Normal Coronary Arteriogram

The syndrome of angina or angina-like chest pain with a normal coronary arteriogram, often termed *syndrome X* (to be differentiated from metabolic syndrome X, characterized by abdominal obesity, hypertriglyceridemia, low HDL cholesterol, insulin resistance, hyperinsulinemia, and hypertension), is an important clinical entity that should be distinguished from classic ischemic heart disease caused by obstructive CAD. Patients with chest pain and normal coronary arteriograms may represent as many as 10% to 20% of those undergoing coronary arteriography because of clinical suspicion of angina. The cause(s) of the syndrome is not conclusively defined and is likely not homogeneous. However, vascular dysfunction and myocardial metabolic abnormalities have been implicated.[224] True myocardial ischemia, reflected in the production of lactate by the myocardium during exercise or pacing, is present in some of these patients; however, others have no metabolic evidence for ischemia as the cause of their discomfort. The incidence of coronary calcification on multislice CT scanning is significantly higher than that of normal controls (53% versus 20%) but lower than that in patients with angina secondary to obstructive CAD (96%). The prognosis of patients with angina and normal or near-normal coronary angiograms is generally more favorable than that for those with angina caused by obstructive atherosclerosis involving the epicardial coronary arteries. However, observational data have indicated that their outcome is not as uniformly excellent as suggested by early cohort studies.[225,226]

It has been postulated that the syndrome of angina pectoris with normal coronary angiograms reflects a number of conditions. Included in syndrome X are patients with endothelial dysfunction or microvascular dysfunction or spasm in whom angina may be the result of ischemia.[224] This condition is frequently termed *microvascular angina*. In others, chest discomfort without ischemia may be caused by abnormal pain perception or sensitivity.[227] Also, IVUS studies have demonstrated anatomic and physiologic heterogeneity of syndrome X, with a spectrum ranging from normal coronary arteries to vessels with intimal thickening and atheromatous plaque but without critical obstructions. It is likely that some patients with syndrome X have a combination of pathobiologic contributors. In addition, it is difficult to distinguish patients with syndrome X in whom chest pain is caused by ischemia from patients with noncardiac pain. Behavioral or psychiatric disorders may be evident.

MICROVASCULAR DYSFUNCTION (INADEQUATE VASODILATOR RESERVE). Patients with chest pain, angiographically normal coronary arteries, and no evidence of large-vessel spasm, even after an acetylcholine challenge, may demonstrate an abnormally decreased capacity to reduce coronary

resistance and increase coronary flow in response to stimuli such as exercise, adenosine, dipyridamole, and atrial pacing.[228] These patients also have an exaggerated response of small coronary vessels to vasoconstrictor stimuli and an impaired response to intracoronary papaverine. Abnormal endothelium-dependent vasoreactivity has been associated with regional myocardial perfusion defects on SPECT and PET imaging. It has been reported that patients with syndrome X also have impaired vasodilator reserve in forearm vessels and airway hyperresponsiveness, which suggests that the smooth muscle of systemic arteries and other organs may be affected, in addition to that of the coronary circulation.

Endothelial dysfunction and endothelial cell activation, reported in patients with syndrome X, may participate in the release of cellular adhesion molecules, proinflammatory cytokines, and constricting mediators that induce changes in the arterial wall, resulting in microvascular dysfunction and higher risk for future development of obstructive CAD. Patients with syndrome X have been observed to have higher levels of circulating intercellular adhesion molecule-1, vasoconstrictor endothelin-1, and the inflammatory marker hsCRP; moreover, the level of hsCRP appears to correlate with the severity of symptoms and burden of ischemic electrocardiographic changes.

EVIDENCE FOR ISCHEMIA. Despite general acceptance that microvascular and/or endothelial dysfunction is present in many patients with syndrome X, whether ischemia is in fact the putative cause of the symptoms in these patients is not clear. Studies of transmyocardial production of lactate have generated mixed results.[224] The development of LV dysfunction and electrocardiographic or scintigraphic abnormalities during exercise in some of these patients supports an ischemic cause. However, stress echocardiography with dobutamine detects regional contraction abnormalities consistent with ischemia in a subset of patients. More sensitive techniques, such as perfusion analysis with CMR, have demonstrated that subendocardial perfusion abnormalities, in particular, may be associated with syndrome X.

ABNORMAL PAIN PERCEPTION. The lack of definitive evidence of ischemia in some patients with syndrome X has focused attention on alternative nonischemic causes of cardiac-related pain, including a decreased threshold for pain perception—the so-called sensitive heart syndrome.[227] This hypersensitivity may result in an awareness of chest pain in response to stimuli such as arterial stretch or changes in heart rate, rhythm, or contractility. A sympathovagal imbalance with sympathetic predominance in some of these patients has also been postulated. At the time of cardiac catheterization, some patients with syndrome X are unusually sensitive to intracardiac instrumentation, with typical chest pain being consistently produced by direct right atrial stimulation and saline infusion. Measurements of regional cerebral blood flow at rest and during chest pain have suggested differential handling of afferent stimuli between patients with syndrome X and those with obstructive CAD.

CLINICAL FEATURES. The syndrome of angina or angina-like chest pain with normal epicardial arteries occurs more frequently in women (see Chap. 81), many of whom are premenopausal, whereas obstructive CAD is found more commonly in men and postmenopausal women.[224] Fewer than half of patients with syndrome X have typical angina pectoris; most have various forms of atypical chest pain. Although the features are frequently atypical, the chest pain may nonetheless be severe and disabling. The condition may have markedly adverse effects on the quality of life, employment, and use of health care resources.

In some patients with minimal or no CAD, an exaggerated preoccupation with personal health is associated with the chest pain, and panic disorder may be responsible in a portion of such patients. Up to two thirds of patients with chest pain and normal coronary arteries have been observed to have psychiatric disorders. Others have reported that the incidence of obstructive CAD is extremely low in patients with atypical chest pain who are anxious and/or depressed. The association between syndrome X and insulin resistance warrants further study.

PHYSICAL AND LABORATORY EXAMINATION. Abnormal physical findings reflecting ischemia, such as a precordial bulge, gallop sound, and the murmur of mitral regurgitation, are uncommon in syndrome X. The resting ECG may be normal, but nonspecific ST-T wave abnormalities are often observed, sometimes occurring in association with the chest pain. Approximately 20% of patients with chest pain and normal coronary arteriograms have positive exercise tests. However, many patients with this syndrome do not complete the exercise test because of fatigue or mild chest discomfort. LV function is usually normal at rest and during stress, unlike the situation in obstructive CAD, in which function often becomes impaired during stress.

PROGNOSIS. Important prognostic information on patients with angina and normal or near-normal coronary arteriograms has been obtained from the CASS Registry. In patients with an ejection fraction of 0.50 or more, the 7-year survival rate was 96% for patients with a normal arteriogram and 92% for those whose arteriogram revealed mild CAD (50% luminal stenosis). Thus, long-term survival of patients with anginal chest pain and normal coronary angiograms is generally excellent, markedly better than in patients with obstructive CAD. Clinical indicators of worse prognosis may be evident. Some but not all studies have indicated that an ischemic response to exercise is associated with increased mortality.[225] Moreover, in women with angina and no obstructive CAD enrolled in the Women's Ischemic Syndrome Evaluation (WISE), persistence of symptoms was associated with a more than twofold higher risk of cardiovascular events.[229] Such patients may be appropriate candidates for formal studies of vascular function and aggressive risk factor modification[224] (see Chap. 81).

MANAGEMENT. In patients with angina-like chest pain syndrome and normal epicardial coronary arteries, noncardiac causes, such as esophageal abnormalities, should be considered. In patients with syndrome X in whom ischemia can be demonstrated by noninvasive stress testing, a trial of anti-ischemic therapy with nitrates, calcium channel blockers, and beta blockers is logical, but the response to this therapy is variable. Perhaps because of the heterogeneity of this population, studies testing these antianginal therapies have produced conflicting results.[224] For example, beta blockers may be most effective in patients with syndrome X who also have evidence of a hyperadrenergic state characterized by increased sympathetic nervous activity (e.g., hypertension, tachycardia, reduced heart rate variability). Sublingual nitroglycerin has shown paradoxical effects on blood flow and exercise tolerance in some studies and beneficial effects in others. Alpha blockers have been demonstrated to be ineffective. Observational studies of calcium antagonists have in general shown disappointing results with respect to amelioration of symptoms.

ACE inhibitors have favorable effects on endothelial function, vascular remodeling, and sympathetic tone that may be relevant to the pathophysiology of syndrome X. Preliminary data studying ACE inhibitors in this population are promising. Similarly, estrogen has been shown to attenuate normal coronary vasomotor responses to acetylcholine, increase coronary blood flow, and potentiate endothelium-dependent vasodilation in postmenopausal women. Studies of estrogen replacement in postmenopausal women with syndrome X have shown improvement in symptoms and/or exercise performance; however, the role of exogenous estrogen in treatment of this group remains in question. Aimed at the altered somatic and visceral pain perception in many patients with syndrome X, imipramine (50 mg) and structured psychological intervention have been reported to be helpful for some patients.[224]

Silent Myocardial Ischemia

The prognostic importance and the mechanisms of silent ischemia have been the subject of considerable interest for almost 30 years. Patients with silent ischemia have been stratified into three categories by Cohn and associates. The first and least common form, type I silent ischemia, occurs in totally asymptomatic patients with obstructive CAD, which may be severe. These patients do not experience angina at any time; some type I patients do not even experience pain in the course of MI. Epidemiologic studies of sudden death (see Chap. 41), as well as clinical and postmortem studies of patients with silent MI and studies of patients with chronic angina pectoris, have suggested that many patients with extensive coronary artery obstruction never experience angina pectoris in any of its recognized forms (stable, unstable, or variant). These patients with type I silent ischemia may be considered to have a defective anginal warning system. Type II silent ischemia is the form that occurs in patients with documented previous MI.

The third and much more frequent form, designated type III silent ischemia, occurs in patients with the usual forms of chronic stable angina, unstable angina, and Prinzmetal angina. When monitored, patients with this form of silent ischemia exhibit some episodes of ischemia associated with chest discomfort and other episodes that are not—that is, episodes of silent (asymptomatic) ischemia. The total ischemic burden in these patients refers to the total period of ischemia, both symptomatic and asymptomatic.

AMBULATORY ELECTROCARDIOGRAPHY. The use of ambulatory electrocardiographic monitoring has led to a greater appreciation of the high frequency of type III silent ischemia, occurring in up to one third of patients with stable angina treated with appropriate therapy. It has become apparent that anginal pain underestimates the frequency of significant cardiac ischemia.[230]

The role of myocardial O_2 demand in the genesis of myocardial ischemia has been evaluated by measuring the heart rate and blood pressure changes preceding silent ischemic events during ambulatory studies. In one series, 92% of all episodes were silent, and 60% to 70% were preceded by significant increases in heart rate or blood pressure. The circadian variations in heart rate and blood pressure also paralleled the increase in silent ischemic events. This and other studies have suggested that increases in myocardial O_2 demand have a significant role in the genesis of silent ischemia, but in other patients reductions in myocardial O_2 supply may make an important contribution to the initiation of symptomatic and asymptomatic episodes. The mechanisms underlying the development of ischemia, as detected by ambulatory electrocardiographic and exercise testing, may be different and, in patients in the ACIP study, concordance between the ambulatory ECG and SPECT was only 50%. For identification of silent ischemia, the two techniques probably complement each other.

Transient ST-segment depression of 0.1 mV or more that lasts longer than 30 seconds is a rare finding in normal subjects. Patients with known CAD show a strong correlation between such transient ST-segment depression and independent measurements of impaired regional myocardial perfusion and ischemia, determined by rubidium-82 uptake as measured by PET. In patients with type III silent ischemia, perfusion defects occur in the same myocardial regions during symptomatic and asymptomatic episodes of ST-segment depression.

Type III silent ischemia is extremely common. Analysis of ambulatory electrocardiographic recordings of patients with CAD who had symptomatic and silent myocardial ischemia has shown that 85% of ambulant ischemic episodes occur without chest pain and 66% of angina reports are unaccompanied by ST-segment depression. Their frequency is such that it has been suggested that overt angina pectoris is merely the "tip of the ischemic iceberg." In patients with stable CAD enrolled 1 to 6 months after hospitalization for an acute ischemic event, only 15% had angina with exercise, but 28% had ST-segment depression and 41% had reversible myocardial perfusion defects on thallium scintigraphy. Episodes of silent ischemia have been estimated to be present in approximately one third of all treated patients with angina, although a higher prevalence has been reported in diabetics (see Chap. 64).[231] Episodes of ST-segment depression, symptomatic and asymptomatic, exhibit a circadian rhythm and are more common in the morning. Asymptomatic nocturnal ST-segment changes are almost invariably an indicator of double- or triple-vessel CAD or left main coronary artery stenosis.

Pharmacologic agents that reduce or abolish episodes of symptomatic ischemia (e.g., nitrates, beta blockers, calcium antagonists) also reduce or abolish episodes of silent ischemia.

MECHANISMS OF SILENT ISCHEMIA. It is not clear why some patients with unequivocal evidence of ischemia do not experience chest pain, whereas others are symptomatic. Differences in peripheral and central neural processing of pain have been proposed as important factors underlying silent ischemia. PET imaging of cerebral blood flow during painful versus silent ischemia has pointed toward differences in handling of afferent signals by the central nervous system. Specifically, overactive gating of afferent signals in the thalamus may reduce the cortical activation necessary for perception of pain from the heart. Autonomic neuropathy has also been implicated as a reason for reduced sensation of pain during ischemia. Although increased release of endorphins may play a role in some patients with silent ischemia, the results of clinical studies are mixed. Some researchers have suggested that anti-inflammatory cytokines are at play in reducing inflammatory processes that may participate in the genesis of cardiac pain.

PROGNOSIS. Although some controversy remains, ample evidence has supported the view that episodes of myocardial ischemia, regardless of whether they are symptomatic or asymptomatic, are of prognostic importance for patients with CAD.[232] In asymptomatic patients (type I), the presence of exercise-induced ST-segment depression has been shown to predict a fourfold to fivefold increase in cardiac mortality in comparison with patients without this finding. Similarly, in patients with stable angina or prior MI, the presence of inducible ischemia evident by ST-segment depression or perfusion abnormalities during exercise testing is associated with unfavorable outcomes, regardless of whether symptoms are present. The strength of this association is greatest when the ischemia is found to occur at a low workload. Several studies evaluating the prognostic implications of silent ischemia on ambulatory monitoring in patients with stable angina (type III) have demonstrated that the presence of myocardial ischemia on the ambulatory ECG, whether silent or symptomatic, is also associated with an adverse cardiac outcome. Moreover, in the ACIP study, in patients treated medically, myocardial ischemia detected by the ambulatory ECG and by an abnormal exercise treadmill test result were each independently associated with adverse cardiac outcomes. However, other studies have not detected a relationship between silent ischemia on ambulatory monitoring and subsequent hard outcomes.

Nevertheless, when the subgroup of patients with ischemia on stress testing is considered, silent ischemia on Holter monitoring is also a significant predictor of subsequent death or MI. In addition, patients with ischemia on the ambulatory ECG are more likely to have multivessel CAD, severe proximal stenoses, and a greater frequency of complex lesion morphology, including intracoronary thrombus, ulceration, and eccentric lesions, than patients without evidence of ischemia on ambulatory monitoring. The presence of severe and complex CAD may partly explain the apparently independent effect of silent ischemia during ambulatory monitoring on prognosis.

Substantial improvements in technology have made long-term ambulatory monitoring for ischemia more convenient and reliable with respect to data quality.[233] Nevertheless, whether the incremental prognostic information provided by adding an ambulatory ECG to a standard stress test justifies the cost of using this modality as a tool for widespread screening remains to be determined, but it is unlikely. The exercise ECG can identify most patients likely to have significant ischemia during their daily activities and remains the most important screening test for significant CAD (see Chap. 14). Many patients with type I silent ischemia have been identified because of an asymptomatic positive exercise ECG obtained following MI. In such patients, with a defective anginal warning system, it is reasonable to assume that asymptomatic ischemia has a significance similar to that of symptomatic ischemia and that their management with respect to disease-modifying preventive therapy, coronary angiography, and revascularization should be similar.

MANAGEMENT. Drugs that are effective for preventing episodes of symptomatic ischemia (e.g., nitrates, calcium antagonists, beta blockers) are also effective for reducing or eliminating episodes of silent ischemia. A number of studies have shown that beta blockers reduce the frequency, duration, and severity of silent ischemia in a dose-dependent fashion. For example, in the Atenolol Silent Ischemia Study Trial (ASIST), 4 weeks of atenolol therapy decreased the number of ischemic episodes detected on ambulatory ECG (from 3.6 to 1.7; $P < 0.001$) and also the average duration (from 30 to 16.4 minutes/48 hours; $P < 0.001$). Coronary revascularization is also effective in reducing the rate of angina and ambulatory ischemia. In the ACIP pilot study, 57% of patients treated with revascularization were free of ischemia at 1 year, compared with 31% and 36% in the ischemia- and angina-guided strategies, respectively ($P < 0.0001$). In the Swiss Interventional Study on Silent Ischemia Type II (SWISSI-II) trial in 201 patients with silent myocardial ischemia who were recovering from acute MI (>2 months), PCI was associated with a significant reduction in late (up to 10-year) mortality as compared with medical therapy,[234] but the medical therapy as used in this study was not as intensive as in the COURAGE and BARI 2D trials, thus making the results of this fairly small study somewhat difficult to interpret. In addition, aggressive secondary prevention with lipid-lowering therapy has also been shown to reduce ischemia on ambulatory monitoring.

Although suppression of ischemia in patients with asymptomatic ischemia appears to be a worthwhile objective, whether treatment should be guided by symptoms or by ischemia as reflected by the ambulatory ECG has not been established. In a study of bisoprolol, nifedipine, and a combination of the two, patients achieving complete eradication of ischemia, symptomatic and asymptomatic, were less likely to suffer death, MI, or angina requiring revascularization. Similarly, amelioration of all symptomatic and asymptomatic ischemia in the ASIST trial conferred an advantage with respect to the primary endpoint of death, resuscitated ventricular tachycardia or ventricular fibrillation, MI, unstable angina, revascularization, or worsening angina. However, in the ACIP trial, no differences in outcome were detected between the groups allocated to ischemia- versus

angina-guided therapy. In contrast, the early benefits of revascularization on ischemia were associated with improved clinical outcomes. Specifically, the rate of death or MI was 12.1% in the angina-guided strategy, 8.8% in the ischemia-guided strategy, and 4.7% in the revascularization strategy, and a strong reduction was also seen in recurrent hospitalizations and the revascularization strategies. Patients who continue to suffer silent ischemia after revascularization may be at increased risk for recurrent cardiac events compared with those who are free of any ischemia.

Heart Failure in Ischemic Heart Disease

Currently, the leading cause of heart failure in developed countries is CAD.[235] In the United States, CAD and its complications account for two thirds to three fourths of all cases of heart failure. In many patients, the progressive nature of heart failure reflects the progressive nature of the underlying CAD. The term *ischemic cardiomyopathy* is used for the clinical syndrome in which one or more of the pathophysiologic features just discussed result in LV dysfunction and heart failure symptoms.[236] This condition is the predominant form of heart failure related to CAD. Additional complications of CAD that may become superimposed on ischemic cardiomyopathy and precipitate heart failure are the development of LV aneurysm and mitral regurgitation caused by papillary muscle dysfunction.

ISCHEMIC CARDIOMYOPATHY. In 1970, Burch and associates first used the term *ischemic cardiomyopathy* to describe the condition in which CAD results in severe myocardial dysfunction, with clinical manifestations often indistinguishable from those of primary dilated cardiomyopathy (see Chap. 68). Symptoms of heart failure caused by ischemic myocardial dysfunction and hibernation, diffuse fibrosis, or multiple MIs, alone or in combination, may dominate the clinical picture of CAD. In some patients with chronic CAD, angina may be the principal clinical manifestation at one time, but later this symptom diminishes or even disappears as heart failure becomes more prominent. Other patients with ischemic cardiomyopathy have no history of angina or MI (type I silent ischemia), and it is in this subgroup that ischemic cardiomyopathy is most often confused with dilated cardiomyopathy.

It is important to recognize hibernating myocardium in patients with ischemic cardiomyopathy because symptoms resulting from chronic LV dysfunction may be incorrectly thought to result from necrotic and scarred myocardium rather than from a reversible ischemic process.[237] Hibernating myocardium may be present in patients with known or suspected CAD with a degree of cardiac dysfunction or heart failure not readily accounted for by previous MIs.

The outlook for patients with ischemic cardiomyopathy treated medically is poor, and revascularization or cardiac transplantation may be considered.[198] The prognosis is particularly poor for patients in whom ischemic cardiomyopathy is caused by multiple MIs, those with associated ventricular arrhythmias, and those with extensive amounts of hibernating myocardium. However, this last group of patients, whose heart failure, even if severe, is caused by large segments of reversibly dysfunctional but viable myocardium, appears to have a significantly better prognosis after revascularization. Revascularization in this group also significantly relieves heart failure symptoms. Thus, the key to management of patients with ischemic cardiomyopathy is to assess the extent of residual viable myocardium with a view to coronary revascularization of viable myocardium. Patients with little or no viable myocardium in whom heart failure is secondary to extensive MI and/or fibrosis should be managed in a manner similar to those with dilated cardiomyopathy (see Chaps. 28 and 68) because their prognosis is poor. By contrast, patients with ischemic cardiomyopathy with extensive multivessel CAD and viable myocardium may derive a survival advantage with CABG surgery, particularly the subset of patients with diabetes.

Additional, more rigorous, adequately sized observational studies and randomized controlled trials are needed to determine the efficacy of revascularization versus medical therapy and to define the role of viability testing. Three such studies are underway—the STICH trial,[204] the Heart Failure Revascularization Trial (HEART), and the PET and Recovery Following Revascularization-2 (PARR-2) study.[198]

LEFT VENTRICULAR ANEURYSM. LV aneurysm is usually defined as a segment of the ventricular wall that exhibits paradoxical (dyskinetic) systolic expansion. Chronic fibrous aneurysms interfere with LV performance principally through loss of contractile tissue. Aneurysms made up largely of a mixture of scar tissue and viable myocardium or of thin scar tissue also impair LV function by a combination of paradoxical expansion and loss of effective contraction.[238] False aneurysms (pseudoaneurysms) represent localized myocardial rupture in which the hemorrhage is limited by pericardial adhesions, and have a mouth that is considerably smaller than the maximal diameter (**Fig. 57-19**). True and false aneurysms may coexist, although the combination is extremely rare.

The frequency of LV aneurysms depends on the incidence of transmural MI and heart failure in the population studied. LV aneurysms and the need for aneurysmectomy have declined dramatically during the last 5 to 10 years in concert with the expanded use of acute reperfusion therapy in evolving MI. More than 80% of LV aneurysms are located anterolaterally near the apex. They are often associated with total occlusion of the LAD coronary artery and a poor collateral blood supply. Approximately 5% to 10% of aneurysms are located posteriorly. Three fourths of patients with aneurysms have multivessel CAD.

Almost 50% of patients with moderate or large aneurysms have symptoms of heart failure, with or without associated angina, approximately 33% have severe angina alone, and approximately 15% have symptomatic ventricular arrhythmias that may be intractable and life-threatening. Mural thrombi are found in almost half of patients with chronic LV aneurysms and can be detected by angiography and two-dimensional echocardiography (see Chap. 15). Systemic embolic events in patients with thrombi and LV aneurysm tend to occur early after MI. In patients with chronic LV aneurysm (documented at least 1 month after MI), subsequent systemic emboli were extremely uncommon (0.35/100 patient-years in patients not receiving anticoagulants).

DETECTION. Clues to the presence of aneurysm include persistent ST-segment elevations on the resting ECG (in the absence of chest pain) and a characteristic bulge of the silhouette of the left ventricle on a chest roentgenogram. Marked calcification of the LV silhouette may be present. These findings, when clear-cut, are relatively specific, but they have limited sensitivity. Radionuclide ventriculography and two-dimensional echocardiography can demonstrate LV aneurysm more readily; the latter is also helpful in distinguishing between true and false aneurysms based on the demonstration of a narrow neck in relation to cavity size in the latter. Color-flow echocardiographic imaging is useful for establishing the diagnosis because flow in and out of the aneurysm, as well as abnormal flow within the aneurysm, can be detected, and subsequent pulsed Doppler imaging can reveal a to-and-fro pattern with characteristic respiratory variation in the peak systolic velocity. CMR may be emerging as the preferred noninvasive technique for the preoperative assessment of LV shape, thinning, and resectability.[238]

LEFT VENTRICULAR ANEURYSMECTOMY. True LV aneurysms do not rupture, and operative excision is carried out to improve the clinical manifestations, most often heart failure but sometimes also angina, embolization, and life-threatening tachyarrhythmias.[238] Coronary revascularization is frequently performed along with aneurysmectomy, especially for patients in whom angina accompanies heart failure.

A large LV aneurysm in a patient with symptoms of heart failure, particularly if angina pectoris is also present, is an indication for surgery. The operative mortality rate for LV aneurysmectomy is approximately 8% (ranging from 2% to 19%), with rates as low as 3% reported in more recent series. Risk factors for early death include poor LV function, triple-vessel CAD, recent MI, presence of mitral regurgitation, and intractable ventricular arrhythmias. The presence of angina pectoris instead of dyspnea as the dominant preoperative symptom is associated with lower operative mortality. Surgery carries a particularly high risk in patients with severe heart failure, a low-output state, and akinesis of the interventricular septum, as assessed by echocardiography. Akinesis or dyskinesia of the posterior basal segment of the left ventricle and significant right coronary artery stenoses are additional risk factors.

Risk factors for late mortality following survival from surgery include incomplete revascularization, impaired systolic function of the basal segments of the ventricle and septum not involved by the aneurysm, the presence of a large aneurysm with a small quantity of residual viable myocardium, and the presence of severe cardiac failure as the initial feature.

Improvement in LV function has been reported in survivors of resection of LV aneurysms. Anterior ventricular restoration has the potential to reverse adverse remodeling, realign contractile fibers, and decrease LV

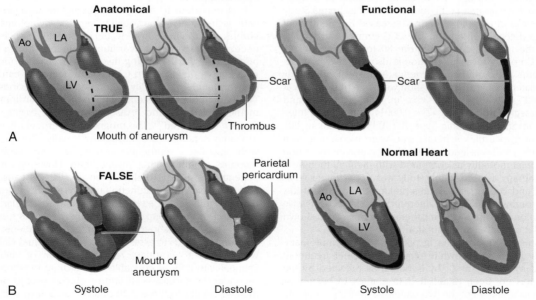

LEFT VENTRICULAR ANEURYSM IN CORONARY HEART DISEASE

FIGURE 57-19 Hearts in systole and diastole with true and false anatomic and functional LV aneurysms and healed MI. A normal heart in systole and diastole is shown for comparison **(inset)**. **A,** A true anatomic LV aneurysm protrudes during both systole and diastole, has a mouth that is as wide as or wider than the maximal diameter, has a wall that was formerly the wall of the left ventricle, and is composed of fibrous tissue with or without residual myocardial fibers. A true aneurysm may or may not contain thrombus and almost never ruptures once the wall is healed. **B,** A false anatomic LV aneurysm protrudes during both systole and diastole, has a mouth that is considerably smaller than the maximal diameter of the aneurysm and represents a myocardial rupture site, has a wall made up of parietal pericardium, almost always contains thrombus, and often ruptures. A functional LV aneurysm protrudes during ventricular systole but not during diastole and consists of fibrous tissue with or without myocardial fibers. Ao = aorta; LA = left atrium; LV = left ventricle. *(From Cabin HS, Roberts WC: Left ventricular aneurysm, intraaneurysmal thrombus, and systemic embolus in coronary heart disease. Chest 77:586, 1980.)*

wall stress. By removing the abnormal mechanical burden, LV aneurysmectomy has been associated with late improvement in overall systolic function and improvement in the performance of regional nonischemic myocardium in zones remote from the LV aneurysm, in addition to improvement in measures of LV relaxation and cardiovascular neuroregulatory mechanisms. A concomitant improvement in exercise performance and clinical symptoms may also occur, particularly in patients who have undergone complete revascularization. In one series of 285 patients, 67% of patients undergoing ventricular reconstruction had an improvement in symptoms, with a survival of 82% at 5 years.[238]

Newer surgical approaches to the repair of LV aneurysms are designed to restore normal LV geometry by using an alternative method of epicardial closure and/or an endocardial patch to divide the area of the aneurysm from the remainder of the LV cavity (see Fig. 57-e3 on website). Favorable clinical and hemodynamic results following the use of these newer techniques have been reported, with 5-year survival rates ranging from 73% to 87.5% and a corresponding improvement in hemodynamics and clinical symptoms.[239] In one series, 88% of patients treated with the endoaneurysmorrhaphy technique were in NYHA Class I or II after a mean follow-up of approximately 3.5 years.

The value of surgical therapy, including surgical ventricular restoration (SVR), for patients with ischemic cardiomyopathy who do not have frank LV aneurysms was tested in the SVR hypothesis evaluation within the STICH trial. In the first report from this study, SVR failed to confer any benefit when added to CABG in patients with heart failure, dilated left ventricles, and severe regional wall motion abnormalities.[240] In this initial analysis, 1000 patients were recruited at 96 clinical sites in 23 countries. To be included, patients had to have an ejection fraction less than 35%, CAD amenable to CABG, and an area of severe regional dysfunction in the LV anterior wall. Patients were randomized to receive CABG alone (n = 499) or CABG plus SVR (n = 501). All participants received intensive evidence-based medical therapy for heart failure. Both surgical interventions improved symptoms of heart failure and exercise capacity, and SVR reduced end-systolic volume index by 20% versus 3% with CABG, at a median follow-up of 4 years; however, no difference was observed between the two groups for combined rates of death or cardiac hospitalization—56% for CABG and 57% for CABG plus SVR. There were no significant differences between surgical treatments for death, cardiac hospitalization, all-cause hospitalization, acute MI, and stroke.

MITRAL REGURGITATION SECONDARY TO CORONARY ARTERY DISEASE.
Mitral regurgitation is an important cause of heart failure in some patients with CAD. Rupture of a papillary muscle or the head of a papillary muscle usually causes severe acute mitral regurgitation in the course of acute MI (see Chaps. 54 and 66). The cause of chronic mitral regurgitation in patients with CAD is multifactorial and the geometric determinants are complex; these include papillary muscle dysfunction from ischemia and fibrosis in conjunction with a wall motion abnormality and changes in LV shape in the region of the papillary muscle and/or dilation of the mitral annulus.[241] Enlargement of the mitral annulus at end-systole is asymmetric, with lengthening primarily involving the posterior annular segments and leading to prolapse of leaflet tissue tethered by the posterior papillary muscle and restriction of leaflet tissue attached to the anterior leaflet. Most patients with chronic CAD and mitral regurgitation have suffered a previous MI. Clinical features that help identify mitral regurgitation secondary to papillary muscle dysfunction as the cause of acute pulmonary edema or of milder symptoms of left-sided failure include a loud systolic murmur and demonstration of a flail mitral valve leaflet on echocardiography.

In some patients with severe mitral regurgitation into a small, noncompliant left atrium, the murmur may be unimpressive or inaudible. Doppler echocardiography is helpful for assessing the severity of the regurgitation (see Chap. 15). As in mitral regurgitation of other causes, the left atrium is not usually greatly enlarged unless mitral regurgitation has been present for more than 6 months. The ECG is nonspecific, and most patients have angiographic evidence of multivessel CAD.

Management

In patients with severe mitral regurgitation, the indications for surgical correction, usually in association with CABG, are fairly clear-cut. Mitral valve repair, as opposed to mitral replacement, is the procedure of choice, but the decision is based on the anatomic characteristics of the structures forming the mitral valve apparatus, urgency of the need for surgery, and severity of LV dysfunction. A more complex and frequently encountered problem involves the indications for mitral valve surgery in patients undergoing CABG in whom the severity of mitral regurgitation is moderate.[241] The decision is based partly on the presence or absence of structural abnormalities of the mitral apparatus and amenability of the valve to repair. Intraoperative transesophageal echocardiography is invaluable for assessing the severity of regurgitation, reparability of the valve, and success of the integrity of the repair after discontinuation of CPB.

The mortality associated with combined CABG and mitral valve placement in the 2005 Society of Thoracic Surgeons data base was approximately 10%. For bypass surgery and mitral valve repair, mortality from 1995 to 2005 was 7% overall, including emergency and reoperative procedures.[186] Predictors of early mortality include the need for replacement versus repair (in some but not all series) but, in addition, may include other variables such as age, comorbid conditions, urgency of surgery, and LV function. Late results are strongly influenced by the pathophysiologic mechanisms underlying mitral regurgitation and are poorer in patients with regurgitation resulting from annular dilation or restrictive leaflet motion than in patients with chordal or papillary muscle rupture. It is encouraging that despite the relatively high operative mortality, late survival of hospital survivors is excellent. In patients with very poor LV function and dilation of the mitral annulus, mitral regurgitation can intensify the severity of LV failure. In such patients, the risk of surgery is high and the long-term benefit is not established,[242] and a trial of intensive medical therapy, including afterload reduction, beta blockade, and biventricular pacing (see Chaps. 28 and 29) may be worthwhile, because favorable remodeling may reduce the severity of mitral regurgitation. For those patients undergoing CABG, the procedural risks associated with combined CABG and mitral valve repair may outweigh the benefit of reduced mitral regurgitation in those at highest perioperative risk.[243] The Cardiothoracic Surgical Trials Network of the National Heart, Lung, and Blood Institute has developed two prospective randomized clinical trials to identify the role of surgery in patients with ischemic mitral regurgitation.[243a]

Cardiac Arrhythmias

In some patients with CAD, cardiac arrhythmias are the dominant clinical manifestation of the disease. Various degrees and forms of ventricular ectopic activity are the most common arrhythmias in patients with CAD, but serious ventricular arrhythmias may be a major component of the clinical findings in other subgroups. The clinical presentation of arrhythmias and their management in patients with CAD are discussed in Chaps. 36 and 37.

Nonatheromatous Coronary Artery Disease

Although atherosclerosis is the most important cause of CAD, other conditions may also be responsible. The most common causes of nonatheromatous CAD resulting in myocardial ischemia are the syndrome of angina-like pain with normal coronary arteriograms (i.e., so-called syndrome X) and Prinzmetal angina (see Chaps. 52 and 56).

Nonatheromatous CAD may result from other diverse abnormalities, including congenital abnormalities in the origin or distribution of the coronary arteries (see Chaps. 21 and 65). The most important of these abnormalities are anomalous origin of a coronary artery (usually the left) from the pulmonary artery, origin of both coronary arteries from either the right or left sinus of Valsalva, and coronary arteriovenous fistula.[244] An anomalous origin of the left main coronary artery or right coronary artery from the aorta, with subsequent coursing between the aorta and pulmonary trunk, is a rare and sometimes fatal coronary arterial anomaly. Coronary anomalies are reported to cause between 12% and 19% of sports-related deaths in U.S. high school and college athletes and account for one third of cardiac anomalies in military recruits with nontraumatic sudden death.[245]

MYOCARDIAL BRIDGING. This cause of systolic compression of the LAD coronary artery is a well-recognized angiographic phenomenon of questionable clinical significance.[246]

CONNECTIVE TISSUE DISORDERS. Several inherited connective tissue disorders are associated with myocardial ischemia (see Chap. 8), including Marfan syndrome (causing aortic and coronary artery dissection),

Hurler syndrome (causing coronary obstruction), homocystinuria (causing coronary artery thrombosis), Ehlers-Danlos syndrome (causing coronary artery dissection), and pseudoxanthoma elasticum (causing accelerated CAD). Kawasaki disease, the mucocutaneous lymph node syndrome, may cause coronary artery aneurysms and ischemic heart disease in children.

SPONTANEOUS CORONARY DISSECTION. This is a rare cause of MI and sudden cardiac death.[247] Chronic dissection manifested as heart failure has been described. In one series, approximately 75% of cases were diagnosed at autopsy and 75% occurred in women, half of which were associated with a postpartum state. Some cases are associated with atherosclerosis. Hypertension has been postulated as a cause of multivessel spontaneous coronary dissection in some patients but, in others, no obvious cause has been identified. In the acute phase, thrombolytic therapy may be dangerous, but early angiography may identify patients who could benefit from stenting or CABG. In survivors of spontaneous coronary artery dissection, the subsequent 3-year mortality was 20%, but complete healing as defined angiographically may lead to a favorable outcome without intervention.

CORONARY VASCULITIS. This condition, resulting from connective tissue diseases or autoimmune forms of vasculitis, including polyarteritis nodosa, giant cell (temporal) arteritis, and scleroderma, has been well described (see Chap. 89). Coronary arteritis is seen at autopsy in about 20% of patients with rheumatoid arthritis but is rarely associated with clinical manifestations. The incidence of CAD is increased in women with systemic lupus erythematosus (SLE). In SLE patients, CAD has been attributed to a vasculitis, immune complex–mediated endothelial damage, and coronary thrombosis from antiphospholipid antibodies, as well as accelerated atherosclerosis. Giant coronary artery aneurysm associated with SLE is an unusual manifestation that has been associated with the development of acute MI, despite therapy. The antiphospholipid syndrome, characterized by arterial and venous thrombosis and associated with the presence of antiphospholipid antibodies, may be associated with MI, angina, and diffuse LV dysfunction.

TAKAYASU ARTERITIS. In rare cases (see Chap. 89), this condition is associated with angina, MI, and cardiac failure in patients younger than 40 years. Coronary blood flow may be decreased by involvement of the ostia or proximal segments of the coronary arteries, but disease in distal coronary segments is rare. The average age at onset of symptoms is 24 years, and the event-free survival rate 10 years after diagnosis is approximately 60%. Luetic aortitis may also produce myocardial ischemia by causing coronary ostial obstruction.

POSTMEDIASTINAL IRRADIATION. The occurrence of CAD and morbid cardiac events in young persons after mediastinal irradiation is highly suggestive of a cause-and-effect relationship. Pathologic changes include adventitial scarring and medial hypertrophy with severe intimal atherosclerotic disease. Radiation injury may be latent and may not be manifested clinically for many years after therapy. Contributory factors include higher doses than those currently administered and the presence of cardiac risk factors. Among patients without risk factors who receive an intermediate total dose of 30 and 40 Gy, the risk of cardiac death and MI is low.

COCAINE. Because of its widespread use, cocaine has become a well-documented cause of chest pain, MI, and sudden cardiac death (see Chap. 73).[248] In a population-based study of sudden death in persons 20 to 40 years old in Olmsted County over a 30-year period, a high prevalence of cocaine abuse was observed in the more recent cohort of young adults who died suddenly. The principal effects of cocaine are mediated by alpha-adrenergic stimulation, which causes an increase in myocardial O_2 demand and a reduction in O_2 supply because of coronary vasoconstriction (see Chap. 52).

OTHER CAUSES OF MYOCARDIAL ISCHEMIA. Myocardial ischemia not caused by coronary atherosclerosis can also result from embolism from infective endocarditis (see Chap. 67), implanted prosthetic cardiac valves (see Chap. 66), calcified aortic valves, mural thrombi, and primary cardiac tumors (see Chap. 74).

Cardiac Transplantation—Associated Coronary Arteriopathy

(See Chaps. 31 and 43.)

REFERENCES

1. Lloyd-Jones D, Adams RJ, Brown TM, et al: Heart disease and stroke statistics—2010 update: A report from the American Heart Association. Circulation 121:e46, 2010.
2. Ford ES, Capewell S: Coronary heart disease mortality among young adults in the U.S. from 1980 through 2002: Concealed leveling of mortality rates. J Am Coll Cardiol 50:2128, 2007.
3. American Heart Association: International Cardiovascular Disease Statistics. Dallas, American Heart Association, 2009.
4. Abidov A, Rozanski A, Hachamovitch R, et al: Prognostic significance of dyspnea in patients referred for cardiac stress testing. N Engl J Med 353:1889, 2005.
5. Kaul P, Naylor CD, Armstrong PW, et al: Assessment of activity status and survival according to the Canadian Cardiovascular Society angina classification. Can J Cardiol 25:e225, 2009.
6. Morrow DA: Cardiovascular risk prediction in patients with stable and unstable coronary heart disease. Circulation 121:2681, 2010.
7. Camici PG, Pagani M: Cardiac nociception. Circulation 114:2309, 2006.
8. Qin C, Du JQ, Tang JS, et al: Bradykinin is involved in the mediation of cardiac nociception during ischemia through upper thoracic spinal neurons. Curr Neurovasc Res 6:89, 2009.
9. Wu ZZ, Pan HL: Role of TRPV1 and intracellular Ca^{2+} in excitation of cardiac sensory neurons by bradykinin. Am J Physiol Regul Integr Comp Physiol 293:R276, 2007.
10. Wang L, Wang DH: TRPV1 gene knockout impairs postischemic recovery in isolated perfused heart in mice. Circulation 112:3617, 2005.
11. Ieda M, Kanazawa H, Ieda Y, et al: Nerve growth factor is critical for cardiac sensory innervation and rescues neuropathy in diabetic hearts. Circulation 114:2351, 2006.
12. Brosius FC 3rd, Hostetter TH, Kelepouris E, et al: Detection of chronic kidney disease in patients with or at increased risk of cardiovascular disease: A science advisory from the American Heart Association Kidney and Cardiovascular Disease Council; the Councils on High Blood Pressure Research, Cardiovascular Disease in the Young, and Epidemiology and Prevention; and the Quality of Care and Outcomes Research Interdisciplinary Working Group: developed in collaboration with the National Kidney Foundation. Circulation 114:1083, 2006.
13. Brunzell JD, Davidson M, Furberg CD, et al: Lipoprotein management in patients with cardiometabolic risk: Consensus conference report from the American Diabetes Association and the American College of Cardiology Foundation. J Am Coll Cardiol 51:1512, 2008.
14. Di Angelantonio E, Sarwar N, Perry P, et al: Major lipids, apolipoproteins, and risk of vascular disease. JAMA 302:1993, 2009.
15. O'Donoghue M, Morrow DA, Sabatine MS, et al: Lipoprotein-associated phospholipase A2 and its association with cardiovascular outcomes in patients with acute coronary syndromes in the PROVE IT-TIMI 22 (PRavastatin Or atorVastatin Evaluation and Infection Therapy-Thrombolysis In Myocardial Infarction) trial. Circulation 113:1745, 2006.
16. Davidson MH, Corson MA, Alberts MJ, et al: Consensus panel recommendation for incorporating lipoprotein-associated phospholipase A2 testing into cardiovascular disease risk assessment guidelines. Am J Cardiol 101:51F, 2008.
17. Serruys PW, Garcia-Garcia HM, Buszman P, et al: Effects of the direct lipoprotein-associated phospholipase A(2) inhibitor darapladib on human coronary atherosclerotic plaque. Circulation 118:1172, 2008.
18. Smith SC Jr, Milani RV, Arnett DK, et al: Atherosclerotic Vascular Disease Conference: Writing Group II: Risk factors. Circulation 109:2613, 2004.
19. Buckley DI, Fu R, Freeman M, et al: C-reactive protein as a risk factor for coronary heart disease: a systematic review and meta-analyses for the U.S. Preventive Services Task Force. Ann Intern Med 151:483, 2009.
20. Greenland P, Lloyd-Jones D: Defining a rational approach to screening for cardiovascular risk in asymptomatic patients. J Am Coll Cardiol 52:330, 2008.
21. Ridker PM, Danielson E, Fonseca FA, et al: Rosuvastatin to prevent vascular events in men and women with elevated C-reactive protein. N Engl J Med 359:2195, 2008.
22. Genest J, McPherson R, Frohlich J, et al: 2009 Canadian Cardiovascular Society/Canadian guidelines for the diagnosis and treatment of dyslipidemia and prevention of cardiovascular disease in the adult—2009 recommendations. Can J Cardiol 25:567, 2009.
23. Morrow DA, Cannon CP, Jesse RL, et al: National Academy of Clinical Biochemistry Laboratory Medicine Practice Guidelines: Clinical characteristics and utilization of biochemical markers in acute coronary syndromes. Clin Chem 53:552, 2007.
24. Daniels LB, Laughlin GA, Clopton P, et al: Minimally elevated cardiac troponin T and elevated N-terminal pro-B-type natriuretic peptide predict mortality in older adults: Results from the Rancho Bernardo Study. J Am Coll Cardiol 52:450, 2008.
25. Omland T, de Lemos JA, Sabatine MS, et al: A sensitive cardiac troponin T assay in stable coronary artery disease. N Engl J Med 361:2538, 2009.
26. Morrow DA, Antman EM: Evaluation of high-sensitivity assays for cardiac troponin. Clin Chem 55:5, 2009.
27. Sabatine MS, Morrow DA, de Lemos JA, et al: Acute changes in circulating natriuretic peptide levels in response to myocardial ischemia. J Am Coll Cardiol 44:1988, 2004.
28. Omland T, Sabatine MS, Jablonski KA, et al: Prognostic value of B-Type natriuretic peptides in patients with stable coronary artery disease: The PEACE Trial. J Am Coll Cardiol 50:205, 2007.
29. Arena R, Myers J, Williams MA, et al: Assessment of functional capacity in clinical and research settings: A scientific statement from the American Heart Association Committee on Exercise, Rehabilitation, and Prevention of the Council on Clinical Cardiology and the Council on Cardiovascular Nursing. Circulation 116:329, 2007.
30. Gibbons RJ: Noninvasive diagnosis and prognosis assessment in chronic coronary artery disease: Stress testing with and without imaging perspective. Circ Cardiovasc Imaging 1:257, 2008.
31. Marcassa C, Bax JJ, Bengel F, et al: Clinical value, cost-effectiveness, and safety of myocardial perfusion scintigraphy: A position statement. Eur Heart J 29:557, 2008.
32. Sicari R, Nihoyannopoulos P, Evangelista A, et al: Stress echocardiography expert consensus statement—Executive Summary: European Association of Echocardiography (EAE) (a registered branch of the ESC). Eur Heart J 30:278, 2009.
33. Lee DC, Johnson NP: Quantification of absolute myocardial blood flow by magnetic resonance perfusion imaging. JACC Cardiovasc Imaging 2:761, 2009.
34. Schwitter J, Wacker CM, van Rossum AC, et al: MR-IMPACT: Comparison of perfusion-cardiac magnetic resonance with single-photon emission computed tomography for the detection of coronary artery disease in a multicentre, multivendor, randomized trial. Eur Heart J 29:480, 2008.
35. Gibbons RJ, Balady GJ, Bricker JT, et al: ACC/AHA 2002 guideline update for exercise testing: Summary article: A report of the American College of Cardiology/American Heart Association Task Force on Practice Guidelines (Committee to Update the 1997 Exercise Testing Guidelines). Circulation 106:1883, 2002.

36. Lauer M, Froelicher ES, Williams M, et al: Exercise testing in asymptomatic adults: A statement for professionals from the American Heart Association Council on Clinical Cardiology, Subcommittee on Exercise, Cardiac Rehabilitation, and Prevention. Circulation 112:771, 2005.

37. Albers AR, Krichaversusky MZ, Balady GJ: Stress testing in patients with diabetes mellitus: Diagnostic and prognostic value. Circulation 113:583, 2006.

38. Di Carli MF, Hachamovitch R: New technology for noninvasive evaluation of coronary artery disease. Circulation 115:1464, 2007.

39. Bluemke DA, Achenbach S, Budoff M, et al: Noninvasive coronary artery imaging: Magnetic resonance angiography and multidetector computed tomography angiography: A scientific statement from the american heart association committee on cardiovascular imaging and intervention of the council on cardiovascular radiology and intervention, and the councils on clinical cardiology and cardiovascular disease in the young. Circulation 118:586, 2008.

40. Greenland P, Bonow RO, Brundage BH, et al: ACCF/AHA 2007 clinical expert consensus document on coronary artery calcium scoring by computed tomography in global cardiovascular risk assessment and in evaluation of patients with chest pain: A report of the American College of Cardiology Foundation Clinical Expert Consensus Task Force (ACCF/AHA Writing Committee to Update the 2000 Expert Consensus Document on Electron Beam Computed Tomography). Circulation 115:402, 2007.

41. Chen J, Krumholz HM: How useful is computed tomography for screening for coronary artery disease? Screening for coronary artery disease with electron-beam computed tomography is not useful. Circulation 113:125, 2006.

41a. Gerber TC, Gibbons RJ: Weighing the risks and benefits of cardiac imaging with ionizing radiation. J Am Coll Cardiol Img 3:528, 2010.

42. Fuster V, Kim RJ: Frontiers in cardiovascular magnetic resonance. Circulation 112:135, 2005.

43. Nicholls SJ, Tuzcu EM, Sipahi I, et al: Intravascular ultrasound in cardiovascular medicine. Circulation 114:e55, 2006.

44. Raffel OC, Merchant FM, Tearney GJ, et al: In vivo association between positive coronary artery remodelling and coronary plaque characteristics assessed by intravascular optical coherence tomography. Eur Heart J 29:1721, 2008.

45. Honda Y, Fitzgerald PJ: Frontiers in intravascular imaging technologies. Circulation 117:2024, 2008.

46. Nichols L, Lagana S, Parwani A: Coronary artery aneurysm: A review and hypothesis regarding etiology. Arch Pathol Lab Med 132:823, 2008.

47. Ishikawa Y, Akasaka Y, Suzuki K, et al: Anatomic properties of myocardial bridge predisposing to myocardial infarction. Circulation 120:376, 2009.

48. Tonino PA, De Bruyne B, Pijls NH, et al: Fractional flow reserve versus angiography for guiding percutaneous coronary intervention. N Engl J Med 360:213, 2009.

49. Beltrame JF, Weekes AJ, Morgan C, et al: The prevalence of weekly angina among patients with chronic stable angina in primary care practices: The Coronary Artery Disease in General Practice (CADENCE) Study. Arch Intern Med 169:1491, 2009.

50. Hemingway H, McCallum A, Shipley M, et al: Incidence and prognostic implications of stable angina pectoris among women and men. JAMA 295:1404, 2006.

51. Steg PG, Bhatt DL, Wilson PW, et al: One-year cardiovascular event rates in outpatients with atherothrombosis. JAMA 297:1197, 2007.

52. Kligfield P, Lauer MS: Exercise electrocardiogram testing: Beyond the ST segment. Circulation 114:2070, 2006.

53. Rosendorff C, Black HR, Cannon CP, et al: Treatment of hypertension in the prevention and management of ischemic heart disease: A scientific statement from the American Heart Association Council for High Blood Pressure Research and the Councils on Clinical Cardiology and Epidemiology and Prevention. Circulation 115:2761, 2007.

54. Chobanian AV: Shattuck Lecture. The hypertension paradox—more uncontrolled disease despite improved therapy. N Engl J Med 361:878, 2009.

54a. The ACCORD Study Group: Effects of intensive blood-pressure control in type 2 diabetes mellitus. N Engl J Med 362:1575, 2010.

55. Schane RE, Glantz SA: Education on the dangers of passive smoking: A cessation strategy past due. Circulation 118:1521, 2008.

56. Kahn R, Robertson RM, Smith R, et al: The impact of prevention on reducing the burden of cardiovascular disease. Circulation 118:576, 2008.

57. Smith SC Jr, Allen J, Blair SN, et al: AHA/ACC guidelines for secondary prevention for patients with coronary and other atherosclerotic vascular disease: 2006 update: Endorsed by the National Heart, Lung, and Blood Institute. Circulation 113:2363, 2006.

58. Nissen SE, Nicholls SJ, Sipahi I, et al: Effect of very high-intensity statin therapy on regression of coronary atherosclerosis: The ASTEROID trial. JAMA 295:1556, 2006.

59. Ballantyne CM, Raichlen JS, Nicholls SJ, et al: Effect of rosuvastatin therapy on coronary artery stenoses assessed by quantitative coronary angiography: A study to evaluate the effect of rosuvastatin on intravascular ultrasound-derived coronary atheroma burden. Circulation 117:2458, 2008.

60. Ray KK, Cannon CP: The potential relevance of the multiple lipid-independent (pleiotropic) effects of statins in the management of acute coronary syndromes. J Am Coll Cardiol 46:1425, 2005.

61. LaRosa JC, Grundy SM, Waters DD, et al: Intensive lipid lowering with atorvastatin in patients with stable coronary disease. N Engl J Med 352:1425, 2005.

62. Pedersen TR, Faergeman O, Kastelein JJ, et al: High-dose atorvastatin versus usual-dose simvastatin for secondary prevention after myocardial infarction: The IDEAL study: A randomized controlled trial. JAMA 294:2437, 2005.

63. Cannon CP, Steinberg BA, Murphy SA, et al: Meta-analysis of cardiovascular outcomes trials comparing intensive versus moderate statin therapy. J Am Coll Cardiol 48:438, 2006.

64. Barter P, Gotto AM, LaRosa JC, et al: HDL cholesterol, very low levels of LDL cholesterol, and cardiovascular events. N Engl J Med 357:1301, 2007.

65. Briel M, Ferreira-Gonzalez I, You JJ, et al: Association between change in high density lipoprotein cholesterol and cardiovascular disease morbidity and mortality: Systematic review and meta-regression analysis. BMJ 338:b92, 2009.

66. deGoma EM, deGoma RL, Rader DJ: Beyond high-density lipoprotein cholesterol levels evaluating high-density lipoprotein function as influenced by novel therapeutic approaches. J Am Coll Cardiol 51:2199, 2008.

67. Nissen SE, Tardif JC, Nicholls SJ, et al: Effect of torcetrapib on the progression of coronary atherosclerosis. N Engl J Med 356:1304, 2007.

68. Tall AR: CETP inhibitors to increase HDL cholesterol levels. N Engl J Med 356:1364, 2007.

69. Nathan DM, Cleary PA, Backlund JY, et al: Intensive diabetes treatment and cardiovascular disease in patients with type 1 diabetes. N Engl J Med 353:2643, 2005.

70. Dormandy JA, Charbonnel B, Eckland DJ, et al: Secondary prevention of macrovascular events in patients with type 2 diabetes in the PROactive Study (PROspective pioglitAzone Clinical Trial In macroVascular Events): A randomised controlled trial. Lancet 366:1279, 2005.

71. Marcus BH, Williams DM, Dubbert PM, et al: Physical activity intervention studies: What we know and what we need to know: A scientific statement from the American Heart Association Council on Nutrition, Physical Activity, and Metabolism (Subcommittee on Physical Activity); Council on Cardiovascular Disease in the Young; and the Interdisciplinary Working Group on Quality of Care and Outcomes Research. Circulation 114:2739, 2006.

72. Wenger NK: Current status of cardiac rehabilitation. J Am Coll Cardiol 51:1619, 2008.

73. Hambrecht R, Walther C, Mobius-Winkler S, et al: Percutaneous coronary angioplasty compared with exercise training in patients with stable coronary artery disease: A randomized trial. Circulation 109:1371, 2004.

74. Mora S, Cook N, Buring JE, et al: Physical activity and reduced risk of cardiovascular events: Potential mediating mechanisms. Circulation 116:2110, 2007.

75. Thompson PD, Franklin BA, Balady GJ, et al: Exercise and acute cardiovascular events placing the risks into perspective: A scientific statement from the American Heart Association Council on Nutrition, Physical Activity, and Metabolism and the Council on Clinical Cardiology. Circulation 115:2358, 2007.

76. Libby P, Ridker PM, Hansson GK, et al: Inflammation in atherosclerosis: From pathophysiology to practice. J Am Coll Cardiol 54:2129, 2009.

77. Ridker PM, Cannon CP, Morrow D, et al: C-reactive protein levels and outcomes after statin therapy. N Engl J Med 352:20, 2005.

78. Morrow DA, de Lemos JA, Sabatine MS, et al: Clinical relevance of C-reactive protein during follow-up of patients with acute coronary syndromes in the Aggrastat-to-Zocor Trial. Circulation 114:281, 2006.

79. Poirier P, Giles TD, Bray GA, et al: Obesity and cardiovascular disease: Pathophysiology, evaluation, and effect of weight loss: An update of the 1997 American Heart Association Scientific Statement on Obesity and Heart Disease from the Obesity Committee of the Council on Nutrition, Physical Activity, and Metabolism. Circulation 113:898, 2006.

80. Gibbons RJ, Abrams J, Chatterjee K, et al: ACC/AHA 2002 guideline update for the management of patients with chronic stable angina—summary article: A report of the American College of Cardiology/American Heart Association Task Force on practice guidelines (Committee on the Management of Patients With Chronic Stable Angina). J Am Coll Cardiol 41:159, 2003.

81. Bhatt DL, Fox KA, Hacke W, et al: Clopidogrel and aspirin versus aspirin alone for the prevention of atherothrombotic events. N Engl J Med 354:1706, 2006.

82. Bhatt DL, Flather MD, Hacke W, et al: Patients with prior myocardial infarction, stroke, or symptomatic peripheral arterial disease in the CHARISMA trial. J Am Coll Cardiol 49:1982, 2007.

83. Morrow DA, Scirica BM, Fox KA, et al: Evaluation of a novel antiplatelet agent for secondary prevention in patients with a history of atherosclerotic disease: Design and rationale for the Thrombin-Receptor Antagonist in Secondary Prevention of Atherothrombotic Ischemic Events (TRA 2 degrees P)-TIMI 50 trial. Am Heart J 158:335, 2009.

84. Go AS, Iribarren C, Chandra M, et al: Statin and beta-blocker therapy and the initial presentation of coronary heart disease. Ann Intern Med 144:229, 2006.

85. Bunch TJ, Muhlestein JB, Bair TL, et al: Effect of beta-blocker therapy on mortality rates and future myocardial infarction rates in patients with coronary artery disease but no history of myocardial infarction or congestive heart failure. Am J Cardiol 95:827, 2005.

86. Sipahi I, Tuzcu EM, Wolski KE, et al: Beta-blockers and progression of coronary atherosclerosis: Pooled analysis of 4 intravascular ultrasonography trials. Ann Intern Med 147:10, 2007.

87. Bangalore S, Messerli FH, Kostis JB, et al: Cardiovascular protection using beta-blockers: A critical review of the evidence. J Am Coll Cardiol 50:563, 2007.

88. Pacanowski MA, Gong Y, Cooper-Dehoff RM, et al: Beta-adrenergic receptor gene polymorphisms and beta-blocker treatment outcomes in hypertension. Clin Pharmacol Ther 84:715, 2008.

89. Al-Mallah MH, Tleyjeh IM, Abdel-Latif AA, et al: Angiotensin-converting enzyme inhibitors in coronary artery disease and preserved left ventricular systolic function: A systematic review and meta-analysis of randomized controlled trials. J Am Coll Cardiol 47:1576, 2006.

90. Braunwald E, Domanski MJ, Fowler SE, et al: Angiotensin-converting enzyme inhibition in stable coronary artery disease. N Engl J Med 351:2058, 2004.

91. Solomon SD, Rice MM, Jablonski KA, et al: Renal function and effectiveness of angiotensin-converting enzyme inhibitor therapy in patients with chronic stable coronary disease in the Prevention of Events with ACE inhibition (PEACE) trial. Circulation 114:26, 2006.

92. Yusuf S, Teo KK, Pogue J, et al: Telmisartan, ramipril, or both in patients at high risk for vascular events. N Engl J Med 358:1547, 2008.

93. Yusuf S, Teo K, Anderson C, et al: Effects of the angiotensin-receptor blocker telmisartan on cardiovascular events in high-risk patients intolerant to angiotensin-converting enzyme inhibitors: A randomised controlled trial. Lancet 372:1174, 2008.

94. Lonn E, Yusuf S, Arnold MJ, et al: Homocysteine lowering with folic acid and B vitamins in vascular disease. N Engl J Med 354:1567, 2006.

95. Bonaa KH, Njolstad I, Ueland PM, et al: Homocysteine lowering and cardiovascular events after acute myocardial infarction. N Engl J Med 354:1578, 2006.

96. Levonen A-L, Vahakangas E, Koponen JK, et al: Antioxidant gene therapy for cardiovascular disease: Current status and future perspectives. Circulation 117:2142, 2008.

97. Rutledge T, Vaccarino V, Johnson BD, et al: Depression and cardiovascular health care costs among women with suspected myocardial ischemia: Prospective results from the WISE (Women's Ischemia Syndrome Evaluation) Study. J Am Coll Cardiol 53:176, 2009.

98. Vaccarino V, Johnson BD, Sheps DS, et al: Depression, inflammation, and incident cardiovascular disease in women with suspected coronary ischemia: The National Heart, Lung, and Blood Institute-sponsored WISE study. J Am Coll Cardiol 50:2044, 2007.

99. Lesperance F, Frasure-Smith N, Koszycki D, et al: Effects of citalopram and interpersonal psychotherapy on depression in patients with coronary artery disease: the Canadian Cardiac Randomized Evaluation of Antidepressant and Psychotherapy Efficacy (CREATE) trial. JAMA 297:367, 2007.

100. Dimsdale JE: Psychological stress and cardiovascular disease. J Am Coll Cardiol 51:1237, 2008.

101. Lichtenstein AH, Appel LJ, Brands M, et al: Diet and lifestyle recommendations revision 2006: A scientific statement from the American Heart Association Nutrition Committee. Circulation 114:82, 2006.

102. Mozaffarian D, Wilson PW, Kannel WB: Beyond established and novel risk factors: Lifestyle risk factors for cardiovascular disease. Circulation 117:3031, 2008.

103. Kostis JB, Jackson G, Rosen R, et al: Sexual dysfunction and cardiac risk (the Second Princeton Consensus Conference). Am J Cardiol 96:85M, 2005.

104. Yang MF, Keng F, He ZX: Nitrate-augmented myocardial perfusion imaging for assessment of myocardial viability: Recent advances. Nucl Med Commun 30:415, 2009.

105. Wenzel P, Schulz E, Gori T, et al: Monitoring white blood cell mitochondrial aldehyde dehydrogenase activity: Implications for nitrate therapy in humans. J Pharmacol Exp Ther 330:63, 2009.

106. Gori T, Parker JD: Nitrate-induced toxicity and preconditioning: A rationale for reconsidering the use of these drugs. J Am Coll Cardiol 52:251, 2008.

107. Thomas GR, DiFabio JM, Gori T, et al: Once daily therapy with isosorbide-5-mononitrate causes endothelial dysfunction in humans: Evidence of a free-radical-mediated mechanism. J Am Coll Cardiol 49:1289, 2007.

108. Munzel T, Wenzel P, Daiber A: Do we still need organic nitrates? J Am Coll Cardiol 49:1296, 2007.

109. Kardas P: Comparison of once daily versus twice daily oral nitrates in stable angina pectoris. Am J Cardiol 94:213, 2004.

110. Jansen R, Cleophas TJ, Zwinderman AH, et al: Chronic nitrate therapy in patients with angina with comorbidity. Am J Ther 13:188, 2006.

111. Munzel T, Daiber A, Mulsch A: Explaining the phenomenon of nitrate tolerance. Circ Res 97:618, 2005.

112. Vlachopoulos C, Ioakeimidis N, Rokkas K, et al: Cardiovascular effects of phosphodiesterase type 5 inhibitors. J Sex Med 6:658, 2009.

113. Frishman WH: Fifty years of beta-adrenergic blockade: A golden era in clinical medicine and molecular pharmacology. Am J Med 121:933, 2008.

114. Egred M, Shaw S, Mohammad B, et al: Under-use of beta-blockers in patients with ischaemic heart disease and concomitant chronic obstructive pulmonary disease. QJM 98:493, 2005.

115. Munzel T, Gori T: Nebivolol: The somewhat-different beta-adrenergic receptor blocker. J Am Coll Cardiol 54:1491, 2009.

116. Cheng JW, Frishman WH, Aronow WS: Updates on cytochrome P450-mediated cardiovascular drug interactions. Am J Ther 16:155, 2009.

117. Lanfear DE, Jones PG, Marsh S, et al: Beta2-adrenergic receptor genotype and survival among patients receiving beta-blocker therapy after an acute coronary syndrome. JAMA 294:1526, 2005.

118. Hassan M, York KM, Li H, et al: Association of beta1-adrenergic receptor genetic polymorphism with mental stress-induced myocardial ischemia in patients with coronary artery disease. Arch Intern Med 168:763, 2008.

119. Liggett SB, Mialet-Perez J, Thaneemit-Chen S, et al: A polymorphism within a conserved beta-1-adrenergic receptor motif alters cardiac function and beta-blocker response in human heart failure. Proc Natl Acad Sci U S A 103:11288, 2006.

120. Ko DT, Hebert PR, Coffey CS, et al: Adverse effects of beta-blocker therapy for patients with heart failure: A quantitative overview of randomized trials. Arch Intern Med 164:1389, 2004.

121. Klapholz M: Beta-blocker use for the stages of heart failure. Mayo Clin Proc 84:718, 2009.

122. Bakris GL, Fonseca V, Katholi RE, et al: Metabolic effects of carvedilol versus metoprolol in patients with type 2 diabetes mellitus and hypertension: A randomized controlled trial. JAMA 292:2227, 2004.

123. Torp-Pedersen C, Metra M, Charlesworth A, et al: Effects of metoprolol and carvedilol on pre-existing and new onset diabetes in patients with chronic heart failure: Data from the Carvedilol Or Metoprolol European Trial (COMET). Heart 93:968, 2007.

124. Frishman WH: Calcium channel blockers: Differences between subclasses. Am J Cardiovasc Drugs 7(Suppl 1):17, 2007.

125. Luscher TF, Pieper M, Tendera M, et al: A randomized placebo-controlled study on the effect of nifedipine on coronary endothelial function and plaque formation in patients with coronary artery disease: The ENCORE II study. Eur Heart J 30:1590, 2009.

126. Nissen SE, Tuzcu EM, Libby P, et al: Effect of antihypertensive agents on cardiovascular events in patients with coronary disease and normal blood pressure: The CAMELOT study: A randomized controlled trial. JAMA 292:2217, 2004.

127. Bangalore S, Parkar S, Messerli FH: Long-acting calcium antagonists in patients with coronary artery disease: A meta-analysis. Am J Med 122:356, 2009.

128. Bangalore S, Messerli FH, Cohen JD, et al: Verapamil-sustained release-based treatment strategy is equivalent to atenolol-based treatment strategy at reducing cardiovascular events in patients with prior myocardial infarction: An INternational VErapamil SR-Trandolapril (INVEST) substudy. Am Heart J 156:241, 2008.

129. Chaitman BR: Ranolazine for the treatment of chronic angina and potential use in other cardiovascular conditions. Circulation 113:2462, 2006.

130. Rousseau MF, Pouleur H, Cocco G, et al: Comparative efficacy of ranolazine versus atenolol for chronic angina pectoris. Am J Cardiol 95:311, 2005.

131. Chaitman BR, Pepine CJ, Parker JO, et al: Effects of ranolazine with atenolol, amlodipine, or diltiazem on exercise tolerance and angina frequency in patients with severe chronic angina: A randomized controlled trial. JAMA 291:309, 2004.

132. Morrow DA, Scirica BM, Karwatowska-Prokopczuk E, et al: Effects of ranolazine on recurrent cardiovascular events in patients with non-ST-elevation acute coronary syndromes: The MERLIN-TIMI 36 randomized trial. JAMA 297:1775, 2007.

133. Wilson SR, Scirica BM, Braunwald E, et al: Efficacy of ranolazine in patients with chronic angina observations from the randomized, double-blind, placebo-controlled MERLIN-TIMI (Metabolic Efficiency With Ranolazine for Less Ischemia in Non-ST-Segment Elevation Acute Coronary Syndromes) 36 Trial. J Am Coll Cardiol 53:1510, 2009.

134. Antzelevitch C, Belardinelli L, Zygmunt AC, et al: Electrophysiological effects of ranolazine, a novel antianginal agent with antiarrhythmic properties. Circulation 110:904, 2004.

135. Scirica BM, Morrow DA, Hod H, et al: Effect of ranolazine, an antianginal agent with novel electrophysiological properties, on the incidence of arrhythmias in patients with non ST-segment elevation acute coronary syndrome: Results from the Metabolic Efficiency With Ranolazine for Less Ischemia in Non ST-Elevation Acute Coronary Syndrome Thrombolysis in

Myocardial Infarction 36 (MERLIN-TIMI 36) randomized controlled trial. Circulation 116:1647, 2007.

136. Morrow DA, Scirica BM, Chaitman BR, et al: Evaluation of the glycometabolic effects of ranolazine in patients with and without diabetes mellitus in the MERLIN-TIMI 36 randomized controlled trial. Circulation 119:2032, 2009.

137. Tardif JC, Ponikowski P, Kahan T: Efficacy of the I(f) current inhibitor ivabradine in patients with chronic stable angina receiving beta-blocker therapy: A 4-month, randomized, placebo-controlled trial. Eur Heart J 30:540, 2009.

138. Tardif JC, Ford I, Tendera M, et al: Efficacy of ivabradine, a new selective I(f) inhibitor, compared with atenolol in patients with chronic stable angina. Eur Heart J 26:2529, 2005.

139. Fox K, Ford I, Steg PG, et al: Ivabradine for patients with stable coronary artery disease and left-ventricular systolic dysfunction (BEAUTIFUL): A randomised, double-blind, placebo-controlled trial. Lancet 372:807, 2008.

140. Fox K, Ford I, Steg PG, et al: Relationship between ivabradine treatment and cardiovascular outcomes in patients with stable coronary artery disease and left ventricular systolic dysfunction with limiting angina: A subgroup analysis of the randomized, controlled BEAUTIFUL trial. Eur Heart J 30:2337, 2009.

141. Simpson D, Wellington K: Nicorandil: A review of its use in the management of stable angina pectoris, including high-risk patients. Drugs 64:1941, 2004.

142. Brown R, Lee A, Welfare M: Nicorandil-induced colonic ulceration. Heart 94:678, 2008.

143. Walker A, McMurray J, Stewart S, et al: Economic evaluation of the impact of nicorandil in angina (IONA) trial. Heart 92:619, 2006.

144. Vicari RM, Chaitman B, Keefe D, et al: Efficacy and safety of fasudil in patients with stable angina: A double-blind, placebo-controlled, phase 2 trial. J Am Coll Cardiol 46:1803, 2005.

145. Morrow DA, Givertz MM: Modulation of myocardial energetics: Emerging evidence for a therapeutic target in cardiovascular disease. Circulation 112:3218, 2005.

146. Eckert S, Horstkotte D: Management of angina pectoris: The role of spinal cord stimulation. Am J Cardiovasc Drugs 9:17, 2009.

147. Eddicks S, Maier-Hauff K, Schenk M, et al: Thoracic spinal cord stimulation improves functional status and relieves symptoms in patients with refractory angina pectoris: The first placebo-controlled randomised study. Heart 93:585, 2007.

148. Manchanda A, Soran O: Enhanced external counterpulsation and future directions: step beyond medical management for patients with angina and heart failure. J Am Coll Cardiol 50:1523, 2007.

149. Soran O, Kennard ED, Kfoury AG, et al: Two-year clinical outcomes after enhanced external counterpulsation (EECP) therapy in patients with refractory angina pectoris and left ventricular dysfunction (report from The International EECP Patient Registry). Am J Cardiol 97:17, 2006.

150. Akhtar M, Wu GF, Du ZM, et al: Effect of external counterpulsation on plasma nitric oxide and endothelin-1 levels. Am J Cardiol 98:28, 2006.

151. Fox K, Garcia MA, Ardissino D, et al: Guidelines on the management of stable angina pectoris: Executive summary: The Task Force on the Management of Stable Angina Pectoris of the European Society of Cardiology. Eur Heart J 27:1341, 2006.

152. Silber S, Albertsson P, Aviles FF, et al: Guidelines for percutaneous coronary interventions. The Task Force for Percutaneous Coronary Interventions of the European Society of Cardiology. Eur Heart J 26:804, 2005.

153. Eagle KA, Guyton RA, Davidoff R, et al: ACC/AHA 2004 guideline update for coronary artery bypass graft surgery: A report of the American College of Cardiology/American Heart Association Task Force on Practice Guidelines (Committee to Update the 1999 Guidelines for Coronary Artery Bypass Graft Surgery). Circulation 110:e340, 2004.

154. Pijls NH, van Schaardenburgh P, Manoharan G, et al: Percutaneous coronary intervention of functionally nonsignificant stenosis: 5-year follow-up of the DEFER Study. J Am Coll Cardiol 49:2105, 2007.

155. Phillips HR, O'Connor CM, Rogers J: Revascularization for heart failure. Am Heart J 153:65, 2007.

156. Tarakji KG, Brunken R, McCarthy PM, et al: Myocardial viability testing and the effect of early intervention in patients with advanced left ventricular systolic dysfunction. Circulation 113:230, 2006.

157. Dixon SR, Grines CL, O'Neill WW: The year in interventional cardiology. J Am Coll Cardiol 53:2080, 2009.

158. Wu C, Hannan EL, Walford G, et al: A risk score to predict in-hospital mortality for percutaneous coronary interventions. J Am Coll Cardiol 47:654, 2006.

159. Boden WE, Taggart DP: Diabetes with coronary disease—a moving target amid evolving therapies? N Engl J Med 360:2570, 2009.

160. Jeremias A, Kleiman NS, Nassif D, et al: Prevalence and prognostic significance of preprocedural cardiac troponin elevation among patients with stable coronary artery disease undergoing percutaneous coronary intervention: Results from the evaluation of drug eluting stents and ischemic events registry. Circulation 118:632, 2008.

161. Pinto Slottow TL, Waksman R: Overview of the 2007 Food and Drug Administration Circulatory System Devices Panel meeting on the endeavor zotarolimus-eluting coronary stent. Circulation 117:1603, 2008.

162. Malenka DJ, Kaplan AV, Lucas FL, et al: Outcomes following coronary stenting in the era of bare-metal versus the era of drug-eluting stents. JAMA 299:2868, 2008.

163. Katritsis DG, Ioannidis JP: Percutaneous coronary intervention versus conservative therapy in nonacute coronary artery disease: A meta-analysis. Circulation 111:2906, 2005.

164. Al Suwaidi J, Holmes DR Jr, Salam AM, et al: Impact of coronary artery stents on mortality and nonfatal myocardial infarction: Meta-analysis of randomized trials comparing a strategy of routine stenting with that of balloon angioplasty. Am Heart J 147:815, 2004.

164a. Brophy JM, Belisle P, Joseph L: Evidence for use of coronary stents: a hierarchical bayesian meta-analysis. Ann Int Med 138:777, 2003.

165. Hueb W, Lopes NH, Gersh BJ, et al: Five-year follow-up of the Medicine, Angioplasty, or Surgery Study (MASS II): A randomized controlled clinical trial of 3 therapeutic strategies for multivessel coronary artery disease. Circulation 115:1082, 2007.

166. Boden WE, O'Rourke RA, Teo KK, et al: Optimal medical therapy with or without PCI for stable coronary disease. N Engl J Med 356:1503, 2007.

167. Boden WE, O'Rourke RA, Teo KK, et al: The evolving pattern of symptomatic coronary artery disease in the United States and Canada: Baseline characteristics of the Clinical Outcomes Utilizing Revascularization and Aggressive DruG Evaluation (COURAGE) trial. Am J Cardiol 99:208, 2007.

168. Shaw LJ, Berman DS, Maron DJ, et al: Optimal medical therapy with or without percutaneous coronary intervention to reduce ischemic burden: Results from the Clinical Outcomes Utilizing Revascularization and Aggressive Drug Evaluation (COURAGE) trial nuclear substudy. Circulation 117:1283, 2008.
169. Gersh BJ, Frye RL: Methods of coronary revascularization—things may not be as they seem. N Engl J Med 352:2235, 2005.
170. Frye RL, August P, Brooks MM, et al: A randomized trial of therapies for type 2 diabetes and coronary artery disease. N Engl J Med 360:2503, 2009.
171. Keenan TD, Abu-Omar Y, Taggart DP: Bypassing the pump: Changing practices in coronary artery surgery. Chest 128:363, 2005.
172. Taggart DP: PCI or CABG in coronary artery disease? Lancet 373:1150, 2009.
173. Argenziano M, Katz M, Bonatti J, et al: Results of the prospective multicenter trial of robotically assisted totally endoscopic coronary artery bypass grafting. Ann Thorac Surg 81:1666, 2006.
174. Verma S, Fedak PW, Weisel RD, et al: Off-pump coronary artery bypass surgery: Fundamentals for the clinical cardiologist. Circulation 109:1206, 2004.
175. Sellke FW, DiMaio JM, Caplan LR, et al: Comparing on-pump and off-pump coronary artery bypass grafting: Numerous studies but few conclusions: A scientific statement from the American Heart Association council on cardiovascular surgery and anesthesia in collaboration with the interdisciplinary working group on quality of care and outcomes research. Circulation 111:2858, 2005.
176. Shroyer AL, Grover FL, Hattler B, et al: On-pump versus off-pump coronary-artery bypass surgery. N Engl J Med 361:1827, 2009.
177. Vassiliades TA Jr, Douglas JS, Morris DC, et al: Integrated coronary revascularization with drug-eluting stents: Immediate and seven-month outcome. J Thorac Cardiovasc Surg 131:956, 2006.
178. Wijeysundera DN, Beattie WS, Djaiani G, et al: Off-pump coronary artery surgery for reducing mortality and morbidity: meta-analysis of randomized and observational studies. J Am Coll Cardiol 46:872, 2005.
179. Jones RH: The year in cardiovascular surgery. J Am Coll Cardiol 47:2094, 2006.
180. Nishida H, Tomizawa Y, Endo M, et al: Survival benefit of exclusive use of in situ arterial conduits over combined use of arterial and vein grafts for multiple coronary artery bypass grafting. Circulation 112:I299, 2005.
181. Baskett RJ, Cafferty FH, Powell SJ, et al: Total arterial revascularization is safe: Multicenter ten-year analysis of 71,470 coronary procedures. Ann Thorac Surg 81:1243, 2006.
182. Lytle BW, Blackstone EH, Sabik JF, et al: The effect of bilateral internal thoracic artery grafting on survival during 20 postoperative years. Ann Thorac Surg 78:2005, 2004.
183. Okrainec K, Platt R, Pilote L, et al: Cardiac medical therapy in patients after undergoing coronary artery bypass graft surgery: A review of randomized controlled trials. J Am Coll Cardiol 45:177, 2005.
184. Stein PD, Schunemann HJ, Dalen JE, et al: Antithrombotic therapy in patients with saphenous vein and internal mammary artery bypass grafts: The Seventh ACCP Conference on Antithrombotic and Thrombolytic Therapy. Chest 126:600S, 2004.
185. Cram P, Rosenthal GE, Vaughan-Sarrazin MS: Cardiac revascularization in specialty and general hospitals. N Engl J Med 352:1454, 2005.
186. Society of Thoracic Surgeons: STS adult cardiac surgery database—Executive Summary. (http://www.sts.org).
187. Shahian DM, Blackstone EH, Edwards FH, et al: Cardiac surgery risk models: A position article. Ann Thorac Surg 78:1868, 2004.
188. Ramsay J, Shernan S, Fitch J, et al: Increased creatine kinase MB level predicts postoperative mortality after cardiac surgery independent of new Q waves. J Thorac Cardiovasc Surg 129:300, 2005.
189. Mangano DT, Miao Y, Tudor IC, et al: Post-reperfusion myocardial infarction: Long-term survival improvement using adenosine regulation with acadesine. J Am Coll Cardiol 48:206, 2006.
190. Dacey LJ, Likosky DS, Leavitt BJ, et al: Perioperative stroke and long-term survival after coronary bypass graft surgery. Ann Thorac Surg 79:532, 2005.
191. Samuels MA: Can cognition survive heart surgery? Circulation 113:2784, 2006.
192. Bar-Yosef S, Anders M, Mackensen GB, et al: Aortic atheroma burden and cognitive dysfunction after coronary artery bypass graft surgery. Ann Thorac Surg 78:1556, 2004.
193. Izhar U, Ad N, Rudis E, et al: When should we discontinue antiarrhythmic therapy for atrial fibrillation after coronary artery bypass grafting? A prospective randomized study. J Thorac Cardiovasc Surg 129:401, 2005.
194. Sedrakyan A, Zhang H, Treasure T, et al: Recursive partitioning-based preoperative risk stratification for atrial fibrillation after coronary artery bypass surgery. Am Heart J 151:720, 2006.
195. Marin F, Pascual DA, Roldan V, et al: Statins and postoperative risk of atrial fibrillation following coronary artery bypass grafting. Am J Cardiol 97:55, 2006.
196. Burns KE, Chu MW, Novick RJ, et al: Perioperative N-acetylcysteine to prevent renal dysfunction in high-risk patients undergoing CABG surgery: A randomized controlled trial. JAMA 294:342, 2005.
197. Topkara VK, Cheema FH, Kesavaramanujam S, et al: Coronary artery bypass grafting in patients with low ejection fraction. Circulation 112:I344, 2005.
198. Chareonthaitawee P, Gersh BJ, Araoz PA, et al: Revascularization in severe left ventricular dysfunction: the role of viability testing. J Am Coll Cardiol 46:567, 2005.
199. Gibbons RJ, Chareonthaitawee P, Bailey KR: Revascularization in systolic heart failure: A difficult decision. Circulation 113:180, 2006.
200. Klocke FJ. Resting blood flow in hypocontractile myocardium: Resolving the controversy. Circulation 112:3222, 2005.
201. Zaglavara T, Pillay T, Karvounis H, et al: Detection of myocardial viability by dobutamine stress echocardiography: Incremental value of diastolic wall thickness measurement. Heart 91:613, 2005.
202. Selvanayagam JB, Kardos A, Francis JM, et al: Value of delayed-enhancement cardiovascular magnetic resonance imaging in predicting myocardial viability after surgical revascularization. Circulation 110:1535, 2004.
203. Rizzello V, Poldermans D, Schinkel AF, et al: Long-term prognostic value of myocardial viability and ischaemia during dobutamine stress echocardiography in patients with ischaemic cardiomyopathy undergoing coronary revascularisation. Heart 92:239, 2006.
204. Velazquez EJ, Lee KL, O'Connor CM, et al: The rationale and design of the Surgical Treatment for Ischemic Heart Failure (STICH) trial. J Thorac Cardiovasc Surg 134:1540, 2007.
205. Jacobs AK: Women, ischemic heart disease, revascularization, and the gender gap: What are we missing? J Am Coll Cardiol 47:S63, 2006.
206. Blankstein R, Ward RP, Arnsdorf M, et al: Female gender is an independent predictor of operative mortality after coronary artery bypass graft surgery: Contemporary analysis of 31 Midwestern hospitals. Circulation 112:I323, 2005.
207. Peterson ED, Alexander KP, Malenka DJ, et al: Multicenter experience in revascularization of very elderly patients. Am Heart J 148:486, 2004.
208. Cooper WA, O'Brien SM, Thourani VH, et al: Impact of renal dysfunction on outcomes of coronary artery bypass surgery: Results from the Society of Thoracic Surgeons National Adult Cardiac Database. Circulation 113:1063, 2006.
209. Hillis GS, Croal BL, Buchan KG, et al: Renal function and outcome from coronary artery bypass grafting: Impact on mortality after a 2.3-year follow-up. Circulation 113:1056, 2006.
210. Flaherty JD, Davidson CJ: Diabetes and coronary revascularization. JAMA 293:1501, 2005.
211. Hannan EL, Wu C, Bennett EV, et al: Risk stratification of in-hospital mortality for coronary artery bypass graft surgery. J Am Coll Cardiol 47:661, 2006.
212. O'Rourke DJ, Quinton HB, Piper W, et al: Survival in patients with peripheral vascular disease after percutaneous coronary intervention and coronary artery bypass graft surgery. Ann Thorac Surg 78:466, 2004.
213. Sabik JF 3rd, Blackstone EH, Gillinov AM, et al: Occurrence and risk factors for reintervention after coronary artery bypass grafting. Circulation 114:I454, 2006.
214. Hannan EL, Racz MJ, Walford G, et al: Long-term outcomes of coronary-artery bypass grafting versus stent implantation. N Engl J Med 352:2174, 2005.
215. Serruys PW, Morice MC, Kappetein AP, et al: Percutaneous coronary intervention versus coronary-artery bypass grafting for severe coronary artery disease. N Engl J Med 360:961, 2009.
216. BARI Investigators: The final 10-year follow-up results from the BARI randomized trial. J Am Coll Cardiol 49:1600, 2007.
217. Barsness GW, Gersh BJ, Brooks MM, et al: Rationale for the revascularization arm of the Bypass Angioplasty Revascularization Investigation 2 Diabetes (BARI 2D) Trial. Am J Cardiol 97:31G, 2006.
218. Hlatky MA, Boothroyd DB, Bravata DM, et al: Coronary artery bypass surgery compared with percutaneous coronary interventions for multivessel disease: A collaborative analysis of individual patient data from ten randomised trials. Lancet 373:1190, 2009.
219. Farkouh ME, Dangas G, Leon MB, et al: Design of the Future REvascularization Evaluation in patients with Diabetes mellitus: Optimal management of Multivessel disease (FREEDOM) Trial. Am Heart J 155:215, 2008.
220. Kushner FG, Hand M, Smith SC Jr, et al: 2009 Focused Updates: ACC/AHA Guidelines for the Management of Patients With ST-Elevation Myocardial Infarction (updating the 2004 Guideline and 2007 Focused Update) and ACC/AHA/SCAI Guidelines on Percutaneous Coronary Intervention (updating the 2005 Guideline and 2007 Focused Update): A report of the American College of Cardiology Foundation/American Heart Association Task Force on Practice Guidelines. Circulation 120:2271, 2009.
221. Hannan EL, Racz M, Holmes DR, et al: Impact of completeness of percutaneous coronary intervention revascularization on long-term outcomes in the stent era. Circulation 113:2406, 2006.
222. Ong AT, Serruys PW, Mohr FW, et al: The SYNergy between percutaneous coronary intervention with TAXus and cardiac surgery (SYNTAX) study: Design, rationale, and run-in phase. Am Heart J 151:1194, 2006.
223. Bridges CR, Horvath KA, Nugent WC, et al: The Society of Thoracic Surgeons practice guideline series: Transmyocardial laser revascularization. Ann Thorac Surg 77:1494, 2004.
224. Bugiardini R, Bairey Merz CN: Angina with "normal" coronary arteries: A changing philosophy. JAMA 293:477, 2005.
225. Johnson BD, Shaw LJ, Buchthal SD, et al: Prognosis in women with myocardial ischemia in the absence of obstructive coronary disease: Results from the National Institutes of Health-National Heart, Lung, and Blood Institute-Sponsored Women's Ischemia Syndrome Evaluation (WISE). Circulation 109:2993, 2004.
226. Bugiardini R: Women, 'non-specific' chest pain, and normal or near-normal coronary angiograms are not synonymous with favourable outcome. Eur Heart J 27:1387, 2006.
227. Valeriani M, Sestito A, Le Pera D, et al: Abnormal cortical pain processing in patients with cardiac syndrome X. Eur Heart J 26:975, 2005.
228. Handberg E, Johnson BD, Arant CB, et al: Impaired coronary vascular reactivity and functional capacity in women: Results from the NHLBI Women's Ischemia Syndrome Evaluation (WISE) Study. J Am Coll Cardiol 47:S44, 2006.
229. Johnson BD, Shaw LJ, Pepine CJ, et al: Persistent chest pain predicts cardiovascular events in women without obstructive coronary artery disease: Results from the NIH-NHLBI-sponsored Women's Ischaemia Syndrome Evaluation (WISE) study. Eur Heart J 27:1408, 2006.
230. Stern S: Symptoms other than chest pain may be important in the diagnosis of "silent ischemia," or "the sounds of silence." Circulation 111:e435, 2005.
231. Gazzaruso C, Solerte SB, De Amici E, et al: Association of the metabolic syndrome and insulin resistance with silent myocardial ischemia in patients with type 2 diabetes mellitus. Am J Cardiol 97:236, 2006.
232. Sajadieh A, Nielsen OW, Rasmussen V, et al: Prevalence and prognostic significance of daily-life silent myocardial ischaemia in middle-aged and elderly subjects with no apparent heart disease. Eur Heart J 26:1402, 2005.
233. Enseleit F, Duru F: Long-term continuous external electrocardiographic recording: A review. Europace 8:255, 2006.
234. Erne P, Schoenenberger AW, Burckhardt D, et al: Effects of percutaneous coronary interventions in silent ischemia after myocardial infarction: The SWISSI II randomized controlled trial. JAMA 297:1985, 2007.
235. Flaherty JD, Bax JJ, De Luca L, et al: Acute heart failure syndromes in patients with coronary artery disease early assessment and treatment. J Am Coll Cardiol 53:254, 2009.
236. Dickstein K, Cohen-Solal A, Filippatos G, et al: ESC guidelines for the diagnosis and treatment of acute and chronic heart failure 2008: The Task Force for the diagnosis and treatment of acute and chronic heart failure 2008 of the European Society of Cardiology. Developed in collaboration with the Heart Failure Association of the ESC (HFA) and endorsed by the European Society of Intensive Care Medicine (ESICM). Eur J Heart Fail 10:933, 2008.

237. Carluccio E, Biagioli P, Alunni G, et al: Patients with hibernating myocardium show altered left ventricular volumes and shape, which revert after revascularization: Evidence that dyssynergy might directly induce cardiac remodeling. J Am Coll Cardiol 47:969, 2006.

238. Mickleborough LL, Merchant N, Ivanov J, et al: Left ventricular reconstruction: Early and late results. J Thorac Cardiovasc Surg 128:27, 2004.

239. Lundblad R, Abdelnoor M, Geiran OR, et al: Surgical repair of postinfarction ventricular septal rupture: Risk factors of early and late death. J Thorac Cardiovasc Surg 137:862, 2009.

240. Jones RH, Velazquez EJ, Michler RE, et al: Coronary bypass surgery with or without surgical ventricular reconstruction. N Engl J Med 360:1705, 2009.

241. Borger MA, Alam A, Murphy PM, et al: Chronic ischemic mitral regurgitation: Repair, replace or rethink? Ann Thorac Surg 81:1153, 2006.

242. Wu AH, Aaronson KD, Bolling SF, et al: Impact of mitral valve annuloplasty on mortality risk in patients with mitral regurgitation and left ventricular systolic dysfunction. J Am Coll Cardiol 45:381, 2005.

243. Kang DH, Kim MJ, Kang SJ, et al: Mitral valve repair versus revascularization alone in the treatment of ischemic mitral regurgitation. Circulation 114:I499, 2006.

243a. Gardner TJ, O'Gara PT. The cardiothoracic surgery network: Randomized clinical trials in the operating room. J Thorac Cardiovasc Surg 139:830, 2010.

244. Rigatelli G, Docali G, Rossi P, et al: Validation of a clinical-significance-based classification of coronary artery anomalies. Angiology 56:25, 2005.

245. Eckart RE, Scoville SL, Campbell CL, et al: Sudden death in young adults: A 25-year review of autopsies in military recruits. Ann Intern Med 141:829, 2004.

246. Alegria JR, Herrmann J, Holmes DR Jr, et al: Myocardial bridging. Eur Heart J 26:1159, 2005.

247. Egred M, Viswanathan G, Davis GK: Myocardial infarction in young adults. Postgrad Med J 81:741, 2005.

248. Jones JH, Weir WB: Cocaine-associated chest pain. Med Clin North Am 89:1323, 2005.

GUIDELINES David A. Morrow and William E. Boden

Chronic Stable Angina

The American College of Cardiology and the American Heart Association (ACC/AHA) updated guidelines for the management of patients with stable chest pain syndromes and known or suspected ischemic heart disease in 2002.[1] Populations addressed by these guidelines include patients with "ischemic equivalents" such as dyspnea or arm pain with exertion and patients with ischemic heart disease who have become asymptomatic, including those who have undergone revascularization procedures. Patients with unstable ischemic syndromes are not included in these guidelines but are instead addressed in guidelines summarized in Chap. 53 Guidelines. As with other ACC/AHA guidelines, indications for interventions are classified into the following four groups:

Class I—for generally accepted indications
Class IIa—when indications are controversial, but the weight of evidence is supportive
Class IIb—when usefulness or efficacy is less well established
Class III—when there is consensus against the usefulness of the intervention

The guidelines use a convention for rating levels of evidence on which recommendations have been based, as follows:

Level A—derived from data from multiple randomized clinical trials
Level B—derived from a single randomized trial or nonrandomized studies
Level C—based on the consensus opinion of experts

OVERVIEW

The ACC/AHA guidelines emphasize the importance of detailed symptom history, focused physical examination, and directed risk factor assessment for patients presenting with chest pain. These data are to be used by the clinician to estimate the probability of significant coronary artery disease (CAD) as low, intermediate, or high. For patients with a low probability of coronary disease (e.g., ≤5%), cardiovascular interventions should be limited, whereas noncardiac causes of chest pain should be evaluated (**Fig. 57G-1**). Recommended initial tests are summarized in **Table 57G-1**. The routine use of chest radiographs or multidetector computed tomography (CT) is not recommended.[2]

For patients with an intermediate or high probability of coronary disease, the clinician should exclude unstable ischemic syndromes and conditions that might exacerbate or cause angina. If these are not present, noninvasive testing should be considered to refine the diagnostic assessment of patients with an intermediate probability of coronary disease and to perform risk stratification for patients with a high probability of coronary disease (**Fig. 57G-2**).

The ACC/AHA guidelines do not mandate exercise testing in all such patients. Pharmacologic imaging studies are recommended for patients who are unable to exercise. Exercise imaging studies are recommended for patients who have had previous coronary revascularization or whose resting electrocardiograms (ECGs) are uninterpretable. Imaging studies are also supported when the clinical evaluation and exercise ECGs have not provided sufficient information to guide management. If the results of noninvasive studies suggest a high risk for complications of coronary heart disease, coronary angiography and revascularization should be considered.

The treatment algorithm recommended by the ACC/AHA guidelines emphasizes the importance of patient education about coronary disease, prevention of ischemia through use of nitrates, beta blockers, and calcium blockers, and prevention of progression of atherosclerosis through risk factor management (**Fig. 57G-3**).

The ACC/AHA guidelines require clarity from the clinician in defining the critical issues for the individual patient. For patients with a chest pain complaint of uncertain cause, the dominant question may be whether coronary artery disease is present or absent (diagnosis). For patients with known or strongly suspected coronary disease, the focus is likely to be on the patient's risk. In these guidelines a specific test may be considered an appropriate option for addressing one or the other of these issues.

The guidelines clearly differentiate between indications for the same tests for the purpose of diagnosis and risk stratification. For example, exercise ECGs are discouraged for establishing diagnosis in patients with a high clinical probability of coronary artery disease on the basis of age, gender, and symptoms (Class IIb indication). However, exercise ECGs are strongly supported as a Class I indication when used to assess prognosis in this same patient population. Thus, interpretation of these guidelines demands rigorous definition of the clinical question at hand.

DIAGNOSIS

Noninvasive Studies

Exercise Electrocardiography

Exercise testing is considered most valuable for diagnosis when the patient's other clinical data suggest an intermediate probability of coronary disease. The ACC/AHA guidelines support the use of exercise ECGs for such patients unless their baseline ECGs show abnormalities likely to render the exercise tracing uninterpretable (**Table 57G-2**). However, exercise ECGs were considered appropriate for patients with complete right bundle branch block or less than 1 mm of ST depression at rest. Use of the exercise test was considered of uncertain value (Class IIb) for patients with high or low pretest probability of coronary disease or those who had less than 1 mm of ST depression and were either using digoxin or had ECG evidence of left ventricular hypertrophy.

Echocardiography

The ACC/AHA guidelines state that "most patients undergoing a diagnostic evaluation for angina do not need an echocardiogram." Echocardiograms are supported to evaluate systolic murmurs suggestive of aortic stenosis or hypertrophic cardiomyopathy and for evaluation of the extent of ischemia when the study can be obtained within 30 minutes after the end of an ischemic episode (**Table 57G-3**). However, routine use of echocardiography for patients with a normal ECG, no history of myocardial infarction, and no evidence of structural heart disease is considered inappropriate (Class III).

Stress Imaging Studies

The ACC/AHA guidelines recommend stress imaging as opposed to exercise ECG in the following: (1) patients who have complete left bundle branch block, electronically paced ventricular rhythm, preexcitation (Wolff-Parkinson-White) syndrome, and other electrocardiographic conduction abnormalities; (2) patients who have more than 1 mm of ST-segment depression at rest including those with left ventricular

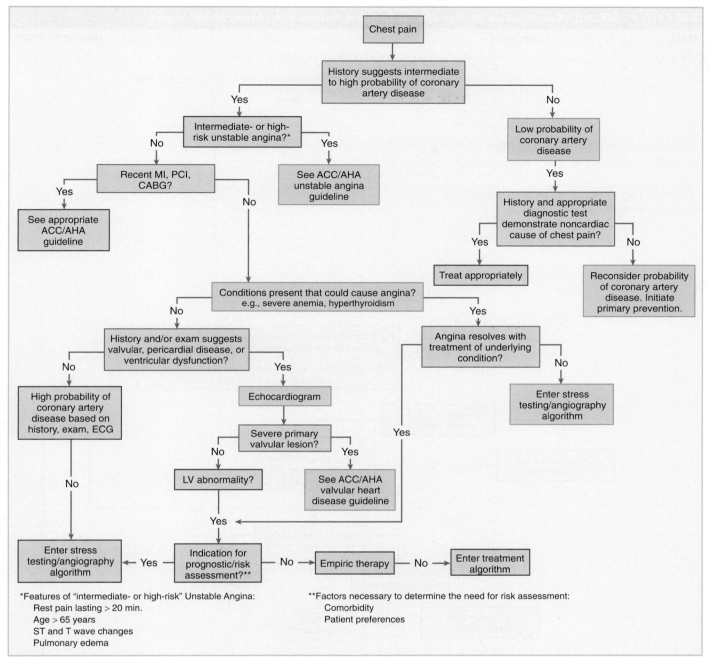

FIGURE 57G-1 Approach to the clinical assessment of chest pain. *(From ACC/AHA 2002 guideline update for the management of patients with chronic stable angina: A report of the American College of Cardiology/American Heart Association Task Force on Practice Guidelines [Committee to Update the 1999 Guidelines for the Management of Patients with Chronic Stable Angina], p 8.) (http://www.acc.org/qualityandscience/clinical/guidelines/stable/stable_clean.pdf.)*

hypertrophy or taking drugs such as digitalis; (3) patients who are unable to exercise to a level high enough to give meaningful results on exercise ECGs; and (4) patients with coronary disease who have undergone prior revascularization, for whom localization of ischemia and establishing the significance of lesions is important.

The guidelines specify that exercise stress testing is preferable to pharmacologic stress testing when the patient can exercise to develop an appropriate level of cardiovascular stress (e.g., 6 to 12 minutes). **Tables 57G-4** and **57G-5** summarize the appropriate indications for stress imaging in patients who are and who are not able to exercise, respectively. As is the case with exercise ECGs, these tests are considered most useful for diagnosis in patients with an intermediate probability of disease.

The guidelines comment on the choice among stress imaging technologies. They conclude that dobutamine perfusion imaging has significant limitations compared with dipyridamole or adenosine perfusion imaging because it does not provoke as great an increase in coronary flow. Therefore, the guidelines recommend that dobutamine be used to provoke ischemia for perfusion imaging only when patients have contraindications to the other agents. In contrast, dobutamine is the agent of choice for pharmacologic stress echocardiography because it enhances myocardial contractile performance and wall motion, which can be observed directly by echocardiography.

Specific Patient Subsets

Although treadmill electrocardiographic testing is less accurate for diagnosis in women than in men, the guidelines note that the diagnostic performance of imaging technologies is also compromised by technical issues (e.g., breast tissue) in women. Therefore, the guidelines conclude

TABLE 57G-1	ACC/AHA Guidelines for Routine Clinical Testing in Patients with Chronic Stable Angina	
CLASS	INDICATION	LEVEL OF EVIDENCE*
I (indicated)	1. Rest ECG in patients without obvious noncardiac cause of chest pain	B
	2. Rest ECG during an episode of chest pain	B
	3. Chest radiograph in patients with signs or symptoms of congestive heart failure, valvular heart disease, pericardial disease, or aortic dissection or aneurysm	B
	4. Hemoglobin	C
	5. Fasting glucose	C
	6. Fasting lipid panel	C
IIa (good supportive evidence)	Chest radiograph in patients with signs or symptoms of pulmonary disease	B
IIb (weak supportive evidence)	1. Chest radiograph in other patients	C
	2. Electron beam CT	B
III (not indicated)	None	

*See guidelines text for definitions of level of evidence.

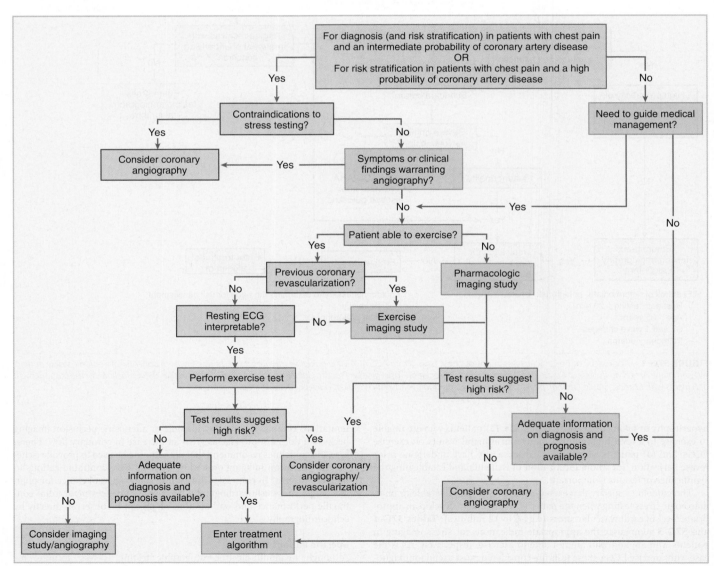

FIGURE 57G-2 Stress testing and angiography in patients with chest pain. *(From ACC/AHA 2002 guideline update for the management of patients with chronic stable angina: A report of the American College of Cardiology/American Heart Association Task Force on Practice Guidelines [Committee to Update the 1999 Guidelines for the Management of Patients with Chronic Stable Angina], p 9.) (http://www.acc.org/qualityandscience/clinical/guidelines/stable/stable_clean.pdf.)*

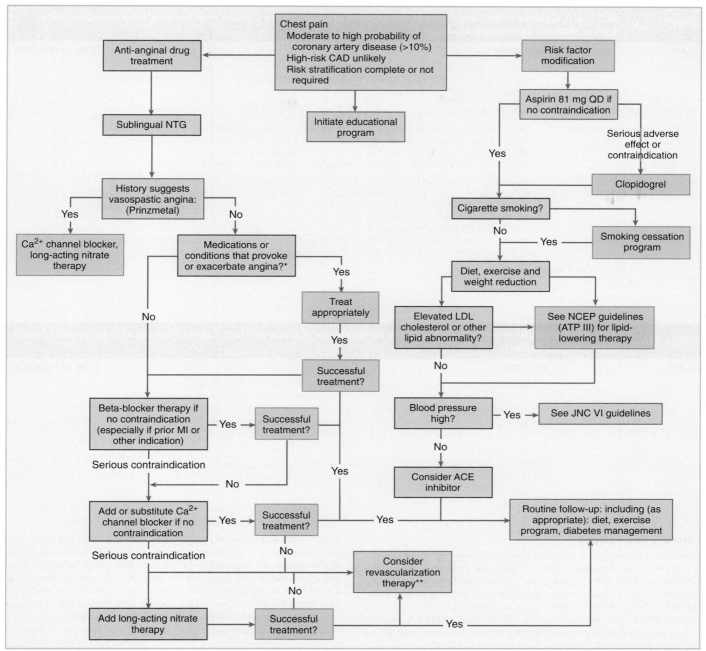

FIGURE 57G-3 Approach to the treatment of chest pain. CAD = coronary artery disease; JNC = Joint National Committee; NCEP = National Cholesterol Education Program; NTG = nitroglycerin. *Conditions that exacerbate or provoke angina are medications (e.g., vasodilators, excessive thyroid replacement, and vasoconstrictors), other cardiac problems (e.g., tachyarrhythmias, bradyarrhythmias, valvular heart disease, especially aortic stenosis), and other medical problems (e.g., hypertrophic cardiomyopathy, profound anemia, uncontrolled hypertension, hyperthyroidism, hypoxemia). **At any point in this process, based on coronary anatomy, severity of anginal symptoms, and patient preferences, it is reasonable to consider evaluation for coronary revascularization. Unless a patient is documented to have left main, triple-vessel, or double-vessel coronary artery disease with significant stenosis of the proximal left anterior descending coronary artery, there is no demonstrated survival advantage associated with revascularization in low-risk patients with chronic stable angina; thus, medical therapy should be attempted in most patients before considering percutaneous coronary intervention or coronary artery bypass grafting. (From ACC/AHA 2002 guideline update for the management of patients with chronic stable angina: A report of the American College of Cardiology/American Heart Association Task Force on Practice Guidelines [Committee to Update the 1999 Guidelines for the Management of Patients with Chronic Stable Angina], p 10.) (http://www.acc.org/qualityandscience/clinical/guidelines/stable/stable_clean.pdf.)

that "there currently are insufficient data to justify replacing standard exercise testing with stress imaging in the initial evaluation of women."

The ACC/AHA guidelines discourage the use of noninvasive testing for coronary disease with and without imaging for asymptomatic patients. No Class I and Class IIa indications exist for exercise testing of asymptomatic patients, and there is just one Class IIb indication (weak support):

asymptomatic patients with possible myocardial ischemia on ambulatory ECG monitoring or with severe coronary calcification on electron beam CT scanning. Myocardial perfusion imaging testing also receives only weak support (Class IIb) for asymptomatic patients who, despite the recommendations of guidelines, had undergone exercise ECGs and who had an intermediate-risk or high-risk Duke treadmill score or an inadequate exercise ECG.

TABLE 57G-2 ACC/AHA Guidelines for Diagnosis of Obstructive Coronary Artery Disease with Exercise Electrocardiographic Testing Without an Imaging Modality

CLASS	INDICATION	LEVEL OF EVIDENCE*
I (indicated)	Patients with intermediate pretest probability of CAD based on age, gender, and symptoms, including those with complete right bundle branch block or <1 mm of ST-segment depression at rest (exceptions are listed in Classes II and III)	B
IIa (good supportive evidence)	Patients with suspected vasospastic angina	C
IIb (weak supportive evidence)	1. Patients with a high pretest probability of CAD by age, gender, and symptoms	B
	2. Patients with a low pretest probability of CAD by age, gender, and symptoms	B
	3. Patients taking digoxin whose ECG has <1 mm of baseline ST-segment depression	B
	4. Patients with ECG criteria for LVH and <1 mm of baseline ST-segment depression	B
III (not indicated)	1. Patients with the following baseline electrocardiographic abnormalities:	
	a. Preexcitation (Wolff-Parkinson-White) syndrome	B
	b. Electronically paced ventricular rhythm	B
	c. >1 mm of ST-segment depression at rest	B
	d. Complete left bundle branch block	B
	2. Patients with an established diagnosis of CAD because of prior myocardial infarction or coronary angiography; however, testing can assess functional capacity and prognosis	

*See guidelines text for definitions of level of evidence.
LVH = left ventricular hypertrophy.

TABLE 57G-3 ACC/AHA Guidelines for Echocardiography for Diagnosis of Cause of Chest Pain in Patients with Suspected Chronic Stable Angina Pectoris

CLASS	INDICATION	LEVEL OF EVIDENCE*
I (indicated)	1. Patients with systolic murmur suggestive of aortic stenosis or hypertrophic cardiomyopathy	C
	2. Evaluation of extent (severity) of ischemia (e.g., LV segmental wall motion abnormality) when the echocardiogram can be obtained during pain or within 30 min after its abatement	C
IIa (good supportive evidence)		
IIb (weak supportive evidence)	Patients with a click or murmur to diagnose mitral valve prolapse	C
III (not indicated)	Patients with a normal ECG, no history of myocardial infarction, and no signs or symptoms suggestive of heart failure, valvular heart disease, or hypertrophic cardiomyopathy	C

*See guidelines text for definitions of level of evidence.

Coronary Angiography

Coronary angiography is a necessary step for the management of patients for whom revascularization with percutaneous coronary intervention (PCI) or coronary artery bypass grafting (CABG) is likely to be beneficial because of a high risk for complications with medical therapy alone. Thus, the ACC/AHA guidelines support coronary angiography for diagnosis in patients with angina who have survived sudden death (**Table 57G-6**). The guidelines consider coronary angiography to be possibly indicated (Class IIa) when patients with chest pain have contraindications to noninvasive testing or such testing is inadequate or likely to be inadequate to guide management.

The committee thought that noninvasive and clinical data are usually sufficient to establish or exclude the diagnosis of coronary disease and that coronary angiography should rarely be used for this purpose. The guidelines assert that coronary angiography is "generally not indicated" for diagnosis in asymptomatic patients. They offer only weak support (Class IIb) for coronary angiography to establish a definitive diagnosis for patients with recurrent hospitalization for chest pain.

RISK STRATIFICATION

The ACC/AHA guidelines emphasize the following four factors that predict survival for patients with coronary artery disease: (1) left ventricular function; (2) anatomic extent and severity of coronary atherosclerosis; (3) presence of recent plaque rupture; and (4) the patient's general health and noncoronary comorbidity.

Assessment of Left Ventricular Function

The guidelines consider assessment of left ventricular function with either echocardiography or radionuclide angiography appropriate (Class I) in patients with symptoms or signs of heart failure, a history of prior myocardial infarction, or pathologic Q waves on the ECG. Echocardiography is also considered appropriate for patients with mitral regurgitation to assess its severity and cause and for patients with complex ventricular arrhythmias to assess left ventricular function. However, the guidelines note that a normal ECG correlates strongly with normal left ventricular function at rest and therefore do not endorse echocardiography as a routine test for patients with a normal ECG, no history of myocardial infarction, and no symptoms or signs of congestive heart failure. They also do not support routine periodic echocardiography for stable patients in whom no new change in therapy is contemplated.

Noninvasive Tests for Ischemia

Exercise testing is recommended for assessment of prognosis for all patients with an intermediate or high probability of coronary artery disease, except those with electrocardiographic abnormalities that compromise interpretation of the exercise tracing and those for which the information is unlikely to alter management (**Table 57G-7**). The committee directly addressed the issue of whether the additional information provided by imaging technologies might make them preferable tests for risk stratification but concluded that the greater costs of these tests could not be justified for most patients. Therefore, the guidelines endorse a stepwise approach in which the exercise ECG is used as the initial test in patients who are not taking digoxin, have a normal rest ECG, and are able to exercise.

The ACC/AHA guidelines support the use of stress testing with echocardiographic or radionuclide imaging to identify the severity of ischemia in patients who have electrocardiographic abnormalities precluding interpretation of the exercise tracing and for patients in whom the functional

TABLE 57G-4	ACC/AHA Guidelines for Cardiac Stress Imaging as Initial Diagnostic Test for Patients with Chronic Stable Angina Who Are Able to Exercise	
CLASS	**INDICATION**	**LEVEL OF EVIDENCE***
I (indicated)	1. Exercise myocardial perfusion imaging or exercise echocardiography in patients with intermediate pretest probability of CAD who have one of the following baseline electrocardiographic abnormalities:	
	a. Preexcitation (Wolff-Parkinson-White) syndrome	B
	b. >1 mm of ST-segment depression at rest	B
	2. Exercise myocardial perfusion imaging or exercise echocardiography in patients with prior revascularization (either PCI or CABG)	B
	3. Adenosine or dipyridamole myocardial perfusion imaging in patients with intermediate pretest probability of CAD and one of the following baseline ECG abnormalities:	
	a. Electronically paced ventricular rhythm	C
	b. Left bundle branch block	B
IIa (good supportive evidence)		
IIb (weak supportive evidence)	1. Exercise myocardial perfusion imaging or exercise echocardiography in patients with low or high probability of CAD who have one of the following baseline ECG abnormalities:	
	a. Preexcitation (Wolff-Parkinson-White) syndrome	B
	b. >1 mm of ST-segment depression	B
	2. Adenosine or dipyridamole myocardial perfusion imaging in patients with low or high probability of CAD and one of the following baseline electrocardiographic abnormalities:	
	a. Electronically paced ventricular rhythm	C
	b. Left bundle branch block	B
	3. Exercise myocardial perfusion imaging or exercise echocardiography in patients with intermediate probability of CAD who have one of the following:	
	a. Digoxin use with <1 mm ST-segment depression on the baseline ECG	B
	b. LVH with <1 mm ST-segment depression on the baseline ECG	B
	4. Exercise myocardial perfusion imaging, exercise echocardiography, adenosine or dipyridamole myocardial perfusion imaging, or dobutamine echocardiography as the initial stress test in a patient with a normal rest ECG who is not taking digoxin	B
	5. Exercise or dobutamine echocardiography in patients with left bundle branch block	C
III (not indicated)		

*See guidelines text for definitions of level of evidence.

TABLE 57G-5	ACC/AHA Guidelines for Cardiac Stress Imaging as Initial Diagnostic Test for Patients with Chronic Stable Angina Who Are Unable to Exercise	
CLASS	**INDICATION**	**LEVEL OF EVIDENCE***
I (indicated)	1. Adenosine or dipyridamole myocardial perfusion imaging or dobutamine echocardiography in patients with intermediate pretest probability of CAD	B
	2. Adenosine or dipyridamole myocardial perfusion imaging or dobutamine echocardiography in patients with prior revascularization (either PCI or CABG)	B
IIa (good supportive evidence)		
IIb (weak supportive evidence)	1. Adenosine or dipyridamole myocardial perfusion imaging or dobutamine echocardiography in patients with low or high probability of CAD in absence of electronically paced ventricular rhythm or left bundle branch block	B
	2. Adenosine or dipyridamole myocardial perfusion imaging in patients with low or high probability of CAD and one of the following baseline ECG abnormalities:	
	a. Electronically paced ventricular rhythm	C
	b. Left bundle branch block	B
	3. Dobutamine echocardiography in patients with left bundle branch block	C
III (not indicated)		

*See guidelines text for definitions of level of evidence.

significance of coronary lesions will guide management (**Tables 57G-8 and 57G-9**). Dipyridamole or adenosine myocardial perfusion imaging is recommended for patients with left bundle branch block or electronically paced ventricular rhythms because of higher rates of false-positive septal perfusion defects with exercise than with dipyridamole or adenosine. Relatively few data exist on the performance of dobutamine echocardiography in this setting, so this approach is not endorsed by the guidelines for patients with left bundle branch block or electronically paced ventricular rhythms. Stress imaging studies are also supported for assessment of the functional significance of coronary lesions in planning PCI.

The guidelines discourage the use of noninvasive testing for risk stratification of patients who have no symptoms of coronary disease. No Class

I or IIa indications exist for the use of cardiac stress imaging as an initial test for risk stratification. Supporting evidence is considered weak for the use of cardiac stress imaging for asymptomatic patients with severe coronary calcification on electron beam CT or who had undergone an exercise ECG and had inadequate tests or intermediate- or high-risk Duke treadmill scores.

Coronary Angiography

In the ACC/AHA guidelines, the decision to proceed to coronary angiography should be based on symptomatic status and risk stratification derived from clinical data and noninvasive test results. The guidelines define noninvasive findings that predict a high (>3%), intermediate (1%

CH
57

TABLE 57G-6 ACC/AHA Guidelines for Coronary Angiography to Establish a Diagnosis in Patients with Suspected Angina*

CLASS	INDICATION	LEVEL OF EVIDENCE[†]
I (indicated)	Patients with known or possible angina pectoris who have survived sudden cardiac death	B
IIa (good supportive evidence)	1. Patients with an uncertain diagnosis after noninvasive testing for whom the benefit of a more certain diagnosis outweighs the risk and cost of coronary angiography	C
	2. Patients who cannot undergo noninvasive testing because of disability, illness, or morbid obesity	C
	3. Patients with an occupational requirement for a definitive diagnosis	C
	4. Patients who because of young age at onset of symptoms, noninvasive imaging, or other clinical parameters are suspected of having a nonatherosclerotic cause for myocardial ischemia (e.g., coronary artery anomaly, Kawasaki disease, primary coronary artery dissection, radiation-induced vasculopathy)	C
	5. Patients in whom coronary artery spasm is suspected and provocative testing may be necessary	C
	6. Patients with high pretest probability of left main or triple-vessel CAD	C
IIb (weak supportive evidence)	1. Patients with recurrent hospitalization for chest pain in whom a definite diagnosis is judged necessary	C
	2. Patients with an overriding desire for a definitive diagnosis and intermediate or high probability of CAD	C
III (not indicated)	1. Patients with significant comorbidity in whom the risk of coronary arteriography outweighs the benefit of the procedure	C
	2. Patients with an overriding personal desire for a definitive diagnosis and a low probability of CAD	C

*Including those with known CAD who have a significant change in anginal symptoms.
†See guidelines text for definitions of level of evidence.

TABLE 57G-7 ACC/AHA Guidelines for Exercise Testing Risk Assessment and Prognosis in Patients with an Intermediate or High Probability of Coronary Artery Disease

CLASS	INDICATION	LEVEL OF EVIDENCE*
I (indicated)	1. Patients undergoing initial evaluation (exceptions are listed below in Classes IIb and III)	B
	2. Patients after a significant change in cardiac symptoms	C
IIa (good supportive evidence)		
IIb (weak supportive evidence)	1. Patients with the following electrocardiographic abnormalities:	
	a. Preexcitation (Wolff-Parkinson-White) syndrome	B
	b. Electronically paced ventricular rhythm	B
	c. >1 mm of ST-segment depression at rest	B
	d. Complete left bundle branch block	B
	2. Patients who have undergone cardiac catheterization to identify ischemia in the distribution of coronary lesion of borderline severity	C
	3. Postrevascularization patients who have a significant change in anginal pattern suggestive of ischemia	C
III (not indicated)	Patients with severe comorbidity likely to limit life expectancy or prevent revascularization	C

*See guidelines text for definitions of level of evidence.

TABLE 57G-8 ACC/AHA Guidelines for Cardiac Stress Imaging as Initial Test for Risk Stratification of Patients with Chronic Stable Angina Who Are Able to Exercise

CLASS	INDICATION	LEVEL OF EVIDENCE*
I (indicated)	1. Exercise myocardial perfusion imaging or exercise echocardiography to identify the extent, severity, and location of ischemia in patients who do not have left bundle branch block or an electronically paced ventricular rhythm, and who have an abnormal rest ECG or are using digoxin	B
	2. Dipyridamole or adenosine myocardial perfusion imaging in patients with left bundle branch block or electronically paced ventricular rhythm	B
	3. Exercise myocardial perfusion imaging or exercise echocardiography to assess the functional significance of coronary lesions (if not already known) when planning PCI	B
IIa (good supportive evidence)		
IIb (weak supportive evidence)	1. Exercise or dobutamine echocardiography in patients with left bundle branch block	C
	2. Exercise, dipyridamole, or adenosine myocardial perfusion imaging, or exercise or dobutamine echocardiography, as the initial test in patients who have a normal rest ECG and are not taking digoxin	B
III (not indicated)	1. Exercise myocardial perfusion imaging in patients with left bundle branch block	C
	2. Exercise, dipyridamole, or adenosine myocardial perfusion imaging, or exercise or dobutamine echocardiography, in patients with severe comorbidity likely to limit life expectation or prevent revascularization	C

*See guidelines text for definitions of level of evidence.

TABLE 57G-9	ACC/AHA Guidelines for Cardiac Stress Imaging as Initial Test for Risk Stratification of Patients with Chronic Stable Angina Who Are Unable to Exercise	
CLASS	**INDICATION**	**LEVEL OF EVIDENCE***
I (indicated)	1. Dipyridamole or adenosine myocardial perfusion imaging or dobutamine echocardiography to identify the extent, severity, and location of ischemia in patients who do not have left bundle branch block or electronically paced ventricular rhythm	B
	2. Dipyridamole or adenosine myocardial perfusion imaging in patients with left bundle branch block or electronically paced ventricular rhythm	B
	3. Dipyridamole or adenosine myocardial perfusion imaging or dobutamine echocardiography to assess the functional significance of coronary lesions (if not already known) when planning PCI	B
IIa (good supportive evidence)		
IIb (weak supportive evidence)	Dobutamine echocardiography in patients with left bundle branch block	C
III (not indicated)	Dipyridamole or adenosine myocardial perfusion imaging or dobutamine echocardiography in patients with severe comorbidity likely to limit life expectation or prevent revascularization	C

*See guidelines text for definitions of level of evidence.

TABLE 57G-10	ACC/AHA Guideline Criteria for Noninvasive Risk Stratification

High Risk (>3% Annual Mortality Rate)
1. Severe resting left ventricular dysfunction (LV ejection fraction [LVEF] < 0.35)
2. High-risk treadmill score (score ≤ −11)
3. Severe exercise left ventricular dysfunction (exercise LVEF < 0.35)
4. Stress-induced large perfusion defect (particularly if anterior)
5. Stress-induced multiple perfusion defects of moderate size
6. Large, fixed perfusion defect with LV dilation or increased lung uptake (thallium-201)
7. Stress-induced moderate perfusion defect with LV dilation or increased lung uptake (thallium-201)
8. Echocardiographic wall motion abnormality (involving more than two segments) developing at low dose of dobutamine (≤10 μg/kg/min) or at low heart rate (<120 beats/min)
9. Stress echocardiographic evidence of extensive ischemia

Intermediate Risk (1%-3% Annual Mortality Rate)
1. Mild or moderate resting LV dysfunction (LVEF = 0.35-0.49)
2. Intermediate-risk treadmill score (−11 < score < 5)
3. Stress-induced moderate perfusion defect without LV dilation or increased lung intake (thallium-201)
4. Limited stress echocardiographic ischemia with a wall motion abnormality only at higher doses of dobutamine involving two segments or less

Low Risk (<1% Annual Mortality Rate)
1. Low-risk treadmill score (score ≥ 5)
2. Normal or small myocardial perfusion defect at rest or with stress*
3. Normal stress echocardiographic wall motion or no change of limited resting wall motion abnormalities during stress*

*Although the published data are limited, patients with these findings will probably not be at low risk in the presence of a high-risk treadmill score or severe resting LV dysfunction (LVEF < 0.35).

From Gibbons RJ, Abrams J, Chatterjee K, et al: ACC/AHA 2002 guideline update for the management of patients with chronic stable angina: A report of the American College of Cardiology/American Heart Association Task Force on Practice Guidelines (Committee to update the 1999 guidelines for the management of patients with chronic stable angina) (http://www.acc.org/clinical/guidelines/stable/stable.pdf).

to 3%), and low (<1%) expected annual mortality rate (**Table 57G-10**). Coronary angiography for risk stratification and as a prelude to intervention is endorsed for patients with high-risk criteria, as well as those with disabling chronic stable angina despite medical therapy or other clinical characteristics suggesting high risk (**Table 57G-11**). The committee considered evidence to be generally supportive (Class IIa) for coronary angiography for patients with milder angina in the setting of left ventricular dysfunction even if they do not have high-risk criteria on noninvasive testing, for asymptomatic patients with high-risk criteria, and for patients whose risk status is uncertain despite noninvasive testing.

Conversely, coronary angiography is discouraged (Class III) for patients who have mild angina and no evidence of ischemia on noninvasive testing or would not undergo revascularization. Only weak support (Class IIb) exists for coronary angiography for patients with mild angina and good left ventricular function in the absence of high-risk criteria on noninvasive testing, for patients with severe angina whose symptoms were controlled with medical therapy, or for patients with mild angina but unacceptable side effects to adequate medical therapy.

TREATMENT

ACC/AHA guidelines for the medical therapy of patients with chronic stable angina are oriented toward preventing myocardial infarction and death and reducing symptoms. When coronary revascularization has been shown to extend life, it is the recommended approach, but in many settings there are a variety of reasonable options including medical therapy, PCI, and CABG. Cost-effectiveness and patient preference are considered important components of the decision making process.

The guidelines assert that the goal of treatment of patients with chronic stable angina should be the complete or almost complete elimination of anginal chest pain and return to normal activities, with minimal side effects. They recommend that the initial treatment of the patient should include all the elements in the following mnemonic:

A = Aspirin and antianginal therapy
B = Beta blocker and blood pressure
C = Cigarette smoking and cholesterol
D = Diet and diabetes
E = Education and exercise

Pharmacologic Therapy

The guidelines emphasize the importance of aspirin and beta blockers for patients with coronary disease in the absence of contraindications (**Table 57G-12**). Absolute contraindications to beta blockers include severe bradycardia, pre-existing high degree of atrioventricular block, sick sinus syndrome, and severe, unstable left ventricular failure. Relative contraindications to beta blockers include asthma and bronchospastic disease, severe depression, and peripheral vascular disease. The guidelines note that most patients with diabetes tolerate beta blockers, although these drugs should be used with caution in patients who require insulin.

Angiotensin-converting enzyme (ACE) inhibitors are recommended (Class I indication) for patients with diabetes, hypertension, chronic kidney disease and/or left ventricular systolic dysfunction, and may be considered for their use in other patients with coronary disease (Class IIa). The guidelines recommend that nitrates and/or calcium antagonists should be used for symptom control but indicate that short-acting dihydropyridine calcium antagonists should be avoided. Low-density lipoprotein cholesterol (LDL-C) should be controlled with a target of less than 100 mg/dL (see later, "Risk Reduction"). Further reduction of LDL-C to less than 70 mg/dL is reasonable (Class IIa).[3]

TABLE 57G-11   ACC/AHA Guidelines for Coronary Angiography for Risk Stratification in Patients with Chronic Stable Angina

CLASS	INDICATION	LEVEL OF EVIDENCE*
I (indicated)	1. Patients with disabling (Canadian Cardiovascular Society [CCS] Classes III and IV) chronic stable angina despite medical therapy	B
	2. Patients with high-risk criteria on noninvasive testing regardless of anginal severity	B
	3. Patients with angina who have survived sudden cardiac death or serious ventricular arrhythmia	B
	4. Patients with angina and symptoms and signs of CHF	C
	5. Patients with clinical characteristics that indicate a high likelihood of severe CAD	C
IIa (good supportive evidence)	1. Patients with significant LV dysfunction (ejection fraction > 0.45), CCS Class I or II angina, and demonstrable ischemia but no high-risk criteria on noninvasive testing	C
	2. Patients with inadequate prognostic information after noninvasive testing	C
	3. Patients with high-risk criteria suggesting ischemia on noninvasive testing	C
IIb (weak supportive evidence)	1. Patients with CCS Class I or II angina, preserved LV function (ejection fraction > 0.45), but no high-risk criteria on noninvasive testing	C
	2. Patients with CCS Class III (not indicated) or IV angina, which improves to Class I or II with medical therapy	C
	3. Patients with CCS Class I or II angina but intolerance (unacceptable side effects) to adequate medical therapy	C
III (not indicated)	1. Patients with CCS Class I or II angina who respond to medical therapy and who have no evidence of ischemia on noninvasive testing	C
	2. Patients who prefer to avoid revascularization	C

*See guidelines text for definitions of level of evidence.
CHF = congestive heart failure.

TABLE 57G-12   ACC/AHA Guidelines for Pharmacotherapy for Chronic Stable Angina

CLASS	INDICATION	LEVEL OF EVIDENCE*
I (indicated)	1. Aspirin in the absence of contraindications	A
	2. Beta blockers as initial therapy in the absence of contraindications in patients with prior myocardial infarction or without prior myocardial infarction	A,B
	3. ACE inhibitor in all patients with CAD who also have diabetes and/or LV systolic dysfunction	A
	4. LDL-lowering therapy in patients with documented or suspected CAD and LDL-C > 130 mg/dL, with a target LDL < 100 mg/dL	A
	5. Sublingual nitroglycerin or nitroglycerin spray for the immediate relief of angina	B
	6. Calcium antagonists† or long-acting nitrates as initial therapy for reduction of symptoms when beta blockers are contraindicated	B
	7. Calcium antagonists† or long-acting nitrates in combination with beta blockers when initial treatment with beta blockers is not successful	B
	8. Calcium antagonists† and long-acting nitrates as a substitute for beta blockers if initial treatment with beta blockers leads to unacceptable side effects	C
IIa (good supportive evidence)	1. Clopidogrel when aspirin is absolutely contraindicated	B
	2. Long-acting nondihydropyridine calcium antagonists† instead of beta blockers as initial therapy	B
	3. In patients with documented or suspected CAD and LDL-C 100-129 mg/dL, several therapeutic options are available:	B
	a. Lifestyle and/or drug therapies to lower LDL to <100 mg/dL; further reduction to <70 mg/dL is reasonable	
	b. Weight reduction and increased physical activity in persons with the metabolic syndrome	
	c. Institution of treatment of other lipid or nonlipid risk factors; consider use of nicotinic acid or fibric acid for elevated triglyceride or low HDL cholesterol levels	
	4. ACE inhibitor in patients with CAD or other vascular disease	B
IIb (weak supportive evidence)	Low-intensity anticoagulation with warfarin in addition to aspirin	B
III (not indicated)	1. Dipyridamole	B
	2. Chelation therapy	B

*See guidelines text for definitions of level of evidence.
†Short-acting dihydropyridine calcium antagonists should be avoided.
LDL = low-density lipoprotein.

Several recommendations about pharmacologic therapy may be altered in future revisions of these guidelines because of further research providing insight into the effects of these agents. Use of dipyridamole or chelation therapy is discouraged.

For asymptomatic patients with known coronary disease (e.g., patients with prior myocardial infarction), the guidelines recommend aspirin and beta blockers in the absence of contraindications and the use of lipid-lowering therapies and ACE inhibitors as described earlier.

Risk Reduction

For patients with chronic stable angina, the ACC/AHA guidelines support intensive management of risk factors, including hypertension (target BP < 130/80 mm Hg),[4] cigarette smoking, diabetes, LDL-C, and obesity (**Table 57G-13**). The guidelines support the use of pharmacologic therapy for patients with LDL levels higher than 130 mg/dL, with a target of 100 mg/dL. Further reduction of LDL-C to less than 70 mg/dL is reasonable (Class IIa).[3] For patients with coronary disease who have an LDL of 100 to

TABLE 57G-13 ACC/AHA Guidelines for Treatment of Risk Factors

CLASS	INDICATION	LEVEL OF EVIDENCE*
I (indicated)	1. Treatment of hypertension according to Joint National Conference VI guidelines	A
	2. Smoking cessation therapy	B
	3. Management of diabetes	C
	4. Comprehensive cardiac rehabilitation program (including exercise)	B
	5. LDL-lowering therapy in patients with documented or suspected CAD and LDL-C ≥ 130 mg/dL, with a target LDL < 100 mg/dL	A
	6. Weight reduction in obese patients in the presence of hypertension, hyperlipidemia, or diabetes mellitus	C
IIa (good supportive evidence)	1. In patients with documented or suspected CAD and LDL-C = 100-129 mg/dL, several therapeutic options are available:	B
	a. Lifestyle and/or drug therapies to lower LDL-C to <100 mg/dL; further reduction to below 70 mg/dL is reasonable	B
	b. Weight reduction and increased physical activity in persons with the metabolic syndrome	B
	c. Institution of treatment of other lipid or nonlipid risk factors; consider use of nicotinic acid or fibric acid for elevated triglyceride or low HDL cholesterol levels	B
	2. Therapy to lower non–HDL-C in patients with documented or suspected CAD and triglyceride > 200 mg/dL, with a target non- HDL-C < 130 mg/dL	B
	3. Weight reduction in obese patients in the absence of hypertension, hyperlipidemia, or diabetes mellitus	C
IIb (weak supportive evidence)	1. Folate therapy in patients with elevated homocysteine levels	C
	2. Identification and appropriate treatment of clinical depression to improve CAD outcomes	C
	3. Interventions directed at psychosocial stress reduction	C
III (not indicated)	1. Initiation of hormone replacement therapy in postmenopausal women to reduce cardiovascular risk	A
	2. Vitamins C and E supplementation	A
	3. Chelation therapy	C
	4. Garlic	C
	5. Acupuncture	C
	6. Coenzyme Q	C

*See guidelines text for definitions of level of evidence.

TABLE 57G-14 Specific Goals for Risk Reduction Strategies in Patients with Chronic Stable Angina

RISK FACTOR OR STRATEGY	GOAL
Smoking	Complete cessation
Blood pressure	130/80 mm Hg*
Lipid management	Primary goal: LDL < 100 mg/dL; further reduction of LDL-C to <70 mg/dL is reasonable (Class IIa) Secondary goal: If triglycerides ≥ 200 mg/dL, then non–HDL-C should be <130 mg/dL
Physical activity	Minimum goal: 30 min, 3 or 4 days/wk Optimal goal: daily
Weight management	BMI: 18.5-24.9 kg/m^2
Diabetes management	HbA1c < 7%
Antiplatelet agents, anticoagulants	All patients—indefinite use of aspirin 75-325 mg/day if not contraindicated. Consider clopidogrel as an alternative if aspirin is contraindicated. Manage warfarin to international normalized ratio = 2.0-3.0 in patients after MI when clinically indicated or for those not able to take aspirin or clopidogrel
ACE inhibitors	Start and continue indefinitely in all patients with LVEF ≤ 40% and in those with hypertension, diabetes, or chronic kidney disease, unless contraindicated. Consider chronic therapy for all other patients with coronary or other vascular disease unless contraindicated. Use as needed to manage blood pressure or symptoms in all other patients
Beta blockers	Start in all postmyocardial infarction and acute patients (arrhythmia, LV dysfunction, inducible ischemia) at 5-28 days. Continue for 6 mo minimum. Observe usual contraindications. Use as needed to manage angina, rhythm, or blood pressure in all patients

BMI = body mass index; CHF = congestive heart failure; HbA1c = hemoglobin A1c.
*Rosendorff C, Black HR, Cannon CP, et al: Treatment of hypertension in the prevention and management of ischemic heart disease: A scientific statement from the American Heart Association Council for High Blood Pressure Research and the Councils on Clinical Cardiology and Epidemiology and Prevention. Circulation 115:2761, 2007.

129 mg/dL, the guidelines consider several options reasonable (Class IIa), including lifestyle modifications and drug therapies.

In changes from prior guidelines, initiation of hormone therapy for the purpose of reducing cardiovascular risk is considered inappropriate (Class III), as is use of vitamins C and E supplementation, chelation therapy, garlic, acupuncture, and coenzyme Q for this purpose. Evidence to support interventions based on lipoprotein (a) and homocysteine levels are considered inconclusive.

Specific goals for key risk reduction interventions are summarized in **Table 57G-14**.

Revascularization

ACC/AHA guidelines for revascularization with PCI or CABG for patients with chronic stable angina focus on improvement of survival for patients with high clinical risk of mortality on medical therapy and on controlling symptoms in patients who have an inadequate quality of life on medical therapy. Recommendations include the use of CABG for patients with significant left main coronary artery disease and in those with triple-vessel disease, particularly those with abnormal left ventricular function (**Table 57G-15**). PCI and CABG are supported for patients with double- and triple-vessel coronary disease who do not have treated diabetes. Revascularization is also supported for patients with single- or double-vessel coronary disease who have a large area of viable myocardium and high-risk criteria on noninvasive testing.

The guidelines discourage the use of PCI or CABG for single- or double-vessel coronary disease without significant proximal left anterior descending (LAD) coronary artery disease if they have mild symptoms or have not received an adequate trial of medical therapy, particularly if noninvasive testing data indicate that they have only a small area of viable myocardium or have no demonstrable ischemia on noninvasive testing. PCI for patients with diabetes is considered a second-choice strategy compared with CABG.

For asymptomatic patients, the guidelines for revascularization with PCI or CABG are identical to those for other patients with chronic stable angina (see Table 57G-15), except that the following indications that were considered Class IIa are regarded as weaker (Class IIb) in asymptomatic patients:

- Use of PCI or CABG for patients with single- or double-vessel CAD without significant proximal LAD disease but with a moderate area of viable myocardium and demonstrable ischemia on noninvasive testing
- Use of PCI or CABG for patients with single-vessel disease with significant proximal LAD disease

Alternative Therapies

The guidelines do not consider alternative therapies to be sufficiently supported by evidence to warrant a Class I indication for patients with chronic stable angina. Surgical laser transmyocardial revascularization is given a Class IIa indication, and enhanced external counterpulsation and spinal cord stimulation are given Class IIb indications.

PATIENT FOLLOW-UP

The ACC/AHA guidelines recommend that patients with chronic stable angina have follow-up evaluations every 4 to 12 months during the first year of therapy; subsequently, annual evaluations are recommended if the patient is stable and reliable enough to call when angina symptoms become worse or other symptoms occur. The guidelines urge restraint in the use of routine testing in follow-up of patients with chronic stable

TABLE 57G-15	ACC/AHA Guidelines for Revascularization with Percutaneous Coronary Intervention and Coronary Artery Bypass Grafting in Patients with Stable Angina	
CLASS	**INDICATION**	**LEVEL OF EVIDENCE***
I (indicated)	1. CABG for patients with significant left main coronary disease	A
	2. CABG for patients with triple-vessel disease. The survival benefit is greater in patients with abnormal LV function (LVEF < 0.50).	A
	3. CABG for patients with double-vessel disease with significant proximal LAD CAD and either abnormal LV function (ejection fraction <50%) or demonstrable ischemia on noninvasive testing	A
	4. PCI for patients with double- or triple-vessel disease with significant proximal LAD CAD, who have anatomy suitable for catheter-based therapy and normal LV function and who do not have treated diabetes	B
	5. PCI or CABG for patients with single- or double-vessel CAD without significant proximal LAD CAD but with a large area of viable myocardium and high-risk criteria on noninvasive testing	B
	6. CABG for patients with single- or double-vessel CAD without significant proximal LAD CAD who have survived sudden cardiac death or sustained ventricular tachycardia	C
	7. In patients with prior PCI, CABG, or PCI for recurrent stenosis associated with a large area of viable myocardium or high-risk criteria on noninvasive testing	C
	8. PCI or CABG for patients who have not been successfully treated by medical therapy and can undergo revascularization with acceptable risk	B
IIa (good supportive evidence)	1. Repeat CABG for patients with multiple saphenous vein graft stenoses, especially when there is significant stenosis of a graft supplying the LAD; it may be appropriate to use PCI for focal saphenous vein graft lesions or multiple stenoses in poor candidates for reoperative surgery.	C
	2. Use of PCI or CABG for patients with single- or double-vessel CAD without significant proximal LAD disease but with a moderate area of viable myocardium and demonstrable ischemia on noninvasive testing	B
	3. Use of PCI or CABG for patients with single-vessel disease with significant proximal LAD disease	B
IIb (weak supportive evidence)	1. Compared with CABG, PCI for patients with double- or triple-vessel disease with significant proximal LAD CAD, who have anatomy suitable for catheter-based therapy and who have treated diabetes or abnormal LV function	B
	2. Use of PCI for patients with significant left main coronary disease who are not candidates for CABG	C
	3. PCI for patients with single- or double-vessel CAD without significant proximal LAD CAD who have survived sudden cardiac death or sustained ventricular tachycardia	C
III (not indicated)	1. Use of PCI or CABG for patients with single- or double-vessel CAD without significant proximal LAD CAD, who have mild symptoms that are unlikely to be caused by myocardial ischemia, or who have not received an adequate trial of medical therapy and a. have only a small area of viable myocardium *or* b. have no demonstrable ischemia on noninvasive testing	C
	2. Use of PCI or CABG for patients with borderline coronary stenoses (50%-60% diameter in locations other than the left main coronary artery) and no demonstrable ischemia on noninvasive testing	C
	3. Use of PCI or CABG for patients with insignificant coronary stenosis (<50% diameter)	C
	4. Use of PCI for patients with significant left main coronary artery disease who are candidates for CABG	B

*See guidelines text for definitions of level of evidence.

TABLE 57G-16 ACC/AHA Guidelines for Echocardiography, Treadmill Exercise Testing, Stress Radionuclide Imaging, Stress Echocardiography Studies, and Coronary Angiography During Patient Follow-up

CLASS	INDICATION	LEVEL OF EVIDENCE*
I (indicated)	1. Chest radiograph for patients with evidence of new or worsening CHF	C
	2. Assessment of LVEF and segmental wall motion by echocardiography or radionuclide imaging in patients with new or worsening CHF or evidence of intervening myocardial infarction by history or ECG	C
	3. Echocardiography for evidence of new or worsening valvular heart disease	C
	4. Treadmill exercise test for patients without prior revascularization who have a significant change in clinical status, are able to exercise, and do not have any of the electrocardiographic abnormalities listed in indication 5	C
	5. Stress radionuclide imaging or stress echocardiography procedures for patients without prior revascularization who have a significant change in clinical status and are unable to exercise or have one of the following electrocardiographic abnormalities: a. Preexcitation (Wolff-Parkinson-White) syndrome b. Electronically paced ventricular rhythm c. >1 mm of ST-segment depression at rest d. Complete left bundle branch block	C
	6. Stress radionuclide imaging or stress echocardiography procedures for patients who have a significant change in clinical status and required a stress imaging procedure on their initial evaluation because of equivocal or intermediate-risk treadmill results	C
	7. Stress radionuclide imaging or stress echocardiography procedures for patients with prior revascularization who have a significant change in clinical status	C
	8. Coronary angiography in patients with marked limitation of ordinary activity (CCS Class III) despite maximal medical therapy	C
IIa (good supportive evidence)		
IIb (weak supportive evidence)	Annual treadmill exercise testing in patients who have no change in clinical status, can exercise, have none of the electrocardiographic abnormalities listed in Class I, indication 5, and have an estimated annual mortality rate > 1%	C
III (not indicated)	1. Echocardiography or radionuclide imaging for assessment of LVEF and segmental wall motion in patients with a normal ECG, no history of MI, and no evidence of CHF	C
	2. Repeat treadmill exercise testing in <3 yr in patients who have no change in clinical status and estimated annual mortality rate <1% on their initial evaluation, as demonstrated by one of the following: a. Low-risk Duke treadmill score (without imaging) b. Low-risk Duke treadmill score with negative imaging c. Normal LV function and normal coronary angiogram d. Normal LV function and insignificant CAD	C
	3. Stress imaging or echocardiographic procedures for patients who have no change in clinical status, a normal rest ECG, are not taking digoxin, are able to exercise, and did not require a stress imaging or echocardiographic procedure on their initial evaluation because of equivocal or intermediate-risk treadmill results	C
	4. Repeat coronary angiography in patients with no change in clinical status, no change on repeat exercise testing or stress imaging, and insignificant CAD on initial evaluation	

*See guidelines text for definitions of level of evidence.

angina if they have not had a change in clinical status (**Table 57G-16**). All the Class I indications for testing are for patients who have had a significant change in clinical status, except for the use of coronary angiography for patients with marked limitations of ordinary activity despite maximal medical therapy.

REFERENCES

1. Gibbons RJ, Abrams J, Chatterjee K, et al: ACC/AHA 2002 guideline update for the management of patients with chronic stable angina—summary article: A report of the American College of Cardiology/American Heart Association Task Force on practice guidelines (Committee on the Management of Patients With Chronic Stable Angina). J Am Coll Cardiol 41:159, 2003.
2. Greenland P, Bonow RO, Brundage BH, et al: ACCF/AHA 2007 clinical expert consensus document on coronary artery calcium scoring by computed tomography in global cardiovascular risk assessment and in evaluation of patients with chest pain: A report of the American College of Cardiology Foundation Clinical Expert Consensus Task Force (ACCF/AHA Writing Committee to Update the 2000 Expert Consensus Document on Electron Beam Computed Tomography). Circulation. 115:402, 2007.
3. Smith SC Jr, Allen J, Blair SN, et al: AHA/ACC guidelines for secondary prevention for patients with coronary and other atherosclerotic vascular disease: 2006 update: Endorsed by the National Heart, Lung, and Blood Institute. Circulation 113:2363, 2006.
4. Rosendorff C, Black HR, Cannon CP, et al: Treatment of hypertension in the prevention and management of ischemic heart disease: A scientific statement from the American Heart Association Council for High Blood Pressure Research and the Councils on Clinical Cardiology and Epidemiology and Prevention. Circulation 115:2761, 2007.

CHAPTER 58 Percutaneous Coronary Intervention

Jeffrey J. Popma and Deepak L. Bhatt

The use of percutaneous coronary intervention (PCI) to treat ischemic coronary artery disease (CAD) has expanded dramatically during the past three decades. In the absence of left main or complex multivessel CAD, PCI is the preferred method of revascularization in the United States for most patients with ischemic CAD. The estimated 1,000,000 PCI procedures performed annually in the United States now exceed the number of coronary artery bypass graft (CABG) procedures.[1] During the past several years, however, the growth of PCI slowed because of the effectiveness of risk factor modification, prevention of restenosis with drug-eluting stents (DES), and better understanding of patients who benefit from revascularization.[2,3] The number of PCIs is expected to grow modestly (1% to 5%) during the next decade because of the aging population and increased frequency of obesity and diabetes in the United States. Other key enablers of the expanded use of PCI in patients with complex CAD include improvements in equipment design (e.g., catheters with lower profile and enhanced deliverability), adjunctive pharmacologic strategies (e.g., adenosine diphosphate receptor antagonists, glycoprotein IIb/IIIa inhibitors, and direct thrombin inhibitors) to improve safety, and better hemodynamic support devices in ultrahigh-risk patients.[4] "Hybrid" procedures for the treatment of CAD and valvular heart disease have also been performed with collaboration of interventional cardiologists and cardiac surgeons.[5,6]

Coronary balloon angioplasty, or percutaneous transluminal coronary angioplasty, was first performed by Andreas Gruentzig in 1977 with use of a fixed-wire balloon catheter. The procedure was initially limited to the less than 10% of patients with symptomatic CAD who had a single, focal, noncalcified lesion of a proximal coronary vessel. As equipment design and operator experience evolved during the next decade, the use of PCI expanded to include an increasing spectrum of coronary anatomy, including multivessel CAD, total occlusions, diseased saphenous vein grafts (SVGs), and patients with acute ST-segment elevation myocardial infarction (STEMI; see Chap. 55), among other complexities. Two limitations prevented the widespread use of balloon angioplasty for CAD: abrupt closure of the treated vessel occurred in 5% to 8% of cases, requiring emergency CABG surgery in 3% to 5% of patients; and restenosis resulted in symptom recurrence in 30% of patients within the ensuing year.

New coronary devices were developed in the late 1980s to improve on the limitations associated with balloon angioplasty. Coronary stents scaffold the inner arterial wall to prevent early and late vascular remodeling. Rotational atherectomy ablates calcific atherosclerotic plaque and was developed as stand-alone therapy for undilatable coronary stenoses or used in combination with coronary stents after calcific plaque ablation. By early 2000, a number of other devices were developed to protect the distal circulation from atherothrombotic embolization (i.e., embolic protection devices). Aspiration and thrombectomy catheters were developed to remove medium and large thrombi from within the coronary artery, thereby preventing distal embolization. The term *percutaneous coronary intervention* now encompasses the broad array of the balloons, stents, and adjunct devices required to perform a safe and effective percutaneous revascularization in complex coronary artery lesions.

This chapter reviews the indications and clinical considerations for the selection of patients for PCI; discusses the current array of coronary devices, antithrombotic therapy, and vascular closure devices used for PCI; and details the short- and long-term outcomes of PCI and requirements for operator and institutional proficiency.

Indications for Percutaneous Coronary Intervention

The major value of percutaneous or surgical coronary revascularization is the relief of symptoms and signs of ischemic CAD (see Chap. 57 and PCI Guidelines). PCI reduces risk of mortality and subsequent myocardial infarction (MI) compared with medical therapy in patients with acute coronary syndromes. However, optimal medical therapy is as effective as PCI in reducing death and MI in patients with stable angina, although symptom relief[2] and ischemia improvement[7] are better with PCI. Improvement in ischemia burden >5% was achieved more often with PCI, and the magnitude of the residual ischemia has been correlated with less frequent death and MI.[7] Further studies comparing the use of coronary arteriography and PCI in patients with moderate degrees of myocardial ischemia are planned (e.g., ISCHEMIA Investigators). Irrespective of the indication for revascularization, it is recommended that PCI be coupled with optimal medical therapy after the procedure, such as hypertension and diabetes control, exercise, and smoking cessation (see Chap. 49). Lipid management is also an important component of optimal medical therapy. Compared with medical therapy alone, CABG prolongs life in certain anatomic subsets, such as in patients with left main disease, three-vessel CAD and reduced ventricular function, or left anterior descending artery disease with involvement of one or two additional vessels irrespective of left ventricular function.[8] The risks and benefits of coronary revascularization need careful review with the patient and family members, and the relative options of PCI, CABG, or optimal medical therapy should be discussed before performance of these procedures. A Task Force of the American College of Cardiology (ACC) and the American Heart Association (AHA) has published guidelines for the performance of PCI and CABG,[8-11] and a multispecialty writing committee has developed appropriateness guidelines for revascularization for a number of clinical and lesion-specific subsets[12] (see PCI Guidelines).

ASYMPTOMATIC PATIENTS OR THOSE WITH MILD ANGINA.
Asymptomatic patients or those who have only mild symptoms are generally best treated with medical therapy unless one or more high-grade lesions subtend a moderate to large area of viable myocardium, the patient prefers to maintain an aggressive lifestyle or has a high-risk occupation, and the procedure can be performed with a high chance of success and low likelihood of complications (see PCI Guidelines).[10,12] Coronary revascularization should not be performed in patients with absent or mild symptoms if only a small area of myocardium is at risk, if no objective evidence of ischemia can be found, or if the likelihood of success is low or the chance of complications is high.[10,12]

PATIENTS WITH MODERATE TO SEVERE ANGINA (see Chap. 57).
Patients with Canadian Cardiovascular Society (CCS) Class III angina, particularly those who are refractory to medical therapy, can benefit from coronary revascularization, provided the lesion subtends a moderate to large area of viable myocardium as determined by noninvasive testing (see PCI Guidelines).[13,14] Patients with recurrent symptoms while receiving medical therapy are candidates for revascularization even if they have a higher risk for an adverse outcome with revascularization. Patients with Class III symptoms should not undergo revascularization without noninvasive evidence of myocardial ischemia or a trial of medical therapy, particularly if only a small region of myocardium is at risk, the likelihood of success is low, or the chance of complications is high.[12]

PATIENTS WITH UNSTABLE ANGINA, NON–ST-SEGMENT ELEVATION MI, AND ST-SEGMENT ELEVATION MI (see Chaps. 55 and 56).
Cardiac catheterization and coronary revascularization in moderate- to high-risk patients who present with unstable angina or non–ST-segment MI (NSTEMI) may improve mortality and reduce the rate of reinfarction.[15] In a meta-analysis of seven trials with 8375 patients observed for up to 2 years, the incidence of all-cause mortality was 4.9% in the early invasive group compared with 6.5% in the conservative group (risk ratio [RR] = 0.75; $P = 0.001$)[16] (**Fig. 58-1**). The 2-year incidence of nonfatal MI was 7.6% in the invasive group versus 9.1% in the conservative group (RR = 0.83; $P = 0.012$).[16] At a mean of 13 months of follow-up, there was a reduction in rehospitalization for unstable angina as well (RR = 0.69; $P < 0.0001$).[16] Current guidelines suggest that an early invasive strategy should be pursued in patients with recurrent ischemia despite therapy, elevated troponin levels, new ST depression, new or worsening symptoms of congestive heart failure, depressed left ventricular function, hemodynamic instability, sustained ventricular tachycardia, or recent PCI or CABG[15] (see PCI Guidelines).

A number of clinical scenarios associated with STEMI, including primary PCI, rescue PCI, facilitated PCI, and PCI after successful thrombolysis, have been published[17] (see PCI Guidelines). Timely PCI in patients with STEMI improves survival compared with medical therapy, provided the PCI is performed within 90 minutes of the patient's arrival to the medical facility, the PCI is performed by a physician who performs PCI on a routine basis, and the hospital has a sufficient PCI volume to support its proficiency. Patients with cardiogenic shock or severe congestive heart failure also benefit from primary PCI, irrespective of their age at presentation.

PATIENTS WITHOUT OPTIONS FOR REVASCULARIZATION.
Patients who suffer from substantial angina yet are poor candidates for conventional revascularization have limited therapeutic options. These patients gen-erally have a single, proximal vessel occlusion that subtends a large amount of myocardium or have undergone one or more prior CABG operations with stenoses or occlusions of the SVGs poorly suited for conventional repeated revascularization. "Limited options" patients represent approximately 4% to 12% of those undergoing coronary angiography; a larger percentage of patients (20% to 30%) have incomplete revascularization because of unsuitable coronary anatomy for surgical or percutaneous techniques.

Creation of new blood vessels in the ischemic tissue with use of laser injury, also known as therapeutic angiogenesis, may provide symptom relief in these patients. Both surgical and percutaneous approaches have been used to improve regional blood flow to the ischemic myocardium in these patients, although these strategies vary with respect to the depth of myocardial injury, the laser-tissue interactions, the presence or absence of guidance, and the number of channels created. Laser therapy has not yet proved efficacious in blinded clinical trials. Enhanced external counterpulsation support may provide improvement of angina in patients with refractory ischemia[18] (see Chap. 57), although the mechanism of benefit by this technique is not clear.[19]

Patient-Specific Considerations for Percutaneous Coronary Intervention
Assessment of the potential risks and benefits of PCI must address five fundamental patient-specific risk factors: extent of jeopardized myocardium, baseline lesion morphology, underlying cardiac function (including left ventricular function, rhythm stability, and coexisting valvular heart disease), presence of renal dysfunction, and pre-existing medical comorbidities that may render the patient at higher risk for PCI. Each of these factors contributes independently to the risk and benefit attributable to PCI. Proper planning for a PCI procedure requires careful attention to each of these factors.

EXTENT OF JEOPARDIZED MYOCARDIUM. The proportion of viable myocardium subtended by the treated coronary artery is the principal consideration in assessing the acute risk of the PCI procedure. PCI interrupts coronary blood flow for a period of seconds to minutes, and the ability of the patient to hemodynamically tolerate a sustained coronary occlusion depends on both the extent of "downstream" viable myocardium and the presence and grade of collaterals to the ischemic region. Although the risk for abrupt closure has been reduced substantially with the availability of coronary stents, when other procedural complications develop, such as a large side branch occlusion, distal embolization, perforation, or no-reflow, there may be rapid clinical deterioration that is proportionate to the extent of jeopardized myocardium. In the unlikely event that out-of-hospital stent thrombosis develops, the clinical sequelae of the episode relate to the extent of myocardium subtended by the occluded stent. Predictors for the occurrence of cardiovascular collapse with a failed PCI include the percentage of myocardium at risk,

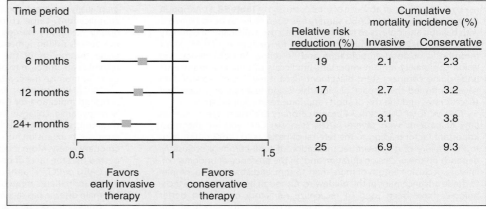

Time period	Relative risk reduction (%)	Cumulative mortality incidence (%)	
		Invasive	Conservative
1 month	19	2.1	2.3
6 months	17	2.7	3.2
12 months	20	3.1	3.8
24+ months	25	6.9	9.3

FIGURE 58-1 In this meta-analysis of the contemporary randomized clinical trials of patients with non–ST-segment elevation acute coronary syndromes, a significant reduction in mortality emerges with longer durations of follow-up with an initial invasive versus conservative approach. *(From Bavry AA, Kumbhani DJ, Rassi AN, et al: Benefit of early invasive therapy in acute coronary syndromes: A meta-analysis of contemporary randomized clinical trials. J Am Coll Cardiol 48:1319, 2006.)*

TABLE 58-1	SCAI Lesion Classification System for Risk Assessment

Type I Lesion (Highest Success Expected; Lowest Risk)
1. Does not meet criteria for C lesion
2. Patent

Type II Lesions
1. Meets any of these criteria for ACC/AHA C lesion
   Diffuse (>2-cm length)
   Excessive tortuosity of proximal segment
   Extremely angulated segments greater than 90 degrees
   Inability to protect major side branches
   Degenerated vein grafts with friable lesions
2. Patent

Type III Lesions
1. Does not meet criteria for C Lesion
2. Occluded

Type IV Lesions (Lowest Success Expected; Highest Risk)
1. Meets any of these criteria for ACC/AHA C lesion
   Diffuse (>2-cm length)
   Excessive tortuosity of proximal segment
   Extremely angulated segments greater than 90 degrees
   Inability to protect major side branches
   Degenerated vein grafts with friable lesions
2. Occluded

Modified from Krone RJ, Shaw RE, Klein LW, et al: Evaluation of the American College of Cardiology/American Heart Association and the Society for Coronary Angiography and Interventions lesion classification system in the current "stent era" of coronary interventions (from the ACC–National Cardiovascular Data Registry). Am J Cardiol 92:389, 2003.

the severity of the baseline stenosis, multivessel CAD, and the presence of diffuse disease.

Whether complete revascularization in patients with multivessel CAD should be performed in a single or staged setting remains controversial. In patients presenting with STEMI, revascularization of only the culprit infarct–related artery is generally recommended,[12] unless there is ongoing cardiogenic shock because of jeopardized myocardium in other regions. In other nonacute situations, the number of vessels treated in a single setting will depend on whether procedural complications have occurred, the length of time required for additional vessel treatment, the underlying renal function, and the general ability of the patient to tolerate long procedures. Staged procedures can be safely performed up to 4 to 8 weeks after the initial procedure. In the setting of NSTEMI, observational data suggest that multivessel versus culprit-only stenting reduces subsequent need for revascularization but does not affect death or MI rates.[20]

BASELINE LESION MORPHOLOGY. Several angiographic findings increase the technical complexity of PCI and elevate the risk for acute and long-term complications. The initial ACC/AHA lesion classification system has been recently refined by the Society for Cardiovascular Angiography and Interventions (SCAI) risk system, which further characterizes risk by the presence or absence of total occlusion[21] (**Table 58-1**). Although the need for emergency CABG surgery has been reduced from 3% to 8% with balloon angioplasty to less than 1% with the availability of coronary stents, they have not eliminated the risk for periprocedural MI, stent thrombosis, or distal embolization and no-reflow. Vessel patency and lesion complexity remain important predictors of outcome in patients undergoing coronary stent placement. Recent reviews of registry data have confirmed the impact of high-risk lesion features on procedural success rates and the risk of short- and long-term complications.

CHRONIC TOTAL OCCLUSIONS. Chronic coronary occlusions are present in 50% of patients with severe (>70% stenosis) CAD and are the most important factor leading to the referral of patients to CABG rather than to PCI. Failure of guidewire recanalization of total coronary occlusions depends on the occlusion duration and on the presence of bridging collaterals, occlusion length of more than 15 mm, and absence of a "nipple" to guide advancement of the guidewire. Although newer guidance technologies have been used to recanalize refractory occlusions, better guidewires and wire techniques have accounted for much of the improvement in crossing success during recent years.[22] Once the chronic total occlusion has been crossed, DES may be used to reduce late clinical recurrence.[23]

SAPHENOUS VEIN GRAFTS. SVG interventions represent approximately 8% of PCI procedures and pose an increased risk of postprocedural MI caused by atheroembolization that occurs during PCI. When no-reflow occurs, administration of arterial vasodilators (e.g., nitroprusside, verapamil, or adenosine) into the SVG may improve the flow into the distal native circulation, but there is still a substantially increased risk for death and MI. More extensive SVG degeneration and bulkier lesions (larger estimated plaque volume) are associated with higher complication rates than SVGs that have less extensive disease. In the setting of "high-risk" SVG anatomy, alternative approaches using the native coronary artery should be pursued whenever possible. Lower rates of restenosis in SVG lesions are found after coronary stent placement than after balloon angioplasty. Although DES may provide even lower angiographic restenosis rates, the current DES are poorly suited to SVGs larger than 4.5 mm in diameter, and bare metal stents (BMS) are preferred in this setting. Embolic protection devices are recommended in patients treated for SVG stenoses to lessen the risk of distal embolization of atherothrombotic debris.

BIFURCATION LESIONS. Optimal management of lesions involving both branches of a coronary bifurcation remains controversial. "Snowplowing" of plaque into the adjacent parent vessel or side branch is a major limitation of conventional balloon angioplasty. Atheroablative devices, such as rotational atherectomy, have only partially reduced this risk. Risk stratification for bifurcation PCI includes assessment of the extent of atherosclerotic disease in both vessels, estimation of the relative vessel size and distribution in the parent vessel and side branch, and determination of the orientation of the vessels to one another. Side branch compromise may also occur in up to 30% of bifurcation lesions without apparent branch vessel disease.

Stent placement in one vessel rather than in both the parent vessel and side branch is generally preferred.[24] In a meta-analysis of six randomized trials including 1642 patients with coronary bifurcation lesions who were randomly selected to undergo PCI by either double or single stenting, there was increased risk of MI with double stenting (RR, 1.78; $P = 0.001$).[24]

When there is extensive disease in both vessels, a number of strategies have been used, including simultaneous kissing stents and "crush," culotte, T stenting, and TAP (T and small protrusion) techniques (**Fig. 58-2**). Irrespective of the bifurcation stenting strategy used, a final "kissing" balloon inflation in the parent vessel and side branch should generally be performed. DES appear to reduce restenosis compared with BMS, but when recurrence develops in patients treated with a DES, it generally occurs at the origin of the side branch. New dedicated bifurcation stents and side branch access main vessel stents are in development.

LESION CALCIFICATION. The presence of extensive coronary calcification poses unique challenges for PCI because calcium in the vessel wall leads to irregular and inflexible lumens and makes the delivery of guidewires, balloons, and stents much more challenging. Extensive coronary calcification also renders the vessel wall rigid, necessitating higher balloon inflation pressures to obtain complete stent expansion and, on occasion, leading to "undilatable" lesions that resist any achievable balloon expansion pressure. Rotational atherectomy effectively ablates vessel wall calcification and facilitates stent delivery and complete stent expansion (**Fig. 58-3**).

THROMBUS. Conventional angiography has poor sensitivity for the detection of coronary thrombus, but the presence of a large, angiographically apparent coronary thrombus heightens risk for procedural complications. Large coronary thrombi may fragment and embolize during PCI or may extrude through gaps between stent struts placed in the vessel, risking lumen compromise or thrombus propagation and acute thrombosis of the treated vessel. In addition, large coronary thrombi can embolize to other coronary branches or vessels or dislodge and compromise the cerebral or other vascular beds (**Fig. 58-4**).

LEFT MAIN CORONARY ARTERY DISEASE. Left main CAD has been an accepted indication for CABG surgery on the basis of the potential for hemodynamic collapse in the setting of acute complications, stent thrombosis, or restenosis involving the body of the left main coronary artery or its extension into the left anterior descending or left circumflex coronary artery. More recent registry and randomized studies have suggested that the rates of death and MI are similar with patients undergoing CABG or PCI,[25,26] although the need for repeated revascularization is higher for patients treated with PCI[3,27-37] (**Table 58-2**). The use of PCI for left main disease has recently been elevated to a Class IIb indication (see PCI Guidelines) pending additional planned randomized study.

UNDERLYING CARDIAC FUNCTION. Left ventricular function is an important predictor of outcome during PCI. For each 10% decrement in resting left ventricular ejection fraction, the risk of in-hospital mortality after PCI increases by approximately twofold. Associated valvular disease or ventricular arrhythmia further increases the risk for PCI in the

FIGURE 58-2 Bifurcation lesion treated with simultaneous kissing stents. **A,** A complex bifurcation lesion involves both the left anterior descending artery (large arrow) and its diagonal branch (small arrow). **B,** After predilation with balloons in both branches, simultaneous inflation of two 3.0 ×18-mm CYPHER stents (Cordis Corp., Bridgewater, NJ) in the left anterior descending and diagonal branches is performed. **C,** Following postdilation of both branches with simultaneous inflations to expand the stents, an excellent angiographic result is obtained.

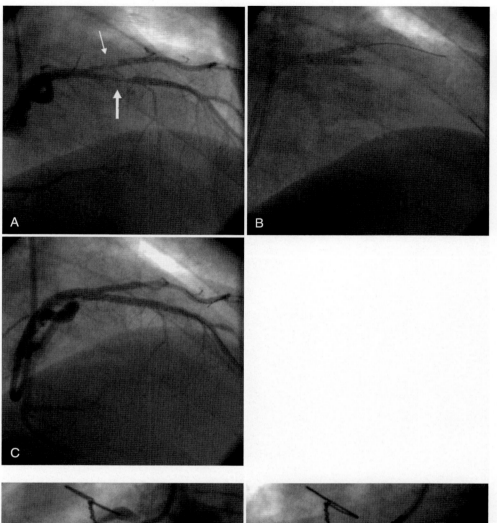

FIGURE 58-3 Rotational atherectomy of an ostial right coronary artery stenosis. **A,** A heavily calcified stenosis of the ostium of the right coronary artery (arrow) precludes conventional balloon angioplasty and stent placement. **B,** A 1.25-mm rotational atherectomy burr (arrow) was advanced to ablate the calcium in the ostium. An additional 1.50-mm rotational atherectomy burr was used to further ablate the calcific plaque. **C,** After predilation with a 2.5-mm balloon, a 3.50 × 23-mm CYPHER stent was advanced and inflated to 16 atm. Note that the guiding catheter is withdrawn (arrow) to allow stent placement just at the origin of the right coronary artery. **D,** An excellent final angiographic result is obtained with no residual stenosis. Note the free reflux of contrast agent from the right coronary artery ostium after stent placement (arrow).

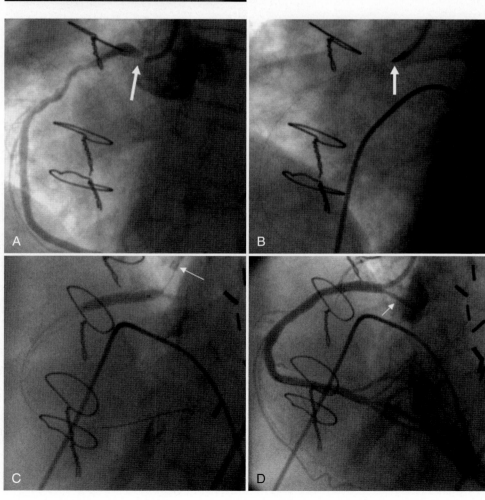

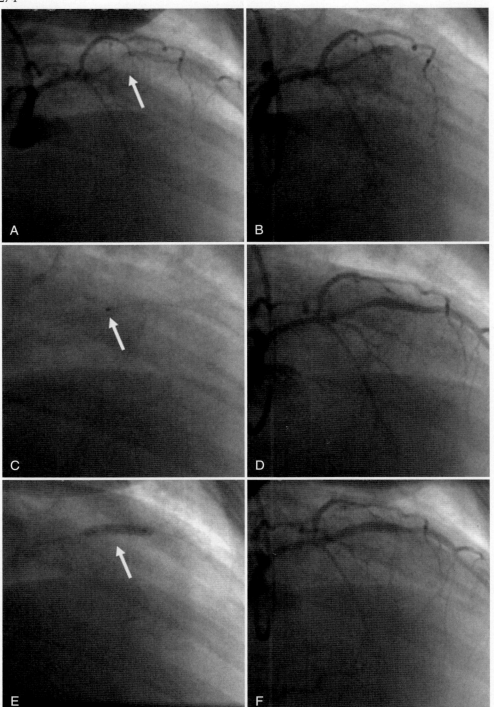

FIGURE 58-4 Aspiration thrombectomy for STEMI. A thrombotic occlusion of the proximal left anterior descending artery is shown (**A,** arrow). There is minimal improvement in flow after a 2.5-mm balloon inflation, with the suspicion of thrombus precluding flow (**B**). An Export catheter is used to remove the thrombus (**C**), and anterograde flow is reestablished and the thrombus is removed (**D**). A 3.0-mm drug-eluting stent was placed (**E**), resulting in no residual stenosis and TIMI 3 flow into the distal vessel (**F**).

that do not effectively reduce left ventricular pressures have been replaced by percutaneous left ventricular assist devices that are positioned in the left atrium (e.g., TandemHeart, CardiacAssist Inc., Pittsburgh, Pa)[39,40] or directly in the left ventricle (Impella LP 2.5, Abiomed Inc., Danvers, Mass)[4,41,42] (**Fig. 58-5**). These devices permit ultrahigh-risk PCI without the risk of hemodynamic collapse during the procedure, although further data are needed to see if they are superior to intra-aortic balloon pumps.

RENAL INSUFFICIENCY. The morbidity and mortality associated with PCI relate directly to the extent of baseline renal disease (see also Chap. 93). Patients with evidence of mild renal dysfunction have a 20% higher risk of death at 1 year after PCI than do patients with preserved renal function.[43] Renal dysfunction after the administration of contrast material during angiography may relate to contrast-induced nephropathy cholesterol embolization syndrome (see Chaps. 61 and 93), or both. The risk of contrast-induced nephropathy is dependent on the dose of the contrast agents used, hydration status at the time of the procedure, pre-existing renal function of the patient, age, hemodynamic stability, anemia, and diabetes. The risk for cholesterol embolization syndrome relates to catheter manipulation in an ascending or descending atherosclerotic aorta that releases cholesterol crystals. Although the risk of hemodialysis is less than 3% in cases of uncomplicated contrast-induced nephropathy, the in-hospital mortality in the setting of hemodialysis exceeds 30%. Mild renal dysfunction after PCI is associated with an increased risk of death up to fourfold at 1 year after PCI compared with patients with preserved renal function.

ASSOCIATED MEDICAL COMORBIDITIES. A number of pre-existing medical conditions may increase short- or long-term risks of PCI and should be considered in evaluation of the risks, benefits, and strategic approach for patients undergoing PCI. Patients with diabetes have higher recurrence rates with BMS and with DES, and a long-term survival benefit was shown in diabetic patients undergoing CABG compared with multivessel balloon angioplasty in an older era (see Chap. 64). Contemporary series have shown no early difference in mortality but a substantial increase in the need for early repeated revascularization.[3] Whether there is a long-term surgical survival benefit with CABG compared with multivessel DES placement is the subject of ongoing studies.

A bleeding diathesis or need for chronic warfarin therapy may preclude the patient from tolerating long-term combination aspirin and clopidogrel therapy after DES placement, thereby placing the patient at higher risk for stent thrombosis. The need for discontinuation of dual antiplatelet therapy before impending noncardiac surgery soon after stent implantation may also predispose to stent thrombosis. In each of these circumstances, BMS placement may be the preferred approach, particularly if the surgery can be deferred for approximately 6 weeks after stent placement.

setting of left ventricular dysfunction. Intra-aortic balloon pump support may be useful when there is severe compromise of left ventricular function (i.e., ejection fraction less than 35%) or when the PCI target lesion supplies a substantial portion of viable myocardium. Routine use of an intra-aortic balloon pump has limited benefit in patients with STEMI,[38] although it is recommended in patients with cardiogenic shock. Other percutaneous cardiopulmonary support devices

TABLE 58-2 Comparative Trials Between Drug-Eluting Stents and Coronary Bypass Surgery in Unprotected Left Main Coronary Revascularization

TRIAL	N	STUDY DURATION	DEATH	MYOCARDIAL INFARCTION	REPEATED REVASCULARIZATION	STROKE	MACCE	COMMENTS
Chieffo[29]	107 PCI 142 CABG	12 months	PCI 2.8% CABG 6.4%	PCI 0.9% CABG 1.4%	PCI 15.8% CABG 3.6%	PCI 0.9% CABG 0.7%	N/A	Significantly lower adjusted death, myocardial infarction, and stroke with PCI versus CABG Significantly lower repeated revascularization with CABG
Lee[28]	50 PCI 123 CABG	12 months	PCI 4.0% CABG 15.0%	N/A	PCI 13.0% CABG 5.0%	N/A	PCI 17.0% CABG 25.0%	Parsonnet score, diabetes, and CABG independent predictors of MACCE
Palmerini[27]	157 PCI 154 CABG	430 days	PCI 13.4% CABG 12.3%	PCI 8.3% CABG 4.5%	PCI 25.5% CABG 2.6%	N/A	N/A	60% of PCI cohort treated with DES Only 68% determined appropriate for either PCI or CABG
Palmerini[30]	98 PCI 161 CABG	2 years	PCI 18.0% CABG 17.0%	PCI 4.0% CABG 6.0%	PCI 25.0% CABG 3.0%	PCI 28.8% CABG 9.4%	N/A	Study limited to patients ≥75 years
Sanmartin[31]	96 PCI 245 DES	12 months	PCI 5.2% CABG 8.4%	PCI 0% CABG 1.3%	PCI 5.2% CABG 0.8%	PCI 0% CABG 0.8%	PCI 10.4% CABG 11.4%	Significantly higher 30-day MACCE with CABG (2.1% versus 9.0%; P = 0.03)
Brener[32]	97 PCI 190 CABG	3 years	PCI 20.0% CABG 15.0%	N/A	N/A	N/A	N/A	57% of PCI cohort treated with DES Higher EuroSCORE and diabetes independent predictors of 3-year mortality
Buszman[33]	Randomized 52 PCI 53 CABG	12 months	PCI 1.9% CABG 7.5%	PCI 1.9% CABG 5.7%	PCI 0% CABG 3.8%	PCI 28.8% CABG 9.4%	PCI 30.8% CABG 24.5%	PCI associated with significant increase in left ventricular ejection fraction at 12 months compared with CABG Trend toward lower mortality with PCI at 28-month follow-up (3 versus 7 events; P = 0.08)
Hsu[34]	20 PCI 39 CABG	12 months	PCI 5.0% CABG 20.5%	PCI 0% CABG 0%	PCI 0% CABG 10.3%	PCI 0% CABG 2.6%	PCI 5.0% CABG 33.3%	50% of PCI cohort treated with DES
Rodes-Cabau[35]	104 PCI 145 CABG	23 ± 16 months	PCI 16.3% CABG 12.4%*	PCI 23.1% CABG 19.3%	PCI 9.6% CABG 4.8%	PCI 8.7% CABG 6.2%	PCI 43.3% CABG 35.2%	Study limited to patients ≥80 years; 48% DES in PCI cohort EuroSCORE independent predictor of MACCE regardless of revascularization strategy
Seung[36]	542 PCI 542 CABG	3 years	PCI 7.9% CABG 7.8%	N/A	PCI 12.6% CABG 2.6%	N/A	PCI 9.3% CABG 9.2%†	Propensity matched analysis of 396 PCI and CABG patient pairs demonstrates no significant difference in death, myocardial infarction, or stroke but significantly higher repeated revascularization with DES
Wu[37]	135 PCI 135 CABG	2 years	PCI 18.0% CABG 5.9%	N/A	PCI 27.4% CABG 5.9%	N/A	N/A	Matched analysis of DES and CABG patients (N = 56 pairs) showed no survival difference and higher repeated revascularization with DES
Serruys[3]	357 PCI 348 CABG	12 months	PCI 4.2% CABG 4.4%	PCI 4.3% CABG 4.1%	PCI 11.8% CABG 6.5%	PCI 0.3% CABG 2.7%	PCI 15.8% CABG 13.7%	No significant differences overall in MACCE or death, myocardial infarction, or stroke PCI associated with significantly higher MACCE in highest SYNTAX tercile

*Cardiovascular death.
†Composite endpoint of death, Q-wave myocardial infarction, or stroke.
MACCE = major adverse cardiac and cerebrovascular events.
Modified from Kandzari DE, Colombo A, Park SJ, et al: Revascularization for unprotected left main disease: Evolution of the evidence basis to redefine treatment standards. J Am Coll Cardiol 54:1576, 2009.

CH 58 PERCUTANEOUS CORONARY INTERVENTION

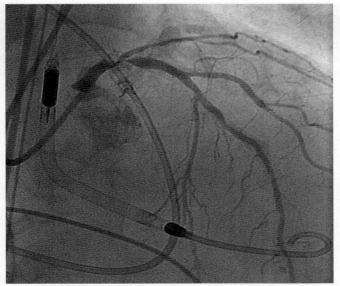

FIGURE 58-5 Impella device position in the left ventricle before left main intervention in a sole remaining artery.

Vascular Access

The most frequently used vascular access sites for PCI include the common femoral artery, the brachial artery, and more recently the radial artery (see Chaps. 20 and 21). The femoral approach (either right or left sided) is the most commonly used vascular access site in the United States and provides the advantages of large vessel size (typically 6 to 8 mm in diameter) and the ability to accommodate larger (>6 French) sheath sizes including intra-aortic balloon pump catheters. In addition, because of the typically straight path from the femoral artery to the ascending aorta, the femoral approach provides excellent guide catheter support and manipulability and access to the venous system through the adjacent femoral vein. Severe peripheral arterial disease, peripheral vascular bypass grafts, and requirement for immobilization after the procedure limit the use of the femoral approach in some patients.

The brachial arterial approach was historically used as the principal alternative to femoral access. However, because the brachial artery provides the only circulation to the forearm and hand (i.e., it is a functional end-artery), any compromise of the brachial artery can lead to severe ischemic complications of the hand.

The radial arterial approach (see Chaps. 20 and 21) has gained in popularity as an alternative to femoral access in patients with significant peripheral vascular disease and particularly in obese patients, in whom direct compression of the radial artery reduces bleeding complications[44,45] (**Table 58-3**). The radial approach provides direct access to the ascending aorta and the unique advantage of allowing immediate mobilization after PCI. An Allen test is useful to assess flow to the hand before radial artery cannulation. Tortuosity of the brachiocephalic trunk may limit the use of the approach in some patients (2% to 3%). The small size of the radial artery limits the size of guiding catheters used during PCI (typically 5F or 6F for women and 7F for men). Transradial access is associated with a generally lower rate (2%) of vascular complications.[46] A meta-analysis has suggested that radial access reduced major bleeding compared with femoral access[47] (**Table 58-4**). A randomized study of 1024 patients undergoing coronary arteriography and PCI found a reduction in major vascular complications (0.58% versus 3.7% in patients accessed by the femoral artery; $P = 0.0008$), albeit at the expense of longer procedure duration and higher radiation exposure.[48] Predictors of failure with the transradial access include age >75 years, prior CABG surgery, and short stature.[49]

TABLE 58-3	Comparison of Radial and Femoral Artery Access	
	FEMORAL	**RADIAL**
Access site bleeding	3%-4%	0%-0.6%
Artery complications	Pseudoaneurysm, retroperitoneal hemorrhage, arteriovenous fistula, painful hematoma	Rare local irritation, pulse loss 3%-9%, forearm hematoma
Patient comfort	Acceptable	Favored
Ambulation	2-4 hours	Immediate
Extra costs	Closure device	Band
Procedure time	Perceived shorter	Perceived longer
Estimated radiation exposure	Perceived shorter	Perceived longer
Access to left internal mammary artery	Easy	Difficult from right radial
Use of artery for CABG	Not applicable	Unknown
Learning curve	Short	Longer
>8F catheter	Acceptable	Maximum 7F (in men)
Peripheral vascular disease, obese	Problematic	Acceptable

Modified from Kern MJ: Cardiac catheterization on the road less traveled. J Am Coll Cardiol Intv 2:1055, 2009.

TABLE 58-4	Outcomes in Radial Versus Femoral Access in Meta-Analysis			
	FEMORAL N/TOTAL (%)	**RADIAL N/ TOTAL (%)**	**ODDS RATIO (95% CI)**	**P VALUE**
Major bleeding	48/2068 (2.3)	13/2390 (0.05)	0.27 (0.16, 0.45)	<0.001
Death, MI, or stroke	71/1874 (3.8)	56/2209 (2.5)	0.71 (0.49, 1.01)	0.058
Death	28/1874 (1.8)	22/1906 (1.2)	0.74 (0.42, 1.30)	0.29
Myocardial infarction	46/1595 (2.9)	39/1931 (2.0)	0.76 (0.49, 1.17)	0.21
Stroke	5/1107 (0.5)	2/1428 (0.1)	0.39 (0.09, 1.75)	0.22
Access site crossover	34/1107 (1.4)	150/2542 (5.9)	3.82 (2.83, 5.15)	<0.001
Inability to cross the lesion with a wire, balloon, or stent during PCI	40/1186 (3.4)	60/1274 (4.7)	1.31 (0.87, 1.96)	0.20

Modified from Jolly SS, Amlani S, Hamon M, et al: Radial versus femoral access for coronary angiography or intervention and the impact on major bleeding and ischemic events: A systematic review and meta-analysis of randomized trials. Am Heart J 157:132, 2009.

Vascular Access Complications

Vascular access site complications occur after 3% to 7% of PCIs and lead to significantly increased length of hospital stay, total costs, and morbidity and mortality.[50] Complications range from relatively minor access site hematomas to life-threatening retroperitoneal bleeds requiring emergent blood transfusion to damage to the vasculature requiring prompt surgical intervention.[51] Factors predisposing patients to an increased risk of serious vascular complications after PCI include age, female gender, larger vascular sheath size, low body mass index, renal insufficiency, and degree of anticoagulation during the procedure. The location of the entry point for transfemoral access predicts the risk and type of vascular complication (see Chap. 20). If the access site is above the level of the inguinal ligament, the risk of retroperitoneal hemorrhage is substantially increased.[51] If the access site is distal to the femoral bifurcation, pseudoaneurysms (0.4%) and arteriovenous fistulas (0.2%) may occur. Major vascular complications of the femoral approach include limb-threatening ischemia (0.1%) and retroperitoneal hemorrhage (0.4%), which are associated with increased risk of death by 2- to 10-fold in the first 30 days after the PCI procedure.[52]

Vascular Closure Devices

Vascular access closure devices were introduced in the mid-1990s as a new way of managing the access site after femoral access procedures. Vascular closure devices reduce the time to ambulation, increase the patient's comfort after PCI, and provide efficiencies of patient flow in the catheterization laboratory.[53-59]

Currently approved vascular closure devices fall into three categories. Sealant devices include collagen- and thrombin-based systems that leave no mechanical anchor inside or outside the vessel. Mechanical closure devices include suture-mediated and nitinol clip–based systems and provide immediate secure closure to the vessel. Hybrid closure devices, such as the dissolvable AngioSeal device (St. Jude Medical, Minneapolis, Minn), use a combination of collagen sealant with an internal mechanical closure to cause rapid hemostasis.[60] Although each device has proved relatively safe and effective, few comparative data permit evaluation of the relative risks and benefits of each device. Two recent meta-analyses concluded that vascular closure devices do not lower the risk of vascular complications compared with manual hemostasis (**Table 58-5**), but infections may occur more often with suture-based closure devices, and occlusions are found more often with hybrid devices.[61,62]

Coronary Devices

During the past three decades, steady improvements in the equipment used for coronary revascularization (e.g., reductions in device profile and improvements in catheter flexibility) have been supplemented with the introduction of periodic "transformational technology," such as coronary stents and more recently DES, which have extended the scope and breadth of clinical practice. The type of lesions amenable to PCI has become progressively more complex during this period, and the outcomes associated with the use of these devices have progressively improved. A brief overview of the currently available coronary devices follows.

Balloon Angioplasty

Balloon angioplasty expands the coronary lumen by stretching and tearing the atherosclerotic plaque and vessel wall and, to a lesser extent, by redistributing atherosclerotic plaque along its longitudinal axis. Elastic recoil of the stretched vessel wall generally leaves a 30% to 35% residual diameter stenosis, and the vessel expansion can result in propagating coronary dissections, leading to abrupt vessel closure in 5% to 8% of patients. Although stand-alone balloon angioplasty is rarely used other than for very small (<2.25 mm) vessels, balloon angioplasty remains integral to PCI for predilation of lesions before stent placement, deployment of coronary stents, and further expansion of stents after deployment.

Most of the enhancements in balloon technology relate to the development of low-profile (deflated diameter = 0.7 mm) balloons that are more trackable through tortuous anatomy and noncompliant balloons that can inflate to pressures in excess of 20 atm without overexpansion or rupture. A modification of balloon angioplasty includes a focused-force dilation in which a scoring blade or guidewire external to the balloon concentrates dilating force and resists balloon slippage during inflation. The Cutting Balloon (Boston Scientific, Natick, Mass) and the AngioScore catheter (AngioScore, Inc., Fremont, Calif) are focused-force balloon angioplasty systems that are currently used in a small minority (less than 5%) of PCIs.

Coronary Atherectomy

Atherectomy refers to removal (rather than simple displacement) of the obstructing atherosclerotic plaque. By removal of plaque or improving lesion wall compliance in calcified or fibrotic lesions, atherectomy can provide a larger final minimal lumen diameter than that achieved by balloon angioplasty alone. Atherectomy was performed

---

TABLE 58-5   Complications Associated with Vascular Closure Devices

AUTHOR	STUDY TYPE	N	ENDPOINT	VASCULAR CLOSURE DEVICE	MANUAL COMPRESSION	P VALUE
Cura[a]	Registry	2918	Vascular complications	2.9%[AS] 3.2%[Per]	3.1%	NS
Dangas[b]	Registry	5093	Surgical repair	2.5%	1.5%	0.03
Resnic[c]	Registry	3027	Vascular complications	3.0%	5.5%	0.002
Dangas[d]	Pooled RCT	2095	Device complications	8.5%	5.9%	0.02
Tavris[53]	ACC Registry	166,680	Vascular complications	1.05-1.48%	1.7%	<0.001
Exaire[54]	TARGET	4736	Transfusions	1.0%	0.8%	NS
Koreny[55]	Meta-analysis	4000	Hematoma	RR = 1.14		NS
Vaitkus[56]	Meta-analysis	5045	Vascular complications	RR = 0.89		<0.05
Nikolsky[57]	Meta-analysis	37,066	Vascular complications	Benefit[AS]		0.06
Applegate[58]	Registry	4699	Vascular complications	1.5%[AS]	1.7%	NS
Arora[58a]	Registry	12,937	Vascular complications	↓ 42%-58%		<0.05

[a]Cura FA, Kapadia SR, L'Allier PL, et al: Safety of femoral closure devices after percutaneous coronary interventions in the era of glycoprotein IIb/IIIa platelet blockade. Am J Cardiol 86:780, 2000.
[b]Dangas G, Mehran R, Kokolis S, et al: Vascular complications after percutaneous coronary interventions following hemostasis with manual compression versus arteriotomy closure devices. J Am Coll Cardiol 38:638, 2001.
[c]Resnic FS, Blake GJ, Ohno-Machado L, et al: Vascular closure devices and the risk of vascular complications after percutaneous coronary intervention in patients receiving glycoprotein IIb-IIIa inhibitors. Am J Cardiol 88:493, 2001.
[d]Dangas G, Mehran R, Fahy M, et al: Complications of vascular closure devices—not yet evidence based [reply]. J Am Coll Cardiol 39:1706, 2002.
ACC = American College of Cardiology; AS = Angioseal; NS = not significant; PER = Perclose; RCT = randomized controlled trials; RR = relative risk ratio.
Modified from Dauerman HL, Applegate RJ, Cohen DJ: Vascular closure devices: The second decade. J Am Coll Cardiol 50:1617, 2007.

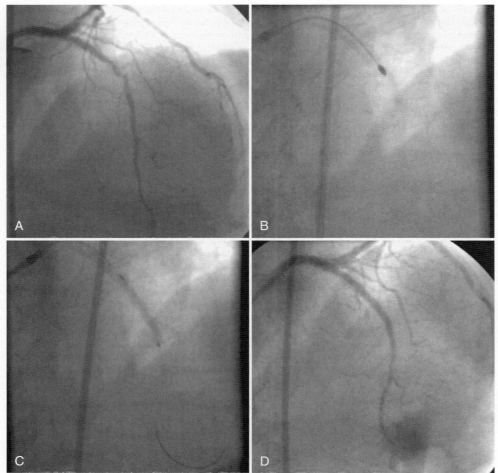

FIGURE 58-6 Rotational atherectomy of an undilatable left anterior descending artery. **A,** A heavily calcified diffuse lesion in the left anterior descending artery is generally considered undilatable by conventional balloon techniques. **B,** A 1.5-mm rotational atherectomy burr revolving at 160,000 rpm is advanced to ablate the calcified lesion. **C,** A 3.0 × 28-mm stent can then be advanced across the blockage and inflated to 16 atm. It is unlikely that full stent expansion could have occurred without pretreatment with rotational atherectomy. **D,** The final angiographic result shows no residual stenosis and normal flow into the distal vessel.

1.5- or 1.75-mm burr to improve lesion compliance (plaque modification) before the lesion is treated definitively by balloon dilation and stent placement. Rotational coronary atherectomy is currently used in less than 5% of PCI procedures (**Fig. 58-6**).

Thrombectomy and Aspiration Devices

The AngioJet rheolytic thrombectomy catheter (Possis Medical, Inc., Minneapolis, Minn) was introduced as a dedicated device for thrombus removal through the dissolution and aspiration of the thrombus. High-speed saline jets within the tip of the catheter create intense local suction by the Venturi effect, pulling surrounding blood, thrombus, and saline into the lumen of the catheter opening, propelling the debris proximally through the catheter lumen. Rheolytic thrombectomy was superior to a prolonged intraluminal urokinase infusion in patients with a large thrombus, but its routine use in patients with STEMI was not associated with improvement in infarct size by single-photon emission computed tomography (SPECT) imaging and may have caused more complications.[63] Rheolytic thrombectomy may still be useful in clinical practice when there is a large angiographic thrombus in a native vessel or SVG.

Newer lower profile aspiration catheters that use 6F and 7F guiding catheters have been developed as alternatives to rheolytic thrombectomy in patients with thrombus-containing lesions. These techniques may be slightly less effective (particularly against partially organized thrombus) than rheolytic thrombectomy, although the risk of distal particulate embolization and device trauma in smaller vessels may be less with these aspiration catheters. In a multicenter study of 1071 patients with STEMI who were randomly assigned to the thrombus-aspiration group or the conventional-PCI group, a myocardial blush grade of 0 or 1 occurred in 17.1% of the patients in the thrombus-aspiration group and in 26.3% of those in the conventional-PCI group (*P* < 0.001).[64] At 30 days, the rate of death in patients with a myocardial blush grade of 0 or 1, 2, and 3 was 5.2%, 2.9%, and 1.0%, respectively (*P* = 0.003), and the rate of adverse events was 14.1%, 8.8%, and 4.2%, respectively (*P* < 0.001).[64] Meta-analysis of the data suggests that simple manual thrombus aspiration before PCI reduces mortality in patients undergoing primary PCI (**Table 58-6** and **Fig. 58-7**)[65] (see PCI Guidelines).

Embolic Protection Devices

The advent of embolic protection systems has reduced the risk of postprocedural adverse events after SVG PCI. Although embolization of atherosclerotic debris was not considered a major complication during the early years of native coronary balloon angioplasty, it is now recognized as one potential cause of distal myocardial necrosis after PCI,[66] particularly in friable SVG lesions. Distal embolization causes postprocedural cardiac enzyme elevation in nearly 20% of cases after SVG PCI, and this enzyme elevation is associated with substantial morbidity and mortality. Numerous additional occlusive and filter-based distal protection systems as well as novel proximal occlusion devices have undergone evaluation and approval for use in SVG interventions. Despite their potential benefit in preventing thromboembolization in patients with STEMI, none of the embolic protection devices has reduced MI size with primary intervention, possibly relating to the high profile of the devices. Embolic protection devices fall into three broad categories: distal occlusion devices, distal embolic filters, and proximal occlusion devices.

in 30% of interventional procedures between 1992 and 1994, but its use fell dramatically with the availability of coronary stents. Less than 5% of current procedures involve the use of atherectomy devices, most often rotational atherectomy in combination with coronary stents.

The most commonly used atherectomy device is rotational coronary atherectomy (Boston Scientific), which removes the atheromatous plaque by the abrasion of inelastic calcified plaque using microscopic (20 to 50 μm) diamond chips on the surface of a rapidly rotating (160,000 rpm) olive-shaped atherectomy burr. This abrasion generates 2- to 5-μm microparticles that pass through the coronary microcirculation for removal by the reticuloendothelial system. Burrs travel over a specialized 0.009-inch guidewire and are available in diameters ranging from 1.25 to 2.50 mm. In the setting of severe calcification, smaller (1.25 mm) burrs can be used initially, followed by larger burrs in 0.25- to 0.50-mm increments up to 70% of the reference vessel diameter. Aggressive rotational coronary atherectomy techniques do not provide a restenosis advantage over more conservative methods and tend to increase acute procedural complications, such as distal embolization or coronary perforation. Rotational atherectomy does not appear to reduce restenosis compared with balloon angioplasty in noncalcified vessels. Current use of rotational atherectomy is reserved for ostial and heavily calcified lesions that cannot be dilated with balloon angioplasty or those that prevent delivery of coronary stents. Rotational coronary atherectomy is generally limited to abrasion of superficial calcification with a single

TABLE 58-6	Clinical Benefits from Reperfusion Device from Meta-Analysis		
	RISK RATIO	**95% CI**	**_P_ VALUE**
Catheter Aspiration Devices			
Mortality	0.63	0.43-0.93	0.018
Myocardial infarction	0.65	0.37-1.12	0.13
Target vessel revascularization	0.83	0.64-1.08	0.16
Stroke	3.43	0.85-14	0.085
MACE	0.76	0.62-0.95	0.013
TIMI blush grade	1.69	1.26-2.28	<0.001
ST-segment resolution	1.41	1.21-1.64	<0.001
Mechanical Thrombectomy Devices			
Mortality	1.93	1.00-3.72	0.05
Myocardial infarction	0.67	0.19-3.01	0.53
Target vessel revascularization	1.14	0.43-3.01	0.79
Stroke	2.67	0.71-10	0.14
MACE	1.64	0.71-1.90	0.55
ST-segment resolution	1.25	0.99-1.58	0.061
Embolic Protection Devices			
Mortality	0.92	0.60-1.40	0.69
Myocardial infarction	0.82	0.44-1.51	0.52
Target vessel revascularization	1.04	0.74-1.47	0.82
Stroke	0.99	0.34-2.92	0.99
MACE	0.95	0.69-1.30	0.73
TIMI blush grade	1.18	1.02-1.38	0.031
ST-segment resolution	1.07	0.98-1.16	0.13

MACE = major adverse cardiac event.

Modified from Bavry AA, Kumbhani DJ, Bhatt DL: Role of adjunctive thrombectomy and embolic protection devices in acute myocardial infarction: A comprehensive meta-analysis of randomized trials. Eur Heart J 29:2989, 2008.

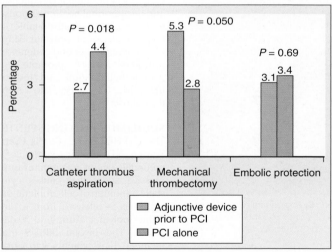

FIGURE 58-7 In this meta-analysis of patients with STEMI undergoing primary PCI, simple manual thrombus aspiration is associated with lower mortality, whereas mechanical aspiration and embolic protection devices are not. *(From Bavry AA, Kumbhani DJ, Bhatt DL: Role of adjunctive thrombectomy and embolic protection devices in acute myocardial infarction: A comprehensive meta-analysis of randomized trials. Eur Heart J 29:2989, 2008.)*

DISTAL OCCLUSION DEVICES. The GuardWire (Medtronic Vascular, Santa Rosa, Calif) is a low-pressure balloon mounted on a hollow guide-wire shaft. The device is passed across the target lesion and inflated with a saline contrast admixture to occlude flow; the debris liberated by intervention remains trapped in the stagnant column of blood and is aspirated with a specially designed aspiration catheter before the occlusion balloon is deflated to restore anterograde flow. Compared with SVG intervention without distal occlusion, use of the GuardWire reduced 30-day major adverse clinical events and no-reflow. The major disadvantage of this device is that blood flow is stopped during SVG intervention while the balloon is inflated.

DISTAL EMBOLIC FILTERS. Distal filters are advanced across the target lesion in their smaller collapsed state, and a retaining sheath is withdrawn, allowing the filters to open and to expand against the vessel wall. The filters then remain in place to catch any liberated embolic material larger than the filter pore size (usually 120 to 150 μm) during intervention. At the end of the intervention, the filters are collapsed by use of a sheath, and the captured embolic material is removed from the body. This type of device has the advantages of maintaining anterograde flow during the procedure and allowing intermittent injection of contrast material to visualize underlying anatomy, but it has the potential disadvantage of allowing the component of debris with a diameter less than the filter pore size to pass (**Fig. 58-8**). Newer filter devices with reduced crossing profiles and more efficient capture of embolic debris have been developed (**Fig. 58-9**).

PROXIMAL OCCLUSION DEVICES. The third type of embolic protection device occludes flow into the vessel with a balloon on the tip of or just beyond the tip of the guiding catheter. Two proximal occlusion devices are currently in use: the Proxis catheter (St. Jude Medical) and Kerberos embolic protection system (Kerberos, Sunnyvale, Calif). With such inflow occlusion, retrograde flow generated by distal collaterals or infusion through a "rinsing" catheter can propel any liberated debris back into the lumen of the guiding catheter. These approaches have the potential advantage of providing embolic protection even before the first wire crosses the target lesion.

Coronary Stents

Coronary stents have emerged as the predominant form of PCI and are currently used in more than 90% of PCI procedures worldwide. Coronary stents scaffold arterial dissection flaps, thereby lowering the incidence of vessel closure and need for emergency CABG surgery, and lessen the frequency of restenosis because of their effect on preventing arterial constriction that is the primary mechanism of restenosis with balloon angioplasty. Despite late clinical improvement compared with balloon angioplasty, restenosis after coronary stent placement occurs in some patients because of excessive intimal hyperplasia within the stent. A number of second-generation balloon-expandable stents were introduced between 1997 and 2003, varying in metallic composition (i.e., cobalt chromium or layered metals versus solid 316 L stainless steel), strut design, stent length, delivery and deployment system, and arterial surface coverage, among other factors. These modifications enhanced flexibility and ease of delivery of the stent while also improving vessel scaffolding and side branch access.

The early use of coronary stents was limited by high (3% to 5%) subacute thrombosis rates, despite aggressive antithrombotic therapy with aspirin (≤325 mg daily), dipyridamole (225 mg daily), and periprocedural low-molecular-weight dextran and an uninterrupted transition from intravenous heparin to oral warfarin. Subacute thrombosis produced profound clinical consequences, resulting in an untoward outcome (e.g., death, MI, or emergency revascularization) in virtually every such patient. Lower frequencies of subacute stent thrombosis (roughly 0.5% to 1.0%) have resulted from use of high-pressure stent deployment and with a drug regimen that includes aspirin and a thienopyridine (e.g., clopidogrel or prasugrel) started just before or after stent placement.

Whereas coronary BMS reduce the incidence of angiographic and clinical restenosis compared with balloon angioplasty, angiographic restenosis (follow-up diameter stenosis >50%) still occurred in 20% to 30% of patients and clinical restenosis (recurrent angina due to restenosis in the treated segment) developed in 10% to 15% of patients in the first year after treatment. Restenosis with BMS occurred more often in patients with small vessels, long lesions, and diabetes mellitus, among other factors. Adjunctive pharmacologic therapy has not prevented restenosis after stent placement.

Several mechanical treatments of in-stent restenosis were attempted, including balloon redilation, removal of in-stent hyperplasia by means of atherectomy, and repeated bare metal stenting. Brachytherapy with use of beta or gamma sources did modestly improve this outcome for in-stent restenosis, but brachytherapy has several limitations, including the requirement for a radiation therapist, a tendency for late "catch-up" restenosis, and the inhibition of endothelialization that markedly

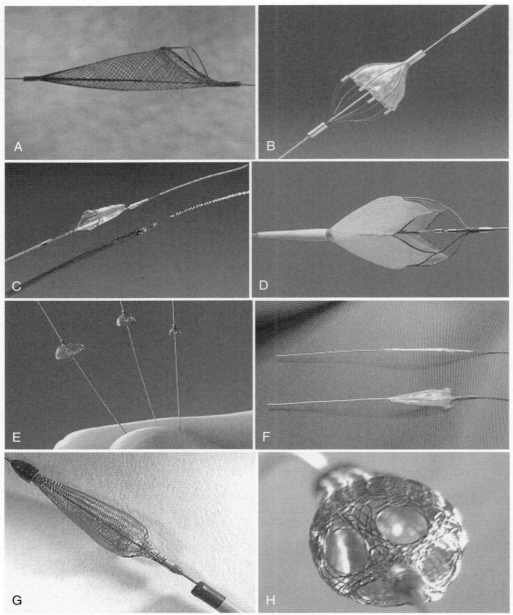

delivery, and the pharmacologic agent employed to limit intimal hyperplasia (**Fig. 58-10**).

DES have proven efficacy in patients with focal, de novo, and "workhorse" lesions that include reference vessel diameters between 2.5 and 3.5 mm and lesion lengths between 15 and 30 mm. Additional randomized trials and registries have also demonstrated the benefit of DES in patients with long (>30 mm) and small (<2.5 mm) vessels, chronic total occlusions, SVG and internal mammary disease, and in-stent restenosis and in patients with STEMI.[69] With the expanded follow-up of patients receiving DES, it has become apparent that DES placement requires extended (up to 1 year) therapy with the combination of aspirin and clopidogrel to prevent stent thrombosis.[70] Moreover, even after 1 year, there is an infrequent (0.2% to 0.6%) annual rate of very late stent thrombosis, warranting a careful discussion of the risks, benefits, and alternative therapies in candidates for PCI.[71] The risk of late and very late stent thrombosis appears related to endothelial dysfunction and an abnormal healing response to the vessel wall attributable to the durable stent polymer. More biocompatible second-generation polymers may promote a re-endothelialization and reduce the risk of very late stent thrombosis.[72]

SIROLIMUS-ELUTING STENTS. The CYPHER stent (Cordis Corp., Warren, NJ) contains sirolimus, a naturally occurring immunosuppressive agent that causes cytostatic inhibition of cell proliferation. Sirolimus is released from a biostable polymer during a 30-day period. The pivotal SIRIUS trial included 1058 patients with workhorse lesions who were randomized to treatment with a

FIGURE 58-8 Filters for distal protection. **A,** The Spider filter (ev3, Minneapolis, Minn). **B,** Angioguard device (Cordis Corp., Warren, NJ). **C,** EPI FilterWire (Boston Scientific, Natick, Mass). **D,** Accunet device (Guidant, Santa Clara, Calif). **E,** MedNova (Abbott, Chicago, Ill). **F,** Rubicon filter (Boston Scientific). **G, H,** The Interceptor filter (Medtronic Vascular, Santa Rosa, Calif) in longitudinal view **(G)** and axial view **(H).**

increases the risk of thrombosis if another stent is implanted in the same vessel segment. Brachytherapy was inferior to DES placement for treatment of restenosis in two randomized studies.[67,68]

BMS are currently used in 10% to 30% of patients undergoing PCI. This is most often due to the inability to take long-term dual antiplatelet therapy; larger (>4.0 mm) vessels, in which the restenosis risk is lower; and acute MI, wherein the issues related to compliance of the patient are more difficult to ascertain.

Drug-Eluting Stents

DES were developed in the early 2000s to provide sustained local delivery of an antiproliferative agent at the site of vessel wall injury. The three components of current DES are the balloon-expandable stent, a durable or resorbable polymer coating that provides sustained drug

sirolimus-eluting stent or a BMS. The primary clinical endpoint of 8-month target vessel failure, composed of target vessel revascularization, death, or MI, was reduced from 21% in patients treated with BMS to 8.6% in patients with sirolimus-eluting stents (P < 0.001). Angiographic restenosis rates were also lower in patients assigned to treatment with the sirolimus-eluting stents within the stent (35.4% with BMS versus 3.2% with sirolimus-eluting stents; P < 0.001) and within the treated segment including 5-mm proximal and distal margins (36.3% with BMS versus 8.9% with sirolimus-eluting stents; P < 0.001). Target vessel revascularization was reduced from 16.6% in BMS to 4.1% in sirolimus-eluting stents (P < 0.001). Reduction in intimal hyperplasia endured for at least 2 years after the procedure. At 5 years, there were significant reductions in target lesion revascularization for sirolimus-eluting stents compared with BMS (cumulative incidence: 12.5% versus 28.8%, respectively; P < 0.001).[73,74] There was no difference in the cumulative incidence of MI or revascularization attributed to

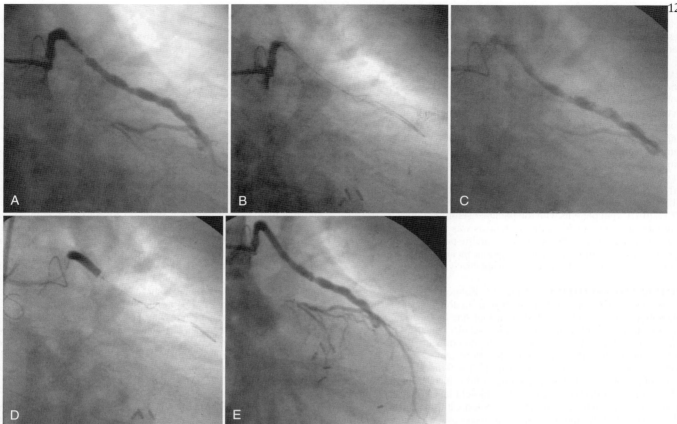

FIGURE 58-9 SVG percutaneous intervention with FilterWire distal protection. **A,** A degenerated SVG to the left anterior descending artery has a stenosis in its proximal segment. **B,** The FilterWire is positioned across the stenosis and deployed against the wall of the SVG. **C,** Flow is shown through the SVG. **D,** A stent is deployed in the proximal segment of the SVG. **E,** The FilterWire is removed, and there is excellent flow into the distal SVG without evidence of distal embolization.

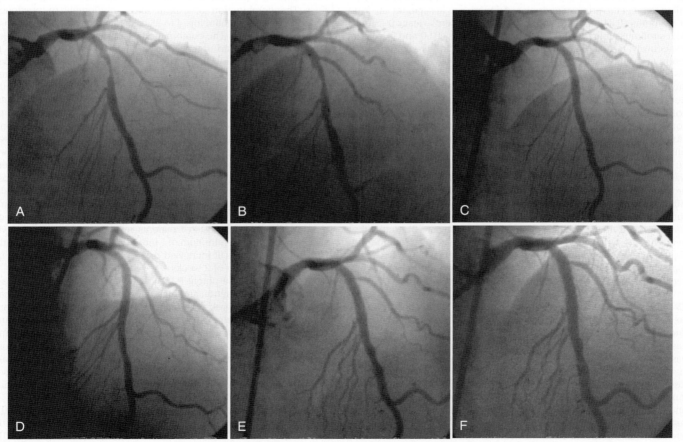

FIGURE 58-10 First-in-human CYPHER stent implantation. **A,** A focal stenosis is shown in the mid left anterior descending artery. **B,** A CYPHER sirolimus-eluting stent is positioned across the stenosis. **C,** There is excellent initial angiographic result and no residual stenosis. Follow-up angiography was performed at 4 months **(D),** 1 year **(E),** and 2 years **(F)** after the procedure without evidence of lumen renarrowing. *(Courtesy of Eduardo Sousa, São Paulo, Brazil.)*

remote segments of the target vessel. Events attributed to the nontarget vessel were frequent and not different for sirolimus-eluting stents versus BMS (25.7% versus 25.8%).[73,74]

PACLITAXEL-ELUTING STENTS. The TAXUS stent (Boston Scientific) is composed of a stainless steel stent platform, a polyolefin polymer derivative, and the microtubular stabilizing agent paclitaxel that has anti-inflammatory effects while also inhibiting both cell migration and division. Paclitaxel release is completed within 30 days of implantation, although a substantial portion (>90%) of the paclitaxel remains within the polymer indefinitely. The pivotal TAXUS IV trial randomly assigned 1314 patients with single de novo coronary lesions to either a TAXUS stent or an identical-appearing BMS. The ischemia-driven target vessel revascularization at 9 months was reduced from 11.3% to 3% and remained significantly reduced at 12 months (from 17.1% to 7.1%) in patients with the paclitaxel-eluting stents ($P < 0.001$). The rate of binary angiographic restenosis was reduced both within the stent (24.4% with BMS versus 5.5% with the paclitaxel-eluting stent; $P < 0.001$) and within the treated segment including 5-mm proximal and distal margins (26.6% and 7.9%, respectively; $P < 0.001$).

ZOTAROLIMUS-ELUTING STENTS. Zotarolimus (previously known as ABT-578) is another rapamycin analogue released from a phosphorylcholine (PC)–coated stent that has been evaluated with use of the Endeavor stent (Medtronic Vascular). In the Endeavor II trial, 1197 patients were assigned to treatment with the Endeavor zotarolimus-eluting PC polymer–coated stent or the same BMS but without the drug or the polymer coating.[75] The 9-month primary endpoint of target vessel failure was reduced from 15.1% with the BMS to 7.9% with the Endeavor ($P < 0.0001$).[75] In-stent late loss was reduced from 1.03 mm to 0.61 mm in patients treated with the Endeavor stent ($P < 0.001$), and the rate of in-segment restenosis was reduced from 35% to 13.2% with the Endeavor stent ($P < 0.0001$). There was a significant reduction associated with the use of the Endeavor stent that persisted to 4 years.[75] The ENDEAVOR III trial compared the Endeavor stent with CYPHER in a 436-patient study (3:1 randomization) and failed to meet the primary endpoint of noninferior in-segment late loss at 8 months (0.34 mm with zotarolimus-eluting stents versus 0.13 mm with sirolimus-eluting stents) with higher late loss (0.60 and 0.15 mm, respectively; $P < 0.001$). There was no significant difference in target lesion revascularization between the two groups (6.3% and 3.5%, respectively; $P = 0.34$). At 3-year follow-up, there was a reduction in the occurrence of death and MI in patients treated with the Endeavor stent but no difference in the occurrence of target vessel revascularization.[76] The Endeavor IV trial, a prospective, randomized, single-blind, controlled trial, compared the safety and efficacy of the zotarolimus-eluting stent with the paclitaxel-eluting stent in 1548 patients with single de novo coronary lesions. The primary endpoint was a composite of cardiac death, MI, or target vessel revascularization, and Endeavor was noninferior to the TAXUS stent. In addition, there were fewer periprocedural MIs with zotarolimus-eluting stents (0.5% versus 2.2%; $P = 0.007$) because of less side branch occlusion in patients with zotarolimus-eluting stents.[77] Although 8-month angiographic restenosis was improved after paclitaxel-eluting stent therapy, at 12 months the frequency of target lesion revascularization was similar comparing zotarolimus- with paclitaxel-eluting stents (4.5% versus 3.8%; $P = 0.228$), especially in those without planned angiographic follow-up (3.6% versus 3.2%; $P = 0.756$), and these results persisted for 2 years.[78]

EVEROLIMUS-ELUTING STENT. The Xience stent (Abbot Vascular, Santa Rosa, Calif) uses the cobalt chromium Vision stent, a durable fluoropolymer, and everolimus, which is a rapamycin analogue that has both immunosuppressive and antiproliferative effects. On the basis of initial studies that evaluated use of an absorbable poly-L-lactic acid polymer, the SPIRIT program has shown reduction in late lumen loss comparable to the CYPHER stent. The SPIRIT III, a prospective, randomized, single-blind, controlled trial, enrolled 1002 patients undergoing PCI in lesions 28 mm or less in length and with reference vessel diameter between 2.5 and 3.75 mm.[79] Angiographic in-segment late loss was significantly less in the everolimus-eluting stent group compared with the paclitaxel group (0.14 mm versus 0.28 mm; $P = 0.004$).[79] The everolimus stent was noninferior to the paclitaxel stent for target vessel failure at 9 months (7.2% versus 9.0%, respectively; $P < 0.001$ for noninferiority).[79] The everolimus stent resulted in significant reductions in composite major adverse cardiac events both at 9 months compared with the paclitaxel stent (4.6% versus 8.1%; $P = 0.03$) and at 1 year (6.0% versus 10.3%; $P = 0.02$) because of fewer MIs and target lesion revascularization procedures.[79]

Antiplatelet Agents (see Chap. 87)

ASPIRIN. Aspirin irreversibly inhibits cyclooxygenase and thus blocks the synthesis of thromboxane A_2, a vasoconstricting agent that promotes platelet aggregation. Aspirin substantially reduces periprocedural MI caused by thrombotic occlusions compared with placebo and has been established as a standard for all patients undergoing PCI. The inhibitory effect of aspirin occurs within 60 minutes, and its effect on platelets lasts for up to 7 days after discontinuation. Although the minimum effective aspirin dosage in the setting of PCI remains uncertain, patients taking daily aspirin should receive 75 to 325 mg aspirin before PCI (see PCI Guidelines). Patients not already taking daily long-term aspirin therapy should be given 300 to 325 mg of aspirin at least 2 hours and preferably 24 hours before PCI is performed. After PCI, in patients without allergy or increased risk of bleeding, aspirin 162 to 325 mg daily should be given for at least 1 month after BMS implantation, 3 months after sirolimus-eluting stent implantation, and 6 months after paclitaxel-eluting stent implantation, after which daily long-term aspirin use should be continued indefinitely at a dose of 75 to 162 mg (see PCI Guidelines).

THIENOPYRIDINE DERIVATIVES. Thienopyridine derivatives cause irreversible platelet inhibition because of their effects on the $P2Y_{12}$ adenosine diphosphate (ADP) receptor that can activate the glycoprotein IIb/IIIa complex. Because aspirin and thienopyridine derivatives have distinct mechanisms of action, their combination inhibits platelet aggregation to a greater extent than either agent alone does. The combination of aspirin and clopidogrel (or previously ticlopidine) was essential for 14 to 28 days to prevent stent thrombosis after BMS placement. The combination of aspirin and clopidogrel also reduces death, MI, and urgent revascularization within 12 months in patients undergoing PCI in the setting of NSTEMI and unstable angina and in those undergoing elective PCI. Recent studies have suggested that a loading dose of 600 mg rather than 300 mg of clopidogrel results in more rapid (<2 hours) platelet inhibition[80,81] and improved clinical outcomes, including lower rates of stent thrombosis. Additional clopidogrel loading with 300 mg or 600 mg may also be used in patients on chronic maintenance clopidogrel therapy.[82] The need for pretreatment with clopidogrel is more controversial, balancing improved clinical outcomes with the potential risk for bleeding should CABG surgery be needed. Current guidelines recommend that a 600-mg loading dose of clopidogrel be administered before or during PCI (see PCI Guidelines). For all post-PCI patients who receive a DES, clopidogrel 75 mg daily should be given for at least 12 months if patients are not at high risk for bleeding. For post-PCI patients receiving a BMS, clopidogrel should be given for a minimum of 1 month and ideally up to 12 months (unless the patient is at increased risk for bleeding; then it should be given for a minimum of 2 weeks) (see PCI Guidelines).

Prasugrel is a more potent $P2Y_{12}$ ADP receptor inhibitor that has a more rapid onset of action and higher levels of platelet inhibition than higher dose clopidogrel.[83] In a study of 13,608 patients with moderate-to high-risk acute coronary syndromes undergoing scheduled PCI and randomly assigned to receive prasugrel (60-mg loading dose and 10-mg daily maintenance dose) or clopidogrel (300-mg loading dose and 75-mg daily maintenance dose) for 6 to 15 months, the primary efficacy endpoint, a composite of death from cardiovascular causes, nonfatal MI, or nonfatal stroke, occurred in 12.1% of patients receiving clopidogrel and 9.9% of patients receiving prasugrel ($P < 0.001$).[84] There were also significant reductions in the prasugrel group in the rates of MI (9.7% for clopidogrel versus 7.4% for prasugrel; $P < 0.001$), urgent target vessel revascularization (3.7% versus 2.5%; $P < 0.001$), and stent thrombosis (2.4% versus 1.1%; $P < 0.001$).[84] On the other hand, major bleeding was observed in 2.4% of patients receiving prasugrel and in 1.8% of patients receiving clopidogrel ($P = 0.03$), with more frequent rates of life-threatening bleeding in the prasugrel group (1.4% versus 0.9% with clopidogrel; $P = 0.01$), including fatal bleeding (0.4% versus 0.1%, respectively; $P = 0.002$).[84,85] Among persons treated with clopidogrel, carriers of reduced-function CYP2C19 alleles had significantly lower levels of active metabolite, diminished platelet inhibition, and higher rates of adverse cardiovascular events.[86] A similar relationship was not found in patients treated with prasugrel. Further research will be necessary to determine if measurement of point-of-care platelet assays of genetic polymorphisms can help in allocating therapy.[87] In patients with an acute coronary syndrome undergoing PCI who are at low bleeding risk, prasugrel 60-mg loading dose should be given as soon as possible after definition of the coronary anatomy and continued for 12 to 15 months after stent placement (see PCI Guidelines).

Ticagrelor, a reversible oral $P2Y_{12}$ receptor antagonist, provides faster, greater, and more consistent ADP-receptor inhibition than clopidogrel.[88] In a multicenter, double-blind trial of 18,624 patients presenting with an acute coronary syndrome, with or without ST-segment elevation, random assignment was made to treatment with ticagrelor (180-mg loading dose, 90 mg twice daily thereafter) or clopidogrel (300- to 600-mg loading dose, 75 mg daily thereafter) for 12 months. The primary endpoint, a composite of death from vascular causes, MI, or stroke at 12 months, occurred in 9.8% of patients receiving ticagrelor and 11.7% of those receiving clopidogrel (hazard ratio, 0.84; $P < 0.001$).[89] There was also a significant reduction in MI alone (5.8% in the ticagrelor group versus 6.9% in the clopidogrel group; $P = 0.005$) and death from vascular causes (4.0% versus 5.1%; $P = 0.001$).[89] No significant difference in the overall rates of major bleeding was found between the ticagrelor and clopidogrel groups (11.6% and 11.2%, respectively; $P = 0.43$), but ticagrelor was associated with a higher rate of major bleeding not related to CABG (4.5% versus 3.8%, $P = 0.03$).[89]

Current evidence suggests that in the absence of risk factors for bleeding, dual antiplatelet therapy should continue for at least 12 months after BMS and DES placement. Prolonged thienopyridine therapy not only reduces late stent thrombosis but also prevents MI by thrombi that complicate plaques remote from the initial intervention. Indefinite aspirin and clopidogrel therapy is recommended in patients receiving brachytherapy, and higher doses (150 mg daily) of chronic clopidogrel are recommended in those patients in whom stent thrombosis may be catastrophic, such as patients with unprotected left main artery stenting or those with stenting of the last remaining vessel if there is less than 50% inhibition of platelet aggregation on platelet assays.[10,11]

GLYCOPROTEIN IIB/IIIA INHIBITORS. Thrombin and collagen are potent platelet agonists that can cause ADP and serotonin release and activate glycoprotein (GP) IIb/IIIa fibrinogen receptors on the platelet surface. Functionally active GP IIb/IIIa serves in the "final common pathway" of platelet aggregation by binding fibrinogen and other adhesive proteins that bridge adjacent platelets. There are three GP IIb/IIIa inhibitors approved for clinical use. Studies supporting the use of these agents during PCI were performed before the widespread use of dual antiplatelet therapy, and the use of these agents has been reevaluated in this context.

Abciximab is a chimeric human-murine monoclonal antibody that irreversibly binds to the platelet GP IIb/IIIa receptor of human platelets. It also binds to the vitronectin ($\alpha_v\beta_3$) receptor found on platelets and vessel wall endothelial and smooth muscle cells. The recommended dosage of abciximab is an intravenous bolus of 0.25 mg/kg, followed by a continuous intravenous infusion of 0.125 µg/kg/min (to a maximum of 10 µg/min) for 12 hours. Abciximab can be safely administered in patients with renal insufficiency, and platelet infusions can reverse the effect of this agent.

Eptifibatide is a cyclic peptide derivative that reversibly binds GP IIb/IIIa. A double eptifibatide bolus, 180 µg/kg boluses 10 minutes apart, and an infusion dose, 2.0 µg/kg/min for 18 to 24 hours, result in sufficient platelet inhibition to prevent ischemic events in patients undergoing PCI. Addition of eptifibatide to clopidogrel, 600-mg loading dose, also results in incremental platelet inhibition. A reduction of the eptifibatide infusion

to 1 µg/kg/min is necessary in patients with a creatinine clearance <50 mL/min. Platelet transfusions do not reverse the platelet inhibition with eptifibatide, although by 4 hours after cessation of the infusion, patients have safely undergone CABG.

Tirofiban, a peptidomimetic small molecule, has also undergone evaluation for its adjunctive benefit during urgent PCI and is inferior to abciximab for the prevention of ischemic events during PCI. The recommended dosage is an initial rate of 0.4 µg/kg/min for 30 minutes and then continued at 0.1 µg/kg/min. Patients with severe renal insufficiency (creatinine clearance <30 mL/min) should receive half the usual rate of infusion. Subsequent studies have suggested that the tirofiban bolus dose given in the initial PCI studies may not have produced optimal antiplatelet effect during PCI, and larger bolus doses can improve the inhibition of platelet aggregation.[90] Tirofiban is generally used for patients with acute coronary syndrome before PCI.

The GP IIb/IIIa inhibitors have demonstrated benefit in improving clinical outcomes within the first 30 days after PCI, primarily by reducing ischemic complications, including periprocedural MI and recurrent ischemia. They are particularly useful in patients with troponin-positive acute coronary syndromes[91] but have no consistent effect on reducing late restenosis. Although GP IIb/IIIa inhibitors differ in their structure, reversibility, and duration, two meta-analyses found no difference between their clinical effects in patients undergoing primary PCI.[92,93] Bleeding is the major risk of GP IIb/IIIa inhibitors, and a downward adjustment of the unfractionated heparin dose has been recommended. GP IIb/IIIa inhibitors are recommended in patients with NSTEMI and unstable angina who are not pretreated with clopidogrel, and it is reasonable to administer them to patients who have a troponin-positive acute coronary syndrome who have also been pretreated with clopidogrel[91] (see PCI Guidelines). Although GP IIb/IIIa inhibitors are recommended in selected patients at the time of PCI, the value of GP IIb/IIIa inhibitors as part of a routine preparatory strategy in patients with STEMI before their transport to the catheterization laboratory has been questioned on the basis of the results of three studies that failed to show benefit of GP IIb/IIIa inhibitors in patients who were pretreated with dual antiplatelet therapy.[90,94,95]

Antithrombin Agents

Unfractionated heparin (see Chap. 87) is the most commonly used thrombin inhibitor during PCI. Point-of-care activated clotting time (ACT) monitoring has facilitated heparin dose titration during PCI, and retrospective studies with balloon angioplasty have related the ACT value to clinical outcome after PCI. An ACT in the range of 350 to 375 seconds provided the lowest composite ischemic event rate, although any level of ACT <250 seconds had no further reductions in ischemic complications with concomitant use of GP IIb/IIIa inhibitors. More recent studies in the thienopyridine era have failed to correlate ischemic outcomes with the level of anticoagulation achieved with unfractionated heparin during coronary stent placement. Weight-adjusted heparin dosing regimens of 50 to 70 IU/kg help avoid "overshooting" the ACT. Sufficient unfractionated heparin should be administered during PCI to achieve an ACT >250 seconds if no GP IIb/IIIa inhibitor is given and >200 seconds if GP IIb/IIIa inhibitors are given. Routine use of intravenous heparin after PCI is no longer indicated. Early sheath removal is encouraged when the ACT falls to less than 150 to 180 seconds (see PCI Guidelines).

LOW-MOLECULAR-WEIGHT HEPARIN (see Chap. 87). Enoxaparin is considered a reasonable alternative to unfractionated heparin in patients with non–ST-segment elevation acute coronary syndromes undergoing PCI (see Chap. 56), but difficulty in monitoring the levels of anticoagulation in the event that PCI is performed has limited its clinical use at many centers.[96] The Superior Yield of the New Strategy of Enoxaparin, Revascularization and Glycoprotein IIb/IIIa Inhibitors (SYNERGY) trial prospectively randomized 10,027 high-risk patients with non–ST-segment elevation acute coronary syndrome with an intended early invasive strategy to treatment with subcutaneous enoxaparin or intravenous unfractionated heparin.[97] The 30-day primary efficacy outcome, a composite clinical endpoint of all-cause death or nonfatal MI, occurred in 14% of patients assigned to enoxaparin and 14.5% of patients assigned to unfractionated heparin. More TIMI (Thrombolysis in Myocardial Infarction) major bleeding was observed in patients treated with enoxaparin (9.1% versus 7.6%; $P = 0.008$). The bleeding risk was highest in those patients who received "crossover" therapy with unfractionated heparin and enoxaparin. When enoxaparin is given before PCI, empiric dose algorithms have been designed to guide additional anticoagulation therapy during PCI. If the last dose of enoxaparin was less than 8 hours before PCI, no additional antithrombin is needed. If the last dose of enoxaparin was given between 8 and 12 hours, a 0.3 mg/kg bolus of intravenous enoxaparin should be given.[97] If the dose was administrated more than 12 hours before PCI, conventional anticoagulation therapy is indicated.

BIVALIRUDIN. Bivalirudin is a direct thrombin inhibitor that has been used as an alternative to unfractionated heparin in patients undergoing PCI. Bivalirudin generally causes fewer bleeding complications than unfractionated heparin because of its shorter half-life (25 minutes) and more predictable bioavailability.[98] Bivalirudin is also accessible to clot-bound thrombin because its anticoagulant effect does not depend on binding with antithrombin. Bivalirudin was not inferior to the combination of unfractionated heparin and a GP IIb/IIIa inhibitor in one trial of 6010 "low-risk" patients in the REPLACE-2 study.[99] In a larger study of 13,819 patients with unstable angina and NSTEMI, bivalirudin alone was compared with bivalirudin with a GP IIb/IIIa inhibitor and heparin with a GP IIb/IIIa inhibitor. With use of a composite ischemia endpoint of death, MI, or unplanned revascularization for ischemia and major bleeding to determine net clinical benefit, bivalirudin alone, compared with heparin plus a GP IIb/IIIa inhibitor, showed noninferiority in the composite ischemia endpoint (7.8% and 7.3%, respectively) and significantly reduced rates of major bleeding (3.0% versus 5.7%; $P < 0.001$), resulting in a better net clinical outcome endpoint (10.1% versus 11.7%; $P = 0.02$).[100] Bivalirudin is considered a reasonable alternative to unfractionated heparin in low-risk patients undergoing PCI and may reduce bleeding complications in higher risk patients with unstable angina and NSTEMI. Bivalirudin may safely be substituted for unfractionated heparin in patients with acute coronary syndromes[101] and is a cost-effective alternative to unfractionated heparin and a GP IIb/IIIa inhibitor.[102] In a randomized study of 3602 patients with STEMI undergoing primary PCI (see Chap. 55), anticoagulation with bivalirudin alone, compared with heparin plus GP IIb/IIIa inhibitors, resulted in significantly reduced 30-day rates of major bleeding and net adverse clinical events, including a lower rate of mortality.[95] Adjunctive clopidogrel should be given as soon as possible (<30 minutes) before PCI in patients with acute coronary syndromes if possible.[103]

FACTOR Xa INHIBITORS. Fondaparinux is a pentasaccharide that has anti-Xa activity without effects on factor IIa and may cause less bleeding when it is used for the treatment of patients with acute coronary syndromes. The OASIS-5 trial randomly assigned 20,078 patients with acute coronary syndromes to receive either fondaparinux (2.5 mg daily) or enoxaparin (1 mg/kg of body weight twice daily) for a mean of 6 days.[104] The occurrence of the 9-day primary study endpoint (death, MI, or refractory ischemia) was similar in the two groups (5.8% with fondaparinux and 5.7% with enoxaparin), although the risk of major bleeding at 9 days was markedly lower with fondaparinux (2.2%) than with enoxaparin (4.1%; $P < 0.001$).[104] This reduction in bleeding was accompanied by an improvement in late mortality in patients treated with fondaparinux. Potential limitations of this approach are the relatively long half-life of fondaparinux and the need for adjunct anticoagulation with heparin during PCI to avoid the occurrence of catheter thrombi. Fondaparinux was not effective in reducing ischemic events in patients undergoing primary PCI for STEMI[105] (see PCI Guidelines).

Outcomes After Percutaneous Coronary Intervention

Procedural success and complication rates are used to measure outcomes after PCI. Early (<30 days) success (e.g., relief of angina; freedom from death, MI, and urgent revascularization) generally relates to the safety and effectiveness of the initial procedure, whereas late (30 days to 1 year) success (e.g., freedom from recurrence of angina, target vessel revascularization, MI, or death) depends on both clinical restenosis and progressive atherosclerosis at remote sites. Substantial improvements in coronary devices (e.g., DES), adjunct antithrombotics used during PCI (e.g., ADP antagonists, GP IIb/IIIa inhibitors, direct thrombin inhibitors), and secondary prevention after PCI (e.g., therapy with lipid-lowering agents, beta-adrenergic blockers, antiplatelet drugs; see Chap. 49) have markedly improved early and late clinical outcomes after PCI over time.[106]

EARLY CLINICAL OUTCOME. Anatomic (or angiographic) success after PCI is defined as the attainment of residual diameter stenosis less than 50%, which is generally associated with at least a 20% improvement in diameter stenosis and relief of ischemia.[10] With the widespread use of coronary stents, the angiographic criterion for success is a 20% stenosis or less when stents are used.[10] Procedural success is defined as angiographic success without the occurrence of major complications (death, MI, or CABG surgery) within 30 days of the procedure. Clinical success is defined as procedural success without the need for urgent repeated PCI or surgical revascularization within the first 30 days of the procedure.[10] A number of clinical, angiographic, and technical variables predict risk of procedural failure in patients undergoing PCI. Major complications include death, MI, or stroke; minor complications include transient ischemic attacks, vascular complications, contrast-induced nephropathy, and a number of angiographic complications (**Table 58-7**).[10]

Mortality

Although mortality after PCI is rare (less than 1%), it is higher in the setting of STEMI, in cardiogenic shock, and in patients who develop an occlusion with prior poor left ventricular function.[10] A number of risk factors for early mortality after PCI have been identified[107-109] (**Table 58-8**).

Myocardial Infarction

Periprocedural MI is one of the most common complications of PCI.[110] Two classification systems were previously used to classify MI after PCI: the World Health Organization (WHO) classification system that defines MI as a total creatine kinase (CK) elevation more than two times normal in association with the elevation of the CK-MB isoform; and a second definition that was more commonly used with evaluations of adjunct pharmacologic agents by the Food and Drug

TABLE 58-7	Variables Associated with Early Failure and Complications After Percutaneous Coronary Intervention

Clinical Variables
Women
Advanced age
Diabetes mellitus
Unstable or Canadian Cardiovascular Society (CCS) Class IV angina
Congestive heart failure
Cardiogenic shock
Renal insufficiency
Preprocedural instability requiring intra-aortic balloon pump support
Preprocedural elevation of C-reactive protein
Multivessel coronary artery disease

Anatomic Variables
Multivessel CAD
Left main disease
Thrombus
SVG intervention
ACC/AHA type B2 and C lesion morphology
Chronic total coronary occlusion

Procedural Factors
A higher final percentage diameter stenosis
Smaller minimal lumen diameter
Presence of a residual dissection or transstenotic pressure gradient

Administration, in which MI was defined as an elevation in CK-MB three times normal or higher after the procedure. A consensus definition for MI has now been reached, in which a cardiac biomarker elevated more than three times normal is used.[111] In clinical practice, asymptomatic CK-MB elevations (<5 times the upper normal limits) occur after 3% to 11% of technically successful PCIs and have little apparent clinical consequence. Larger degrees of myonecrosis (CK-MB ≥5 times the upper normal limits) predict higher 1-year mortality rates and should be considered a periprocedural MI. Many of these clinically silent infarcts may reflect a higher atherosclerotic burden in patients who suffer such events. Troponin T and I elevations occur more commonly than CK-MB elevations, but their prognostic significance over that of the CK-MB elevation is not known. Spontaneous MI after PCI has much more prognostic importance than periprocedural enzyme elevation.[112]

Urgent Revascularization

Emergent or urgent CABG surgery after PCI is now uncommon and, in the era of coronary stents, results from catastrophic complications during PCI, such as coronary perforation or severe dissection and abrupt closure. Chest pain after PCI is relatively common, and its evaluation requires an immediate 12-lead electrocardiogram. Recurrent ischemia after PCI manifested by chest pain, electrocardiographic abnormalities, and elevation of cardiac biomarkers may occur as a result of acute or subacute stent thrombosis, residual dissections, plaque prolapse, side branch occlusion, or thrombus at the treatment site or may relate to residual disease not treated with the initial procedure. In the presence of suspected recurrent ischemia, coronary arteriography is the most expeditious way to identify the cause of the residual ischemia.

Angiographic Complications

A number of complications may occur during PCI and, depending on their severity and duration, may result in periprocedural MI. If coronary dissections that extend deeper into the media or adventitia begin to compromise the true lumen of the vessel, clinical ischemia may develop (**Fig. 58-11**). Whereas most intraprocedural dissections can be treated promptly with stenting, significant residual dissections of the treated artery occur in 1.7% of patients. These residual dissections

TABLE 58-8	Factors Associated with Early Mortality After Percutaneous Coronary Intervention

Clinical Variables
Advanced age
Female gender
Diabetes mellitus
Chronic lung disease
Prior myocardial infarction
Impairment of left ventricular function
Renal dysfunction
Cardiogenic shock
Salvage, urgent, or emergent PCI

Anatomic Variables
Multivessel CAD
Left main disease
Proximal left anterior descending disease
Large area of myocardium at risk
PCI of artery supplying collaterals to large artery
Higher SCAI lesion classification

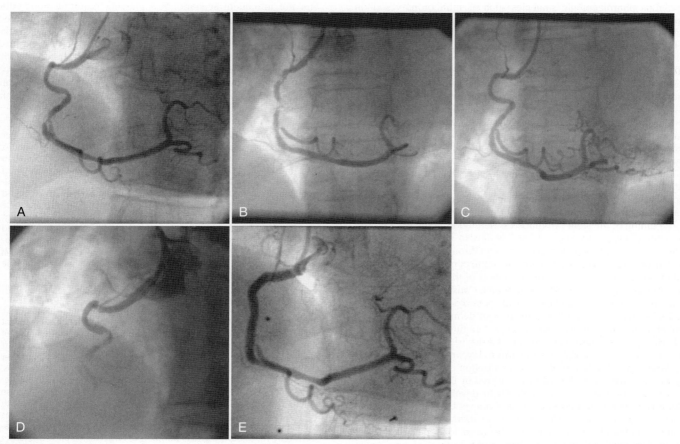

FIGURE 58-11 Abrupt closure after coronary stent placement. **A,** An extremely tortuous right coronary artery has a stenosis in its midportion. **B,** After crossing with a coronary guidewire, there is marked straightening of the vessel. **C,** After a stent is placed and the guidewire is removed, there is an excellent result. **D,** Abrupt closure develops because of a guide catheter dissection, resulting in typical chest pain and ST-segment elevation. **E,** Coronary stents are placed to "bail out" the severe coronary dissection, and normal flow is reestablished to the vessel. Without the availability of coronary stents, it is highly likely that coronary artery bypass graft surgery would have been needed to reverse the abrupt closure event.

CH
58

raise the risk of postprocedure MI, need for emergent CABG surgery, and stent thrombosis and increase mortality threefold.[113] In addition to barotrauma-induced dissections, guiding catheter dissections represent another mechanism for disruption of the coronary vessel and compromise of distal flow.

Coronary perforation develops in 0.2% to 0.5% of patients undergoing PCI and is more common with atheroablative devices and hydrophilic wires than with balloon angioplasty or with conventional guidewires. Depending on the rate of flow through the vessel perforation, cardiac tamponade and hemodynamic collapse can occur within minutes, requiring immediate recognition and treatment of the perforation. Strategies to control coronary perforations include reversal of intraprocedural anticoagulation and prolonged inflation (at least 10 minutes) of an oversized balloon at low pressure at the site of the perforation to encourage sealing of the tear in the vessel. Management strategies for perforations include the use of perfusion balloons, which provide for a small amount of distal perfusion, and polytetrafluoroethylene (PTFE)–covered stents, which may control free perforations, in addition to decompression of the pericardial pressure with prompt pericardiocentesis. Approximately one third of cases of PCI-associated coronary artery perforation require emergent cardiac surgery.

No-reflow, defined as reduced anterograde perfusion in the absence of a flow-limiting stenosis, occurs in up to 2% to 3% of PCI procedures, typically occurring during interventions on degenerated SVGs, during rotational atherectomy, and during acute MI interventions.[114] No-reflow is likely to be caused by distal embolization of atheromatous and thrombotic debris dislodged by balloon inflation, atherectomy, or stent implantation. Once it occurs, no-reflow can cause severe short- and long-term consequences including a fivefold increased risk of periprocedural MI and threefold increased risk of death. Although numerous pharmacologic strategies such as intracoronary sodium nitroprusside have been used to treat no-reflow, their efficacy in reducing the frequency of subsequent adverse events remains debated.

STENT THROMBOSIS. With the routine use of high-pressure stent postdilation and dual antiplatelet therapy after stent implantation, the rate of stent thrombosis has declined to approximately 1% within the first year after stenting. A number of clinical, angiographic, and procedural factors predispose to its occurrence. Lesion-specific factors that increase the likelihood of stent thrombosis include a residual dissection at the margin of the stent, impaired flow into or out of the stent, small stent diameters (<3 mm), long stent lengths, and treatment of an acute MI, among other factors. Noncompliance of the patient with dual antiplatelet therapy, resistance to the antiplatelet effects of aspirin and clopidogrel, and hypercoagulability may also play important roles in the development of stent thrombosis (**Table 58-9**).

The timing of the stent thrombosis is defined as acute (<24 hours), subacute (24 hours to 30 days), late (30 days to 1 year), and very late (after 1 year). Traditional definitions of stent thrombosis have included only those episodes associated with an acute coronary syndrome and angiographic or pathologic demonstration of thrombosis within the stent or its margins. The Academic Research Consortium has proposed new criteria for documentation of all possible stent thrombosis in clinical studies, including the categories of definite stent thrombosis, probable stent thrombosis, and possible stent thrombosis.[115]

Early reports suggested an incremental risk (0.2% to 0.5% per year) of very late stent thrombosis occurring 1 year or more after DES implantation.[116] Inhibition of endothelialization caused by the potent antiproliferative effect of the drugs delivered by DES may significantly prolong the period of risk for patients to develop stent thrombosis. Although concerning, these events have not yet been shown to cause a significant increase in late morbidity or mortality, probably owing to the benefits of DES in reducing the need for repeated revascularization procedures and the avoidance of the complications associated with the development of in-stent restenosis.[117-120] Ongoing evaluation of the long-term safety of DES has engendered intense investigation, with efforts focused on determining whether patient- and lesion-specific risk factors (such as insensitivity to aspirin or

TABLE 58-9 Variables Associated with Stent Thrombosis
Clinical Variables
Acute myocardial infarction
Clopidogrel noncompliance and discontinuation
Clopidogrel bioavailability
Diabetes mellitus
Renal failure
Congestive heart failure
Prior radiation brachytherapy
Anatomic Variables
Long lesions
Smaller vessels
Multivessel disease
Acute myocardial infarction
Bifurcation lesions
Procedural Factors
Stent underexpansion
Incomplete wall apposition
Residual inflow and outflow disease
Margin dissections
Crush technique
Overlapping stent
Polymer materials

thienopyridine derivatives) may contribute, whether these risks are device- or drug-specific phenomena, and whether prolonged dual antiplatelet therapy may ameliorate these risks. Preliminary data suggest that second-generation DES have lower rates of stent thrombosis than the first-generation DES.

The not infrequent scenario of a patient's requiring noncardiac surgery in the weeks after PCI can markedly increase the risk of stent thrombosis. Studies of outcomes in patients undergoing noncardiac surgery soon after PCI with BMS have documented stent thrombosis occurring in up to 8% of patients in the first 2 weeks after PCI, with risks declining to baseline rates by 8 weeks. This increased risk probably results from the frequent cessation of thienopyridine therapy before surgery as well as the hypercoagulable state in the perioperative period.

LATE CLINICAL OUTCOMES. Ischemic events within the first year after PCI result from one of three processes. Lumen renarrowing that requires repeated revascularization (i.e., target lesion revascularization) occurs in 20% to 30% of patients undergoing balloon angioplasty because of reparative arterial constriction, also known as negative remodeling. Clinical restenosis after stent implantation is less common (10% to 20%) and is attributable to intimal hyperplasia within the stent. Clinical recurrence caused by restenosis is least common (3% to 5%) after DES placement because of focal tissue growth within the stent or at its margins. A second cause of clinical events after PCI is the progression of coronary atherosclerosis at a site remote from that treated earlier by PCI. Death and MI can also result from sudden rupture of a plaque that is remote from the site of the initial intervention.

These processes can be partially distinguished by the timing of their occurrence. Clinical restenosis resulting from lumen renarrowing at the site of PCI generally develops within the first 6 to 9 months after PCI, whereas death and MI due to plaque instability may occur at any point after PCI at a low but constant rate (1% to 2% risk per year). Predictors of higher risk of all-cause late mortality include advanced age, reduced left ventricular function, congestive heart failure, diabetes mellitus, number of diseased vessels, inoperable disease, and severe comorbid conditions. A 95% 10-year survival rate can be expected in patients with single-vessel CAD, and an 80% survival rate after PCI can be achieved in those with multivessel CAD. In a 5-year follow-up study of patients treated with the TAXUS stent, target vessel revascularization during the first year was driven by target lesion revascularization, and target vessel revascularization after 1 year involved similar numbers of target lesion and non–target lesion revascularization events, primarily due to the progression of atherosclerotic disease.[121] The annualized hazard ratio for non–target lesion revascularization and other major adverse events (including death, MI, and stent thrombosis) was relatively constant beyond 1 year and not significantly different between paclitaxel-eluting stents and BMS.[121]

Outcomes Benchmarking and Procedural Volumes

Along with CABG surgery, PCI ranks among the most studied of all procedures in the United States. National structured outcomes registries such as the National Heart, Lung and Blood Institute (NHLBI) Dynamic Registry[122-126] and the ACC National Cardiovascular Data Registry (NCDR) have been examined.[9,127-130] The NCDR CathPCI Registry also provides contemporary risk-adjusted outcomes benchmarking to hundreds of participating institutions. Participants in such national, regional, or state-wide outcomes reporting initiatives can compare their risk-adjusted clinical outcomes with institutions of similar patient mix and size. The detailed nature of these data sets, in which the data collected span the range of patient clinical characteristics, lesion descriptors, and device level information, provides centers with a comprehensive comparison of their practice patterns and outcomes compared with peer institutions. More than 50% of hospitals in the United States participate in the NCDR CathPCI Registry. It is recommended that centers performing PCI participate in a prospective quality assessment and outcomes registry (see PCI Guidelines).

Current guidelines recommend that physicians undergo a 3-year comprehensive cardiac training program with 12 months of training in diagnostic catheterization, during which the trainee performs 300 diagnostic catheterizations, including 200 as the primary operator.[131] Interventional training requires a fourth year of training, including more than 250 interventional procedures but not more than 600, a level that is also required for physicians to be eligible for the American Board of Internal Medicine certifying examination in interventional cardiology.

The guidelines favor performance of PCI by higher volume operators, defined as those performing more than 75 procedures per year at high-volume centers, defined as those in which more than 400 procedures are performed each year. These recommendations are based on the ongoing observation that higher volume operators have lower adverse event rates than lower volume operators.[132,133] In one analysis of 1338 PCIs performed in the United States and Canada, operators with fewer than 100 cases per year had higher rates of 30-day death, MI, or target vessel revascularization (13.2% versus 8.7%; $P = 0.18$) and large MI (7.7% versus 3.3%; $P = 0.06$) than those with 100 or more cases per year.[133] However, a recent analysis of primary PCI found no relationship between hospital PCI volume and mortality in hospitals participating in a quality improvement initiative.[134]

Although PCI has traditionally been performed at centers that offer on-site surgical back-up, more recent analyses have shown that PCI can be performed for STEMI and elective PCI safely, provided PCI is performed by high-volume operators with minimal institutional volumes requirements.[9,135] Off-site PCI is best suited for underserved areas that are geographically far removed from major centers.[136]

Institutions must have a system for quality measurement and improvement that includes valid peer review. The guidelines recommend that quality assessment reviews take into consideration risk adjustment, statistical power, and national benchmark statistics. They should also include tabulation of adverse event rates for comparison with benchmark values and case review of complicated procedures and some uncomplicated procedures.

Future Directions

After three decades of rapid growth and dissemination of coronary interventional techniques and the associated dramatic refinement in the devices used for revascularization, there are still many challenges remaining for the percutaneous treatment of CAD. Ongoing large-scale multicenter randomized trials will assess the safety and efficacy of PCI with DES for patients with unprotected left main coronary artery stenosis and for patients with diabetes and multivessel CAD. Additional technologies are currently in clinical testing for the treatment of complex bifurcation stenosis with use of dedicated bifurcation stent systems. Better techniques to treat chronic total occlusions are being developed.

Continued evolution of drug-eluting design will attempt to optimize effective early endothelialization of the stented segment without sacrificing the long-term benefits of DES in terms of reducing target lesion revascularization.

Determination of the optimal duration of antiplatelet therapy after DES deployment requires further study. Bioabsorbable stents, produced from bioerodable polymers or magnesium alloys, show promise as a mechanism of providing short-term scaffolding to prevent abrupt closure of the vessel and leaving nothing permanent in the vessel wall after 6 months, thereby potentially reducing the risks of stent thrombosis.

Early investigation into myocardial regeneration after acute MI by percutaneous delivery of autologous stem cell or progenitor cell lines has generated great interest in the potential of such therapies to improve myocardial recovery. Continued refinement of ventricular support devices offers hope for myocardial recovery in the setting of severe myocardial dysfunction.

ACKNOWLEDGMENTS

The authors acknowledge Donald Baim, MD, and Fred Resnic, MD, for their prior contribution to this chapter and Thomas Lee, MD, for his prior contribution to the Guidelines section.

REFERENCES

1. Lloyd-Jones D, Adams RJ, Brown TM, et al: Heart disease and stroke statistics—2010 update. A report from the American Heart Association. Circulation 121:948, 2010.
2. Boden WE, O'Rourke RA, Teo KK, et al: Optimal medical therapy with or without PCI for stable coronary disease. N Engl J Med 356:1503, 2007.
3. Serruys PW, Morice MC, Kappetein AP, et al: Percutaneous coronary intervention versus coronary-artery bypass grafting for severe coronary artery disease. N Engl J Med 360:961, 2009.
4. Henriques JP, Remmelink M, Baan J Jr, et al: Safety and feasibility of elective high-risk percutaneous coronary intervention procedures with left ventricular support of the Impella Recover LP 2.5. Am J Cardiol 97:990, 2006.
5. Byrne JG, Leacche M, Unic D, et al: Staged initial percutaneous coronary intervention followed by valve surgery ("hybrid approach") for patients with complex coronary and valve disease. J Am Coll Cardiol 45:14, 2005.
6. Popma JJ, Nathan S, Hagberg RC, Khabbaz KR: Hybrid myocardial revascularization: An integrated approach to coronary revascularization. Catheter Cardiovasc Interv 75(Suppl 1):S28, 2010.

Indications for Percutaneous Coronary Intervention

7. Shaw LJ, Berman DS, Maron DJ, et al: Optimal medical therapy with or without percutaneous coronary intervention to reduce ischemic burden: Results from the Clinical Outcomes Utilizing Revascularization and Aggressive Drug Evaluation (COURAGE) trial nuclear substudy. Circulation 117:1283, 2008.
8. Eagle KA, Guyton RA, Davidoff R, et al: ACC/AHA 2004 guideline update for coronary artery bypass graft surgery: Summary article: A report of the American College of Cardiology/American Heart Association Task Force on Practice Guidelines (Committee to Update the 1999 Guidelines for Coronary Artery Bypass Graft Surgery). Circulation 110:1168, 2004.
9. Kutcher MA, Klein LW, Ou FS, et al: Percutaneous coronary interventions in facilities without cardiac surgery on site: A report from the National Cardiovascular Data Registry (NCDR). J Am Coll Cardiol 54:16, 2009.
10. Smith SC Jr, Feldman TE, Hirshfeld JW Jr, et al: ACC/AHA/SCAI 2005 Guideline Update for Percutaneous Coronary Intervention—summary article: A report of the American College of Cardiology/American Heart Association Task Force on Practice Guidelines (ACC/AHA/SCAI Writing Committee to Update the 2001 Guidelines for Percutaneous Coronary Intervention). Circulation 113:156, 2006.
11. King SB 3rd, Smith SC Jr, Hirshfeld JW Jr, et al: 2007 Focused Update of the ACC/AHA/SCAI 2005 Guideline Update for Percutaneous Coronary Intervention: A report of the American College of Cardiology/American Heart Association Task Force on Practice Guidelines: 2007 Writing Group to Review New Evidence and Update the ACC/AHA/SCAI 2005 Guideline Update for Percutaneous Coronary Intervention, Writing on Behalf of the 2005 Writing Committee. Circulation 117:261, 2008.
12. Patel MR, Dehmer GJ, Hirshfeld JW, et al: ACCF/SCAI/STS/AATS/AHA/ASNC 2009 Appropriateness Criteria for Coronary Revascularization: A report by the American College of Cardiology Foundation Appropriateness Criteria Task Force, Society for Cardiovascular Angiography and Interventions, Society of Thoracic Surgeons, American Association for Thoracic Surgery, American Heart Association, and the American Society of Nuclear Cardiology Endorsed by the American Society of Echocardiography, the Heart Failure Society of America, and the Society of Cardiovascular Computed Tomography. J Am Coll Cardiol 53:530, 2009.
13. Smith SC Jr, Feldman TE, Hirshfeld JW Jr, et al: ACC/AHA/SCAI 2005 guideline update for percutaneous coronary intervention: A report of the American College of Cardiology/American Heart Association Task Force on Practice Guidelines (ACC/AHA/SCAI Writing Committee to Update the 2001 Guidelines for Percutaneous Coronary Intervention). J Am Coll Cardiol 47:e1, 2006.
14. King SB 3rd, Smith SC Jr, Hirshfeld JW Jr, et al: 2007 focused update of the ACC/AHA/SCAI 2005 guideline update for percutaneous coronary intervention: A report of the American College of Cardiology/American Heart Association Task Force on Practice guidelines. J Am Coll Cardiol 51:172, 2008.
15. Antman EM, Hand M, Armstrong PW, et al: 2007 Focused Update of the ACC/AHA 2004 Guidelines for the Management of Patients With ST-Elevation Myocardial Infarction: A report of the American College of Cardiology/American Heart Association Task Force on Practice Guidelines: Developed in collaboration with the Canadian Cardiovascular Society endorsed by the American Academy of Family Physicians: 2007 Writing Group to Review New Evidence and Update the ACC/AHA 2004 Guidelines for the Management of Patients With ST-Elevation Myocardial Infarction, Writing on Behalf of the 2004 Writing Committee. Circulation 117:296, 2008.
16. Bavry AA, Kumbhani DJ, Rassi AN, et al: Benefit of early invasive therapy in acute coronary syndromes: A meta-analysis of contemporary randomized clinical trials. J Am Coll Cardiol 48:1319, 2006.

CH 58 PERCUTANEOUS CORONARY INTERVENTION

17. Kushner FG, Hand M, Smith SC Jr, et al: 2009 Focused Updates: ACC/AHA Guidelines for the Management of Patients With ST-Elevation Myocardial Infarction (updating the 2004 Guideline and 2007 Focused Update) and ACC/AHA/SCAI Guidelines on Percutaneous Coronary Intervention (updating the 2005 Guideline and 2007 Focused Update): A report of the American College of Cardiology Foundation/American Heart Association Task Force on Practice Guidelines. Circulation 120:2271, 2009.

18. Cohn PF: Enhanced external counterpulsation for the treatment of angina pectoris. Prog Cardiovasc Dis 49:88, 2006.

19. Nichols WW, Estrada JC, Braith RW, et al: Enhanced external counterpulsation treatment improves arterial wall properties and wave reflection characteristics in patients with refractory angina. J Am Coll Cardiol 48:1208, 2006.

20. Shishehbor MH, Lauer MS, Singh IM, et al: In unstable angina or non–ST-segment acute coronary syndrome, should patients with multivessel coronary artery disease undergo multivessel or culprit-only stenting? J Am Coll Cardiol 49:849, 2007.

21. Krone RJ, Shaw RE, Klein LW, et al: Evaluation of the American College of Cardiology/American Heart Association and the Society for Coronary Angiography and Interventions lesion classification system in the current "stent era" of coronary interventions (from the ACC–National Cardiovascular Data Registry). Am J Cardiol 92:389, 2003.

22. Thompson CA, Jayne JE, Robb JF, et al: Retrograde techniques and the impact of operator volume on percutaneous intervention for coronary chronic total occlusions an early U.S. experience. J Am Coll Cardiol Intv 2:834, 2009.

23. Migliorini A, Moschi G, Vergara R, et al: Drug-eluting stent–supported percutaneous coronary intervention for chronic total coronary occlusion. Catheter Cardiovasc Interv 67:344, 2006.

24. Katritsis D, Siontis G, Ioannidis J: Double versus single stenting for coronary bifurcation lesions: A meta-analysis. Circ Cardiovasc Interv 2:409, 2009.

25. Tamburino C, Angiolillo DJ, Capranzano P, et al: Long-term clinical outcomes after drug-eluting stent implantation in unprotected left main coronary artery disease. Catheter Cardiovasc Interv 73:291, 2009.

26. Kandzari DE, Colombo A, Park SJ, et al: Revascularization for unprotected left main disease: Evolution of the evidence basis to redefine treatment standards. J Am Coll Cardiol 54:1576, 2009.

27. Palmerini T, Marzocchi A, Marrozzini C, et al: Comparison between coronary angioplasty and coronary artery bypass surgery for the treatment of unprotected left main coronary artery stenosis (the Bologna Registry). Am J Cardiol 98:54, 2006.

28. Lee MS, Kapoor N, Jamal F, et al: Comparison of coronary artery bypass surgery with percutaneous coronary intervention with drug-eluting stents for unprotected left main coronary artery disease. J Am Coll Cardiol 47:864, 2006.

29. Chieffo A, Morici N, Maisano F, et al: Percutaneous treatment with drug-eluting stent implantation versus bypass surgery for unprotected left main stenosis: A single-center experience. Circulation 113:2542, 2006.

30. Palmerini T, Barlocco F, Santarelli A, et al: A comparison between coronary artery bypass grafting surgery and drug eluting stent for the treatment of unprotected left main coronary artery disease in elderly patients (aged > or =75 years). Eur Heart J 28:2714, 2007.

31. Sanmartin M, Baz JA, Claro R, et al: Comparison of drug-eluting stents versus surgery for unprotected left main coronary artery disease. Am J Cardiol 100:970, 2007.

32. Brener SJ, Galla JM, Bryant R 3rd, et al: Comparison of percutaneous versus surgical revascularization of severe unprotected left main coronary stenosis in matched patients. Am J Cardiol 101:169, 2008.

33. Buszman PE, Kiesz SR, Bochenek A, et al: Acute and late outcomes of unprotected left main stenting in comparison with surgical revascularization. J Am Coll Cardiol 51:538, 2008.

34. Hsu JT, Chu CM, Chang ST, et al: Percutaneous coronary intervention versus coronary artery bypass graft surgery for the treatment of unprotected left main coronary artery stenosis: In-hospital and one year outcome after emergent and elective treatments. Int Heart J 49:355, 2008.

35. Rodes-Cabau J, Deblois J, Bertrand OF, et al: Nonrandomized comparison of coronary artery bypass surgery and percutaneous coronary intervention for the treatment of unprotected left main coronary artery disease in octogenarians. Circulation 118:2374, 2008.

36. Seung KB, Park DW, Kim YH, et al: Stents versus coronary-artery bypass grafting for left main coronary artery disease. N Engl J Med 358:1781, 2008.

37. Wu C, Hannan EL, Walford G, et al: Utilization and outcomes of unprotected left main coronary artery stenting and coronary artery bypass graft surgery. Ann Thorac Surg 86:1153, 2008.

38. Sjauw KD, Engstrom AE, Vis MM, et al: A systematic review and meta-analysis of intra-aortic balloon pump therapy in ST-elevation myocardial infarction: Should we change the guidelines? Eur Heart J 30:459, 2009.

39. Vranckx P, Otten A, Schultz C, et al: Assisted circulation using the TandemHeart, percutaneous transseptal left ventricular assist device, during percutaneous aortic valve implantation: The Rotterdam experience. EuroIntervention 5:465, 2009.

40. Vranckx P, Schultz CJ, Valgimigli M, et al: Assisted circulation using the TandemHeart during very high-risk PCI of the unprotected left main coronary artery in patients declined for CABG. Catheter Cardiovasc Interv 74:302, 2009.

41. Dixon SR, Henriques JP, Mauri L, et al: A prospective feasibility trial investigating the use of the Impella 2.5 system in patients undergoing high-risk percutaneous coronary intervention (the PROTECT I Trial): Initial U.S. experience. J Am Coll Cardiol Intv 2:91, 2009.

42. Lam K, Sjauw KD, Henriques JP, et al: Improved microcirculation in patients with an acute ST-elevation myocardial infarction treated with the Impella LP2.5 percutaneous left ventricular assist device. Clin Res Cardiol 98:311, 2009.

43. McCullough P: Outcomes of contrast-induced nephropathy: Experience in patients undergoing cardiovascular intervention. Catheter Cardiovasc Interv 67:335, 2006.

Vascular Access

44. Vavalle JP, Rao SV: The association between the transradial approach for percutaneous coronary interventions and bleeding. J Invasive Cardiol 21(Suppl A):21A, 2009.

45. Kern MJ: Cardiac catheterization on the road less traveled. J Am Coll Cardiol Intv 2:1055, 2009.

46. Eichhofer J, Horlick E, Ivanov J, et al: Decreased complication rates using the transradial compared to the transfemoral approach in percutaneous coronary intervention in the era of routine stenting and glycoprotein platelet IIb/IIIa inhibitor use: A large single-center experience. Am Heart J 156:864, 2008.

47. Jolly SS, Amlani S, Hamon M, et al: Radial versus femoral access for coronary angiography or intervention and the impact on major bleeding and ischemic events: A systematic review and meta-analysis of randomized trials. Am Heart J 157:132, 2009.

48. Brueck M, Bandorski D, Kramer W, et al: A randomized comparison of transradial versus transfemoral approach for coronary angiography and angioplasty. J Am Coll Cardiol Intv 2:1047, 2009.

49. Degghani P, Mohammad A, Bajaj R, et al: Mechanism and predictors of failed transradial approach for percutaneous coronary interventions. J Am Coll Cardiol Intv 2:1057, 2009.

50. Kugelmass AD, Cohen DJ, Brown PP, et al: Hospital resources consumed in treating complications associated with percutaneous coronary interventions. Am J Cardiol 97:322, 2006.

51. Ellis SG, Bhatt D, Kapadia S, et al: Correlates and outcomes of retroperitoneal hemorrhage complicating percutaneous coronary intervention. Catheter Cardiovasc Interv 67:541, 2006.

52. Eikelboom JW, Mehta SR, Anand SS, et al: Adverse impact of bleeding on prognosis in patients with acute coronary syndromes. Circulation 114:774, 2006.

53. Tavris DR, Gallauresi BA, Lin B, et al: Risk of local adverse events following cardiac catheterization by hemostasis device use and gender. J Invasive Cardiol 16:459, 2004.

54. Exaire JE, Dauerman HL, Topol EJ, et al: Triple antiplatelet therapy does not increase femoral access bleeding with vascular closure devices. Am Heart J 147:31, 2004.

55. Koreny M, Riedmuller E, Nikfardjam M, et al: Arterial puncture closing devices compared with standard manual compression after cardiac catheterization: Systematic review and meta-analysis. JAMA 291:350, 2004.

56. Vaitkus PT: A meta-analysis of percutaneous vascular closure devices after diagnostic catheterization and percutaneous coronary intervention. J Invasive Cardiol 16:243, 2004.

57. Nikolsky E, Mehran R, Halkin A, et al: Vascular complications associated with arteriotomy closure devices in patients undergoing percutaneous coronary procedures: A meta-analysis. J Am Coll Cardiol 44:1200, 2004.

58. Applegate RJ, Sacrinty M, Kutcher MA, et al: Vascular complications with newer generations of angioseal vascular closure devices. J Interv Cardiol 19:67, 2006.

58a. Arora N, Matheny ME, Sepke C, Resnic FS: A propensity analysis of the risk of vascular complications after cardiac catheterization procedures with the use of vascular closure devices. Am Heart J 153:606, 2007.

59. Dauerman HL, Applegate RJ, Cohen DJ: Vascular closure devices: The second decade. J Am Coll Cardiol 50:1617, 2007.

60. Wong SC, Bachinsky W, Cambier P, et al: A randomized comparison of a novel bioabsorbable vascular closure device versus manual compression in the achievement of hemostasis after percutaneous femoral procedures: The ECLIPSE (Ensure's Vascular Closure Device Speeds Hemostasis Trial). J Am Coll Cardiol Intv 2:785, 2009.

61. Chhatriwalla AK, Bhatt DL: You can't keep a good man (or woman) down. J Invasive Cardiol 18:109, 2006.

62. Chhatriwalla AK, Bhatt DL: Walk this way: Early ambulation after cardiac catheterization—good for the patient and the health care system. Mayo Clin Proc 81:1535, 2006.

Coronary Devices

63. Ali A, Cox D, Dib N, et al: Rheolytic thrombectomy with percutaneous coronary intervention for infarct size reduction in acute myocardial infarction: 30-day results from a multicenter randomized study. J Am Coll Cardiol 48:244, 2006.

64. Svilaas T, Vlaar PJ, van der Horst IC, et al: Thrombus aspiration during primary percutaneous coronary intervention. N Engl J Med 358:557, 2008.

65. Bavry AA, Kumbhani DJ, Bhatt DL: Role of adjunctive thrombectomy and embolic protection devices in acute myocardial infarction: A comprehensive meta-analysis of randomized trials. Eur Heart J 29:2989, 2008.

66. Mauri L, Rogers C, Baim DS: Devices for distal protection during percutaneous coronary revascularization. Circulation 113:2651, 2006.

67. Holmes DR Jr, Teirstein P, Satler L, et al: Sirolimus-eluting stents vs vascular brachytherapy for in-stent restenosis within bare-metal stents: The SISR randomized trial. JAMA 295:1264, 2006.

68. Stone GW, Ellis SG, O'Shaughnessy CD, et al: Paclitaxel-eluting stents vs vascular brachytherapy for in-stent restenosis within bare-metal stents: The TAXUS V ISR randomized trial. JAMA 295:1253, 2006.

69. Stone GW, Lansky AJ, Pocock SJ, et al: Paclitaxel-eluting stents versus bare-metal stents in acute myocardial infarction. N Engl J Med 360:1946, 2009.

70. Chhatriwalla AK, Bhatt DL: Should dual antiplatelet therapy after drug-eluting stents be continued for more than 1 year? Dual antiplatelet therapy after drug-eluting stents should be continued for more than one year and preferably indefinitely. Circ Cardiovasc Interv 1:217, 2008.

71. Bavry AA, Kumbhani DJ, Helton TJ, et al: Late thrombosis of drug-eluting stents: A meta-analysis of randomized clinical trials. Am J Med 119:1056, 2006.

72. Pendyala LK, Yin X, Li J, et al: The first-generation drug-eluting stents and coronary endothelial function. J Am Coll Cardiol Intv 2:1169, 2009.

73. Caixeta A, Leon MB, Lansky AJ, et al: 5-Year clinical outcomes after sirolimus-eluting stent implantation insights from a patient-level pooled analysis of 4 randomized trials comparing sirolimus-eluting stents with bare-metal stents. J Am Coll Cardiol 54:894, 2009.

74. Weisz G, Leon MB, Holmes DR Jr, et al: Five-year follow-up after sirolimus-eluting stent implantation results of the SIRIUS (Sirolimus-Eluting Stent in De-Novo Native Coronary Lesions) trial. J Am Coll Cardiol 53:1488, 2009.

75. Eisenstein E, Wijns W, Fajadet J, et al: Long-term clinical and economic analysis of the Endeavor drug-eluting stent versus the Driver bare metal stent. J Am Coll Cardiol Intv 2:1178, 2009.

76. Eisenstein EL, Leon MB, Kandzari DE, et al: Long-term clinical and economic analysis of the Endeavor zotarolimus-eluting stent versus the Cypher sirolimus-eluting stent. J Am Coll Cardiol Intv 2:1199, 2009.

77. Popma JJ, Mauri L, O'Shaughnessy C, et al: Frequency and clinical consequences associated with sidebranch occlusion during stent implantation using zotarolimus-eluting and paclitaxel-eluting coronary stents. Circ Cardiovasc Interv 2:133, 2009.

78. Leon MB, Kandzari DE, Eisenstein EL, et al: Late safety, efficacy, and cost-effectiveness of a zotarolimus-eluting stent compared with a paclitaxel-eluting stent in patients with de novo coronary lesions. J Am Coll Cardiol Intv 2:1208, 2009.

79. Stone GW, Midei M, Newman W, et al: Comparison of an everolimus-eluting stent and a paclitaxel-eluting stent in patients with coronary artery disease: A randomized trial. JAMA 299:190, 2008.

Antiplatelet Agents

80. Cuisset T, Frere C, Quilici J, et al: Benefit of a 600-mg loading dose of clopidogrel on platelet reactivity and clinical outcomes in patients with non–ST-segment elevation acute coronary syndrome undergoing coronary stenting. J Am Coll Cardiol 48:1339, 2006.

81. Montalescot G, Sideris G, Meuleman C, et al: A randomized comparison of high clopidogrel loading doses in patients with non–ST-segment elevation acute coronary syndromes: The ALBION (Assessment of the Best Loading Dose of Clopidogrel to Blunt Platelet Activation, Inflammation and Ongoing Necrosis) trial. J Am Coll Cardiol 48:931, 2006.

82. Mehta SR, Bassand JP, Chrolavicius S, et al: Design and rationale of CURRENT-OASIS 7: A randomized, 2 × 2 factorial trial evaluating optimal dosing strategies for clopidogrel and aspirin in patients with ST and non–ST-elevation acute coronary syndromes managed with an early invasive strategy. Am Heart J 156:1080, 2008.

83. Wiviott SD, Trenk D, Frelinger AL, et al: Prasugrel compared with high loading- and maintenance-dose clopidogrel in patients with planned percutaneous coronary intervention: The Prasugrel in Comparison to Clopidogrel for Inhibition of Platelet Activation and Aggregation-Thrombolysis in Myocardial Infarction 44 trial. Circulation 116:2923, 2007.

84. Wiviott SD, Braunwald E, McCabe CH, et al: Prasugrel versus clopidogrel in patients with acute coronary syndromes. N Engl J Med 357:2001, 2007.

85. Bhatt DL: Intensifying platelet inhibition—navigating between Scylla and Charybdis. N Engl J Med 357:2078, 2007.

86. Mega JL, Close SL, Wiviott SD, et al: Cytochrome P450 genetic polymorphisms and the response to prasugrel: Relationship to pharmacokinetic, pharmacodynamic, and clinical outcomes. Circulation 119:2553, 2009.

87. Bhatt DL: Prasugrel in clinical practice. N Engl J Med 361:940, 2009.

88. James S, Akerblom A, Cannon CP, et al: Comparison of ticagrelor, the first reversible oral P2Y$_{12}$ receptor antagonist, with clopidogrel in patients with acute coronary syndromes: Rationale, design, and baseline characteristics of the PLATelet inhibition and patient Outcomes (PLATO) trial. Am Heart J 157:599, 2009.

89. Wallentin L, Becker RC, Budaj A, et al: Ticagrelor versus clopidogrel in patients with acute coronary syndromes. N Engl J Med 361:1045, 2009.

90. Van't Hof AW, Ten Berg J, Heestermans T, et al: Prehospital initiation of tirofiban in patients with ST-elevation myocardial infarction undergoing primary angioplasty (On-TIME 2): A multicentre, double-blind, randomised controlled trial. Lancet 372:537, 2008.

91. Kastrati A, Mehilli J, Neumann FJ, et al: Abciximab in patients with acute coronary syndromes undergoing percutaneous coronary intervention after clopidogrel pretreatment: The ISAR-REACT 2 randomized trial. JAMA 295:1531, 2006.

92. Gurm HS, Tamhane U, Meier P, et al: A comparison of abciximab and small-molecule glycoprotein IIb/IIIa inhibitors in patients undergoing primary percutaneous coronary intervention: A meta-analysis of contemporary randomized controlled trials. Circ Cardiovasc Interv 2:230, 2009.

93. De Luca G, Ucci G, Cassetti E, et al: Benefits from small molecule administration as compared with abciximab among patients with ST-segment elevation myocardial infarction treated with primary angioplasty: A meta-analysis. J Am Coll Cardiol 3:166, 2009.

94. Mehilli J, Kastrati A, Schulz S, et al: Abciximab in patients with acute ST-segment-elevation myocardial infarction undergoing primary percutaneous coronary intervention after clopidogrel loading: A randomized double-blind trial. Circulation 119:1933, 2009.

95. Stone GW, Witzenbichler B, Guagliumi G, et al: Bivalirudin during primary PCI in acute myocardial infarction. N Engl J Med 358:2218, 2008.

Antithrombin Agents

96. Gurm HS, Eagle KA: Use of anticoagulants in ST-segment elevation myocardial infarction patients; a focus on low-molecular-weight heparin. Cardiovasc Drugs Ther 22:59, 2008.

97. Ferguson JJ, Califf RM, Antman EM, et al: Enoxaparin vs unfractionated heparin in high-risk patients with non–ST-segment elevation acute coronary syndromes managed with an intended early invasive strategy: Primary results of the SYNERGY randomized trial. JAMA 292:45, 2004.

98. Kastrati A, Neumann FJ, Mehilli J, et al: Bivalirudin versus unfractionated heparin during percutaneous coronary intervention. N Engl J Med 359:688, 2008.

99. Lincoff AM, Bittl JA, Harrington RA, et al: Bivalirudin and provisional glycoprotein IIb/IIIa blockade compared with heparin and planned glycoprotein IIb/IIIa blockade during percutaneous coronary intervention: REPLACE-2 randomized trial. JAMA 289:853, 2003.

100. Stone G, McLaurin B, Cox D, et al: Bivalirudin for patients with acute coronary syndromes. N Engl J Med 355:2203, 2006.

101. White HD, Chew DP, Hoekstra JW, et al: Safety and efficacy of switching from either unfractionated heparin or enoxaparin to bivalirudin in patients with non–ST-segment elevation acute coronary syndromes managed with an invasive strategy: Results from the ACUITY (Acute Catheterization and Urgent Intervention Triage strategY) trial. J Am Coll Cardiol 51:1734, 2008.

102. Pinto DS, Stone GW, Shi C, et al: Economic evaluation of bivalirudin with or without glycoprotein IIb/IIIa inhibition versus heparin with routine glycoprotein IIb/IIIa inhibition for early invasive management of acute coronary syndromes. J Am Coll Cardiol 52:1758, 2008.

103. Lincoff AM, Steinhubl SR, Manoukian SV, et al: Influence of timing of clopidogrel treatment on the efficacy and safety of bivalirudin in patients with non–ST-segment elevation acute coronary syndromes undergoing percutaneous coronary intervention: An analysis of the ACUITY (Acute Catheterization and Urgent Intervention Triage strategY) trial. J Am Coll Cardiol Intv 1:639, 2008.

104. Yusuf S, Mehta SR, Chrolavicius S, et al: Comparison of fondaparinux and enoxaparin in acute coronary syndromes. N Engl J Med 354:1464, 2006.

105. Yusuf S, Mehta SR, Chrolavicius S, et al: Effects of fondaparinux on mortality and reinfarction in patients with acute ST-segment elevation myocardial infarction: The OASIS-6 randomized trial. JAMA 295:1519, 2006.

Outcomes After Percutaneous Coronary Intervention

106. Williams DO, Abbott JD, Kip KE: Outcomes of 6906 patients undergoing percutaneous coronary intervention in the era of drug-eluting stents: Report of the DEScover Registry. Circulation 114:2154, 2006.

107. Hannan EL, Wu C, Bennett EV, et al: Risk index for predicting in-hospital mortality for cardiac valve surgery. Ann Thorac Surg 83:921, 2007.

108. MacKenzie TA, Malenka DJ, Olmstead EM, et al: Prediction of survival after coronary revascularization: Modeling short-term, mid-term, and long-term survival. Ann Thorac Surg 87:463, 2009.

109. Hamburger JN, Walsh SJ, Khurana R, et al: Percutaneous coronary intervention and 30-day mortality: The British Columbia PCI risk score. Catheter Cardiovasc Interv 74:377, 2009.

110. Bhatt DL, Topol EJ: Does creatinine kinase–MB elevation after percutaneous coronary intervention predict outcomes in 2005? Periprocedural cardiac enzyme elevation predicts adverse outcomes. Circulation 112:906, 2005.

111. Thygesen K, Alpert JS, White HD, et al: Universal definition of myocardial infarction. Circulation 116:2634, 2007.

112. Prasad A, Gersh BJ, Bertrand ME, et al: Prognostic significance of periprocedural versus spontaneously occurring myocardial infarction after percutaneous coronary intervention in patients with acute coronary syndromes: An analysis from the ACUITY (Acute Catheterization and Urgent Intervention Triage Strategy) trial. J Am Coll Cardiol 54:477, 2009.

113. Javaid A, Buch AN, Satler LF, et al: Management and outcomes of coronary artery perforation during percutaneous coronary intervention. Am J Cardiol 98:911, 2006.

114. Harding SA: The role of vasodilators in the prevention and treatment of no-reflow following percutaneous coronary intervention. Heart 92:1191, 2006.

115. Cutlip DE, Windecker S, Mehran R, et al: Clinical end points in coronary stent trials: A case for standardized definitions. Circulation 115:2344, 2007.

116. Mauri L, Hsieh WH, Massaro JM, et al: Stent thrombosis in randomized clinical trials of drug-eluting stents. N Engl J Med 356:1020, 2007.

117. Bavry AA, Bhatt DL: Appropriate use of drug-eluting stents: Balancing the reduction in restenosis with the concern of late thrombosis. Lancet 371:2134, 2008.

118. Chen MS, John JM, Chew DP, et al: Bare metal stent restenosis is not a benign clinical entity. Am Heart J 151:1260, 2006.

119. Sarkees ML, Bavry AA, Galla JM, et al: Bare metal stent thrombosis 13 years after implantation. Cardiovasc Revasc Med 10:58, 2009.

120. Roukoz H, Bavry AA, Sarkees ML, et al: Comprehensive meta-analysis on drug-eluting stents versus bare-metal stents during extended follow-up. Am J Med 122:581, 2009.

121. Leon MB, Allocco DJ, Dawkins KD, et al: Late clinical events after drug-eluting stents: The interplay between stent-related and natural history-driven events. J Am Coll Cardiol Intv 2:504, 2009.

122. Mulukutla SR, Vlachos HA, Marroquin OC, et al: Impact of drug-eluting stents among insulin-treated diabetic patients: A report from the National Heart, Lung, and Blood Institute Dynamic Registry. J Am Coll Cardiol Intv 1:139, 2008.

123. Srinivas VS, Selzer F, Wilensky RL, et al: Completeness of revascularization for multivessel coronary artery disease and its effect on one-year outcome: A report from the NHLBI Dynamic Registry. J Interv Cardiol 20:373, 2007.

124. Abbott JD, Voss MR, Nakamura M, et al: Unrestricted use of drug-eluting stents compared with bare-metal stents in routine clinical practice: Findings from the National Heart, Lung, and Blood Institute Dynamic Registry. J Am Coll Cardiol 50:2029, 2007.

125. Abbott JD, Ahmed HN, Vlachos HA, et al: Comparison of outcome in patients with ST-elevation versus non–ST-elevation acute myocardial infarction treated with percutaneous coronary intervention (from the National Heart, Lung, and Blood Institute Dynamic Registry). Am J Cardiol 100:190, 2007.

126. Abbott JD, Vlachos HA, Selzer F, et al: Gender-based outcomes in percutaneous coronary intervention with drug-eluting stents (from the National Heart, Lung, and Blood Institute Dynamic Registry). Am J Cardiol 99:626, 2007.

127. Frutkin AD, Lindsey JB, Mehta SK, et al: Drug-eluting stents and the use of percutaneous coronary intervention among patients with class I indications for coronary artery bypass surgery undergoing index revascularization: Analysis from the NCDR (National Cardiovascular Data Registry). J Am Coll Cardiol Intv 2:614, 2009.

128. Diercks DB, Kontos MC, Chen AY, et al: Utilization and impact of pre-hospital electrocardiograms for patients with acute ST-segment elevation myocardial infarction: Data from the NCDR (National Cardiovascular Data Registry) ACTION (Acute Coronary Treatment and Intervention Outcomes Network) Registry. J Am Coll Cardiol 53:161, 2009.

129. Akhter N, Milford-Beland S, Roe MT, et al: Gender differences among patients with acute coronary syndromes undergoing percutaneous coronary intervention in the American College of Cardiology–National Cardiovascular Data Registry (ACC-NCDR). Am Heart J 157:141, 2009.

130. Wang TY, Peterson ED, Dai D, et al: Patterns of cardiac marker surveillance after elective percutaneous coronary intervention and implications for the use of periprocedural myocardial infarction as a quality metric: A report from the National Cardiovascular Data Registry (NCDR). J Am Coll Cardiol 51:2068, 2008.

131. Beller GA, Bonow RO, Fuster V: ACCF 2008 Recommendations for Training in Adult Cardiovascular Medicine Core Cardiovascular Training (COCATS 3). Revision of the 2002 COCATS training statement. J Am Coll Cardiol 51:335, 2008.

132. Kansagra SM, Curtis LH, Anstrom KJ, et al: Trends in operator and hospital procedure volume and outcomes for percutaneous transluminal coronary angioplasty, 1996 to 2001. Am J Cardiol 99:339, 2007.

133. Madan M, Nikhil J, Hellkamp AS, et al: Effect of operator and institutional volume on clinical outcomes after percutaneous coronary interventions performed in Canada and the United States: A brief report from the Enhanced Suppression of the Platelet glycoprotein IIb/IIIa Receptor with Integrilin Therapy (ESPRIT) study. Can J Cardiol 25:e269, 2009.

134. Pottenger BC, Diercks DB, Bhatt DL: Regionalization of care for ST-segment elevation myocardial infarction: Is it too soon? Ann Emerg Med 52:677, 2008.

135. Singh M, Gersh BJ, Lennon RJ, et al: Outcomes of a system-wide protocol for elective and nonelective coronary angioplasty at sites without on-site surgery: The Mayo Clinic experience. Mayo Clin Proc 84:501, 2009.

136. Kumbhani DJ, Cannon CP, Fonarow GC, et al: Association of hospital primary angioplasty volume in ST-segment elevation myocardial infarction with quality and outcomes. JAMA 302:2207, 2009.

GUIDELINES JEFFREY J. POPMA AND DEEPAK L. BHATT

Percutaneous Coronary Intervention

The American College of Cardiology/American Heart Association (ACC/AHA) published their initial guidelines for the performance of percutaneous coronary intervention (PCI) in 2001[1] and have since provided a series of focused updates that revised selected recommendations on the basis of the ever-expanding clinical evidence base and evolving practice patterns.[2-4] In aggregate, these guidelines have provided clinicians with the tools required to enhance their clinical decision making in patients undergoing percutaneous revascularization.

Like other ACC/AHA guidelines, these use the standard ACC/AHA classification system for indications:

Class I: conditions for which there is evidence and/or general agreement that the test is useful and effective

Class II: conditions for which there is conflicting evidence and/or a divergence of opinion about the usefulness or efficacy of performing the test

Class IIa: weight of evidence or opinion is in favor of usefulness or efficacy

Class IIb: usefulness or efficacy is less well established by evidence/opinion

Class III: conditions for which there is evidence and/or general agreement that the test is not useful or effective and in some cases may be harmful

Three levels are used to rate the evidence on which recommendations have been based.

Level A: recommendations are derived from data from multiple randomized clinical trials.

Level B: recommendations are derived from a single randomized trial or nonrandomized studies.

Level C: recommendations are based on the consensus opinion of experts.

CLINICAL PRESENTATION

Guidelines relevant to the use of PCI for stable ischemic heart disease (**Table 58G-1**), unstable angina with ST elevation myocardial infarction (UA/NSTEMI) (**Table 58G-2**), and ST elevation myocardial infarction (STEMI) (**Table 58G-3**) are provided. Guidelines are also included for patients undergoing PCI with left main stenoses or prior coronary bypass surgery, for patients with acute myocardial infarction complicated by thrombus, and for those undergoing drug-eluting stent placement (**Table 58G-4**).

TABLE 58G-1	ACC/AHA Recommendations for Percutaneous Coronary Intervention in Patients with Stable Coronary Artery Disease[2-4]		
INDICATION	**CLASS**	**RECOMMENDATION**	**LOE**
Asymptomatic ischemia or CCS Class I or II angina	Class IIa	Patients with one or more significant lesions in 1 or 2 coronary arteries suitable for PCI with a high likelihood of success and a low risk of morbidity and mortality. The vessels to be dilated must subtend a moderate to large area of viable myocardium or be associated with a moderate to severe degree of ischemia on noninvasive testing.	B
		Recurrent stenosis after PCI with a large area of viable myocardium or high-risk criteria on noninvasive testing	C
		Significant left main CAD (>50% diameter stenosis) in patients who are candidates for revascularization but are not eligible for CABG	B
	Class IIb	Effectiveness of PCI for patients with 2- or 3-vessel CAD with significant proximal LAD disease who are otherwise eligible for CABG with one arterial conduit and who have treated diabetes or abnormal LV function is not well established	B
		Nonproximal LAD stenosis that subtends a moderate area of viable myocardium and ischemia on noninvasive testing	C
	Class III	Not recommended in patients with one or more of the following: • Only a small area of viable myocardium at risk • No objective evidence of ischemia • Lesions that have a low likelihood of successful dilation • Mild symptoms that are unlikely to be due to myocardial ischemia • Factors associated with increased risk of morbidity or mortality • Left main disease and eligibility for CABG • Insignificant disease (<50% coronary stenosis)	C
CCS Class III angina	Class IIa	Patients with single-vessel or multivessel CAD who are undergoing medical therapy and who have one or more significant lesions in one or more coronary arteries suitable for PCI with a high likelihood of success and low risk of morbidity or mortality	B
		Patients with single-vessel or multivessel CAD who are undergoing medical therapy with focal saphenous vein graft lesions or multiple stenoses and are poor candidates for reoperative surgery	C
		Patients with significant left main CAD (>50% diameter stenosis) who are candidates for revascularization but are not eligible for CABG	B
	Class IIb	Patients with single-vessel or multivessel CAD who are undergoing medical therapy and who have one or more lesions to be dilated with a reduced likelihood of success	B
		Patients with no evidence of ischemia on noninvasive testing or who are undergoing medical therapy and have 2- or 3-vessel CAD with significant proximal LAD stenosis and treated diabetes or abnormal LV function	B
	Class III	Not recommended for patients with single-vessel or multivessel CAD, no evidence of myocardial injury or ischemia on objective testing, and no trial of medical therapy or who have one of the following: • Only a small area of myocardium at risk • All lesions or the culprit lesion to be dilated with morphology that conveys a low likelihood of success • A high risk of procedure-related morbidity or mortality • Insignificant disease (<50% coronary stenosis) • Significant left main CAD and candidacy for CABG	C

CABG = coronary artery bypass graft surgery; CAD = coronary artery disease; CCS = Canadian Cardiovascular Society; LAD = left anterior descending coronary artery; LOE = level of evidence; LV = left ventricular; PCI = percutaneous coronary intervention.

TABLE 58G-2	ACC/AHA Recommendations for Percutaneous Coronary Intervention in Patients with Unstable Angina or NSTEMI[2-4]		
INDICATION	CLASS	RECOMMENDATION	LOE
Unstable angina or non–ST-segment myocardial infarction	Class I	Early invasive PCI strategy for patients who have no serious comorbidity and who have coronary lesions amenable to PCI and who have characteristics for invasive therapy	A
		Patients with 1- or 2- vessel CAD with or without significant proximal LAD disease but with a large area of viable myocardium and high-risk criteria on noninvasive testing[3]	B
		Patients with multivessel CAD with suitable coronary anatomy, normal LV function, and without diabetes mellitus	A
		An intravenous platelet GP IIb/IIIa inhibitor is useful in UA/NSTEMI patients undergoing PCI.	A
		An early invasive strategy (i.e., diagnostic angiography with intent to perform PCI) is indicated in patients who have refractory angina or hemodynamic or electrical instability (without serious comorbidities or contraindications to such procedures).	B
		Patients selected for an invasive approach should receive dual antiplatelet therapy.	A
		• Aspirin should be initiated on presentation.	A
		• The recommended second agent is clopidogrel (before or at the time of PCI) or prasugrel (at the time of PCI).	A / B
	Class IIa	Patients with focal saphenous vein graft lesions or multiple stenoses who are undergoing medical therapy and who are poor candidates for reoperative surgery	C
		Patients with 1- or 2-vessel CAD with or without significant proximal LAD disease but with a moderate area of viable myocardium and ischemia on noninvasive testing	B
		Patients with 1-vessel CAD with significant proximal LAD disease	B
		Patients with significant left main CAD (>50% diameter stenosis) who are candidates for revascularization but are not eligible for CABG or who require emergency intervention at angiography for hemodynamic instability	B
		It is reasonable for initially stabilized high-risk patients with GRACE (Global Registry of Acute Coronary Events) risk score above 140 to undergo an early invasive strategy within 12 to 24 hours of admission. For patients not at high risk, an early invasive approach is also reasonable.	B
	Class IIb	Patients with 1-vessel or multivessel CAD, in the absence of high-risk features associated with UA/NSTEMI, who are undergoing medical therapy and who have one or more lesions to be dilated with a reduced likelihood of success	B
		Patients who are undergoing medical therapy who have 2- or 3-vessel CAD, significant proximal LAD disease, and treated diabetes or abnormal LV function, with anatomy suitable for catheter-based therapy	B
		In initially stabilized patients, an initially conservative (i.e., a selectively invasive) strategy may be considered as a treatment strategy for patients (without serious comorbidities or contraindications to such procedures) who have an elevated risk for clinical events including those who are troponin positive.	B
		The decision to implement an initial conservative (versus initial invasive) strategy may be made by considering physician and patient preference.	C
	Class III	Not recommended for patients with 1- or 2-vessel CAD without significant proximal LAD disease with no current symptoms or symptoms that are unlikely to be due to myocardial ischemia and who have no ischemia on noninvasive testing	C
		In the absence of high-risk features associated with UA/NSTEMI, PCI is not recommended for patients with UA/NSTEMI who have single-vessel or multivessel CAD and no trial of medical therapy or who have 1 or more of the following:	C
		• Only a small area of myocardium at risk	C
		• All lesions or the culprit lesion to be dilated with morphology that conveys a low likelihood of success	C
		• A high risk of procedure-related morbidity or mortality	C
		• Insignificant disease (<50% coronary stenosis)	B
		• Significant left main CAD and candidacy for CABG	B
		A PCI strategy in stable patients with persistently occluded infarct-related coronary arteries after NSTEMI is not indicated.	B

CABG = coronary artery bypass graft surgery; CAD = coronary artery disease; GP = glycoprotein; LAD = left anterior descending coronary artery; LOE = level of evidence; LV = left ventricular; NSTEMI = non–ST-segment elevation myocardial infarction; PCI = percutaneous coronary intervention; UA = unstable angina.

CH 58

PERCUTANEOUS CORONARY INTERVENTION

TABLE 58G-3 ACC/AHA Recommendations for Percutaneous Coronary Intervention in Patients with STEMI[2-5]

INDICATION	CLASS	RECOMMENDATION	LOE
ST-segment myocardial infarction	Class I	If immediately available, primary PCI should be performed in patients with STEMI (including true posterior MI) or MI with new or presumably new left bundle branch block who can undergo PCI of the infarct artery within 12 hours of symptom onset, if performed in a timely fashion (balloon inflation goal within 90 minutes of presentation) by persons skilled in the procedure (individuals who perform more than 75 PCI procedures per year, ideally at least 11 PCIs per year for STEMI). The procedure should be supported by experienced personnel in an appropriate laboratory environment (one that performs more than 200 PCI procedures per year, of which at least 36 are primary PCI for STEMI, and that has cardiac surgery capability).	A
		Primary PCI should be performed as quickly as possible, with a goal of a medical contact-to-balloon or door-to-balloon time within 90 minutes.	B
		Primary PCI should be performed in patients with severe congestive heart failure and/or pulmonary edema (Killip Class III) and onset of symptoms within 12 hours. The medical contact-to-balloon or door-to-balloon time should be as short as possible (i.e., goal within 90 minutes).	B
	Class IIa	It is reasonable to perform primary PCI for patients with onset of symptoms within the prior 12 to 24 hours and 1 or more of the following: • Severe congestive heart failure • Hemodynamic or electrical instability • Evidence of persistent ischemia	C
	Class IIb	The benefit of primary PCI for STEMI patients eligible for fibrinolysis when performed by an operator who performs fewer than 75 PCI procedures per year (or fewer than 11 PCIs for STEMI per year) is not well established.	C
	Class III	Elective PCI should not be performed in a non–infarct-related artery at the time of primary PCI of the infarct-related artery in patients without hemodynamic compromise.	C
		Primary PCI should not be performed in asymptomatic patients more than 12 hours after onset of STEMI who are hemodynamically and electrically stable.	C
PCI in fibrinolytic-ineligible patients	Class I	Primary PCI should be performed in fibrinolytic-ineligible patients who present with STEMI within 12 hours of symptom onset.	C
	Class IIa	It is reasonable to perform primary PCI for fibrinolytic-ineligible patients with onset of symptoms within the prior 12 to 24 hours and 1 or more of the following: • Severe congestive heart failure • Hemodynamic or electrical instability • Evidence of persistent ischemia	C
Facilitated PCI	Class IIb	Patients who are not at high risk who receive fibrinolytic therapy as primary reperfusion therapy at a non–PCI-capable facility may be considered for transfer as soon as possible to a PCI-capable facility where PCI can be performed either when needed or as a pharmacoinvasive strategy. Consideration should be given to initiating a preparatory antithrombotic (anticoagulant plus antiplatelet) regimen before and during patient transfer to the catheterization laboratory.	C
	Class III	A planned reperfusion strategy using full-dose fibrinolytic therapy followed by immediate PCI may be harmful.	C
Rescue PCI	Class I	A strategy of coronary angiography with intent to perform PCI (or emergency CABG) is recommended for patients who have received fibrinolytic therapy and have any of the following:	
		• Cardiogenic shock in patients younger than 75 years who are suitable candidates for revascularization	B
		• Severe congestive heart failure and/or pulmonary edema (Killip Class III)	B
		• Hemodynamically compromising ventricular arrhythmias	C
	Class IIa	A strategy of coronary angiography with intent to perform PCI (or emergency CABG) is reasonable in patients 75 years of age or older who have received fibrinolytic therapy and are in cardiogenic shock, provided they are suitable candidates for revascularization.	B
		It is reasonable to perform rescue PCI for patients with 1 or more of the following: • Hemodynamic or electrical instability • Persistent ischemic symptoms	C
		A strategy of coronary angiography with intent to perform rescue PCI is reasonable for patients in whom fibrinolytic therapy has failed (ST-segment elevation <50% resolved after 90 minutes following initiation of fibrinolytic therapy in the lead showing the worst initial elevation) and a moderate or large area of myocardium is at risk (anterior MI, inferior MI with right ventricular involvement or precordial ST-segment depression).	B
	Class III	A strategy of coronary angiography with intent to perform PCI (or emergency CABG) is not recommended in patients who have received fibrinolytic therapy if further invasive management is contraindicated or the patient or designee does not wish further invasive care.	C

TABLE 58G-3 ACC/AHA Recommendations for Percutaneous Coronary Intervention in Patients with STEMI[2-5]—cont'd

INDICATION	CLASS	RECOMMENDATION	LOE
PCI after successful fibrinolysis or for patients not undergoing primary reperfusion	Class I	In patients whose anatomy is suitable, PCI should be performed when there is objective evidence of recurrent MI.	C
		In patients whose anatomy is suitable, PCI should be performed for moderate or severe spontaneous or provokable myocardial ischemia during recovery from STEMI.	C
		In patients whose anatomy is suitable, PCI should be performed for cardiogenic shock or hemodynamic instability.	C
	Class IIa	It is reasonable to perform routine PCI in patients with LV ejection fraction ≤0.40, heart failure, or serious ventricular arrhythmias.	C
		It is reasonable to perform PCI when there is documented clinical heart failure during the acute episode, even though subsequent evaluation shows preserved LV function (LV ejection fraction >0.40).	C
	Class IIb	PCI of a hemodynamically significant stenosis in a patent infarct artery longer than 24 hours after STEMI may be considered as part of an invasive strategy.	B
	Class III	PCI of a totally occluded infarct artery longer than 24 hours after STEMI is not recommended in asymptomatic patients with 1- or 2-vessel disease if they are hemodynamically and electrically stable and do not have evidence of severe ischemia.	C
Cardiogenic shock	Class I	Primary PCI should be performed for patients younger than 75 years with ST elevation or presumably new left bundle branch block who develop shock within 36 hours of MI and are suitable for revascularization that can be performed within 18 hours of shock, unless further support is futile because of the patient's wishes or contraindications/unsuitability for further invasive care.	A
	Class IIa	Primary PCI is reasonable for selected patients 75 years or older with ST elevation or left bundle branch block or who develop shock within 36 hours of MI and are suitable for revascularization that can be performed within 18 hours of shock. Patients with good prior functional status who are suitable for revascularization and agree to invasive care may be selected for such an invasive strategy.	B

CABG = coronary artery bypass graft surgery; LOE = level of evidence; LV = left ventricular; MI = myocardial infarction; PCI = percutaneous coronary intervention; STEMI = ST-segment elevation myocardial infarction.

TABLE 58G-4 ACC/AHA Recommendations for Percutaneous Coronary Intervention in Specific Clinical Circumstances[2-4]

INDICATION	CLASS	RECOMMENDATION	LOE
Prior coronary artery bypass surgery	Class I	When technically feasible, PCI should be performed in patients with early ischemia (usually within 30 days) after CABG.*	B
		It is recommended that distal embolic protection devices be used when technically feasible in patients undergoing PCI to saphenous vein grafts.	B
	Class IIa	Patients with ischemia that occurs 1 to 3 years after CABG and who have preserved LV function with discrete lesions in graft conduits*	B
		Patients with disabling angina secondary to new disease in a native coronary circulation after CABG. (If angina is not typical, objective evidence of ischemia should be obtained.*)	B
		Patients with diseased vein grafts more than 3 years after CABG	B
		When technically feasible in patients with a patent left internal mammary artery graft who have clinically significant obstructions in other vessels*	C
	Class III	Not recommended in patients with prior CABG for chronic total vein graft occlusions	B
		Not recommended in patients who have multiple target lesions with prior CABG and who have multivessel disease, failure of multiple saphenous vein grafts, and impaired LV function unless repeated CABG poses excessive risk due to severe comorbid conditions	B
Left main	Class IIb	PCI of the left main coronary artery with stents as an alternative to CABG may be considered in patients with anatomic conditions that are associated with a low risk of PCI procedural complications and clinical conditions that predict an increased risk of adverse surgical outcomes.	B

TABLE 58G-4 ACC/AHA Recommendations for Percutaneous Coronary Intervention in Specific Clinical Circumstances[2-5]—cont'd

INDICATION	CLASS	RECOMMENDATION	LOE
Aspiration thrombectomy	Class IIa	Aspiration thrombectomy is reasonable for patients undergoing primary PCI.	B
Drug-eluting stent	Class I	A DES should be considered as an alternative to a BMS in those patients for whom clinical trials indicate a favorable effectiveness/safety profile.	A
		Before implanting a DES, the interventional cardiologist should discuss with the patient the need for and duration of dual antiplatelet therapy and confirm the patient's ability to comply with the recommended therapy for DES.	C
		In patients who are undergoing preparation for PCI and are likely to require invasive or surgical procedures for which dual antiplatelet therapy must be interrupted during the next 12 months, consideration should be given to implantation of a BMS or performance of balloon angioplasty with a provisional stent implantation instead of the routine use of a DES.	B
	Class IIa	It is reasonable to use a DES as an alternative to a BMS for primary PCI in STEMI.	B
	Class IIb	A DES may be considered for clinical and anatomic settings in which the efficacy/safety profile appears favorable in STEMI.	B
Contrast medium	Class I	In patients with chronic kidney disease undergoing angiography who are not undergoing chronic dialysis, either an isosmolar contrast medium	A
		or a low-molecular-weight contrast medium other than ioxaglate or iohexol is indicated.	B

*Note: Elective PCI should not be performed at institutions that do not provide on-site cardiac surgery.
BMS = bare metal stent; CABG = coronary artery bypass graft surgery; DES = drug-eluting stent; LOE = level of evidence; LV = left ventricular; MI = myocardial infarction; PCI = percutaneous coronary intervention; STEMI = ST-segment elevation myocardial infarction.

ADJUNCTIVE PHARMACOTHERAPY

The expanding number of antiplatelet and antithrombotic agents available for use during PCI has provided clinicians with a number of competing therapeutic options. Guidelines for antithrombotic therapy during (**Table 58G-5**) and after (**Table 58G-6**) PCI are provided. There is also an increasing awareness that providing optimal medical therapy after PCI is mandatory, including secondary risk factor modifications with lipid-lowering therapy (see Chap. 49).

APPROPRIATENESS CRITERIA FOR PERCUTANEOUS CORONARY INTERVENTION

An ongoing challenge for the application of guidelines to clinical practice is the creation of relevant clinical scenarios that the clinician faces on a daily basis and the construction of expert opinion for the appropriateness of revascularization based on the integration of the clinical presentation, noninvasive testing, coronary anatomy, and intensiveness of medical therapy. Appropriateness criteria for revascularization have been published with a consensus opinion of interventionalists, cardiac surgeons, and noninvasive cardiologists.[6] Risk stratification for cardiac events was established (**Table 58G-7**), and a series of clinical scenarios were graded on a scale of 1 to 9 on the basis of the following appropriateness definitions:

Score 7-9: Appropriate (A) when the expected benefits, in terms of survival or health outcomes (symptoms, functional status, and/or quality of life), exceed the expected negative consequences of the procedure.

Score 4-6: Uncertain (U) for the indication provided, meaning coronary revascularization may be acceptable and may be a reasonable approach for the indication but with uncertainty, implying that more research and/or patient information is needed to further classify the indication.

Score 1-3: Inappropriate (I) for the indication provided, meaning coronary revascularization is not generally acceptable and is not a reasonable approach for the indication and is unlikely to improve the patient's health outcomes or survival.

The appropriateness for revascularization in various manifestations of acute coronary syndromes is listed in **Table 58G-8**. In general, the guidelines support a prominent role for revascularization in patients with acute coronary syndrome. The criteria for stable coronary artery disease are based on extent of coronary artery disease, complexity of coronary anatomy, severity of angina, degree of ischemia, and extent of antianginal medical therapy (**Tables 58G-9 to 58G-11**). These key factors must be weighed before deciding on the appropriateness of revascularization. Patients with prior coronary artery bypass grafting (CABG) who require repeated revascularization merit special consideration, as the risks of repeated bypass surgery are higher than with the initial surgery. In patients with prior CABG, the guidelines recommend revascularization for severe angina (Canadian Class III or IV), especially with large areas or ischemia and when medical therapy has already been maximized. The appropriate mode of revascularization by PCI versus CABG for various anatomic subsets incorporates diabetic status and left ventricular status into the decision making. Importantly, three-vessel disease is categorized as having uncertain appropriateness for PCI, even in the absence of diabetes and depressed left ventricular function (**Table 58G-12**). Similarly, isolated left main stenosis is deemed inappropriate for treatment by PCI. These last two evaluations are controversial, as a substantial amount of data supports PCI in these two scenarios, with a large number of such procedures already performed worldwide.

GUIDELINES FOR TRAINING

The guidelines recommend that physicians undergo a 3-year comprehensive cardiac training program before dedicated interventional training in an accredited program. Interventional training requires a fourth year of training, including more than 250 interventional procedures, a level that is required for physicians to be eligible for the American Board of Internal Medicine certifying examination in interventional cardiology.[7,8] Maintenance of certification requires performance of 150 procedures in the 2 years before the 10-year certification lapses, in addition to retaking of the added qualification examination in interventional cardiology.

TABLE 58G-5 ACC/AHA Recommendations for Medical Therapy During Percutaneous Coronary Intervention[2-4]

INDICATION	CLASS	RECOMMENDATION	LOE
Aspirin	Class I	Patients already taking daily long-term ASA therapy should take 75 to 325 mg of ASA before PCI is performed.	A
		Patients not already taking daily long-term ASA therapy should be given 300 to 325 mg of ASA at least 2 hours and preferably 24 hours before PCI is performed.	C
Clopidogrel/prasugrel	Class I	A loading dose of clopidogrel, generally 600 mg, should be administered before or when PCI is performed.	C
		When a loading dose of clopidogrel is administered, a regimen of more than 300 mg is reasonable to achieve higher levels of antiplatelet activity more rapidly, but the efficacy and safety compared with a 300-mg loading dose are less established.	C
		In patients undergoing PCI within 12 to 24 hours of receiving fibrinolytic therapy, a clopidogrel oral loading dose of 300 mg may be considered.	C
		A loading dose of thienopyridine is recommended for STEMI patients for whom PCI is planned. Regimens should be one of the following:	
		• At least 300 to 600 mg of clopidogrel should be given as early as possible before or at the time of primary or nonprimary PCI.	C
		• Prasugrel 60 mg should be given as soon as possible for primary PCI.	B
		For STEMI patients undergoing nonprimary PCI, the following regimens are recommended:	
		• If the patient has received fibrinolytic therapy and has been given clopidogrel, clopidogrel should be continued as the thienopyridine of choice.	C
		• If the patient has received fibrinolytic therapy without a thienopyridine, a loading dose of 300 to 600 mg of clopidogrel should be given as the thienopyridine of choice.	C
		• If the patient did not receive fibrinolytic therapy, either a loading dose of 300 to 600 mg of clopidogrel should be given or, once the coronary anatomy is known and PCI is planned, a loading dose of 60 mg of prasugrel should be given promptly and no later than 1 hour after the PCI.	B
	Class III	In STEMI patients with a prior history of stroke and transient ischemic attack for whom primary PCI is planned, prasugrel is not recommended as part of a dual antiplatelet therapy regimen.	C
GP IIb/IIIa inhibitors	Class IIa	In patients with UA/NSTEMI undergoing PCI with clopidogrel administration, it is reasonable to administer a GP IIb/IIIa inhibitor (abciximab, eptifibatide, or tirofiban).	B
		In patients undergoing elective PCI with stent placement, it is reasonable to administer a GP IIb/IIIa inhibitor (abciximab, eptifibatide, or tirofiban).	B
		It is reasonable to start treatment with GP IIb/IIIa receptor antagonists at the time of primary PCI (with or without stenting) in selected patients with STEMI. GP IIb/IIIa inhibitors include	
		• Abciximab	A
		• Tirofiban	B
		• Eptifibatide	C
	Class IIb	The usefulness of GP IIb/IIIa receptor antagonists (as part of a preparatory pharmacologic strategy for patients with STEMI before their arrival in the cardiac catheterization laboratory for angiography and PCI) is uncertain.	B
Unfractionated heparin	Class I	UFH should be administered to patients undergoing PCI.	C
		For prior treatment with UFH, administer additional boluses of UFH as needed to support the procedure, taking into account whether GP IIb/IIIa receptor antagonists have been administered.	C
		For patients proceeding to primary PCI who have been treated with aspirin, a thienopyridine, and UFH, additional boluses of UFH should be administered as needed to maintain therapeutic activated clotting time levels, taking into account whether GP IIb/IIIa receptor antagonists have been administered.	C
Bivalirudin	Class I	For patients with heparin-induced thrombocytopenia, it is recommended that bivalirudin or argatroban be used to replace heparin.	B
		For patients proceeding to primary PCI who have been treated with aspirin and a thienopyridine, recommended supportive anticoagulation includes bivalirudin with or without prior treatment with UFH.	B
	Class IIa	It is reasonable to use bivalirudin as an alternative to UFH and GP IIb/IIIa antagonists in low-risk patients undergoing elective PCI.	B
		In STEMI patients undergoing PCI who are at high risk of bleeding, bivalirudin anticoagulation is reasonable.	B
Enoxaparin	Class I	For prior treatment with enoxaparin, if the last subcutaneous dose was administered at least 8 to 12 hours earlier, an IV dose of 0.3 mg/kg of enoxaparin should be given; if the last subcutaneous dose was administered within the prior 8 hours, no additional enoxaparin should be given.	B
	Class IIa	Low-molecular-weight heparin is a reasonable alternative to UFH in patients with UA/NSTEMI undergoing PCI.	B
	Class IIb	Low-molecular-weight heparin may be considered as an alternative to UFH in patients with STEMI undergoing PCI.	B
Fondaparinux	Class I	For prior treatment with fondaparinux, administer additional intravenous treatment with an anticoagulant possessing anti-IIa activity, taking into account whether GP IIb/IIIa receptor antagonists have been administered.	C
		Because of the risk of catheter thrombosis, fondaparinux should not be used as the sole anticoagulant to support PCI. An additional anticoagulant with anti-IIa activity should be administered.	C

ASA = aspirin; GP = glycoprotein; LOE = level of evidence; NSTEMI = non–ST-segment elevation myocardial infarction; PCI = percutaneous coronary intervention; STEMI = ST-segment elevation myocardial infarction; UA = unstable angina; UFH = unfractionated heparin.

CH 58

PERCUTANEOUS CORONARY INTERVENTION

TABLE 58G-6 ACC/AHA Recommendations for Medical Therapy After Percutaneous Coronary Intervention[2-4]

INDICATION	CLASS	RECOMMENDATION	LOE
Aspirin	Class I	In patients without allergy or increased risk of bleeding, aspirin 162 to 325 mg daily should be given for at least 1 month after BMS implantation, 3 months after sirolimus-eluting stent implantation, and 6 months after paclitaxel-eluting stent implantation, after which long-term aspirin use should be continued indefinitely at a dose of 75 to 162 mg daily.	B
	Class IIa	In patients for whom the physician is concerned about risk of bleeding, lower dose 75 to 162 mg of aspirin is reasonable during the initial period after stent implantation.	C
Clopidogrel/prasugrel: elective PCI	Class I	For all post-PCI patients who receive a DES, clopidogrel 75 mg daily should be given for at least 12 months if patients are not at high risk of bleeding. For post-PCI patients receiving a BMS, clopidogrel should be given for a minimum of 1 month and ideally up to 12 months (unless the patient is at increased risk of bleeding; then it should be given for a minimum of 2 weeks).	B
Clopidogrel/prasugrel: STEMI and unstable angina/NSTEMI	Class I	The duration of thienopyridine therapy should be as follows: • In patients receiving a stent (BMS or DES) during PCI for ACS, clopidogrel 75 mg daily or prasugrel 10 mg daily should be given for at least 12 months.	B
		• If the risk of morbidity because of bleeding outweighs the anticipated benefit afforded by thienopyridine therapy, earlier discontinuation should be considered.	C
		In patients in whom subacute thrombosis may be catastrophic or lethal (unprotected left main, bifurcating left main, or last patent coronary vessel), platelet aggregation studies may be considered and the dose of clopidogrel increased to 150 mg/day if less than 50% inhibition of platelet aggregation is demonstrated.	C
		In patients taking a thienopyridine in whom CABG is planned and can be delayed, it is recommended that the drug be discontinued to allow dissipation of the antiplatelet effect. The period of withdrawal should be	
		• At least 5 days in patients receiving clopidogrel	B
		• At least 7 days in patients receiving prasugrel	C
		unless the need for revascularization and/or the net benefit of the thienopyridine outweighs the potential risks of excess bleeding	C
	Class IIa	Continuation of clopidogrel or prasugrel beyond 15 months may be considered in patients undergoing DES placement.	B
	Class IIb	For all post-PCI nonstented STEMI patients, treatment with clopidogrel should continue for at least 14 days.	C
		Long-term maintenance therapy (e.g., 1 year) with clopidogrel (75 mg/day orally) is reasonable in STEMI and non-STEMI patients who undergo PCI without reperfusion therapy.	C
		It is reasonable that patients undergoing brachytherapy be given daily clopidogrel 75 mg indefinitely and daily aspirin 75 to 325 mg indefinitely unless there is significant risk for bleeding.	C

ACS = acute coronary syndrome; BMS = bare metal stent; CABG = coronary artery bypass graft surgery; DES = drug-eluting stent; LOE = level of evidence; NSTEMI = non–ST-segment elevation myocardial infarction; PCI = percutaneous coronary intervention; STEMI = ST-segment elevation myocardial infarction.

TABLE 58G-7 Noninvasive Risk Stratification

High Risk (>3% annual mortality rate)
Severe resting left ventricular dysfunction (LVEF <35%)
High-risk treadmill score (score ≤ −11)
Severe exercise left ventricular dysfunction (exercise LVEF <35%)
Stress-induced large perfusion defect (particularly if anterior)
Stress-induced multiple perfusion defects of moderate size
Large, fixed perfusion defect with left ventricular dilation or increased lung uptake (thallium-201)
Stress-induced moderate perfusion defect with left ventricular dilation or increased lung uptake (thallium-201)
Echocardiographic wall motion abnormality (involving more than two segments) developing at low-dose dobutamine (≤10 mg/kg/min) or at a low heart rate (<120 beats/min)
Stress echocardiographic evidence of extensive ischemia

Intermediate Risk (1%-3% annual mortality rate)
Mild to moderate resting left ventricular dysfunction (LVEF = 35%-49%)
Intermediate-risk treadmill score (score > −11 to < 5)
Stress-induced moderate perfusion defect without LV dilation or increased lung uptake (thallium-201)
Limited stress echocardiographic ischemia with a wall motion abnormality only at higher doses of dobutamine involving two segments or less

Low Risk (<1% annual mortality rate)
Low-risk treadmill score (score ≥5)
Normal or small myocardial perfusion defect at rest or with stress
Normal stress echocardiographic wall motion or no change or limited resting wall motion abnormalities during stress

Modified from Patel MR, Dehmer GJ, Hirshfeld JW, et al: ACCF/SCAI/STS/AATS/AHA/ASNC 2009 Appropriateness Criteria for Coronary Revascularization: A Report of the American College of Cardiology Foundation Appropriateness Criteria Task Force, Society for Cardiovascular Angiography and Interventions, Society of Thoracic Surgeons, American Association for Thoracic Surgery, American Heart Association, and the American Society of Nuclear Cardiology: Endorsed by the American Society of Echocardiography, the Heart Failure Society of America, and the Society of Cardiovascular Computed Tomography. J Am Coll Cardiol 53:530, 2009.

TABLE 58G-8 Appropriateness Criteria for Revascularization in Patients with Acute Coronary Syndromes

INDICATION		APPROPRIATENESS SCORE (1-9)
1.	• STEMI • Onset of symptoms within the prior 12 to 24 hours • Severe HF, persistent ischemic symptoms, or hemodynamic or electrical instability present	A (9)
2.	• STEMI • Onset of symptoms within the prior 12 to 24 hours • Severe HF, persistent ischemic symptoms, or hemodynamic or electrical instability present	A (9)
3.	• STEMI • Greater than 12 hours from symptom onset • Asymptomatic; no hemodynamic instability and no electrical instability	I (3)
4.	• STEMI with presumed successful treatment with fibrinolysis • Evidence of HF, recurrent ischemia, or unstable ventricular arrhythmias present • One-vessel CAD, presumed to be the culprit artery	A (9)
5.	• STEMI with presumed successful treatment with fibrinolysis • Asymptomatic; no HF or no recurrent ischemic symptoms, or no unstable ventricular arrhythmias • Normal LVEF • One-vessel CAD presumed to be the culprit artery	U (5)
6.	• STEMI with presumed successful treatment with fibrinolysis • Asymptomatic; no HF, no recurrent ischemic symptoms, or no unstable ventricular arrhythmias at time of presentation • Depressed LVEF • Three-vessel CAD • Elective/semi-elective revascularization	A (8)
7.	• STEMI with successful treatment of the culprit artery by primary PCI or fibrinolysis • Asymptomatic; no HF, no evidence of recurrent or provokable ischemia or no unstable ventricular arrhythmias during index hospitalization • Normal LVEF • Revascularization of a non-infarct related artery during index hospitalization	I (2)
8.	• STEMI or NSTEMI and successful PCI of culprit artery during index hospitalization • Symptoms of recurrent myocardial ischemia and/or high-risk findings on noninvasive stress testing performed after index hospitalization • Revascularization of 1 or more additional coronary arteries	A (8)
9.	• UA/NSTEMI and high-risk features for short-term risk of death or nonfatal MI • Revascularization of the presumed culprit artery	A (9)
10.	• UA/NSTEMI and high-risk features for short-term risk of death or nonfatal MI • Revascularization of multiple coronary arteries when the culprit artery cannot be clearly determined	A (9)
11.	• Patients with acute myocardial infarction (STEMI or NSTEMI) • Evidence of cardiogenic shock • Revascularization of 1 or more coronary arteries	A (8)

CAD = coronary artery disease; HF = heart failure; LVEF = left ventricular ejection fraction; MI = myocardial infarction; NSTEMI = non–ST-segment elevation myocardial infarction; PCI = percutaneous coronary intervention; STEMI = ST-segment elevation myocardial infarction; UA = unstable angina.
From Patel MR, Dehmer GJ, Hirshfeld JW, et al: ACCF/SCAI/STS/AATS/AHA/ASNC 2009 Appropriateness Criteria for Coronary Revascularization: A Report of the American College of Cardiology Foundation Appropriateness Criteria Task Force, Society for Cardiovascular Angiography and Interventions, Society of Thoracic Surgeons, American Association for Thoracic Surgery, American Heart Association, and the American Society of Nuclear Cardiology: Endorsed by the American Society of Echocardiography, the Heart Failure Society of America, and the Society of Cardiovascular Computed Tomography. J Am Coll Cardiol 53:530, 2009.

TABLE 58G-9 Low-Risk Findings on Noninvasive Testing and Asymptomatic Patients

SYMPTOMS MEDICAL THERAPY	CTO OF 1 VESSEL; NO OTHER DISEASE	1 OR 2 VESSELS; NO OTHER DISEASE; NO PROXIMAL LAD	1-VESSEL DISEASE OF PROXIMAL LAD	2-VESSEL DISEASE WITH PROXIMAL LAD	3-VESSEL DISEASE; NO LEFT MAIN DISEASE
Class III or IV Maximum treatment	U	A	A	A	A
Class I or II Maximum treatment	U	U	A	A	A
Asymptomatic Maximum treatment	I	I	U	U	U
Class III or IV No or minimal treatment	I	U	A	A	A
Class I or II No or minimal treatment	I	I	U	U	U
Asymptomatic No or minimal treatment	I	I	U	U	U

TABLE 58G-9 Low-Risk Findings on Noninvasive Testing and Asymptomatic Patients—cont'd

EXERCISE STRESS TEST MEDICAL THERAPY	CTO OF 1 VESSEL; NO OTHER DISEASE	1 OR 2 VESSELS; NO OTHER DISEASE; NO PROXIMAL LAD	1-VESSEL DISEASE OF PROXIMAL LAD	2-VESSEL DISEASE WITH PROXIMAL LAD	3-VESSEL DISEASE; NO LEFT MAIN DISEASE
High risk Maximum treatment	U	A	A	A	A
High risk No or minimal treatment	U	U	A	A	A
Intermediate risk Maximum treatment	U	U	U	U	A
Intermediate risk No or minimal treatment	I	I	U	U	A
Low risk Maximum treatment	I	I	U	U	U
Low risk No or minimal treatment	I	I	U	U	U

CTO = chronic total occlusion; LAD = left anterior descending coronary artery.
Modified from Patel MR, Dehmer GJ, Hirshfeld JW, et al: ACCF/SCAI/STS/AATS/AHA/ASNC 2009 Appropriateness Criteria for Coronary Revascularization: A Report of the American College of Cardiology Foundation Appropriateness Criteria Task Force, Society for Cardiovascular Angiography and Interventions, Society of Thoracic Surgeons, American Association for Thoracic Surgery, American Heart Association, and the American Society of Nuclear Cardiology: Endorsed by the American Society of Echocardiography, the Heart Failure Society of America, and the Society of Cardiovascular Computed Tomography. J Am Coll Cardiol 53:530, 2009.

TABLE 58G-10 Intermediate-Risk Findings on Noninvasive Study and CCS Class I or II Angina

SYMPTOMS MEDICAL THERAPY	CTO OF 1 VESSEL; NO OTHER DISEASE	1 OR 2 VESSELS; NO OTHER DISEASE; NO PROXIMAL LAD	1-VESSEL DISEASE OF PROXIMAL LAD	2-VESSEL DISEASE WITH PROXIMAL LAD	3-VESSEL DISEASE; NO LEFT MAIN DISEASE
Class III or IV Maximum treatment	A	A	A	A	A
Class I or II Maximum treatment	U	A	A	A	A
Asymptomatic Maximum treatment	U	U	U	U	A
Class III or IV No or minimal treatment	U	U	A	A	A
Class I or II No or minimal treatment	U	U	U	A	A
Asymptomatic No or minimal treatment	I	I	U	U	A

EXERCISE STRESS TEST MEDICAL THERAPY	CTO OF 1 VESSEL; NO OTHER DISEASE	1 OR 2 VESSELS; NO OTHER DISEASE; NO PROXIMAL LAD	1-VESSEL DISEASE OF PROXIMAL LAD	2-VESSEL DISEASE WITH PROXIMAL LAD	3-VESSEL DISEASE; NO LEFT MAIN DISEASE
High risk Maximum treatment	A	A	A	A	A
High risk No or minimal treatment	U	A	A	A	A
Intermediate risk Maximum treatment	U	A	A	A	A
Intermediate risk No or minimal treatment	U	U	U	U	A
Low risk Maximum treatment	U	U	A	A	A
Low risk No or minimal treatment	I	I	U	U	U

CCS = Canadian Cardiovascular Society; CTO = chronic total occlusion; LAD = left anterior descending coronary artery.
Modified from Patel MR, Dehmer GJ, Hirshfeld JW, et al: ACCF/SCAI/STS/AATS/AHA/ASNC 2009 Appropriateness Criteria for Coronary Revascularization: A Report of the American College of Cardiology Foundation Appropriateness Criteria Task Force, Society for Cardiovascular Angiography and Interventions, Society of Thoracic Surgeons, American Association for Thoracic Surgery, American Heart Association, and the American Society of Nuclear Cardiology: Endorsed by the American Society of Echocardiography, the Heart Failure Society of America, and the Society of Cardiovascular Computed Tomography. J Am Coll Cardiol 53:530, 2009.

TABLE 58G-11 High-Risk Findings on Noninvasive Study and CCS Class III or IV Angina

SYMPTOMS MEDICAL THERAPY	CTO OF 1 VESSEL; NO OTHER DISEASE	1 OR 2 VESSELS; NO OTHER DISEASE; NO PROXIMAL LAD	1-VESSEL DISEASE OF PROXIMAL LAD	2-VESSEL DISEASE WITH PROXIMAL LAD	3-VESSEL DISEASE; NO LEFT MAIN DISEASE
Class III or IV Maximum treatment	A	A	A	A	A
Class I or II Maximum treatment	A	A	A	A	A
Asymptomatic Maximum treatment	U	A	A	A	A
Class III or IV No or minimal treatment	A	A	A	A	A
Class I or II No or minimal treatment	U	A	A	A	A
Asymptomatic No or minimal treatment	U	U	A	A	A

EXERCISE STRESS TEST MEDICAL THERAPY	CTO OF 1 VESSEL; NO OTHER DISEASE	1 OR 2 VESSELS; NO OTHER DISEASE; NO PROXIMAL LAD	1-VESSEL DISEASE OF PROXIMAL LAD	2-VESSEL DISEASE WITH PROXIMAL LAD	3-VESSEL DISEASE; NO LEFT MAIN DISEASE
High risk Maximum treatment	A	A	A	A	A
High risk No or minimal treatment	A	A	A	A	A
Intermediate risk Maximum treatment	A	A	A	A	A
Intermediate risk No or minimal treatment	U	U	A	A	A
Low risk Maximum treatment	U	A	A	A	A
Low risk No or minimal treatment	I	U	A	A	A

CCS = Canadian Cardiovascular Society; CTO = chronic total occlusion; LAD = left anterior descending coronary artery.
Modified from Patel MR, Dehmer GJ, Hirshfeld JW, et al: ACCF/SCAI/STS/AATS/AHA/ASNC 2009 Appropriateness Criteria for Coronary Revascularization: A Report of the American College of Cardiology Foundation Appropriateness Criteria Task Force, Society for Cardiovascular Angiography and Interventions, Society of Thoracic Surgeons, American Association for Thoracic Surgery, American Heart Association, and the American Society of Nuclear Cardiology: Endorsed by the American Society of Echocardiography, the Heart Failure Society of America, and the Society of Cardiovascular Computed Tomography. J Am Coll Cardiol 53:530, 2009.

TABLE 58G-12 Appropriateness of Coronary Artery Bypass Surgery and Percutaneous Coronary Intervention

	CABG			PCI		
	NO DIABETES AND NORMAL LVEF	DIABETES	DEPRESSED LVEF	NO DIABETES AND NORMAL LVEF	DIABETES	DEPRESSED LVEF
Two-vessel coronary artery disease with proximal LAD stenosis	A	A	A	A	A	A
Three-vessel coronary artery disease	A	A	A	U	U	U
Isolated left main stenosis	A	A	A	I	I	I
Left main stenosis and additional coronary artery disease	A	A	A	I	I	I

CABG = coronary artery bypass graft surgery; LAD = left anterior descending coronary artery; LVEF = left ventricular ejection fraction; PCI = percutaneous coronary intervention.
Modified from Patel MR, Dehmer GJ, Hirshfeld JW, et al: ACCF/SCAI/STS/AATS/AHA/ASNC 2009 Appropriateness Criteria for Coronary Revascularization: A Report of the American College of Cardiology Foundation Appropriateness Criteria Task Force, Society for Cardiovascular Angiography and Interventions, Society of Thoracic Surgeons, American Association for Thoracic Surgery, American Heart Association, and the American Society of Nuclear Cardiology: Endorsed by the American Society of Echocardiography, the Heart Failure Society of America, and the Society of Cardiovascular Computed Tomography. J Am Coll Cardiol 53:530, 2009.

REFERENCES

1. Smith SC Jr, Dove JT, Jacobs AK, et al: ACC/AHA guidelines for percutaneous coronary intervention (revision of the 1993 PTCA guidelines)—executive summary: A report of the American College of Cardiology/American Heart Association task force on practice guidelines (Committee to revise the 1993 guidelines for percutaneous transluminal coronary angioplasty) endorsed by the Society for Cardiac Angiography and Interventions. Circulation 103:3019, 2001.

2. Smith SC Jr, Feldman TE, Hirshfeld JW Jr, et al: ACC/AHA/SCAI 2005 guideline update for percutaneous coronary intervention: A report of the American College of Cardiology/American Heart Association Task Force on Practice Guidelines (ACC/AHA/SCAI Writing Committee to Update the 2001 Guidelines for Percutaneous Coronary Intervention). J Am Coll Cardiol 47:e1, 2006.

3. King SB 3rd, Smith SC Jr, Hirshfeld JW Jr, et al: 2007 Focused Update of the ACC/AHA/SCAI 2005 Guideline Update for Percutaneous Coronary Intervention: A report of the American College of Cardiology/American Heart Association Task Force on Practice Guidelines: 2007 Writing Group to Review New Evidence and Update the ACC/AHA/SCAI 2005 Guideline Update for Percutaneous Coronary Intervention, Writing on Behalf of the 2005 Writing Committee. Circulation 117:261, 2008.

4. Kushner FG, Hand M, Smith SC Jr, et al: 2009 Focused Updates: ACC/AHA Guidelines for the Management of Patients With ST-Elevation Myocardial Infarction (updating the 2004 Guideline and 2007 Focused Update) and ACC/AHA/SCAI Guidelines on Percutaneous Coronary Intervention (updating the 2005 Guideline and 2007 Focused Update): A report of the American College of Cardiology Foundation/American Heart Association Task Force on Practice Guidelines. Circulation 120:2271, 2009.

5. Antman EM, Anbe DT, Armstrong PW, et al: ACC/AHA guidelines for the management of patients with ST-elevation myocardial infarction: A report of the American College of Cardiology/American Heart Association Task Force on Practice Guidelines (Committee to Revise the 1999 Guidelines for the Management of Patients with Acute Myocardial Infarction). Circulation 110:e82, 2004.

6. Patel MR, Dehmer GJ, Hirshfeld JW, et al: ACCF/SCAI/STS/AATS/AHA/ ASNC 2009 Appropriateness Criteria for Coronary Revascularization: A Report of the American College of Cardiology Foundation Appropriateness Criteria Task Force, Society for Cardiovascular Angiography and Interventions, Society of Thoracic Surgeons, American Association for Thoracic Surgery, American Heart Association, and the American Society of Nuclear Cardiology: Endorsed by the American Society of Echocardiography, the Heart Failure Society of America, and the Society of Cardiovascular Computed Tomography. J Am Coll Cardiol 53:530, 2009.

7. American Board of Internal Medicine: Interventional Cardiology Policies. American Board of Internal Medicine 2010. Available at: http://www.abim.org/certification/policies/imss/icard.aspx#tpr. Accessed January 10, 2010.

8. American Board of Internal Medicine: Interventional Cardiology Policies. American Board of Internal Medicine 2010. Available at: http:// www.abim.org/specialty/icard.aspx. Accessed January 10, 2010.

CHAPTER **59** # Percutaneous Therapies for Structural Heart Disease in Adults

John G. Webb

This chapter will review transcatheter interventional therapy of structural heart disease in adults. Although the focus is primarily on acquired conditions, some conditions that are not acquired typically become apparent in adulthood and will also be briefly reviewed here.

Non-Valvular Therapies

Patent Foramen Ovale

The foramen ovale, which allows blood flow across the atrial septum in utero, normally closes shortly after birth as pulmonary blood flow increases and the flaplike septum primum is forced against the septum secundum. However, in approximately 25% of adults, closure of the foramen ovale is not complete. The presence of a patent foramen ovale (PFO) has been implicated in paradoxical embolism, cryptogenic stroke, platypnea-orthodeoxia syndrome, arterial gas embolism in decompression illness, high-altitude pulmonary edema, and migraine.[1,2]

Several lines of evidence suggest a role in the pathogenesis of cryptogenic stroke, including documented instances of paradoxical embolism of venous thrombi into the arterial system, a higher than expected incidence of PFO in stroke patients with otherwise unexplained stroke or who are young, and a lower than expected incidence of recurrent stroke after PFO closure. Factors that appear to increase the risk of paradoxical embolism include the presence of a large transatrial shunt at rest, a mobile atrial septal aneurysm, and elevated right atrial pressures. Several lines of evidence also suggest a role in the pathogenesis of migraine, particularly in patients with aura. These include a high incidence of PFO in migraine sufferers, a reduction in migraine frequency and severity following PFO closure for stroke, and anecdotal reports of marked benefit.

Percutaneous PFO closure involves femoral venous access and passage of a long sheath into the right atrium and through the defect into the left atrium. A large number of occlusion devices are available, some of which are shown in **Figure 59-1**. A double-umbrella or double-disk device is most often used. A left atrial disk is first introduced into the left atrium and withdrawn against the septum primum. Withdrawal of the sheath then releases the waist and right atrial disk elements. Most operators use transesophageal or intracardiac echocardiographic guidance in addition to fluoroscopy to confirm positioning, and the device is then released.[3,4]

Serious complications are rare in the hands of experienced operators, but may include cardiac perforation or embolization of thrombus or air, or of the device itself. Episodic atrial fibrillation may occur in up to 5% of patients in the first weeks after implantation, but tends to resolve spontaneously. Late cardiac perforation caused by device erosion is a rare late occurrence.

The indications for PFO closure for the prevention of recurrent thromboembolic stroke remain controversial. However, the low rate of serious complications and multiple nonrandomized studies suggesting a reduction in recurrent thromboembolic events have led to widespread adoption of this therapy, particularly for patients who have failed a trial of anticoagulation. PFO closure is a definitive treatment for systemic deoxygenation syndromes involving right-to-left shunts across a PFO and for documented paradoxical arterial embolism in the setting of venous thrombosis. The randomized Migraine Intervention with StarFlex Technology (MIST) trial has suggested a possible role for PFO closure in patients with refractory migraine, although further evaluation is needed.[5]

Atrial Septal Defect

Although patients with atrial septal defects (ASDs) often remain asymptomatic until early adulthood, they may present at any age with exertional dyspnea, fatigue, right ventricular failure, pulmonary hypertension, atrial arrhythmias, or paradoxical embolism (see Chap. 65). The functional significance of an ASD is primarily determined by the presence of right atrial or ventricular enlargement in the presence of an echocardiographic defect diameter larger than 10 mm or documentation of an elevated left-to-right shunt ratio ($Q_p/Q_s > 1.5:1$), determined from oxygen saturation at the time of catheterization.

Ostium secundum ASDs involve the fossa ovalis and account for approximately two thirds of all ASDs. Less common are ostium primum ASDs, typically associated with mitral valve or ventricular septal anomalies, and sinus venosus ASDs, typically involving the junction of the right atrium and superior vena cava. Ostium secundum ASDs are often well suited to percutaneous repair, whereas primum and sinus venosus ASDs generally are not. Surgical repair is generally favored in the presence of additional intracardiac anomalies, deficient rims over a large portion of the circumference of the defect, very large ASDs (diameter > 35 to 40 mm) or proximity to the atrioventricular valves.[3]

The most common device used for percutaneous closure is the Amplatzer ASO atrial septal occluder, consisting of two self-expanding nitinol disks, with each containing embedded synthetic fabric patches and joined by a central waist (**Fig. 59-2**). A device with a waist diameter slightly larger than the defect is selected to be occlusive and to center the device. The procedural approach to percutaneous ASD closure is similar to that for PFO closure. However, the variable size of ASDs requires more accurate sizing, which often involves inflating a calibrated sizing balloon within the defect to aid in measurement. Technical complexities are common, particularly when ASDs are large or multiple, are adjacent to other cardiac structures, or have deficient rims.

Successful defect closure is commonly associated with an improvement in functional class, exercise capacity, and often by a reduction in right heart chamber size and normalization of intracardiac pressures. Complications from ASD closure are rare, but may include device embolization, atrial arrhythmias, stroke, chamber perforation, and exacerbation of headaches. Late and potentially catastrophic device erosion through the atrial or aortic wall may rarely occur, usually as a consequence of device under- or oversizing. Thrombus

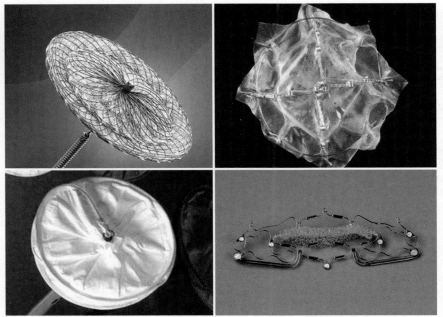

FIGURE 59-1 Patent foramen ovale occluders. **Clockwise from upper left:** (1) Amplatzer PFO occluder (AGA Medical, Plymouth, Minn) fashioned of two nitinol alloy disks, each with embedded fabric and connected by a central waist; (2) BioSTAR device (NMT Medical, Boston), which incorporates biodegradable collagenous disks fashioned similarly to its predecessors, the CardioSEAL and StarFlex devices; (3) Coherex device (Coherex Medical, Salt Lake City), which stretches the defect in one dimension while approximating the edges of the defect; and (4) Helex device (WL Gore & Associates, Newark, Del) with a single spiral coil of nitinol wire covered in fabric.

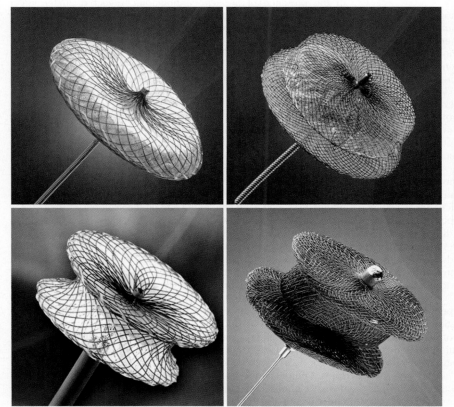

FIGURE 59-2   Clockwise from upper left: Amplatzer devices (AGA Medical) designed to occlude an atrial septal defect, left atrial appendage, paravalvular leak, and ventricular septal defect.

formation on the atrial disks may occur, with the potential for thromboembolism.

Ventricular Septal Defects

Acquired ventricular septal defects (VSDs) in adults are relatively rare. They can occur as a consequence of trauma or cardiac surgery, although the most common association is with infarction.[6] Postinfarction rupture of the interventricular septum complicates approximately 0.2% of patients, typically between days 2 to 7, when the large necrotic zone weakens and ruptures (see Chap. 55). Defects that develop in this setting are often irregular, serpiginous, sometimes multiple, and prone to further expansion with time or manipulation. Cardiogenic shock is the norm and mortality exceeds 90% if left untreated. Even in patients undergoing emergent surgical patch exclusion of the VSD, reported mortality ranges from 30 to 60%. Percutaneous closure of postinfarction VSDs has been accomplished with various devices, although usually a specialized Amplatzer occluder is used (see Fig. 59-2).[4] An experienced operator can generally implant an occluder safely, but success is variable, residual leaks are common, and mortality caused by progressive shock remains high.[6,7] The choice between surgical and percutaneous options must take into account the relative risks, likelihood of successful closure, and the need for additional revascularization or valve procedures.[1]

Left Atrial Appendage

Atrial fibrillation is the most common cause of cardioembolic stroke, with an annual stroke rate of approximately 5% (see Chap. 40). Although warfarin may reduce the risk of stroke, its narrow therapeutic range, variable dosing, monitoring requirements, and reported risk of major bleeding rates of 2% to 7%/ year are limitations. Most thromboemboli caused by atrial fibrillation appear to originate in the left atrial appendage (LAA) and surgical exclusion of the appendage at the time of cardiac surgery is believed to reduce the risk of subsequent cardioembolic stroke. The feasibility and efficacy of percutaneous LAA exclusion was demonstrated with a prototypic percutaneous LAA occlusion system (PLAATO).[8] Most experience has been with the subsequent Watchman device (Atritech, Plymouth, Minn), incorporating a self-expanding nitinol frame, barbs for fixation, and a polyester fabric cover (**Fig. 59-3**). In the randomized PROTECT-AF trial, LAA exclusion appeared noninferior to warfarin therapy for stroke prevention.[9] However, short-term complications were increased in this early experience, particularly pericardial effusions caused by transseptal access. LAA occlusion may be a reasonable option in patients intolerant to, or who have failed, warfarin. Long-term safety and efficacy remain to be established.[10]

Paravalvular Leak

Paravalvular regurgitation after valve replacement surgery may occur as a consequence of an incomplete seal between the sewing ring of the prosthetic valve and the annulus (see Chap. 66). Annular calcification, infection, and technical factors may predispose to paravalvular dehiscence. Most small leaks that develop early after surgery seal spontaneously, and most that do not require no treatment. However, when regurgitation is severe, congestive heart failure may result, and hemolysis may occur in the presence of high-velocity left ventricular to left atrial jets associated with mitral leaks, even when relatively small.

The great majority of symptomatic leaks occur in association with mitral valves and, much more rarely, in association with aortic valves. Reoperation for such leaks is associated with significant morbidity and mortality, as well as a high likelihood of recurrent leaks.

Percutaneous closure of paravalvular leaks may be achievable in many patients.[11-13] To date, the role of percutaneous closure has been limited by technical difficulty and modest efficacy. However, recent advances in imaging (particularly three-dimensional transesophageal echocardiography; see Chap. 15), technique (steerable catheters, apical access), and availability of newer closure devices specifically designed for paravalvular leaks offer increasing clinical efficacy.[4] A large number of devices have been used to occlude paravalvular leaks. Most of this experience has been with round plugs designed for closure of a septal defect or patent ductus arteriosus (see Chap. 65). Problems, although rare, include device embolization, interference with mechanical leaflets, and incomplete closure, with worsening of hemolysis. Newer devices specifically designed for the typical crescenteric shape of paravalvular defects (Amplatzer Vascular Plug III) may offer safer and more effective sealing (see Fig. 59-2). Regardless of which device is used, the defect must first be imaged and cannulated using transesophageal echocardiographic and fluoroscopic imaging. Aortic and some mitral leaks can be cannulated retrograde from the aorta. However, most mitral leaks require a transseptal puncture to access the left atrium, after which cannulation of the leak may be a difficult and lengthy process. Direct puncture of the left ventricle with percutaneous or minithoracotomy access has been found to facilitate access to mitral paravalvular leaks (**Fig. 59-4**).

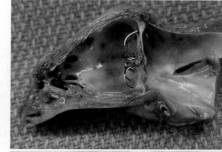
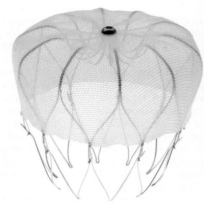
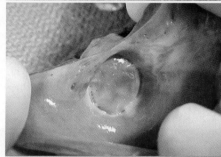

FIGURE 59-3 Left atrial appendage closure with the Watchman device (Atritech, Plymouth, Minn) at 45 days in an animal model.

Septal Ablation

Asymmetric hypertrophy of the basal interventricular septum and systolic anterior motion (SAM) of the anterior mitral leaflet (AML) may result in severe obstruction of the left ventricular outflow tract (LVOT) in patients with hypertrophic cardiomyopathy (see Chap. 69). Surgical myectomy has an established role in the palliation of severely symptomatic patients. More recently, percutaneous chemical ablation of the basal septum has been demonstrated to offer similar benefit in selected patients.[14]

Typically, the first septal perforator branch of the left anterior descending artery provides the blood supply to the anterior two thirds of the basal septum (**Fig. 59-5**). This branch is identified angiographically and cannulated. Selective injection of contrast allows demarcation of the area perfused by the chosen artery and echocardiographic confirmation that this is adjacent to the area of mitral valve–septal contact and maximal flow acceleration.[3] A small amount of absolute alcohol (1 to 2 mL) is injected slowly through the central lumen of a balloon catheter, during which the balloon is kept inflated to prevent reflux of alcohol back into the left anterior descending artery. Transient chest discomfort typically accompanies the controlled infarction that occurs.[15,16] Ethanol ablation results in coagulative necrosis of the septal perforator artery and adjacent myocardium. There is typically an immediate reduction in left ventricular systolic function, but diastolic function improves as the LVOT gradient is reduced. A gradual further reduction in gradient commonly occurs over a period of months as the infarcted ventricular septum thins.

Conduction abnormalities may occur as a consequence of temporary or permanent damage to septal conduction tissue. QRS lengthening, first-degree atrioventricular (AV) block, and new bundle branch blocks are common (see Chap. 69). Because complete heart block may occur, a temporary transvenous pacemaker lead is placed prior to the procedure, and permanent pacemaker implantation may be required in approximately 10% of patients. Serious myocardial injury may occur if ethanol refluxes into the left anterior

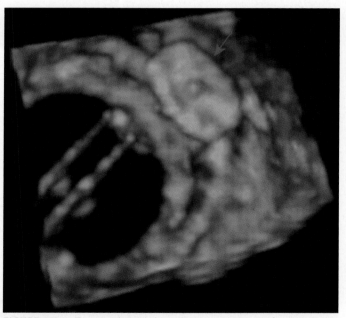

FIGURE 59-4 Transesophageal three-dimensional image of mitral double leaflet mechanical valve. An Amplatzer vascular plug III (AGA Medical) *(arrow)* was implanted to occlude a paravalvular leak using a transapical puncture.

descending artery or passes through septal collaterals to remote areas. Although periprocedural arrhythmias may occur, an increase in late arrhythmias has not been observed. In a pooled analysis of 42 published studies, with a mean follow-up of approximately 1 year, there was a decrease in resting LVOT gradient from 65 to 16 mm Hg, provocable gradient from 125 to 32 mm Hg, and basal septal diameter from 20.9 to 13.9 mm. This was associated with significant improvement in functional class, exercise capacity, and peak oxygen consumption. Mean 30-day mortality was 1.5%.[17]

Valvular Therapies

Mitral Balloon Valvotomy

Percutaneous valvotomy using inflatable balloon catheters was first developed as a therapeutic option for congenital pulmonary and aortic valvular stenosis almost 30 years ago. Percutaneous mitral balloon valvotomy has subsequently become a mainstay of the management of rheumatic mitral stenosis (see Chap. 66). In the past, closed or open commissurotomy (after the advent of cardiopulmonary bypass) was the mainstay of therapy for rheumatic mitral stenosis. However, in the early 1980s, several techniques of mitral balloon valvotomy were developed incorporating single or double cylindrical balloons, and even a mechanical dilator. Currently, this procedure is most often performed using transseptal access to the left atrium and a balloon catheter developed by a Japanese surgeon, Kanji Inoue. The dumbbell-shaped Inoue balloon catheter allows stable and sequential dilation of the stenotic mitral valve (see Fig. 66-24). Although rheumatic valvular disease is increasingly rare in the developed countries, it remains common in less developed countries, where mitral balloon valvotomy remains a common procedure.[18]

A favorable response to mitral dilation is predicated on the presence of fused mitral commissures, as seen in rheumatic disease. Dilation is relatively ineffective in the absence of commissural fusion. Dilation of congenital, prosthetic, or calcific stenosis is generally ineffective and the risk of severe regurgitation generally contraindicates this procedure. Patient selection for mitral valvotomy is largely based on echocardiographic assessment of the mitral valve apparatus.[3] The most widely used tool is the echocardiographic Wilkins score, which attempts to consider the anatomic characteristics of the leaflets, commissures, and chordal apparatus (**Table 59-1**).[19] This system assigns a point value from 1 to 4 for each of the following: (1) leaflet calcification; (2) leaflet mobility; (3) leaflet thickness; and (4) subvalvular apparatus degeneration. A score less than 8 suggests a favorable response to valvotomy (see Fig. 66-26), whereas a score of 9 to 16 suggests that surgical replacement may be needed. Even in the presence of a low score, adverse baseline factors to be considered include increasing severity of regurgitation, advanced age, prior commissurotomy, absence of commissural fusion, and presence of commissural calcification.[4]

A favorable result is evidenced by a reduction in mean transmitral gradient from more than 10 to less than 5 mm Hg, without development of severe mitral regurgitation. Complications, although uncommon, may include pericardial tamponade as a consequence of transseptal puncture, stroke caused by thromboembolism, and severe mitral regurgitation. Consequently, contraindications to valvotomy include anticoagulation, left atrial thrombus, and unfavorable valve anatomy, which might predispose to mitral regurgitation. Multiple lines of evidence, including randomized comparisons with open surgical commissurotomy, have demonstrated that the procedure can be performed with a relatively low rate of complications and a durable benefit (**Table 59-2**). Freedom from restenosis has been reported to be approximately 85% at 5 years, comparable to that for open surgical commissurotomy (see Fig. 66-25). When restenosis does occur, redilation may often be feasible.

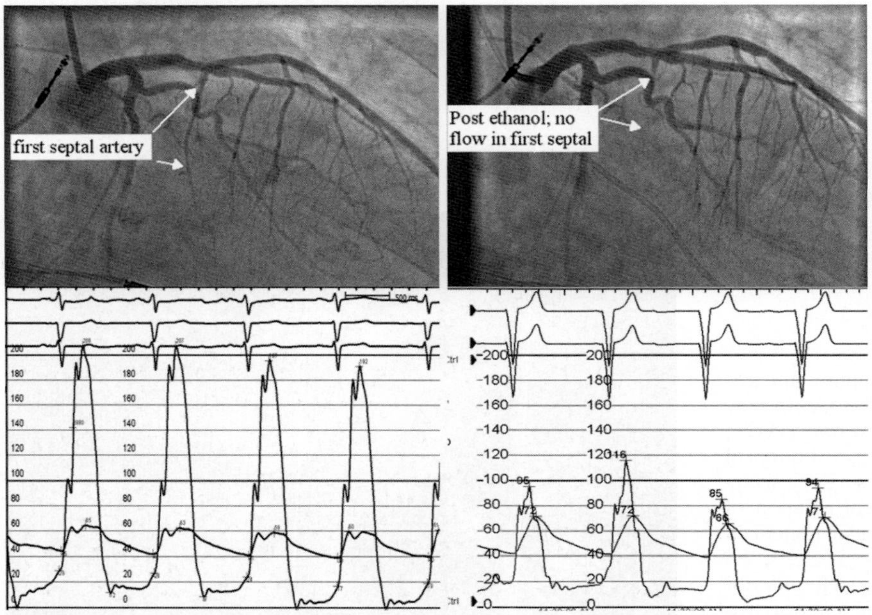

Aortic Balloon Valvotomy

Percutaneous aortic balloon valvotomy for degenerative aortic stenosis was initially described in 1985. Initial enthusiasm was tempered by reports documenting significant risk, limited benefit, and lack of durability.[20] Periprocedural complications included stroke in 1% to 3% of patients, severe aortic regurgitation in 1% to 2%, access site injury in 5% to 20%, and in-hospital mortality of 5% to 10%. More recent

FIGURE 59-5 Septal ablation for obstructive hypertrophic cardiomyopathy. **Left,** Large pressure gradient between the left ventricle and aorta. A large proximal septal perforating artery is identified. **Right,** Following selective injection of ethanol, there is no flow within the septal artery and the gradient is dramatically reduced.

TABLE 59-1	Echocardiographic Determinants of Suitability for Mitral Balloon Valvotomy.			
GRADE	MOBILITY	THICKENING	CALCIFICATION	SUBVALVULAR THICKENING
1	Highly mobile valve with only leaflet tips restricted	Minimal thickening just below the mitral leaflets	Leaflets almost normal in thickness (4-5 mm)	Single area of increased echo brightness
2	Leaflet mid and base portions have normal mobility	Thickening of chordal structures, extending up to one third of chordal length	Midleaflets normal, considerable thickening of margins (5-8 mm)	Scattered areas of brightness confined to leaflet margins
3	Valve continues to move forward in diastole, mainly from the base	Thickening, extending to the distal third of the chords	Thickening extending through entire leaflet (5-8 mm)	Brightness extending into midportion of the leaflets
4	No or minimal forward movement of the leaflets in diastole	Extensive thickening and shortening of all chordal structures, extending down to the papillary muscles	Considerable thickening of all leaflet tissue (>8-10 mm)	Extensive brightness throughout much of the leaflet tissue

From Wilkins GT, Weyman AE, Abascal AM, et al: Percutaneous balloon dilation of the mitral valve: An analysis of echocardiographic variables related to outcome and the mechanism of dilatation. Br Heart J 60:299, 1988.

TABLE 59-2 Indications for Percutaneous Mitral Balloon Valvotomy

Class I

1. Percutaneous mitral balloon valvotomy is effective for symptomatic patients (NYHA functional Class II, III, or IV), with moderate or severe mitral stenosis (MS)* and valve morphology favorable for percutaneous mitral balloon valvotomy in the absence of left atrial thrombus or moderate to severe MR (level of evidence: A).
2. Percutaneous mitral balloon valvotomy is effective for asymptomatic patients with moderate or severe MS* and valve morphology that is favorable for percutaneous mitral balloon valvotomy who have pulmonary hypertension (pulmonary artery systolic pressure > 50 mm Hg at rest or > 60 mm Hg with exercise) in the absence of left atrial thrombus or moderate to severe mitral regurgitation (MR) (level of evidence: C).

Class IIa

Percutaneous mitral balloon valvotomy is reasonable for patients with moderate or severe MS* who have a nonpliable calcified valve, are in NYHA functional Class III or IV, and are either not candidates for surgery or are at high risk for surgery (level of evidence: C).

Class IIb

1. Percutaneous mitral balloon valvotomy may be considered for asymptomatic patients with moderate or severe MS* and valve morphology favorable for percutaneous mitral balloon valvotomy who have new onset of atrial fibrillation in the absence of left atrial thrombus or moderate to severe MR (level of evidence: C).
2. Percutaneous mitral balloon valvotomy may be considered for symptomatic patients (NYHA functional Class II, III, or IV) with mitral valve (MV) area greater than 1.5 cm² if there is evidence of hemodynamically significant MS based on pulmonary artery systolic pressure higher than 60 mm Hg, pulmonary artery wedge pressure of 25 mm Hg or more, or mean MV gradient higher than 15 mm Hg during exercise (level of evidence: C).
3. Percutaneous mitral balloon valvotomy may be considered as an alternative to surgery for patients with moderate or severe MS who have a nonpliable calcified valve and are in NYHA Class III or IV (level of evidence: C).

Class III

1. Percutaneous mitral balloon valvotomy is not indicated for patients with mild MS (level of evidence: C).
2. Percutaneous mitral balloon valvotomy should not be performed in patients with moderate to severe MR or left atrial thrombus (level of evidence: C).

From Bonow RO, Carabello BA, Chatterjee K, et al: 2008 focused update incorporated into the ACC/AHA 2006 guidelines for the management of patients with valvular heart disease: A report of the American College of Cardiology/American Heart Association Task Force on Practice Guidelines (Writing Committee to Revise the 1998 Guidelines for the Management of Patients With Valvular Heart Disease). J Am Coll Cardiol 52:e1, 2008.

TABLE 59-3 Indications for Aortic Balloon Valvulotomy.

Class IIb

1. Aortic balloon valvotomy might be reasonable as a bridge to surgery in hemodynamically unstable adult patients with aortic stenosis (AS) who are at high risk for aortic valve replacement (AVR) (level of evidence: C).
2. Aortic balloon valvotomy might be reasonable for palliation in adult patients with AS in whom AVR cannot be performed because of serious comorbid conditions (level of evidence: C).

Class III

Aortic balloon valvotomy is not recommended as an alternative to AVR in adult patients with AS; certain younger adults without valve calcification may be an exception (level of evidence: B).

From Bonow RO, Carabello BA, Chatterjee K, et al: 2008 focused update incorporated into the ACC/AHA 2006 guidelines for the management of patients with valvular heart disease: A report of the American College of Cardiology/American Heart Association Task Force on Practice Guidelines (Writing Committee to Revise the 1998 Guidelines for the Management of Patients With Valvular Heart Disease). J Am Coll Cardiol 52:e1, 2008.

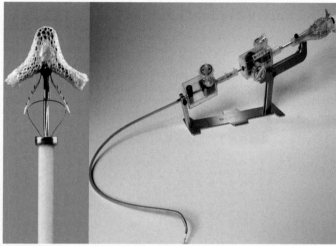

FIGURE 59-6 MitraClip and delivery system (Abbott Laboratories, Abbott Park, Ill).

Current American College of Cardiology/American Heart Association (ACC/AHA) guidelines recognize the possibility that aortic balloon valvotomy may have a limited therapeutic role (**Table 59-3**).[24] Valvotomy remains a Class I therapeutic option in young patients with congenital aortic stenosis. Class IIB recommendations include the following: (1) a bridge to surgery in hemodynamically unstable patients who are at high risk for surgery; and (2) for palliation in adult patients in whom surgery cannot be performed because of serious comorbid conditions. More recently, balloon valvotomy has found an expanded role as part of a transcatheter aortic valve implantation strategy.

Mitral Valve Repair

The potential for less invasive repair of the mitral valve without the need for open heart surgery has generated considerable interest. For the most part, these new approaches are modeled after established surgical strategies (see Chap. 66). The relatively simple but, in selected patients, effective surgical repair originally described by Alfieri can be reproduced percutaneously. Using transesophageal echocardiographic and fluoroscopic guidance, the anterior and posterior mitral leaflets are approximated with a small clip (MitraClip, Abbott Laboratories, Abbott Park, Ill) resulting in a double-orifice or edge to edge repair (**Fig. 59-6**).[4] Although initially intended for structural mitral regurgitation caused by prolapse, the procedure has also proven effective in patients with functional regurgitation and central malcoaptation.[25,26] Success is associated with a sustained, sometimes marked, clinical benefit and a reduction in left ventricular dimensions.[27-30] Potential concerns with respect to a percutaneous edge to edge procedure relate to long-term durability, the potential requirement for adjunctive annuloplasty, and the implications for subsequent surgical repair. The outcome of the now completed pivotal EVEREST II trial, randomized

reports have suggested improving outcomes with technical advances and increased experience.[21,22]

Aortic valvotomy may offer modest clinical benefit (see Chap. 66). Most reports have shown that balloon valvotomy in patients with critical aortic stenosis results in significant residual stenosis with valve areas typically between 0.7 and 1 cm². In the largest series to date, valve area increased less than 0.4 cm² in 77% of patients. Unfortunately, the clinical benefit of aortic balloon valvotomy is not durable. Restenosis, with loss of symptomatic benefit, occurs in approximately 50% of patients by 6 months and in most by 1 year.[21] Pathologic data has shown that balloon valvotomy improves leaflet mobility by fracturing calcified nodules and creating cleavage planes within collagenous stroma. Restenosis appears to occur as a result of granulation tissue, fibrosis, and active osteoblast-mediated calcification. Procedural improvements do not appear to have increased this durability. However, it does appear that external beam radiation early following aortic balloon valvotomy may reduce the rate of restenosis.[23]

Reported survival at 1 year following aortic balloon valvotomy ranges from 38% to 75% and at 2 years is 28% to 60%, comparable to survival in older patients with untreated aortic stenosis. Because balloon valvotomy may offer early benefit but has limited durability, repeat valvotomy has been proposed as a palliative approach.[21] Although repeat aortic balloon valvotomy is reported to provide symptomatic benefit with repeated dilation, the durability and degree of benefit appear to be progressively reduced.

to MitraClip or surgical therapy, will help define the appropriate role for this procedure.

Percutaneous mitral annuloplasty remains investigational at present. Various coronary sinus implants, such as the MONARC (Edwards Lifesciences, Irvine, Calif) and CARILLON (Cardiac Dimensions, Kirkland, Wash) devices, have been evaluated; the objective is to displace the adjacent posterior mitral annulus anteriorly, thus improving leaflet coaptation. Concerns relate to the suboptimal and variable relationship between the coronary sinus and mitral annulus, possibility of left circumflex coronary artery compression, and modest efficacy. Other more direct approaches to modification of the mitral annulus, such as suture plication of the posterior mitral annulus from the left ventricle (Accucinch, Guided Delivery Systems, Santa Clara, Calif) are under active investigation. Although implantation of a valved stent within the native mitral valve is problematic because of the complexities of the mitral apparatus, a number of groups are pursuing transcatheter mitral valve replacement.

Pulmonary Valve Implantation

The use of valved conduits to reconstruct the right ventricular outflow tract in patients with congenital heart disease has allowed most of these patients to survive to adulthood (see Chap. 65). However, calcification leading to valve stenosis and/or regurgitation invariably occurs, often requiring multiple open heart operations over a lifetime. Balloon valvotomy may offer some palliation.[31] Stenting these conduits may relieve stenosis and delay the need for surgery, but the development

of free pulmonary regurgitation results in progressive right ventricular dysfunction. Bonhoeffer and colleagues[32] and Zahn and associates[33] have demonstrated the possibility of percutaneous catheter implantation of stented valves in these pulmonary conduits. This initial experience was with a bovine jugular venous valve sutured inside a balloon-expandable stent (Melody, Medtronic, Minneapolis; **Fig. 59-7**).[33a] Late stent fracture with this device has been common, although generally well tolerated. Recently, the bovine pericardial balloon-expandable SAPIEN aortic valve has been used in the pulmonary position.[34]

Aortic Valve Implantation

Early experience with percutaneous valve implantation for aortic stenosis used an antegrade delivery technique with femoral vein access followed by a transseptal puncture to allow passage through the left atrium, mitral valve, and left ventricle.[35] However widespread application required the development of a reproducible transarterial procedure; with which aortic valve implantation has grown rapidly in popularity (**Fig. 59-8**).[36]

Currently, two valve systems are widely available (**Fig. 59-9**)—the balloon-expandable SAPIEN valve (Edwards Lifesciences, Irvine, Calif) and the self-expanding CoreValve device (Medtronic, Minneapolis). The SAPIEN valve consists of a stainless steel balloon-expandable stent frame to which bovine pericardial leaflets and a synthetic fabric sealing cuff to prevent paravalvular leaks are attached. The subsequently developed SAPIEN XT valve uses a cobalt chromium alloy frame with other features to facilitate its use, with a low-profile delivery system.[37] The CoreValve ReValving System (Medtronic) incorporates a self-expanding nitinol alloy frame constrained within a delivery sheath. As the sheath is withdrawn, the frame expands to assume its predetermined shape. The lower portion of the frame, with its sealing cuff, is positioned within the aortic annulus, displacing the native leaflets. The middle portion contains a trileaflet porcine pericardial valve. The upper portion extends above the coronaries to anchor the prosthesis against the ascending aorta.[38,39]

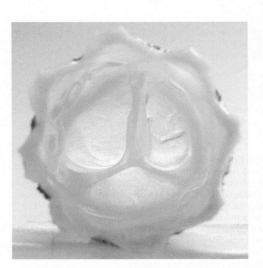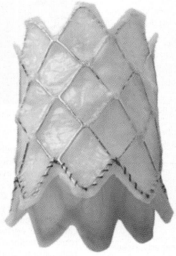

Although initial arterial procedures required a femoral artery cutdown, percutaneous access and closure are becoming the norm using various pre-closure suture techniques. In the presence of small or diseased femoral arteries, direct access to the left ventricle through an intercostal incision (transapical approach) or to the subclavian artery through an axillary incision has been widely used.[40]

The hemodynamic characteristics of current transcatheter valves compare favorably with surgical valves (see Chap. 66). Valvular regurgitation is rare. However, paravalvular regurgitation is common, although for the most part relatively mild and well tolerated. Clinical hemolysis has not been reported. Clinically significant paravalvular leaks may sometimes occur because of poor sealing as a consequence of prosthesis undersizing or poor alignment. If severe, this may require redilation, implantation of a second overlapping valve or, rarely, surgical replacement.

FIGURE 59-7 Transcatheter pulmonary valve implant. The Melody valve (Medtronic, Minneapolis) is constructed of a balloon-expandable metallic frame and a bovine jugular venous valve.

Arterial injury has been the major cause of morbidity and mortality complicating transarterial aortic valve implantation. Consequently, detailed iliofemoral angiography and multislice computed tomography have become routine components of the screening process; a major focus of ongoing development has been to reduce the profile of delivery systems. AV block may occur because of compression of the conduction system as it passes through the periaortic septum. Predisposing factors may include preexisting conduction

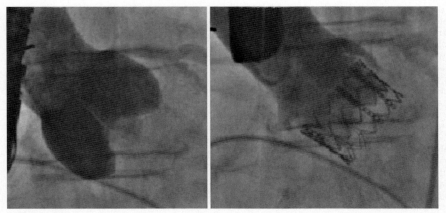

FIGURE 59-8 Aortic root angiogram in a patient with aortic stenosis before **(left)** and after **(right)** implantation of a SAPIEN valve (Edwards Lifesciences, Irvine, Calif).

abnormalities, prosthesis oversizing, and extension of the prosthesis into the outflow tract. Permanent pacemakers are required in 5% to 30% of patients, varying with the valve type implanted and local practice. Coronary obstruction may rarely occur when a bulky native leaflet is displaced over the left main coronary ostium (<1%), and stroke may occur because of embolization from the native valve or aortic arch (1% to 4%).[38,39,41,42]

Current transcatheter valves appear sufficiently durable to provide benefit in the mostly elderly patients with comorbid conditions who are currently considered candidates.[41] Accelerated wear testing has demonstrated in vitro durability longer than 10 years and late structural valve failure has not been reported, although clinical follow-up remains limited. Whether durability is sufficient for patients with greater longevity and less comorbidity remains to be determined. However, the feasibility of transcatheter valve implantation in failing aortic, pulmonary, tricuspid, and mitral bioprosthetic surgical valves has recently been demonstrated.[43] Repeat valve in valve implants appear likely to prove to be a commonly used modality for managing late valve failure when this occurs.

Multiple single and multicenter high-risk registries have documented survival rates higher than predicted with conventional surgery and associated with a reduction in morbidity.[38,39,41,44] The large randomized North American PARTNER trial compared the Edwards SAPIEN valve to medical management (including balloon valvotomy) in patients considered to be at too high risk for surgical valve replacement and demonstrated substantial reduction in death and hospitalization with transcatheter valve implantation associated with significant improvement in symptoms.[44a] This study will have a major impact on defining the role of transcatheter aortic valve implantation.[45]

Surgical aortic valve replacement remains the current standard of care for symptomatic aortic stenosis because of a large body of favorable experience. In the absence of more studies, transcatheter aortic valve implantation is currently recommended only for patients in whom the risks of surgical morbidity or mortality are high. Logistic EuroSCORE estimates (www.euroscore.org) of a 30-day mortality exceeding 20% or Society of Thoracic Surgeons (STS) estimates (www.sts.org) exceeding 10% have been widely used to determine high surgical risk. However, both risk models commonly overestimate surgical risk in surgical candidates, but underestimate risk in patients with many important comorbidities, such as porcelain aorta, multivalve disease, and frailty, for whom clinical data allowing incorporation into these risk models is lacking. Moreover, the reduced morbidity of a transcatheter procedure may be more important to many older patients than the potential for reduced mortality. Often, the opinion of an experienced surgeon is the best estimate of risk.[46]

Future Perspectives

Percutaneous closure of intracardiac defects is now relatively common. Transcatheter valve implantation is rapidly becoming routine for the management of aortic and pulmonary valve disease, and may play a prominent role in the management of degenerated bioprosthetic valves. It appears likely that edge to edge repair for mitral regurgitation and left atrial appendage exclusion for atrial fibrillation may become widely accepted therapeutic options. New transcatheter procedures for chronic heart failure are on the horizon. Transcatheter approaches to adult structural heart disease have seen dramatic advances over the past decade, and this trend appears likely to continue.

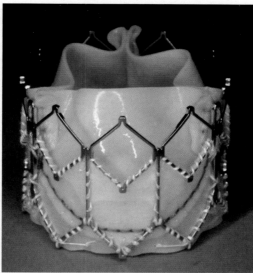 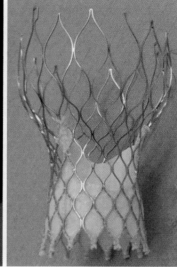

FIGURE 59-9 Transcatheter aortic valves. **Left,** SAPIEN XT valve (Edwards Lifesciences). **Right,** CoreValve (Medtronic).

REFERENCES

Closure Devices

1. Kim MS, Klein AJ, Carroll JD: Transcatheter closure of intracardiac defects in adults. J Interv Cardiol 20:524, 2007.

2. Kedia G, Tobis J, Lee MS: Patent foramen ovale: Clinical manifestations and treatment. Rev Cardiovasc Med 9:168, 2008.

3. Kim SS, Hijazi ZM, Lang RM, Knight BP: The use of intracardiac echocardiography and other intracardiac imaging tools to guide noncoronary cardiac interventions. J Am Coll Cardiol 53:2117, 2009.

4. Silvestry FE, Kerber RE, Brook MM, et al: Echocardiography-guided interventions. J Am Soc Echocardiogr 22:213, 2009.

5. Dowson A, Mullen MJ, Peatfield R, et al: Migraine intervention with STARFlex Technology (MIST) trial: A prospective, multicenter, double-blind, sham-controlled trial to evaluate the effectiveness of patent foramen ovale closure with STARFlex septal repair implant to resolve refractory migraine headache. Circulation 117:1397, 2008.

6. Martinez MW, Mookadam F, Sun Y, et al: Transcatheter closure of ischemic and post-traumatic ventricular septal ruptures. Cathet Cardiovasc Interv 69:403, 2007.

7. Butera G, Chessa M, Carminati M: Percutaneous closure of ventricular septal defects. State of the art. J Cardiovasc Med 8:39, 2007.

8. Sievert H, Bayard YL: Percutaneous closure of the left atrial appendage: A major step forward. JACC Cardiovasc Interv 2:601, 2009.

9. Holmes DR, Reddy VY, Turi ZG, et al: Percutaneous closure of the left atrial appendage versus warfarin therapy for prevention of stroke in patients with atrial fibrillation: A randomized non-inferiority trial. Lancet 374:534, 2009.

10. McCabe DJH, Kinsella JA, Tobin WO: Left atrial appendage occlusion in non-valvular atrial fibrillation. Lancet 374:504, 2009.

Paravalvular Leaks

11. Pate GE, Al Zubaidi A, Chandavimol M, et al: Percutaneous closure of prosthetic paravalvular leaks: Case series and review. Catheter Cardiovasc Interv 68:528, 2006.

12. Pate GE, Thompson CR, Munt BI, Webb JG: Techniques for percutaneous closure of prosthetic paravalvular leaks. Cathet Cardiovasc Interv 67:158, 2006.

13. Hein R, Wunderlich N, Wilson N, Sievert H: New concepts in transcatheter closure of paravalvular leaks. Future Cardiology 4:373, 2008.

Septal Ablation

14. Fifer MA: Most fully informed patients choose septal ablation over septal myectomy. Circulation 116:207, 2007.

15. Sorajja P, Valeti U, Nishimura RA, et al: Outcome of alcohol septal ablation for obstructive hypertrophic cardiomyopathy. Circulation 118:131, 2008.

16. van der Lee C, Scholzel B, ten Berg JM, et al: Usefulness of clinical, echocardiographic, and procedural characteristics to predict outcome after percutaneous transluminal septal myocardial ablation. Am J Cardiol 101:1315, 2008.

17. Alam M, Dokainsh H, Lakkis N: Alcohol septal ablation for hypertrophic obstructive cardiomyopathy: A systematic review of published studies. J Interv Cardiol 19:319, 2006.

Mitral Balloon Valvotomy

18. Nobuyoshi M, Arita T, Shirai S, et al: Percutaneous balloon mitral valvuloplasty: A review. Circulation 119:e211, 2009.

19. Wilkins GT, Weyman AE, Abascal AM, et al: Percutaneous balloon dilation of the mitral valve: An analysis of echocardiographic variables related to outcome and the mechanism of dilatation. Br Heart J 60:299,1988.

Aortic Balloon Valvotomy

20. Boone RH, Webb J: Nonsurgical aortic valve therapy: Balloon valvuloplasty and transcatheter aortic valve replacement. In Yusuf S, Cairns, J, Camm J, et al (eds): Evidence-Based Cardiology. 3rd ed. Oxford, Blackwell Publishing, 2010, pp 896-912.

21. Agarwal A, Kini AS, Attanti S, et al: Results of repeat balloon valvuloplasty for treatment of aortic stenosis in patients aged 59 to 104 years. Am J Cardiol 95:43, 2005.

22. Klein A, Lee K, Gera A, et al: Long-term mortality, cause of death, and temporal trends in complications after percutaneous aortic balloon valvuloplasty for calcific aortic stenosis. J Interv Cardiol 19:269, 2006.

23. Pedersen WR, Block P, Feldman T: The iCoapsys Repair System for the percutaneous treatment of functional mitral insufficiency (http://www.northshore.org/uploadedfiles/cardiology/forphysicians/InterventionalRadiology/5_2006_IntCardioArticle2.pdf).
24. Bonow RO, Carabello BA, Chatterjee K, et al: 2008 focused update incorporated into the ACC/AHA 2006 guidelines for the management of patients with valvular heart disease: A report of the American College of Cardiology/American Heart Association Task Force on Practice Guidelines (Writing Committee to Revise the 1998 Guidelines for the Management of Patients With Valvular Heart Disease). J Am Coll Cardiol 52:e1, 2008.

Mitral Valve Repair

25. Foster E, Wasserman HS, Gray W, et al: Quantitative assessment of severity of mitral regurgitation by serial echocardiography in a multicenter clinical trial of percutaneous mitral valve repair. Am J Cardiol 100:1577, 2007.
26. Feldman T: EVEREST Registry (Endovascular Valve Edge-to-edge REpair Studies). Reduction in mitral regurgitation 12 months following percutaneous mitral valve repair. Clin Cardiol 30:416, 2007.
27. Herrmann HC, Kar S, Fail P, et al: Stability of mitral valve area and gradient following percutaneous repair of mitral regurgitation with the Mitraclip device. J Am Coll Cardiol 51(Suppl B):79, 2008.
28. Feldman T , Kar S, Rinaldi M, et al: Percutanesous mitral repair with the MitraClip system. J Am Coll Cardiol 54:686, 2009.
29. Silvestry FE, Rodriguez LL, Herrmann HC, et al: Echocardiographic guidance and assessment of percutaneous repair for mitral regurgitation with the Evalve MitraClip: Lessons learned from EVEREST I. J Am Soc Echocardiogr 20:1131, 2007.
30. Feldman T, Glower D: Patient selection for percutaneous mitral valve repair: Insight from early clinical trial applications. Nat Clin Pract Cardiovasc Med 5:84, 2008.

Pulmonary Valve Implantation

31. Rao PS: Percutaneous balloon pulmonary valvuloplasty: State of the art. Cathet Cardiovasc Interv 69:747, 2007.
32. Bonhoeffer P, Boudjemline Y, Qureshi SA, et al: Percutaneous insertion of the pulmonary valve. J Am Coll Cardiol 39:1664, 2002.
33. Zahn EM, Hellenbrand WE, Lock JE, McElhinney DB: Implantation of the Melody transcatheter pulmonary valve in patients with a dysfunctional right ventricular outflow tract conduit. J Am Coll Cardiol 54:1722, 2009.
33a. McElhinney DB, Hellenbrand WE, Zahn EM, et al: Short-term outcomes after transcatheter pulmonary valve placement in the expanded multicenter US Melody valve trial. Circulation 122:507, 2010.

34. Boone RH, Webb JG, Horlick E, et al: Transcatheter pulmonary valve implantation using the Edwards SAPIEN transcatheter heart valve (THV). Cathet Cardiovasc Interv 75:286, 2010.

Aortic Valve Implantation

35. Eltchaninoff H, Zajarias A, Tron C, Litzlerb PY, et al: Transcatheter aortic valve implantation: Technical aspects, results and indications. Arch Cardiovasc Dis 101:126, 2008.
36. Webb JG, Chandavimol M, Thompson C, et al: Percutaneous aortic valve implantation retrograde from the femoral artery. Circulation 113:842, 2006.
37. Nietlispach F, Wijesinghe N, Wood D, Carere RG, Webb JG. Current balloon-expandable transcatheter heart valve and delivery systems. Cathet Cardiovasc Intv. 75:295,2010.
38. Grube E, Buellesfeld L, Mueller R, et al: Progress and current status of percutaneous aortic valve replacement: results of three device generations of the CoreValve revalving system. Circ Cardiovasc Intervent 1:167, 2008.
39. Piazza N, Grube E, Gerckens U, et al: Procedural and 30-day outcomes following transcatheter aortic valve implantation using the third generation (18Fr) CoreValve ReValving System: Results from the multicentre, expanded evaluation registry 1-year following CE mark approval. EuroInterv 4:242, 2008.
40. Wong D, Ye J, Cheung A, et al: Technical considerations to avoid pitfalls during transapical aortic valve implantation. J Thorac Cardiovasc Surg 140:196, 2010.
41. Webb JG, Altwegg L, Boone RH, et al: Transcatheter aortic valve implantation: Impact on clinical and valve-related outcomes. Circulation 119:3009, 2009.
42. Masson JB, Kovac J, Schuler G, et al: Transcatheter aortic valve implantation: review of the nature, management and avoidance of procedural complications. JACC Cardiovasc Interv 2:811, 2009.
43. Webb JG, Wood DA, Ye J, et al: Transcatheter valve-in-valve implantation for failed bioprosthetic valves. Circulation 121:1848, 2010.
44. Thomas M, Schymik G, Walter T, et al: 30-day results of the SOURCE Registry: A European registry of transcatheter aortic valve implantation using the Edwards SAPIEN valve. Circulation122:62, 2010.
44a. Leon MB, Smith CR, Mack Met al: Transcatheter aortic-valve implantation for aortic stenosis in patients who cannot undergo surgery. N Engl J Med 2010 [E-pub ahead of print Sep. 22 (10.1056/NEJMoa1008232].
45. Zuckerman BD, Saperstein W, Swain JA: The FDA role in the development of percutaneous valve technology. EuroInterv Suppl A 1:A75, 2006.
46. Dewey TM, Brown D, Ryan WH, et al: Reliability of risk algorithms in predicting early and late operative outcomes in high-risk patients undergoing aortic valve replacement. J Thorac Cardiovasc Surg 135:180, 2008.

CHAPTER **60** # Diseases of the Aorta

Alan C. Braverman, Robert W. Thompson, and Luis A. Sanchez

The Normal Aorta

Anatomy and Physiology

The aorta, the body's largest artery, extends from the aortic valve in the chest to the midabdomen, where it bifurcates into the common iliac arteries. Along its course the aorta is divided anatomically into thoracic and abdominal components. The thoracic aorta is further subdivided into the ascending, arch, and descending segments and the abdominal aorta into the suprarenal and infrarenal segments.

The ascending thoracic aorta has two distinct portions. The lower portion is the aortic root, which begins at the level of the aortic valve and extends to the sinotubular junction. The aortic root supports the bases of the three aortic valve leaflets, which bulge outward into the sinuses of Valsalva to allow for full valve cusp excursion during systole. The right and left coronary artery origins arise from within the sinuses of Valsalva. The upper portion of the ascending aorta begins at the sinotubular junction and rises to join the aortic arch. The proximal portion of ascending aorta lies within the pericardial cavity, anterior to the pulmonary artery bifurcation. The aortic arch gives rise to the arch vessels, innominate artery, left common carotid artery, and left subclavian artery.

The descending thoracic aorta begins just past the origin of the left subclavian artery. The point at which the aortic arch joins the descending aorta is called the aortic isthmus and is marked by the location of the ligamentum arteriosum. The aortic isthmus is especially vulnerable to deceleration trauma, because at this site, the relatively mobile portion of the aorta—the ascending aorta and arch—becomes relatively fixed to the thoracic cage. The descending aorta gradually courses downward, where it gives rise to paired intercostal arteries from the posterior aortic wall at each level of the spine. At its distal extent, the thoracic aorta passes through the diaphragm, usually at the level of the 12th thoracic vertebra, and becomes the abdominal aorta.

The abdominal aorta continues downward, giving rise to the celiac axis and the superior mesenteric artery from its anterior wall, followed within several centimeters by the posterolateral origins of the right and left renal arteries. This segment of the aorta is described as the suprarenal or visceral segment. The infrarenal aorta continues along the anterior surface of the lumbar spine, where it gives origin to the paired lumbar artery braches from its posterior wall. The aorta ends by bifurcation into common iliac arteries, usually at the level of the fourth lumbar vertebra.

MICROSCOPIC STRUCTURE. The aortic wall is comprised of three layers—the innermost tunica intima, which contacts the blood through its thin layer of endothelium, the musculoelastic tunica media, which is the thickest layer of the aortic wall, and the fibrous tunica adventitia, which forms its outermost layer (see Chap. 43). The intima consists of endothelial cells and the immediate subendothelial space, and is demarcated from the media by the internal elastic lamina. The media contains concentric layers of elastic fibers alternating with vascular smooth muscle cells (SMCs), with each layer of elastin and SMC constituting a lamellar unit of medial structure. In addition to SMCs, the aortic media normally contains a small number of fibroblasts, mast cells, and other cell types and, although dominated by elastic fibers, the extracellular matrix of the media includes collagen fibers, proteoglycans, and glycosaminoglycans. The microscopic architecture of the media gives the aorta its circumferential resilience (elasticity), necessary to resist hemodynamic stress. The outer portion of the aortic media is delineated from the adventitial layer by the external elastic lamina, which is normally thinner than the internal elastic lamina. The aortic adventitia is composed of a loose network of collagen fibers and fibroblasts, as well as small nerves and capillary-sized blood vessels. The adventitial collagen fibers ultimately govern the tensile strength of the aortic wall.

The human ascending aorta normally contains approximately 55 to 60 elastic lamellae, with a gradual decrease in the number of elastic lamellae down the length of the aorta to approximately 26 at the aortic bifurcation. Despite this regional variation in medial thickness, there appears to be a relatively consistent relationship between the number of elastic lamellae and the estimated amount of hemodynamic stress placed on the vessel wall, except for in the infrarenal aorta, with fewer elastic lamellae than predicted for its hemodynamic load.

Oxygen and nutrients reach the aortic wall by simple diffusion from the lumen, at least in segments of the aorta that contain up to about 29 elastic lamellae. In the proximal aortic segments that contain a greater number of elastic lamellae, additional nutrient supply is provided by an independent network of microvessels, the vasa vasorum, which extends from the adventitia to the outer layers of the elastic media. The outer third of the aortic media in the thoracic aorta contains many vasa vasorum, but the infrarenal aorta normally lacks an independent microvascular supply.

The compliance of the aortic wall under normal conditions results from the reversible extension of the elastic lamellar units in the media. This extensibility derives primarily from the properties of elastic fibers, whereas SMCs make only a minor contribution. At mechanical strain levels that exceed the extensile capacity of medial elastic fibers, the aortic tensile strength becomes dependent on the collagen fiber meshwork of the media and adventitia. Although not functionally significant under normal circumstances or in systemic hypertension, the dependence on adventitial collagen in accommodating greater hemodynamic stress is an important feature of abdominal aortic aneurysms (AAAs), where estimates of wall tension within the dilated segment may exceed that in the normal aorta by several orders of magnitude. In AAAs, collagen fibers are reorganized to accommodate higher degrees of tensile stress. In addition, there is evidence that aneurysmal dilation is accompanied by an active process characterized by a marked increase in collagen production. Surgical experience has shown that much of the inner arterial wall (endothelium and tunica media) can be removed, as is performed during an endarterectomy, without resulting in aneurysmal dilation. This observation illustrates that the structures conferring resistance aneurysmal dilation reside principally within the outer aspect of the media and the adventitia.

PHYSIOLOGY. The aorta is responsible for transmitting pulsatile arterial blood pressure to all points in the arterial tree, a function that depends on its properties as an elastic conduit. The aortic wall therefore requires properties of resilience to cyclic deformation, resistance to structural failure, and durability. The biomechanical properties attributable to elastin and collagen in the media and adventitia serve these demands. The aortic wall pressure-diameter relationship is nonlinear, demonstrating a more distensible component at lower pressures and a stiffer component at higher pressures, with the transition from distensible to stiff behavior occurring at pressures above 80 mm Hg. Thus, the more distensible elastin is the principal load bearer at low pressures and small distentions, whereas at higher pressures and large distentions, both elastin and the stiffer collagen are load bearing.

It is important to point out that the pressure-diameter curve of the aorta becomes less steep with increasing age (i.e., the aorta stiffens and aortic diameter increases). One explanation for this is an increase in the collagen-to-elastin ratio because of an age-related decrease in elastin and a simultaneous increase in collagen. Another factor is a gradual alteration of aortic wall architecture with age, characterized by progressively disordered medial elastic fibers and lamellae displaying thinning, splitting, and fragmentation in older individuals. A third factor is an increase in aortic wall thickness with age because of increased deposition of collagen and proteoglycan, as well as age-related calcification of elastic fibers. Finally, atherosclerotic changes are associated with aging, and may contribute to aortic wall stiffening. In addition to the direct effects of aortic wall plaque, stiffening may occur through compensatory increases in distensibility in areas free of disease (i.e., expansive arterial wall remodeling).

Evaluation of the Aorta

The only location in which the aorta can normally be palpated is in the midabdomen, where in some individuals (depending on body habitus) it may be detected on deep palpation adjacent to the spine. Plain radiography is insensitive for evaluating the thoracic and abdominal aorta. Much more diagnostic detail regarding the aorta is obtained through imaging modalities, such as ultrasound (including echocardiography), computed tomography (CT) and CT angiography, magnetic resonance imaging (MRI), or aortography.

Aortic Aneurysms

The term *aortic aneurysm* refers to a pathologic segment of aortic dilation that has a propensity to expand and rupture. The extent of aortic dilation required to be considered aneurysmal is debated, but one criterion is an increase in diameter at least 50% greater than that expected for the same aortic segment in unaffected individuals of the same age and sex. Aortic aneurysms are usually described in terms of their size, location, morphology, and etiology. Size criteria are usually focused on cross-sectional diameter, as measured in imaging studies. Aortic aneurysms are either fusiform or saccular. Fusiform aneurysms are most common and are characterized by a general symmetric dilation with a fairly uniform shape involving the entire aortic wall circumference. Saccular aneurysms exhibit localized dilation involving only a portion of the aortic wall circumference, appearing as a focal outpouching. These lesions represent true aneurysms in that the aortic wall is intact but dilated, involving all layers of aortic structure. In contrast, pseudoaneurysms (false aneurysms) represent lesions in which there has been bleeding through the aortic wall, resulting in a contained periaortic hematoma in continuity with the aortic lumen. These lesions may result from trauma or from contained rupture of an aortic aneurysm, dissection, or penetrating ulcer.

Abdominal Aortic Aneurysms

AAAs are defined by an increase in size of the abdominal aorta to more than 3.0 cm in diameter. AAAs occur in 3% to 9% of men older than 50 years and are the most common form of aortic aneurysms. Most AAAs arise in the infrarenal aorta (**Fig. 60-1**), but up to 10% may

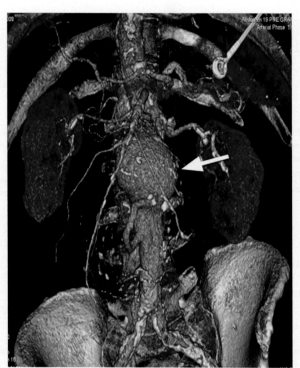

FIGURE 60-1 Three-dimensional reconstruction of a CT scan in a patient with an infrarenal abdominal aortic aneurysm (arrow).

involve the pararenal or visceral aorta, and some extend into the thoracoabdominal segment. The overall incidence of AAAs appears to have increased steadily over the past several decades. AAAs are approximately five times more prevalent in men than in women, and the incidence strongly associates with age, with most occurring in those older than 60 years. AAAs strongly associate with cigarette smoking; current and former smokers have a fivefold increase in risk compared with nonsmokers. Additional risk factors include emphysema, hypertension, and hyperlipidemia. Up to 20% of patients with AAAs describe a family history of aortic aneurysms, suggesting an inherited predisposition in some cohorts. AAAs are a multifactorial disease of aging without a known specific cause.

PATHOGENESIS. Aneurysm formation closely associates with chronic aortic wall inflammation, increased local expression of proteinases, and degradation of connective tissue proteins.[1] Aneurysmal dilation and rupture result from mechanical failure of medial elastin and adventitial collagen, the fibrillar matrix proteins normally responsible for maintaining aortic wall tensile strength, resilience, and structural integrity. Infiltration of the aortic wall by inflammatory cells occurs commonly in AAAs. In contrast to occlusive atherosclerosis, in which inflammation concentrates within the diseased intimal plaque, the distribution of inflammatory cells is transmural in AAAs, with dense focal infiltrates and scattered inflammatory cells centered within the elastic media and adventitia. In some patients with inflammatory AAAs, this process extends to the periaortic retroperitoneal tissues. Because inflammatory cells can elaborate matrix-degrading enzymes thought to be involved in medial degeneration, this process may be responsible for aneurysmal dilation and rupture.

Although the initial events responsible for inflammatory cell recruitment into the aortic media are unknown, they may include signals elaborated by medial SMCs in response to hemodynamic stress and/or ischemia, autoimmune processes, or an extension of intimal atherosclerosis. AAA tissues produce a large number of chemotactic peptides, including chemokines and biologically active products released during matrix degradation that could amplify the mononuclear inflammatory response. The tissue environment of AAAs also includes proinflammatory cytokines capable of stimulating macrophage expression of connective tissue proteinases, such as tumor necrosis factor-α, interleukin-1β, interleukin-6, and interferon-γ. Direct cell-to-cell interactions may be another local mechanism amplifying macrophage proteinase production. Although a response to foreign antigens or microbial infection has been postulated in the development of AAAs, the chronic inflammation in aneurysm tissue also exhibits features of an autoimmune response. AAA tissues thereby contain focal infiltrates of T and B lymphocytes, as well as large amounts of immunoglobulin, which is reactive with a number of matrix protein-related antigens. Whereas the autoimmune response in AAAs suggests a primary mechanism of disease, this response may represent a secondary consequence of extensive matrix degradation, leading to exposure of previously hidden epitopes and amplifying aortic wall inflammation.

Loss of medial elastin both morphologically and biochemically occurs consistently in AAAs. Experimental studies have demonstrated that damage to the elastic lamellae leads to aneurysmal dilation and tortuosity. Because elastin is extremely durable, and its degradation requires the activity of potent substrate-specific enzymes, the elastolytic proteinases produced within aneurysm tissues probably play a critical role in aneurysm development. Experimental studies have shown that maintenance of aortic wall tensile strength is principally attributable to interstitial collagen, and that AAAs are generally associated with an increase in collagen content. This finding manifests clinically as increased wall stiffness, exhibited by aortic aneurysms and elevations in type III procollagen fragments, which can be measured in the plasma as a marker of collagen turnover. Increased collagen production may thereby help preserve the dilated aneurysm wall, whereas enzymes that can initiate cleavage of interstitial collagens are an important factor in rapid aneurysm expansion and rupture.

The most prominent elastin- and collagen-degrading enzymes produced in human AAA tissues are matrix metalloproteinases (MMPs). MMPs degrade a broad range of matrix proteins, with four exhibiting specific activity against elastin (72-kDa gelatinase type IV collagenase [MMP-2], matrilysin [MMP-7], 92-kDa gelatinase type IV collagenase [MMP-9], and macrophage metalloelastase [MMP-12]). At least three MMPs can initiate the degradation of intact fibrillar collagen (MMP-1, MMP-8, and MMP-13), and several others act against denatured collagen (gelatin). Cellular production of MMPs is closely regulated at the level of gene transcription, and most MMPs are secreted into the extracellular space as inactive proenzymes; once secreted, pro-MMPs are regulated by local factors in the pericellular environment, such as proteases that mediate their extracellular activation, oxidative protein modifications, and interaction with secreted tissue inhibitors of metalloproteinases (TIMPs) and other proteinase scavengers.

MMP-9 has an especially important role in human and experimental AAAs. Aneurysm tissue contains abundant MMP-9, and mice lacking expression of MMP-9 show suppression of experimental AAAs. Moreover, treatment of experimental animals with tetracyclines and other MMP inhibitors has consistently suppressed aneurysm development in almost every animal model tested. Other experimental interventions found to suppress AAAs, such as treatment with statins and anti-inflammatory agents, induce a decrease in aortic tissue MMP-9. These observations have suggested the use of doxycycline and other MMP-inhibiting agents as therapeutic approaches to suppress the progression of aneurysmal degeneration in patients with small AAAs.

The development and natural history of AAAs involves a balance between degradative and reparative processes. Because vascular SMCs normally produce elastin and collagen during aortic development, and SMCs are the dominant cell type within the elastic media, SMCs are ideally positioned to mediate connective tissue repair within AAAs. Human AAAs show a pronounced depletion of medial SMCs. Mechanisms underlying the loss of SMCs in AAAs include apoptotic cell death, which may be initiated by medial ischemia, signaling molecules prevalent in AAA tissue, or cellular immune responses. Medial SMC ischemia may also participate in aneurysmal degeneration, because in the absence of vasa vasorum, the nutrient supply to the media depends on diffusion from the aortic lumen, a process jeopardized by intimal thickening and atherosclerotic plaques.

CLINICAL FEATURES. AAAs develop insidiously over a period of several years and rarely cause symptoms in the absence of distal thromboembolism, rapid expansion, or overt rupture. Although large AAAs are at substantial risk of rupture and thereby attract most clinical attention, the vast majority of AAAs are small. Most AAAs are thereby detected by screening, or as an incidental finding on imaging studies performed for other purposes.

Physical examination is notoriously inaccurate in the detection of AAAs, but abdominal palpation may reveal a pulsatile epigastric or periumbilical mass, particularly in relatively thin patients with large aneurysms. Mural thrombus associated with AAAs may lead to thromboembolism, which may be the presenting symptom in 2% to 5% of patients. Because AAAs are frequently associated with peripheral artery aneurysms, physical examination should also include palpation of the femoral and popliteal arteries.

DIAGNOSTIC IMAGING

Ultrasound

Abdominal ultrasound can detect AAAs with a high degree of accuracy, with sensitivities and specificities that approach 100%. Abdominal ultrasound is preferred in screening for AAAs because it is also inexpensive, noninvasive, and avoids radiation exposure. In approximately 2% to 3% of patients, visualization of the infrarenal aorta by ultrasound may be limited by overlying bowel gas or obesity, and alternate imaging studies are necessary. Abdominal ultrasound is also used for serial measurements of AAA size during follow-up surveillance of patients with small AAAs. Because the accuracy of ultrasound-derived aneurysm diameter measurements is not as great as those obtained by CT or MRI, many recommend the use of ultrasound for follow-up of AAAs up to 4.5 cm in diameter, with the use of alternative modalities for larger AAAs. The wide availability of ultrasound has suggested its use in emergency room detection of ruptured AAAs. Despite reports indicating a high degree of accuracy, up to half of ruptured AAAs may be missed in the emergency setting.

Computed Tomography

Abdominal CT is extremely accurate for the detection of AAAs and measurement of aneurysmal diameter (**Fig. 60-2**). Particularly when combined with radiographic contrast enhancement, thin-slice techniques, and three-dimensional reconstructions with measurements

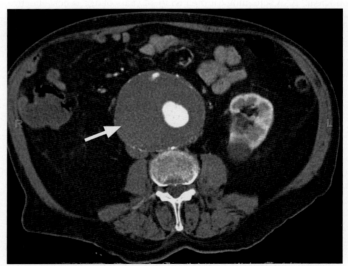

FIGURE 60-2 Contrast CT scan of a large, thrombus-filled abdominal aortic aneurysm (arrow). Contrast fills the lumen of the aneurysm.

obtained perpendicular to the center line of the aorta, CT angiography (CTA) is more accurate than ultrasound and has superseded the need for catheter-based aortography in preoperative planning. CTA is especially useful for demonstrating the extent of aneurysm disease; the relationship of the AAA to the renal, visceral, and iliac arteries; and patterns of mural thrombus, calcification, or coexisting occlusive atherosclerosis that might influence surgical AAA repair. CT imaging is also preferred for the assessment of unusual variants of AAAs, such as inflammatory AAAs and mycotic aneurysms, and AAAs associated with anatomic variations, such as vena cava or renal vein anomalies and pelvic or horseshoe kidneys.

Magnetic Resonance Aortography

Like CT imaging, magnetic resonance aortography (MRA) is extremely accurate for the detection of AAAs, the measurement of aneurysm diameter, and the delineation of aortic anatomy for planning treatment. MRA has the distinct advantage of avoiding exposure to radiation and iodine-based contrast materials. Although MRA is preferred in some centers, where it may be readily available, in most institutions CT imaging remains the preferred imaging modality for the evaluation of AAAs.

As noted, CT angiography now generally supersedes aortography, which is rarely used in this setting. For patients undergoing endovascular AAA repair, aortography is one of the initial steps in the operative procedure. It is also used in subsequent interventions following AAA stent-graft repair, such as embolization of lumbar or iliac artery branches. An unsuspected AAA may occasionally be identified during transfemoral angiography performed for another reason (e.g., cardiac catheterization). The characteristics of an AAA include an enlarged abdominal aortic segment, marked by calcification and occlusion of lumbar branch vessels. The aortic lumen may or may not appear enlarged because of the presence of mural thrombus.

SCREENING. Screening for AAAs with ultrasound, coupled with repair for AAAs above a given size threshold, can reduce AAA-related deaths.[2] The overall incidence of screening-detected AAAs ranges from 1:1000 in adults younger than 60 years of age to 7:1000 in those in their mid-60s, but may be as high as 10% in the presence of risk factors such as older age, male sex, smoking, family history, history of other aneurysms, hypertension, atherosclerotic diseases, and hypercholesterolemia. In asymptomatic U.S. veterans 50 to 79 years of age participating in the Aneurysm Detection and Management Trial, 66% of AAAs identified by screening were smaller than 4.0 cm in diameter. Randomized trials have demonstrated that AAA screening is associated with a 50% reduction in AAA rupture and a 50% decrease in aneurysm-related mortality. Whereas overall there was a 6% reduction in mortality, the presence of a significant reduction in all-cause mortality remains unclear.[3] AAA screening for men 65 to 74 years of age is cost-effective, but the cost-effectiveness of screening for AAAs in women remains debated. Whereas the prevalence of AAAs is lower in women than in men, AAAs occur about 10 years later in women, and the rupture rate and mortality of AAA rupture are both higher. In 2005, the U.S. Preventative Services Task Force reported a recommendation for one-time ultrasound screening for AAA for men 65 to 75 years of age with a history of smoking.[4] The Society for Vascular Surgery also recommends AAA screening in men and women with a family history of AAAs.[5]

GENETICS AND MOLECULAR GENETICS. Several well-defined but relatively uncommon genetic disorders are associated with aortic aneurysms, typically involving the ascending thoracic aorta, but less commonly the abdominal aorta, including Marfan syndrome (MFS), Loeys-Dietz syndrome (LDS), and vascular Ehlers-Danlos syndrome (see later, "Thoracic Aortic Aneurysms"). Up to 20% of patients with an infrarenal AAA describe a family history of AAAs, suggesting an inherited component. A number of genetic variants appear to link with AAAs through analysis of single nucleotide polymorphisms (SNPs) in relatively large populations. One example is a common sequence variant on chromosome 9p21 (rs10757278-G) that is associated with a 31% increased risk of AAAs, as well as increased risks for intracranial aneurysms.[6] Although further work is needed to help validate these findings in additional populations, broader use of genome-wide screening will undoubtedly help identify additional SNPs associated with AAAs.

NATURAL HISTORY. AAAs usually gradually expand over a period of years, and eventually rupture. The risk of AAA rupture is closely correlated with aneurysm size, with the 5-year risk of rupture being approximately 5% for AAAs 3.0 to 4.0 cm in diameter, 10% to 20% for AAAs 4.0 to 5.5 cm in diameter, and 30% to 40% for AAAs 5.5 to 6.0 cm in diameter.[5] The risk of rupture for AAAs larger than 6.0 cm in diameter rises even more rapidly, exceeding 80% for AAAs larger than 7.0 cm. The average rate of aneurysm expansion is approximately 0.3 to 0.5 cm/year, although there is considerable individual variation. Not all AAAs follow a linear or consistent rate of expansion, and many factors may influence AAA growth patterns. Thus, whereas some patients have stable AAAs that grow slowly for many years, others can have a stable AAA size for many years followed by a sudden increase within a short period of time.

Ruptured Abdominal Aortic Aneurysm

Symptoms directly attributable to AAAs usually occur with overt aneurysm rupture or rapid recent expansion presumed to indicate impending rupture. Rupture of an AAA into the peritoneal cavity results in rapid hemorrhage, with severe abdominal pain and cardiovascular collapse because of exsanguination. Rupture into the retroperitoneum may result in a temporarily contained periaortic hematoma, with severe abdominal or back pain that may radiate into the flank or groin. A tender pulsatile abdominal or flank mass is often present, along with hypotension or loss of consciousness. An estimated 30% to 50% of patients with ruptured AAAs die before reaching a hospital, and an additional 30% to 40% die after reaching a hospital but before operative treatment.[5] Whereas immediate surgical treatment is necessary for all ruptured AAAs, the operative mortality rate after rupture is 40% to 50%. Recent evidence has indicated that the mortality rate for repair of ruptured AAAs can be markedly diminished by the use of endovascular repair as compared with open surgical techniques.[7] Hemodynamically stable patients presenting with symptomatic but unruptured AAAs should undergo CT to determine whether rupture has occurred. In the absence of rupture, in some cases it may be prudent to delay surgical repair for 4 to 24 hours until optimal conditions can be achieved, with the patient closely monitored.

MANAGEMENT

Medical Therapy

Patients with small AAAs can be safely observed with imaging surveillance and little risk of rupture and, in general, AAA repair is reserved for aneurysms at least 5.0 to 5.5 cm in diameter.[8] For those with AAAs 3.0 to 4.0 cm in diameter, the rate of growth is less than 10% per year, and annual imaging with abdominal ultrasound is recommended. For those with AAAs larger than 4.0 cm in diameter, variability in growth is greater, so that imaging is recommended at 6-month intervals. For those with AAAs larger than 4.5 cm in diameter, CT may be preferred over ultrasound for more accurate measurement of AAA size.

For patients with small AAAs undergoing imaging surveillance, several steps may help minimize the risk of aneurysm expansion and improve overall health. The most important of these is smoking cessation, because there is strong evidence that ongoing tobacco use is associated with more rapid rates of AAA expansion and rupture. Appropriate management should also be undertaken for hypertension, hyperlipidemia and, diabetes. Almost all patients with small AAAs should take a statin, based on the presence of coexisting atherosclerotic disease, and although randomized data are lacking, these medications may suppress AAA growth.[9] Animal model data have demonstrated a favorable influence of angiotensin-converting enzyme (ACE) inhibitors or angiotensin receptor blockers (ARBs), but interpretable data in humans with AAAs are not yet available. Patients with small AAAs should be encouraged to exercise regularly, because moderate physical activity does not adversely influence the risk of rupture and may even limit the rate of AAA growth.

EXPERIMENTAL THERAPY. Based on laboratory research conducted over the past two decades, interest has accelerated in the potential use of medical (pharmacologic) therapies to suppress the growth rate of small AAAs, thereby reducing the need for surgical repair.[8] One of the earliest approaches suggested was the use of beta-adrenergic receptor blockers (beta blockers) to diminish mechanical stress on the aortic wall. Although several reports have indicated successful use of propranolol in animal models of AAAs, two large clinical trials have demonstrated no benefit to propranolol treatment in patients with small AAAs.[8] A second approach is to suppress proteinases involved in extracellular matrix degradation through the use of doxycycline as a MMP inhibitor. Treatment with doxycycline suppresses or prevents AAAs in a spectrum of animal models in association with MMP inhibition, particularly of MMP-9. Doxycycline is well tolerated by patients with small AAAs, in whom it also appears to decrease MMP activities in aneurysmal aortic tissue and in the circulation. Further clinical investigation is needed to determine whether doxycycline treatment can reduce the rate of AAA expansion. A third experimental approach is the use of angiotensin receptor antagonists, such as losartan, as a means to modify aortic wall connective tissue metabolism. Treatment with losartan suppresses aneurysm formation in mouse models of Marfan syndrome. Because losartan and other ARBs are also effective in other animal models of AAAs, it will be important to determine whether ARBs are useful in suppressing the growth of AAAs in humans.

SURGERY. The decision to repair an asymptomatic AAA electively is based on life expectancy and the estimated risk of rupture, balanced against the estimated risks of AAA repair. Factors significantly influencing operative morbidity and mortality include coronary artery disease (the leading cause of early and late mortality after AAA repair), chronic kidney disease, chronic pulmonary disease, and diabetes mellitus.[5] Thus, evaluation for these conditions is warranted before elective AAA repair, along with optimization of perioperative status wherever possible.

Because many patients with AAAs have underlying coronary artery disease, and postoperative myocardial infarction has a substantial risk of death or later cardiovascular events, special attention is directed toward coronary disease prior to elective AAA repair. Although guidelines to minimize perioperative cardiac risk have been recently updated (see Chap. 85), the first step is to identify those patients with an active cardiac condition that warrants urgent treatment or even precludes repair. In the absence of an active cardiac condition, further noninvasive testing is only indicated if it will change management, in accord with current guidelines. Some patients benefit from preoperative coronary ischemic evaluation and treatment. Perioperative medical management to reduce cardiac risks in patients undergoing AAA repair may include titrated administration of beta blockers, and treatment with statins and/or aspirin, in accord with the individual patient's risk factors and medical findings.[5,9]

Invasive treatment for AAAs can be performed by one of two general approaches—open surgical repair (OSR) or endovascular aneurysm repair (EVAR). The selection of approach depends on the individual anatomy and on secondary factors, such as patient age and estimated risks for anesthesia and surgery.[10]

TECHNIQUES AND OUTCOMES. For open surgical repair (OSR) of infrarenal AAAs, the abdominal aorta may be approached through a transperitoneal exposure, using a full midline laparotomy incision, or a left retroperitoneal exposure. A tube or bifurcated prosthetic graft is attached with suture directly to the proximal aorta, followed by sutured anastomosis to the distal aorta (tube graft) or common iliac arteries (bifurcation graft). Following restoration of lower extremity flow through the aortic graft, the aneurysm sac is sewn together to prevent contact between the prosthetic graft and the gastrointestinal tract. The operative mortality rate for conventional OSR ranges from 1% to 4% in reports from single-institution centers of excellence, whereas mortality rates in statewide or national data bases range from 4% to 8%. Operative complication rates range from 10% to 30% and include morbidity related to cardiac, pulmonary, and renal complications, as well as colonic ischemia. Based on recent evidence that outcomes for OSR are related to hospital and surgeon volumes, there has been a trend to recommend that OSR for AAAs be performed at centers with demonstrable operative mortality rates less than 5%.

A number of late complications may develop during long-term follow-up after OSR for AAAs. The most significant of these include problems related to the abdominal incision, para-anastomotic aneurysms (including false aneurysms secondary to suture line disruptions and true aneurysms secondary to proximal aortic degeneration), graft infection, graft-enteric erosions or fistula, and graft limb occlusions with lower extremity ischemia. Annual clinical follow-up and CT at 5-year intervals are generally recommended after open AAA repair.

ENDOVASCULAR ABDOMINAL AORTIC ANEURYSM REPAIR. For patients with suitable anatomy, endovascular aortic aneurysm repair (EVAR) offers a less invasive alternative than open surgical repair (see Chap. 63). EVAR is performed in the operating room or angiographic suite under fluoroscopic guidance, and most patients are discharged within 24 hours. There are currently five U.S. Food and Drug Administration (FDA)-approved endografts commercially available, each with its own design and method of fixation to the aortic wall. The Open Versus Endovascular Repair (OVER) Veterans Affairs Cooperative Study Group randomized 881 veterans 49 years of age or older with a minimum aneurysm diameter of 5.0 cm. The perioperative mortality was lower for endovascular repair compared with open repair (0.5% to 3.0%).[11] High-risk patients can also benefit from endovascular repair. Using high-risk criteria from five multicenter investigational device exemption clinical trials, 565 EVAR patients and 61 open surgical controls were identified. The 30-day operative mortality was 2.9% in EVAR and 5.1% in the open surgical group (P = 0.32). The aneurysm-related death rate after EVAR was 3.0% at 1 year and 4.2% at 4 years compared with 5.1% at both time points for the open surgical group (P = 0.58). The overall survival at 4 years after EVAR was 56% versus 66% in the open surgical group (P = 0.23). After treatment, EVAR successfully prevented rupture in 99.5% at 1 year and 97.2% at 4 years.[12] Patients with ruptured aneurysms also benefit significantly from endovascular repair. In evaluating 27,750 hospital discharges for ruptured AAA, EVAR had a lower overall in-hospital mortality than open surgical repair (32% to 41%; P < 0.0001).[13] Data from 13 centers were collected on 1037 patients treated by EVAR and 763 patient treated by open surgical repair. The overall 30-day mortality in all EVAR patients was 21%. In centers performing EVAR whenever possible, almost 50% of patients underwent EVAR. The 30-day mortality rates for these centers were 20% for EVAR compared with 36% for open surgical repair.[14] With appropriate patient selection and accurate graft deployment, low perioperative mortality rates (~1%) and complication rates (10% to 15%) can be achieved irrespective of the endograft used. These results have led to the increased application of EVAR to patients with AAAs that have suitable anatomy. The options of endovascular and open surgical repair with their advantages and disadvantages currently are considered in medically fit patients with suitable anatomy. Most patients select endovascular treatment because of its early perioperative advantages and its less invasive nature.

The development of endoleaks (incomplete exclusion of blood flow from the aneurysm sac) can complicate EVAR. In addition, various other late complications (e.g., endograft migration, limb thrombosis, and implant-related complications such as fractures, component separation, and fabric tears) and graft infection can occur. Long-term radiographic surveillance is essential following EVAR. Imaging with contrast-enhanced CTA is typically performed at 1 month, at 6 months, and annually post–device implantation. A reduced surveillance regimen may be appropriate in cases in which there is early success with newer devices, but this approach has not been validated in a randomized prospective trial setting. In patients for whom contrast use is prohibited (e.g., renal insufficiency, allergy), duplex ultrasound may be combined with noncontrast CT for complete evaluation.

Thoracic Aortic Aneurysms

Thoracic aortic aneurysms (TAAs) occur much less commonly than AAAs, with an estimated incidence of at least 10/100,000 person-years.[15] TAAs may involve the ascending arch and/or the descending aorta. Their cause, natural history, and treatment varies, depending on their location. Ascending aortic aneurysms are most common (~60%), followed by aneurysms of the descending aorta (~35%) and arch (<10%). The term *thoracoabdominal aortic aneurysm* refers to descending thoracic aneurysms that extend distally to involve the abdominal aorta. *Annuloaortic ectasia*, an enlargement of the aorta at the sinuses of Valsalva with normal aortic dimensions above the sinotubular junction, often occurs in genetically triggered aortic diseases.

CAUSES AND PATHOGENESIS. Aneurysms involving the aortic root and ascending aorta can be genetically triggered, degenerative or atherosclerotic, inflammatory, or can result from infectious diseases (see Table 60-e1 on website). Cystic medial degeneration (CMD) describes degeneration and fragmentation of elastic fibers, smooth muscle cell loss, increase in collagen deposition, and replacement with interstitial cysts of mucoid appearing basophilic-staining ground substance (see Fig. 60-e1 on website). CMD of the aorta is present in MFS and many other genetically triggered TAA diseases. In addition, aging associates with some degree of CMD, a process that may be accelerated by hypertension. These changes cause progressive weakening of the aortic wall, leading to dilation and aneurysm formation.

Genetically Triggered Thoracic Aortic Aneurysm Diseases

There are many disorders of the thoracic aorta with an underlying genetic trigger, some of which associate with widespread syndromic features, whereas others associate with thoracic aortic disease alone (see Chap. 8). These include MFS, LDS, vascular Ehlers-Danlos syndrome (vEDS), familial thoracic aortic aneurysm and dissection syndrome (FTAA/D), bicuspid aortic valve (BAV) disease, Turner syndrome (TS), and the aortopathy associated with many congenital heart diseases.

MFS, an autosomal dominant disorder of connective tissue, is caused by abnormal fibrillin-1 resulting from mutations in the *FBN1* gene. In addition to directing elastogenesis and providing structural support to tissues, fibrillin-1 interacts with latent transforming growth factor-β (TGF-β)–binding proteins and controls TGF-β activation and signaling. Mutations in *FBN1* result in abnormal elastin content and function in the aortic wall. Aortic dilation in MFS involves the sinuses of Valsalva (**Fig. 60-3**; see Video 60-1 on website and Fig. 15-81), with the ascending aorta above the sinotubular junction usually being normal in dimension. Angiotensin is important in TGF-β signaling and blocking TGF-β, whether by neutralizing antibody or by the angiotensin II type I receptor blocker (ARB), losartan, attenuating or preventing aortic aneurysm formation in genetically engineered Marfan mice with abnormal fibrillin. In Marfan children with very aggressive aortic disease, ARB therapy resulted in a dramatic stabilization of aortic root size. A trial of beta blockade versus ARB therapy (losartan) in MFS is being conducted to examine the effects of these agents on aortic growth.

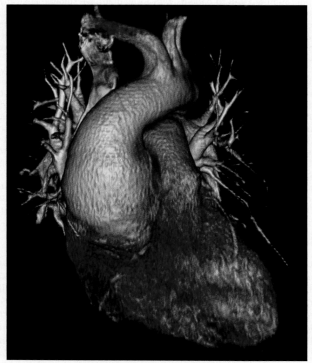

FIGURE 60-3 Three-dimensional CT reconstruction of an aortic root aneurysm in a patient with Marfan syndrome. *(Courtesy of Dr. Kristopher Cummings, Washington University School of Medicine, St. Louis.)*

LDS, an autosomal dominant disorder caused by mutations in *TGFBR1* and *TGFBR2*, is associated with craniofacial features (hypertelorism, bifid-broad uvula, cleft palate, craniosynostosis), arterial tortuosity, and aneurysms and dissections of the aorta and branch vessels.[16] Excess TGF-β signaling is suggested in the diseased tissues of LDS. Importantly, LDS has a much more aggressive vascular phenotype than MFS, and prophylactic aortic surgery at a smaller aortic root dimension is recommended.[17]

Mutations in *COL3A1* leading to abnormal collagen synthesis cause vEDS, an autosomal dominant condition that may be associated with aortic aneurysm and dissection. Individuals with vEDS are at risk for sudden death from spontaneous arterial dissection and rupture, often involving medium-sized arteries. Aortic root involvement is less common, with the descending and abdominal aorta and aortic branch vessels more frequently involved. Unlike MFS and LDS, the abnormal arteries in vEDS are friable, making surgical repair difficult and complicated, with increased risk.

Ascending TAAs, in the absence of other genetic syndromes, may be familial and associated with CMD. When TAA and dissection (TAAD) occur in the absence of other syndromic features, it is often inherited as an autosomal dominant trait with decreased penetrance and variable expression, a disorder known as familial TAAD.[18] Pedigree studies have emphasized the familial nature of TAA disease, highlighting the variable age of onset and variable expression in these families. An inherited pattern for TAA is present in 20% of TAA patients.[19] Among familial TAAD kindreds, 66% had TAAs, 25% had AAAs, and 8% had cerebral aneurysms. Several genes associated with TAAD have been identified to date, including *FBN1*, *TGFBR1*, *TGFBR2*, *MYH11*, and *ACTA2*. Whereas TGF-β signaling abnormalities underlie the pathogenesis in *FBN1*, *TGFBR1*, and *TGFBR2* mutations, defects in SMC contractile function leading to aortic aneurysm and dissection are related to *MYH11* and *ACTA2* mutations. Fibrillin-1 microfibrils may be a component of the mechanotransduction system of vascular SMCs, linking fibrillin-1 in the matrix to intracellular actin filaments. In most families with TAAD, the disorder is autosomal dominant, with decreased penetrance and variable expression with respect to the age of onset of aortic disease, location of the aneurysm, and degree of aortic enlargement prior to dissection. Histopathology of the aortic tissue in TAAD reveals CMD. Imaging of the aorta in family members often reveals asymptomatic aneurysms, and the incidence of aortic disease increases with advancing age. Decreased penetrance complicates the evaluation in this disorder. Some family members with TAAD have associated bicuspid aortic valve (BAV), cerebral aneurysm, and/or patent ductus arteriosus (PDA). *ACTA2* mutations have associated with livedo reticularis, iris flocculi, PDA, and BAV.[20] *MYH11* mutations may be associated with PDA and livedo reticularis. First-degree relatives of the individual with unexplained TAA or dissection should undergo thoracic aortic imaging. If a mutation in a gene associated with TAA or dissection is found, first-degree relatives should undergo testing for the same gene mutation.

BAV affects approximately 1% of the population and may associate with abnormalities of the aorta, including ascending aortic aneurysm, coarctation of the aorta, and aortic dissection (see Chaps. 65 and 66). The aortopathy associated with BAV is one of the most common causes of ascending aortic aneurysm. Ascending aortic dilation is not caused by poststenotic dilation, but instead relates to underlying abnormalities of the aortic media. Ascending aortic aneurysm associated with BAV may occur without associated aortic stenosis or regurgitation, and may occur late after aortic valve replacement. Compared with patients with tricuspid aortic valves, those with BAVs have larger aortic dimensions, even in childhood.[21] The aortic enlargement in BAV often arises in the proximal to mid-ascending aorta, emphasizing the importance of visualizing the entire extent of the ascending aorta in BAV patients to evaluate for aneurysms above the sinotubular junction (**Fig. 60-4**).

CMD underlies the aortic aneurysm and risk of dissection associated with BAV, and has been demonstrated in the aortic wall of patients with BAV, even without significant aneurysm formation.[21] Compared with tricuspid aortic valve aneurysms, patients with BAV aneurysms exhibit a distinct pattern of CMD, increased apoptosis, increased MMP-2 activity, and greater expression of death-promoting mediators by infiltrating lymphocytes.[21] Fibrillin-1 content is reduced in BAV aortas, compared with that seen in tricuspid aortic valve aortas. Polymorphisms in MMP-9 may play a role in thoracic aortic aneurysms and dissections in certain individuals.

BAV and ascending aortic aneurysm may be familial and associate with the risk of aortic dissection, inherited as an autosomal dominant

ATHEROSCLEROTIC ANEURYSMS. Atherosclerotic aneurysms are less common in the ascending aorta and associate with diffuse aortic atherosclerosis. Isolated arch aneurysms (see Fig. 60-e2 on website) are unusual and may be caused by atherosclerosis, penetrating aortic ulcers, CMD, and, rarely, by syphilis or other infections. The major cause of descending aortic aneurysms is atherosclerosis. These aneurysms tend to originate just distal to the origin of the left subclavian artery and may be either fusiform or saccular. They may extend into the abdominal aorta (thoracoabdominal aneurysm) or coexist with abdominal aortic aneurysms.

SYPHILIS. Cardiovascular syphilis occurs in the tertiary stage and typically involves the ascending aorta and arch. Aortitis is rarely seen today because of antibiotic treatment of syphilis early in its course. Cardiovascular syphilis usually occurs with a latency of at least 10 to 25 years. During secondary syphilis, direct invasion by spirochetes into the aortic wall occurs. The inflammatory response causes destructive changes in the muscular and elastic tissue, with fibrous and calcific degeneration. Pathologic features include lymphocytic and plasma cell inflammation in the adventitia, with a classic appearance of a "tree bark" or wrinkled appearance of the aortic intima. Progressive weakening of the aortic wall, with resultant aneurysm formation of the ascending aorta, occurs in 40% of cases. Other features of tertiary syphilis involving the heart include aortic valvulitis with aortic regurgitation in 29% of cases, and coronary ostial stenosis in approximately 30% of cases.

Infectious aortitis is discussed later in this chapter (see "Bacterial Infections of the Aorta"). Other causes of thoracic aortic aneurysms include noninfectious aortitis, such as that associated with large vessel vasculitis (giant cell arteritis), and other vasculitides, as well as idiopathic aortitis. Noninfectious aortitis may underlie aortic aneurysms in 2% to 8% of TAAs and is discussed in other chapters. Chap. 76 discusses aortic trauma.

CLINICAL MANIFESTATIONS. Most patients with TAAs are asymptomatic, with the aneurysm discovered incidentally by chest radiography, echocardiography, CT, or MRI. Occasionally, physical findings such as aortic regurgitation lead to further imaging and diagnosis of the TAA (see Fig. 18-20). Symptoms from TAAs usually relate to a local mass effect, progressive aortic regurgitation and heart failure from aortic root dilation, or systemic embolization caused by mural thrombus or atheroembolism. Obstruction of the superior vena cava or innominate vein may occur from ascending aorta or arch aneurysms. TAAs may compress the trachea, bronchus, or esophagus, leading to dyspnea, bronchospasm, cough, hemoptysis, dysphagia, or hematemesis. Persistent chest or back pain may occur because of a direct mass effect from the TAA, with compression of the intrathoracic structures or erosion into adjacent bones.

The most serious complications of TAAs are rupture and dissection. Aortic rupture leads to sudden severe chest or back pain (see Fig. 60-e3 on website). Rupture into the pleural cavity (usually left) or into the mediastinum causes hypotension. Rupture into the esophagus leads to hematemesis from an aortoesophageal fistula; rupture into the bronchus or trachea causes hemoptysis. Infected TAAs are associated more commonly with fistulas. Acute aortic expansion, contained rupture, and pseudoaneurysm can cause severe chest or back pain. Thoracic aortic dissection is more common than rupture and is discussed later.

DIAGNOSIS. Many TAAs are evident on chest radiographs (**Fig. 60-5**; see Fig. 16-9) with features including a widened mediastinum, prominent aortic knob, or displaced trachea. Importantly, smaller aneurysms, especially saccular ones, may not be visible on a chest radiograph. Aneurysms involving the sinuses of Valsalva and aortic root are often hidden behind the sternum, mediastinal structures, and vertebrae, and they may not be visualized on chest radiographs. Aortic tortuosity and unfolding in older patients may also mimic or mask TAA. Therefore, chest radiographs cannot exclude the diagnosis of TAA.

Transthoracic echocardiography is an excellent modality for imaging the aortic root (see Fig. 60-4A; also see Fig, 60-e4 and Video 60-1 on website), and can visualize TAAs involving the sinuses of Valsalva (see Figs. 15-81 and 15-82) and often of the proximal ascending aorta, arch, and proximal descending aorta. Other modalities are better suited to diagnose and characterize arch and descending TAAs. Transesophageal echocardiography (TEE) (see Chap. 15) can image almost

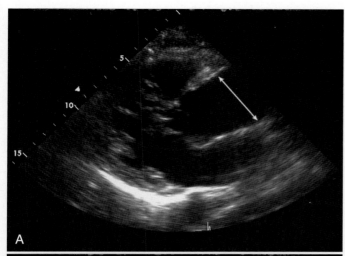

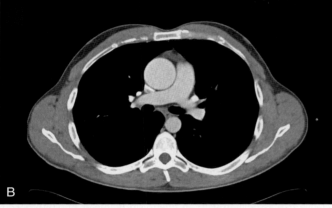

FIGURE 60-4   A, Transthoracic echocardiogram of a dilated ascending aorta in a patient with bicuspid aortic valve. Note that the dilation continues above the sinotubular junction into the ascending aorta. **B,** CT scan of a dilated ascending aorta at the level of the pulmonary artery in the same patient. *(From Braverman AC, Beardslee M: Bicuspid aortic valve. In Otto C, Bonow R [eds]: Valvular Heart Disease: A Companion to Braunwald's Heart Disease. Philadelphia, Saunders/Elsevier, 2009, pp 169-186.)*

pattern with variable expressivity and incomplete penetrance. Altered TGF-β signaling has been hypothesized in BAV aneurysm disease.[22] Potential loci at 15q, 18q, 5q, and 13q have been suggested for BAV and aortic aneurysm. *NOTCH1* mutations have been found in a small number of families with BAV and ascending aortic aneurysms and associate with aortic valve calcification.[21] First-degree relatives of the patient with BAV may have aortic dilation and/or abnormal aortic elastic properties, even in the absence of BAV.[23] All family members should undergo evaluation for BAV and ascending aortic aneurysm.

Turner syndrome (TS), affecting 1 in 2000 live-born girls (see Chap. 65), results from a complete or partial loss of a second sex chromosome (XO, Xp). Approximately 50% of TS patients have cardiovascular defects, including BAV in approximately 20% and coarctation of the aorta in approximately 12%.[24] Aortic dilation occurs in TS and is associated with CMD. TGF-β signaling may also play a role in this process. TS patients have an estimated 100-fold greater risk of aortic dissection compared with age-matched controls. Because TS patients have short stature, ascending aortic dimensions should be evaluated in relation to body-surface area. TS patients have increased aortic diameter relative to body-surface area. Prophylactic aortic root replacement should be considered in TS when the absolute aortic dimension exceeds 3.5 cm or the aortic root size index exceeds 2.5 cm/m².

CMD can occur in several types of congenital heart disease in addition to BAV, including coarctation of the aorta, transposition of the great vessels, ventricular septal defect, and tetralogy of Fallot (TOF). In TOF, aortic dilation is associated with male sex, with a longer time interval from palliation to definitive repair, and with pulmonary atresia and right-sided aortic arch, and may lead to aortic regurgitation, aortic aneurysm formation, and aortic dissection.[25]

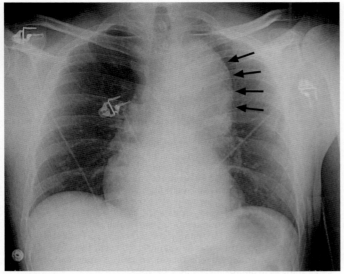

FIGURE 60-5 Chest radiograph demonstrating a large descending thoracic aortic aneurysm (arrows).

the entire thoracic aorta well and has become widely used for the detection of aortic dissection and to characterize aortic atherosclerosis.

CT (see Fig. 60-e5 on website) and MRA are preferred over aortography in most cases of TAA to define aortic and branch vessel anatomy (see Chaps. 18 and 19). In the setting of a tortuous aorta, axial images alone may be misleading and may overstate the true dimension of the aorta. When the axial images cut through the descending aorta at a plane that is off-axis, it results in a falsely large aortic diameter. Multidetector computed tomography (MDCT) angiography allows reconstruction of the axial data into three-dimensional images (i.e., CT angiography), and the aorta may be measured in a true cross section, obtaining an accurate diameter (**Fig. 60-6**). CTA and contrast-enhanced MRA are highly accurate for the evaluation and follow-up of patients undergoing endovascular TAA therapy.

The use of biomarkers to detect aneurysms in the general population and to monitor the disease activity of thoracic aortic aneurysm is an area of immense interest. Studying RNA expression patterns in the blood of patients with TAA, Elefteriades and coworkers[26] have found that a 41-SNP panel predicts whether a patient has had an aneurysm with over 80% accuracy.

NATURAL HISTORY. Many factors influence the natural history of TAA, most importantly the underlying cause. Genetically triggered TAAs behave differently than atherosclerotic aneurysms. The location and size of the TAA also affect its growth rate and likelihood of rupture or dissection. Surgery is generally recommended when the TAA reaches a certain size threshold in an appropriate candidate.[26-28] Patients considered inoperable have often been older or had significant morbidities. Endovascular therapy is changing the demographics of these subgroups.

TAAs are relatively indolent, with a growth rate of 0.07 to 0.2 cm/year and marked individual variability.[26-28] Larger aneurysms grow at a more rapid rate than smaller ones. In a study of 304 patients with TAAs at least 3.5 cm in size followed for more than 31 months, the mean rate of growth of TAAs was 0.1 cm/year.[27] Aneurysms of the descending aorta had a much greater growth rate (0.19 cm/year) than those of the ascending aorta (0.07 cm/year), and dissected TAAs grew more rapidly (0.14 cm/year) than those without dissection (0.09 cm/year). Patients with MFS had a more rapid growth rate than non-Marfan patients. The size of the aorta affects growth rate and risk of rupture and dissection. The mean rate of rupture or dissection was 2% per year for aneurysms smaller than 5.0 cm in diameter; 3% per year for aneurysms 5.0 to 5.9 cm, and 7% per year for aneurysms 6.0 cm or larger. In an analysis of the predictors of dissection or rupture, the

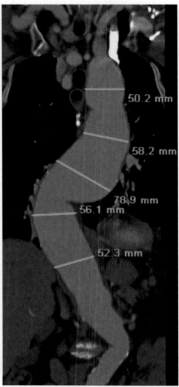

FIGURE 60-6 CT scan reconstruction of a thoracic aortic aneurysm, with measurements orthogonal to the long axis included.

relative risk associated with an aneurysm diameter of 5.0 to 5.9 cm was 2.5, with an aneurysm diameter of 6.0 cm or larger was 5.2, with Marfan syndrome was 3.7, and with female sex was 2.9.

Risk factors for increased growth and rupture of TAAs include increasing age, female sex, chronic obstructive pulmonary disease, hypertension, cigarette smoking, rapid aneurysm growth, pain, aortic dissection, and a positive family history of TAAs.[28] Aortic diameter is the most important risk factor for aneurysm rupture, dissection, and death. In large data bases, sharp hinge points in the aortic size, at which rupture or dissection risk increases markedly, has been reported at 6.0 cm in the ascending aorta and 7.0 cm in the descending aorta.[26] In the Yale Center for Aortic Disease experience, the median aortic diameter at the time of dissection or rupture of the ascending aorta or arch was 6.0 cm. For ascending aortic aneurysms larger than 6.0 cm, the risk of rupture, dissection, or death was 15.6%.[26,29] Sex and body-surface area may also help to predict aneurysm complications. Patients presenting with an aortic size index (ASI) less than 2.75 cm/m² had a complication rate of 4%; those with an ASI between 2.75 and 4.25 cm/m² had event rates of approximately 8%, and those with an ASI more than 4.25 cm/m² had an event rate of 20% to 25%.[29] BAV ascending aortic aneurysms have a higher growth rate (0.19 cm/year) than do aneurysms in patients with a tricuspid aortic valve (0.13 cm/year).[30]

In the International Registry of Acute Aortic Dissection (IRAD), there were 68 cases of dissection in those younger than 40 years of age, including 9% with BAV and 12% with prior aortic surgery.[31] The average size of the ascending aorta at the time of dissection in this group was 5.4 ± 1.8 cm. In the Yale experience of 70 ascending TAAs associated with BAV, 6 patients (8.6%) suffered aortic dissection or rupture in follow-up, with the average size of the ascending aorta at the time of dissection measuring 5.2 cm.[30]

In general, surgical intervention is recommended when the ascending aortic diameter reaches 5.5 cm, or 5.0 cm in the setting of BAV aneurysm.[21,26,30] Patients undergoing aortic valve repair or replacement, who have an aortic root or ascending aorta larger than 4.5 cm, should be considered for concomitant aortic replacement.[32] In the setting of other genetically triggered TAA syndromes, different size thresholds exist regarding the timing of prophylactic aortic root replacement. In MFS and with FTAA/D, surgery is recommended when the ascending aorta reaches 5.0 cm, although some recommend surgery at 4.5 to 5.0 cm. In adults with LDS, prophylactic surgery has been recommended when the aortic root reaches 4.0 cm.[17] In the 2010 Guidelines for the Diagnosis and Management of Patients with Thoracic Aortic Disease, surgical repair in adults with LDS has been recommended at a slightly larger aortic dimension—larger than 4.2 cm by TEE (internal diameter) or larger than 4.4 to 4.6 cm by CT or MRI (external diameter).[32] However, aortic dissection has occurred in LDS patients at smaller aortic dimensions, and one must make take this into account when deciding about the timing of surgery for each individual. In one large series, more severe craniofacial abnormalities correlated with more aggressive cardiovascular disease.[16] In TS, prophylactic surgery has been recommended when the ascending aorta is 3.5 cm or larger, or 2.5 cm/m² or larger.[24] The timing of surgical intervention also depends on factors such as family history, rate of aneurysm growth, body size, coexisting aortic valve disease, requirement for heart surgery for another condition, comorbid conditions, and patient and physician preference. The importance of body size is further emphasized in the recent guidelines. If the maximal cross-sectional area (in cm²) of the ascending aorta or root divided by the patient's height in meters exceeds a ratio of 10, surgical repair is reasonable.[32] Patients with descending TAAs larger than 5.5 cm should be considered for open or endovascular repair, whereas surgical repair of thoracoabdominal aortic aneurysm is generally recommended when the aortic diameter exceeds 6.0 cm.[32] Rupture or acute dissection are the major, and often fatal, complications of TAAs (see Fig. 60-e3 on website). Less than 50% of patients with rupture may arrive at the hospital alive; mortality at 24 hours reaches 75%. Acute dissection is discussed later in this chapter.

MANAGEMENT

SURGICAL TREATMENT

ASCENDING THORACIC AORTIC ANEURYSMS. The treatment of ascending aortic aneurysms involves resection and grafting of the ascending aorta and, when needed, concomitant replacement of the aortic valve and coronary revascularization. Cardiopulmonary bypass is necessary for the removal of ascending aortic aneurysms, and partial bypass to support the circulation distal to the aneurysm while the aortic site being repaired is cross-clamped is often advisable when resecting descending TAAs. TAAs are generally resected and replaced with an appropriately sized prosthetic sleeve. The use of a composite graft consisting of a Dacron tube with a prosthetic aortic valve sewn into one end (composite aortic repair, or modified Bentall procedure) is generally the method of choice in treating ascending TAAs that involve the root and are associated with significant aortic valve disease. The valve and graft are sewn directly into the aortic annulus, and the coronary arteries are then reimplanted into the Dacron aortic graft. For elective aneurysm resection, the risk of death or stroke ranges from 1% to 5%, depending on the disease, patient population, and surgical experience.[28] The risk for morbidity and mortality increases with the need for arch dissection. For patients with structurally normal aortic valve leaflets, and patients whose aortic regurgitation is secondary to dilation of the root, it may be possible to perform a valve-sparing root replacement by reimplanting the native valve within a Dacron graft or by remodeling the aortic root (**Fig. 60-7**; see Fig. 66-17). The reimplantation technique is preferable to the remodeling technique because the annulus is stabilized, preventing aortic dilation and late aortic regurgitation. In a series of 220 patients undergoing valve-sparing root replacement, the 10-year survival was 88%, with freedom from moderate to severe aortic regurgitation at 10 years being 85% in all patients, but 94% after reimplantation and 75% after remodeling.[33]

When younger patients have a dilated aortic root but the aortic valve cannot be spared, an alternative to a composite aortic graft is a pulmonary autograft (the Ross procedure) (see Chap. 66). This approach involves replacing the patient's native aortic valve and root with the patient's own pulmonary root, which is transplanted into the aortic position. The pulmonary root is then replaced with a cryopreserved homograft root. The Ross procedure does carry risks of late autograft aneurysm formation and should not be used for genetically triggered aortic root diseases. The Ross procedure is controversial in the setting of BAV disease.[21,34] Another surgical alternative to a composite graft is the use

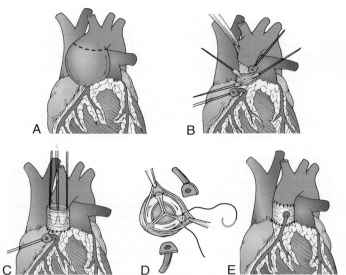

FIGURE 60-7 Valve-sparing aortic root reconstruction (modified David procedure). **A,** The large root and ascending aortic aneurysm. Step 1 is the initial aortotomy to visualize the aortic valve. Step 2 identifies the lines of incision in the root, marking the commissural posts and coronary artery buttons. **B,** Resected ascending aorta and root pathology after incisions have been made, as detailed in **A**. Note the preserved aortic leaflets. **C,** Commissural posts and associated leaflets are inserted within the cylinder of the aortic graft (reimplantation technique). **D,** Commissural posts are resuspended within the aortic graft. **E,** Coronary buttons are reimplanted between the commissural posts, thus completing the valve-sparing aortic root resection. As shown in this figure, the aortic annulus is situated within the graft itself. *(From Patel MJ, Deeb GM: Ascending and arch aorta: Pathology, natural history, and treatment. Circulation 118:188, 2008.)*

of cryopreserved aortic allografts (cadaveric aortic root and proximal ascending aorta), but durability issues limit this choice.

AORTIC ARCH ANEURYSMS. Aortic arch aneurysms are more difficult to manage because reconstruction of the aortic arch vessels requires interruption of blood flow to the arch vessels.[28] In some cases, a proximal hemiarch resection is performed; the arch vessels are left intact, with the descending aorta as a roof and the remaining arch replaced. Extended arch resection can be performed with removal of the entire arch tissue using bypasses constructed to each great vessel or with reimplantation of an island of arch tissue, including the great vessel origins. There are several methods for cerebral protection during arch surgery. Deep hypothermic circulatory arrest reduces cerebral metabolism during arch surgery and has been a traditional method. Adjunctive retrograde cerebral perfusion and selective antegrade cerebral perfusion have been performed to allow less neurologic injury during prolonged circulatory arrest. If the aneurysm extends partially into the descending thoracic aorta, which often occurs, the polyester graft is extended as an elephant trunk into the descending portion of the aneurysm and a secondary procedure is needed to complete the repair. In this procedure, the distal anastomosis is created to the midportion of a graft. The distal edge of this graft is within the lumen of the distal aorta and thus can be retrieved without arch manipulation. The treatment of arch aneurysms is associated with higher morbidity and mortality rates compared with the treatment of ascending aortic aneurysms, with a 5% to 7% risk of death and a 2% to 5% risk of stroke.[28] Endovascular techniques using currently approved endovascular devices and extra-anatomic reconstructions have been increasingly used to treat complex cases—such as patients with aortic arch aneurysms—and completion of elephant trunk procedures have helped to avoid second-stage procedures.

DESCENDING THORACIC ANEURYSMS. The treatment of descending TAAs includes resection and grafting of the aneurysmal segment with a polyester graft. The procedures are commonly performed with partial femorofemoral bypass and a pump oxygenator or atriofemoral bypass to maintain retrograde perfusion to critical arterial branches. Aneurysms of the descending aorta can be treated with a perioperative mortality of less than 10% and a paraplegia rate of approximately 2%.[35,36] Five-year survival after descending TAA resection approaches 70%.

Endovascular devices have been developed and approved for the treatment of patients with TAAs that have the appropriate anatomy to accommodate the currently approved devices. These devices can be used to treat patients who are not candidates for open surgical repair and any other patients who have good proximal and distal landing zones for the endovascular device (see later, "Endovascular Repair of Thoracic Aneurysms").

THORACOABDOMINAL ANEURYSMS. Thoracoabdominal aneurysms can extend from the subclavian artery to the iliac vessels. The treatment of thoracoabdominal aneurysms includes the resection and grafting of the involved segment of the aorta with a polyester graft. The procedure is extremely complex and is usually performed through an extensive thoracoabdominal incision, with transthoracic access to the thoracic aorta and retroperitoneal access to the abdominal aorta. It is usually carried out with atriofemoral bypass to maintain retrograde perfusion of the lower extremities and the mesenteric vessels. At the time of direct reconstruction of the mesenteric and renal vessels, selective cannulation of each vessel with a balloon catheter that maintains perfusion from the bypass pump is often used to diminish the warm ischemia time of these organs. Additionally, cerebrospinal fluid (CSF) drainage and other techniques are performed, such as for thoracic aneurysms, to diminish the risk of paraplegia and paraparesis. The perioperative mortality rate for good-risk patients is 8% to 12%, with a paraplegia rate less than 6% in experienced hands.[35,36] Alternative procedures have been developed to use endovascular techniques for the treatment of patients with thoracoabdominal aneurysms. Debranching procedures or extra-anatomic bypasses can revascularize the mesenteric and renal vessels from the iliac arteries in a retrograde fashion or the descending thoracic aorta above the aneurysm being treated. The aneurysm can be excluded with currently available endovascular thoracic devices. Unfortunately, these procedures can involve substantial periprocedural morbidity and mortality, and have been used to treat patients who are not candidates for the standard thoracoabdominal procedure. Branched devices to accommodate the mesenteric and renal branches have been used to treat small numbers of patients with thoracoabdominal aneurysms, with early success. Future improvements with branched endovascular devices will likely allow us to treat patients with thoracoabdominal aneurysms and have lower morbidity and mortality rates.

ENDOVASCULAR REPAIR OF THORACIC ANEURYSMS. An alternative approach to the open surgical management of TAAs is the use of transluminally placed endovascular grafts. This technique has the advantage of being far less invasive than open thoracic surgery, and it entails lower periprocedural morbidity and mortality rates. The aortic anatomy must be favorable, however, with proximal and distal landing zones at least 20 mm in length and diameters that accommodate the available endovascular devices. Over the past decade, devices have been developed and evaluated for the treatment of descending thoracic aortic aneurysms, with the approval of the first device, the TAG thoracic graft (W.L. Gore and Associates, Newark, Del) in 2005. Since then, the application of these techniques to patients with TAAs has grown rapidly, and two other devices have been approved in the United States (the Talent endovascular graft [Medtronic Vascular, Santa Rosa, Calif], and the TX2 endovascular graft [Cook Medical, Bloomington, Ind]). The results of the three prospective trials comparing endovascular repair to open surgical repair in good-risk patients that led to the approval of these devices have shown that endovascular repair of anatomically suitable TAAs and large penetrating ulcers has significantly lower perioperative morbidity and mortality rates when compared with open surgical repair. In the TAG trial, the perioperative major morbidity rates for endovascular repair compared with open-surgical repair were 37.5% versus 63% ($P < 0.05$), and the mortality rates were 1.4% versus 11.7% ($P < 0.05$).[37] All three prospective trials had excellent endovascular results, with rates of successful device delivery and deployment of approximately 98%, 30-day all-cause mortality rates of 1.5% to 2.1%, 12-month all-cause mortality rates of 8% to 16%, and 12-month aneurysm-related mortality rates of 2.9% to 5.8%.[37-39] Endovascular repair of TAA is associated with a lower rate of paraplegia and paraparesis, 2.9% compared with 11.7% in the open surgical group in the TAG trial. All trials had a very low paraplegia-paraparesis rate (1.3% to 3.0%) and a rate of perioperative stroke comparable to open surgical repair (2.5% to 4.0%). Endovascular TAA repair can be complicated by endovascular graft migration and endoleaks. Fortunately, these complications are relatively rare in patients with appropriate aortic anatomy. In the prospective trials, the 12-month migration rates were 1.9% to 3.9%, endoleak rates were 3.9% to 12.2%, and secondary intervention rates were 1.3% to 6.5%. Long-term follow up is necessary to understand better the results of these interventions.

Unfortunately, the curvilinear nature of the ascending aorta and transverse arch makes application of these techniques and currently available devices very challenging in these proximal segments. Nevertheless, because of the very low morbidity and mortality associated with endovascular repair of thoracic aneurysms, as well as the encouraging early results, the techniques are being applied to patients with more complex aortic anatomy. Hybrid techniques using extra-anatomic bypass procedures have been developed to gain or create an appropriate proximal landing and seal zone for the endovascular graft in the aortic arch or ascending aorta without the need for major open thoracic surgery. A left subclavian artery transposition or left carotid to subclavian bypass can allow attachment and seal of an endovascular graft across the takeoff of the subclavian artery without occlusion of that vessel. In the early experiences with endovascular devices, the left subclavian artery was only reconstructed before endovascular repair in patients who had a dominant left vertebral artery and those who had a coronary reconstruction using the left mammary artery. Recent reviews have suggested that subclavian artery occlusion without reconstruction is associated with an increased risk for cerebrovascular complications, including stroke, that can be avoided with a reconstruction prior to endovascular exclusion of the subclavian artery.[40] A right to left carotid-carotid bypass can be performed if the takeoff of the left common carotid artery needs to be excluded for endovascular repair of an arch aneurysm. If all the branches of the aortic arch need to be excluded for appropriate endovascular repair of an arch aneurysm, a few options exist for the hybrid management of these patients. A complete extra-anatomic aortic arch debranching can be performed obtaining inflow from one or both femoral arteries (femoral to axillary bypasses) and reconstructing the arch branches, with subsequent carotid and subclavian bypasses as necessary. Femoral-based reconstructions have been described but rarely performed, because the cerebral circulation would be based on a femoral to axillary bypass that has questionable long-term patency rates. Other options for patients with complex arch aneurysms require a median sternotomy and direct access to the ascending aorta. One option is to perform an elephant trunk procedure under cardiopulmonary arrest, suturing a prosthetic graft to the healthy portion of the ascending aorta and aortic arch and leaving the branches of the aortic arch intact. This method creates a proximal attachment zone of a predetermined length and diameter that can be extended distally with an endovascular graft to complete the aneurysm repair. This technique avoids bypasses to the arch vessels that may fail in the long term but requires a more complex open surgical graft placement that many aneurysm patients might not tolerate due to their medical and surgical comorbidities. Bypasses to all the aortic arch branches can also be performed from the proximal ascending aortic arch, in selected patients, leaving a healthy portion in the ascending aorta for attachment and seal of an endovascular graft. This procedure does not require aortic cross clamping or cardiopulmonary arrest and is likely associated with lower perioperative morbidity; it is a good option for select patients with aortic arch aneurysms. These hybrid techniques have broadened the application of currently available endovascular devices for patients with complex aneurysms of the thoracic aorta. Precurved and branch devices are being developed that will help treat patients with complex thoracic and thoracoabdominal aneurysms with even lower morbidity and mortality rates, as well as low long-term failure and reintervention rates.

Open and endovascular repairs of TAAs are associated with a variety of complications. Patients who undergo aneurysm treatment likely have some degree of cardiac and pulmonary disease and are thus susceptible to cardiopulmonary complications. Patients who undergo treatment of aneurysms of the ascending aorta and aortic arch are additionally at risk for cerebrovascular complications. A variety of bypass techniques are used to limit the risk of hypoperfusion during the procedure. Thoracic and thoracoabdominal aneurysms are also associated with renal dysfunction and spinal cord dysfunction with the development of paraparesis or paraplegia. Spinal cord CSF drainage has been used in combination with a mean arterial pressure of at least 70 mm Hg to diminish the rate of spinal cord complications to less than 5% in large published series.[36]

Endovascular grafts have particular complications. Material fatigue and endovascular graft migration are fortunately rare with currently available endovascular thoracic devices; endoleaks are the most common complication. Type I endoleaks are associated with reperfusion and pressurization of the aneurysm sac from the proximal or distal end of the graft. Type III endoleaks are caused by separation of endograft components. Types I and III endoleaks require treatment to avoid continued aneurysmal growth and potential rupture. Type II endoleaks are rare and associate with persistent flow from intercostal branches; they rarely require reintervention, because most of them seal during long-term observation.

Medical Management

Because risk factors for TAA formation and rupture include hypertension and cigarette smoking, treating hypertension and smoking cessation are important tenets of management. Long-term surveillance of the aorta with imaging is imperative (see Table 60-e2 on website). Beta blockers are recommended for patients with MFS. Although there have been no randomized trials, beta blockers are often recommended for non-Marfan patients with TAAs and for patients after aneurysm repair. Lifestyle modification is necessary for those with TAAs, including awareness of the condition and risk for aortic dissection and rupture. Avoidance of strenuous physical activity, especially isometric exercise and weightlifting, is important. Pregnancy is associated with an increased risk of aortic dissection in MFS and related disorders, and management strategies must encompass this risk. Because TGF-β signaling is related to the pathogenesis of MFS, and probably LDS, drugs that affect this signaling pathway, such as ARBs, may provide benefit in these conditions. Results of clinical trials of ARBs and matrix metalloproteinase inhibitors, such as doxycycline, are needed to confirm any benefit in humans. Because many diseases that lead to TAAs are familial and have a genetic trigger, it is important to screen for TAAs in first-degree relatives of the patient with a thoracic aneurysm.

Aortic Dissection

Acute aortic dissection is the most common catastrophic event affecting the aorta, with an estimated annual incidence of approximately 5 to 30 per million.[41] In a necropsy series, the prevalence of aortic dissection ranged from 0.2% to 0.8%.[42] The early mortality rate in acute aortic dissection is very high, with a mortality rate up to 1% to 2% per hour reported in the first several hours after dissection occurs.[43] Aortic dissection occurs at least twice as frequently in men than in women.[40] Ascending aortic dissection occurs most commonly between 50 and 60 years of age, whereas descending aortic dissection is more common in older individuals, peaking at 60 to 70 years of age. Because dissection is far less common than other conditions associated with chest or back pain, a high index of suspicion of acute aortic dissection must be maintained when evaluating the patient with unexplained chest or back pain or a syndrome complex compatible with this diagnosis. Improved survival requires immediate recognition of the disorder and timely institution of medical and/or surgical therapy.

There are two main hypotheses for acute aortic dissection (see Fig. 60-e6 on website). The first is that an aortic dissection may be related to a primary tear in the aortic intima, with blood from the aortic lumen penetrating into the diseased media, leading to dissection and creating the true and false lumen. The second main hypothesis is that a primary rupture of the vasa vasorum leads to hemorrhage in the aortic wall, with subsequent intimal disruption, creating the intimal tear and aortic dissection. The pressure of the pulsatile blood within the aortic wall after dissection leads to extension of the dissection. Aortic dissections usually propagate in an antegrade direction related to the pressure pulse from the aortic blood, but occasionally extend in a retrograde direction. The dissection flap may be localized or may spiral the entire length of the aorta. Arterial pressure and shear forces may lead to further tears in the intimal flap (the inner portion of the dissected aortic wall), producing exit sites or additional entry sites for blood flow into the false lumen. Distention of the false lumen with blood causes the intimal flap to compress the true lumen, narrowing its caliber and distorting its shape, which leads to malperfusion. Classic aortic dissection (see earlier) occurs in approximately 80% to 90% of acute aortic syndromes. The variants of aortic dissection, aortic intramural hematoma, and penetrating atherosclerotic ulcers (**Fig. 60-8**), are discussed later.

CLASSIFICATION. There are two major classification schemes of aortic dissection, based on the location of the dissection—the DeBakey and Stanford classifications (**Fig. 60-9** and **Table 60-1**). The DeBakey classification system divides dissections into types I, II, and III. DeBakey type I dissections originate in the ascending aorta

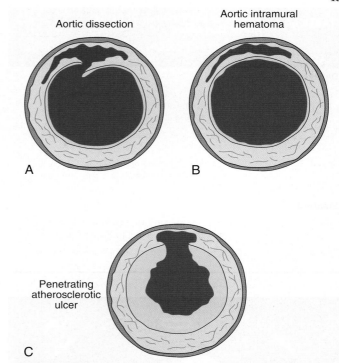

FIGURE 60-8 Acute aortic syndromes. **A,** Classic aortic dissection. **B,** Aortic intramural hematoma. **C,** Penetrating atherosclerotic aortic ulcer.

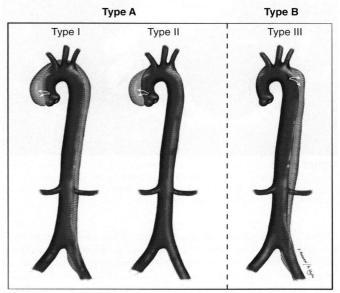

FIGURE 60-9 Classification schemes of acute aortic dissection.

and extend at least to the aortic arch and often to the descending aorta, frequently all the way to the iliac arteries (**Fig. 60-10**). DeBakey type II dissections involve the ascending aorta alone. DeBakey type III dissections begin in the descending aorta, usually just distal to the left subclavian artery. Type III dissections may be classified further, depending on whether the dissection stops above the diaphragm (IIIa) or extends below the diaphragm (IIIb). Infrequently, a type III dissection may propagate in a retrograde manner into the arch and ascending aorta. The Stanford classification categorizes dissections into types A and B, based on whether the ascending aorta is involved. Stanford type A dissections involve the ascending aorta, with or without extension into the descending aorta, and Stanford type B dissections are those that do not involve the ascending aorta.

TABLE 60-1 Classification Schemes of Acute Aortic Dissection

CLASSIFICATION	SITE OF ORIGIN AND EXTENT OF AORTIC INVOLVEMENT
DeBakey	
Type I	Originates in the ascending aorta and extends at least to the aortic arch and often to the descending aorta (and beyond)
Type II	Originates in the ascending aorta; confined to this segment
Type III	Originates in the descending aorta, usually just distal to the left subclavian artery, and extends distally
Stanford	
Type A	Dissections that involve the ascending aorta (with or without extension into the descending aorta)
Type B	Dissections that do not involve the ascending aorta

TABLE 60-2 Risk Factors for Aortic Dissection

Hypertension
Genetically triggered thoracic aortic disease
• Marfan syndrome
• Bicuspid aortic valve
• Loeys-Dietz syndrome
• Hereditary thoracic aortic aneurysm or dissection
• Vascular Ehlers-Danlos syndrome
Congenital diseases or syndromes
• Coarctation of the aorta
• Turner syndrome
• Tetralogy of Fallot
Atherosclerosis
• Penetrating atherosclerotic ulcer
Trauma, blunt or iatrogenic
• Catheter or stent
• Intra-aortic balloon pump
• Aortic or vascular surgery
• Motor vehicle accident
• Coronary artery bypass surgery or aortic valve replacement
Cocaine use
Inflammatory or infectious disease
• Giant cell arteritis
• Takayasu arteritis
• Behçet disease
• Aortitis
• Syphilis
Pregnancy

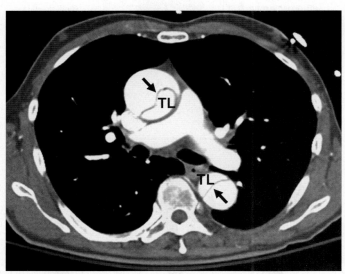

FIGURE 60-10 Contrast CT scan demonstrating acute type A aortic dissection with enlargement of the ascending aorta and intimal flaps (arrows) in the ascending and descending aorta. Both the true lumen (TL) and false lumen are opacified with contrast in this example.

Most ascending aortic dissections begin within a few centimeters of the aortic valve, and most descending aortic dissections have their origin just distal to the left subclavian artery. Approximately 65% of intimal tears occur in the ascending aorta, 30% in the descending aorta, less than 10% in the aortic arch, and approximately 1% in the abdominal aorta. The treatment depends on the site, with emergency surgery recommended for acute type A dissections and initial medical therapy for type B dissections. Aortic dissection is also classified according to its duration, being acute when present for less than 2 weeks and chronic when present for more than 2 weeks. The morbidity and mortality rates of acute dissection are highest in the first 2 weeks, especially within the first 24 hours.

CAUSES AND PATHOGENESIS. Several conditions predispose the aorta to dissection (**Table 60-2**), with most resulting from disruption of the normal architecture and integrity of the aortic wall. Approximately 75% of all patients with aortic dissection have hypertension, which promotes aortic intimal thickening, calcification, and adventitial fibrosis. These structural changes can affect the elastic properties of the arterial wall, increasing stiffness and predisposing to aneurysm or dissection, but hypertension alone usually does not associate with aortic root dilation. Genetically-triggered thoracic aortic syndromes,

congenital heart diseases, atherosclerosis, inflammatory vascular diseases, cocaine use, and iatrogenic causes are also risk factors for aortic dissection. CMD is the most common underlying factor in aortic dissection (see Fig. 60-e1 on website). Any disease process that undermines the integrity of the elastic or muscular components of the media predisposes the aorta to dissection (see earlier discussion in TAA section). CMD is an underlying pathophysiologic feature of several genetically triggered disorders of connective tissue, including MFS, LDS, FTAA/D syndrome, and vEDS, and is also common among patients with a congenital BAV (see Table 60-e3 on website). Excessive signaling in the TGF-β pathway and abnormalities in SMC contractile element function may underlie certain aortic dissections.[18] Patients with MFS have a high risk for aortic root aneurysm, especially type A aortic dissection. Although only present in approximately 1 in 5000 individuals, MFS accounts for approximately 5% of all aortic dissections.[31,41]

CMD may accompany many other conditions and factors affecting the aorta, including aging and hypertension. Although hypertension is a very common disorder, the vast majority of hypertensive patients, even severely hypertensive ones, never suffer TAA or dissection. Whether the preponderance of cases of aortic dissection will eventually be related to an underlying genetic trigger is yet unknown, and is the subject of active investigation. Among the 464 patients in the IRAD, hypertension was present in 72%, atherosclerosis in 31%, known aortic aneurysm in 16%, prior aortic dissection in 6%, prior cardiac surgery in 18% (including aortic valve replacement [AVR] in 5% and coronary artery bypass grafting [CABG] in 4%), and iatrogenic dissection in 4%.[41]

When encountering a young patient with aortic dissection, one must consider genetically triggered aortic disease (e.g., MFS, LDS, vEDS, FTAA/D, BAV, TS), pregnancy, cocaine use, congenital heart disease (coarctation of the aorta, tetralogy of Fallot), and prior AVR. The mortality rate for acute dissection is no different for those younger than 40 years of age compared with those older than 40 years of age.[31]

A BAV is an often underrecognized risk factor for ascending aortic aneurysm and dissection and is present in 5% to 7% of aortic dissections, even more commonly among ascending dissections in younger patients. Aortic dissection may occur in the setting of a BAV that functions normally and, importantly, may occur years after BAV replacement.[21] Other congenital disorders associated with dissection include unicuspid aortic valve, supravalvular aortic stenosis, coarctation of the aorta, and TS. Weightlifting, especially in the setting of underlying aortic dilation, may be associated with acute aortic dissection.[26]

Rarely, aortic dissection complicates arteritis involving the aorta, particularly giant cell arteritis. Nonspecific aortitis, Takayasu arteritis, and Behçet disease have all been associated with aortic dissection (see Chap. 89). Syphilitic aortitis is a rare cause of dissection. Cocaine abuse accounts for less than 1% of aortic dissection and is associated with crack cocaine use. Cocaine-related dissection is most typical in young, African American, and hypertensive men who smoke cigarettes.[44] Underlying elastic medial abnormalities and severe sheer forces related to hypertension and tachycardia may play a role.

Aortic dissection can occur during pregnancy or the postpartum period (see Chap. 82). The relationship between pregnancy and aortic dissection is difficult to reconcile based on hemodynamic factors alone. When pregnancy-related dissection occurs, one must diligently search for an underlying genetic trigger, such as mutations in *FBN1*, *TGFBR1*, *TGFBR2*, *ACTA2*, and *MYH11*. Dissections during pregnancy typically occur in the third trimester, but occasionally occur in the early postpartum period. In addition to hemodynamic factors, hormonal changes in aortic wall composition have been described. Women with MFS, LDS, FTAA/D syndrome, vEDS, TS, and BAV with a dilated aorta have increased risk for acute aortic dissection during pregnancy. In MFS, the risk of type A dissection is greatest when the aortic root is enlarged; it has been estimated at 1% when the aortic diameter is smaller than 40 mm and at 10% in high-risk patients (aortic diameter > 40 mm, rapid dilation, or previous dissection of the aorta).[45] Postpartum type B aortic dissection has occurred in MFS, even in the setting of a relatively normal descending aortic dimension, and has occurred late after aortic root repair.

Blunt aortic trauma usually leads to localized tears, periaortic hematomas, or frank aortic transection, and only rarely causes classic aortic dissection. Iatrogenic trauma accounts for approximately 4% of aortic dissections.[41] Intra-arterial catheterization, stent placement, and the insertion of intra-aortic balloon pumps may induce aortic dissection related to intimal disruption. Retrograde ascending aortic dissection occurs in approximately 1% of patients undergoing thoracic endovascular aortic repair (TEVAR) for acute or chronic type B aortic dissection, and associates with a 40% mortality rate.[46] Cardiac surgery also entails a very small risk (0.12% to 0.16%) of acute aortic dissection.[47] But aortic dissection may occur late (months to years) after cardiac surgery. Of cardiac surgical patients, those undergoing AVR and those with prior aortic aneurysm or dissection have the highest risk for aortic dissection as a late complication. Persistent abnormalities of the aortic wall, such as the aortopathy seen with BAV, untreated or recurrent dissection, and injuries to the aortic wall and intima related to cross clamping, suture lines, or cannulation during surgery, account for the increased risk of subsequent aortic dissection.

Individuals with TAA are at risk for aortic dissection, with increased risk of dissection and rupture as aneurysm size increases,[29] but many aortic dissections occur in patients without severely dilated aortic dimensions. Of 591 type A aortic dissections in the IRAD, the maximum aortic diameter averaged 5.3 cm, with 349 patients (59%) having aortic diameters smaller than 5.5 cm and 229 patients (40%) having aortic diameters smaller than 5.0 cm.[48] In a series of 177 non-Marfan patients with tricuspid aortic valves with acute type A aortic dissection, 62% of patients had a maximum aortic diameter smaller than 5.5 cm, 42% had a maximum aortic diameter smaller than 5.0 cm, and more than 20% had a maximum aortic diameter smaller than 4.5 cm, at the time of dissection.[49] Thus, the absolute size of the aorta is not the only factor important in triggering acute dissection. Age, sex, body size, and rate of aortic growth also play a role. Underlying genetic triggers may lead to dissection at differing aortic sizes. The mechanisms responsible for individual susceptibility for acute dissection at a certain aortic size are poorly understood. Mechanical factors and aortic curvature may also affect risk of dissection and location of entry tears.[50] The biomechanical properties (distensibility and wall stress) of the aorta may be assessed noninvasively, and studies are in progress to aid in the prediction of patients at increased risk of aortic complications.[26]

CLINICAL MANIFESTATIONS. (see Chaps. 12 and 53)

Symptoms

The symptoms of aortic dissection can be variable and may mimic those of more common conditions, emphasizing the importance of a high index of suspicion. The most common symptom of acute aortic dissection is pain, which is present in up to 96% of cases.[41] The pain is typically severe and of sudden onset, being at maximum intensity at its inception. This pattern contrasts with the pain of myocardial infarction, which usually has a crescendo-like onset and is not as intense. The pain is often accompanied by a "sense of doom" and may force the patient to writhe in distress or pace restlessly in an attempt to gain relief. The quality of the pain is most commonly described as "sharp" or "severe," and adjectives such as "tearing," "ripping," or "stabbing" are used in about half the cases. Cataclysmic descriptors that are suggestive of aortic dissection, such as being "stabbed in the chest with a knife" or "hit in the back with a baseball bat" are sometimes reported. Some aortic dissections present with chest burning, pressure, or pleuritic discomfort; in others, the symptoms related to a complication from the dissection dominate the clinical scenario, and the pain is not mentioned or is downplayed. In some instances (<5%), no pain is reported at all. Those with painless dissections are often found to have chronic dissections, significant neurologic symptoms, or heart failure dominating their presentation.

The pain of acute aortic dissection is migratory in approximately 17% of patients, tending to follow the path of the dissection through the aorta.[41] The pain of dissection may radiate from chest to back or vise versa. The presence of any pain in the neck, throat, jaw, or head predicts involvement of the ascending aorta (and often the great vessels), whereas pain in the back, abdomen, or lower extremities usually indicates descending aortic involvement.

Other clinical features at initial evaluation, occurring with or without associated chest pain, may include congestive heart failure (7%), syncope (9%), acute stroke (6%), acute myocardial infarction, ischemic peripheral neuropathy, paraplegia, and cardiac arrest or sudden death.[39] Acute congestive heart failure in this setting is usually caused by acute severe aortic regurgitation because of the ascending aortic dissection (see Chap. 66). Syncope is much more common in ascending aortic dissection and is usually associated with hemopericardium, rupture, or stroke. Patients with aortic dissection may have abdominal pain and, on occasion, develop severe nausea and vomiting related to abdominal visceral involvement. These symptoms may delay diagnosis and increase mortality rate.[51] Painless aortic dissection was reported in 6% of patients in one study and was more commonly associated with diabetes, prior aortic aneurysm, and prior cardiac surgery.[52] Painless aortic dissections present with syncope in one third, heart failure in 20%, and stroke in 11%, and are associated with a higher mortality rate (33%).

PHYSICAL FINDINGS. The physical examination findings in acute aortic dissection vary widely, ranging from almost unremarkable to cardiac arrest from hemopericardium or rupture. The findings may demonstrate complications related to the dissection such as aortic regurgitation, abnormal peripheral pulses (see Chap. 12), stroke, or heart failure. Such findings must heighten one's clinical suspicion of aortic dissection. The absence of these findings, however, does not exclude dissection and should not dissuade one from pursuing the diagnosis when suspected. Hypertension is present in approximately 70% of patients with acute aortic dissection. Although most patients with type B dissections are hypertensive, many patients with type A dissections are normotensive or hypotensive on presentation.[41] Hypotension complicating acute dissection is usually the result of cardiac tamponade, acute aortic rupture, or heart failure related to acute severe aortic regurgitation. Hypotension is associated with altered mental status and neurologic deficits; visceral, limb, and myocardial ischemia; and death in 55% of patients.[42] Dissection involving the brachiocephalic vessels may result in pseudohypotension, an inaccurate measurement of blood pressure caused by compromise of the brachial artery circulation.

The physical findings most typically associated with aortic dissection—pulse deficits, aortic regurgitation, and neurologic manifestations—are more characteristic of ascending than descending dissection. Acute chest or back pain associated with these findings strongly suggest the possibility of aortic dissection. In the IRAD, pulse deficit was reported in 19% of type A and only 9% of type B dissections.[41] When acute lower extremity vascular insufficiency occurs and

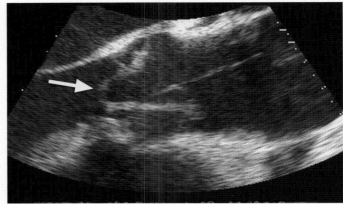

FIGURE 60-12 Transesophageal echocardiogram demonstrating ascending aortic dissection. Prolapse of the dissection flap across the aortic valve into the left ventricular outflow tract (arrow) leads to severe aortic regurgitation.

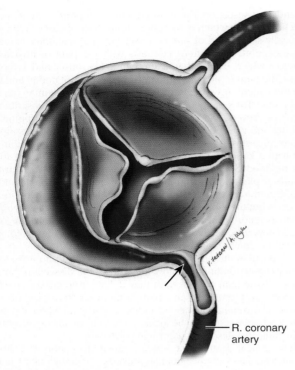

R. coronary artery

FIGURE 60-11 Aortic regurgitation complicating acute type A aortic dissection. The dissection flap distorts the normal aortic leaflet alignment, leading to malcoaptation of the aortic valve and subsequent aortic regurgitation. In this example, the dissection flap extends into the ostium of the right coronary artery (arrow).

is not relieved with emergency embolectomy, one should consider the possibility of acute dissection. Vascular insufficiency related to aortic dissection may result from the dissection flap propagating into a branch artery, leading to compression of the true lumen by the distended false lumen and limiting blood flow, or from obstruction of flow into the orifice of the artery by a mobile intimal flap. The pulse deficits may be intermittent because the intimal flap movement sporadically obstructs the arterial orifice or because of distal reentry of blood into the true lumen, which decompresses the false channel. Acute limb ischemia, a marker for more extensive and severe dissection, is associated with a threefold increase in mortality in type B dissection.[53]

Aortic regurgitation is an important diagnostic feature in type A aortic dissection (**Fig. 60-11**). The diastolic murmur of aortic regurgitation accompanying acute chest pain should make one suspect aortic dissection. The murmur of aortic regurgitation is present in 44% of type A dissections and 12% of type B dissections.[41] When aortic regurgitation accompanies type B dissection, this usually indicates coexisting aortic valve disease, aortic root aneurysm, or retrograde dissection. The murmur of aortic regurgitation can vary in intensity, depending on the blood pressure and degree of heart failure and, in some cases, may be inaudible. Aortic regurgitation complicating type A dissection may lead to acute decompensated heart failure (see Chap. 66).

Several mechanisms may explain acute aortic regurgitation in the setting of type A aortic dissection. First, there may be incomplete coaptation of the aortic leaflets because of concurrent dilation of the aortic root and annulus, leading to central aortic regurgitation. Second, and most commonly, the dissection may lead to aortic leaflet prolapse because of the dissection flap into the aortic leaflets or commissures, or from distortion of proper leaflet alignment by an asymmetric dissection flap, leading to eccentric aortic regurgitation (see Fig. 60-11 and Videos 60-2 and 60-3 on website). Third, an extensive or circumferential dehiscing intimal flap may prolapse into the left ventricular outflow tract during diastole, interfere with valve coaptation, and cause severe aortic regurgitation (**Fig. 60-12**; see Videos 60-4 and

60-5 on website).[54] Additionally, there may be preexisting aortic regurgitation related to underlying aortic root aneurysm or BAV.

Neurologic manifestations occur in 17% to 40% of aortic dissections, more commonly in type A dissections. Variability in incidence likely results from a failure to record a detailed neurologic examination in such critically ill patients. The findings may be evanescent, with rapid improvement related to transient arterial occlusion. Syncope, painless aortic dissection, and dissections with predominantly neurologic symptoms may lead to difficulty or delay in diagnosis. Neurologic syndromes include persistent or transient ischemic stroke, spinal cord ischemia, ischemic neuropathy, and hypoxic encephalopathy. These are related to malperfusion to one or more branches supplying the brain, spinal cord, or peripheral nerves (see Table 60-e4 on website).[55] Ischemic stroke occurs in approximately 6% of ascending dissections and more commonly in the left hemisphere, because the left-sided arch vessels are more susceptible to the advancing false lumen.[41,55] Syncope is relatively common in aortic dissection, affecting 9% in one large series (13%, type A; 4%, type B) and may occur without pain or other neurologic findings.[41] Syncope may be related to acute hypotension caused by cardiac tamponade or aortic rupture, cerebral vessel obstruction, or activation of cerebral baroreceptors. It is important to consider aortic dissection in the differential diagnosis in cases of unexplained syncope. Less common neurologic manifestations of dissection include seizures, transient global amnesia, ischemic neuropathy, disturbances of consciousness and coma, and paraparesis or paraplegia related to spinal cord ischemia. Some studies have failed to identify brain malperfusion as an independent risk factor for an adverse outcome after surgical repair,[41,55,56] whereas other reports have associated cerebral malperfusion with poor outcomes.[57]

Acute myocardial infarction, related to involvement of the dissection flap into the ostium of a coronary artery, occurs in 1% to 2% of acute type A aortic dissections, and was more commonly reported in older series.[43] This usually involves the right coronary artery (see Fig. 60-11), leading to acute inferior myocardial infarction. Because coronary ischemia and myocardial infarction are much more common than aortic dissection, when acute infarction complicates acute dissection, the diagnosis of dissection might not be considered. This type of patient may be taken emergently to the catheterization laboratory, and the acute dissection may be recognized only after angiography. Not only does the time delay increase morbidity and mortality, but the use of antiplatelet, anticoagulant, and thrombolytic therapy may have disastrous consequences, including cardiac tamponade and death. Aortic dissection always should be considered in the differential diagnosis of patients presenting with acute infarction, particularly inferior infarction, especially when their risk factors, symptoms, or examination are compatible with this diagnosis.

Types A and B dissections may extend into the abdominal aorta, leading to vascular complications involving one or more branch

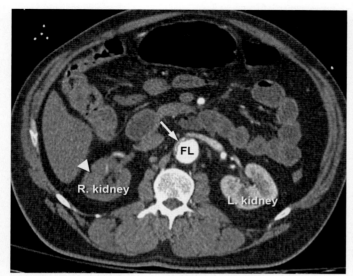

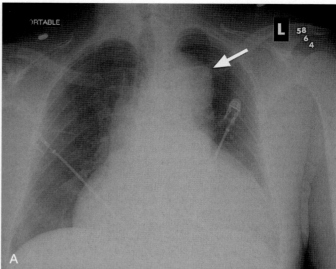

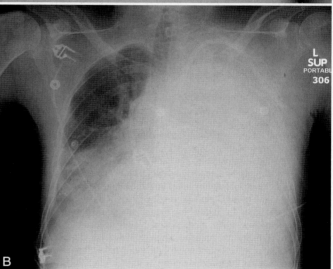

FIGURE 60-13 Contrast CT scan of aortic dissection with malperfusion to the right kidney (arrowhead), which demonstrates less opacification with contrast than the left kidney. The left kidney fills from the collapsed and underfilled true lumen (arrow). The false lumen (FL) is larger than the true lumen.

vessels. Renal artery involvement occurs in at least 5% to 10% of patients and may lead to renal ischemia, infarction, renal insufficiency, or refractory hypertension (**Fig. 60-13**). Mesenteric ischemia or infarction, complications associated with a high level of morbidity and mortality, occurs in approximately 5% of aortic dissections and are associated with acute limb ischemia and renal ischemia.[53] A high index of suspicion is required for this diagnosis, and identifying and correcting visceral malperfusion may improve outcomes. Aortic dissection may extend into the iliac arteries and cause diminished femoral pulses (12%) and acute lower extremity ischemia. Acute limb ischemia and malperfusion syndromes are associated with extensive and severe dissection and a higher mortality rate.[57]

Additional clinical manifestations of aortic dissection include the presence of left-sided pleural effusion, usually related to an inflammatory response. On occasion, acute hemothorax occurs from rupture, contained rupture, or leaking of the descending aortic dissection (**Fig. 60-14**). Type A aortic dissection may present with acute pericarditis, including characteristic electrocardiographic changes (see Chap. 75). Isolated abdominal aortic dissection is rare, accounting for approximately 1% of dissections, and is associated with an existing AAA or has an iatrogenic cause. Acute abdominal pain, mesenteric ischemia, and limb ischemia are more common in this subset of dissections.[58] Rare clinical manifestations of aortic dissection include hoarseness, upper airway obstruction, dysphagia, superior vena cava syndrome, pulsatile neck or abdominal masses, hematemesis (from rupture into the esophagus), hemoptysis (from rupture into the trachea or bronchus), ischemic pancreatitis, and unexplained fever (from the inflammatory reaction).

Aortic dissection may not be considered during the evaluation of a patient with chest, back, or abdominal pain. The signs and symptoms associated with aortic dissection are highly variable and depend on the underlying cause and extent and involvement of the heart and branch vessels from the dissection. Dissection may mimic many other more common disorders, including pleurisy, pericarditis, pulmonary embolism, coronary ischemia, stroke, esophageal disease, gastric gallbladder or pancreatic disease, and acute mesenteric or limb ischemia. In some cases, the diagnosis is immediately suspected on presentation, whereas at other times the diagnosis is made when imaging studies are performed for another reason. Thus, one of the most important factors in making the diagnosis of aortic dissection is a high index of suspicion.

FIGURE 60-14 Chest radiograph in aortic dissection. **A,** Widened mediastinum with abnormal aortic knob and enlarged cardiac silhouette is present. **B,** Acute hemothorax occurred from rupture of the aortic dissection, with rapid opacification of the left hemithorax.

CHRONOBIOLOGY. Like other cardiovascular disorders, aortic dissection demonstrates significant circadian and seasonal or monthly variations. In the IRAD, the onset of aortic dissection was most common in the morning. There was a seasonal variation also, with more dissections being reported in the winter and fewest in the summer. Chronobiologic periodicity may be explained by changes in sympathetic tone and hemorrheologic properties of the blood.[42]

LABORATORY FINDINGS. The chest radiograph may be the first clue to the diagnosis of aortic dissection (see Fig. 60-14 and Fig. 60-e7 on website), but the findings on the chest radiograph are nonspecific, subject to interobserver variability and, in many cases, completely normal. The dissected aorta may not be dilated, and its image between the sternum and vertebrae may not be displaced or widened on the chest radiograph. The most common abnormality seen on a chest radiograph in cases of aortic dissection is an abnormal aortic contour or widening of the aortic silhouette, which appears in 80% to 90% of cases (83%, type A; 72%, type B).[41] Nonspecific widening of the superior mediastinum may be present. If calcification of the aortic knob is present, one may detect a separation of the intimal calcification from the outer aortic soft tissue border by more than 0.5 to 1.0 cm—the calcium sign (see Fig. 60-e8 on website). Comparison of the current chest radiograph with a previous study may reveal acute changes in the aortic or mediastinal silhouettes that would otherwise have gone unrecognized. Pleural effusions are reported in approximately 20% of dissections. Most effusions relate to an inflammatory reaction, but acute hemothorax may occur from aortic rupture (see Fig. 60-14). Most patients with aortic dissection will have an abnormal chest radiograph, but 12% to 15% have normal chest radiographs. Thus, a normal chest radiograph cannot exclude the presence of an aortic dissection.

The electrocardiographic findings in patients with aortic dissection are nonspecific, but may indicate acute complications such as myocardial ischemia or infarction related to coronary artery involvement, or low-voltage QRS complexes (or rarely, acute pericarditis) related to hemopericardium. Three quarters of electrocardiograms (ECGs) on dissection are normal or demonstrate nonspecific ST-segment or T wave changes, and 25% have left ventricular hypertrophy.[41] Acute myocardial infarction is present in 1% to 2% of type A dissections. These are particularly dangerous because the presence of acute coronary ischemia may lead the clinician away from the evaluation of dissection.

Biomarkers

Biomarkers could reliably diagnose or exclude acute aortic dissection. Release of smooth muscle proteins, soluble elastin fragments, and myosin heavy chain and creatine kinase BB isoforms have been reported after aortic dissection.[59] These assays have limited usefulness because of sensitivity, specificity, or time delay, and are not currently available clinically.

D-dimer levels are elevated in pulmonary embolism and can rise in aortic dissection. In a prospective study, D-dimer levels were markedly elevated in patients proven to have aortic dissection (and pulmonary embolism).[59] A D-dimer level higher than 1600 ng/mL within the first 6 hours of presentation showed a positive likelihood ratio of 12.8, suggesting that this test may be useful for identifying patients with a high probability of acute aortic dissection. In patients within the first 24 hours of onset, a D-dimer level less than 500 ng/mL had a negative likelihood ratio of 0.07 and a negative predictive value of 95%. The D-dimer assay may be useful for ruling out acute aortic dissection in this time window, with a diagnostic performance similar to that reported for pulmonary embolism. An elevated D-dimer level may assist clinicians in risk-stratifying patients presenting with chest pain or dyspnea for appropriate imaging. D-dimer levels, however, may not be as useful in various forms of acute aortic syndromes. The patency of the false lumen affects D-dimer levels in acute dissection. In addition, the dissection variants, aortic intramural hematoma and penetrating aortic ulcer, may not have elevated D-dimer levels. Moreover, patients may present more than 24 hours after symptom onset, affecting D-dimer levels. More studies are required to determine the sensitivity and specificity of this assay in acute aortic syndromes, and how best to integrate D-dimer testing into the diagnostic algorithm of aortic dissection.

DIAGNOSTIC IMAGING. When aortic dissection is suspected, it is imperative to confirm the diagnosis quickly and accurately. Diagnostic methods include contrast-enhanced CT, MRI, transthoracic and transesophageal echocardiography (TEE), and aortography. Each modality has advantages and disadvantages with respect to diagnostic accuracy, speed, convenience, and risk. The choice of imaging study often depends on local availability and expertise, with contrast-enhanced CT and TEE being the most commonly performed. Many patients undergo multiple studies in the diagnostic evaluation of suspected aortic dissection. If the probability of dissection is very high, a second diagnostic test should be performed if the first test is negative or nondiagnostic.

When comparing imaging modalities, one must consider the diagnostic information required (see Table 60-e5 on website). Most importantly, the study must confirm the diagnosis of aortic dissection and its variants (intramural hematoma and penetrating atherosclerotic ulcer). Second, it must determine the location of the dissection and whether the dissection involves the ascending aorta (type A) or is confined to

the descending aorta or arch. Additional useful information includes anatomic features and complications related to the dissection, including its extent, sites of entry and reentry, presence of thrombus in the false lumen, branch vessel involvement, presence and severity of aortic regurgitation, presence or absence of pericardial effusion and hemopericardium, any coronary artery involvement by the intimal flap, and any signs of rupture or leaking.

Computed Tomography

Contrast-enhanced CT scanning has become the most commonly used modality in evaluating aortic dissection (see Chap. 19). It is best performed as an electrocardiographically gated CT on a multidetector (16 or more) row scanner, which may eliminate aortic pulsation artifacts. On CT, an aortic dissection is diagnosed by the presence of two distinct lumens with a visible intimal flap, which is seen in most cases, or by the detection of two lumens by their differing rates of opacification with contrast (see Fig. 60-10). If the false lumen is completely thrombosed, it demonstrates low attenuation. Acute aortic intramural hematoma, a dissection variant discussed later, demonstrates only a thickened aortic wall with high attenuation on noncontrast CT and no entry tears or visible intimal flap. Spiral (helical) contrast CT allows for three-dimensional reconstruction to evaluate the dissection and branch vessels with enhanced anatomic definition (**Fig. 60-15**) and is critical for decision making, especially when planning endovascular repair (see Fig. 60-e9 on website). Contrast CT is highly accurate for diagnosing aortic dissection, with a sensitivity and specificity of 95% to 98% being reported.

CT scanning does require intravenous contrast; without contrast enhancement, aortic dissection may go undetected (see Fig. 60-e10 on website). CT is also useful for identifying thrombus (partial or complete) in the false lumen, pericardial effusion, hemopericardium, periaortic hematoma, aortic rupture, and branch vessel involvement, and blood supply from the true and false lumens (see Fig. 60-13). Major limitations to CT include the inability to evaluate the coronary arteries and aortic valve reliably, motion artifact related to cardiac movement, streak artifact related to implanted devices, and

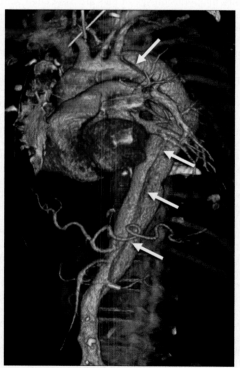

FIGURE 60-15 Three-dimensional CT reconstruction of a type B aortic dissection. The intimal flap is denoted by the arrows.

complications associated with the use of iodinating contrast agents, especially in renal failure.

Magnetic Resonance Imaging

MRI is a highly accurate noninvasive technique for evaluating aortic dissection (see Chap. 18), which does not require intravenous iodinated contrast or ionizing radiation (see Fig. 60-e11 on website). MRI is capable of multiplanar imaging with three-dimensional reconstruction and cine MRI to visualize blood flow, differentiating slow flow and clot and detecting aortic regurgitation. Most MRI protocols involve techniques to assess branch vessel morphology combined with contrast-enhanced MRA. Studies have demonstrated a high sensitivity (95% to 100%) and specificity (94% to 98%) for the detection of aortic dissection. Contrast-enhanced MRI using intravenous gadolinium is highly accurate for the evaluation of dissection and branch vessel involvement. Like CT, MRI may detect pericardial effusion, aortic rupture, entry and exit points, and intramural hematoma with high levels of accuracy. MRA may detect and quantify aortic regurgitation. MRI has important limitations in acute aortic dissection. First, MRI is contraindicated in patients with certain implantable devices (e.g., pacemaker, defibrillator) and other metallic implants. Additionally, MRI has limited availability on an emergency basis in many hospitals and emergency rooms and takes longer for image acquisition than CT. Gadolinium contrast should not be used in those with renal impairment. MRI is rarely used as the initial test for diagnostic evaluation of acute dissection. However, because of the imaging detail and lack of ionizing radiation, MRI is particularly attractive for the long-term follow-up of aortic dissection.

Echocardiography

Echocardiography is well suited for the evaluation of patients with suspected aortic dissection because it is readily available in most hospitals and is noninvasive and quick to perform, and the full examination can be completed at the bedside (see Chap. 15). The echocardiographic finding considered diagnostic of an aortic dissection is the presence of an undulating intimal flap within the aortic lumen that separates the true and false channels (see Fig. 15-84; see Videos 60-6, 60-7, and 60-8 on website). Reverberations and other artifacts can cause linear echodensities within the aortic lumen that mimic aortic dissection. In cases in which the false lumen is thrombosed, displacement of intimal calcification or thickening of the aortic wall may suggest aortic dissection.

TRANSTHORACIC ECHOCARDIOGRAPHY. Transthoracic echocardiography (TTE) is less sensitive (59% to 83%) and less specific (63% to 93%) for the diagnosis of aortic dissection than other modalities (see Fig. 60-e12 and Videos 60-9, 60-10, and 60-11 on website). Thus, it has limited usefulness in the diagnosis of aortic dissection. TTE may demonstrate an intimal flap, thickened aortic wall, aortic regurgitation, and pericardial effusion or tamponade. It has a sensitivity of 78% to 100% for type A aortic dissection, but only 31% to 55% in type B dissection; therefore, a negative TTE does not exclude acute aortic dissection. If dissection is suspected, TTE should not be chosen as a first test for evaluation because a delay in diagnosis may occur. In the emergency setting, however, TTE may be performed rapidly and can help assess features complicating dissection, such as aortic regurgitation, pericardial effusion and tamponade, and associated wall motion abnormalities.

TRANSESOPHAGEAL ECHOCARDIOGRAPHY. TEE is highly accurate for the evaluation and diagnosis of acute aortic dissection (sensitivity of ~98% and specificity of 94% to 97% (**Fig. 60-16**; see Videos 60-2 to 60-8 on website; see Fig. 15-84). The distal ascending aorta and proximal aortic arch may not be well visualized by TEE, but the remaining thoracic aortic segments are well visualized. Adequate sedation is important to avoid a hypertensive response to the procedure, often related to patient discomfort. TEE is less sensitive for detecting the intimal tear (see Fig. 60-e13 and Video 60-12 on website), but it is 100% sensitive in detecting aortic regurgitation complicating dissection and may define its mechanism (see Fig. 60-12 and Videos 60-2 to 60-5 on website).[54] Additionally, TEE provides information about wall motion and left ventricular function and the presence or absence of

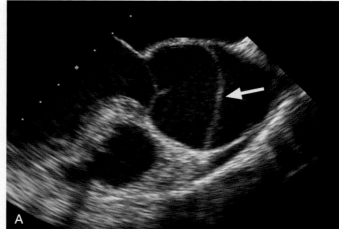
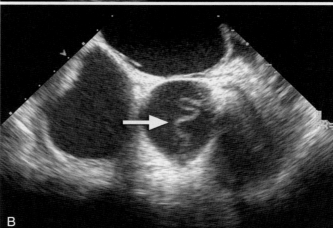

FIGURE 60-16 Transesophageal echocardiogram in acute aortic dissection. **A,** Acute type A dissection in a patient with Marfan syndrome. The dissection flap (arrow) is present in the dilated aortic root. **B,** Serpiginous intimal flap (arrow) immediately distal to the aortic valve in a patient with a type A aortic dissection.

pericardial effusion. TEE allows visualization of the coronary ostia and determination of whether they arise from the true or false lumen and whether the dissection extends into the coronary artery.

Aortography

Aortography is now rarely used for the diagnosis of acute aortic dissection; it is currently used most often for anatomic imaging and planning before endovascular therapy. Aortography has limited availability in the emergency setting and carries risk because of the procedure itself and the time required to assemble an angiography team. The diagnosis of dissection by aortography is based on imaging the two lumens or an intimal flap (see Fig. 60-e14 on website). Other features may include an undulating deformation of the aortic lumen, aortic wall thickening, branch vessel involvement, and aortic regurgitation. Compared with other imaging modalities, aortography is less accurate in the diagnosis of aortic dissection (sensitivity, 90%; specificity, 94%). A false-negative aortogram may be obtained in the setting of false lumen thrombosis, equal and simultaneous opacification of true and false lumina, and an aortic intramural hematoma.

Selecting an Imaging Modality

Because of its high level of sensitivity and specificity and availability on an emergency basis, contrast CT is usually the test of first choice for the diagnosis of aortic dissection. The risk of contrast nephropathy often complicates the decision about which test to perform, especially in emergency rooms or hospitals in which TEE or MRI is unavailable. It is important to remember than a noncontrast CT scan may fail to diagnose aortic dissection (see Fig. 60-e10 on website). If TEE or MRI is not available on an urgent basis, one must weigh the risks of intravenous contrast versus the potentially fatal consequences of failing to diagnose aortic dissection. A TTE may occasionally diagnose acute ascending aortic dissection, and if there is any concern about time delay for the other imaging modalities to be performed, an emergency bedside TTE may be useful. A negative TTE, however, does not exclude aortic dissection.

In the IRAD, CT was the most commonly used initial imaging study (63%), whereas TEE was used as the initial study in 32% of cases.[41] MRI is less available on an emergent basis, requires a longer time for imaging acquisition and processing, and poses potential risk because of restricted monitoring and accessibility to the patient during imaging. Aortography requires an angiography team and is subject to the risks associated with an invasive procedure, including time delay and intravenous contrast. The diagnostic approach to the patient with suspected aortic dissection must be based on each institution's available resources and expertise, and the rapidity and accuracy with which procedures may be performed.

Role of Coronary Angiography

Routine coronary angiography is not recommended before surgery for acute type A aortic dissection because of concern about delay in emergency surgery.[57,60] Coronary artery involvement in aortic dissection may have various causes. The aortic dissection flap may obstruct the orifice of the coronary artery, leading to coronary ischemia or infarction. Additionally, the dissection flap may propagate down the coronary artery for a variable length, leading to obstruction of flow (see Fig. 60-11), or the patient may have coexisting atherosclerotic coronary artery disease. The presence of occlusive coronary artery disease has been identified in approximately 20% of patients with ascending dissection. At present, preoperative catheterization is only infrequently performed before emergency ascending aortic dissection repair, being carried out in only 10% of patients in one recent report.[60] In IRAD, approximately 10% of patients with acute type A dissection underwent coronary angiography. Preoperative identification of coronary disease by catheterization has not proved to alter survival in patients with acute aortic dissection. In addition to the time delay incurred, coronary angiography may be technically difficult in the setting of dissection. Arterial access may fail to gain entry into the true lumen. Potential complications of catheterization include catheter or guidewire injury to the aorta, leading to an extension of the dissection or perforation of the aorta.

In specific patients, further evaluation for coronary artery disease or coronary artery involvement before aortic dissection surgery may be indicated. Individuals with a history of coronary disease, prior coronary artery bypass surgery, and those with acute ischemic electrocardiographic changes are subgroups in which this decision is usually contemplated. Usually, coronary artery involvement by the dissection may be identified and rectified at surgery, so angiography is not required. One has to make individual decisions based on the specific circumstances. These patients must be hemodynamically stable to be candidates for preoperative cardiac catheterization. The presence of cardiac tamponade and aortic rupture are contraindications to coronary angiography.

Direct inspection of the coronary ostia may be performed once the aorta has been opened at surgery, and any obstruction or involvement of the coronary arteries by the dissection process may then be corrected. TEE may evaluate the ostia of the coronary arteries before surgery or intraoperatively and may assess wall motion, suggesting ischemia. Additionally, coronary atherosclerosis may be identified intraoperatively by inspection, probing, or palpation of the coronary arteries. There is very limited experience in intraoperative coronary angiography in aortic dissection.

MANAGEMENT. The goals of medical management are to stabilize the patient, control pain, lower blood pressure, and reduce the rate of rise or force (dP/dt) of left ventricular ejection. These measures are

undertaken immediately while the patient is undergoing diagnostic evaluation. Lowering blood pressure may help prevent further propagation of the dissection and lessen risk of aortic rupture. Aortic dissection is a highly lethal condition. Early literature reported that more than 25% of untreated individuals with acute dissection died in the first 24 hours, 50% died within the first week, and more than 75% died within the first month.[43] Emergency surgery improves survival in acute type A dissections, whereas initial medical therapy is recommended for acute type B dissections. Patients with acute aortic dissection require urgent multidisciplinary evaluation and management. They should be transferred emergently to a tertiary medical center with access to cardiovascular surgery, vascular surgery, interventional radiology, and cardiology. Surgical consultation is recommended, regardless of the anatomic location of the dissection.[32]

Surgical therapy for type A aortic dissection has dramatically improved survival for this lethal condition. The goals of surgical therapy are to treat or prevent the common complications of dissection, such as cardiac tamponade, aortic regurgitation, aortic rupture, stroke, and visceral ischemia. The immediate surgical goals are as follows: (1) excise the intimal tear; (2) obliterate the false channel by oversewing the edges of the aorta; and (3) reconstitute the aorta directly, or more commonly with placement of an interposition graft. In type A dissection, aortic regurgitation is also treated by resuspension of the aortic valve leaflets or by prosthetic aortic valve replacement.

Blood Pressure Reduction

Reduction of systolic blood pressure to levels of approximately 100 to 120 mm Hg, or the lowest level appropriate for adequate perfusion to vital organs, is recommended. Beta-blocking agents should be administered, regardless of whether systolic hypertension is present, with a goal of attaining a heart rate of 60 beats/min or lower. For rapid administration of agents to reduce the rate of rise of ventricular force (dP/dt) and stress on the aorta, intravenous beta blockers should be given. The short-acting beta blocker esmolol is often the first choice, and is given as an initial bolus of 500 μg/kg and then a continuous infusion of 50 to 200 μg/kg/min. Labetolol is an alpha- and beta-adrenergic blocker and may be administered intravenously in the acute setting or orally. Labetolol is given at an initial dose of 20 mg IV over 2 minutes, and then at a dose of 40 to 80 mg IV every 15 minutes (maximum dose 300 mg), until an adequate response is achieved. Labetolol is then given by continuous intravenous infusion at a rate of 2 to 8 mg/min. Propranolol and metoprolol may be used intravenously or orally for acute aortic dissection. When acute severe aortic regurgitation complicates aortic dissection, caution should be exercised with beta blocker use.[32]

When beta blockers are contraindicated, one may consider the calcium channel blockers verapamil or diltiazem. These agents have negative inotropic and chronotropic effects and may be administered intravenously, making them advantageous in the acute setting. Intravenous diltiazem is given as 0.25 mg/kg over 2 minutes and then continued as an infusion at a rate of 5 to 15 mg/hr, depending on the effect.

Sodium nitroprusside leads to a rapid reduction of blood pressure, but when used alone may lead to an increase in dP/dt, which could contribute to propagation of the dissection. In the setting of acute aortic dissection, sodium nitroprusside must be used together with beta blockade. Sodium nitroprusside is initiated with a dose of 20 μg/min, with titration to 0.5 to 5 μg/kg/min as required. Caution must be exercised in the setting of renal insufficiency or prolonged use. Because of the risk of cyanide toxicity, nitroprusside is used only for short periods.

Often, multiple agents are required for adequate blood pressure and heart rate control in acute aortic dissection. Intravenous ACE inhibitors (such as IV enalaprilat) and intravenous nitroglycerin may be useful.

When the patient with acute dissection has hypertension that is refractory or difficult to control, there are many considerations. First, the patient may have underlying severe hypertension and may have gone without medications, with medication withdrawal playing a role, especially beta blockers or clonidine. Uncontrolled pain may exacerbate hypertension. Additionally, acute cocaine use may lead to tachycardia and hypertension. Finally, the patient may have renal artery involvement by the dissection flap, leading to hypertension. Renal artery hypertension due to the dissection process may respond favorably to ACE inhibitor therapy, and in some cases requires endovascular therapy. When the patient with suspected aortic dissection has significant hypotension, rapid volume expansion should be considered, given the possible presence of cardiac tamponade or aortic rupture with hemorrhage into the mediastinum, pleural space, or abdomen.

Management of Cardiac Tamponade (See Chap. 75)

Cardiac tamponade, occurring in 19% of acute type A dissections, is one of the most common mechanisms for death in this disorder (**Fig. 60-17**).[61] Patients with tamponade are more likely to present with hypotension, syncope, or altered mental status. The in-hospital mortality rate among patients with cardiac tamponade is twice as high as that among those without tamponade (54% versus 25%). Because hemodynamic instability with hypotension often complicates hemopericardium in acute dissection, pericardiocentesis is commonly considered as initial therapy in this condition, to attempt to stabilize these patients before surgery. But sudden death from pulseless electrical activity has been reported minutes after pericardiocentesis in this setting. The relative increase in intra-aortic pressure that occurs after pericardiocentesis may lead to a reopening or resurgence of blood under pressure from the false channel into the pericardial space, resulting in acute hemorrhage and fatal cardiac tamponade. Therefore, in the relatively stable patient with acute type A dissection and cardiac tamponade, the risks of pericardiocentesis likely outweigh its benefits. The initial strategy should be to proceed emergently to the operating room for open surgical repair of the aorta and drainage of the pericardium under direct visualization, but when managing such a patient, with pulseless electrical activity or refractory hypotension, an attempt at resuscitation with pericardiocentesis may be lifesaving. In this case, one should attempt to aspirate only enough pericardial fluid to stabilize the patient, and then proceed to emergency surgery. Reports of successful pericardiocentesis in acute type A intramural hematoma from the Asian population have suggested that this may be effective in this subset of acute aortic syndrome[32] (see later, "Aortic Intramural Hematoma").

Definitive Therapy

Definitive therapy for acute aortic dissection includes emergency surgery for all patients with acute ascending aortic dissection who are considered surgical candidates. Patients with acute type A aortic dissection are at risk of progression of the disease, including aortic rupture, aortic regurgitation with heart failure, stroke, cardiac tamponade, and visceral ischemia. Compared with medical therapy, immediate surgical treatment improves survival in acute type A aortic dissection. In the IRAD, the mortality rate of patients with type A aortic dissection undergoing surgery was 26%, and was 58% for those treated medically (typically because of advanced age and comorbid conditions) (**Fig. 60-18**).[41] Thus, almost 25% of patients with acute ascending aortic dissection will die, even after presenting to centers with extensive experience with aortic dissection. Other single-center series have reported even lower mortality rates for surgical patients.[60,62] In the IRAD, 526 patients underwent surgical treatment for acute ascending aortic dissection, and the mortality rate was variable, depending on risk factors present preoperatively. In patients considered unstable (e.g., with shock, congestive heart failure, cardiac tamponade, myocardial infarction, renal failure, or mesenteric ischemia), the mortality rate was 31% versus 17% for those considered stable.[42,56] Independent predictors for operative mortality included prior aortic valve replacement, migrating chest pain, hypotension, shock or cardiac tamponade, and limb ischemia. Mortality for patients with a preoperative malperfusion syndrome in

type A dissection was fivefold greater (30% versus 6%) than for those without malperfusion.

A bedside preoperative and postoperative risk prediction tool of mortality has been developed to understand better the expected risks of surgery in acute type A aortic dissection (**Table 60-3**).[63] Intraoperative variables, including hypotension, right ventricular dysfunction, and surgical aspects (CABG, partial arch resection), are also used in obtaining a postoperative score (see Table 60-e6 on website). One may use these data to estimate an individual's expected mortality rate with acute type A aortic dissection (**Fig. 60-19**; see Fig. 60-e15 on website).

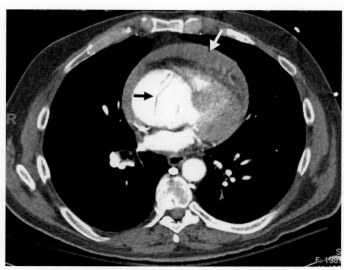

FIGURE 60-17 Contrast CT scan of acute type A aortic dissection (black arrow), with associated hemopericardium (white arrow).

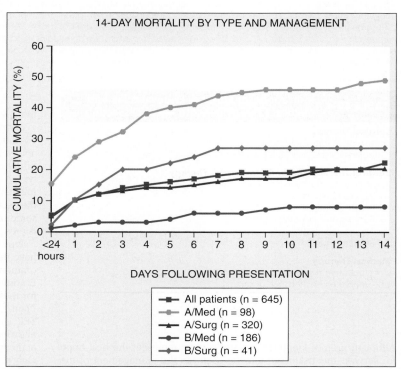

FIGURE 60-18 Two-week mortality rates for acute aortic dissection according to dissection type and medical or surgical treatment. (*From Hagan PG, Nienaber CA, Isselbacher EM, et al: The International Registry of Acute Aortic Dissection [IRAD]: New insights into an old disease. JAMA 283:897, 2000.*)

TABLE 60-3 Preoperative Prediction Model of Surgical Mortality Risk

VARIABLE	OVERALL TYPE A (%)	AMONG SURVIVORS (%)	AMONG DEATH (%)	COEFFICIENT	SCORE ASSIGNED	P VALUE	ODDS RATIO, DEATH (95% CI)
Age ≥ 70 yr	27.3	24.1	37.4	0.68	0.7	<0.01	1.98 (1.19-3.29)
History of aortic valve replacement	4.5	3.8	6.6	1.44	1.5	<0.01	4.21 (1.56-.34)
Presenting hypotension, shock, or tamponade	28.8	22.4	49.0	1.17	1.2	<0.01	3.23 (1.95-5.37)
Migrating chest pain	13.8	12.1	19.3	0.88	0.9	<0.01	2.42 (1.32-4.45)
Preoperative cardiac tamponade	15.5	11.7	28.2	0.97	1.0	<0.01	2.65 (1.48-4.75)
Any pulse deficit	28.6	25.7	37.8	0.56	0.6	0.03	1.75 (1.06-2.88)

From Rampoldi V, Trimarchi S, Eagle KA, et al: Simple risk models to predict surgical mortality in acute type A aortic dissection: The International Registry of Acute Aortic Dissection score. Ann Thorac Surg 83:55, 2007.

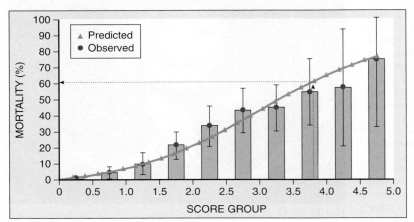

FIGURE 60-19 Observed versus model probabilities of death by preoperative score. This example is of a 77-year-old woman with migrating chest pain, preoperative cardiac tamponade, a pulse deficit, and ST-segment elevation. Her model score is 0.7 (age > 70 years) + 0.9 (migratory chest pain) + 1.0 (preoperative cardiac tamponade) + 0.6 (pulse deficit) + 0.6 (ST-segment elevation). Total score = 3.8 and estimated surgical mortality risk is 61%. *(From Rampoldi V, Trimarchi S, Eagle, KA, et al: Simple risk models to predict surgical mortality in acute type A aortic dissection: The International Registry of Acute Aortic Dissection score. Ann Thorac Surg 83:55, 2007.)*

TABLE 60-4 Indications for Surgical, Endovascular, and Medical Therapy in Acute Aortic Dissection

Surgical Therapy
Acute type A aortic dissection
Retrograde dissection into the ascending aorta

Surgical Therapy and/or Endovascular Therapy
Acute type B aortic dissection complicated by:
• Visceral ischemia
• Limb ischemia
• Rupture or impending rupture
• Aneurysmal dilation
• Refractory pain

Medical Therapy
Uncomplicated type B aortic dissection
Uncomplicated isolated arch dissection

Although prompt identification and surgery represent the best hope for survival, this risk score may be useful in the management of the truly moribund patient who, regardless of surgery, has a very poor chance of survival.

Patients with acute type B aortic dissection have a lower risk of early death than those with acute type A dissection. In the IRAD, the mortality rate of patients with type B dissection treated medically was 10.7% (see Fig. 60-18). However, most series of acute aortic descending dissection have reported a mortality rate of 25% to 50% for those requiring surgery. In patients with uncomplicated type B dissection, the in-hospital mortality rate is very low.[64] However, complicated type B dissection carries a much higher mortality rate, especially when accompanied by shock or malperfusion. In the IRAD, surgery was performed in 20% of type B dissections, with a mortality rate of 31%.[41] Independent predictors for surgical mortality in type B dissection include age older than 70 years and preoperative shock or hypotension. In a series of 129 acute type B aortic dissections treated with the strategy of initial medical therapy, the in-hospital mortality rate was 10%; it was 19% when early vascular intervention was required, and 8% when medical management was maintained.[65] This series and other large retrospective series have demonstrated that in general, initial medical therapy provides an outcome superior to that of initial surgical therapy for uncomplicated type B aortic dissection. Typical indications for surgical or endovascular intervention in type B aortic dissection are complications that develop, such as visceral or limb ischemia, aortic rupture or impending rupture, rapid expansion of the aortic diameter, uncontrollable pain, or retrograde extension of the dissection into the ascending aorta (**Table 60-4**). Often, endovascular therapy for certain complications may be preferred.[66]

Primary arch dissections are uncommon, and management of this condition requires individualization. Mortality for surgical repair of acute arch dissection has been reported as 15% to 29%. If involvement of the ascending aorta is present, then the dissection is classified as type A and emergency surgery is recommended. Many recommend initial medical therapy for primary arch dissections that do not involve the ascending aorta, whereas others advocate emergency surgery for some primary arch dissections, especially if aneurysmal enlargement is present.

Type B dissections that extend retrograde into the transverse arch have been managed variably. For most, initial medical therapy is recommended. In the IRAD population of almost 500 patients with type B aortic dissections, 25% had aortic arch involvement, and mortality for these patients was no different from those without arch involvement.[67] In one series, when extension into the arch is observed, a TEE is performed to characterize the intimal flap and aortic tear, allowing exclusion of ascending aortic involvement.[65] In this series, acute type B dissections with arch involvement were managed medically, and 7% in that subpopulation had cerebral complications.

Surgical Management

Generally accepted indications for definitive surgical therapy are summarized in Table 60-4. Operative therapy for acute aortic dissection is technically very demanding. The aortic wall is thin and friable, and Teflon felt and pledgeted sutures are used to buttress the wall and prevent sutures from tearing through the fragile aortic wall.

TYPE A AORTIC DISSECTION. Open surgery, performed as expediently as possible, is the treatment of choice for ascending aortic dissection to prevent life-threatening complications.[28,41,66] The early mortality rate for surgical treatment in acute type A dissection is typically approximately 25%, whereas single-center experience is often lower.[60] A median sternotomy is routinely performed, and cannulation for cardiopulmonary bypass usually involves the axillary or femoral approach to avoid trauma to the weakened aortic wall. Surgical therapy includes excision of the intimal tear when possible, obliteration of entry into the false lumen proximally and distally, and interposition graft replacement of the ascending aorta. Most patients can be treated by obliteration of the false lumen by placement of Teflon felt as a neomedium and resuspension of the native aortic valve. When aortic regurgitation complicates dissection, repair of the aortic wall and decompression of the false lumen and resuspension of the commissures usually restore valve competence. When aortic leaflet disease precludes repair, aortic valve replacement and associated ascending aortic replacement are indicated. When the sinuses are significantly dilated, composite valve and root replacement is often performed using the modified Bentall procedure. When the aortic root and sinuses are dilated but the aortic leaflets are normal, many have achieved success by performing a valve-sparing root replacement, typically using the reimplantation technique (see Fig. 60-7).[33] At present, no data support the use of endovascular repair for type A dissection. Arch replacement using deep hypothermic circulatory arrest is also performed if the aortic arch is aneurysmal or ruptured or has a primary arch tear at the time of surgical treatment, and is done for some patients with genetically triggered aneurysm syndromes.[68]

TYPE B AORTIC DISSECTION. The treatment of patients with type B aortic dissections is currently evolving with the increased use of endovascular devices. In general, stable patients with uncomplicated type B dissections should be treated medically because of the high mortality rates associated with surgery.[15,41,68] Patients with complicated type B aortic dissections caused by aortic rupture, intractable chest or back pain, and/or visceral ischemia resulting from aortic branch vessel involvement require an intervention, but open surgical repair is associated with high mortality rates. Endovascular techniques have been increasingly used to treat this patient population, with encouraging results (**Fig. 60-20**).

Aortic fenestration techniques with or without additional aortic branch stenting have been used with reasonable success for the treatment of patients with aortic branch vessel involvement and malperfusion syndromes. The first technique is balloon fenestration of the intimal flap, which allows blood to flow from the false lumen into the true lumen, thereby decompressing the distended false lumen. The second technique involves percutaneous stenting of an affected arterial branch whose flow has been compromised by the dissection process. Recently, Patel and colleagues[69] reported the treatment of 69 patients over a period of 10 years, with a 30-day mortality rate of 17%. The freedom from aortic rupture or open surgical repair rates were 80% at 1 year, 68% at 5 years, and 54% at 8 years. These endovascular techniques can address some complications of type B dissections, but are associated with a high rate of conversion to open surgery in the long term.

Endovascular grafts have the potential to treat most, if not all, complications of type B dissections, with relatively low morbidity and mortality rates. The rationale behind this technique is that covering the area of the primary intimal tear with the endovascular graft redirects flow to the true lumen and promotes false lumen thrombosis, allowing aortic remodeling (**Fig. 60-21**).[65] This treatment often corrects branch vessel ischemia and is useful in the treatment of enlarging symptomatic dissections and ruptured aortas. STABLE and other trials are starting to evaluate prospectively the treatment of acute complicated type B dissections with endovascular grafts. The persistence of a perfused false lumen, which can occur in up to two thirds of patients treated, is concerning, as it can lead to reinterventions and surgical conversions. The Petticoat technique, in which the entry point is sealed

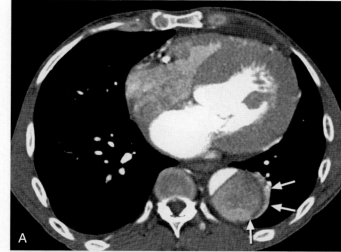

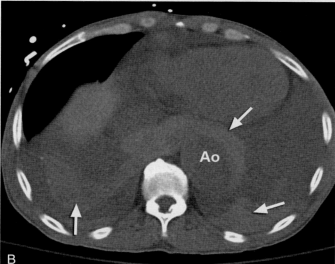

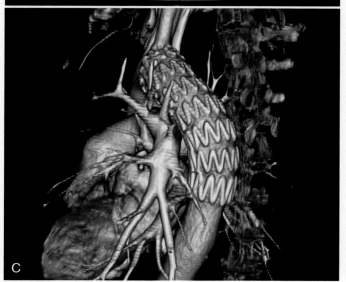

FIGURE 60-20 Rupture of a type B aortic dissection. **A,** Contrast CT scan demonstrating early leaking of blood from the dilated false lumen (arrows). The small true lumen is densely opacified with contrast. **B,** Noncontrast CT scan demonstrating acute hemorrhage from the ruptured type B dissection. **C,** Three-dimensional reconstruction of the descending thoracic aorta after emergency endovascular repair of the ruptured aortic dissection. Ao = aorta.

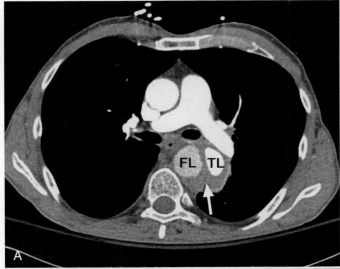

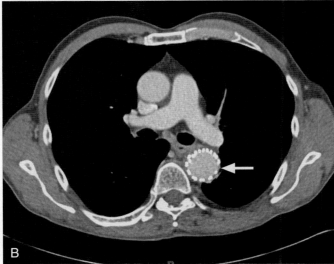

FIGURE 60-21 **A,** Type B aortic dissection with partial thrombosis of the false lumen (arrow). **B,** After endovascular repair of the type B dissection, the false lumen (arrow) has collapsed and remodeled and is no longer visualized. FL = false lumen; TL = true lumen.

with an endograft and the remaining thoracic and potentially the abdominal aorta is stented open, may address this problem.[70] This technique can decrease the chance of true lumen collapse, enhance aortic remodeling, and promote false lumen thrombosis. In addition, various methods of hybrid approaches to the surgical and endovascular repair of dissections involving the arch and descending aorta are being studied, with promising early results but no long-term data as of yet.

Patients with uncomplicated type B aortic dissections are at risk for long-term complications of aneurysm formation, late rupture, and dissection. Whether early endovascular grafting of the uncomplicated type B dissection will change this natural history is under investigation. The first comparison study between endovascular and open surgical repair for patients with subacute or chronic descending thoracic aortic dissections has reported periprocedural mortality rates of 0% and 33% for the endovascular and surgical groups, respectively.[68] This initial experience led to the organization of the INSTEAD trial in Europe, randomizing 140 patients with stable, uncomplicated, chronic type B dissections to endovascular grafting versus medical therapy. At 2 years, there was no significant difference in all-cause mortality,[71] but patients treated with endovascular grafts had a significantly higher

rate of aortic remodeling and false lumen thrombosis compared with the medically treated group. The ADSORB trial is enrolling patients with acute uncomplicated type B dissections and will examine various endpoints, including false lumen thrombosis and the prevention of aortic dilation and rupture. The indications for endovascular therapy are evolving and must be balanced against the advances in open therapy, especially when performed by highly skilled surgical teams.

Definitive Medical Management

Hypertension is common in the setting of acute dissection and is related to underlying hypertension, renal artery involvement, pain, or systemic inflammation accompanying the dissection process. Difficult to control or refractory hypertension is not usually considered as an indication for surgical repair of type B dissection. Whereas many patients require multiple antihypertensive agents to control blood pressure acutely, blood pressure often falls over the first several days as the inflammatory response resolves. When severe hypertension persists or there are signs of renal ischemia, one should evaluate the patient for renal artery involvement. It is important to follow the patient closely for malperfusion syndromes involving the viscera or extremities and for evidence of aortic rupture. Mesenteric ischemia may be difficult to recognize, and identification of this serious complication requires vigilance.

LONG-TERM THERAPY AND FOLLOW-UP. Short- and long-term survival in type A aortic dissections has ranged from 52% to 94% at 1 year and 45% to 88% at 5 years.[72] The 10-year actuarial survival rate among patients with acute aortic dissection who survive initial hospitalization has been between 30% and 60% in various studies. In a single-center study of long-term follow-up after type A aortic dissection, 10-year survival was 55% and 20-year survival was 30%.[60]

Among 303 patients who survived acute type A aortic dissection to hospital discharge, 273 were treated surgically and 30 were treated medically. With a mean follow-up of 2.8 years, the survival for patients treated surgically was 96% ± 2% at 1 year and 90% ± 4% at 3 years, versus 89% ± 12% at 1 year and 69% ± 20% at 3 years without surgery.[72] During the 5-year follow-up period, patients managed surgically had a significantly lower mortality rate of 14%, versus 37% for those treated medically. Predictors of increased mortality rate in follow-up include age older than 70 years, renal or cardiac failure, prior cardiac surgery, stroke, and Marfan syndrome.

Medically treated patients with type A aortic dissection have a very high mortality rate, with death rates in excess of 50% reported early after presentation. Little information exists in the literature about the natural history and management of chronic type A aortic dissection. There are some reports of dismal survival with medical therapy alone, even in those who survive initial hospitalization. A few patients are discovered in the subacute stage, and surgery is recommended for them. On occasion, however, patients are discovered incidentally to have a chronic type A dissection in the evaluation of aortic regurgitation or a dilated ascending aorta. Most have advocated surgical treatment for all appropriate candidates with chronic type A dissection, whereas some have reserved surgery for those with aneurysmal dilation of the ascending aorta, aortic regurgitation, or relatively young age. In the IRAD experience, two thirds of patients who survived hospitalization for acute type A aortic dissection with medical therapy alone were still alive at 3 years.[70] In-hospital mortality rate for surgical therapy of chronic type A aortic dissection has ranged from 8% to 17%, depending on the series. Long-term survival after surgical repair of chronic type A aortic dissection has been reported at 42% to 71% at 12 years, depending on whether operative mortality is included and the extent of the dissection.[73]

The long-term survival rates in acute type B dissection have varied, with reports ranging from 56% to 92% at 1 year and from 48% to 82% at 5 years.[74] These studies have included single-center reports with heterogeneous enrollment criteria and lack of endovascular therapy. Nonetheless, the long-term follow-up after type B aortic dissection is worse than that of type A dissection, with about one in four patients dying within 3 years. Studies have demonstrated that many deaths in follow-up are related to subsequent aortic complications, such as rupture, extension of the dissection, and risks of subsequent aortic and vascular surgery. An IRAD study reported the 3-year survival rates for those patients discharged after initial hospitalization for acute type B aortic dissection. The survival for patients treated medically, surgically, or with endovascular therapy were 78% ± 7%, 83% ± 19%, and 76% ± 25%, respectively.[75] Independent predictors of increased mortality in follow-up included in-hospital hypotension or shock, pleural effusion, renal failure, history of atherosclerosis or prior aneurysm, and female sex.

Tenets of long-term management after aortic dissection include the following: (1) medical therapy, including antihypertensive therapy; (2) screening the individual and first-degree relatives for genetically triggered disorders associated with aortic dissection; (3) serial imaging of the aorta over time; (4) lifestyle modifications; and (5) education.

One important goal in long-term management after dissection is treating hypertension, with a blood pressure goal of less than 120/80 mm Hg in most individuals. Studies have demonstrated a dramatic increase in late morbidity and mortality in dissection patients with poorly controlled hypertension. Beta blockers are the drugs of first choice because of their effect on aortic stress and dP/dt, and are recommended even in the absence of hypertension. ARBs, by antagonizing TGF-β, have demonstrated benefit in a mouse model of Marfan syndrome and are the subject of investigation in people with Marfan syndrome. A Japanese trial in patients with hypertension and other types of heart disease has demonstrated a reduction in aortic dissection in patients treated with the ARB valsartan.[32] Whether these or alternative antihypertensive agents have a special role in management after dissection is unknown. Smoking cessation and risk factor modification for atherosclerotic disease are also important in management.

Although most patients who experience acute aortic dissection have underlying hypertension, only a small fraction of hypertensive patients ever suffer a dissection. Many with dissection will eventually be found to have a genetic trigger for the aortic disease. Some have syndromic features recognized as MFS or LDS. Features of these disorders should be sought on examination. The recognition of dural ectasia in the lumbosacral spine on the CT or MRI scan will often provide a clue to such a genetically triggered disorder. Some patients will have an underlying BAV, a condition that is familial in almost 10% of cases. Others will have familial thoracic aortic aneurysm or dissection syndromes. Comprehensive family studies have recognized that almost one in five individuals with a TAA or dissection will have another first-degree relative with thoracic aortic disease.[19] Thus, it is important to evaluate the patient with aortic dissection for a genetically triggered disorder and to evaluate and image first-degree relatives for the presence of familial thoracic aortic disease.[32]

Long-term management after dissection also includes regular imaging of the aorta and its branches for complications (see Fig. 60-e16 on website). Up to one third of patients require additional surgery on the aorta or its branches in the first several years after dissection to address aneurysm formation at the site of dissection, recurrent dissection, rupture, aneurysm formation at a remote site, graft dehiscence or pseudoaneurysm formation, aortic valve regurgitation, or infection. Typical protocols for follow-up after acute dissection include cross-sectional imaging with CT or MRI at 1 to 3, 6, 12, 18, and 24 months, with variability depending on the size of the aorta and changes in aortic dimension over time (see Table 60-e2 on website). One advantage of MRI for long-term follow-up is the avoidance of repeated radiation exposure. Reevaluation at least yearly thereafter is important to survey for aneurysmal dilation or false lumen expansion.

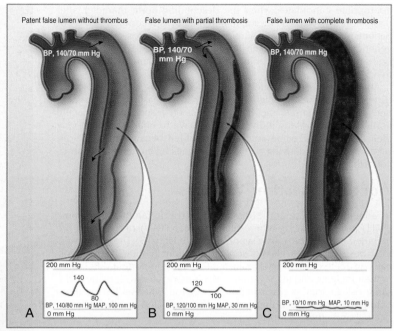

FIGURE 60-22 Conceptual model of risk according to the status of the false lumen. The figure shows a proposed model of the physiologic consequences of false lumen patency or thrombosis, based on hemodynamic studies in ex vivo models and in patients with aortic dissection. **A,** Type B aortic dissection with patent proximal and patent distal reentry tears in the absence of thrombus. The blood pressure tracing shows systolic, diastolic, and mean arterial pressures in the false lumen similar to the pressures in the true lumen. **B,** Type B aortic dissection with a patent entry tear and partial thrombosis that occupies the inner circumference of the false lumen and obstructs the reentry tears, forming a blind sac. The blood pressure tracing shows diastolic and mean arterial pressures in the false lumen that exceed the pressures seen in **A,** with identical pressures in the true lumen. **C,** Type B aortic dissection with a false lumen filled with thrombus and no longer communicating with the true lumen. The pressure within the false lumen is likely to be low and nonpulsatile. BP = blood pressure; MAP = mean arterial pressure. *(From Tsai TT, Evangelista A, Nienaber CA, et al; International Registry of Acute Aortic Dissection: Partial thrombosis of the false lumen in patients with acute type B aortic dissection. N Engl J Med 357:349, 2007.)*

The status of the false lumen is a significant predictor of late outcomes after acute type B aortic dissection.[75] Aortic dilation and patency of the false lumen are associated with subsequent aneurysmal dilation and late complications. Patients with partial false lumen thrombosis (see Fig. 60-21 and Fig. 19-23A) have higher mortality rates at follow-up than patients with completely patent or completely thrombosed false lumen. Increased pressure may occur in the false lumen in the setting of partial thrombosis because of lack of distal reentry tears, leading to subsequent expansion and increased risk of rupture. Additionally, false lumen thrombus may cause arterial wall hypoxemia, resulting in localized wall weakening (**Fig. 60-22**). Whether endovascular intervention used as a primary therapy for certain patients with uncomplicated type B dissection will alter their natural history is unknown. To date, studies of subacute and chronic type B dissections have not found established benefit of prophylactic endovascular stent placement.[71]

Many late deaths following surgery for aortic dissection result from rupture of the aorta at the site of prior dissection or another aneurysm at a remote site (see Fig. 60-20 and Fig. 19-23A). The proximal descending aorta is the most common site of aneurysmal enlargement.[76] Aneurysms related to false lumen expansion have relatively thin walls and have a higher risk of rupture than atheromatous aneurysms. Thus, continued surveillance of the entire aorta and surgical treatment (or endovascular, when appropriate) of aneurysms at appropriate size thresholds is important for long-term survival. The timing of surgical repair for aneurysmal involvement of the residual aorta depends on several factors, including age and general medical condition of the individual, comorbidities, underlying disease process, rate of aneurysmal enlargement, and absolute size of the aorta. In general, for appropriate candidates, when the descending aorta diameter after dissection exceeds 5.5 cm, surgical treatment is recommended.[32] For patients at relatively lower surgical risk and for those with certain genetically triggered thoracic aortic aneurysms and dissection diseases, repair may be appropriate when the aortic diameter exceeds 5.0 to 5.5 cm.

After aortic dissection, lifestyle modifications are necessary. Isometric activities, including weightlifting, leads to increased blood pressure and aortic wall stress, and have rarely been associated with acute aortic dissection. Many individuals will have to change jobs, modify their type of work, or be considered disabled because of aortic dissection and/or underlying aortic disease causing limitations on physical activity.

Aortic Dissection Variants

In addition to acute aortic dissection, aortic intramural hematoma (IMH) and penetrating atherosclerotic ulcer (PAU) of the aorta are included in the acute aortic syndromes (see Fig. 60-8). These disorders may be identical to classic aortic dissection in their presentation, causing acute chest or back pain, but they have important differences in their imaging and management. IMH is associated with many of the same risk factors as classic aortic dissection, whereas PAU is more common in the descending aorta and is associated with heavy calcification and atherosclerosis.

Aortic Intramural Hematoma

In approximately 5% to 25% of cases of acute aortic syndrome, a hematoma develops within the medial layer of the aortic wall with no evidence of an intimal flap or false lumen visualized by imaging study, surgery, or autopsy. These noncommunicating dissections are labeled as aortic IMH. Most consider IMH to be the result of a primary rupture of the vasa vasorum leading to mural hemorrhage. When an aortic atheromatous plaque ruptures into the media—that is, a PAU—a secondary IMH often accompanies the acute ulceration. PAU with IMH formation is a separate entity than a spontaneous IMH (see later).

IMH is an important variant of aortic dissection and must be recognized. In the IRAD experience, approximately 6% of aortic dissections were classified as IMH.[77] In Asian studies, approximately 25% of acute aortic syndromes are IMHs.[78] Compared with classic aortic dissection, patients with IMH are older and more likely to have descending aortic involvement.

IMHs may be localized or may propagate the length of the aorta. They are classified as type A or B, using the same classification scheme as for classic aortic dissection. The presenting symptoms and risk factors associated with IMH resemble those of aortic dissection, with acute chest and/or back pain predominating. The proximity of the intramural hemorrhage to the adventitia may explain the frequent coexistence of pleural and pericardial effusion and underlie the higher risk of subsequent aortic rupture associated with IMH. Ascending IMH may lead to aortic regurgitation, hemopericardium, or rupture, but because there is no intimal flap or false lumen, stroke and visceral ischemia appear less common. There may be a geographic difference in incidence, because IMH is a more common diagnosis among acute aortic syndromes in Asian countries than in Western countries.[79]

Imaging studies that can diagnose IMH include TEE, CT, and MRI. TEE features of IMH include focal crescentic or circumferential aortic wall thickening, eccentric aortic lumen, displaced intimal calcification, and areas of echolucency within the aortic wall (**Fig. 60-23**; see Video 60-13 on website; see Fig. 15-85). There is no evidence of an intimal flap, false lumen, or flow in the aortic wall. The aortic wall thickness in IMH ranges from 5 to 25 mm. On noncontrast CT, IMH appears as an area of high attenuation in the wall of the aorta (see Fig. 60-e17 on website), whereas on contrast CT, the aortic wall demonstrates low attenuation because no contrast enters the wall (**Fig. 60-24**; see Fig. 19-23B). MRI demonstrates focal thickening of the aortic wall with phase contrast cine and gradient echo demonstrating no flow in the aortic wall (see Fig. 60-e18 on website). High signal intensity on

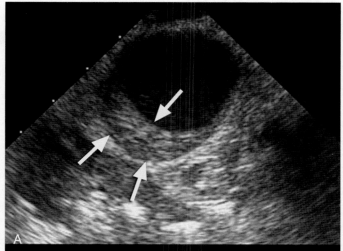

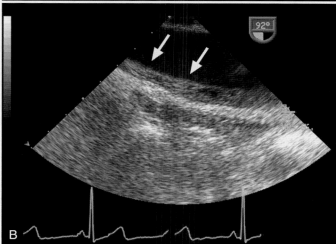

FIGURE 60-23 Transesophageal echocardiographic images of acute type B IMH (arrows). **A,** Short-axis views of the descending aorta demonstrating typical crescentic thickening of the aortic wall in IMH. **B,** Longitudinal views of the aorta demonstrating IMH (arrows).

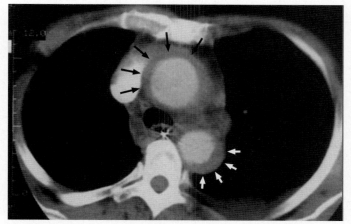

FIGURE 60-24 Contrast CT scan demonstrating type A IMH of the aorta. Note the circumferential hematoma involving the ascending aorta (black arrows) and the crescentic hematoma involving the descending aorta (white arrows).

T2-weighted imaging may be visualized related to blood in the aortic wall in acute IMH, but signal intensity varies, depending on the age of the hemorrhage. Aortography has a poor sensitivity to detect IMH, because this disease involves the aortic wall and not the lumen.

Distinct from an aneurysm with mural thrombus, the IMH has a smooth lumen and curvilinear wall (see Figs. 60-23 and 60-24). In certain cases, it may be difficult to differentiate IMH from aortic dissection with thrombosis of the false lumen, mural thrombus within an aortic aneurysm, or severe aortic atherosclerosis. By TEE, identifying the intima, which is often calcified and echodense, is helpful in this distinction. Thickening beneath the intima is suggestive of IMH, whereas thickening above the intima (on the luminal side) occurs with mural thrombus formation in an aneurysm. In contrast to aortic atherosclerosis, IMH typically is not associated with diffuse irregularities of the aortic intima surface, unless accompanying a penetrating ulcer.

IMH may have several fates: (1) progression to acute, classic aortic dissection or aortic rupture; (2) complete resolution of the hematoma with no evidence of the disorder on follow-up imaging; (3) persistence without progression of the hematoma; or (4) progressive aortic dilation and aneurysm formation.

Early studies from Western Europe and the United States have reported that patients with type A IMH were at high risk for complications, including aortic dissection (25% to 50%), hemopericardium, and rupture, with a mortality in excess of 30% with medical therapy alone.[77,79] In a review of 160 patients from 11 studies, mortality for type A IMH treated medically was almost 50% and was 24% when treated surgically. Type B IMH is associated with a lower mortality rate, 10% to 13% with medical therapy and 15% with surgical repair. These data have led most authorities to recommend emergency cardiac surgery in type A IMH and initial medical therapy in type B IMH. Cardiac surgery in type B IMH is reserved for complications such as progression, impending rupture, or rupture. Descending IMH may progress to frank dissection and late aneurysm formation, or may also reabsorb completely (see Fig. 60-e19 on website).

Reports from Japan and South Korea have suggested much different approaches for the management of type A IMH—medical therapy, serial imaging, and careful observation, with prolonged hospitalization as an initial strategy.[78] In a series of 101 patients with type A IMH from Korea, 16 patients underwent emergency surgery for hemodynamic instability, whereas 85 patients had initial medical therapy.[79] Medically treated patients underwent weekly imaging studies, prolonged hospitalization, and delayed surgery in 29% of patients at a median of 27 days, with a mortality rate of 4%. Predictors of adverse outcomes in these patients included syncope, enlarged aortic diameter (>55 mm), and increased hematoma thickness (>16 mm).

With this approach, however, many patients with type A IMH have progressed to frank dissection, hemopericardium, or rupture requiring emergency surgery (see Fig. 60-e20 on website). In a pooled analysis of 309 type A IMH cases, clinical outcomes were available for 160 patients from North America (NA) and Europe and for 149 patients from Asia.[79] The Asian population was usually treated with initial medical therapy. The overall mortality was lower (9%) for the Asian group compared with the NA-European group (21%). The Asian group also had a lower mortality for patients treated medically compared with the NA-European group. The mortality rates for patients undergoing early surgery for type A IMH were lower in the NA-European group than the Asian group.

Important differences in IMH in these different geographic regions may influence outcomes. IMH causes more frequent acute aortic syndromes in Asia compared with NA-Europe. This variation may be related to more subtle cases being recognized in Asia or because of genetic or environmental issues. In a pooled analysis, those sent for early surgery had lower in-hospital mortality (10%) than those with early medical treatment (18%). In a prior meta-analysis of 143 cases of type A IMH, early surgery associated with a lower mortality than did medical therapy (14% versus 36%, respectively).[79] In the Asian population treated medically, rates of pericardial tamponade were four times more common, and progression to frank aortic dissection was twice as frequent as in NA-European patients. With the strategy of medical

therapy for ascending IMH, 30% of those initially treated medically, and more than 50% of IMH overall, eventually underwent surgical repair.[78-80] The IRAD population included 23 patients with ascending IMH. Progression to aortic dissection occurred in 16%, and the mortality rate for type A IMH was 39%.[77] In a series of 36 type A IMHs, 7 patients underwent immediate surgery, 28 underwent initial medical therapy with subsequent conversion to surgical repair (33% of these progressed to acute dissection), and 1 was treated medically, with resolution of the IMH.[81]

Given the potential for unpredictable and catastrophic complications, most authorities continue to recommend immediate surgical therapy for type A IMH in patients at reasonable risk and at experienced surgical centers, and medical management for type B IMH.[77] Management of localized arch IMH must be individualized, with some advocating initial medical therapy for this group.[78] Patients with IMH require continued surveillance after surgery and while on medical therapy for type B IMH. Complete resolution of type B IMH has been described in more than 50% in some series, whereas others have led to frank dissection, rupture, or late aneurysm formation.[82] In one series of type B IMH, almost one third of cases were referred for surgical repair, initially or in follow-up.[83] Although information is limited, predictors of resolution of type B hematoma have included younger age, smaller aortic diameters (<4 to 4.5 cm), hematoma thickness (<1 cm), and postoperative beta blocker use.

Penetrating Atherosclerotic Ulcer

PAU (penetrating aortic ulcer) is a condition in which an atherosclerotic lesion penetrates the internal elastic lamina into the media, often associated with a variable degree of intramural hematoma formation.[83] PAU may lead to pseudoaneurysm formation, aortic rupture, or late aneurysm (**Fig. 60-25**). Aortic ulcers may be single or multiple and range from 5 mm to 25 mm in diameter and 4 mm to 30 mm in depth. PAUs can occur throughout the aorta, but are more common in the thoracic and abdominal aorta than in the arch or ascending aorta.

The incidence of PAU is unknown. Among symptomatic patients with suspected acute aortic syndrome, PAUs are present in 2% to 8%.[83] Patients with PAU are typically older and hypertensive, with multiple coronary risk factors and coexisting vascular disease. Many patients have concomitant aneurysmal dilation of the aorta elsewhere. Whereas up to 25% of PAUs are found incidentally on imaging studies, typical symptoms of PAU include acute chest or back pain, similar in description to those of classic aortic dissection. Because acute PAU may have a higher propensity to rupture, it is imperative to recognize this condition. Although PAU may lead to aortic dissection, most patients do not have aortic regurgitation, pulse deficits, or visceral ischemia.

Imaging techniques for PAU include aortography, CT, MRI, and TEE. Although aortography is no longer the preferred method for diagnosis, the ulcer-like appearance on angiography gave this entity its name. Findings on CT include focal aortic ulceration, associated IMH, and a calcified displaced intima (**Fig. 60-26**). Typically, there is a crater-like outpouching with irregular edges in the setting of heavy atherosclerosis (see Fig. 60-e21 on website). CT findings may also demonstrate pleural effusions, mediastinal hemorrhage, coexisting aneurysms, contained rupture, pseudoaneurysm, and frank rupture (see Fig. 60-24). Approximately 80% of patients have some degree of IMH formation.[83] When PAU occurs with aortic dissection, the dissection often involves a short segment of aorta and has a thick intimal flap. MRI findings in PAU include localized areas of high signal intensity in the aorta wall consistent with IMH, focal intimal thickening, and ulcer-like projections. TEE demonstrates aortic atherosclerosis with focal ulceration of the intima and can demonstrate complications.

The natural history of PAU is uncertain, and descriptions in the literature vary depending on patient selection. A PAU may stabilize or lead to complications, including IMH, distal embolization, aortic rupture, pseudoaneurysm (contained rupture), aortic dissection, and development of a saccular or fusiform aneurysm. In one study, the annual growth rate of PAU was 0.31 cm/year. Some studies have reported gradual aortic enlargement and a low incidence of acute or

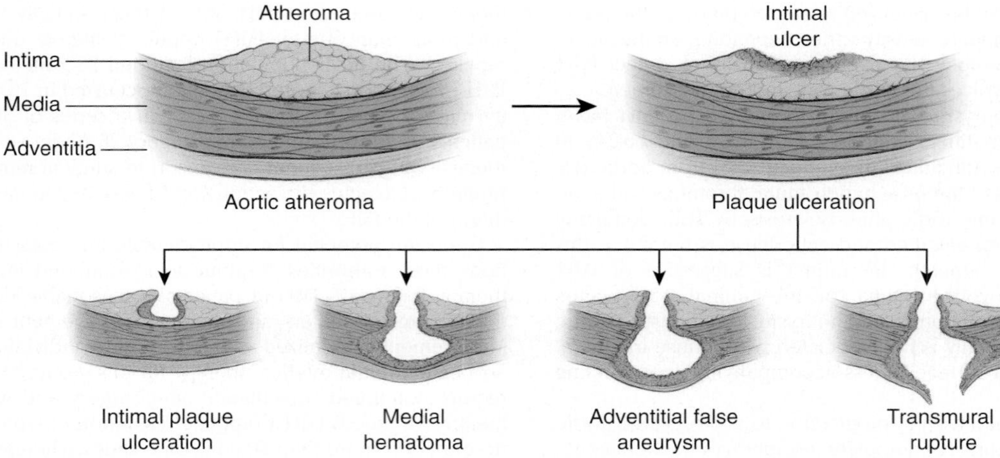

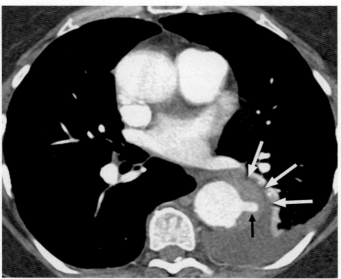

Atheroma

Intima

Media

Adventitia

Aortic atheroma

Intimal ulcer

Plaque ulceration

Intimal plaque ulceration | Medial hematoma | Adventitial false aneurysm | Transmural rupture

FIGURE 60-25 Evolution of a penetrating atherosclerotic ulcer of the aorta. Once an intimal ulcer has formed, it may then progress to a variable length. Penetration through the intima causes a medial hematoma, whereas penetration through the media leads to the formation of a pseudoaneurysm, and perforation through the adventitial layer results in an aortic rupture. *(From Stanson AW, Kazmier FJ, Hollier LH, et al: Penetrating atherosclerotic ulcers of the thoracic aorta: Natural history and clinicopathologic correlations. Ann Vasc Surg 1:15, 1986.)*

FIGURE 60-26 Contrast CT scan of a penetrating atherosclerotic ulcer of the aorta. Note the ulcer-like projection (black arrow) from the aortic lumen in the proximal descending aorta and the associated intramural hematoma (white arrows). A small pleural effusion is also present. *(Courtesy of Dr. Sanjeev Bhalla, Washington University School of Medicine, St. Louis.)*

life-threatening complications, whereas others have reported a high incidence of acute complications.[82,84] In a report of 26 patients with PAU, more than one third presented with rupture, 46% had ascending involvement, and two thirds underwent surgical repair.[82] In another series of 107 PAU patients, only 2% involved the ascending aorta, 9% presented with rupture, and 72% were treated medically. Only rupture at presentation and maximum aortic diameter predicted failure of medical therapy, defined as death from an aortic cause or caused by aortic surgery.

The management of the patient with PAU must be individualized. In general, patients with ascending PAUs are treated with surgical resection. Stable patients with type B PAUs may be managed medically, with strict follow-up and serial imaging. Patients with refractory or recurrent pain have increased risk of disease progression. Those with a rapid increase in aortic dimension are at risk for rupture and should

be treated surgically or with endovascular stent grafts. Indications for surgery or endovascular therapy may include features on imaging that include interval development of hemorrhage, periaortic hematoma, expanding pseudoaneurysm, and rupture. Other predictors of progression of disease include increasing aortic wall thickness, ulcer craters more than 20 mm in diameter or 10 mm in depth, increasing aortic hematoma, and increasing pleural effusion. In a retrospective review, one third of patients with PAU required surgical repair during follow-up for complications.[82] Many have recommended a more aggressive approach to type B PAU than classic type B dissection because of concern of increased risk of rupture.[84]

Because of the relatively focal aortic segment involved in PAU, this acute aortic syndrome may be suitable for endovascular therapy in many cases (see Fig. 60-e22A and 60-e22B on website).[66,82] Patients with PAU are usually older, with multiple comorbidities, which increases their risk for open surgical repair. In a series of 19 patients with complications related to PAU (including aortic rupture in seven patients, aneurysmal enlargement > 55 mm in nine patients, rapid expansion > 10 mm/year, and recurrent pain in three patients), endovascular stent-graft implantation was successful in 95%.[84]

Bacterial Infections of the Aorta

Infected aortic aneurysms are a rare but lethal condition comprising less than 1% of all aneurysms undergoing operation.[85] Although the disease may be insidious in onset, it may also have a fulminant course, with frequent aneurysm rupture (>50%) and a high mortality rate (>25% to 50%). Even in the current era, with medical therapy alone, in-hospital mortality exceeds 50%. The treatment involves aneurysm resection, débridement of infected soft tissues, antibiotics, and arterial reconstruction. Most patients receive in situ aortic grafting, and others undergo extra-anatomic bypass. Endovascular repair has been performed selectively in high-risk patients.[86] The cause of infected aneurysms is most commonly related to direct invasion of circulating microorganisms into an atherosclerotic or disrupted arterial wall. Contiguous spread of microbes from adjacent infection may occur and, occasionally, septic embolization from bacterial endocarditis may seed the aorta, resulting in septic aneurysm formation.

Most patients with an infected aortic aneurysm are symptomatic, with fever, abdominal, back, or chest pain, and a pulsatile tender mass being pathognomonic. But this classic triad is only present in the minority of patients. Patients are febrile, have leukocytosis, and have a high erythrocyte sedimentation rate. Symptoms that arise from involvement of adjacent organs include odynophagia, hematemesis, and hemoptysis. Most patients have positive blood cultures, but in some patients the organism is established only at the time of operative repair with culture and Gram stain of the aortic wall. The average patient in most series is in his or her 70s, and many patients have comorbidities, including diabetes and chronic disease, an underlying immunocompromised state, or chronic steroid therapy. Many have recently undergone gastrointestinal operations or invasive procedures. Infected aneurysms most commonly involve the infrarenal aorta, with the paravisceral and juxtarenal aorta involved less commonly. Infected thoracic aortic aneurysms are rare, most commonly affecting the descending aorta, and usually present with rupture or pseudoaneurysm.[87] Infections of prosthetic aortic grafts occur in 1% to 2% of such reconstructions and present with abdominal or back pain and fever. Aortic graft-enteric erosion or fistula occur in 50%.[85,88]

The most common microorganisms associated with infected aortic aneurysms include *Staphylococcus aureus* and *Salmonella* species, but almost any organism may be responsible. *Escherichia coli*, *Streptococcus* species, *Neisseria* species, and gram-negative bacilli and fungi have been associated. Although *Salmonella* may infect an underlying atherosclerotic aortic aneurysm, this microbe may directly penetrate an intact intima of a normal aortic wall, leading to arteritis and aneurysm formation. Thus, one should always be suspicious of underlying aortic seeding when *Salmonella* bacteremia is present.

CT, MRI, and aortography may be diagnostic in infected aortic aneurysms, with most series describing saccular aneurysms in 70% to 90% and fusiform aneurysms in 10% to 30%.[88] Features on CT scan include disruption of calcification, irregular wall thickening, periaortic mass, rim enhancement, and periaortic stranding. The presence of gas and vertebral body erosion are highly suggestive of infection. Other findings may include periaortic hematoma and associated dissecting aneurysm.[89] Aortocaval or aortoenteric fistulae may complicate infected aneurysms. The aorta is typically enlarged and aneurysmal on diagnosis but, importantly, the aorta is not always significantly dilated on presentation. These aneurysms may be rapidly expanding and have a propensity to rupture—hence, the importance of diagnosis. Because most descending or abdominal aneurysms are atherosclerotic, the lack of calcium in an involved aorta may suggest an infected aneurysm.[89] MRI features of infected aneurysms include soft tissue mass, stranding fluid retention, and rim enhancement. Imaging studies with indium-111–labelled white blood cells have been used in some cases.

The natural history of infected aortic aneurysms is that of expansion and eventual rupture, often with rapid progression. *Salmonella* and other gram-negative infections have a greater tendency for early rupture and death. Overall mortality from infected aortic aneurysms has been reported to be in excess of 50% with medical therapy alone.

The treatment of infected abdominal aortic aneurysms involves excision or exclusion of infected aortic tissue, in situ or extra-anatomic bypass of the aorta and branches, débridement of infected periaortic tissues, and prolonged antibiotic therapy. In the past, most operations included extra-anatomic bypass because of concern about the risk of postoperative aortic graft infection. Many infected aneurysms are in locations not amenable to conventional extra-anatomic reconstruction. In general, when infrarenal aortic aneurysms are associated with extensive aortic and periaortic purulence, extra-anatomic bypass is performed. In situ bypass is more commonly performed in the setting of suprarenal aneurysms or infrarenal aneurysms with minimal purulence. Recent surgical series have reported operative mortality of 12% to 21%.[85,87,88]

In a series of 43 patients with infected aneurysms, 53% had ruptured at the time of surgery, with 60% located at or above the renal arteries. The average aneurysm size was 5.9 cm (range, 3 to 12 cm), and most had periaortic extension of infection. In this series, 85% of patients underwent in situ prosthetic graft placement and 15% had extra-anatomic bypass. The operative mortality was 21%. Antibiotics were continued for 1 to 6 months in 60%, and for life in many.[85] In a series of 32 patients with infected aortic aneurysms, 25 patients underwent open repair with a mortality rate of 12%, compared with 57% on medical therapy alone.[87] Because many patients are considered at high risk of complications of surgery for infected aortic aneurysms, some have advocated endovascular repair as an option for those who

are not suitable for open repair, either as a bridge to open repair or as definitive therapy.[86]

Prosthetic stent-graft infections are uncommon, with true incidence unknown. *Staphylococcus*, *Streptococcus*, and *Enterococcus* species are the most common microorganism involved. Risk factors include wound infections, immunosuppression, diabetes, and intestinal ischemia. Pseudoaneurysm and aneurysm expansion and rupture may occur. Treatment includes removal of the infected stent-graft. Axillofemoral bypass with total graft excision and oversewing of the aorta stump has been the traditional repair, but more recently, in situ prosthetic reconstruction has had a more favorable outcome in selected cases. Operative mortality is reported at approximately 10% to 15%, with graft reinfections complicating approximately 10%.[88]

Primary Tumors of the Aorta

Aortic tumors are rare and almost always malignant. They typically present with embolism or arterial obstruction and are often not suspected until histologic analysis reveals malignancy. In one literature review, the average age was 60 years, with a male predominance.[90] Risk factors for aortic tumors are unknown, with prior radiation, prosthetic grafts, and atherosclerosis being hypothesized. Locations of these tumors include the descending thoracic aorta (35%), abdominal aorta (27%), thoracoabdominal aorta (27%), and ascending aorta and arch (11%).[90] Presenting symptoms include pain, embolism, intermittent claudication, renovascular hypertension, and visceral ischemia. Less commonly, these tumors present as stroke, hemorrhagic complications, or invasion of adjacent structures. Aortic tumors fall into three groups—intraluminal (polypoid), intimal, and adventitial (mural). Intraluminal and intimal tumors are the most common. These tumors spread along the aortic inner wall and may appear polypoid on imaging. They may present with acute arterial embolization, with the embolus being a mixture of tumor and thrombus, or lead to arterial obstruction or involvement of visceral arteries. Widely metastatic emboli may occur. Adventitial (mural) tumors are rare and grow to involve periaortic tissue and adjacent organs.

Aortic tumors are of mesenchymal origin and include intimal sarcoma (21%), malignant fibrous histiocytoma (15%), angiosarcoma (26%), leiomyosarcoma (15%), and undifferentiated sarcoma. The diagnosis is usually made by pathologic examination of tumor emboli or at surgery or autopsy, and metastatic spread is present in most patients at diagnosis. Aortography findings are nonspecific and imitate an aneurysm or mural thrombus. Intimal tumors may be detected by CT (**Fig. 60-27**), but the findings may mimic those of protruding atheroma. MRI is considered most reliable for diagnosis and may differentiate between tumor and atheromatous material. TEE has been useful in some cases. If no metastases are present, resection with prosthetic graft replacement is recommended. Because of difficulties in achieving wide margins, local recurrence of tumor may occur. Palliative treatment of obstructive tumors has included endarterectomy, endovascular grafts, and extra-anatomic bypass. Chemotherapy and radiation have been used in some cases, with limited success. The average survival has been about 1 year, with adventitial (mural) tumors having a better prognosis than intimal tumors. In surgically treated patients, 3-year survival has been reported at 16%.[90]

Future Perspectives

Because of dedicated individuals across multiple disciplines, remarkable discovery and progress have occurred in the understanding of aortic disease. Basic and translational research with experimental and animal models of aneurysms and genetically triggered aortic syndromes have led to enhanced understanding of the pathophysiologic events underlying these disorders. This knowledge may lead to direct clinical application with pharmacologic interventions that may well change the course of these diseases. Advances in biomarker development hold promise in identifying disease activity, disease progression, and response to therapy. New biomarkers may allow the rapid identification of patients with a high likelihood of acute aortic dissection.

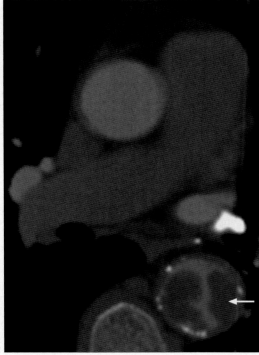

FIGURE 60-27 Contrast CT scan demonstrating an intimal tumor of the descending aorta (arrow). The tumor has the appearance of an intraluminal filling defect with septations.

Advances in imaging the aorta structurally and functionally, using techniques to understand biomechanical forces and biologic activity in the aortic wall, hold promise in following patients with aortic disease. These techniques may allow better individual decision making about the timing of preventive intervention.

Finally, rapid advances in surgical and endovascular therapy have revolutionized the management of complex aortic disease, greatly reducing the morbidity and mortality rates of elective and emergency procedures.

ACKNOWLEDGMENT

The authors gratefully acknowledge the contributions of Dr. Eric Isselbacher to previous versions of this chapter in earlier editions of this text.

REFERENCES

Abdominal Aortic Aneurysms

1. Golledge J, Norman PE: Pathophysiology of abdominal aortic aneurysm relevant to improvements in patients' management. Curr Opin Cardiol 24:532, 2009.
2. Kim LG, P Scott RA, Ashton HA, Thompson SG; Multicentre Aneurysm Screening Study Group: A sustained mortality benefit from screening for abdominal aortic aneurysm. Ann Intern Med 146:699, 2007.
3. Cosford PA, Leng GC: Screening for abdominal aortic aneurysm. Cochrane Database Syst Rev (2):CD002945, 2007.
4. Fleming C, Whitlock EP, Beil TL, Lederle FA: Screening for abdominal aortic aneurysm: A best-evidence systematic review for the U.S. Preventive Services Task Force. Ann Intern Med 142:203, 2005.
5. Chaikof EL, Brewster DC, Dalman RL, et al: The care of patients with an abdominal aortic aneurysm: The Society for Vascular Surgery practice guidelines. J Vasc Surg 50(Suppl):S2, 2009.
6. Helgadottir A, Thorleifsson G, Magnusson KP, et al: The same sequence variant on 9p21 associates with myocardial infarction, abdominal aortic aneurysm and intracranial aneurysm. Nat Genet 40:217, 2008.
7. Rayt HS, Sutton AJ, London NJ, et al: A systematic review and meta-analysis of endovascular repair (EVAR) for ruptured abdominal aortic aneurysm. Eur J Vasc Endovasc Surg 36:536, 2008.
8. Baxter BT, Terrin MC, Dalman RL: Medical management of small abdominal aortic aneurysms. Circulation 117:1883, 2008.
9. Sukhija R, Aronow WS, Sandhu R, et al: Mortality and size of abdominal aortic aneurysm at long-term follow-up of patients not treated surgically and treated with and without statins. Am J Cardiol 97:279, 2006.
10. Schermerhorn ML, O'Malley AJ, Jhaveri A, et al: Endovascular vs. open repair of abdominal aortic aneurysms in the Medicare population. N Engl J Med 358:464, 2008.
11. Lederle FA, Freischlag JA, Kyriakides TC, et al: Open Versus Endovascular Repair (OVER) Veterans Affairs Cooperative Study Group. Outcomes following endovascular vs open repair of abdominal aortic aneurysm: A randomized trial. JAMA 302:1535, 2009.
12. Sicard GA, Zwolak RM, Sidawy AN, et al: Endovascular abdominal aortic aneurysm repair: Long-term outcome measures in patients at high risk for open surgery. J Vasc Surg 44:229, 2006.
13. McPhee J, Eslami MH, Arous EJ, et al: Endovascular treatment of ruptured abdominal aortic aneurysms in the United States (2001-2006): A significant survival benefit over open repair is independently associated with increased institutional volume. J Vasc Surg 49:817, 2009.
14. Veith FJ, Lachat M, Mayer D, et al: Collected world and single center experience with endovascular treatment of ruptured abdominal aortic aneurysms. Ann Surg 250:818, 2009.

Thoracic Aortic Aneurysms

15. Ramanath VS, Oh JK, Sundt TM, Eagle KA: Acute aortic syndromes and thoracic aortic aneurysm. Mayo Clin Proc 84:465, 2009.
16. Loeys BL, Schwarze U, Holm T, et al: Aneurysm syndromes caused by mutations in the TGF-β receptor. N Engl J Med 355:788, 2006.
17. Williams JA, Loeys BL, Nwakanma LU, et al: Early surgical experience with Loeys-Dietz: A new syndrome of aggressive thoracic aortic aneurysm disease. Ann Thorac Surg 83:S757, 2007.
18. Milewicz DM, Guo DG, Tran-Fadulu V, et al: Genetic basis of thoracic aortic aneurysms and dissections: Focus on smooth muscle cell contractile dysfunction. Annu Rev Genomics Hum Genet 9:283, 2008.
19. Albornoz G, Coady MA, Roberts M, et al: Familial thoracic aortic aneurysms and dissections: Incidence, modes of inheritance, and phenotypic patterns. Ann Thorac Surg 82:1400, 2006.
20. Guo DC, Pannu H, Papke CL, et al: Mutations in smooth muscle α-actin (ACTA2) lead to thoracic aortic aneurysms and dissections. Nat Genet 39:1488, 2007.
21. Braverman AC, Beardslee MA: The bicuspid aortic valve. In Otto C, Bonow R (eds): Valvular Heart Disease: A Companion to Braunwald's Heart Disease. Philadelphia, Saunders Elsevier, 2009, pp 169-186.
22. Loscalzo ML, Goh D, Loeys B, et al: Familial thoracic aortic dilation and bicommissural aortic valve: A prospective analysis of the natural history and inheritance. Am J Med Genet A 143A:1960, 2007.
23. Biner S, Rafique AM, Ray I, et al: Aortopathy is prevalent in relatives of bicuspid aortic valve patients. J Am Coll Cardiol 53:2288, 2009.
24. Bondy CA: Aortic dissection in Turner syndrome. Curr Opin Cardiol 23:519, 2008.
25. Tan JL, Gatzoulis MA, Ho SY: Aortic root disease in tetralogy of Fallot. Curr Opin Cardiol 1:569, 2007.
26. Elefteriades JA, Farkas EA: Thoracic aortic aneurysm. Clinical pertinent controversies and uncertainties. J Am Coll Cardiol 55:841, 2010.
27. Davies RR, Goldstein LJ, Coady MA, et al: Yearly rupture or dissection rates for thoracic aortic aneurysms: Simple prediction based on size. Ann Thorac Surg 2002;73:17-27
28. Patel HJ, Deeb GM: Ascending and arch aorta: Pathology, natural history, and treatment. Circulation 118:188, 2008.
29. Davies RR, Gallo A, Coady MA, et al: Novel measurement of relative aortic size predicts rupture of thoracic aortic aneurysms. Ann Thorac Surg 81:169, 2006.
30. Davies RR, Kaple RK, Mandapati D, et al: Natural history of ascending aortic aneurysms in the setting of an unreplaced bicuspid aortic valve. Ann Thorac Surg 83:1338, 2007.
31. Januzzi JL, Isselbacher EM, Fattori R, et al: Characterizing the young patient with aortic dissection: Results from the International Registry of Acute Aortic Dissection (IRAD). J Am Coll Cardiol 43:665, 2004.
32. Hiratzka LF, Bakris GL, Beckman JA, et al: 2010 ACCF/AHA/AATS/ACR/ASA/SCA/ SCAI/SIR/STS/ SVM guidelines for the diagnosis and management of patients with Thoracic Aortic Disease: A report of the American College of Cardiology Foundation/American Heart Association Task Force on Practice Guidelines, American Association for Thoracic Surgery, American College of Radiology, American Stroke Association, Society of Cardiovascular Anesthesiologists, Society for Cardiovascular Angiography and Interventions, Society of Interventional Radiology, Society of Thoracic Surgeons, and Society for Vascular Medicine. Circulation 121:e266, 2010.
33. Fazel SS, David TE: Aortic valve-sparing operations for aortic root and ascending aortic aneurysms. Curr Opin Cardiol 22: 497, 2007.
34. Luciani GB, Mazzucco A: Aortic root disease after the Ross procedure. Curr Opin Cardiol 21:555, 2006.
35. Elefteriades JA, Botta DM: Indications for the treatment of thoracic aortic aneurysms. Surg Clin North Am 89:845, 2009.
36. Estrera AL, Miller CC 3rd, Chen EP, et al: Descending thoracic aortic aneurysm repair: 12-year experience using distal aortic perfusion and cerebrospinal fluid drainage. Ann Thor Surg 80:1290, 2005.
37. Makaroun MS, Dillavou ED, Kee ST, et al: Endovascular treatment of thoracic aortic aneurysms: Results of the phase II multicenter trial of the Gore TAG thoracic endoprosthesis. J Vasc Surg 41:1, 2005.
38. Fairman RM, Criado F, Farber M, et al: Pivotal results of the Medtronic vascular talent thoracic stent graft system: The Valor Trial. J Vasc Surg 48:546, 2008.
39. Matsumura JS, Cambria RP, Dake MD, et al: International controlled clinical trial of the thoracic endovascular aneurysm repair with the Zenith TX2 endovascular graft: 1 year results. J Vasc Surg 47:247, 2008.
40. Rizvi AZ, Murad MH, Fairman RM, et al: The effect of left subclavian artery coverage on morbidity and mortality in patients undergoing endovascular thoracic aortic interventions: A systematic review and meta-analysis. J Vasc Surg 50:1159, 2009.

Aortic Dissection

41. Hagan PG, Nienaber CA, Isselbacher EM, et al: International Registry of Acute Aortic Dissection (IRAD): New insights from an old disease. JAMA 283:897, 2000.
42. Tsai TT, Trimarchi S, Neinaber CA: Acute aortic dissection: Perspectives from the international registry of acute aortic dissection (IRAD). Eur J Vasc Endovasc Surg 37:149, 2009.
43. Hirst AE Jr, Johns VJ Jr, Kime SW Jr: Dissecting aneurysm of the aorta: A review of 505 cases. Medicine (Baltimore) 37:217, 1958.
44. Hsue PY, Salinas C, Bolger AF, et al: Acute aortic dissection induced by crack cocaine. Circulation 105:1592, 2002.

45. Goland S, Elkayam U: Cardiovascular problems in pregnant women with Marfan syndrome. Circulation 119:619, 2009.

46. Eggebrecht H, Thompson M, Rousseau H, et al: Retrograde ascending aortic dissection during or after thoracic aortic stent-graft placement: Insight from the European registry on endovascular aortic repair complications. Circulation 120(Suppl):S276, 2009.

47. Collins JS, Evangelista A, Nienaber CA, et al: Differences in clinical presentation, management, and outcomes of acute type A aortic dissection in patients with and without previous cardiac surgery. Circulation 110 (Suppl II):II-237, 2004.

48. Pape LA, Tsai TT, Isselbacher EM, et al: Aortic diameter >5.5 cm is not a good predictor of type A aortic dissection. Observations from the international registry of acute aortic dissection. Circulation 116:1120, 2007.

49. Parish LM, Gorman JH III, Kahn S, et al: Aortic size in acute type A dissection: Implications for preventative ascending aortic replacement. Eur J Cardiothorac Surg 35:941, 2009.

50. Poullis M, Warwick R, Oo A, Poole RJ: Ascending aortic curvature as an independent risk factor for type A aortic dissection, and ascending aortic aneurysm formation: A mathematical model. Eur J Cardiovasc Surg 33:995, 2008.

51. Upchurch GR, Nienaber C, Fattori R, et al: Acute aortic dissection presenting with primarily abdominal pain: A rare manifestation of a deadly disease. Ann Vasc Surg 19:367, 2005.

52. Park SW, Hutchinson S, Mehta RH, et al: Association of painless aortic dissection with increased mortality. Mayo Clin Proc 79:1252, 2004.

53. Henke PK, Williams DM, Upchurch GR Jr, et al: Acute limb ischemia associated with type B aortic dissection: Clinical relevance and therapy. Surgery 140:532, 2006.

54. Chow JL, Marian ER, Liang D: Transesophageal echocardiography assessment of severe aortic regurgitation in type A aortic dissection caused by a prolapsed circumferential intimal flap. J Cardiothorac Vasc Anesth 21:85, 2007.

55. Gaul C, Dietrich W, Erbguth FJ: Neurologic symptoms in acute aortic dissection: A challenge for neurologists. Cerebrovasc Dis 26:1, 2008.

56. Trimarchi S, Nienaber CA, Rampoldi V, et al: Contemporary results of surgery in acute type A aortic dissection: The international registry of acute aortic dissection experience. J Thorac Cardiovasc Surg 129:112, 2005.

57. Geirsson A, Szeto Wilson Y, Pochettino A, et al: Significance of malperfusion syndromes prior to contemporary surgical repair for acute type A dissection: Outcomes and need for additional revascularizations. Eur J Cardiothorac Surg 32:255, 2007.

58. Trimarchi S, Tsai T, Eagle KA, et al: Acute abdominal aortic dissection: insight from the international registry of acute aortic dissection (IRAD). J Vasc Surg 46:913, 2007.

59. Suzuki T, Distante A, Zizza A, et al: Diagnosis of acute aortic dissection by D-dimer: The international registry of acute aortic dissection substudy on biomarkers (IRAD-bio) experience. Circulation 119:2702, 2009.

60. Stevens LM, Madsen JC, Isselbacher EM, et al: Surgical management and long-term outcomes of acute ascending aortic dissection. J Thorac Cardiovasc Surg 138:1349, 2009.

61. Gilon D, Mehta RH, Oh JK, et al: Characteristics and in-hospital outcomes of patients with cardiac tamponade complicating type A acute aortic dissection. Am J Cardiol 103:1029, 2009.

62. Geirsson A, Szeto WY, Pochettino A, et al: Significance of malperfusion syndromes prior to contemporary surgical repair for acute type A dissection: Outcomes and need for additional revascularizations. Eur J Cardiothorac Surg 32:255, 2007.

63. Rampoldi V, Trimarchi S, Eagle, KA, et al: Simple risk models to predict surgical mortality in acute type A aortic dissection: The International Registry of Acute Aortic Dissection score. Ann Thorac Surg 83:55, 2007.

64. Trimarchi S, Nienaber CA, Rampoldi V, et al: Role and results of surgery in acute type B aortic dissection. Insights from the international registry of acute aortic dissection (IRAD). Circulation 114(Suppl I):1-357, 2006.

65. Estrera AL, Miller CC, Safi HJ, et al: Outcomes of medical management of acute type B aortic dissection. Circulation 114(Supp I):I-384, 2006.

66. Svensson LG, Kouchoukos NT, Miller DC, et al: Expert consensus document on the treatment of descending thoracic aortic disease using endovascular stent-grafts. Ann Thorac Surg 85:(Suppl):1, 2008.

67. Tsai TT, Isselbacher EM, Trimarchi S, et al: Acute type B aortic dissection: Does aortic arch involvement affect management and outcomes? Insights from the International Registry of Acute Aortic Dissection (IRAD). Circulation 116:I-150, 2007.

68. Lin PH, Huynh TT, Kougias P, et al: Descending thoracic aortic dissection: Evaluation and management in the era of endovascular technology. Vasc Endovasc Surg 43:5, 2009.

69. Patel HJ, Williams DM, Meerkov M, et al: Long-term results of percutaneous management of malperfusion in acute Type B aortic dissection: Implications of thoracic aortic endovascular repair. J Thorac Cardiovasc Surg 38:300, 2009.

70. Nienaber CA, Kische S, Zeller T, et al: Provisional extension to induce complete attachment after stent-graft placement in type B aortic dissection: The PETTICOAT concept. J Endovasc Ther 13:738, 2006.

71. Nienaber CA, Rousseau H, Eggbrecht H, et al: Randomized comparison of strategies for type B aortic dissection. The Investigation of STEnt grafts in Aortic Dissection (INSTEAD) Trial. Circulation 120:2519, 2009.

72. Tsai TT, Evangelista A, Nienaber CA, et al: Long-term survival in patients presenting with type A acute aortic dissection. Insights from the International Registry of Acute Aortic Dissection. Circulation 114(Suppl I):I-350, 2006.

73. Jault F, Rama A, Lievre L, et al: Chronic dissection of the ascending aorta: Surgical results during a 20-year period. Eur J Cardiothorac Surg 29:1041, 2006.

74. Tsai TT, Fattori R, Trimarchi S, et al: Long-term survival in patients presenting with type B acute aortic dissection. Insights from the international registry of acute aortic dissection. Circulation 114:2226, 2006.

75. Tsai TT, Evangelista A, Nienaber CA, et al: Partial thrombosis of the false lumen in patients with acute type B dissection. N Engl J Med 357:349, 2007.

76. Song JK, Kim S, Kim J, et al: Long-term predictors of descending aorta aneurysmal change in patients with aortic dissection. J Am Coll Cardiol 50:799, 2007.

77. Evangelista A, Mukherjee D, Mehta RH, et al: Acute intramural hematoma of the aorta. Circulation 111:1063, 2005.

78. Song JK, Yim JH, Ahn JM, Kim DH, et al: Outcomes of patients with acute type A intramural hematoma. Circulation 120:2046, 2009.

79. Pelzel JM, Braverman AC, Hirsch AT, Harris KM: International heterogeneity in diagnostic frequency and clinical outcomes of ascending aortic intramural hematoma. J Am Soc Echo 20:1260, 2007.

80. Moizumi Y, Komatsu T, Motoyoshi N, Tabayashi K: Clinical features and long-term outcome of type A and type B intramural hematoma. J Thorac Cardiovasc Surg 127:421, 2004.

81. Kitai T, Kaji S, Tani T, et al: Clinical outcomes of medical therapy and timely operation in initially diagnosed type A intramural hematoma: a 20 year experience. Circulation 120(Suppl):S292, 2009.

82. Estrera A, Miller C 3rd, Lee TY, et al: Acute type A intramural hematoma: Analysis of current management strategy. Circulation 120(Suppl):S287, 2009.

83. Sundt TM: Intramural hematoma and penetrating atherosclerotic ulcer of the aorta. Ann Thorac Surg 83:S835, 2007.

84. Botta L, Buttazzi K, Russo V, et al: Endovascular repair for penetrating atherosclerotic ulcers of the descending aorta: Early and mid-term results. Ann Thorac Surg 85:987, 2008.

85. Oderich GS, Panneton JM, Bower TC et al: Infected aortic aneurysms: Aggressive presentation, complicated early outcome, but durable results. J Vasc Surg 34:900, 2001.

86. Patel HJ, Williams DM, Upchurch GR Jr, et al: Late outcomes of endovascular aortic repair for the infected thoracic aorta. Ann Thorac Surg 87:1366, 2009.

87. Hsu RB, Lin FY: Infected aneurysm of the thoracic aorta. J Vasc Surg 47:270, 2008.

88. Oderich GS, Bower TC, Cherry KJ Jr, et al: Evolution from axillofemoral to in situ prosthetic reconstruction for the treatment of aortic graft infections at a single center. J Vasc Surg 43:1166, 2006.

89. Lin MP, Chang SC, Wu RH, et al: A comparison of computed tomography, magnetic resonance imaging, and digital subtraction angiography findings in the diagnosis of infected aortic aneurysm. J Comput Assist Tomogr 32:616, 2008.

Primary Tumors of the Aorta

90. Chiche L, Mongredien B, Brocheriou I, Kieffer E: Primary tumors of the thoracoabdominal aorta: Surgical treatment of 5 patients and review of the literature. Ann Vasc Surg 17:354, 2003.

CHAPTER 61 Peripheral Artery Diseases

Mark A. Creager and Peter Libby

Peripheral artery disease (PAD) generally refers to a disorder that obstructs the blood supply to the lower or upper extremities.[1] Most commonly caused by atherosclerosis, it may also result from thrombosis, embolism, vasculitis, fibromuscular dysplasia, or entrapment. The term *peripheral vascular disease* is less specific because it encompasses a group of diseases affecting blood vessels, including other atherosclerotic conditions such as renal artery disease and carotid artery disease, as well as vasculitides, vasospasm, venous thrombosis, venous insufficiency, and lymphatic disorders.

PAD correlates strongly with risk of major cardiovascular events, as it frequently associates with coronary and cerebral atherosclerosis.[2] Moreover, symptoms of PAD, including intermittent claudication, jeopardize quality of life and independence for many patients. PAD is commonly underdiagnosed and undertreated; thus, practitioners of cardiology have increasing interest in its diagnosis and management. This chapter provides a framework for the diagnosis and management of the patient with PAD.

Epidemiology

The prevalence of PAD varies according to the population studied, the diagnostic method used, and whether symptoms are included to derive estimates. Most epidemiologic studies have used a noninvasive measurement, the ankle-brachial index (ABI), to diagnose PAD. The ABI is the ratio of the ankle to brachial systolic blood pressure (described in greater detail later). The prevalence of PAD based on abnormal ABI ranges from approximately 4% among persons 40 years of age and older to 15% to 20% among those 65 years of age and older.[3-6] PAD prevalence is greater in men than in women in some studies, and greater in blacks than in non-Hispanic whites.[7] In the Multi-Ethnic Study of Atherosclerosis (MESA), the odds for development of PAD were 1.47 times higher in blacks than in non-Hispanic whites, whereas it was less than 0.5 times higher in Hispanics and Chinese.[8] These aggregate data indicate that some 8 to 10 million individuals in the United States have PAD.

Questionnaires specifically designed to elicit symptoms of intermittent claudication can assess the prevalence of symptomatic disease in these populations. Estimates vary by age and sex but generally indicate that only 10% to 30% of patients with PAD have claudication. Overall, the estimated prevalence of claudication ranges from 1.0% to 4.5% of a population older than 40 years.[6,9] The prevalence and incidence of claudication increase with age and are greater in men than in women in most studies (**Fig. 61-1**).[3,6,9,10] Less information exists about the incidence of critical limb ischemia, but it is estimated at 400 to 450 per million population per year.[6] The incidence of amputation ranges from 112 to 250 per million population per year.

Risk Factors for Peripheral Artery Disease

(see Chap. 44)

The well-known modifiable risk factors associated with coronary atherosclerosis also contribute to atherosclerosis of the peripheral circulation. Cigarette smoking, diabetes mellitus, dyslipidemia, and hypertension increase the risk of PAD[11] (**Table 61-1**). Data from observational studies indicate a twofold to threefold increase in the risk for development of PAD in smokers.[6] Approximately 84% to 90% of patients with claudication are current or former smokers.[12] Progression of disease to critical limb ischemia and limb loss is more likely to occur in patients who continue to smoke than in those who stop. Smoking can even increase the risk for development of PAD more than it does coronary artery disease (CAD). Current smoking dose-dependently correlates with the presence of PAD in both men and women, and smoking cessation lowers PAD risk.[13] Patients with diabetes mellitus often have extensive and severe PAD and a greater propensity for arterial calcification.[14,15] Involvement of the femoral and popliteal arteries resembles that of nondiabetic persons, but distal disease affecting the tibial and peroneal arteries occurs more frequently. The risk for development of PAD increases twofold to fourfold in patients with diabetes mellitus.[6,16] Among patients with PAD, diabetic patients are more likely to have an amputation than are nondiabetic patients.

Abnormalities in lipid metabolism also associate with an increased prevalence of PAD. Elevations in total or low-density lipoprotein (LDL) cholesterol increase the risk for development of PAD and claudication in most studies. Hypertriglyceridemia independently predicts risk for

PAD.[16] Some epidemiologic studies have found a link between hypertension and PAD.[17] Insulin resistance is associated with a greater prevalence of PAD.[18] Chronic kidney disease also increases the risk for development of PAD.[19] The risk for development of PAD and intermittent claudication increases progressively with the burden of contributing factors. Contemporary views of atherogenesis emphasize inflammation as a link between risk factors and the formation and complication of lesions. Strong evidence supports the concept that the pathobiology of PAD also involves inflammation. Classic studies associated high levels of fibrinogen with risk not only for coronary events but also for the development of PAD. Current analyses suggest that adjustment for the trigger of the acute-phase response, interleukin-6, or for inflammatory markers, such as C-reactive protein, eliminates the risk for PAD associated with fibrinogen.[20] Thus, the elevated fibrinogen levels in PAD may reflect inflammation as much as or more than a procoagulant effect. Considerable evidence links leukocytes, the crucial cellular mediators of the inflammatory response, with the development of PAD. Levels of the soluble forms of leukocyte adhesion molecules correlate with the development and extent of PAD and with the risk of complications.[21-25] Levels of C-reactive protein and of monocytes in peripheral blood independently associate with PAD, consistent with a role for innate immunity and chronic inflammation in its pathogenesis.[23,26] Conversely, serum bilirubin, an endogenous antioxidant with anti-inflammatory properties, associates with reduced PAD prevalence.[27] Inflammation provides the mechanistic link between many of the common risk factors for atherosclerosis and the pathophysiologic processes in the arterial wall that lead to PAD. Ongoing studies will determine whether biomarkers of inflammation add to traditional risk factors in gauging susceptibility to PAD.

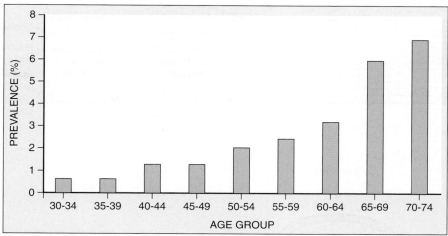

FIGURE 61-1 Age-related prevalence of intermittent claudication, derived from large population-based studies. *(From Norgren L, Hiatt WR, Dormandy JA, et al: Inter-Society Consensus for the Management of Peripheral Arterial Disease [TASC II]. Eur J Vasc Endovasc Surg 33:S1, 2007.)*

Pathophysiology of Peripheral Artery Disease

Pathophysiologic considerations in patients with PAD must take into account the balance of circulatory supply of nutrients to the skeletal muscle and the oxygen and nutrient demand of the skeletal muscle (**Table 61-2**). Intermittent claudication occurs when skeletal muscle oxygen demand during effort exceeds blood oxygen supply and results from activation of local sensory receptors by accumulation of lactate or other metabolites. Patients with intermittent claudication may have single or multiple occlusive lesions in the arteries supplying the limb. Blood flow and leg oxygen consumption are normal at rest, but the obstructive lesions limit blood flow and oxygen delivery so that the metabolic needs of the exercising muscle during exercise outstrip the available supply of oxygen and nutrients. Patients with critical limb ischemia typically have multiple occlusive lesions that often affect proximal and distal limb arteries. As a result, even the resting blood supply diminishes and cannot meet the nutritional needs of the limb.

Factors Regulating Blood Supply (see Chap. 52)

The primary determinant of inadequate blood supply to an extremity is a flow-limiting lesion of a conduit artery (**Fig. 61-2**). Flow through an artery is directly proportional to perfusion pressure and inversely proportional to vascular resistance. If atherosclerosis causes a stenosis, flow through the artery is reduced, as described in Poiseuille's equation:

$$Q = \frac{\Delta P \pi r^4}{8 \eta l}$$

where ΔP is the pressure gradient across the stenosis, r is the radius of the residual lumen, η is blood viscosity, and l is the length of the vessel affected by the stenosis. As the severity of a stenotic lesion increases, flow becomes progressively reduced. The pressure gradient across the stenosis increases in a nonlinear manner, emphasizing the importance of a stenosis at high blood flow rates. Usually, a blood pressure gradient

TABLE 61-1 Odds Ratio of Peripheral Artery Disease in Persons with Risk Factors

RISK FACTOR	ODDS RATIO (95% CONFIDENCE INTERVAL)
Cigarette smoking	4.46 (2.25-8.84)
Diabetes mellitus	2.71 (1.03-7.12)
Hypertension	1.75 (0.97-3.13)
Hypercholesterolemia	1.68 (1.09-2.57)
Hyperhomocysteinemia	1.92 (0.95-3.88)
Chronic kidney disease	2.00 (1.08-3.70)
Insulin resistance	2.06 (1.10-4.00)
C-reactive protein	2.20 (1.30-3.60)

Data derived from reports of the National Health and Nutrition Examination (Selvin E, Erlinger TP: Prevalence of and risk factors for peripheral arterial disease in the United States: Results from the National Health and Nutrition Examination Survey, 1999-2000. Circulation 110:738, 2004; Pande RL, Perlstein TS, Beckman JA, Creager MA: Association of insulin resistance and inflammation with peripheral arterial disease: The National Health and Nutrition Examination Survey, 1999 to 2004. Circulation 118:33, 2008; O'Hare AM, Glidden DV, Fox CS, Hsu CY: High prevalence of peripheral arterial disease in persons with renal insufficiency: Results from the National Health and Nutrition Examination Survey 1999-2000. Circulation 109:320, 2004; Guallar E, Silbergeld EK, Navas-Acien A, et al: Confounding of the relation between homocysteine and peripheral arterial disease by lead, cadmium, and renal function. Am J Epidemiol 163:700, 2006.)

TABLE 61-2 Pathophysiologic Considerations in Peripheral Artery Disease

Factors Regulating Blood Supply to Limb

Flow-limiting lesion (stenosis severity, inadequate collateral vessels)

Impaired vasodilation (decreased nitric oxide and reduced responsiveness to vasodilators)

Accentuated vasoconstriction (thromboxane, serotonin, angiotensin II, endothelin, norepinephrine)

Abnormal rheology (reduced red blood cell deformability, increased leukocyte adhesivity, platelet aggregation, microthrombosis, increased fibrinogen)

Altered Skeletal Muscle Structure and Function

Axonal denervation of skeletal muscle

Loss of type II, glycolytic fast-twitch fibers

Impaired mitochondrial enzymatic activity

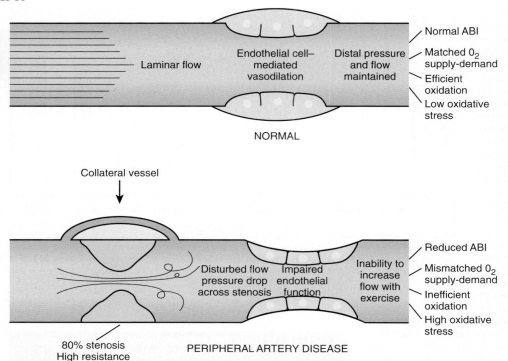

FIGURE 61-2 Pathophysiology of intermittent claudication. In healthy arteries **(top)**, flow is laminar and endothelial function is normal; therefore, blood flow and oxygen delivery match muscle metabolic demand at rest and during exercise. Muscle metabolism is efficient, resulting in low oxidative stress. In contrast, in peripheral artery disease **(bottom)**, the arterial stenosis results in disturbed flow, and the loss of kinetic energy results in a pressure drop across the stenosis. Collateral vessels have high resistance and only partially compensate for the arterial stenosis. In addition, endothelial function is impaired, resulting in further loss of vascular function. These changes limit the blood flow response to exercise, resulting in a mismatch of oxygen delivery to muscle metabolic demand. Changes in skeletal muscle metabolism further compromise the efficient generation of high-energy phosphates. Oxidant stress, the result of inefficient oxidation, further impairs endothelial function and muscle metabolism. *(From Hiatt WR, Brass EP: Pathophysiology of intermittent claudication. In Creager MA, Dzau VJ, Loscalzo J [eds]: Vascular Medicine. A Companion to Braunwald's Heart Disease. Philadelphia, Elsevier, 2006.)*

exists at rest if the stenosis reduces the lumen diameter by more than 50% because as distorted flow develops, kinetic energy is lost. A stenosis that does not cause a pressure gradient at rest may cause one during exercise, when blood flow increases from higher cardiac output and vascular resistance decreases. Thus, as flow through a stenosis increases, distal perfusion pressure drops. As the metabolic demand of exercising muscle outstrips its blood supply, local metabolites (including adenosine, nitric oxide, potassium, and hydrogen ion) accumulate, and peripheral resistance vessels dilate. Perfusion pressure then drops further because the stenosis limits flow. In addition, intramuscular pressure rises during exercise and may exceed the arterial pressure distal to an occlusion, causing blood flow to cease. Flow through collateral blood vessels can usually meet the resting metabolic needs of the skeletal muscle tissue at rest but does not suffice during exercise.

Functional abnormalities in vasomotor reactivity also may interfere with blood flow. Vasodilator capability of both conduit and resistance vessels is reduced in patients with peripheral atherosclerosis. Normally, arteries dilate in response to pharmacologic and biochemical stimuli, such as acetylcholine, serotonin, thrombin, and bradykinin, as well as to shear stress induced by increases in blood flow. This vasodilator response results from the release of biologically active substances from the endothelium, particularly nitric oxide (see Chap. 48). The vascular relaxation of a conduit vessel that occurs after a flow stimulus, such as that induced by exercise, may facilitate the delivery of blood to exercising muscles in healthy persons. Endothelium-dependent vasodilation subsequent to flow or pharmacologic stimuli is impaired in the atherosclerotic femoral arteries and calf resistance vessels of patients with PAD. This failure of vasodilation might prevent an increase in nutritive blood supply to exercising muscle because endothelium-derived nitric oxide can contribute to hyperemic blood volume after an ischemic stimulus. It is not known whether vasodilator function with respect to prostacyclin, adenosine, or ion channels is abnormal in atherosclerotic peripheral arteries. Endogenous vasoconstrictor substances, such as prostanoids and other lipid mediators, thrombin, serotonin, angiotensin II, endothelin, and norepinephrine, may interfere with vasodilation.

Abnormalities in the microcirculation contribute to the pathophysiology of critical limb ischemia. Patients with severe limb ischemia have a reduced number of perfused skin capillaries. Other potential causes of decreased capillary perfusion in this condition include reduced red blood cell deformability, increased leukocyte adhesivity, platelet aggregates, fibrinogen, microvascular thrombosis, excessive vasoconstriction, and interstitial edema. Intravascular pressure may also decrease because of precapillary arteriolar dilation due to locally released vasoactive metabolites.[28]

Skeletal Muscle Structure and Metabolic Function

Electrophysiologic and histopathologic examination has found evidence of partial axonal denervation of the skeletal muscle in legs affected by PAD. There is preservation of type I, oxidative slow-twitch fibers but a loss of type II, or glycolytic, fast-twitch fibers in the skeletal muscle of patients with PAD.[10] The loss of type II fibers correlates with decreased muscle strength and reduced exercise capacity. In skeletal muscle distal to PAD, there is a shift to anaerobic metabolism earlier during exercise, and it persists longer after cessation of exercise. Patients with claudication have increased lactate release and accumulation of acylcarnitines during exercise and slowed oxygen desaturation kinetics, indicative of ineffective oxidative metabolism.[29,30] Moreover, mitochondrial respiratory activity and phosphocreatine and adenosine triphosphate recovery time are delayed in the calf muscles of PAD patients, as assessed after submaximal exercise by ^{31}P magnetic resonance spectroscopy.[31]

Clinical Presentation

Symptoms

The cardinal symptoms of PAD include intermittent claudication and rest pain. The term *claudication* is derived from the Latin word *claudicare*, "to limp." Intermittent claudication refers to a pain, ache, sense of fatigue, or other discomfort that occurs in the affected muscle group with exercise, particularly walking, and resolves with rest. The location of the symptom often relates to the site of the most proximal stenosis. Buttock, hip, or thigh claudication typically occurs in patients with obstruction of the aorta and iliac arteries. Calf claudication characterizes femoral or popliteal artery stenoses. The gastrocnemius muscle consumes more oxygen during walking than other muscle groups in the leg and hence causes the most frequent symptom reported by patients. Ankle or foot claudication occurs in patients with tibial and peroneal artery disease. Similarly, stenoses of the subclavian, axillary, or brachial arteries may cause shoulder, biceps, or forearm claudication, respectively. Symptoms should resolve several minutes after cessation of effort. Calf and thigh pain that occurs at rest, such as nocturnal cramps, should not be confused with claudication and is not a symptom of PAD. The history obtained from persons reporting claudication should note the walking distance, speed, and incline that precipitate claudication. This baseline assessment evaluates disability and provides an initial qualitative measure with which to determine stability, improvement, or deterioration during subsequent encounters with the patient. Symptoms other than claudication can limit functional capacity.[32] Patients with PAD walk more slowly and have less walking endurance than patients who do not have PAD.[33]

Several questionnaires have been developed to assess the presence and severity of claudication. The Rose Questionnaire was developed initially to diagnose both angina and intermittent claudication in epidemiologic surveys. It questions whether the patient develops pain in either calf with walking and whether the pain occurs at rest, while walking at an ordinary or hurried pace, or on walking uphill. There have been several modifications to this questionnaire, including the Edinburgh Claudication Questionnaire and the San Diego Claudication Questionnaire,[34] both of which are more sensitive and specific than a physician's diagnosis of intermittent claudication based on walking distance, walking speed, and nature of symptoms. Another validated instrument, the Walking Impairment Questionnaire, asks a series of questions and develops a point score based on walking distance, walking speed, and nature of symptoms.[35]

Symptoms resembling limb claudication occasionally result from nonatherosclerotic causes of arterial occlusive disease (**Table 61-3**). These other causes include arterial embolism; vasculitides such as thromboangiitis obliterans, Takayasu arteritis, and giant cell arteritis; aortic coarctation; fibromuscular dysplasia; irradiation; endofibrosis of the external iliac artery; and extravascular compression due to arterial entrapment or adventitial cyst (see Chap. 89). Several nonvascular causes of exertional leg pain should be considered in patients who present with symptoms suggestive of intermittent claudication (see Table 61-3). Lumbosacral radiculopathy resulting from degenerative joint disease, spinal stenosis, and herniated discs can cause pain in the buttock, hip, thigh, calf, or foot with walking, often after very short distances, or even with standing. This symptom has been called neurogenic pseudoclaudication. Lumbosacral spine disease and PAD both preferentially affect the elderly and hence may coexist in the same individual. Arthritis of the hips and knees also provokes leg pain with walking. Typically, the pain localizes to the affected joint and can be elicited on physical examination through palpation and range-of-motion maneuvers. Exertional compartment syndrome is most often seen in athletes with large calf muscles; increased tissue pressure during exercise limits microvascular flow and results in calf pain or tightness. Symptoms improve after cessation of exercise. Rarely, skeletal muscle disorders such as myositis can cause exertional leg pain. Muscle tenderness, an abnormal neuromuscular examination finding, elevated skeletal muscle enzyme levels, and a normal pulse examination finding should distinguish myositis from PAD. McArdle syndrome, in which there is a deficiency of skeletal muscle phosphorylase, can cause symptoms mimicking the claudication of PAD. Patients with chronic venous insufficiency sometimes report leg discomfort with exertion, which is designated venous claudication. Venous hypertension during exercise increases arterial resistance in the affected limb and limits blood flow. In the case of venous insufficiency, elevated extravascular pressure caused by interstitial edema further diminishes capillary perfusion. A physical examination demonstrating peripheral edema, venous stasis pigmentation, and occasionally venous varicosities will identify this unusual cause of exertional leg pain.

Symptoms may occur at rest in patients with critical limb ischemia. Typically, patients complain of pain or paresthesias in the foot or toes of the affected extremity. This discomfort worsens on leg elevation and improves with leg dependency, as might be anticipated by the effect of gravity on perfusion pressure. The pain can be particularly severe at sites of skin fissuring, ulceration, or necrosis. Often the skin is very sensitive, and even the weight of bedclothes or sheets elicits pain. Patients may sit on the edge of the bed and dangle their legs to alleviate the discomfort. Patients with ischemic or diabetic neuropathy can experience little or no pain despite the presence of severe ischemia.

Critical limb and digital ischemia can result from arterial occlusions other than those caused by atherosclerosis. These include conditions such as thromboangiitis obliterans, vasculitides such as systemic lupus erythematosus or scleroderma, vasospasm, atheromatous embolism, and acute arterial occlusion caused by thrombosis or embolism (see later). Acute gouty arthritis, trauma, and sensory neuropathy such as that caused by diabetes mellitus, lumbosacral radiculopathies, and complex regional pain syndrome (previously known as reflex sympathetic dystrophy) can cause foot pain. Leg ulcers also occur in patients with venous insufficiency and sensory neuropathy, particularly that related to diabetes. These ulcers are easily distinguished from those caused by arterial disease. The ulcer of venous insufficiency usually localizes near the medial malleolus and has an irregular border and a pink base with granulation tissue. Ulcers due to venous disease produce milder pain than those caused by arterial disease. Neurotrophic ulcers occur where there is pressure or trauma, usually on the sole of the foot. These ulcers are deep, frequently infected, and usually not painful because of the loss of sensation (**Fig. 61-3**).

TABLE 61-3 Differential Diagnosis of Exertional Leg Pain

Vascular Causes
Atherosclerosis
Thrombosis
Embolism
Vasculitis
   Thromboangiitis obliterans
   Takayasu arteritis
   Giant cell arteritis
Aortic coarctation
Fibromuscular dysplasia
Irradiation
Endofibrosis of the external iliac artery
Extravascular compression
   Arterial entrapment (e.g., popliteal artery entrapment, thoracic outlet syndrome)
   Adventitial cysts

Nonvascular Causes
Lumbosacral radiculopathy
   Degenerative arthritis
   Spinal stenosis
   Herniated disc
Arthritis
   Hips, knees
Venous insufficiency
Myositis
McArdle syndrome

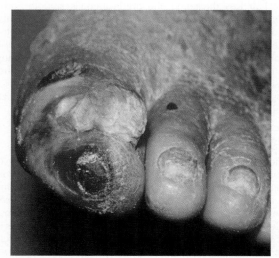

FIGURE 61-3 A typical arterial ulcer. It is a discrete, circumscribed, necrotic ulcer, located on the great toe.

TABLE 61-4	Fontaine Classification of Peripheral Artery Disease
STAGE	**SYMPTOMS**
I	Asymptomatic
II	Intermittent claudication
IIa	Pain free, claudication walking >200 m
IIb	Pain free, claudication walking <200 m
III	Rest and nocturnal pain
IV	Necrosis, gangrene

TABLE 61-5	Clinical Categories of Chronic Limb Ischemia	
GRADE	**CATEGORY**	**CLINICAL DESCRIPTION**
	0	Asymptomatic, not hemodynamically correct
I	1	Mild claudication
	2	Moderate claudication
	3	Severe claudication
II	4	Ischemic rest pain
	5	Minor tissue loss: nonhealing ulcer, focal gangrene with diffuse pedal ulcer
III	6	Major tissue loss extending above transmetatarsal level, functional foot no longer salvageable

Modified from Rutherford RB, Baker JD, Ernst C, et al: Recommended standards for reports dealing with lower extremity ischemia: Revised version. J Vasc Surg 26:517, 1997.

Physical Findings

The complete cardiovascular examination includes palpation of pulses and auscultation of accessible arteries for bruits (see also Fig. 12-4). Pulse abnormalities and bruits increase the likelihood of PAD.[36] Readily palpable pulses in healthy individuals include the brachial, radial, and ulnar arteries of the upper extremities and the femoral, popliteal, dorsalis pedis, and posterior tibial arteries of the lower extremities. The aorta also can be palpated in thin people. A decreased or absent pulse provides insight into the location of arterial stenoses. For example, a normal right femoral pulse but absent left femoral pulse suggests the presence of left iliofemoral arterial stenosis. A normal femoral artery pulse but absent popliteal artery pulse would indicate a stenosis in the superficial femoral artery or proximal popliteal artery. Similarly, disease of the anterior and posterior tibial arteries can be inferred when the popliteal artery pulse is present but the dorsalis pedis and posterior tibial pulses, respectively, are not palpable. Bruits often indicate accelerated blood flow velocity and flow disturbance at sites of stenosis. A stethoscope should be used to auscultate the supraclavicular and infraclavicular fossae for evidence of subclavian artery stenosis; the abdomen, flank, and pelvis for evidence of stenoses in the aorta and its branch vessels; and each groin for evidence of femoral artery stenoses. Pallor can be elicited on the soles of the feet of some patients with PAD by performing a maneuver in which the feet are elevated above the level of the heart and the calf muscles are exercised by repeated dorsiflexion and plantar flexion of the ankle. The legs are then placed in the dependent position, and the time to the onset of hyperemia and venous distention is measured. Each of these variables depends on the rate of blood flow, which in turn reflects the severity of stenosis and adequacy of collateral vessels.

The legs of patients with chronic aortoiliac disease may show muscle atrophy. Additional signs of chronic low-grade ischemia include hair loss, thickened and brittle toenails, smooth and shiny skin, and subcutaneous fat atrophy of the digital pads. Patients with severe limb ischemia have cool skin and may also have petechiae, persistent cyanosis or pallor, dependent rubor, pedal edema resulting from prolonged dependency, skin fissures, ulceration, or gangrene. Ulcers due to PAD typically have a pale base with irregular borders and usually involve the tips of the toes or the heel of the foot or develop at sites of pressure (Fig. 61-3). These ulcers vary in size and may be as small as 3 to 5 mm.

Categorization

Classification of patients with PAD depends on the severity of the symptoms and abnormalities detected on physical examination. Categorization of the clinical manifestations of PAD improves communication among professionals caring for these patients and provides a structure for defining guidelines for therapeutic interventions. Fontaine described one widely used scheme that classified patients in one of four stages progressing from asymptomatic to critical limb ischemia (**Table 61-4**). Several professional vascular societies have adopted a contemporary, more descriptive classification that includes asymptomatic patients, three grades of claudication, and three grades of

critical limb ischemia ranging from rest pain alone to minor and major tissue loss (**Table 61-5**).[37]

Testing in Peripheral Artery Disease

Segmental Pressure Measurement

The measurement of systolic blood pressure along selected segments of each extremity furnishes one of the simplest and most useful noninvasive tests to evaluate the presence and severity of stenoses in the peripheral arteries. In the lower extremities, pneumatic cuffs are placed on the upper and lower portions of the thigh, on the calf, above the ankle, and often over the metatarsal area of the foot. Likewise, for the upper extremities, pneumatic cuffs are placed on the upper arm over the biceps, on the forearm below the elbow, and at the wrist. Systolic blood pressure at each respective limb segment is measured by first inflating the pneumatic cuff to suprasystolic pressure, then determining the pressure at which blood flow occurs during cuff deflation. The onset of flow is assessed by placing a Doppler ultrasound flow probe over an artery distal to the cuff. In the lower extremities, it is most convenient to place the Doppler probe on the foot over the posterior tibial artery, as it courses inferior and posterior to the medial malleolus, or over the dorsalis pedis artery on the dorsum of the metatarsal arch. In the upper extremities, the Doppler probe can be placed over the brachial artery in the antecubital fossa or over the radial and ulnar arteries at the wrist.

Left ventricular contraction imparts kinetic energy to blood, which is maintained throughout the large and medium-sized vessels. Systolic blood pressure may be higher in the more distal vessels than in the aorta and proximal vessels because of amplification and reflection of blood pressure waves. A stenosis can cause loss of pressure energy, as a result of increased frictional forces and flow disturbance at the site of the stenosis. Approximately 90% of the cross-sectional area of the aorta must be narrowed before a pressure gradient develops. In smaller vessels, such as the iliac and femoral arteries, a 70% to 90% decrease in cross-sectional area will cause a resting pressure gradient sufficient to decrease systolic blood pressure distal to the stenosis. Taking into consideration the precision of this noninvasive method and the variability in blood pressure during even short periods, a blood pressure gradient in excess of 20 mm Hg between successive cuffs is generally used as evidence of arterial stenosis in the lower extremity, whereas a gradient of 10 mm Hg indicates a stenosis between sequential cuffs in the upper extremity. Systolic blood pressure in the toes and fingers approximates 60% of the systolic blood pressure at the ankle and wrist, respectively, as pressure diminishes further in the smaller distal vessels.

Figure 61-4 gives examples of leg segmental pressure measurements in a patient with bilateral calf claudication. In the right leg, there are pressure gradients between the upper and lower thigh and between the calf and ankle. These gradients indicate stenoses in the superficial femoral artery and in the tibioperoneal arteries. In the left leg, pressure gradients between the upper and lower thigh, between

gauge the severity of PAD. Patients with symptoms of leg claudication often have ABIs ranging from 0.5 to 0.8, and patients with critical limb ischemia usually have an ABI of less than 0.5. The ABI correlates inversely with walking distance and speed. Fewer than 40% of patients whose ABI is less than 0.40 can complete a 6-minute walk.[38] In patients with skin ulcerations, an ankle pressure of less than 55 mm Hg would predict poor ulcer healing. One limitation of leg blood pressure recordings is that they cannot be used reliably in patients with calcified vessels, as might occur in persons with diabetes mellitus or renal insufficiency. The calcified vessel cannot be compressed during inflation of the pneumatic cuff, and therefore the Doppler probe indicates continuous blood flow, even when the pressure exceeds 250 mm Hg.

Treadmill Exercise Testing

Treadmill exercise testing can evaluate the clinical significance of peripheral artery stenoses and provide objective evidence of the patient's walking capacity. The claudication onset time is defined as the time at which symptoms of claudication first develop, and the peak walking time is when the patient is no longer able to continue walking because of severe leg discomfort. This standardized and more objective measurement of walking capacity supplements the patient's history and provides a quantitative assessment of his or her disability, as well as a metric for monitoring therapeutic interventions.

Treadmill exercise protocols use a motorized treadmill that incorporates fixed or progressive speeds and angles of incline. A fixed workload test usually maintains a constant grade of 12% and speed of 1.5 to 2.0 miles per hour. A progressive, or graded, treadmill protocol typically maintains a constant speed of 2 miles per hour while the grade is gradually increased by 2% every 2 to 3 minutes. Reproducibility of repeated treadmill test results is reportedly better with progressive than with constant grade protocols.[39]

Treadmill testing can determine whether arterial stenoses contribute to the patient's symptoms of exertional leg pain. During exercise, blood flow through a stenosis increases as vascular resistance falls in the exercising muscle. According to Poiseuille's equation, described previously, the pressure gradient across the stenosis increases in direct proportion to flow. Thus, ankle and brachial systolic blood pressures are measured under resting conditions before treadmill exercise, within 1 minute after exercise, and repeatedly until baseline values are reestablished. Normally, the blood pressure increase that occurs during exercise should be the same in both the upper and lower extremities, maintaining a constant ABI of 1.0 or greater. In the presence of peripheral artery stenoses, the ABI decreases because the increase in blood pressure observed in the arm is not matched by a comparable increase in ankle blood pressure. A 25% or greater decrease in ABI after exercise in a patient whose walking capacity is limited by claudication is considered diagnostic, implicating PAD as a cause of the patient's symptoms.

Many patients with PAD also have coronary atherosclerosis. The addition of cardiac monitoring to the exercise protocol may provide adjunctive information about the presence of myocardial ischemia. A workload sufficient to increase myocardial oxygen demand and to provoke myocardial ischemia may not be achieved in patients whose exercise capacity is limited by claudication. Nonetheless, electrocardiographic changes, particularly during low levels of treadmill exercise, may provide evidence of severe CAD.

Pulse Volume Recording

The pulse volume recording graphically illustrates the volumetric change in a segment of the limb that occurs with each pulse. Plethysmographic instruments, typically using strain gauges or pneumatic cuffs, can transduce volumetric changes in the limb, which can be displayed on a graphic recorder. These transducers are strategically placed along the limb to record the pulse volume in its different segments, such as the thigh, calf, ankle, metatarsal region, and toes or the upper arm, forearm, and fingers. The normal pulse volume contour depends on both local arterial pressure and vascular wall distensibility and resembles a blood pressure waveform. It consists of a sharp

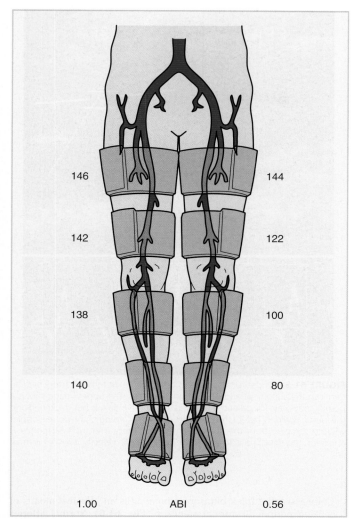

FIGURE 61-4 Segmental pressure measurements in a patient with left calf intermittent claudication. Pressure gradient is present between the left upper and lower thigh cuffs, lower thigh and calf cuffs, and calf and ankle cuffs, consistent with multisegmental disease affecting the femoral-popliteal and tibial arteries. The left ankle-brachial index is 0.56, which is abnormal. The segmental pressure measurements and ankle-brachial index in the right leg are normal.

the lower thigh and calf, and between the calf and ankle indicate stenoses in the superficial femoral and popliteal arteries and in the tibioperoneal arteries.

Ankle-Brachial Index

Determination of the ABI furnishes a simplified application of leg segmental blood pressure measurements readily used at the bedside (see Fig. 61-4 and Fig. 12-4). This index is the ratio of the systolic blood pressure measured at the ankle to the systolic blood pressure measured at the brachial artery. A pneumatic cuff placed around the ankle is inflated to suprasystolic pressure and subsequently deflated while the onset of flow is detected with a Doppler ultrasound probe placed over the dorsalis pedis and posterior tibial arteries, thus denoting ankle systolic blood pressure. Brachial artery systolic pressure can be assessed in a routine manner, with use of either a stethoscope to listen for the first Korotkoff sound or a Doppler probe to listen for the onset of flow during cuff deflation. The normal ABI should be 1.0 or greater; recognizing the variability intrinsic to sequential blood pressure measurements, however, an ABI of less than 0.90 is considered abnormal and is 90% to 95% sensitive and 98% to 100% specific for angiographically verified peripheral arterial stenosis.[6] The ABI is often used to

systolic upstroke rising rapidly to a peak, a dicrotic notch, and a concave downslope that drops off gradually toward the baseline. The contour of the pulse wave changes distal to a stenosis, with loss of the dicrotic notch, a slower rate of rise, a more rounded peak, and a slower descent. The amplitude becomes lower with increasing severity of disease, and the pulse wave may not be recordable at all in the critically ischemic limb. Segmental analysis of the pulse wave may indicate the location of an arterial stenosis, which is likely to be sited in the artery between a normal and an abnormal pulse volume recording. The pulse volume wave also provides information about the integrity of blood flow when blood pressure measurements cannot be accurately obtained because of noncompressible vessels.

Doppler Ultrasonography

Continuous-wave and pulsed-wave Doppler systems transmit and receive high-frequency ultrasound signals. The Doppler frequency shift caused by moving red blood cells varies directly with the velocity of blood flow. Typically, the perceived frequency shift is between 1 and 20 kHz and is within the audible range of the human ear. Therefore, placement of a Doppler probe along an artery enables the examiner to hear whether blood flow is present and the vessel is patent. Processing and graphic recording of the Doppler signal permit a more detailed analysis of the frequency components.

Doppler instruments can be used without or with gray-scale imaging to evaluate an artery for the presence of stenoses. The Doppler probe is positioned at approximately a 60-degree angle over the common femoral, superficial femoral, popliteal, dorsalis pedis, and posterior tibial arteries. The normal Doppler waveform has three components: a rapid forward flow component during systole, a transient flow reversal during early diastole, and a slow anterograde component during late diastole. The Doppler waveform becomes altered if the probe is placed distal to an arterial stenosis and is characterized by deceleration of systolic flow, loss of the early diastolic reversal, and diminished peak frequencies. Arteries in a limb with critical ischemia may not show any Doppler frequency shift. As with pulse volume recordings, a change from a normal to an abnormal Doppler waveform as the artery is interrogated more distally provides inferential evidence of the location of a stenosis.

Duplex Ultrasound Imaging

Duplex ultrasound imaging provides a direct, noninvasive means of assessing both the anatomic characteristics of peripheral arteries and the functional significance of arterial stenoses. The methodology incorporates gray-scale B-mode ultrasound imaging, pulsed Doppler velocity measurements, and color coding of the Doppler-shift information (**Fig. 61-5**). Real-time ultrasonography scanners emit and receive high-frequency sound waves, typically ranging from 2 to 10 MHz, to construct an image. The acoustic properties of the vascular wall differ from those of the surrounding tissue, enabling them to be imaged easily. Atherosclerotic plaque may be present and visible on gray-scale images. Pulsed-wave Doppler systems emit ultrasound beams at precise times and can therefore sample the reflected ultrasound waves at specific depths, enabling the examiner to determine the blood cell velocity within the lumen of the artery. Positioning the pulsed Doppler beam at a known angle, the examiner can calculate blood flow velocity according to the equation

$$Df = 2VF\cos\theta/C$$

where Df is the frequency shift, V is the velocity, F is the frequency of the transmitted sound, θ is the angle between the transmitted sound and the velocity vector, and C is the velocity of sound and tissue. For optimal measurements, the angle of the pulsed Doppler beam should be less than 60 degrees. With color Doppler, the frequency shift information within the entire field sampled by the ultrasound beam can be superimposed on the gray-scale image. This approach provides a composite real-time display of flow velocity within the vessel.

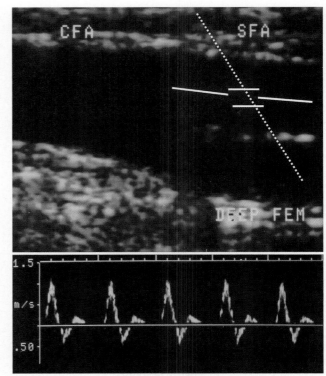

FIGURE 61-5 Duplex ultrasonogram of the common femoral artery bifurcation into the superficial and deep femoral arteries. The upper image shows a normal gray-scale image of the artery in which the intima is not thickened and the lumen is widely patent. The lower image is a recording of the pulse Doppler velocity sampled from the superficial femoral artery. The triphasic profile is apparent, the envelope is thin, and the peak systolic velocity is within normal limits.

Color-assisted duplex ultrasound imaging is an effective means of localizing peripheral arterial stenoses (**Fig. 61-6**). Normal arteries have laminar flow, with the highest velocity at the center of the artery. The corresponding color image is usually homogeneous, with relatively constant hue and intensity. In the presence of an arterial stenosis, blood flow velocity increases through the narrowed lumen. As the velocity increases, there is progressive desaturation of the color display, and flow disturbance distal to the stenosis causes changes in hue and color. Pulsed Doppler velocity measurements can be made along the length of the artery and particularly at areas of flow abnormalities suggested by the color images. A twofold or greater increase in peak systolic velocity at the site of an atherosclerotic plaque indicates a 50% or greater stenosis (see Fig. 61-6). A threefold increase in velocity suggests 75% or greater stenosis. An occluded artery generates no Doppler signal. With contrast angiography as a reference standard, duplex ultrasound imaging for identification of sites of arterial stenoses has approximately 89% to 99% specificity and 80% to 98% sensitivity.[40]

Magnetic Resonance Angiography

Magnetic resonance angiography (MRA) can visualize noninvasively the aorta and the peripheral arteries (see Chaps. 18 and 60). The resolution of the vascular anatomy with gadolinium-enhanced MRA approaches that of conventional contrast digital subtraction angiography (**Fig. 61-7**). Comparative studies have reported excellent interobserver agreement, sensitivity of 93% to 100%, and specificity of 96% to 100% for the aorta, iliac, femoropopliteal, and tibioperoneal arteries.[40-42] MRA currently has greatest utility for the evaluation of symptomatic patients to assist decision making before endovascular and surgical intervention or in patients at risk for renal, allergic, or other complications during conventional angiography.

Computed Tomographic Angiography

Computed tomographic angiography (CTA) uses intravenous administration of radiocontrast material to opacify and visualize the aorta and peripheral arteries (see Chap. 19). New computed tomography scanners use multidetector technology to acquire cross-sectional images. This advance permits imaging of peripheral arteries with excellent spatial resolution during a relatively short time, with a reduced amount of radiocontrast material (**Fig. 61-8**).[43] Images can be displayed in three dimensions and rotated to optimize visualization of arterial stenoses. Compared with conventional contrast angiography, the sensitivity and specificity for stenoses greater than 50% or occlusion reported for CTA using multiple detector technology are 95% (95% CI, 92% to 97%) and 96% (95% CI, 93% to 97%), respectively.[44] CTA offers an advantage over MRA in that it can be used in patients with stents, metal clips, and pacemakers, although it has the disadvantage of requiring radiocontrast and ionizing radiation.

Contrast Angiography

Conventional angiography, using a radioiodinated or other contrast agent, can aid in the evaluation of the arterial anatomy before a revascularization procedure. It still has occasional utility when the diagnosis is in doubt. Most contemporary angiography laboratories

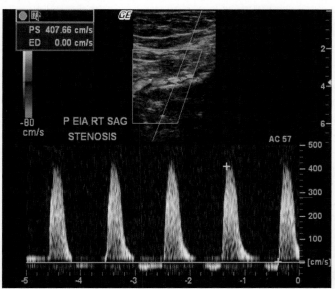

FIGURE 61-6 Duplex ultrasonogram of the external iliac artery. The **upper image** shows a color image of the artery in which there is heterogeneity and desaturation of color, indicative of high-velocity flow through a stenosis. The **lower image** is a recording of the pulse Doppler velocity sampled from the right external iliac artery. The peak velocity of 350 cm/sec is elevated. These features are consistent with a significant stenosis.

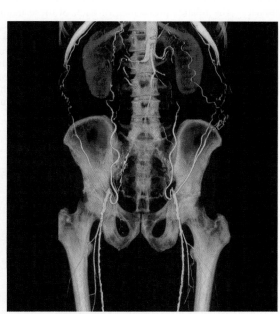

FIGURE 61-8 Computed tomographic angiogram of a patient with complete occlusion of the aorta and both iliac arteries. There is reconstitution of the common femoral arteries. *(Courtesy of the 3D and Image Processing Center of Brigham and Women's Hospital, Boston, Mass.)*

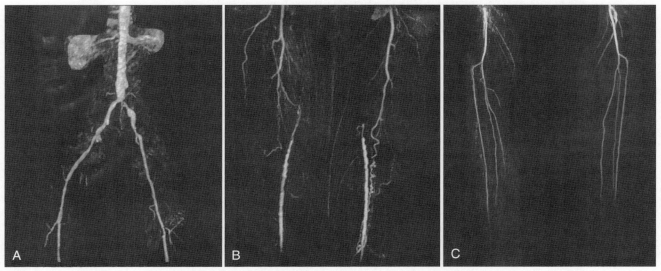

FIGURE 61-7 Gadolinium-enhanced two-dimensional magnetic resonance angiogram of the aorta and both legs, extending from the thighs to above the ankle. **A,** Aortoiliac atherosclerosis with stenosed left common iliac artery. **B,** Bilateral superficial femoral artery occlusion with reconstitution of the distal portion of the right and left superficial femoral arteries. **C,** The anterior tibial, posterior tibial, and peroneal arteries, which are patent in each leg.

use digital subtraction techniques after intra-arterial administration of contrast material to enhance resolution. Injection of the radiocontrast material into the aorta permits visualization of the aorta and iliac arteries, and injection of contrast material into the iliofemoral segment of the involved leg permits optimal visualization of the femoral, popliteal, tibial, and peroneal arteries (**Fig. 61-9**). In patients with aortic occlusion, catheterization of the femoral arteries is not feasible. The aorta can be approached by brachial or axillary artery cannulation or, if necessary, directly by a translumbar approach.

Prognosis

Patients with PAD have an increased risk for adverse cardiovascular events, as well as the risk of limb loss and impaired quality of life.[2,9,11,33] Patients with PAD frequently have concomitant CAD and cerebrovascular disease.[6,9] The relative prevalence of each of these manifestations of atherosclerosis depends in part on the diagnostic criteria used to establish their diagnosis. Patients with abnormal ABIs are twofold to fourfold more likely than those with normal ABIs to have a history of myocardial infarction (MI), angina, congestive heart failure, or cerebrovascular ischemia.[6,9] Coronary calcium scores and carotid artery intima-media thickness are greater in patients with PAD than in those without PAD.[45] Angiographically significant CAD occurs in approximately 60% to 80% of patients with PAD,[9] and 15% to 25% of patients with PAD have significant carotid artery stenoses as detected by duplex ultrasonography. Two international registries have detected a high coprevalence of CAD and cerebrovascular disease in patients with PAD. In the Reduction of Atherothrombosis for Continued Health (REACH) registry, 62% of patients had either or both coronary and cerebrovascular disease.[46] Approximately 25% of the patients with PAD had a history of MI, 30% had angina, 16% had a prior stroke, and 15% had a prior transient ischemic attack. In the AGATHA (A Global Atherothrombosis Assessment) registry, approximately 50% of patients with PAD had established CAD, and 50% had prior stroke, transient ischemic attack, or carotid artery revascularization.[47] The specificity of an abnormal ABI to predict future cardiovascular events is approximately 90%.[48] The risk of death from cardiovascular causes increases 2.5- to 6-fold in patients with PAD, and their annual mortality rate is 4.3% to 4.9%.[6,9,49] The risk of death is greatest in those with the most severe PAD, and mortality correlates with decreasing ABI (**Fig. 61-10**).[50-52] Approximately 25% of patients with critical limb ischemia die within 1 year, and the 1-year mortality rate among patients who have undergone amputation for PAD may be as high as 45%.[6]

Approximately 25% of patients with claudication develop worsening symptoms. Moreover, mobility loss occurs more commonly in patients with PAD than in those without PAD, even among patients who do not

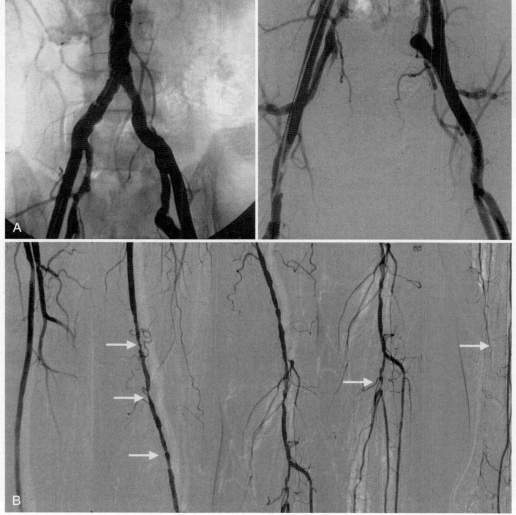

FIGURE 61-9 Angiogram of a patient with disabling left calf claudication. **A,** The aorta and bilateral common iliac arteries are patent. **B,** The left superficial femoral artery has multiple stenotic lesions (arrows). There is a significant stenosis of the left tibioperoneal trunk and left posterior tibial artery (arrows).

have classic symptoms of claudication.[32] Clinical progression to critical limb ischemia occurs in 7% to 9% of patients with claudication in the first year after diagnosis and in approximately 2% to 3% each year thereafter.[6,9,53] Both smoking and diabetes mellitus independently predict progression of disease.[6,9] The risk of amputation in those with diabetes mellitus is at least 12-fold higher than in nondiabetic persons.[54]

Treatment

The goal for treatment of PAD is reduction in cardiovascular morbidity and mortality, as well as improvement in quality of life by decreasing symptoms of claudication, eliminating rest pain, and preserving limb viability. Therapeutic considerations therefore include risk factor modification by lifestyle measures and pharmacologic therapy to reduce the risk of adverse cardiovascular events, such as MI, stroke, and death. Symptoms of claudication can improve with pharmacotherapy or exercise rehabilitation. Optimal management of critical limb ischemia often includes endovascular interventions or surgical reconstruction to improve blood supply and to maintain limb viability. Revascularization is also indicated in some patients with disabling symptoms of claudication that persist despite exercise therapy and pharmacotherapy.[6,9]

Risk Factor Modification

(see Chaps. 47 and 49)

Lipid-lowering therapy can reduce the risk of adverse cardiovascular events (see Chap. 47). The Heart Protection Study found that lipid-lowering therapy with simvastatin reduced the risk of adverse cardiovascular outcomes by 25% in patients with atherosclerosis, including more than 6700 patients with PAD (**Fig. 61-11**).[55] Pooled results from 17 lipid-lowering trials found that lipid-lowering therapy reduced the risk of cardiovascular events in patients with PAD by 26%.[56] Thus, patients with PAD should receive diet and drug therapy to achieve a target LDL-cholesterol level of 100 mg/dL or less.[9] Also, several prospective trials have found that statins improve walking distance in patients with PAD.[57-59] In the Treatment of Peripheral Atherosclerotic Disease with Moderate or Intensive Lipid Lowering (TREADMILL) trial, atorvastatin (80 mg) increased pain-free walking distance by more than 60%, compared with a 38% increase with placebo (**Fig. 61-12**).[58] Additional trials support these findings.[60] Also, patients treated with statins have superior leg functioning, as assessed by walking speed and distance, compared with those not treated.[61] It is not known whether other lipid-lowering therapies (such as niacin, ezetimibe, or fibrates) reduce the risk for cardiovascular events in patients with PAD. In the Fenofibrate and Event Lowering Intervention in Diabetes (FIELD) study, fenofibrate reduced the risk of minor amputation, primarily among patients who did not have known PAD.[62]

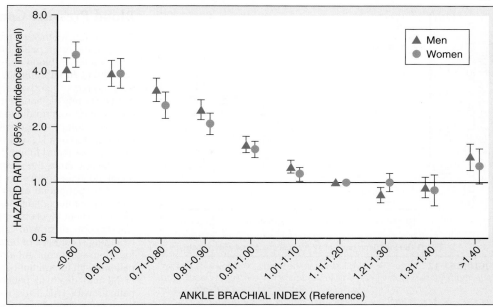

FIGURE 61-10 Association of ABI with all-cause mortality in a meta-analysis of 16 cohort studies. *(From Fowkes FG, Murray GD, Butcher I, et al: Ankle brachial index combined with Framingham Risk Score to predict cardiovascular events and mortality: A meta-analysis. JAMA 300:197, 2008.)*

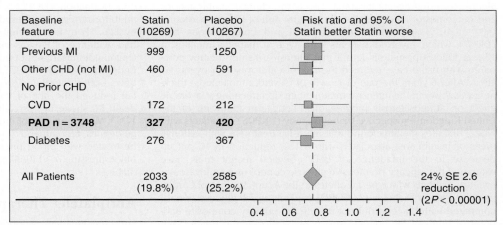

FIGURE 61-11 Relative risk of adverse cardiovascular events in participants of the Heart Protection Study, based on treatment with statin or placebo. Included in this study were 6700 patients with PAD, including 3748 patients who had no prior coronary heart disease (CHD), in whom there was an approximate 24% risk reduction of vascular events. CVD = cardiovascular disease; MI = myocardial infarction. *(From MRC/BHF Heart Protection Study of cholesterol lowering with simvastatin in 20,536 high-risk individuals: A randomized placebo-controlled trial. Lancet 360:7, 2002.)*

Smoking Cessation

Prospective trials examining the benefits of smoking cessation are lacking, but observational evidence unequivocally shows that cigarette smoking increases the risk of atherosclerosis and its clinical sequelae. Nonsmokers with PAD have lower rates of MI and mortality than those who have smoked or continue to smoke, and PAD patients who discontinue smoking have approximately twice the 5-year survival rate of those who continue to smoke.[12] Smoking cessation also lowers the risk for the development of critical limb ischemia. In addition to frequent physician advice, pharmacologic interventions that effectively promote smoking cessation include nicotine replacement therapy, bupropion, and varenicline.[63,64]

Treatment of Diabetes (see Chap. 64)

Aggressive treatment of diabetes decreases the risk for microangiopathic events such as nephropathy and retinopathy, but current data

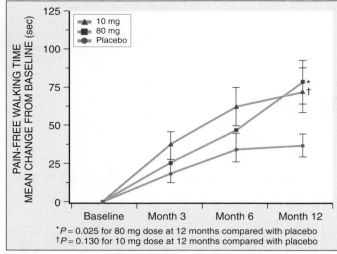

FIGURE 61-12 In the TREADMILL study, lipid-lowering therapy with atorvastatin improved pain-free walking time in patients with intermittent claudication. *(From Mohler ER III, Hiatt WR, Creager MA: Cholesterol reduction with atorvastatin improves walking distance in patients with arterial artery disease. Circulation 108:1481, 2003.)*

fail to support the notion that aggressive treatment of diabetes with glucose-lowering agents favorably affects the clinical manifestations and outcomes of atherosclerosis in general and of PAD in particular (see Chap. 64). In the Diabetes Control and Complications Trial (DCCT), which involved patients with type 1 diabetes mellitus, a 13-year follow-up analysis found that intensive insulin therapy, compared with usual care, reduced the risk of cardiovascular events by 42%.[65] After 6 years, the rate of growth of carotid intima-media thickness was lower in the intensive treatment group, indicating a favorable effect on atherosclerosis progression.[66] Long-term follow-up of the United Kingdom Prospective Diabetes Study (UKPDS) of patients with type 2 diabetes mellitus found that intensive treatment with sulfonylureas or insulin was associated with a 15% reduction in MI but no decrease in the incidence of PAD.[67] Several recent trials have examined the efficacy of intensive glucose control on cardiovascular events in patients with type 2 diabetes. In the Action to Control Cardiovascular Risk in Diabetes (ACCORD) study, intensive glucose control compared with placebo did not reduce the primary composite endpoint of nonfatal MI, nonfatal stroke, or cardiovascular death,[68] but intensive glucose control increased the risk of death and decreased the risk of nonfatal MI, which were secondary outcome measures. In the ADVANCE study, intensive glucose control reduced microvascular events, primarily the incidence of nephropathy, but did not affect macrovascular events, notably cardiovascular death.[69] In the Veterans Affairs Diabetes Trial (VADT), intensive glucose control did not affect the primary composite endpoint of MI, stroke, cardiovascular death, congestive heart failure, revascularization, and amputation for ischemic gangrene.[70] The PROactive (Prospective Pioglitazone Clinical Trial in Macrovascular Events) study assessed the effect of pioglitazone versus placebo on a broad range of cardiovascular endpoints in patients with type 2 diabetes and established atherosclerosis, including CAD, cerebrovascular disease, and PAD, and found no significant benefit of pioglitazone on the primary outcome.[71] Among patients with no PAD at baseline, composite primary and secondary event rates were less with pioglitazone than with placebo treatment. In the PAD patients, however, pioglitazone did not affect these cardiovascular events in patients with PAD.[72] A meta-analysis of five prospective randomized controlled trials found that intensive glycemic control resulted in a 17% reduction in events of nonfatal MI and a 15% reduction in coronary heart disease events, but it had no significant effect on stroke or all-cause mortality.[73] Current guidelines recommend that patients with PAD and diabetes be treated with glucose-lowering agents to achieve a hemoglobin A1c of <7.0%.[9,74]

Blood Pressure Control

Antihypertensive therapy reduces the risk of stroke, CAD, and vascular death. In the Appropriate Blood Pressure Control in Diabetes (ABCD) trial, intensive blood pressure control to levels approximating 128/75 mm Hg substantially reduced cardiovascular events compared with moderate blood pressure control in patients with PAD.[75] In the ACCORD study of patients with diabetes at high risk for cardiovascular events, there was no difference in cardiovascular outcomes between intensive antihypertensive therapy to achieve a systolic blood pressure less than 120 mm Hg and standard therapy to a target systolic blood pressure less than 140 mm Hg.[76] It is not known whether antihypertensive therapy limits the progression of PAD. Treatment of hypertension might decrease perfusion pressure to extremities already compromised by peripheral artery stenoses. In addition, concern has been raised about the potential adverse affects of beta-adrenergic receptor blockers (beta blockers) on peripheral blood flow and symptoms of claudication or critical limb ischemia. A recent systematic review including six studies of beta blocker therapy compared with placebo found no significant impairment on walking capacity in a total of 119 patients with intermittent claudication.[77] Beta blockers reduce the risk of MI and death in patients with CAD, a problem affecting many patients with PAD. Thus, if clinically indicated for other conditions, these drugs should not be withheld in patients with PAD. The balance of evidence supports the treatment of hypertension in patients with PAD according to established clinical guidelines (see Chap. 46).[78]

Angiotensin-converting enzyme inhibitors reduce cardiovascular events in patients with atherosclerosis. In the Heart Outcomes Prevention Evaluation (HOPE) study, the angiotensin-converting enzyme inhibitor ramipril decreased the risk for vascular death, MI, or stroke by 22%.[79] Forty-four percent of the patients enrolled in the HOPE trial had evidence of PAD, as manifested by an ABI less than 0.9. In the Ongoing Telmisartan Alone and in Combination with Ramipril Global Endpoint Trial (ONTARGET) of patients with vascular disease or diabetes, both ramipril and the angiotensin receptor antagonist telmisartan reduced the rate of the composite endpoint of cardiovascular death, MI, stroke, or hospitalization for heart failure by approximately 17%.[80] More than 13% of the patients in ONTARGET had PAD. Current guidelines recommend that patients with PAD and hypertension be treated with blood pressure–lowering agents to achieve a target blood pressure of <140/90 mm Hg, or <130/80 mm Hg in patients with diabetes.[9]

Antiplatelet Therapy (see Chap. 87)

Substantial evidence supports the use of antiplatelet agents to reduce adverse cardiovascular outcomes in patients with atherosclerosis. A meta-analysis that included approximately 135,000 high-risk patients with atherosclerosis, including those with acute and prior MI, stroke, or transient cerebrovascular ischemia, and other high-risk groups including those with PAD, found that antiplatelet therapy yielded a 22% reduction in subsequent vascular death, MI, or stroke.[81] Among the 9214 patients with PAD, included in this analysis, antiplatelet therapy reduced the risk of MI, stroke, or death by 22%. The majority of the PAD trials in this report, however, included antiplatelet therapy other than aspirin. A recent meta-analysis that included 18 prospective, randomized controlled trials, comprising 5269 persons with PAD, found that aspirin therapy compared with placebo was not associated with significant reductions in all-cause or cardiovascular mortality, MI, or major bleeding.[82] Included in this analysis was the Prevention of Progression of Arterial Disease and Diabetes (POPADAD) trial of diabetic patients with asymptomatic PAD, which found that aspirin did not decrease the risk of a composite primary endpoint including death from coronary heart disease or stroke, nonfatal MI or stroke, or amputation above the ankle for critical limb ischemia.[83] Within the Aspirin for Asymptomatic Atherosclerosis trial, in the 3350 participants with ABI ≤0.95, aspirin (100 mg daily) did not significantly reduce vascular events (**Fig. 61-13**).[84] The Clopidogrel versus Aspirin in Patients at Risk of Ischemic Events (CAPRIE) trial compared clopidogrel with aspirin for efficacy in preventing ischemic events in patients with recent MI,

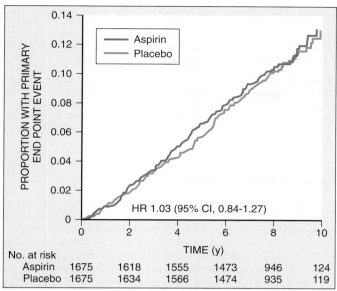

FIGURE 61-13 The primary endpoint event according to treatment group and duration of follow-up in the subset of participants in the Aspirin for Asymptomatic Atherosclerosis Trial with ABI ≤0.95 (fatal or nonfatal coronary event, stroke, or revascularization). CI indicates confidence interval; HR, hazard ratio. *(From Fowkes FG, Price JF, Stewart MC, et al: Aspirin for prevention of cardiovascular events in a general population screened for a low ankle brachial index: A randomized controlled trial. JAMA 303:841, 2010.)*

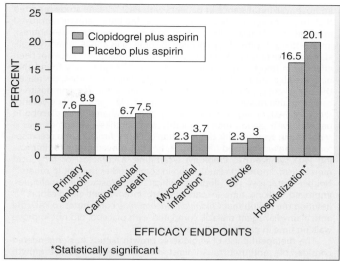

FIGURE 61-14 The effect of clopidogrel plus aspirin versus placebo plus aspirin on the rate of the composite endpoint (cardiovascular death, myocardial infarction, or stroke), cardiovascular death, myocardial infarction, stroke, and hospitalization (for unstable angina, transient ischemic attack, or revascularization procedure). *(From Cacoub PP, Bhatt DL, Steg PG, et al: Patients with peripheral arterial disease in the CHARISMA trial. Eur Heart J 30:192, 2009.)*

recent ischemic stroke, or PAD. Overall, there was an 8.7% relative risk reduction for MI, ischemic stroke, or vascular death in the group treated with clopidogrel.[85] Notably, among the 6452 patients in the PAD subgroup, clopidogrel treatment reduced adverse cardiovascular events by 23.8%. The Clopidogrel for High Atherothrombotic Risk and Ischemic Stabilization, Management, and Avoidance (CHARISMA) trial compared the efficacy of dual antiplatelet therapy with clopidogrel plus aspirin to aspirin alone in patients with established CAD, cerebrovascular disease, or PAD, as well as in patients with multiple atherosclerotic risk factors.[86] Overall, dual antiplatelet therapy produced no significant benefit compared with aspirin alone on the primary efficacy endpoint, a composite of MI, stroke, or cardiovascular death. Among the 3096 patients with PAD in the CHARISMA trial, dual antiplatelet therapy reduced the rates of MI and hospitalization for ischemic events (**Fig. 61-14**).[87] The Warfarin Antiplatelet Vascular Evaluation (WAVE) trial compared combination antiplatelet and oral anticoagulant therapy with antiplatelet therapy alone in patients with PAD.[88] There was no significant difference between the two treatments on the primary composite endpoint of MI, stroke, or cardiovascular death, but life-threatening bleeding occurred more frequently in patients receiving combination antiplatelet and anticoagulant therapy.

Current guidelines recommend that patients with PAD be treated with an antiplatelet drug, such as aspirin or clopidogrel.[9] Oral anticoagulation with warfarin is not recommended to reduce cardiovascular events in patients with PAD because it is no more effective than antiplatelet therapy and confers a higher risk of bleeding. Antiplatelet therapy also prevents occlusion in the peripheral circulation after revascularization procedures. Of approximately 3000 patients with peripheral arterial procedures previously analyzed by the Antiplatelet Trialists Collaboration, the odds reduction for arterial or graft occlusion by antiplatelet therapy (primarily aspirin or aspirin plus dipyridamole) was 43%.

Pharmacotherapy

The development of effective pharmacotherapy for symptoms of PAD has lagged substantially behind drug treatment for CAD. Most studies of vasodilator therapy have failed to demonstrate any efficacy in patients with intermittent claudication. Several pathophysiologic explanations may account for the failure of vasodilator therapy in patients with PAD. During exercise, resistance vessels distal to a stenosis dilate in response to ischemia. Vasodilators would have minimal if any effect on these endogenously dilated vessels but would decrease resistance in other vessels and create a relative steal phenomenon, reducing blood flow and perfusion pressure to the affected leg. Moreover, in contrast to their effects on myocardial oxygen consumption in patients with CAD (due to afterload reduction), vasodilators do not reduce skeletal muscle oxygen demand.

The U.S. Food and Drug Administration (FDA) has approved two drugs, pentoxifylline (Trental) and cilostazol (Pletal), for the treatment of claudication in patients with PAD. Licensing bodies in Europe, Asia, and South America have approved additional drugs. Pentoxifylline is a xanthine derivative used to treat patients with intermittent claudication. Its action may be mediated through its hemorheologic properties, including its ability to decrease blood viscosity and to improve erythrocyte flexibility. It may have anti-inflammatory and antiproliferative effects. Pentoxifylline has marginal efficacy,[6,9] increasing maximum walking distance by only 14% compared with placebo in one study.[89] Cilostazol is a quinolinone derivative that inhibits phosphodiesterase 3, thereby decreasing cyclic adenosine monophosphate degradation and increasing its concentration in platelets and blood vessels. Although cilostazol inhibits platelet aggregation and causes vasodilation in experimental animals, its mechanism of action in patients with PAD is not known. Several trials have reported that cilostazol improves absolute claudication distance by 40% to 50% compared with placebo (**Fig. 61-15**).[90,91] Quality of life measures, assessed by the Medical Outcomes Scale (SF-36) and Walking Impairment Questionnaire, also demonstrated improvement. An FDA advisory stated that cilostazol should not be used in patients with congestive heart failure because other phosphodiesterase 3 inhibitors have been shown to decrease survival in these patients. A long-term safety trial found that cilostazol compared with placebo did not increase the risk of total or cardiovascular mortality, but the study was limited because more than 60% of patients discontinued treatment before study completion.[92]

Other classes of drugs—including statins, angiotensin-converting enzyme inhibitors, serotonin (5-HT₂) antagonists, alpha-adrenergic antagonists, L-arginine, carnitine derivatives, vasodilator prostaglandins, antibiotics, and angiogenic growth factors—have been studied or are currently under investigation for treatment of either claudication or critical limb ischemia. As noted previously, three trials have found that statins improve walking distance in patients with PAD.[57-59] One study reported that the angiotensin-converting enzyme inhibitor ramipril improved maximal claudication time.[93] Naftidrofuryl, a serotonin antagonist, improved symptoms of claudication in some trials and is currently available for use in Europe.[6] Selective serotonin 2A antagonists have not been effective in improving claudication distance.[94,95] One study found that buflomedil, a drug with adrenoceptor antagonist properties, decreased the risk of critical cardiovascular events—defined as the composite of cardiovascular death, nonfatal MI, nonfatal stroke, symptomatic deterioration of PAD, or leg amputation—by 26% compared with placebo in patients with claudication.[96] Notable among these outcomes was a reduction in symptomatic deterioration of PAD. L-Arginine, the precursor for endothelium-derived nitric oxide, has not proved useful for improving PAD symptoms.[97] Propionyl L-carnitine, a cofactor for fatty acid metabolism, improved claudication in some studies but not in others.[98] Neither beraprost nor iloprost, which are prostacyclin analogues, improved walking time in patients with intermittent claudication.[89,99] Refuting the notion that *Chlamydia pneumoniae* contributes to PAD, the antichlamydial agent rifalazil, compared with placebo, did not improve walking time in patients with claudication.[100]

The therapeutic use of angiogenic growth factors has engendered considerable enthusiasm. Administration of basic fibroblast growth factor and vascular endothelial growth factor as protein or gene therapy increases collateral blood vessel development, capillary number, and blood flow in experimental models of hindlimb ischemia. Preliminary

studies of gene therapy with hypoxia-inducible factor 1α, hepatocyte growth factor, and fibroblast growth factor 1 have yielded encouraging findings in patients with critical limb ischemia.[101-103] Placebo-controlled clinical trials of angiogenic growth factors, such as vascular endothelial growth factor and hypoxia inducible factor 1α, in patients with claudication have failed to show improvement in walking time.[104,105] Stem cell–based therapies for PAD, including intra-arterial and intramuscular administration of peripheral and bone marrow–derived stem cells to induce angiogenesis, improved ABI, rest pain, and pain-free walking time and prevented amputation in patients with chronic limb ischemia in initial reports.[106-109] These findings require confirmation with additional clinical trials.

Exercise Rehabilitation (see Chaps. 50 and 83)

Supervised exercise rehabilitation programs improve symptoms of claudication in patients with PAD. Meta-analyses of controlled studies of exercise rehabilitation found that supervised walking programs increase the average maximal distance walked by 50% to 200% (**Fig. 61-16**).[110] The greatest benefit occurred when sessions were at least 30 minutes in duration, when sessions occurred at least three times per week for 6 months, and when walking was the mode of exercise. Leg strength training also improves walking time, although not as much as treadmill exercise training.[111] Postulated mechanisms through which exercise training improves claudication include the formation of collateral vessels and improvement in endothelium-dependent vasodilation, hemorheology, muscle structure and metabolism, and walking efficiency.[112,113] Studies in experimental hindlimb ischemia have suggested that regular exercise increases the development of collateral blood vessels.[112] Exercise increases the expression of angiogenic factors, particularly in hypoxic tissue.[114,115] Exercise training may improve endothelium-dependent vasodilation in patients with PAD, as it does in patients with coronary atherosclerosis.[116] Improvement in calf blood flow has not been demonstrated consistently in patients with claudication after exercise training, although one study found that maximal calf blood flow increased commensurate with improvement in walking distance.[112,117] To date, no imaging studies have demonstrated increased collateral blood vessels after exercise training in patients with PAD.

The benefits of exercise training in patients with PAD may result from changes in skeletal muscle structure or function, such as increased muscle mitochondrial enzyme activity, oxidative metabolism, and ATP production rate. In patients with PAD, improvement in exercise performance is associated with a decrease in plasma and skeletal muscle short-chain acylcarnitine concentrations, which

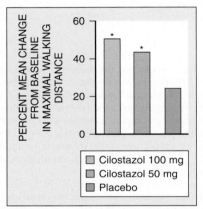

FIGURE 61-15 The effect of cilostazol compared with placebo on maximal walking distance, based on a meta-analysis of nine randomized trials. *(Modified from Pande RL, Hiatt WR, Zhang P, et al: A pooled analysis of the durability and predictors of treatment response of cilostazol in patients with intermittent claudication. Vasc Med 15:181, 2010.)*

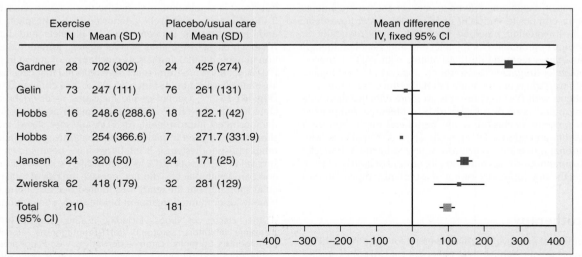

FIGURE 61-16 A meta-analysis of the effect of exercise training versus usual care on maximum walking distance in patients with intermittent claudication. *(From Watson L, Ellis B, Leng GC: Exercise for intermittent claudication. Cochrane Database Syst Rev [4]:CD000990, 2008.)*

indicates improvement in oxidative metabolism and increased peak oxygen consumption. Higher physical activity levels in patients with PAD are associated with greater calf muscle area and density.[38] Training may also enhance biomechanical performance, enabling patients to walk more efficiently with less energy expenditure. Current guidelines recommend that patients with intermittent claudication undergo supervised exercise rehabilitation as initial therapy. Supervised exercise training should consist of 30- to 45-minute sessions, at least three times per week, for a minimum of 12 weeks.[9]

Percutaneous Transluminal Angioplasty and Stents (see Chap. 63)

Peripheral catheter-based interventions are indicated for patients with lifestyle-limiting claudication, despite a trial of exercise rehabilitation or pharmacotherapy.[6,9,118] Endovascular intervention should be considered in symptomatic patients with clinical evidence of inflow disease, manifested by buttock or thigh claudication and diminished femoral pulses. Patients with critical limb ischemia whose anatomy is amenable to catheter-based therapy should also receive endovascular intervention.

Peripheral Artery Surgery

Surgical revascularization generally improves quality of life in patients with disabling claudication on maximal medical therapy and is indicated to relieve rest pain and to preserve limb viability in patients with critical limb ischemia that is not amenable to percutaneous interventions. The specific operation must take into account the anatomic location of the arterial lesions and the presence of comorbid conditions. The surgical procedure is planned after identification of the arterial obstruction by imaging, ensuring that there is sufficient arterial inflow to and outflow from the graft to maintain patency. A preoperative evaluation to assess the risk of vascular surgery should be performed because many of these patients have coexisting CAD. Guidelines for this evaluation exist (see Chap. 85).[119]

Aorto-bifemoral bypass is the most frequent operation for patients with aortoiliac disease. Typically, a knitted or woven prosthesis made of Dacron or polytetrafluoroethylene (PTFE) is anastomosed proximally to the aorta and distally to each common femoral artery. On occasion, the iliac artery is used for the distal anastomosis to maintain anterograde flow into at least one hypogastric artery.

Extra-anatomic surgical reconstructive procedures for aortoiliac disease include axillo-bifemoral bypass, ilio-bifemoral bypass, and femoral-femoral bypass. These bypass grafts, made of Dacron or PTFE, circumvent the aorta and iliac arteries and are generally used in high-risk patients with critical limb ischemia. Long-term patency rates are inferior to those of aorto-bifemoral bypass procedures. Five-year patency rates range from 50% to 70% for axillo-bifemoral bypass operations and from 70% to 80% for femoral-femoral bypass grafts.[9] The operative mortality rate for extra-anatomic bypass procedures is 3% to 5% and reflects, in part, the serious comorbid conditions and advanced atherosclerosis of many of the patients who undergo these procedures.

Reconstructive surgery for infrainguinal arterial disease includes femoral-popliteal and femoral-tibial or femoral-peroneal artery bypass. In situ or reversed autologous saphenous veins or synthetic grafts made of PTFE are used for the infrainguinal bypass. Patency rates for autologous saphenous vein bypass grafts exceed those with PTFE grafts,[6,9] and patency rates are better for grafts in which the distal anastomosis is placed in the popliteal artery above the knee, compared with below the knee.[6] Five-year primary patency rates for femoral-popliteal reconstruction in patients with claudication are approximately 80% and 75% for autogenous vein grafts or PTFE grafts, respectively, and approximately 65% and 45%, respectively, in patients with critical limb ischemia. For femoral below-knee bypass, including tibioperoneal artery reconstruction, the 5-year patency rates for saphenous vein grafts in patients with claudication or critical limb ischemia are comparable to those for femoral-popliteal above-knee grafts (60%

to 80%). The 5-year patency rate for PTFE grafts in the infrapopliteal position is considerably lower, approximating 65% in patients with claudication and 33% in patients with critical limb ischemia. The operative mortality rate for infrainguinal bypass operations is 1% to 2%.

Graft stenoses can result from technical errors at the time of surgery, such as retained valve cuffs or intimal flap or valvotome injury; from fibrous intimal hyperplasia, usually within 6 months of surgery; or from atherosclerosis, usually occurring within the vein graft at least 1 to 2 years after surgery. Institution of graft surveillance protocols with the use of color-assisted duplex ultrasonography has enabled the identification of graft stenoses, prompting graft revision and avoiding complete graft failure.[9] Graft outcome is improved as a result of routine ultrasonographic surveillance. Antithrombotic agents, including antiplatelet drugs and coumarin derivatives, also improve graft patency. Several studies have suggested that antiplatelet drugs may be more effective in preserving synthetic grafts, whereas coumarin derivatives may be more effective for vein bypass grafts.[120-122]

Algorithm for Treatment of the Symptomatic Leg

Figure 61-17 provides a management algorithm for the treatment of intermittent claudication.

Vasculitis (see Chap. 89)

Thromboangiitis Obliterans

Thromboangiitis obliterans (TAO) is a segmental vasculitis that affects the distal arteries, veins, and nerves of the upper and lower extremities. It typically occurs in young persons who smoke.[123]

Pathology and Pathogenesis

TAO primarily affects the medium and small vessels of the arms, including the radial, ulnar, palmar, and digital arteries, and their counterparts in the legs, including the tibial, peroneal, plantar, and digital arteries. Involvement can extend to the cerebral, coronary, renal, mesenteric, aortoiliac, and pulmonary arteries.[123] The pathologic findings include an occlusive, highly cellular thrombus incorporating polymorphonuclear leukocytes, microabscesses, and occasionally multinucleated giant cells. The inflammatory infiltrate can also affect the vascular wall, but the internal elastic membrane remains intact. In the chronic phase of the disease, the thrombus becomes organized and the vascular wall becomes fibrotic.

The precise cause of TAO is not known. Tobacco use or exposure is present in virtually every patient. Potential immunologic mechanisms include increased cellular sensitivity to types I and III collagen and the presence of antiendothelial cell antibodies. CD4 T cells have been identified in cellular infiltrates of vessels of patients with TAO.[123,124] Decreased endothelium-dependent vasodilation to acetylcholine can occur in both affected and unaffected limbs of patients with TAO, raising the possibility that reduced bioavailability of nitric oxide contributes to the disorder.[124]

Clinical Presentation

The prevalence of TAO is greater in Asia than in North America or western Europe. In the United States, TAO occurs in approximately 13 per 100,000 population.[123,124] Most patients develop symptoms before 45 years of age, and 75% to 90% are men. Patients can have claudication of the hands, forearms, feet, or calves. The majority of patients with TAO present with rest pain and digital ulcerations; often, more than one extremity is affected. Raynaud phenomenon occurs in approximately 45% of patients, and superficial thrombophlebitis,

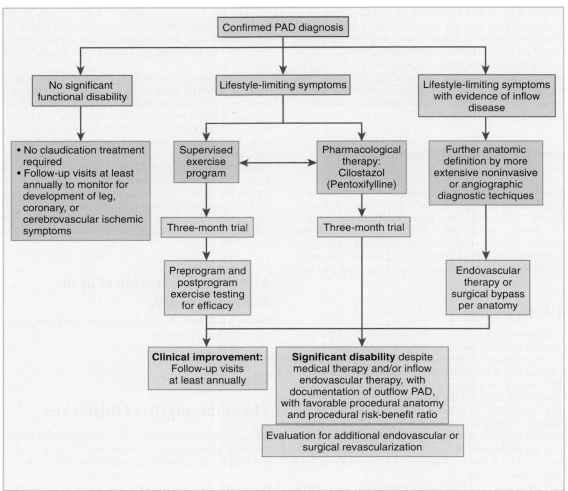

FIGURE 61-17 Management algorithm for the treatment of symptomatic PAD. *(From Hirsch AT, Haskal ZJ, Hertzer NR, et al: ACC/AHA 2005 guidelines for the management of patients with peripheral arterial disease [lower extremity, renal, mesenteric, and abdominal aortic]: Executive summary a collaborative report from the American Association for Vascular Surgery/Society for Vascular Surgery, Society for Cardiovascular Angiography and Interventions, Society for Vascular Medicine and Biology, Society of Interventional Radiology, and the ACC/AHA Task Force on Practice Guidelines [Writing Committee to Develop Guidelines for the Management of Patients With Peripheral Arterial Disease] endorsed by the American Association of Cardiovascular and Pulmonary Rehabilitation; National Heart, Lung, and Blood Institute; Society for Vascular Nursing; TransAtlantic Inter-Society Consensus; and Vascular Disease Foundation. J Am Coll Cardiol 47:1239, 2006.)*

which may be migratory, occurs in approximately 40%. The risk of amputation within 5 years is approximately 25%.[125]

The radial, ulnar, dorsalis pedis, and posterior tibial pulses may be absent if the corresponding vessel is involved. The clinical characteristics of critical limb ischemia and ischemic digital ulcerations are described earlier in this chapter. The Allen test result is abnormal in two thirds of patients. To perform the Allen test, both radial and ulnar arteries are compressed while the hand is clenched and then opened. This maneuver causes palmar blanching. Release of compression from either pulse should normally produce palmar erythema if the palmar arches are patent. If these are occluded, pallor persists on the side where compression is maintained. The distal aspects of the extremities may have discrete, tender, erythematous subcutaneous cords, indicating a superficial thrombophlebitis.

Diagnosis

No specific laboratory tests, other than biopsy, can diagnose TAO. Most tests, therefore, aim to exclude other diseases that might have similar clinical presentations, including autoimmune diseases such as scleroderma or systemic lupus erythematosus, hypercoagulable states, diabetes, and acute arterial occlusion due to embolism. Acute-phase indicators, such as the erythrocyte sedimentation rate or C-reactive protein, are usually normal. Serum immunologic markers, including antinuclear antibodies and rheumatoid factor, should not be present, and serum complement levels should be normal. If it is clinically indicated, a proximal source of embolism should be excluded by cardiac and vascular ultrasonography or by computed tomography, magnetic resonance angiography, or conventional arteriography. Arteriography of an affected limb supports the diagnosis of TAO if there is segmental occlusion of small and medium arteries, absence of atherosclerosis, and corkscrew collateral vessels circumventing the occlusion (**Fig. 61-18**). These same findings, however, can occur in patients with scleroderma, systemic lupus erythematosus, mixed connective tissue disease, and antiphospholipid antibody syndrome. The conclusive test is a biopsy showing the classic pathologic findings. This procedure is rarely indicated, and biopsy sites may fail to heal because of severe ischemia. The diagnosis, therefore, usually depends on an age at onset of younger than 45 years, a history of tobacco use, physical examination demonstrating distal limb ischemia, exclusion of other diseases, and if necessary, angiographic demonstration of typical lesions.

Treatment

The cornerstone of treatment is cessation of tobacco use. Patients without gangrene who stop smoking rarely require amputation.[123,125] In contrast, one or more amputations may ultimately be required in 40% to 45% of patients with TAO who continue to smoke.

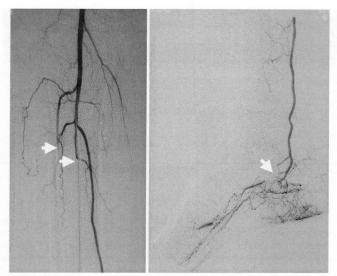

FIGURE 61-18 Angiogram of a young woman with thromboangiitis obliterans. The **left panel** demonstrates occlusion of the anterior tibial and peroneal arteries (arrows). The **right panel** demonstrates an occlusion of the distal portion of the posterior tibial artery (arrow) with bridging collateral vessels.

There is no definitive drug therapy for limb ischemia in patients with TAO. Vascular reconstructive surgery is usually not a viable option because of the segmental nature of this disease and the involvement of distal vessels. An autogenous saphenous vein bypass graft can be considered if a target vessel for the distal anastomosis is available. Long-term patency rates are better in ex-smokers than in smokers.[126]

Takayasu Arteritis and Giant Cell Arteritis (see Chap. 89)

Fibromuscular Dysplasia

Fibromuscular dysplasia is a disease of medium and large arteries. It typically affects the renal and carotid arteries. It may affect the arteries supplying the leg, particularly the iliac arteries and less so the femoral, popliteal, tibial, and peroneal arteries.[127] Fibromuscular dysplasia is a rare cause of either intermittent claudication or critical limb ischemia. It most often occurs in young white women but can occur at any age in both sexes. The histopathologic examination shows fibroplasia that most often affects the media but can involve the intima or adventitia. The histologic classification of fibromuscular dysplasia includes the medial subtypes (medial fibroplasia, perimedial fibroplasia, and medial hyperplasia) as well as intimal fibroplasia and adventitial hyperplasia.[10,127] Depending on the histopathologic type, stenosis results from hyperplasia of fibrous or muscular components of the vessel wall. Angiography demonstrates a beaded appearance of arteries affected by medial and perimedial fibroplasia and focal or tubular stenosis in arteries affected by intimal fibroplasia. Symptomatic patients should be treated with percutaneous transluminal angioplasty.

Popliteal Artery Entrapment Syndrome

Popliteal artery entrapment syndrome is an uncommon cause of intermittent claudication. It occurs when an anatomic variation in the configuration or insertion of the medial head of the gastrocnemius muscle compresses the popliteal artery.[128,129] The popliteus muscle can also compress the popliteal artery and cause this syndrome. Popliteal artery entrapment is bilateral in approximately one third of affected patients. It should be suspected when a young, typically athletic, usually male person presents with claudication. Potential consequences include popliteal artery thrombosis, embolism, and aneurysm formation.

The peripheral pulse examination findings may be normal unless provocative maneuvers are performed. Walking or repeated ankle dorsiflexion and plantar flexion maneuvers may cause attenuation or disappearance of pedal pulses and a decrease in the ABI in patients with popliteal artery entrapment. Imaging studies, such as duplex ultrasonography, computed tomography, and magnetic resonance angiography or conventional angiography, performed at rest and during ankle flexion maneuvers, can confirm the diagnosis. Magnetic resonance and computed tomography imaging will also provide information about the relationship of the gastrocnemius muscle to the popliteal artery.

Treatment of popliteal artery entrapment syndrome involves release of the popliteal artery. This may require division and reattachment of the medial head of the gastrocnemius muscle. On occasion, if the popliteal artery is occluded, surgical bypass is required.

Acute Limb Ischemia

Acute limb ischemia occurs when an arterial occlusion suddenly reduces blood flow to the arm or leg. The metabolic needs of the tissue outstrip perfusion, placing limb viability in jeopardy. The clinical presentation of patients with acute limb ischemia relates to the location of the arterial occlusion and the resulting decrease in blood flow. Depending on the severity of ischemia, patients may note disabling claudication or pain at rest. Pain may develop during a short period and is manifested in the affected extremity distal to the site of obstruction. It is not necessarily confined to the foot or toes, or hand or fingers, as is usually the case in chronic limb ischemia. Concurrent ischemia of peripheral nerves causes sensory loss and motor dysfunction. The physical findings can include absence of pulses distal to the occlusion, cool skin, pallor, delayed capillary return and venous filling, diminished or absent sensory perception, and muscle weakness or paralysis. This constellation of symptoms and signs is often recalled as the five *p*'s: pain, pulselessness, pallor, paresthesias, and paralysis.

Prognosis

Patients presenting with acute limb ischemia usually have comorbid cardiovascular disorders, which may even be responsible for the ischemia. This population therefore has a poor long-term outcome. The 5-year survival rate after acute limb ischemia caused by thrombosis approximates 45%, and after embolism, it is less than 20%.[6] The 1-month survival rate in persons older than 75 years with acute limb ischemia is approximately 40%.[130] The risk of limb loss depends on the severity of the ischemia and the elapsed time before a revascularization procedure is performed.

A classification scheme that takes into consideration the severity of ischemia and the viability of the limb, along with related neurologic findings and Doppler signals, has been developed by the Society for Vascular Surgery and the International Society for Cardiovascular Surgery (**Table 61-6**).[37] A viable limb, category I, is not immediately threatened, has neither sensory nor motor abnormalities, and has blood flow detectable by Doppler interrogation. Threatened viability, category II, indicates that the severity of ischemia will cause limb loss unless the blood supply is restored promptly. The category is subdivided into marginally and immediately threatened limbs, the latter characterized by pain, sensory deficits, and muscle weakness. Doppler interrogation cannot detect arterial blood flow. Irreversible limb ischemia leading to tissue loss and requiring amputation, category III, is characterized by loss of sensation, paralysis, and the absence of Doppler-detected blood flow in both arteries and veins distal to the occlusion.

Pathogenesis

The causes of acute limb ischemia include arterial embolism, thrombosis in situ, dissection, and trauma. Most arterial emboli arise from thrombotic sources in the heart. Atrial fibrillation complicating valvular heart disease, congestive heart failure, CAD, and hypertension accounts

TABLE 61-6	**Clinical Categories of Acute Limb Ischemia**					
			FINDINGS		DOPPLER SIGNALS	
CATEGORY	DESCRIPTION/PROGNOSIS	SENSORY LOSS	MUSCLE WEAKNESS	ARTERIAL	VENOUS
I. Viable	Not immediately threatened	None	None	Audible	Audible

II. Threatened
  a. Marginally
  b. Immediately
	
	Salvageable if promptly treated
	Salvageable with immediate
	  revascularization
		
		Minimal (toes) or none
		More than toes, rest pain
			
			None
			Mild, moderate
				
				(Often) inaudible
				(Usually) inaudible
					
					Audible
					Audible

III. Irreversible	Major tissue loss or permanent nerve damage inevitable	Profound, anesthetic	Profound, paralysis (rigor)	Inaudible	Inaudible

Modified from Rutherford RB, Baker JD, Ernst C, et al: Recommended standards for reports dealing with lower extremity ischemia: Revised version. J Vasc Surg 26:517, 1997.

for approximately 50% of cardiac emboli to the limbs. Other sources include rheumatic or prosthetic cardiac valves, ventricular thrombus resulting from MI or left ventricular aneurysm, paradoxical embolism of venous thrombi through the intra-atrial or intraventricular communications, and cardiac tumors such as left atrial myxomas. Aneurysms of the aorta or peripheral arteries may harbor thrombi, which subsequently embolize to more distal arterial sites, usually lodging at branch points where the artery decreases in size.

Thrombosis in situ occurs in atherosclerotic peripheral arteries, infrainguinal bypass grafts, peripheral artery aneurysms, and normal arteries of patients with hypercoagulable states. In patients with peripheral atherosclerosis, thrombosis in situ may complicate plaque rupture, causing acute arterial occlusion and limb ischemia, in a manner analogous to that which occurs in coronary arteries in patients with acute MI. Thrombosis complicating popliteal artery aneurysms is a much more common complication than rupture and may account for 10% of cases of acute limb ischemia in elderly men.[6] One of the most common causes of acute limb ischemia is thrombotic occlusion of an infrainguinal bypass graft, as discussed previously. Acute thrombotic occlusion of a normal artery is unusual but may occur in patients with acquired thrombophilic disorders, such as antiphospholipid antibody syndrome, heparin-induced thrombocytopenia, disseminated intravascular coagulation, and myeloproliferative diseases. There is limited evidence that inherited thrombophilic disorders such as activated protein C resistance (factor V Leiden), prothrombin G20210 gene mutation, or deficiencies of antithrombin III and protein C and S increase the risk of acute peripheral arterial thrombosis.

Diagnostic Tests

The history and physical examination usually establish the diagnosis of acute limb ischemia. Time available for diagnostic tests is often limited, and tests should not delay urgent revascularization procedures if limb viability is immediately threatened. The pressure in the affected limb and corresponding ABI can be measured if flow is detectable by Doppler ultrasonography. A Doppler probe can interrogate the presence of blood flow in peripheral arteries, particularly when pulses are not palpable. Color-assisted duplex ultrasonography can determine the site of occlusion. It is particularly applicable to evaluate the patency of infrainguinal bypass grafts. Magnetic resonance, computed tomography, and conventional contrast arteriography can demonstrate the site of occlusion and provide an anatomic guide for revascularization.

Treatment

Analgesic medications should be administered to reduce pain. For patients with acute leg ischemia, the bed should be positioned such that the feet are lower than chest level, thereby increasing limb perfusion pressure by gravitational effects. This goal can be accomplished by putting blocks under the posts at the head of the bed. Efforts should be made to reduce pressure on the heels, on bone prominences, and between the toes by appropriate placement of soft material on the bed (such as sheepskin) and between the toes (such as lamb's wool). The

room should be kept warm to prevent cold-induced cutaneous vasoconstriction.

Heparin should be administered intravenously as soon as the diagnosis of acute limb ischemia is made. The dose should be sufficient to increase the partial thromboplastin time by 1.5 to 2.5 times control values to prevent thrombus propagation or recurrent embolism. It is not known whether low-molecular-weight heparin is as effective as unfractionated heparin in patients with acute limb ischemia.

Revascularization is indicated when the viability of the limb is threatened or when symptoms of ischemia persist. Options for revascularization include intra-arterial thrombolytic therapy, percutaneous mechanical thrombectomy, and surgical revascularization. Catheter-directed intra-arterial thrombolysis is an initial treatment option for patients presenting with either category I or II acute limb ischemia, if there is no contraindication to thrombolysis.[131] Catheter-based thrombolysis can also be considered for patients who are considered at high risk for surgical intervention. Long-term patency after thrombolysis is greater in patients with category I and II critical limb ischemia than in those with category III ischemia, greater in native arteries than in grafts, and greater in vein grafts than in prosthetic grafts.[132] Identification and repair of a graft stenosis after successful thrombolysis improve long-term graft patency. Thrombolytic regimens have employed streptokinase, urokinase, recombinant tissue plasminogen activator, reteplase, and tenecteplase. The duration of catheter-based thrombolytic therapy should generally not exceed 48 hours to achieve optimal benefit and to limit the risk of bleeding. It is not known whether adjuvant use of platelet glycoprotein IIb/IIIa inhibitors shortens thrombolysis time or improves outcome.[133] Percutaneous, catheter-based mechanical thrombectomy, with devices that apply hydrodynamic forces or rotating baskets, can be used alone or in addition to pharmacologic thrombolysis to treat patients with acute limb ischemia. Surgical thromboembolectomy is no longer common.[134] Surgical reconstruction, bypassing the occluded area, is an option for restoration of blood flow to an ischemic limb. These techniques were discussed previously in this chapter.

Five prospective randomized trials, comprising 1283 patients, have compared the benefits and risks of thrombolysis and surgical reconstruction in patients presenting with acute limb ischemia.[135] Overall, there was no difference in the rate of death or amputation during 1 year between the two interventions, although the risk of major bleeding within 30 days was greater in patients receiving thrombolysis. The findings from the individual trials suggest that catheter-based thrombolysis is an appropriate initial option in patients with category I and IIa acute limb ischemia of less than 14 days' duration, especially those with thrombosed bypass grafts, whereas surgical revascularization is more appropriate for those with category IIb and III acute limb ischemia and in those whose symptoms have lasted for more than 14 days (**Fig. 61-19**).[136]

Atheroembolism

Atheroembolism refers to the occlusion of arteries resulting from detachment and embolization of atheromatous debris, including fibrin, platelets, cholesterol crystals, and calcium fragments. Other terms include atherogenic embolism and cholesterol embolism. Atheroemboli originate most frequently from shaggy protruding atheromas of the aorta and less frequently from atherosclerotic branch arteries. The atheroemboli typically occlude small downstream arteries and arterioles of the extremities, brain, eye, kidneys, or mesentery.[137,138] The prevalence of atheroembolism in the general population is not known. Most affected individuals are men older than 60 years with clinical evidence of atherosclerosis.

Pathogenesis

The risk of atheroembolism is greatest in patients with aortic atherosclerosis characterized by large protruding atheromas (**Fig. 61-20**). Large aortic plaques identified by ultrasonography strongly associate with previous embolic disease.[137] Similarly, identification of large protruding atheromas by transesophageal ultrasound predicts future embolic events.[137,139] Atheroemboli typically occlude arterioles and small arteries. Approximately 50% of atheroemboli involve vessels in the lower extremities. Catheter manipulation causes a large proportion of atheroemboli, affecting approximately 1% to 2% of patients undergoing endovascular procedures.[138,140] Similarly, surgical manipulation of the aorta during cardiac or vascular operations may precipitate atheroembolism. Controversy remains as to whether anticoagulants or thrombolytic drugs contribute to atheroembolism.[139] Recent clinical trials of anticoagulant drugs have found a relatively low incidence of atheroembolism in patients with large aortic plaques.[137]

Clinical Presentation

The most notable clinical features of atheroembolism to the extremities include painful cyanotic toes, called blue toe syndrome (**Fig. 61-21**). Livedo reticularis occurs in approximately 50% of patients. Local areas of erythematous or violaceous

discoloration may be present on the lateral aspects of the feet and the soles, and also on the calves. Other findings include digital and foot ulcerations, nodules, purpura, and petechiae. Pedal pulses are typically present because the emboli tend to lodge in the more distal digital arteries and arterioles. Symptoms and signs indicating additional organ involvement with atheroemboli should be sought. Funduscopy can visualize Hollenhorst plaques in patients with visual loss secondary to retinal ischemia or infarction. Renal involvement, manifested by increased blood pressure and azotemia, commonly occurs in patients with peripheral atheroemboli. Patients also sometimes show evidence of mesenteric or bladder ischemia and splenic infarction.

The clinical setting and findings are usually sufficient for diagnosis of atheroembolism, but some of the manifestations of

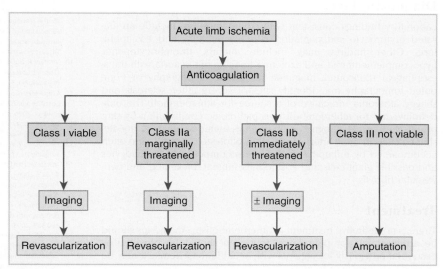

FIGURE 61-19 Management algorithm for the treatment of acute limb ischemia. *(Modified from Norgren L, Hiatt WR, Dormandy JA, et al: Inter-Society Consensus for the Management of Peripheral Arterial Disease [TASC II]. J Vasc Surg 45[Suppl S]:S5, 2007.)*

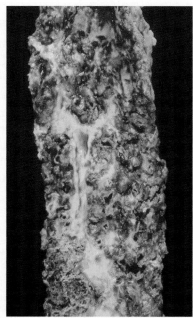

FIGURE 61-20 Atherosclerotic aorta of a patient with atheroemboli. There are multiple, protruding, shaggy atheromas with superimposed mural thrombi. *(Courtesy of R.N. Mitchell, MD, PhD, Department of Pathology, Brigham and Women's Hospital, Boston, Mass.)*

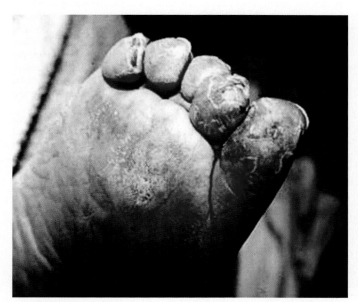

FIGURE 61-21 Atheroemboli to the foot or "blue toe syndrome." There is cyanotic discoloration of toes, with localized areas of violaceous discoloration. *(Modified from Beckman JA, Creager MA: Peripheral arterial disease: Clinical evaluation. In Creager MA, Dzau VJ, Loscalzo J [eds]: Vascular Medicine: A Companion to Braunwald's Heart Disease. Philadelphia, Elsevier, 2006, p 259.)*

atheroemboli may be present with other diseases. As discussed previously, critical limb ischemia occurs in patients with severe peripheral atherosclerosis, and acute limb ischemia is a consequence of thromboembolism, each of which would be characterized by an abnormal pulse examination. Hypersensitivity vasculitides secondary to connective tissue diseases, infections, drugs, polyarteritis nodosa, or cryoglobulinemia, for example, may be manifested with multisystem organ damage and cutaneous findings of purpura, ulcers, and digital ischemia similar to those resulting from atheroemboli (see Chap. 89). Procoagulant disorders such as antiphospholipid antibody syndrome, heparin-induced thrombocytopenia, and myeloproliferative disorders such as essential thrombocythemia can cause digital artery thrombosis with resultant digital ischemia, cyanosis, and ulceration.

Diagnostic Tests

Laboratory findings consistent with atheroembolism include an elevated erythrocyte sedimentation rate, eosinophilia, and eosinophiluria. Other findings may include anemia, thrombocytopenia, hypocomplementemia, and azotemia. Imaging of the aorta with transesophageal ultrasound, magnetic resonance angiography, or computed tomography may identify sites of severe atherosclerosis and shaggy atheroma indicative of a source for atheroemboli. The only definitive test for atheroembolism is pathologic confirmation by skin or muscle biopsy. Pathognomonic findings include elongated needle-shaped clefts in small arteries, caused by cholesterol crystals and often accompanied by inflammatory infiltrates composed of lymphocytes and possibly giant cells and eosinophils, intimal thickening, and perivascular fibrosis.

Treatment

There is no definitive treatment of atheroembolism. Analgesics should be administered for pain. Local foot care should be provided as described previously for patients with acute limb ischemia. It may be necessary to excise or to amputate necrotic areas.

Patients with this condition are subject to recurrent atheroembolic events. Risk factor modification, such as lipid-lowering therapy with statins and smoking cessation, can favorably affect overall outcome from atherosclerosis, but whether such intervention will prevent recurrent atheroembolism is unknown. The use of antiplatelet drugs to prevent recurrent atheroembolism remains controversial. It is reasonable, however, to administer antiplatelet agents even in the absence of strong clinical evidence of efficacy, because the agents will prevent other adverse cardiovascular events in patients with atherosclerosis. The use of warfarin also engenders controversy, and some investigators have even suggested that anticoagulants precipitate atheroemboli, whereas others have found that warfarin reduces atheroembolic events, particularly in patients with mobile aortic atheroma.[139] The use of corticosteroids to treat atheroembolism also is controversial.

Surgical removal of the source should be considered in patients with atheroembolism, particularly in those in whom it recurs. Surgical procedures include excision and replacement of affected portions of the aorta, endarterectomy, and bypass operations. Operative intervention is targeted to the site of the aorta and iliac or femoral arteries where there is aneurysm formation or obvious shaggy friable atherosclerotic plaque. Often, the aorta is diffusely affected by severe atherosclerosis, and it is not possible to identify the precise segment that is responsible for atheroembolism. In addition, many of these patients are elderly and have coexisting CAD, which increases the risk of major vascular operations. Endovascular placement of stents and stent grafts to prevent recurrent atheroembolism has been reported in several small case series.[138]

REFERENCES

Epidemiology

1. Hiatt WR, Goldstone J, Smith SC Jr, et al: Atherosclerotic Peripheral Vascular Disease Symposium II: Nomenclature for vascular diseases. Circulation 118:2826, 2008.

2. Steg PG, Bhatt DL, Wilson PW, et al: One-year cardiovascular event rates in outpatients with atherothrombosis. JAMA 297:1197, 2007.

3. Criqui MH: Peripheral arterial disease—epidemiological aspects. Vasc Med 6(Suppl):3, 2001.

4. Diehm C, Schuster A, Allenberg JR, et al: High prevalence of peripheral arterial disease and co-morbidity in 6880 primary care patients: Cross-sectional study. Atherosclerosis 172:95, 2004.

5. Selvin E, Erlinger TP: Prevalence of and risk factors for peripheral arterial disease in the United States: Results from the National Health and Nutrition Examination Survey, 1999-2000. Circulation 110:738, 2004.

6. Norgren L, Hiatt WR, Dormandy JA, et al: Inter-Society Consensus for the Management of Peripheral Arterial Disease (TASC II). J Vasc Surg 45(Suppl S):S5, 2007.

7. Criqui MH, Vargas V, Denenberg JO, et al: Ethnicity and peripheral arterial disease: The San Diego Population Study. Circulation 112:2703, 2005.

8. Allison MA, Criqui MH, McClelland RL, et al: The effect of novel cardiovascular risk factors on the ethnic-specific odds for peripheral arterial disease in the Multi-Ethnic Study of Atherosclerosis (MESA). J Am Coll Cardiol 48:1190, 2006.

9. Hirsch AT, Haskal ZJ, Hertzer NR, et al: ACC/AHA 2005 guidelines for the management of patients with peripheral arterial disease (lower extremity, renal, mesenteric, and abdominal aortic): Executive summary a collaborative report from the American Association for Vascular Surgery/Society for Vascular Surgery, Society for Cardiovascular Angiography and Interventions, Society for Vascular Medicine and Biology, Society of Interventional Radiology, and the ACC/AHA Task Force on Practice Guidelines (Writing Committee to Develop Guidelines for the Management of Patients With Peripheral Arterial Disease) endorsed by the American Association of Cardiovascular and Pulmonary Rehabilitation; National Heart, Lung, and Blood Institute; Society for Vascular Nursing; TransAtlantic Inter-Society Consensus; and Vascular Disease Foundation. J Am Coll Cardiol 47:1239, 2006.

10. Virmani R, Burke AP, Taylor AJ: Congenital malformations of the vasculature. In Creager MA, Dzau VJ, Loscalzo J (eds): Vascular Medicine: A Companion to Braunwald's Heart Disease. Philadelphia, Elsevier, 2006, pp 934-960.

11. Criqui MH, Ninomiya J: The epidemiology of peripheral arterial disease. In Creager MA, Dzau VJ, Loscalzo J (eds): Vascular Medicine: A Companion to Braunwald's Heart Disease. Philadelphia, Elsevier, 2006, pp 223-238.

12. Lu JT, Creager MA: The relationship of cigarette smoking to peripheral arterial disease. Rev Cardiovasc Med 5:189, 2004.

13. He Y, Jiang Y, Wang J, et al: Prevalence of peripheral arterial disease and its association with smoking in a population-based study in Beijing, China. J Vasc Surg 44:333, 2006.

14. Marso SP, Hiatt WR: Peripheral arterial disease in patients with diabetes. J Am Coll Cardiol 47:921, 2006.

15. Aboyans V, Criqui MH, Denenberg JO, et al: Risk factors for progression of peripheral arterial disease in large and small vessels. Circulation 113:2623, 2006.

16. Wattanakit K, Folsom AR, Selvin E, et al: Risk factors for peripheral arterial disease incidence in persons with diabetes: The Atherosclerosis Risk in Communities (ARIC) Study. Atherosclerosis 180:389, 2005.

17. Olin JW: Hypertension and peripheral arterial disease. Vasc Med 10:241, 2005.

18. Pande RL, Perlstein TS, Beckman JA, Creager MA: Association of insulin resistance and inflammation with peripheral arterial disease: The National Health and Nutrition Examination Survey, 1999 to 2004. Circulation 118:33, 2008.

19. Wattanakit K, Folsom AR, Selvin E, et al: Kidney function and risk of peripheral arterial disease: Results from the Atherosclerosis Risk in Communities (ARIC) Study. J Am Soc Nephrol 18:629, 2007.

20. Tzoulaki I, Murray GD, Lee AJ, et al: C-reactive protein, interleukin-6, and soluble adhesion molecules as predictors of progressive peripheral atherosclerosis in the general population: Edinburgh Artery Study. Circulation 112:976, 2005.

21. Barani J, Nilsson JA, Mattiasson I, et al: Inflammatory mediators are associated with 1-year mortality in critical limb ischemia. J Vasc Surg 42:75, 2005.

22. Brevetti G, Schiano V, Chiariello M: Cellular adhesion molecules and peripheral arterial disease. Vasc Med 11:39, 2006.

23. Wildman RP, Muntner P, Chen J, et al: Relation of inflammation to peripheral arterial disease in the national health and nutrition examination survey, 1999-2002. Am J Cardiol 96:1579, 2005.

24. Owens CD, Ridker PM, Belkin M, et al: Elevated C-reactive protein levels are associated with postoperative events in patients undergoing lower extremity vein bypass surgery. J Vasc Surg 45:2, 2007.

25. Pradhan AD, Shrivastava S, Cook NR, et al: Symptomatic peripheral arterial disease in women: Nontraditional biomarkers of elevated risk. Circulation 117:823, 2008.

26. Nasir K, Guallar E, Navas-Acien A, et al: Relationship of monocyte count and peripheral arterial disease: Results from the National Health and Nutrition Examination Survey 1999-2002. Arterioscler Thromb Vasc Biol 25:1966, 2005.

27. Perlstein TS, Pande RL, Beckman JA, Creager MA: Serum total bilirubin level and prevalent lower-extremity peripheral arterial disease: National Health and Nutrition Examination Survey (NHANES) 1999 to 2004. Arterioscler Thromb Vasc Biol 28:166, 2008.

28. Hiatt WR, Brass EP: Pathophysiology of claudication. In Creager MA (ed): Peripheral Arterial Disease. 2nd ed. London, Remedica, 2008, pp 49-70.

29. Hiatt WR, Brass EP: Pathophysiology of intermittent claudication. In Creager MA, Dzau VJ, Loscalzo J (eds): Vascular Medicine: A Companion to Braunwald's Heart Disease. Philadelphia, Elsevier, 2006, pp 239-247.

30. Bauer TA, Brass EP, Barstow TJ, Hiatt WR: Skeletal muscle StO$_2$ kinetics are slowed during low work rate calf exercise in peripheral arterial disease. Eur J Appl Physiol 100:143, 2007.

31. Isbell DC, Berr SS, Toledano AY, et al: Delayed calf muscle phosphocreatine recovery after exercise identifies peripheral arterial disease. J Am Coll Cardiol 47:2289, 2006.

Clinical Presentation

32. McDermott MM, Liu K, Greenland P, et al: Functional decline in peripheral arterial disease: Associations with the ankle brachial index and leg symptoms. JAMA 292:453, 2004 .

33. McDermott MM, Hoff F, Ferrucci L, et al: Lower extremity ischemia, calf skeletal muscle characteristics, and functional impairment in peripheral arterial disease. J Am Geriatr Soc 55:400, 2007.

34. Golomb BA, Criqui MH: Epidemiology. In Creager MA (ed): Peripheral Arterial Disease. 2nd ed. London, Remedica, 2008, pp 1-21.

35. Coyne KS, Margolis MK, Gilchrist KA, et al: Evaluating effects of method of administration on Walking Impairment Questionnaire. J Vasc Surg 38:296, 2003.
36. Khan NA, Rahim SA, Anand SS, et al: Does the clinical examination predict lower extremity peripheral arterial disease? JAMA 295:536, 2006.
37. Rutherford RB, Baker JD, Ernst C, et al: Recommended standards for reports dealing with lower extremity ischemia: Revised version. J Vasc Surg 26:517, 1997.

Testing in Peripheral Arterial Drsease

38. McDermott MM, Guralnik JM, Ferrucci L, et al: Physical activity, walking exercise, and calf skeletal muscle characteristics in patients with peripheral arterial disease. J Vasc Surg 46:87, 2007.
39. Chaudhry H, Holland A, Dormandy J: Comparison of graded versus constant treadmill test protocols for quantifying intermittent claudication. Vasc Med 2:93, 1997.
40. Collins R, Cranny G, Burch J, et al: A systematic review of duplex ultrasound, magnetic resonance angiography and computed tomography angiography for the diagnosis and assessment of symptomatic, lower limb peripheral arterial disease. Health Technol Assess 11:iii, xi, 1, 2007.
41. Ouwendijk R, Kock MC, Visser K, et al: Interobserver agreement for the interpretation of contrast-enhanced 3D MR angiography and MDCT angiography in peripheral arterial disease. AJR Am J Roentgenol 185:1261, 2005.
42. Ouwendijk R, de Vries M, Pattynama PM, et al: Imaging peripheral arterial disease: A randomized controlled trial comparing contrast-enhanced MR angiography and multi-detector row CT angiography. Radiology 236:1094, 2005.
43. Flohr TG, Schaller S, Stierstorfer K, et al: Multi-detector row CT systems and image-reconstruction techniques. Radiology 235:756, 2005.
44. Met R, Bipat S, Legemate DA, et al: Diagnostic performance of computed tomography angiography in peripheral arterial disease: A systematic review and meta-analysis. JAMA 301:415, 2009.

Prognosis

45. McDermott MM, Liu K, Criqui MH, et al: Ankle-brachial index and subclinical cardiac and carotid disease: The multi-ethnic study of atherosclerosis. Am J Epidemiol 162:33, 2005.
46. Cacoub PP, Abola MT, Baumgartner I, et al: Cardiovascular risk factor control and outcomes in peripheral artery disease patients in the Reduction of Atherothrombosis for Continued Health (REACH) Registry. Atherosclerosis 204:e86, 2009.
47. Fowkes FG, Low LP, Tuta S, Kozak J: Ankle-brachial index and extent of atherothrombosis in 8891 patients with or at risk of vascular disease: Results of the international AGATHA study. Eur Heart J 27:1861, 2006.
48. Doobay AV, Anand SS: Sensitivity and specificity of the ankle-brachial index to predict future cardiovascular outcomes: A systematic review. Arterioscler Thromb Vasc Biol 25:1463, 2005.
49. Fowkes FG, Murray GD, Butcher I, et al: Ankle brachial index combined with Framingham Risk Score to predict cardiovascular events and mortality: A meta-analysis. JAMA 300:197, 2008.
50. O'Hare AM, Katz R, Shlipak MG, et al: Mortality and cardiovascular risk across the ankle-arm index spectrum: Results from the Cardiovascular Health Study. Circulation 113:388, 2006.
51. Resnick HE, Lindsay RS, McDermott MM, et al: Relationship of high and low ankle brachial index to all-cause and cardiovascular disease mortality: The Strong Heart Study. Circulation 109:733, 2004.
52. Criqui MH, Ninomiya JK, Wingard DL, et al: Progression of peripheral arterial disease predicts cardiovascular disease morbidity and mortality. J Am Coll Cardiol 52:1736, 2008.
53. Aquino R, Johnnides C, Makaroun M, et al: Natural history of claudication: Long-term serial follow-up study of 1244 claudicants. J Vasc Surg 34:962, 2001.
54. Fosse S, Hartemann-Heurtier A, Jacqueminet S, et al: Incidence and characteristics of lower limb amputations in people with diabetes. Diabet Med 26:391, 2009.

Treatment

55. Randomized trial of the effects of cholesterol-lowering with simvastatin on peripheral vascular and other major vascular outcomes in 20,536 people with peripheral arterial disease and other high-risk conditions. J Vasc Surg 45:645; discussion 653, 2007.
56. Aung PP, Maxwell HG, Jepson RG, et al: Lipid-lowering for peripheral arterial disease of the lower limb. Cochrane Database Syst Rev (4):CD000123, 2007.
57. Aronow WS, Nayak D, Woodworth S, Ahn C: Effect of simvastatin versus placebo on treadmill exercise time until the onset of intermittent claudication in older patients with peripheral arterial disease at six months and at one year after treatment. Am J Cardiol 92:711, 2003.
58. Mohler ER 3rd, Hiatt WR, Creager MA: Cholesterol reduction with atorvastatin improves walking distance in patients with peripheral arterial disease. Circulation 108:1481, 2003.
59. Mondillo S, Ballo P, Barbati R, et al: Effects of simvastatin on walking performance and symptoms of intermittent claudication in hypercholesterolemic patients with peripheral vascular disease. Am J Med 114:359, 2003.
60. Momsen AH, Jensen MB, Norager CB, et al: Drug therapy for improving walking distance in intermittent claudication: A systematic review and meta-analysis of robust randomised controlled studies. Eur J Vasc Endovasc Surg 38:463, 2009 .
61. McDermott MM, Guralnik JM, Greenland P, et al: Statin use and leg functioning in patients with and without lower-extremity peripheral arterial disease. Circulation 107:757, 2003.
62. Rajamani K, Colman PG, Li LP, et al: Effect of fenofibrate on amputation events in people with type 2 diabetes mellitus (FIELD study): A prespecified analysis of a randomised controlled trial. Lancet 373:1780, 2009.
63. Gonzales D, Rennard SI, Nides M, et al: Varenicline, an α4β2 nicotinic acetylcholine receptor partial agonist, vs sustained-release bupropion and placebo for smoking cessation: A randomized controlled trial. JAMA 296:47, 2006.
64. Jorenby DE, Hays JT, Rigotti NA, et al: Efficacy of varenicline, an α4β2 nicotinic acetylcholine receptor partial agonist, vs placebo or sustained-release bupropion for smoking cessation: A randomized controlled trial. JAMA 296:56, 2006.
65. Nathan DM, Cleary PA, Backlund JY, et al: Intensive diabetes treatment and cardiovascular disease in patients with type 1 diabetes. N Engl J Med 353:2643, 2005.
66. Nathan DM, Lachin J, Cleary P, et al: Intensive diabetes therapy and carotid intima-media thickness in type 1 diabetes mellitus. N Engl J Med 348:2294, 2003.
67. Holman RR, Paul SK, Bethel MA, et al: 10-year follow-up of intensive glucose control in type 2 diabetes. N Engl J Med 359:1577, 2008.
68. Gerstein HC, Miller ME, Byington RP, et al: Effects of intensive glucose lowering in type 2 diabetes. N Engl J Med 358:2545, 2008.
69. Patel A, MacMahon S, Chalmers J, et al: Intensive blood glucose control and vascular outcomes in patients with type 2 diabetes. N Engl J Med 358:2560, 2008.
70. Duckworth W, Abraira C, Moritz T, et al: Glucose control and vascular complications in veterans with type 2 diabetes. N Engl J Med 360:129, 2009.
71. Dormandy JA, Charbonnel B, Eckland DJ, et al: Secondary prevention of macrovascular events in patients with type 2 diabetes in the PROactive Study (PROspective pioglitAzone Clinical Trial In macroVascular Events): A randomised controlled trial. Lancet 366:1279, 2005.
72. Dormandy JA, Betteridge DJ, Schernthaner G, et al: Impact of peripheral arterial disease in patients with diabetes—results from PROactive (PROactive 11). Atherosclerosis 202:272, 2009.
73. Ray KK, Seshasai SR, Wijesuriya S, et al: Effect of intensive control of glucose on cardiovascular outcomes and death in patients with diabetes mellitus: A meta-analysis of randomised controlled trials. Lancet 373:1765, 2009.
74. Skyler JS, Bergenstal R, Bonow RO, et al: Intensive glycemic control and the prevention of cardiovascular events: Implications of the ACCORD, ADVANCE, and VA diabetes trials: A position statement of the American Diabetes Association and a scientific statement of the American College of Cardiology Foundation and the American Heart Association. Circulation 119:351, 2009.
75. Mehler PS, Coll JR, Estacio R, et al: Intensive blood pressure control reduces the risk of cardiovascular events in patients with peripheral arterial disease and type 2 diabetes. Circulation 107:753, 2003.
76. The ACCORD Study Group: Effects of intensive blood-pressure control in type 2 diabetes mellitus. N Engl J Med 362:1575, 2010.
77. Paravastu SC, Mendonca D, Da Silva A: Beta blockers for peripheral arterial disease. Cochrane Database Syst Rev (4):CD005508, 2008.
78. Chobanian AV, Bakris GL, Black HR, et al: The Seventh Report of the Joint National Committee on Prevention, Detection, Evaluation, and Treatment of High Blood Pressure: The JNC 7 report. JAMA 289:2560, 2003.
79. Bosch J, Lonn E, Pogue J, et al: Long-term effects of ramipril on cardiovascular events and on diabetes: Results of the HOPE study extension. Circulation 112:1339, 2005.
80. Yusuf S, Teo KK, Pogue J, et al: Telmisartan, ramipril, or both in patients at high risk for vascular events. N Engl J Med 358:1547, 2008.
81. Collaborative meta-analysis of randomised trials of antiplatelet therapy for prevention of death, myocardial infarction, and stroke in high risk patients. BMJ 324:71, 2002.
82. Berger JS, Krantz MJ, Kittelson JM, Hiatt WR: Aspirin for the prevention of cardiovascular events in patients with peripheral artery disease: A meta-analysis of randomized trials. JAMA 301:1909, 2009.
83. Belch J, MacCuish A, Campbell I, et al: The prevention of progression of arterial disease and diabetes (POPADAD) trial: Factorial randomised placebo controlled trial of aspirin and antioxidants in patients with diabetes and asymptomatic peripheral arterial disease. BMJ 337:a1840, 2008.
84. Fowkes FG, Price JF, Stewart MC, et al: Aspirin for prevention of cardiovascular events in a general population screened for a low ankle brachial index: A randomized controlled trial. JAMA 303:841, 2010.
85. A randomised, blinded, trial of clopidogrel versus aspirin in patients at risk of ischaemic events (CAPRIE). CAPRIE Steering Committee. Lancet 348:1329, 1996.
86. Bhatt DL, Fox KA, Hacke W, et al: Clopidogrel and aspirin versus aspirin alone for the prevention of atherothrombotic events. N Engl J Med 354:1706, 2006.
87. Cacoub PP, Bhatt DL, Steg PG, et al: Patients with peripheral arterial disease in the CHARISMA trial. Eur Heart J 30:192, 2009.
88. Anand S, Yusuf S, Xie C, et al: Oral anticoagulant and antiplatelet therapy and peripheral arterial disease. N Engl J Med 357:217, 2007.
89. Creager MA, Pande RL, Hiatt WR: A randomized trial of iloprost in patients with intermittent claudication. Vasc Med 13:5, 2008.
90. Robless P, Mikhailidis DP, Stansby GP: Cilostazol for peripheral arterial disease. Cochrane Database Syst Rev (1):CD003748, 2007.
91. Pande RL, Hiatt WR, Zhang P, et al: A pooled analysis of the durability and predictors of treatment response of cilostazol in patients with intermittent claudication. Vasc Med 15:181, 2010.
92. Hiatt WR, Money SR, Brass EP: Long-term safety of cilostazol in patients with peripheral artery disease: The CASTLE study (Cilostazol: A Study in Long-term Effects). J Vasc Surg 47:330, 2008.
93. Ahimastos AA, Lawler A, Reid CM, et al: Brief communication: Ramipril markedly improves walking ability in patients with peripheral arterial disease: A randomized trial. Ann Intern Med 144:660, 2006.
94. Hiatt WR, Hirsch AT, Cooke JP, et al: Randomized trial of AT-1015 for treatment of intermittent claudication. A novel 5-hydroxytryptamine antagonist with no evidence of efficacy. Vasc Med 9:18, 2004.
95. Norgren L, Jawien A, Matyas L, et al: Sarpogrelate, a 5-hT2A receptor antagonist in intermittent claudication. A phase II European study. Vasc Med 11:75, 2006.
96. Leizorovicz A, Becker F: Oral buflomedil in the prevention of cardiovascular events in patients with peripheral arterial obstructive disease: A randomized, placebo-controlled, 4-year study. Circulation 117:816, 2008.
97. Wilson AM, Harada R, Nair N, et al: L-Arginine supplementation in peripheral arterial disease: No benefit and possible harm. Circulation 116:188, 2007.
98. Hiatt WR: Carnitine and peripheral arterial disease. Ann N Y Acad Sci 1033:92, 2004.
99. Mohler ER 3rd, Hiatt WR, Olin JW, et al: Treatment of intermittent claudication with beraprost sodium, an orally active prostaglandin I_2 analogue: A double-blinded, randomized, controlled trial. J Am Coll Cardiol 41:1679, 2003.
100. Jaff MR, Dale RA, Creager MA, et al: Anti-chlamydial antibiotic therapy for symptom improvement in peripheral artery disease: Prospective evaluation of rifalazil effect on vascular symptoms of intermittent claudication and other endpoints in *Chlamydia pneumoniae* seropositive patients (PROVIDENCE-1). Circulation 119:452, 2009.

101. Rajagopalan S, Olin J, Deitcher S, et al: Use of a constitutively active hypoxia-inducible factor-1α transgene as a therapeutic strategy in no-option critical limb ischemia patients: Phase I dose-escalation experience. Circulation 115:1234, 2007.

102. Nikol S, Baumgartner I, Van Belle E, et al: Therapeutic angiogenesis with intramuscular NV1FGF improves amputation-free survival in patients with critical limb ischemia. Mol Ther 16:972, 2008.

103. Powell RJ, Simons M, Mendelsohn FO, et al: Results of a double-blind, placebo-controlled study to assess the safety of intramuscular injection of hepatocyte growth factor plasmid to improve limb perfusion in patients with critical limb ischemia. Circulation 118:58, 2008.

104. Rajagopalan S, Mohler ER 3rd, Lederman RJ, et al: Regional angiogenesis with vascular endothelial growth factor in peripheral arterial disease: A phase II randomized, double-blind, controlled study of adenoviral delivery of vascular endothelial growth factor 121 in patients with disabling intermittent claudication. Circulation 108:1933, 2003.

105. Creager MA: Treatment of intermittent claudication with hypoxia-inducible factor-1α. Paper presented at Late Breaking Clinical Trials Session of the American College of Cardiology 58th Annual Scientific Sessions; March 2009; Orlando, Florida.

106. Bartsch T, Brehm M, Zeus T, et al: Transplantation of autologous mononuclear bone marrow stem cells in patients with peripheral arterial disease (the TAM-PAD study). Clin Res Cardiol 96:891, 2007.

107. Burt RK, Loh Y, Pearce W, et al: Clinical applications of blood-derived and marrow-derived stem cells for nonmalignant diseases. JAMA 299:925, 2008.

108. Burt RK, Testori A, Oyama Y, et al: Autologous peripheral blood CD133⁺ cell implantation for limb salvage in patients with critical limb ischemia. Bone Marrow Transplant 45:111, 2010.

109. Matoba S, Tatsumi T, Murohara T, et al: Long-term clinical outcome after intramuscular implantation of bone marrow mononuclear cells (Therapeutic Angiogenesis by Cell Transplantation [TACT] trial) in patients with chronic limb ischemia. Am Heart J 156:1010, 2008.

110. Watson L, Ellis B, Leng GC: Exercise for intermittent claudication. Cochrane Database Syst Rev (4):CD000990, 2008.

111. McDermott MM, Ades P, Guralnik JM, et al: Treadmill exercise and resistance training in patients with peripheral arterial disease with and without intermittent claudication: A randomized controlled trial. JAMA 301:165, 2009.

112. Stewart KJ, Hiatt WR, Regensteiner JG, Hirsch AT: Exercise training for claudication. N Engl J Med 347:1941, 2002.

113. Brass EP, Hiatt WR, Green S: Skeletal muscle metabolic changes in peripheral arterial disease contribute to exercise intolerance: A point-counterpoint discussion. Vasc Med 9:293, 2004.

114. Sandri M, Adams V, Gielen S, et al: Effects of exercise and ischemia on mobilization and functional activation of blood-derived progenitor cells in patients with ischemic syndromes: Results of 3 randomized studies. Circulation 111:3391, 2005.

115. Arany Z, Foo SY, Ma Y, et al: HIF-independent regulation of VEGF and angiogenesis by the transcriptional coactivator PGC-1α. Nature 451:1008, 2008.

116. Hambrecht R, Adams V, Erbs S, et al: Regular physical activity improves endothelial function in patients with coronary artery disease by increasing phosphorylation of endothelial nitric oxide synthase. Circulation 107:3152, 2003.

117. Gardner AW, Katzel LI, Sorkin JD, et al: Exercise rehabilitation improves functional outcomes and peripheral circulation in patients with intermittent claudication: A randomized controlled trial. J Am Geriatr Soc 49:755, 2001.

118. White CJ, Gray WA: Endovascular therapies for peripheral arterial disease: An evidence-based review. Circulation 116:2203, 2007.

119. Fleisher LA, Beckman JA, Brown KA, et al: ACC/AHA 2007 Guidelines on Perioperative Cardiovascular Evaluation and Care for Noncardiac Surgery: Executive Summary: A Report of the American College of Cardiology/American Heart Association Task Force on Practice Guidelines (Writing Committee to Revise the 2002 Guidelines on Perioperative Cardiovascular Evaluation for Noncardiac Surgery): Developed in Collaboration With the American Society of Echocardiography, American Society of Nuclear Cardiology, Heart Rhythm Society, Society of Cardiovascular Anesthesiologists, Society for Cardiovascular Angiography and Interventions, Society for Vascular Medicine and Biology, and Society for Vascular Surgery. Circulation 116:1971, 2007.

120. Dorffler-Melly J, Buller HR, Koopman MM, Prins MH: Antithrombotic agents for preventing thrombosis after infrainguinal arterial bypass surgery. Cochrane Database Syst Rev (4):CD000536, 2003.

Thromboangitis, Obliterans, Fibromuscular Dysplasia, and Popliteal Artery Entrapment Syndrome

121. Dorffler-Melly J, Koopman MM, Adam DJ, et al: Antiplatelet agents for preventing thrombosis after peripheral arterial bypass surgery. Cochrane Database Syst Rev (3):CD000535, 2003.

122. Brown J, Lethaby A, Maxwell H, et al: Antiplatelet agents for preventing thrombosis after peripheral arterial bypass surgery. Cochrane Database Syst Rev (4):CD000535, 2008.

123. Olin JW: Thromboangiitis obliterans (Buerger's disease). In Creager MA, Dzau VJ, Loscalzo J (eds): Vascular Medicine: A Companion to Braunwald's Heart Disease. Philadelphia, Elsevier, 2006, pp 641-656.

124. Olin JW, Shih A: Thromboangiitis obliterans (Buerger's disease). Curr Opin Rheumatol 18:18, 2006.

125. Cooper LT, Tse TS, Mikhail MA, et al: Long-term survival and amputation risk in thromboangiitis obliterans (Buerger's disease). J Am Coll Cardiol 44:2410, 2004.

126. Sasajima T, Kubo Y, Inaba M, et al: Role of infrainguinal bypass in Buerger's disease: An eighteen-year experience. Eur J Vasc Endovasc Surg 13:186, 1997.

127. Slovut DP, Olin JW: Fibromuscular dysplasia. N Engl J Med 350:1862, 2004.

128. Rigberg DA, Freischlag JA, Machleder HE: Vascular compression syndromes. In Creager MA, Dzau VJ, Loscalzo J (eds): Vascular Medicine: A Companion to Braunwald's Heart Disease. Philadelphia, Elsevier, 2006, pp 920-933.

129. Korngold EC, Jaff MR: Unusual causes of intermittent claudication: Popliteal artery entrapment syndrome, cystic adventitial disease, fibromuscular dysplasia, and endofibrosis. Curr Treat Options Cardiovasc Med 11:156, 2009.

Acute Limb Ischemia

130. Braithwaite BD, Davies B, Birch PA, et al: Management of acute leg ischaemia in the elderly. Br J Surg 85:217, 1998.

131. Ouriel K: Acute arterial occlusion. In Creager MA, Dzau VJ, Loscalzo J (eds): Vascular Medicine: A Companion to Braunwald's Heart Disease. Philadelphia, Elsevier, 2006, pp 669-676.

132. Thrombolysis in the management of lower limb peripheral arterial occlusion—a consensus document. J Vasc Interv Radiol 14(pt 2):S337, 2003.

133. Kessel DO, Berridge DC, Robertson I: Infusion techniques for peripheral arterial thrombolysis. Cochrane Database Syst Rev (1):CD000985, 2004.

134. Dormandy J, Heeck L, Vig S: Acute limb ischemia. Semin Vasc Surg 12:148, 1999.

135. Berridge DC, Kessel D, Robertson I: Surgery versus thrombolysis for acute limb ischaemia: Initial management. Cochrane Database Syst Rev (3):CD002784, 2002.

136. Sobel M, Verhaeghe R: Antithrombotic therapy for peripheral artery occlusive disease: American College of Chest Physicians Evidence-Based Clinical Practice Guidelines (8th Edition). Chest 133(Suppl):815S, 2008.

Artheroembolism

137. Tunick PA, Kronzon I: Atheroembolism. In Creager MA, Dzau VJ, Loscalzo J (eds): Vascular Medicine: A Companion to Braunwald's Heart Disease. Philadelphia, Elsevier, 2006, pp 677-687.

138. Liew YP, Bartholomew JR: Atheromatous embolization. Vasc Med 10:309, 2005.

139. Molisse TA, Tunick PA, Kronzon I: Complications of aortic atherosclerosis: Atheroemboli and thromboemboli. Curr Treat Options Cardiovasc Med 9:137, 2007.

140. Fukumoto Y, Tsutsui H, Tsuchihashi M, et al: The incidence and risk factors of cholesterol embolization syndrome, a complication of cardiac catheterization: A prospective study. J Am Coll Cardiol 42:211, 2003.

CHAPTER **62** # Prevention and Management of Stroke

Larry B. Goldstein

Each year, more than 795,000 Americans have strokes and more than 150,000 die, making stroke the country's third leading cause of death.[1] More than 25% of stroke survivors older than 65 years of age are institutionalized 6 months later. Stroke disproportionately affects minority populations (see Chap. 2). Over 60% of stroke-related deaths occur in women, and women have greater poststroke disability than men (see Chap. 81). Advancing age is a major risk factor for stroke, but more than one third of strokes occur in persons younger than 65 years of age, and even children can be affected. Many of the risk factors for stroke overlap with those of cardiac and peripheral vascular disease (consistent with the concept of global risk), yet stroke represents a variety of conditions and can reflect a diverse set of pathophysiologic processes, and specific therapeutic interventions can confer levels of benefit and risk that differ from those for other forms of vascular disease. This discussion focuses on therapeutic interventions for stroke prevention and treatment of particular relevance to cardiologists. The American Stroke Association and American Heart Association have provided detailed, current, evidence-based guidelines for the primary prevention of ischemic stroke,[2] prevention of ischemic stroke in patients with prior stroke or transient ischemic attack,[3,4] and early management of patients with ischemic stroke, including the use of thrombolytic therapy.[5-7]

Medical Therapy for Stroke Prevention

Approximately 77% of strokes are first events, making primary prevention of paramount importance.[1] Prevention of recurrent events is also critical. Depending on age and race or ethnicity, approximately 10% to 30% of survivors will have a second stroke within 5 years. The period soon after the stroke entails the highest rate of recurrence. The risk of ischemic stroke after a transient ischemic attack (TIA, a condition frequently misdiagnosed, that has been defined as a brief episode of neurologic dysfunction that results from focal brain or retinal ischemia, with clinical symptoms that typically last less than 1 hour and with no radiologic evidence of infarction) is as high as 10.5% over 90 days, with the highest risk over the first week.[3] The ABCD[2] score is helpful in assessing the short-term risk of stroke in patients with TIA (**Table 62-1**).[8] The risk of stroke within 2 days is low (1%) in those with a score of 0 to 3, moderate (4%) in those with a score of 4 or 5, and high (8%) in those with a score of 6 or 7. The risks and benefits of therapeutic interventions differ for primary and secondary stroke prevention.

Platelet Antiaggregants

PRIMARY PREVENTION. The use of antiplatelet agents for primary stroke prevention requires consideration in the context of the patient's global risk for cardiovascular events and stroke. No evidence has shown that antiplatelet therapy reduces stroke in persons at low risk.[2]

The benefit of aspirin for primary cardiovascular prophylaxis outweighs its associated risk of bleeding complications in persons with a

10-year risk of coronary heart events of 6% to 10%, but does not reduce stroke risk even in men, and aspirin is not recommended for this purpose.[2] Although the Women's Health Study found no reduction in its prespecified primary endpoint (nonfatal myocardial infarction [MI], nonfatal stroke, or cardiovascular death) with aspirin (100 mg on alternate days), stroke fell 17%, although the risk of bleeding increased.[9] This benefit accrued primarily in women at elevated stroke risk because of other factors (e.g., hypertension, diabetes). Thus, aspirin may be considered for women whose risk of stroke outweighs its associated bleeding risk. Evidence does not support the benefit of any other antiplatelet agent in reducing the risk of a first stroke.

Anticoagulation is generally recommended for stroke prevention in patients with atrial fibrillation who are at high risk of systemic embolization (see later and Chap. 40).[2] Aspirin plus clopidogrel may decrease the risk of major vascular events (MVEs, predominately stroke) and stroke (**Fig. 62-1**) as compared with aspirin alone in patients with atrial fibrillation judged not to be candidates for anticoagulation, but the combination increases the risk of major bleeding complications—so there was no overall net benefit (MVEs decreased 0.8%/year, major hemorrhages increased 0.7%/year; relative risk [RR], 0.97; 95% confidence interval [CI], 0.89 to 1.06; $P = 0.54$).[10]

SECONDARY PREVENTION. Aspirin (lowest effective dose compared with placebo is 50 mg/day) lowers the risk of recurrent stroke in persons with a noncardioembolic ischemic stroke by approximately 18%.[3] Sustained-release dipyridamole (200 mg twice daily) is as effective as aspirin in reducing the risk of recurrent stroke, with a further reduction (approximately 37%) when the two drugs are combined.[11] Aspirin–sustained-release dipyridamole is available in the United States in a fixed-dose combination (25 mg aspirin plus 200 mg dipyridamole) given twice daily. Cardiologists often worry that dipyridamole might increase the risk of cardiac ischemia, but clinical trials have not substantiated this reservation. There is also concern that the total dose of aspirin (50 mg/day), although effective for secondary stroke prophylaxis, is below the dose shown to be effective for cardiac prophylaxis. To address this potential limitation, a small additional dose of aspirin can be added (e.g., 81 mg/day) to the fixed combination of aspirin-dipyridamole.

Clopidogrel monotherapy given to patients with a history of MI, stroke, or symptomatic peripheral arterial disease reduces the combined risk of MI, stroke, or vascular death as compared with aspirin by 8.7%.[3] Although based on a potentially underpowered subgroup analysis, there is no evidence of a significant reduction in stroke among those with prior stroke. There was no reduction in a composite endpoint of MI, stroke, or cardiovascular death in patients with cardiovascular disease (including stroke) or multiple risk factors with aspirin plus clopidogrel as compared with aspirin alone.[12] When tested directly in patients with stroke, the combination of aspirin and clopidogrel increased bleeding complications without reducing ischemic stroke.[13] Aspirin and clopidogrel should not be used in combination for stroke prophylaxis in patients at high risk or in patients with recent stroke.

TABLE 62-1	Short-Term Risk of Stroke After Transient Ischemic Attack: ABCD² Score	
FACTOR		**POINTS**
Age ≧ 60 years		1
BP ≧ 140/90 mm Hg		1
Clinical features		
• Speech deficit, no weakness		1
• Unilateral weakness		2
Diabetes		1
Duration (minutes)		
• 0-59		1
• ≧60		2

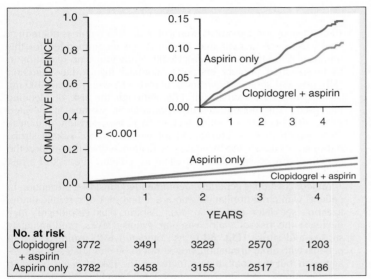

No. at risk

Clopidogrel + aspirin	3772	3491	3229	2570	1203
Aspirin only	3782	3458	3155	2517	1186

FIGURE 62-1 Clopidogrel plus aspirin versus aspirin alone in patients with atrial fibrillation judged not to be candidates for anticoagulation and risk of stroke. *(From ACTIVE Investigators: Effect of clopidogrel added to aspirin in patients with atrial fibrillation. N Engl J Med 360:2066, 2009.)*

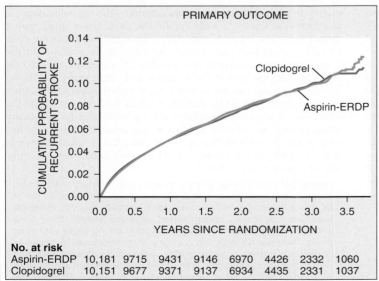

No. at risk

Aspirin-ERDP	10,181	9715	9431	9146	6970	4426	2332	1060
Clopidogrel	10,151	9677	9371	9137	6934	4435	2331	1037

FIGURE 62-2 Clopidogrel versus aspirin plus extended-release dipyridamole (ERDP) for secondary stroke prevention. The primary outcome is time to first recurrent stroke. *(From Sacco RL, Diener HC, Yusuf S, et al: Aspirin and extended-release dipyridamole versus clopidogrel for recurrent stroke. N Engl J Med 359:1238, 2008.)*

A direct comparison found that aspirin plus dipyridamole was comparable to clopidogrel monotherapy for secondary stroke prevention in patients with noncardioembolic stroke (**Fig. 62-2**).[14] Aspirin, aspirin plus sustained-release dipyridamole, and clopidogrel are reasonable options for secondary prevention in these types of patients.[4]

Anticoagulation

PRIMARY PREVENTION. The use of long-term anticoagulation to reduce the risk of a first cardiogenic embolism in patients at increased risk caused by conditions such as mechanical heart valves, atrial fibrillation, and cardiomyopathy is addressed in Chaps. 28, 40, and 66. The combination of aspirin and clopidogrel is inferior to warfarin for stroke prevention in patients with atrial fibrillation (**Fig. 62-3**).[15]

SECONDARY PREVENTION. The evidence supporting the use of anticoagulation for prevention of recurrent stroke in patients without atrial fibrillation or other high-risk cardiogenic sources is uncertain, or the evidence suggests that the benefit does not outweigh the risk of warfarin-associated bleeding complications.

For patients with noncardioembolic stroke, the Warfarin-Aspirin Recurrent Stroke Study (WARSS) directly compared warfarin (international normalized ratio [INR], 2 to 3) and aspirin (325 mg/day).[16] There was a nonsignificant advantage associated with aspirin treatment (17.8% rate of recurrent stroke or death for warfarin, versus 16.0% for aspirin, $P = 0.25$; **Fig. 62-4**). Given the increased costs and monitoring associated with warfarin, there is no reason to use this drug for this purpose.

Although based on a post hoc analysis, data from WARSS also evaluated the problem of what has been termed *aspirin failures*. This term is used variably to refer to patients taking aspirin who have no measurable platelet antiaggregant effect, or to patients who have a recurrent ischemic event such as stroke despite treatment. The latter definition was used in the WARSS analysis. Of the patients who had a history of stroke before the study index stroke, those taking aspirin before randomization (i.e., aspirin failures) and randomized to receive aspirin had a 31.8% rate of recurrent stroke as compared with a 16.9% rate in those who were randomized to aspirin but had not been taking aspirin before randomization (i.e., the rate of recurrent stroke was higher in those who had failed aspirin). The rate of recurrent stroke, however, was 29% in those who had failed aspirin and were randomized to warfarin. Therefore, based on the data from WARSS, despite a high rate of recurrent stroke in patients failing aspirin who subsequently received aspirin, treatment with warfarin showed no advantage. No data show that patients who fail aspirin benefit from an alternative antiplatelet regimen.

A retrospective data analysis has suggested that patients with symptomatic, intracranial, large-vessel stenotic disease benefited from warfarin as compared with aspirin.[17] This hypothesis was subsequently tested in the Warfarin-Aspirin Symptomatic Intracranial Disease (WASID) trial comparing warfarin (INR, 2 to 3) with aspirin (1300 mg/day).[18] The rate of recurrent ischemic stroke, intracerebral hemorrhage, or nonstroke vascular death did not differ between the two treatment regimens (22% with warfarin versus 21% with aspirin; $P = 0.83$), but there was a higher rate of major hemorrhages with warfarin (8.3% versus 3.2%; $P = 0.01$). Because of a lack of efficacy and higher rate of bleeding complications, warfarin should generally not be used for patients with symptomatic large-vessel intracranial stenotic disease. Angioplasty and stenting may also be considered for patients with this condition who fail medical therapy, but no prospective randomized trial has compared this approach with medical therapy.

Although a patent foramen ovale (PFO, with or without an atrial septal aneurysm) is found more commonly in young patients with cryptogenic stroke, optimal medical therapy for secondary stroke prophylaxis is uncertain, and randomized trials assessing the potential benefits of endovascular closure as compared with medical therapy are underway (see Chap. 59). Uncertainty about appropriate management exists in part because of the unclear relationship between the presence of PFO (whether large or small, and with or without an atrial septal aneurysm) and the risk of recurrent stroke and death. A systematic literature review of 129 articles identified four meeting minimal quality criteria and found, as compared with those without a PFO, that there was no significant increase in recurrent stroke or death for those with PFO (odds ratio [OR], 0.95; 95% CI, 0.62 to 1.44), small PFO (OR, 1.23; 95% CI, 0.76 to 2.00), large PFO (OR, 0.59; 95% CI, 0.28 to 1.24), or combined PFO and atrial septal aneurysm (OR, 2.10; 95% CI, 0.86 to 5.06).[19] This finding agrees with the results of the subsequently reported PFO in Cryptogenic Stroke Study (PICSS) that found almost identical rates of recurrent stroke or death, regardless of the presence of a PFO.[20] Essentially, no prospective randomized trials have compared antiplatelet and anticoagulant therapy in this setting, and PICSS found almost identical rates of recurrent stroke or death with aspirin or warfarin in those with and without a PFO.

Patients with low ejection fraction (EF) congestive heart failure are also at risk for systemic embolization, but data from large prospective randomized trials were previously unavailable to determine optimal antithrombotic therapy. The Warfarin and Antiplatelet Therapy in Chronic Heart Failure (WATCH) trial compared open-label warfarin (target INR, 2.5 to 3.0) with double-blind treatment with clopidogrel or aspirin in patients in sinus rhythm with chronic congestive heart failure (EF < 35%).[21] There were no differences between warfarin and aspirin (hazard ratio [HR], 0.98; 95% CI, 0.86 to 1.12; $P = 0.77$), between warfarin and clopidogrel (HR, 0.89; 95% CI, 0.68 to 1.16; $P = 0.39$), or between clopidogrel and aspirin (HR, 1.08; 95% CI, 0.83 to 1.40; $P = 0.57$) for the primary outcome (time to nonfatal stroke, nonfatal MI, or death). There was also no evidence that warfarin is superior to aspirin or that clopidogrel is superior to aspirin for stroke prevention in patients with low ejection fraction congestive heart failure.

The various inherited (e.g., protein C, protein S, antithrombin III deficiency, factor V Leiden, prothrombin G20210A mutation) and acquired (e.g., lupus anticoagulant, anticardiolipin, or antiphospholipid antibodies) coagulopathies are more commonly associated with venous as compared with arterial thromboses (see Chap. 87).[3] Although occasionally these disorders associate with ischemic stroke, particularly in children or young adults, causal relationships remain controversial. For example, in another substudy of the WARSS trial, the Antiphospholipid Antibody Stroke Study (APASS), 41% of 1770 subjects were positive for one or more antiphospholipid antibodies.[22] Rates of recurrent thromboembolic events were somewhat higher for those who were antiphospholipid antibody–positive, but there was no difference for those antibody-positive patients who were treated with warfarin as compared with aspirin. Patients with venous thromboembolic events who have an underlying coagulopathy, or those with stroke or TIA otherwise fulfilling the criteria for the antiphospholipid antibody syndrome (venous and arterial occlusive disease in multiple organs, miscarriages, and livedo reticularis) are appropriately treated with warfarin. Because coagulopathies, especially the genetic forms listed, are more commonly associated with venous thromboses, cryptogenic stroke in this setting should prompt an evaluation for sources of paradoxical embolism. The yield of magnetic resonance imaging (MRI) of the pelvic and lower extremities is higher than with ultrasound, and should be considered in patients with a presumed paradoxical embolus.[23] Those with arterial stroke who are found to have only elevated antiphospholipid antibody levels may reasonably be treated with aspirin.

HMG-CoA Reductase Inhibitors (Statins)

(See Chaps. 47 and 49.)

PRIMARY PREVENTION. Statins not only reduce cardiac events, but also the risk of a first stroke in patients at risk (**Fig. 62-5**). A

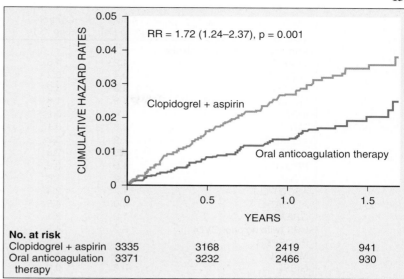

FIGURE 62-3 Clopidogrel plus aspirin versus anticoagulation in patients with atrial fibrillation and risk of stroke. *(From the Active Writing Group of the ACTIVE Investigators; Connolly S, Pogue J, Hart R, et al: Clopidogrel plus aspirin versus oral anticoagulation for atrial fibrillation in the Atrial Fibrillation Clopidogrel Trial with Irbesartan for prevention of Vascular Events (ACTIVE W): A randomised controlled trial. Lancet 367:1903, 2006.)*

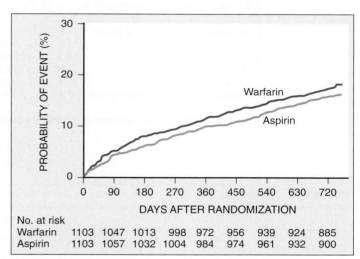

FIGURE 62-4 Kaplan-Meier analyses of the time to recurrent ischemic stroke or death according to treatment assignment. *(From Mohr JP, Thompson JL, Lazar RM, et al: A comparison of warfarin and aspirin for the prevention of recurrent ischemic stroke. N Engl J Med 345:1444, 2001.)*

meta-analysis of randomized trials of statins including 165,792 subjects found that each 40-mg/dL decrease in low-density lipoprotein (LDL) cholesterol was associated with a 21.1% (95% CI, 6.3 to 33.5%; $P = 0.009$) reduction in the risk of a first stroke (**Fig. 62-6**).[24]

Some studies have shown a reduction in the risk of first stroke with statin treatment among diabetics,[25,26] hypertensives,[27] and older adults.[28] The Justification for the Use of Statins in Prevention: An Intervention Trial Evaluating Rosuvastatin (JUPITER) evaluated the effect of a statin in persons with an elevated (more than 2 mg/dL) high sensitivity C-reactive protein level, but with LDL cholesterol below 130 mg/dL (see Chap. 47).[29] Statin treatment resulted in a 44% reduction in the time to the primary endpoint (combined risk of MI, stroke, arterial revascularization, hospitalization for unstable angina, or death from cardiovascular causes [HR, 0.56; 95% CI, 0.46 to 0.69; $P < 0.00001$] including an approximate 50% reduction in stroke (**Fig. 62-7**). The implications of the results of the trial for patient management have engendered debate.[30]

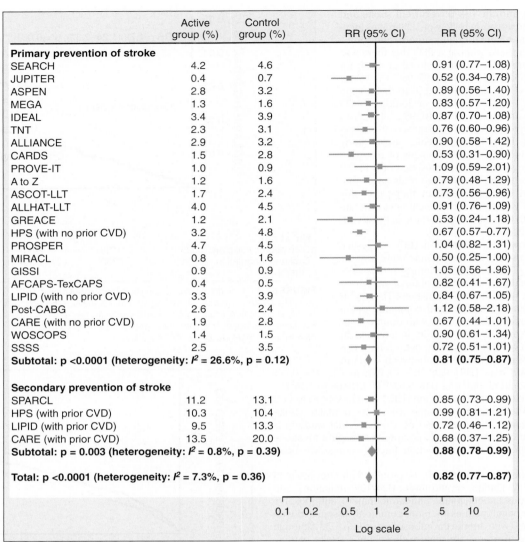

	Active group (%)	Control group (%)	RR (95% CI)	RR (95% CI)
Primary prevention of stroke				
SEARCH	4.2	4.6		0.91 (0.77–1.08)
JUPITER	0.4	0.7		0.52 (0.34–0.78)
ASPEN	2.8	3.2		0.89 (0.56–1.40)
MEGA	1.3	1.6		0.83 (0.57–1.20)
IDEAL	3.4	3.9		0.87 (0.70–1.08)
TNT	2.3	3.1		0.76 (0.60–0.96)
ALLIANCE	2.9	3.2		0.90 (0.58–1.42)
CARDS	1.5	2.8		0.53 (0.31–0.90)
PROVE-IT	1.0	0.9		1.09 (0.59–2.01)
A to Z	1.2	1.6		0.79 (0.48–1.29)
ASCOT-LLT	1.7	2.4		0.73 (0.56–0.96)
ALLHAT-LLT	4.0	4.5		0.91 (0.76–1.09)
GREACE	1.2	2.1		0.53 (0.24–1.18)
HPS (with no prior CVD)	3.2	4.8		0.67 (0.57–0.77)
PROSPER	4.7	4.5		1.04 (0.82–1.31)
MIRACL	0.8	1.6		0.50 (0.25–1.00)
GISSI	0.9	0.9		1.05 (0.56–1.96)
AFCAPS-TexCAPS	0.4	0.5		0.82 (0.41–1.67)
LIPID (with no prior CVD)	3.3	3.9		0.84 (0.67–1.05)
Post-CABG	2.6	2.4		1.12 (0.58–2.18)
CARE (with no prior CVD)	1.9	2.8		0.67 (0.44–1.01)
WOSCOPS	1.4	1.5		0.90 (0.61–1.34)
SSSS	2.5	3.5		0.72 (0.51–1.01)
Subtotal: p <0.0001 (heterogeneity: I^2 = 26.6%, p = 0.12)				**0.81 (0.75–0.87)**
Secondary prevention of stroke				
SPARCL	11.2	13.1		0.85 (0.73–0.99)
HPS (with prior CVD)	10.3	10.4		0.99 (0.81–1.21)
LIPID (with prior CVD)	9.5	13.3		0.72 (0.46–1.12)
CARE (with prior CVD)	13.5	20.0		0.68 (0.37–1.25)
Subtotal: p = 0.003 (heterogeneity: I^2 = 0.8%, p = 0.39)				**0.88 (0.78–0.99)**
Total: p <0.0001 (heterogeneity: I^2 = 7.3%, p = 0.36)				**0.82 (0.77–0.87)**

0.1   0.2   0.5   1   2   5   10

Log scale

FIGURE 62-5 Meta-analysis of the effects of statins on stroke prevention. Results are from 24 trials with 165,792 patients with fatal and nonfatal stroke. *(From Amarenco P, Labreuche J: Lipid management in the prevention of stroke: Review and updated meta-analysis of statins for stroke prevention. Lancet Neurol 8:453, 2009; data on LIPID and CARE with or without prior CVD from Vergouwen MD, de Haan RJ, Vermeulen M, Roos YB: Statin treatment and the occurrence of hemorrhagic stroke in patients with a history of cerebrovascular disease. Stroke 39:497, 2008.)*

SECONDARY PREVENTION. In contrast to the large amount of data showing a reduction in the risk of a first stroke in patients with coronary heart disease (CHD) or at high CHD risk who are treated with a statin, until recently there has been no evidence that treatment with a statin reduces the risk of a second stroke. The Heart Protection Study (HPS) included 3280 subjects with a history of stroke (including 1820 with stroke and no history of CHD) who were treated with a statin or placebo.[31] Among those with a prior history of stroke, statin treatment reduced the frequency of MVEs (e.g., MI, stroke, revascularization procedure, or vascular death) by 20%, but did not lower the risk of recurrent stroke (occurring in 10.5% in those treated with placebo versus 10.4% in those treated with the statin). Among several plausible reasons for the lack of effect on recurrent stroke, the most important might be that patients were randomized an average of approximately 4 years after the index event. Most recurrent strokes occur within the first few years, so those randomized in the HPS were at relatively low risk of recurrent stroke.

The Stroke Prevention with Aggressive Reduction in Cholesterol Levels (SPARCL) trial randomized over 4700 subjects who were within 6 months of a noncardioembolic stroke or TIA and with no known CHD to high-dose statin or placebo, for a primary endpoint of the first occurrence of a nonfatal or fatal stroke.[32] Those randomized to high-dose statin treatment had a 16% relative reduction in nonfatal or fatal stroke, as well as a 35% relative reduction in major coronary events. Added to the previous data on prevention of a first stroke, SPARCL showed that treatment with a high-dose statin can reduce the risk of recurrent stroke after a stroke or TIA (**Fig. 62-8**). On the basis of this trial, statin therapy with intensive lipid-lowering effects is recommended for patients with atherosclerotic ischemic stroke or TIA and without known CHD to reduce the risk of stroke and cardiovascular events.[4] The results suggest that noncardioembolic stroke might be considered as a CHD equivalent because of the dramatic reduction in CHD events, despite the subjects having no known CHD at the time of randomization.

Antihypertensives (see Chap. 46)

PRIMARY PREVENTION. Hypertension is one of the most important treatable risk factors for both ischemic stroke and parenchymal intracerebral hemorrhage. The Seventh Report of the Joint National Committee on Prevention, Detection, Evaluation, and Treatment of High Blood Pressure (JNC 7) has provided comprehensive,

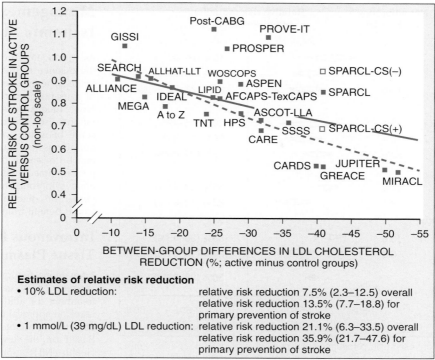

FIGURE 62-6 Cholesterol lowering with statins and stroke risk. Inverse variance-weighted regression lines have been plotted after including all 24 trials (165,792 patients; solid line) and after excluding trials with clearly identified groups of patients in secondary stroke prevention (SPARCL; HPS, LIPID, and CARE subgroups with previous cerebrovascular disease; dashed line). The underlying causes of stroke are important when considering the association between lipid and stroke risk, so the SPARCL results are also shown in accordance with the presence or absence of documented CS. The data for the SEARCH trial were presented at the 2008 American Heart Association meeting. CS = carotid stenosis. *(From Amarenco P, Labreuche J: Lipid management in the prevention of stroke: Review and updated meta-analysis of statins for stroke prevention. Lancet Neurol 8:453, 2009.)*

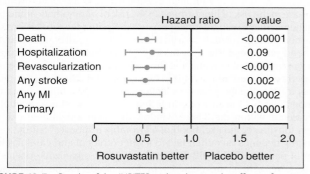

FIGURE 62-7 Results of the JUPITER trial evaluating the effects of statin treatment in patients with high-sensitivity C-reactive protein (hs-CRP) > 2 mg/dL and no other indication for statin therapy. Numbers indicate point estimate; horizontal lines indicate 95% CI. *(From Goldstein LB: JUPITER and the world of stroke medicine. Lancet Neurol 8:130, 2009; data from Ridker PM: Rosuvastatin in the primary prevention of cardiovascular disease among patients with low levels of low-density lipoprotein cholesterol and elevated high-sensitivity C-reactive protein: Rationale and design of the JUPITER trial. Circulation 108:2292, 2003.)*

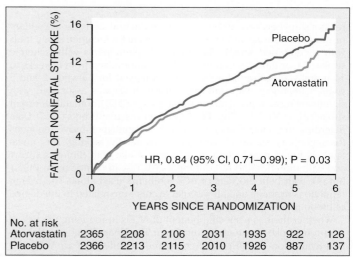

FIGURE 62-8 Kaplan-Meier curve for stroke or TIA in SPARCL. The data report an intention-to-treat analysis with prespecified adjustments for geographic region, entry event, time since entry event, sex, and baseline age for the first occurrence of a fatal or nonfatal stroke or TIA. *(From Amarenco P, Bogousslavsky J, Callahan A III, et al: High-dose atorvastatin after stroke or transient ischemic attack. N Engl J Med 355:549, 2006.)*

evidence-based guidelines for the classification and treatment of hypertension, reiterated in the current American Stroke Association Primary Stroke Prevention Guidelines.[2,33] Both guidelines support individualization of the choice of a specific antihypertensive regimen, and suggest that the reduction in blood pressure is generally more important than the specific agent(s) used to achieve this goal. A meta-analysis of randomized controlled trials comparing antihypertensive drugs with placebo or no treatment on stroke, including more than 73,500 participants and almost 2900 stroke events, found similar risk reductions for angiotensin-converting enzyme (ACE) inhibitors (28%), beta-adrenergic receptor blockers (beta blockers) or diuretics (35%),

and calcium channel antagonists (39%), corresponding to blood pressure reductions of 5/2, 13/6 and 10/5 mm Hg, respectively (**Fig. 62-9**).[34]

SECONDARY PREVENTION. Only limited data directly address the role of blood pressure treatment in secondary prevention for those with a history of stroke or TIA. A systematic review focused on the

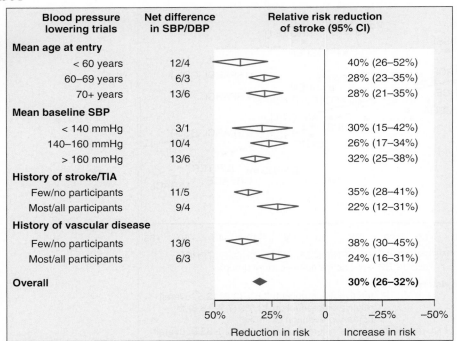

Blood pressure lowering trials	Net difference in SBP/DBP	Relative risk reduction of stroke (95% CI)	
Mean age at entry			
< 60 years	12/4		40% (26–52%)
60–69 years	6/3		28% (23–35%)
70+ years	13/6		28% (21–35%)
Mean baseline SBP			
< 140 mmHg	3/1		30% (15–42%)
140–160 mmHg	10/4		26% (17–34%)
> 160 mmHg	13/6		32% (25–38%)
History of stroke/TIA			
Few/no participants	11/5		35% (28–41%)
Most/all participants	9/4		22% (12–31%)
History of vascular disease			
Few/no participants	13/6		38% (30–45%)
Most/all participants	6/3		24% (16–31%)
Overall			**30% (26–32%)**

50%   25%   0   −25%   −50%

Reduction in risk   Increase in risk

FIGURE 62-9 Randomized controlled trials comparing antihypertensive drugs with a placebo (or no treatment) by subgroup. The meta-analyses of blood pressure–lowering trials were stratified into subgroups on the basis of mean age of trial participants at entry, baseline systolic blood pressure level, and whether trial participants predominantly had a history of stroke-TIA or vascular disease. The diamonds are centered on the pooled estimate of effect and represent a 95% CI. The solid diamond represents the pooled relative risk and 95% CI for all contributing trials. BP = blood pressure; DBP = diastolic blood pressure; SBP = systolic blood pressure. *(From Lawes CM, Bennett DA, Feigin FL, Rodgers A: Blood pressure and stroke: An overview of published reviews. Stroke 35:1024, 2004.)*

relationship between blood pressure reduction and the secondary prevention of stroke and other vascular events; it included seven trials with a combined sample size of 15,527 participants with ischemic stroke, TIA, or intracerebral hemorrhage randomized from 3 weeks to 14 months after the index event and followed for between 2 and 5 years.[35] Treatment with antihypertensive drugs was associated with significant reductions in all recurrent strokes (24%), nonfatal recurrent stroke (21%), MI (21%; **Fig. 62-10**), and all vascular events (21%). Data regarding the relative benefits of specific antihypertensive regimens for secondary stroke prevention are generally lacking. This meta-analysis found a reduction in recurrent stroke with diuretics (32%), and with diuretics and ACE inhibitors (ACEIs) in combination (45%), but not with beta blockers or ACE inhibitors used alone. The overall reductions in stroke and all vascular events were related to the degree of blood pressure lowering.

Whether there is a specific benefit of ACEIs in reducing the risk of recurrent stroke also remains uncertain. The Heart Outcomes Prevention Evaluation (HOPE) study compared the effects of an ACEI with placebo in high-risk persons and found a 24% risk reduction in the risk of stroke, MI, or vascular death among the 1013 patients with a history of stroke or TIA.[3] The Perindopril Protection Against Recurrent Stroke Study (PROGRESS) tested the effects of a blood pressure–lowering regimen, including an ACEI, in 6105 patients with stroke or TIA within the prior 5 years.[3] Randomization was stratified by intention to use single (ACEI) or combination (ACEI plus the diuretic indapamide) therapy in hypertensive (>160 mm Hg systolic or >90 mm Hg diastolic) and nonhypertensive patients. The combination (lowering blood pressure by an average of 12/5 mm Hg) reduced the risk of recurrent stroke by 43% and of major vascular events by 40% in both the hypertensive and normotensive groups. However, there was no significant benefit of either antihypertensive given alone. The choice of a specific antihypertensive regimen should be guided by specific patient characteristics and comorbid conditions.

Management of Acute Ischemic Stroke

As with acute coronary syndromes, time is of the essence in the treatment of patients with acute ischemic stroke. Stroke has a large variety of causative factors and potential pathophysiologic mechanisms that critically influence the rational use of secondary preventive therapies, some of which were reviewed earlier. Some conditions may cause symptoms and signs that can be mistaken for those of a stroke. In the period immediately following the onset of ischemic symptoms, however, evaluation should center on determining whether the patient would benefit from reperfusion therapy.

Intravenous Recombinant Tissue Plasminogen Activator

Intravenous recombinant tissue plasminogen activator (rt-PA) is currently the only specific treatment for acute ischemic stroke that has received approval from the FDA. The treatment aims to lyse a clot occluding a cerebral artery. Based on the pivotal National Institutes of Health (NIH)–sponsored randomized clinical trial, treatment of appropriate patients is associated with an approximate 13% absolute (32% relative) increase in the proportion of patients free of disability 3 months later.[6] Benefits are similar for patients with small penetrating artery distribution ischemic stroke and for those with occlusion of larger intracranial arteries. Although treatment is also associated with an increase in the risk of hemorrhage (6.4% risk of symptomatic intracerebral hemorrhage with treatment versus 0.6% with placebo; 2.9% risk of fatal hemorrhage versus 0.3% with placebo), the overall benefit includes these adverse events. The drug must be given within 3 hours of the onset of symptoms, which means that the patient must generally arrive at a properly equipped and organized hospital within 2 hours of symptom onset to have the necessary evaluations (including a brain computed tomography [CT] scan to exclude hemorrhage or other conditions) completed. Within the 3-hour window, the sooner treatment can be given, the greater the likelihood of a favorable response.[36] Safest use of the drug depends on adherence to a strict protocol and careful selection of patients (**Table 62-2**). Development of organized systems of stroke care has been advocated to perform rapidly the necessary clinical evaluations, to minimize delays in treatment, to institute other interventions associated with improved outcomes, and ensure that patients receive appropriate secondary prevention.[37]

Secondary analyses of prior thrombolytic trials have suggested a benefit, albeit reduced, with treatment up to 4 to 5 hours after symptom onset.[36] This hypothesis was tested in a separate clinical trial that included restrictions in addition to those of the NIH-sponsored three-hour trial (see Table 62-2).[38] Treatment resulted in an increase in the proportion of patients with excellent outcomes (Rankin index, 0 to 1) after 3 months (52.4% versus 45.2% with placebo; OR, for global favorable outcome, 1.28; 95% CI, 1.00 to 1.65). Although not FDA-approved, guidelines have been modified to extend treatment to this restricted group of patients who can be treated between 3 to 4.5 hours of symptom onset, but stress that treatment must be given as soon as possible after symptom onset to derive the greatest benefit.[7]

Up to one third of patients may have early arterial reocclusion after intravenous thrombolysis.[6] One study has suggested that clot lysis might be facilitated by concomitant exposure to ultrasound provided by transcranial Doppler, which can also be used to monitor clot dissolution.[39] A prospective trial is evaluating the usefulness of this approach.

Endovascular Therapy

Endovascular approaches that are catheter-based for acute reperfusion have the theoretical advantages of allowing for direct clot visualization and localized rather than systemic administration of thrombolytics, as well as the opportunity for mechanical clot disruption. No prospective randomized trials have directly compared endovascular therapy with intravenous rt-PA. In addition, endovascular therapy can only be accomplished in centers with immediate access to neurovascular interventionalists, is not generally feasible in patients with distal arterial occlusions, and might entail longer times to reperfusion (e.g., related to the need for access to an interventional suite, catheter placement time).

Prospective randomized data comparing intra-arterial thrombolysis with non-thrombolytic medical therapy have come primarily from a single clinical trial.[6] This study evaluated intra-arterial thrombolysis with prourokinase in patients within 6 hours of angiographically proven proximal middle cerebral artery occlusion, and found a significant improvement in 3-month outcome (40% of treated versus 25% of control patients had little or no disability), despite a trend toward an increase in symptomatic intracerebral hemorrhages (10% versus 2%, respectively). Prourokinase has not been approved by the FDA and is not currently available in the United States. Intra-arterial rt-PA is commonly used for this purpose in patients who do not qualify for treatment with intravenous rt-PA (usually because of arriving at the hospital too late) and otherwise fulfills the inclusion

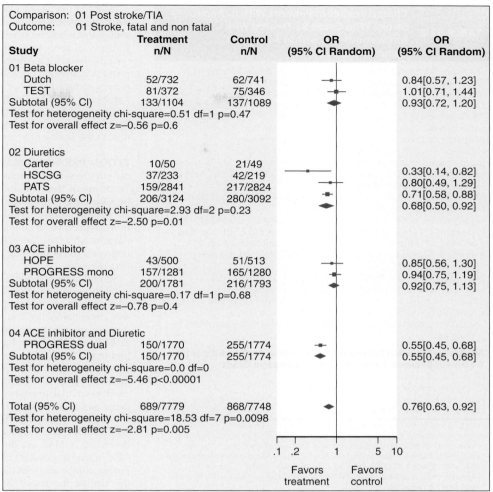

FIGURE 62-10 Forrest plot of the effect of antihypertensive therapy in patients with prior stroke or TIA on subsequent fatal and nonfatal stroke. *(From Rashid P, Leonardi-Bee J, Bath P: Blood pressure reduction and secondary prevention of stroke and other vascular events: A systematic review. Stroke 34:2741, 2003.)*

criteria for the prourokinase trial cited. In addition to patients with middle cerebral artery occlusions up to 6 hours earlier, based on case series data, selected patients with basilar artery occlusion up to 12 hours or longer may also be treated with this approach. Several ongoing studies are evaluating intra-arterial thrombolysis with rt-PA, but the FDA has not yet approved this approach.

Mechanical clot retrieval has the theoretical advantage of avoiding the bleeding risk associated with thrombolytic drugs. The MERCI clot retriever was the first approved by the FDA for the removal of blood clots from brain blood vessels, but not as a specific treatment for acute stroke. This approval was based on the results of a noncontrolled case series involving 151 enrolled patients (141 of whom could be treated) with proximal (internal carotid, middle cerebral, or vertebrobasilar) arterial occlusions within 6 hours (mean, 4.3 hours to catheterization).[40] Recanalization was achieved in 48%, of whom 30% died or had a second stroke or MI within 30 days. Approximately 30% died within 90 days, but 46% of those surviving at 90 days had little or no disability. Procedural complications occurred in 13% (six arterial perforations, four arterial dissections, three cases of embolization to another artery, three subarachnoid hemorrhages, and three groin hematomas), with 28% having asymptomatic intracerebral hemorrhages and 8% symptomatic hemorrhages. The frequency of parenchymal hemorrhages might at first seem surprising; however, the arterial endothelium can be subject to ischemia-related damage, and reperfusion of a damaged artery (with or without a thrombolytic) can lead to bleeding. This study had no concurrent controls, leaving open whether outcomes would be similar, better, or worse than with other reperfusion treatments. Other devices have since been approved, also based on case series lacking concurrent controls. The approach has the same logistic limitations as endovascular thrombolytic therapy, but does offer the possibility of treatment for selected patients

who cannot be treated with a thrombolytic drug (e.g., patients already anticoagulated, having a recent operation or invasive procedure, or having an embolus complicating cardiac or other catheterization after the catheter sheath has been removed).

Other Measures for Stroke Treatment

Several other important questions often arise concerning the management of patients with acute ischemic stroke and other interventions that are generally used, even without definitive supporting data.

ANTICOAGULATION AND ANTIPLATELET THERAPY. The indications for acute anticoagulation of patients with ischemic stroke are extremely limited. The most recent American Heart Association/American Academy of Neurology guidelines specifically discourage emergent anticoagulation with the goal of improving neurologic outcomes or preventing early recurrent stroke in patients with acute ischemic stroke because of a high risk of intracranial bleeding complications, and do not recommend the initiation of anticoagulant therapy within 24 hours of treatment with intravenously administered rt-PA.[41] Patients with atrial fibrillation–associated stroke benefit from long-term anticoagulation, unless contraindicated because of high bleeding risk (e.g., prior intracerebral hemorrhage, falls). The risk of early recurrence in patients with stroke related to atrial fibrillation is generally low (approximately 0.3 to 0.5%/day for the first 2 weeks), so the timing of the initiation of anticoagulation needs to be balanced

TABLE 62-2 **Characteristics of Patients With Ischemic Stroke Who Could Be Treated With Intravenous-tPA within 3 Hours of Symptom Onset**

Diagnosis of ischemic stroke causing measurable neurologic deficit
The neurologic signs should not be clearing spontaneously.
The neurologic signs should not be minor and isolated.
Caution should be exercised in treating a patient with major deficits.
The symptoms of stroke should not be suggestive of subarachnoid hemorrhage.
Onset of symptoms < 3 hours before beginning treatment
No head trauma or prior stroke in the previous 3 months
No myocardial infarction in the previous 3 months
No gastrointestinal or urinary tract hemorrhage in the previous 21 days
No major surgery in the previous 14 days
No arterial puncture at a noncompressible site in the previous 7 days
No history of previous intracranial hemorrhage
Blood pressure not elevated (systolic > 185 mm Hg; diastolic > 110 mm Hg)
No evidence of active bleeding or acute trauma (fracture) on examination
Not taking an oral anticoagulant, or if anticoagulant being taken, INR< 1.7
If receiving heparin in previous 48 hr, aPTT must be in normal range
Platelet count > 100,000 mm^3
Blood glucose concentration > 50 mg/dL (2.7 mmol/liter)
No seizure with postictal residual neurologic impairments
CT does not show a multilobar infarction (hypodensity one third of cerebral hemisphere).
The patient and/or family understands the potential risks and benefits of treatment.

Additional Exclusion Criteria for Patients Who Are Candidates for Treatment Between 3 and 4.5 Hours of Symptom Onset
Older than 80 years
Taking oral anticoagulants regardless of INR
NIHSS score > 25
History of both prior stroke and diabetes

aPTT = activated partial thromboplastin time; NIHSS = NIH stroke scale.
Modified from Adams HP, Adams R, Del Zoppo G, Goldstein LB: Guidelines for the early management of patients with ischemic stroke: 2005 guidelines update. A scientific statement from the Stroke Council of the American Heart Association/American Stroke Association. Stroke 36:916, 2005; and Del Zoppo G, Saver J, Jauch EC, Adams HP: Expansion of the time window for treatment of acute ischemic stroke with intravenous tissue plasminogen activator. Stroke 40:2945, 2009.

against the risk of bleeding. Those with large strokes and those with uncontrolled hypertension generally have the highest risk of spontaneous hemorrhagic transformation of an ischemic stroke.

The use of anticoagulants in patients with stroke related to infective endocarditis is problematic (see Chap. 67). Systemic embolization occurs in 22% to 50% of patients with infective endocarditis, with up to 65% of emboli affecting the central nervous system; most of these (90%) involve the middle cerebral artery.[42] There is no demonstrated benefit for anticoagulation in patients with native valve endocarditis, and it is generally not recommended for at least the first 2 weeks of antibiotic therapy in patients with stroke related to *Staphylococcus aureus* prosthetic valve endocarditis. Of particular concern is the possible development of mycotic intracranial aneurysms. These are often multiple and can be asymptomatic, associated with focal neurologic signs, or can affect distal branches of the middle cerebral artery, associated with signs and symptoms of subarachnoid hemorrhage or a sterile meningitis. Although CT angiography in patients without renal insufficiency or MR angiography can be useful screening tests in patients with symptoms suggesting the presence of a mycotic aneurysm, because distal portions of the artery are most commonly affected, catheter angiography is the gold standard for the detection of these lesions; distal portions of the middle cerebral artery can be difficult to visualize by CT or MR angiography. The management of patients with intracranial mycotic aneurysms is complex; many regress with antibiotic treatment. Depending on a variety of factors, surgical clipping or endovascular obliteration can also be considered. Anticoagulation is generally avoided in patients with known mycotic aneurysms because of their propensity to rupture.

As noted, the use of antiplatelet agents reduces the risk of recurrent stroke in patients with a history of ischemic stroke or TIA. In the acute setting, there may be benefit from treatment with aspirin begun within 48 hours of acute ischemic stroke (these platelet antiaggregant drugs are prohibited for the first 24 hours in patients treated with intravenous rt-PA). A combined analysis of two relevant trials has found that treatment with aspirin (160 or 325 mg daily) is associated with a small but statistically significant reduction of nine (±three) fewer deaths or nonfatal strokes/1000 treated patients.[41] There remain no data showing the benefit of any other platelet antiaggregant, given alone or in combination, in the setting of acute ischemic stroke.

BLOOD PRESSURE MANAGEMENT. Management of blood pressure in the setting of acute ischemic stroke remains largely empiric.[6] Treatment of elevated blood pressure in patients who might otherwise be candidates for intravenous rt-PA differs from that of patients who are not thrombolytic candidates, and follows a specific protocol. Relatively aggressive treatment for elevated blood pressure is used for patients who have been treated with a thrombolytic because of an increased risk of bleeding complications associated with uncontrolled hypertension.

Several lines of evidence suggest cautious blood pressure management in nonthrombolytic-treated patients with acute ischemic stroke who do not have malignant hypertension (i.e., patients with hypertensive encephalopathy, aortic dissection, acute renal failure, acute pulmonary edema, acute myocardial infarction, or blood pressures > 220/120 mm Hg).[6] Cerebral autoregulation maintains constant cerebral blood flow (CBF) despite fluctuations in systemic blood pressure (see Chaps. 45 and 46). CBF is determined by the cerebral perfusion pressure (generally the mean arterial pressure, MAP) divided by the cerebrovascular resistance (CVR).[43] As reflected by this relationship, decreases in MAP lead to dilation of cerebral arterioles (decreased CVR), thereby keeping CBF constant. The local acidosis that accompanies brain ischemia leads to maximal vasodilatation. As a result, decreases in MAP are directly reflected in changes in local CBF (if CVR remains constant). Therefore, lowering blood pressure may further compromise an already ischemic brain, potentially increasing the size of the stroke. If treatment is necessary, precipitous drops should be avoided.

Stroke after Percutaneous Coronary Intervention and Thrombolytic Treatment for Myocardial Infarction

Although occurring infrequently, stroke can be a major complication of percutaneous coronary intervention (PCI) (see Chap. 58). The same principles outlined for the management of acute stroke in other settings apply. If neurologic symptoms are recognized while the catheter sheath is still in place, the patient might be treated with intravenous rt-PA, provided that all the other inclusion criteria are met and there are no other contraindications to the therapy. If symptoms are first noted after the catheter sheath has been removed, then the patient could be evaluated for catheter-based endovascular treatment. It is important to have a system in place to ensure the rapid evaluation and treatment of patients with stroke after PCI.

Intracerebral hemorrhage following thrombolytic administration for acute myocardial MI is another serious treatment-related complication (see Chap. 55). The infusion should be stopped and heparin discontinued for any patient developing acute neurologic symptoms. Because these symptoms might result from hemorrhage or ischemia, a brain imaging study is mandatory before proceeding with further treatment. Treatments to reduce the amount of thrombolytic-associated intracerebral hemorrhage once it has occurred are not well established. The administration of cryoprecipitate and/or fresh-frozen plasma has been advocated. Those with brainstem compression related to cerebellar hemorrhage may benefit from surgical evacuation of the hematoma. Patients should be transferred to a setting with expertise in neurologic intensive care as soon as feasible.

REFERENCES

1. Lloyd-Jones D, Adams R, Carnethon M, et al: Heart disease and stroke statistics—2009 update: A report from the American Heart Association Statistics Committee and Stroke Statistics Subcommittee. Circulation 119:480, 2009.

Guidelines

2. Goldstein LB, Adams R, Alberts MJ, et al: Primary prevention of ischemic stroke: A guideline from the American Heart Association/American Stroke Association Stroke Council. Stroke 37:1583, 2006.
3. Sacco RL, Adams R, Albers G, et al: Guidelines for prevention of stroke in patients with ischemic stroke or transient ischemic attack. A statement for healthcare professionals from the American Heart Association/ American Stroke Association Council on Stroke. Stroke 37:577, 2006.
4. Adams RJ, Albers G, Alberts MJ, et al: Update to the AHA/ASA recommendations for the prevention of stroke in patients with stroke and transient ischemic attack. Stroke 39:1647, 2008.
5. Adams HP, Adams RJ, Brott T, et al: Guidelines for the early management of patients with ischemic stroke: A scientific statement from the Stroke Council of the American Stroke Association. Stroke 34:1056, 2003.
6. Adams HP, Adams R, Del Zoppo G, Goldstein LB: Guidelines for the early management of patients with ischemic stroke: 2005 guidelines update. A scientific statement from the Stroke Council of the American Heart Association/American Stroke Association. Stroke 36:916, 2005.
7. Del Zoppo G, Saver J, Jauch EC, Adams HP: Expansion of the time window for treatment of acute ischemic stroke with intravenous tissue plasminogen activator. Stroke 40:2945, 2009.

Medical Therapy for Stroke Prevention

8. Johnston SC, Rothwell PM, Nguyen-Huynh MN, et al: Validation and refinement of scores to predict very early stroke risk after transient ischaemic attack. Lancet 369:283, 2007.
9. Ridker PM, Cook NR, Lee I-M, et al: A randomized trial of low-dose aspirin in the primary prevention of cardiovascular disease in women. N Engl J Med 352:1293, 2005.
10. ACTIVE Investigators: Effect of clopidogrel added to aspirin in patients with atrial fibrillation. N Engl J Med 360:2066, 2009.
11. ESPRIT Study Group: Aspirin plus dipyridamole versus aspirin alone after cerebral ischaemia of arterial origin (ESPRIT): Randomised controlled trial. Lancet 367:1665, 2006.
12. Bhatt DL, Fox KA, Hacke W, et al: Clopidogrel and aspirin versus aspirin alone for the prevention of atherothrombotic events. N Engl J Med 354:1706, 2006.
13. Diener H-C, Bogousslavsky J, Brass LM, et al: Aspirin and clopidogrel compared with clopidogrel alone after recent ischaemic stroke or transient ischaemic attack in high-risk patients (MATCH): Randomised, double-blind, placebo-controlled trial. Lancet 364:331, 2004.
14. Sacco RL, Diener HC, Yusuf S, et al: Aspirin and extended-release dipyridamole versus clopidogrel for recurrent stroke. N Engl J Med 359:1238, 2008.
15. Active Writing Group of the ACTIVE Investigators: Clopidogrel plus aspirin versus oral anticoagulation for atrial fibrillation in the Atrial fibrillation Clopidogrel Trial with Irbesartan for prevention of Vascular Events (ACTIVE W): A randomised controlled trial. Lancet 367:1903, 2006.
16. Mohr JP, Thompson JLP, Lazar RM, et al: Comparison of warfarin and aspirin for the prevention of recurrent ischemic stroke. N Engl J Med 345:1444, 2001.
17. Chimowitz MI, Kokkinos J, Strong J, et al: The Warfarin-Aspirin Symptomatic Intracranial Disease study. Neurology 45:1488, 1995.
18. Chimowitz MI, Lynn MJ, Howlett-Smith H, et al: Comparison of warfarin and aspirin for symptomatic intracranial arterial stenosis. N Engl J Med 352:1305, 2005.
19. Messé SR, Silverman IE, Kizer JR, et al: Practice parameter: Recurrent stroke with patent foramen ovale and atrial septal aneurysm: Report of the Quality Standards Subcommittee of the American Academy of Neurology. Neurology 62:1042, 2004.
20. Homma S, Sacco RL, Di Tullio MR, et al: Effect of medical treatment in stroke patients with patent foramen ovale: Patent Foramen Ovale in Cryptogenic Stroke Study. Circulation 105:2625, 2002.
21. Massie BM, Collins JF, Ammon SE, et al: Randomized trial of warfarin, aspirin, and clopidogrel in patients with chronic heart failure: The Warfarin and Antiplatelet Therapy in Chronic Heart Failure (WATCH) Trial. Circulation 119:1616, 2009.

22. Levine SR, Brey RL, Tilley BC, et al: Antiphospholipid antibodies and subsequent thrombo-occlusive events in patients with ischemic stroke. JAMA 291:576, 2004.
23. Cramer SC, Rordorf G, Maki JH, et al: Increased pelvic vein thrombi in cryptogenic stroke. Results of the Paradoxical Emboli from Large Veins in Ischemic Stroke (PELVIS) study. Stroke 35:46, 2004.
24. Amarenco P, Labreuche J: Lipid management in the prevention of stroke: Review and updated meta-analysis of statins for stroke prevention. Lancet Neurol 8:453, 2009.
25. Collins R, Armitage J, Parish S, et al; Heart Protection Study Collaborative Group: MRC/BHF Heart Protection Study of cholesterol-lowering with simvastatin in 5963 people with diabetes: A randomized placebo-controlled trial. Lancet 361:2005, 2003.
26. Colhoun HM, Betteridge DJ, Durrington PN, et al: Primary prevention of cardiovascular disease with atorvastatin in type 2 diabetes in the Collaborative Atorvastatin Diabetes Study (CARDS): Multicentre randomised placebo-controlled trial. Lancet 364:685, 2004.
27. Sever PS, Dahlof B, Poulter NR, et al: Prevention of coronary and stroke events with atorvastatin in hypertensive patients who have average or lower-than-average cholesterol concentrations, in the Anglo-Scandinavian Cardiac Outcomes Trial—Lipid Lowering Arm (ASCOT-LLA): A multicentre randomised controlled trial. Lancet 361:1149, 2003.
28. Shepherd J, Blauw GJ, Murphy MB, et al: Pravastatin in elderly individuals at risk of vascular disease (PROSPER): A randomised controlled trial. Lancet 360:1623, 2002.
29. Ridker PM, Danielson E, Fonseca FAH, et al: Rosuvastatin to prevent vascular events in men and women with elevated C-reactive protein. N Engl J Med 359:2195, 2009.
30. Goldstein LB: JUPITER and the world of stroke medicine. Lancet Neurol 8:130, 2009.
31. Collins R, Armitage J, Parish S, et al: Effects of cholesterol-lowering with simvastatin on stroke and other major vascular events in 20536 people with cerebrovascular disease or other high-risk conditions. Lancet 363:757, 2004.
32. Amarenco P, Bogousslavsky J, Callahan AS, et al: Design and baseline characteristics of the stroke prevention by aggressive reduction in cholesterol levels (SPARCL) study. Cerebrovasc Dis 16:389, 2003.
33. Chobanian AV, Bakris GL, Black HR, et al: The Seventh Report of the Joint National Committee on Prevention, Detection, Evaluation, and Treatment of High Blood Pressure: The JNC 7 report. JAMA 289:2560, 2003.
34. Lawes CMM, Bennett DA, Feigin VL, Rodgers A: Blood pressure and stroke. An overview of published reviews. Stroke 35:776, 2004.
35. Rashid P, Leonardi-Bee J, Bath P: Blood pressure reduction and secondary prevention of stroke and other vascular events: a systematic review. Stroke 34:2741, 2003.

Management of Acute Ischemic Stroke

36. Hacke W, Donnan G, Fieschi C, et al: Association of outcome with early stroke treatment: Pooled analysis of ATLANTIS, ECASS, and NINDS rt-PA stroke trials. Lancet 363:768, 2004.
37. Schwamm LH, Pancioli A, Acker JE 3rd, et al: Recommendations for the establishment of stroke systems of care: Recommendations from the American Stroke Association's Task Force on the Development of Stroke Systems. Circulation 111:1078, 2005.
38. Hacke W, Kaste M, Bluhmki E, et al: Thrombolysis with alteplase 3 to 4.5 hours after acute ischemic stroke. N Engl J Med 359:1317, 2008.
39. Alexandrov AV, Molina CA, Grotta JC, et al: Ultrasound-enhanced systemic thrombolysis for acute ischemic stroke. N Engl J Med 351:2170, 2004.
40. Smith WS, Sung G, Starkman S, et al: Safety and efficacy of mechanical embolectomy in acute ischemic stroke: Results of the MERCI trial. Stroke 36:1432, 2005.
41. Coull BM, Williams LS, Goldstein LB, et al: Anticoagulants and antiplatelet agents in acute ischemic stroke. Report of the Joint Stroke Guideline Development Committee of the American Academy of Neurology and the American Stroke Association. Neurology 59:13, 2002.
42. Baddour LM, Wilson WR, Bayer AS, et al: Infective endocarditis: diagnosis, antimicrobial therapy, and management of complications. Circulation 111:e394, 2005.
43. Goldstein LB: Blood pressure management in patients with acute ischemic stroke. Hypertension 43:137, 2004.

CH
62
PREVENTION AND MANAGEMENT OF STROKE

CHAPTER **63**

Endovascular Treatment of Noncoronary Obstructive Vascular Disease

Andrew C. Eisenhauer, Christopher J. White, and Deepak L. Bhatt

Noncoronary, peripheral vascular disease encompasses a very broad range of arterial, venous, and lymphatic diseases. This chapter focuses on percutaneous, catheter-based, endovascular treatment of atherosclerotic peripheral arterial disease (upper and lower extremity, renal, mesenteric, aortic arch vessels, carotid and vertebral arteries) and venous disease. Recognition is increasing that atherosclerotic peripheral arterial disease (PAD) has a high prevalence and clinical importance (see Chap. 61). As the population ages, the number of people with both symptomatic and asymptomatic PAD increases. Physicians and patients are becoming more aware of the ramifications of PAD, including its associated morbidity and mortality. Revascularization strategies are shifting from open surgery to percutaneous or endovascular procedures. Percutaneous transluminal angioplasty (PTA) was initially developed as a treatment for PAD. Recent improvements in technology have generally led to better and much more reliable clinical results. These advances in technology have combined with patient demand for less invasive therapies and revolutionized revascularization therapies for PAD. The widespread availability of high-resolution noninvasive diagnostic imaging, capable of accurately identifying pathology and arterial obstructions that are amenable to less invasive treatment, has further enabled percutaneous therapies for symptomatic PAD.

Although historically, the primary method of revascularization therapy for PAD has involved surgery, percutaneous catheter-based or endovascular therapies now provide patients with a less invasive and equally effective modality for the treatment of atheromatous disease in almost all vascular territories. Effective therapies for arterial aneurysmal disease and venous conditions are currently available and offer advantages over surgical treatments. The American College of Cardiology (ACC) and American Heart Association (AHA) guidelines and recommendations for the diagnosis and treatment of atherosclerotic peripheral arterial disease have recently been published.[1] To provide optimal therapy, clinicians must understand the specific disease state being managed and consider the full range of treatment options. In complicated cases, the patient will benefit from the input of those in vascular-related specialties.

Endovascular Therapy for Atherosclerotic Peripheral Artery Disease

Atherosclerotic Lower Extremity Disease

Lower extremity intermittent claudication is caused by stenosis or occlusion of the iliac, femoral-popliteal, or tibioperoneal vessels (see Chap. 61). Claudication is an exertion-related discomfort affecting specific muscle groups and is relieved with rest. Symptoms affect the muscle groups below the level of the arterial narrowing. For example, vascular blockages (occlusions or stenoses) of the iliac vessels typically cause hip, thigh, and calf pain, whereas femoral and popliteal artery obstructions cause symptoms in the calf and foot muscles. Patients with typical symptoms of intermittent claudication represent fewer than 20% of patients with objective evidence of PAD. The clinician must distinguish pseudoclaudication (discomfort from spinal stenosis, compartment syndromes, venous congestion, or arthritis) from claudication (**Table 63-1**).

The initial therapy for patients with claudication should be atherosclerosis risk factor modification, antiplatelet therapy, and supervised exercise training (see Chap. 61). Because patients with claudication progress to limb-threatening ischemia uncommonly, revascularization is reserved for those patients who have failed a trial of medical therapy, or those with lifestyle-limiting symptoms and favorable anatomy for revascularization. Patients with more advanced disease—that is, vocation-limiting claudication or limb-threatening ischemia (rest pain, nonhealing ulcers, or gangrene)—require a more aggressive approach and are considered candidates for revascularization.

Therapy in patients with claudication aims to relieve symptoms, resulting in an increased walking distance and improvement in quality of life. A durable revascularization solution is important, because symptoms will likely return if restenosis occurs. In contrast, in patients with limb-threatening ischemia, the goal of therapy is limb salvage. The best treatment option will offer a high success rate for restoration of pulsatile flow to the distal limb, with a low procedural morbidity. Less blood flow is required to maintain tissue integrity than to heal a wound; restenosis will generally not result in recurrent limb-threatening ischemia without a subsequent reinjury to the limb. For the clinician caring for patients with lower extremity vascular disease, it is important to weigh improvement in functional capacity and quality of life, as well as long-term results, when considering revascularization.

Basic noninvasive testing includes determining the ankle-brachial index (ABI) at rest and potentially after exercise. Pulse volume recordings with segmental Doppler pressures are helpful in confirming the presence of obstructive disease and estimating its level and severity (see Chaps. 12 and 61). Normal ABIs at rest may miss significant aortoiliac disease, so if clinical suspicion is high, exercise ABIs should be determined. In general, lower extremity angiography is reserved for patients who meet criteria for revascularization, if suitable anatomy is found. Magnetic resonance angiography (MRA) and computed tomography angiography (CTA) enable remarkable noninvasive definition of the vascular anatomy; invasive angiography confirms the diagnosis and helps formulate a strategy and approach to revascularization. For

TABLE 63-1 Intermittent Claudication Versus Pseudoclaudication

FEATURE	INTERMITTENT CLAUDICATION	PSEUDOCLAUDICATION
Character of discomfort	Cramping, tightness, or tiredness	Same or tingling, weakness, clumsiness
Location of discomfort	Buttock, hip, thigh, calf, foot	Same
Exercise induced	Yes	Yes or no
Distance to claudication	Same each time	Variable
Occurs with standing	No	Yes
Relief	Stop walking	Often must sit or change body position

critical limb ischemia, anatomic definition is required in almost all cases to plan therapy. For claudication, imaging should be performed as outlined in **Figure 63-1**.

The probability of clinical success and the technical approach to percutaneous revascularization will vary according to anatomic site. These aspects are best considered separately for aortoiliac, femoropopliteal, and tibioperoneal segments.

AORTOILIAC OBSTRUCTIVE DISEASE. Ischemia producing lesions (stenosis or occlusion) of the aorta and iliac vessels is most commonly atherosclerotic in origin and treatment for both sites, typically referred to as inflow vessels to the leg, is similar. Lower extremity vascular disease frequently involves multiple levels. Patients with aortoiliac occlusive disease will often also have femoral and/or tibial disease. In patients with claudication and multilevel disease, correction of any hemodynamically significant inflow lesions may be undertaken as the first stage in revascularization. Aorto-iliac revascularization will often result in symptomatic improvement, by increasing inflow to the limb, and thus collateral blood flow to the distal extremity.

The preferred mode of revascularization of the aortoiliac vessels has shifted from predominantly surgical to almost completely catheter-based percutaneous therapies. This change is based on the less invasive nature of PTA and the excellent rate of clinical success, which now rivals surgical bypass for many patients. The primary use of stents, as opposed to balloon angioplasty alone, has become the clinical standard of care in the aortoiliac vessels.

Treatment

Because experience has suggested that when excellent angiographic and hemodynamic results are obtained from PTA alone, patency rates and clinical success rates at 2 years are similar to stent placement. Some interventionalists favor a strategy of provisional stenting, wherein stents are reserved for cases of failed balloon angioplasty, but many patients ultimately receive stents. The immediate success rate and 4-year patency are superior for stents versus PTA alone. Longer lesions, diffuse disease, and occlusions, in particular, will likely benefit from primary stenting. The current guidelines recommend primary stent placement in the iliac arteries.[1] As is the case with all revascularization techniques, limited or compromised runoff seems to predict higher failure rates. For the subset of patients with stenotic or occlusive disease that involves the terminal aorta and compromises the origins of the common iliac arteries, the preferred

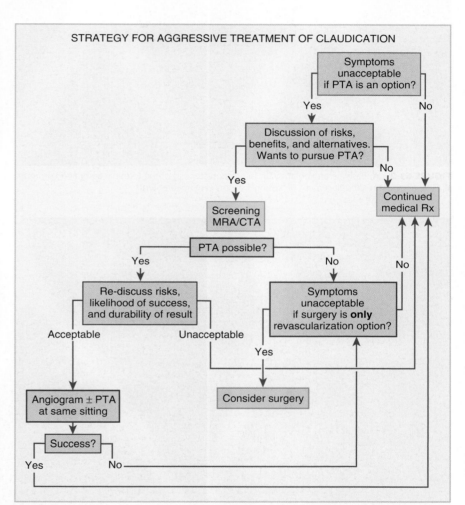

FIGURE 63-1 Strategy for aggressive treatment of claudication. The strategy is based on assessment of symptoms and frank discussion with patients about the risks and benefits of available therapies. Currently, noninvasive diagnostic imaging is used not to make a diagnosis but to ascertain the anatomic suitability for intervention and to assess the patient's procedural risk profile. Rx = treatment. See Figure 61-17 for a management scheme for less lifestyle-limiting claudication.

therapy is placement of "kissing" balloon-expandable stents (**Fig. 63-2**).

Finally, with regard to the composition of stent selected, there is no advantage of self-expanding nitinol over balloon-expandable stainless steel.[2] Balloon expandable stents offer stronger radial force and more precise placement, whereas self-expanding stents offer flexible diameters that accommodate a tapering and sometimes tortuous vessel.

The most serious complications of endovascular aortoiliac repair remain distal embolizations, with rates reportedly as high as 7%, although most operators' experience suggests lower rates of significant

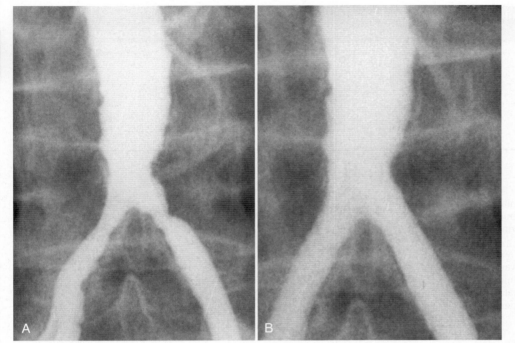

FIGURE 63-2 **A,** Baseline angiogram with bifurcation stenosis of the terminal aorta and common iliac arteries. **B,** Final angiogram after placement of "kissing" balloon-expandable stents.

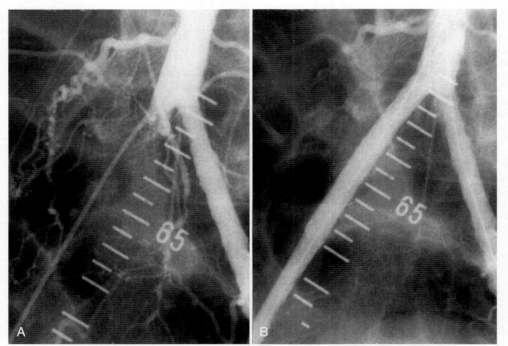

FIGURE 63-3 **A,** Occlusion of right common iliac artery. **B,** Recanalization and stent placement of right common iliac artery.

reconstruction, with less risk and at reduced cost. In the small percentage of patients in whom patency cannot be maintained, surgery remains a feasible option. The availability of these effective, less invasive techniques has lowered the threshold for performing intervention in patients with aortoiliac disease who are disabled by claudication or limb ischemia. Technical success and durability of results remain high (**Table 63-2**).[3-18]

FEMOROPOPLITEAL OBSTRUCTIVE DISEASE. Because the results of endovascular therapy for the superficial femoral artery (SFA) or popliteal artery differ little, this chapter will consider their indications and results together. The SFA, particularly within the adductor canal of the thigh, has a propensity to accumulate atherosclerotic plaque. Procedural success for femoropopliteal recanalization now exceeds 90%. The advent of hydrophilic guidewires and reentry catheters, including those with ultrasound guidance, has greatly enhanced the ability to traverse femoropopliteal occlusions.

Despite such technologic advances, the rate of restenosis remains more than twofold that for iliac disease and far exceeds what would be expected, considering the size (mean lumen diameter, 5 to 6 mm) of the SFA. A variety of adjunct technologies have been attempted to improve long-term patency. Cryotherapy, cutting balloons, and debulking devices such as directional atherectomy, excimer laser, and rotational atherectomy, although sometimes providing a better immediate angiographic result, have not demonstrated a reduction in restenosis in any controlled comparative trials.[19]

Treatment

Multiple small trials failed to demonstrate an advantage for first-generation stent placement over PTA in the femoropopliteal vessels, until more collective experience demonstrated that stents have superior long-term patency compared with PTA. Good clinical evidence from a randomized trial by Schillinger and colleagues[20] has indicated that a strategy of primary stent placement in the femoropopliteal

embolization. Arterial perforation or rupture is rare. Covered stents, or stent grafts, are available for treating vessel rupture. Based on these improved outcomes, percutaneous treatment is generally attempted for short occlusions and for longer iliac stenosis or occlusions that are technically suitable (**Fig. 63-3**). Total occlusions of the abdominal aorta are more often treated surgically, although thrombolysis followed by PTA remains an option.

In summary, primary stent placement represents appropriate first-line therapy for aortoiliac obstructive disease. Stent placement offers high procedural success and durability similar to that of surgical vessels yields superior patency rates and functional outcomes compared with provisional stent placement (i.e., placement of stents for failed PTA). Restenosis at 1 year was 63% in the PTA group, but 37% in the stent arm. Functionally, both walking distance and ABI were increased significantly in the stent arm compared with the PTA group. These benefits accrued, even though 32% of the PTA group crossed over and received a stent after a suboptimal balloon angioplasty result.

A second trial by Krankenberg and associates[21] randomized 244 patients with relatively discrete SFA lesions (mean length, 45 mm) to

TABLE 63-2 Evolution of Results of Iliac Artery Stent Placement*

STUDY (YEAR)	NO. OF PATIENTS TREATED	NO. OF LESIONS STENTED	TOTAL OCCLUSIONS (%)	TECHNICAL SUCCESS (%)	ABI BEFORE	ABI AFTER	MEAN LESION LENGTH (cm)	STENT(S) USED	PRIMARY PATENCY AT 2 yr (%)	CUMULATIVE PATENCY AT 2 yr (%)
Reyes et al (1997)[3]	59	61	100	92	0.51	0.9	10	SES	73	88
Dyet (1997)[4]	72	72	100	93	NA	NA	6.7	BES, SES	85	85
Murphy et al (1998)[5]	65	90	31	97	0.62	0.9	5.6	BES, SES	69	80
Tetteroo et al (1998)[6]	143	187	9	NA	0.78	NA	NA	BES	NA	71.3
Powell et al (2000)[7]	87	210	NA	97	0.56	0.75	NA	Various	43	72
Saha et al (2001)[8]	50	61	4	97	NA	NA	NA	BES, SES	97	100
Timaran et al (2001)[9]	189	247	NA	97	NA	NA	NA	BES, SES	NA	—
Haulon et al (2002)[10]	106	212	NA	100	NA	NA	NA	BES, SES	79.4	97.7
Siskin et al (2002)[11]	42	59	8.5	95	0.68	0.99	NA	BES, SES	72	88
Mohamed et al (2002)[12]	24	48	42	100	NA	NA	5.2	BES, SES	58	84
Reekers et al (2002)[13]	126	143	10	100	0.67	0.92	3.3	BES	84†	89†
Funovics et al (2002)[14]	78	94	100	96	NA	NA	6.2	Various	74.5	88.8
Hans et al (2008)[15]	40	68	48	95	0.55/0.52‡	0.82/0.77‡	NA	Various	69	89
Kashyap et al (2008)[16]	83	127	59	96	0.36	0.82	NA	Various	74	97
Sixt et al (2008)[17]	375	354	26	97	0.36	NA	4.9	Various	86†	98†
Uberol et al (2009)[18]				98						—
	2233									

BES = balloon-expandable stainless steel; SES = self-expanding stainless steel; SEN = self-expanding nitinol; SESG = self-expanding stent graft; — = not assessed or reported.
*Historical and contemporary results of iliac artery stent placement. The difficulty in interpreting the literature is that these reports of experience include patients with widely varying degrees of disease and incorporate a variety of stent types and techniques. Nevertheless, cumulative 2-year patency is approximately 90% in most series.
†At 12 months.
‡Separate report for right and left legs.

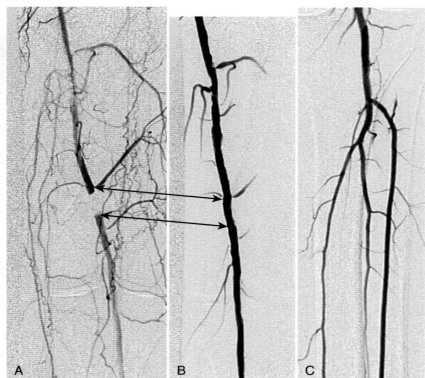

FIGURE 63-4 Result of recanalization and balloon dilation of a short-segment femoropopliteal occlusion. **A,** Digital subtraction angiogram illustrating the area of total occlusion and comparing it with that in **B,** which shows the results of balloon dilation only. Both areas are indicated by the double-ended black arrows. **C,** Intact three-vessel runoff without evidence of distal embolization.

general, multiple modalities have been used successfully to treat a wide variety of femoropopliteal lesions in multiple series (**Table 63-3**). [20,26-42]

When weighing the risks and benefits of invasive therapy, each patient and lesion requires individual consideration. When comparing medical therapy with revascularization, quality-of-life measures for treatment of claudication have suggested that PTA is more effective than exercise alone, with a cost-effectiveness ratio generally within the acceptable range. If one compares surgery to PTA in patients with claudication, remembering that late patency is the key to long-term symptom relief, PTA emerges as the preferred strategy if the 5-year patency rate for PTA is more than 30%. An initial endovascular approach may also benefit patients with critical limb ischemia and femoropopliteal vascular disease. [43] In a large (N = 452) randomized trial, a surgery-first strategy, was compared with a PTA-first strategy, with follow-up over 5 years. PTA and surgery resulted in similar outcomes for amputation-free survival, and PTA was less expensive, leading to a recommendation for a PTA-first strategy when feasible.

To summarize, in many cases, surgery or interventional techniques can ameliorate symptoms. The decision about which is the most appropriate therapy can be made by the patient and physician, taking into account the risks and discomforts of the proposed procedure, its probable durability and reproducibility, the degree to which a procedure closes the door to other therapies, the degree of lifestyle limitation, and the individual patient's tolerance for risk.

The treatment of symptomatic femoropopliteal disease should favor a percutaneous approach over an open surgical procedure, and provisional stent placement appears to be the preferred strategy. Controversy exists about the correct approach for longer lesions (>10 cm) and chronic total occlusions. The advent of fracture-resistant stent designs, better recanalization techniques for occlusions, and perhaps the future development of effective drug-eluting stents, holds promise for further enhancements in the future.

balloon angioplasty or primary stent placement. Only 11% of the PTA patients crossed over to receive a stent, which improves the validity of the intention-to-treat analysis that showed no restenosis benefit for stent over PTA. The major difference between the Schillinger and Krankenburg trials was lesion length. The stent group in both trials had restenosis rates ranging from 30% to 39%, whereas the PTA restenosis rate in the long lesions was 67%, compared with only 38% for the shorter SFA lesions. A current meta-analysis of 10 randomized controlled trials included data on 1442 limbs, with an average length lesion similar to the Krankenberg trial (stent, 45.8 mm; PTA, 43.3 mm). No benefit was found for primary stent placement over provisional stent placement for SFA lesions. Thus, longer SFA lesions and total occlusions are more likely to benefit from primary stenting, whereas more discrete stenoses do just as well with PTA.

Two recently published multicenter randomized controlled trials in 87 and 154 patients have demonstrated significant benefit for paclitaxel-coated balloons compared with controls out to 18 and 24 months. [22,23] The next step will be a study of drug-coated balloons with provisional stenting, compared with drug-coated balloons with primary stenting.

The use of endovascular approaches to recanalize and stent diffuse femoropopliteal disease is reemerging (**Figs. 63-4 to 63-7**). With the success of drug-eluting coronary stents, strong interest has been rekindled in the development of stent coatings such as rapamycin for lower extremity use. In a randomized series of long-segment SFA disease patients, the results for those receiving rapamycin-coated nitinol self-expanding stents were no different than those in the bare-metal stent control group. [24] One concern raised in this trial was a high incidence of stent fractures, which appear to be related to restenosis. [25] After a period of study, fracture-resistant stent designs and modified coatings are emerging. Recent reports of paclitaxel-coated self-expanding stents are more favorable, with few fractures and preserved results at 12 and 24 months. [26] So far, the results of drug-eluting stents in the lower limbs have been mixed, but this work remains in its preliminary stages. In

TIBIOPERONEAL OBSTRUCTIVE DISEASE. PAD often involves multiple levels, from proximal to distal, in the extremity. When disease affects the proximal vessels, the infrapopliteal arteries often also have significant occlusive disease (anterior tibial, peroneal, and posterior tibial). Similarly, when tibioperoneal narrowing is present, proximal disease probably coexists. A symptomatic lesion is rarely isolated to a single vessel below the knee. Revascularization strategies for below-knee lesions must take into account the extent, severity, and distribution of disease in more proximal vessels.

For patients with claudication and multilevel disease, correction of inflow obstructive disease in a proximal vessel may be sufficient for symptom relief. This differs from critical limb ischemia, which usually requires restoration of uninterrupted (pulsatile flow) patency to at least one vessel to the foot to heal the lesion. In the absence of severe and flow-limiting proximal disease, significant disease of all three crural vessels is usually required to provoke symptomatic calf claudication or higher grades of ischemia (rest pain or tissue loss).

Treatment

Historically, revascularization of tibioperoneal vessels has been reserved for patients with critical limb ischemia. Endovascular approaches are rapidly replacing traditional surgical bypass. Technologic advances and the use of coronary equipment allow for routine and uncomplicated access to the infrapopliteal vessels. Numerous reports have confirmed the feasibility, safety, and efficacy of tibioperoneal PTA. Primary success rates are generally 80% to 95%, and cumulative 2-year patency rates can approximate 75% (**Table 63-4**). [44-53] Limb salvage rates for percutaneous intervention can rival those of surgical

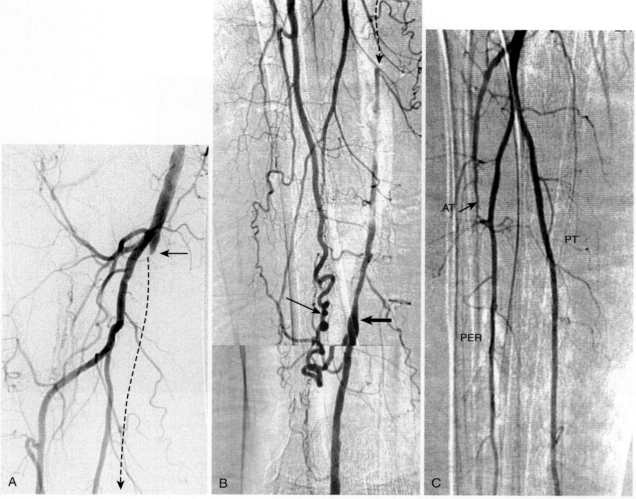

FIGURE 63-5   Long-segment chronic total occlusion. In contrast to the short-segment disease in Figure 63-4, this lesion requires recanalization from the origin of the SFA (**A,** solid arrow) along the path of the SFA (dashed arrow), continuing to the level of the most significant collateral inflow (**B,** thin arrow) and reconstitution of the vessel (**B,** thick arrow). **C,** Crural vessels and occlusion of the anterior tibial (AT) with patent peroneal (PER) and posterior tibial (PT) runoff.

reconstruction. PTA can also effectively salvage ischemic limbs in diabetic patients with small-vessel disease.[54,55]

For tibioperoneal PTA, focal stenoses have the best outcomes, and patients with fewer than five separate lesions have a higher success rate. The success of endovascular therapy is measured by relief of rest pain, healing of ulcers, and avoiding amputation, and not necessarily by long-term vessel patency. It requires more oxygenated blood to heal a wound than to maintain tissue integrity.

The safe and effective revascularization of tibioperoneal vessels with the percutaneous approach in this higher risk cohort has changed the management of patients with critical limb ischemia. When anatomically feasible, a strategy of PTA first is a reasonable and appropriate strategy for revascularization in all patients, even those with low surgical risk for infrapopliteal bypass (**Figs. 63-8 and 63-9**).[43]

The changing approach to revascularization also relates to the indications for intervention in patients with symptomatic but less critical tibioperoneal disease. The threshold for revascularization had traditionally been very high, largely because of the risk of the surgical approach. The availability of effective, less-invasive options permits a lower threshold for intervention. Specifically, in the subset of patients who claudicate solely because of infrapopliteal disease, PTA offers favorable acute and intermediate-term patency and clinical results. Such a strategy should be limited to patients who have severe symptoms (Rutherford category 3) and straightforward anatomy.

Infrapopliteal PTA may also help claudicants undergoing proximal revascularization, either with surgery or PTA, with severely impaired runoff. When tibial outflow is a major determinant of long-term patency, recanalizing the runoff vessels may provide benefit.

In summary, optimal management of patients with lower extremity arterial occlusive disease and associated symptoms requires the input of practitioners knowledgeable about the capabilities of percutaneous and surgical revascularization. A strategy of PTA first should be considered if the anatomy is favorable and is certainly preferable to primary amputation.[56] The physician must explain the risks, potential symptomatic benefit, and durability of the proposed intervention. For patients with claudication, there is little evidence that early and aggressive revascularization alters the natural history of lower extremity occlusive disease. Thus, treatment should be guided by the patient's degree of functional impairment.

Limb-threatening ischemia, in contrast, requires prompt treatment, using the modality that will provide the most complete revascularization with the lowest procedural risk. The principal of restoring straight line pulsatile flow to the extremity affected by diffuse disease or long-segment femoropopliteal obstruction may be accomplished with traditional bypass surgery or an endovascular approach. Current evidence supports a PTA-first approach, in selected patients with limb-threatening ischemia and obstructive infrainguinal PAD.[43] As the short and long-term outcomes of catheter-based interventions continue to improve, these endovascular techniques will assume an even more

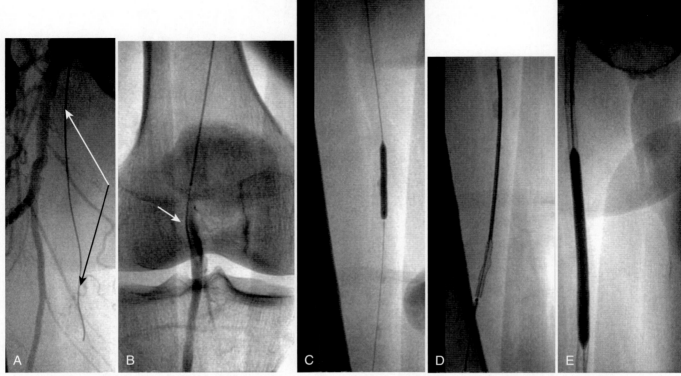

FIGURE 63-6 **A,** Recanalization of this lesion was accomplished from the contralateral approach, using a hydrophilic guidewire advanced into the occluded segment (arrows). **B,** Once the guidewire is free in the distal vessel, a small catheter is passed over the wire and a contrast agent is injected to confirm the intravascular position (arrow). This is followed by predilation **(C),** self-expanding stent placement from distal to proximal **(D),** and finally postdilation to the appropriate size **(E).**

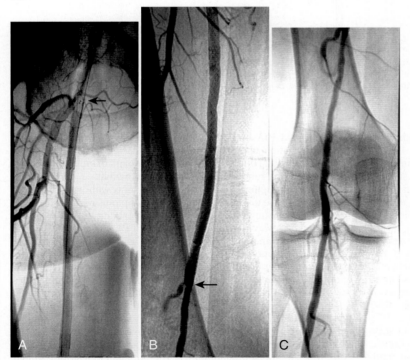

FIGURE 63-7 Recanalization of this long-segment occlusion and stenting from the origin of the SFA in **A** (arrow) to the level of collateral reconstitution in **B** (arrow) resulted in reconstitution of the normal anatomy, **(C),** return of pedal pulses, and healing of digital ulcers. Care was taken to preserve the collateral vessel ostia so that in the event of restenosis, collateral pathways could be reestablished. This anatomy should be contrasted with total occlusion of the SFA but short-segment disease, shown in Figure 63-4. These cases illustrate the anatomic variations that commonly occur and emphasize the difficulty in characterizing the true extent of disease in patients with total occlusions of this vessel.

prominent role in the treatment of patients presenting with claudication or critical limb ischemia.

Regardless of initial treatment strategy, optimum long-term outcome requires diligent follow-up and intrinsic risk factor management. Although surveillance strategies for surgical bypass grafts exist, formal guidelines for monitoring patients following percutaneous therapy are lacking. Pending such guidelines, these individuals should undergo regular evaluation, including clinical examination of the affected limb and performance of duplex sonographic studies.

Atherosclerotic Renal Artery Disease

RENAL ARTERY STENOSIS. Atherosclerosis of the renal artery resulting in renal artery stenosis (RAS) associates with increased cardiovascular events and mortality (see Chap. 93). Assessment of a general population by renal duplex ultrasound in individuals older than 65 years of age has revealed an approximately 7% prevalence of RAS, which increases to 20% to 30% in high-risk populations (e.g., patients with known atherosclerotic vascular disease). Atherosclerotic RAS is a progressive disease associated with a loss of renal mass over time, despite control of hypertension. Progression of RAS to occlusion is more likely with more severe (>60%) lesions and may occur at a rate of up to 20%/year.

Atherosclerotic RAS is an important cause of renal insufficiency, refractory hypertension, and cardiac destabilization syndromes (unstable angina and flash pulmonary edema). Unilateral RAS manifests clinically as a vasoconstrictor-mediated hypertension, whereas bilateral RAS causes hypertension caused by volume overload. Up to 20% of patients older than 50 years of age entering renal dialysis

TABLE 63-3 Evolution of Results of Femoropopliteal Artery Stenting*

STUDY (YEAR)	NO. OF LESIONS	TOTAL OCCLUSIONS (%)	TECHNICAL SUCCESS (%)	ABI BEFORE	ABI AFTER	MEAN LESION LENGTH (cm)	DEVICES USED	PRIMARY SUCCESS (%)†	CUMULATIVE DURATION (MO)	SUCCESS (%)†	DURATION (mo)
Gray et al (1997)[27]	58	NA	NA	0.48	0.71	16.5	SES, BES	22	24	46	24
Martin (1999)[28]	NA	6	100	NA	NA	NA	PTA	NA	–	57	24
Kessel et al (1999)[29]	NA	–	95	0.6	1	17	SG	29	12	64	12
Conroy et al (2000)[30]	61	100	100	NA	NA¶	13.5	SES, BES	47	12	79	12
Cheng et al (2001)[31]	69	NA	92	NA	NA	13.8	SEN, SES	52.8	24	72.1	24
Gordon et al (2001)[32]	71	100	NA	0.59	0.86	14.4	SES	38.2	24	76.2	24
Scheinert et al (2001)[33]	411	100	83	0.62	NA	19.4	LPTA, SEN	33.6†	12	75.9	12
Lofberg et al (2001)[34]	121	47	88	NA	NA	NA	PTA	27	60	34	60
Bauermeister (2001)[35]	NA	100	100	0.25	0.87	22	SG§	73.2	12	82.6	12
Duda et al (2002)[36]	36	57	100	NA	NA	8.5	DEN/SEN	100/77	6	NA	–
Steinkamp et al (2002)[37]	312	100	91.7	0.56	0.88	7.5	LPTA, SEN	61.5	24	90.2	24
Gray et al (2002)[38]	NA	84	88	0.54	0.84	6.2	LPTA	33	24	75	24
Jamsen et al (2002)[39]	218	NA	83.5	NA	NA	NA	PTA	25	60	4.1	60
Cho et al (2003)[40]	40	100	100	0.61	0.93	NA	SEN	NA	–	NA	–
Becquemin et al (2003)[41]	277	NA	90	0.52	NA	2.5	BES vs. PTA	65/67‡	12	NA	–
Jahnke et al (2003)[42]	63	83	100	0.54	0.89	10.9	SG	74.1	24	83.2	24
Duda et al (2005)[24]	57	65	—	0.61	0.87	81.5	DEN vs. SEN	20.7/17.9	18	NA	–
Schillinger et al (2006)[20]	104	35	100	0.58	0.84	13.2	SEN vs. PTA	37/63	12	NA	–
Dake (2009)[26]	843	—	—	—	—	—	DEN	82	24	78 (EFS)	24

*Summary of reports of femoropopliteal interventions from the literature. A wide variety of anatomic situations are represented here, including many with chronic long-segment total occlusions. Of note is that primary patency of 2 years, when reported, is considerably lower than that for iliac interventions, yet cumulative patency ranges from approximately 75% to 90%. This emphasizes the need for both postprocedure surveillance and consideration of the performance of a femoral intervention when embarking on a course of therapy.
†Clinical or objective patency.
‡Angiographic patency (<50% stenosis) in mandatory stent group versus PTA with selective stenting group.
§Devices placed surgically.
¶Average increase of 0.26.
BES = balloon-expandable stainless steel; DEN = drug-eluting nitinol; EFS = event-free survival; LPTA = excimer laser-assisted PTA; NA = not assessed or reported; PTA = percutaneous transluminal (balloon) angioplasty; SEN = self-expanding nitinol; SES = self-expanding stainless steel; SG = stent graft.

TABLE 63-4 Evolution of Results of Tibioperoneal Artery Interventions

STUDY (YEAR)*	NO. OF PATIENTS TREATED	NO. OF LESIONS TREATED	TOTAL OCCLUSION (%)	TECHNICAL SUCCESS (%)	ABI BEFORE	ABI AFTER	MEAN LESION LENGTH (cm)	PRIMARY DEVICE	PRIMARY PATENCY (%)	DURATION (MO)	CUMULATIVE PATENCY (%)	DURATION (mo)	EVENT-FREE SURVIVAL (%)	DURATION (mo)	LIMB SALVAGE (%)	DURATION (mo)
Sivananthan et al (1994)[44]	38	73	24	96	—	—	—	PTA	—	—	—	—	—	—	—	—
Varty et al (1995)[45]	38	40	17	98	0.55	0.84	1	PTA	59	24	68	24	—	—	77	12
Dorros et al (1998)[46]	312	657	27	98	—	—	—	PTA	—	—	—	—	—	—	—	—
Desgranges et al (2000)[47]	33	—	—	82	—	—	—	PTA	66	12	77	12	94	12	91	12
Soder et al (2000)[48]	60	72	35	84/61†	—	—	—	PTA	68/48†	10	56	18	—	—	80	18
Dorros et al (2001)[49]	235	529	28.9	92	—	—	—	PTA	—	—	—	—	31	60	91	60
Tsetis et al (2002)[50]	12	13	100	92.3	0.35	0.68	7	VPTA	—	—	—	—	—	—	—	—
Feiring et al (2004)[51]	82	92	—	94	0.32	0.9	—	SE	—	—	—	—	92	12	96	12
Giles et al (2008)[52]	163	176	29	93	—	—	—	PTA	24	24	61	24	35	24	—	24
Sioablis et al (2009)[53]	75	153	24.2	98.7	—	—	5.5	DES	36	36	—	—	78	36	84	36

*Selected recent literature on tibial artery interventions. Most reports are of single-center experience and procedural results.
†Stenosis or occlusion.
DES = drug-eluting stent; PTA = percutaneous transluminal (balloon) angioplasty; VPTA = vibrational PTA; — = not assessed or reported.

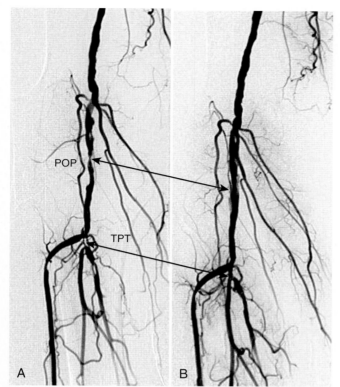

FIGURE 63-8 Intervention in tibial disease. Lesions in the below-knee popliteal artery (POP; **A**) and in the very short tibioperoneal trunk (TPT; **B**) were identified and successfully treated with PTA.

hemodynamically significant stenosis, defined as the following: (1) 50% diameter or larger stenosis, with a systolic translesional gradient (measured with a 5Fr or smaller catheter or pressure wire) of 20 mm Hg or more or a mean pressure gradient of 10 mm Hg or more; (2) 70% diameter or larger stenosis by quantitative angiographic methods; or (3) 70% diameter or larger stenosis by intravascular ultrasound measurement.[57]

Although PTA alone remains the treatment of choice for fibromuscular dysplasia (FMD) lesions, primary stent placement for atherosclerotic RAS is the current standard of care (**Fig. 63-12**).[1] Stents have been proven to yield more predictable and hemodynamically favorable results in renal revascularization, and studies have suggested that restenosis rates for renal stenting are generally very low (**Table 63-7**).[58-65]

The strongest predictor of late renal stent patency is acute gain, or maximizing the stent lumen. Larger diameter (≥6 mm) renal arteries have lower restenosis rates than smaller (<4.5 mm) vessels. Long-term follow-up has suggested primary patency rates of approximately 80% to 85% and secondary patency rates of more than 90%. Almost all in-stent restenosis occurs during the first year after stent implantation, with restenosis later than 2 years an unusual occurrence.

Despite technical success rates in excess of 95% using stents, angiographic stenosis does not predict clinical benefit (**Table 63-8**).[58-61,63-66] This implies that either the renal artery stenosis is not causally related to the hypertension, or the successful revascularization procedure did not relieve the renal hypoperfusion. A major difficulty in predicting a treatment response in patients with renovascular disease is that they commonly have other nephrotoxic conditions that could confound their response to revascularization, such as diabetes, essential hypertension, atheroemboli, and medication-related insults.

Patient Selection

Analogous to the coronary technique of fractional flow reserve (FFR), the renal fractional flow reserve serves as a lesion-specific functional assessment of a renal artery stenosis (see Chap. 52). Consistent with the unpredictable clinical results, quantitative angiography correlates poorly with hemodynamic gradients (peak, mean, and hyperemic), whereas an excellent correlation has been shown for the renal FFR and the baseline pressure gradient.[67] Renal FFR, determined in 17 patients with poorly controlled hypertension, correlated with clinical improvement. An abnormal renal FFR (<0.8) predicted blood pressure improvement (86%), compared with a 30% improvement if the FFR was normal ($P = 0.04$).[68]

Brain natriuretic peptide (BNP) promotes diuresis, natriuresis, and arterial vasodilation; antagonizes the renin-angiotensin system and angiotensin II; and may serve as a biomarker of response to renal revascularization. In 27 patients with uncontrolled hypertension and RAS (≥70% diameter stenosis), hypertension improved in 77% of those with elevated BNP levels, compared with 0 of 5 patients with a baseline BNP of 80 pg/mL or less ($P = 0.001$). If BNP levels decreased to more than 30% after successful stent placement, 94% (16 of 17) had improvement in their blood pressure control.[69]

The renal artery resistive index (RI), measured noninvasively by Doppler ultrasound, may also stratify patients likely to respond to renal intervention. Data conflict, however, regarding the ability of RI to predict treatment response in patients with RAS. A retrospective study in which most patients were treated with balloon angioplasty, not stents, has suggested that an elevated RI is associated with a low probability of improved blood pressure or renal function after revascularization.[70] In a prospective study of renal stent placement in 241 patients, however, patients with an abnormal RI experienced blood pressure response and renal functional improvement at 1 year after renal arterial intervention (**Figs. 63-13 and 63-14**).[71] The preponderance of evidence and scientific quality of the latter studies favors the conclusion that an elevated RI should not preclude the performance of renal artery intervention for obstructive RAS.

Several clinical trials have demonstrated that successful renal artery stent placement improves or stabilizes renal function in patients with atherosclerotic renovascular renal insufficiency. Patients with renal insufficiency and hemodynamically significant RAS improve after

programs in the United States have atherosclerotic RAS (ischemic nephropathy) as the cause of their renal failure. The 2-, 5-, and 10-year survival rates are about 60%, 20%, and 5%, respectively, for dialysis-dependent patients with RAS. The mortality risk depends on the severity of RAS (**Table 63-5**). The median survival for dialysis patients with atherosclerotic RAS was 25 months, compared with 133 months for patients with polycystic kidney disease. Clearly, the early diagnosis of RAS and the prevention of end-stage renal disease (ESRD) is an important goal.

Diagnosis

Clinical clues to the diagnosis of RAS (**Table 63-6**) include the onset of diastolic hypertension after 55 years of age refractory or malignant hypertension, resistant hypertension in a previously well-controlled patient, and/or an increasing serum creatinine level. These should alert the clinician and prompt further diagnostic testing (**Figs. 63-10 and 63-11**). Imaging best diagnoses RAS. Duplex renal artery ultrasound, CTA, and MRA are all recommended as noninvasive screening tests for patients suspected of having RAS.[1] Invasive renal angiography is recommended when the clinical suspicion is high and noninvasive testing is inconclusive or inconsistent with the clinical evidence. Some advocate renal angiography at the time of cardiac catheterization or peripheral vascular angiography for patients who are at increased risk for RAS. Screening modalities that are no longer recommended include captopril renal scintigraphy, measurement of plasma renin activity (with or without captopril stimulation), and selective renal vein renin measurements.

Treatment

After establishing the anatomic diagnosis of RAS, one must consider the most appropriate management. The goals of treatment include blood pressure control, preserving or improving renal function, and reducing the risk of flash pulmonary edema, refractory heart failure, and difficult to control angina pectoris. The indications for revascularization require the presence of clinical findings related to RAS with a

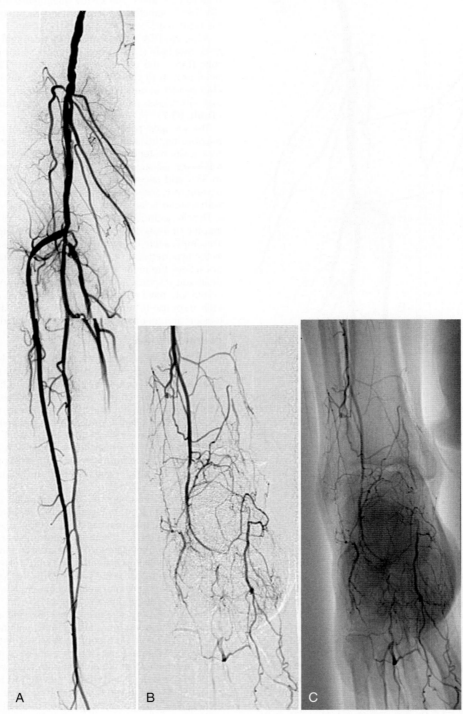

FIGURE 63-9 **A,** Composite angiogram from the patient depicted in Figure 63-8 demonstrating the intact anterior tibial runoff in the calf. The peroneal normally attenuates by the level of the malleoli and, in this case, the posterior tibial is also occluded. **B, C,** Pedal circulation in digital subtraction angiography and native views. Although straight line flow to the foot was reconstituted and the patient's ulcers healed, the evident diffuse small-vessel disease in the pedal vessels still places the foot in long-term jeopardy. Careful surveillance and compulsive continuing medical management are critical for this group of patients, even in the context of technical procedural success.

stent placement. Successful renal artery stent placement can significantly slow the progression of renal failure. Calculation of the mean slope of the reciprocal of serum creatinine levels before and after stent placement shows a fourfold slowing in the progression of renal insufficiency after renal artery stent placement. One of the best predictors

TABLE 63-5 Severity of Renal Artery Stenosis and Survival

SEVERITY OF RAS	4-YEAR SURVIVAL
No RAS	90%
50% to 75%	70%
76% to 95%	68%
> 95%	48%

Modified from Conlon PJ, Little MA, Pieper K, Mark DB: Severity of renal vascular disease predicts mortality in patients undergoing coronary angiography. Kidney Int 60:1490, 2001.

TABLE 63-6 Clinical Predictors of Renal Artery Stenosis

1. Onset of hypertension in patients ≤30 yr or >55 yr
2. Malignant, accelerated, or resistant hypertension
3. Unexplained renal dysfunction
4. Development of azotemia or worsening renal function after ACE inhibitor or ARB
5. "Flash" pulmonary edema
6. Atrophic kidney or size discrepancy between kidneys of >1.5 cm
7. Multivessel coronary disease or peripheral arterial disease

Modified from Hirsch AT, Haskal ZJ, Hertzer NR, et al: ACC/AHA 2005 guidelines for the management of patients with peripheral arterial disease (lower extremity, renal, mesenteric, and abdominal aortic): Executive summary: A collaborative report from the American Association for Vascular Surgery/Society for Vascular Surgery, Society for Cardiovascular Angiography and Interventions, Society for Vascular Medicine and Biology, Society of Interventional Radiology, and the ACC/AHA Task Force on Practice Guidelines (Writing Committee to Develop Guidelines for the Management of Patients with Peripheral Arterial Disease) endorsed by the American Association of Cardiovascular and Pulmonary Rehabilitation; National Heart, Lung and Blood Institute; Society for Vascular Nursing; TransAtlantic Inter-Society Consensus; and Vascular Disease Foundation. J Am Coll Cardiol 47:1239, 2006.

of improvement in renal function following percutaneous revascularization is a rapid rate of decline in renal function immediately prior to intervention, suggesting that the rapid decline in renal function reflects a more acute injury, which is more likely to be reversible.[72] Alternatively, approximately 20% of patients who undergo renal intervention will have a decline or worsening in their renal function. One contributing factor may be atheroembolism, resulting from the trauma to the bulky aortic plaque (**Fig. 63-15**). Work is ongoing to adapt embolic protection for renal interventions.[73]

Unilateral Renal Artery Stenosis and Nephropathy

Traditional teaching holds that unilateral RAS does not cause ischemic nephropathy when the contralateral renal artery is patent. However, revascularization of unilateral RAS can improve or stabilize renal function. Revascularization of unilateral RAS can result in measurable improvement in the split renal function of the stenotic kidney. Restoring flow to the stenotic kidney can reverse the hyperfiltration of the nonstenotic kidney, resulting in decreased proteinuria. Thus, in patients with abnormal renal function, treatment of unilateral RAS may improve and/or stabilize renal function.

Percutaneous treatment of renovascular disease, in summary, offers a safe and effective therapy that is preferable to open surgical revascularization. Renal artery stenting can ameliorate hypertension and improve or stabilize renal function, and may delay the need for hemodialysis in appropriately selected patients. Finally, the advent of distal protection devices to limit atheroembolic complications may further improve safety and renal parenchymal preservation. The current recommended systematic approach to the investigation and treatment of this condition is outlined in Figures 63-10 and 63-11. Despite many reports of clinical success in selected and carefully chosen patient groups, the enthusiasm for widespread treatment of mild or moderate renovascular disease has waned. Recent published data from the ASTRAL trial, in which patients were randomized to revascularization versus continued medical therapy alone, did not show a clear benefit of renal revascularization,[65] although its design and conclusions have been criticized.[74] The ongoing CORAL trial is randomizing patients with RAS to renal stenting versus medical therapy alone to determine whether an even broader population might benefit from revascularization.[75]

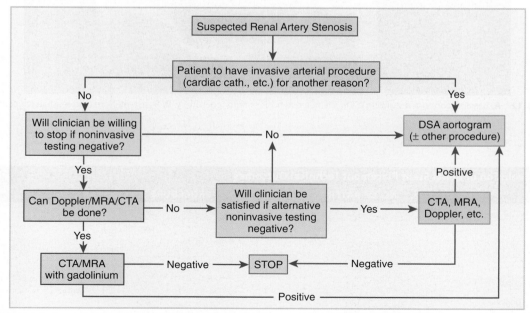

FIGURE 63-10 Approach to the anatomic evaluation of RAS. Once stenosis is suspected, if the patient is to have another invasive arterial procedure, noninvasive imaging is deferred and low-volume DSA is performed at the time of that procedure. In other cases, the clinician should assess whether a negative noninvasive test would be sufficient evidence to acquit the renal arteries. If so, noninvasive testing should be performed. If not, consideration should be given to DSA and selective angiography. Cath = catheterization.

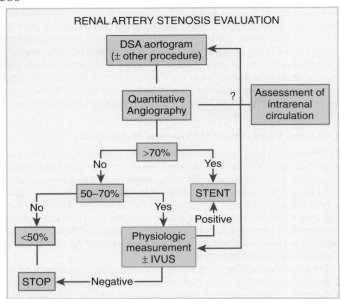

RENAL ARTERY STENOSIS EVALUATION

FIGURE 63-11 Approach to the angiographic evaluation and treatment of renal artery stenosis. Once DSA is performed, confirming the presence of renovascular disease, quantitative angiography and objective evaluation of the severity of stenosis should be performed. Very severe (>70% diameter stenosis) lesions are subjected to revascularization, and mild lesions (<50% diameter stenosis) are not. We believe that the intermediate lesion should be assessed with physiologic evaluation and/or additional anatomic documentation of severity, such as intravascular ultrasound (IVUS) or fractional flow reserve. The absence of translesional flow acceleration or a pressure gradient should mitigate the desire to intervene (see Fig. 45-14).

Chronic Mesenteric Ischemia

The clinical syndrome of chronic mesenteric ischemia (CMI) is surprisingly uncommon, given the high frequency of atherosclerotic disease of the aorta and the common finding of aorto-ostial stenosis of the visceral vessels.[76] The mesenteric circulation consists of the celiac trunk, the superior mesenteric artery (SMA), and the inferior mesenteric artery (IMA). The rarity of this clinical syndrome probably reflects the redundancy of the visceral circulation with multiple pathways from the SMA and IMA. Females are disproportionately affected (70%), and the classic presentation is postprandial abdominal discomfort; patients with CMI typically avoid food and usually have significant weight loss. Even in advanced cases, multiple other causes of the weight loss and abdominal pain are often entertained before intestinal angina comes into focus as the diagnosis of exclusion. Significant obstruction of two or more of these vessels usually underlies classic symptoms. Endoscopic findings suggest bowel ischemia, although single-vessel disease, usually of the SMA, can sometimes cause CMI, particularly if collateral connections have been disrupted by prior abdominal surgery.

Diagnosis

The relatively common application of CTA and MRA for these abdominal symptoms now enables the anatomic diagnosis without invasive angiography. Invasive angiography is useful for diagnosis, but requires a lateral aortogram to visualize the ostia of the mesenteric vessels (**Figs. 63-16 and 63-17**). When the symptoms are typical, the anatomic findings severe, and the alternative pathologic explanations few, the diagnosis is confirmed and revascularization is in order. As might be expected, however, this patient group has a high incidence of coronary artery disease and the surgical mortality and morbidity ranges from 5% to 8%, with the highest incidence of complications occurring in older patients.

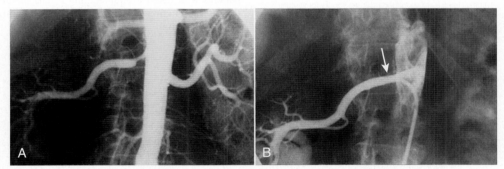

FIGURE 63-12 **A,** Baseline aortogram showing ≥70% diameter stenosis of right renal artery. **B,** Poststent. Note mild residual narrowing (arrow).

TABLE 63-7   Evolution of Renal Stent Placement Technical Outcomes

STUDY (YEAR)	NO. OF ARTERIES	PROCEDURE SUCCESS (%)	RESTENOSIS
White et al (1997)[58]	133	99	18.8
Blum et al (1997)[59]	74	100	11.0
Tuttle et al (1998)[60]	148	98	14.0
Henry et al (1999)[61]	209	99	11.4
van de Ven et al (1999)[62]	43	90	14.0
Rocha-Singh et al (1999)[63]	180	97	12.0
Lederman et al (2001)[64]	358	100	21.0
Wheatley et al (2009)[65]	335	95	NR

NR = not reported.

TABLE 63-8   Blood Pressure Response to Renal Artery Stenting

STUDY (YEAR)	NO. OF PATIENTS	ARTERIES	CURED (%)	IMPROVED (%)	BENEFIT (%)
Blum et al 1997[59]	68	74	16	62	78
Tuttle et al (1998)[60]	129	148	2	55	57
Henry et al (1999)[61]	210	244	19	61	78
Rocha-Singh et al (1999)[63]	150	180	6	50	56
Dorros et al (1993)[66]	76	92	7	52	59
White et al (1997)[58]	100	133	NR	76	76
Lederman et al (2001)[64]	261	NR	<1	70	70

NR = not reported.

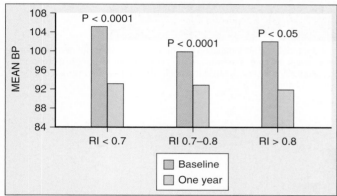

FIGURE 63-13   Blood pressure (BP) response in patients with normal RI (<0.7), moderate elevation (RI = 0.7-0.8), and severe nephrosclerosis (>0.8) at 1 year after stent placement. *(Data from Zeller T, Frank U, Müller C, et al: Predictors of improved renal function after percutaneous stent-supported angioplasty of severe atherosclerotic ostial renal artery stenosis. Circulation 108:2244, 2003.)*

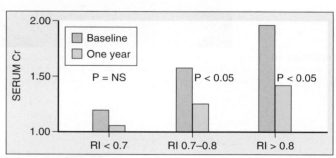

FIGURE 63-14   Renal function change in patients with normal RI (<0.7), moderate elevation (RI = 0.7-0.8), and severe nephrosclerosis (>0.8) at 1 year after stent placement. Cr = creatinine. *(Data from Zeller T, Frank U, Müller C, et al: Predictors of improved renal function after percutaneous stent-supported angioplasty of severe atherosclerotic ostial renal artery stenosis. Circulation 108:2244, 2003.)*

Treatment

Obstructions of the visceral vessels resemble those of the renal arteries. The technical considerations for PTA and stent placement are similar to those for renal artery intervention. The endovascular approach circumvents the need for general anesthesia and the operative trauma associated with open surgery, and may result in a lower acute mortality and morbidity.[77,78]

Because of the relative infrequency of this disease, there are no comparative trials of surgery versus endovascular treatment for CMI. Interpretation of the literature, which reports successful case series of surgical and interventional treatment, is confounded by the obvious case selection and other inherent biases. Interventional treatment offers an alternative for the management of chronic visceral ischemia that may have advantages over surgery, especially for those patients of advanced age or with additional increased risk of morbidity and mortality (see Fig. 63-17).

The single largest series of endovascular therapy for CMI was recently reported, with a technical success rate of 96% and symptom relief in 88% of 63 patients (79 vessels).[79] At a mean follow-up of 38 ± 15 months, 17% had recurrence of symptoms but none developed

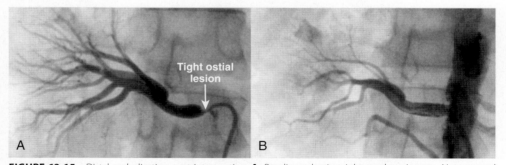

FIGURE 63-15   Distal embolization post intervention: **A,** Baseline selective right renal angiogram. Note normal cortical vessels. **B,** Poststent. Note the absence of distal filling because of atheroembolization.

acute mesenteric ischemia, and all underwent successful revascularization without complication. Follow-up was carried out in 90% of patients and 90% of the vessels with angiographic CT, conventional angiography, or Duplex ultrasound, showing an in-stent restenosis rate of 29%.

In summary, although no prospective controlled data compare outcomes of balloon angioplasty versus stent placement for the treatment of mesenteric arterial stenoses, recent studies have suggested that endovascular stent placement confers immediate and long-term results superior to balloon angioplasty alone. Therefore,

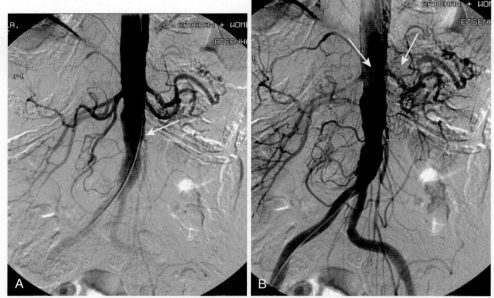

FIGURE 63-16 Visceral angiogram from a patient with postprandial abdominal pain, weight loss, and abdominal bruits. This projection does not demonstrate the origins of the celiac or superior mesenteric arteries. **A,** Early in the run, however, the thin arrow indicates a stenosis at the origin of the inferior mesenteric artery. **B,** Then, from a later frame, the origins of the renal arteries are seen (arrows); although potentially not seen in absolute profile, they appear unobstructed.

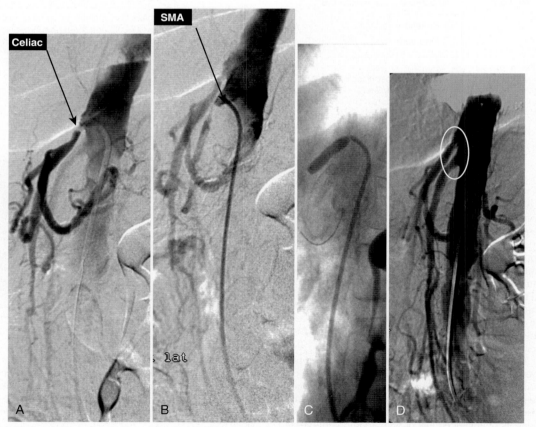

FIGURE 63-17 Selective evaluation of the celiac arteries and SMA in the lateral projection of the patient in Figure 63-16. **A, B,** Both these vessels proved to be critically stenosed. **C,** They were treated interventionally, restoring wide patency to both, as outlined in **D.** The patient's symptoms abated and she began to gain weight.

stent revascularization should be the percutaneous treatment of choice.

Brachiocephalic and Subclavian Obstructive Disease

Once considered relatively rare, brachiocephalic and subclavian artery obstructions have received increased attention recently because of the use of internal mammary conduits for coronary bypass surgery. Asymptomatic differences in systolic arm pressures (≥10 mm Hg) are the most common presentation of brachiocephalic or subclavian stenosis. Subclavian steal syndrome arises because of reversal of flow in the vertebral artery as blood is shunted to the upper extremity circulation. Vertebrobasilar symptoms of dizziness, syncope, and vertigo are most common, along with upper extremity claudication of the ipsilateral limb. In coronary subclavian steal, there is reversal of flow within the left internal mammary artery because of proximal subclavian stenosis. These patients often come to clinical attention with myocardial ischemia. Although conservative therapy offers some clinical improvement, the problem usually requires relief of the anatomic obstruction.

Treatment

Balloon angioplasty for subclavian artery stenosis was described in the early 1980s, with subsequent reports showing acute success and patency rates at follow-up comparable to those of surgery. Furthermore, there was a low rate of complications and infrequent mortality. There was initial concern about the potential for distal embolization and stroke, uncertain long-term patency, and difficulty in treating total occlusions. With continued improvements in anesthetic and operative technique, short hospital stays, and early discharge, many practitioners continue to regard surgery as the standard against which endovascular methods must be compared.

Clinical data regarding long-term patency of the subclavian or brachiocephalic vessels are limited (**Fig. 63-18**). An evaluation of the reports of surgery versus angioplasty or stenting of this condition has described technical success (with the planned procedure yielding target lesion revascularization and survival to discharge), patient death, stroke, and patency of the treated segment.[80] There was no uniformity or standardization for evaluating or reporting complications in the studies in which stenting was performed; however, adverse events were reported in approximately 6% of patients.

Similarly, the overall incidence of postprocedure complications, such as vascular access bleeding, hemorrhage, pseudoaneurysm, transfusion, or contrast-mediated transient renal insufficiency, is not known. Technical success has been reported in 97% of cases. No strokes or deaths occurred. Follow-up data were available in about two thirds of cases at a mean of 16.8 months. Occlusion or restenosis was found in less than 10%.[80] Additional reports of subclavian stent placement continue to suggest that perioperative strokes are uncommon and the results are favorable.[81] There have been some concerns not only about long-term patency, but also about durability of the stent because of strut fracture at the site of flexion and compression.

A European series reviewed 115 patients with subclavian disease who were treated percutaneously.[82] Successful revascularization was achieved in 98% of patients. There were no periprocedural deaths, but 1 patient had a transient ischemic attack from the left vertebral artery and 2 patients had emboli—1 to the renal artery and 1 to the mesenteric artery. All 3 patients recovered completely from these events. Whereas patency rates were significantly higher at 1 year in the stent group, compared with those treated only with angioplasty (95% versus 76%), by 4 years of follow-up there was more restenosis in the stent patients.[82] Another recent report[83] on 170 symptomatic patients with 177 subclavian and innominate arteries treated with catheter-based stent therapy had a procedure success rate of 98.3%, no mortalities occurred within 30 days, and the periprocedural stroke rate was less than 1%. At 3 years of follow-up, 82% of patients remained asymptomatic, with a primary patency rate of 83% and a secondary patency rate of 96%.

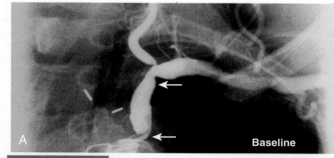
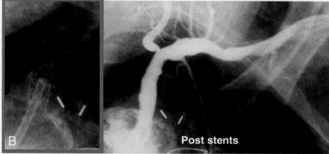
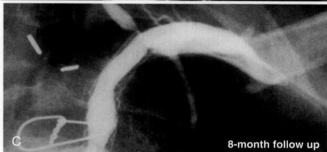

FIGURE 63-18 **A,** Baseline angiogram of a left subclavian artery with a tight proximal stenosis and a moderate stenosis just proximal to the vertebral artery. **B,** After placement of two balloon expandable stents. Note the position of the stents in the inset. **C,** Follow-up angiogram at 8 months with patent stents.

In summary, it is unlikely that a large well-designed trial comparing surgical and interventional treatment of patients with brachiocephalic and subclavian disease will be carried out because of the relative infrequency of this disease. At present, experience and examination of the literature support the consideration of a primary percutaneous approach in most patients with symptomatic obstructive disease.

Carotid and Vertebral Disease

CAROTID ARTERY DISEASE. Slightly more than 50% of the 731,000 strokes/year in the United States result from extracranial atherosclerotic carotid artery disease. Stroke is the leading cause of disability and the third leading cause of death after coronary artery disease and cancer in the United States (see Chap. 62). Atherosclerotic extracranial carotid artery disease usually causes symptoms as a result of embolic events. In contrast to acute coronary syndromes, a minority of ischemic strokes are caused by thrombotic occlusion.

The two internal carotid arteries and two vertebral arteries come together at the base of the skull to form the circle of Willis, which is an ideal anastomotic network. In theory, a single vessel could supply the circulatory needs of the entire brain. However, although a circle of Willis is present in every brain, there is a huge amount of individual variability, and fewer than half are complete.

Cerebrovascular events are classified as transient ischemic attacks (TIAs) if they are transient and do not result in an infarction, or as strokes if they cause an acute infarction[84] (see Chap. 62). Patients with a TIA have a 1 in 20 (5%) chance of stroke within 30 days, and almost 25% will have a recurrent cerebrovascular event within 1 year. Hemispheric symptoms refer to a single carotid distribution, typically causing contralateral hemiparesis or hemiparesthesia, aphasia, and/or ipsilateral monocular blindness (amaurosis fugax). Nonhemispheric symptoms include dysarthria, diplopia, vertigo, syncope, and/or transient confusion.

Noninvasive Imaging

Doppler ultrasound of the carotid arteries is cost-effective, accurate, and reproducible. Blood flow velocity measurements translate into estimates of lesion severity that have clinical relevance. There is controversy regarding the ability of ultrasound imaging to serve as the sole imaging criteria to select patients for carotid revascularization and, although ultrasound is an excellent screening tool, its accuracy in a community setting has been debated. However, many patients are revascularized based solely on their carotid ultrasound findings. MRA and CTA are being used to image the extracranial carotid arteries and intracerebral vessels (**Fig. 63-19**). The images can be reconstructed into noninvasive angiograms that have the advantage of imaging the circle of Willis with excellent resolution and clarity. If the ultrasound, MRA, and CTA results agree, many proceed directly to revascularization without angiography if the clinical indications are also appropriate.

Invasive Angiography

All the revascularization trials that have informed carotid artery treatment decisions have used angiographic criteria for patient selection. Digital subtraction angiography (DSA) is the gold standard for the diagnosis of vascular pathology of the aortic arch, cervical, and cerebral vessels (**Fig. 63-20**). Invasive angiography can cause adverse events, including a 0.5% stroke rate.

Surgical Treatment

Treatment of carotid artery disease aims to prevent disabling stroke and death. All therapeutic modalities should be judged ultimately on their ability to achieve these endpoints rather than surrogates. For revascularization to benefit patients, the strokes prevented by the procedure must exceed the strokes caused by the procedure. Similarly, procedure-related mortality cannot obliterate the late benefit of surgery. This concept is important, because the longer patients live after a revascularization procedure, the greater the benefit they will enjoy.

Very old or very ill patients may not live long enough to justify placing them at risk of a procedure-related death.[85]

Carotid endarterectomy (CEA) is an established surgical procedure for stroke prevention in patients with extracranial carotid artery disease (**Table 63-9**). Randomized controlled trials in selected populations have demonstrated benefit in both symptomatic (>50%) and asymptomatic (≥60%) patients for stroke prevention with CEA compared with medical therapy.[86]

The applicability of these surgical trial results to daily patient outcomes has generated controversy. Results in the Medicare population have not been as good as those reported in the trials. The AHA expert consensus panel suggested that indications for CEA include good surgical risk candidates with symptoms related to a 50% or greater stenosis, and asymptomatic patients with an 80% or greater stenosis; however, the perioperative risk of stroke and death should not exceed 3% for asymptomatic patients, 6% for symptomatic patients, or 10% for repeat CEA.[87]

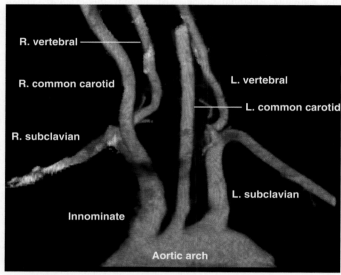

FIGURE 63-19 CTA depiction of aortic arch and arch vessels.

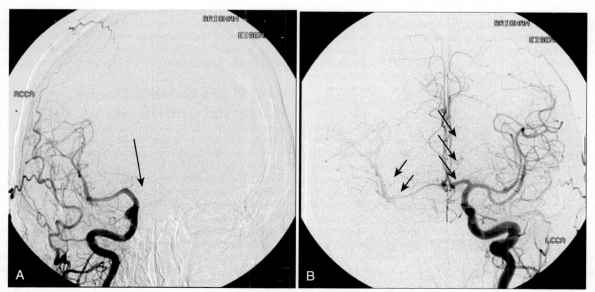

FIGURE 63-20 Corresponding anteroposterior (Townes) view of the right **(A)** and left **(B)** intracranial carotid angiograms. **A,** Perfusion of the right middle cerebral territory only. No flow is seen into the anterior cerebral vessel, the expected location of which is delineated by the arrow. **B,** Injection of the left carotid artery, demonstrating filling of both hemispheres, including the right anterior cerebral (three long arrows) and middle cerebral (two short arrows) territories.

TABLE 63-9 Carotid Surgery Versus Medical Therapy Trials

TRIAL	MEDICAL RISK OF STROKE (%)	CEA RISK OF STROKE (%)	PERIOPERATIVE 30-DAY INCIDENCE OF STROKE AND DEATH (%)
NASCET, 70%-99%	25.1	8.9	5.8
NASCET, 50%-69%	16.2	11.3	7.1
ECST, 70%-99%	16.8	10.3	7.5
ACAS, ≥60%	11.0	5.1	2.3
ACST, ≥60%	11.0	3.8	3.1

ACAS = Asymptomatic Carotid Atherosclerosis Study; ACST = Asymptomatic Carotid Surgery Trial; ECST = European Carotid Surgery Trial; NASCET = North American Symptomatic Carotid Endarterectomy Trial.

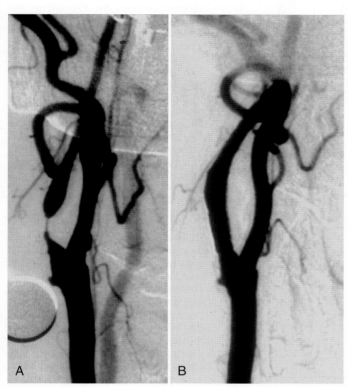

FIGURE 63-21 A, Baseline selective carotid angiogram showing critical stenosis of the internal carotid artery. The external carotid is identified as the vessel that gives off branches. **B,** Following stent deployment.

Catheter-Based Treatment

Carotid artery stent (CAS) placement has evolved over the past 20 years to become an accepted method for treating selected patients (**Fig. 63-21**).[88] Self-expanding stents are used to avoid stent deformation and compression. Concern over the potential release of atheroemboli has led to the development of several emboli protection systems, including the following: (1) distal balloon occlusion with aspiration[89]; (2) proximal occlusion with aspiration[90]; and (3) distal filter systems.[91]

Several large contemporary, nonrandomized, prospective registry studies (e.g., BEACH, ARCHeR 2, SECuRITY) have investigated the safety and efficacy of CAS, with embolic protection in symptomatic and asymptomatic patients at increased risk for surgical treatment.[92-96] All these trials have met their targets for safety and efficacy (**Fig. 63-22**).

The Stenting and Angioplasty with Protection in Patients at High Risk for Endarterectomy (SAPPHIRE) trial was a randomized controlled trial that compared CAS with distal emboli protection to CEA in patients at increased risk for CEA.[97] A total of 747 patients were entered into the trial, with 159 randomized to CAS with distal protection and 151 randomized to CEA. An additional 406 patients were refused surgery and were treated in a stent registry, but only 7 patients were refused CAS and were treated in a surgery registry.

In the randomized patients, the 30-day incidence of stroke, death, or myocardial infarction was lower for CAS (4.8%) than for CEA (9.6%; $P = 0.14$). The CEA group also had cranial nerve injuries (5.3%), which were not seen in the CAS group. The 1-year combined endpoint for the CAS group was 12%, compared with 20.1% ($P = 0.048$) in the CEA group (**Fig. 63-23**). This trial met the criteria for noninferiority, and led to the first U.S. Food and Drug Administration (FDA) approval of a carotid stent. This randomized trial provides compelling evidence that CAS with distal protection is the procedure of choice for patients at increased risk for carotid surgery.

Recently, three large peer-reviewed reports considered CAS in high-surgical-risk postmarket surveillance trials reporting on more than 8000 patients treated outside the clinical investigational setting. The Stenting and Angioplasty with Protection of Patients with High Risk for Endarterectomy World-Wide (SAPPHIRE WW) postmarket approval registry trial evaluated 30-day outcomes after CAS in high-surgical-risk patients.[98] Independent neurologic assessment was used for outcomes assessment. The investigators reported 30-day safety and efficacy outcomes in 2001 symptomatic and asymptomatic high-surgical-risk patients (anatomic = 716; comorbid = 918; both = 327) treated by carotid stent operators with varying clinical experience. Approximately 72% were asymptomatic and 28% were symptomatic. The criteria for anatomic or comorbid surgical risk features were based on the FDA labeling for the devices. The primary endpoint of composite adverse outcomes included combined stroke (based on independent neurologic assessment using the National Institutes of Health Stroke Scale [NIHSS] and Rankin scale), death, and myocardial infarction. The overall independently adjudicated 30-day stroke and death rate for CAS in the high-surgical-risk patients was 4.0%. In the asymptomatic SAPPHIRE WW patients, the adverse outcome rate was 1.8% in the anatomic subgroup and 3.0% in the comorbid subgroup, within the 3% limit required by the AHA Expert Consensus group. For symptomatic patients, the overall adverse event rate was again lower than the 6% rate described by the AHA consensus document—4.5% for the anatomic subgroup, which rose to 8.3% in the comorbid high-risk group. This study involved almost 350 sites and operators with a wide variety of experience, suggesting that the outcomes from prior premarket approval (PMA) trials are generalizable.

Two other large postmarket registry trials, EXACT and CAPTURE-2, reported on more than 6000 high-surgical-risk patients treated by CAS operators with varying levels of experience in large prospective, multicenter registries (EXACT, $N = 2145$; CAPTURE-2, $N = 4175$).[99] Both trials included independent neurologic assessment of outcomes to reinforce the rigor for ascertaining adverse events. The overall incidence of 30-day stroke and death for the EXACT patients was 4.1%, and for the CAPTURE-2 patients it was only 3.4%. Importantly, for patients who would have been comparable to patients included in the 2006 AHA published guidelines (<80 years), the CAS results met the threshold recommendations for 30-day stroke and death rates for symptomatic patients (≥50% stenosis) at 5.3% (benchmark for CEA, ≤6%), and for

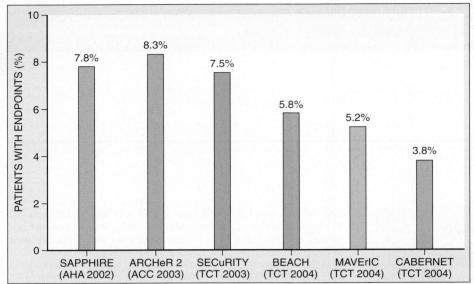

FIGURE 63-22 Bar graph showing 30-day composite endpoint (stroke, death, myocardial infarction) for U.S. carotid stent trials.

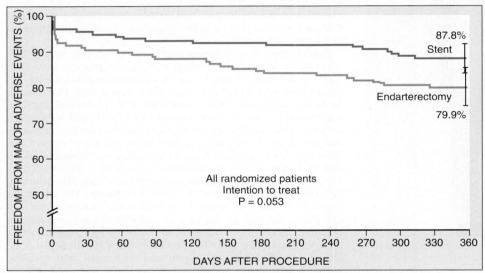

FIGURE 63-23 Outcome at 1 year for freedom from major adverse events, showing superiority for carotid stent over carotid surgery in randomized patients by intention to treat in the SAPPHIRE trial. *(From Yadav JS, Wholey MH, Kuntz RE, et al: Protected carotid-artery stenting versus endarterectomy in high-risk patients. N Engl J Med 351:1493, 2004.)*

6.38% among those who had endarterectomy.[102] The SPACE study actually demonstrated superior (log rank, $P = 0.001$) outcomes in average- or low-surgical-risk patients for CAS compared with CEA for patients 68 years of age or younger.[103] These two trials reflect the current controversies in carotid revascularization, the interpretation of which depends on the bias of the reader.

The International Carotid Stent Study (ICSS) randomized 1713 usual-risk patients to CAS ($N = 855$) versus CEA ($N = 858$).[104] The primary endpoint for the trial, disabling stroke or death, was no different between the two groups, but there was an excess of nondisabling strokes and fatal strokes in the CAS arm. These three European trials (EVA-3S, SPACE, and ICSS) all contain a significant bias against CAS by allowing very inexperienced operators to be tutored in the technique while enrolling patients and requiring emboli protection devices. These two issues, which did not occur in the Carotid Revascularization Endarterectomy versus Stenting Trial (CREST), contributed to the excess in strokes seen in the CAS arm.

Currently, CREST is widely viewed as the definitive comparison of these two techniques of carotid revascularization.[105] This study randomized over 2500 patients with significant carotid stenosis to stenting with embolic protection or surgery. More than one third were female, and more than 50% of the population consisted of symptomatic patients. There was no difference in the primary endpoint of periprocedural stroke, myocardial infarction, death, or postprocedural ipsilateral stroke up to 4 years (7.2% versus 6.8%; $P = 0.51$). There were significantly more myocardial infarctions with surgery and significantly more strokes with carotid stenting, although no significant difference in periprocedural major strokes. Of note, the periprocedural event rates were remarkably low in both arms of the study. As expected, periprocedural cranial nerve palsies were significantly lower with carotid stenting (0.3% versus 4.8%; $P < 0.0001$). There was no evidence of differential efficacy based on sex or symptomatic status. There was, however, an interaction by age that appeared significant, such that carotid stenting provided superior results in patients younger than 70 years of age, whereas those older than 70 years of age appeared to have better results with surgery. Further research is needed to define the optimal treatment of older patients,[85] but the results of CREST have shown that when performed by well-trained operators, carotid stenting with embolic protection and carotid surgery both provide excellent periprocedural outcomes and freedom from ipsilateral stroke. The choice of which form of revascularization is best likely depends on patient characteristics and individual preferences, which for many patients will be carotid stenting. At present, the moderate viewpoint is that the techniques are not very different, and that much still remains to be learned about their safe and effective applications.

Current indications for carotid artery stent placement are both in symptomatic (diameter > 50%) and asymptomatic (diameter ≥ 60% to

asymptomatic patients (≥80% stenosis) at 2.9% (benchmark for CEA, ≤ 3%).

Four randomized trials of CEA versus CAS in usual-surgical-risk patients have been reported. The Endarterectomy versus Stenting in Patients with Symptomatic Severe Carotid Stenosis (EVA-3S) trial compared CAS with a variety of techniques and variable cerebral embolic protection with CEA. The results showed statistically lower rates of stroke and death at 6 months in the endarterectomy group.[100,101] This trial was carried out by experienced vascular surgeons and inexperienced interventionalists, and it used a much wider variety of techniques for CAS than other trials.

The 30-day results of the Stent-Supported Percutaneous Angioplasty versus Endarterectomy of the Carotid Artery versus Endarterectomy (SPACE) trial showed no difference in stroke or death, but it enrolled too few patients to demonstrate noninferiority of carotid stenting compared with endarterectomy. The rate of ipsilateral stroke or death was 6.84% among patients who underwent carotid stenting, compared with

TABLE 63-10	Factors Associated with Increased Risk of Complications from Carotid Artery Stent Placement

- Tortuous aortic arch
- Platelet or clotting disorder
- Difficult vascular access
- Lesion or vessel calcification
- Visible thrombus
- Advanced age (>75-80 yr)*

*Risk of cerebrovascular accident (CVA) with CAS increased and risk of myocardial infarction (MI) with CEA increased.

TABLE 63-11	Factors Associated with Increased Risk from Carotid Artery Surgery

Anatomic Criteria
- High cervical or intrathoracic lesion
- Prior neck surgery or radiation therapy
- Contralateral carotid artery occlusion
- Prior ipsilateral CEA
- Contralateral laryngeal nerve palsy
- Tracheostomy

Medical Comorbidities
- Age > 80 yr*
- Class III or IV congestive heart failure
- Class III or IV angina pectoris
- Left main coronary disease
- Two- or three-vessel coronary artery disease
- Need for open heart surgery
- Ejection fraction ≤30%
- Recent myocardial infarction
- Severe chronic obstructive lung disease

*Risk of CVA with CAS increased and risk of MI with CEA increased.

80%) stenoses in patients at increased risk for carotid surgery who are anatomically good candidates for CAS (**Table 63-10**). Currently, patients who do not meet high-surgical-risk criteria (**Table 63-11**) should have their treatment individualized and may be offered surgery[106] or stenting. Trials and registries are continuing to enroll low-surgical-risk patients and are hoping to readdress the issue of whether prophylactic medical therapy, which itself is improving, may be equivalent or superior to stenting and/or endarterectomy for asymptomatic patients. The best patient care will continue to require knowledge, skill, and the best application of the physician's judgment.

VERTEBRAL ARTERY DISEASE. People can tolerate ligature of one of the two vertebral arteries well, making the clinical presentation of vertebrobasilar insufficiency infrequent. Atherosclerotic occlusive disease of the origin of both vertebral arteries is the most common clinical lesion culprit; however, other combinations of carotid, subclavian, and innominate stenoses can compromise the posterior circulation and precipitate symptoms of vertebrobasilar insufficiency. In patients presenting with symptoms of cerebrovascular disease, 40% will have evidence of at least vertebral stenosis and 10% will have a vertebral occlusion. Of those with posterior circulation symptoms (e.g., dizziness, ataxia, drop attacks, or diplopia), up to 35% will have a stroke within 5 years.

Treatment

Although initial treatment with platelet inhibitors and anticoagulants is warranted, arch and four-vessel study (CTA, MRA, or DSA) is indicated if posterior circulation symptoms continue despite medical management. Surgical therapy is difficult and associated with significant perioperative morbidity. Transection of the vertebral artery above the stenosis and reimplantation into the ipsilateral subclavian or carotid artery, vertebral artery endarterectomy, or vein patch angioplasty are the surgical techniques for treatment of this disease.

In one series, 174 patients undergoing proximal vertebral artery reconstruction had no in-hospital deaths, and reported complications were as follows: recurrent laryngeal nerve palsy, 2%; Horner's syndrome, 15%; lymphocele, 4%; chylothorax, 0.5%; and immediate thrombosis, 1%. Secondary patency rates were 95% and 91% at 5 and 10 years, respectively. Seventy-five patients undergoing reconstruction of the distal vertebral artery had a mortality rate of 4% and an immediate graft thrombosis rate of 8%. Secondary patency rates for distal vertebral artery reconstruction were 87% and 82% at 5 and 10 years, respectively. Mortality rates for surgical treatment of this disease are acceptable, but excessive morbidity restricts this technique from widespread use for the treatment of vertebral artery disease. Percutaneous treatment of this disease is not associated with the excessive morbidity that accompanies surgical correction.

The safety and efficacy of stent placement in treating atherosclerotic vertebral artery disease has been demonstrated by Jenkins and coworkers,[107] who reported 105 consecutive symptomatic patients treated with stents (112 arteries, 71% male) for extracranial (91%) and intracranial (9%) vertebral artery stenosis (VAS). Of these, 57 patients (54%) had bilateral VAS, 71 patients (68%) had concomitant carotid disease, and 43 patients (41%) had a prior stroke. Procedural and clinical success was achieved in 105 patients (100%) and 95 patients (90.5%), respectively (**Fig 63-24**). At 1-year follow-up in 87 patients (82.9%), 69 patients (79.3%) remained symptom-free. At 1 year, 6 patients (5.7%) had died and 5 patients (5%) had a posterior circulation stroke. Target vessel revascularization occurred in 7.4% at 1 year. At a median follow-up of 29.1 months, 13.1% had target vessel revascularization, 71.4% were alive, and 70.5% remained symptom-free.

Concern about the risk of distal embolization of debris renders debulking devices inappropriate for use in the cerebral circulation. Because the most common location for vertebral artery stenoses is at or near its origin from the subclavian artery, considerable recoil often accompanies PTA alone. Embolic protection devices have been used, although whether they improve outcomes remains uncertain.

Endoluminal stenting of vertebral artery lesions is safe and effective with a durable result, as evidenced by the low recurrence rate. Primary stent placement is an attractive treatment option for atherosclerotic vertebral artery disease.

Obstructive Venous Disease

Extremity Deep Venous Thrombosis

Unlike atherosclerotic arterial obstructive disease, the major presenting obstructive element in venous obstruction is thrombus (see Chaps. 77 and 87). Thus, dissolution or removal of the offending thrombus is the most evident goal of interventions for extremity venous thrombosis. However, underlying the thrombus is almost always a predisposing factor, such as a hypercoagulable state, external obstruction, venous stricture, scarring, or an indwelling foreign body. As a result, the treatment of venous thrombosis is comprised not only of the removal of the thrombus but also an attempt to correct the underlying cause.

Treatment

For most patients, anticoagulation and/or thrombolytic therapy are the mainstays of therapy (see Chaps. 77 and 87). Both systemic and catheter-directed thrombolysis have achieved some success (**Fig. 63-25**). Mechanical thrombectomy, balloon venoplasty, and stenting have all been reported, but evidence supporting the use of catheter-directed therapy is limited.

Because of the possibility of a reduction in the incidence of post-thrombotic syndrome with lysis compared with anticoagulation alone, and because of the possibility of reduced major bleeding, catheter-directed therapy seems reasonable in patients at higher risk for the complications of systemic lysis and in those who have a large thrombus burden and/or a high risk of developing a post-thrombotic syndrome. In addition, more interventional concepts are emerging. There are reports of experience with rheolytic thrombectomy[108] or mechanical clot disruption. The ATTRACT trial will randomize patients with DVT to medical therapy with anticoagulation or catheter-directed therapy.[109] Additional experience with stents suggests that in patients

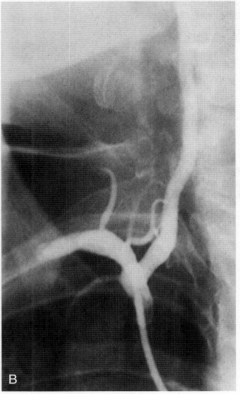

FIGURE 63-24 **A,** Angiogram of a tight stenosis at the ostium of the right vertebral artery (arrow). **B,** After balloon-expandable stent placement.

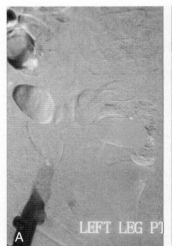
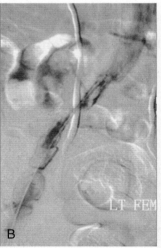
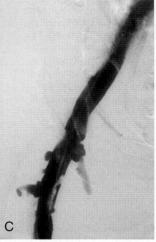

FIGURE 63-25 Venogram of the left femoral vein after gaining access at the popliteal vein with ultrasound guidance. The patient is lying face down on the table to allow access to the popliteal vein. **A,** Baseline shows occlusion of the left femoral vein. **B,** Multiholed catheter across the venous occlusion; the administration of lytic agents is started. **C,** 4 hours after lysis following PTA and placement of a self-expanding stent to restore patency.

Central Venous Obstruction

SUPERIOR VENA CAVA SYNDROME. Superior vena cava (SVC) syndrome results from the obstruction of the blood flow in the superior vena cava. Pathologic processes from contiguous structures can compress or directly invade the SVC. Superimposed venous thrombosis may contribute to the development of SVC syndrome in up to 50% of patients. Historically, SVC syndrome was most frequently caused by direct tumor compression (see Chap. 90). The use of indwelling venous access catheters, coupled with the improved survival of chemotherapy patients, has increased the occurrence of nonmalignant SVC syndrome in patients following cure of their cancer. The explosion in the use of the automatic implantable cardioverter-defibrillator (AICD) and sophisticated multilead pacing systems has increased the incidence and recognition of this condition.

Percutaneous Treatment

Medical and surgical options for the treatment of superior vena cava obstruction are well established (see Chap. 90). Since the initial description of successful percutaneous treatment of SVC syndrome in the adult, the use of angioplasty alone was limited by a high rate of initial failure and early restenosis because of recoil of the highly elastic SVC wall. Stenting therefore quickly gained acceptance in this area of vascular intervention after its introduction in the 1980s. Stenting in malignant SVC syndrome results in rapid improvement of symptoms. Patients report almost immediate resolution of headache, visual disturbances, and other central nervous system symptoms. Dyspnea, cough, and edema usually resolve within 1 to 3 days, but occasionally may take up to 1 week. Stenting results in complete resolution of symptoms in most patients with malignant SVC syndrome. In the largest series,[110] 76 consecutive patients with SVC syndrome were treated with stents and compared with historical controls of patients treated with radiation. Procedural success was 100%, and all patients had improvement of symptoms within 48 hours. Of patients treated with a stent, 90% had no symptoms of SVC obstruction at the time of death, compared with 12% of patients treated with radiation. The recurrence rate of SVC syndrome after percutaneous intervention has been reported to vary widely, occurring in up to 45% of patients. This variability likely results from diverse mechanisms. Acute stent thrombosis can develop shortly after stent placement in patients on insufficient anticoagulation or antiplatelet therapy; tumor ingrowth through stent struts or intimal

prevent postphlebitic syndromes is appropriate based on individual circumstances.

in whom there is residual venous obstruction from scarring or external compression, relief of that obstruction with self-expanding stents may be important to maintain venous patency and prevent recurrent thrombosis. This is particularly true after relief of the initial insult, such as an indwelling port infusion catheter. Balloon venoplasty is also increasingly used to provide temporary relief of venous obstruction to facilitate the placement of transvenous pacing and/or defibrillator leads.

The mainstay of venous thrombosis of the extremities is anticoagulation. However, the selective application of catheter-based thrombolysis, thrombectomy, and venous stenting to relieve symptoms and help

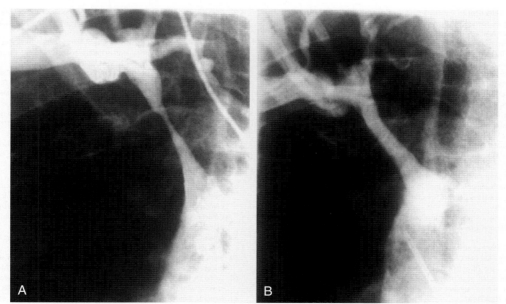

FIGURE 63-26 SVC syndrome and its treatment. **A,** Baseline venogram showing a tight stenosis of the SVC, which was crossed with a 0.035-in. guidewire from the femoral vein. The stenosis was predilated with a balloon and a large self-expanding stent was then placed to overcome recoil. **B,** Final venogram.

hyperplasia or fibrous scarring can occur. Stent length oversizing may prevent recurrence of SVC syndrome because of stent edge overgrowth, but may increase the risk of SVC stent thrombosis or restenosis. Patients with total SVC occlusion have the highest recurrence rate of SVC syndrome, but repeat procedures in these patients are uniformly successful; additional stent placement, angioplasty, and/or thrombolysis can be used alone or in combination.[111]

In the developed world, SVC syndrome of nonmalignant cause (benign SVC syndrome) is usually iatrogenic in origin, most frequently as a result of indwelling intravenous catheters and pacing leads. Complications of pacemaker lead placement, such as venous thrombosis or stenosis, occur in up to 30% of patients. Only a few patients become symptomatic, but the presence of multiple leads, retention of severed lead(s), and previous lead infection may increase the risk of SVC syndrome. The largest series of percutaneous therapy in benign SVC syndrome included 16 patients.[112] In this series, 10 patients had SVC syndrome because of the indwelling catheter, 2 because of the pacemaker wire, and 1 each because of goiter, fibrous mediastinitis, heart-lung transplantation, and spontaneous thrombosis. The patency rate in 13 patients who were followed for a mean of 17 months was 85%. Similar results can be expected in patients with SVC syndrome associated with central venous infusion catheters. Ideally, interventional treatment should also include removal of the inciting lead or catheter. Combination laser sheath extraction of pacemaker and defibrillator leads followed by venous angioplasty and stenting with subsequent lead reimplantation can be performed successfully.

Superior vena cava stenting is a low-risk procedure that provides fast and durable symptomatic relief in malignant caval obstruction, often in combination with chemotherapy or radiation. It provides patients with the benefit of life prolongation together with effective symptom control. In patients with SVC syndrome of nonmalignant cause, based on mid-term follow-up results, stenting is the treatment of choice (**Fig. 63-26**). Surgical therapy should be reserved for patients with benign SVC syndrome refractory to percutaneous therapy. Only a few patients become truly refractory; most patients with recurrent SVC syndrome can undergo repeated percutaneous intervention.

Conclusion

Although the specific tools and techniques vary, the theme of endovascular intervention is similar across many vascular territories. In general, vascular stenting has become the mainstay of percutaneous revascularization for relief of symptoms. The challenge for the future will be to continue to improve the long-term durability of endovascular therapy and to explore its potential for preventing the complications of progressive vascular disease.

REFERENCES

1. Hirsch AT, Haskal ZJ, Hertzer NR, et al: ACC/AHA 2005 guidelines for the management of patients with peripheral arterial disease (lower extremity, renal, mesenteric, and abdominal aortic): Executive summary: A collaborative report from the American Association for Vascular Surgery/Society for Vascular Surgery, Society for Cardiovascular Angiography and Interventions, Society for Vascular Medicine and Biology, Society of Interventional Radiology, and the ACC/AHA Task Force on Practice Guidelines (Writing Committee to Develop Guidelines for the Management of Patients With Peripheral Arterial Disease) endorsed by the American Association of Cardiovascular and Pulmonary Rehabilitation; National Heart, Lung and Blood Institute; Society for Vascular Nursing; TransAtlantic Inter-Society Consensus; and Vascular Disease Foundation. J Am Coll Cardiol 47:1239, 2006.

Atherosclerotic Lower Extremity Disease

2. Ponec D, Jaff MR, Swischuk J, et al: The nitinol SMART stent vs wallstent for suboptimal iliac artery angioplasty: The CRISP US trial results. J Vasc Interv Radiol 9:911, 2004.
3. Reyes R, Maynar M, Lopera J, et al: Treatment of chronic iliac artery occlusions with guide wire recanalization and primary stent placement. J Vasc Interv Radiol 8:1049, 1997.
4. Dyet JF: Endovascular stents in the arterial system—current status. Clin Radiol 52:83, 1997.
5. Murphy TP, Khwaja AA, Webb MS: Aortoiliac stent placement in patients treated for intermittent claudication. J Vasc Interv Radiol 9:421, 1998.
6. Tetteroo E, van der Graaf Y, Bosch JL, et al: Randomised comparison of primary stent placement versus primary angioplasty followed by selective stent placement in patients with iliac artery occlusive disease. Lancet 351:1153, 1998.
7. Powell RJ, Fillinger M, Bettmann M, et al: The durability of endovascular treatment of multisegment iliac occlusive disease. J Vasc Surg 31:1178, 2000.
8. Saha S, Gibson M, Magee TR, et al: Early results of retrograde transpopliteal angioplasty of iliofemoral lesions. Cardiovasc Intervent Radiol 24:378, 2001.
9. Timaran CH, Stevens SL, Freeman MB, Goldman MH: External iliac and common iliac artery angioplasty and stenting in men and women. J Vasc Surg 34:440, 2001.
10. Haulon S, Mounier-Véhier C, Gaxotte V, et al: Percutaneous reconstruction of the aortoiliac bifurcation with the "kissing stents" technique: Long-term follow-up in 106 patients. J Endovasc Ther 9:363, 2002.
11. Siskin GP, Englander M, Roddy S, et al: Results of iliac artery stent placement in patients younger than 50 years of age. J Vasc Interv Radiol 13:785, 2002.
12. Mohamed F, Sarkar B, Timmons G, et al: Outcome of "kissing stents" for aortoiliac atherosclerotic disease, including the effect on the non-diseased contralateral iliac limb. Cardiovasc Intervent Radiol 25:472, 2002.
13. Reekers JA, Vorwerk D, Rousseau H, et al: Results of a European multicentre iliac stent trial with a flexible balloon expandable stent. Eur J Vasc Endovasc Surg 24:511, 2002.
14. Funovics MA, Lackner B, Cejna M, et al: Predictors of long-term results after treatment of iliac artery obliteration by transluminal angioplasty and stent deployment. Cardiovasc Intervent Radiol 25:397, 2002.
15. Hans SS, DeSantis D, Siddiqui R, Khoury M: Results of endovascular therapy and aortobifemoral grafting for Transatlantic Inter-Society type C and D aortoiliac occlusive disease. Surgery 144:583, 2008.

16. Kashyap VS, Pavkov ML, Bena JF, et al: The management of severe aortoiliac occlusive disease: Endovascular therapy rivals open reconstruction. J Vasc Surg 48:1451, 2008.
17. Sixt S, Alawied AK, Rastan A, et al: Acute and long-term outcome of endovascular therapy for aortoiliac occlusive lesions stratified according to the TASC classification: A single-center experience. J Endovasc Ther 15:408, 2008.
18. Uberoi R, Milburn S, Moss J, et al: British Society of Interventional Radiology Iliac Artery Angioplasty-Stent Registry III. Cardiovasc Intervent Radiol 32:887, 2009.
19. Amighi J, Schillinger M, Dick P, et al: De novo superficial femoropopliteal artery lesions: peripheral cutting balloon angioplasty and restenosis rates—randomized controlled trial. Radiology 247:267, 2008.
20. Schillinger M, Sabeti S, Loewe C, et al: Balloon angioplasty versus implantation of nitinol stents in the superficial femoral artery. N Engl J Med 354:1879, 2006.
21. Krankenberg H, Schlüter M, Steinkamp HJ, et al: Nitinol stent implantation versus percutaneous transluminal angioplasty in superficial femoral artery lesions up to 10 cm in length: The femoral artery stenting trial (FAST). Circulation 116:285, 2007.
22. Tepe G, Zeller T, Albrecht T, et al: Local delivery of paclitaxel to inhibit restenosis during angioplasty of the leg. N Engl J Med 358:689, 2008.
23. Werk M, Langner S, Reinkensmeier B, et al: Inhibition of restenosis in femoropopliteal arteries: paclitaxel-coated versus uncoated balloon: Femoral paclitaxel randomized pilot trial. Circulation 118:1358, 2008.
24. Duda SH, Bosiers M, Lammer J, et al: Sirolimus-eluting versus bare nitinol stent for obstructive superficial femoral artery disease: The SIROCCO II trial. J Vasc Interv Radiol 16:331, 2005.
25. Scheinert D, Scheinert S, Sax J, et al: Prevalence and clinical impact of stent fractures after femoropopliteal stenting. J Am Coll Cardiol 45:312, 2005.
26. Dake M: Interim report on the Zilver PTX clinical study. J Vasc Surg 50:447, 2009.
27. Gray BH, Sullivan TM, Childs MB, et al: High incidence of restenosis/reocclusion of stents in the percutaneous treatment of long-segment superficial femoral artery disease after suboptimal angioplasty. J Vasc Surg 25:74, 1997.
28. Martin DR, Katz SG, Kohl RD, Qian D: Percutaneous transluminal angioplasty of infrainguinal vessels. Ann Vasc Surg 13:184, 1999.
29. Kessel DO, Wijesinghe LD, Robertson I, et al: Endovascular stent-grafts for superficial femoral artery disease: Results of 1-year follow-up. J Vasc Interv Radiol 10:289, 1999.
30. Conroy RM, Gordon IL, Tobis JM, et al: Angioplasty and stent placement in chronic occlusion of the superficial femoral artery: Technique and results. J Vasc Interv Radiol 11:1009, 2000.
31. Cheng SW, Ting AC, Wong J: Endovascular stenting of superficial femoral artery stenosis and occlusions: Results and risk factor analysis. Cardiovasc Surg 9:133, 2001.
32. Gordon IL, Conroy RM, Arefi M, et al: Three-year outcome of endovascular treatment of superficial femoral artery occlusion. Arch Surg 136:221, 2001.
33. Scheinert D, Laird JR Jr, Schröder M, et al: Excimer laser-assisted recanalization of long, chronic superficial femoral artery occlusions. J Endovasc Ther 8:156, 2001.
34. Löfberg AM, Karacagil S, Ljungman C, et al: Percutaneous transluminal angioplasty of the femoropopliteal arteries in limbs with chronic critical lower limb ischemia. J Vasc Surg 34:114, 2001.
35. Bauermeister G: Endovascular stent-grafting in the treatment of superficial femoral artery occlusive disease. J Endovasc Ther 8:315, 2001.
36. Duda SH, Pusich B, Richter G, et al: Sirolimus-eluting stents for the treatment of obstructive superficial femoral artery disease: Six-month results. Circulation 106:1505, 2002.
37. Steinkamp HJ, Wissgott C, Rademaker J, et al: Short (1-10 cm) superficial femoral artery occlusions: Results of treatment with excimer laser angioplasty. Cardiovasc Intervent Radiol 25:388, 2002.
38. Gray BH, Laird JR, Ansel GM, Shuck JW: Complex endovascular treatment for critical limb ischemia in poor surgical candidates: A pilot study. J Endovasc Ther 9:599, 2002.
39. Jämsén TS, Manninen HI, Jaakkola PA, Matsi PJ: Long-term outcome of patients with claudication after balloon angioplasty of the femoropopliteal arteries. Radiology 225:345, 2002.
40. Cho L, Roffi M, Mukherjee D, et al: Superficial femoral artery occlusion: Nitinol stents achieve better flow and reduce the need for medications than balloon angioplasty alone. J Inv Cardiol 15:198, 2003.
41. Becquemin JP, Favre JP, Marzelle J, et al: Systematic versus selective stent placement after superficial femoral artery balloon angioplasty: A multicenter prospective randomized study. J Vasc Surg 37:487, 2003.
42. Jahnke T, Andresen R, Müller-Hülsbeck S, et al: Hemobahn stent-grafts for treatment of femoropopliteal arterial obstructions: Midterm results of a prospective trial. J Vasc Interv Radiol 14:41, 2003.
43. Adam DJ, Beard JD, Cleveland T, et al: Bypass versus angioplasty in severe ischaemia of the leg (BASIL): Multicentre, randomised controlled trial. Lancet 366:1925, 2005.
44. Sivananthan UM, Browne TF, Thorley PJ, Rees MR: Percutaneous transluminal angioplasty of the tibial arteries. Br J Surg 81:1282, 1994.
45. Varty K, Bolia A, Naylor AR, et al: Infrapopliteal percutaneous transluminal angioplasty: A safe and successful procedure. Eur J Vasc Endovasc Surg 9:341, 1995.
46. Dorros G, Jaff MR, Murphy KJ, Mathiak L: The acute outcome of tibioperoneal vessel angioplasty in 417 cases with claudication and critical limb ischemia. Cathet Cardiovasc Diagn 45:251, 1998.
47. Desgranges P, Kobeiter K, d'Audiffret A, et al: Acute occlusion of popliteal and/or tibial arteries: The value of percutaneous treatment. Eur J Vasc Endovasc Surg 20:138, 2000.
48. Söder HK, Manninen HI, Jaakkola P, et al: Prospective trial of infrapopliteal artery balloon angioplasty for critical limb ischemia: Angiographic and clinical results. J Vasc Interv Radiol 11:1021, 2000.
49. Dorros G, Jaff MR, Dorros AM, et al: Tibioperoneal (outflow lesion) angioplasty can be used as primary treatment in 235 patients with critical limb ischemia: Five-year follow-up. Circulation 104:2057, 2001.
50. Tsetis DK, Michalis LK, Rees MR, et al: Vibrational angioplasty in the treatment of chronic infrapopliteal arterial occlusions: Preliminary experience. J Endovasc Ther 9:889, 2002.
51. Feiring AJ, Wesolowski AA, Lade S: Primary stent-supported angioplasty for treatment of below-knee critical limb ischemia and severe claudication: Early and one-year outcomes. J Am Coll Cardiol 44:2307, 2004.
52. Giles KA, Pomposelli FB, Spence TL, et al: Infrapopliteal angioplasty for critical limb ischemia: Relation of TransAtlantic InterSociety Consensus class to outcome in 176 limbs. J Vasc Surg 48:128, 2008.
53. Siablis D, Karnabatidis D, Katsanos K, et al: Infrapopliteal application of sirolimus-eluting versus bare metal stents for critical limb ischemia: Analysis of long-term angiographic and clinical outcome. J Vasc Interv Radiol 20:1141, 2009.
54. Faglia E, Mantero M, Caminiti M, et al: Extensive use of peripheral angioplasty, particularly infrapopliteal, in the treatment of ischaemic diabetic foot ulcers: Clinical results of a multicentric study of 221 consecutive diabetic subjects. J Intern Med 252:225, 2002.
55. Faglia E, Dalla Paola L, Clerici G, et al: Peripheral angioplasty as the first-choice revascularization procedure in diabetic patients with critical limb ischemia: Prospective study of 993 consecutive patients hospitalized and followed between 1999 and 2003. Eur J Vasc Endovasc Surg 29:620, 2005.
56. Tefera G, Hoch J, Turnipseed WD: Limb-salvage angioplasty in vascular surgery practice. J Vasc Surg 41:988-993.

Atherosclerotic Renal Artery Disease

57. Rundback JH, Sacks D, Kent KC, et al: AHA Councils on Cardiovascular Radiology, High Blood Pressure Research, Kidney in Cardiovascular Disease, Cardio-Thoracic and Vascular Surgery, and Clinical Cardiology, and the Society of Interventional Radiology FDA Device Forum Committee: Guidelines for the reporting of renal artery revascularization in clinical trials. American Heart Association. Circulation 106:1572, 2002.
58. White CJ, Ramee SR, Collins TJ, et al: Renal artery stent placement: Utility in lesions difficult to treat with balloon angioplasty. J Am Coll Cardiol 30:1445, 1997.
59. Blum U, Krumme B, Flügel P, et al: Treatment of ostial renal-artery stenoses with vascular endoprostheses after unsuccessful balloon angioplasty. N Engl J Med 336:459, 1997.
60. Tuttle KR, Chouinard RF, Webber JT, et al: Treatment of atherosclerotic ostial renal artery stenosis with the intravascular stent. Am J Kidney Dis 32:611, 1998.
61. Henry M, Amor M, Henry I, et al: Stents in the treatment of renal artery stenosis: Long-term follow-up. J Endovasc Surg 6:42, 1999.
62. van de Ven PJ, Kaatee R, Beutler JJ, et al: Arterial stenting and balloon angioplasty in ostial atherosclerotic renovascular disease: a randomised trial. Lancet 353:282, 1999.
63. Rocha-Singh KJ, Mishkel GJ, Katholi RE, et al: Clinical predictors of improved long-term blood pressure control after successful stenting of hypertensive patients with obstructive renal artery atherosclerosis. Catheter Cardiovasc Interv 47:167, 1999.
64. Lederman RJ, Mendelsohn FO, Santos R, et al: Primary renal artery stenting: Characteristics and outcomes after 363 procedures. Am Heart J 142:314, 2001.
65. ASTRAL Investigators: Revascularization versus medical therapy for renal-artery stenosis. N Engl J Med 361:1953, 2009.
66. Dorros G, Prince C, Mathiak L: Stenting of a renal artery stenosis achieves better relief of the obstructive lesion than balloon angioplasty. Cathet Cardiovasc Diagn 29:191, 1993.
67. Subramanian R, White CJ, Rosenfield K, et al: Renal fractional flow reserve: A hemodynamic evaluation of moderate renal artery stenoses. Catheter Cardiovasc Interv 64:480, 2005.
68. Mitchell JA, Subramanian R, Stewart R, White CJ: Pressure-derived renal fractional flow reserve with clinical outcomes following intervention. Catheter Cardiovasc Interv 65:135, 2005.
69. Silva JA, Chan AW, White CJ, et al: Elevated brain natriuretic peptide predicts blood pressure response after stent revascularization in patients with renal artery stenosis. Circulation 111:328, 2005.
70. Radermacher J, Chavan A, Bleck J, et al: Use of Doppler ultrasonography to predict the outcome of therapy for renal-artery stenosis. N Eng J Med 344:410, 2001.
71. Zeller T, Frank U, Müller C, et al: Predictors of improved renal function after percutaneous stent-supported angioplasty of severe atherosclerotic ostial renal artery stenosis. Circulation 108:2244, 2003.
72. Muray S, Martín M, Amoedo ML, et al: Rapid decline in renal function reflects reversibility and predicts the outcome after angioplasty in renal artery stenosis. Am J Kidney Dis 39:60, 2002.
73. White CJ: Catheter-based therapy for atherosclerotic renal artery stenosis. Circulation 113:1464, 2006.
74. Dworkin LD, Cooper CJ: Clinical practice. Renal-artery stenosis. N Engl J Med 361:1972, 2009.
75. National Heart, Lung and Blood Institute: Benefits of Medical Therapy Plus Stenting for Renal Atherosclerotic Lesions (CORAL), 2010 (http://clinicaltrials.gov/ct2/show/NCT00081731).

Chronic Mesenteric Disease

76. Hansen KJ, Wilson DB, Craven TE, et al: Mesenteric artery disease in the elderly. J Vasc Surg 40:45, 2004.
77. Cercueil JP, Weiller M, Tatou E, et al: Chronic mesenteric ischemia: Imaging and percutaneous treatment. Radiographics 22:863, 2002.
78. Matsumoto AH, Angle JF, Spinosa DJ, et al: Percutaneous transluminal angioplasty and stenting in the treatment of chronic mesenteric ischemia: Results and long-term followup. J Am Coll Surg 194(1 Suppl):S22, 2002.
79. Silva JA, White CJ, Collins TJ, et al: Endovascular therapy for chronic mesenteric ischemia. J Am Coll Cardiol 47:944, 2006.

Brachiocephalic and Subclavian Obstructive Disease

80. Eisenhauer AC, Shaw JA: Atherosclerotic subclavian artery disease and revascularization. *In* Abella G (ed): Peripheral Vascular Disease: Basic Diagnostic and Therapeutic Approaches. Philadelphia, Lippincott Williams & Wilkins, 2004, pp 283:294.
81. Amor M, Eid-Lidt G, Chati Z, Wilentz JR: Endovascular treatment of the subclavian artery: Stent implantation with or without predilatation. Catheter Cardiovasc Interv 63:364, 2004.
82. Schillinger M, Haumer M, Schillinger S, et al: Risk stratification for subclavian artery angioplasty: Is there an increased rate of restenosis after stent implantation? J Endovasc Ther 8:550, 2001.
83. Patel SN, White CJ, Collins TJ, et al: Catheter-based treatment of the subclavian and innominate arteries. Catheter Cardiovasc Interv 71:963, 2008.

Carotid and Vertebral Disease

84. Easton JD, Saver JL, Albers GW, et al: Definition and evaluation of transient ischemic attack: A scientific statement for healthcare professionals from the American Heart Association/

American Stroke Association Stroke Council; Council on Cardiovascular Surgery and Anesthesia; Council on Cardiovascular Radiology and Intervention; Council on Cardiovascular Nursing; and the Interdisciplinary Council on Peripheral Vascular Disease. The American Academy of Neurology affirms the value of this statement as an educational tool for neurologists. Stroke 40:2276, 2009.

85. Belkin M, Bhatt DL: Carotid stenting in the elderly: Is 80 the new 60? Circulation 119:2302, 2009.

86. MRC Asymptomatic Carotid Surgery Trial (ACST) Collaborative Group: Prevention of disabling and fatal strokes by successful carotid endarterectomy in patients without recent neurological symptoms: Randomised controlled trial. Lancet 363:1491, 2004.

87. Biller J, Feinberg WM, Castaldo JE, et al: Guidelines for carotid endarterectomy: A statement for healthcare professionals from a Special Writing Group of the Stroke Council, American Heart Association. Circulation 97:501, 1998.

88. Helton TJ, Bavry AA, Rajagopal V, et al: The optimal treatment of carotid atherosclerosis: A 2008 update and literature review. Postgrad Med 120:103, 2008.

89. Henry M, Amor M, Henry I, et al: Carotid stenting with cerebral protection: First clinical experience using the PercuSurge GuardWire system. J Endovasc Surg 6:321, 1999.

90. Grunwald IQ, Dorenbeck U, Axmann C, et al: Proximal protection systems using carotid artery stent. Radiologe 44:998, 2004.

91. Müller-Hülsbeck S, Jahnke T, Liess C, et al: Comparison of various cerebral protection devices used for carotid artery stent placement: An in vitro experiment. J Vasc Interv Radiol 14:613, 2003.

92. Gray W: Two-year composite endpoint results for the Archer Trials: Acculink for revascularization of carotids in high risk patients. Am J Cardiol 94(Suppl 6A):62E, 2004.

93. Gray WA: A cardiologist in the carotids. J Am Coll Cardiol 43:1602, 2004.

94. White CJ, for the Beach Investigators: 30 day outcomes of carotid wallstent and filterwire EX/EZ distal protection system placement for treatment of high surgical risk patients. J Am Coll Cardiol 45(Suppl A):28A, 2005.

95. Whitlow P: Security: More good data for protected carotid stenting in high-risk surgical patients, 2003 (http://www.medscape.com/viewarticle/461721_print).

96. Ramee S, Higashida R: Evaluation of the Medtronic self-expanding carotid stent system with distal protection in the treatment of carotid artery stenosis. Am J Cardiol 94(Suppl 6A):61E, 2004.

97. Yadav JS, Wholey MH, Kuntz RE, et al: Protected carotid-artery stenting versus endarterectomy in high-risk patients. N Engl J Med 351:1493, 2004.

98. Massop D, Dave R, Metzger C, et al: Stenting and angioplasty with protection in patients at high-risk for endarterectomy: SAPPHIRE Worldwide Registry first 2,001 patients. Catheter Cardiovasc Interv 73:129, 2009.

99. Gray WA, Chaturvedi S, Verta P: Thirty-day outcomes for carotid artery stenting in 6320 patients from 2 prospective, multicenter, high-surgical-risk registries. Circ Cardiovasc Interv 2:159, 2009.

100. Mas JL, Chatellier G, Beyssen B, et al: Endarterectomy versus stenting in patients with symptomatic severe carotid stenosis. N Engl J Med 355:1660, 2006.

101. Furlan AJ: Carotid-artery stenting—case open or closed? N Engl J Med 355:1726, 2006.

102. SPACE Collaborative Group; Ringleb PA, Allenberg J, Brückmann H, et al: 30 day results from the SPACE trial of stent-protected angioplasty versus carotid endarterectomy in symptomatic patients: A randomised non-inferiority trial. Lancet 368:1239, 2006.

103. Stingele R, Berger J, Alfke K, et al: Clinical and angiographic risk factors for stroke and death within 30 days after carotid endarterectomy and stent-protected angioplasty: A subanalysis of the SPACE study. Lancet Neurol 7:216, 2008.

104. International Carotid Stenting Study investigators: Carotid artery stenting compared with endarterectomy in patients with symptomatic carotid stenosis (International Carotid Stenting Study): An interim analysis of a randomised controlled trial. Lancet 375:985, 2010.

105. Brott T, Roubin GS, Howard G: The randomized carotid revascularization endarterectomy versus stenting trial (CREST): Primary results. Presented at the American Stroke Association's International Stroke Conference, A29: Plenary Session II: Late-Breaking Science. San Diego, Calif, February 2009.

106. Coward LJ, Featherstone RL, Brown MM: Safety and efficacy of endovascular treatment of carotid artery stenosis compared with carotid endarterectomy: A Cochrane systematic review of the randomized evidence. Stroke 36:905, 2005.

107. Jenkins JS, Patel SN, White CJ, et al: Endovascular stenting for vertebral artery stenosis. J Am Coll Cardiol 55:538, 2010.

Obstructive Venous Disease

108. Kasirajan K, Gray B, Beavers FP, et al: Rheolytic thrombectomy in the management of acute and subacute limb-threatening ischemia. J Vasc Interv Radiol 12:413, 2001.

109. Washington University School of Medicine: Acute Venous Thrombosis: Thrombus Removal With Adjunctive Catheter-Directed Thrombolysis (ATTRACT), 2010 (http://clinicaltrials.gov/ct2/show/NCT00790335).

110. Nicholson AA, Ettles DF, Arnold A, et al: Treatment of malignant superior vena cava obstruction: Metal stents or radiation therapy. J Vasc Interv Radiol 8:781, 1997.

111. Schifferdecker B, Shaw JA, Piemonte TC, Eisenhauer AC: Nonmalignant superior vena cava syndrome: pathophysiology and management. Catheter Cardiovasc Interv 65:416, 2005.

112. Kee ST, Kinoshita L, Razavi MK, et al: Superior vena cava syndrome: Treatment with catheter-directed thrombolysis and endovascular stent placement. Radiology 206:187, 1998.

CHAPTER 64 Diabetes and the Cardiovascular System

Darren K. McGuire

Scope of the Problem

Diabetes Mellitus

Diabetes mellitus is a group of diseases characterized by insufficient production of insulin or by the failure to respond appropriately to insulin, resulting in hyperglycemia. The diagnostic criteria are summarized in **Table 64-1**.[1] Importantly, new to the diagnostic criteria in 2010, a glycosylated hemoglobin (A1c) level ≥6.5% has been added. Diabetes is typically classified as type 2 diabetes, characterized by relative insulin deficiency with a backdrop of insulin resistance and representing >90% of all diabetes cases, or type 1 diabetes, characterized by absolute insulin deficiency.

Diabetes is among the most common chronic diseases in the world, affecting an estimated 180 million people in 2008.[2] Confounding this high global burden is the increasing incidence and prevalence of type 2 diabetes, driven by increasing population age, obesity, and physical inactivity (see Chaps. 1 and 44), as well as by the increasing longevity of patients with diabetes; estimates project that more than 360 million persons will be affected by diabetes by 2030 (**Fig. 64-1**).

Whereas much attention historically has focused on the prevention and treatment of microvascular disease complications of diabetes (i.e., retinopathy, nephropathy, and neuropathy), cardiovascular disease (CVD) remains the principal morbidity and driver of mortality in the setting of diabetes—most commonly in the form of coronary heart disease (CHD), but also in the incremental risk associated with diabetes for cerebrovascular disease, peripheral vascular disease, and heart failure. For these reasons, continual efforts toward mitigating the risk of CVD in diabetes remain a global public health imperative.

Atherosclerosis

Compared with nondiabetic individuals, patients with diabetes have a twofold to fourfold increased risk for development and dying of CHD (**Fig. 64-2**).[3] Whereas older studies have suggested a diabetes-associated CVD risk similar to that observed among nondiabetic patients with a prior myocardial infarction (MI)—that is, a "coronary disease equivalent"—more recent observations from clinical trials including patients with diabetes suggest a substantially lower CHD risk, most likely reflecting the effectiveness of contemporary therapeutic interventions.[4-6]

Diabetes is associated with an increased risk for MI; and across the spectrum of acute coronary syndrome (ACS) events, in which diabetes may affect more than one in three patients,[7] patients with diabetes have worse CVD outcomes after ACS events (**Fig. 64-3**; see Chaps. 54

to 56).[8] Despite overall improvements in outcomes during the past several decades for patients with and without diabetes, the gradient of risk associated with diabetes persists (**Fig. 64-4**).[8] Furthermore, the graded association of increased risk observed with diabetes in the setting of ACS events extends to glucose values in the range well below the diabetes threshold, whether it is analyzed by glucose values at the time of presentation or those observed throughout hospitalization (**Fig. 64-5**).[9]

In addition to CHD, diabetes increases the risks of stroke and peripheral arterial disease. The diagnosis of diabetes portends a twofold increased stroke risk compared with nondiabetic individuals (see Chap. 62), with hyperglycemia affecting approximately one in three patients with acute stroke, associated with a twofold to sixfold increased risk for adverse clinical outcomes after stroke.[10] Among patients with symptomatic peripheral arterial disease, diabetes prevalence ranges from 20% to 30% and accounts for approximately 50% of all lower extremity amputations (see Chap. 61).[11]

Heart Failure

In the ambulatory setting, diabetes associates independently with a twofold to fivefold increased risk of heart failure (HF) compared with those without diabetes, comprising both systolic and diastolic HF, and diabetes patients have worse outcomes once HF has developed.[12] In addition, diabetes is associated with an increased HF risk in the setting of ACS events.[13] The increased risk of HF observed in diabetes is multifactorial, caused by ischemic, metabolic, and functional myocardial perturbations.[14]

Coronary Heart Disease in the Patient with Diabetes

Mechanistic Considerations Linking Diabetes and Atherosclerosis

Traditional CHD risk factors such as hypertension, dyslipidemia, and adiposity cluster in patients with impaired glucose tolerance or diabetes, and each condition directly influences atherosclerotic disease risk (see Chaps. 44 to 47). However, this clustering does not completely account for the increased risk observed among patients with diabetes, with numerous other implicated mechanisms (**Table 64-2**).[15]

The pathobiologic attribution of hyperglycemia to CVD risk per se remains poorly understood; but given the clear associations between severity of hyperglycemia and CVD risk in both type 1 and type 2 diabetes (sharing hyperglycemia as the common pathophysiologic

TABLE 64-1	American Diabetes Association Diagnostic Criteria for Diabetes Mellitus[1]

Fasting plasma glucose ≥ 7.0 mmol/liter (126 mg/dL)
   or
2-hour plasma glucose ≥ 11.1 mmol/liter (200 mg/dL) during standardized 75-g oral glucose tolerance test
   or
Symptoms of hyperglycemia plus nonfasting plasma glucose ≥ 11.1 mmol/liter
   or
A1c ≥ 6.5% (200 mg/dL)

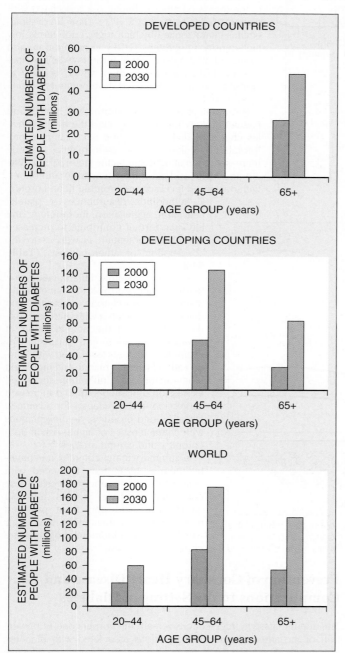

FIGURE 64-1 Estimated number of adults with diabetes in 2000 and projected for 2030 stratified by age group, with projections for the overall global population and by developed and developing country categories. *(From Wild S, Roglic G, Green A, et al: Global prevalence of diabetes: Estimates for the year 2000 and projections for 2030. Diabetes Care 27:1047, 2004.)*

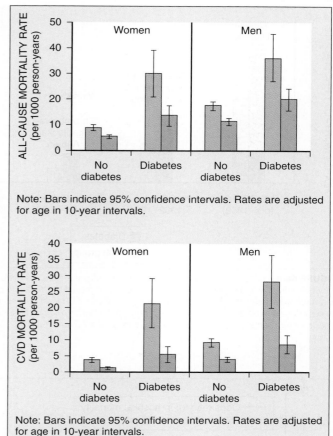

Note: Bars indicate 95% confidence intervals. Rates are adjusted for age in 10-year intervals.

FIGURE 64-2 Age-adjusted all-cause **(top)** and CVD **(bottom)** mortality rates among participants with and without diabetes mellitus by sex and time period. Pink bars represent earlier time period (1950 to 1975); blue bars represent later time period (1976 to 2001). *(From Preis SR, Hwang SJ, Coady S, et al: Trends in all-cause and cardiovascular disease mortality among women and men with and without diabetes mellitus in the Framingham Heart Study, 1950 to 2005. Circulation 119:1728, 2009.)*

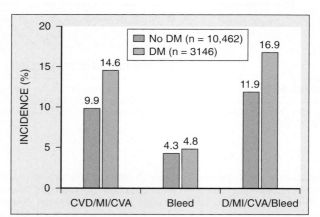

FIGURE 64-3 Adverse clinical outcomes after acute coronary syndromes during more than 1 year of follow-up, according to diabetes status, among patients participating in the TRITON–TIMI 38 randomized trial.[8] CVA = cerebrovascular accident; CVD = cardiovascular death; D = death; DM = diabetes mellitus; MI = myocardial infarction.

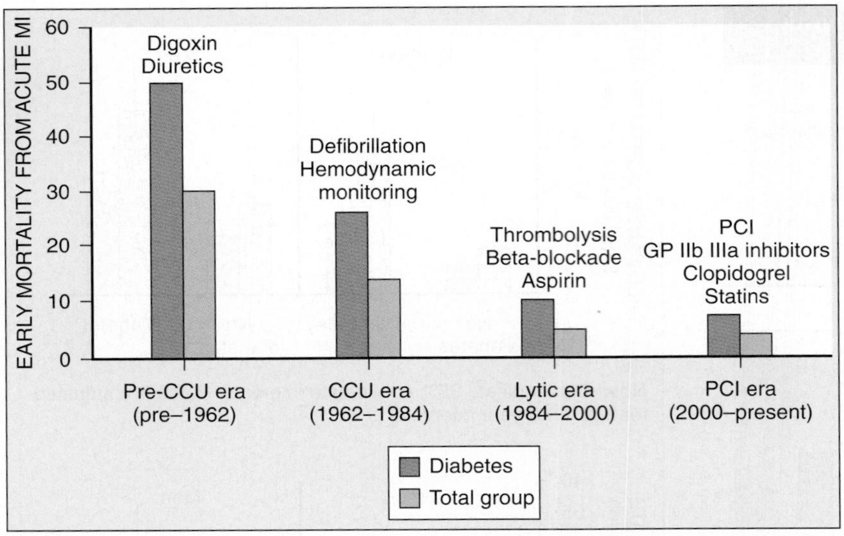

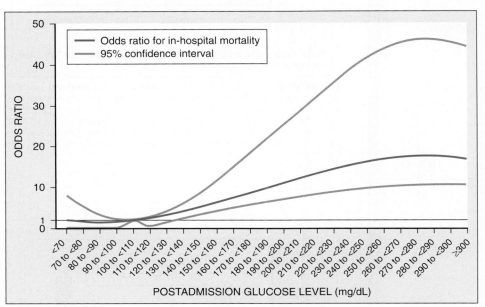

FIGURE 64-4 People with diabetes have an increased prevalence of atherosclerosis and coronary heart disease and experience higher morbidity and mortality after acute coronary syndrome and myocardial infarction than do people without diabetes. CCU = coronary care unit; GP = glycoprotein; PCI = percutaneous coronary intervention. *(Modified from Braunwald E: Cardiovascular medicine at the turn of the millennium: Triumphs, concerns, and opportunities. N Engl J Med 337:1360, 1997.)*

FIGURE 64-5 Postadmission glucose levels and mortality in the entire patient cohort after multivariable adjustment (to convert glucose to millimoles per liter, multiply by 0.0555). *(From Kosiborod M, Inzucchi SE, Krumholz HM, et al: Glucose normalization and outcomes in patients with acute myocardial infarction. Arch Intern Med 169:438, 2009.)*

The myriad mechanisms contributing to endothelial dysfunction include abnormal nitric oxide biology, increased endothelin and angiotensin II, and reduced prostacyclin activity, all of which contribute to abnormal control of blood flow. In the setting of ACS events, no-reflow after percutaneous intervention reflecting acute endothelial dysfunction occurs more commonly in the presence of diabetes or hyperglycemia and may contribute to increased myocardial jeopardy, resulting in larger infarcts, increased arrhythmia, and worse systolic function.

Abnormalities in lipid metabolism also contribute to the increased atherosclerotic risk associated with diabetes (see Chaps. 44 and 47).[17] Diabetic dyslipidemia is characterized by high triglyceride levels, low high-density lipoprotein (HDL) concentration, and increased atherogenic small dense low-density lipoprotein (LDL) particles, each of which is likely to contribute to the accelerated development and progression of atherosclerosis.

Perturbations in the proteo-fibrinolytic system and platelet biology further compound the direct vascular effects of diabetes, yielding a constitutive prothrombotic milieu.[18] These abnormalities include increased circulating tissue factor, factor VII, von Willebrand factor, and plasminogen activator inhibitor 1, with decreased levels of antithrombin III and protein C. In addition, disturbances of platelet activation, aggregation, morphology, and life span further contribute to increased thrombotic potential, as well as to the acceleration of atherosclerosis (**Table 64-3**).

Increased systemic inflammation portends an increased risk for diabetes and diabetic atherosclerotic disease,[19] and diabetes is associated with increased oxidative stress and the accumulation of advanced glycation end products. For example, diabetes is associated with lipid-rich atherosclerotic plaque and increased inflammatory cell infiltration, increased expression of tissue factor, and increased expression of the receptor for advanced glycation end products, yielding plaques with characteristics of higher risk in both coronary and carotid arteries.[15,20]

In summary, many complex mechanistic theories have been advanced with regard to diabetic atherosclerosis. These considerations have yielded an avid investigative field and have provided myriad potential therapeutic targets for which drug development programs are currently under way.

Prevention of Coronary Heart Disease and Its Complications in the Setting of Diabetes

Therapeutic lifestyle interventions remain the cornerstone of prevention of the atherosclerotic complications associated with diabetes; therapeutic targets similar to those reviewed in Chap. 49 are effective both for the prevention of type 2 diabetes and for the mitigation of atherosclerotic risk in the setting of diabetes. As recommended by the American Diabetes Association (ADA) and the American Heart Association (AHA), overarching therapeutic lifestyle targets include smoking abstinence, at least 150 minutes of moderate-intensity aerobic activity weekly, and medical nutrition therapy recommendations for weight control and dietary composition.[21,22]

disturbance), hyperglycemia is likely to directly influence atherosclerosis development, progression, and instability.[15] The principal vascular perturbations linked to hyperglycemia include endothelial dysfunction, vascular effects of advanced glycation end products, adverse effects of circulating free fatty acids, and increased systemic inflammation. In addition, the pernicious effects of hypoglycemia complicating diabetes therapy, the sympathovagal imbalance due to diabetic autonomic neuropathy, and the vascular effects of constitutive exposure to excess insulin may further contribute to atherosclerotic risk.

Endothelial dysfunction, a hallmark of diabetic vascular disease,[16] is associated with increased hypertension and adverse CVD outcomes.

TABLE 64-2	Examples of Mechanisms Implicated in Diabetic Vascular Disease
Endothelium	↑ NF-κβ activation
	↓ Nitric oxide production
	↓ Prostacyclin bioavailability
	↑ Endothelin 1 activity
	↑ Angiotensin II activity
	↑ Cyclooxygenase 2 activity
	↑ Thromboxane A₂ activity
	↑ Reactive oxygen species
	↑ Lipid peroxidation products
	↓ Endothelium-dependent relaxation
	↑ RAGE expression
Vascular smooth muscle cells and vascular matrix	↑ Proliferation and migration into intima
	↑ Increased matrix degradation
	Altered matrix components
Inflammation	↑ IL-1β, IL-6, CD36, MCP-1
	↑ ICAMs, VCAMs, and selectins
	↑ Activity of protein kinase C
	↑ AGEs and AGE/RAGE interactions

AGEs = advanced glycation end products; ICAMs = intracellular adhesion molecules; IL = interleukin; MCP = monocyte chemoattractant protein; NF = nuclear factor; RAGE = receptor for advanced glycation end products; VCAMs = vascular cell adhesion molecules.
Modified from Orasanu G, Plutzky J: The pathologic continuum of diabetic vascular disease. J Am Coll Cardiol 53:S35, 2009.

TABLE 64-3	Perturbations of Platelet Structure and Function Associated with Diabetes
Reduced membrane fluidity	
Altered Ca²⁺ and Mg²⁺ homeostasis	
Increased arachidonic acid metabolism	
Increased thromboxane A₂ synthesis	
Decreased nitric oxide and prostacyclin production	
Decreased antioxidant levels	
Increased expression of activation-dependent adhesion molecules (e.g., glycoprotein IIb/IIIa, P-selectin)	
Increased platelet microparticle formation	
Increased platelet turnover	

Modified from Colwell JA, Nesto RW: The platelet in diabetes: Focus on prevention of ischemic events. Diabetes Care 26:2181, 2003.

Beyond lifestyle, a number of pharmacologic strategies have proven effective for CVD risk reduction in diabetes and are recommended for routine prescription for patients with diabetes.[21,22] Such interventions include intensive blood pressure and lipid management, consideration for angiotensin-converting enzyme (ACE) inhibitors independent of blood pressure, and daily antiplatelet therapy for patients with prevalent CVD or increased primary risk. In the context of these evidence-based CVD interventions, the accumulated data regarding the effects of glucose control on CVD risk mitigation remain less robust.[23,24]

LIPID THERAPY. Insulin resistance and type 2 diabetes are associated with a characteristic pattern of dyslipidemia, reviewed in detail in Chap. 47. Each component of diabetic lipid abnormality independently associates with adverse cardiovascular outcomes, including increased small dense LDL particles, increased apolipoprotein B concentration, increased triglycerides, and decreased HDL cholesterol.[17] Despite extensive research in modifying triglyceride and HDL cholesterol levels with a variety of pharmacologic agents, however, the net influence on CVD risk of these strategies remains uncertain, and the modification of LDL cholesterol remains the cornerstone of therapeutic lipid intervention in patients with diabetes.[22]

STATIN THERAPY. Contemporary guidelines for the management of diabetic dyslipidemia focus on the use of statin medications,[21,22] based on results from randomized clinical trials enrolling large numbers of patients with diabetes and supported by a recent meta-analysis yielding estimates of numbers needed to treat to prevent major adverse CVD complications in the setting of diabetes: 39 for primary prevention and 19 among patients with prevalent CVD.[25] Recommendations from many contemporary professional societies do not require elevation of LDL cholesterol as a requisite for the initiation of a statin; instead they use the aggregate risk assessment recommending statins for all patients with diabetes older than 40 years of age with one or more other CVD factors, or younger in the setting of prevalent CVD or clustering of CVD risk, endorsing the lower target of LDL <100 mg/dL or 35% to 40% reduction from baseline.[21] In addition, considering diabetes as a coronary disease risk equivalent, an optional target for LDL cholesterol of <70 mg/dL should be considered for patients with diabetes.[22]

Once LDL cholesterol targets have been achieved through lifestyle modification and statin therapy, the principal secondary therapeutic lipid target for patients with diabetes who have persistent fasting triglyceride elevation >200 mg/dL is non–HDL cholesterol (i.e., total cholesterol − HDL cholesterol = non–HDL cholesterol). Therapeutic targets for this parameter are 30 mg/dL higher than the corresponding LDL cholesterol target for the individual patient.[22] The preferred method to achieve the

secondary non-HDL target is by intensification of statin monotherapy as tolerated, with the secondary option to add another lipid-modifying agent such as niacin, fish oil, ezetimibe, bile acid binders, or fibric acid derivatives. The net CVD efficacy and overall safety associated with add-on therapy, however, remain poorly defined. Large-scale randomized clinical trials are currently under way, assessing the addition of fibrates, niacin, and omega-3 fatty acids.

OMEGA-3 FATTY ACIDS. (see Chap. 48) Given the principal lipid effect of long-chain omega-3 fatty acids (predominantly fish oil preparations in clinical use) of lowering circulating triglycerides by up to 40%, such therapy holds particular promise in the treatment of diabetic dyslipidemia. In addition, in the absence of reported interactions with statins, fish oil is particularly attractive as an add-on therapy to statins if incremental triglyceride reduction is desired once LDL targets have been achieved with statin medication. Fish oil has minimal effects on HDL and total cholesterol and modestly raises LDL with no adverse glycemic effects in patients with diabetes, despite early concerns to the contrary.[17] In addition, a series of randomized clinical trials have demonstrated beneficial effects on CVD outcomes with fish oil, such as data from a subanalysis of 4565 patients with impaired fasting glucose or diabetes participating in the Japan EPA Lipid Intervention Study (JELIS), a randomized trial comparing treatment with 1800 mg of eicosapentaenoic acid (EPA) plus simvastatin daily versus simvastatin alone.[26] In this subset, EPA treatment conferred a 22% risk reduction ($P = 0.048$) for major adverse CVD events compared with simvastatin alone. On the basis of the accumulated data, fish oil has emerged as the primary consideration for add-on therapy in patients with diabetes who do not achieve non-HDL targets with maximally tolerated statin monotherapy.

FIBRIC ACID DERIVATIVES (FIBRATES). Fibrates are agonists of the nuclear transcriptional regulator peroxisome proliferator–activated receptor (PPAR) α that lower triglycerides and modestly increase HDL cholesterol. Although they favorably affect two of the fundamental abnormalities of diabetic dyslipidemia, the net CVD effects of this class of drugs remain uncertain. Randomized trials of gemfibrozil versus placebo have demonstrated efficacy among subjects with diabetes, but these trials were executed before the use of statins became prevalent in the populations studied, and the use of gemfibrozil with statins is limited by an increased risk of myopathy.[17,27] More recently, the Fenofibrate Intervention and Event Lowering in Diabetes (FIELD) trial evaluated the CVD effect of fenofibrate versus placebo in a population of 9795 patients with type 2 diabetes and failed to demonstrate a statistically significant reduction in the primary endpoint of coronary death or nonfatal MI, despite accumulating 544 primary outcome events for evaluation (5.2% versus 5.9%; HR = 0.89; 95% CI, 0.75-1.05).[28] The interpretation of this trial is confounded by the prevalent drop-in of statin use in the placebo arm, which may have contributed to the negative results; but in the present era, when statins are indicated for all patients eligible for the FIELD trial, the trial results have limited generalizability and challenge the utility of fenofibrate add-on therapy for CVD risk mitigation. In the more recently completed ACCORD-Lipid trial that included 5518 patients with type 2 diabetes at high cardiovascular risk, fenofibrate, compared with placebo each added to simvastatin background therapy, likewise failed to yield significant improvements on major adverse cardiovascular outcomes, despite the accumulation of 601 primary endpoint events of CV death, MI, and stroke.[29]

In summary, fibrates remain an option for patients with intolerance to statin medications, for isolated hypertriglyceridemia in diabetic patients at otherwise low CVD risk, and as add-on therapy to maximally tolerated statin monotherapy when patients do not achieve therapeutic targets (noting some increased myopathy risk).

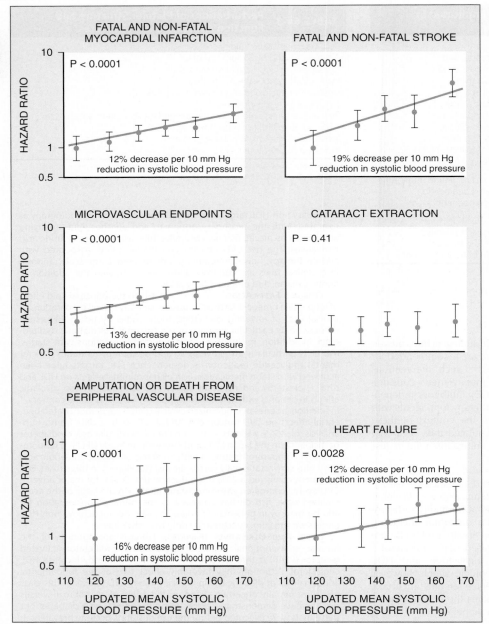

FATAL AND NON-FATAL
MYOCARDIAL INFARCTION

P < 0.0001

12% decrease per 10 mm Hg
reduction in systolic blood pressure

FATAL AND NON-FATAL STROKE

P < 0.0001

19% decrease per 10 mm Hg
reduction in systolic blood pressure

MICROVASCULAR ENDPOINTS

P < 0.0001

13% decrease per 10 mm Hg
reduction in systolic blood pressure

CATARACT EXTRACTION

P = 0.41

AMPUTATION OR DEATH FROM
PERIPHERAL VASCULAR DISEASE

P < 0.0001

16% decrease per 10 mm Hg
reduction in systolic blood pressure

HEART FAILURE

P = 0.0028

12% decrease per 10 mm Hg
reduction in systolic blood pressure

UPDATED MEAN SYSTOLIC
BLOOD PRESSURE (mm Hg)

UPDATED MEAN SYSTOLIC
BLOOD PRESSURE (mm Hg)

FIGURE 64-6 Hazard rates (95% confidence intervals as floating absolute risks) as estimate of association between category of updated mean systolic blood pressure and myocardial infarction, stroke, and heart failure, with log linear scales. Reference category (hazard ratio 1.0) is systolic blood pressure <120 mm Hg for myocardial infarction and <130 mm Hg for stroke and heart failure; *P* value reflects contribution of systolic blood pressure to multivariate model. Data adjusted for age at diagnosis of diabetes, ethnic group, smoking status, presence of albuminuria, hemoglobin A1c, high- and low-density lipoprotein cholesterol, and triglyceride. *(Modified from Adler AI, Stratton IM, Neil HA, et al: Association of systolic blood pressure with macrovascular and microvascular complications of type 2 diabetes [UKPDS 36]: Prospective observational study. BMJ 321:412, 2000.)*

comprising 3300 patients with vascular disease and atherogenic dyslipidemia; and the Heart Protection Study 2-Treatment of HDL to Reduce the Incidence of Vascular Events (HPS2-THRIVE) trial, coordinated by the Oxford University Clinical Trial Service Unit, that has completed enrollment of over 25,000 patients with CVD.

Like fibrates, niacin remains an option for patients with intolerance to statin medications, for isolated hypertriglyceridemia in diabetic patients with an otherwise low CVD risk, and as add-on therapy to maximally tolerated statin monotherapy when patients do not achieve therapeutic targets.

HYPERTENSION. (see Chap. 46) Hypertension affects approximately 70% of diabetic patients (twice the rate observed in nondiabetic subjects), with a steep graded association between blood pressure and adverse cardiovascular outcomes (**Fig. 64-6**). In this context, numerous classes of antihypertensive medications reduce diabetic CVD risk,[29a] and given the potent benefits for both macrovascular and microvascular disease complications, blood pressure management is of principal importance in this high-risk population. Furthermore, blood pressure targets for patients with diabetes are more aggressive than for the overall population, with a goal of <130/80 mm Hg.[21,22]

ANTAGONISTS OF THE RENIN-ANGIOTENSIN-ALDOSTERONE SYSTEM (RAAS). ACE inhibitors and angiotensin II receptor blockers (ARBs) have become keystones of therapy for hypertension in diabetes because of their broadly demonstrated favorable effects on diabetic nephropathy and CVD outcomes, as well as their modest favorable effects on measures of glucose metabolism.[21,22,29a,30]

ACE INHIBITORS. The recommendation for ACE inhibitors as first-line hypertension therapy in the setting of diabetes is supported by data from randomized trials of patients with and without hypertension. For example, in the Heart Outcomes Prevention Evaluation (HOPE) study, which compared ramipril versus placebo among patients at increased risk for CVD, ramipril was superior to placebo in the diabetes subset of 3577 HOPE patients for the primary outcome of cardiovascular death, MI, and stroke (25% RRR; *P* = 0.004) and for overt nephropathy (24% RRR; *P* = 0.027). Similar observations derive from the diabetes subanalysis of the EUROPA trial, which tested perindopril versus placebo; the point estimate of treatment effect with perindopril, compared with placebo, of 19% relative risk reduction among the 1502 participants with diabetes was similar to the 20% risk reduction observed in the overall trial. On the basis of these results and support from a meta-analysis of reported trials, ACE inhibitors are the first-line treatment for hypertension in the setting of diabetes and should be considered for all diabetic patients with prevalent CVD or a clustering of CVD risk factors.[21,22]

ANGIOTENSIN II RECEPTOR BLOCKERS. Cardiovascular outcomes data for ARBs are much less robust than for ACE inhibitors and are particularly lacking for patients with diabetes. The Telmisartan Randomized AssessmeNt Study in ACE iNtolerant subjects with cardiovascular Disease (TRANSCEND) trial enrolled 5926 patients with intolerance to ACE inhibitors, randomized to telmisartan 80 mg daily versus placebo, including 2118 patients with diabetes.[31] In the overall trial, telmisartan failed to achieve statistical superiority over placebo in reducing the primary

NIACIN. Niacin is a potent modulator of lipid metabolism (although the mechanism of action remains poorly understood) and has the greatest effect among currently available drugs on increasing HDL-cholesterol while also lowering triglycerides. However, the net CVD effects and safety of niacin, especially in the context of background statin therapy, remain to be determined.[17,27] As with fibrates, the accumulated data set regarding the net CVD effects of niacin remains limited by small studies with substantial dropout rates; a recent meta-analysis estimated a 27% relative risk reduction associated with niacin in the absence of statin background therapy.[27] The incremental CVD efficacy and safety of niacin added to simvastatin therapy, compared with simvastatin alone, are presently being evaluated in two large, ongoing randomized trials: the National Heart, Lung, and Blood Institute (NHLBI)–sponsored Atherothrombosis Intervention in Metabolic Syndrome with Low HDL/High Triglycerides and Impact on Global Health Outcomes (AIM HIGH) trial, composite of CVD death, MI, stroke, or HF hospitalization (HR = 0.92; 95% CI, 0.81-1.05), but it significantly reduced the secondary composite of CV death, MI, or stroke (HR = 0.87; 95% CI, 0.76-1.00). Although the results in the subgroup with diabetes lacked statistical power, the point estimates of effect for both the primary and key secondary outcomes were markedly attenuated in the subset with diabetes. Although guidelines from the ADA and AHA have endorsed ARBs and ACE inhibitors with similar levels of recommendation,[21,22] such recommendations for ARB use are based almost entirely on trials assessing ARB effects on intermediate outcomes, especially intermediate measures of nephropathy, with little evidence available with regard to CVD outcomes—excepting demonstrated superiority in the randomized trial meta-analysis of ARBs compared with non–RAAS-blocking drugs in the prevention of HF among patients with diabetes.[29a] Therefore, ARBs should be considered second-line therapy, and their use reserved for those patients who cannot tolerate ACE inhibitors because of cough, angioedema, or rash.

CALCIUM CHANNEL BLOCKERS. Dihydropyridine calcium channel blockers, such as nifedipine, nitrendipine, nisoldipine, and amlodipine, are well tolerated and effective at lowering blood pressure. Analyses of diabetes subsets of randomized clinical trials have suggested CVD clinical benefits of a magnitude similar to or greater than those observed in the nondiabetic cohorts, including evaluations of nitrendipine, nisoldipine, and amlodipine.[29a] In active controlled comparisons, amlodipine has been proven superior to hydrochlorothiazide when it is added to a background of benazepril therapy,[32] but in randomized trials directly comparing the efficacy of calcium channel blockers versus ACE inhibitors, superior outcomes were observed with ACE inhibitors.

BETA BLOCKERS. Antagonists of the beta-adrenergic receptors (beta blockers) are another key component of effective CVD risk reduction in diabetes. Early in the course of clinical use, beta blockers were considered relatively contraindicated in the setting of diabetes because of concerns about masking hypoglycemia symptoms and adverse effects on glucose and lipid metabolism. These concerns have been mitigated by the results of CVD outcomes trials supporting the benefit of beta blockers for patients with diabetes in the chronic ambulatory setting[33] and in the post-ACS population.[34] In addition, the metabolic effects of various beta blockers differ, which suggests improved metabolic parameters with noncardioselective beta blockers that also have alpha receptor–blocking properties; the clinical relevance of these differential effects remains to be determined. The utility of beta blockers in the treatment of patients with diabetes has most recently been supported by a meta-analysis of randomized clinical trials.[29a]

THIAZIDE DIURETICS. Concern about the adverse glycometabolic effects of the thiazide diuretic class of medications—including hydrochlorothiazide, chlorthalidone, indapamide, and bendroflumethiazide—has resulted in some degree of hesitancy to use these medications in the setting of diabetes or in patients at increased risk for development of diabetes. However, randomized trials of thiazide diuretics that included substantial numbers of patients with diabetes have consistently demonstrated CVD benefits despite their adverse metabolic effects. In a subanalysis of the Antihypertensive and Lipid-Lowering Treatment to Prevent Heart Attack Trial (ALLHAT), the CVD effects of chlorthalidone compared with both lisinopril and amlodipine were similar in patients with diabetes or impaired fasting glucose, despite modest but statistically significant increases in incident diabetes associated with chlorthalidone.[35] A meta-analysis of randomized trials further supported the benefits of thiazide diuretics in the treatment of patients with diabetes.[29a]

COMBINATION THERAPY FOR HYPERTENSION. In addition to demonstrated efficacy with individual drugs, a number of studies have also demonstrated the benefits of combination therapy in patients with diabetes. In the Action in Diabetes and Vascular disease: preterAx and diamicroN-MR Controlled Evaluation (ADVANCE) trial, which compared combination therapy with perindopril and indapamide versus placebo in 11,140 patients with type 2 diabetes,[36] the combination therapy was associated with a 9% relative reduction in a composite primary outcome combining microvascular and macrovascular disease endpoints, compared with placebo. In the Anglo-Scandinavian Cardiac Outcomes Trial–Blood Pressure Lowering Arm (ASCOT-BPLA),[37] which randomized treatment to amlodipine with perindopril added as needed versus atenolol with bendroflumethiazide added as needed, the amlodipine-perindopril combination yielded a significant 13% relative risk reduction (P = 0.028) in major CVD outcomes in the 923 patients with diabetes, compared with atenolol-bendroflumethiazide. Finally, in the Avoiding Cardiovascular Events through Combination Therapy in Patients Living with Systolic Hypertension (ACCOMPLISH) trial,[32] in which all patients were treated with benazepril, with randomization to add-on amlodipine versus add-on hydrochlorothiazide, treatment with benazepril-amlodipine versus benazepril-hydrochlorothiazide was associated with

a 21% reduction in CVD outcomes among the 6946 patients with diabetes (60.4% of the study cohort; P = 0.003). Therefore, in combination with thiazide diuretics and with amlodipine, ACE inhibitors are associated with improved CVD outcomes, with the combination with amlodipine proving superior in head-to-head comparison.

BLOOD PRESSURE TARGETS FOR PATIENTS WITH DIABETES. Given the incremental CVD risk associated with hypertension in DM, and the clearly demonstrated graded association between magnitude of blood pressure reduction and CVD clinical risk reduction, patients with DM have been identified as a special population warranting more aggressive than usual blood pressure control, with targets for patients with DM of <130/80 mm Hg being endorsed by a number of professional guidelines.[21,37a,37b] These recommendations, based largely on epidemiologic data, have been supported by observations of more recent randomized clinical trials. In the Hypertension Optimal Treatment (HOT) trial, participants with elevated diastolic blood pressure were randomized to treatment to three different targets: 90, 85, and 80 mm Hg.[37c] While the overall trial failed to demonstrate significant differences by intensity of blood pressure treatment, a post hoc analysis of the subset of patients with DM exhibited a significant intensity-dependent reduction in CVD, including a 50% relative risk reduction for major adverse CVD events in the group with the lowest compared with the highest blood pressure target. Likewise, the average systolic blood pressure achieved in the diabetic subset of HOPE (139/77 mm Hg) and in the ADVANCE trial (136/73 mm Hg) provide further support for the safety and efficacy of such intensified blood pressure targets in the high-risk population of patients with DM. More recently, results were reported from the NHLBI-sponsored Action to Control Cardiovascular Risk in Diabetes (ACCORD) trial, in which 4733 patients with type 2 diabetes at high cardiovascular risk were randomized to treatment to systolic blood pressure goals of <120 mm Hg versus <140 mm Hg.[37d] In a comparison of the more intensive versus less intensive arm, the point estimate of a 12% relative risk reduction in the primary composite endpoint of CV death, MI, and stroke failed to achieve statistical significance (HR = 0.88; 95% CI, 0.73-1.06); more intensive control was associated with a significant 41% reduction in stroke (HR = 0.59; 95% CI, 0.39-0.89). Of note, at the time of randomization, when clinical guidelines endorsed systolic blood pressure targets of <130/80 mm Hg, the average blood pressure at study entry was 139/76 mm Hg in this high-risk cohort. During the trial, the average blood pressure achieved in the <120 mm Hg arm was 119.3 mm Hg, contrasted with an average of 133.5 mm Hg in the patients randomized to a target of <140 mm Hg requiring an average of 3.4 and 2.3 medications, respectively. Therefore, though the trial failed to prove the benefit of more intensive blood pressure control than contemporary targets, the blood pressure achieved in the less intensive group fell quite close to such targets, and in the context of favorable secondary outcomes with no prohibitive safety signals observed, the present target of <130/80 mm Hg seems prudent, with no clear imperative to target more aggressive control.

Antihypertensive Therapy Summary

In summary, five classes of medications have substantial evidence basis for CVD efficacy in the setting of diabetes, including ACE inhibitors, calcium channel blockers, beta blockers, thiazide diuretics, and ARBs. In addition, evidence supports an aggressive blood pressure target of <130/80 mm Hg for patients with diabetes to achieve optimal CVD risk mitigation, with most patients requiring a combination of multiple blood pressure medications to achieve such targets.

ANTIPLATELET THERAPY. As discussed earlier, patients with diabetes have a number of aberrations of platelet structure, function, and activity, yielding in aggregate a prothrombotic milieu. On the basis of these observations, much interest and investigation have been focused on optimizing antiplatelet therapy for this high-risk cohort of patients.

Aspirin Therapy

The ADA and AHA presently recommend daily aspirin (75 to 162 mg/day) for all patients with diabetes who have prevalent CVD or for primary prevention in all patients older than 40 years with additional CVD risk factors (or younger in the presence of prevalent CVD risk).[21,22] Whereas these recommendations are supported by a substantial evidence base in the setting of secondary CVD risk modification,[38] they have been challenged to some degree by the absence of statistically significant benefits observed in two recent meta-analyses of primary prevention with aspirin in patients with diabetes,[38,39] and uncertainties remain about the optimal population of patients to treat and the optimal dose of aspirin to use for patients with diabetes.[18] In addition to the spectrum of platelet abnormalities associated with diabetes, absolute or relative aspirin resistance may occur in up to 40% of patients with diabetes, with increasing prevalence associated with poor metabolic control.[40]

On the basis of this ongoing uncertainty with regard to the role of aspirin in the setting of primary CVD risk prevention in type 2 diabetes, two large-scale randomized clinical trials are currently under way. A Study of Cardiovascular Events In Diabetes (ASCEND) plans to enroll 10,000 patients with type 1 or type 2 diabetes without CVD, randomized factorially to treatment with 100 mg acetylsalicylic acid (ASA) daily versus placebo or with omega-3 fatty acid 1 g daily versus placebo, with a primary endpoint of major adverse cardiovascular events (http://www.ctsu.ox.ac.uk/ascend/). The Aspirin and Simvastatin Combination for Cardiovascular Events Prevention Trial in Diabetes (ACCEPT-D) plans to enroll 4700 patients with type 1 or type 2 diabetes to receive 100 mg ASA plus simvastatin versus simvastatin alone in a prospective, open-label, blinded endpoint evaluation (PROBE) design trial to assess the cardiovascular efficacy of ASA in primary prevention for patients with diabetes that has been treated with statins.[41]

In summary, until further evidence becomes available, the present recommendations—as outlined by guidelines from diabetes and cardiovascular professional societies—remain the most evidence-based approach. Daily aspirin (75 to 162 mg) is recommended for all patients with diabetes who have prevalent CVD, or increased CVD risk assessed by >50 years of age for men and >60 years of age for women with additional CVD risk factors present.[21,22]

Thienopyridines

In aggregate, the epidemiologic, mechanistic, and primary or secondary prevention clinical trial data support the hypothesis that patients with type 2 diabetes may require more aggressive antiplatelet treatment to yield commensurate antiplatelet effects to affect CVD risk reduction, and that more aggressive antiplatelet dosing in this setting may not increment bleeding risk. The thienopyridines irreversibly bind to $P2Y_{12}$ ADP receptors and inhibit ADP-induced activation of glycoprotein (GP) IIb/IIIa, preventing the binding of fibrinogen and platelet thrombus formation, thus yielding more potent antiplatelet effects than achieved with aspirin alone.

Observations from trials of the thienopyridines clopidogrel and prasugrel provide support for the concept of incremental efficacy in diabetes with more potent platelet inhibition in the chronic ambulatory setting and, as reviewed later in this chapter, in the setting of ACS.[18] In the CAPRIE trial, which compared outcomes in patients with non–ST-segment elevation MI, ischemic stroke, or established peripheral artery disease randomized to treatment with aspirin versus clopidogrel, 3866 patients with diabetes were enrolled. In the subset of patients with diabetes, the 12.5% reduction in major adverse CVD events with clopidogrel versus aspirin was comparable to the effect observed in the overall study cohort. Given the incremental expense of clopidogrel and its associated increment in bleeding risk, however, this strategy is not routinely recommended over the use of aspirin alone for most patients.

Diabetes is associated with an increased prevalence of resistance to clopidogrel, a prodrug requiring metabolic conversion that appears to be impaired in diabetes, resulting in decreased circulating active metabolite.[42,43] These observations have led some investigators to explore the effects of increased dosing of clopidogrel in patients with diabetes, with preliminary data suggesting increased antiplatelet effects with such a strategy.[43] However, the net clinical safety and efficacy of increased dosing of clopidogrel requires further evaluation before application in clinical practice.

GLUCOSE MANAGEMENT. For the treatment of hyperglycemia associated with diabetes, there are numerous drug classes comprising oral and injectable glucose-lowering medications approved for clinical use (**Table 64-4**). These drugs work by stimulating endogenous insulin release, impairing hepatic glucose production, improving the body's response to insulin, or delaying intestinal carbohydrate absorption.

Cardiovascular Effects of Selected Drugs for Diabetes

To date, the approval of drugs for diabetes has been based almost exclusively on the demonstration of proof of concept for efficacy of glucose lowering without requirement of demonstration of efficacy on clinical outcomes. The regulatory landscape for diabetes drugs has recently undergone major changes, such that all future diabetes drugs (and probably those currently on the market) will be required to demonstrate designated margins of CVD safety to achieve or to maintain regulatory approval, leading to a rapid proliferation of clinical trials under way or in planning to assess CVD outcomes associated with these therapies.[44] In this context, few data are available with regard to the net CVD safety and efficacy of such medications, and current management strategies and guidelines remain grounded on the proven microvascular disease benefits demonstrated with glucose control.[21,45]

METFORMIN. Metformin, in the biguanide class, lowers blood glucose primarily by decreasing hepatic glucose output and with some improvement in insulin sensitivity.[46] In addition to improved glucose control, metformin is also associated with weight reduction, favorable effects on lipid parameters, improved coagulation profiles, and low risk for hypoglycemia. In the United Kingdom Prospective Diabetes Study (UKPDS) of various glucose-lowering strategies in a population of patients with newly diagnosed type 2 diabetes, patients who were overweight at study entry were eligible to randomization to metformin therapy in addition to the other treatments, which included sulfonylureas, insulin, and usual care. Those treated with metformin had statistically superior outcomes for all diabetes endpoints, MI, and all-cause mortality compared with either of the other two drug treatment strategies or with usual care.[4]

Delaying the regulatory approval of metformin in the United States and hindering its clinical uptake were concerns about its potential to cause lactic acidosis, based primarily on observations with the earlier use of another biguanide, phenformin, that clearly caused lactic acidemia and was removed from the market on that basis. In response to this concern, metformin has been contraindicated for use in the setting of renal compromise including chronic kidney disease (CKD), for 48 to 72 hours after the administration of iodinated contrast material, and in symptomatic HF. However, in the context of widespread global use of metformin for more than five decades and a substantial aggregated data base of comparative clinical trials, no convincing signal for increased lactic acidemia has been observed.[47] Whereas the CKD and contrast agent exposure contraindications remain in the product label, with their relevance remaining uncertain, the contraindication for use in HF was recently removed on the basis of demonstrated clinical safety.[46]

On the basis of safety, tolerability, low hypoglycemia risk, outcomes data, and relatively low cost of the generic medication, metformin should be the first-line drug for type 2 diabetes in the absence of CKD contraindications.[21,46] It is the only oral therapy routinely recommended to be continued once insulin therapy has been initiated.

SULFONYLUREAS. Sulfonylurea medications, in clinical use since 1950, are the oldest oral glucose-lowering drugs. They lower glucose by augmenting insulin release through inhibition of ATP-dependent potassium (K_{ATP}) channels in pancreatic beta cells. Although these drugs are typically well tolerated and are relatively potent, their use results in the highest rate of hypoglycemia of any available oral drug and is associated with weight gain. Whereas tolbutamide, a first-generation sulfonylurea, was shown to increase cardiovascular risk and mortality in an early randomized trial,[48] no such adverse cardiovascular safety signals have emerged from subsequent trials with randomized assignment to second- and third-generation sulfonylureas. On the basis of the extensive clinical experience, the availability of low-cost generics, and the efficacy of glucose control demonstrated in a number of clinical trials, sulfonylureas have been endorsed as a second-line drug (after metformin) for the treatment of type 2 diabetes.[45]

Some concerns persist about the use of sulfonylureas in CVD cohorts, driven by the weight gain associated with the drugs, the increased risk for hypoglycemia and commensurate stimulation of the

TABLE 64-4   Glucose-Lowering Medications for Type 2 Diabetes Mellitus

AGENT	MECHANISM OF ACTION	EXPECTED A1C REDUCTION	ADVERSE EFFECTS	CARDIOVASCULAR ISSUES
Sulfonylureas Glyburide Glipizide Glimepiride Gliclazide Chlorpropamide Tolbutamide	Bind to sulfonylurea receptors on pancreatic islet beta cells, closing K_{ATP} channels, stimulating insulin release Relatively long duration of action	~1%-2%	Hypoglycemia Weight gain	Hypoglycemia may precipitate ischemia, arrhythmia Cardiac K_{ATP} channel closure may impair ischemic preconditioning
Meglitinides Repaglinide Nateglinide	Bind to sulfonylurea receptors on pancreatic islet beta cells, closing K_{ATP} channels, stimulating insulin release Relatively short duration of action	~1%-2%	Hypoglycemia Weight gain	Hypoglycemia may precipitate ischemia, arrhythmia Cardiac K_{ATP} channel closure may impair ischemic preconditioning
Biguanides Metformin	Decrease hepatic glucose production	~1%-2%	Diarrhea, nausea Lactic acidosis Decreases B_{12} levels	May improve CVD outcomes[105] Should not be used in acute or unstable HF because of lactic acidosis risk
α-Glucosidase inhibitors Acarbose Miglitol	Slow gut carbohydrate absorption	~0.5%-1.0%	Gas, bloating	Improves postprandial glucose excursions, which are more tightly associated with CVD than fasting glucose May reduce MI risk[106]
Thiazolidinediones Rosiglitazone Pioglitazone	Activate the nuclear receptor PPAR-γ, increasing peripheral insulin sensitivity Also reduces hepatic glucose production	~1%-1.5%	Weight gain Edema ? Bone loss in women	May precipitate clinical HF in predisposed individuals Contraindicated in NYHA Class III-IV HF (because of fluid retention); not recommended in Class II HF[107] Pioglitazone may reduce MI, stroke risk[51] Rosiglitazone may increase MI risk[108]
Incretin modulators GLP-1 mimetics Exenatide	Increase glucose-dependent insulin secretion, decrease glucagon secretion, and delay gastric emptying	~1%	Nausea, vomiting	Very preliminary data suggest possible benefit in patients with cardiomyopathy[109]
Dipeptidyl peptidase 4 inhibitors Sitagliptin Saxagliptin	Inhibit degradation of endogenous GLP-1 (and GIP-1), thereby enhancing the effects of these incretins	~0.6%-0.8%	—	—
Amylin analogues Pramlintide	Decrease glucagon secretion and delay gastric emptying	~0.4%-0.6%	Nausea, vomiting	—
Insulins Glargine, Detemir NPH, Lente Regular Lispro, Aspart, Glulisine Premixed Inhaled	Increase insulin supply	No limit (theoretically)	Hypoglycemia Weight gain Edema (at high doses)	Retrospective data in HF suggest worse clinical outcomes in HF patients who require and are treated with insulin

CVD = cardiovascular disease; GLP-1 = glucagon-like peptide 1; GIP-1 = glucose-dependent insulinotropic peptide; HF = heart failure; MI = myocardial infarction; NPH = neutral protamine Hagedorn.

Reprinted from Inzucchi SE, McGuire DK: New drugs for the treatment of diabetes: Part II: Incretin-based therapy and beyond. Circulation 117:574, 2008.

adrenergic stress-response system with potential adverse CVD effects,[46] and their potential to inhibit ischemic preconditioning via blockade of myocardial K_{ATP} channels.[49] In experimental MI, activation of myocardial K_{ATP} channels reduces infarct size, an effect termed ischemic preconditioning, that is blocked by sulfonylureas. The relevance of these observations to humans remains poorly understood[49] but is one potential explanation of the increased MI case-fatality rate observed in the more intensively treated patients of the ACCORD trial (summarized later), a conjecture that remains speculative, with limited ability to analyze outcomes according to drugs used in that trial.[5] Observations from the UKPDS trial counter the likelihood of such an effect, as an intensive glucose control policy with two different sulfonylureas—chlorpropamide and glyburide—yielded similar MI and cardiovascular death outcomes, as did insulin in a trial that accumulated 595 MI events.[48] On the basis of these concerns, sulfonylureas that are relatively specific for pancreatic K_{ATP} channels have been developed,[49] although no cardiovascular clinical outcomes trials have yet been executed to evaluate the cardiovascular safety and efficacy resulting from such evolution of the class.

THIAZOLIDINEDIONES. Thiazolidinediones (i.e., rosiglitazone and pioglitazone) decrease glucose levels in type 2 diabetes by increasing the insulin sensitivity of target tissues and induce a wide variety of nonglycemic effects mediated through activation of the nuclear receptor PPAR-γ, including a number of favorable effects on intermediate markers of CVD risk and disease, leading to much interest in their effects on CVD morbidity and mortality.[50] In the Prospective Pioglitazone Clinical Trial in Macrovascular Events (PROactive study), the first randomized trial designed to assess the effect of any glucose-lowering medication on cardiovascular clinical outcomes, treatment with pioglitazone significantly reduced the composite endpoint of all-cause mortality, nonfatal MI, and stroke compared with placebo in patients with type 2 diabetes and prevalent CVD at study entry, treated during a 34.5-month follow-up, although the effect on the primary endpoint was not significant.[51] In contrast, rosiglitazone may increase CVD risk—and, specifically, increase MI risk (**Fig. 64-7**).[50,52] Though the data are not definitive, the signal for increased MI risk with rosiglitazone has led to severe product-label restrictions for use in the United States and withdrawal of the drug from the European market.

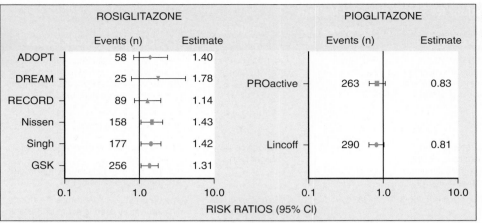

FIGURE 64-7 Relative risk of myocardial infarction associated with rosiglitazone **(left)** and pioglitazone **(right)** versus comparator in randomized clinical trials and meta-analyses. *(Modified from Rohatgi A, McGuire DK. Effects of the thiazolidinedione medications on micro- and macrovascular complications in patients with diabetes—update 2008. Cardiovasc Drugs Ther 22:233, 2008.)*

diabetes,[44] numerous randomized CVD clinical outcomes trials are currently under way or in advanced planning.

Cardiovascular Effects of Intensive Glucose Control Strategies

UKPDS[4,48] randomized 5102 patients with newly diagnosed type 2 diabetes to intensive glucose control with sulfonyl-urea or insulin compared with diet alone; those overweight at study entry (n = 795) could also be randomized in the intensive arm to receive metformin. In the insulin and sulfonylurea analyses, achieving A1c levels of 7.0% versus 7.9% during an average of 10 years, intensive control decreased risk for a composite endpoint of all diabetes-related complications (RRR = 12%; P = 0.029) and significantly improved microvascular disease risk (RRR = 25%; P = 0.01). Whereas a trend toward decreased risk of MI was observed with intensive control (14.8% versus 16.8%; P = 0.052), stroke was numerically increased, although the difference was not statistically significant (5.6% versus 5.2%; P = 0.52). In overweight subjects, metformin had better glucose control (A1c 7.4% versus 8.0%) as well as significantly improved risk for MI (RRR = 39%; P = 0.01) and for all-cause mortality (RRR = 36%; P = 0.011). These observations have recently been extended by the publication of results derived from long-term post-trial follow-up of the UKPDS trial cohort, with an average duration of 10 years after completion of the trial,[4] during which glucose control converged rapidly after the study treatment discontinuation. These analyses reveal a significantly reduced risk for MI in those originally randomized to intensive control, both in the insulin and sulfonylurea group (RRR = 15%; P = 0.01) and in the metformin group (RRR = 33%; P = 0.005).

More recently, the results from three trials assessing the CVD effects of more intensive glucose control among patients with type 2 diabetes at high CVD risk have become available (**Table 64-5**).[5,6,55] Comprising

Both available thiazolidinediones increase the risk for peripheral edema, with a small but consistent increase in risk for new or worsening HF.[50] On that basis, the product labels for both agents caution against their use in patients with HF, with a contraindication for initiation in patients with New York Heart Association (NYHA) Class III or IV HF.[53] Although the mechanism of the observed increase in edema and HF remains unclear, it appears to be primarily due to increased renal sodium reclamation and plasma volume expansion, with no evidence to date of pernicious cardiac effects of these drugs.[50,53a]

OTHER GLUCOSE-LOWERING MEDICATIONS. Few data are available with regard to the CVD effects of other glucose-lowering medications.[46] Suggested CVD benefits with insulin derive from selected trials including both type 2 and type 1 diabetes, but these studies all had limited statistical power to assess such effects.[4,54] On this backdrop, and in the wake of increased regulatory scrutiny with regard to safety and efficacy assessment of drugs being developed for

TABLE 64-5	Baseline Characteristics and Main Results from Three Large Randomized Cardiovascular Trials in Patients with Type 2 Diabetes Mellitus					
	ACCORD		**ADVANCE**		**VADT**	
N	10,251		11,140		1791	
Age (mean, years)	62		66		60	
BMI (mean, kg/m²)	32		28		31	
Follow-up (mean, years)	3.5		5		5.6	
A1c target	<6.0% versus 7.0%-7.9%		≤6.5% versus "standard"		<6% versus 8%-9%	
Baseline A1c (mean)	8.3%		7.5%		9.4%	
Endpoint A1c (mean)	Intensive 6.4%	Standard 7.5%	Intensive 6.43%	Standard 7.0%	Intensive 6.9%	Standard 8.4%
Severe hypoglycemic events	Intensive 10.5%	Standard 3.5%	Intensive 2.7%	Standard 1.5%	Intensive 8.5%	Standard 2.1%
Weight change	Intensive +3.5 kg	Standard +0.4 kg	Intensive −0.1 kg	Standard −1.0 kg	Intensive +8.1 kg	Standard +4.1 kg
Major macrovascular or microvascular event	Not reported		0.9 (0.82-0.98), P = 0.01		0.88 (0.74-1.05), P = 0.14	
Nonfatal MI/stroke, CV death	HR 0.9 (0.78-1.04), P = 0.16		0.94 (0.84-1.06), P = 0.32		Not reported	
All-cause mortality	HR 1.22 (1.01-1.46), P = 0.04		0.93 (0.83-1.06), P = 0.28		1.07 (0.81-1.42), P = 0.62	
Nonfatal MI	HR 0.76 (0.62-0.92), P = 0.004		0.98 (0.77-1.22), P = NS		0.82 (059-1.14), P = 0.24	

ACCORD = Action to Control Cardiovascular Risk in Diabetes trial[5]; ADVANCE = Action in Diabetes and Vascular disease: preterAx and diamicroN-MR Controlled Evaluation trial[6];
A1c = glycosylated hemoglobin; BMI = body mass index; CV = cardiovascular; MI = myocardial infarction; VADT = Veterans Affairs Diabetes Trial[55].
From Gore MO, Inzucchi SE, McGuire DK. *In* Prevention of Cardiovascular Disease: Companion to Braunwald's Heart Disease. Philadelphia, Elsevier, 2010.

more than 23,000 patients treated on study protocol from 3 to 5 years, all three trials showed no significant CVD benefit of intensified glucose control.

The ACCORD trial compared intensive versus standard glucose control in 10,251 patients with type 2 diabetes who were at high CVD risk, achieving A1c contrast of 6.4% versus 7.5%.[5] This trial was stopped early at the recommendation of the Data Safety Monitoring Committee because of an excess of all-cause mortality (257 versus 203 events; $P =$ 0.04) in the intensively treated group, with no significant difference observed in the primary composite CVD endpoint of cardiovascular death, MI, and stroke (HR = 0.90; 95% CI, 0.78-1.04). The explanation for the incremental mortality remains unresolved; possible explanations currently being explored include increased hypoglycemia precipitating cardiovascular death, pernicious effects of specific drugs or drug combinations, and a chance finding in the context of the other recently reported trials. More than 75% of the intensively treated patients were treated with insulin during the trial, and most patients were prescribed three or more oral agents simultaneously; in the absence of randomization to specific therapies, post hoc analysis of cause is especially difficult.

The ADVANCE trial enrolled 11,140 patients with type 2 diabetes who had CVD, microvascular disease, or another vascular risk factor at study entry. The patients were randomized to intensive versus standard glucose control with gliclazide plus other drugs in the intensive arm, compared with other drugs in the standard control group.[6] Similar to the ACCORD trial, the ADVANCE trial failed to achieve statistically significant improvement in the composite CVD outcome of cardiovascular death, MI, and stroke with intensive control (achieved A1c 6.4% versus 7.0%), despite the ascertainment of 1147 events (10.0% versus 10.6%; RRR = 6%; 95% CI, −6% to 16%).

In the Veterans Affairs Diabetes Trial (VADT), 1791 U.S. veterans with type 2 diabetes and inadequate glucose control were randomized to intensive versus standard glucose control. Despite a wide separation in glucose control values (A1c 6.9% versus 8.4%) and ascertainment of 499 primary major adverse cardiovascular events, this trial also failed to demonstrate significant improvement in cardiovascular outcomes with intensive control (29.5% versus 33.5%; $P = 0.14$).

From post hoc analyses of each of these recent trials, and supported by the long-term observations reported from UKPDS of patients with newly diagnosed diabetes at study entry, the concept has emerged that more intensive glycemic control may both be safer and have more favorable cardiovascular effects when it is used in patients earlier in the course of diabetes, particularly among those without prevalent CVD. This hypothesis requires confirmation in additional clinical trials.

In summary, whereas these recent randomized trials failed to demonstrate significant incremental cardiovascular benefits with more intensive glucose control, the analyses of the primary composite endpoints for each trial revealed point estimates of relative risk reductions ranging from 6% to 12%, each with upper 95% confidence limits ranging from 1.04 to 1.06. Such results provide significant assurance of a margin of cardiovascular safety with more intensive glucose control, supported by a recently published meta-analysis of the available data, demonstrating statistically significant reductions in MI (HR = 0.83; 95% CI, 0.75-0.93), with no significant effects on stroke (HR = 0.93; 95% CI, 0.81-1.06) or all-cause mortality (HR = 1.02; 95% CI, 0.87-1.19).[24] These observed upper confidence limits are well within the noninferiority margins recently adopted as acceptable by U.S. and European regulatory agencies for diabetes drug registration[44] to exclude the upper noninferiority confidence limit of 1.3 (or no greater than 30% worse than comparator) for cardiovascular safety.

Comparative Effectiveness of Insulin Provision Versus Insulin Sensitization

In a randomized trial comparing two strategies for glucose control (as opposed to different intensities), the Bypass Angioplasty Revascularization Investigation 2 Diabetes (BARI 2D) trial enrolled patients with type 2 diabetes and prevalent obstructive coronary disease, randomized to insulin provision therapy (IP; insulin or sulfonylurea) versus insulin sensitization (IS; metformin or thiazolidinedione), with a factorial randomization to prompt revascularization with intensive medical therapy versus intensive medical therapy alone.[56] Comprising a sample of 2368 patients with the co-primary endpoints of all-cause mortality

and the composite of cardiovascular death, MI, and stroke (major adverse cardiovascular events [MACE]), and with an average study treatment duration of 5.3 years, there was no statistical difference between the two glucose treatment strategies in either of the primary endpoints, in the context of a difference in achieved A1c of 0.5% favoring IS (7.0% versus 7.5%; $P < 0.001$). All-cause mortality occurred in 115 patients in the IP group versus 117 in the IS group (11.8% versus 12.1%; $P = 0.89$), and the primary MACE composite occurred in 218 versus 238 patients (22.3% versus 24.6%; $P = 0.13$). Peripheral edema was more common in the IS group (56.6% versus 51.9%; $P = 0.02$), and hypoglycemia was much more common in the IP group (53.3% versus 73.8%; $P < 0.001$). Confounding interpretation of this trial, however, was the nearly exclusive use of rosiglitazone as the thiazolidinedione treatment, given its uncertain cardiovascular effects (as outlined earlier) and a relatively high rate of crossover treatment between the randomized groups—especially in the IS group, requiring the addition of sulfonylurea or insulin to maintain targeted glucose control.

Summary of Glucose Management

In the context of these recently accumulated data, the ADA, the AHA, and the American College of Cardiology (ACC) continue to endorse a treatment target for glucose control in diabetes of A1c <7%,[23] based predominantly on microvascular disease mitigation with acknowledged uncertainty regarding the effects of intensive glucose control on CVD risk and with little evidence from a CVD standpoint to support a lower target. Similar targets have been endorsed in a consensus statement from the ADA and the European Association for the Study of Diabetes, with recommendations for drug therapies summarized in their published algorithm (**Fig. 64-8**).[45] Key among these recommendations is the use of metformin as foundation therapy in all patients without contraindications, and combination therapy including the early use of insulin to achieve A1c targets expeditiously. From a CVD standpoint, the early use of metformin is justifiable, but recommendations beyond that are less certain. Among other considerations are the demonstrated CVD benefits of pioglitazone and continued uncertainty with rosiglitazone; the risk of weight gain, peripheral edema, and HF observed with thiazolidinediones; the risk of hypoglycemia and weight gain with both insulin and insulin secretagogues; and the limited data regarding cardiovascular safety and efficacy of other diabetes medications currently available.

Acute Coronary Syndromes

Given the high risk associated with diabetes in the setting of ACS, much investigation has focused on this population. In general, as endorsed by the most recent ACS guidelines,[34] the treatment of patients with diabetes should mimic that of the overall population (see Chaps. 54 to 56). Some specific therapies also are recommended in patients with diabetes.

INSULIN AND GLUCOSE CONTROL. The myocardium preferentially metabolizes free fatty acids under physiologic conditions,[14] but it can also metabolize a variety of substrates during periods of stress (such as ischemia), and glucose is principal among these. Countering the metabolic switch to glucose metabolism during ischemia, the myocardium develops a relative insulin resistance, underpinning extensive research into metabolic modulation of the ischemic myocardium, with insulin as the primary focus of investigation.[57] However, it is critical to differentiate study results deriving from protocols designed to deliver high-dose insulin supported by exogenous glucose administration (i.e., glucose-insulin-potassium or GIK therapy), comprising virtually the entirety of data in this area, contrasted with the evaluation of insulin administration to achieve targeted glucose control, for which no large-scale clinical outcomes trials exist to date (**Table 64-6**).

Glucose-Insulin-Potassium Therapy

The use of insulin for ACS was first described in 1963 by Sodi-Pallares, with the intention of facilitating potassium flux in the ischemic myocardium, the so-called polarizing therapy. After decades of investigation, this combination of glucose, insulin, and potassium has become

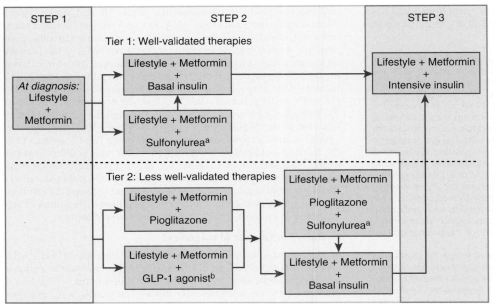

STEP 1	STEP 2	STEP 3
	Tier 1: Well-validated therapies	
At diagnosis: Lifestyle + Metformin	Lifestyle + Metformin + Basal insulin	Lifestyle + Metformin + Intensive insulin
	Lifestyle + Metformin + Sulfonylurea[a]	
	Tier 2: Less well-validated therapies	Lifestyle + Metformin + Pioglitazone + Sulfonylurea[a]
	Lifestyle + Metformin + Pioglitazone	
	Lifestyle + Metformin + GLP-1 agonist[b]	Lifestyle + Metformin + Basal insulin

[a]Sulfonylureas other than glibenclamide (glyburide) or chlorpropamide.
[b]Insufficient clinical use to be confident regarding safety.

FIGURE 64-8 Algorithm for the metabolic management of type 2 diabetes. Reinforce lifestyle interventions at every visit. Check A1c every 3 months until A1c is <7%, and then at least every 6 months. Interventions should be changed if A1c is ≥7%. *(From Nathan DM, Buse JB, Davidson MB, et al: Medical management of hyperglycaemia in type 2 diabetes mellitus: A consensus algorithm for the initiation and adjustment of therapy: A consensus statement from the American Diabetes Association and the European Association for the Study of Diabetes. Diabetologia 52:17, 2009.)*

known as GIK therapy, and the focus of attention has shifted from the polarizing effects to the direct effects of insulin, including promotion of myocardial glucose oxidation, reduction of circulating nonesterified free fatty acids that may contribute to myocardial injury through an increased oxygen demand associated with free fatty acid metabolism and resultant accumulation of toxic free fatty acid metabolites, improved coagulation parameters, and anti-inflammatory effects (**Fig. 64-9**).[58] Despite these proposed mechanistic benefits of GIK therapy and the suggestion of clinical benefit derived from numerous small trials,[57] the strategy recently has been proven futile in a trial comprising 20,201 patients with MI, randomized to GIK therapy versus usual care and accumulating 1980 mortality events—demonstrating no benefit of GIK therapy compared with usual care (10.0% versus 9.7%; HR = 1.03; 95% CI, 0.95-1.13).[59] The GIK therapy protocol specifies high-dose insulin supported by glucose administration to maintain modest levels of hyperglycemia (to avoid hypoglycemia), notably contrasted with targeting tight glucose control with insulin (see Table 64-6).

Targeted Glucose Control

To date, no large-scale clinical trial has assessed the effect of intensive glucose control in the setting of ACS events. The Diabetes Mellitus Insulin-Glucose Infusion in Acute Myocardial Infarction (DIGAMI) trial enrolled 620 patients with hyperglycemia at presentation with MI, randomized to insulin infusion acutely followed by multidose subcutaneous insulin injection compared with usual care, demonstrating significant mortality reduction in the insulin-treated group during long-term follow-up.[60] DIGAMI, however, used an acute infusion of high-dose insulin (5 units/hour), coupled with intravenous glucose administration with protocol targeted hyperglycemia ranging from 126 to 198 mg/dL, a GIK insulin dosing protocol that has been used in each subsequent GIK trial (see Table 64-6). Often misinterpreted as a trial of intensive glucose control, this study has been cited as the basis of guideline recommendations for intensive glucose control in the management of ACS events since 2004, advocating normalization or near-normalization of blood glucose concentration.[34,61] However, in the wake of numerous randomized trials in noncardiac intensive care unit (ICU) populations demonstrating, at best, no benefit and, at worst, increased mortality associated with insulin infusions to normalize blood glucose concentration (**Table 64-7**),[62-66] professional guidelines have evolved substantially toward much more conservative targets in the care of patients with ACS events, recommending insulin infusion to achieve targets of <180 mg/dL.[67,68]

The risk of hypoglycemia associated with intensive glucose control in acutely ill patients remains an important concern, with an incidence of severe hypoglycemia as high as 19% observed in the recently reported trials. This concern may be especially important in the treatment of ACS events, in which the counter–hormone response associated with hypoglycemia may be particularly deleterious to ischemic and infarcting myocardium. Data from observational studies have shown increased risk associated with hypoglycemia among ACS cohorts,[69,70] but it remains unclear whether hypoglycemia is simply a marker of disease severity or contributes to adverse outcomes.[71] In the Normoglycemia in Intensive Care Evaluation–Survival Using Glucose Algorithm Regulation (NICE-SUGAR) trial,[66] the incidence of hypoglycemia associated with the insulin infusion was the lowest (6.8%) of all the trials reported, yet it is the only trial to demonstrate statistically significant increased mortality with intensive glycemic control in the ICU setting, raising the possibility that alternative mechanisms may mediate the adverse effects of the insulin infusion. The importance of

TABLE 64-6	**Summary of Selected Randomized Trials Assessing the Effect of Insulin Infusion on Major Adverse Cardiovascular Outcomes Among Patients with Acute Coronary Syndrome Events**					
	DIGAMI	**ECLA**	**GIPS**	**CREATE**	**HI-5**	**POL-GIK**
N	620	407	940	20,000+	240	954
Dose (units/hr)	5	1.4/5.2	5	5	2.0	1.3→0.8
Infusion	24-72 hr	24 hr	8-12 hr	24 hr	24 hr	24 hr
Glucose target	126-198	126-198	126-198	126-198	72-180	(<300)
Results	↓ Mortality	↓ Mortality	↓ Mortality*	Neutral	↑ Mortality*	↑ Mortality

*Not significant.
DIGAMI = Diabetes Mellitus Insulin-Glucose Infusion in Acute Myocardial Infarction trial[60]; ECLA = Estudios Cardiológicos Latinoamérica glucose-insulin-potassium pilot trial[110]; GIPS = glucose-insulin-potassium study[111]; CREATE = Clinical Trial of REviparin and Metabolic Modulation in Acute Myocardial Infarction Treatment Evaluation[59]; Hi-5 = The Hyperglycemia: Intensive Insulin Infusion in Infarction study[112]; Pol-GIK = The Poland glucose-insulin-potassium trial[113]; units/hr = units per hour of intravenous insulin.

this observation is that the ability to avoid excess hypoglycemia should no longer be justification for the continued use of insulin infusions targeting tight glycemic control.

Few of the reported trials assessing targeted glucose control in ICU settings included patients with ACS events, and therefore the generalizability of the observations remains uncertain. In this context, and with the paucity of data in the ACS setting, a more conservative approach to glucose management should be used for patients with ACS events than has previously been recommended. The most recently recommended glucose targets of <180 mg/dL are reasonable, based on existing data.[67,68]

ANTIPLATELET DRUGS. Aspirin therapy is effective in an ACS setting, including in patients with diabetes. However, because of the aberrations of platelet function associated with diabetes, significant interest and investigation have centered on the unique potential for more intensive antiplatelet therapies to be especially beneficial in patients with diabetes who are experiencing ACS events. Support for this concept derives from clinical trial data of thienopyridine medications and GP IIb/IIIa antagonists.

Thienopyridines

The incremental efficacy of adding thienopyridines (clopidogrel or prasugrel) to aspirin therapy in the treatment of ACS has been demonstrated in randomized clinical trials that included significant enrollment of patients with diabetes.[18,72] In the Clopidogrel in Unstable Angina to Prevent Recurrent Events (CURE) trial, which included 2840 patients with diabetes, the estimate of treatment benefit of clopidogrel in this subpopulation of 15% relative risk reduction was numerically similar to the overall trial results (14.2% versus 16.7%; $P > 0.05$). More recently, prasugrel (a third-generation thienopyridine) added to aspirin therapy, compared with aspirin alone, demonstrated significantly reduced CVD risk in the diabetes subset of the Trial to Assess Improvement in Therapeutic Outcomes by Optimizing Platelet Inhibition With Prasugrel–Thrombolysis In Myocardial Infarction 38 (TRITON–TIMI 38) trial, including patients with ACS undergoing a primary invasive management strategy (12.2% versus 17.0%; $P < 0.001$).[8] Most notably, the incremental CVD risk-benefit with prasugrel within the diabetes subset did not entail a significant increase in major bleeding complications (2.6% versus 2.5%). In aggregate, these observations support the incremental benefits of thienopyridine treatment added to aspirin therapy in diabetes patients with ACS events, and they should be part of routine clinical management.

Glycoprotein IIb/IIIa Blockers

The GP IIb/IIIa inhibitors potently inhibit platelet aggregation (see Chap. 87). In current clinical practice, eptifibatide and tirofiban are approved for use in the setting of ACS; abciximab is approved for percutaneous coronary intervention (PCI) but not specifically for ACS. On the basis of results from a meta-analysis of the GP IIb/IIIa antagonists trials for the treatment of ACS events, demonstrating a significant mortality benefit with GP IIb/IIIa blockers in the subset with diabetes but not in the nondiabetic subjects,[18] the use of GP IIb/IIIa antagonists for patients with diabetes suffering an ACS event is a level I (A) recommendation in the ACC/AHA guidelines.[34]

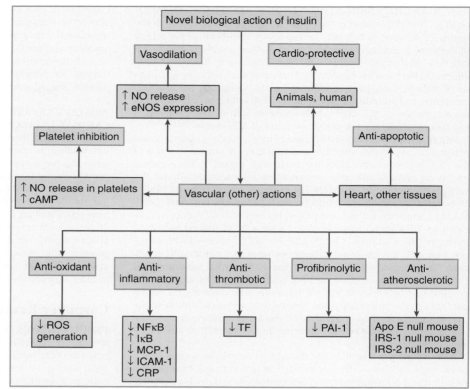

FIGURE 64-9 Novel biologic effects of insulin. CRP = C-reactive protein; cAMP = cyclic adenosine monophosphate; eNOS = endothelial nitric oxide synthase; Iκß = inhibitor of nuclear factor κß; ICAM = intercellular adhesion molecule; MCP = monocyte chemotactic protein; NFκB = nuclear factor κß; NO = nitric oxide; PAI-1 = plasmin activator inhibitor type 1; ROS = reactive oxygen species; TF = tissue factor. *(Modified from Dandona P, Aljada A, Chaudhuri A, et al: Metabolic syndrome: A comprehensive perspective based on interactions between obesity, diabetes, and inflammation. Circulation 111:1448, 2005.)*

TABLE 64-7 Summary of Randomized Trials Comparing Normalization of Blood Glucose Concentration with Insulin Infusion, Compared with Standard of Care in a Variety of Intensive Care Unit Settings

STUDY	POPULATION	GLUCOSE TARGET	PRIMARY ENDPOINT	RESULT	HYPOGLYCEMIA
Van den Berghe—1	SICU (n = 1548)	80-110 versus 180-200	ICU death	42% RRR	7.2% (<40 mg/dL)
Van den Berghe—2	MICU (n = 1200)	80-110 versus 180-215	Hospital death	No difference	18.7% (mean 32 mg/dL)
VISEP*	MICU, sepsis (n = 488)	80-110 versus 180-200	28-day death	↑ Mortality trend	17.0% (<40 mg/dL)
GIST-UK*	Stroke ICU (n = 933)	72-126 versus usual care	90-day death	No difference	15.7% (<70 mg/dL)
European Glucontrol*	MICU (n = 1101)	80-110 versus 140-180	Hospital death	↑ Mortality trend	8.6% (<40 mg/dL)
NICE-SUGAR	MICU	81-108 versus <180	90-day death	14% ↑ Mortality	6.8% (<40 mg/dL)

*Stopped early/futility.

Van den Berghe—1 = trial of intensive insulin in the SICU[114]; Van den Berghe—2 = trial of intensive insulin in the MICU[62]; VISEP = Efficacy of Volume Substitution and Insulin Therapy in Severe Sepsis trial[63]; GIST-UK = UK Glucose Insulin in Stroke Trial[64]; European Glucontrol = Glucontrol study[65]; NICE-SUGAR = Normoglycemia in Intensive Care Evaluation–Survival Using Glucose Algorithm Regulation[66]; SICU = surgical intensive care unit; MICU = medical intensive care unit; RRR = relative risk reduction.

RENIN-ANGIOTENSIN-ALDOSTERONE SYSTEM ANTAGONISTS. The ACE inhibitors have a number of favorable effects in the setting of ACS events that may be especially beneficial in the setting of diabetes, including ventricular structure and function, endothelial function, fibrinolytic system, and metabolic and neurohormonal effects. On the basis of observational data and analyses from subanalysis of diabetic patients in randomized trials, beneficial effects on HF incidence and mortality appear greater in the setting of diabetes. Thus, the routine use of ACE inhibitors for patients with diabetes is a level I (A) recommendation across the spectrum of ACS events.[34,61]

Whereas the effects of the ARB class of medications on intermediate markers of myocardial structure and function are similar to those of the ACE inhibitors, the evidence basis with regard to their overall effects on clinical outcomes remains less robust, especially for the subset of patients with diabetes. For example, in the Optimal Trial in Myocardial Infarction with Angiotensin II Antagonist Losartan (OPTIMAAL), a randomized trial comprising patients with MI events complicated by HF, losartan was associated with a trend toward increased mortality (RR = 1.13; 95% CI, 0.99-1.28; $P = 0.07$) compared with captopril, although the observed differences were not statistically significant.[73] In contrast, in the Valsartan in Acute Myocardial Infarction Trial (VALIANT), which enrolled patients within 10 days of an acute MI complicated by HF, including 3400 patients with diabetes, no significant difference in mortality was observed between patients randomized to treatment with captopril and those treated with valsartan, with effects in the diabetes subset mirroring those observed in the overall study cohort.[74]

Aldosterone was traditionally thought to contribute to the pathophysiologic process of HF only through its action to increase sodium retention and potassium excretion. But aldosterone may also stimulate directly the production of inflammatory mediators, cause myocardial fibrosis, and promote endothelial dysfunction and vascular stiffening, and the role of aldosterone blockade in the setting of ACS has been a subject of recent investigation.[75] In the Eplerenone Post–Acute Myocardial Infarction Heart Failure Efficacy and Survival Study (EPHESUS) trial, the mineralocorticoid-selective aldosterone antagonist eplerenone was compared with placebo, added to optimal therapy, in a population of 6632 MI patients with decreased ejection fraction who had either clinical HF or, in the absence of manifest HF, diabetes.[76] In the overall study cohort, treatment with eplerenone compared with placebo reduced the risk of cardiovascular death by 17% (RR = 0.83; 95% CI, 0.72, 0.94), with numerically similar observations in the subset of 2232 patients with diabetes. On the basis of this trial, the use of an aldosterone antagonist for patients with diabetes and reduced ejection fraction after MI is recommended across the spectrum of ACS events,[34,61] with the important caveat that such therapy should not be used in patients with impaired renal function (creatinine >2.0 mg/dL) or hyperkalemia (>5.0 mEq/liter). In addition, serial monitoring of potassium concentration is recommended for patients with diabetes, given the high prevalence of type 4 renal tubular acidosis in the diabetes population.

BETA-ADRENERGIC BLOCKING AGENTS. As discussed earlier, despite evidence of their incremental effectiveness in the treatment of patients with diabetes after ACS events, beta blockers continue to be underprescribed in this group.[77] As discussed in the previous section on hypertension, such observations are likely to have resulted in part from the ongoing perception of relative contraindications in the setting of diabetes because of metabolic effects. To the contrary, beta blockers have magnified benefits in post-ACS care of the diabetic patient,[78] probably owing to several factors. Beta blockers can help restore sympathovagal balance in diabetic patients with autonomic neuropathy and may decrease fatty acid use within the myocardium, thus reducing oxygen demand. Therefore, they should be prescribed for all patients after ACS events, independent of diabetes status, unless other contraindications exist.[34,61]

PRIMARY INVASIVE STRATEGY FOR NON–ST ELEVATION ACUTE CORONARY SYNDROMES. (See Chap. 56.) In randomized trials comparing primary invasive versus noninvasive strategies for

treatment of ACS events, the subsets of patients with diabetes have derived benefits similar to or greater than those of nondiabetic patients associated with a primary invasive management strategy, although mortality and reinfarction were still higher in the groups with diabetes in both treatment arms.[34] Despite these benefits, a primary invasive strategy for patients with diabetes continues to be underused in patients with ACS events.[77]

PRIMARY REPERFUSION THERAPY FOR ST ELEVATION MYOCARDIAL INFARCTION. (See Chap. 55.) Early in the development of thrombolytic therapy, concern arose about the potential for such intervention to cause retinal hemorrhage in patients with diabetes, given the prevalence of background diabetic retinopathy. Such concerns have not been borne out in analyses of diabetic subsets in the randomized trials of thrombolytics, with the group with diabetes deriving much greater absolute benefit compared with nondiabetic patients.[79] Similarly, analyses from trials of primary angioplasty suggest greater benefit among patients with diabetes, with primary angioplasty proving superior to thrombolysis in patients with diabetes.[80] Therefore, patients with diabetes should undergo reperfusion therapy in the absence of other contraindications, preferentially with a strategy of primary angioplasty when it is available.

Coronary Revascularization Considerations

PERCUTANEOUS CORONARY INTERVENTION. The optimal strategy of coronary revascularization for patients with diabetes remains controversial (see Chap. 57). Although diabetic and nondiabetic patients have similar rates of initial angioplasty success, diabetic patients have higher restenosis rates after percutaneous transluminal coronary angioplasty (PTCA) and worse long-term outcomes.[81] The mechanism underlying the increased restenosis rate in diabetes after coronary intervention is unclear. A variety of metabolic and anatomic abnormalities associated with diabetes and a greater degree of plaque burden may contribute to restenosis in diabetic patients.

Although drug-eluting stents have reduced the need for target lesion revascularization in diabetic patients,[82] diabetic patients still have more restenosis (see Chap. 58).[81] Most trials have included relatively few patients with diabetes and have excluded patients with multivessel disease. Despite these limitations, the favorable outcomes with drug-eluting stents compared with bare metal stents in the high-risk subset of patients with diabetes supports their preferential use.

The GP IIb/IIIa antagonists have demonstrated similar or increased efficacy in the setting of PCI in patients with diabetes compared with nondiabetic patients, including a suggestion of improved long-term mortality in diabetic patients treated with abciximab.[83] Given the relatively small sample sizes of diabetic patients participating in the reported studies, however, the power to evaluate fully this treatment interaction with diabetes status is limited, and these drugs should be considered adjunctive therapy for PCI in the presence or absence of diabetes.

CORONARY ARTERY BYPASS GRAFT SURGERY. Most studies comparing outcomes in diabetic and nondiabetic patients undergoing coronary artery bypass graft (CABG) surgery show an increased risk of postoperative death and 30-day and long-term mortality, and an increased need for subsequent reoperation in the diabetic population.[81] Although diabetic patients have a worse risk profile, tend to be older, and have more extensive coronary artery disease and poorer left ventricular function than do nondiabetic patients, their higher long-term mortality does not depend entirely on these factors and continues to diverge from that of nondiabetic patients during long-term follow-up, a difference that probably reflects accelerated disease progression in both bypassed and untreated coronary vessels.

Perioperative Glucose Control

The utility of intensive glucose control for the improvement of outcomes among patients undergoing cardiac surgery has been extensively studied, including assessment of longitudinal cohort studies[84] and randomized trial comparisons.[85] The Society of Thoracic Surgeons recently has published guideline recommendations for the perioperative glucose management of patients undergoing cardiac surgery,[86] advocating insulin infusions for patients with or without diabetes to maintain glucose ≤180 mg/dL, with a more stringent target of ≤150 mg/dL advocated for those patients with anticipated ICU stays exceeding 3 days.

CORONARY ARTERY BYPASS GRAFT VERSUS PERCUTANEOUS CORONARY INTERVENTION. In general, randomized trials comparing PTCA with CABG have reported similar outcomes. However, in patients with diabetes, CABG yields superior mortality outcomes compared with PCI, with incremental benefit associated with increasing severity of underlying coronary artery disease.[81,87] This interaction of the mode of revascularization with diabetes status was first observed in the Bypass Angioplasty Revascularization Investigation (BARI) trial, which compared balloon angioplasty with bypass surgery in patients with multivessel coronary disease (see Chap. 57). Whereas the outcomes were comparable in the overall trial and in the subset of patients without diabetes, patients with diabetes had a significantly lower mortality in the bypass arm compared with angioplasty (19% versus 34%; $P < 0.003$), prompting an NHLBI clinical alert advocating CABG over angioplasty for all such diabetic patients.[81] Subsequently, despite the widespread availability of drug-eluting stents and other advances in devices, techniques, and adjunctive pharmacotherapy, the mortality benefit of CABG over PCI remains, and it continues to be recommended as the preferred mode of revascularization for patients with diabetes and multivessel coronary disease.[87]

REVASCULARIZATION VERSUS OPTIMAL MEDICAL THERAPY. In the BARI 2D trial, 2368 patients with type 2 diabetes and obstructive coronary artery disease were randomized to receive prompt revascularization plus intensive medical therapy for CVD risk reduction compared with intensive medical therapy alone.[56] The mode of revascularization was left to the discretion of the treating physician and was determined before randomization, with randomization stratified by the planned mode of revascularization. During 5 years of study follow-up, the overall mortality rates between the two groups did not differ significantly—11.7% in those undergoing revascularization and 12.2% in those treated with intensive medical therapy alone ($P = 0.97$). In secondary analyses stratified according to the mode of revascularization, all cardiovascular outcomes were statistically similar between the PCI and medical therapy groups, but CABG compared with medical therapy was associated with a significant reduction in major adverse cardiovascular events (22.4% versus 30.5%; $P = 0.01$). These data provide support for a primary strategy of intensive medical therapy, as well as additional suggestion of the benefit of bypass surgery, although direct comparisons between PCI and CABG are not possible from this study design.

Applying Coronary Heart Disease Risk Reduction to Practice

Whereas myriad lifestyle and pharmacologic interventions can improve CVD risk of diabetes in the chronic and the acute setting, clinical use of such therapies remains suboptimal,[77,88,89] probably contributing to a portion of the excess CVD risk associated with diabetes. Systematic application of global CVD risk modification to patients with diabetes measurably improves CVD outcomes. For example, in a large registry study in Germany, total hospital mortality of diabetic patients hospitalized for MI declined from 29% in 1999 to 17% in 2001, and mortality within 24 hours of admission fell from 16% to 4% during the same period.[90] This reduction was associated with the increased use of therapeutic approaches (e.g., coronary angiography, stenting, antiplatelet therapy) in diabetic patients during this period. Similarly, in the chronic stable population, in a randomized trial comprising a cohort of patients with diabetes and increased CVD risk defined by the presence of albuminuria, an intensive strategy of global CVD risk modification (including intensive lifestyle, glucose, lipid, and blood pressure interventions) reduced major CVD events by 50% compared with usual care.[91]

Although much of the gap between the outcomes evidence and its clinical application remains poorly understood, some contributing factors may pertain. For example, patients with diabetes have been commonly denied beta blockers because of concerns about their adverse effects on glucose measures and lipid metabolism and the potential masking of symptoms of hypoglycemia. As discussed previously, however, numerous studies have demonstrated clinical benefits of beta blockers among diabetes cohorts similar to or exceeding those observed in the nondiabetic population.[33] Underuse of antiplatelet and anticoagulant therapies has been attributed to concerns for increased risk for retinal hemorrhage, yet these concerns have not been borne out in clinical trials.[48] Therefore, continued diligence to the application of evidence-based therapies with proven benefit in the diabetes population remains a key public health imperative.

Heart Failure in the Patient with Diabetes (see Chaps. 25 to 28)

Scope of the Problem

HF is the pathophysiologic state in which the heart cannot maintain cardiac output sufficient to meet the metabolic needs of the body. Although MI and hypertension are the most common risk factors associated with HF, diabetes mellitus and measures of insulin resistance before the development of diabetes are also strong and independent risk factors for HF, with associated twofold to fivefold increased risk.[12,14] In addition, once HF is present, diabetes portends especially adverse prognosis for subsequent morbidity and mortality, with estimates of relative increases in mortality hazard ranging from 30% to 60% based on subanalyses of data from a series of randomized clinical trials.[13,92] Given these observations, improved understanding of the pathobiologic underpinnings linking diabetes with HF and optimization of strategies for the prevention and treatment of HF in this population remain key public health considerations.

Mechanistic Considerations

Diabetic and nondiabetic subjects share common causes of HF, such as ischemic heart disease, hypertension, left ventricular hypertrophy, atrial fibrillation, and valvular disease. The incremental HF risk with diabetes is not completely attributable to these common risk factors, however, suggesting increased myocardial vulnerability in the setting of diabetes and probable synergistic effects between such factors and diabetes that increase HF risk, yielding the concept of "diabetic cardiomyopathy." The pathologic underpinnings of abnormal cardiac structure and function in diabetes remain poorly understood (**Table 64-8**).

ISCHEMIC HEART DISEASE AND HYPERTENSION. Given the high prevalence in patients with diabetes, ischemic heart disease remains the principal risk factor for HF in patients with diabetes both in the chronic ambulatory setting and after ACS events. In addition to the burden of coronary atherosclerosis, other contributors to this

TABLE 64-8 Pathophysiologic Abnormalities Associated with Cardiac Dysfunction, Congestive Heart Failure, and Adverse Outcomes in Diabetes

Sympathetic nervous system activation
Renin-angiotensin system activation
Increased sodium and free water retention
Decreased vascular compliance
Elevated endothelin levels (in diabetes)
Loss of "dipping" nocturnal blood pressure pattern
Increased free fatty acid levels
Dysregulated myocardial glucose and fatty acid metabolism
Increased left ventricular hypertrophy or mass via myocyte hypertrophy
Deposition of advanced glycation end products in extracellular matrix
Increased cardiac fibrosis
Increased cardiac steatosis

increased risk may include increased prevalence of silent or atypical symptoms of ischemia delaying diagnosis and intervention, suboptimal use of therapeutic interventions, disturbed sympathovagal balance, prothrombotic milieu that may attenuate benefit of antithrombotic therapies, impaired coronary endothelial function, and disordered ischemic myocardial metabolism.[14,93] In aggregate, these effects and others probably increase ischemic burden, increase infarct size, and adversely affect remodeling in the setting of ischemic heart disease and ACS events. Affecting both ischemic heart disease and HF risk, hypertension prevalence exceeds 70% in populations with diabetes. Among patients with type 2 diabetes, HF risk increases 12% for every increment of 10 mm Hg in systolic blood pressure (see Fig. 64-6).[94]

MYOCARDIAL METABOLISM AND STRUCTURE. (see Chap. 24) The direct effects of hyperglycemia and insulin resistance on myocardial cellular metabolism may contribute to cardiac dysfunction in diabetes,[14] with altered energy substrate supply and impairment of metabolic substrate switching under conditions of stress. The myocardium uses predominantly free fatty acids under aerobic conditions but increasingly shifts to glycolysis and pyruvate oxidation during ischemia (**Fig. 64-10**). In the diabetic heart, insulin resistance impairs such substrate switching and glucose transport into cells, resulting in anaerobic fatty acid oxidation and compromising the efficiency of myocardial energetics, as well as generating pernicious oxidative byproducts. Systemic free fatty acid excess, combined with cellular dysregulation of lipid metabolism in type 2 diabetes, contributes to accumulation of myocellular triglyceride (myocardial steatosis), resulting in further perturbations of myocyte metabolism and inducing apoptosis due to lipotoxicity, in addition to the adverse influence of cardiac mechanical function attributable to the increased myocardial mass.[95,96]

Diabetes causes a variety of morphologic changes in the myocardium, with abnormalities in myocytes, extracellular matrix, and microvasculature.[14] Whereas such abnormalities are commonly present across causes of cardiomyopathy, they tend to be more common and more severe in the setting of diabetes. In addition, more specific to diabetes, the myocardial accumulation of advanced glycation end products (AGEs)—which are products of macromolecules, the formation and accumulation of which depend on the severity of hyperglycemia—may contribute to HF risk. Deposition of AGEs within the myocardial extracellular matrix adversely affects both systolic and diastolic cardiac function, largely attributable to AGE cross-linking of matrix collagen.[97]

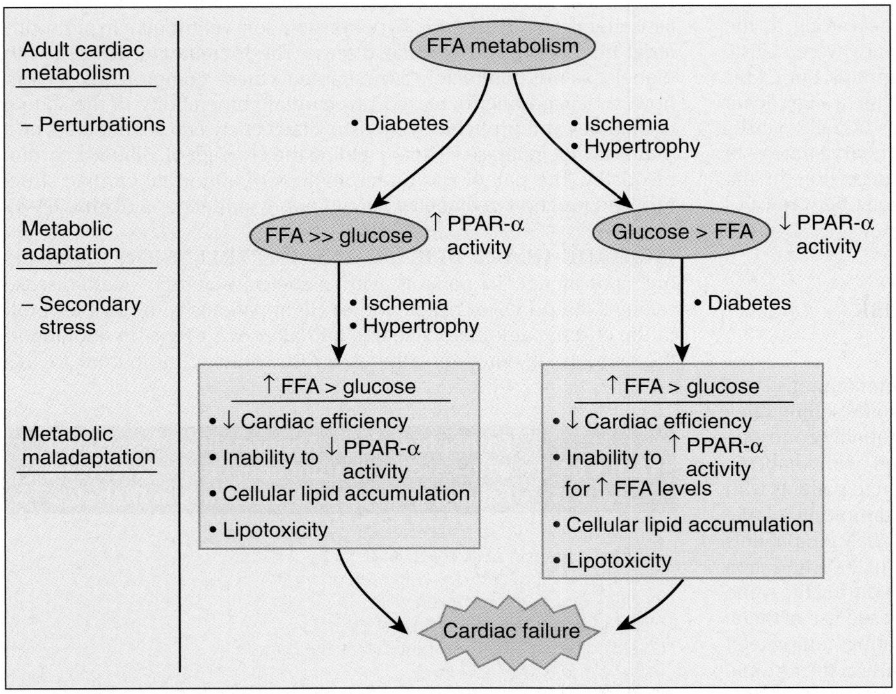

Prevention and Management of Heart Failure in Diabetes

The goals of prevention and treatment of HF in diabetic patients resemble those in nondiabetic patients: preservation of myocardial function, relief of pulmonary congestion, slowing of the progression of the disease, and prolongation of survival. In general, drug therapies for HF evaluated in the overall population of patients with risk and disease generally have similar if not better efficacy in patients with diabetes compared with those without diabetes (see Chap. 28).[98]

MODULATION OF THE RENIN-ANGIOTENSIN-ALDOSTERONE SYSTEM. Whereas diabetes patients were underrepresented in early studies of ACE inhibitors in HF cohorts, yielding little insight into specific effects in diabetes, more recent studies have enrolled increasingly higher numbers of patients with diabetes, demonstrating marked benefit of ACE inhibitors in patients with diabetes for the prevention and treatment of HF.[29a] Meta-analysis of the effect of ACE inhibitors for primary prevention of HF in high-risk cohorts of patients with diabetes demonstrates an 18% relative risk reduction (HR = 0.82; 95% CI, 0.69-0.98).[29a] Likewise, in a meta-analysis of trials comprising patients with moderate to severe systolic dysfunction, ACE inhibitors compared with placebo were associated with a significant mortality benefit among patients with diabetes (RR = 0.84; 95% CI, 0.7-1.0),[99] numerically similar to that observed among the nondiabetic group. Therefore, ACE inhibitors should be first-line therapy for the prevention and treatment of HF in patients with diabetes.[100]

Fewer data are available regarding the effect of ARBs for the prevention and treatment of HF among patients with diabetes. In the context of primary prevention of HF in patients with diabetes, in a meta-analysis of placebo-controlled trials, ARBs were associated with significant reduction for incident HF commensurate with the treatment effect observed with ACE inhibitors (HR = 0.70; 95% CI, 0.59-0.83).[29a] In the treatment of patients with prevalent HF, the data for the ARB class of medications are less consistent.[29a] On the basis of accumulated data, ARBs may be considered alternatives to ACE inhibitors for the prevention and treatment of HF,[100] with losartan having the most rigorous data for HF prevention, and both candesartan and valsartan having been proven effective in the setting of prevalent HF with decreased ejection fraction.

The effect of aldosterone antagonists (e.g., spironolactone and eplerenone) among patients with diabetes and systolic HF has not been extensively studied. In the EPHESUS randomized trial of 6632 patients with acute MI and decreased ejection fraction complicating acute MI who had either clinical HF or prevalent diabetes, eplerenone was associated with a significant 15% reduction in all-cause mortality in the overall study (HR = 0.85; 95% CI, 0.75-0.96), with similar observations in the diabetes subset of 2122 patients. On the basis of these results, eplerenone is recommended for all patients with diabetes and acute MI with decreased ejection fraction, except in the presence of contraindications such as renal insufficiency or hyperkalemia, as described before.[34]

FIGURE 64-10 Schematic summary of cardiac adaptive and maladaptive metabolic modifications occurring in response to diabetes with or without superimposed ischemia or hypertrophy, culminating in overt cardiomyopathy. FFA = free fatty acid; PPAR-α = peroxisome proliferator–activated receptor α. *(From Saunders J, Mathewkutty S, Drazner MH, McGuire DK: Cardiomyopathy in type 2 diabetes: Update on pathophysiological mechanisms. Herz 33:184, 2008.)*

BETA-ADRENERGIC BLOCKING AGENTS. Beta blockers and diuretic medications have been demonstrated to significantly reduce incident HF among patients with diabetes.[29a] In addition, a number of beta blockers, including metoprolol succinate, carvedilol, and bisoprolol, have demonstrated benefit in the setting of HF with systolic dysfunction (see Chap. 28), and these effects appear to be similar independent of diabetes status.[98,99] Carvedilol may offer advantages in diabetic patients because of its favorable effects on insulin sensitivity and plasma lipid profiles,[101] but the clinical relevance of these observations remains uncertain. In summary, all beta blockers proven effective in the treatment of HF appear to yield similar effects in patients with diabetes.[100]

GLUCOSE MANAGEMENT. Poor glycemic control is associated with the risk for development of HF in diabetes, with the association stronger in women than in men. Whether dysglycemia is causal or is simply associated as a marker of underlying CVD risk remains poorly understood.[12] No trials to date have rigorously assessed the effect of targeting glucose control to any specific therapeutic targets, or the comparative effect of existing therapies alone or in combination with regard to their influence on major adverse HF events. Therefore, the role of glucose control in the prevention and treatment of HF remains poorly understood, and pending further data, patients with HF should be treated to the same A1c goals as the overall population of patients with diabetes, with a target of A1c <7%.[23]

Some specific considerations warrant attention with regard to drugs and strategies used to treat hyperglycemia in the setting of HF.[46] Drugs with a propensity to precipitate hypoglycemia, especially sulfonylureas and exogenous insulin administration, should be used with some caution, as the stress response to hypoglycemia stimulates the neurohormonal axis that has been linked to clinical adversity in the setting of HF. Thiazolidinedione medications have a propensity to increase plasma volume and to precipitate incident or worsening HF, and their use is cautioned for patients with any degree of HF and contraindicated for initiation in patients with NYHA Class III or IV HF.[50] Whereas the modulators of the incretin axis that have most recently come to clinical use, including incretin mimetics and dipeptidyl peptidase 4 inhibitors, appear to have some favorable effects on a variety of intermediate markers associated with myocardial dysfunction and HF, research and clinical experience remain limited with regard to their overall safety and efficacy in cardiovascular cohorts, including those at risk for HF or with HF.[46]

Metformin has been contraindicated in the setting of HF on the basis of concern about the development of lactic acidosis resulting from observations of its predecessor phenformin, which was withdrawn from clinical use because of this risk. Extensive surveillance of metformin in widespread global use for decades and approved for use in the United States in 1995, as well as meta-analysis of existing comparative clinical trials, has yielded no signal for lactic acidosis with metformin, with estimates suggesting an incidence of no more than 1 in 300,000 patient-years of exposure.[47] Given this information, as well as a number of observational studies in populations with HF yielding no signal of lactic acidosis risk and suggesting net clinical benefit,[102,103] the boxed product label contraindicating metformin use in the setting of HF has been removed, retaining a caution for use specifically in the setting of acute or decompensated HF.[46] The best available evidence supports consideration of the use of metformin in patients with stable and compensated HF, especially in the context of the available CVD outcomes data, low risk of hypoglycemia, low cost, and tolerability profile.

Insulin therapy remains an option in patients failing conventional oral glucose-lowering therapies; some concern persists with regard to effects in patients with HF on the basis of observational analyses, in which the effect of insulin cannot be resolved from the confounding and incremental risk based on underlying disease severity of those patients treated with insulin.[104] Plausibility exists, however, whereby insulin may exacerbate signs and symptoms of HF by its effects of increasing renal sodium reclamation, contributing to increased intravascular volume.[46] Nonetheless, in HF patients failing to achieve acceptable A1c targets with oral agents, insulin remains an acceptable option.

In summary, HF is common among patients with diabetes, and in addition to usual pathologic contributors to HF in common with the overall population, numerous metabolic and pathologic abnormalities associated with diabetes may explain the increased HF risk and inform drug development efforts toward new therapeutic targets. Whereas the safety and efficacy of drugs and strategies of glucose control in patients with HF remain uncertain, the bulk of the evidence accumulated for the broader therapeutic arsenal for HF treatment in the overall population suggests that patients with diabetes derive at least as much and often more benefit from such evidence-based therapies. Therefore, in addition to ongoing research in this area, clinical efforts should focus on the optimal application of existing risk-mitigating therapies in patients with diabetes and HF.

Summary and Future Directions

Overall, diabetes increases risk for virtually all CVD complications and, most notably, atherosclerotic vascular disease and HF. Virtually all the advances in the care of patients at risk for CVD complications during the past few decades apply to patients with diabetes, with similar or even greater benefit in this high-risk population. Nonetheless, the gradient of risk associated with diabetes persists. Further progress requires continued efforts in two domains. First, increased and optimal application of the existing evidence for CVD risk reduction has paramount importance, with studies consistently demonstrating a substantial gap between the accumulated evidence and its application in patients with diabetes. Second, continued investigation into specific therapies and strategies targeting the unique risks for CVD associated with diabetes remains a critical global public health imperative. In that light, driven largely by the regulatory evolution toward requiring CVD safety and efficacy evaluations for all drugs developed for diabetes management, a proliferation of randomized CVD clinical outcomes trials is currently under way or under development, providing great promise for the future management of diabetic CVD.

ACKNOWLEDGMENT

The author gratefully acknowledges the contributions of Dr. Richard W. Nesto to previous versions of this chapter in earlier editions of this text.

REFERENCES

General

1. American Diabetes Association: Diagnosis and classification of diabetes mellitus. Diabetes Care 33(Suppl 1):S62, 2010.
2. Wild S, Roglic G, Green A, et al: Global prevalence of diabetes: Estimates for the year 2000 and projections for 2030. Diabetes Care 27:1047, 2004.
3. Preis SR, Hwang SJ, Coady S, et al: Trends in all-cause and cardiovascular disease mortality among women and men with and without diabetes mellitus in the Framingham Heart Study, 1950 to 2005. Circulation 119:1728, 2009.
4. Holman RR, Paul SK, Bethel MA, et al: 10-year follow-up of intensive glucose control in type 2 diabetes. N Engl J Med 359:1577, 2008.
5. Gerstein HC, Miller ME, Byington RP, et al: Effects of intensive glucose lowering in type 2 diabetes. N Engl J Med 358:2545, 2008.
6. Patel A, MacMahon S, Chalmers J, et al: Intensive blood glucose control and vascular outcomes in patients with type 2 diabetes. N Engl J Med 358:2560, 2008.
7. Fang J, Alderman MH: Impact of the increasing burden of diabetes on acute myocardial infarction in New York City: 1990-2000. Diabetes 55:768, 2006.
8. Wiviott SD, Braunwald E, Angiolillo DJ, et al: Greater clinical benefit of more intensive oral antiplatelet therapy with prasugrel in patients with diabetes mellitus in the trial to assess improvement in therapeutic outcomes by optimizing platelet inhibition with prasugrel–Thrombolysis in Myocardial Infarction 38. Circulation 118:1626, 2008.
9. Kosiborod M, Inzucchi SE, Krumholz HM, et al: Glucose normalization and outcomes in patients with acute myocardial infarction. Arch Intern Med 169:438, 2009.
10. Martini SR, Kent TA: Hyperglycemia in acute ischemic stroke: A vascular perspective. J Cereb Blood Flow Metab 27:435, 2007.
11. Canavan RJ, Unwin NC, Kelly WF, Connolly VM: Diabetes- and nondiabetes-related lower extremity amputation incidence before and after the introduction of better organized diabetes foot care: Continuous longitudinal monitoring using a standard method. Diabetes Care 31:459, 2008.
12. Aguilar D: Management of type 2 diabetes in patients with heart failure. Curr Treat Options Cardiovasc Med 10:465, 2008.
13. Aguilar D, Solomon SD, Kober L, et al: Newly diagnosed and previously known diabetes mellitus and 1-year outcomes of acute myocardial infarction: The VALsartan In Acute myocardial iNfarcTion (VALIANT) trial. Circulation 110:1572, 2004.
14. Saunders J, Mathewkutty S, Drazner MH, McGuire DK: Cardiomyopathy in type 2 diabetes: Update on pathophysiological mechanisms. Herz 33:184, 2008.

15. Orasanu G, Plutzky J: The pathologic continuum of diabetic vascular disease. J Am Coll Cardiol 53:S35, 2009.

16. Rask-Madsen C, King GL: Mechanisms of disease: Endothelial dysfunction in insulin resistance and diabetes. Nat Clin Pract Endocrinol Metab 3:46, 2007.

17. Khera A, McGuire DK: Management of diabetic dyslipidemia: Need for reappraisal of the goals. Am J Cardiovasc Drugs 5:83, 2005.

18. Mathewkutty S, McGuire DK: Platelet perturbations in diabetes: Implications for cardiovascular disease risk and treatment. Expert Rev Cardiovasc Ther 7:541, 2009.

19. Libby P, Plutzky J: Inflammation in diabetes mellitus: Role of peroxisome proliferator–activated receptor-alpha and peroxisome proliferator–activated receptor-gamma agonists. Am J Cardiol 99:27B, 2007.

20. Lindsey JB, Cipollone F, Abdullah SM, McGuire DK: Receptor for advanced glycation end-products (RAGE) and soluble RAGE (sRAGE): Cardiovascular implications. Diab Vasc Dis Res 6:7, 2009.

21. American Diabetes Association: Standards of medical care in diabetes—2010. Diabetes Care 33(Suppl 1):S11, 2010.

22. Pignone M, Alberts MJ, Colwell JA, et al: Aspirin for primary prevention of cardiovascular events in people with diabetes: A position statement of the American Diabetes Association, a scientific statement of the American Heart Association, and an expert consensus document of the American College of Cardiology Foundation. Circulation 121:2694, 2010.

23. Skyler JS, Bergenstal R, Bonow RO, et al: Intensive glycemic control and the prevention of cardiovascular events: Implications of the ACCORD, ADVANCE, and VA Diabetes Trials: A position statement of the American Diabetes Association and a Scientific Statement of the American College of Cardiology Foundation and the American Heart Association. J Am Coll Cardiol 53:298, 2009.

Risk Factor Control

24. Ray KK, Seshasai SR, Wijesuriya S, et al: Effect of intensive control of glucose on cardiovascular outcomes and death in patients with diabetes mellitus: A meta-analysis of randomised controlled trials. Lancet 373:1765, 2009.

25. Kearney PM, Blackwell L, Collins R, et al: Efficacy of cholesterol-lowering therapy in 18,686 people with diabetes in 14 randomised trials of statins: A meta-analysis. Lancet 371: 117, 2008.

26. Oikawa S, Yokoyama M, Origasa H, et al: Suppressive effect of EPA on the incidence of coronary events in hypercholesterolemia with impaired glucose metabolism: Sub-analysis of the Japan EPA Lipid Intervention Study (JELIS). Atherosclerosis 206:535, 2009.

27. Birjmohun RS, Hutten BA, Kastelein JJ, Stroes ES: Efficacy and safety of high-density lipoprotein cholesterol–increasing compounds: A meta-analysis of randomized controlled trials. J Am Coll Cardiol 45:185, 2005.

28. Keech A, Simes RJ, Barter P, et al: Effects of long-term fenofibrate therapy on cardiovascular events in 9795 people with type 2 diabetes mellitus (the FIELD study): Randomised controlled trial. Lancet 366:1849, 2005.

29. Ginsberg HN, Elam MB, Lovato LC, et al: Effects of combination lipid therapy in type 2 diabetes mellitus. N Engl J Med 362:1563, 2010.

29a. Turnbull F, Neal B, Algert C, et al: Effects of different blood pressure–lowering regimens on major cardiovascular events in individuals with and without diabetes mellitus: Results of prospectively designed overviews of randomized trials. Arch Intern Med 165: 1410, 2005.

30. McGuire DK, Winterfield JR, Rytlewski JA, Ferrannini E: Blocking the renin-angiotensin-aldosterone system to prevent diabetes mellitus. Diab Vasc Dis Res 5:59, 2008.

31. Yusuf S, Teo K, Anderson C, et al: Effects of the angiotensin-receptor blocker telmisartan on cardiovascular events in high-risk patients intolerant to angiotensin-converting enzyme inhibitors: A randomised controlled trial. Lancet 372:1174, 2008.

32. Jamerson K, Weber MA, Bakris GL, et al: Benazepril plus amlodipine or hydrochlorothiazide for hypertension in high-risk patients. N Engl J Med 359:2417, 2008.

33. Holman RR, Paul SK, Bethel MA, et al: Long-term follow-up after tight control of blood pressure in type 2 diabetes. N Engl J Med 359:1565, 2008.

34. Anderson JL, Adams CD, Antman EM, et al: ACC/AHA 2007 guidelines for the management of patients with unstable angina/non ST-elevation myocardial infarction: A report of the American College of Cardiology/American Heart Association Task Force on Practice Guidelines (Writing Committee to Revise the 2002 Guidelines for the Management of Patients With Unstable Angina/Non ST-Elevation Myocardial Infarction): developed in collaboration with the American College of Emergency Physicians, the Society for Cardiovascular Angiography and Interventions, and the Society of Thoracic Surgeons: endorsed by the American Association of Cardiovascular and Pulmonary Rehabilitation and the Society for Academic Emergency Medicine. Circulation 116:e148, 2007.

35. Barzilay JI, Davis BR, Cutler JA, et al: Fasting glucose levels and incident diabetes mellitus in older nondiabetic adults randomized to receive 3 different classes of antihypertensive treatment: A report from the Antihypertensive and Lipid-Lowering Treatment to Prevent Heart Attack Trial (ALLHAT). Arch Intern Med 166:2191, 2006.

36. Patel A, MacMahon S, Chalmers J, et al: Effects of a fixed combination of perindopril and indapamide on macrovascular and microvascular outcomes in patients with type 2 diabetes mellitus (the ADVANCE trial): A randomised controlled trial. Lancet 370:829, 2007.

37. Dahlof B, Sever PS, Poulter NR, et al: Prevention of cardiovascular events with an antihypertensive regimen of amlodipine adding perindopril as required versus atenolol adding bendroflumethiazide as required, in the Anglo-Scandinavian Cardiac Outcomes Trial–Blood Pressure Lowering Arm (ASCOT-BPLA): A multicentre randomised controlled trial. Lancet 366:895, 2005.

37a. Buse JB, Ginsberg HN, Bakris GL, et al: Primary prevention of cardiovascular diseases in people with diabetes mellitus: a scientific statement from the American Heart Association and the American Diabetes Association. Circulation 115:114, 2007.

37b. Chobanian AV, Bakris GL, Black HR, et al: The Seventh Report of the Joint National Committee on Prevention, Detection, Evaluation, and Treatment of High Blood Pressure: The JNC 7 report. JAMA 289:2560, 2003.

37c. Hansson L, Zanchetti A, Carruthers SG, et al: Effects of intensive blood-pressure lowering and low-dose aspirin in patients with hypertension: Principal results of th Hypertension Optimal Treatment (HOT) randomised trial. HOT Study Group. Lancet 351:1755, 1998.

37d. Cushman WC, Evans GW, Byington RP, et al: Effects of intensive blood-pressure control in type 2 diabetes mellitus. N Engl J Med 362:1575, 2010.

38. Baigent C, Blackwell L, Collins R, et al: Aspirin in the primary and secondary prevention of vascular disease: Collaborative meta-analysis of individual participant data from randomised trials. Lancet 373:1849, 2009.

39. De Berardis G, Sacco M, Strippoli GF, et al: Aspirin for primary prevention of cardiovascular events in people with diabetes: Meta-analysis of randomised controlled trials. BMJ 339:b4531, 2009.

40. Fateh-Moghadam S, Plockinger U, Cabeza N, et al: Prevalence of aspirin resistance in patients with type 2 diabetes. Acta Diabetol 42:99, 2005.

41. De Berardis G, Sacco M, Evangelista V, et al: Aspirin and Simvastatin Combination for Cardiovascular Events Prevention Trial in Diabetes (ACCEPT-D): Design of a randomized study of the efficacy of low-dose aspirin in the prevention of cardiovascular events in subjects with diabetes mellitus treated with statins. Trials 8:21, 2007.

42. Erlinge D, Varenhorst C, Braun OO, et al: Patients with poor responsiveness to thienopyridine treatment or with diabetes have lower levels of circulating active metabolite, but their platelets respond normally to active metabolite added ex vivo. J Am Coll Cardiol 52:1968, 2008.

43. Angiolillo DJ, Capranzano P, Desai B, et al: Impact of P2Y$_{12}$ inhibitory effects induced by clopidogrel on platelet procoagulant activity in type 2 diabetes mellitus patients. Thromb Res 124:318, 2009.

Glycemic Control

44. Gore MO, McGuire DK: Cardiovascular disease and type 2 diabetes mellitus: Regulating glucose and regulating drugs. Curr Cardiol Rep 11:258, 2009.

45. Nathan DM, Buse JB, Davidson MB, et al: Medical management of hyperglycaemia in type 2 diabetes mellitus: A consensus algorithm for the initiation and adjustment of therapy: A consensus statement from the American Diabetes Association and the European Association for the Study of Diabetes. Diabetologia 52:17, 2009.

46. Inzucchi SE, McGuire DK: New drugs for the treatment of diabetes: Part II: Incretin-based therapy and beyond. Circulation 117:574, 2008.

47. Salpeter S, Greyber E, Pasternak G, Salpeter E: Risk of fatal and nonfatal lactic acidosis with metformin use in type 2 diabetes mellitus. Cochrane Database Syst Rev (1):CD002967, 2006.

48. Stancoven A, McGuire DK: Preventing macrovascular complications in type 2 diabetes mellitus: Glucose control and beyond. Am J Cardiol 99:5H, 2007.

49. Quast U, Stephan D, Bieger S, Russ U: The impact of ATP-sensitive K$^+$ channel subtype selectivity of insulin secretagogues for the coronary vasculature and the myocardium. Diabetes 53(Suppl 3):S156, 2004.

50. McGuire DK, Inzucchi SE: New drugs for the treatment of diabetes mellitus: Part I: Thiazolidinediones and their evolving cardiovascular implications. Circulation 117:440, 2008.

51. Dormandy JA, Charbonnel B, Eckland DJ, et al: Secondary prevention of macrovascular events in patients with type 2 diabetes in the PROactive Study (PROspective pioglitAzone Clinical Trial In macroVascular Events): A randomised controlled trial. Lancet 366:1279, 2005.

52. Rohatgi A, McGuire DK: Effects of the thiazolidinedione medications on micro- and macrovascular complications in patients with diabetes—update 2008. Cardiovasc Drugs Ther 22:233, 2008.

53. Nathan DM, Buse JB, Davidson MB, et al: Management of hyperglycemia in type 2 diabetes: A consensus algorithm for the initiation and adjustment of therapy: Update regarding thiazolidinediones: A consensus statement from the American Diabetes Association and the European Association for the Study of Diabetes. Diabetes Care 31:173, 2008.

53a. McGuire DK, Abdullah SM, See R, et al: Randomized comparison of the effects of rosiglitazone vs. placebo on peak integrated cardiovascular performance, cardiac structure, and function. Eur Heart J 31:2262, 2010.

54. Nathan DM, Cleary PA, Backlund JY, et al: Intensive diabetes treatment and cardiovascular disease in patients with type 1 diabetes. N Engl J Med 353:2643, 2005.

55. Duckworth W, Abraira C, Moritz T, et al: Glucose control and vascular complications in veterans with type 2 diabetes. N Engl J Med 360:129, 2009.

56. Frye RL, August P, Brooks MM, et al: A randomized trial of therapies for type 2 diabetes and coronary artery disease. N Engl J Med 360:2503, 2009.

Acute Coronary Syndromes and Cardiac Surgery

57. Gnaim CI, McGuire DK: Glucose-insulin-potassium therapy for acute myocardial infarction: What goes around comes around. Am Heart J 148:924, 2004.

58. Dandona P, Aljada A, Chaudhuri A, et al: Metabolic syndrome: A comprehensive perspective based on interactions between obesity, diabetes, and inflammation. Circulation 111:1448, 2005.

59. Mehta SR, Yusuf S, Diaz R, et al: Effect of glucose-insulin-potassium infusion on mortality in patients with acute ST-segment elevation myocardial infarction: The CREATE-ECLA randomized controlled trial. JAMA 293:437, 2005.

60. Malmberg K: Prospective randomised study of intensive insulin treatment on long term survival after acute myocardial infarction in patients with diabetes mellitus. DIGAMI (Diabetes Mellitus, Insulin Glucose Infusion in Acute Myocardial Infarction) Study Group. BMJ 314:1512, 1997.

61. Antman EM, Anbe DT, Armstrong PW, et al: ACC/AHA guidelines for the management of patients with ST-elevation myocardial infarction: A report of the American College of Cardiology/American Heart Association Task Force on Practice Guidelines (Committee to Revise the 1999 Guidelines for the Management of Patients with Acute Myocardial Infarction). Circulation 110:e82, 2004.

62. Van den Berghe G, Wilmer A, Hermans G, et al: Intensive insulin therapy in the medical ICU. N Engl J Med 354:449, 2006.

63. Brunkhorst FM, Engel C, Bloos F, et al: Intensive insulin therapy and pentastarch resuscitation in severe sepsis. N Engl J Med 358:125, 2008.

64. Gray CS, Hildreth AJ, Sandercock PA, et al: Glucose-potassium-insulin infusions in the management of post-stroke hyperglycaemia: The UK Glucose Insulin in Stroke Trial (GIST-UK). Lancet Neurol 6:397, 2007.

65. Preiser JC, Devos P, Ruiz-Santana S, et al: A prospective randomised multi-centre controlled trial on tight glucose control by intensive insulin therapy in adult intensive care units: The Glucontrol study. Intensive Care Med 35:1738, 2009.

66. Finfer S, Chittock DR, Su SY, et al: Intensive versus conventional glucose control in critically ill patients. N Engl J Med 360:1283, 2009.

67. Deedwania P, Kosiborod M, Barrett E, et al: Hyperglycemia and acute coronary syndrome: A scientific statement from the American Heart Association Diabetes Committee of the Council on Nutrition, Physical Activity, and Metabolism. Circulation 117:1610, 2008.

68. Kushner FG, Hand M, Smith SC Jr, et al: 2009 Focused Updates: ACC/AHA Guidelines for the Management of Patients With ST-Elevation Myocardial Infarction (Updating the 2004 Guideline and 2007 Focused Update) and ACC/AHA/SCAI Guidelines on Percutaneous Coronary Intervention (Updating the 2005 Guideline and 2007 Focused Update). A Report of the American College of Cardiology Foundation/American Heart Association Task Force on Practice Guidelines. Circulation 120:2271, 2009.

69. Svensson AM, McGuire DK, Abrahamsson P, Dellborg M: Association between hyper- and hypoglycaemia and 2 year all-cause mortality risk in diabetic patients with acute coronary events. Eur Heart J 26:1255, 2005.

70. Pinto DS, Skolnick AH, Kirtane AJ, et al: U-shaped relationship of blood glucose with adverse outcomes among patients with ST-segment elevation myocardial infarction. J Am Coll Cardiol 46:178, 2005.

71. Kosiborod M, Inzucchi SE, Goyal A, et al: Relationship between spontaneous and iatrogenic hypoglycemia and mortality in patients hospitalized with acute myocardial infarction. JAMA 301:1556, 2009.

72. Wiviott SD, Braunwald E, McCabe CH, et al: Prasugrel versus clopidogrel in patients with acute coronary syndromes. N Engl J Med 357:2001, 2007.

73. Dickstein K, Kjekshus J: Effects of losartan and captopril on mortality and morbidity in high-risk patients after acute myocardial infarction: The OPTIMAAL randomised trial. Optimal Trial in Myocardial Infarction with Angiotensin II Antagonist Losartan. Lancet 360:752, 2002.

74. Pfeffer MA, McMurray JJ, Velazquez EJ, et al: Valsartan, captopril, or both in myocardial infarction complicated by heart failure, left ventricular dysfunction, or both. N Engl J Med 349:1893, 2003.

75. Brandimarte F, Blair JE, Manuchehry A, et al: Aldosterone receptor blockade in patients with left ventricular systolic dysfunction following acute myocardial infarction. Cardiol Clin 26:91, vii, 2008.

76. Pitt B, Remme W, Zannad F, et al: Eplerenone, a selective aldosterone blocker, in patients with left ventricular dysfunction after myocardial infarction. N Engl J Med 348:1309, 2003.

77. Brogan GX Jr, Peterson ED, Mulgund J, et al: Treatment disparities in the care of patients with and without diabetes presenting with non–ST-segment elevation acute coronary syndromes. Diabetes Care 29:9, 2006.

78. McDonald CG, Majumdar SR, Mahon JL, Johnson JA: The effectiveness of beta-blockers after myocardial infarction in patients with type 2 diabetes. Diabetes Care 28:2113, 2005.

79. Collet JP, Montalescot G: The acute reperfusion management of STEMI in patients with impaired glucose tolerance and type 2 diabetes. Diab Vasc Dis Res 2:136, 2005.

80. Timmer JR, Ottervanger JP, de Boer MJ, et al: Primary percutaneous coronary intervention compared with fibrinolysis for myocardial infarction in diabetes mellitus: Results from the Primary Coronary Angioplasty vs Thrombolysis-2 trial. Arch Intern Med 167:1353, 2007.

81. Flaherty JD, Davidson CJ: Diabetes and coronary revascularization. JAMA 293:1501, 2005.

82. Garg P, Normand SL, Silbaugh TS, et al: Drug-eluting or bare-metal stenting in patients with diabetes mellitus: Results from the Massachusetts Data Analysis Center Registry. Circulation 118:2277, 2008.

83. Smith SC Jr, Feldman TE, Hirshfeld JW Jr, et al: ACC/AHA/SCAI 2005 guideline update for percutaneous coronary intervention: A report of the American College of Cardiology/American Heart Association Task Force on Practice Guidelines (ACC/AHA/SCAI Writing Committee to Update 2001 Guidelines for Percutaneous Coronary Intervention). Circulation 113:e166, 2006.

84. Furnary AP, Wu Y: Clinical effects of hyperglycemia in the cardiac surgery population: The Portland Diabetic Project. Endocr Pract 12(Suppl 3):22, 2006.

85. Van den Berghe G: Does intensive insulin therapy during cardiac surgery improve postoperative outcome? Nat Clin Pract Endocrinol Metab 3:630, 2007.

86. Lazar HL, McDonnell M, Chipkin SR, et al: The Society of Thoracic Surgeons practice guideline series: Blood glucose management during adult cardiac surgery. Ann Thorac Surg 87:663, 2009.

87. Hlatky MA, Boothroyd DB, Bravata DM, et al: Coronary artery bypass surgery compared with percutaneous coronary interventions for multivessel disease: A collaborative analysis of individual patient data from ten randomised trials. Lancet 373:1190, 2009.

Heart Failure

88. Das SR, Vaeth PA, Stanek HG, et al: Increased cardiovascular risk associated with diabetes in Dallas County. Am Heart J 151:1087, 2006.

89. Saydah SH, Fradkin J, Cowie CC: Poor control of risk factors for vascular disease among adults with previously diagnosed diabetes. JAMA 291:335, 2004.

90. Schnell O, Schafer O, Kleybrink S, et al: Intensification of therapeutic approaches reduces mortality in diabetic patients with acute myocardial infarction: The Munich registry. Diabetes Care 27:455, 2004.

91. Gaede P, Lund-Andersen H, Parving HH, Pedersen O: Effect of a multifactorial intervention on mortality in type 2 diabetes. N Engl J Med 358:580, 2008.

92. Pocock SJ, Wang D, Pfeffer MA, et al: Predictors of mortality and morbidity in patients with chronic heart failure. Eur Heart J 27:65, 2006.

93. Prior JO, Quinones MJ, Hernandez-Pampaloni M, et al: Coronary circulatory dysfunction in insulin resistance, impaired glucose tolerance, and type 2 diabetes mellitus. Circulation 111:2291, 2005.

94. Adler AI, Stratton IM, Neil HA, et al: Association of systolic blood pressure with macrovascular and microvascular complications of type 2 diabetes (UKPDS 36): Prospective observational study. BMJ 321:412, 2000.

95. Saunders SA, Wallymhamed M, Macfarlane IA: Improvements in glycaemic control and cardiovascular risk factors in a cohort of patients with type 1 diabetes over a 5-year period. QJM 102:29, 2009.

96. McGavock JM, Victor RG, Unger RH, Szczepaniak LS: Adiposity of the heart, revisited. Ann Intern Med 144:517, 2006.

97. Zieman S, Kass D: Advanced glycation end product cross-linking: Pathophysiologic role and therapeutic target in cardiovascular disease. Congest Heart Fail 10:144, 2004.

98. Masoudi FA, Inzucchi SE: Diabetes mellitus and heart failure: Epidemiology, mechanisms, and pharmacotherapy. Am J Cardiol 99:113B, 2007.

99. Shekelle PG, Rich MW, Morton SC, et al: Efficacy of angiotensin-converting enzyme inhibitors and beta-blockers in the management of left ventricular systolic dysfunction according to race, gender, and diabetic status: A meta-analysis of major clinical trials. J Am Coll Cardiol 41:1529, 2003.

100. Hunt SA, Abraham WT, Chin MH, et al: 2009 focused update incorporated into the ACC/AHA 2005 Guidelines for the Diagnosis and Management of Heart Failure in Adults: A report of the American College of Cardiology Foundation/American Heart Association Task Force on Practice Guidelines: Developed in collaboration with the International Society for Heart and Lung Transplantation. Circulation 119:e391, 2009.

101. Bakris GL, Fonseca V, Katholi RE, et al: Metabolic effects of carvedilol vs metoprolol in patients with type 2 diabetes mellitus and hypertension: A randomized controlled trial. JAMA 292:2227, 2004.

102. Masoudi FA, Inzucchi SE, Wang Y, et al: Thiazolidinediones, metformin, and outcomes in older patients with diabetes and heart failure: An observational study. Circulation 111:583, 2005.

103. Eurich DT, Majumdar SR, McAlister FA, et al: Improved clinical outcomes associated with metformin in patients with diabetes and heart failure. Diabetes Care 28:2345, 2005.

104. Smooke S, Horwich TB, Fonarow GC: Insulin-treated diabetes is associated with a marked increase in mortality in patients with advanced heart failure. Am Heart J 149:168, 2005.

105. UK Prospective Diabetes Study (UKPDS) Group: Effect of intensive blood-glucose control with metformin on complications in overweight patients with type 2 diabetes (UKPDS 34). Lancet 352:854, 1998.

106. Chiasson JL, Josse RG, Gomis R, et al: Acarbose treatment and the risk of cardiovascular disease and hypertension in patients with impaired glucose tolerance: The STOP-NIDDM trial. JAMA 290:486, 2003.

107. Nesto RW, Bell D, Bonow RO, et al: Thiazolidinedione use, fluid retention, and congestive heart failure: A consensus statement from the American Heart Association and American Diabetes Association. Circulation 108:2941, 2003.

108. Nissen SE, Wolski K: Effect of rosiglitazone on the risk of myocardial infarction and death from cardiovascular causes. N Engl J Med 356:2457, 2007.

109. Nikolaidis LA, Mankad S, Sokos GG, et al: Effects of glucagon-like peptide-1 in patients with acute myocardial infarction and left ventricular dysfunction after successful reperfusion. Circulation 109:962, 2004.

110. Diaz R, Paolasso EA, Piegas LS, et al: Metabolic modulation of acute myocardial infarction. The ECLA (Cardiológicos Latinoamérica) Collaborative Group. Circulation 98:2227, 1998.

111. van der Horst IC, Zijlstra F, van't Hof AW, et al: Glucose-insulin-potassium infusion in patients treated with primary angioplasty for acute myocardial infarction: The glucose-insulin-potassium study: A randomized trial. J Am Coll Cardiol 42:784, 2003.

112. Cheung NW, Wong VW, McLean M: The Hyperglycemia: Intensive Insulin Infusion in Infarction (HI-5) study: A randomized controlled trial of insulin infusion therapy for myocardial infarction. Diabetes Care 29:765, 2006.

113. Ceremuzynski L, Budaj A, Czepiel A, et al: Low-dose glucose-insulin-potassium is ineffective in acute myocardial infarction: Results of a randomized multicenter Pol-GIK trial. Cardiovasc Drugs Ther 13:191, 1999.

114. van den Berghe G, Wouters P, Weekers F, et al: Intensive insulin therapy in the critically ill patients. N Engl J Med 345:1359, 2001.

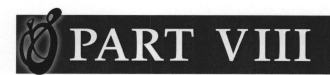

PART VIII

DISEASES OF THE HEART, PERICARDIUM, AND PULMONARY VASCULATURE BED

CHAPTER **65**

Congenital Heart Disease

Gary D. Webb, Jeffrey F. Smallhorn, Judith Therrien, and Andrew N. Redington

This chapter has been written for the practicing cardiologist and is compatible with the existing expert management recommendations[1] for the care of adult patients with congenital cardiac defects. Additional information can be found in other sources.[2] *Congenital cardiovascular disease* is defined as an abnormality in cardiocirculatory structure or function that is present at birth, even if it is discovered much later. Congenital cardiovascular malformations usually result from altered embryonic development of a normal structure or failure of such a structure to progress beyond an early stage of embryonic or fetal development. The aberrant patterns of flow created by an anatomic defect can, in turn, significantly influence the structural and functional development of the remainder of the circulation. For instance, the presence in utero of mitral atresia can prohibit normal development of the left ventricle, aortic valve, and ascending aorta. Similarly, constriction of the fetal ductus arteriosus can result in right ventricular dilation and tricuspid regurgitation in the fetus and newborn, contribute importantly to the development of pulmonary arterial aneurysms in the presence of a ventricular septal defect (VSD) and absent pulmonary valve, or result in an alteration in the number and caliber of fetal and newborn pulmonary vascular resistance vessels.

Postnatal events can markedly influence the clinical presentation of a specific "isolated" malformation. Infants with Ebstein malformation of the tricuspid valve may improve dramatically as the magnitude of tricuspid regurgitation diminishes with the normal fall in pulmonary vascular resistance after birth; and infants with pulmonary atresia or severe stenosis may not become cyanotic until normal spontaneous closure of a patent ductus arteriosus (PDA) occurs. Ductal constriction many days after birth also may be a central factor in some infants in the development of coarctation of the aorta. Still later in life, patients with a VSD may experience spontaneous closure of the abnormal communication or can develop right ventricular outflow tract obstruction, aortic regurgitation, or pulmonary vascular obstructive

disease. These selected examples serve to emphasize that anatomic and physiologic changes in the heart and circulation can continue indefinitely from prenatal life in association with any specific congenital cardiocirculatory lesion.

INCIDENCE. The true incidence of congenital cardiovascular malformations is difficult to determine accurately, partly because of difficulties in definition. About 0.8% of live births are complicated by a cardiovascular malformation. This figure does not take into account what may be the two most common cardiac anomalies: the congenital, functionally normal bicuspid aortic valve and prolapse of the mitral valve.

Specific defects can show a definite gender preponderance. PDA, Ebstein anomaly of the tricuspid valve, and atrial septal defect (ASD) are more common in females, whereas aortic valve stenosis, coarctation of the aorta, hypoplastic left heart syndrome, pulmonary and tricuspid atresia, and transposition of the great arteries (TGA) are more common in males.

Extracardiac anomalies occur in about 25% of infants with significant cardiac disease, and their presence may significantly increase mortality. The extracardiac anomalies are often multiple. One third of infants with both cardiac and extracardiac anomalies have some established syndrome.

ADULT PATIENT. Thanks to the great successes of pediatric cardiac care, the overall number of adult patients with congenital heart disease (CHD) is now greater than the number of pediatric cases. In 2000, there were about 485,000 American adults with moderately complex to very complex CHD. There were another 300,000 patients with simple forms of CHD, for a total population of 785,000 adult CHD patients in the United States. The 485,000 patients with moderately to very complex CHD are at significant risk of premature mortality, reoperation, or future complications of their conditions and their treatments. Many patients, especially those with moderately to very complex conditions, should see a specialist. At present, there are not enough such practitioners or facilities to always make this possible. Adult patients should have been taught in adolescence about their condition, their future outlook, and the

TABLE 65-1 Types of Simple Congenital Heart Disease in Adult Patients*

Native Disease
Isolated congenital aortic valve disease
Isolated congenital mitral valve disease (except parachute valve, cleft leaflet)
Isolated patent foramen ovale or small atrial septal defect
Isolated small ventricular septal defect (no associated lesions)
Mild pulmonic stenosis

Repaired Conditions
Previously ligated or occluded ductus arteriosus
Repaired secundum or sinus venosus atrial septal defect without residua
Repaired ventricular septal defect without residua

*These patients can usually be cared for in the general medical community.
From Webb G, Williams R, Alpert J, et al: 32nd Bethesda Conference: Care of the Adult with Congenital Heart Disease, October 2-3, 2000. J Am Coll Cardiol 37:1161, 2001.

TABLE 65-2 Types of Congenital Heart Disease of Moderate Severity in Adult Patients*

Aorto–left ventricular fistulas
Anomalous pulmonary venous drainage, partial or total
Atrioventricular septal defects (partial or complete)
Coarctation of the aorta
Ebstein anomaly
Infundibular right ventricular outflow obstruction of significance
Ostium primum atrial septal defect
Patent ductus arteriosus (not closed)
Pulmonary valve regurgitation (moderate to severe)
Pulmonic valve stenosis (moderate to severe)
Sinus of Valsalva fistula or aneurysm
Sinus venosus atrial septal defect
Subvalvular or supravalvular aortic stenosis (except HOCM)
Tetralogy of Fallot
Ventricular septal defect with the following:
  Absent valve or valves
  Aortic regurgitation
  Coarctation of the aorta
  Mitral disease
  Right ventricular outflow tract obstruction
  Straddling tricuspid or mitral valve
  Subaortic stenosis

*These patients should be seen periodically at regional adult congenital heart disease centers.
HOCM = hypertrophic obstructive cardiomyopathy.
From Webb G, Williams R, Alpert J, et al: 32nd Bethesda Conference: Care of the Adult with Congenital Heart Disease, October 2-3, 2000. J Am Coll Cardiol 37:1161, 2001.

TABLE 65-3 Types of Congenital Heart Disease of Great Complexity in Adult Patients*

Conduits, valved or nonvalved
Cyanotic congenital heart (all forms)
Double-outlet ventricle
Eisenmenger syndrome
Fontan procedure
Mitral atresia
Single ventricle (also called double inlet or outlet, common or primitive)
Pulmonary atresia (all forms)
Pulmonary vascular obstructive diseases
Transposition of the great arteries
Tricuspid atresia
Truncus arteriosus or hemitruncus
Other abnormalities of atrioventricular or ventriculoarterial connection not included above (i.e., crisscross heart, isomerism, heterotaxy syndromes, ventricular inversion)

*These patients should be seen regularly at adult congenital heart disease centers.
From Webb G, Williams R, Alpert J, et al: 32nd Bethesda Conference: Care of the Adult with Congenital Heart Disease, October 2-3, 2000. J Am Coll Cardiol 37:1161, 2001.

qualified staff has relevant training, experience, and equipment. Ideally, patient care should be multidisciplinary. Special cardiology and echocardiography skills are essential, but individuals with other special training, experience, and interest should also be accessible. These include congenital heart surgeons and their teams, nurses, reproductive health staff, mental health professionals, medical imaging specialists, respiratory consultants, and others.

ETIOLOGY

Congenital cardiac malformations can occur with mendelian inheritance directly as a result of a genetic abnormality, be strongly associated with an underlying genetic disorder (e.g., trisomy), be related directly to the effect of an environmental toxin (e.g., alcohol), or result from an interaction between multifactorial genetic and environmental influences too complex to allow a single definition of cause (e.g., CHARGE syndrome; see Syndromes in Congenital Heart Disease later). The last group is shrinking as genetic research identifies new genetic abnormalities underlying many conditions.

GENETIC. A single gene mutation can be causative in the familial forms of ASD with prolonged atrioventricular (AV) conduction; mitral valve prolapse; VSD; congenital heart block; situs inversus; pulmonary hypertension; and the syndromes of Noonan, LEOPARD, Ellis–van Creveld, and Kartagener (see Syndromes in Congenital Heart Disease later). The genes responsible for several defects have now been identified (e.g., long-QT syndrome, Holt-Oram syndrome, Marfan syndrome, hypertrophic cardiomyopathy, supravalvular aortic stenosis), and contiguous gene defects on the long arm of chromosome 22 underlie the conotruncal malformations of DiGeorge and velocardiofacial syndromes. However, at present, less than 15% of all cardiac malformations can be accounted for by chromosomal aberrations or genetic mutations or transmission (see Chaps. 7 to 9).

It is interesting, but unexplained, that several different gene defects may lead to the same cardiac malformation (e.g., atrioventricular septal defect). Furthermore, the finding that, with some exceptions, only one of a pair of monozygotic twins is affected by CHD indicates that most cardiovascular malformations are not inherited in a simple manner. However, this observation may have led, in the past, to an underestimation of the genetic contribution because most recent twin studies reveal more than double the incidence of heart defects in monozygotic twins but usually in only one of the pair. Family studies indicate a 2-fold to 10-fold increase in the incidence of CHD in siblings of affected patients or in the offspring of an affected parent. Malformations are often concordant or partially concordant within families. Routine fetal cardiac screening of subsequent pregnancies should be performed in such circumstances.

ENVIRONMENTAL. Maternal rubella, ingestion of thalidomide and isotretinoin early during gestation, and chronic maternal alcohol abuse are environmental insults known to interfere with normal cardiogenesis in humans. Rubella syndrome consists of cataracts; deafness; microcephaly; and, either singly or in combination, PDA, pulmonary valve or arterial stenosis, and ASD. Thalidomide exposure is associated with major limb deformities and, occasionally, with cardiac malformations without a predilection for a specific lesion. Tricuspid valve anomalies are associated with ingestion of lithium during pregnancy. The fetal alcohol syndrome consists of microcephaly, micrognathia, microphthalmia, prenatal

possibility of further surgery and complications if appropriate, and they also should have been advised about their responsibilities in ensuring self-care and professional surveillance. Copies of operative reports should accompany patients being transferred for adult care, along with other key documents from the pediatric file.

Table 65-1 lists the types of simple CHD in adult patients which are suitable for community care. **Tables 65-2 and 65-3** show the diagnoses for adults with moderately complex and very complex CHD. Patients with moderately complex and very complex CHD should be monitored throughout their lives.

CHD in the adult is not simply a continuation of the childhood experience. The patterns of many lesions change in adult life. Arrhythmias are more frequent and of a different character (see Chap. 39). Cardiac chambers often enlarge, and ventricles tend to develop systolic dysfunction. Bioprosthetic valves, prone to early failure in childhood, last longer when they are implanted at an older age. The comorbidities that tend to develop in adult life often become important factors needing attention. As a result, the needs of these adult CHD patients are often best met by a physician or a team familiar with both pediatric and adult cardiology issues. Congenital heart surgery and interventional catheterization procedures should be performed at centers with adequate surgical and institutional volumes of congenital heart cases at any age.

Echocardiographic studies, diagnostic heart catheterizations, electrophysiologic studies, and cardiac magnetic resonance (CMR) and other imaging of complex cases (see Chaps. 15 to 20) are best done where

growth retardation, developmental delay, and cardiac defects (often defects of the ventricular septum) in about 45% of affected infants.

PREVENTION

Physicians who treat pregnant women (see Chap. 82) should be aware of the effects of known teratogens as well as drugs (e.g., angiotensin-converting enzyme [ACE] inhibition and fetal renal development) that may have a functional rather than a structural damaging influence on the fetal and newborn heart and circulation. They should also recognize that for many drugs, information about their teratogenic potential is inadequate. Similarly, appropriate radiologic equipment and techniques for reducing gonadal and fetal radiation exposure should always be used to reduce the hazards of this potential cause of birth defects.

Detection of genetic abnormalities during fetal life is becoming an increasing reality. Fetal cells are obtained from amniotic fluid or chorionic villus biopsy. Many fetuses in whom CHD is detected will undergo genetic testing, and fetal echocardiography is frequently indicated when a chromosomal abnormality is diagnosed for other reasons. Many social, religious, and legal considerations influence whether termination of pregnancy is performed under these circumstances, but the improved outcomes for even the most complex CHDs frequently argue against the cardiac condition being used as the sole reason. Immunization of children with rubella vaccine has been one of the most effective preventive strategies against fetal rubella syndrome and its associated congenital cardiac abnormalities.

ANATOMY AND EMBRYOLOGY
Embryology

NORMAL CARDIAC DEVELOPMENT. During the first month of gestation, the primitive, straight cardiac tube is formed, comprising the sinuatrium (most cephalad), the primitive ventricle, the bulbus cordis, and the truncus arteriosus (most caudad) in series. In the second month of gestation, there is rightward looping of the heart tube. By the end of the fifth week, parts of the ventricles are visible and the left ventricle supports most of the circumference of the AV canal. The superior and inferior cushions fuse by the sixth week into the left and right AV junctions. Migration of the AV canal to the right and of the ventricular septum to the left serves to align each ventricle with its appropriate AV valve. At the distal end of the cardiac tube, the bulbus cordis divides into a subaortic muscular conus and a subpulmonary muscular conus; the subpulmonary conus elongates and the subaortic conus resorbs, allowing the aorta to move posteriorly and to connect with the left ventricle.

ABNORMAL DEVELOPMENT. A host of anomalies can result from defects in this basic developmental pattern. Double-inlet left ventricle is observed if the tricuspid orifice does not align over the right ventricle. The various types of persistent truncus arteriosus result from failure of the truncus to divide into main pulmonary artery and aorta. Double-outlet anomalies of the right ventricle are produced by failure of either the subpulmonary or subaortic conus to resorb, whereas resorption of the subpulmonary instead of the subaortic conus may lead to TGA.

ATRIA. The primitive sinuatrium is separated into right and left atria by the downgrowth from its roof of the septum primum toward the AV canal, fusing with the cushions. Numerous perforations form in the anterosuperior portion of the septum primum. After this, there is a superior infolding of the roof of the atria, which has traditionally been called the septum secundum. The remnant of the septum primum forms the fossa ovalis.

Fusion of the endocardial cushions anteriorly and posteriorly divides the AV canal into tricuspid and mitral inlets. The inferior portion of the atrial septum, the superior portion of the ventricular septum, and portions of the septal leaflet of the tricuspid and aortic leaflet of the mitral valve are formed from the endocardial cushions. The posterior or mural leaflet of the mitral valve is mainly formed from a sheet of AV myocardium that protrudes into the lumen of the ventricle, rather than by delamination, as was previously thought. The integrity of the atrial septum depends on growth of the septum primum and the superior infolding and proper fusion of the endocardial cushions. ASDs and various degrees of AV defect are the result of developmental deficiencies of this process.

VENTRICLES. Partitioning of the ventricles occurs as cephalic growth of the main ventricular septum results in its fusion with the endocardial cushions and the infundibular or conus septum. Defects in the ventricular septum may occur because of a deficiency of septal substance; malalignment of septal components in different planes, preventing their fusion; or an overly long conus, keeping the septal components apart. Isolated defects probably result from the first mechanism, whereas the last two appear to generate the VSDs in tetralogy of Fallot and transposition complexes.

PULMONARY VEINS. These structures arise from the primitive foregut and are drained early in embryogenesis by channels from the splanchnic plexus to the cardinal and umbilicovitteline veins. When the pulmonary vein is first recognized as a channel entering the heart, it is a solitary structure, entering the atrial component close to the AV junction. After closure of the interventricular communication, the pulmonary veins migrate to the roof of the left atrium. This communicates with the splanchnic plexus, establishing pulmonary venous drainage to the left atrium. The umbilicovitteline and anterior cardinal vein communications atrophy as the common pulmonary vein is incorporated into the left atrium. Anomalous pulmonary venous connections to the umbilicovitteline (portal) venous system or to the cardinal system (superior vena cava) result from failure of the common pulmonary vein to develop or to establish communications to the splanchnic plexus.

GREAT ARTERIES. The truncus arteriosus is connected to the dorsal aorta in the embryo by six pairs of aortic arches. Partition of the truncus arteriosus into two great arteries is a result of the fusion of tissue arising from the back wall of the vessel and the truncus septum. Rotation of the truncus coils the aortopulmonary septum and creates the normal spiral relation between aorta and pulmonary artery. Semilunar valves and their related sinuses are created by absorption and hollowing out of tissue at the distal side of the truncus ridges. Aortopulmonary septal defect and persistent truncus arteriosus represent various degrees of partitioning failure.

Although the six aortic arches appear sequentially, portions of the arch system and dorsal aorta disappear at different times during embryogenesis. The first, second, and fifth sets of paired arches regress completely. The proximal portions of the sixth arches become the right and left pulmonary arteries, and the distal left sixth arch becomes the ductus arteriosus. The third aortic arch forms the connection between internal and external carotid arteries, and the left fourth arch becomes the arterial segment between left carotid and subclavian arteries. The proximal portion of the right subclavian artery forms from the right fourth arch. An abnormality in regression of the arch system in a number of sites can produce a wide variety of arch anomalies, whereas a failure of regression usually results in a double aortic arch malformation.

Normal Cardiac Anatomy

The key to understanding CHD is an appreciation of the segmental approach to the diagnosis of both simple and complex lesions.

CARDIAC SITUS. This refers to the status of the atrial appendages. The normal left atrial appendage is a finger-like structure with a narrow base and no guarding crista. On the other hand, the right atrial appendage is broad based and has a guarding crista and pectinate muscles. *Situs solitus* or *inversus* refers to hearts with both a morphologic left and right atrium. *Situs ambiguus* refers to hearts with two morphologic left or right atrial appendages. These are dealt with in the section on isomerism and have implications with regard to associated intracardiac and extracardiac abnormalities.

ATRIOVENTRICULAR CONNECTIONS. This refers to the connections between the atria and ventricles. The AV connections are said to be concordant if the morphologic left atrium is connected to a morphologic left ventricle via the mitral valve, with the morphologic right atrium connecting to the morphologic right ventricle via a tricuspid valve. They are said to be discordant in other circumstances, such as in congenitally corrected TGA (cc-TGA).

VENTRICULOARTERIAL CONNECTIONS. This refers to the connections between the semilunar valve and the ventricles. Ventriculoarterial concordance occurs when the morphologic left ventricle is connected to the aorta and the morphologic right ventricle is connected to the pulmonary artery. Ventriculoarterial discordance occurs when the morphologic left ventricle is connected to the pulmonary artery, with the aorta being connected to the morphologic right ventricle. Double-outlet right ventricle occurs when more than 50% of both great arteries is connected to the morphologic right ventricle. A single-outlet heart has only one great artery connected to the heart.

ATRIA. The assignment of either a morphologic left or right atrium is determined by the morphology of the atrial appendages and not by the status of the systemic or pulmonary venous drainage. The right atrial appendage is broad and triangular; the left is smaller and finger-like. The internal architecture is the key feature to an accurate diagnosis, with the right having extensive pectinate muscles, unlike its left counterpart. Although the pulmonary veins usually drain to a morphologic left atrium and the systemic veins drain into a morphologic right atrium, this is not always the case.

ATRIOVENTRICULAR VALVES. The morphologic mitral valve is a bileaflet valve with the anterior or aortic leaflet in fibrous continuity with the noncoronary cusp of the aortic valve. The mitral valve leaflets are supported by two papillary muscle groups located in the antero-lateral and posteromedial positions. Each papillary muscle supports the adjacent part of both valve leaflets, with considerable variation in the morphology of the papillary muscles.

The tricuspid valve is a trileaflet valve, although it can frequently be difficult to identify all three leaflets because of variability in the anteroposterior commissure. With close inspection, the commissural chordae that arise from the papillary muscles may permit the identification of the three leaflets. The three leaflets occupy a septal anterior, superior, and inferior position. The commissures between the leaflets are the anterior septal, anterior inferior, and inferior. The papillary muscles supporting the valve leaflets arise mostly from the trabecula septomarginalis and its apical ramifications.

MORPHOLOGIC RIGHT VENTRICLE. The morphologic right ventricle is a triangular structure with an inlet, trabecular, and outlet component. The inlet component of the right ventricle has attachments from the septal leaflet of the tricuspid valve. Inferior to this is the moderator band, which arises at the base of the trabecula septomarginalis, with extensive trabeculations toward the apex of the right ventricle. The outlet component of the right ventricle consists of a fusion of three structures (i.e., the infundibular septum separating the aortic from the pulmonary valve, the ventriculoinfundibular fold separating the tricuspid valve from the pulmonary valve, and finally the anterior and posterior limbs of the trabecula septomarginalis).

MORPHOLOGIC LEFT VENTRICLE. The morphologic left ventricle is an elliptical structure with a fine trabecular pattern, with absent septal attachments of the mitral valve in the normal heart. It consists of an inlet portion containing the mitral valve and a tension apparatus, with an apical trabecular zone that is characterized by fine trabeculations and an outlet zone that supports the aortic valve.

SEMILUNAR VALVES. The aortic valve is a trileaflet valve with the left and right cusps giving rise to the left and right coronary arteries, respectively; the noncoronary cusp lacks a coronary artery connection. Of note, the noncoronary cusp is in fibrous continuity with the anterior leaflet of the mitral valve. The aortic valve has a semilunar attachment to the junction of the ventricular outlet and its great arteries. The aortic cusps have a main core of fibrous tissue with endocardial linings on each surface. The cusps are thickened at the midpoint to form a nodule. The characteristics of the pulmonary valve are similar to those of its aortic counterpart, noting the absence of the coronary ostia arising at the superior portion of the sinuses.

AORTIC ARCH AND PULMONARY ARTERIES. In the normal heart, the aortic arch usually points to the left, with the first branch, the innominate artery, giving rise to the right carotid and subclavian arteries. In general, the left carotid and left subclavian arteries arise separately from the aortic arch. By definition, the ascending aorta is proximal to the origin of the innominate artery, with the transverse aortic arch being from the innominate artery to the origin of the left subclavian artery. The aortic isthmus is the area between the left subclavian artery and a PDA or ligamentum arteriosum.

SYSTEMIC VENOUS CONNECTIONS. In the normal heart, the left and right innominate veins form the superior caval vein, which connects to the roof of the right atrium. The inferior caval vein connects to the inferior portion of the morphologic right atrium, with hepatic veins joining the inferior caval vein before its insertion into the atrium. The coronary veins drain into the flow of the coronary sinus, with the latter running in the posterior AV groove and terminating in the right atrium. The inferior caval vein is guarded by the eustachian valve, which may vary in size among hearts.

PULMONARY VENOUS DRAINAGE IN THE NORMAL HEART. The pulmonary veins drain to the left-sided atrium. Usually three pulmonary veins arise from the trilobed right lung and two pulmonary veins from the bilobed left lung. The pulmonary veins drain into the left atrium in superior and inferior locations. There is a short segment of extraparenchymal pulmonary vein before it disappears into the adjacent hila of the lungs.

Fetal and Transitional Circulations (Fig. 65-1)

CHD is being diagnosed with increasing frequency during fetal life. Our ability to modify the evolution of structural (by fetal intervention) and physiologic (by drug therapy) heart disease is increasing. Knowledge of the changes in cardiovascular structure, function, and metabolism that occur during fetal development is perhaps more important today than at any time in the past.

FETAL CIRCULATORY PATHWAYS. Dynamic alterations occur in the circulation during the transition from fetal to neonatal life when the lungs take over the function of gas exchange from the placenta. The fetal circulation consists of parallel pulmonary and systemic pathways in contrast to the "in-series" circuit of the normal postnatal circulation. Oxygenated blood returns from the placenta through the umbilical vein and enters the portal venous system. A variable amount of this stream bypasses the hepatic microcirculation and enters the inferior vena cava by way of the ductus venosus. Inferior vena caval blood is from the

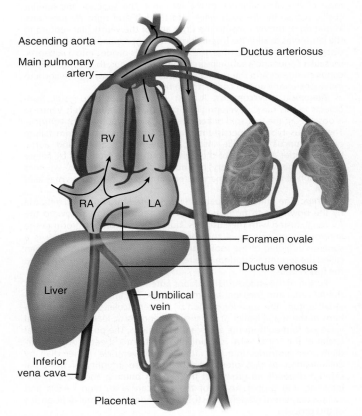

FIGURE 65-1 The fetal circulation, with arrows indicating the directions of flow. A fraction of umbilical venous blood enters the ductus venosus and bypasses the liver. This relatively highly oxygenated blood flows across the foramen ovale to the left side of the heart, preferentially perfusing the coronary arteries, head, and upper trunk. The output of the right ventricle flows preferentially across the ductus arteriosus and circulates to the placenta as well as to the abdominal viscera and lower trunk. *(Courtesy of Dr. David Teitel.)*

ductus venosus, hepatic veins, and lower body venous drainage and is partly deflected across the foramen ovale into the left atrium. Because of a streaming effect, almost all superior vena caval blood passes directly through the tricuspid valve, entering the right ventricle. Most of the blood that reaches the right ventricle bypasses the high-resistance, unexpanded lungs and passes through the ductus arteriosus into the descending aorta. The right ventricle contributes about 55% and the left ventricle 45% to the total fetal cardiac output. The major portion of blood ejected from the left ventricle supplies the brain and upper body, with lesser flow to the coronary arteries; the balance passes across the aortic isthmus to the descending aorta, where it joins with the large stream from the ductus arteriosus before flowing to the lower body and back to the placenta.

FETAL PULMONARY CIRCULATION. In fetal life, the alveoli are fluid filled, and the pulmonary arteries and arterioles have relatively thick walls and a small lumen, similar to arteries in the systemic circulation. The low pulmonary blood flow in the fetus (7% to 10% of the total cardiac output) is the result of high pulmonary vascular resistance. Fetal pulmonary vessels are highly reactive to changes in oxygen tension or in the pH of blood perfusing them as well as to a number of other physiologic and pharmacologic influences.

EFFECTS OF CARDIAC MALFORMATIONS ON THE FETUS. Although fetal somatic growth may be unimpaired, the hemodynamic effects of many cardiac malformations can alter the development and structure of the fetal heart and circulation. For example, although lesions associated with left-to-right shunts in postnatal life rarely influence fetal cardiac size and function, regurgitant AV valves can lead to chamber dilation, hydrops, and fetal death. Ventricular obstructive lesions (e.g., aortic valve stenosis) may variably lead to hypertrophy, dilation, and failure. The secondary effects of congenital lesions are also important. Reduced flow through the left side of the heart can result in aortic hypoplasia and coarctation. Reduced anterograde pulmonary blood flow is associated with pulmonary artery hypoplasia. These effects rarely affect the fetal circulation overtly, however, and often only become exposed as problems after birth as the ductus arteriosus closes.

FUNCTION OF THE FETAL HEART. Compared with the adult heart, the fetal and newborn heart is unique with respect to its ultrastructural appearance, its mechanical and biochemical properties, and its autonomic innervation. During late fetal and early neonatal development, there is maturation of the excitation-contraction coupling process and changes in the biochemical composition of the heart's energy-using myofibrillar proteins and of adenosine triphosphate and creatine phosphate energy-producing proteins. Moreover, fetal and neonatal myocardial cells are small in diameter and reduced in density so that the immature heart contains relatively more noncontractile mass (primarily mitochondria, nuclei, and surface membranes) than later in postnatal life. As a result, force generation and the extent and velocity of shortening are decreased, and stiffness and water content of ventricular myocardium are increased in the fetal and early newborn periods. The fetal heart is surrounded by fluid-filled rather than air-filled lungs. As a result, the fetal and neonatal heart has limited ability to increase cardiac output in the presence of either a volume load or a lesion that increases resistance to emptying. Ultimately, cardiac output is much more dependent on changes in heart rate, explaining why bradycardia is so poorly tolerated by the fetal circulation. Tachycardia can also rapidly lead to heart failure in the fetus, whether it is due to the hemodynamic issues discussed earlier or a manifestation of energy substrate use.

CHANGES AT BIRTH. Inflation of the lungs at the first inspiration produces a marked reduction in pulmonary vascular resistance. The reduced extravascular pressure and increased alveolar oxygen content, as fluid is removed from the lungs and replaced by air, lead to pulmonary vasodilation and recruitment. As a result, pulmonary artery pressure falls, and pulmonary blood flow increases greatly, raising left atrial pressure and closing the flap valve of the foramen ovale. Conversely, systemic vascular resistance rises. This is related to loss of the low-resistance placental circulation and gradual closure of the ductus arteriosus. It is also related to a sudden increase in arterial blood oxygen tension, subsequent to the lack of mixing of oxygenated and deoxygenated blood that characterizes the fetal milieu. In healthy, mature infants, the ductus arteriosus is profoundly constricted at 10 to 15 hours and is closed functionally by 72 hours, with total anatomic closure following within a few weeks by a process of thrombosis, intimal proliferation, and fibrosis. Preterm infants have a high incidence of persistent patency of the ductus arteriosus because of an immaturity of those mechanisms responsible for constriction.

The ductus venosus, ductus arteriosus, and foramen ovale remain potential channels for blood flow after birth. Thus, persistent patency of the ductus venosus is capitalized on during balloon atrial septostomy performed through the umbilical vein. Lesions producing right or left atrial volume or pressure overload can stretch the foramen ovale and render incompetent the flap valve mechanism for its closure. Anomalies that depend on patency of the ductus arteriosus for preservation of pulmonary or systemic blood flow may remain latent until the ductus arteriosus constricts. A common example is the rapid intensification of cyanosis observed in infants with tetralogy of Fallot when the magnitude of pulmonary hypoperfusion is unmasked by spontaneous closure of the ductus arteriosus. Moreover, increasing evidence shows that ductal constriction is a key factor in the postnatal development of coarctation of the aorta and is clearly the most important factor governing the presentation in babies with a duct-dependent systemic circulation. The management of these conditions is discussed in the appropriate sections later.

NEONATE AND INFANT. Most management decisions in patients with significant CHD occur during the first few months of life. An increase in the prenatal diagnosis of major congenital heart defects has resulted in earlier admission and intervention in the neonate with CHD. These neonates are, in general, healthier than in the past because of the administration of prostaglandins at the time of delivery, thus maintaining hemodynamic stability. With improved surgery and interventional catheterization techniques, many of these neonates undergo intervention within the first days or weeks of life. Indeed, there has been a trend toward complete repair in the neonate and young infant because of an improvement in myocardial preservation and surgical techniques. In most major cardiac centers, the surgical mortality for this age group is in the range of 2% to 4%, which is an improvement on the results of the past, when a palliative procedure often preceded a complete repair.

With increasing experience in this age group, the focus has now shifted from mortality to morbidity. Because the expectation is that most of these neonates and young infants will survive into their adult years, their neurodevelopmental outcome has become as important as the results of the cardiac intervention.[3] It is also being recognized that systemic venous obstruction is a major cause of ongoing morbidity, being directly related to the use of central and peripheral lines in the immediate postoperative period.

CHILD AND ADOLESCENT. The rapid somatic growth rates of infancy and adolescence are periods of rapid hemodynamic change. Stenotic lesions that may be relatively slowly progressive throughout early childhood need more frequent surveillance during adolescence. Childhood and adolescence is a time to begin educating patients, not just their parents, about their heart disease and the responsibilities that go with it. Issues such as the need for compliance with medications, avoidance of smoking and illicit drug use, and pregnancy and contraception counseling are by no means exclusively issues of the adult with CHD and increasingly require discussion in the pediatric cardiac clinic.

Indeed, the early teenage years should be regarded as part of the transition process before transfer to adult follow-up. The management of the older adolescent and follow-up of adults with newly discovered or previously treated CHD is a burgeoning new subspecialty that will require careful planning to ensure adequate resources for the increasing number of adult "graduates" of pediatric programs. A coordinated approach with specialists in an affiliated adult congenital clinic is clearly desirable.

ADULT. Patients, and often family members, should understand their cardiac condition in terms of both what has been done so far and what could happen in the future. This is important for a young patient graduating into the adult world. Patients need information and should become partners in their own care.

Potential long-term complications in adults with CHD (such as arrhythmias, ventricular failure, conduit obstruction, and endocarditis) should be explained to patients who are at relatively high risk. The possible need for future therapy—medical (antiarrhythmics, anticoagulation, heart failure therapy), catheter based (valve dilation, stents, arrhythmia ablation), or surgical (redo surgery, transplantation)—should be discussed if the patient may require treatment in the short or intermediate future. Day-to-day issues of concern for these young adults need to be addressed, such as exercise prescriptions, driving restrictions, and traveling limitations. Many young people with CHD need advice about career choices, entering the work force, insurability, and life expectancy.

Many will want to start a family, and reproductive issues will need to be addressed. Discussion of appropriate contraception methods for any given patient should be offered.[4] Counseling before conception as to the risk to the mother and the fetus for any given pregnancy should be done by specialized physicians. They will take into account the maternal cardiac anatomy, maternal functional status, maternal life expectancy, risk of CHD transmission to the offspring, and risk of premature birth. High-risk patients (e.g., Marfan with aortic root dilation, severe pulmonary hypertension, New York Heart Association [NYHA] Class III or IV, and severe aortic stenosis) should be advised against pregnancy. Intermediate-risk patients (e.g., cyanotic, mechanical valve and other warfarin-requiring patients, moderate left ventricular outflow tract obstruction, moderate to severe left ventricular dysfunction) need to know that pregnancy, although possible, may be complicated and that they will require careful follow-up.

Last but not least, comorbidities such as obesity, smoking, high blood pressure, diabetes, and high cholesterol add new levels of complexity to these adults as they age and must be part of the mandate of the patient's cardiologist.

Pathologic Consequences of Congenital Cardiac Lesions

Congestive Heart Failure (see Chaps. 25 to 30)

Although the basic mechanisms of cardiac failure are similar for all ages, the common causes, the time of onset, and often the approach to treatment vary with age (see Chaps. 31 to 34 and Chap. 80). Fetal echocardiography now allows the diagnosis of intrauterine cardiac failure. The cardinal findings of fetal heart failure are scalp edema, ascites, pericardial effusion, and decreased fetal movements. In preterm infants, especially of less than 1500 g birth weight, persistent patency of the ductus arteriosus is the most common cause of cardiac decompensation, and other forms of structural heart disease are rare. In full-term newborns, the earliest important causes of heart failure are the hypoplastic left heart and aortic coarctation syndromes, sustained tachyarrhythmia, cerebral or hepatic arteriovenous fistula, and myocarditis. Among the lesions commonly producing heart failure beyond age 1 to 2 weeks, when diminished pulmonary vascular resistance allows substantial left-to-right shunting, are VSDs and AV septal defects, TGA, truncus arteriosus, and total anomalous pulmonary venous connection. Infants younger than 1 year who have cardiac malformations account for 80% to 90% of pediatric patients who develop congestive failure. In older children, heart failure is often due to acquired disease or is a complication of open heart surgical procedures. In the acquired category are rheumatic and endomyocardial diseases, infective endocarditis, hematologic and nutritional disorders, and severe cardiac arrhythmias.

The distinction between left-sided and right-sided heart failure is less obvious in infants than in older children or adults. Conversely, augmented filling or elevated pressure of the right ventricle in infants reduces left ventricular compliance disproportionately compared with older children or adults and gives rise to signs of both systemic and pulmonary venous congestion.

Care of infants with heart failure must include careful consideration of the underlying structural or functional disturbance. The general aims of treatment are to achieve an increase in cardiac performance, to augment peripheral perfusion, and to decrease pulmonary and systemic venous congestion. In many conditions, medical management cannot control the effects of the abnormal loads imposed by a host of congenital cardiac lesions. Under these circumstances, cardiac diagnosis and interventional catheter or operative intervention may be urgently required.

Congestive heart failure is not common in adult congenital heart practice, although prevention of myocardial dysfunction is a common concern. The adult patient with CHD may develop heart failure in the presence of a substrate (e.g., myocardial dysfunction, valvular regurgitation) and a precipitant (e.g., sustained arrhythmia, pregnancy, hyperthyroidism). Patients prone to congestive failure include those with longstanding volume loads (e.g., valvular regurgitation and left-to-right shunts) and those with a primary depression of myocardial function (e.g., systemic right ventricles, ventricles damaged during surgery or because of late treatment of ventricular overload). Treatment depends on a clear understanding of the elements contributing to decompensation and addressing each of the treatable components. The greatest success is achieved when the main elements can be eliminated. When this is not possible, standard palliative adult heart failure regimens are applied and may include ACE inhibitors,

angiotensin receptor blockers, beta blockers, diuretics, resynchronization pacing, transplantation, or other novel therapies.

CHD accounts for 40% of pediatric heart transplants but only 2% of adult heart transplants.[5] Adult CHD heart transplant recipients have a mean survival of 11 years, similar to that of patients with other forms of heart disease. Patients who have had Fontan surgery tend to have worse outcomes, presumably because they have multiorgan disease.[6] About one third of heart-lung transplants are done for CHD. Three-year survival is about 50% and better in patients with Eisenmenger syndrome.

Cyanosis

DEFINITION. Central cyanosis refers to arterial oxygen desaturation resulting from the shunting or mixing of systemic venous blood into the arterial circulation. The magnitude of shunting or mixing and the amount of pulmonary blood flow determine the severity of desaturation.

MORPHOLOGY. Cardiac defects that result in central cyanosis can be divided into two categories: (1) those with increased pulmonary blood flow and (2) those with decreased pulmonary blood flow (**Table 65-4**).

PATHOPHYSIOLOGY. Hypoxemia increases renal production of erythropoietin, which in turn stimulates bone marrow production of circulating red blood cells, enhancing oxygen-carrying capacity. Secondary erythrocytosis should be present in all cyanotic patients because it is a physiologic response to tissue hypoxia. The improved tissue oxygenation that results from this adaptation may be sufficient to reach a new equilibrium at a higher hematocrit. However, adaptive failure can occur if the increased whole blood viscosity rises so much that it impairs oxygen delivery.

CLINICAL FEATURES

Hyperviscosity Syndrome

Erythrocytosis, by virtue of increasing whole blood viscosity, can cause hyperviscosity symptoms including headaches, faintness, dizziness, fatigue, altered mentation, visual disturbances, paresthesias, tinnitus, and myalgias. Iron deficiency, a common finding in cyanotic adult patients if repeated phlebotomies or excessive bleeding occurs, may cause hyperviscosity symptoms at hematocrit levels well below 65%.

Hematologic

Hemostatic abnormalities have been documented in cyanotic patients with erythrocytosis and can occur in up to 20% of patients. A bleeding tendency can be mild and superficial, leading to easy bruising, skin petechiae, and mucosal bleeding, or it can be moderate or life-threatening with hemoptysis or intracranial, gastrointestinal, or postoperative bleeding. Elevated prothrombin and partial thromboplastin times, decreased factor levels (factors V, VII, VIII, and IX), qualitative and quantitative platelet disorders, increased fibrinolysis, and systemic endothelial dysfunction from increased shear stress have all been implicated.[7]

TABLE 65-4 Cardiac Defects Causing Central Cyanosis	
Transposition of the great arteries	**E**bstein anomaly
Tetralogy of Fallot	**E**isenmenger physiology
Tricuspid atresia	Critical pulmonary stenosis or atresia
Truncus arteriosus	Functionally single ventricle
Total anomalous pulmonary venous return	
Note five T's and two E's.	

Central Nervous System

Neurologic complications including cerebral hemorrhage can occur secondary to hemostatic defects and can be seen in patients taking anticoagulants. Patients with right-to-left shunts may be at risk for paradoxical cerebral emboli, especially if they are iron deficient. A brain abscess should be suspected in a cyanotic patient with a new or different headache or new neurologic symptoms. Air filters should be used in peripheral and central venous lines in cyanotic patients to avoid paradoxical emboli through a right-to-left shunt.

Renal

Renal dysfunction can be manifested as proteinuria, hyperuricemia, or renal failure. Pathologic studies at the level of the glomeruli show evidence of vascular abnormalities as well as increased cellularity and fibrosis. Hyperuricemia is common and is thought to be due mainly to the decreased reabsorption of uric acid rather than to overproduction with erythrocytosis. Urate nephropathy, uric acid nephrolithiasis, and gouty arthritis may occur.

Arthritic

Rheumatologic complications include gout and, especially, hypertrophic osteoarthropathy, which is thought to be responsible for the arthralgias and bone pain affecting up to one third of patients. In patients with right-to-left shunting, megakaryocytes released from the bone marrow can bypass the lung. The entrapment of megakaryocytes in the systemic arterioles and capillaries induces the release of platelet-derived growth factor, promoting local cell proliferation. New osseous formation with periostitis ensues and gives rise to arthralgia and bone pain.

Coronary Arteries

Patients with central cyanosis display dilated coronaries with no obstruction. Their level of total cholesterol is also lower than that of the general population.[8]

INTERVENTIONAL OPTIONS AND OUTCOMES

Physiologic Repair

Physiologic repair results in total or near-total anatomic and physiologic separation of the pulmonary and systemic circulations in complex cyanotic lesions that leads to relief of cyanosis. Such procedures should be performed whenever feasible.

Palliative Surgical Intervention

Palliative surgical interventions can be performed in patients with cyanotic lesions to increase pulmonary blood flow while allowing cyanosis to persist. Palliative surgical shunts are summarized in **Table 65-5**. Blalock-Taussig, central, and Glenn (also called cavopulmonary) shunts are still in use today. Blalock-Taussig shunts seldom have caused pulmonary hypertension compared with central shunts and are less likely to cause pulmonary artery distortion. Glenn shunts have the advantage of increasing pulmonary flow without imposing a volume load on the systemic ventricle. Glenn shunts require low pulmonary

---

TABLE 65-5 Palliative Systemic to Pulmonary Shunts

Arterial
Blalock-Taussig shunt (subclavian artery to pulmonary artery)
  Classic: end-to-side, no or reduced ipsilateral arm pulses
  Current: side-to-side tubular grafts, preserved arm pulses
Central shunt (side-to-side tubular graft, aorta to pulmonary artery)
Potts shunt (descending aorta to left pulmonary artery)
Waterston shunt (ascending aorta to right pulmonary artery)

Venous
Glenn shunt (superior vena cava to ipsilateral pulmonary artery without cardiac or other pulmonary artery connection)
Bidirectional cavopulmonary (Glenn) shunt (end-to-side superior vena cava to left pulmonary artery and right pulmonary artery shunt)

---

artery pressures to work, and they may be associated with the development over time of pulmonary arteriovenous fistulas, which can worsen cyanosis.

Transplantation (see Chap. 31)

Transplantation of heart, one or both lungs with surgical cardiac repair, and heart-lung transplantation have been performed in cyanotic patients with or without palliation who were no longer candidates for other forms of intervention. Pulmonary vascular obstructive disease precludes isolated heart transplantation. An increasing number of CHD patients with previous palliation and ventricular failure are successfully undergoing cardiac transplantation.[5] Timing of transplantation in these patients remains difficult.

OTHER MANAGEMENT

Phlebotomy

The goal of phlebotomy is symptom control. When patients have troubling symptoms of hyperviscosity, are iron replete (normal mean corpuscular volume, hematocrit >65%), and are not dehydrated, removal of 250 to 500 mL of blood during 30 to 45 minutes should be performed with concomitant quantitative volume replacement. The procedure may be repeated every 24 hours until symptomatic improvement occurs or the hemoglobin level has fallen below 18 to 19 g/dL. Phlebotomy is not indicated for asymptomatic patients.

Iron Replacement

If iron deficiency anemia is found, iron supplements should be prescribed. Cyanotic patients should avoid iron deficiency, which can cause functional deterioration and is associated with an increased risk of stroke.

Bleeding Diathesis

Platelet transfusions, fresh frozen plasma, vitamin K, cryoprecipitate, and desmopressin can be used to treat severe bleeding. Given the inherent tendency to bleed, aspirin, heparin, and warfarin should be avoided in the cyanotic patient unless the risks of treatment are outweighed by the risks of nontreatment. Likewise, nonsteroidal anti-inflammatory drugs should be avoided to prevent bleeding.

Gouty Arthritis

Symptomatic hyperuricemia and gouty arthritis can be treated as needed with colchicine, probenecid, or allopurinol.

REPRODUCTIVE ISSUES. Pregnancy in cyanotic CHD (excluding Eisenmenger syndrome) results in a 32% incidence of maternal cardiovascular complications and a 37% incidence of fetal prematurity. Pregnant women with a resting oxygen saturation greater than 85% fare better than do women with an oxygen saturation less than 85%.

FOLLOW-UP. All cyanotic patients should be observed by a CHD cardiologist, and particular attention should be paid to the following: underlying heart condition; symptoms of hyperviscosity; systemic complications of cyanosis; change in exercise tolerance; change in saturation levels; and prophylaxis against endocarditis, influenza, and pneumococcal infections. The clinician should remember to measure oxygen saturation only after the patient has been resting for at least 5 minutes. In stable cyanotic patients, yearly follow-up is recommended and should include annual influenza vaccination, periodic pneumococcal vaccination, yearly blood work (complete blood count, ferritin, clotting profile, renal function, uric acid), and regular echocardiographic Doppler studies. Home oxygen therapy may have a role in increasing oxygen saturation through its pulmonary vasodilatory effect, but clinical indications and outcomes are not clear.[9]

Pulmonary Hypertension

Pulmonary hypertension is a common accompaniment of many congenital cardiac lesions,[10] and the status of the pulmonary vascular bed is often the principal determinant of the clinical manifestations, the course, and whether corrective treatment is feasible (see Chap. 78). Recent consensus statements provide important information on this general topic.[11,12] Increases in pulmonary arterial pressure result from elevations of pulmonary blood flow or resistance, the latter sometimes caused by an increase in vascular tone but usually the result of underdevelopment or obstructive or obliterative structural changes within the pulmonary vascular bed. Although pulmonary hypertension usually affects the entire pulmonary vascular bed, it may occur focally. For example, unilateral pulmonary hypertension may occur in an overshunted lung (the other lung perhaps protected and fed by a cavopulmonary Glenn shunt) or in lung segments supplied by aortopulmonary collateral flow.

Pulmonary vascular resistance normally falls rapidly immediately after birth because of the onset of ventilation and subsequent pulmonary vasodilation. Subsequently, the medial smooth muscle of pulmonary arterial resistance vessels thins gradually. In infants with large aortopulmonary or ventricular communications, this process is often delayed by several months, at which time levels of pulmonary vascular resistance are still somewhat elevated. In patients with high pulmonary arterial pressures from birth, failure of normal growth of the pulmonary circulation may occur, and anatomic changes in the pulmonary vessels in the form of proliferation of intimal cells and intimal and medial thickening often progress, so in an older child or adult, vascular resistance ultimately may become relatively fixed by obliterative changes in the pulmonary vascular bed. The causes of pulmonary vascular obstructive disease remain unknown, although increased pulmonary arterial blood pressure, elevated pulmonary venous pressure, erythrocytosis, systemic hypoxia, acidemia, and the nature of the bronchial circulation have been implicated. Quite likely, injury to pulmonary vascular endothelial cells initiates a cascade of events that involves the release or activation of factors that alter the extracellular matrix, induces hypertrophy, causes proliferation of vascular smooth muscle cells, and promotes connective tissue protein synthesis. Considered together, these may permanently alter vessel structure and function.

MECHANISMS OF DEVELOPMENT. Intimal damage appears to be related to shear stresses because endothelial cell damage occurs at high shear rates. A reduction in pulmonary arteriolar lumen size due to either thickened medial muscle or vasoconstriction increases the velocity of flow. Shear stress also increases as blood viscosity rises; therefore, infants with hypoxemia and high hematocrit levels as well as increased pulmonary blood flow are at increased risk for development of pulmonary vascular disease. In patients with left-to-right shunts, pulmonary arterial hypertension, if it is not present in infancy or childhood, may never occur or may not develop until the third or fourth decade or later. Once developed, intimal proliferative changes with hyalinization and fibrosis are not reversible by repair of the underlying cardiac defect. In severe pulmonary vascular obstructive disease, arteriovenous malformations may develop and predispose to massive hemoptysis.

Most vexing is the variability among patients with the same or similar cardiac lesions in both the time of appearance and the rate of progression of the pulmonary vascular obstructive process. Although genetic influences may be operative (an example is the apparent acceleration of pulmonary vascular disease in patients with CHD and trisomy 21), evidence is now accumulating for important prenatal and postnatal modifiers of the pulmonary vascular bed that appear, at least in part, to be lesion dependent. Thus, a quantitative variability exists in the pulmonary vascular bed related to the number, not just the size and wall structure, of arterial vessels within the pulmonary circulation.

Modeling of the blood vessels occurs proximal to and within terminal bronchioles (preacinar and intra-acinar vessels, respectively) continuously from before birth. The intra-acinar vessels, in particular, increase in size and number from late fetal life throughout childhood, with minimal muscularization of their walls. The ensuing increase in the cross-sectional area of the pulmonary arterial circulation allows the cardiac output to rise substantially without an increase in pulmonary arterial pressure. If, however, the presence of a cardiac lesion interferes with the normal growth and multiplication of these peripheral arteries, the resulting elevation of pulmonary vascular resistance may first be related to failure of the intra-acinar pulmonary circulation to develop fully and then secondarily to the morphologic changes of obliterative vascular disease: medial thickening, intimal proliferation, hyalinization and fibrosis, angiomatoid and plexiform lesions, and, ultimately, arterial necrosis.

Eisenmenger Syndrome

DEFINITION. Eisenmenger syndrome, a term coined by Paul Wood, is defined as pulmonary vascular obstructive disease that develops as a consequence of a large preexisting left-to-right shunt such that pulmonary artery pressures approach systemic levels and the direction of the flow becomes bidirectional or right-to-left. Congenital heart defects that can result in Eisenmenger syndrome include simple defects, such as ASD, VSD, and PDA, as well as more complex defects, such as AV septal defect, truncus arteriosus, aortopulmonary window, and univentricular heart. The high pulmonary vascular resistance is usually established in infancy (by the age of 2 years, except in ASD) and is sometimes present from birth.

NATURAL HISTORY OF THE UNREPAIRED PATIENT. Patients with defects that allow free communication between the pulmonary and systemic circuits at the aortic or ventricular levels usually have a fairly healthy childhood and gradually become overtly cyanotic during their second or third decade. Exercise intolerance (dyspnea and fatigue) is proportional to the degree of hypoxemia or cyanosis. In the absence of complications, these patients generally have an excellent to good functional capacity up to their third decade and thereafter usually experience a slowly progressive decline in their physical abilities. Most patients survive to adulthood, with a reported 77% and 42% survival rate at 15 and 25 years of age, respectively.

Congestive heart failure in patients with Eisenmenger syndrome usually occurs after 40 years of age. The most common modes of death are sudden death (≈30%; see Chap. 41), congestive heart failure (≈25%), and pulmonary hemorrhage (≈15%). Pregnancy, perioperative mortality after noncardiac surgery, and infectious causes (brain abscesses and endocarditis) account for most of the remainder.

CLINICAL MANIFESTATIONS. Patients can present with the following complications: those related to the cyanotic state; palpitations in nearly half the patients (atrial fibrillation or flutter in 35%, ventricular tachycardia in up to 10%); hemoptysis in about 20%; pulmonary thromboembolism, angina, syncope, and endocarditis in about 10% each; and congestive heart failure. Hemoptysis is usually due to bleeding bronchial vessels or pulmonary infarction. Physical examination reveals central cyanosis and clubbing of the nailbeds. Patients with Eisenmenger PDA can have pink nailbeds on the right (>left) hand and cyanosis and clubbing of both feet, so-called differential cyanosis. This occurs because venous blood shunts through the ductus and enters the aorta distal to the subclavian arteries. The jugular venous pressure in patients with Eisenmenger syndrome can be normal or elevated, especially with prominent v waves when tricuspid regurgitation is present. Signs of pulmonary hypertension—right ventricular heave, palpable and loud P_2, and right-sided S_4—are typically present. In many patients, a pulmonary ejection click and a soft and scratchy systolic ejection murmur, attributable to dilation of the pulmonary trunk, and a high-pitched decrescendo diastolic murmur of pulmonary regurgitation (Graham Steell) are audible. Peripheral edema is absent until right-sided heart failure ensues.

LABORATORY INVESTIGATIONS
ELECTROCARDIOGRAPHY. Peaked P waves consistent with right atrial overload and evidence of right ventricular hypertrophy with right-axis deviation are the rule. Atrial arrhythmias can be present.

CHEST RADIOGRAPHY. Dilated central pulmonary arteries with rapid tapering of the peripheral pulmonary vasculature are the radiographic hallmarks of Eisenmenger syndrome. Pulmonary artery calcification may be seen and is diagnostic of longstanding pulmonary hypertension. Eisenmenger syndrome due to VSD or PDA usually has a normal or slightly increased cardiothoracic ratio. Eisenmenger syndrome due to an ASD typically has a large cardiothoracic ratio because of right atrial and ventricular dilation, along with an inconspicuous aorta. Calcification of the duct may be seen in Eisenmenger PDA.

ECHOCARDIOGRAPHY. The intracardiac defect should be seen readily along with bidirectional shunting. A pulmonary hypertensive PDA is not easily seen. Evidence of pulmonary hypertension is found. Assessment of pulmonary right ventricular function adds prognostic value.

CARDIAC CATHETERIZATION. Cardiac catheterization not only provides direct measurement of the pulmonary artery pressure, documenting the existence of severe pulmonary hypertension, but also can allow assessment of reactivity of the pulmonary vasculature. Administration of pulmonary arterial vasodilators (oxygen, nitric oxide, prostaglandin I_2 [epoprostenol]) can discriminate patients in whom surgical repair is contraindicated and those with reversible pulmonary hypertension who may benefit from surgical repair. Radiographic contrast material may cause hypotension and worsening cyanosis and should be used cautiously.

OPEN LUNG BIOPSY. Open lung biopsy should be considered only when reversibility of the pulmonary hypertension is uncertain from the hemodynamic data. An expert opinion will be necessary to determine the severity of the changes, often by use of the Heath-Edwards classification.

INDICATIONS FOR INTERVENTION. The underlying principle of clinical management in patients with Eisenmenger syndrome is to avoid any factors that may destabilize the delicately balanced physiology. In general, an approach of nonintervention has been traditionally recommended, although research in the treatment of pulmonary hypertension may alter this approach in the future.[13] The main interventions, therefore, are directed toward prevention of complications (e.g., influenza vaccine and pneumococcal vaccine to reduce the morbidity of respiratory infections) or restoration of the physiologic balance (e.g., iron replacement for iron deficiency, antiarrhythmic management of atrial arrhythmias, diuretics for right-sided heart failure). As a general rule, the first episode of hemoptysis should be considered an indication for investigation. Bed rest is usually recommended; and although it is usually self-limited, each such episode should be regarded as potentially life-threatening, and a treatable cause should be sought. When patients are seriously incapacitated from severe hypoxemia or congestive heart failure, the main intervention available is lung transplantation (plus repair of the cardiac defect) or, with somewhat better results, heart-lung transplantation. This is generally reserved for individuals without contraindications who are thought to have a 1-year survival of less than 50%. Such assessment is fraught with difficulty because of the unpredictability of the time course of the disease and the risk of sudden death.

Noncardiac surgery should be performed only when it is absolutely necessary because of its high associated mortality. Eisenmenger syndrome patients are particularly vulnerable to alterations in hemodynamics induced by anesthesia or surgery, such as a minor decrease in systemic vascular resistance that can increase right-to-left shunting and possibly potentiate cardiovascular collapse. Local anesthesia should be used whenever possible. Avoidance of prolonged fasting and especially dehydration, use of antibiotic prophylaxis when appropriate, and careful intraoperative monitoring are recommended. The choice of general versus epidural-spinal anesthesia is controversial. An experienced cardiac anesthetist with an understanding of Eisenmenger syndrome physiology should administer anesthesia. Additional risks of surgery include excessive bleeding, postoperative arrhythmias, and deep venous thrombosis with paradoxical emboli. An air filter or "bubble trap" should be used for most intravenous lines in cyanotic patients. Early ambulation is recommended. Postoperative care in an intensive care unit setting is optimal.

INTERVENTIONAL OPTIONS AND OUTCOMES

Oxygen

Supplemental nocturnal oxygen has recently been shown to have no impact on exercise capacity or on survival in adult patients with Eisenmenger syndrome. Supplemental oxygen during commercial air travel is often recommended, but the scientific basis for this recommendation is lacking.

Transplantation

Lung transplantation may be undertaken in association with repair of existing cardiovascular defects. Alternatively, heart-lung transplantation may be required if the intracardiac anatomy is not correctable. The 3-year survival rate after heart-lung transplantation for CHD is 50%.[14] The subgroup of patients with Eisenmenger syndrome may do better, with a 50% 5-year survival. These procedures offer the best hope to individuals with end-stage CHD who are confronting death and have an intolerable quality of life.

Medical Therapy

ENDOTHELIN RECEPTOR ANTAGONISTS. A randomized trial of a nonselective endothelin receptor antagonist (bosentan) in patients with Eisenmenger syndrome[15] showed that pulse oximetry was not reduced. Compared with placebo, bosentan reduced the pulmonary vascular resistance index and pulmonary artery pressure and improved 6-minute walk and functional class. A smaller observational study of bosentan 125 mg twice a day in nine Eisenmenger patients showed an improvement in functional class and increased resting oxygen saturation levels.[16] In another study, bosentan was less effective in patients with Down syndrome.[17]

PHOSPHODIESTERASE INHIBITORS. Sildenafil (Viagra), in a large double-blind, placebo-controlled study administered in varying doses to 278 patients with symptomatic pulmonary arterial hypertension of different causes, improved the 6-minute walk distance (maintained for the 1 year of the trial), increased functional class, and modestly improved pulmonary arterial pressures and cardiac output.[18] A second randomized, placebo-controlled, double-blind crossover study of a smaller group of patients produced similar improvements.[19] Additional experience has recently been reported,[20,21] and the importance of considering safety issues in treating these patients has been highlighted.[22]

FOLLOW-UP. Education of the patient is critical. Avoidance of over-the-counter medications, dehydration, smoking, high-altitude exposure, and excessive physical activity should be stressed. Avoidance of pregnancy is of paramount importance. Annual influenza vaccination, a single dose of pneumococcal vaccine, and use of endocarditis prophylaxis together with proper skin hygiene (avoidance of nail biting) are recommended. A yearly assessment of complete blood cell count and uric acid, creatinine, and ferritin levels should be done to monitor treatable causes of deterioration.

Cardiac Arrhythmias (see Chaps. 35 to 39)

In teenagers and young adults, most arrhythmias (see Chap. 39) are in association with previously repaired CHD. Arrhythmias can be a major clinical challenge in adolescent and adult congenital heart patients. They are the most frequent reason for emergency department visits and hospital admissions, and they are usually recurrent and may worsen or become less responsive to treatment with time. Treatment may be challenging.

ATRIAL ARRHYTHMIAS. Atrial flutter and, to a lesser degree, atrial fibrillation are most common. Atrial flutter tends to reflect right atrial abnormalities, and atrial fibrillation, left atrial abnormalities. Atrial flutter in such patients is often atypical in appearance and behavior and is better called intra-atrial reentrant tachycardia. Recognition of atrial flutter can be difficult, and the observer must be vigilant in recognizing 2:1 conduction masquerading as sinus rhythm. Recurrence is likely and should not necessarily be assumed to represent failure of the management strategy. The conditions in which atrial flutter is most likely are Mustard or Senning repairs of TGA, repaired or unrepaired ASDs, repaired tetralogy of Fallot, Ebstein anomaly of the tricuspid valve, and after a Fontan operation. Atrial flutter may reflect hemodynamic deterioration in patients who have had Mustard, Senning, tetralogy of Fallot, or Fontan repairs. Its arrival is usually associated with more symptoms and functional limitation.

The pharmaceutical agents most commonly used in therapy are warfarin, beta blockers, amiodarone, sotalol, propafenone, and digoxin. As a rule, patients with good ventricular function can receive sotalol or propafenone, whereas those with depressed ventricular function should receive amiodarone. Other therapies including pacemakers, ablative procedures, and innovative surgery are being both applied and refined. Sustained ventricular tachycardia or ventricular fibrillation occurs less often, usually in the setting of ventricular dilation, dysfunction, and scarring. Although sudden death is common in several conditions, the mechanism is poorly understood.

VENTRICULAR TACHYCARDIA. This arrhythmia can be seen as a manifestation of proarrhythmic effects of various agents in patients with acute myocardial injury or infarction, and in CHD patients with severe ventricular dysfunction. In particular, sustained ventricular tachycardia has been seen in patients with repaired tetralogy of Fallot as a manifestation of hemodynamic problems requiring repair, as a reflection of right ventricular dilation and dysfunction, and in relation to ventricular scarring.

SUDDEN DEATH. In contrast to adults, children seldom die suddenly and unexpectedly of cardiovascular disease. Nonetheless, sudden death has been reported with arrhythmias, aortic stenosis, hypertrophic obstructive cardiomyopathy, primary pulmonary hypertension, Eisenmenger syndrome, myocarditis, congenital complete heart block, and primary endocardial fibroelastosis and when there are certain anomalies of the coronary arteries. Sudden death is more frequent in older patients with postoperative heart disease, particularly after atrial switch procedures and repair of tetralogy of Fallot.

ATRIOVENTRICULAR BLOCK. First-degree AV block is commonly seen in patients with AV septal defects, Ebstein anomaly, complete TGA (D-TGA), and in the older ASD patient. Complete heart block may develop spontaneously in patients with cc-TGA and may develop postoperatively in these and other patients. When pacing is required, epicardial leads are usually placed in cyanotic patients. Many adult patients with CHD are prone to problems of vascular access because of prior surgeries and pacing leads.

Infective Endocarditis (see Chap. 67)

Infective endocarditis complicating CHD is uncommon before 2 years of age, except in the immediate postoperative period. Recent guidelines for endocarditis prophylaxis have substantially altered clinical practice.[23,24] Maintenance of excellent oral hygiene is encouraged most strongly. Antibiotic prophylaxis before dental procedures is recommended for patients with prosthetic heart valves or prosthetic material used for cardiac valve repair; for patients with a prior history of infective endocarditis, persistently cyanotic CHD, or residual defects that are adjacent to a prosthetic patch or prosthetic device; for the first 6 months after placement of prosthetic material or device for CHD; and for cardiac transplant recipients who develop cardiac valvulopathy.

Chest Pain (see Chap. 53)

Angina pectoris is an uncommon symptom of cardiac disease in young infants and children, although it probably explains the irritability and crying during or after feeding in babies with coronary ischemia resulting from anomalous origin of the coronary artery from the pulmonary artery. In older children and young adults with severe left or right ventricular outflow tract obstruction and pulmonary hypertension, chest pain commonly occurs with or follows effort and may be identical to effort angina of coronary artery disease in older adults. A sensation of chest discomfort or cardiac awareness is frequently interpreted as pain by the parents of children with cardiac arrhythmias. Careful questioning serves to identify palpitations rather than pain as the symptom and often elicits an additional history of anxiety, pallor, and sweating. Pain caused by pericarditis is commonly of acute onset and associated with fever, and it can be identified by specific physical, radiographic, and echocardiographic findings. Most commonly, late postoperative chest pain is musculoskeletal in origin and may be reproduced on upper extremity movement or by palpation. Finally, children and adults may suffer chest pain of nonspecific form as a result of anxiety, with or without hyperventilation.

Syndromes in Congenital Heart Disease

ALCAPA SYNDROME. The acronym stands for *a*nomalous *l*eft *c*oronary *a*rtery *a*rising from the *p*ulmonary *a*rtery. It is also called Bland-White-Garland syndrome.

ALAGILLE SYNDROME. This is a hereditary syndrome consisting of intrahepatic cholestasis, characteristic facies, butterfly-like vertebral anomalies, and varying degrees of peripheral pulmonary artery stenoses or diffuse hypoplasia of the pulmonary artery and its branches. It is associated with a deletion in chromosome 20p.

DIGEORGE SYNDROME. This syndrome is caused by a microdeletion at chromosome 22q11, resulting in a wide clinical spectrum. It was previously referred to as CATCH 22 syndrome, with CATCH standing for *c*ardiac defect, *a*bnormal facies, *t*hymic hypoplasia, *c*left palate, and *h*ypocalcemia. Cardiac defects include conotruncal defects such as interrupted aortic arch, tetralogy of Fallot, truncus arteriosus, and double-outlet right ventricle. This umbrella grouping also encompasses patients with velocardiofacial syndrome.

CHARGE ASSOCIATION. This anomaly is characterized by the presence of coloboma or choanal atresia and three of the following defects: CHD, nervous system anomaly or mental retardation, genital abnormalities, ear abnormality, or deafness. Congenital heart defects seen in the CHARGE association are tetralogy of Fallot with or without other cardiac defects, AV septal defect, double-outlet right ventricle, double-inlet left ventricle, TGA, interrupted aortic arch, and others.

DOWN SYNDROME. This is the most common genetic malformation and is caused by trisomy 21. Most of the patients (95%) have complete trisomy of chromosome 21; some have translocation or mosaic forms. The phenotype is diagnostic (short stature, characteristic facial appearance, mental retardation, brachydactyly, atlantoaxial instability, and thyroid and white blood cell disorders). Congenital heart defects are frequent (40%), with AV septal defect, VSD, and PDA being the most common. Patients with Down syndrome are prone to earlier and more severe pulmonary vascular disease than otherwise expected as a result of the lesions identified. Hypothyroidism is common in later life, and patients should be screened intermittently.

ELLIS–VAN CREVELD SYNDROME. This is an autosomal recessive syndrome in which common atrium, primum ASD, and partial AV septal defects are the most common cardiac lesions.

HOLT-ORAM SYNDROME. This is an autosomal dominant syndrome consisting of radial abnormalities of the forearm and hand associated with secundum ASD (most common), VSD, or, rarely, other cardiac malformations.

LEOPARD SYNDROME. This autosomal dominant condition is a close cousin of Noonan syndrome and shares a similar genetic substrate (deletion of the *PTPN11* gene). It includes *l*entigines, *e*lectrocardiographic abnormalities, *o*cular hypertelorism, *p*ulmonary stenosis, *a*bnormal genitalia, *r*etardation of growth, and *d*eafness. Rarely, cardiomyopathy or complex CHD may be present.

NOONAN SYNDROME. This is an autosomal dominant syndrome, phenotypically somewhat similar to Turner syndrome but with a normal chromosomal complement. Noonan syndrome is associated with congenital cardiac anomalies, especially dysplastic pulmonary valve stenosis, pulmonary artery stenosis, and ASD. Hypertrophic cardiomyopathy is less common. Congenital lymphedema is a commonly associated anomaly that may be unrecognized.

RUBELLA SYNDROME. This is a wide spectrum of malformations caused by rubella infection early in pregnancy, including cataracts, retinopathy, deafness, CHD, bone lesions, and mental retardation. The spectrum of congenital heart lesions is wide and includes pulmonary artery stenosis, PDA, tetralogy of Fallot, and VSD.

SCIMITAR SYNDROME. This is a constellation of anomalies including total or partial anomalous pulmonary venous connection (PAPVC) of the right lung to the inferior vena cava, often associated with hypoplasia of the right lung and right pulmonary artery. The lower portion of the right lung (sequestered lobe) tends to receive its arterial supply from the abdominal aorta. The name of the syndrome derives from the appearance on the posteroanterior chest radiograph of the shadow formed by the anomalous pulmonary venous connection that resembles a Turkish sword or scimitar (see Fig. 18-19).

SHONE COMPLEX (SYNDROME). This is an association of multiple levels of left ventricular inflow and outflow obstruction (subvalvular and valvular left ventricular outflow tract obstruction, coarctation of the aorta, and mitral stenosis [parachute mitral valve and supramitral ring]).

TURNER SYNDROME. This is a clinical syndrome due to the 45 XO karyotype in about 50% of cases, with various other X chromosome abnormalities in the remainder. There is a characteristic but variable phenotype and an association with congenital cardiac anomalies, especially postductal coarctation of the aorta and other left-sided obstructive lesions, as well as PAPVC without ASD. The female phenotype varies with the age at presentation and is somewhat similar to that of Noonan syndrome.

WILLIAMS SYNDROME. This is a congenital syndrome frequently associated with inherited or sporadic mutations of 7q11.23. It is associated with intellectual deficit, infantile hypercalcemia, characteristic phenotype, and CHD, especially supravalvular aortic stenosis and multiple peripheral pulmonary stenoses. An identical vascular phenotype is sometimes seen in otherwise phenotypically and intellectually normal families.

Evaluation of the Patient with Congenital Heart Disease

Physical Examination

Although the advances in technology have profoundly improved our diagnostic abilities, there is still a role for detailed clinical examination in the assessment and follow-up of patients with unrepaired, palliated, and repaired CHD. The relevant findings pertaining to specific abnormalities are outlined in the appropriate sections that follow, but some general principles bear consideration (see Chap. 12).

PHYSICAL ASSESSMENT. The presence of characteristic facial or somatic features of an underlying syndrome may be a strong clue to the type of heart disease (e.g., Williams, Noonan, Down) at any age. Central cyanosis can be difficult to diagnose clinically when it is mild but should be actively excluded by oximetry in any patient with suspected CHD. One should assess both cardiac and visceral situs and not assume that the heart will be left sided. Careful surveillance of the chest wall for scars is also important in older patients and adults, who do not always know or report the type and sequence of their surgical interventions. The thin chest wall of children and many young adults with CHD assists the detection of chamber enlargement by palpation as well as the detection of systolic or diastolic thrills.

The infant or child with hemodynamically significant heart disease may show signs of failure to thrive (underweight, small, or both). The weight and height should therefore be plotted sequentially against normal growth curves appropriate to race, sex, and underlying syndrome (e.g., Down syndrome growth chart). The manifestations of "heart failure" vary with age and the underlying problem. In children, peripheral edema is rare, but intercostal recession, nasal flaring, and grunting with respiration are signs of congestive heart failure. In small children, an excellent barometer of cardiac function is liver size and pulsatility, reflecting right atrial pressure, right ventricular filling time, and diastolic dysfunction or tricuspid regurgitation. The jugular venous pressure is difficult to assess in young children but is a fundamental part of the examination of the older child, teenager, and adult.

Examination of the upper and lower limb peripheral pulses is important at any age. Delay, absence, or reduction of a pulse is an important clue to the presence of arterial obstruction and its site. The left brachial pulse is often compromised by surgery for coarctation, and blood pressure measurements should not be taken in only the left arm. Similarly, other palliative procedures (Blalock-Taussig shunt, interposition grafts) may affect either or both upper limb pulses. Assessment of the femoral and carotid pulses in addition to the upper limb pulses is important in such patients. Just as in acquired disease, the pulse volume and character also provide important information about the severity of obstructive or regurgitant left-sided heart disease. A low-volume pulse (usually with a narrow pulse pressure) reflects a low cardiac output. Pulsus alternans signifies severe systemic ventricular dysfunction. Pulsus paradoxus points to cardiac tamponade. In adolescents and adults, the jugular venous pressure examination is often important. It may indicate cardiac decompensation, cardiac chamber hypertrophy or restriction, valvular regurgitation or stenosis, arrhythmia or conduction disturbance, cardiac tamponade, pericardial constriction, and other phenomena.

AUSCULTATION. The rules of auscultation also follow those developed for acquired heart disease. However, cardiac and vascular malposition may significantly affect the appreciation of heart sounds and murmurs. For example, in TGA treated by an atrial switch procedure, the aorta remains anterior to the pulmonary artery. Consequently, the aortic component of the second sound can be exceptionally loud, and the pulmonary component may be virtually inaudible, making it difficult to estimate the pulmonary artery pressure clinically under such circumstances. Conversely, when there is a valved conduit between the right ventricle and pulmonary artery, the pulmonary closure sound may be extremely loud, even though the pulmonary artery diastolic pressure is low. This is because the conduit is frequently adherent to the chest wall, assisting sound transmission to the stethoscope placed close to it. Calcification of semilunar valves is relatively unusual in childhood and early adult life, making the differentiation of valve stenosis from subvalve or supravalve narrowing, by the presence of an ejection click, more precise in these patients. The differentiation of multiple murmurs is sometimes a challenge. Systolic or diastolic murmurs in an individual may have several causes, and supplementary clinical information may be required to establish their significance in some cases. Auscultation over the entire anterior and posterior chest wall is important. The continuous murmurs of aorto-aortic collateral arteries in coarctation may be audible only between the shoulder blades posteriorly, for example; similarly, a localized distal pulmonary artery stenosis or an aortopulmonary collateral artery may be detected only in a localized area of the chest wall, particularly in adults.

Electrocardiography

The electrocardiogram (ECG; see Chap. 13) remains an important tool in the assessment of CHD. Heart rhythm and rate as well as AV conduction can be evaluated. The dominant theme that runs through ECGs in CHD is the prevalence of right-sided heart disease. This often takes the form of right-axis deviation along with right atrial and right ventricular hypertrophy. Right ventricular hypertrophy may reflect pulmonary hypertension, right ventricular outflow tract obstruction, or a subaortic right ventricle. Incomplete right bundle branch block often indicates right ventricular hypertrophy due to pressure (e.g., pulmonary hypertension or pulmonary stenosis) or volume (e.g., ASD) overload. Right ventricular volume overload is likely when the r' in V_1 is less than 7 mm. Very wide QRS complexes should be seen as possible manifestations of dilated and dysfunctional ventricles, most specifically in patients with repaired tetralogy, complete right bundle branch block, and severe pulmonary regurgitation. The ECG may be uninterpretable in patients with abnormal cardiac or visceral situs unless it is clear where the leads were placed.

Atrial flutter (often in an atypical form, so-called intra-atrial reentrant tachycardia) is much more common in young patients than is atrial fibrillation. First-degree block is often seen in AV septal defects, cc-TGA, and Ebstein anomaly. Complete heart block is most often seen in patients with cc-TGA as well as in those with older VSD repairs.

Left atrial overload may reflect increased pulmonary blood flow as well as AV valve dysfunction and myocardial failure. Left-axis deviation should make one think of AV septal defect, a univentricular heart, and a hypoplastic right ventricle. Deep Q waves in the left chest leads can be caused by left ventricular volume overload in a young person with aortic or mitral regurgitation. Pathologic Q waves can be evidence of the anomalous origin of the left coronary from the pulmonary artery.

Chest Radiography

The chest radiograph (see Chap. 16) is another valuable tool for the discerning physician caring for patients with congenital heart defects. Although more recent technologies have rightly attracted much attention, there is value in learning how to interpret the chest radiograph. Some teaching points can be made that may anchor the interpretation of chest radiographs of some CHD patients. The following sections provide a number of clinical and radiographic differential diagnoses.

CRITERIA FOR SHUNT VASCULARITY (see Fig. 16-14). These include (1) uniformly distributed vascular markings with absence of the normal lower lobe vascular predominance, (2) right descending pulmonary artery diameter that exceeds 17 mm, and (3) pulmonary artery branch that is larger than its accompanying bronchus (best noted in the right parahilar area). Prominent vascularity is apparent only if the pulmonary-to-systemic flow ratio is greater than 1.5 : 1. As a rule, cardiac enlargement usually implies a shunt greater than 2.5:1. Anemia, pregnancy, thyrotoxicosis, and a pulmonary AV fistula may mimic shunt vascularity.

CYANOTIC PATIENTS WITH SHUNT VASCULARITY. This group includes single ventricle with transposition, persistent truncus arteriosus, tricuspid atresia without significant pulmonary outflow obstruction, total anomalous pulmonary venous connection, double-outlet right ventricle, and a common atrium.

CYANOTIC PATIENTS WITH A VSD AND NORMAL OR DECREASED PULMONARY VASCULARITY. This group includes tetralogy of Fallot, tricuspid atresia with pulmonary stenosis, single ventricle and pulmonary stenosis, D-TGA with pulmonary stenosis, cc-TGA with pulmonary stenosis, double-outlet right ventricle with pulmonary stenosis, pulmonary atresia, and asplenia syndrome.

CAUSES OF RETROSTERNAL FILLING ON LATERAL CHEST RADIOGRAPH. These include right ventricular dilation, TGA, ascending aortic aneurysm, and noncardiovascular masses (e.g., lymphoma, thymoma, teratoma, thyroid).

CAUSES OF A STRAIGHT LEFT-SIDED HEART BORDER. These include right ventricular dilation, left atrial dilation, cc-TGA, pericardial effusion, Ebstein anomaly, and congenital absence of the left pericardium.

CARDIOVASCULAR DISEASES ASSOCIATED WITH SCOLIOSIS. These include cyanotic CHD, Eisenmenger syndrome, Marfan syndrome, and occasionally mitral prolapse.

CAUSES OF LARGE CENTRAL PULMONARY ARTERIES. These include increased pulmonary flow (main pulmonary artery and branches), increased pulmonary pressure (main pulmonary artery and branches), pulmonary stenosis (main and left pulmonary artery), and idiopathic dilation of the pulmonary artery (main pulmonary artery).

SITUS SOLITUS WITH CARDIAC DEXTROVERSION. Situs solitus with cardiac dextroversion is associated with CHD in more than 90% of cases. Up to 80% have a congenitally corrected transposition with a high incidence of associated VSD, pulmonary stenosis, and tricuspid atresia. Situs inversus with dextrocardia carries a low incidence of CHD, whereas situs inversus with levocardia is virtually always associated with severe CHD.

Cardiovascular Magnetic Resonance Imaging

CMR (see Chap. 18) in adolescents and adults with CHD has become of ever-increasing importance in the past decade. CMR can circumvent the echocardiographic problem of suboptimal visualization of the heart in adult patients, especially those who have had surgery. This technique can now generate information never previously available and do so more easily and more accurately than by other means. New magnetic resonance image acquisition methods are faster and provide improved temporal and spatial resolution. Major advances in hardware design, new pulse sequences, and faster image reconstruction techniques now permit rapid high-resolution imaging of complex cardiovascular anatomy. CMR can produce quantitative measures of ventricular volumes, mass, and ejection fraction. CMR can quantify blood flow in any vessel.

CMR is of particular value when transthoracic echocardiography cannot provide the needed diagnostic information; as an alternative to diagnostic cardiac catheterization; and for its unique capabilities, such as tissue imaging, myocardial tagging, and vessel-specific flow quantification. The value of CMR over echocardiography in the evaluation of the right ventricle is becoming increasingly appreciated. The capability of CMR to assess the right ventricle is of great importance because the right ventricle is a key component of many of the more complex CHD lesions. In addition, CMR can evaluate valve regurgitation, postoperative systemic and pulmonary venous pathways, Fontan pathways, and the great vessels. CMR should be considered the main imaging modality in adolescents and adults with repaired tetralogy of Fallot, TGA, Fontan procedure, and diseases of the aorta. In the near future, we will see real-time CMR to allow magnetic resonance–guided interventional procedures and molecular imaging that will further expand the capabilities of CMR.

Transthoracic Echocardiography (see Chap. 15)

FETAL ECHOCARDIOGRAPHY

General Considerations

Fetal echocardiography has graduated from being a special area of interest to some pediatric cardiologists to one of standard care. As early as 16 weeks' gestation, excellent images of the fetal cardiac structures can be obtained by the transabdominal route, along with an appreciation of cardiac and placental physiology through the use of Doppler technology. Transvaginal ultrasound is a newer approach that permits the echocardiographer to obtain images at approximately 13 to 14 weeks' gestation. Data are beginning to emerge as to the benefit of this approach, although current opinion would support a follow-up cardiac screen at 18 weeks' gestation. Although it has some application for cases with a higher risk of recurrent CHD (e.g., obstructive left-sided lesions), its accuracy has yet to be determined. This is in part due to the limited number of views that are possible because of a relatively fixed position of the transducer. Although there are specific indications for fetal echocardiographic scanning, the highest number of cases arise from anatomic or functional abnormalities detected at routine obstetric screening. A routine anatomic screen has become a standard of care in many obstetric practices throughout the world. As a result, there has been a tremendous push by pediatric fetal echocardiographers to improve the standard of routine screening of the prenatal heart. A rapid rise has occurred in the number of abnormalities that are detected by general obstetric ultrasonographers and subsequently referred in a timely manner to the pediatric cardiologist and echocardiographer. Nevertheless, the routine detection rate in unselected populations is still less than 50%.

Impact of Fetal Echocardiography

Most major structural congenital heart defects are now accurately categorized through fetal echocardiography. Once the abnormalities are identified, families and obstetric caregivers can be counseled as to the impact of the abnormality on both the fetus and the family. Decisions appropriate to the individual family and fetus can then be made. Although termination of pregnancy is one of the consequences of prenatal diagnosis, it is not the main objective. In fact, data are starting to appear in the literature indicating that prenatal diagnosis of some major cardiac malformations has a direct impact on outcome, from a survival, morbidity, and cost standpoint. This is in part due to the fact that when a prenatal diagnosis is made, subsequent caregivers are prepared for the immediate postnatal effects of the defect. For example, in hypoplastic left heart syndrome and other duct-dependent lesions, prostaglandin E_1 can be started immediately after birth, in a hospital within or attached to a pediatric cardiology facility.

Fetal echocardiography has also permitted an improved understanding of the evolution of certain congenital cardiac malformations. For example, although the fetal heart is fully formed by the time a prenatal scan is performed, tremendous growth of the cardiac structures still must occur. Therefore, in some circumstances, a cardiac chamber that may appear only mildly hypoplastic at 16 weeks' gestation may be profoundly affected at the time of birth. This has a major impact on the management of the newborn as well as on the counseling process at 16 weeks' gestation.

Direct Fetal Intervention

The next step is direct intervention for specific cardiac lesions. This has initially involved obstructive lesions, thus far mainly being limited to the left ventricle.[25] The rationale behind this therapy is based on the notion that the relief of obstructive outflow tract lesions will permit growth of the affected ventricle, potentially changing a neonatal pathway from univentricular to biventricular. Cardiac surgery to the fetus is also a future option, and indeed there is already a considerable amount of research on the impact of this in fetal animal models.

SEGMENTAL APPROACH TO ECHOCARDIOGRAPHY IN CONGENITAL HEART DISEASE. The following four echocardiographic steps of segmental analysis are crucial in any patient with CHD. Starting from a standard subcostal view, one should determine the position of the apex, the situs of the atria, and the atrioventricular and ventriculo-arterial relationships.

1. *Apex position.* From a standard subcostal view, determine if the apex of the heart is pointing to the right (dextrocardia), to the left (levocardia), or to the middle (mesocardia).

2. *Situs of the atria* (**Fig. 65-2**). The right and left atria differ morphologically with regard to their appendages. A morphologic right atrium has a broad right atrial appendage, whereas a morphologic left atrium has a narrow left atrial appendage. Right and left atrial appendages, however, are difficult to visualize by transthoracic echocardiography, and one often has to rely on abdominal situs to determine the atrial situs. Atrial situs follows abdominal situs in about 70% to 80% of the cases. From a standard subcostal view with the probe pointing at a right angle to the spine, one can visualize the abdominal aorta as well as the inferior vena cava and the spine at the back. When the aorta is to the left of the spine and the inferior vena cava to the right of the spine, there is abdominal situs solitus and, in all probability, corresponding atrial situs solitus (meaning the morphologic right atrium is on the right side and the morphologic left atrium is on the left side). When the aorta is to the right of the spine and the inferior vena cava is to the left of the spine, there is abdominal situs inversus and, in all probability, corresponding atrial situs inversus (morphologic right atrium on the left side and morphologic left atrium on the right side). When both the aorta and inferior vena cava are to the left of the spine, there is abdominal and atrial left isomerism (two morphologic left atria). When both the aorta and inferior vena cava are to the right of the spine, there is abdominal and atrial right isomerism (two morphologic right atria).

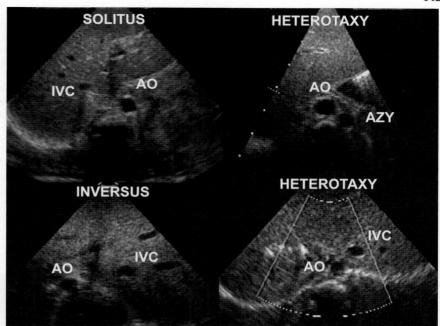

FIGURE 65-2 Montage of the different types of situs as seen by a subcostal echocardiographic scan. Note that situs solitus and inversus are just the mirror image of each other. The upper right picture is in the setting of heterotaxy with an interrupted intrahepatic inferior vena cava, with azygos continuation on the left. This is seen more frequently in left atrial isomerism. The lower right picture is also in the setting of heterotaxy with an intrahepatic inferior vena cava that is positioned closer to the aorta than in solitus or inversus. Note also the midline liver. This pattern is seen more commonly in right atrial isomerism. AO = aorta; AZY = azygos; IVC = inferior vena cava.

3. *Atrioventricular relationship.* Once the situs of the atria is determined, one must assess the position of the ventricles in relation to the atria. The morphologic right ventricle has four characteristic features that distinguish it from the morphologic left ventricle: a trabeculated apex, a moderator band, a septal attachment of the tricuspid valve, and a lower (apical) insertion of the tricuspid valve. The tricuspid valve is always attached to the morphologic right ventricle. The morphologic left ventricle has the following characteristics: a smooth apex, no moderator band, no septal attachment of the mitral valve, and a higher (basal) insertion of the mitral valve. The mitral valve is always attached to the morphologic left ventricle. Once the position of the ventricles is determined, one can then establish the AV relationship. When the morphologic right atrium empties into the morphologic right ventricle and the morphologic left atrium empties into the morphologic left ventricle, there is AV concordance. When the morphologic right atrium empties into the morphologic left ventricle and the morphologic left atrium empties into the morphologic right ventricle, there is AV discordance. When both atria predominantly empty into one ventricle (right or left), the AV connection is called a double-inlet.

4. *Ventriculoarterial relationship.* Once the AV relationship has been determined, one should assess the position of the great arteries in relation to the ventricles. The pulmonary artery can be distinguished by its early branching pattern into the left and right pulmonary arteries; the pulmonary valve is always attached to the pulmonary artery. Similarly, the aorta can be distinguished by its "candy cane" shape and the takeoff of its three head and neck vessels (innominate, carotid, and subclavian arteries). The aortic valve is always attached to the aorta. Once the position of the great arteries is determined, one can then establish the ventriculoarterial relationship. When the morphologic right ventricle ejects into the pulmonary artery and the morphologic left ventricle ejects into the aorta, there is ventriculoarterial concordance. When the morphologic right ventricle ejects into the aorta and the morphologic left ventricle ejects into the pulmonary artery, there is ventriculoarterial

discordance. When more than 50% of both great arteries exit from one ventricle (right or left), this is called a double-outlet (right or left) ventricle.

Once segmental analysis has been completed, one can then proceed to the usual echocardiographic windows to determine the nature of the specific lesions as well as their hemodynamic relevance.

ECHOCARDIOGRAPHY IN THE NEONATE AND INFANT. Echocardiography is of immense value in differentiating between heart disease and lung disease in newborns. Indeed, it has become the standard for the diagnosis of virtually all cardiovascular malformations. Most neonates and infants needing intervention are now referred directly after ultrasound study for repair, without intervening cardiac catheterization. It is simpler to list those lesions for which it cannot be used as the sole mode of investigation before a management decision is made. For example, in pulmonary atresia and VSD with multiple aortopulmonary collaterals, echocardiography is used as an adjunct to angiocardiography. Echocardiography provides details about the intracardiac disease, whereas angiocardiography is necessary to delineate the sources of pulmonary blood supply. In pulmonary atresia with intact ventricular septum, the presence or absence of a right ventricle–dependent coronary circulation is best assessed by angiocardiography. Apart from these two lesions, there are few other preoperative decisions that cannot be made by echocardiography alone in the newborn and infant. Postoperative management is different, particularly for those defects that are on a Fontan track, when precise hemodynamic measurements are of key importance in the decision process.

Transesophageal echocardiography (TEE) is usually unnecessary for the preoperative evaluation of the neonate or infant with heart disease. This technique has now become a standard in the immediate postoperative period for the evaluation of residual anatomic or functional abnormalities. Newer techniques, such as tissue Doppler and three-dimensional echocardiography, are being applied to this age group and will be used more widely in the future.

ECHOCARDIOGRAPHY IN THE OLDER CHILD AND ADOLES-CENT. This technique still plays a key role in the diagnosis and follow-up of the older child and adolescent with congenital or acquired heart disease. Because many of the patients underwent surgery in the neonatal or infant period, they often have suboptimal ultrasound windows that necessitate other modes of investigation, especially magnetic resonance angiography. The application of newer technologies, such as tissue Doppler and three-dimensional echocardiography, is already possible in this population and provides additional information that has thus far not been obtainable from standard techniques. For example, force-frequency relationships have been obtained in postoperative patients to try to predict optimal heart rates for maintaining maximum cardiac efficiency. On the other hand, three-dimensional echocardiography can provide new insights into congenital and acquired heart disease[26] that have not been possible from standard two-dimensional techniques. Despite the new information from this technique, it is still limited by the quality of the transthoracic window, which is more of a problem in the older and previously repaired patient. This limitation has been partially overcome by the recent introduction of a real-time three-dimensional TEE matrix array probe, which can be used in children with a weight of >16 to 18 kg (**Fig. 65-3**).

ECHOCARDIOGRAPHY IN THE ADULT. Advances in cardiac ultrasonography now allow comprehensive noninvasive assessment of cardiovascular structure and function in adults with CHD. Because of its widespread availability, easy use, and quick interpretation, transthoracic echocardiography remains the technique of choice for the initial diagnosis and for follow-up in adults with CHD. The general initial approach to the diagnosis of CHD by transthoracic echocardiography starts with a segmental approach to ascertain the relative position of the various cardiac chambers. Once the segmental approach has been completed, a more lesion-specific approach can then be carried out, as discussed in the individual lesion sections.

Transesophageal Echocardiography

DIAGNOSTIC ASSESSMENT. TEE offers a better two-dimensional resolution than transthoracic echocardiography. This is especially important in adult patients with multiple previous cardiac operations, when adequate transthoracic windows are often difficult to obtain.

TEE should be used whenever transthoracic echocardiography does not provide adequate two-dimensional, color, or Doppler information. The addition of real-time three-dimensional TEE has opened up a new window in this age group.[13] TEE should be considered in the setting of the conditions discussed in the following sections.

SECUNDUM ATRIAL SEPTAL DEFECT. Use TEE for assessment of device closure feasibility, measurement of ASD size, assessment of adequacy of margins for device anchoring, and ruling out of anomalous pulmonary venous connection. This information can be enhanced by real-time three-dimensional imaging, which provides precise anatomic detail of the ASD.

MITRAL REGURGITATION. Use TEE for preoperative evaluation of mitral valve leaflet morphology and suitability for mitral valve repair versus replacement. Real-time three-dimensional TEE is rapidly becoming the reference standard for evaluation of mitral valve form and function before surgical or catheter intervention.[13]

EBSTEIN ANOMALY. Use TEE for preoperative assessment of tricuspid valve morphology and the potential for tricuspid valve repair.

FONTAN. Use TEE when a right atrial clot is suspected on clinical grounds or by transthoracic echocardiography or when circuit obstruction is suspected.

BEFORE CARDIOVERSION. For any patient who is not anticoagulated, presenting with atrial flutter or fibrillation longer than 24 hours, TEE should be performed before chemical or electrical cardioversion. Patients with a Fontan

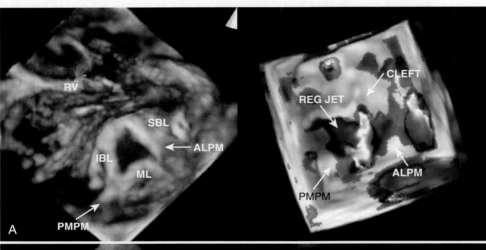

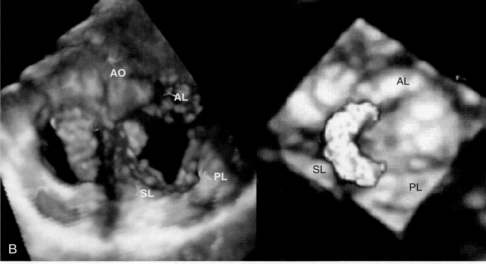

FIGURE 65-3 A, This montage is from a child with an atrioventricular septal defect with left atrioventricular valve regurgitation. This was acquired by real-time three-dimensional echocardiography from the transthoracic approach. The valve is viewed from beneath and the three leaflets that constitute the left atrioventricular valve can be clearly identified. The image on the right, also viewed from below, demonstrates the left atrioventricular valve regurgitation that originates at the cleft, directed toward the inferior bridging leaflet and mural leaflet commissure. ALPM = anterolateral papillary muscle; IBL = inferior bridging leaflet; ML = mural leaflet; PMPM = posteromedial papillary muscle; RV = right ventricle; SBL = superior bridging leaflet. **B,** These images were obtained with the real-time transesophageal three-dimensional probe in an adolescent. They demonstrate the tricuspid valve, as seen from above in a surgical view, with evidence of a cleft in the septal leaflet, which is the site of regurgitation seen in the right-hand image. Note the detail with the regurgitation involving the coaptation of the whole septal leaflet. AO = aorta; AL = anterior leaflet; PL = posterior leaflet; SL = septal leaflet.

circuit should undergo TEE irrespective of the duration of atrial tachyarrhythmia to rule out a right or left atrial thrombus.

GUIDANCE OF THERAPEUTIC INTERVENTION. Both standard two-dimensional TEE and, more recently, real-time three-dimensional TEE can be instrumental in helping guide therapy at the time of transcatheter or surgical procedures. TEE is particularly helpful in the following situations.

PERCUTANEOUS DEVICE CLOSURE. TEE is performed at the time of transcatheter ASD closure to assist ASD stretched balloon sizing and device deployment, unless intracardiac echocardiography (see later) is available.

INTRAOPERATIVE AND POSTOPERATIVE ASSESSMENT. TEE is often required for the intraoperative and postoperative assessment of the adult patient undergoing congenital cardiac surgery. It has a particular role in the intraoperative assessment of adequacy of valve repair. A TEE service by an experienced echocardiographer is an essential requirement for centers performing adult congenital cardiac surgery.

Three-Dimensional Echocardiography

DIAGNOSTIC ASSESSMENT. Three-dimensional echocardiography has advanced from the research arena to a clinical tool with the advent of transthoracic and transesophageal real-time systems.[13] Although much of it still depends on an adequate transthoracic window, this is readily overcome in the adult population through the application of real-time three-dimensional TEE techniques. Indeed, for mitral valve assessment, this technique has already established itself as the standard before intervention (**Fig. 65-4**).[14] In addition, this technique can be used to improve the accuracy of left ventricular volume calculation by echocardiography.[27,28]

Intracardiac Echocardiography

Intracardiac echocardiography (ICE) uses lower frequency transducers that have been miniaturized and mounted into catheters capable of percutaneous insertion into the heart.[29] ICE not only provides high-resolution two-dimensional and hemodynamic data with full Doppler capabilities but also eliminates the need for general anesthesia, which is often required for TEE.

CURRENT APPLICATIONS

PERCUTANEOUS ASD DEVICE CLOSURE. ICE supports percutaneous ASD device closure by adequately sizing the defect and assisting device positioning while avoiding the need for general anesthesia. More recently, real-time three-dimensional TEE is being used not only to assess the size and suitability for ASD device closure but to monitor the procedure, either in an interventional setting or surgically by use of robotic procedures.[30]

ELECTROPHYSIOLOGIC STUDIES. ICE assists electrophysiologic procedures by guiding transseptal puncture, enabling endocardial visualization, and ensuring electrode-tissue contact at the time of ablative procedures. More recently, a forward-looking imaging and ablation probe has been developed, which would enable precise localization of energy delivery to an arrhythmogenic focus[31] (see Chap. 36).

Cardiac Catheterization

With the development of cross-sectional echocardiography and the subsequent introduction of CMR and fast computed tomography (CT) methods, truly diagnostic cardiac catheterization (see Chap. 20) is becoming a thing of the past for both children and adults. "Diagnostic" catheterization is reserved for resolving unanswered questions from the less-invasive techniques and measuring hemodynamics. A good example of this is the assessment of major aortopulmonary collateral arteries in tetralogy of Fallot with pulmonary atresia; their presence and distribution may be shown beautifully by magnetic resonance angiography, but cardiac catheterization may be required to demonstrate the presence of communications with the central pulmonary arteries and to measure the pressure within them. There is no adequate substitute for cardiac catheterization to measure ventricular end-diastolic pressures or pulmonary artery pressures and resistance with the precision required to plan for or to assess the Fontan circulation. Furthermore, diagnostic testing may also be needed to evaluate possible coronary artery disease, especially before heart surgery in the adult.

THERAPEUTIC CATHETERIZATION. Balloon atrial septostomy was the first catheter intervention that proved useful in treating heart disease, and it remains the standard initial palliation in many infants with D-TGA. Many transcatheter techniques are now used successfully to treat CHD: blade atrial septostomy; device or coil closure of PDA; closure of ASD and patent foramen ovale; transluminal balloon dilation of pulmonary and aortic valve stenosis; radiofrequency perforation of pulmonary valve atresia; balloon-expandable intravascular stents for right ventricular outflow tract, pulmonary artery, aortic coarctation, and other vascular stenoses; and device occlusion of unwanted collateral vessels and AV fistulas. These have all become treatments of choice in centers with these capabilities. Some are universally accepted as the standard of care (e.g., balloon pulmonary valvuloplasty), whereas debate continues for other interventions (e.g., unrepaired coarctation). One of the most exciting recent developments has been that of transcatheter valved stents for the treatment of right ventricular outflow stenosis and regurgitation in patients with congenital defects, which has led to an explosion of transcatheter valve techniques for acquired disease.

Going along with the extraordinary expansion of interventional techniques for the treatment of structural abnormalities, ablative techniques for the treatment of tachycardias are now performed routinely in centers with congenital heart electrophysiology programs and are crucial to the management of the adult with repaired and unrepaired CHD, in whom arrhythmias are such a burden in terms of their morbidity as well as a significant cause of late mortality.

The indications, outcomes, and current status of each of these techniques are discussed in detail in the sections concerning specific lesions.

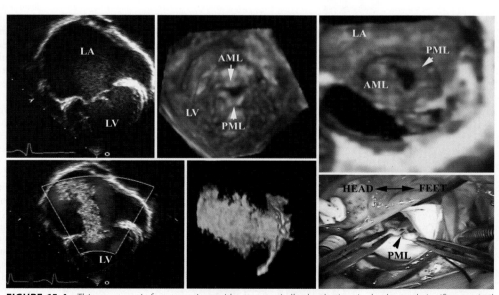

FIGURE 65-4 This montage is from a patient with a congenitally dysplastic mitral valve and significant mitral valve regurgitation. The two left-hand images show the transthoracic four-chamber view during systole. Note the large central jet of regurgitation. The upper middle panel is a real-time three-dimensional image of the mitral valve as seen from below. Note the tethered posterior leaflet. The lower middle panel shows the three-dimensional regurgitant jet. The upper right-hand panel views the mitral valve from above. Note the poor coaptation of the two leaflets. The lower right-hand panel is the surgical view of the valve that demonstrates the tethering of the posterior leaflet. AML = anterior mitral leaflet; LA = left atrium; LV = left ventricle; PML = posterior mitral leaflet.

Specific Cardiac Defects

Left-to-Right Shunts

Atrial Septal Defect

MORPHOLOGY. Four types of ASDs or interatrial communications exist: ostium primum, ostium secundum, sinus venosus, and coronary sinus defects (**Fig. 65-5**). (Ostium primum is discussed in the section on AV septal defect.) Ostium secundum defects occur from either excessive resorption of the septum primum or deficient growth of the septum secundum and are occasionally associated with anomalous pulmonary venous connection (<10%). Sinus venosus defects of the superior vena cava type occur at the cardiac junction of the superior vena cava, giving rise to a superior vena cava connected to both atria, and are almost always associated with anomalous pulmonary venous connection (right » left). Sinus venosus–inferior vena cava defects are very uncommon and abut the junction of the inferior vena cava, inferior to the fossa ovalis. Coronary sinus septal defects are rare and

arise from an opening of its wall with the left atrium, allowing left-to-right atrial shunting.

PATHOPHYSIOLOGY. In any type of ASD, the degree of left-to-right atrial shunting depends on the size of the defect and the relative diastolic filling properties of the two ventricles. Any condition causing reduced left ventricular compliance (e.g., systemic hypertension, cardiomyopathy, myocardial infarction) or increased left atrial pressure (mitral stenosis or regurgitation) tends to increase the left-to-right shunt. If similar forces are present in the right side of the heart, this will diminish the left-to-right shunt and promote right-to-left shunting.

NATURAL HISTORY. A large ASD (pulmonary artery blood flow relative to systemic blood flow [Q_p/Q_s] > 2.0:1.0) may cause congestive heart failure and failure to thrive in an infant or child. An undetected ASD with a significant shunt (Q_p/Q_s > 1.5:1.0) probably causes symptoms over time in adolescence or adulthood, and symptomatic patients usually become progressively more physically limited as they age. Effort dyspnea is seen in about 30% of patients by the third decade and in more than 75% of patients by the fifth decade. Supraventricular arrhythmias (atrial fibrillation or flutter) and right-sided heart failure develop by 40 years of age in about 10% of patients and become more prevalent with aging. Paradoxical embolism resulting in a transient ischemic attack or stroke can call attention to the diagnosis. The development of pulmonary hypertension, although probably not as common as originally thought, can occur at an early age.[32] If pulmonary hypertension is severe, a second causative diagnosis should be sought. Life expectancy is clearly reduced in ASD patients, although not as severely as was quoted in earlier papers because only patients with large ASDs were described.

CLINICAL FEATURES

Pediatrics

Most children are asymptomatic, and the diagnosis is made after the discovery of a murmur. On occasion, increased pulmonary blood flow may be so great that congestive heart failure, recurrent chest infections, chronic wheezing, or even pulmonary hypertension may necessitate closure in infancy. Spontaneous closure of an ASD may occur within the first year of life. Even quite substantial defects diagnosed in the neonatal period (>7 mm) may reduce in size and not require later intervention. Thus, in asymptomatic children with an isolated secundum ASD, intervention is usually deferred so that elective device closure becomes an option if indicated.

Adults

The most common presenting symptoms in adults are exercise intolerance (exertional dyspnea and fatigue) and palpitations (typically from atrial flutter, atrial fibrillation, or sick sinus syndrome). Right ventricular failure can be the presenting symptom in older patients. The presence of cyanosis should alert one to the possibility of shunt reversal and Eisenmenger syndrome or, alternatively, to a prominent eustachian valve directing inferior vena cava flow to the left atrium via a secundum ASD or sinus venosus ASD of the inferior vena cava type.

On examination, there is "left atrialization" of the jugular venous pressure (A wave = V wave). A hyperdynamic right ventricular impulse may be

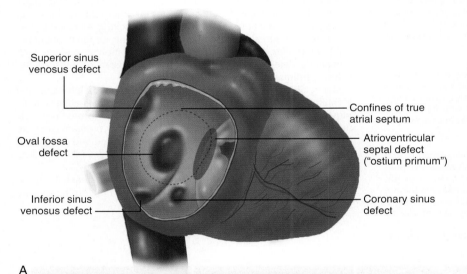

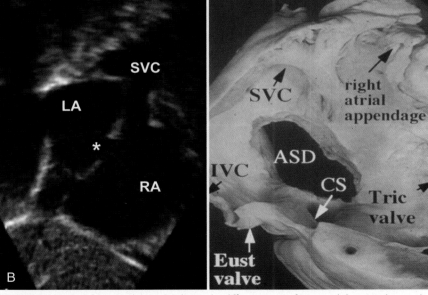

FIGURE 65-5 A, Schematic diagram outlining the different types of interatrial shunting that can be encountered. Note that only the central defect is suitable for device closure. **B,** Subcostal right anterior oblique view of a secundum atrial septal defect (asterisk) that is suitable for device closure. The right panel is a specimen as seen in a similar view, outlining the landmarks of the defect.

felt at the left sternal border at the end of expiration or in the subxiphoid area on deep inspiration. A dilated pulmonary artery trunk may be palpated in the second left intercostal space. A wide and fixed split of S_2 is the auscultatory hallmark of ASD, although it is not always present. A systolic ejection murmur, usually grade 2 and often scratchy, is best heard at the second left intercostal space, and a mid-diastolic rumble, from increased flow through the tricuspid valve, may be present at the left lower sternal border. When right ventricular failure occurs, a pansystolic murmur of tricuspid regurgitation is usual.

LABORATORY INVESTIGATIONS

ELECTROCARDIOGRAPHY. Sinus rhythm or atrial fibrillation or flutter may be present. The QRS axis is typically rightward in secundum ASD. Negative P waves in the inferior leads indicate a low atrial pacemaker often seen in sinus venosus–superior vena cava defects, which are located in the area of the sinoatrial node and render it deficient. Complete right bundle branch block appears as a function of age. Tall R or R′ waves in V_1 often indicate pulmonary hypertension.

CHEST RADIOGRAPHY. The classic radiographic features are of cardiomegaly (from right atrial and ventricular enlargement), dilated central pulmonary arteries with pulmonary plethora indicating increased pulmonary flow, and a small aortic knuckle (reflecting a chronic low cardiac output state).

ECHOCARDIOGRAPHY. Transthoracic echocardiography documents the type and size (defect diameter) of the ASD (see Figs. 15-95, 15-96, and 15-97), the direction of the shunt (Fig. 65-5B), and sometimes the presence of anomalous pulmonary venous return. The functional importance of the defect can be estimated by the size of the right ventricle (see Fig. 15-94), the presence or absence of right ventricular volume overload (paradoxical septal motion), and the estimation of Q_p/Q_s. Indirect measurement of the pulmonary artery pressure can be obtained from the Doppler velocity of the tricuspid regurgitation jet. TEE permits better visualization of the interatrial septum and is usually required when device closure is contemplated, partly to ensure that pulmonary venous drainage is normal. ICE can be used instead of TEE during device closure to help guide device insertion, reducing the fluoroscopy and procedural time and forgoing the need for general anesthesia.[33]

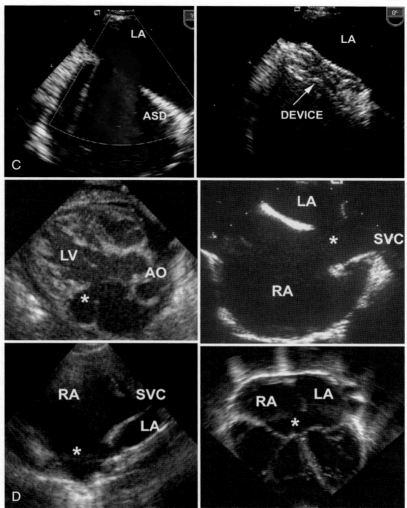

FIGURE 65-5, cont'd C, Transesophageal echocardiogram with color flow before device closure (left) and after release of an Amplatzer device (right). **D,** Montage of interatrial communications that are not atrial septal defects (asterisks) and therefore not suitable for device closure. The upper left is a coronary sinus defect due to unroofing; the top right is a superior sinus venosus defect; the bottom left is an inferior sinus venosus defect; and the bottom right is an atrial septal defect in the setting of an atrioventricular septal defect. AO = aorta; ASD = atrial septal defect; CS = coronary sinus; Eust = eustachian; IVC = inferior vena cava; LA = left atrium; LV = left ventricle; RA = right atrium; SVC = superior vena cava; Tric = tricuspid.

INDICATIONS FOR INTERVENTION. In asymptomatic children, the decision to intervene is based on the presence of right-sided heart dilation and a significant ASD (>5 mm) that shows no sign of spontaneous closure. Shunt fractions are now rarely measured and are reserved for "borderline" cases. Hemodynamically insignificant ASDs ($Q_p/Q_s < 1.5$) do not require closure, with the possible exception of trying to prevent paradoxical emboli in older patients after a stroke. "Significant" ASDs ($Q_p/Q_s > 1.5$, or ASDs associated with right ventricular volume overload) should be closed, especially if device closure is available and appropriate. For patients with pulmonary hypertension (pulmonary artery pressure > ⅔ systemic arterial blood pressure or pulmonary arteriolar resistance > ⅔ systemic arteriolar resistance), closure can be recommended if there is a net left-to-right shunt of at least 1.5:1 or evidence of pulmonary artery reactivity on challenge with a pulmonary vasodilator (e.g., oxygen or nitric oxide).

Device Closure

Device closure of secundum ASDs percutaneously under fluoroscopy and TEE or with intracardiac echocardiographic guidance is the therapy of choice when appropriate (Fig. 65-5C). Indications for device closure are the same as for surgical closure, but the selection criteria are stricter. Depending on the device, this technique is available only for patients with a secundum ASD with a stretched diameter of less than 41 mm and with adequate rims to enable secure deployment of the device. Anomalous pulmonary venous connection or proximity of the defect to the AV valves or coronary sinus or systemic venous drainage usually precludes the use of this technique. It is a safe and effective procedure in experienced hands, with major complications (e.g., device embolization, atrial perforation, thrombus formation[34]) occurring in less than 1% of patients and clinical closure achieved in more than 90% of patients. Device closure of an ASD improves functional status in symptomatic patients and exercise capacity in asymptomatic and symptomatic patients. Intermediate follow-up data have proved ASD device closure to be safe and effective,[35] with better preservation of right ventricular function[36] and lower complication rates than with surgery.[37]

Surgery

Device closure is not an option for those with sinus venosus or ostium primum defects or with secundum defects with unsuitable anatomy. Surgical closure of ASDs can be performed by primary suture closure or by use of a pericardial or synthetic patch. The procedure is usually performed through a midline sternotomy, but the availability of an inframammary or minithoracotomy approach to a typical secundum ASD should be made known to cosmetically sensitive patients. Surgical mortality in the adult without pulmonary hypertension should be less than 1%. Surgical closure of an ASD improves functional status and exercise capacity in symptomatic patients and improves (but usually does not normalize) survival and improves or eliminates congestive heart failure, especially when patients are operated on at an earlier age. However, surgical closure of ASD in adult life does not prevent atrial fibrillation or flutter or stroke, especially when patients are operated on after the age of 40 years. The role of a concomitant Cox maze procedure in patients with a prior history of atrial flutter or fibrillation should be considered[38] (see Chaps. 37 and 39).

REPRODUCTIVE ISSUES. Pregnancy is well tolerated in patients after ASD closure (see Chap. 82). Pregnancy is also well tolerated in women with unrepaired ASDs, but the risk of paradoxical embolism is increased (still only to a very low risk) during pregnancy and in the postpartum period. Pregnancy is contraindicated in Eisenmenger syndrome because of the high maternal (≈50%) and fetal (≈60%) mortality.

FOLLOW-UP. Most children with isolated secundum defect can be discharged to the care of their family physician 6 months after complete closure is confirmed, no matter whether it is surgical or by device. After device closure, patients require 6 months of aspirin and endocarditis prophylaxis until the device endothelializes, after which, assuming there is no residual shunt, they do not require any special precautions or endocarditis prophylaxis. Patients with sinus venosus defect are at risk for development of caval or pulmonary vein stenosis and should be kept under intermittent review. Patients who have had surgical or device repair as adults, patients with atrial arrhythmias preoperatively or postoperatively, and patients with ventricular dysfunction should remain under long-term cardiology surveillance.

Patent Foramen Ovale

ANATOMY. The foramen ovale is a tunnel-like space between the overlying septum secundum and septum primum and typically closes in 75% of people at birth by fusion of the septum primum and secundum. In utero, the foramen ovale is necessary for blood flow across the fetal atrial septum. Oxygenated blood from the placenta returns to the inferior vena cava, crosses the foramen ovale, and enters the systemic circulation. In about 25% of people, a patent foramen ovale (PFO) persists into adulthood. PFOs may be associated with atrial septal aneurysms (a redundancy of the interatrial septum), eustachian valves (a remnant of the sinus venosus valve), and Chiari networks (filamentous strands in the right atrium).

PATHOPHYSIOLOGY. PFOs have recently been scrutinized for their implication in the mechanism of cryptogenic stroke. Many of the basic tenets linking PFO and stroke seem plausible but have not been demonstrated. The current views may be summarized as follows. PFOs may serve either as a conduit for paradoxical embolization from the venous side to the systemic circulation or, because of their tunnel-like structure and propensity to stagnant flow, as a nidus for in situ thrombus formation. Variation in PFO size, right atrial anatomy, varying hemodynamic conditions, and occurrence of venous thrombi may all contribute to the chances of paradoxical embolization. The risk of a cryptogenic stroke seems increased for larger PFOs. The presence of an interatrial septal aneurysm in combination with a PFO also increases the risk of an adverse event, perhaps because of increased in situ thrombus formation in the aneurysmal tissue or simply because PFOs associated with an interatrial septal aneurysm tend to be larger. Eustachian valves and a Chiari network may direct blood flow from the inferior vena cava toward the atrial septum, encouraging right-to-left shunting in the presence of an interatrial communication. Physiologic (Valsalva maneuvers) and pathologic conditions increasing right ventricular pressure will raise the right atrial pressure, favoring right-to-left shunting. Finally, pelvic vein thrombi are found more frequently in young patients with cryptogenic stroke than in patients with a known cause of stroke[39] and may provide the source of venous thrombi.

PFOs have also been implicated in the pathophysiologic mechanism of decompression sickness (arterial gas embolism from the venous side) as well as more recently in the pathogenesis of migraine headaches.[40] Platypnea-orthodeoxia syndrome (dyspnea and arterial desaturation in the upright position, which improves on lying down) has also been attributed to the presence of a PFO.

CLINICAL IMPACT. The cause-and-effect relationship between PFO and cryptogenic stroke is still tentative and needs clarification. The recent body of literature would suggest a strong association, if not a causative link, especially in younger patients. Indeed, young patients with cryptogenic stroke have a significantly higher incidence of PFO (36% to 54%) than normal controls (15% to 25%). The association is more controversial in the population of older patients. Older patients often have more risk factors for stroke, and the causative role of a PFO in these patients is more difficult to establish.

When a patient presents with a stroke and a PFO is discovered, the usual causes of stroke must first be eliminated. Potential causes of stroke include carotid artery disease, ascending aortic atherosclerosis, atrial fibrillation, neurovascular abnormalities, and prothrombotic tendencies. If, after an exhaustive investigation (see later), no other cause of the stroke can be found, the PFO may be seen to have possibly had a causative role. The diagnosis of a PFO as a cause of cryptogenic stroke is, at best, a diagnosis of exclusion.

INVESTIGATIONS. A PFO is usually detected by transthoracic echocardiography, transesophageal echocardiography, or transcranial Doppler study. Transesophageal echocardiography is the most sensitive test, especially when it is performed with contrast media injected during a cough or Valsalva maneuver (see Fig. 15-17). A PFO is judged to be present if microbubbles are seen in the left-sided cardiac chambers within three cardiac cycles from the maximum right atrial opacification.

Screening for prothrombotic states (e.g., protein C or S deficiency, antithrombin III, or lupus anticoagulant), atrial fibrillation, significant carotid atherosclerosis by carotid Doppler imaging, and neurovascular abnormalities by brain magnetic resonance angiography must be undertaken in each patient before a PFO can be considered a possible culprit.

THERAPEUTIC OPTIONS. Once the presumptive diagnosis of a cryptogenic stroke caused by a PFO is determined, treatment modalities to prevent recurrent events include antiplatelet or anticoagulant agents, percutaneous device closure (see Fig. 59-1),[41,42] and surgical PFO closure. Medical therapy for secondary prevention of stroke with warfarin or antiplatelet agents is often used as "first-line" therapy with similar efficacy, a yearly recurrence rate of about 2%. Patients with PFO and atrial septal aneurysm who have had strokes seem to be at higher risk of recurrent stroke (as high as 15% per year), and a preventive strategy other than aspirin or warfarin should perhaps be considered. Device closure is safe and seems effective, with a recurrence rate of stroke between 0% and 3.8% per year (see Chap. 59). Surgical closure of PFO is usually performed when cardiac surgery is required for other reasons.

Recent nonrandomized trials comparing anticoagulation and antiplatelet treatment showed a lower risk of recurrent events with anticoagulation.[41,42] Regarding medical management after a cryptogenic stroke, the available nonrandomized trials support anticoagulation for patients with PFO and atrial septal aneurysm and at least antiplatelet treatment for patients with PFO without atrial septal aneurysm. The recurrence rate of stroke after transcatheter closure of PFO is lower compared with trials that used medical treatment. For patients with atrial septal aneurysm or those with recurrent cryptogenic ischemic events, closure of the PFO should be considered to provide a lower recurrence rate of ischemic events and to avoid the bleeding risk associated with long-term anticoagulation.[43]

Randomized clinical trials comparing various treatment options are necessary before definitive recommendations for the optimal treatment of cryptogenic stroke can be made.

Atrioventricular Septal Defect

TERMINOLOGY. The terms *atrioventricular septal defect, atrioventricular canal defect,* and *endocardial cushion defect* can be used interchangeably to describe this group of defects. The variable components of these lesions are explained in the following sections.

MORPHOLOGY. The basic morphology of AV septal defect is common to all types and is independent of the presence or absence of an ASD or VSD. These common features (**Figs. 65-6** and **65-7**) are absence of the muscular AV septum (resulting in the AV valves being at the same level on echocardiographic examination), inlet/outlet disproportion (resulting in an elongated left ventricular outflow tract, the so-called goose-neck deformity), abnormal lateral rotation of the posteromedial papillary muscle, and abnormal configuration of the AV valves. The left AV valve is a trileaflet valve made of superior and inferior bridging leaflets separated by a mural leaflet. The space between the superior and inferior leaflets as they bridge the interventricular septum is called the cleft in the left AV valve. The bridging leaflets may be completely adherent to the crest of the interventricular septum, free floating, or attached by chordal apparatus.

PARTITIONED VERSUS COMPLETE ATRIOVENTRICULAR SEPTAL DEFECTS. A partitioned orifice is one in which the superior and inferior leaflets are joined by a connecting tongue of tissue as they bridge the interventricular septum. This partitions the valve into separate left and right orifices. A common AV valve orifice is one in which there is no such connecting tongue, resulting in one large orifice that encompasses the left- and right-sided components. Interatrial (ostium primum) and interventricular defects are common in AV septal defect.

The left ventricular outflow tract is elongated and predisposes to subaortic stenosis. The papillary muscles are closer together than normal. The term *unbalanced AV septal defect* refers to cases in which one ventricle is hypoplastic. This is seen more commonly in patients with heterotaxy and those with left-sided obstructive defects.

PATHOPHYSIOLOGY

NATIVE. The pathophysiology of an isolated shunt at atrial level (commonly referred to as a primum ASD) is similar to that of a large secundum ASD, with unrestricted left-to-right shunting through the primum ASD, leading to right-sided atrial and ventricular volume overload. Chronic left AV valve regurgitation may produce left-sided ventricular and atrial volume overload. Complete AV septal defect has a greater degree of left-to-right shunting from the primum ASD as well as the nonrestrictive VSD, which triggers earlier left ventricular dilation and a greater degree of pulmonary hypertension.

AFTER CORRECTION. Residual significant left AV valve regurgitation may occur and cause significant left atrial as well as left ventricular dilation. Left AV valve stenosis from overzealous repair of the valve may also occur. The long, narrow left ventricular outflow tract of AV septal defect promotes left ventricular outflow tract obstruction and leads to subaortic stenosis in about 5% of patients.

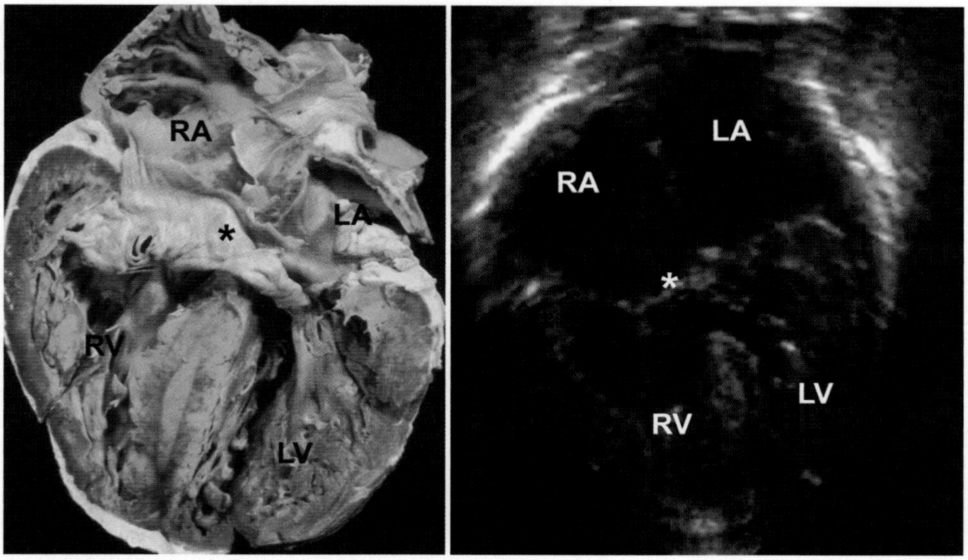

NATURAL HISTORY. Patients with an isolated primum ASD have a course similar to that of those with large secundum ASDs, although symptoms may appear sooner when significant left AV valve regurgitation is present. Patients may be asymptomatic until their third or fourth decade, but progressive symptoms related to congestive heart failure, atrial arrhythmias, complete heart block, and variable degrees of pulmonary hypertension develop in virtually all of them by the fifth decade.

Most patients with complete AV septal defect have had surgical repair in infancy. Infants present with dyspnea, congestive heart failure, and failure to thrive. When presenting unrepaired, most adults have established pulmonary vascular disease. Patients with Down syndrome have a propensity for development of pulmonary hypertension at an even earlier age than do other patients with AV septal defect.

CLINICAL ISSUES

Down Syndrome

Down syndrome occurs in 35% of patients with AV septal defect. These patients more commonly have a complete AV septal defect with a common AV valve orifice and a large associated VSD. They often present in infancy with pulmonary hypertension. Clinical features are cardiomegaly, right ventricular heave, and pulmonary outflow tract murmur. If associated AV valve regurgitation exists, there is a pansystolic murmur.

FIGURE 65-6 Apical four-chamber view in a complete atrioventricular septal defect with a common atrioventricular valve orifice (asterisk). Note the large interatrial and interventricular communications and the large free-floating superior bridging leaflet. LA = left atrium; LV = left ventricle; RA = right atrium; RV = right ventricle.

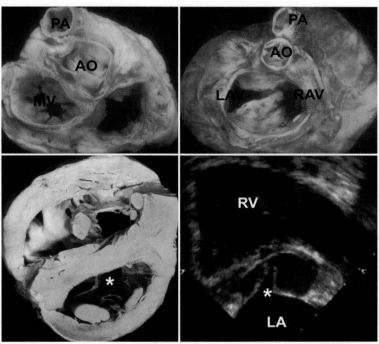

FIGURE 65-7 Montage comparing the normal atrioventricular junction with that seen in an atrioventricular septal defect. The upper left picture is the normal atrioventricular junction as seen from above. Note the normal morphology of the mitral and tricuspid valves, with the aorta wedged between them. The upper right picture is a similar view in an atrioventricular septal defect. Note the unwedged aorta, the trileaflet left atrioventricular valve, and the cleft between the superior and inferior bridging leaflets. The lower left picture is a specimen of an atrioventricular septal defect demonstrating the cleft. The lower right picture is an echocardiogram showing the cleft. AO = aorta; LA = left atrium; LAV = left atrioventricular valve; MV = mitral valve; PA = pulmonary artery; RAV = right atrioventricular valve; RV = right ventricle; TV = tricuspid valve.

Non—Down Syndrome

Clinical presentation depends on the presence and size of the ASD and the VSD and on the competence of the left AV valve. A large left-to-right shunt gives rise to symptoms of heart failure (exertional dyspnea or fatigue) or pulmonary vascular disease (exertional syncope, cyanosis). In adulthood, palpitations from atrial arrhythmias are common. Cardiac findings on physical examination for patients with an isolated shunt at atrial level are similar to those of patients with secundum ASD, with the important addition of a prominent left ventricular apex and pansystolic murmur when significant left AV valve regurgitation is present. Cases with a primum ASD and a restrictive VSD have similar findings but with the addition of a pansystolic VSD murmur heard best at the left sternal border. Complete AV septal defects have a single S_1 (common AV valve), a mid-diastolic murmur from augmented AV valve inflow, and findings of pulmonary hypertension or a right-to-left shunt.

LABORATORY INVESTIGATIONS

ELECTROCARDIOGRAPHY. Most patients have left-axis deviation. Complete AV block and atrial fibrillation or flutter can be present in older patients. Partial or complete right bundle branch block is usually associated with right ventricular dilation or prior surgery.

CHEST RADIOGRAPHY. If the defect is unrepaired, this demonstrates cardiomegaly with right atrial and right ventricular prominence with increased pulmonary vascular markings. In those cases with a small interatrial communication and important left AV valve regurgitation, there is cardiomegaly due to left ventricular enlargement and normal pulmonary vascular markings. Findings of Eisenmenger syndrome are also possible. When the defect has been repaired, the study may be normal with sternal wires.

ECHOCARDIOGRAPHY. This has replaced angiography in assessing virtually all cases with AV septal defect. The cardinal and common features discussed in the morphology section are readily recognized by echocardiography. In the four-chamber view, the AV valves appear at the same level, irrespective of the presence or absence of a VSD. The typical inferior ASD and the posteriorly positioned VSD will be sought. The degree of associated AV valve regurgitation, the left-to-right shunt, and the estimated right ventricular systolic pressure should be determined. When the right AV valve is used to assess right ventricular pressure, care must be taken to ensure that the jet is not contaminated by an obligatory left ventricle to right atrial shunt.

CARDIAC CATHETERIZATION. In general, this technique has been replaced by echocardiography for the evaluation of patients with an AV septal defect. The one role it still has is in the evaluation of the patient who presents late and may have associated pulmonary vascular or coronary disease.

INDICATIONS FOR INTERVENTION. The patient with an unrepaired or newly diagnosed AV septal defect and significant hemodynamic defects requires surgical repair. Equally, patients with persistent left AV valve regurgitation (or stenosis from previous repair) causing symptoms, atrial arrhythmia, or deterioration in ventricular function, and patients with significant subaortic obstruction (a mean gradient >50 mm Hg at rest) require surgical intervention.

In the presence of severe pulmonary hypertension (pulmonary artery pressure > ⅔ systemic blood pressure or pulmonary arteriolar resistance > ⅔ systemic arteriolar resistance), there must be a net left-to-right shunt of at least 1.5:1 or evidence of pulmonary artery reactivity on challenge with a pulmonary vasodilator (e.g., oxygen, nitric oxide, prostaglandins).

INTERVENTIONAL OPTIONS AND OUTCOMES

Isolated Shunt at Atrial Level (Primum Atrial Septal Defect)

Pericardial patch closure of the primum ASD with concomitant suture (with or without annuloplasty) of the "cleft" left AV valve is usually performed. When left AV valve repair is not possible, replacement may be necessary. In the short term, the results of repair of partial AV septal defect are similar to those after closure of secundum ASD, but sequelae of left AV ("mitral") valve regurgitation,[44,45] subaortic stenosis, and AV block may develop or progress.

Complete Atrioventricular Septal Defect

The "staged approach" (pulmonary artery banding followed by intracardiac repair) has been supplanted by primary intracardiac repair in infancy. The goals of intracardiac repair are ventricular and atrial septation with adequate mitral and tricuspid reconstruction. Both single- and double-patch techniques to close ASDs and VSDs have been described with comparable results. On occasion, left AV valve replacement is necessary when valve repair is not possible. The intermediate results of repair of complete AV septal defect are good for Down syndrome patients as well as for non—Down syndrome patients,[46,47] with problems similar to those of partial AV septal defect.

REPRODUCTIVE ISSUES. Pregnancy is well tolerated in patients with complete repair and no significant residual lesions. Women in NYHA Classes I and II with unrepaired, isolated primum ASD usually tolerate pregnancy well. Pregnancy is contraindicated in Eisenmenger syndrome because of the high maternal (≈50%) and fetal (≈60%) mortality.

FOLLOW-UP ISSUES. All patients require periodic follow-up by an expert cardiologist because of the possibility of postoperative complications, which include patch dehiscence or residual septal defects (1%), development of complete heart block (3%), late atrial fibrillation or flutter, significant left AV valve dysfunction (10%), and subaortic stenosis (5% to 10%). Left AV valve regurgitation requires reoperation in at least 10% of patients. Subaortic stenosis develops or progresses in 5% to 10% of patients after repair, particularly in patients with primum ASD, especially if the left AV ("mitral") valve has been replaced. Particular attention should be paid to those patients with pulmonary hypertension preoperatively. Antibiotic prophylaxis is necessary only in the first 6 months after surgery unless there is residual patch leak or a prosthetic valve.

Isolated Ventricular Septal Defect

MORPHOLOGY. The ventricular septum can be divided into three major components—inlet, trabecular, and outlet—all abutting on a small membranous septum lying just underneath the aortic valve. VSDs (**Fig. 65-8**) are classified into three main categories according to their location and margins (**Fig. 65-9**). Muscular VSDs are bordered entirely by myocardium and can be trabecular, inlet, or outlet in location. Membranous VSDs often have inlet, outlet, or trabecular extension and are bordered in part by fibrous continuity between the leaflets of an AV valve and an arterial valve. Doubly committed subarterial VSDs are more common in Asian patients, are situated in the outlet septum, and are bordered by fibrous continuity of the aortic and pulmonary valves. This section deals with VSDs occurring in isolation from major associated cardiac anomalies.

PATHOPHYSIOLOGY. A restrictive VSD is a defect that produces a significant pressure gradient between the left ventricle and the right ventricle (pulmonary-to-aortic systolic pressure ratio < 0.3) and is accompanied by a small (≤1.4:1) shunt. A moderately restrictive VSD is accompanied by a moderate shunt (Q_p/Q_s of 1.4 to 2.2:1) with a pulmonary-to-aortic systolic pressure ratio less than 0.66. A large or nonrestrictive VSD is accompanied by a large shunt (Q_p/Q_s > 2.2) and a pulmonary-to-aortic systolic pressure ratio greater than 0.66. An Eisenmenger VSD has a systolic pressure ratio of 1 and Q_p/Q_s less than 1:1 or a net right-to-left shunt.

NATURAL HISTORY. A restrictive VSD does not cause significant hemodynamic derangement and may close spontaneously during childhood and sometimes in adult life. A perimembranous defect in an immediately subaortic position, or any doubly committed VSD, may be associated with progressive aortic regurgitation. Late development of subaortic and subpulmonary stenosis (see section on double-chambered right ventricle) and the formation of a left ventricular to right atrial shunt are well described and should be excluded at follow-up. A moderately restrictive VSD imposes a hemodynamic burden on the left ventricle, which leads to left atrial and ventricular dilation and dysfunction as well as a variable increase in pulmonary vascular resistance. A large or nonrestrictive VSD features left ventricular volume overload early in life with a progressive rise in pulmonary artery pressure and a fall in left-to-right shunting. In turn, this leads to higher pulmonary vascular resistance and eventually to Eisenmenger syndrome.

CLINICAL FEATURES

Pediatrics

Neonatal presentation with a murmur is increasingly frequent. Most of these patients have a restrictive defect, and the murmur becomes apparent only as the pulmonary vascular resistance falls. Paradoxically, those infants with large nonrestrictive defects tend to present later. This is because equalization of pressures across the defect obviates the generation of a pansystolic murmur. Instead, pulmonary blood flow increases progressively as the pulmonary vascular resistance falls. Presentation with breathlessness, congestive heart failure, and failure to thrive in the second and third months of life are usual. At that time, a pulmonary ejection murmur and a mitral rumble may be heard, reflecting increased pulmonary flow and pulmonary venous return. Cyanosis is rare in early childhood, and if it is present, other causes of a raised pulmonary vascular resistance should be excluded (e.g., mitral stenosis or coexisting lung disease).

Medical management of the symptomatic infant is directed at improving symptoms before surgery or "buying time" while spontaneous closure or diminution in size occurs. Treatment with diuretics is universally accepted, and increasingly, the successful use of ACE inhibition is being reported.

Adults

Most adult patients with a small restrictive VSD are asymptomatic. Physical examination reveals a harsh or high-frequency pansystolic murmur, usually grade 3 to 4/6, heard with maximal intensity at the left sternal border in the third or fourth intercostal space. Patients with a moderately restrictive VSD often present with dyspnea in adult life, perhaps triggered by atrial fibrillation. Physical examination typically reveals a displaced cardiac apex with a similar pansystolic murmur as well as an apical diastolic rumble and third heart sound at the apex from the increased flow through the mitral valve. Patients with large nonrestrictive Eisenmenger VSDs present as adults with central cyanosis and clubbing of the nailbeds. Signs of pulmonary hypertension—a right ventricular heave, a palpable and loud P_2, and a right-sided S_4—are typically present. A pulmonary ejection click, a soft and scratchy systolic ejection murmur, and a high-pitched decrescendo diastolic murmur of pulmonary regurgitation (Graham Steell) may be audible. Peripheral edema usually reflects right-sided heart failure.

LABORATORY INVESTIGATIONS

ELECTROCARDIOGRAPHY. The ECG mirrors the size of the shunt and the degree of pulmonary hypertension. Small, restrictive VSDs usually produce a normal tracing. Moderate-sized VSDs produce a broad, notched P wave characteristic of left atrial overload as well as evidence of left ventricular volume overload, namely, deep Q and tall R waves with tall T waves in leads V_5 and V_6 and perhaps eventually atrial fibrillation. After repair, the ECG is usually normal with right bundle branch block.

CHEST RADIOGRAPHY. The chest radiograph reflects the magnitude of the shunt as well as the degree of pulmonary hypertension. A moderate-sized shunt causes signs of left ventricular dilation with some pulmonary plethora.

ECHOCARDIOGRAPHY. (See Figs. 15-97 and 15-98.) Transthoracic echocardiography can identify the location, size, and hemodynamic consequences of the VSD as well as any associated lesions (aortic regurgitation, right ventricular outflow tract obstruction, or left ventricular outflow tract obstruction).

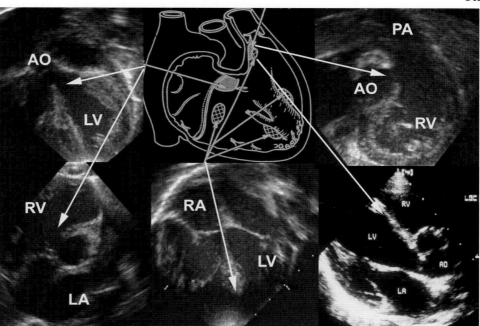

FIGURE 65-8 Montage of the different types of ventricular septal defects. The central diagram outlines the location of the various types of defects as seen from the right ventricle. The two left images show a perimembranous ventricular septal defect as seen in the five-chamber and short-axis views. Note that the defect is roofed by the aorta and is next to the tricuspid valve. The bottom middle echocardiogram is a muscular apical defect. The upper right image is a right anterior oblique view in a doubly committed ventricular septal defect. The lower right image is a short-axis view showing an outlet ventricular septal defect with prolapse of the right coronary cusp. AO = aorta; LA = left atrium; LV = left ventricle; PA = pulmonary artery; RA = right atrium; RV = right ventricle.

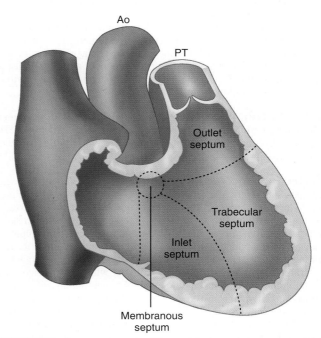

FIGURE 65-9 Four components of the ventricular septum shown here from the right ventricular aspect are now described by Anderson and associates as inlet and outlet components of the right ventricle because these areas do not correspond to septal structures as initially suggested. Ao = aorta; PT = pulmonary trunk. *(Modified from Anderson RH, Becker AE, Lucchese E, et al: Morphology of Congenital Heart Disease. Baltimore, University Park Press, 1983.)*

CARDIAC CATHETERIZATION. Cardiac catheterization may be required when the hemodynamic significance of a VSD is questioned or when assessment of pulmonary artery pressures and resistances is necessary. In some centers, therapeutic catheterization is performed for percutaneous closure (see later).

INDICATIONS FOR INTERVENTION. The presence of a significant VSD (the symptomatic patient shows a $Q_p/Q_s > 1.5:1$, pulmonary artery systolic pressure > 50 mm Hg, increased left ventricular and left atrial size, or deteriorating left ventricular function) in the absence of irreversible pulmonary hypertension warrants surgical closure. If severe pulmonary hypertension (see ASD section) is present, closure is seldom feasible. Other relative indications for VSD closure are the presence of a perimembranous or outlet VSD with more than mild aortic regurgitation and a history of recurrent endocarditis.

In children, a nonrestrictive VSD and a smaller VSD with significant symptoms failing to respond to medication are indications for surgical or device closure. Elective surgery is usually performed between 3 and 9 months of age. Some patients have pulmonary hypertension. If pulmonary arteriolar resistance is less than 7 Wood units, closure can be safely undertaken if there is a net left-to-right shunt of at least 1.5:1 or strong evidence of pulmonary reactivity on challenge with a pulmonary vasodilator (oxygen, nitric oxide).

INTERVENTIONAL OPTIONS AND OUTCOMES

Surgery

Surgical closure by direct suture or with a patch has been used for more than 50 years with a low perioperative mortality—even in adults—and a high closure rate. Patch leaks are not uncommon but seldom need reoperation. Late sinus node disease may occur.[48]

Device Closure

Successful transcatheter device closure of trabecular (muscular) and perimembranous VSDs has been reported. Trabecular VSDs have proven more amenable to this technique because of their relatively straightforward anatomy and muscular rim to which the device attaches well and, as such, result in excellent closure rates with a low procedural mortality.[49,50] Immediate as well as short-term results are good. The closure of a perimembranous VSD is technically more challenging because of its proximity to valve structures, and careful selection of patients is required. It should be performed only in centers with appropriate expertise. Short-term follow-up data show complete closure in 96% of patients, with the development of aortic or tricuspid regurgitation or the development of complete heart block in less than 5% of patients.[50] No long-term follow-up data are available yet.

REPRODUCTIVE ISSUES. Pregnancy is well tolerated in women with small or moderate VSDs and in women with repaired VSDs. Pregnancy is contraindicated in Eisenmenger syndrome because of high maternal (≈50%) and fetal (≈60%) mortality.

FOLLOW-UP. For patients with good to excellent functional class and good left ventricular function before surgical closure, life expectancy after surgical correction is close to normal.[48] The risk of progressive aortic regurgitation is reduced after surgery, as is the risk of endocarditis, unless a residual VSD persists. Yearly cardiac evaluation is suggested for patients with right ventricular outflow tract obstruction, left ventricular outflow tract obstruction, and aortic regurgitation not undergoing surgical repair; for patients with Eisenmenger syndrome; and for adults with significant atrial or ventricular arrhythmias. Cardiac surveillance is also recommended for patients who had late repair of moderate or large defects, which are often associated with left ventricular impairment and elevated pulmonary artery pressure at the time of surgery.

Patent Ductus Arteriosus

MORPHOLOGY. The ductus arteriosus derives from the left sixth primitive aortic arch and connects the proximal left pulmonary artery to the descending aorta, just distal to the left subclavian artery.

PATHOPHYSIOLOGY. The ductus is widely patent in the normal fetus, carrying unoxygenated blood from the right ventricle through the descending aorta to the placenta, where the blood is oxygenated. Functional closure of the ductus from vasoconstriction occurs shortly after a term birth, whereas anatomic closure from intimal proliferation and fibrosis takes several weeks to be completed. Some patients have "ductus-dependent" physiology as neonates. This means their circulation depends on the ductus for pulmonary blood flow, such as in severe aortic coarctation, hypoplastic left heart syndrome, and sometimes D-TGA. If spontaneous closure of the ductus occurs in such neonates, clinical deterioration and death usually follow.

Isolated PDAs, the subject of this section, are often categorized according to the degree of left-to-right shunting, which is determined by both the size and length of the duct and the difference between systemic and pulmonary vascular resistances, as follows:
- Silent: tiny PDA detected only by nonclinical means (usually echocardiography)
- Small: continuous murmur common; $Q_p/Q_s < 1.5:1$
- Moderate: continuous murmur common; Q_p/Q_s of 1.5 to 2.2:1
- Large: continuous murmur present; $Q_p/Q_s > 2.2:1$
- Eisenmenger: continuous murmur absent; substantial pulmonary hypertension, differential hypoxemia, and differential cyanosis (pink fingers, blue toes)

NATURAL HISTORY

Premature Infants

Patency of a ductus arteriosus is common in a preterm infant who lacks the normal mechanisms for postnatal ductal closure because of immaturity. A PDA is thus an expected finding in a premature infant, and delayed spontaneous closure of the ductus may be anticipated if the infant does not succumb to other problems.

Full-Term Infants

In a full-term newborn, patency of a ductus is a true congenital malformation. On occasion, some full-term newborns have persistent patency of the ductus arteriosus because their relative hypoxemia contributes to vasodilation of the channel. This includes infants born at high altitude; those with congenital malformations causing hypoxemia; or malformations in which ductal flow supplies the systemic circulation, such as hypoplastic left heart syndrome, interrupted aortic arch, or aortic coarctation.

Children and Adults

Children and adults with silent PDAs are detected by nonclinical means, usually echocardiography, and face virtually no long-term complications. An exception occurs if the patient's murmur is inaudible because of obesity or other somatic factors. A small ductus accompanied by a small shunt does not cause a significant hemodynamic derangement but may predispose to endarteritis,[51] especially when a murmur is present. A moderate-sized duct and shunt pose a volume load on the left atrium and ventricle with resultant left ventricular dilation and dysfunction and perhaps eventual atrial fibrillation. A large duct results initially in left ventricular volume overload but develops a progressive rise in pulmonary artery pressures and eventually irreversible pulmonary vascular changes by 2 years of age.

CLINICAL FEATURES

Premature Infants

Most preterm infants with a birth weight less than 1500 g have a PDA, and about one third have a large enough shunt to cause significant cardiopulmonary deterioration. Clinical findings in these patients include bounding peripheral pulses, infraclavicular and interscapular systolic murmur (occasionally a continuous murmur), precordial hyperactivity, hepatomegaly, and either multiple episodes of apnea and bradycardia or ventilator dependence.

Full-Term Infants, Children, and Adults

A small audible duct usually causes no symptoms but may rarely be manifested as an endovascular infection. Physical examination may reveal a grade 1 or 2 continuous murmur peaking in late systole and best heard in the first or second left intercostal space. Patients with a moderate-sized duct may present with dyspnea or palpitations from atrial arrhythmias. A louder continuous or "machinery" murmur in the first or second left intercostal space is typically accompanied by a wide systemic pulse pressure from aortic diastolic runoff into the pulmonary trunk and signs of left ventricular volume overload, such as a displaced left ventricular apex and sometimes a left-sided S_3 (meaningful in adults only). With a moderate degree of pulmonary hypertension, the diastolic component of the murmur disappears, leaving a systolic murmur. Adults with a large uncorrected PDA eventually present with a short systolic ejection murmur, hypoxemia in the feet more than in the hands (differential cyanosis), and Eisenmenger physiology.

LABORATORY INVESTIGATIONS IN PREMATURE INFANTS

ELECTROCARDIOGRAPHY. This may be normal or demonstrate right or left ventricular hypertrophy or both, depending on the amount of left-to-right shunting and the degree of associated pulmonary hypertension.

CHEST RADIOGRAPHY. This may demonstrate cardiomegaly and increased pulmonary vascular markings that may be difficult to interpret in the setting of hyaline membrane disease.

ECHOCARDIOGRAPHY. This is the key to diagnosis. The ductus arteriosus can be imaged in its entirety and its size estimated. Doppler study demonstrates the shunt and permits an accurate assessment of mean pulmonary artery pressure. This is achieved by calculating the mean left-to-right spectral trace and subtracting it from the mean blood pressure. Measurements of the left atrial and left ventricular size provide indirect evidence of the magnitude of left-to-right shunting.

LABORATORY INVESTIGATIONS IN FULL-TERM INFANTS, CHILDREN, AND ADULTS

ELECTROCARDIOGRAPHY. The ECG reflects the size and degree of shunting occurring through the duct. A small duct produces a normal ECG. A moderate duct may show left ventricular volume overload with broad, notched P waves together with deep Q waves, tall R waves, and peaked T waves in V_5 and V_6. A large duct with Eisenmenger physiology produces findings of right ventricular hypertrophy.

CHEST RADIOGRAPHY. A small duct produces a normal chest radiograph. A moderate-sized duct causes moderate cardiomegaly with left-sided heart enlargement, a prominent aortic knuckle, and increased pulmonary perfusion. Ring calcification of the ductus may be seen through the soft tissue density of the aortic arch or pulmonary trunk in older adults. The large PDA produces an Eisenmenger appearance with a prominent aortic knuckle.

ECHOCARDIOGRAPHY. (See Fig. 15-99.) This determines the presence, size, and degree of shunting and the physiologic consequences of the shunt. The PDA is seen with difficulty in an Eisenmenger context. A bubble study shows the communication.

INDICATIONS FOR INTERVENTION

Premature Infants

Treatment of preterm infants with a PDA varies with the magnitude of shunting and the severity of hyaline membrane disease because the ductus may contribute importantly to mortality in infants with respiratory distress syndrome. Intervention in an asymptomatic infant with a small left-to-right shunt is unnecessary because the PDA almost invariably undergoes spontaneous closure. Those infants who demonstrate unmistakable signs of a significant ductal left-to-right shunt during the course of the respiratory distress syndrome are often unresponsive to medical measures to control congestive heart failure and require closure of the PDA to survive. These infants are best treated by pharmacologic inhibition of prostaglandin synthesis with indomethacin or ibuprofen to constrict and to close the ductus. Surgical ligation is required in the estimated 10% of infants who are unresponsive to indomethacin.

Full-Term Infants

In the clinical settings in which the ductus preserves pulmonary blood flow, the inevitable spontaneous closure of the vessel is associated with profound clinical deterioration and often death. Undesirable ductal closure may be reversed medically within the first 4 or 5 days of life by an infusion of prostaglandin E$_1$. By dilation of the constricted ductus arteriosus, a temporary increase should occur in arterial blood oxygen tension and saturation and correct acidemia.

Children and Adults

There is no debate about the desirability of closing a hemodynamically important PDA. There is debate about the merits of closing an inaudible or small PDA strictly to reduce the risk of endarteritis. In the presence of severe pulmonary hypertension (see ASD earlier), closure is seldom indicated. Contraindications to ductal closure include irreversible pulmonary hypertension and active endarteritis.

INTERVENTIONAL OPTIONS AND OUTCOMES

Transcatheter Treatment (Fig. 65-10)

During the past 20 years, the efficacy and safety of transcatheter device closure for ducts smaller than 8 mm have been established, with complete ductal closure achieved in more than 85% of patients by 1 year after device placement at a mortality rate of less than 1%. In centers with appropriate resources and experience, transcatheter device occlusion should be the method of choice for ductal closure.[52]

Surgical Treatment

Surgical closure, by ductal ligation or division, has been performed for more than 50 years with a marginally greater closure rate than by device closure but with somewhat greater morbidity and mortality. Immediate clinical closure (no shunt audible on physical examination) is achieved in more than 95% of patients. Surgical closure is a low-risk procedure in children. Surgical mortality in adults is 1% to 3.5% and relates to the presence of pulmonary arterial hypertension and difficult ductal morphology (calcified or aneurysmal) often seen in adults. Surgical closure should be reserved for those in whom the PDA is too large for device closure or at centers without access to device closure.

REPRODUCTIVE ISSUES. Pregnancy is well tolerated in women with silent and small PDAs and in patients who were asymptomatic before pregnancy. In the woman with a hemodynamically important PDA, pregnancy may precipitate or worsen heart failure. Pregnancy is contraindicated in Eisenmenger syndrome because of the high maternal ($\approx$50%) and fetal ($\approx$60%) mortality.

FOLLOW-UP. Patients with device occlusion or after surgical closure should be examined periodically for possible recanalization. Silent residual shunts may be found by transthoracic echocardiography. Endocarditis prophylaxis is recommended for 6 months after PDA device closure or for life if any residual defect persists. Patients with a silent or small PDA probably do not require endocarditis prophylaxis or follow-up.

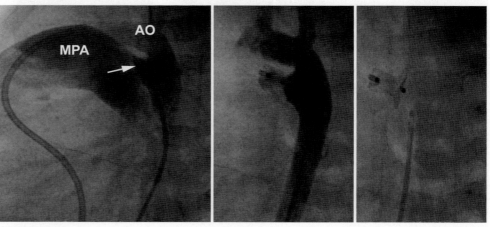

FIGURE 65-10 Montage of a patent arterial duct (arrow), before and after device occlusion. AO = aorta; MPA = main pulmonary artery.

Persistent Truncus Arteriosus

MORPHOLOGY. Persistent truncus arteriosus is an anomaly in which a single vessel forms the outlet of both ventricles and gives rise to the systemic, pulmonary, and coronary arteries. It is always accompanied by a VSD and frequently with a right-sided aortic arch. The truncal valve is usually tricuspid but is quadricuspid in about one third of patients. Truncal valve regurgitation and truncal valve stenosis are each seen in 10% to 15% of patients. There can be a single coronary artery.

Truncus malformations can be classified either anatomically according to the mode of origin of pulmonary vessels from the common trunk or from a functional point of view on the basis of the magnitude of blood flow to the lungs. In the common type (type I) of truncus arteriosus, a partially separate pulmonary trunk of variable length exists and gives rise to left and right pulmonary arteries. In type II, each pulmonary artery arises separately but close to the other from the posterior aspect of the truncus. In type III, each pulmonary artery arises from the lateral aspect of the truncus. Less commonly, one pulmonary artery branch may be absent, with aortopulmonary collateral arteries supplying the lung that does not receive a pulmonary artery branch from the truncus.

PATHOPHYSIOLOGY. Pulmonary blood flow is governed by the size of the pulmonary arteries and the pulmonary vascular resistance. In infancy, pulmonary blood flow is usually excessive because pulmonary vascular resistance is not greatly increased. Thus, in the neonate, only minimal cyanosis is present. With time, pulmonary vascular resistance increases, relieving the left ventricular volume load but at the price of increasing cyanosis. When pulmonary vascular resistance reaches systemic levels, Eisenmenger physiology and bidirectional shunting occur. Significant truncal valve regurgitation produces a volume load on both right and left ventricles because of the biventricular origin of the truncal artery.

NATURAL HISTORY. Most deaths from congestive heart failure occur before 1 year of age. Unrepaired patients who survive past 1 year most likely present with established pulmonary hypertension. The prevalence of truncal valve regurgitation increases with age, causing biventricular heart failure and increasing susceptibility to endocarditis.

CLINICAL FEATURES

Pediatrics

Infants with truncus arteriosus usually present with mild cyanosis coexisting with the cardiac findings of a large left-to-right shunt. This is the result of excessive pulmonary blood flow due to a low pulmonary vascular resistance. Symptoms of heart failure and poor physical development usually appear in the first weeks or months of life. The most frequent physical findings include cardiomegaly, collapsing peripheral pulses, loud single second heart sound, harsh systolic murmur preceded by an ejection click, and low-pitched mid-diastolic rumbling murmur and bounding pulses. A decrescendo diastolic murmur suggests associated truncal valve regurgitation.

DiGeorge syndrome may be seen with truncus arteriosus. Facial dysmorphism, high incidence of extracardiac malformations (particularly of the limbs, kidneys, and intestine), atrophy or absence of the thymus gland, T-lymphocyte deficiency, and predilection to infection also may be features of the clinical presentation.

The physical findings are different if pulmonary blood flow is restricted by a high pulmonary vascular resistance. Cyanosis is prominent, and only a short systolic murmur may be heard in association with an ejection click. Pulmonary vascular obstruction usually does not restrict pulmonary blood flow before 1 year of age.

Adults

Adults presenting with an unrepaired truncus arteriosus have Eisenmenger syndrome and its typical findings.

LABORATORY INVESTIGATIONS (UNREPAIRED)

ELECTROCARDIOGRAPHY. This demonstrates biventricular hypertrophy with strain as the pulmonary resistance rises.

CHEST RADIOGRAPHY. This demonstrates cardiomegaly with prominent pulmonary arterial markings and unusually high hilar areas. A right aortic arch occurs in 50% of cases.

ECHOCARDIOGRAPHY (**Fig. 65-11**). In most cases, two-dimensional echocardiography provides a complete diagnosis. The study should demonstrate the overriding truncal root, the origin of the pulmonary arteries, the number of truncal cusps, the origin of the coronary arteries, the functional status of the truncal valve, and the size of the VSD.

CARDIAC CATHETERIZATION AND ANGIOGRAPHY. This is rarely necessary and in fact carries a risk of both morbidity and mortality. In general, significant arterial desaturation in the absence of branch pulmonary artery stenosis indicates that the lesion cannot be repaired.

INDICATIONS FOR INTERVENTION. Early surgical intervention is indicated in all cases within the first 2 months of life. In the presence of severe pulmonary hypertension (see ASD section), surgical intervention is usually not performed.

INTERVENTIONAL OPTIONS AND OUTCOMES. Operation consists of closure of the VSD, leaving the aorta arising from the left ventricle; excision of the pulmonary arteries from their truncus origin; and placement of a valve-containing prosthetic conduit or aortic homograft valve conduit between the right ventricle and the pulmonary arteries to establish circulatory continuity. Truncal valve insufficiency is a challenging problem and may require valve replacement or repair.

Important risk factors for perioperative death are severe truncal valve regurgitation, interrupted aortic arch, coronary artery anomalies, and age at initial operation older than 100 days. Patients with only one pulmonary artery are especially prone to early development of severe pulmonary vascular disease.

REPRODUCTIVE ISSUES. Patients with a repaired truncus arteriosus and no hemodynamically important residual lesions should tolerate pregnancy well. Patients with significant conduit obstruction or important truncal valve regurgitation need pre-pregnancy counseling, with consideration of correction of the lesions before pregnancy and careful follow-up throughout pregnancy. Pregnancy is contraindicated in patients with Eisenmenger syndrome, given its 50% maternal mortality.

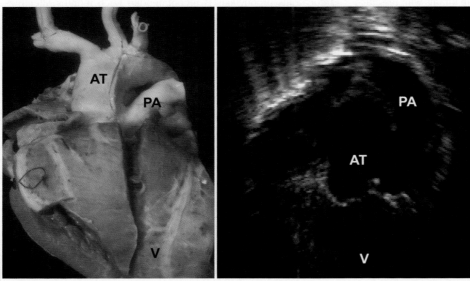

FIGURE 65-11 View of the origin of the pulmonary artery in truncus arteriosus. Note the lateral origin of the pulmonary artery. AT = ascending trunk; PA = pulmonary artery; V = ventricle.

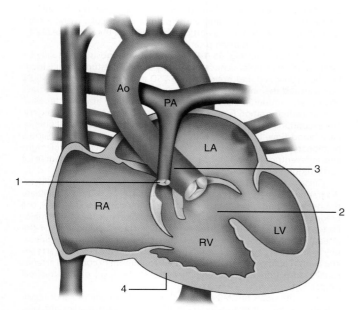

FIGURE 65-12 Diagrammatic representation of tetralogy of Fallot: 1, pulmonary stenosis; 2, ventricular septal defect; 3, overriding aorta; 4, right ventricle hypertrophy. Ao = aorta; LA = left atrium; LV = left ventricle; PA = pulmonary artery; RA = right atrium; RV = right ventricle. *(From Mullins CE, Mayer DC: Congenital Heart Disease: A Diagrammatic Atlas. New York, Wiley-Liss, 1988.)*

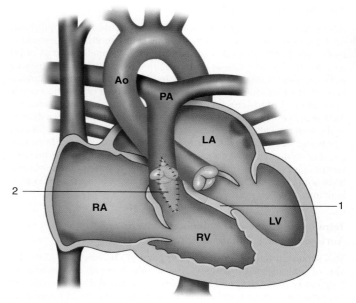

FIGURE 65-13 Diagrammatic representation of the surgical repair of tetralogy of Fallot: 1, patch closure of ventricular septal defect; 2, right ventricular outflow–main pulmonary artery outflow patch (transannular patch). Ao = aorta; LA = left atrium; LV = left ventricle; PA = pulmonary artery; RA = right atrium; RV = right ventricle. *(From Mullins CE, Mayer DC: Congenital Heart Disease: A Diagrammatic Atlas. New York, Wiley-Liss, 1988.)*

FOLLOW-UP. Patients operated on early (<1 year of age) generally do well. However, conduit change is often indicated within the first few years after repair as the patient outgrows its size. Those cases with significant truncal valve stenosis or regurgitation may eventually require truncal valve replacement. Patients operated on late (>1 year of age) require careful follow-up for any signs of pulmonary hypertension progression. Endocarditis prophylaxis is required in all patients.

Cyanotic Heart Disease

Tetralogy of Fallot (Including Tetralogy with Pulmonary Atresia)

MORPHOLOGY (Figs. 65-12 and 65-13). The four components of tetralogy of Fallot are an outlet VSD, obstruction to right ventricular outflow, overriding of the aorta (>50%), and right ventricular hypertrophy. The fundamental abnormality contributing to each of these features is anterior and cephalad deviation of the outlet septum, which is malaligned with respect to the trabecular septum. Thus, tetralogy may occur in the setting of double-outlet right ventricle (aortic override >50%) and may coexist with an AV septal defect, for example. Right ventricular outflow tract obstruction is variable. Often, a stenotic, bicuspid pulmonary valve with supravalvular hypoplasia exists. The dominant site of obstruction is usually at the subvalve level. In some cases, the outflow tract is atretic, and the heart can be diagnosed as having tetralogy of Fallot with pulmonary atresia (also known as complex pulmonary atresia when major aortopulmonary collateral arteries are present). The management and outcome of patients with major aortopulmonary collateral arteries are significantly different from those of patients with less extreme forms of tetralogy and are discussed separately.

ASSOCIATED ANOMALIES. A right aortic arch occurs in about 25% of patients, and abnormalities of the course of the coronary arteries occur in approximately 5%. In the most common anomaly, the anterior descending artery originates from the right coronary artery and courses anteriorly to cross the infundibulum of the right ventricle. Absent pulmonary valve syndrome is a rare form of tetralogy in which stenosis and regurgitation of the right ventricular outflow tract are due to a markedly stenotic pulmonary valve ring with poorly formed or absent valve leaflets. The pulmonary arteries are usually markedly dilated or aneurysmal and may produce airway compression at birth, a poor prognostic feature.

PATHOPHYSIOLOGY. In the absence of alternative sources of pulmonary blood flow, the degree of cyanosis reflects the severity of right ventricular outflow tract obstruction and the level of systemic vascular resistance. There is right-to-left shunting across the VSD. A tetralogy "spell" is an acute fall in arterial saturation, and it may be life-threatening. Its treatment is aimed at relieving obstruction and increasing systemic resistance. Relief of hypoxia with oxygen and morphine, intravenous propranolol, and systemic vasoconstriction (e.g., squatting, knee-chest position, vasoconstrictor drugs) usually reverses the cyanosis.

NATURAL HISTORY. Progressive hypoxemia in the first years of life is expected. Survival to adult life is rare without palliation or correction. The presence of additional sources of blood supply (see later) modifies the rate of progression of cyanosis and its complications.

CLINICAL FEATURES

Unrepaired Patients

Variable cyanosis exists. A right ventricular impulse and systolic thrill are often palpable along the left sternal border. An early systolic ejection sound that is aortic in origin may be heard at the lower left sternal border and apex; the second heart sound is usually single. The intensity and duration of the systolic ejection murmur vary inversely with the severity of subvalve obstruction, the opposite of the relation that exists in patients with pulmonary valve stenosis. With extreme outflow tract stenosis or pulmonary atresia and during an attack of paroxysmal hypoxemia, no murmur or only a short, faint murmur may be detected. A continuous murmur faintly audible over the anterior or posterior chest reflects flow through aortopulmonary collateral vessels or a duct.

After Surgery, Palliated

Progressive cyanosis with its complications can result from worsening right ventricular outflow tract obstruction, gradual stenosis and occlusion of palliative aortopulmonary shunts, or the development of pulmonary hypertension (sometimes seen after Waterston or Potts shunts). Progressive aortic dilation and aortic regurgitation are becoming increasingly recognized. Central cyanosis and clubbing are invariably present.

After Surgery, Repaired

After intracardiac repair, more than 85% of patients are asymptomatic on follow-up, although objective testing will usually demonstrate a reduction in maximal exercise performance. Palpitations from atrial and ventricular arrhythmias and exertional dyspnea from progressive right ventricular dilation secondary to chronic pulmonary regurgitation or severe residual right ventricular outflow tract obstruction occur in 10% to 15% of patients within 20 years after initial repair. An ascending aortic aneurysm and progressive aortic regurgitation from a dilated aortic root may also be present. A parasternal right ventricular lift and a soft and delayed P$_2$ with a low-pitched diastolic murmur from pulmonary regurgitation may exist. A systolic ejection murmur from right ventricular outflow tract obstruction, a high-pitched diastolic murmur from aortic regurgitation, and a pansystolic murmur from a VSD patch leak may also be heard.

Tetralogy of Fallot with Pulmonary Atresia and Major Aortopulmonary Collateral Arteries

This subgroup represents one of the greatest challenges in CHD. The aim of unifocalization surgery is to amalgamate all the sources of pulmonary blood flow and to establish unobstructed right ventricular to pulmonary artery continuity while achieving a normal pulmonary artery pressure and a closed ventricular septum. When this is not possible, a combined interventional catheterization and surgical approach may be indicated. Balloon dilation and stenting of stenosed arteries and anastomoses can "rehabilitate" segmental supply and allow subsequent VSD closure or, if it is already closed, reduce right ventricular pressure.

LABORATORY INVESTIGATIONS

ELECTROCARDIOGRAPHY. Right-axis deviation with right ventricular and right atrial hypertrophy is common. In adults with repaired tetralogy of Fallot, a complete right bundle branch block after repair has been the rule. QRS width may reflect the degree of right ventricular dilation and, when extreme (>180 milliseconds) or rapidly progressive, may be a risk factor for sustained ventricular tachycardia and sudden death.

CHEST RADIOGRAPHY. Characteristically, there is a normal-sized, boot-shaped heart *(coeur en sabot)* with prominence of the right ventricle and a concavity in the region of the underdeveloped right ventricular outflow tract and main pulmonary artery. The pulmonary vascular markings are typically diminished, and the aortic arch may be on the right side (25%). The ascending aorta is often prominent.

ECHOCARDIOGRAPHY (**Fig. 65-14**). A complete diagnosis can usually be established by Doppler echocardiography alone. The study should identify the malaligned and nonrestrictive VSD and overriding aorta (>50% override) and the presence and degree of right ventricular outflow tract obstruction (infundibular, valvular, or pulmonary arterial stenosis). Cardiac catheterization is now rarely required before corrective surgery. The exception to this rule is when there are additional sources of pulmonary blood flow. In patients with repaired tetralogy of Fallot, residual pulmonary stenosis and regurgitation (see Fig. 66-42), residual VSD, right and left ventricular size and function, aortic root size, and degree of aortic regurgitation should be assessed.

CARDIAC CATHETERIZATION AND ANGIOCARDIOGRAPHY. Although echocardiography, magnetic resonance angiography, and fast CT may delineate the presence and proximal course of the pulmonary blood vessels, the preoperative assessment of tetralogy with pulmonary atresia with major aortopulmonary collateral arteries usually includes delineation of the arterial supply to both lungs by selective catheterization and angiography to show the course and segmental supply from the collateral arteries and central pulmonary arteries. Major aortopulmonary collateral arteries usually arise from the descending aorta at the level of the tracheal bifurcation.

CMR. The goals of CMR examination after tetralogy of Fallot repair include the quantitative assessment of left and particularly right ventricular volumes, stroke volumes, and ejection fraction; imaging of the anatomy of the right ventricular outflow tract, pulmonary arteries, aorta, and aortopulmonary collaterals; and quantification of pulmonary, aortic, and tricuspid regurgitation (see Fig. 66-42).

INDICATIONS FOR INTERVENTION

Children

Symptomatic infants are now repaired at any age, and elective repair in asymptomatic infants during the first 6 months is advocated by many. This is often at the expense of a transannular patch enlargement of the right ventricular outflow tract, which is a risk factor for later reintervention. Marked hypoplasia of the pulmonary arteries, small body size, and prematurity are relative contraindications for early corrective operation, and these patients may be successfully palliated by balloon dilation of the right ventricular outflow tract (with or without stenting) and pulmonary arteries.

Adults, Unrepaired

For unrepaired adults, surgical repair is still recommended because the results are gratifying and the operative risk is comparable to that of pediatric series, provided there is no serious coexisting morbidity.

Palliated

Palliation was seldom intended as a permanent treatment strategy, and most of these patients should undergo surgical repair. In particular, palliated patients with increasing cyanosis and erythrocytosis (from gradual shunt stenosis or development of pulmonary hypertension), left ventricular dilation, or aneurysm formation in the shunt should undergo intracardiac repair with takedown of the shunt unless irreversible pulmonary hypertension has developed.

Repaired

The following situations *may* warrant intervention after repair: a residual VSD with a shunt greater than 1.5:1; residual pulmonary stenosis (either the native right ventricular outflow or valved conduit if one is present) with right ventricular systolic pressure two thirds or more of

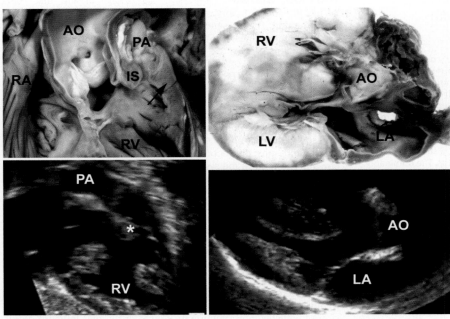

FIGURE 65-14 Montage of tetralogy of Fallot. The two left images are in the right anterior oblique view that demonstrates the anteriorly deviated infundibular septum (asterisk) and the ventricular septal defect. The arrow on the specimen points to the hypertrophied septoparietal trabeculations. The right images demonstrate the overriding aorta and the ventricular septal defect. AO = aorta; IS = infundibular septum; LA = left atrium; PA = pulmonary artery; RA = right atrium; RV = right ventricle.

systemic pressure; or severe pulmonary regurgitation associated with substantial right ventricular dilation or dysfunction (i.e., right ventricular diastolic volume index >150 to 170 mL/m^2 or a right ventricular ejection fraction <45%),[53,54] exercise intolerance, or sustained arrhythmias. The coexistence of substantial left ventricular dysfunction or a QRS duration >180 milliseconds offers additional support when other indications are present. The development of major cardiac arrhythmias, most commonly atrial flutter or fibrillation or sustained ventricular tachycardia, usually reflects hemodynamic deterioration and should be treated accordingly. Surgery is occasionally necessary for significant aortic regurgitation associated with symptoms or progressive left ventricular dilation and for aortic root enlargement of 55 mm or more.[55] Rapid enlargement of a right ventricular outflow tract aneurysm needs surgical attention.

INTERVENTIONAL OPTIONS

Surgery

Reparative surgery involves closure of the VSD with a Dacron patch and relief of the right ventricular outflow tract obstruction. The latter may involve resection of infundibular muscle and insertion of a right ventricular outflow tract or transannular patch—a patch across the pulmonary valve annulus that disrupts the integrity of the pulmonary valve and causes important pulmonary regurgitation. When an anomalous coronary artery crosses the right ventricular outflow tract and precludes a patch, an extracardiac conduit is placed between the right ventricle and pulmonary artery, bypassing the right ventricular outflow tract obstruction. A PFO or secundum ASD may be closed. Additional treatable lesions, such as muscular VSDs, PDAs, and aortopulmonary collaterals, should also be addressed at the time of surgery.

Reoperation is necessary in 10% to 15% of patients after reparative surgery during a 20-year follow-up. For persistent right ventricular outflow tract obstruction, resection of residual infundibular stenosis or placement of a right ventricular outflow or transannular patch, with or without pulmonary arterioplasty, can be performed. On occasion, an extracardiac valved conduit may be necessary. Pulmonary valve replacement (either homograft or xenograft) is used to treat severe pulmonary regurgitation. Concomitant tricuspid valve annuloplasty may be performed for moderate or severe tricuspid regurgitation. Concomitant cryoablation may be performed at the time of surgery for patients with preexisting atrial or ventricular arrhythmias.

Transcatheter

Percutaneous pulmonary valve replacement can be performed with mortality similar to that of surgical pulmonary valve replacement and favorable hemodynamic short- and intermediate-term results with less morbidity to the patient,[56,57] but it should be done only in adult CHD centers with expertise in the procedure.[57] At present, these therapies are reserved primarily for those patients with circumferential right ventricle–pulmonary artery conduits (i.e., homografts, valved conduits) measuring ≤22 mm.[58] Significant branch pulmonary artery stenosis can be managed with balloon dilation and usually stent insertion.

Implantable Cardioverter-Defibrillator (see Chap. 38)

The selection of appropriate candidates for primary prevention implantable-cardioverter defibrillators (ICDs) remains controversial. ICDs are probably most beneficial in "high-risk patients" (e.g., prior palliative shunt, QRS >180 milliseconds, inducible ventricular tachycardia, and left ventricular dysfunction) and are probably best reserved for those with a high annual risk (≥3.5% per year) of sudden cardiac death. When a patient presents with ventricular tachycardia and no underlying significant hemodynamic lesion, ICD implantation should be considered a secondary prevention measure.

INTERVENTIONAL OUTCOMES. The overall survival of patients who have had initial operative repair is excellent, provided the VSD has been closed and the right ventricular outflow tract obstruction has been relieved. A 25-year survival of 94% has been reported. Pulmonary valve replacement for chronic pulmonary regurgitation or right ventricular outflow tract obstruction after initial intracardiac repair can be done safely with a mortality rate of 1%. Pulmonary valve replacement, when it is performed for significant pulmonary regurgitation, leads to an improvement in exercise tolerance as well as favorable right ventricular remodeling. Sudden death can occur. Ventricular tachycardia can arise at the site of the right ventriculotomy, from VSD patch sutures, or from the right ventricular outflow tract. Patients at high risk for sudden death include those with right ventricular dilation and a QRS duration of 180 milliseconds or more on the ECG. Moderate to severe left ventricular dysfunction is another risk factor for sudden death. The reported incidence of sudden death is approximately 5%, which accounts for approximately one third of late deaths during the first 20 years of follow-up.

FOLLOW-UP. All patients should have expert cardiology follow-up every 1 to 2 years.

Fontan Procedure–Requiring Lesions

The next four sections describe lesions usually or often treated with a Fontan procedure. These include tricuspid atresia, hypoplastic left heart syndrome, double-inlet ventricle, and isomerism. *Fontan procedure* has become a generic term to describe a palliative surgical procedure that redirects the systemic venous return directly to the pulmonary arteries without passing through a subpulmonary ventricle. It is performed in patients having a "functionally single" ventricle or when a biventricular intracardiac repair is not possible, even though there are two good-sized ventricles. Although it is undoubtedly imperfect, the Fontan circuit restores an in-series pulmonary-to-systemic circulation, removing the chronic volume load of the systemic ventricle previously supporting a parallel circuit of pulmonary and systemic circulations. The earliest iteration of the Fontan procedure was a simple "atriopulmonary" connection, whereby the right atrium or its appendage was anastomosed to the pulmonary arteries. Because of the long-term problems of atrial dilation, arrhythmia, and thrombosis, this procedure has been abandoned in favor of hemodynamically superior versions. In the early 1990s, the total cavopulmonary anastomosis or lateral tunnel Fontan was introduced. This consisted of a direct, end-to-side superior cavopulmonary anastomosis (bidirectional Glenn operation) in combination with an intra-atrial baffle or tube connection of the inferior vena cava to the underside of the confluent pulmonary arteries. More recently, the inferior vena cava has been directed to the pulmonary arteries via an extracardiac conduit, completely excluding the atrium from the circuit. It remains to be seen whether these modifications will have the desired effect of reducing late morbidity, and all patients will require regular and careful review in special centers.

Tricuspid Atresia (Absent Right Atrioventricular Connection)

MORPHOLOGY. Classic tricuspid atresia is best described as absence of the right AV connection (**Figs. 65-15** and **65-16**). Consequently, there must be an ASD. There is usually hypoplasia of the morphologic right ventricle, which communicates to the dominant ventricle via a VSD. Patients may be subdivided into those with concordant ventriculoarterial connections and normally related great arteries (70% to 80% of cases) and those with discordant connections, in which the aorta arises from the small right ventricle and is fed via the VSD. Associated lesions in the latter group include subaortic stenosis and aortic arch anomalies.

PATHOPHYSIOLOGY. The clinical picture and management are dominated by issues related to the ventriculoarterial connections. All patients have "mixing" of atrial blood, and thus their degree of cyanosis is governed by the amount of pulmonary blood flow and systemic venous saturations. Patients with concordant ventriculoarterial connections tend to be more cyanosed (depending on the size of the VSD), whereas those with discordant connections are pinker and tend to develop heart failure (because the unobstructed pulmonary circulation arises directly from the left ventricle). Some present with a critical reduction of systemic blood flow because of obstruction at the VSD or associated aortic arch anomalies and behave much like hypoplastic left heart syndrome.

LABORATORY INVESTIGATIONS

ELECTROCARDIOGRAPHY. Left-axis deviation, right atrial enlargement, and left ventricular hypertrophy often occur. Left atrial enlargement may be present if pulmonary flow is high.

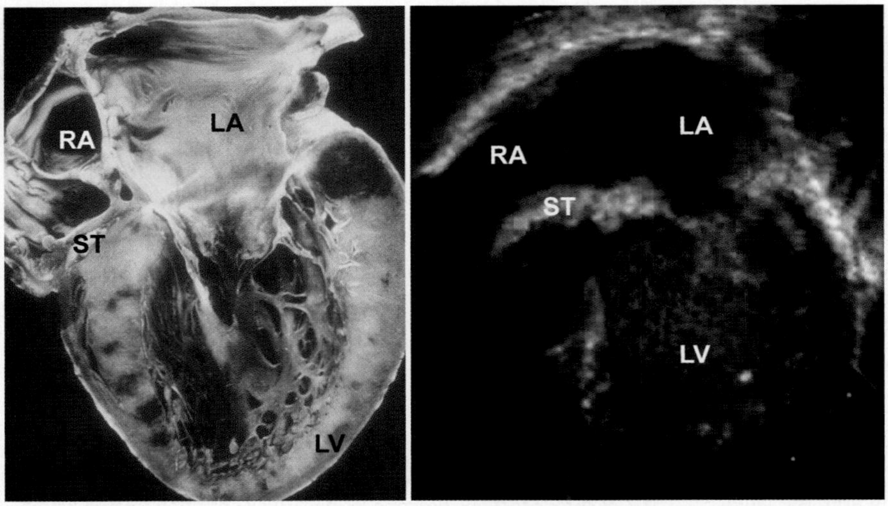

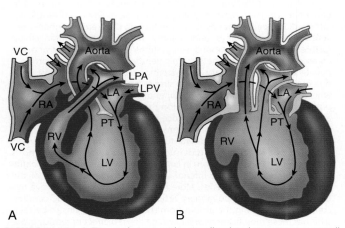

FIGURE 65-15 Apical four-chamber view in univentricular connection of left ventricular type with absent right connection (tricuspid atresia). Note the wedge of sulcus tissue in the floor of the right atrium. LA = left atrium; LV = left ventricle; RA = right atrium; ST = sulcus tissue.

is no subaortic narrowing to a full Norwood stage 1 procedure in those presenting with severe stenosis and a hypoplastic ascending aorta and arch.

The aim of early palliation is to prepare for a Fontan procedure. This should be performed only when there is good ventricular function, unobstructed systemic blood flow, and minimal AV valve regurgitation. Candidates for these corrective procedures must also have a low pulmonary resistance, a mean pulmonary artery pressure less than 15 mm Hg, and pulmonary arteries of adequate size.

Hypoplastic Left Heart Syndrome

DEFINITION. Hypoplastic left heart syndrome is a generic term used to describe a group of closely related cardiac anomalies characterized by underdevelopment of the left cardiac chambers, in association with atresia or stenosis of the aortic or the mitral orifice and hypoplasia of the aorta. The term should be restricted to those with normally connected hearts with concordant atrioventricular and ventriculoarterial connections. Hypoplastic left heart syndrome (**Fig. 65-17**) is characterized by duct-dependent systemic blood flow and so tends to present with severe symptoms within the first week of life, as ductal constriction occurs. Untreated, the disease is almost uniformly fatal in infancy. In the past, many infants would present with severe acidemic circulatory collapse, but this is becoming less frequent as fetal ultrasound screening for cardiac

FIGURE 65-16 **A,** Tricuspid atresia with normally related great arteries, a small ventricular septal defect, diminutive right ventricular chamber, and narrowed outflow tract. **B,** An example of tricuspid atresia and complete transposition of the great arteries in which the left ventricular chamber is essentially a common ventricle, with the aorta arising from an infundibular component (RV) of the common ventricle. LA = left atrium; LPA = left pulmonary artery; LPV = left pulmonary vein; LV = left ventricle; PT = pulmonary trunk; RA = right atrium; RV = right ventricle; VC = vena cava. (**A** and **B** modified from Edwards JE, Burchell HB: Congenital tricuspid atresia: Classification. Med Clin North Am 33:1177, 1949.)

CHEST RADIOGRAPHY. Situs solitus, levocardia, and a left-sided aortic arch usually occur. The heart size and pulmonary vascular markings vary with the amount of pulmonary blood flow. The main pulmonary trunk is inapparent. A right aortic arch exists in 25% of patients.

ECHOCARDIOGRAPHY. This establishes the full segmental diagnosis. The size of the ASD, VSD, and aortic arch must be carefully assessed.

CARDIAC CATHETERIZATION. This is rarely required for initial diagnosis or management. It can be useful to assess the degree of subaortic stenosis (by assessing the change in left ventricle to aortic pressure gradient while performing an isoprenaline or dobutamine challenge) and is usually performed to measure the pulmonary artery pressure and resistance before venopulmonary connections.

MANAGEMENT OPTIONS. In those with concordant ventriculoarterial connections and severe cyanosis, a systemic to pulmonary shunt is performed in the first 6 to 8 weeks of life, and in older children, a primary bidirectional Glenn procedure can be considered. In infants with discordant arterial connections, early palliation ranges from pulmonary artery banding to reduce pulmonary blood flow when there

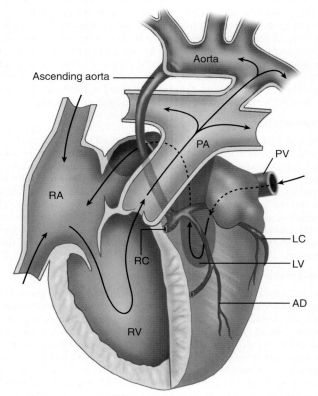

FIGURE 65-17 Hypoplastic left heart with aortic hypoplasia, aortic valve atresia, and a hypoplastic mitral valve and left ventricle. AD = anterior descending; LC = left circumflex; LV = left ventricle; PA = pulmonary artery; PV = pulmonary vein; RA = right atrium; RC = right coronary artery; RV = right ventricle. (From Neufeld HN, Adams P Jr, Edwards JE, et al: Diagnosis of aortic atresia by retrograde aortography. Circulation 25:278, 1962.)

anomalies becomes more generally available and successful. Fetal diagnosis allows a planned delivery and institution of prostaglandin therapy from birth and has now been proven to reduce subsequent preoperative morbidity and perioperative mortality during the first stage of surgical repair.

PATHOPHYSIOLOGY. It remains uncertain whether hypoplastic left heart syndrome reflects a primary myocardial disease or is a consequence of a structural or hemodynamic abnormality. There is no doubt that in some patients, an apparently isolated dilated cardiomyopathy in early fetal life may evolve (as a result of a subsequent lack of left ventricular growth) into hypoplastic left heart syndrome later in gestation. Congenital structural abnormalities clearly play a significant role as well. This is exemplified by the effect of isolated valvular stenosis to produce a continuum of hypoplastic left heart syndrome to critical aortic stenosis with a normal-sized left ventricle. Therefore, hypoplastic left heart syndrome is likely to be multifactorial in origin.

CLINICAL FEATURES. The diagnosis should be considered in any infant with the sudden onset of circulatory collapse and severe lactic acidosis. As such, it must be distinguished from neonatal sepsis and metabolic disorders. Until it is excluded, any child presenting in this way should be treated with prostaglandin, which may have a dramatically positive effect if there is an underlying cardiac abnormality and little effect if there is not.

LABORATORY INVESTIGATIONS
ELECTROCARDIOGRAPHY. This frequently shows right-axis deviation, right atrial and ventricular enlargement, and ST and T wave abnormalities in the left precordial leads.
CHEST RADIOGRAPHY. This usually shows some cardiac enlargement shortly after birth; but with clinical deterioration, there may be marked cardiomegaly and increased pulmonary venous and arterial vascular markings.
ECHOCARDIOGRAPHY (**Fig. 65-18**). Cross-sectional echocardiography provides a full segmental diagnosis. In its classic form, the left ventricular cavity is small, with a diminutive mitral valve. The myocardium may be thinned or be of normal thickness, but the endocardium is usually thickened, consistent with endocardial fibroelastosis. There may be fistulous communications between the left ventricular cavity and the coronary arteries, a feature much more likely when the mitral valve is patent rather than atretic. The aortic root is usually diminutive, less than 4 to 5 mm in diameter at the level of the sinuses of Valsalva and narrowed in its ascending portion. The aortic arch is usually larger, but there is often a juxtaductal coarctation. The duct varies in size according to treatment, and assessment of this and the size of the interatrial communication is crucial to management. There may be profound desaturation and rapid demise (because of a combination of reduced pulmonary blood flow and pulmonary edema) in children with an intact atrial septum or restrictive PFO.

MANAGEMENT OPTIONS. Early treatment with prostaglandin is mandatory. Those presenting in shock require paralysis, mechanical ventilation, and inotropic support. Crucial to management of these patients is maintenance of a balanced pulmonary and systemic blood flow. The cardiac output is fixed and is distributed according to the relative magnitude of the systemic and pulmonary vascular resistance. Thus, measures to elevate the pulmonary resistance (by imposing hypercapnia or by alveolar hypoxia) and to reduce the systemic resistance (using vasodilators) are frequently required.

Surgical Treatment

Staged surgical management now provides long-term palliation to most patients with hypoplastic left heart syndrome. The first stage, often referred to as the Norwood procedure, now has many versions, but its essence is the creation of an unobstructed communication between the right ventricle and an unobstructed aorta. The right ventricular to aortic connection is accomplished by direct connection between the transected proximal pulmonary trunk and ascending aorta, usually with a patch extending around the augmented aortic arch. Pulmonary blood flow is established via a systemic to pulmonary shunt or the more recently introduced right ventricle to pulmonary artery conduit. The PDA is ligated, and a large interatrial communication is created. Early results of this procedure were poor, but survival rates higher than 85% have recently been published. Institutional variations, the interval mortality, and those unsuitable to progress to stage 2 must also be taken into account, however, and in some centers, the preferred operation is cardiac transplantation.

Stage 2 consists of an end-to-side superior vena cava to pulmonary artery connection (bidirectional Glenn procedure) or a hemi-Fontan (incorporating the roof of the atrium into the pulmonary artery anastomosis). This is performed at approximately 6 months of age as an intermediate step before stage 3, a Fontan operation. A newer innovation is the so-called hybrid procedure, whereby at the first stage each pulmonary artery is banded separately and a stent is placed, by the interventional cardiologist, to maintain ductal patency either directly via the main pulmonary artery in concert with the surgeon or percutaneously. The second stage combines the surgical aortopulmonary anastomosis with the bidirectional Glenn procedure. It remains to be seen whether this approach confers a survival or physiologic advantage.

ADULT ISSUES. The survivors of the earliest attempts at staged Norwood palliation are just now entering adult life. Their issues are likely to be common to all late survivors of Fontan palliation with a systemic right ventricle.

Double-Inlet Ventricle

DEFINITION. Double-inlet connection falls under the umbrella of univentricular AV connections. These hearts are defined by having more than 50% of each AV connection connected to a dominant ventricle. In practice, this usually means that the whole of one and more than 50% of the alternative junction is connected to either a left or right ventricle. When there is a common junction, more than 75% of the junction must be connected to the dominant ventricle.

MORPHOLOGY. In about 75% of patients, the dominant ventricle is a left ventricle that is separated from the right ventricle by a VSD. In 20%, the dominant ventricle is a right ventricle, and the small, incomplete ventricle is of left ventricular apical morphology. In only 5% of cases is there truly only one ventricle in the ventricular mass. In double-inlet left ventricle, the most common ventriculoarterial connection is discordant. Thus, the aorta arises from the small right ventricle and is fed via the VSD, and the generally unobstructed pulmonary artery arises from the left ventricle. Aortic and aortic arch anomalies are frequent in these patients.

PATHOPHYSIOLOGY. The basic circulatory physiology of double-inlet left ventricle is identical to that of tricuspid atresia. Common mixing of systemic and pulmonary venous blood occurs, and the blood is then ejected from the left ventricle into the pulmonary artery (with discordant connections) or aorta (with concordant connections). In the former, the

CH
65

CONGENITAL HEART DISEASE

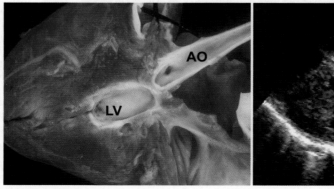

FIGURE 65-18 Long-axis view of the left ventricle and aorta in hypoplastic left heart syndrome. Note the associated endocardial fibroelastosis in the specimen. AO = aorta, LV = left ventricle.

blood must pass through the VSD to gain egress to the aorta. Subaortic stenosis, aortic hypoplasia, and arch anomalies are therefore common. In double-inlet right ventricle, it is those patients with concordant ventriculoarterial connections who are at particular risk of systemic outflow obstruction. One or the other or both of the two AV valves (when present) may be stenotic, atretic, or regurgitant. Under these circumstances, the integrity of the atrial septum becomes important. If there is left or right atrial outflow obstruction, a septectomy or septostomy will be required.

CLINICAL FEATURES. When there is critical reduction of systemic outflow, infants may be duct dependent and present with acidemic shock. Conversely, when pulmonary blood flow is reduced, presentation may be with severe cyanosis or with duct-dependent pulmonary blood flow. Other patients may not present in the neonatal period and will develop heart failure because of increased pulmonary blood flow. Patients undergo the same surgical algorithms as those with tricuspid atresia and so ultimately will undergo a Fontan operation. Their clinical issues are typical of any patient after this procedure.

LABORATORY INVESTIGATIONS
ELECTROCARDIOGRAPHY. This is highly variable. Ventricular hypertrophy appropriate to the dominant ventricle is expected.
CHEST RADIOGRAPHY. This is similarly variable and rarely diagnostic.
ECHOCARDIOGRAPHY (**Fig. 65-19**). A full segmental diagnosis should be possible in all patients. Particular attention should be paid to defining AV valve anomalies and the presence and anatomy of any subaortic obstruction. This may develop, even if it is not present at birth, and should be part of the routine surveillance of these patients.

INDICATIONS AND OPTIONS FOR INTERVENTION. Survival without intervention may be prolonged, but at the expense of increasing cyanosis (when there is restriction to pulmonary blood flow) or pulmonary vascular disease (when there is unrestricted pulmonary blood flow). Those born with restricted systemic blood flow require urgent surgical intervention, usually undergoing a Norwood-type repair to establish the pulmonary valve as the unobstructed systemic outflow tract. Pulmonary artery banding is offered only to those infants with pulmonary overcirculation, heart failure, and unobstructed systemic outflow. Subsequently, and sometimes as the primary procedure, a bidirectional Glenn anastomosis is performed as a prelude to a Fontan procedure.

FOLLOW-UP. These patients should be reviewed frequently and in a center conversant with the issues of the Fontan operation.

Isomerism

DEFINITION. For the purposes of illustrating the cardiac manifestations, isomerism describes the situation in which both atrial appendages have either left or right anatomic features (i.e., bilateral right or bilateral left atrial appendages).

MORPHOLOGY. Experts have made many attempts to describe hearts with complex abnormalities of visceral and atrial situs, whereby normal lateralization is lost. Terms such as *heterotaxy, asplenia,* and *polysplenia* fail to adequately describe either the visceral or cardiac manifestations with enough precision. The left atrial appendage is characterized by its tubular shape and pectinate muscles confined to the appendage. The pectinate muscles of the triangular right atrial appendage extend from its broad junction with the atrium to extend around the vestibule or AV junction. Thus, the arrangement of the atria (usual, mirror image, right or left isomerism) can be defined independently of the venous anatomy.

In left isomerism, it is not unusual to have a biventricular AV connection, with separate AV junctions. A common junction (with an AV septal defect) is seen in approximately 30% of cases of left isomerism and more than 90% of hearts with right isomerism. Concordant ventriculoarterial connections predominate in left isomerism, and a double-outlet right ventricle with an anterior aorta is most frequently seen when there is right isomerism. The venous connections are variable. These variations significantly affect the clinical and interventional management of these patients.

Isomerism of the Right Atrial Appendages

CLINICAL FEATURES. Bilateral "right-sidedness" results in a pattern of visceral abnormalities sometimes described as asplenia syndrome. The liver is midline, and both lungs are trilobed with symmetrically short bronchi on the chest radiograph; the spleen is hypoplastic or absent, which mandates immunization against pneumococcal infection and continuous penicillin prophylaxis against gram-positive sepsis. The diagnosis can be inferred from the bronchial pattern on the chest radiograph but most often is established by cross-sectional echocardiography because of early presentation with severe CHD. Abdominal scanning shows ipsilateral arrangement of the aorta and an anterior inferior vena cava. The intracardiac anatomy is most often that of an AV septal defect with varying degrees of right ventricular dominance, and there is frequently an associated double-outlet right ventricle with an anterior aorta and subpulmonary stenosis or atresia. Thus, cyanosis is the most common presentation. The inferior vena cava may connect to either right atrium, and superior venae cavae are often lateralized and separate. It is the pulmonary venous drainage that is crucial to the presentation and outcome of these children. By definition, the pulmonary veins are draining anomalously to one or other right atrium, but this is frequently indirect or obstructed. Adequate repair of this is fundamental to the outcome of these children, who almost uniformly ultimately require a Fontan procedure.

MANAGEMENT OPTIONS AND OUTCOMES. Initial palliation is usually directed toward regulating pulmonary blood flow and dealing with anomalies of pulmonary venous connection. Subsequently, these patients (even when there are equal-sized ventricles) are treated along a Fontan algorithm. This is because repair of complete AV septal defect in the setting of abnormal ventriculoarterial connections is technically difficult or impossible. Thus, a unilateral or bilateral superior cavopulmonary anastomosis is performed at approximately 6 months of age, followed when possible by a Fontan procedure at 2 to 4 years of age.

The long-term outcome of surgery for right isomerism, however, has been poor. Improved early palliation and a staged approach toward the Fontan procedure have led to improved results. The prognosis for these infants, particularly when there is obstruction to pulmonary venous return, must remain guarded.

Isomerism of the Left Atrial Appendages

CLINICAL FEATURES. These patients have bilateral "left-sidedness." Hence, they have two left lungs and bronchi, tend to have

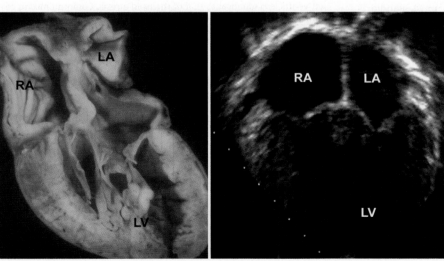

FIGURE 65-19 Apical four-chamber view in a double-inlet univentricular connection of left ventricular type with two atrioventricular valves. LA = left atrium; LV = left ventricle; RA = right atrium.

polysplenia, and frequently have malrotation of the gut. The cardiac abnormalities tend to be less severe than those of right isomerism. These patients are particularly prone to development of atrial arrhythmias because the normal sinoatrial node is a right atrial structure and is usually absent in these patients. The ECG often shows an abnormal P wave axis, or wandering pacemaker. Complete heart block may also occur. The anatomic diagnosis is usually established by echocardiography. The abdominal great vessels are both to the right or left of the spine, as with right isomerism; but in left isomerism, the vein is a posterior azygos vein that continues to connect to a left- or right-sided superior vena cava. The intrahepatic inferior vena cava is absent in 90%, and under these circumstances, the hepatic veins drain directly to the atria. The pulmonary venous connection needs to be defined precisely before any surgical intervention. Pulmonary arteriovenous malformations are not infrequently seen in patients with left isomerism. These can lead to cyanosis in unrepaired or repaired patients. The intracardiac anatomy varies from essentially normal to complex. Again, AV septal defect (partial and complete) is overrepresented but with less frequent ventricular imbalance and abnormalities of ventriculo-arterial connection.

MANAGEMENT OPTIONS. A biventricular repair is achieved in many more of these patients, albeit with the need for complex atrial baffle surgery to separate the systemic and pulmonary venous returns. The long-term outcome for patients with left isomerism is therefore much better than that for patients with right isomerism. The issues are much like those related to the type of surgery, but monitoring for arrhythmia needs to be even more intense than usual.

The Fontan Patient (Fig. 65-20)

BACKGROUND. As stated in the introduction to this section, the uncertain nature of the Fontan circulation and the frequency of its failure require that all patients be followed up regularly in a specialized center for CHD, and new symptoms should prompt early reevaluation in such a center.

Since its description for the surgical management of tricuspid atresia in 1971, the Fontan procedure has become the definitive palliative surgical treatment when a biventricular repair is not possible. The principle is diversion of the systemic venous return directly to the pulmonary arteries without passing through a sub-pulmonary ventricle. Over the years, many modifications of the original procedure have been described and performed, namely, direct atriopulmonary connection, total cavopulmonary connection, and extracardiac conduit. Fenestration (4- to 5-mm diameter) of the Fontan circuit into the left atrium is sometimes performed at the time of surgery in high-risk patients, permitting right-to-left shunting and decompression of the Fontan circuit.

PATHOPHYSIOLOGY. Elevation of the central venous pressure and a reduced cardiac output (sometimes at rest but always on exercise) are inevitable consequences of the Fontan procedure. Small adverse changes in ventricular function (particularly diastolic) or circuit efficiency (elevated pulmonary resistance, obstruction, thrombosis) and the onset of arrhythmia all potentially lead to major symptomatic deterioration.

Although it is reasonable to describe patients after the Fontan procedure as existing in a form of chronic heart failure (since their right atrial pressure must be high), this is seldom due to marked systolic dysfunction. Indeed, a

small elevation in ventricular diastolic pressure may be much more harmful. Thus, it may be incorrect to treat these patients with traditional heart failure medications. In a randomized, blinded placebo-controlled study, ACE inhibition failed to improve functional performance, and some indices worsened.

The more "streamlined" Fontan circulations (total cavopulmonary anastomosis, extracardiac conduit) that exclude the right atrium from the circulation have demonstrably better fluid dynamic properties and improved functional performance. Physical obstruction at surgical anastomoses, distal pulmonary arteries, or pulmonary veins (often due to compression by a dilated right atrium) reduces circulatory efficiency, however. Similarly, elevated pulmonary arteriolar resistances have adverse effects. This is because the pulmonary vascular resistance is the single biggest contributor to impairment of venous return and elevation of venous pressure. Relatively little is known about pulmonary vascular resistance late after the procedure, but it has been shown to be elevated in a significant number of patients and to be reactive to inhaled nitric oxide, suggesting pulmonary endothelial dysfunction. Recently, beneficial effects on exercise performance were shown with sildenafil treatment, but this remains to be confirmed in larger studies.

CLINICAL FEATURES. The majority of patients (≈90%) present in functional Class I or II at 5 years' follow-up after a Fontan procedure. Progressive deterioration of functional status with time is the rule. Supraventricular arrhythmias such as atrial tachycardia, flutter, and fibrillation are common. Physical examination in an otherwise uncomplicated patient reveals an elevated, usually nonpulsatile jugular venous pulse, a quiet apex, a normal S_1, and a single S_2 (the pulmonary artery having been tied off). A heart murmur should not be present, and its identification may suggest the presence of systemic AV valve regurgitation or subaortic obstruction. Generalized edema and ascites may be a sign of protein-losing enteropathy (see later).

COMPLICATIONS AND SEQUELAE

Arrhythmia (see Chap. 39)

Although often associated with marked symptomatic decline, atrial arrhythmias tend to reflect the consequences of the abnormalities of ventricular function and circulatory efficiency described earlier. The

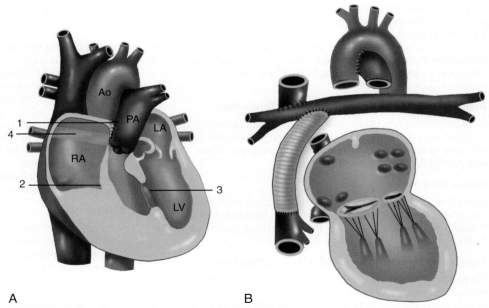

A   B

FIGURE 65-20 Modification of the Fontan operation. **A,** Direct atriopulmonary connection (1) for tricuspid valve atresia (2); ventricular septal defect, oversewn (3); patch closure of atrial septal defect (4). **B,** Extracardiac conduit made of a Dacron graft bypassing the right atrium, connecting the inferior vena cava to the inferior aspect of the right pulmonary artery. Superior vena cava is anastomosed to the superior aspect of the right pulmonary artery. Ao = aorta; LA = left atrium; LV = left ventricle; PA = pulmonary artery; RA = right atrium. (**A** from Mullins CE, Mayer DC: Congenital Heart Disease: A Diagrammatic Atlas. New York, Wiley-Liss, 1988. **B** from Marcelletti C: Inferior vena cava–pulmonary artery extracardiac conduit: A new form of right heart bypass. J Thorac Cardiovasc Surg 100:228, 1990.)

massively dilated right atrium after an atriopulmonary connection is commonly associated with atrial flutter and fibrillation (15% to 20% at 5 years' follow-up).[59] Atrial flutter or fibrillation carries significant morbidity, can be associated with profound hemodynamic deterioration, and needs prompt medical attention. The combination of atrial incisions and multiple suture lines at the time of Fontan surgery along with increased right atrial pressure and size probably explains the high incidence of atrial arrhythmias in such patients. Patients at greater risk for atrial tachyarrhythmias are those who were operated on at an older age, with poor ventricular function, systemic AV valve regurgitation, or increased pulmonary artery pressure. It has been suggested that the exclusion of the right atrium from elevated systemic venous pressure (as in total cavopulmonary connections or extracardiac conduits) leads to a decrease in the incidence of atrial arrhythmias. This apparent benefit may, however, be due exclusively to the shorter length of follow-up in this group of patients. Sinus node dysfunction and complete heart block can occur and require pacemaker insertion.

Thrombosis and Stroke

The reported incidence of thromboembolic complications in the Fontan circuit varies from 6% to 25%, depending on the diagnostic method used and the length of follow-up. Thrombus formation may relate to the presence of supraventricular arrhythmias, right atrial dilation, right atrial "smoke," and the artificial material used to construct the Fontan circuit. Systemic arterial embolism in patients with and without a fenestrated Fontan has also been reported. Protein C deficiency has been reported in these patients and may explain in part their propensity to thromboembolism. There is continuing debate as to the role of anticoagulation, antiplatelet therapy, or both in the long-term management of these patients, but most receive some form of therapy.

Protein-Losing Enteropathy

Protein-losing enteropathy, defined as severe loss of serum protein into the intestine, occurs in 4% to 13% of patients after a Fontan procedure.[60] Patients present with generalized edema, ascites, pleural effusion, or chronic diarrhea. Protein-losing enteropathy is thought to result principally from chronically elevated systemic venous pressure causing intestinal lymphangiectasia with consequent loss of albumin, protein, lymphocytes, and immunoglobulin into the gastrointestinal tract. The diagnosis is confirmed by the findings of low serum albumin and protein concentrations, low plasma alpha$_1$-antitrypsin level and lymphocyte counts, and, most important, high alpha$_1$-antitrypsin stool clearance. It carries a dismal prognosis, with a 5-year survival of 46% to 59%.

Right Pulmonary Vein Compression or Obstruction

Right pulmonary vein obstruction or compression can occur from the enlarged right atrium or atrial baffle bulging into the left atrium and can lead to a vicious spiral of increased pulmonary artery pressure with further dilation of the right atrium.

Fontan Obstruction

Stenosis or partial obstruction of the Fontan connection leads to exercise intolerance, atrial tachyarrhythmias, and right-sided heart failure. Sudden total obstruction (usually thrombotic) can present as sudden death.

Ventricular Dysfunction and Valvular Regurgitation

Progressive deterioration of systemic ventricular function, with or without progressive AV valve regurgitation, is common. Patients with morphologic systemic right ventricles may fare less well than those with morphologic left ventricles.

Hepatic Dysfunction

Mildly raised hepatic transaminase levels from hepatic congestion are frequent but seldom clinically important. Cirrhosis due to chronic venous hypertension is increasingly recognized, and monitoring for complications of cirrhosis should be initiated.[61]

Cyanosis

Worsening cyanosis may relate to worsening of ventricular function, the development of venous collateral channels draining to the left atrium, or the development of pulmonary arteriovenous malformations (especially if a classic Glenn procedure remains as part of the Fontan circulation). In Fontan patients with cirrhosis, the hepatopulmonary syndrome may occur.[62]

LABORATORY INVESTIGATIONS

ELECTROCARDIOGRAPHY. Sinus rhythm, atrial flutter, junctional rhythm, or complete heart block may be present. The QRS complex reflects the basic underlying cardiac anomaly. In patients with tricuspid atresia, left-axis deviation is the norm. In patients with univentricular hearts, the conduction pattern varies widely and depends on the morphology and relative position of the rudimentary chamber.

CHEST RADIOGRAPHY. Mild bulging of the right lower heart border from a dilated right atrium is often seen in patients with an atriopulmonary connection.

ECHOCARDIOGRAPHY. The presence or absence of right atrial stasis, thrombus, patency of a fenestration, and Fontan circuit obstruction should be sought. Superior and inferior venae cavae biphasic and pulmonary artery triphasic flow patterns suggest unobstructed flow in the Fontan circuit, whereas a mean gradient between the Fontan circuit and the pulmonary artery of 2 mm Hg or more may represent significant obstruction. Assessment of the pulmonary venous flow pattern is important in detecting pulmonary vein obstruction (right pulmonary vein > left pulmonary vein) sometimes caused by an enlarged right atrium. Concomitant assessment of systemic ventricular function and AV valve regurgitation can be readily accomplished. TEE may be required if there is inadequate visualization of the Fontan anastomosis or to exclude thrombus in the right atrium.

CMR. The objectives of CMR in Fontan patients include assessment of the pathways from the systemic veins to the pulmonary arteries for obstruction and thrombus; detection of Fontan baffle fenestration or leaks; evaluation of the pulmonary veins for compression; assessment of systemic ventricular volume, mass, and ejection fraction; imaging of the systemic ventricular outflow tract for obstruction; and quantitative assessment of the AV and semilunar valves for regurgitation, of the aorta for obstruction or an aneurysm, and for aortopulmonary, systemic venous, or systemic to pulmonary venous collateral vessels.

DIAGNOSTIC CATHETERIZATION. Complete heart catheterization is advised if surgical reintervention is planned or if adequate assessment of the hemodynamics is not obtained by noninvasive means.

MANAGEMENT OPTIONS AND OUTCOMES. Selection of patients is of utmost importance and has a major impact on clinical outcome. Long-term survival in "ideal" candidates is 81% at 10 years, compared with 60% to 71% in "all comers." Death occurs mostly from congestive heart failure and atrial arrhythmias. The Fontan procedure remains a palliative, not curative, procedure. A more radical approach to the failing atriopulmonary Fontan circulation, including surgical revision of the circuit to an extracardiac conduit, in combination with a Cox maze procedure and, frequently, simultaneous epicardial pacemaker insertion, has recently been shown to provide good early palliation. Ultimately, cardiac transplantation may be required by some of these patients, although outcomes are less favorable in such patients.[5,6]

Arrhythmias

Atrial tachyarrhythmias are difficult to manage and should quickly raise the thought of long-term warfarin therapy. When atrial flutter or fibrillation is present, an underlying hemodynamic cause should always be sought, and, in particular, evidence for obstruction of the Fontan circuit needs to be excluded. Prompt attempts should be made to restore sinus rhythm. Antiarrhythmic medications, alone or combined with an epicardial antitachycardia pacing device, and radiofrequency catheter ablation techniques have had limited success (see Chap. 39). Surgical conversion from an atriopulmonary Fontan to a total cavopulmonary connection with concomitant atrial cryoablation therapy at the time of surgery has been reported with good short-term success.[63] Epicardial pacemaker insertion for sinus node dysfunction or complete heart block may be necessary. Epicardial AV sequential pacing should be employed whenever possible (see Chap. 38).

Anticoagulant Therapy

The use of prophylactic long-term anticoagulation is contentious. Experts recommend that patients with a history of documented arrhythmias, fenestration in the Fontan connection, or spontaneous contrast (smoke) in the right atrium on echocardiography be anticoagulated. For established thrombus, thrombolytic therapy versus surgical removal of the clot and conversion of the Fontan circuit have been described, both with high mortality rates.

Protein-Losing Enteropathy

Treatment modalities include a low-fat, high-protein, medium-chain triglyceride diet to reduce intestinal lymphatic production; albumin infusions to increase intravascular osmotic pressure; and the introduction of diuretics, afterload-reducing agents, and positive inotropic agents to lower central venous pressure. Most often, these therapies are ineffective and should not be continued if indeed they are tried at all. Catheter-based interventions such as balloon dilation of pathway obstruction or creation of an atrial fenestration and surgical interventions from conversion or takedown of the Fontan circuit to cardiac transplantation have also been advocated. Other reportedly effective treatment modalities include subcutaneous heparin, octreotide treatment, and steroid therapy. All therapies have a similar failure rate of about 50%.

Right Pulmonary Vein Compression or Obstruction

When this is hemodynamically significant, Fontan conversion to a total cavopulmonary connection or extracardiac conduit may be recommended.

Fontan Obstruction

Surgical revision of an obstructed right atrium to pulmonary artery or superior and inferior venae cavae to pulmonary artery connections is recommended, usually to an extracardiac Fontan. Alternatively, balloon angioplasty with or without stenting may be used when it is appropriate and feasible.

Ventricular Failure and Valvular Regurgitation

ACE inhibitors are of unproven benefit, do not appear to enhance exercise capacity, and may cause clinical deterioration in Fontan patients. Patients with systemic AV valve regurgitation may require AV valve repair or replacement. Cardiac transplantation should also be considered.

Cyanosis

In the setting of a fenestrated Fontan, surgical or preferably transcatheter closure of the fenestration can be attempted. Pulmonary arteriovenous fistulas from a classic Glenn shunt may be improved by surgical conversion to a bidirectional Glenn connection.

FOLLOW-UP. Close and expert follow-up is recommended, with particular attention to ventricular function and systemic AV valve regurgitation. The development of atrial tachyarrhythmia should instigate a search for possible obstruction at the Fontan anastomosis, right pulmonary vein obstruction, or thrombus within the right atrium.

Total Anomalous Pulmonary Venous Connection

DEFINITION. This describes the situation in which all pulmonary veins fail to connect directly to the morphologic left atrium. As a result, all of the systemic and pulmonary venous return usually drains to the right atrium, albeit by varied routes.

MORPHOLOGY (Fig. 65-21). The anatomic varieties of total anomalous pulmonary venous connection may be subdivided according to the path of the abnormal drainage. The anomalous connection is most often supradiaphragmatic, connecting via a vertical vein to the left brachiocephalic vein, directly to the right atrium, to the coronary sinus, or directly to the superior vena cava. In about 10% to 15%, the pathway is below the diaphragm. The anomalous trunk then connects into the portal vein or one of its tributaries, the ductus venosus, or, rarely, the hepatic or other abdominal veins.

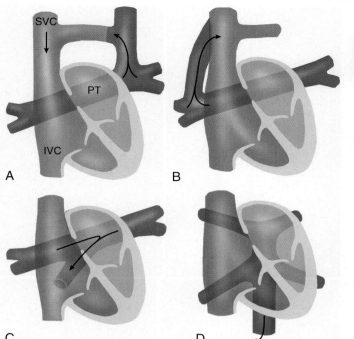

FIGURE 65-21 Anatomic types of total anomalous pulmonary venous return: supracardiac, in which the pulmonary veins drain either via the vertical vein to the anomalous vein (**A**) or directly to the superior vena cava (SVC) with the orifice close to the orifice of the azygos vein (**B**); drainage into the right atrium via the coronary sinus (**C**); infracardiac drainage (**D**) via a vertical vein into the portal vein or the inferior vena cava (IVC). PT = pulmonary trunk. (*A to D from Stark J, deLeval M: Surgery for Congenital Heart Defects. 2nd ed. Philadelphia, WB Saunders, 1994, p 330.*)

PATHOPHYSIOLOGY. The physiologic consequences and, accordingly, the clinical picture depend on the size of the interatrial communication and the degree of obstruction elsewhere within the pathway. When the interatrial communication is small, systemic blood flow is severely limited with right-sided heart failure. Obstruction to pulmonary venous return and pulmonary venous hypertension are invariably present in patients with infradiaphragmatic anomalous pulmonary venous connection.

NATURAL HISTORY. Most patients with total anomalous pulmonary venous connection have symptoms during the first year of life, and 80% die before 1 year of age if they are not treated. The presence of obstruction in the pulmonary venous pathway or at the atrial septum leads to earlier presentation. When the obstruction is severe, neonatal presentation with severe cyanosis and cardiovascular collapse may occur. This is incompatible with survival without urgent surgical intervention.

CLINICAL FEATURES. Symptomatic infants with total anomalous pulmonary venous connection present with signs of heart failure or cyanosis. Infants with pulmonary venous obstruction present with the early onset of severe dyspnea, pulmonary edema, cyanosis, and right-sided heart failure. Without obstruction, cyanosis may be minimal and go undetected. On auscultation, there is usually a fixed, widely split second heart sound with an accentuated pulmonic component.

LABORATORY INVESTIGATIONS

ELECTROCARDIOGRAPHY. This usually shows right-axis deviation and right atrial and right ventricular hypertrophy.

CHEST RADIOGRAPHY. In the unrepaired patient, this usually shows cardiomegaly with increased pulmonary blood flow. The right atrium and ventricle are dilated and hypertrophied, and the pulmonary artery segment is enlarged. The so-called figure-of-8 or "snowman" heart is due to enlargement of the heart and the presence of a dilated right superior vena cava, innominate vein, and left vertical vein.

ECHOCARDIOGRAPHY (**Fig. 65-22**). This usually shows marked enlargement of the right ventricle and a small left atrium. Demonstration of the

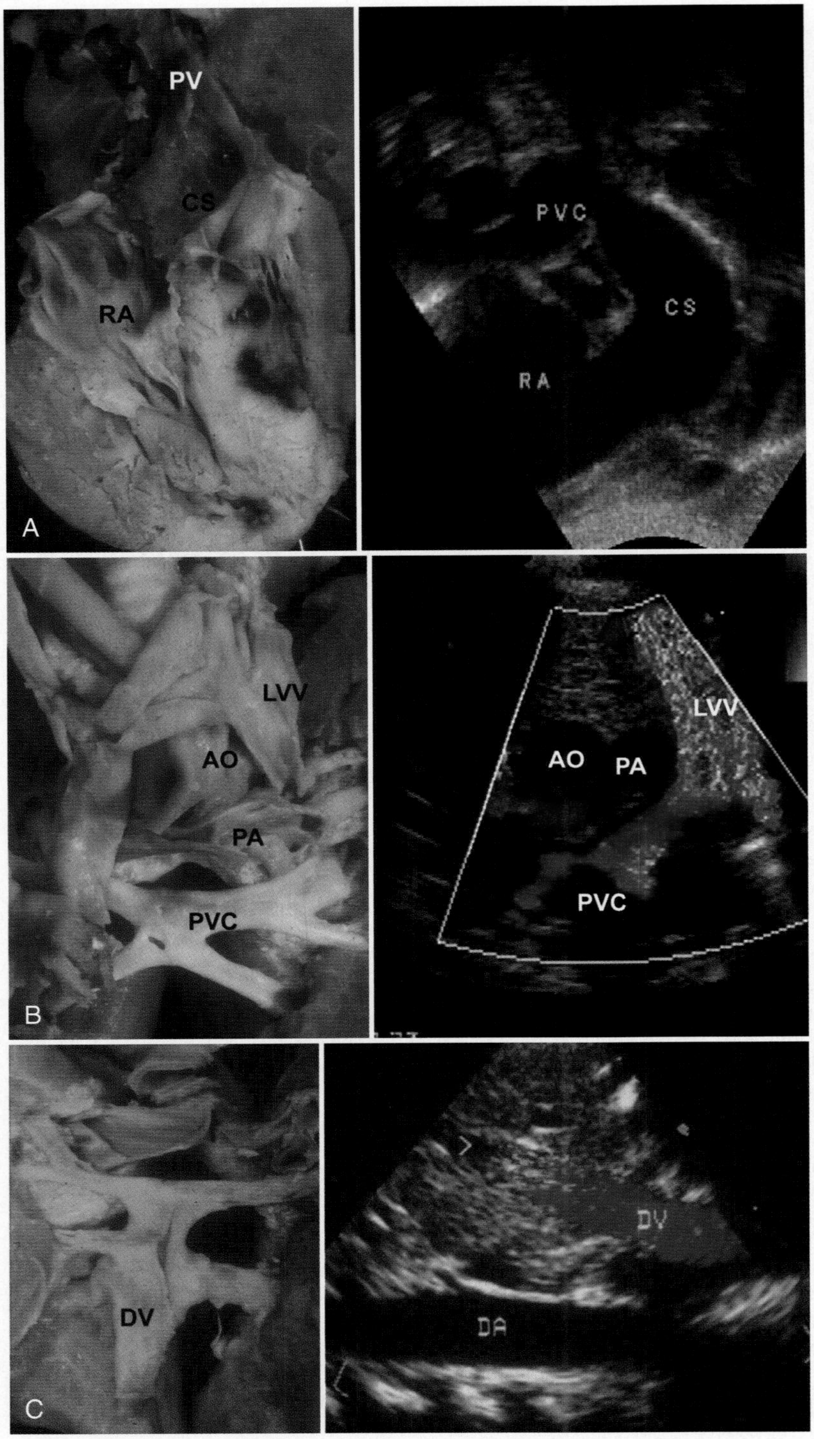

FIGURE 65-22 A, Subcostal view demonstrating total anomalous pulmonary drainage to the coronary sinus. Note the dilated coronary sinus in both images. The echocardiogram also demonstrates an associated confluence that connects to the coronary sinus. **B,** Suprasternal view demonstrating total anomalous pulmonary venous drainage to a left vertical vein. Note the direction of flow in the vertical vein that differentiates it from a left superior vena cava. **C,** Total anomalous pulmonary venous drainage below the diaphragm. The specimen shows the pulmonary veins as they enter the confluence, whereas the echocardiogram demonstrates the descending veins as they enter the liver. Note that the direction of flow is away from the heart. AO = aorta; CS = coronary sinus; DA = descending aorta; DV = descending vein; LVV = left vertical vein; PA = pulmonary artery; PV = pulmonary vein; PVC = pulmonary venous confluence; RA = right atrium.

entire pathway of pulmonary venous drainage is usually possible, and cardiac catheterization (which may be hazardous) is almost never performed now. An echo-free space representing the pulmonary venous confluence can usually be seen behind the left atrium. The drainage of all four pulmonary veins and their connections must be identified.

CMR. Although it is not often used, especially in infants, CMR may be helpful in delineation of the site of connections of total anomalous pulmonary venous return, when there are multiple mixed sites, in older children, and for detection of stenosis in postoperative patients.

INDICATIONS FOR INTERVENTION. Medical therapy, other than mechanical ventilation, has a limited role in the symptomatic infant, and corrective surgery should be performed as soon as possible. In asymptomatic children without pulmonary hypertension, surgery can be deferred to 3 to 6 months of age.

INTERVENTIONAL OPTIONS AND OUTCOMES. An urgent balloon atrial septostomy is occasionally required to increase systemic blood flow before surgery. Otherwise, interventional catheterization is restricted to attempts at relief of postoperative pulmonary venous stenosis, although this is often unrewarding. Historically, surgical repair of restenosis was also disappointing. However, the sutureless technique, whereby the pulmonary veins are opened widely into the retroatrial space, has markedly improved the results of such surgery. Adult patients have almost always had surgical repair in childhood. As a rule, they function normally and are not too prone to arrhythmias or other problems. They are seen as low- to moderate-risk adults.

FOLLOW-UP. Early follow-up should be frequent and aimed at early detection of stenosis of the pulmonary veins or the surgical anastomosis. If it is not present within the first year, stenosis is rare, but annual follow-up during childhood is required.

Transposition Complexes

The key anatomic feature that characterizes this group of diagnoses is ventriculoarterial discordance. This is most commonly seen in the context of AV concordance, also known as complete transposition or D-TGA. The second condition that is discussed in this section is the combination of ventriculoarterial discordance with AV discordance, commonly referred to as congenitally corrected TGA or L-TGA. More complicated arrangements are not considered here.

Complete Transposition of the Great Arteries

DEFINITION AND NATURAL HISTORY. This is a common and potentially lethal form of heart disease in newborns and infants. The malformation consists of the origin of the aorta from the morphologic right ventricle and that of the pulmonary artery from the morphologic left ventricle. Consequently, the pulmonary and systemic circulations are connected in parallel rather than the normal in-series connection. In one circuit, systemic venous blood passes to the right atrium, to the right ventricle, and then to the aorta. In the other, pulmonary venous blood passes through the left atrium and ventricle to the pulmonary artery. This situation is incompatible with life unless mixing of the two circuits occurs.

Approximately two thirds of patients have no major associated abnormalities (simple transposition), and one third have associated abnormalities (complex transposition). The most common associated abnormalities are VSD and pulmonary or subpulmonary stenosis. It is increasingly being diagnosed in utero. Without treatment, about 30% of these infants die within the first week of life, and 90% die within the first year.

MORPHOLOGY. Some communication between the two circulations must exist after birth to sustain life. Almost all patients have an interatrial communication, blood flow across which governs the amount of desaturation. Two thirds have a PDA, and about one third have an associated VSD.

PATHOPHYSIOLOGY. The degree of tissue hypoxia, the nature of the associated cardiovascular anomalies, and the anatomic and functional status of the pulmonary vascular bed determine the clinical course. The anatomic arrangement results in two separate and parallel circulations. The systemic arterial oxygen saturation is governed by the amount of blood exchanged between the two circulations. Infants with D-TGA are particularly susceptible to the early development of pulmonary vascular obstructive disease even in the absence of a PDA and even with an intact ventricular septum.

CLINICAL FEATURES

Pediatric

The average birth weight and size of infants born with complete TGA are greater than normal. The usual clinical manifestations are dyspnea and cyanosis from birth, progressive hypoxemia, and congestive heart failure. The most severe cyanosis and hypoxemia are observed in infants who have only a small PFO or ductus arteriosus and an intact ventricular septum or in those infants with relatively reduced pulmonary blood flow because of left ventricular outflow tract obstruction. With a large ASD or PDA or large VSD, cyanosis can be minimal, and heart failure is usually the dominant problem after the first few weeks of life. Cardiac murmurs are of little diagnostic significance.

The two-dimensional echocardiogram should establish the complete diagnosis, including the coronary artery pattern. Prenatal detection is possible and favorably modifies neonatal morbidity and mortality. Ultrasound imaging has become a standard procedure to guide catheter placement and manipulation during balloon atrial septostomy and to assess the anatomic adequacy of the septostomy.

MANAGEMENT OPTIONS. Maintenance of ductal patency by prostaglandin E_1 in the early neonatal period improves the arterial saturation by enhancing mixing at atrial level. This is usually as a prelude to the creation or enlargement of an interatrial communication by a balloon or blade atrial septostomy. Surgical atrial septectomy is seldom required now.

Surgery

Although balloon atrial septostomy is often lifesaving, it is palliative and anticipates "corrective" surgery. Atrial redirection procedures were developed in the 1950s and 1960s but were replaced by the arterial switch operation, which became widely adopted in the 1980s.

Atrial Switch (Fig. 65-23)

The most common surgical procedure in patients who are currently adults is the atrial switch operation. Patients will have had either a Mustard or a Senning procedure. Blood is redirected at the atrial level by a baffle made of Dacron or pericardium (Mustard operation) or atrial flaps (Senning operation), achieving physiologic correction. Systemic venous return is diverted through the mitral valve into the subpulmonary left ventricle, and the pulmonary venous return is rerouted through the tricuspid valve into the subaortic right ventricle. By virtue of this repair, the morphologic right ventricle supports the systemic circulation.

Palliative Atrial Switch

Uncommonly, in patients with a large VSD and established pulmonary vascular disease, a palliative atrial switch operation is done to improve oxygenation. The VSD is left open or enlarged at the time of atrial baffle surgery. These patients resemble patients with Eisenmenger VSDs and should be managed as such.

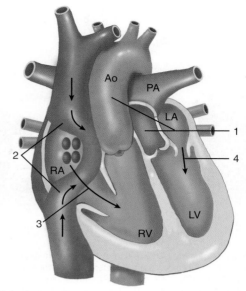

FIGURE 65-23 Diagrammatic representation of atrial switch surgery (Mustard or Senning procedure). Superior vena cava and inferior vena cava blood is redirected into the morphologic left ventricle (LV), which pumps blood into the pulmonary artery (PA), whereas the pulmonary venous blood flow is rerouted to the morphologic right ventricle (RV), which empties into the aorta (Ao). RA = right atrium; LA = left atrium; 1, transposition of the great arteries; 2, atrial baffles; 3, pulmonary vein blood flow through tricuspid valve to right ventricle; 4, inferior vena cava and superior vena cava blood flow through mitral valve to left ventricle. *(From Mullins CE, Mayer DC: Congenital Heart Disease: A Diagrammatic Atlas. New York, Wiley-Liss, 1988.)*

Arterial Switch Operation (Fig. 65-24)

In this operation, the arterial trunks are transected and reanastomosed to the contralateral root. If a VSD is present, it is closed. The coronary arteries must be transposed to the neoaorta. This is the most challenging part of the procedure and accounts for most of the mortality. Nonetheless, this rate has fallen to less than 2% in most large centers. The major advantages of the arterial switch procedure, compared with the atrial switch procedure, are restoration of the left ventricle as the systemic pump and the potential for long-term maintenance of sinus rhythm.

Follow-up studies after the arterial switch operation have demonstrated good left ventricular function and normal exercise capacity. Potential sequelae of the operation include coronary occlusion, supravalvular pulmonary stenosis (which may be treated by either reoperation or balloon angioplasty), supravalvular aortic stenosis, ascending aortic aneurysms, and neoaortic regurgitation (usually mild).[64-66] Long-term patency and growth of the coronary arteries appear satisfactory.

Rastelli Procedure

Infants with TGA plus a VSD and left ventricular outflow tract obstruction may require an early systemic–pulmonary artery shunt when a pronounced diminution in pulmonary blood flow exists. A later corrective procedure for these patients bypasses the left ventricular outflow obstruction with an extracardiac prosthetic conduit between the right ventricle and the distal end of a divided pulmonary artery and uses an intracardiac ventricular baffle to tunnel the left ventricle to the aorta (Rastelli procedure).

MANAGEMENT OUTCOMES

Atrial Switch

After atrial baffle surgery, most patients who reach adulthood are in NYHA Classes I and II, but abnormalities of ventricular filling, due to the abnormal atrial pathways, may be of more direct importance to functional capacity than right ventricular performance issues in many.

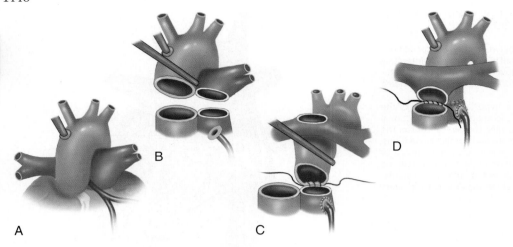

A

B

C

D

FIGURE 65-24 Complete transposition of the great arteries, corrected by a modified arterial switch operation. The aorta and pulmonary artery are transected **(A)**, and the orifices of the coronary arteries are excised with a rim of adjacent aortic wall **(B).** The aorta is brought under the bifurcation of the pulmonary artery, and the pulmonary artery and the aorta are anastomosed without necessitating graft interposition. The coronary arteries are transferred to the pulmonary artery **(C).** The mobilized pulmonary artery is directly anastomosed to the proximal aortic stump **(D).** (*A to D from Stark J, deLeval M: Surgery for Congenital Heart Defects. New York, Grune & Stratton, 1983, p 379.*)

Some present with symptoms of congestive heart failure (2% to 15%). Echocardiographic evidence of moderate or severe systemic right ventricular dysfunction is present in up to 40% of patients. Relative right ventricular ischemia (supply-demand mismatch) is thought to perhaps play a role in systemic right ventricular dysfunction. More than mild systemic tricuspid regurgitation is present in 10% to 40%, both reflecting and exacerbating right ventricular dysfunction. Palpitations and near-syncope or syncope from rhythm disturbances are fairly common. Atrial flutter occurs in 20% of patients by 20 years of age, and sinus node dysfunction is seen in half of the patients by that time. These rhythm disturbances are a consequence of direct and indirect atrial and sinus node damage at the time of atrial baffle surgery.

A shortened life expectancy is the rule, with 70% to 80% survival at 20 to 30 years' follow-up. Patients with complex TGA in general fare much worse than those with simple TGA. Sudden cardiac death can occur in these patients and may relate to systemic right ventricular dysfunction, the presence of atrial flutter, and pulmonary hypertension. Significant pulmonary vascular disease can develop over time and relates to older age at the time of atrial switch operation, particularly in patients with a substantial VSD as well as in those with longstanding left-to-right shunts through a baffle leak. Superior vena cava or inferior vena cava baffle obstruction often goes undetected because collateral drainage through the azygos vein prevents systemic venous congestion. Pulmonary venous baffle obstruction causes elevated pulmonary artery pressure, and patients can present with dyspnea and pulmonary venous congestive features.

Physical examination of a patient whose condition is otherwise uncomplicated reveals a right ventricular parasternal lift, a normal S_1, a single S_2 (P_2 is not heard because of its posterior location), a pansystolic murmur from tricuspid regurgitation if it is present (best heard at the left lower sternal border, but not increasing with inspiration), and a right-sided S_4 when severe systemic ventricular dysfunction is present.

Arterial Switch

Data on long-term complications in adults who have undergone the arterial switch procedure are emerging. The development of progressive neoaortic valve regurgitation from neoaortic root dilation is the most common long-term sequela. It is time dependent and as such requires periodic follow-up.[65,66] Supra–neopulmonary artery stenosis is a frequent finding but rarely has clinical consequences. The development of ostial coronary artery disease has also been described in some patients.[64] Arrhythmia promises to be less of a problem in this

group of patients. Cardiac examination in uncomplicated patients is normal.

Rastelli Procedure

Progressive right ventricular to pulmonary artery conduit obstruction can cause exercise intolerance or right ventricular angina. Left ventricular tunnel obstruction can present as exertional dyspnea or syncope. Conduit replacement or transcatheter stent or stent-valve implantation is inevitably required in surviving patients.[67] Physical examination in uncomplicated patients reveals, in contrast to those after atrial switch, no right ventricular lift, an ejection systolic murmur from the conduit, and two components to the S_2.

LABORATORY INVESTIGATIONS

ELECTROCARDIOGRAPHY. Sinus bradycardia or junctional rhythm (without a right atrial overload pattern) with evidence of marked right ventricular hypertrophy is characteristically present in patients after the atrial switch procedure. The ECG is typically normal in patients after the arterial switch procedure. The ECG typically shows right bundle branch block after a Rastelli procedure.

CHEST RADIOGRAPHY. On the posteroanterior film, a narrow vascular pedicle with an oblong cardiac silhouette ("egg on side") is typically seen in patients after the atrial switch procedure. On the lateral view, the anterior aorta may be seen to fill the retrosternal space. For the arterial switch, normal mediastinal borders are present despite the Lecompte maneuver. After the Rastelli procedure, the chest radiograph may be normal unless the conduit becomes calcified.

ECHOCARDIOGRAPHY. After the atrial switch procedure, parallel great arteries are the hallmark of TGA (**Fig. 65-25**). They are best visualized from a parasternal long-axis view (running side by side) or from a parasternal short-axis view (seen en face, with the aorta anterior and rightward). Qualitative assessment of systemic right ventricular function, the degree of tricuspid regurgitation, and the presence or absence of subpulmonary left ventricular obstruction (dynamic or fixed) is important. Assessment of baffle leak or obstruction (**Fig. 65-26**) is best done with color and Doppler flow imaging. Normal baffle flow should be phasic in nature and vary with respiration, with a peak velocity less than 1 m/sec. After arterial switch, neoaortic valve regurgitation, supra–neopulmonary valve stenosis, and segmental wall motion abnormality from ischemia due to coronary ostial stenosis should be sought. In patients who have undergone the Rastelli operation, left ventricular to aorta tunnel obstruction as well as right ventricular to pulmonary artery conduit degeneration (stenosis or regurgitation) must be assessed.

CMR. The major role of CMR in patients with atrial switch is to evaluate the baffles and systemic right ventricular volume and ejection fraction. As a rule, CMR reports better right ventricular size and function than does echocardiography. For patients who are claustrophobic or have a pacemaker, CT angiography may serve as a substitute.

CARDIAC CATHETERIZATION. Diagnostic cardiac catheterization may be required to assess the presence or severity of systemic or pulmonary baffle obstruction, baffle leak, and pulmonary hypertension; coronary ostial stenosis; or tunnel or conduit obstruction when it is not diagnosed by noninvasive means.

INDICATIONS FOR REINTERVENTION. After the atrial switch procedure, severe symptomatic right ventricular dysfunction may warrant surgical treatment in the form of a two-stage arterial switch procedure[68] or cardiac transplantation. Tricuspid valve repair or replacement is rarely performed for severe systemic (tricuspid) AV valve regurgitation, particularly if it is due to a flail leaflet or cusp perforation and provided right ventricular function is adequate. A baffle leak resulting in a significant left-to-right shunt (>1.5:1), any right-to-left shunt, or attributable symptoms require surgical or transcatheter closure. Superior vena cava or inferior vena cava pathway obstruction may require intervention. Superior vena cava stenosis is usually benign, whereas inferior vena cava stenosis may have greater hemodynamic consequences, depending on the adequacy of alternative routes of venous return, usually via the azygos vein to the superior vena cava. Balloon dilation of superior vena cava or inferior vena cava stenosis is an option in expert hands. Stenting usually relieves the stenosis completely.

Pathway obstruction after the Senning operation is usually more amenable to balloon dilation and stenting. Pulmonary venous obstruction, although usually seen early and reoperated on in childhood, may present in adulthood. Symptomatic bradycardia warrants permanent pacemaker implantation, whereas tachyarrhythmias may require catheter ablation, an antitachycardia pacemaker device, or medical therapy. After an atrial switch, transvenous pacing leads must traverse the upper limb of the baffle to enter the morphologic left ventricle. Active fixation is required because coarse trabeculation is absent in the morphologic left ventricle. Transvenous pacing should be avoided in patients with residual intracardiac communications because paradoxical emboli can occur.[69]

After an arterial switch procedure, significant right ventricular outflow tract obstruction at any level (gradient > 50 mm Hg or right-to-left ventricular pressure ratio > 0.6) may require surgical or catheter augmentation of the right ventricular outflow tract. Myocardial ischemia from coronary artery obstruction may require coronary artery bypass grafting, preferably with arterial conduits. Significant neoaortic valve regurgitation may warrant aortic valve replacement.

In patients who have had the Rastelli procedure, significant right ventricle to pulmonary artery conduit stenosis (>50 mm Hg withdrawal gradient or mean echo gradient) or significant regurgitation necessitates intervention. Subaortic obstruction across the left ventricle to aorta tunnel necessitates left ventricle to aorta baffle reconstruction. A significant residual VSD (shunt >1.5:1) may require surgical closure.

REINTERVENTION OPTIONS

Medical Therapy

In patients with an atrial switch, the role of afterload reduction with ACE inhibitors, angiotensin receptor blockers,[70,71] or beta blockade[72,73] to preserve systemic right ventricular function is unknown.

Two-Stage Arterial Switch and Cardiac Transplantation

Patients with symptomatic, severe systemic (right) ventricular dysfunction with or without severe systemic (tricuspid) AV valve regurgitation, following an atrial switch procedure, may require consideration of a conversion procedure to an arterial switch (two-stage arterial switch) or heart transplantation. The two-stage arterial switch, or switch-conversion procedure, consists of banding the pulmonary artery in the first stage to induce subpulmonary left ventricular hypertrophy and to "train" the left ventricle to support systemic pressure. Once left ventricular systolic pressure is more than 75% of systemic pressure and the left ventricular mass is considered adequate, in the second stage the atrial baffles and the pulmonary band are taken down, the atrial septum is reconstructed, and the great arteries are switched, leaving the morphologic left ventricle as the systemic ventricle. This procedure is still experimental in adults, with few data available to assess its short- and long-term efficacy.

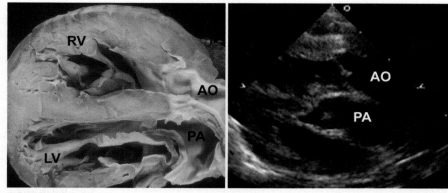

FIGURE 65-25 Parasternal long-axis view in transposition of the great arteries. Note the parallel nature of the aorta and pulmonary artery. AO = aorta; LV = left ventricle; PA = pulmonary artery; RV = right ventricle.

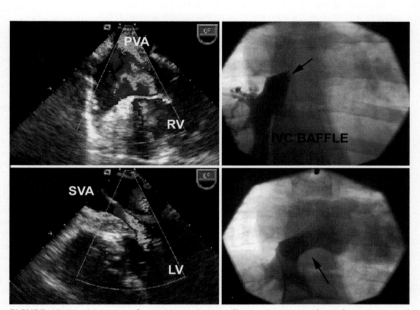

FIGURE 65-26 Montage of post-Mustard cases. The angiogram in the right upper panel shows complete obstruction of the inferior limb of the systemic venous baffle, whereas the lower right panel is the same case after stenting. The upper left image is a transesophageal echocardiogram showing the pulmonary venous baffle with some mild flow acceleration in its midpoint. The lower left panel shows the systemic venous baffle at its left ventricular end. IVC = inferior vena cava; LV = left ventricle; PVA = pulmonary venous atrium; RV = right ventricle; SVA = systemic venous atrium.

REPRODUCTIVE ISSUES. Severe systemic ventricular dysfunction or intractable arrhythmias may be a contraindication to pregnancy, and baffle obstruction should, ideally, be relieved before pregnancy. Women who have had an atrial switch usually tolerate pregnancy well, but about 15% will develop worsening right ventricular function or tricuspid regurgitation during the pregnancy. In half of these cases, the problem does not improve after delivery.[74]

FOLLOW-UP. Regular follow-up by physicians with special expertise in CHD is recommended.

Atrial Switch

Serial follow-up of systemic right ventricular function is warranted. Asymptomatic baffle obstruction should be sought with echocardiography or CMR. Regular Holter monitoring is recommended to diagnose unacceptable bradyarrhythmias or tachyarrhythmias.

Arterial Switch and Rastelli Procedure

Regular follow-up with echocardiography is recommended.

Congenitally Corrected Transposition of the Great Arteries

DEFINITION. The term *congenitally corrected transposition of the great arteries* describes hearts in which there are discordant AV connections in combination with discordant ventriculoarterial connections.

MORPHOLOGY (Fig. 65-27). cc-TGA is a rare condition, accounting for less than 1% of all CHD. When there is the usual atrial arrangement, systemic venous blood passes from the right atrium through a mitral valve to a left ventricle and then to the posteriorly located pulmonary artery. Pulmonary venous blood passes from the left atrium through a tricuspid valve to a left-sided right ventricle and then to an anterior, left-sided aorta. The circulation is thus "physiologically" corrected, but the morphologic right ventricle supports the systemic circulation. Associated anomalies occur in up to 95% of patients and consist of VSD (75%), pulmonary or subpulmonary stenosis (75%), and left-sided (tricuspid and often Ebstein-like) valve anomalies (>75%).

Because of the inherently abnormal conduction system, 5% of patients with cc-TGA are born with congenital complete heart block.

PATHOPHYSIOLOGY. Patients with no associated abnormalities (isolated cc-TGA) can exceptionally survive until the seventh or eighth decade. Progressive systemic (tricuspid) AV valve regurgitation and systemic (right) ventricular dysfunction tend to occur from the fourth decade onward, whereas atrial tachyarrhythmias are more common from the fifth decade onward. In addition to those born with congenital complete heart block, acquired complete AV block continues to develop at a rate of 2% per year, concentrated mainly at the time of cardiac surgery. Patients with associated anomalies (VSD, pulmonary stenosis, left-sided [tricuspid] valve anomaly) often have undergone surgical palliation (systemic to pulmonary artery shunt for cyanosis) or repair of the associated anomalies (see section on surgical procedures), but a significant number of patients are naturally balanced by a combination of their VSD and subpulmonary left ventricular outflow tract obstruction. Although cyanosed, they often remain well, with no intervention for many years.

CLINICAL FEATURES

Unrepaired

Patients with no associated defects can be asymptomatic until late adulthood. Dyspnea, exercise intolerance from developing congestive heart

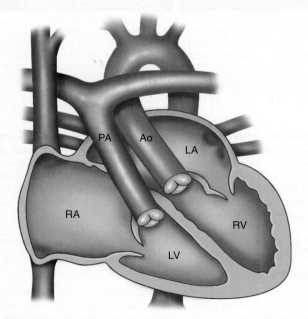

FIGURE 65-27 Diagrammatic representation of congenitally corrected transposition of the great arteries. Ao = aorta; LA = left atrium; LV = left ventricle; PA = pulmonary artery; RA = right atrium; RV = right ventricle. *(From Mullins CE, Mayer DC: Congenital Heart Disease: A Diagrammatic Atlas. New York, Wiley-Liss, 1988.)*

failure, and palpitations from supraventricular arrhythmias most often arise in the fifth decade. Patients with well-balanced VSD and pulmonary stenosis can present with paradoxical emboli or cyanosis, especially if pulmonary stenosis is severe. Physical examination of a patient whose condition is otherwise uncomplicated reveals a somewhat more medial apex due to the side-by-side orientation of the two ventricles. The A_2 is often palpable in the second left intercostal space because of the anterior location of the aorta. A single S_2 (A_2) is heard, with P_2 often being silent because of its posterior location. The murmur of an associated VSD or of left AV valve regurgitation may be heard. The murmur of pulmonary stenosis radiates upward and to the right, given the rightward direction of the main pulmonary artery. If there is complete heart block, cannon *a* waves with an S_1 of variable intensity are present.

VSD Patch and Left Ventricular to Pulmonary Artery Conduit Repair

Most patients are in functional Class I at 5 to 10 years after surgery despite the common development of systemic tricuspid regurgitation and systemic right ventricular dysfunction after surgical repair. Dyspnea, exercise intolerance, and palpitations from supraventricular arrhythmia often occur in the fourth decade. Complete heart block may complicate surgery in an additional 25%. Physical examination reflects the basic cardiac malformation with or without residual coexisting anomalies.

LABORATORY INVESTIGATIONS

ELECTROCARDIOGRAPHY. An abnormal direction of initial (septal) depolarization from right to left causes reversal of the precordial Q wave pattern (Q waves are often present in the right precordial leads and absent in the left). First-degree AV block occurs in about 50%, and complete AV block occurs in up to 25% of patients. Atrial arrhythmias may be seen.

CHEST RADIOGRAPHY. Chest radiography characteristically reveals absence of the normal pulmonary artery segment in favor of a smooth convexity of the left supracardiac border produced by the left-sided ascending aorta. The main pulmonary trunk is medially displaced and absent from the cardiac silhouette; the right pulmonary hilum is often prominent and elevated compared with the left, producing a right-sided "waterfall" appearance.

ECHOCARDIOGRAPHY (**Fig. 65-28;** see Fig. 15-93B). Echocardiography permits the identification of the basic malformation as well as of any associated anomalies. The right-sided morphologic left ventricle is characterized by its smooth endocardial surface and is guarded by a bileaflet AV (mitral) valve with no direct septal attachment. The morphologic right ventricle is recognized by its apical trabeculation and moderator band and is guarded by a trileaflet apically displaced AV valve (tricuspid valve) with direct attachment to the septum. The AV valves therefore show reversed offsetting, a strong clue to the diagnosis. Ebstein-like malformation of the left (tricuspid) AV valve is defined by excessive (>8 mm/m² body surface area) apical displacement of the left (tricuspid) AV valve, with or without dysplasia.

CMR. The major role of CMR in cc-TGA patients is to evaluate the systemic right ventricular volume and ejection fraction. It does so better than echocardiography can at present. For claustrophobic or pacemaker patients, high-quality radionuclide angiography or CT angiography with volume estimates may serve as a substitute. CMR can evaluate other issues as well, including conduit function and AV valve regurgitation.

CARDIAC CATHETERIZATION. This is rarely required for diagnosis but may be indicated before surgical repair to demonstrate the coronary artery anatomy as well as ventricular end-diastolic and pulmonary artery pressures.

INDICATIONS FOR INTERVENTION AND REINTERVENTION. If moderate or severe systemic (tricuspid, left) AV valve regurgitation develops, valve replacement should be considered. Left AV valve replacement should be performed before systemic right ventricular function deteriorates, namely, at an ejection fraction of 45% or more. When tricuspid regurgitation is associated with poor systemic (right) ventricular function, the double-switch procedure should perhaps be considered, although its role remains controversial.[75] Patients with end-stage symptomatic heart failure should be referred for cardiac transplantation. The presence of a hemodynamically significant VSD ($Q_p/Q_s > 1.5:1$) or residual VSD with significant native or postsurgical (conduit) pulmonary outflow tract stenosis (echo mean or catheter gradient > 50 mm Hg) may require surgical correction, although the latter is sometimes best left alone as it can maintain a neutral septal position and minimize tricuspid regurgitation. Left AV valve replacement at the time of VSD and pulmonary stenosis surgery should be considered if concomitant left AV valve regurgitation is present. Pacemaker implantation is usual when complete AV block is present. The optimal pacing modality is DDD. Active fixation electrodes are required because of the lack of apical trabeculation in the morphologic left ventricle. Transvenous pacing should be avoided if there are intracardiac shunts because paradoxical emboli may occur.[69] Epicardial leads are preferred under these circumstances.

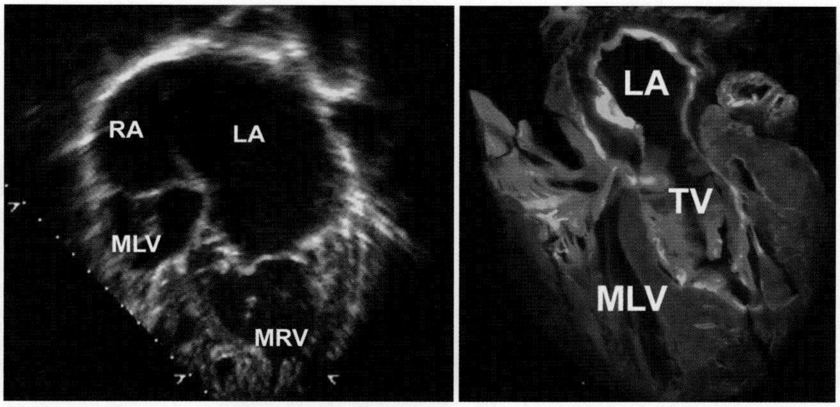

FIGURE 65-28 Four-chamber view in congenitally corrected transposition with dysplasia and displacement of the morphologic left-sided tricuspid valve. LA = left atrium; MLV = morphologic left ventricle; MRV = morphologic right ventricle; RA = right atrium; TV = tricuspid valve.

INTERVENTIONAL OPTIONS

Medical Therapy

ACE inhibitor or beta blocker therapy for patients with systemic ventricular dysfunction may be intuitive, but the role of such agents has not yet been demonstrated conclusively.[70,71,73]

Conduit Replacement or Repair

This is inevitably required in survivors of this type of initial surgery. Fortunately, it is now possible in some patients and in many countries to repair a failing conduit with a percutaneously delivered stented valve.[58]

Tricuspid Valve Replacement

For significant regurgitation, this is preferable to tricuspid valve repair. Valve repair is usually unsuccessful because of the abnormal, often Ebstein-like anatomy of the valve.

Double-Switch Procedure

This procedure has been successfully performed in children and carefully selected adults. It should be considered for patients with severe tricuspid regurgitation and systemic ventricular dysfunction.[75] Its purpose is to relocate the left ventricle into the systemic circulation and the right ventricle into the pulmonary circulation, achieving physiologic correction. An atrial switch procedure (Mustard or Senning), together with either an arterial switch procedure (when pulmonary stenosis is not present) or a Rastelli-type repair, the so-called Ilbawi procedure (left ventricle tunneled to aorta and right ventricle to pulmonary artery valved conduit when VSD and pulmonary stenosis are present), can be performed after adequate left ventricular retraining, leaving the regurgitant tricuspid valve and failing right ventricle on the pulmonary side.

Cardiac Transplantation

Patients with deteriorating systemic (right) ventricular function should be treated aggressively with medical therapy but may need to be considered for transplantation.

INTERVENTIONAL OUTCOMES. After conduit repair and VSD patching, the median survival of patients reaching adulthood is 40 years. The usual causes of death are sudden (presumed arrhythmic) and, more commonly, progressive systemic right ventricular dysfunction with systemic (tricuspid) AV valve regurgitation. The major predictor of poor outcome is the presence of left AV (tricuspid) valve regurgitation. Reoperation is common (15% to 25%), with left AV valve replacement usually being the primary reason. Data in adults who have had the double-switch procedure are lacking, and this procedure should be considered experimental in this population of patients.

FOLLOW-UP. All patients should have at least annual cardiology follow-up with an expert in the care of patients with congenital cardiac defects. Regular assessment of systemic (tricuspid) AV valve regurgitation by serial echocardiographic studies and systemic ventricular function by CMR or radionuclide angiography should be done. Holter recording can be useful if paroxysmal atrial arrhythmias or transient complete AV block is suspected.

Double-Outlet Right Ventricle

DEFINITION. The term *double-outlet right ventricle* describes hearts in which more than 50% of each semilunar valve arises from the morphologic right ventricle. It may coexist with any form of atrial arrangement or AV connection and is independent of infundibular (conal) anatomy.

MORPHOLOGY (Fig. 65-29). Few morphologic descriptors have invoked more discussion and controversy than double-outlet right ventricle. The definition given earlier is flawed but pragmatic. To some extent, this anatomic definition is less important than the understanding of the relationship between the great vessels and the VSD and the anatomy of the outlets to the great vessels, both of which are crucial determinants of clinical presentation and management.

CLINICAL FEATURES. Three main categories of double-outlet right ventricle exist: (1) double-outlet right ventricle with a subaortic VSD, (2) double-outlet right ventricle with a subpulmonary VSD, and (3) double-outlet right ventricle with a noncommitted VSD.

The position of the infundibular septum further modifies the hemodynamics. Taking double-outlet right ventricle with a subaortic VSD as an example, in which the aorta and its semilunar valve are closest to or overriding the trabecular septum, anterior deviation of the outlet septum causes subpulmonary stenosis, and the clinical scenario and management algorithm are similar or identical to those of tetralogy of Fallot. Conversely, if the outlet septum is deviated posteriorly, there will be subaortic stenosis, often with a coexisting abnormality of the aortic arch. The presentation and management of this variation are therefore entirely different. If there is no deviation of the outlet septum and no outlet obstruction, the clinical scenario will be that of a simple VSD. Double-outlet right ventricle with a subpulmonary VSD (Taussig-Bing anomaly) can be considered along with TGA. This is because the usual position of the pulmonary artery (posterior and leftward to the aorta) means that the streaming of deoxygenated and oxygenated blood is similar to that of transposition, even though most of the pulmonary valve is connected to the right ventricle. Anterior deviation of the outlet septum causes subaortic stenosis and aortic anomalies, and posterior deviation causes subpulmonary stenosis and limits pulmonary blood flow. It is also important to recognize double-outlet right ventricle with a noncommitted VSD. This defines hearts in which the VSD is remote from the outlets, making surgical management particularly difficult.

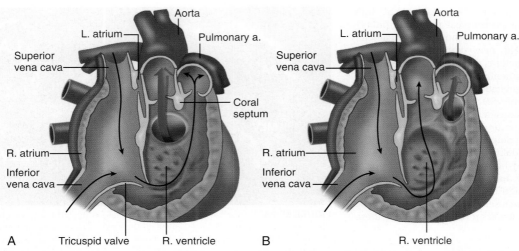

FIGURE 65-29 Double-outlet right ventricle with side-by-side relation of great arteries is illustrated in both panels. **A,** A subaortic ventricular septal defect below the crista supraventricularis favors delivery of left ventricular blood to the aorta. **B,** Subpulmonary location of the ventricular septal defect above the crista favors streaming to the pulmonary trunk. (**A** and **B** from Castañeda A, Jonas RA, Mayer JE, et al: Cardiac Surgery of the Neonate and Infant. Philadelphia, WB Saunders, 1994, p 446.)

ASSOCIATED LESIONS. More than half of patients with double-outlet right ventricles have associated anomalies of the AV valves. Mitral valve stenosis or atresia associated with a hypoplastic left ventricle is common. Ebstein anomaly of the tricuspid valve, complete AV septal defect, and overriding or straddling of either AV valve may occur.

LABORATORY INVESTIGATIONS. Because of the diversity of underlying anatomies, discussion of the electrocardiographic and radiographic features is not included here.

ECHOCARDIOGRAPHY. This is the mainstay of diagnosis. The commitment of the semilunar valves to the ventricles is ascertained. When it is present, deviation of the outlet septum beneath a semilunar valve probably has implications for downstream development of the great vessels. For example, when there is subaortic stenosis, the echocardiographic examination is incomplete until abnormalities of the aortic arch have been excluded. Preoperative evaluation must also take into account potential AV valve anomalies and straddling, in particular.

INDICATIONS FOR INTERVENTION. The goals of operative treatment are to establish continuity between the left ventricle and aorta, to create adequate right ventricle to pulmonary continuity, and to repair associated lesions. Palliative surgery is reserved for those in whom biventricular repair is not possible and in those with markedly reduced pulmonary blood flow. In the latter, an aortopulmonary shunt may be placed to temporize before complete correction. For the remainder, complete repair is now performed as a primary procedure in the majority. In double-outlet right ventricle with a subaortic VSD, repair is accomplished by creation of an intraventricular baffle that conducts left ventricular blood to the aorta. If there is coexisting subpulmonary stenosis, the repair is similar to that of tetralogy of Fallot. When the VSD is subpulmonary, but without subpulmonary stenosis, repair is accomplished by closure of the VSD and arterial switch. Subpulmonary stenosis is frequently present in a double-outlet right ventricle with a subpulmonary VSD. In these cases, the aorta is connected to the left ventricle by an intraventricular baffle, and a right ventricle to pulmonary artery conduit is placed to complete the repair (Rastelli procedure). Classic surgical approaches cannot be used when the VSD is remote and uncommitted to either semilunar orifice. On occasion, the VSD can be baffled toward the aorta, but when this is not possible, the right ventricle may be used as the systemic ventricle. This requires a Mustard or Senning atrial redirection procedure, closure of the VSD, and placement of a conduit between the left ventricle and the pulmonary trunk.

INTERVENTIONAL OPTIONS AND OUTCOMES. The late follow-up of the surgical procedures described earlier (e.g., tetralogy

of Fallot repair, arterial switch, Rastelli procedure) tends to be less satisfactory when there is a double-outlet right ventricle than when surgery is performed for more classic indications. The development of subaortic stenosis is more likely because of the abnormal geometry of the left ventricular outflow tract that often results after correction. Similarly, right ventricle to pulmonary artery conduit obstruction is more likely because of the spatial difficulties imposed on placement of the conduit with respect to the position on the right ventricle and the sternum. Because of these considerations, the options for catheter interventions are often fairly limited. However, recurrent arch obstruction and distal pulmonary artery obstruction are amenable to balloon dilation with or without stenting.

FOLLOW-UP. All of these patients require at least annual review by a CHD cardiologist.

Ebstein Anomaly

MORPHOLOGY (Fig. 65-30). The common feature in all cases of Ebstein anomaly is apical displacement of the septal tricuspid leaflet in conjunction with leaflet dysplasia. Many but not all have associated displacement of the posterior mural leaflet, with the anterior leaflet never being displaced. Although the anterior leaflet is never displaced apically, it may be adherent to the free wall of the right ventricle, causing right ventricular outflow tract obstruction. The displacement of the tricuspid valve results in "atrialization" (functioning as an atrial chamber) of the inflow tract of the right ventricle and consequently produces a variably small functional right ventricle. Associated anomalies include PFO or ASD in approximately 50% of patients; accessory conduction pathways in 25% (usually right sided); and, occasionally, varying degrees of right ventricular outflow tract obstruction, VSD, aortic coarctation, PDA, or mitral valve disease. Left ventricular abnormalities resembling noncompaction syndrome have also been described.

PATHOPHYSIOLOGY. Varying degrees of tricuspid regurgitation (or exceptionally tricuspid stenosis) result from the abnormal tricuspid leaflet morphology with consequent further right atrial enlargement. Right ventricular volume overload from significant tricuspid regurgitation and infundibular dilation can also be present. Right-to-left shunting through a PFO or ASD occurs if the right atrial pressure exceeds the left atrial pressure (which is often the case when severe tricuspid regurgitation is present).

NATURAL HISTORY. The natural history of patients with Ebstein anomaly depends on its severity. When the tricuspid valve deformity and dysfunction are extreme, death in utero from hydrops fetalis is the norm. When the tricuspid valve deformity is severe, symptoms usually develop in newborn infants. Patients with moderate tricuspid valve deformity and dysfunction usually develop symptoms during late

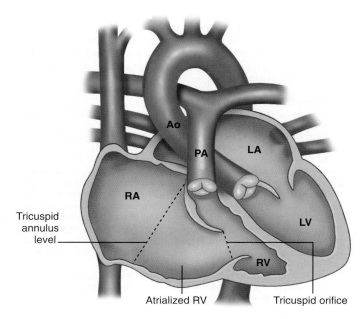

FIGURE 65-30 Diagrammatic representation of Ebstein anomaly. Ao = aorta; LA = left atrium; LV = left ventricle; PA = pulmonary artery; RA = right atrium; RV = right ventricle. (*From Mullins CE, Mayer DC: Congenital Heart Disease: A Diagrammatic Atlas. New York, Wiley-Liss, 1988.*)

adolescence or young adult life. Adults with Ebstein anomaly can occasionally remain asymptomatic throughout their lives if the anomaly is mild; exceptional survival to the ninth decade has been reported.

CLINICAL ISSUES

Pediatrics

With severe tricuspid valve deformity, newborns and infants present with failure to thrive and right-sided congestive heart failure. Most other pediatric patients who present after the neonatal period remain asymptomatic until late adolescence or early adult life.

Adults

Most adult patients present with exercise intolerance (exertional dyspnea and fatigue), palpitations of supraventricular origin, or cyanosis from a right-to-left shunt at atrial level. On occasion, a paradoxical embolus resulting in a transient ischemic attack or stroke can call attention to the diagnosis. Right-sided cardiac failure from severe tricuspid regurgitation and right ventricular dysfunction is possible. Sudden death (presumed to be arrhythmic in nature) is described. Physical examination typically reveals an unimpressive jugular venous pressure because of the large and compliant right atrium and atrialized right ventricle, a widely split S_1 with a loud tricuspid component (the "sail sound"), a widely split S_2 from a right bundle branch block, and a right-sided third heart sound. A pansystolic murmur increasing on inspiration from tricuspid regurgitation is best heard at the lower left sternal border. Cyanosis from a right-to-left shunt at the atrial level may or may not be present.

LABORATORY INVESTIGATIONS

ELECTROCARDIOGRAPHY. The electrocardiographic presentation of Ebstein anomaly varies widely (see Chap. 13). Low voltage is typical. Peaked P waves in leads II and V_1 reflect right atrial enlargement. The PR interval is usually prolonged, but a short PR interval and a delta wave from early activation through an accessory pathway can be present. An rsr′ pattern consistent with right ventricular conduction

delay is typically seen in lead V_1, and right bundle branch block is common in adults. Atrial flutter and fibrillation are common. The ECG may be normal.

CHEST RADIOGRAPHY. A rightward convexity from an enlarged right atrium and atrialized right ventricle coupled with a leftward convexity from a dilated infundibulum gives the heart a "water bottle" appearance on the chest radiograph. Cardiomegaly, highly variable in degree, is the rule. The aorta and the pulmonary trunk are inconspicuous. The pulmonary vasculature is usually normal to reduced.

ECHOCARDIOGRAPHY (**Fig. 65-31**; see Fig. 15-93A). The diagnosis of Ebstein anomaly is usually made by echocardiography. Apical displacement of the septal leaflet of the tricuspid valve by 8 mm/m² or more, combined with an elongated sail-like appearance of the anterior leaflet, confirms the diagnosis. The size of the atrialized portion of the right ventricle (identified between the tricuspid annulus and the ventricular attachment of the tricuspid valve leaflets) and the systolic performance of the functional right ventricle can be estimated. The degree of tricuspid regurgitation (and more rarely stenosis) can be assessed. Associated defects such as ASDs as well as the presence and direction of shunting can also be identified.

ANGIOGRAPHY. Cardiac catheterization is required mainly when concomitant coronary artery disease is suspected and to determine if pulmonary artery pressures are elevated. When it is performed, selective right ventricular angiography shows the extent of tricuspid valve displacement, the size of the functional right ventricle, and configuration of its outflow tract.

CMR. This investigation can offer insights into functional right ventricular volume and function.

INDICATIONS FOR INTERVENTION. Indications for intervention include substantial cyanosis, right-sided heart failure, poor functional capacity, and perhaps the occurrence of paradoxical emboli. Recurrent supraventricular arrhythmias not controlled by medical or ablation therapy and asymptomatic substantial cardiomegaly (cardiothoracic ratio > 65%) are relative indications.

INTERVENTIONAL OPTIONS. Tricuspid valve repair, when feasible, is preferable to tricuspid valve replacement. The feasibility of tricuspid valve repair depends primarily on the experience and skill of the surgeon as well as on the adequacy of the anterior leaflet of the tricuspid valve to form a monocusp valve. Tricuspid valve repair is possible when the edges of the anterior leaflet of the tricuspid valve are not severely tethered down to the myocardium and when the functional right ventricle is of adequate size (>35% of the total right ventricle). If the tricuspid valve is irreparable, valve replacement will be necessary, usually with a bioprosthetic tricuspid valve.[76]

For high-risk patients (those with severe tricuspid regurgitation, an inadequate functional right ventricle [because of size or function], or chronic supraventricular arrhythmias), a bidirectional

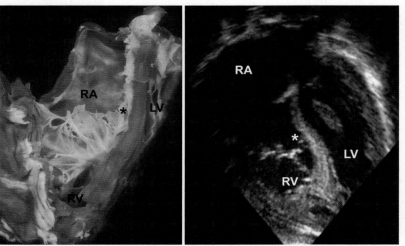

FIGURE 65-31 Apical four-chamber view in Ebstein malformation of the tricuspid valve. Note the significant displacement of the septal tricuspid valve leaflet (asterisk), with associated valve dysplasia. LV = left ventricle; RA = right atrium; RV = right ventricle.

cavopulmonary connection can be added to reduce right ventricular preload if pulmonary artery pressures are low.[77] On occasion, a Fontan operation may be the best option in patients with tricuspid stenosis or a hypoplastic right ventricle.[78] A concomitant right atrial or biatrial maze procedure at the time of surgery should be considered in patients with chronic atrial flutter or fibrillation.[79] If an accessory pathway is present, this should be mapped and obliterated either at the time of surgical repair or preoperatively in the catheterization laboratory. An atrial communication, if present, should be closed. In occasional patients with a resting oxygen saturation >90% and exercise intolerance due to worsening hypoxemia, closure of the PFO or ASD may be indicated without addressing the tricuspid valve itself.

With satisfactory valve repair, with or without plication of the atrialized right ventricle or bidirectional cavopulmonary connection, the medium-term prognosis is excellent. Late arrhythmias can occur.[80] With valve replacement, results are less satisfactory. Valve re-replacement may be necessary because of a failing bioprosthesis or a thrombosed mechanical valve.[76]

REPRODUCTIVE ISSUES. In the absence of maternal cyanosis, right-sided heart failure, or arrhythmias, pregnancy is usually well tolerated.

FOLLOW-UP. All patients with Ebstein anomaly should have regular follow-up, the frequency being dictated by the severity of their disease. Particular attention should be paid to patients with cyanosis, substantial cardiomegaly, poor right ventricular function, and recurrent atrial arrhythmias. Patients with substantial tricuspid regurgitation after tricuspid valve repair need close follow-up, as do patients with recurrent atrial arrhythmias, degenerating bioprostheses, or dysfunctional mechanical valves.

Valvular and Vascular Conditions

(see Chaps. 60, 61, and 66)

LEFT VENTRICULAR OUTFLOW TRACT LESIONS
(Fig. 65-32)

Coarctation of the Aorta

Aortic arch obstruction can be divided into (1) localized coarctation close to a PDA or ligamentum, (2) tubular hypoplasia of some part of the aortic arch system, and (3) aortic arch interruption.

Localized Aortic Coarctation

MORPHOLOGY. This lesion consists of a localized shelf in the posterolateral aortic wall opposite the ductus arteriosus. A neonatal presentation is more often associated with a shelf plus transverse aortic arch and isthmic hypoplasia, whereas with a later presentation, these areas are larger.

CLINICAL FEATURES. Coarctation occurs two to five times more commonly in males, and there is a high degree of association with gonadal dysgenesis (Turner syndrome) and bicuspid aortic valve. Other common associated anomalies include VSD and mitral stenosis or regurgitation. Additional lesions have an impact on outcome.

Neonates

Rapid, severe obstruction in infancy is a prominent cause of left ventricular failure and systemic hypoperfusion. Heart failure in this setting is due to a sudden increase in left ventricular wall stress after closure of the arterial duct. Substantial left-to-right shunting across a PFO and pulmonary venous hypertension secondary to heart failure cause pulmonary arterial hypertension. Because little or no aortic obstruction existed during fetal life, the collateral circulation in the newborn period is often poorly developed. In these infants, peripheral pulses are characteristically weak throughout the body until left ventricular function is improved with medical management; a significant pressure difference then develops between the arms and the legs, allowing detection of a pulse discrepancy. Cardiac murmurs are nonspecific in infancy and are commonly derived from associated lesions.

LABORATORY INVESTIGATIONS

ELECTROCARDIOGRAPHY. The ECG shows right-axis deviation and right ventricular hypertrophy.

CHEST RADIOGRAPHY. This shows generalized cardiomegaly and pulmonary arterial and venous engorgement.

ECHOCARDIOGRAPHY (**Fig. 65-33A**). This demonstrates the posterior shelf and the degree of associated isthmic or transverse arch hypoplasia. Doppler echocardiography is helpful if the ductus is closed or partially restrictive and demonstrates a high-velocity jet during systole and diastole. On the other hand, if the ductus is widely patent, the usual right-to-left shunting makes the Doppler assessment invalid because the distal pressure then reflects the high pulmonary artery pressure. With associated tubular hypoplasia, Doppler-derived gradients provide higher and less reliable values compared with those obtained by blood pressure or catheterization measurements.

MAGNETIC RESONANCE ANGIOGRAPHY. Although this is the gold standard for evaluation of the aortic arch in the older child and adult, it is usually unnecessary in the neonate and infant.

MANAGEMENT. Management usually involves prostaglandin therapy in an attempt to reopen or to maintain patency of a ductus arteriosus. After prostaglandin E_1 infusion to dilate the ductus arteriosus, the pressure difference may be obliterated across the site of coarctation because the fetal flow pattern is reestablished. This has the additional benefit of improving renal perfusion, which in turn helps reverse the frequently associated metabolic acidosis.

INTERVENTION. Intervention in this age group usually involves surgical relief of the obstruction with excision of the area of coarctation and extended end-to-end repair or end-to-side anastomosis with absorbable sutures to allow remodeling of the aorta with time. Subclavian flap aortoplasty, which was employed extensively in the past, is now less popular than the earlier-mentioned procedures. Experts generally believe that balloon dilation does not play a role in management in this age group because there is a lower rate of medium-term success.[81] Early surgery is associated with a lower incidence of

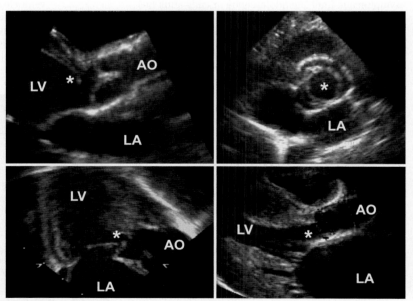

FIGURE 65-32 Montage demonstrating the different types of left ventricular outflow tract obstruction (asterisks). The upper left image shows isolated fibromuscular obstruction; the upper right, stenosis due to a bicuspid aortic valve; the lower left, obstruction because of chordal apparatus from the anterior mitral leaflet; and the lower right, obstruction due to tunnel narrowing at the valve, annular, and subvalve level. AO = aorta; LA = left atrium; LV = left ventricle.

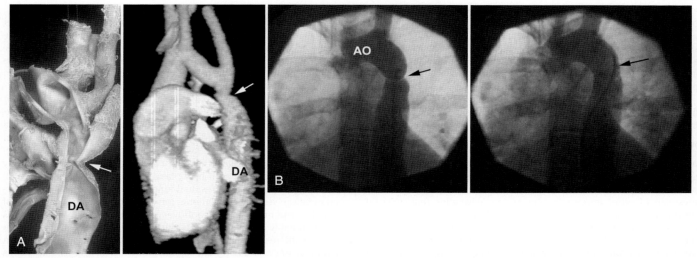

FIGURE 65-33 A, Montage of a coarctation of the aorta. The left image is a specimen that shows the site of the posterior shelf, as outlined by the arrow. The right image is from a CMR examination and shows the posterior shelf and some associated transverse arch hypoplasia. **B,** Angiogram of a coarctation of the aorta, before and after stenting. AO, aorta; DA, descending aorta.

long-term hypertension. At time of presentation, transverse arch and isthmal hypoplasia are frequent associations; however, subsequent growth appears to occur, even in neonates weighing less than 2.5 kg.[82]

Infants and Children

PRESENTATION. Most infants and children with isolated coarctation are asymptomatic, with the findings of reduced femoral pulses and hypertension being detected during routine medical care of the pediatric patient. Heart failure is uncommon because the left ventricle has a chance to become hypertrophied, thus maintaining a normal wall stress. Complaints of headache, cold extremities, and claudication with exercise may be noted in the older child and adolescent.

A midsystolic murmur over the anterior chest, back, and spinous processes is most frequent, becoming continuous if the lumen is sufficiently narrowed to result in a high-velocity jet across the lesion throughout the cardiac cycle. Additional systolic and continuous murmurs over the lateral thoracic wall may reflect increased flow through dilated and tortuous collateral vessels, which are commonly not heard until later childhood.

LABORATORY INVESTIGATIONS

ELECTROCARDIOGRAPHY. This reveals left ventricular hypertrophy of various degrees, depending on the height of arterial pressure above the obstruction and the patient's age. Coexisting right ventricular hypertrophy usually implies a complicated lesion.

CHEST RADIOGRAPHY. The characteristic posteroanterior film feature is the so-called figure-3 configuration of the proximal descending thoracic aorta due to both prestenotic and poststenotic dilation. Rib notching (unilateral or bilateral, second to ninth ribs) is present in 50% of cases. Rib notching is unilateral if the right or left subclavian arteries arise from the aorta distal to the coarctation. Rib notching is noted as an erosion of the undersurface of a posterior rib, usually at its outer third, with a sclerotic margin.

ECHOCARDIOGRAPHY. This demonstrates a posterior shelf, a well-expanded isthmus and transverse aortic arch (in most cases), and a high-velocity continuous jet through the coarctation site. Interestingly, a slow upstroke is observed on the abdominal aortic velocity profile compared with that seen in the ascending aorta.

CMR. This provides detailed information in this age group and may be performed before intervention, particularly if balloon dilation is the treatment of choice. This is the best tool for postintervention imaging and has become routine in many centers.

ANGIOCARDIOGRAPHY. This is reserved for delineating the coarctation at the time of balloon dilation. Primary management in those cases with a well-expanded isthmus and transverse aortic arch invariably involves balloon dilation.

INTERVENTION. Balloon dilation is the current technique in many centers,[83] with surgery being reserved for cases with associated arch hypoplasia. Extended end-to-end anastomosis is the currently favored surgical approach, with patch augmentation being reserved for cases with significant arch hypoplasia.

Paradoxical hypertension of short duration is often noted in the immediate postoperative period, a phenomenon much less common after balloon angioplasty. A resetting of carotid baroreceptors and increased catecholamine secretion appear to be responsible for the initial phase of postoperative systemic hypertension, with a later, second phase of prolonged elevation of systolic and particularly diastolic blood pressure related to activation of the renin-angiotensin system. A necrotizing panarteritis of the small vessels of the gastrointestinal tract of uncertain cause occasionally complicates the course of recovery.

Recoarctation

The risk of recurrent narrowing after repair of coarctation in infancy is 5% to 10%. Such narrowing is best screened for with Doppler ultrasonography, with CMR being the gold standard for imaging. Clinical decisions to intervene are usually based on a cuff blood pressure difference between the right arm and leg (for a left aortic arch and normal innominate artery). Although there are no hard and fast rules for absolute blood pressure difference, it has been common practice to reintervene when the blood pressure difference is more than 25 to 30 mm Hg in the presence of systemic hypertension. Although Doppler measurements can detect a recurrent obstruction, this technique provides an overestimation of the blood pressure–measured gradients because of the phenomenon of pressure recovery. Recoarctation is usually addressed with balloon dilation if the obstruction is relatively localized. In the presence of long-segment narrowings, surgical intervention may be necessary, with the use of patch augmentation of the hypoplastic segment. In the adolescent or adult, balloon-expandable stents are routinely employed with good success (see Fig. 65-33B). This has the advantage of avoiding the risk of potential spinal cord damage perisurgery in patients with poorly developed collaterals.

Long-term Complications

In patients who survive the first 2 years of life without an intervention, complications of juxtaductal coarctation are uncommon before the second or third decade. The chief hazards to patients with coarctation result from severe hypertension and include the development of cerebral aneurysms and hemorrhage, hypertensive encephalopathy, rupture of the aorta, left ventricular failure, and infective endocarditis. In patients with coarctation repaired, systemic hypertension in the absence of residual coarctation has been observed in resting or exercise-stressed patients postoperatively and appears to be related to the duration of preoperative hypertension as well as the architecture of the aortic arch segments.[84] These patients also have abnormalities of vascular reactivity, as demonstrated by flow-mediated studies. Increased left ventricular mass is observed, even in the absence of a residual arm-leg gradient. Life-long observation is desirable because of the late onset of hypertension in some postoperative patients.

In those who have undergone balloon dilation of a native coarctation, the incidence of aneurysm formation at the coarctation site is on the order of 7%.[85]

Adults

Although much of the previous material is also relevant to the adult, there are some differences in the issues faced by adult patients. *Complex coarctation* is used to describe coarctation in the presence of other important intracardiac anomalies (e.g., VSD, left ventricular outflow tract obstruction, and mitral stenosis) and is usually detected in infancy. *Simple coarctation* refers to coarctation in the absence of such lesions. It is the most common form detected de novo in adults. Associated abnormalities include bicuspid aortic valve in most cases (80%), intracranial aneurysms (most commonly of the circle of Willis) in 2% to 10%, and acquired intercostal artery aneurysms. One definition of *significant coarctation* requires a gradient greater than 20 mm Hg across the coarctation site at angiography with or without proximal systemic hypertension. A second definition of significant coarctation requires the presence of proximal hypertension in the company of echocardiographic or angiographic evidence of aortic coarctation. If there is an extensive collateral circulation (see Fig. 82-4), there may be minimal or no pressure gradient and acquired aortic atresia.

Death in patients who do not undergo repair is usually due to heart failure (usually older than 30 years), coronary artery disease, aortic rupture or dissection, concomitant aortic valve disease, infective endarteritis or endocarditis, or cerebral hemorrhage.[86] Of Turner syndrome patients, 35% have aortic coarctation.

CLINICAL FEATURES. Patients can be asymptomatic, or they can present with minimal symptoms of epistaxis, headache, and leg weakness on exertion or more serious symptoms of congestive heart failure, angina, aortic stenosis, aortic dissection, or unexplained intracerebral hemorrhage. Leg claudication (pain) is rare unless there is concomitant abdominal aortic coarctation. A thorough clinical examination reveals upper limb systemic hypertension as well as a differential systolic blood pressure of at least 10 mm Hg (brachial > popliteal artery pressure). Radial-femoral pulse delay is evident unless significant aortic regurgitation coexists. Auscultation may reveal an interscapular systolic murmur emanating from the coarctation site and a widespread crescendo-decrescendo continuous murmur throughout the chest wall from intercostal collateral arteries. Funduscopic examination can reveal "corkscrew" tortuosity of retinal arterioles.

INTERVENTIONAL OUTCOMES
Surgical

After surgical repair of simple coarctation, the obstruction is usually relieved, with minimal mortality (1%). Paraplegia due to spinal cord ischemia is uncommon (0.4%) and may occur in patients who do not have well-developed collateral circulation. The prevalence of recoarctation reported in the literature varies widely from 7% to 60% but is probably about 10%,[87] depending on the definition used, the length of follow-up, and the age at surgery. The appropriateness of the surgical repair for a given anatomy is probably the main factor dictating the chance of recoarctation rather than the type of surgical repair itself. True aneurysm formation at the site of coarctation repair is also a well-recognized entity, with a reported incidence between 2% and 27%. Aneurysms are particularly common after Dacron patch aortoplasty and usually occur in the native aorta opposite the patch.[88] Late dissection at the repair site is rare, but false aneurysms, usually at the suture line, can occur. Long-term follow-up after surgical correction of coarctation of the aorta still reveals an increased incidence of premature cardiovascular disease and death.

Transcatheter

After balloon dilation (see Fig. 65-33B), aortic dissection, restenosis, and aneurysm formation at the site of coarctation have been documented. These complications have been reduced with the now increasing if not exclusive use of primary stenting in the adults with native coarctation as well as recoarctation.[89] The significance of aneurysm formation is often unknown, and longer term data are necessary.

Prior hypertension resolves in up to 50% of patients but may recur later in life, especially if the intervention is performed at an older age. In some of these patients, this may be essential hypertension, but a hemodynamic basis should be sought and blood pressure control should be attained. Systolic hypertension is also common with exercise and is not a surrogate marker for recoarctation of the aorta. It may be related to residual arch hypoplasia or to increased renin and catecholamine activity from residual functional abnormalities of the precoarctation vessels. The criteria for and significance of exertional systolic hypertension are controversial. Late cerebrovascular events occur, notably in those patients undergoing repair as adults and in those with residual hypertension. Endocarditis or endarteritis can occur at the coarctation site or on intracardiac lesions; and if this occurs at the coarctation site, embolic manifestations are restricted to the legs.

FOLLOW-UP. All patients should have a follow-up examination every 1 to 3 years. Particular attention should be directed toward residual hypertension, heart failure, intracardiac disease (such as an associated bicuspid aortic valve (see Chap. 66), which can become stenotic or regurgitant later in life), or an ascending aortopathy sometimes seen in the presence of bicuspid aortic valve. Complications at the site of repair, such as restenosis and aneurysm formation, should also be sought by clinical examination, chest radiography, echocardiography, and periodic CMR or CT scanning. Patients with Dacron patch repair should probably undergo CMR or spiral CT examination every 3 to 5 years or so to detect subclinical aneurysm formation. Hemoptysis from a leaking or ruptured aneurysm is a serious complication requiring immediate investigation and surgery. New or unusual headaches raise the possibility of berry aneurysms.

Aortic Arch Hypoplasia

MORPHOLOGY. The aortic isthmus, the portion of the aorta between the left subclavian artery and the ductus arteriosus, should be narrowed in the fetus and newborn. The lumen of the aortic isthmus is about two thirds that of the ascending and descending portions of the aorta until age 6 to 9 months, when the physiologic narrowing disappears. Pathologic tubular hypoplasia of the aortic arch usually is noted in the aortic isthmus and is most commonly associated with presentation of aortic coarctation in the newborn period. Despite this, in a small group of cases, the arch obstruction is due primarily to tubular hypoplasia, usually involving both the aortic isthmus and transverse aortic arch (between the innominate and subclavian arteries). These cases usually present early in life with findings similar to those with a severe coarctation of the aorta. As with the latter, they are duct dependent and may also be associated with other left-sided obstructive lesions.

MANAGEMENT OPTIONS. Provided the other left-sided structures are formed well enough to sustain life, the management involves arch reconstruction with a patch, in a fashion similar to those cases undergoing a Norwood procedure for hypoplastic left heart syndrome. If the left-sided structures are hypoplastic, palliative surgery with a Norwood procedure and cardiac transplantation are the two treatments of choice.

Complex Coarctation

In some instances, the coarctation of the aorta is part of a more complex spectrum of lesions. This can be seen in cases with double-outlet right ventricle, cc-TGA, D-TGA, functionally single ventricle, truncus arteriosus, and AV septal defect. In these cases, the decision process involves not only the coarctation repair but the management of the associated lesions. The current trend is to complete repair of the intracardiac lesion at the same time as the arch repair.

Aortic Arch Interruption

Aortic arch interruption is a rare and usually lethal anomaly. Unless it is treated surgically, almost all infants die within the first month of life. Interruptions distal to the left subclavian artery (type A) occur with almost equal frequency to interruptions distal to the left common carotid artery (type B). The right subclavian artery is of variable origin, frequently arising from the descending aortic segment distal to the interruption. The clinical presentation resembles that in tubular hypoplasia or severe coarctation of the aorta with a PDA.

Virtually all patients have associated intracardiac anomalies. A PDA almost always connects the main pulmonary artery with the descending aorta. Patients with interrupted aortic arch typically have either a VSD (80% to 90% of cases) or an aortopulmonary window (10% to 20%). Because the ductus arteriosus provides lower body blood flow, its spontaneous constriction results in profound clinical deterioration. The latter may be temporarily managed by prostaglandin E_1 infusion. Other complex intracardiac malformations, such as TGA, aortopulmonary window, and truncus arteriosus, are common.

CLINICAL FEATURES. An association with the genetic 22q11 deletion DiGeorge syndrome is frequent. The major clinical problem is severe congestive heart failure as a consequence of volume overload of the left ventricle from an associated intracardiac left-to-right shunt and of pressure overload imposed by systemic hypertension. Absent upper and lower limb pulses, with a palpable superficial temporal pulse, is a helpful clue to the diagnosis.

LABORATORY INVESTIGATIONS
ELECTROCARDIOGRAPHY. This demonstrates right ventricular hypertrophy with right-axis deviation and ST-T wave changes.
CHEST RADIOGRAPHY. Cardiomegaly is noted with increased pulmonary markings and pulmonary edema.
ECHOCARDIOGRAPHY. This is the gold standard for the diagnosis of aortic arch interruption and associated lesions. The VSD can be characterized, as can the degree of left ventricular outflow tract obstruction.

MANAGEMENT. The perioperative clinical condition of most patients can be improved by intensive medical management with mechanical ventilation, inotropic support, and prostaglandin infusion. There has been increasing success with complete primary repair in infancy as the procedure of choice. In some cases in which the left ventricular outflow tract obstruction is thought to be too severe for standard primary repair, a Norwood procedure is initially performed. This is followed by a complete repair by tunneling the left ventricle through the VSD to the new aorta and placement of a right ventricle to pulmonary artery conduit.

OUTCOME. The medium- and long-term outcomes are reasonable, but there may be a need for reintervention for left ventricular outflow tract obstruction and recurrent arch obstruction.[90]

Sinus of Valsalva Aneurysm and Fistula

MORPHOLOGY. The malformation consists of a separation, or lack of fusion, between the media of the aorta and the annulus fibrosus of the aortic valve. The receiving chamber of a right aortic sinus aortocardiac fistula is usually the right ventricle, but occasionally, when the noncoronary cusp is involved, the fistula drains into the right atrium. From 5% to 15% of aneurysms originate in the posterior or noncoronary sinus. The left aortic sinus is seldom involved. Associated anomalies are common and include a VSD, bicuspid aortic valve, and aortic coarctation.

CLINICAL FEATURES. The deficiency in the aortic media appears to be congenital. Reports in infants are exceedingly rare and are infrequent in children because progressive aneurysmal dilation of the weakened area develops but may not be recognized until the third or fourth decade of life, when rupture into a cardiac chamber occurs. A congenital aneurysm of an aortic sinus of Valsalva, particularly the right coronary sinus, is an uncommon anomaly that occurs three times more often in males. An unruptured aneurysm usually does not produce a hemodynamic abnormality. Rarely, myocardial ischemia may be caused by coronary arterial compression. Rupture is often of abrupt onset, causes chest pain, and creates continuous arteriovenous shunting and acute volume loading of both right and left heart chambers, which promptly results in heart failure. An additional complication is infective endocarditis, which may originate either on the edges of the aneurysm or on those areas in the right side of the heart that are traumatized by the jetlike stream of blood flowing through the fistula.

This anomaly should be suspected in a patient with a combination of chest pain of sudden onset, resting or exertional dyspnea, bounding pulses, and a loud, superficial, continuous murmur accentuated in diastole when the fistula opens into the right ventricle as well as a thrill along the right or left lower sternal border. The physical findings can be difficult to distinguish from those produced by a coronary arteriovenous fistula.

LABORATORY INVESTIGATIONS
ELECTROCARDIOGRAPHY. This may show biventricular hypertrophy, or it may be normal.
CHEST RADIOGRAPHY. This may demonstrate generalized cardiomegaly and usually heart failure.
ECHOCARDIOGRAPHY. Studies based on two-dimensional and pulsed Doppler echocardiography may detect the walls of the aneurysm and disturbed flow within the aneurysm or at the site of perforation. TEE may provide more precise information than the transthoracic approach.
CARDIAC CATHETERIZATION. This reveals a left-to-right shunt at the ventricular or, less commonly, the atrial level. The diagnosis may be established definitively by retrograde thoracic aortography.

MANAGEMENT OPTIONS AND OUTCOMES. Preoperative medical management consists of measures to relieve cardiac failure and to treat coexistent arrhythmias or endocarditis, if present. At operation, the aneurysm is closed and amputated, and the aortic wall is reunited with the heart, either by direct suture or with a prosthesis. All efforts should be made to preserve the aortic valve in children because patch closure of the defect combined with prosthetic valve replacement greatly increases the risk of operation in small patients. Device closure of the ruptured aneurysm has also been attempted.

Vascular Rings

MORPHOLOGY. The term *vascular ring* is used for those aortic arch or pulmonary artery malformations that exhibit an abnormal relation with the esophagus and trachea, often causing dysphagia or respiratory symptoms.

DOUBLE AORTIC ARCH (**Fig. 65-34**). The most common vascular ring is produced by a double aortic arch in which both the right and left fourth embryonic aortic arches persist. In the most common type of double aortic arch, there is a left ligamentum arteriosum or occasionally a ductus arteriosus. Although both arches may be patent at the time of diagnosis, invariably the left arch distal to the left subclavian artery is atretic and is connected to the descending aorta by a fibrous remnant that completes the ring. When both arches are patent, the right arch is usually larger than the left. This usually occurs as an isolated lesion, with the respiratory symptoms being caused by tracheal compression and frequently associated laryngomalacia, usually in the neonate and young infant.

RIGHT AORTIC ARCH. A right aortic arch with a left ductus or ligamentum arteriosum connecting the left pulmonary artery and the upper part of the descending aorta is the next most important vascular ring seen. Although all cases with this lesion have a vascular ring, not all cases are symptomatic. Indeed, those patients who are symptomatic usually have an associated diverticulum of Kommerell. This is a large outpouching at the distal takeoff of the left subclavian artery from the descending aorta. It is the combination of the diverticulum and the ring that causes the airway compression.

ANOMALOUS ORIGIN OF A RIGHT SUBCLAVIAN ARTERY. Anomalous origin of a right subclavian artery is one of the most common abnormalities of the aortic arch. Although the aberrant right subclavian artery runs posterior to the esophagus, it does not form a vascular ring unless there is an associated right-sided ductus or ligamentum to complete the ring. During adulthood, about 5% of patients with an aberrant right subclavian artery (and a left ductus) develop symptoms due to rigidity of the aberrant vessel.

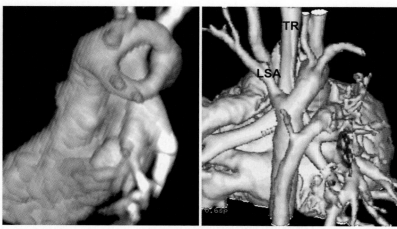

FIGURE 65-34 The left image is a three-dimensional reconstruction of a double aortic arch from a CMR examination. The right image is from an aberrant left subclavian artery as seen by spiral CT. LSA = left subclavian artery; TR = trachea.

RETROESOPHAGEAL DESCENDING AORTA. This is a rarer but more problematic type of vascular ring. In this setting, there may be either an ascending left and descending right aorta or an ascending right and descending left aorta. The retroesophageal component of the descending aorta causes the tracheal compression, in conjunction with the left- or right-sided ligamentum.

PULMONARY ARTERY SLING. This is usually made up of the left pulmonary artery arising from the right pulmonary artery and runs posterior to the trachea but anterior to the esophagus. This is usually seen in isolation and is associated with significant hypoplasia of the bronchial tree, which is the predominant cause of the airway symptoms.

CLINICAL FEATURES. The symptoms produced by vascular rings depend on the tightness of anatomic constriction of the trachea and esophagus and consist principally of respiratory difficulties including stridor, cyanosis (especially with feeding), and dysphagia. Not all patients with a vascular ring are symptomatic, and cases with an aberrant left subclavian artery are frequently detected at the time of evaluation for associated CHD. Although most patients with a true ring and some airway compression present early in life, others present later with dysphagia; others escape diagnosis forever.

LABORATORY INVESTIGATIONS

ELECTROCARDIOGRAPHY. This appears normal unless associated cardiovascular anomalies are present.

CHEST RADIOGRAPHY. If there is evidence of a right aortic arch in a symptomatic patient, a vascular ring should be suspected. In some instances, there is evidence of some airway narrowing. The barium esophagogram is a useful screening procedure. Prominent posterior indentation of the esophagus is observed in many of the common vascular ring arrangements, although the pulmonary artery vascular sling produces an anterior indentation.

ECHOCARDIOGRAPHY. Echocardiography is a sensitive tool for evaluation of the laterality of the aortic arch, including a detailed assessment of the associated brachiocephalic vessels. In general, if there is normal branching of the innominate artery, to the right for a left aortic arch and to the left for a right, along with the correct "sideness" of the descending aorta, a vascular ring can be excluded. *Most cases with a double aortic arch* have a dominant right arch, with the descending aorta appearing to dip posteriorly as it runs behind the esophagus. A patent ductus or ligamentum can usually be identified by echocardiography. When both arches are patent, a frontal plane sweep from inferior to superior demonstrates both patent arches as well as their brachiocephalic vessels. *A right aortic arch with an aberrant left subclavian artery* is suspected when it is not possible to identify normal branching of the left-sided innominate artery. *A retroesophageal descending aorta* should be suspected when the ascending aorta and its brachiocephalic arteries are readily identified but there is difficulty in identifying the descending aorta as it traverses behind the esophagus. *A left pulmonary artery sling* is suspected when the normal branching pattern of pulmonary arteries cannot be identified. In this setting, color Doppler study permits the identification of the left pulmonary artery as it arises from the right pulmonary artery and runs in a posterior and leftward direction.

CMR AND CT. CMR and CT play a major role in the evaluation of patients with a vascular ring. In fact, CMR has become the gold standard for the evaluation of the aorta and its branches. The only disadvantage for infants is that general anesthesia is often required for a successful examination to be achieved. On the other hand, spiral CT is a technique that is fast and provides better definition of the affected airways; this technique is particularly valuable for patients with a pulmonary artery sling, in which the vascular ring plays a secondary role to the airway abnormalities. The advantages of these techniques are that, unlike echocardiography, they permit a precise assessment of the more posterior vascular structures and their relationships to the esophagus and airways. These techniques are particularly valuable in the more complex forms, such as a retroesophageal descending aorta.

MANAGEMENT OPTIONS AND OUTCOMES. The severity of symptoms and the anatomy of the malformation are the most important factors in determining treatment. Patients, particularly infants, with respiratory obstruction require prompt surgical intervention. A left thoracotomy is the surgical approach in most patients with a vascular ring. For the most common vascular rings, such as double aortic arch and aberrant left subclavian artery, the combination of chest radiography, barium swallow study, and echocardiography is all that is necessary before surgical intervention.

Operative repair of the double aortic arch requires division of the minor arch (usually the left) and the ligamentum. Patients with a right aortic arch and a left ductus or ligamentum arteriosum require division of the ductus or ligamentum or ligation and division of the left subclavian artery, which is the posterior component of the ring. Video-assisted thoracoscopy holds promise as an alternative to open thoracotomy for management. In patients with a pulmonary artery vascular sling, operation consists of detachment of the left pulmonary artery at its origin and anastomosis to the main pulmonary artery directly or by way of a conduit with its proximal end brought anterior to the trachea. The addition of tracheal narrowing that requires surgical intervention adds to the mortality in this group of patients, as does the association with intracardiac malformations.[91]

Congenital Aortic Valve Stenosis

GENERAL CONSIDERATIONS. We deal here only with this condition in newborns and children because the adult presentation is described in Chap. 66. Congenital aortic valve stenosis is a relatively common anomaly. Congenital aortic valve stenosis occurs much more frequently in males, with a gender ratio of 4:1. Associated cardiovascular anomalies have been noted in up to 20% of patients. PDA and coarctation of the aorta occur most frequently with aortic valve stenosis; all three of these lesions may coexist.

MORPHOLOGY. The basic malformation consists of thickening of valve tissue with various degrees of commissural fusion. The valve is most commonly bicuspid. In some patients, the stenotic aortic valve is unicuspid and dome shaped, with no or one lateral attachment to the aorta at the level of the orifice. In infants and young children with severe aortic stenosis, the aortic valve annulus may be relatively underdeveloped. This lesion forms a continuum with the hypoplastic left heart syndrome and the aortic atresia and hypoplasia complexes. Secondary calcification of the valve is rare in childhood. When the obstruction is hemodynamically significant, concentric hypertrophy of the left ventricular wall and dilation of the ascending aorta occur.

NEONATAL PRESENTATION. The newborn presentation is often similar to that seen with other obstructive left-sided lesions, such as coarctation of the aorta and interrupted aortic arch. The infant presents with heart failure and depends on ductal patency for survival. An association with varying degrees of left ventricular hypoplasia, mitral valve abnormalities, and endocardial fibroelastosis occurs frequently. With the advent of good prenatal screening, many are detected before birth, with deliveries being performed in a high-risk obstetric unit attached to a congenital heart facility. The decision process around single versus biventricular repair is a complex one and beyond the scope of this chapter. Suffice it to say that this still poses a challenge in the newborn period.[92]

Clinical Findings

Newborns generally have weak pulses throughout, signs of heart failure, and often little in the way of murmurs, despite the severe left ventricular outflow tract obstruction.

LABORATORY INVESTIGATIONS

ELECTROCARDIOGRAPHY. An ECG usually shows right ventricular dominance with evidence of diffuse ST wave changes due to left ventricular strain.

CHEST RADIOGRAPHY. Chest radiography usually shows cardiomegaly due to a large right ventricle and varying degrees of pulmonary edema.

ECHOCARDIOGRAPHY. Echocardiography is currently the diagnostic test of choice. It usually shows a poorly contracting left ventricle with varying degrees of endocardial fibroelastosis and frequently hypoplasia of the left ventricle and aortic root. Doppler assessment of gradients is often unreliable because of poor left ventricular function. Right ventricular hypertension and tricuspid valve regurgitation are common associated findings.

Management

Prostaglandin therapy is instituted in this population of patients to maintain the fetal circulation with retrograde ductal flow that permits coronary and cerebral perfusion. The nature of further treatment depends on whether the left ventricle and aortic root are believed to be of a sufficient size to support a biventricular repair. If so, balloon dilation is rapidly becoming the treatment of choice, although surgical intervention is still preferred by some. If the left-sided heart structures are believed to be too small to sustain life, either cardiac transplantation or a Norwood procedure can be undertaken.

PRESENTATION BEYOND THE NEWBORN PERIOD. The diagnosis is invariably made after the detection of a murmur. On occasion, heart failure ensues, usually in the first 1 to 2 months of life, when there is a rapid progression of the obstruction and lack of left ventricular mass to maintain a normal wall stress. Natural history studies performed several years ago demonstrated that more rapid progression of aortic valve stenosis is more likely to happen within the first 2 years of life, after which the rate of progressive obstruction is more uniform.

Clinical Findings

In general, the children are asymptomatic, having normal peripheral pulses if the stenosis is less severe and low-volume, slow-rising pulses when it progresses. Exercise fatigue and chest pain are rare complaints and occur only when the stenosis is severe. With severe stenosis, there is a systolic thrill in the same area that can also be felt in the suprasternal notch and carotid arteries. Beyond the newborn period, there is usually an ejection click at the apex that precedes the murmur. The second heart sound is usually normal in children. An ejection systolic murmur is heard along the left sternal border, with radiation into the right infraclavicular area. Associated aortic regurgitation may be heard.

LABORATORY INVESTIGATIONS

ELECTROCARDIOGRAPHY. Left ventricular hypertrophy with or without strain is the hallmark feature.

CHEST RADIOGRAPHY. Overall heart size is normal or the degree of enlargement is slight in most children with congenital aortic valve stenosis.

ECHOCARDIOGRAPHY. Two-dimensional echocardiography provides detailed information about the morphology of the valve, the left ventricular function, and the presence of associated left-sided lesions. Doppler echocardiography can be used to determine the severity of stenosis and the presence or absence of associated aortic regurgitation. Doppler study provides peak instantaneous gradients that are higher than the peak-to-peak gradients determined from cardiac catheterization. The importance of this lies in the fact that the natural history studies and clinical decision making have thus far been based on peak-to-peak catheterization gradients in the infant, child, and adolescent. Valve areas are usually not calculated in this age group because there are no good data to support their use in pediatric patients. Mean gradients as derived from Doppler study and catheterization correlate closely, but again, no

data support their use in clinical decision making. Some data convert the Doppler-derived mean gradients to peak to peak, with the addition of the pulse pressure as obtained from blood pressure measurements. Whatever absolute number is chosen to work with, the additional finding of left ventricular hypertrophy on electrocardiography and echocardiography provides supportive data about timing for intervention. The pediatric community generally agrees that a peak-to-peak gradient of 60 mm Hg or more probably warrants intervention.

CARDIAC CATHETERIZATION. Cardiac catheterization is now rarely used to establish the site and severity of obstruction to left ventricular outflow. Instead, catheterization is undertaken when therapeutic interventional balloon aortic valvuloplasty is indicated.

Management Options

In this era, balloon dilation has almost completely replaced primary surgical valvotomy in children.

FOLLOW-UP. Follow-up studies indicate that aortic valvotomy is a safe and effective means of palliative treatment with excellent relief of symptoms. Aortic insufficiency can occasionally be progressive and require valve replacement. Moreover, after commissurotomy, the valve leaflets remain somewhat deformed, and further degenerative changes including calcification will likely lead to significant stenosis in later years. Thus, prosthetic aortic valve replacement is required in approximately 35% of patients within 15 to 20 years of the original operation. For those children and adolescents requiring aortic valve replacement, the surgical options include replacement with a mechanical aortic valve, an aortic homograft, and a pulmonary autograft in the aortic position. Accumulating evidence shows that the pulmonary autograft may ultimately be preferable to the aortic homograft. In the pulmonary autograft, called the Ross procedure, the patient's pulmonary valve is removed and used to replace the diseased aortic valve, and the right ventricular outflow tract is reconstructed with a pulmonary valve homograft. This approach appears to confer a survival advantage in the younger age group, in whom repeated mechanical valve replacement is associated with an increased mortality.[63] Despite this advantage, caution is necessary when it is applied to patients with bicuspid aortic valve and aortic regurgitation. This is due to associated aortic root dilation, which is inherent to this lesion and may complicate the long-term reliability of the Ross procedure. This surgical approach can be applied from neonatal through adult life. Neither homografts nor autografts require anticoagulation.

Subaortic Stenosis

MORPHOLOGY

DISCRETE FIBROMUSCULAR. This lesion consists of a ridge or fibrous ring encircling the left ventricular outflow tract at varying distances from the aortic valve. The subvalvular fibrous process usually extends onto the aortic valve cusps and almost always makes contact with the ventricular aspect of the anterior mitral leaflet at its base. In other cases with fibrous discontinuity between the mitral and aortic valves, it forms more of a tunnel obstruction.

FOCAL MUSCULAR. Rarely there is no fibrous element but rather a focal muscular obstruction on the crest of the interventricular septum, which differs from typical cases with hypertrophic cardiomyopathy.

HYPOPLASIA OF THE LEFT VENTRICULAR OUTFLOW TRACT. In some cases, valvular and subvalvular aortic stenoses coexist with hypoplasia of the aortic valve annulus and thickened valve leaflets, producing a tunnel-like narrowing of the left ventricular outflow tract. Additional findings often include a small ascending aorta.

DISCRETE SUBAORTIC STENOSIS AND VSD. This combination is frequently encountered in the pediatric age group, with the fibromuscular component often being absent at the initial echocardiographic evaluation. The association should be suspected in VSDs with some associated anterior malalignment of the aorta and a more acute aortoseptal angle. These hearts frequently develop subpulmonary stenosis. In a different subset of patients with aortic arch interruption and a VSD, there is muscular subaortic stenosis due to posterior deviation of the infundibular septum.

COMPLEX SUBAORTIC STENOSIS. Various anatomic lesions other than a discrete ridge may produce subaortic stenosis. Among these are abnormal adherence of the anterior leaflet of the mitral valve to the septum and the presence in the left ventricular outflow tract of accessory endocardial cushion tissue. These are frequently associated with a "cleft in the anterior mitral valve leaflet," which is to be differentiated from that seen in an AV septal defect. These types of obstruction are seen more commonly in those cases with abnormalities of the ventriculoarterial connection in association with a VSD (e.g., double-outlet right ventricle, transposition, VSD).

CLINICAL FEATURES. These types of obstruction are usually identified as secondary lesions in those cases with associated VSDs, with or without abnormalities of the ventriculoarterial connections or aortic arch obstruction. In general, the substrate for left ventricular outflow tract obstruction is present, although actual physiologic obstruction is absent in some cases. In other cases, the patients are referred for evaluation because of a systolic murmur. In cases with a gradient across the left ventricular outflow tract, there is an ejection systolic murmur heard along the lower left sternal border with the absence of an ejection click.

LABORATORY INVESTIGATIONS

ELECTROCARDIOGRAPHY. In those with associated defects, the ECG reflects the major abnormality rather than the associated left ventricular outflow tract obstruction. With isolated forms of left ventricular outflow tract obstruction, there may be left ventricular hypertrophy when the obstruction is significant.

CHEST RADIOGRAPHY. This is usually unhelpful in these cases.

ECHOCARDIOGRAPHY. Echocardiography is the standard diagnostic tool in this lesion. Not only can it permit an accurate delineation of the mechanisms of obstruction, but it provides detailed data about associated lesions. In all forms, the parasternal long-axis view is key to providing an accurate diagnosis. The presence of mitral aortic discontinuity, the relationship of a fibromuscular ridge to the aortic valve, the presence of accessory obstructive tissue, and the dimensions of the aortic annulus and root are well imaged in this view. In addition, color flow mapping permits the identification of associated aortic valve regurgitation and provides hemodynamic evidence of the site of onset of obstruction. The extension of a fibromuscular ridge onto the anterior mitral leaflet is best appreciated in the apical five-chamber view. This also provides the best site for pulsed or continuous-wave Doppler assessment of the maximum gradient across the left ventricular outflow tract. In the older patient, TEE plays an important role in delineating the pathologic process. Real-time three-dimensional echocardiography provides additional information, particularly in cases with complex mechanisms of left ventricular outflow tract obstruction (**Fig. 65-35**).

CARDIAC CATHETERIZATION. This technique is no longer of importance in evaluating this lesion. Although balloon dilation has been attempted, it is generally believed that this is a surgical lesion.

CMR. In general, CMR is unnecessary unless there are problems obtaining the needed information by echocardiography.

INTERVENTIONAL OPTIONS. Surgical intervention is indicated either at the time of the repair of the underlying primary lesion or in those cases with discrete obstruction when the obstruction is severe enough to raise concerns.

Discrete Subaortic Stenosis (Fibrous and Muscular)

The rate of progression is varied and may be slow. In general, the approach to the latter group has been to intervene when there is a mean echo gradient across the left ventricular outflow tract of greater than 30 mm Hg to avoid future aortic leaflet damage. Surgery involves a fibromyectomy, with care to avoid damage to the aortic valve or creation of a traumatic VSD. There is a recurrence rate of subaortic stenosis requiring reoperation in up to 20% of cases.[93] In some cases, the recurrence is in the form of a fibrous ridge; in others, there is acquired disease of the aortic valve in the form of stenosis or regurgitation. Reoperation may involve just repeated resection of a recurrent fibrous ridge, or it may involve surgery for the aortic valve in those cases with significant aortic regurgitation.

Complex Forms of Left Ventricular Outflow Tract Obstruction and an Intact Ventricular Septum

In cases with an intact ventricular septum, the indications for intervention are similar to those in cases with discrete obstruction. The difference lies in the fact that the surgical approach must be modified

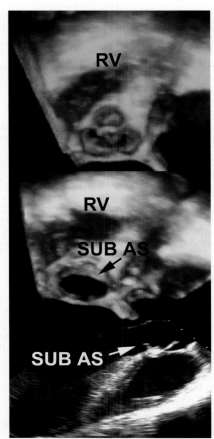

FIGURE 65-35 This montage is from a case with left ventricular outflow tract obstruction, as seen by transesophageal echocardiography in both the two- and three-dimensional modes. **Upper panel,** surgical view of the aortic valve demonstrating the three aortic leaflets. **Middle panel,** is the same case with the aortic valve open. Note the subaortic membrane that is crescentic in shape *(black arrow).* **Bottom panel,** the image seen by two-dimensional echocardiography shows only part of the shelf. RV = right ventricle, SUB AS = subaortic stenosis.

according to the underlying pathologic process. Resection of any fibromuscular component or accessory tissue (provided it is not a primary support mechanism for the mitral valve), a valve-sparing Konno operation, and, in those cases with a hypoplastic aortic annulus, a classic Konno procedure with aortic valve replacement are the potential surgical options.

Left Ventricular Outflow Tract Obstruction and Complex Forms of CHD

In general, surgery to the left ventricular outflow tract is part of the general repair of the lesion and is not dependent on the precise degree of obstruction across this site.

OUTCOMES. Immediate complications related to surgery include complete AV block, creation of a VSD, and mitral regurgitation from intraoperative damage to the mitral valve apparatus. Long-term complications include recurrence of fibromuscular subvalvular left ventricular outflow tract obstruction (up to 20%).[93] Clinically important aortic regurgitation is not uncommon (up to 25% of patients). In some cases with predominant acquired aortic valve stenosis, balloon dilation has been the treatment of choice.

FOLLOW-UP. Particular attention should be paid to patients with residual or recurrent subaortic stenosis and those with an associated bicuspid aortic valve or important aortic regurgitation because they are most likely to require surgery eventually. Reoperation is more likely in cases with complex forms of obstruction, younger age at operation, and incomplete relief of obstruction at the initial procedure.[65] Patients with bioprosthetic aortic valves in the aortic position (after the Konno procedure) or the pulmonary position (after the Ross-Konno procedure) need close follow-up. Endocarditis prophylaxis should be used for prosthetic valves or in the presence of any residual lesions.

Supravalvular Aortic Stenosis

MORPHOLOGY. Three anatomic types of supravalvular aortic stenosis are recognized, although some patients may have findings of more than one type. Most common is the hourglass type, in which marked thickening and disorganization of the aortic media produce a constricting annular ridge at the superior margin of the sinuses of Valsalva. The membranous type is the result of a fibrous or fibromuscular semicircular diaphragm with a small central opening stretched across the lumen of the aorta. Diffuse hypoplasia of the ascending aorta characterizes the third type.

Because the coronary arteries arise proximal to the site of outflow obstruction in supravalvular aortic stenosis, they are subjected to the elevated pressure that exists within the left ventricle. These vessels are often dilated and tortuous, and premature coronary arteriosclerosis has been described. Moreover, if the free edges of some or all of the aortic cusps adhere to the site of supravalvular stenosis, coronary artery inflow may be compromised. The left ventricle may have a "ballerina foot" configuration, which can result in muscular left ventricular outflow tract obstruction, particularly in association with significant supravalvular obstruction.

CLINICAL FEATURES. The clinical picture of supravalvular obstruction differs in major respects from that observed in the other forms of aortic stenosis. Chief among these differences is the association of supravalvular aortic stenosis with idiopathic infantile hypercalcemia, a disease that occurs in the first years of life and can be associated with deranged vitamin D metabolism.

Williams Syndrome

The designation *supravalvular aortic stenosis syndrome, Williams syndrome,* or *Williams-Beuren syndrome* has been applied to the distinctive picture produced by the coexistence of the cardiac features in the setting of a multisystem disorder. Beyond infancy in these patients, a challenge with vitamin D or calcium-loading tests unmasks abnormalities in the regulation of circulating 25-hydroxyvitamin D. Infants with Williams syndrome often exhibit feeding difficulties, failure to thrive, and gastrointestinal problems in the form of vomiting, constipation, and colic. The entire spectrum of clinical manifestations includes auditory hyperacusis,

inguinal hernia, hoarse voice, and a typical personality that is outgoing and engaging. Other manifestations of this syndrome include intellectual impairment, "elfin facies," narrowing of peripheral systemic and pulmonary arteries, strabismus, and abnormalities of dental development consisting of microdontia, enamel hypoplasia, and malocclusion.

Many medical conditions can complicate the course of Williams syndrome, including systemic hypertension, gastrointestinal problems, and urinary tract abnormalities. In an older child or adult, progressive joint limitation and hypertonia may become a problem. Adult patients are usually handicapped by their developmental disabilities.

Williams syndrome was previously considered to be nonfamilial; however, a number of families in which parent-to-child transmission of Williams syndrome has occurred have now been identified. All of these families show a parent and child to be affected with Williams syndrome, including one instance of male-to-male transmission. This supports autosomal dominant inheritance as the likely pattern, with most cases of Williams syndrome probably occurring as the result of a new mutation. New information indicates that a genetic defect for supravalvular aortic stenosis is located in the same chromosomal subunit as elastin on chromosome 7q11.23. Elastin is an important component of the arterial wall, but precisely how mutations in elastin genes cause the phenotypes of supravalvular aortic stenosis is not known.

FAMILIAL AUTOSOMAL DOMINANT PRESENTATION. On occasion, the aortic anomaly and peripheral pulmonary arterial stenosis are also found in familial and sporadic forms not associated with the other features of the syndrome. Affected patients have normal intelligence and are normal in facial appearance. Genetic studies suggest that when the anomaly is familial, it is transmitted as autosomal dominant with variable expression. Some family members may have peripheral pulmonary stenosis either as an isolated lesion or in combination with the supravalvular aortic anomaly.

CLINICAL FEATURES. Patients with Williams syndrome are intellectually challenged (**Fig. 65-36**). The typical appearance is similar to that of the elfin facies observed in the severe form of idiopathic infantile hypercalcemia and is characterized by a high prominent forehead, stellate or lacy iris patterns, epicanthal folds, underdeveloped bridge of the nose and mandible, overhanging upper lip, strabismus, and anomalies of dentition. Recognition of this distinctive appearance, even in infancy, should alert the physician to the possibility of underlying multisystem disease. In addition, a positive family history in a patient with a normal appearance and clinical signs suggesting left ventricular outflow obstruction should lead to the suspicion of either supravalvular aortic stenosis or hypertrophic obstructive cardiomyopathy.

Prior studies of the natural history of the principal vascular lesions in these patients—supravalvular aortic stenosis and peripheral pulmonary artery stenosis—indicate that the aortic lesion is usually progressive, with an increase in the intensity of obstruction related often to poor growth of the ascending aorta. This has recently been questioned in a longitudinal single-center study, in which those with smaller gradients at presentation appeared to have evidence of regression of their

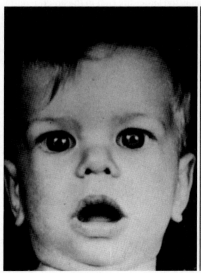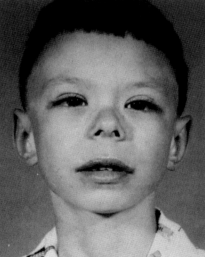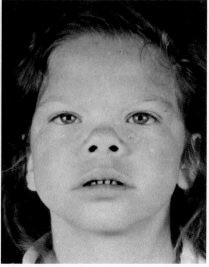

FIGURE 65-36 Typical elfin facies in three patients with supravalvular aortic stenosis. (*From Friedman WF, Kirkpatrick SE: Congenital aortic stenosis. In Adams FH, Emmanouilides GC, Riemenschneider TA, et al [eds]: Moss' Heart Disease in Infants, Children, and Adolescents. 4th ed. Baltimore, Williams & Wilkins, 1989.)*

stenosis.[94] Those with pulmonary branch stenosis, whether associated with the aortic lesion or not, tend to show no change or a reduction in right ventricular pressure with time.

With few exceptions, the major physical findings resemble those observed in patients with aortic valve stenosis. Among these exceptions are an accentuation of aortic valve closure due to elevated pressure in the aorta proximal to the stenosis, an absent ejection click, and the especially prominent transmission of a thrill and murmur into the jugular notch and along the carotid vessels. The narrowing of the peripheral pulmonary arteries may produce a late systolic or continuous murmur heard best in the lung fields and is usually accentuated by inspiration. Another hallmark of supravalvular aortic stenosis is that the systolic pressure in the right arm is usually higher than in the left arm. This pulse disparity may relate to the tendency of a jet stream to adhere to a vessel wall (Coanda effect) and selective streaming of blood into the innominate artery.

LABORATORY INVESTIGATIONS

ELECTROCARDIOGRAPHY. This usually reveals left ventricular hypertrophy when the obstruction is severe. Biventricular or even right ventricular hypertrophy may be found if there is significant narrowing of peripheral pulmonary arteries.

CHEST RADIOGRAPHY. In contrast to valvular and discrete subvalvular aortic stenosis, dilation of the ascending aorta is absent.

ECHOCARDIOGRAPHY. This is a valuable technique to localize the site of obstruction to the supravalvular area. Most often, the sinuses of Valsalva are dilated, and the ascending aorta and arch appear small or of normal size. The diameter of the aortic annulus is always greater than that of the sinotubular junction. Doppler examination determines the location of obstruction but usually overestimates the gradient compared with that obtained at cardiac catheterization. This results from the obstruction being lengthy, and the Doppler gradient is overestimated because of the phenomenon of pressure recovery.

ANGIOCARDIOGRAPHY. In most cases, this is necessary to define an accurate hemodynamic gradient across the left ventricular outflow tract as well as to determine the status of the coronary arteries. It also usually involves an assessment of the branch pulmonary arteries as well as the brachiocephalic, renal, and mesenteric arteries, all of which can be stenotic. Because of the nature of the anatomic defect, transcatheter balloon angioplasty, with or without stenting, is not an effective treatment option.

INTERVENTIONAL OPTIONS AND OUTCOMES. Surgical intervention for supravalvular aortic stenosis has been successful in most cases with good medium- and long-term results.[95] A variety of surgical procedures may be performed, all of which are tailored to the type of pathologic change. The use of a Y patch, resection with end-to-end anastomosis, and a Ross procedure are the main techniques employed. Additional procedures including coronary bypass of ostial stenosis, aortic valvuloplasty, and subaortic resection may be necessary in some cases.

The cardiac prognosis is good, with some patients requiring further surgery for recurrent supravalvular stenosis. As peripheral pulmonary artery stenosis tends to improve with time, there is a reluctance to attempt intervention, either surgical or by balloon angioplasty. Long-term behavioral and intellectual problems persist.

CONGENITAL MITRAL VALVE ANOMALIES
Congenital Mitral Stenosis

MORPHOLOGY. Anatomic types of mitral stenosis include the parachute deformity of the valve, in which shortened chordae tendineae converge and insert into a single large papillary muscle; thickened leaflets with shortening and fusion of the chordae tendineae; anomalous arcade of obstructing papillary muscles; accessory mitral valve tissue; and supravalvular circumferential ridge or "ring" of connective tissue arising at the base of the atrial aspect of the mitral leaflets. Associated cardiac defects are common and include endocardial fibroelastosis, coarctation of the aorta, PDA, and left ventricular outflow tract obstruction. An association between persistence of the left superior vena cava and obstructive left-sided lesions also exists.

CLINICAL FEATURES. In most cases, the findings are incidental at the time of evaluation of another left-sided obstructive lesion, such as coarctation of the aorta or aortic valve stenosis. The classic

auscultatory findings seen with rheumatic mitral valve stenosis are often absent in the congenital form. Typical findings include a normal S_1, a mid-diastolic murmur with or without some presystolic accentuation, and no opening snap.

LABORATORY INVESTIGATIONS

ELECTROCARDIOGRAPHY. In milder forms, this is usually normal, or there may be left atrial overload, with or without right ventricular hypertrophy due to associated pulmonary hypertension.

CHEST RADIOGRAPHY. This is normal in milder forms, with evidence of pulmonary edema in those cases with more severe obstruction.

ECHOCARDIOGRAPHY. Two-dimensional and more recently three-dimensional echocardiography, combined with Doppler studies, usually provides a complete analysis of the anatomy and function of congenital mitral stenosis. The status of the papillary muscles is best appreciated in the precordial short-axis view. If two papillary muscles are present, they are usually closer together than is seen in the normal heart. The precordial long-axis view permits identification of a supravalvular mitral ring as well as the degree of mobility of the valve leaflets. Color flow Doppler allows identification of the level of the obstruction as well as the presence of mitral valve regurgitation. Pulsed or continuous-wave Doppler provides an accurate assessment of the mean gradient across the mitral valve. The advantage of the pressure half-time lies in the fact that it is independent of cardiac output, unlike the mean gradient across the mitral valve. Because of the more rapid heart rates in children, the pressure half-time is of less value.

INTERVENTIONAL OPTIONS AND OUTCOMES. In asymptomatic cases, clinical and echocardiographic follow-up is all that is necessary. The presence of a single papillary muscle in itself does not predict progressive stenosis.[96] If the patient starts to develop pulmonary hypertension or symptoms, surgical intervention is usually indicated. Mitral valve balloon dilation is not as successful as it is in rheumatic mitral valve stenosis.[97] Surgery usually involves removal of a supramitral ring if it is present, splitting papillary muscles and fused chordal apparatus in those cases with more common forms of congenital mitral stenosis. In general, surgical intervention provides temporary relief, with many surgical cases requiring valve replacement later in life.

Congenital Mitral Regurgitation

MORPHOLOGY

ISOLATED CONGENITAL MITRAL VALVE REGURGITATION. This is usually either due to an isolated cleft of the anterior mitral valve leaflet or the result of leaflet dysplasia. In these cases, there is evidence of shortened chordae in conjunction with dysplastic valve leaflets. In those with an isolated mitral valve *cleft*, the deficiency in the anterior mitral leaflet points toward the left ventricular outflow tract, unlike those cases with an AV septal defect. In general, the larger the cleft in the anterior mitral leaflet, the greater the degree of regurgitation.

In cases with a *dysplastic* mitral valve, the chordal apparatus is shortened with varying degrees of dysplasia of the leaflets. Other anatomic lesions, such as mitral valve arcade resulting in regurgitation, are usually part of a more generalized abnormality of the left side of the heart.

Complex Congenital Mitral Valve Regurgitation

This is seen more frequently in association with abnormalities of the ventriculoarterial connection, such as double-outlet right ventricle, transposition and VSD, and corrected transposition. In the first two, it is frequent to have a cleft in the anterior mitral valve leaflet with some chordal support apparatus that renders the valve less regurgitant than in those cases with an isolated cleft. In cc-TGA, the morphologic mitral valve may have an associated cleft, be dysplastic, or have multiple papillary muscles, all of which increase the tendency for it to be regurgitant.

CLINICAL FEATURES. The presence of symptoms relates to the severity of the regurgitation in cases in which the pathologic change is isolated to the valve. Exercise intolerance, combined with a pansystolic murmur at the apex, with or without a mid-diastolic murmur, is the cardinal clinical feature.

LABORATORY INVESTIGATIONS

ELECTROCARDIOGRAPHY. This is either normal or demonstrates left atrial and left ventricular hypertrophy.

CHEST RADIOGRAPHY. This demonstrates cardiomegaly predominantly involving the left ventricle and atrium.

ECHOCARDIOGRAPHY. Doppler and two-dimensional echocardiography provide an accurate evaluation of the mechanisms and degree of valvular regurgitation. The cleft in the anterior mitral valve leaflet is best seen in the precordial short-axis view, pointing toward the left ventricular outflow tract. Patients with a dysplastic mitral valve lack mobility of the valve leaflets and have shortened chordae. Color Doppler interrogation helps in locating the site of regurgitation. The severity of regurgitation is assessed in the standard fashion. Three-dimensional echocardiography permits a comprehensive evaluation of the mechanisms of regurgitation, with additional information being obtained about commissural length, leaflet area, and sites of regurgitation from color flow Doppler.[98]

ANGIOCARDIOGRAPHY AND MRI. These procedures are seldom helpful in management planning.

INTERVENTIONAL OPTIONS AND OUTCOMES. This depends on the severity of regurgitation and its impact on left ventricular function. Surgery should not be delayed until the patients become symptomatic. Surgery involves suture of an isolated cleft, with or without associated commissuroplasties. In those cases with a dysplastic mitral valve, leaflet extension in conjunction with an annuloplasty and commissuroplasty usually results in effective control of the regurgitation in the short and medium term.[99,100] Despite this, many of these patients require a mitral valve replacement at some stage in the future. Attempted surgical repair, rather than replacement, is important in the pediatric age group because it permits temporary relief that allows the child to grow, such that future surgery can be done into a larger mitral annulus. When it is required, mitral valve replacement has had a good short- and medium-term outcome in cases in which repair is not possible.

RIGHT VENTRICULAR OUTFLOW TRACT LESIONS

Peripheral Pulmonary Artery Stenosis (Fig. 65-37)

Right ventricular outflow tract is a term that applies to patients with both peripheral pulmonary artery stenosis and an intact ventricular septum. It excludes those with an associated VSD, which is dealt with in the sections on tetralogy of Fallot and pulmonary atresia with a VSD. Also excluded is Noonan syndrome, which is dealt with in the subsequent section on pulmonary valve stenosis.

ETIOLOGY

RUBELLA SYNDROME. The most important cause of significant pulmonary artery stenoses producing symptoms in newborns used to be intrauterine rubella infection. Other cardiovascular malformations commonly found in association with congenital rubella include PDA, pulmonary

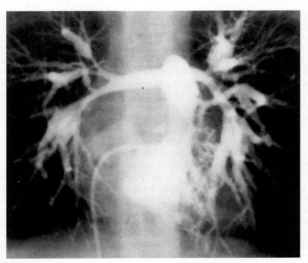

FIGURE 65-37 Right ventricular angiocardiogram showing numerous sites of peripheral pulmonic stenosis and poststenotic dilation of the peripheral pulmonic arteries.

valve stenosis, and ASD. Generalized systemic arterial stenotic lesions also may be a feature of the rubella embryopathy, which may involve large and medium-sized vessels such as the aorta and coronary, cerebral, mesenteric, and renal arteries. Cardiovascular lesions are but one manifestation of intrauterine rubella infection because cataracts, microphthalmia, deafness, thrombocytopenia, hepatitis, and blood dyscrasias are also common. The clinical picture in infants with rubella syndrome depends on the severity of the cardiovascular lesions and the associated abnormalities.

WILLIAMS SYNDROME. Peripheral pulmonary artery stenosis is also associated with supravalvular aortic stenosis in patients with Williams syndrome, which is discussed in the section on supravalvular aortic stenosis.

ALAGILLE SYNDROME. Peripheral pulmonary artery stenosis is a component of this syndrome, with some cases having a *JAG1* mutation.

ISOLATED BRANCH PULMONARY ARTERY STENOSIS. This is encountered mainly in the proximal left pulmonary artery and is invariably related to a sling of ductal tissue that causes stenosis when the ductus arteriosus closes after birth. In most cases, this is fairly mild, but a significant obstruction resulting in failure of distal growth of the left pulmonary artery may also be seen.

MORPHOLOGY. Apart from the isolated form mentioned earlier, the stenoses are usually diffuse and bilateral and extend into the mediastinal, hilar, and intraparenchymal pulmonary arteries.

CLINICAL FEATURES. The degree of obstruction is the principal determinant of clinical severity. The type of obstruction determines the feasibility of intervention. Most patients are asymptomatic. An ejection systolic murmur heard at the upper left sternal border and well transmitted to the axilla and back is most common. No pulmonary ejection click is heard. The pulmonic component of the second heart sound may be accentuated and is loud only if there is proximal pulmonary hypertension. A continuous murmur is often audible in patients with significant branch stenosis. The murmurs in the lung fields are typically increased by inspiration.

LABORATORY INVESTIGATIONS

ELECTROCARDIOGRAPHY. Right ventricular hypertrophy is seen when obstruction is severe. Left-axis deviation with counterclockwise orientation of the frontal QRS vector is common in rubella syndrome and when there is also supravalvular aortic stenosis.

CHEST RADIOGRAPHY. Mild or moderate stenosis usually produces normal findings. Detectable differences in vascularity between regions of the lungs or dilated pulmonary artery segments are uncommon. When obstruction is bilateral and severe, right atrial and ventricular enlargement may be seen.

ECHOCARDIOGRAPHY. Echocardiography is helpful in making the diagnosis and excluding associated lesions; however, it is limited in its ability to image the distal pulmonary arteries beyond the hilum of the lung. Right ventricular pressure assessment may be predicted if there is associated tricuspid valve regurgitation.

CMR AND SPIRAL CT. These are valuable diagnostic tests because they permit a more distal evaluation of the branch pulmonary arteries. The advantage of spiral CT in young children is that it can be performed without the need for heavy sedation or even general anesthesia. Although most patients require cardiac catheterization and angiography, these other techniques are excellent for the initial evaluation and for following the progress of the lesions.

RADIONUCLIDE QUANTITATIVE LUNG PERFUSION SCAN. This is valuable in cases with unilateral stenosis to determine whether intervention is necessary. Similar flow estimates can now be obtained by CMR.

CARDIAC CATHETERIZATION AND ANGIOCARDIOGRAPHY. This permits the assessment of right ventricular pressure and the pressures in the pulmonary arterial tree. Angiocardiography is the key to precise assessment of the extent and severity of the stenoses.

INTERVENTIONAL OPTIONS AND OUTCOMES. For those cases with isolated left pulmonary artery stenosis in which there is less than 30% of flow to the lung, balloon dilation with or without stent insertion is effective in relieving the obstruction. In those cases with more diffuse bilateral stenoses, the indications for intervention depend on the right ventricular pressure. As the natural history of diffuse peripheral pulmonary artery stenosis in Williams syndrome is one of potential regression over time, intervention is in general reserved for those cases with systemic or suprasystemic right ventricular pressure. Intervention also depends in part on the extent of the stenosis and the dilation capability of the lesions, with or without stenting. In some cases, several attempts at dilation are required to achieve any improvement in vessel caliber. High-pressure balloons are usually necessary, but some lesions cannot be dilated even with such balloons. Recently, improved results have been reported with use of "cutting" balloons, which may assist dilation in an otherwise

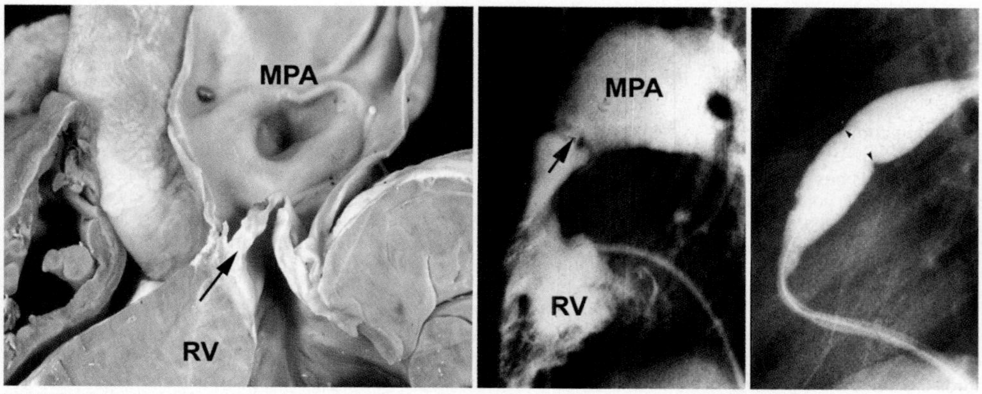

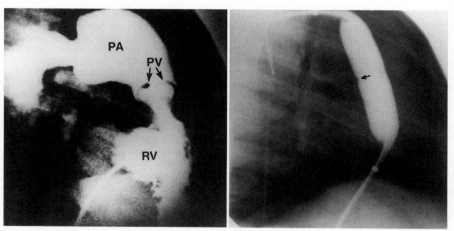

FIGURE 65-38 Montage of pulmonary valve stenosis demonstrating typical pathology (**left,** arrow) with a thickened pulmonary valve and obstruction due to commissural fusion. Note the poststenotic dilation. The angiogram demonstrates a case before (**middle,** arrow) and during (**right**) balloon dilation. MPA = main pulmonary artery; RV = right ventricle.

FIGURE 65-39   Left, Right ventriculogram (RV) in the lateral projection from a patient with valvular pulmonic stenosis. The pulmonary valve (PV) is thickened and domes in systole (arrows). Poststenotic dilation of the pulmonary artery (PA) is seen. **Right,** Successful balloon valvuloplasty shows almost complete disappearance of the stenotic waist (arrow). *(Courtesy of Dr. Thomas G. DiSessa.)*

undilatable stenosis. As a rule, surgery has little to offer those patients with diffuse peripheral pulmonary artery stenoses and can indeed make the situation worse.

Supravalvular Right Ventricular Outflow Tract Obstruction

Supravalvular right ventricular outflow tract obstruction seldom occurs in isolation. It can occur in tetralogy of Fallot, Williams syndrome, Noonan syndrome, VSD, or arteriohepatic dysplasia (Alagille syndrome). Supravalvular right ventricular outflow tract obstruction can progress in severity and should be monitored. Dilation of the pulmonary trunk is not a feature of subvalvular and supravalvular right ventricular outflow tract obstruction. Intervention is recommended when the peak gradient across the right ventricular outflow tract is more than 50 mm Hg at rest or when the patient is symptomatic.

Pulmonary Stenosis with Intact Ventricular Septum (Figs. 65-38 and 65-39)

This lesion exists as a continuum, ranging from isolated valvular stenosis to complete atresia of the pulmonary outflow tract. Two modes of presentation exist. The first is manifested in the neonatal period, usually with associated disease of the tricuspid valve, right ventricle, or coronary arteries. The second mode of presentation is beyond the neonatal period, when the valvular stenosis is usually isolated. Some cases with severe stenosis diagnosed in utero can present with valvular atresia at the time of birth.

MORPHOLOGY. The pulmonary valve may vary from a well-formed trileaflet valve with varying degrees of commissural fusion to an imperforate membrane. If stenosis is present, the right ventricle is usually of normal size or only mildly hypoplastic. Patients with an imperforate valve and a patent infundibulum invariably have a larger right ventricular

volume than do patients with both infundibular and valve atresia.

CLINICAL FEATURES

NEONATE WITH CRITICAL PULMONARY VALVE STENOSIS. The neonate presents with central cyanosis due to right-to-left shunting at the atrial level and depends on a prostaglandin infusion to maintain the patency of the ductus arteriosus. Auscultatory findings include a single second heart sound, no ejection click, and a murmur that, when present, is due to tricuspid valve regurgitation.

INFANT AND CHILD. In cases beyond the newborn period, the referral is usually for the assessment of a cardiac murmur. This may be detected within the first few weeks of life, more commonly at the routine 6-week postnatal visit or later. These patients usually have an ejection click and a second heart sound that moves with respiration but with a soft pulmonary component. An ejection murmur of varying intensity and duration is heard best in the pulmonary area.

ADULT. Adults with isolated mild to moderate right ventricular outflow tract obstruction of any type usually have no symptoms. Patients with severe right ventricular outflow tract obstruction may present with exertional fatigue, dyspnea, lightheadedness, and chest discomfort (right ventricular angina). Physical examination may reveal a prominent jugular *a* wave, a right ventricular lift, and possibly a thrill in the second left intercostal space. Auscultation reveals a normal S_1, a single or split S_2 with a diminished P_2 (unless the obstruction is supravalvular, in which case the intensity of the P_2 is normal or increased), and a systolic ejection murmur best heard in the second left intercostal space. When the pulmonary valve is thin and pliable, a systolic ejection click will be heard, which decreases on inspiration. As the severity of the pulmonary stenosis progresses, the interval between S_1 and the systolic ejection click becomes shorter, S_2 becomes widely split, P_2 diminishes or disappears, and the systolic ejection murmur lengthens and peaks later in systole, often extending beyond A_2. An ejection click seldom occurs with dysplastic pulmonary stenosis. Cyanosis may be present when a PFO or ASD permits right-to-left shunting.

Adult patients with trivial and mild valvular right ventricular outflow tract obstruction do not become worse with time. Moderate valvular right ventricular outflow tract obstruction can progress in 20% of unrepaired patients, especially in adults because of calcification of the valve, and may require intervention. Some of these patients can also become symptomatic, particularly in later life, because of atrial arrhythmias resulting from right atrial pressure overload and tricuspid regurgitation. Patients with severe valvular right ventricular outflow tract obstruction will have had balloon or surgical valvotomy to survive to adult life. Long-term survival in patients with repaired pulmonary valve stenosis is similar to that of the general population, with good to excellent functional class at long-term follow-up in most patients. A few patients have severe pulmonary regurgitation.

LABORATORY INVESTIGATIONS

ELECTROCARDIOGRAPHY. In the newborn period, this may show left-axis deviation and left ventricular dominance in cases with significant right ventricular hypoplasia. Other patients may have a normal QRS axis. Right atrial overload is present in those with increased right atrial pressure. In the infant, child, and adult, the findings depend on the severity of the stenosis. In milder cases, the ECG should be normal. As the stenosis progresses, evidence of right ventricular hypertrophy appears. Severe stenosis is seen in the form of a tall R wave in lead V_4R or V_1 with a deep S wave in V_6. A tall QR wave in the right precordial leads with T wave inversion and ST-segment depression (right ventricular "strain") reflects severe stenosis. When an rSR′ pattern is observed in lead V_1 (20% of patients), lower right ventricular pressures are found than in patients with a pure R wave of equal amplitude. Right atrial overload is associated with moderate to severe pulmonary stenosis.

CHEST RADIOGRAPHY. In the neonate, this demonstrates pulmonary oligemia with a prominent right-sided heart border in those with associated tricuspid valve regurgitation. In the infant, child, and adult with mild or moderate pulmonary stenosis, chest radiography often shows a heart of normal size and normal pulmonary vascularity. Poststenotic dilation of the main and left pulmonary arteries is often seen. Right atrial and right ventricular enlargement is observed in patients with severe obstruction and right ventricular failure. The pulmonary vascularity is usually normal in the absence of a right-to-left atrial shunt but may be reduced in patients with severe stenosis and right ventricular failure.

ECHOCARDIOGRAPHY. Combined two-dimensional echocardiographic and continuous-wave Doppler examination characterizes the anatomic valve abnormality and its severity and has essentially eliminated the requirement for diagnostic cardiac catheterization. Although maximum instantaneous gradients have traditionally been used to select patients for balloon valvuloplasty, recent data would suggest the contrary. Mean Doppler gradients appear to correlate better with catheter-derived peak-peak gradients, with a value of 50 mm Hg being the cut point for intervention.[101] Invasive studies are currently used for balloon valvuloplasty.

Right ventricular size is currently best assessed indirectly from the tricuspid annular dimension. In the absence of a VSD, there is an excellent correlation between the two. Right ventricular pressure can be assessed indirectly from the tricuspid regurgitation gradient. Tricuspid valve morphology and function and the status of the interatrial septum need to be addressed.

INTERVENTIONAL OPTIONS AND OUTCOMES

NEONATE. In the neonate, prostaglandin E$_1$ is instituted in cases with ductal dependency. After this, balloon dilation is performed in those with stenosis, whereas radiofrequency perforation in conjunction with dilation may be undertaken in those with pulmonary valve atresia. If relief of the obstruction is successful, the prostaglandins are slowly discontinued to determine if the right ventricle is large enough to support the circulation. If not, a systemic to pulmonary artery shunt is necessary early in the management. In cases with a normal-sized right ventricle, no further therapy is usually necessary in the future because there is a low recurrence rate of stenosis. Newborns with isolated pulmonary stenosis do well after relief of the stenosis.[102]

INFANT AND OLDER CHILD. Balloon dilation of the pulmonary valve is the therapeutic procedure of choice with excellent short- and medium-term results.

ADULTS. Balloon valvuloplasty is recommended when the gradient across the right ventricular outflow tract is greater than 50 mm Hg at rest[2] or when the patient is symptomatic.

Despite the excellent survival results from the second natural history study (survival after surgical valvotomy of 95.7% compared with sex-matched controls of 96.6%), recent long-term data suggest that this population of patients faces ongoing challenges. After a mean follow-up period of 33 years, 53% of patients had required further intervention and 38% had either atrial or ventricular arrhythmias.[103]

Dysplastic Pulmonary Valve Stenosis

MORPHOLOGY. In pulmonary valve stenosis due to valvular dysplasia, the obstruction is caused not by commissural fusion but by a combination of thickened and dysplastic pulmonary valve leaflets in combination with varying degrees of supravalvular pulmonary stenosis. The supravalvular stenosis is classically at the distal part of pulmonary valve sinuses, and there is usually no poststenotic pulmonary artery dilation. This entity is associated with Noonan syndrome, which in turn may be associated with hypertrophic cardiomyopathy.

CLINICAL FEATURES. In most cases, the diagnosis is made either during an evaluation of a systolic murmur or in a child with dysmorphic features who is undergoing clinical evaluation. Children with Noonan syndrome have short stature, webbed necks, and broad-shaped chests in a fashion similar to Turner syndrome. Although this syndrome does not have an associated chromosomal abnormality, it may be familial and affects both sexes equally. A unique association in the newborn is pulmonary lymphangiectasia. The auscultatory finding that differentiates dysplastic valves from simple pulmonary valve stenosis is the lack of an ejection click. The other features of the murmur are similar to those described in pulmonary valve stenosis.

LABORATORY INVESTIGATIONS

ELECTROCARDIOGRAPHY. The ECG is helpful in that patients with dysplastic pulmonary stenosis frequently have a leftward QRS axis, particularly in association with hypertrophic cardiomyopathy. The remainder of the ECG is similar to that seen in pulmonary valve stenosis.

CHEST RADIOGRAPHY. The findings are similar to typical pulmonary valve stenosis, apart from the lack of poststenotic pulmonary trunk dilation,

even in the presence of severe obstruction. In those with pulmonary lymphangiectasia, the chest radiograph has a ground-glass appearance, which can be difficult to differentiate from pulmonary venous obstruction.

ECHOCARDIOGRAPHY. This demonstrates a thickened fleshy pulmonary valve, lack of poststenotic dilation, and varying degrees of supravalvular pulmonary stenosis. The associated diagnosis of hypertrophic cardiomyopathy can be confirmed or excluded. If the initial echocardiogram does not demonstrate hypertrophic cardiomyopathy, further studies should be performed throughout childhood and adolescence, particularly in cases with left-axis deviation.

INTERVENTIONAL OPTIONS AND OUTCOMES

CARDIAC CATHETERIZATION AND ANGIOGRAPHY. Although the results of balloon valvuloplasty are less rewarding than in those with stenosis due to commissural fusion, it is worth attempting this before considering surgical intervention. Success has been varied, with many cases having some reduction in gradient that can delay surgery.

SURGICAL INTERVENTION. If balloon valvuloplasty fails, surgical intervention is indicated. This usually involves a partial valvectomy in conjunction with patch repair of the supravalvular stenosis.

OUTCOMES. Adequate relief of the right ventricular outflow tract obstruction results in an excellent outlook. The greatest long-term risk factor is the presence of hypertrophic cardiomyopathy.

Subpulmonary Right Ventricular Outflow Tract Obstruction (Anomalous Muscle Bundles or a Double-Chambered Right Ventricle)

MORPHOLOGY. A double-chambered right ventricle is formed by right ventricular obstruction due to anomalous muscle bundles. Although this can occur in isolation, it is more frequently part of a combination of lesions that includes right ventricular muscle bundles, a perimembranous-outlet VSD, and subaortic stenosis with or without aortic valve prolapse.

CLINICAL FEATURES. Most cases are discovered incidentally during the evaluation of a VSD. In some cases, there may be only an ejection systolic murmur. If the obstruction is isolated, there is an ejection systolic murmur that is heard best in the upper left sternal border. If the VSD is the predominant lesion, the right ventricular outflow tract murmur may not be appreciated. Before the routine use of echocardiography, the diagnosis was often made during follow-up for a VSD when the pansystolic murmur decreased in intensity and a systolic ejection murmur emerged. The patients are usually pink unless there is progression of the subpulmonary stenosis in the setting of a VSD. The diagnosis may be more problematic in adults.

LABORATORY INVESTIGATIONS

ELECTROCARDIOGRAPHY. The ECG is similar to that of those with isolated pulmonary valve stenosis beyond the newborn period. In cases with a nonrestrictive VSD and mild subpulmonary stenosis, the ECG typically shows biventricular hypertrophy due to a left-to-right shunt and associated pulmonary hypertension. If the stenosis is more severe, right ventricular hypertrophy will be seen. Those with a restrictive VSD may have a normal ECG or left ventricular hypertrophy, which is replaced with right ventricular hypertrophy if the subpulmonary stenosis increases in severity.

CHEST RADIOGRAPHY. This is usually normal in those with isolated subpulmonary stenosis, whereas those with a VSD may have either increased or reduced pulmonary blood flow, depending on the severity of the obstruction.

ECHOCARDIOGRAPHY. Doppler and two-dimensional echocardiography usually provide a complete diagnosis. The level of subpulmonary obstruction is appreciated best in a combination of subcostal right anterior oblique and precordial short-axis views. These views permit the identification of the relationship of the VSD to the muscle bundles as well as the degree of anterior malalignment of the infundibular septum in those with a VSD. The precordial short-axis view is the best position to evaluate the presence of possible subaortic stenosis and aortic cusp prolapse. Color and pulsed or continuous-wave Doppler evaluation usually allows differentiation of the VSD flow jet from that originating from the muscle bundles. This permits an accurate assessment of the hemodynamic effect of the subpulmonary obstruction.

CARDIAC CATHETERIZATION AND ANGIOCARDIOGRAPHY. This technique is rarely necessary. In older patients in whom the echocardiographic images of the subpulmonary region may be suboptimal, a combination of magnetic resonance angiography and echocardiography is all that is generally necessary.

MANAGEMENT OPTIONS AND OUTCOMES. Management is dictated by the severity of the subpulmonary stenosis and the presence of associated defects. In patients with isolated subpulmonary stenosis, surgery is indicated when the right ventricular pressure is more than 60% of systemic. This involves resection of the muscle bundles through the right atrium. For those cases with an associated VSD, the decision is based on the size of the VSD, the degree of associated subaortic stenosis, the presence of aortic valve prolapse, and the severity of the subpulmonary stenosis. These patients tend to have a progressive disease, so many cases that are followed up conservatively for several years will eventually require surgery. In general, the outcome is excellent with a low rate of recurrence after surgical resection of obstructive muscle bundles. Infrequently, recurrence of the subaortic obstruction may occur.

Miscellaneous Lesions

Cor Triatriatum

MORPHOLOGY. In this malformation, failure of resorption of the common pulmonary vein results in a left atrium divided by an abnormal fibromuscular diaphragm into a posterosuperior chamber receiving the pulmonary veins and an anteroinferior chamber giving rise to the left atrial appendage and leading to the mitral orifice. The communication between the divided atrial chambers may be large, small, or absent, depending on the size of the opening in the diaphragm, which determines the degree of obstruction to pulmonary venous return. Elevations of both pulmonary venous pressure and pulmonary vascular resistance may result in severe pulmonary artery hypertension.

CLINICAL FEATURES. Cor triatriatum may be detected as an incidental finding in a patient who has echocardiography for another reason. In general, this represents the unobstructed form that requires no early intervention. Cases with more severe obstruction present in a fashion similar to patients with congenital pulmonary vein stenosis.

LABORATORY INVESTIGATIONS

ELECTROCARDIOGRAPHY. In unobstructed cases, this is normal. In those with significant obstruction, there is right ventricular hypertrophy due to the associated pulmonary hypertension.

CHEST RADIOGRAPHY. This may be normal in those with mild obstruction or who demonstrate pulmonary edema in those with significant obstruction.

ECHOCARDIOGRAPHY. The diagnosis is established by two-dimensional echocardiography or TEE, with further insight from three-dimensional reconstruction. The obstructive diaphragm is visualized in the parasternal long- and short-axis and four-chamber views and can be distinguished from a supravalvular mitral ring by its position superior to the left atrial appendage, which forms part of the distal chamber. Also present is diastolic fluttering of the mitral leaflets and high-velocity flow detected by Doppler examination in the distal atrial chamber and at the mitral orifice.

CARDIAC CATHETERIZATION AND ANGIOCARDIOGRAPHY. This technique is usually unnecessary since the advent of echocardiography and CMR.

MANAGEMENT OPTIONS AND OUTCOMES. Surgical resection of the membrane is the treatment of choice for patients with significant obstruction. This results in symptom relief and a reduction of pulmonary artery pressure. In general, the outcome after surgery is good. With the advent of more routine echocardiography, a subset of cases with typical but nonobstructive forms has been recognized. Thus far, these cases appear to remain asymptomatic, with an infrequent need for surgical intervention.

Pulmonary Vein Stenosis

Congenital pulmonary vein stenosis may occur as a focal stenosis at the atrial junction or generalized hypoplasia of one or more pulmonary veins. The incidence of associated cardiac malformations, including VSD, ASD, tetralogy of Fallot, tricuspid and mitral atresia, and AV septal defect, is extremely high. In other cases, the pulmonary vein stenosis is acquired after surgical intervention for total anomalous pulmonary venous connection. Children frequently present with recurrent respiratory infections, whereas adults exhibit exercise intolerance. Pulmonary hypertension is one of the consequences of pulmonary vein stenosis, whether it is congenital or acquired. In cases with unilateral pulmonary vein stenosis, clinical symptoms are frequently absent because there is pulmonary blood flow redistribution away from the affected lung.

LABORATORY INVESTIGATIONS

ELECTROCARDIOGRAPHY. The ECG is usually normal unless there is evidence of pulmonary hypertension, in which case right ventricular hypertrophy may be seen.

CHEST RADIOGRAPHY. With unilateral pulmonary vein stenosis, there is oligemia of the affected lung and increased flow to the contralateral side. If the obstruction is bilateral, pulmonary edema is seen.

ECHOCARDIOGRAPHY. This can usually exclude or confirm the diagnosis of pulmonary vein stenosis. Assessment of pulmonary artery pressure

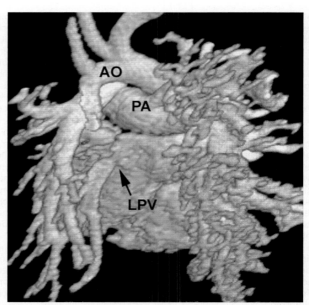

FIGURE 65-40 Three-dimensional CMR demonstrating stenosis of the left lower lobe pulmonary vein. AO = aorta; LPV = left pulmonary vein; PA = pulmonary artery.

from tricuspid or pulmonary valve regurgitation is possible. Doppler color flow assessment of the right- and left-sided pulmonary veins is the best screening tool. If there is evidence of turbulence or aliasing in the color flow pattern, spectral analysis with pulsed Doppler will help confirm the diagnosis. Usually, pulmonary venous flow is low velocity and phasic. If the pattern is high velocity and turbulent, there is disturbed pulmonary venous flow. Absolute Doppler gradients may or may not be helpful for two reasons. First, the absolute velocity depends on the amount of pulmonary blood flow to that segment of lung. Second, it is often difficult to obtain a parallel line of interrogation of the pulmonary veins that will affect gradient assessment. The absolute velocity is less important than the diagnosis of pulmonary vein stenosis and its effect on pulmonary artery pressure.

CMR (**Fig. 65-40**). This technique has now become the gold standard for the diagnosis of pulmonary vein stenosis. This permits a detailed assessment of the pulmonary veins. Velocity assessment is now possible, although this is in the actual veins themselves rather than at the venoatrial junction, which is the site assessed by Doppler echocardiography.

CARDIAC CATHETERIZATION AND ANGIOGRAPHY. In general, a combination of echocardiography and CMR makes invasive procedures unnecessary.

MANAGEMENT OPTIONS AND OUTCOMES. If the patient has unilateral pulmonary vein stenosis and normal pulmonary artery pressure, no treatment may be necessary. Continued follow-up is important because this is often a progressive disease that can subsequently affect both sides. In cases with bilateral stenoses, the outlook in the past was believed to be hopeless, with virtually 100% mortality. Stents usually provided only temporary relief. More recently, a pericardial reflection procedure using native tissue has resulted in some early success in this lesion. This involves use of native atrial tissue to form a pocket around the surgically resected stenotic region.

Partial Anomalous Pulmonary Venous Connection

MORPHOLOGY. This refers to conditions in which part or all of one lung drains to a site other than the left atrium. Sinus venosus defects are associated with PAPVC typically from the right upper and middle lobe pulmonary veins to the superior vena cava. PAPVC may be directed to a left vertical vein, to the superior vena cava at the level of or above the right pulmonary artery, to the azygos vein, or to the coronary sinus. PAPVC to the inferior vena cava (scimitar syndrome) may have associated hypoplasia of the right lung, pulmonary sequestration, and abnormal collateral supply to the sequestered segment. It can be seen in some patients (<10%) with a secundum ASD as well as in association with many other forms of CHD. PAPVC to the right atrium has the pulmonary veins lying in the normal position; however, there is deviation of the septum primum to the left with absence of the septum secundum. This type of lesion is seen more frequently in hearts with visceral heterotaxy.

CLINICAL FEATURES. In the absence of associated anomalies, the physiologic disturbance is determined by the number of anomalous veins and their site of connection, the presence and size of an ASD, and the state of the pulmonary vascular bed. In the usual patient with isolated partial pulmonary venous connection, the hemodynamic state and physical findings are similar to those in ASD.

LABORATORY INVESTIGATIONS

ELECTROCARDIOGRAPHY. In isolated cases, findings similar to a secundum ASD may be seen.

CHEST RADIOGRAPHY. Isolated cases show cardiomegaly involving the right ventricle with increased pulmonary vascular markings. In scimitar syndrome, there is typically right lung hypoplasia, with a secondary shift of the heart into the right thorax and a right-sided scimitar sign that represents the anomalous pulmonary vein.

ECHOCARDIOGRAPHY. If there is a significant left-to-right shunt, there is right ventricular volume overload with paradoxical interventricular septal motion. A dilated coronary sinus is seen in PAPVC to the coronary sinus. In scimitar syndrome, the abnormal pulmonary vein can be seen from the subcostal position during evaluation of the inferior vena cava. Associated stenosis of the pulmonary vein may exist. The suprasternal position permits identification of a left vertical vein, and in general it is possible in children to identify the number of connecting veins on that side. Abnormal venous drainage to the right superior vena cava may be more difficult to identify unless a systematic approach is undertaken. The suprasternal frontal plane view allows the identification of veins that connect just above the right pulmonary artery. Those that connect just behind the right pulmonary artery, into either the superior vena cava or the azygos, can be identified with a right anterior oblique view of the superior vena cava, whether from the subcostal position or a high right parasternal location. In adults, TEE may also be useful in detecting PAPVC.

CMR. Although TEE can be used with a considerable degree of accuracy in older patients with a poorer ultrasound window, it is less invasive to obtain the data by CMR. This provides superb images of the connecting veins that can be seen more distally to their connections with the hilum of the lung. The pulmonary-to-systemic flow ratio can be calculated, obviating the need for hemodynamic evaluation. The pulmonary-to-systemic flow ratio can also be calculated by radionuclide techniques.

MANAGEMENT OPTIONS. In cases with a volume-loaded right ventricle, surgical intervention should be considered. Surgery is not necessary when a single anomalously draining vein has not produced right ventricular volume loading. Surgery is typically performed at a time similar to an ASD repair, at approximately 3 to 5 years of age. The type of surgery depends on the location of the drainage but in general consists of reconnection of the abnormal veins to the left atrium, either directly in the case of a left vertical vein or by a baffle in most other instances. In scimitar syndrome, occlusion of the collateral arteries as well as redirection of the pulmonary veins may be necessary.

OUTCOMES. In general, patients with repaired PAPVC have a good outcome similar to that of patients with an isolated ASD. What is unclear is the exact patency rate of the veins that are reconnected or baffled back to the left atrium. Patients with scimitar syndrome fare well if the lesion is relatively isolated but do poorly if there is significant associated intracardiac disease.

Pulmonary Arteriovenous Fistula

Abnormal development of the pulmonary arteries and veins in a common vascular complex is responsible for this congenital anomaly. A variable number of pulmonary arteries communicate directly with branches of the pulmonary veins. Most patients have an associated Weber-Osler-Rendu syndrome; associated problems include bronchiectasis and other malformations of the bronchial tree as well as absence of the right lower lobe. Pulmonary arteriovenous fistulas may also complicate classic Glenn shunts used in the palliation of cyanotic CHD and are believed to be due to the absence of "hepatic factor" in the venous blood feeding the superior vena cava–pulmonary artery connection. Hepatopulmonary syndrome may also be associated with substantial right-to-left intrapulmonary shunting.[62] The amount of right-to-left shunting depends on the extent of the fistulous communications and may result in cyanosis. Paradoxical emboli or a brain abscess may result and cause major neurologic deficits. Patients with hereditary hemorrhagic telangiectasia are often anemic because of repeated blood loss and may have less obvious cyanosis because of anemia. Systolic and continuous murmurs may be audible over areas of the fistula. Rounded opacities of various sizes in one or both lungs on chest radiography may suggest the presence of the lesion.

LABORATORY INVESTIGATIONS. Echocardiography is helpful in the initial diagnostic process with the use of a saline contrast injection into a systemic vein. With pulmonary arteriovenous malformations, there is early pulmonary venous return to the left atrium, but not as quickly as

for patients with a PFO or ASD and right-to-left atrial shunting. More recently, CT and CMR techniques have provided valuable diagnostic information. Pulmonary angiography reveals the site and extent of the abnormal communication.

MANAGEMENT OPTIONS. Unless the lesions are widespread throughout both lungs, surgical treatment aimed at removal of the lesions with preservation of healthy lung tissue is commonly indicated to avoid the complications of massive hemorrhage, bacterial endocarditis, and rupture of arteriovenous aneurysms. Transcatheter balloon or plug or coil occlusion embolotherapy may prove to be the therapeutic procedure of choice in some patients.

Coronary Arteriovenous Fistula

MORPHOLOGY. A coronary arteriovenous fistula is a communication between one of the coronary arteries and a cardiac chamber or vein. The right coronary artery (or its branches) is the site of the fistula in about 55% of patients; the left coronary artery is involved in about 35%; and both coronary arteries are involved in a few. Connections between the coronary system and a cardiac chamber appear to represent persistence of embryonic intertrabecular spaces and sinusoids. Most of these fistulas drain into the right ventricle, the right atrium, or the coronary sinus. Coronary to pulmonary artery fistulas are an occasional and usually incidental finding in the adult coronary angiography suite.

CLINICAL FEATURES. The shunt through the fistula is usually small, and myocardial blood flow is not compromised. Potential complications include pulmonary hypertension and congestive heart failure if a large left-to-right shunt exists, bacterial endocarditis, rupture or thrombosis of the fistula or of an associated arterial aneurysm, and myocardial ischemia distal to the fistula due to a "myocardial steal."

Most pediatric patients are asymptomatic and are referred because of a cardiac murmur that is loud, superficial, and continuous at the lower or midsternal border. The site of maximal intensity of the murmur is related to the site of drainage and is usually away from the second left intercostal space, the classic site of the continuous murmur of persistent ductus arteriosus.

LABORATORY INVESTIGATIONS

ELECTROCARDIOGRAPHY. This is usually normal unless there is a large left-to-right shunt.

CHEST RADIOGRAPHY. Radiographic findings are often normal and seldom show selective chamber enlargement.

ECHOCARDIOGRAPHY. Coronary artery fistulas are now recognized with a high degree of accuracy with the advent of routine coronary artery evaluation during most pediatric echocardiography examinations. A significantly enlarged feeding coronary artery can be detected, and the entire course and site of entry of the arteriovenous fistula can be traced by Doppler color flow mapping. The shunt entry site is characterized by a continuous turbulent systolic and diastolic flow pattern. Multiplane TEE also accurately defines the origin, course, and drainage site of the fistula.

CARDIAC CATHETERIZATION AND ANGIOCARDIOGRAPHY. If echocardiography demonstrates a significant coronary artery fistula, hemodynamic evaluation is warranted. Standard retrograde thoracic aortography, balloon occlusion angiography of the aortic root with a 45-degree caudal tilt of the frontal camera ("laid-back" aortogram), or coronary arteriography can be used reliably to identify the size and anatomic features of the fistulous track.

MANAGEMENT OPTIONS AND OUTCOMES. Small fistulas have an excellent long-term prognosis. Untreated larger fistulas may predispose the individual to premature coronary artery disease in the affected vessel. Coil embolization at the time of cardiac catheterization is rapidly becoming the treatment of choice. Surgical treatment is still required in some instances.

REFERENCES

1. Warnes CA, Williams RG, Bashore TM, et al: ACC/AHA 2008 guidelines for the management of adults with congenital heart disease: A report of the American College of Cardiology/American Heart Association Task Force on Practice Guidelines (Writing Committee to Develop Guidelines on the Management of Adults With Congenital Heart Disease). Developed in Collaboration With the American Society of Echocardiography, Heart Rhythm Society, International Society for Adult Congenital Heart Disease, Society for Cardiovascular Angiography and Interventions, and Society of Thoracic Surgeons. J Am Coll Cardiol 52:e1, 2008.
2. Gatzoulis MA, Webb GD, Daubeney PEF: Diagnosis and Management of Adult Congenital Heart Disease. Edinburgh, Churchill Livingstone, 2003.

Anatomy and Embryology

3. Bird GL, Jeffries HE, Licht DJ, et al: Neurological complications associated with the treatment of patients with congenital cardiac disease: Consensus definitions from the Multi-Societal Database Committee for Pediatric and Congenital Heart Disease. Cardiol Young 18(Suppl 2):234, 2008.

4. Thorne S, MacGregor A, Nelson-Piercy C: Risks of contraception and pregnancy in heart disease. Heart 92:1520, 2006.

Pathologic Consequences of Congenital Cardiac Lesions

5. Hosseinpour AR, Cullen S, Tsang VT: Transplantation for adults with congenital heart disease. Eur J Cardiothorac Surg 30:508, 2006.
6. Lamour JM, Kanter KR, Naftel DC, et al: The effect of age, diagnosis, and previous surgery in children and adults undergoing heart transplantation for congenital heart disease. J Am Coll Cardiol 54:160, 2009.

Cyanosis

7. Oechslin E, Kiowski W, Schindler R, et al: Systemic endothelial dysfunction in adults with cyanotic congenital heart disease. Circulation 112:1106, 2005.
8. Fyfe A, Perloff JK, Niwa K, et al: Cyanotic congenital heart disease and coronary artery atherogenesis. Am J Cardiol 96:283, 2005.
9. Walker F, Mullen MJ, Woods SJ, Webb GD: Acute effects of 40% oxygen supplementation in adults with cyanotic congenital heart disease. Heart 90:1073, 2004.

Pulmonary Hypertension

10. Duffels MG, Engelfriet PM, Berger RM, et al: Pulmonary arterial hypertension in congenital heart disease: An epidemiologic perspective from a Dutch registry. Int J Cardiol 120:198, 2007.
11. McLaughlin VV, Archer SL, Badesch DB, et al: ACCF/AHA 2009 expert consensus document on pulmonary hypertension a report of the American College of Cardiology Foundation Task Force on Expert Consensus Documents and the American Heart Association developed in collaboration with the American College of Chest Physicians; American Thoracic Society, Inc.; and the Pulmonary Hypertension Association. J Am Coll Cardiol 53:1573, 2009.
12. Consensus statement on the management of pulmonary hypertension in clinical practice in the UK and Ireland. Thorax 63(Suppl 2):ii1, 2008.
13. Beghetti M, Galie N: Eisenmenger syndrome a clinical perspective in a new therapeutic era of pulmonary arterial hypertension. J Am Coll Cardiol 53:733, 2009.
14. Trulock EP, Christie JD, Edwards LB, et al: Registry of the International Society for Heart and Lung Transplantation: Twenty-fourth official adult lung and heart-lung transplantation report—2007. J Heart Lung Transplant 26:782, 2007.
15. Galie N, Beghetti M, Gatzoulis MA, et al: Bosentan therapy in patients with Eisenmenger syndrome: A multicenter, double-blind, randomized, placebo-controlled study. Circulation 114:48, 2006.
16. Christensen DD, McConnell ME, Book WM, Mahle WT: Initial experience with bosentan therapy in patients with the Eisenmenger syndrome. Am J Cardiol 94:261, 2004.
17. Duffels MG, Vis JC, van Loon RL, et al: Effect of bosentan on exercise capacity and quality of life in adults with pulmonary arterial hypertension associated with congenital heart disease with and without Down's syndrome. Am J Cardiol 103:1309, 2009.
18. Galie N, Ghofrani HA, Torbicki A, et al: Sildenafil citrate therapy for pulmonary arterial hypertension. N Engl J Med 353:2148, 2005.
19. Singh TP, Rohit M, Grover A, et al: A randomized, placebo-controlled, double-blind, crossover study to evaluate the efficacy of oral sildenafil therapy in severe pulmonary artery hypertension. Am Heart J 151:851.e1, 2006.
20. Garg N, Sharma MK, Sinha N: Role of oral sildenafil in severe pulmonary arterial hypertension: Clinical efficacy and dose response relationship. Int J Cardiol 120:306, 2007.
21. Chau EM, Fan KY, Chow WH: Effects of chronic sildenafil in patients with Eisenmenger syndrome versus idiopathic pulmonary arterial hypertension. Int J Cardiol 120:301, 2007.
22. Wort SJ: Sildenafil in Eisenmenger syndrome: Safety first. Int J Cardiol 120:314, 2007.

Infective Endocarditis

23. Wilson W, Taubert KA, Gewitz M, et al: Prevention of infective endocarditis: Guidelines from the American Heart Association: A guideline from the American Heart Association Rheumatic Fever, Endocarditis and Kawasaki Disease Committee, Council on Cardiovascular Disease in the Young, and the Council on Clinical Cardiology, Council on Cardiovascular Surgery and Anesthesia, and the Quality of Care and Outcomes Research Interdisciplinary Working Group. J Am Dent Assoc 139(Suppl):3S, 2008.
24. Gould FK, Elliott TS, Foweraker J, et al: Guidelines for the prevention of endocarditis: Report of the Working Party of the British Society for Antimicrobial Chemotherapy. J Antimicrob Chemother 57:1035, 2006.

Evaluation of the Patient with Congenital Heart Disease

25. Makikallio K, McElhinney DB, Levine JC, et al: Fetal aortic valve stenosis and the evolution of hypoplastic left heart syndrome: Patient selection for fetal intervention. Circulation 113:1401, 2006.
26. Barrea C, Levasseur S, Roman K, et al: Three-dimensional echocardiography improves the understanding of left atrioventricular valve morphology and function in atrioventricular septal defects undergoing patch augmentation. J Thorac Cardiovasc Surg 129:746, 2005.
27. Sawada SG, Thomaides A: Three-dimensional stress echocardiography: The promise and limitations of volumetric imaging. Curr Opin Cardiol 24:426, 2009.
28. van den Bosch AE, Robbers-Visser D, Krenning BJ, et al: Real-time transthoracic three-dimensional echocardiographic assessment of left ventricular volume and ejection fraction in congenital heart disease. J Am Soc Echocardiogr 19:1, 2006.
29. Awad SM, Cao QL, Hijazi ZM: Intracardiac echocardiography for the guidance of percutaneous procedures. Curr Cardiol Rep 11:210, 2009.
30. Suematsu Y, Kiaii B, Bainbridge DT, et al: Robotic-assisted closure of atrial septal defect under real-time three-dimensional echo guide: In vitro study. Eur J Cardiothorac Surg 32:573, 2007.
31. Stephens DN, O'Donnell M, Thomenius K, et al: Experimental studies with a 9F forward-looking intracardiac imaging and ablation catheter. J Ultrasound Med 28:207, 2009.
32. Roberts KE, McElroy JJ, Wong WP, et al: BMPR2 mutations in pulmonary arterial hypertension with congenital heart disease. Eur Respir J 24:371, 2004.
33. Boccalandro F, Baptista E, Muench A, et al: Comparison of intracardiac echocardiography versus transesophageal echocardiography guidance for percutaneous transcatheter closure of atrial septal defect. Am J Cardiol 93:437, 2004.
34. Krumsdorf U, Ostermayer S, Billinger K, et al: Incidence and clinical course of thrombus formation on atrial septal defect and patient foramen ovale closure devices in 1,000 consecutive patients. J Am Coll Cardiol 43:302, 2004.
35. Masura J, Gavora P, Podnar T: Long-term outcome of transcatheter secundum-type atrial septal defect closure using Amplatzer septal occluders. J Am Coll Cardiol 45:505, 2005.
36. Cheung YF, Lun KS, Chau AK: Doppler tissue imaging analysis of ventricular function after surgical and transcatheter closure of atrial septal defect. Am J Cardiol 93:375, 2004.
37. Butera G, Carminati M, Chessa M, et al: Percutaneous versus surgical closure of secundum atrial septal defect: Comparison of early results and complications. Am Heart J 151:228, 2006.
38. Silversides CK, Siu SC, McLaughlin PR, et al: Symptomatic atrial arrhythmias and transcatheter closure of atrial septal defects in adult patients. Heart 90:1194, 2004.
39. Cramer SC, Rordorf G, Maki JH, et al: Increased pelvic vein thrombi in cryptogenic stroke: Results of the Paradoxical Emboli from Large Veins in Ischemic Stroke (PELVIS) study. Stroke 35:46, 2004.
40. Beda RD, Gill EA Jr: Patent foramen ovale: Does it play a role in the pathophysiology of migraine headache? Cardiol Clin 23:91, 2005.
41. Windecker S, Wahl A, Nedeltchev K, et al: Comparison of medical treatment with percutaneous closure of patent foramen ovale in patients with cryptogenic stroke. J Am Coll Cardiol 44:750, 2004.
42. Schuchlenz HW, Weihs W, Berghold A, et al: Secondary prevention after cryptogenic cerebrovascular events in patients with patent foramen ovale. Int J Cardiol 101:77, 2005.
43. Wohrle J: Closure of patent foramen ovale after cryptogenic stroke. Lancet 368:350, 2006.
44. Ten Harkel AD, Cromme-Dijkhuis AH, Heinerman BC, et al: Development of left atrioventricular valve regurgitation after correction of atrioventricular septal defect. Ann Thorac Surg 79:607, 2005.
45. Murashita T, Kubota T, Oba J, et al: Left atrioventricular valve regurgitation after repair of incomplete atrioventricular septal defect. Ann Thorac Surg 77:2157, 2004.
46. Masuda M, Kado H, Tanoue Y, et al: Does Down syndrome affect the long-term results of complete atrioventricular septal defect when the defect is repaired during the first year of life? Eur J Cardiothorac Surg 27:405, 2005.
47. Frid C, Bjorkhem G, Jonzon A, et al: Long-term survival in children with atrioventricular septal defect and common atrioventricular valvar orifice in Sweden. Cardiol Young 14:24, 2004.
48. Roos-Hesselink JW, Meijboom FJ, Spitaels SE, et al: Outcome of patients after surgical closure of ventricular septal defect at young age: Longitudinal follow-up of 22-34 years. Eur Heart J 25:1057, 2004.
49. Thanopoulos BD, Rigby ML: Outcome of transcatheter closure of muscular ventricular septal defects with the Amplatzer ventricular septal defect occluder. Heart 91:513, 2005.
50. Carminati M, Butera G, Chessa M, et al: Transcatheter closure of congenital ventricular septal defect with Amplatzer septal occluders. Am J Cardiol 96:52L, 2005.
51. Sadiq M, Latif F, Ur-Rehman A: Analysis of infective endarteritis in patent ductus arteriosus. Am J Cardiol 93:513, 2004.
52. Moore JW, Levi DS, Moore SD, et al: Interventional treatment of patent ductus arteriosus in 2004. Catheter Cardiovasc Interv 64:91, 2005.

Cyanotic Heart Disease

53. Oosterhof T, van Straten A, Vliegen HW, et al: Preoperative thresholds for pulmonary valve replacement in patients with corrected tetralogy of Fallot using cardiovascular magnetic resonance. Circulation 116:545, 2007.
54. Knauth AL, Gauvreau K, Powell AJ, et al: Ventricular size and function assessed by cardiac MRI predict major adverse clinical outcomes late after tetralogy of Fallot repair. Heart 94:211, 2008.
55. Yetman AT, Graham T: The dilated aorta in patients with congenital cardiac defects. J Am Coll Cardiol 53:461, 2009.
56. Lurz P, Coats L, Khambadkone S, et al: Percutaneous pulmonary valve implantation: Impact of evolving technology and learning curve on clinical outcome. Circulation 117:1964, 2008.
57. Lurz P, Bonhoeffer P, Taylor AM: Percutaneous pulmonary valve implantation: An update. Expert Rev Cardiovasc Ther 7:823, 2009.
58. Khambadkone S, Bonhoeffer P: Percutaneous pulmonary valve implantation. Semin Thorac Cardiovasc Surg Pediatr Card Surg Annu 23, 2006.
59. Wong T, Davlouros PA, Li W, et al: Mechano-electrical interaction late after Fontan operation: Relation between P-wave duration and dispersion, right atrial size, and atrial arrhythmias. Circulation 109:2319, 2004.
60. Rychik J: Protein-losing enteropathy after Fontan operation. Congenit Heart Dis 2:288, 2007.
61. Kiesewetter CH, Sheron N, Vettukattill JJ, et al: Hepatic changes in the failing Fontan circulation. Heart 93:579, 2007.
62. Rodriguez-Roisin R, Krowka MJ: Hepatopulmonary syndrome—a liver-induced lung vascular disorder. N Engl J Med 358:2378, 2008.
63. Mavroudis C, Backer CL, Deal BJ: Late reoperations for Fontan patients: State of the art invited review. Eur J Cardiothorac Surg 34:1034, 2008.
64. Prandstetter C, Hofer A, Lechner E, et al: Early and mid-term outcome of the arterial switch operation in 114 consecutive patients: A single centre experience. Clin Res Cardiol 96:723, 2007.
65. Bove T, De Meulder F, Vandenplas G, et al: Midterm assessment of the reconstructed arteries after the arterial switch operation. Ann Thorac Surg 85:823, 2008.
66. Lange R, Cleuziou J, Horer J, et al: Risk factors for aortic insufficiency and aortic valve replacement after the arterial switch operation. Eur J Cardiothorac Surg 34:711, 2008.
67. Horer J, Schreiber C, Dworak E, et al: Long-term results after the Rastelli repair for transposition of the great arteries. Ann Thorac Surg 83:2169, 2007.
68. Benzaquen BS, Webb GD, Colman JM, Therrien J: Arterial switch operation after Mustard procedures in adult patients with transposition of the great arteries: Is it time to revise our strategy? Am Heart J 147:E8, 2004.
69. Khairy P, Landzberg MJ, Gatzoulis MA, et al: Transvenous pacing leads and systemic thromboemboli in patients with intracardiac shunts: A multicenter study. Circulation 113:2391, 2006.
70. Dore A, Houde C, Chan KL, et al: Angiotensin receptor blockade and exercise capacity in adults with systemic right ventricles: A multicenter, randomized, placebo-controlled clinical trial. Circulation 112:2411, 2005.

71. Therrien J, Provost Y, Harrison J, et al: Effect of angiotensin receptor blockade on systemic right ventricular function and size: A small, randomized, placebo-controlled study. Int J Cardiol 129:187, 2008.

72. Doughan AR, McConnell ME, Book WM: Effect of beta blockers (carvedilol or metoprolol XL) in patients with transposition of great arteries and dysfunction of the systemic right ventricle. Am J Cardiol 99:704, 2007.

73. Josephson CB, Howlett JG, Jackson SD, et al: A case series of systemic right ventricular dysfunction post atrial switch for simple D-transposition of the great arteries: The impact of beta-blockade. Can J Cardiol 22:769, 2006.

74. Guedes A, Mercier LA, Leduc L, et al: Impact of pregnancy on the systemic right ventricle after a Mustard operation for transposition of the great arteries. J Am Coll Cardiol 44:433, 2004.

75. Quinn DW, McGuirk SP, Metha C, et al: The morphologic left ventricle that requires training by means of pulmonary artery banding before the double-switch procedure for congenitally corrected transposition of the great arteries is at risk of late dysfunction. J Thorac Cardiovasc Surg 135:1137, 2008.

76. Brown ML, Dearani JA, Danielson GK, et al: Comparison of the outcome of porcine bioprosthetic versus mechanical prosthetic replacement of the tricuspid valve in the Ebstein anomaly. Am J Cardiol 103:555, 2009.

77. Quinonez LG, Dearani JA, Puga FJ, et al: Results of the 1.5-ventricle repair for Ebstein anomaly and the failing right ventricle. J Thorac Cardiovasc Surg 133:1303, 2007.

78. Dearani JA, Danielson GK: Surgical management of Ebstein's anomaly in the adult. Semin Thorac Cardiovasc Surg 17:148, 2005.

79. Khositseth A, Danielson GK, Dearani JA, et al: Supraventricular tachyarrhythmias in Ebstein anomaly: Management and outcome. J Thorac Cardiovasc Surg 128:826, 2004.

80. Brown ML, Dearani JA, Danielson GK, et al: Functional status after operation for Ebstein anomaly: The Mayo Clinic experience. J Am Coll Cardiol 52:460, 2008.

Valvular and Vascular Conditions

81. Fiore AC, Fischer LK, Schwartz T, et al: Comparison of angioplasty and surgery for neonatal aortic coarctation. Ann Thorac Surg 80:1659, 2005.

82. Karamlou T, Bernasconi A, Jaeggi E, et al: Factors associated with arch reintervention and growth of the aortic arch after coarctation repair in neonates weighing less than 2.5 kg. J Thorac Cardiovasc Surg 137:1163, 2009.

83. Wong D, Benson LN, Van Arsdell GS, et al: Balloon angioplasty is preferred to surgery for aortic coarctation. Cardiol Young 18:79, 2008.

84. Ou P, Celermajer DS, Raisky O, et al: Angular (Gothic) aortic arch leads to enhanced systolic wave reflection, central aortic stiffness, and increased left ventricular mass late after aortic coarctation repair: Evaluation with magnetic resonance flow mapping. J Thorac Cardiovasc Surg 135:62, 2008.

85. Fawzy ME, Fathala A, Osman A, et al: Twenty-two years of follow-up results of balloon angioplasty for discreet native coarctation of the aorta in adolescents and adults. Am Heart J 156:910, 2008.

86. Oliver JM, Gallego P, Gonzalez A, et al: Risk factors for aortic complications in adults with coarctation of the aorta. J Am Coll Cardiol 44:1641, 2004.

87. Hager A, Kanz S, Kaemmerer H, et al: Coarctation Long-term Assessment (COALA): Significance of arterial hypertension in a cohort of 404 patients up to 27 years after surgical repair of isolated coarctation of the aorta, even in the absence of restenosis and prosthetic material. J Thorac Cardiovasc Surg 134:738, 2007.

88. Pacini D, Bergonzini M, Loforte A, et al: Aneurysms after coarctation repair associated with hypoplastic aortic arch: Surgical management through median sternotomy. Ann Thorac Surg 81:758, 2006.

89. Tzifa A, Ewert P, Brzezinska-Rajszys G, et al: Covered Cheatham-platinum stents for aortic coarctation: Early and intermediate-term results. J Am Coll Cardiol 47:1457, 2006.

90. Suzuki T, Ohye RG, Devaney EJ, et al: Selective management of the left ventricular outflow tract for repair of interrupted aortic arch with ventricular septal defect: Management of left ventricular outflow tract obstruction. J Thorac Cardiovasc Surg 131:779, 2006.

91. Chiu PP, Rusan M, Williams WG, et al: Long-term outcomes of clinically significant vascular rings associated with congenital tracheal stenosis. J Pediatr Surg 41:335, 2006.

92. Hickey EJ, Caldarone CA, Blackstone EH, et al: Critical left ventricular outflow tract obstruction: The disproportionate impact of biventricular repair in borderline cases. J Thorac Cardiovasc Surg 134:1429, 2007.

93. Dodge-Khatami A, Schmid M, Rousson V, et al: Risk factors for reoperation after relief of congenital subaortic stenosis. Eur J Cardiothorac Surg 33:885, 2008.

94. Hickey EJ, Jung G, Williams WG, et al: Congenital supravalvular aortic stenosis: Defining surgical and nonsurgical outcomes. Ann Thorac Surg 86:1919, 2008.

95. Scott DJ, Campbell DN, Clarke DR, et al: Twenty-year surgical experience with congenital supravalvar aortic stenosis. Ann Thorac Surg 87:1501, 2009.

96. Schaverien MV, Freedom RM, McCrindle BW: Independent factors associated with outcomes of parachute mitral valve in 84 patients. Circulation 109:2309, 2004.

97. McElhinney DB, Sherwood MC, Keane JF, et al: Current management of severe congenital mitral stenosis: Outcomes of transcatheter and surgical therapy in 108 infants and children. Circulation 112:707, 2005.

98. Macnab A, Jenkins NP, Ewington I, et al: A method for the morphological analysis of the regurgitant mitral valve using three dimensional echocardiography. Heart 90:771, 2004.

99. Oppido G, Davies B, McMullan DM, et al: Surgical treatment of congenital mitral valve disease: Midterm results of a repair-oriented policy. J Thorac Cardiovasc Surg 135:1313, 2008.

100. Chauvaud S: Congenital mitral valve surgery: Techniques and results. Curr Opin Cardiol 21:95, 2006.

101. Silvilairat S, Cabalka AK, Cetta F, et al: Echocardiographic assessment of isolated pulmonary valve stenosis: Which outpatient Doppler gradient has the most clinical validity? J Am Soc Echocardiogr 18:1137, 2005.

102. Karagoz T, Asoh K, Hickey E, et al: Balloon dilation of pulmonary valve stenosis in infants less than 3 kg: A 20-year experience. Catheter Cardiovasc Interv 74:753, 2009.

103. Earing MG, Connolly HM, Dearani JA, et al: Long-term follow-up of patients after surgical treatment for isolated pulmonary valve stenosis. Mayo Clin Proc 80:871, 2005.

CHAPTER 66 **Valvular Heart Disease**

Catherine M. Otto and Robert O. Bonow

Valvular heart disease accounts for 10% to 20% of all cardiac surgical procedures in the United States. The primary causes of valve disease are age-associated calcific valve changes and inherited or congenital conditions (e.g., a bicuspid aortic valve or myxomatous mitral valve disease). The prevalence of rheumatic valve disease now is very low in the United States and Europe because of primary prevention of rheumatic fever, although rheumatic valve disease remains prevalent in the developing world (see Chap. 88). About two thirds of all heart valve operations are for aortic valve replacement (AVR), most often for aortic stenosis (AS). Mitral valve surgery is most often performed for mitral regurgitation (MR) because most patients with mitral stenosis (MS) are treated by a percutaneous approach.[1,2] In addition to patients with severe valve disease that eventually requires mechanical intervention, there is a larger group of patients with mild to moderate disease who need accurate diagnosis and appropriate medical management.

Aortic Valve Disease

Aortic Stenosis

CAUSES AND PATHOLOGY. Obstruction to left ventricular (LV) outflow is localized most commonly at the aortic valve and is discussed in this section. However, obstruction may also occur above the valve (supravalvular stenosis) or below the valve (discrete subvalvular stenosis; see Chap. 65), or it may be caused by hypertrophic cardiomyopathy (HCM; see Chap. 69). Valvular AS has three principal causes—a congenital bicuspid valve with superimposed calcification, calcification of a normal trileaflet valve, and rheumatic disease (**Fig. 66-1**). In a U.S. series of 933 patients undergoing AVR for AS, a bicuspid valve was present in more than 50% including two thirds of those younger than 70 years and 40% of those older than 70 years.[3]

In addition, AS may be caused by a congenital valve stenosis presenting in infancy or childhood. Rarely, AS is caused by severe atherosclerosis of the aorta and aortic valve; this form of AS occurs most frequently in patients with severe hypercholesterolemia and is observed in children with homozygous type II hyperlipoproteinemia. Rheumatoid involvement of the valve is a rare cause of AS and results in nodular thickening of the valve leaflets and involvement of the proximal portion of the aorta. Ochronosis with alkaptonuria is another rare cause of AS.

Congenital Aortic Valve Disease

Congenital malformations of the aortic valve may be unicuspid, bicuspid, or tricuspid, or there may be a dome-shaped diaphragm (see Chap. 65). Unicuspid valves produce severe obstruction in infancy and are the most frequent malformations found in fatal valvular AS in children

younger than 1 year. Congenitally bicuspid valves may be stenotic with commissural fusion at birth, but more often they are not responsible for serious narrowing of the aortic orifice during childhood.[4-6] A subset of patients with a bicuspid aortic valve develops significant aortic regurgitation (AR) requiring valve surgery in young adulthood. However, most patients have normal valve function until late in life, when superimposed calcific changes result in valve obstruction (see later,"Bicuspid Aortic Valve Disease").

Calcific Aortic Valve Disease

Age-related calcific (formerly termed *senile* or *degenerative*) AS of a congenital bicuspid or normal trileaflet valve is now the most common cause of AS in adults. In a population-based echocardiographic study, 2% of persons 65 years of age or older had frank calcific AS (see Chap. 80), whereas 29% exhibited age-related aortic valve sclerosis without stenosis, defined by Otto and colleagues[7,7a] as irregular thickening of the aortic valve leaflets detected by echocardiography without significant obstruction. Aortic sclerosis is the initial stage of calcific valve disease and, even in the absence of valve obstruction, is associated with a 50% increased risk of cardiovascular death and myocardial infarction.[8-10]

Although once considered to represent the result of years of normal mechanical stress on an otherwise normal valve, the evolving concept is that the disease process represents proliferative and inflammatory changes, with lipid accumulation, upregulation of angiotensin-converting enzyme (ACE) activity, increased oxidative stress, and infiltration of macrophages and T lymphocytes (**Fig. 66-2**),[11-15] ultimately leading to bone formation[16] in a manner similar, but not identical, to vascular calcification. Progressive calcification, initially along the flexion lines at their bases, leads to immobilization of the cusps. A high prevalence of calcific AS also exists in patients with Paget disease of bone and end-stage renal disease.

Age-related calcific AS shares common risk factors with mitral annular calcification, and the two conditions often coexist. Genetic polymorphisms have been linked to the presence of calcific AS, including the vitamin D receptor, interleukin-10 alleles, and the apolipoprotein E4 allele. Familial clustering of calcific AS also has been described, suggesting a possible genetic predisposition to valve calcification.[17-19] The risk factors for the development of calcific AS are similar to those for vascular atherosclerosis—elevated serum levels of low-density lipoprotein (LDL) cholesterol and lipoprotein(a) [Lp(a)], diabetes, smoking, and hypertension.[7,7a,10,20] Calcific AS has also been linked to inflammatory markers and components of the metabolic syndrome.[21,22] Retrospective studies have linked treatment with 3-hydroxy-3-methylglutaryl-coenzyme A (HMG-CoA) reductase (statin) medications with a lower rate of progression of calcific AS, and this effect has been demonstrated in animal models of hypercholesterolemia.[14,23] Hence there is growing consensus that "degenerative" calcific AS

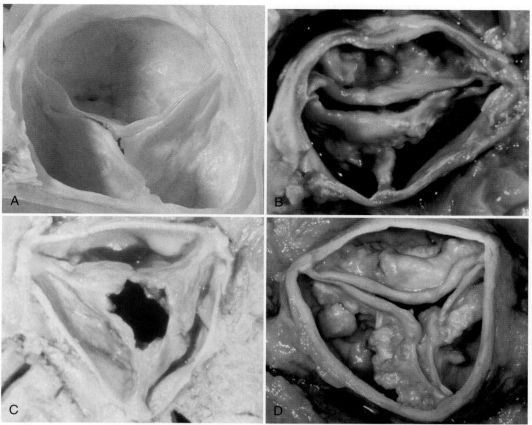

FIGURE 66-1 Major types of aortic valve stenosis. **A,** Normal aortic valve. **B,** Congenital bicuspid aortic stenosis. A false raphe is present at 6 o'clock. **C,** Rheumatic aortic stenosis. The commissures are fused with a fixed central orifice. **D,** Calcific degenerative aortic stenosis. (**A,** *From Manabe H, Yutani C [eds]: Atlas of Valvular Heart Disease. Singapore, Churchill Livingstone, 1998, pp 6, 131;* **B, C, D,** *Courtesy of Dr. William C. Roberts, Baylor University Medical Center, Dallas, Tex.*)

shares many pathophysiologic features with atherosclerosis and that specific pathways might be targeted to prevent or retard disease progression.[11,16,24]

However, no benefit was seen in a small prospective randomized trial of atorvastatin versus placebo, despite a significant lowering of serum LDL levels, in patients with relatively advanced calcific AS,[25] and a subsequent prospective study in patients with less severe AS demonstrated only a slight reduction in the rate of progression of AS with rosuvastatin.[26] The Simvastatin and Ezetimibe for Aortic Stenosis (SEAS) Trial[27] and the Aortic Stenosis Progression Observation: Measuring Effects of Rosuvastatin (ASTRONOMER) Trial[28] randomized 1800 and 269 adults, respectively, with mild to moderate AS to intensive lipid-lowering therapy versus placebo. These studies convincingly showed no improvement in mortality, time to valve replacement, or rate of AS progression in the treatment versus placebo groups. Current interest is focused on other disease pathways in calcific valve disease that may be amenable to medical therapy.[16,29]

Rheumatic Aortic Stenosis

Rheumatic AS results from adhesions and fusions of the commissures and cusps and vascularization of the leaflets of the valve ring, leading to retraction and stiffening of the free borders of the cusps. Calcific nodules develop on both surfaces, and the orifice is reduced to a small round or triangular opening (see Fig. 66-1C). As a consequence, the rheumatic valve is often regurgitant, as well as stenotic. Patients with rheumatic AS invariability have rheumatic involvement of the mitral valve (see Chap. 88). With the decline in rheumatic fever in developed nations, rheumatic AS is decreasing in frequency, although it continues to be a major problem on a worldwide basis.

PATHOPHYSIOLOGY. In adults with AS, outflow obstruction usually develops and increases gradually over a prolonged period (**Fig. 66-3**). In infants and children with congenital AS, the valve orifice shows little change as the child grows, thereby intensifying the relative obstruction gradually. LV function can be well maintained in experimentally produced, gradually developing subcoronary AS in animals. In the experimental model, as well as in children and adults with chronic severe AS, LV output is maintained by the presence of LV hypertrophy, which may sustain a large pressure gradient across the aortic valve for many years without a reduction in cardiac output, LV dilation, or development of symptoms.

Severe obstruction to LV outflow is usually characterized by the following: (1) an aortic jet velocity greater than 4 m/sec; (2) a mean systolic pressure gradient exceeding 40 mm Hg in the presence of a normal cardiac output; or (3) an effective aortic orifice (calculated by the continuity equation; see Chap. 15) less than approximately 1.0 cm^2 in an average-sized adult (i.e., <0.6 cm^2/m^2 of body surface area, approximately 25% of the normal aortic orifice of 3.0 to 4.0 cm^2). An aortic valve orifice of 1.0 to 1.5 cm^2 is considered moderate stenosis, and an orifice of 1.5 to 2.0 cm^2 is referred to as mild stenosis[1,30,30a] (**Table 66-1**). However, the degree of stenosis associated with symptom onset varies among patients, and there is no single number that defines severe or critical AS in an individual patient. Clinical decisions are based on consideration of symptom status and the LV response to chronic pressure overload, in conjunction with hemodynamic severity. In some cases, additional measures of hemodynamic severity, such as stroke work loss or valvular impedance, or evaluation with changing loading conditions (e.g., dobutamine stress) or with exercise, are necessary to evaluate disease severity fully.[31-33a]

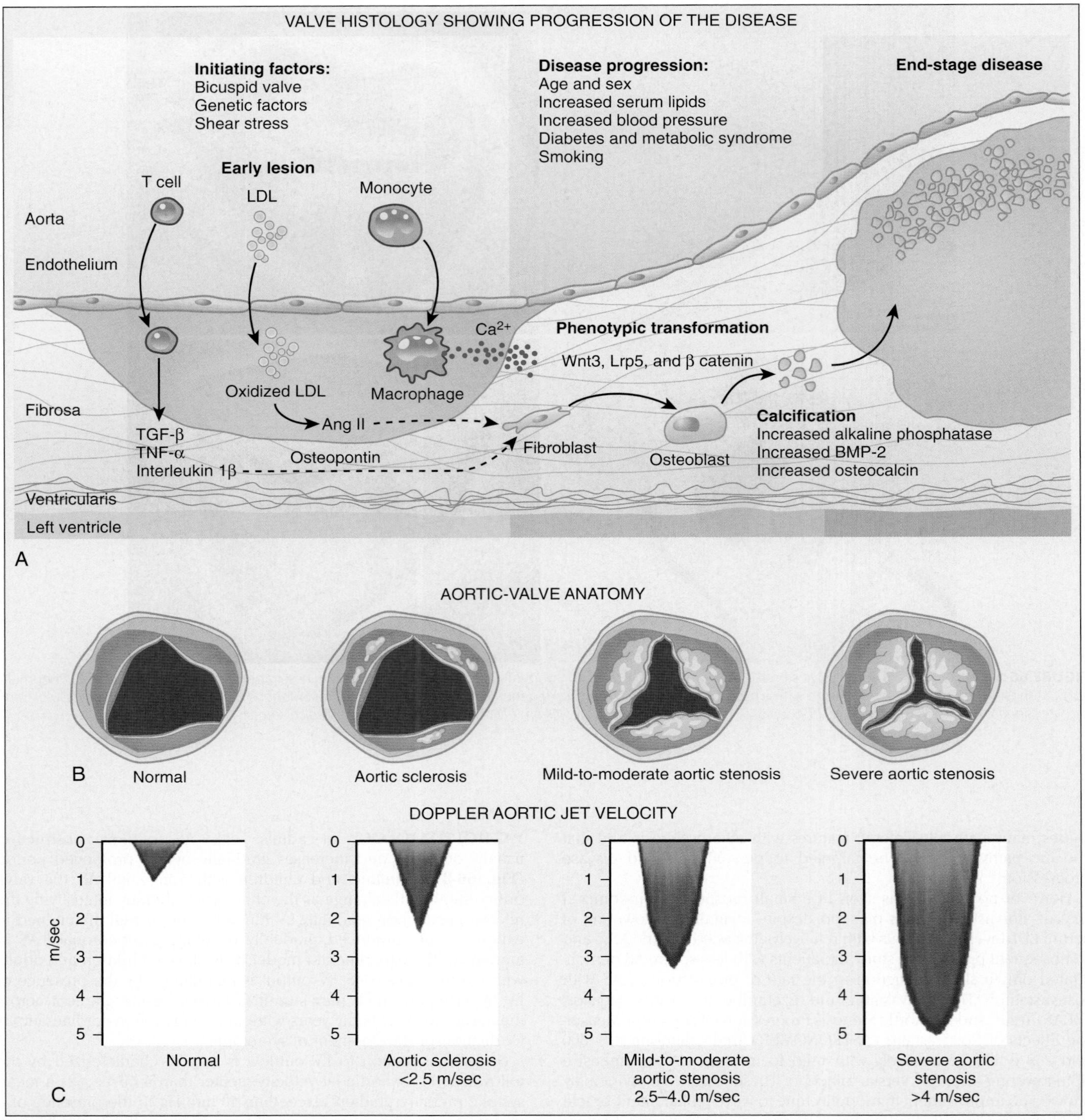

FIGURE 66-2 Disease progression in calcific aortic stenosis, showing changes in aortic valve histologic features, leaflet opening in systole, and Doppler velocities. **A,** The histology of the early lesion is characterized by a subendothelial accumulation of oxidized LDL, production of angiotensin (Ang) II, and inflammation with T lymphocytes and macrophages. Disease progression occurs by several mechanisms, including local production of proteins, such as osteopontin, osteocalcin, and bone morphogenic protein 2 (BMP-2), which mediate tissue calcification; activation of inflammatory signaling pathways, including tumor necrosis factor (TNF), tumor growth factor-β (TGF-β), the complement system, C-reactive protein, and interleukin-1β; and changes in tissue matrix, including the accumulation of tenascin C, and upregulation of matrix metalloproteinase 2 and alkaline phosphatase activity. In addition, leaflet fibroblasts undergo phenotypic transformation into osteoblasts, regulated by the Wnt3-Lrp5-β catenin signaling pathway. Microscopic accumulations of extracellular calcification (Ca²⁺) are present early in the disease process, with progressive calcification as the disease progresses and areas of frank bone formation in end-stage disease. **B,** The corresponding changes in aortic valve anatomy are viewed from the aortic side with the valve open in systole. **C,** Corresponding changes in Doppler aortic jet velocity. *(From Otto CM: Calcific aortic stenosis—time to look more closely at the valve. N Engl J Med 359:1395, 2008.)*

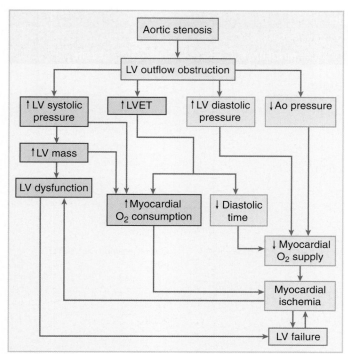

FIGURE 66-3 Pathophysiology of aortic stenosis. LV outflow obstruction results in an increased LV systolic pressure, increased LV ejection time (LVET), increased LV diastolic pressure, and decreased aortic (Ao) pressure. Increased LV systolic pressure with LV volume overload increases LV mass, which may lead to LV dysfunction and failure. Increased LV systolic pressure, LV mass, and LVET increase myocardial oxygen (O_2) consumption. Increased LVET results in a decrease of diastolic time (myocardial perfusion time). Increased LV diastolic pressure and decreased Ao diastolic pressure decrease coronary perfusion pressure. Decreased diastolic time and coronary perfusion pressure decrease myocardial O_2 supply. Increased myocardial O_2 consumption and decreased myocardial O_2 supply produce myocardial ischemia, which further deteriorates LV function. *(From Boudoulas H, Gravanis MB: Valvular heart disease. In Gravanis MB [ed]: Cardiovascular Disorders: Pathogenesis and Pathophysiology. St. Louis, CV Mosby, 1993, p 64.)*

Chronic pressure overload typically results in concentric LV hypertrophy, with increased wall thickness and a normal chamber size. The increased wall thickness allows normalization of wall stress (afterload) so that LV contractile function is maintained. However, the increased myocardial cell mass and increased interstitial fibrosis result in diastolic dysfunction, which may persist even after relief of AS. Gender differences in the LV response to AS have been reported, with women more frequently exhibiting normal LV performance and a smaller, thicker walled, concentrically hypertrophied left ventricle with diastolic dysfunction (see later) and normal or even subnormal systolic wall stress. Men more frequently have eccentric LV hypertrophy, excessive systolic wall stress, systolic dysfunction, and chamber dilation.

The LV changes caused by chronic pressure overload are reflected in the LV and left atrial pressure waveforms and Doppler velocity curves. As contraction of the left ventricle becomes progressively more isometric, the LV pressure pulse exhibits a rounded, rather than flattened, summit and the Doppler velocity curve exhibits a progressively later systolic peak. The elevated LV end-diastolic pressure and the corresponding Doppler changes in LV filling, which are characteristic of severe AS, reflect delayed relaxation and eventually decreased compliance of the hypertrophied LV wall. In patients with severe AS, large *a* waves usually appear in the left atrial pressure pulse and Doppler LV filling curve because of the combination of enhanced contraction of a hypertrophied left atrium and diminished LV compliance. Atrial contraction plays a particularly important role in filling of the left ventricle in AS. It raises LV end-diastolic pressure without causing a concomitant

elevation of mean left atrial pressure. This "booster pump" function of the left atrium prevents the pulmonary venous and capillary pressures from rising to levels that would produce pulmonary congestion, whereas at the same time maintaining LV end-diastolic pressure at the elevated level necessary for effective contraction of the hypertrophied left ventricle. These changes in diastolic function are reflected in the Doppler parameter of LV filling and noninvasive measures of diastolic function, such as strain and strain rate (see Chap. 15). Loss of appropriately timed, vigorous atrial contraction, as occurs in atrial fibrillation (AF) or atrioventricular dissociation, may result in rapid clinical deterioration in patients with severe AS.

Systemic vascular resistance also contributes to total LV afterload in adults with AS. Concurrent hypertension increases total LV load and may affect the evaluation of AS severity.[34] Mild pulmonary hypertension is present is about one third of adults with AS because of the chronic elevation of LV end-diastolic pressure; more severe pulmonary hypertension is seen in about 15% of AS patients.

Exercise physiology is abnormal in adults with moderate to severe AS, and even asymptomatic patients have a reduced exercise tolerance. Although cardiac output at rest is within normal limits, the normal increase in cardiac output with exercise is blunted and is mediated primarily by increased heart rate, with little change in stroke volume. Even though stroke volume is unchanged, transvalvular flow rate increases because of the shortened systolic ejection period so that aortic jet velocity and transvalvular gradient increase proportionally. Prior to symptom onset, valve area increases slightly with exercise (by 0.2 cm^2 on average) but as AS becomes more severe and symptoms are imminent, valve area becomes fixed, resulting in an even greater rise in jet velocity and pressure gradient with exercise. At this point, there is an abnormal blood pressure response to exercise (rise in systolic blood pressure < 10 mm Hg), signifying severe valve obstruction.

MYOCARDIAL FUNCTION IN AORTIC STENOSIS. When the aorta is suddenly constricted in experimental animals, LV pressure rises, wall stress increases significantly, and both the extent and velocity of shortening decline. As noted in Chap. 24, the development of LV hypertrophy is one of the principal mechanisms whereby the heart adapts to such an increased hemodynamic burden. The increased systolic wall stress induced by AS leads to parallel replication of sarcomeres and concentric hypertrophy. The increase in LV wall thickness is often sufficient to counterbalance the increased pressure so that peak systolic wall tension returns to normal, or remains normal, if the obstruction develops slowly. An inverse correlation between wall stress and ejection fraction has been described in patients with AS. This suggests that the depressed ejection fraction and velocity of fiber shortening that occur in some patients are a consequence of inadequate wall thickening, resulting in afterload mismatch. In others, the lower ejection fraction is secondary to a true depression of contractility; in this group, surgical treatment is less effective. Thus, both increased afterload and altered contractility are operative to varying extents in depressing LV performance. To evaluate myocardial function in patients with AS, ejection phase indices, such as ejection fraction and myocardial fiber shortening, should be related to the existing wall tension.

DIASTOLIC PROPERTIES. Although LV hypertrophy is a key adaptive mechanism to the pressure load imposed by AS, it has an adverse pathophysiologic consequence (i.e., it increases diastolic stiffness; see Chaps. 24 and 30). As a result, greater intracavitary pressure is required for LV filling. Some patients with AS manifest an increase in stiffness of the left ventricle (increased chamber stiffness) simply because of increased muscle mass with no alteration in the diastolic properties of each unit of myocardium (normal muscle stiffness); others exhibit increases in chamber and muscle stiffness. This increased stiffness, however produced, contributes to the elevation of LV diastolic filling pressure at any level of ventricular diastolic volume. Diastolic dysfunction may revert toward normal with regression of hypertrophy following surgical relief of AS, but some degree of long-term diastolic dysfunction typically persists.

ISCHEMIA. In patients with AS, coronary blood flow at rest is elevated in absolute terms but is normal when corrections are made for myocardial mass. Reduced coronary blood flow reserve may produce inadequate myocardial oxygenation in patients with severe AS, even in the absence of coronary artery disease. The hypertrophied LV muscle mass, increased systolic pressure, and prolongation of ejection all elevate myocardial oxygen consumption. The abnormally heightened pressure

TABLE 66-1 Classification of the Severity of Valve Disease in Adults

VALVE DISEASE	MILD	MODERATE	SEVERE
		Severity	
Aortic Stenosis			
Jet velocity (m/sec)	<3.0	3.0-4.0	>4.0
Mean gradient (mm Hg)*	<25	25-40	>40
Valve area (cm²)	>1.5	1.0-1.5	<1.0
Valve area index (cm²/m²)			<0.6
Mitral Stenosis			
Mean gradient (mm Hg)*	<5	5-10	>10
Pulmonary artery systolic pressure (mm Hg)	<30	30-50	>50
Valve area (cm²)	>1.5	1.0-1.5	<1.0
Aortic Regurgitation			
Qualitative			
Angiographic grade	1+	2+	3-4+
Color Doppler jet width	Central jet, width < 25% of LVOT	> Mild but no signs of severe AR	Central jet, width >65% LVOT
Doppler vena contracta width (cm)	<0.3	0.3-0.6	>0.6
Quantitative (cath or echo)			
Regurgitant volume (mL/beat)	<30	30-59	≥60
Regurgitant fraction (%)	<30	30-49	≥50
Regurgitant orifice area (cm²)	<0.10	0.10-0.29	≥0.30
Additional Essential Criteria			
Left ventricular size			Increased
Mitral Regurgitation			
Qualitative			
Angiographic grade	1+	2+	3-4+
Color Doppler jet area	Small, central jet (<4 cm² or <20% LA area)	Signs of MR > mild present, but no criteria for severe MR	Vena contracta width >0.7 cm with large central MR jet (area >40% of LA area) or with a wall-impinging jet of any size, swirling in LA
Doppler vena contracta width (cm)	<0.3	0.3–0.69	≥0.70
Quantitative (cath or echo)			
Regurgitant volume (mL/beat)	<30	30-59	≥60
Regurgitant fraction (%)	<30	30-49	≥50
Regurgitant orifice area (cm²)	<0.20	0.2-0.39	≥0.40
Additional Essential Criteria			
Left atrial size			Enlarged
Left ventricular size			Enlarged
Right-Sided Valve Disease			
Severe tricuspid stenosis		Valve area <1.0 cm²	
Severe tricuspid regurgitation		Vena contracta width >0.7 cm and systolic flow reversal in hepatic veins	
Severe pulmonic stenosis		Jet velocity >4 m/sec or maximum gradient >60 mm Hg	
Severe pulmonic regurgitation		Color jet fills outflow tract	
		Dense continuous wave Doppler signal with a steep deceleration slope	

*Valve gradients are flow-dependent and, when used as estimates of severity of valve stenosis, should be assessed with knowledge of cardiac output or forward flow across the valve.
LA = left atrial, left atrium; LVOT = left ventricular outflow tract.
From Zoghbi WA, Enriquez-Sarano M, Foster E, et al: Recommendations for evaluation of the severity of native valvular regurgitation with two-dimensional and Doppler echocardiography. J Am Soc Echocardiogr 16:777, 2003; and from Bonow RO, Carabello BA, Chatterjee K, et al: ACC/AHA 2006 guidelines for the management of patients with valvular heart disease: A report of the American College of Cardiology/American Heart Association Task Force on Practice Guidelines (writing Committee to Revise the 1998 guidelines for the management of patients with valvular heart disease) developed in collaboration with the Society of Cardiovascular Anesthesiologists endorsed by the Society for Cardiovascular Angiography and Interventions and the Society of Thoracic Surgeons. J Am Coll Cardiol 48:e1, 2006.

compressing the coronary arteries may exceed the coronary perfusion pressure and the shortening of diastole interferes with coronary blood flow, thus leading to an imbalance between myocardial oxygen supply and demand (see Fig. 66-3). Myocardial perfusion is also impaired by the relative decrease in myocardial capillary density as myocardial mass increases and by the elevation of LV end-diastolic pressure, which lowers the aortic-LV pressure gradient in diastole (i.e., the coronary perfusion pressure gradient). This underperfusion may be responsible for the development of subendocardial ischemia, especially when oxygen demand is increased or the diastolic filling period is reduced (e.g., tachycardia, anemia, infection, pregnancy).

CLINICAL PRESENTATION

Symptoms

The cardinal manifestations of acquired AS are exertional dyspnea, angina, syncope, and ultimately heart failure.[31,35] Many patients now are diagnosed before symptom onset on the basis of the finding of a systolic murmur on physical examination, with confirmation of the diagnosis by echocardiography. Symptoms typically occur at age 50 to 70 years with bicuspid aortic valve stenosis and in those older than 70 years with calcific stenosis of a trileaflet valve, although even in this age group about 40% of AS patients have a congenital bicuspid valve.[3]

The most common clinical presentation in patients with a known diagnosis of AS who are followed prospectively is a gradual decrease in exercise tolerance, fatigue, or dyspnea on exertion. The mechanism of exertional dyspnea may be LV diastolic dysfunction, with an excessive rise in end-diastolic pressure leading to pulmonary congestion. Alternatively, exertional symptoms may be a result of the limited ability to increase cardiac output with exercise. More severe exertional dyspnea, with orthopnea, paroxysmal nocturnal dyspnea, and pulmonary edema reflects varying degrees of pulmonary venous hypertension. These are relatively late symptoms in patients with AS, and intervention now is typically undertaken before this disease stage.

Angina occurs in approximately two thirds of patients with severe AS, about 50% of whom have associated significant coronary artery obstruction. It usually resembles the angina observed in patients with coronary artery disease (see Chap. 53) in that it is commonly precipitated by exertion and relieved by rest. In patients without coronary artery disease, angina results from the combination of the increased oxygen needs of hypertrophied myocardium and reduction of oxygen delivery secondary to the excessive compression of coronary vessels. In patients with coronary artery disease, angina is caused by a combination of epicardial coronary artery obstruction and the oxygen imbalance characteristic of AS. Very rarely, angina results from calcium emboli to the coronary vascular bed.

Syncope is most commonly caused by the reduced cerebral perfusion that occurs during exertion when arterial pressure declines consequent to systemic vasodilation in the presence of a fixed cardiac output. Syncope has also been attributed to malfunction of the baroreceptor mechanism in severe AS (see Chap. 94), as well as to a vasodepressor response to a greatly elevated LV systolic pressure during exercise. Premonitory symptoms of syncope are common. Exertional hypotension may also be manifested as graying out spells or dizziness on effort. Syncope at rest may be caused by transient AF with loss of the atrial contribution to LV filling, which causes a precipitous decline in cardiac output, or to transient atrioventricular block caused by extension of the calcification of the valve into the conduction system.

Other late findings in patients with isolated AS include AF, pulmonary hypertension, and systemic venous hypertension. Although AS may be responsible for sudden death (see Chap. 41), this usually occurs in patients who had previously been symptomatic.

Gastrointestinal bleeding may develop in patients with severe AS, often associated with angiodysplasia (most commonly of the right colon) or other vascular malformations. This complication arises from shear stress–induced platelet aggregation with a reduction in high-molecular-weight multimers of von Willebrand factor and increases in proteolytic subunit fragments. These abnormalities correlate with the severity of AS and are correctable by AVR.

Infective endocarditis is a greater risk in younger patients with milder valvular deformity than in older patients with rocklike calcific aortic deformities. Cerebral emboli resulting in stroke or transient ischemic attacks may be caused by microthrombi on thickened bicuspid valves. Calcific AS may cause embolization of calcium to various organs, including the heart, kidneys, and brain.

PHYSICAL EXAMINATION. The key features of the physical examination in patients with AS are palpation of the carotid upstroke, evaluation of the systolic murmur, assessment of splitting of the second heart sound, and examination for signs of heart failure (see Chap. 12).

The carotid upstroke directly reflects the arterial pressure waveform. The expected finding with severe AS is a slow-rising, late-peaking, low-amplitude carotid pulse, the parvus and tardus carotid impulse (**Fig. 66-4**). When present, this finding is specific for severe AS. However, many adults with AS have concurrent conditions, such as AR or systemic hypertension, that affect the arterial pressure curve and the carotid impulse. Thus, an apparently normal carotid impulse is not reliable for excluding the diagnosis of severe AS. Similarly, blood pressure is not a helpful method for evaluation of AS severity. When severe AS is present, systolic blood pressure and pulse pressures may be

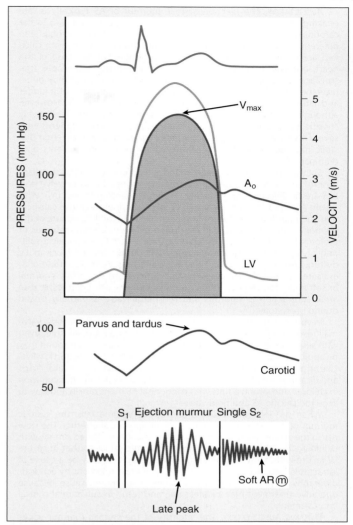

FIGURE 66-4 Relationship between LV and aortic (Ao) pressures and the Doppler aortic stenosis velocity curve (in red). The pressure difference between the left ventricle and aorta in systole is four times the velocity squared (the Bernoulli equation). Thus, a maximum velocity (V_{max}) of 4.3 m/sec corresponds to a maximum LV to Ao pressure difference of 74 mm Hg and a mean systolic gradient of 44 mm Hg. On physical examination, the slow rate of rise and delayed peak in the carotid pulse (or parvus and tardus) matches the contour of the aortic pressure waveform. The murmur corresponds to the Doppler velocity curve with a harsh crescendo-decrescendo late-peaking systolic murmur, best heard at the aortic region (upper right sternal border). Often, a soft, high-pitched diastolic decrescendo murmur of aortic regurgitation also is appreciated.

reduced. However, in patients with associated AR or in older patients with an inelastic arterial bed, systolic and pulse pressures may be normal or even increased. With severe AS, radiation of the murmur to the carotids may result in a palpable thrill or carotid shudder.

The cardiac impulse is sustained and becomes displaced inferiorly and laterally with LV failure. Presystolic distention of the left ventricle (i.e., a prominent precordial *a* wave) is often visible and palpable. A hyperdynamic left ventricle suggests concomitant AR and/or MR. A systolic thrill is usually best appreciated when the patient leans forward during full expiration. It is palpated most readily in the second right intercostal space or suprasternal notch and is frequently transmitted along the carotid arteries. A systolic thrill is specific, but not sensitive, for severe AS.

AUSCULTATION. The ejection systolic murmur of AS typically is late peaking and heard best at the base of the heart, with radiation to the carotids (see Fig. 66-4). Cessation of the murmur before A_2 is helpful in differentiation from a pansystolic mitral murmur. In patients with calcified aortic valves, the systolic murmur is loudest at the base of the heart, but high-frequency components may radiate to the apex (the so-called Gallavardin phenomenon), in which the murmur may be so prominent that it is mistaken for the murmur of MR. In general, a louder and later peaking murmur indicates more severe stenosis. However, although a systolic murmur of grade 3 intensity or greater is relatively specific for severe AS, this finding is insensitive and many patients with severe AS have only a grade 2 murmur. High-pitched decrescendo diastolic murmurs secondary to AR are common in many patients with dominant AS.

Splitting of the second heart sound is helpful in excluding the diagnosis of severe AS because normal splitting implies the aortic valve leaflets are flexible enough to create an audible closing sound (A_2). With severe AS, the second heart sound (S_2) may be single because calcification and immobility of the aortic valve make A_2 inaudible, closure of the pulmonic valve (P_2) is buried in the prolonged aortic ejection murmur, or prolongation of LV systole makes A_2 coincide with P_2. Paradoxical splitting of S_2, which suggests associated left bundle branch block or LV dysfunction, may also occur. Thus, in older adults, normal splitting of S_2 indicates a low likelihood of severe AS. The first heart sound (S_1) is normal or soft and a fourth heart sound (S_4) is prominent, presumably because atrial contraction is vigorous and the mitral valve is partially closed during presystole.

In young patients with congenital AS (see Chap. 65), the flexible valve may result in an accentuated A_2 so that S_2 may be normally split, even with severe valve obstruction. In addition, an aortic ejection sound may be audible because of the halting upward movement of the aortic valve. Like an audible A_2, this sound is dependent on mobility of the valve cusps and disappears when they become severely calcified. Thus, it is common in children and young adults with congenital AS but is rare in adults with acquired calcific AS and rigid valves.

When the left ventricle fails and stroke volume falls, the systolic murmur of AS becomes softer; rarely, it disappears altogether. The slow rise in the arterial pulse is more difficult to recognize. Stated simply, with LV failure, the clinical picture changes from typical AS to that of severe LV failure with a low cardiac output. Thus, occult AS may be a cause of intractable heart failure, and severe AS should be ruled out by echocardiography in patients with heart failure of unknown cause because operative treatment may be lifesaving and result in substantial clinical improvement.

DYNAMIC AUSCULTATION. The intensity of the systolic murmur varies from beat to beat when the duration of diastolic filling varies, as in AF or following a premature contraction. This characteristic is helpful in differentiating AS from MR, in which the murmur is usually unaffected. The murmur of valvular AS is augmented by squatting, which increases stroke volume. It is reduced in intensity during the strain of the Valsalva maneuver and when standing, which reduce transvalvular flow.

Echocardiography

Echocardiography is the standard approach for evaluating and following patients with AS and selecting them for operation (see Chap. 15 and Figs. 15-36 to 15-38, and 15-43 to 15-45).

Echocardiographic imaging allows accurate definition of valve anatomy, including the cause of AS and the severity of valve calcification, and sometimes allows direct imaging of the orifice area.[30,36] Echocardiographic imaging also is invaluable for the evaluation of LV hypertrophy and systolic function, with calculation of the ejection fraction, and for measurement of aortic root dimensions and detection of associated mitral valve disease.[37]

Doppler echocardiography allows measurement of the transaortic jet velocity, which is the most useful measure for following disease severity and predicting clinical outcome. The effective orifice area is calculated using the continuity equation, and mean transaortic pressure gradient is calculated using the modified Bernoulli equation (see Fig. 15-38).[37,38] Both valve area and pressure gradient calculations from Doppler data have been well validated compared with invasive hemodynamics and in terms of their ability to predict clinical outcome. However, the accuracy of these measures requires an experienced laboratory with meticulous attention to technical details.

The combination of pulsed, continuous wave and color flow Doppler echocardiography is helpful in detecting and determining the severity of AR (which coexists in about 75% of patients with predominant AS) and in estimating pulmonary artery pressure. In some patients, additional measures of AS severity may be necessary, such as correction for poststenotic pressure recovery or transesophageal imaging of valve anatomy.[31,39] Evaluation of AS severity is affected by the presence of systemic hypertension so that reevaluation after blood pressure control may be necessary.[34] In patients with LV dysfunction and low cardiac output, assessing the severity of AS can be enhanced by assessing hemodynamic changes during dobutamine infusion (see later).

OTHER DIAGNOSTIC EVALUATION MODALITIES

ELECTROCARDIOGRAPHY. The principal electrocardiographic change is LV hypertrophy (see Chap. 13), which is found in approximately 85% of patients with severe AS. The absence of LV hypertrophy does not exclude the presence of critical AS, and the correlation between the absolute electrocardiographic voltages in precordial leads and the severity of obstruction is poor in adults but good in children with congenital AS. T wave inversion and ST-segment depression in leads with upright QRS complexes are common. There is evidence of left atrial enlargement in more than 80% of patients with severe isolated AS. AF occurs in only 10% to 15% of AS patients. The extension of calcific infiltrates from the aortic valve into the conduction system may cause various forms and degrees of atrioventricular and intraventricular block in 5% of patients with calcific AS. Such conduction defects are more common in patients who have associated mitral annular calcification.

RADIOGRAPHY. On chest radiography (see Figs. 16-10 and 16-23), the heart is usually of normal size or slightly enlarged, with a rounding of the LV border and apex, unless regurgitation or LV failure is present and causes substantial cardiomegaly. Dilation of the ascending aorta is a common finding, particularly in patients with a bicuspid aortic valve. Calcification of the aortic valve is found in almost all adults with hemodynamically significant AS but is rarely visible on the chest radiograph, although readily detected by fluoroscopy or cardiac computed tomography (CT; see Fig. 19-21). The left atrium may be slightly enlarged in patients with severe AS, and there may be radiologic signs of pulmonary venous hypertension. However, when left atrial enlargement is marked, the presence of associated mitral valvular disease should be suspected.

CARDIAC CATHETERIZATION AND ANGIOGRAPHY. In almost all patients, the echocardiographic examination provides the important hemodynamic information required for patient management, and cardiac catheterization is now recommended only when noninvasive tests are inconclusive, when clinical and echocardiographic findings are discrepant, and for coronary angiography prior to surgical intervention.[1,2,40] Hemodynamic or echocardiographic assessment of AS severity at rest and with dobutamine is reasonable when AS is associated with low cardiac output and impaired LV function (see later).

CHEST COMPUTED TOMOGRAPHY. In addition to assessing aortic valve calcification, CT (see Chap. 19) is useful for evaluating aortic dilation in patients with evidence of aortic root disease by echocardiography or chest radiography. Measurement of aortic dimensions at several levels, including the sinuses of Valsalva, sinotubular junction, and ascending aorta, is necessary for clinical decision making and surgical planning.

CARDIAC MAGNETIC RESONANCE. Cardiac magnetic resonance (CMR) is useful for assessing LV volume, function, and mass, especially in settings in which this information cannot be obtained readily from echocardiography (see Chap. 18). AS severity also can be quantitated by CMR, although this approach is not widely used.[41]

DISEASE COURSE

Clinical Outcome

ASYMPTOMATIC PATIENTS. The severity of outflow tract obstruction gradually increases over 10 to 15 years, so there is a long latent period during which stenosis severity is only mild to moderate and clinical outcomes are similar to those of age-matched normal patients.[42] In patients with mild valve thickening but no obstruction to outflow (e.g., aortic sclerosis), 16% will develop valve obstruction at 1 year of follow-up, but only 2.5% will develop severe valve obstruction at an average of 8 years after the diagnosis of aortic sclerosis.

Once moderate to severe AS is present, prognosis remains excellent as long as the patient remains asymptomatic.[43] However, retrospective studies of survival in adults with severe AS diagnosed by echocardiography emphasize the progressive nature of the disease and the need

TABLE 66-2   Clinical Outcomes in Prospective Studies of Asymptomatic Aortic Stenosis in Adults

STUDY (YEAR)	NO. OF PATIENTS	SEVERITY OF AORTIC STENOSIS	AGE (YR)	MEAN FOLLOW-UP	EVENT-FREE SURVIVAL WITHOUT SYMPTOMS
Kelly et al (1988)	51	$V_{max} > 3.6$ m/sec	63 ± 8	5-25 mo	Overall: 59% at 15 mo
Pellikka et al (1990)	113	$V_{max} \geq 4.0$ m/sec	40-94	20 mo	Overall: 86% at 1 yr; 62% at 2 yr
Kennedy et al (1991)	66	AVA = 0.7-1.2 cm^2	67 ± 10	35 mo	Overall: 59% at 4 yr
Otto et al (1997)	123	$V_{max} > 2.6$ m/sec	63 ± 16	2.5 ± 1.4 yr	Overall: 93 ± 5% at 1 yr; 62 ± 8% at 3 yr; 26 ± 10% at 5 yr *Subgroups:* $V_{max} < 3$ m/sec, 84% ± 16% at 2 yr; V_{max} 3-4 m/sec, 66% ± 13% at 2 yr; $V_{max} > 4$ m/sec, 21% ± 18% at 2 yr
Rosenhek et al (2000)	128	$V_{max} > 4.0$ m/sec	60 ± 18	22 ± 18 mo	Overall: 67 ± 5% at 1 yr; 56 ± 55% at 2 yr; 33 ± 5% at 4 yr *Subgroups:* No or mild Ca^{++}, 75% ± 9% at 4 yr; Mod-severe Ca^{++}, 20% ± 5% at 4 yr
Amato et al (2001)	66	AVA ≥ 1.0 cm^2	18-80 (50 ± 15)	15 ± 12 mo	Overall: 57% at 1 yr; 38% at 2 yr *Subgroups:* AVA ≥ 0.7 cm^2, 72% at 2 yr; AVA < 0.7 cm^2, 21% at 2 yr; Negative exercise test 85% at 2 yr; Positive exercise test* 19% at 2 yr
Das et al (2005)	125	AVA < 1.4 cm^2	56-74 (mean, 65)	12 mo	Overall: 71% at 1 yr *Subgroups:* AVA ≥ 1.2 cm^2, 100% at 1 yr; AVA ≤ 0.8 cm^2, 46% at 1 yr; No symptoms on exercise test,* 89% at 1 yr; Symptoms on exercise test, 49% at 1 yr
Pellikka et al (2005)	622	V_{max} 4.0 ≥ m/sec	72 ± 11	5.4 ± 4.0 yr	Overall: 82% at 1 yr; 67% at 2 yr; 33% at 5 yr
Monin et al (2009)	211	V_{max} = 3.5-4.4 (mean, 4.1) m/sec	63-77 (mean, 72)	21 mo	Risk score = $2V_{max}$ + 1.5 ln$_{BNP}$ + 1.5 (if female)† 24 mo event rate < 10% in lowest risk quartile compared with >75% in highest risk quartile (score > 15)

*Positive exercise test = symptoms, abnormal ST-segment response, or abnormal blood pressure response (less than 20 mmHg increase) with exercise.
$^†V_{max}$ measured in m/sec.
AVA = aortic valve area; BNP = blood natriuretic peptide level (pg/mL); Ca^{++} = aortic valve calcification; ln = logarithm; Mod = moderate; V_{max} = maximum aortic velocity.
From Bonow RO, Carabello BA, Chatterjee K, et al: ACC/AHA 2006 guidelines for the management of patients with valvular heart disease: A report of the American College of Cardiology/ American Heart Association Task Force on Practice Guidelines (writing Committee to Revise the 1998 guidelines for the management of patients with valvular heart disease) developed in collaboration with the Society of Cardiovascular Anesthesiologists endorsed by the Society for Cardiovascular Angiography and Interventions and the Society of Thoracic Surgeons. J Am Coll Cardiol 48:e1, 2006.
Data from Kelly TA, Rothbart RM, Cooper CM, et al: Comparison of outcome of symptomatic to symptomatic patients older that 20 years of age with valvular aortic stenosis. Am J Cardiol 61:123,1988; Pellikka PA, Nishimura RA, Bailey KR, Tajik AJ: The natural history of adults with asymptomatic, hemodynamically significant aortic stenosis. J Am Coll Cardiol 15:1012, 1990; Kennedy KD, Nishimura RA, Holmes DRJ, Bailey KR: Natural history of moderate aortic stenosis. J Am Coll Cardiol 17:313, 1991; Otto CM, Burwash IG, Legget ME, et al: A prospective study of asymptomatic valvular aortic stenosis: Clinical, echocardiographic, and exercise predictors of outcome. Circulation 95:2262, 1997; Rosenhek R, Binder T, Porenta G, et al: Predictors of outcome in severe asymptomatic aortic valve stenosis. N Engl J Med 343:611, 2000; Amato MC, Moffa PJ, Werner KE, Ramires JA: Treatment decision in asymptomatic aortic valve stenosis: Role of exercise testing. Heart 86:381, 2001; Das P, Rimington H, Chambers J: Exercise testing to stratify risk in aortic stenosis. Eur Heart J 26:1309, 2005; Pellikka PA, Sarano ME, Nishimura RA, et al: Outcome of 622 adults with asymptomatic, hemodynamically significant aortic stenosis during prolonged follow-up. Circulation 111:3290, 2005; and Monin JL, Lancellotti P, Monchi M, et al: Risk score for predicting outcome in patients with asymptomatic aortic stenosis. Circulation 120:69, 2009.)

for close follow-up.[44] Although stenosis severity on average is more severe in symptomatic versus asymptomatic patients, there is marked overlap in all measures of severity between these two groups. Prospective studies evaluating the rate of progression to symptomatic AS in initially asymptomatic patients are summarized in **Table 66-2**. The strongest predictor of progression to symptoms is the Doppler aortic jet velocity.[45,46,46a] Survival free of symptoms is 84% at 2 years when jet velocity is less than 3 m/sec compared with only 21% when jet velocity is greater than 4 m/sec (**Fig. 66-5**).[31] In adults with severe AS (Doppler velocity > 4 m/sec), outcome can be further predicted by the magnitude of the Doppler velocity and also by the severity of aortic valve calcification.[47,47a] Event-free survival at 5 years is 75% ± 9% in those with little valve calcification compared with 20% ± 5% in those with moderate to severe valve calcification. Retrospective studies have reported some cases of sudden death in apparently asymptomatic adults with severe AS. However, more recent prospective studies have suggested that sudden death in asymptomatic patients is very unlikely, with an estimated risk of less than 1%/year.[46]

SYMPTOMATIC PATIENTS. Once even mild symptoms are present, survival is poor unless outflow obstruction is relieved. Survival curves derived from older retrospective studies show that the interval from the onset of symptoms to the time of death is approximately 2 years in patients with heart failure, 3 years in those with syncope, and 5 years in those with angina. More recent series have confirmed this poor prognosis, with an average survival of only 1 to 3 years after symptom onset.[48] Among symptomatic patients with severe AS, the outlook is poorest when the left ventricle has failed and the cardiac output and transvalvular gradient are both low. The risk of sudden death is high with symptomatic severe AS, so these patients should be promptly referred for surgical intervention. In patients who do not undergo surgical intervention, recurrent hospitalizations for angina and decompensated heart failure are common.

Hemodynamic Progression

The average rate of hemodynamic progression is an annual decrease in aortic valve area of 0.12 cm^2/year,[31] an increase in aortic jet velocity of 0.32 m/sec/year, and an increase in mean gradient of 7 mm Hg/year. However, the rate of progression is highly variable and difficult to predict in individual patients. In clinical studies, the factors associated with more rapid hemodynamic progression included older age, more severe leaflet calcification, renal insufficiency, hypertension, smoking, and hyperlipidemia. The role of genetic factors remains unclear.

Because of the variability in hemodynamic severity at symptom onset and because many patients fail to recognize symptom onset resulting from the insidious rate of disease progression, both exercise testing (see Table 66-2)[32,49,50] and serum brain natriuretic peptide

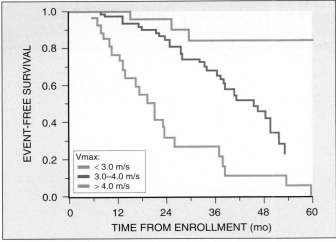

FIGURE 66-5 Natural history of asymptomatic patients with aortic stenosis. Initial aortic jet velocity (Vmax) stratifies patients according to the likelihood that symptoms requiring valve replacement will develop over time. Most events in this series were the onset of symptoms warranting aortic valve replacement. *(From Otto CM, Burwarsh IG, Legget ME, et al: A prospective study of asymptomatic valvular aortic stenosis: Clinical, echocardiographic, and exercise predictors of outcome. Circulation 95:2262, 1997.)*

(BNP) levels[51-53a] have been evaluated as measures of disease progression and predictors of symptom onset. Clearly, patients who develop symptoms on treadmill exercise or who have a decrease in blood pressure with exertion show evidence of severe symptomatic disease. An elevated BNP level may be helpful when symptoms are equivocal or when stenosis severity is only moderate, but the role of BNP in evaluation of disease progression has not been fully defined.

MANAGEMENT

Medical Treatment

The most important principle in the management of adults with AS is patient education regarding the disease course and typical symptoms.[31,39] Patients should be advised to promptly report the development of any symptoms possibly related to AS. Patients with severe AS should be cautioned to avoid vigorous athletic sports and physical activity.[54] However, such restrictions do not apply to patients with mild obstruction. Although medical therapy has not been shown to affect disease progression, adults with AS (as with any other adult) should be evaluated and treated for conventional coronary disease risk factors, as per established guidelines.

Echocardiography is recommended for the initial diagnosis and assessment of AS severity, assessment of LV hypertrophy and systolic function, reevaluation in patients with changing signs or symptoms, and reevaluation annually for severe AS, every 1 to 2 years for moderate AS, and every 3 to 5 years for mild AS.[1,2] Because patients may tailor their lifestyle to minimize symptoms or may ascribe fatigue and dyspnea to deconditioning or aging, they may not recognize early symptoms as important warning signals, although these symptoms often can be elicited by a careful history. Exercise testing may be helpful in apparently asymptomatic patients to detect covert symptoms, limited exercise capacity, or an abnormal blood pressure response.[31] Exercise stress testing should be absolutely avoided in symptomatic patients.

Symptomatic patients with severe AS are usually operative candidates because medical therapy has little to offer. However, medical therapy may be necessary for patients considered to be inoperable, usually because of comorbid conditions that preclude surgery. Some of these patients may be candidates for transcatheter valve implantation, but others will not be candidates for or will decline this procedure. Although diuretics are beneficial when there is abnormal accumulation of fluid, they must be used with caution because hypovolemia may reduce the elevated LV end-diastolic pressure, lower cardiac output, and produce orthostatic hypotension. ACE inhibitors should be used with caution but are beneficial in treating patients with symptomatic LV systolic dysfunction who are not candidates for surgery. They should be initiated at low doses and increased slowly to target doses, avoiding hypotension. Beta-adrenergic blockers can depress myocardial function and induce LV failure, and should be avoided in patients with AS.

AF or atrial flutter occurs in less than 10% of patients with severe AS, perhaps because of the late occurrence of left atrial enlargement in this condition. When such an arrhythmia is observed in a patient with AS, the possibility of associated mitral valvular disease should be considered. When AF occurs, the rapid ventricular rate may cause angina pectoris. The loss of the atrial contribution to ventricular filling and a sudden fall in cardiac output may cause serious hypotension. Therefore, AF should be treated promptly, usually with cardioversion. New-onset AF in a previously asymptomatic patient with severe AS may be a marker of impending symptom onset.

Management of concurrent cardiac conditions, such as hypertension and coronary disease, is complicated in patients with asymptomatic AS by the concern that the vasodilatory effects of medications may not be offset by a compensatory increase in cardiac output. Despite this concern, AS patients should receive appropriate treatment for concurrent disease, although medications should be started at low doses and slowly titrated upward, with close monitoring of blood pressure and symptoms. Adults with asymptomatic severe AS can undergo noncardiac surgery and pregnancy, with careful hemodynamic monitoring and optimization of loading conditions. However, when stenosis is very severe, elective AVR prior to noncardiac surgery or a planned pregnancy may be considered.[55]

Surgical Treatment

CHILDREN. In the adolescent or young adult with severe congenital AS, balloon aortic valvotomy is recommended for all symptomatic patients and asymptomatic patients with a transvalvular gradient higher than 60 mm Hg or electrocardiographic ST-segment changes at rest or with exercise.[56] The same indications are appropriate for surgical intervention, although balloon valvotomy is probably preferable at experienced centers. At surgery, simple commissural incision under direct vision usually leads to substantial hemodynamic improvement with low risk (i.e., mortality rate < 1%; see Chap. 65). Despite the salutary hemodynamic results following percutaneous or surgical valvotomy, the valve is not rendered entirely normal anatomically. The turbulent blood flow through the valve may subsequently lead to further deformation, calcification, development of regurgitation, and restenosis after 10 to 20 years, often requiring reoperation and valve replacement later.

ADULTS. AVR is recommended for adults with symptomatic severe AS, even if symptoms are mild. Despite this clear guideline recommendation,[1,2] many patients with symptomatic AS are not referred appropriately for surgery, even when the operative risk is low.[48,57] AVR also is recommended for severe AS with an ejection fraction less than 50% and for patients with severe asymptomatic AS who are undergoing coronary bypass grafting (CABG) or other forms of heart surgery (**Fig. 66-6**).[1,2,58,59] In addition, AVR may be considered for apparently asymptomatic patients with severe AS when exercise testing provokes symptoms or a fall in blood pressure. In asymptomatic patients with severe AS and a low operative risk, AVR may be considered when markers of rapid disease progression are present (e.g., severe valve calcification) or when AS is very severe, depending on patient preferences regarding the risk of earlier intervention versus careful monitoring with intervention promptly at symptom onset. Coronary angiography should be performed before valve replacement in most adults with AS.

Surgical AVR is the procedure of choice for relief of outflow obstruction in adults with valvular AS. Surgical repair is not feasible because attempts at débridement of valve calcification have not been successful. Balloon aortic valvotomy has only a modest hemodynamic effect in patients with calcific AS and does not favorably affect long-term outcome. Thus, balloon aortic valvotomy is not recommended as an alternate to AVR for calcific AS. In selected cases, balloon valvotomy might be reasonable as a bridge to surgery in unstable patients or as a palliative procedure when surgery is very high risk. Transcatheter aortic

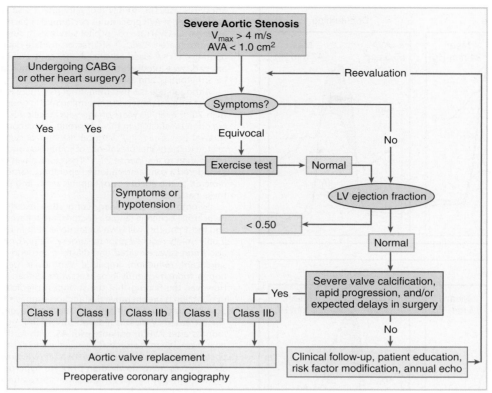

FIGURE 66-6 Management strategy for patients with severe aortic stenosis. Preoperative coronary angiography should be performed routinely as determined by age, symptoms, and coronary risk factors. Cardiac catheterization and angiography may also be helpful when there is discordance between clinical findings and echocardiography. AVA = aortic valve area; BP = blood pressure; V$_{max}$ = maximal velocity across aortic valve by Doppler echocardiography. *(From Bonow RO, Carabello BA, Chatterjee K, et al: ACC/AHA 2006 guidelines for the management of patients with valvular heart disease: A report of the American College of Cardiology/American Heart Association Task Force on Practice Guidelines [writing committee to revise the 1998 Guidelines for the Management of Patients With Valvular Heart Disease]: Developed in collaboration with the Society of Cardiovascular Anesthesiologists: Endorsed by the Society for Cardiovascular Angiography and Interventions and the Society of Thoracic Surgeons. Circulation 114:e84, 2006.)*

valve implantation (TAVI) by a percutaneous or transapical approach is a rapidly evolving technology that is available in Europe and under investigation in the US for seriously ill patients who are not candidates for conventional surgery.[60-64a] In the Canadian multicenter registry of TAVI in 339 patients, the procedure was successful in 93% with a 30 day mortality of 10%. At a median followup of 8 months, overall mortality was 22%, and the procedure was effective in both frail elderly adults and in those with a porcelain aorta.[60,63] The US randomized prospective PARTNER trial, comparing TAVI with medical therapy (including balloon valvotomy) in patients considered to be at too high risk for conventional AVR, demonstrated substantial reduction in death and hospitalization with TAVI, associated with significant improvement in symptoms.[64a]

AORTIC STENOSIS WITH LEFT VENTRICULAR DYSFUNCTION. Surgical risk is higher in patients with impaired LV function (ejection fraction < 35%).[32,65-68] However, their prognosis is extremely poor without operation, overall survival is improved with AVR, and many patients in this group have significant clinical and functional recovery following AVR. Hence, AVR should generally be offered to these patients. Even octogenarians with LV dysfunction can have improved survival after AVR, although their operative risks are higher. Exceptions are patients with advanced congestive heart failure or LV dysfunction that can be related to previous myocardial infarction rather than to AS. In acutely ill patients with decompensated heart failure, nitroprusside has been reported to be safe and effective for improving hemodynamics rapidly and may be used in bridging critically ill patients to AVR. The role of TAVI for severe AS with significant LV systolic dysfunction has not been studied.

AORTIC STENOSIS WITH LOW GRADIENT AND LOW CARDIAC OUTPUT. Patients with critical AS, severe LV dysfunction, and low cardiac output (and hence a low transvalvular pressure gradient) often create diagnostic dilemmas for the clinician because their clinical presentation and hemodynamic data may be indistinguishable from those of patients with a dilated cardiomyopathy and a calcified valve that is not stenotic.[38,65] Low-flow, low-gradient AS is defined as a valve area smaller than 1.0 cm^2, LV ejection fraction less than 40% and mean gradient less than 30 to 40 mm Hg. Because aortic valve velocities and estimates of aortic valve area are dependent on flow, an important method for distinguishing between those with severe AS versus those with primary LV dysfunction is to reassess hemodynamics during transient increases in flow, usually by increasing cardiac output with dobutamine while measuring hemodynamics with Doppler or invasive approaches. (**Fig. 66-7**; see Fig. 15-45).[69,70] Severe AS is present if there is an increase in aortic velocity to at least 4 m/sec at any flow rate, with a valve area less than 1.0 cm^2; AS is not severe if the valve area is increased to more than 1.0 cm^2.[30] Dobutamine echocardiography also provides evidence of myocardial contractile reserve (an increase in stroke volume or ejection fraction > 20% from baseline), which is an important predictor of operative risk, improvement in LV function, and survival after AVR in these patients. However, even in patients with a lack of contractile reserve, AVR should be considered if the mean gradient is over 20 mm Hg because survival after AVR is better (≈50% at 5 years) than with medical therapy.[66,67]

RESULTS. Successful replacement of the aortic valve results in substantial clinical and hemodynamic improvement in patients with AS, AR, or combined lesions. In patients without frank LV failure, the operative risk ranges from 2% to 5% in most centers[71] and, in patients younger than 70 years, the operative risk has been reported to be as low as 1%. The STS National Database Committee has reported an overall operative mortality rate of 3.2% in 67,292 patients undergoing isolated AVR and 5.6% in 66,074 patients undergoing AVR and coronary artery bypass grafting (**Table 66-3**).[72,73] Risk factors associated with a higher mortality rate include a high New York Heart Association (NYHA) class, impairment of LV function, advanced age, and the presence of associated coronary

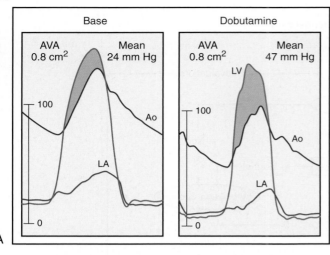

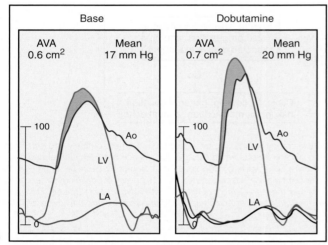

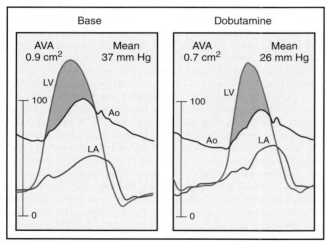

FIGURE 66-7 Hemodynamic tracings from three patients with left ventricular dysfunction, low cardiac output, and low aortic valve gradient, demonstrating three different responses to dobutamine. **A,** Increase in cardiac output and in mean aortic valve gradient from 24 to 47 mm Hg. Aortic valve area (AVA) remained 0.8 cm². This patient underwent successful valve replacement. **B,** Increase in cardiac output and minimal increase in mean pressure gradient from 17 to 20 mm Hg. The final calculated aortic valve area was 0.7 cm². The patient was found to have only minimal AS at the time of surgery. **C,** No change in cardiac output, with decrease in mean pressure gradient from 37 to 26 mm Hg in response to dobutamine. The test was terminated because of hypotension. The patient was found to have severe AS at the time of surgery. Ao = aortic; LA = left atrial; LV = left ventricular. (*From Nishimura RA, Grantham A, Connolly HM, et al: Low-output, low-gradient aortic stenosis in patients with depressed ventricular systolic function: The clinical utility of the dobutamine challenge in the catheterization laboratory. Circulation 106:809, 2002.*)

artery disease. The 30-day mortality rate is also significantly related to the number of AVR procedures performed at each hospital.[74] The 10-year actuarial survival rate of hospital survivors in surgically treated patients is approximately 85%.[75,76] Risk factors for late death include higher preoperative NYHA class, advanced age, concomitant untreated coronary artery disease, preoperative impaired LV function, preoperative ventricular arrhythmias, and associated significant AR.[77-80]

Although age is a determinant of risk, there is increasing experience at most surgical centers in performing AVR in symptomatic patients older than 70 or even 80 years of age with calcific AS.[81,81a] The results of AVR are often satisfactory in this age group, with improved quality of life and survival (see Chap. 80). Surgical risk and postoperative morbidity are related to the higher prevalence of comorbid conditions in older patients, rather than to age per se.[75,82,82a] Therefore, advanced age should not be considered a contraindication to operation. Particular attention must be directed to the adequacy of hepatic, renal, and pulmonary functions in these patients.

Symptoms of pulmonary congestion (exertional dyspnea) and of myocardial ischemia (angina pectoris) are relieved in almost all patients, and most patients will have an improvement in exercise tolerance, even if only mildly reduced prior to surgery. Hemodynamic results of AVR are also impressive; elevated end-diastolic and end-systolic volumes show significant reduction. Impaired ventricular performance returns to normal more frequently in patients with AS than in those with AR or MR. However, the finding that the strongest predictor of postoperative LV dysfunction is preoperative dysfunction suggests that patients should, if possible, be operated on before LV function becomes seriously impaired. The increased LV mass is reduced toward (but not to) normal within 18 months after AVR in patients with AS, with further reduction over the next several years. Coronary flow reserve and diastolic function also demonstrate considerable improvement after AVR. However, interstitial fibrosis regresses more slowly than myocyte hypertrophy, so that diastolic dysfunction may persist for years after successful valve replacement.

When operation is carried out in patients with critical AS, frank LV failure, depressed ejection fraction, or low cardiac output (and hence a reduced transaortic pressure gradient), the operative risk is higher, and the mortality rate ranges from 8% to 20% , depending on the skill of the surgical team and the severity of heart failure. Obviously, performing surgery before heart failure develops is desirable, but emergency operation, even in patients with severe heart failure, is sometimes lifesaving. In view of the extremely poor prognosis of such patients who are treated medically, unless serious comorbid conditions exist that preclude surgery, there is usually little choice but to advise immediate mechanical relief of obstruction.

In patients with AS and obstructive coronary artery disease—a relatively common combination—AVR and myocardial revascularization should be performed together. Although the risk of AVR is increased when accompanied by CABG (see Table 66-3), the surgical risk increases even more when severe coronary artery disease is left untreated. The ability to avoid serious myocardial ischemia in the perioperative period is a major factor that has served to reduce operative mortality in these patients. Characteristics of patients that have been shown to increase the risk of AVR, as reported in different series, are shown in **Table 66-4**.

Aortic Regurgitation

CAUSES AND PATHOLOGY. AR may be caused by primary disease of the aortic valve leaflets and/or the wall of the aortic root (**Fig. 66-8**).[83-85] Among patients with isolated AR who undergo valve replacement, the percentage with aortic root disease has been increasing steadily during the past few decades; it now represents the most common cause and accounts for more than 50% of all such patients in some series.

Valvular Disease

Primary valvular causes of AR include the following: calcific AS in older patients, in whom some degree (usually mild) of AR is present (in 75% of patients); infective endocarditis (see Chap. 67), in which the infection may destroy or cause perforation of a leaflet, or the vegetations may interfere with proper coaptation of the cusps; and trauma that results in a tear of the ascending aorta, in which loss of commissural support can cause prolapse of an aortic cusp. Although the most common complication of a congenitally bicuspid valve in adults is stenosis, incomplete closure and/or prolapse of a bicuspid valve may also cause isolated regurgitation or a combination of stenosis and regurgitation.[6] Rheumatic fever remains a common cause of primary

TABLE 66-3 Operative Mortality Rates Following Valve Replacement and Repair (2002-2006 STS Data Base)*

OPERATIVE CATEGORY	NUMBER	OPERATIVE MORTALITY (%)	CVA (%)	RENAL FAILURE (%)	PROLONGED VENTILATION (%)	REOPERATION (%)	ANY ADVERSE EVENT (%)	PROLONGED LENGTH OF STAY (%)
AVR	67,292	3.2	1.5	4.1	10.9	8.0	17.4	7.9
AVR + CABG	66,074	5.6	2.7	7.6	17.6	10.7	26.3	12.7
MVR	21,229	5.7	2.1	6.4	18.9	11.5	26.7	15.3
MVR + CABG	13.663	11.6	3.7	13.6	32.7	16.6	43.2	24.0
MV repair	21,238	1.6	1.4	2.6	7.3	6.3	12.7	5.5
MV repair + CABG	21,924	7.4	3.1	10.3	25.0	12.6	33.5	17.8

*Operative mortality = death during hospitalization or within 30 days of valve surgery. Other endpoints are during initial hospitalization for valve surgery: CVA = permanent stroke (neurologic deficit persisting > 72 hr); Renal Failure = new need for dialysis, increase in serum creatinine level to > 2.0 mg/dL or increase to twice preoperative baseline; Prolonged Ventilation = need for ventilatory support > 24 hours postoperatively; Reoperation = reoperation during initial hospitalization; Any Adverse Event = any of the above endpoints plus deep sternal wound infection (occurred in <1%); Prolonged length of stay = postoperative hospitalization > 14 days.

Data from Shahian DM, O'Brien SM, Filardo G, et al: The Society of Thoracic Surgeons 2008 cardiac surgery risk models: Part 3—valve plus coronary artery bypass grafting surgery. Ann Thorac Surg 88:S43, 2009; and O'Brien SM, Shahian DM, Filardo G, et al: The Society of Thoracic Surgeons 2008 cardiac surgery risk models: Part 2—isolated valve surgery. Ann Thorac Surg 88:S23, 2009.

TABLE 66-4 Predictors of Poor Outcome After Aortic Valve Replacement for Aortic Stenosis

- Advanced age (>70 yr)
- Female gender
- Emergent surgery
- Coronary artery disease
- Previous CABG
- Hypertension
- Left ventricular dysfunction (ejection fraction <45% or 50%)
- Heart failure
- Atrial fibrillation
- Concurrent mitral valve replacement or repair
- Renal failure

disease of the aortic valve that leads to regurgitation. The cusps become infiltrated with fibrous tissues and retract a process that prevents cusp apposition during diastole; this usually leads to regurgitation into the left ventricle through a defect in the center of the valve (see Fig. 66-1C). The associated fusion of the commissures may restrict the opening of the valve, resulting in combined AS and AR; some associated mitral valve involvement is also common. Progressive AR may occur in patients with a large ventricular septal defect, as well as in patients with membranous subaortic stenosis (see Chap. 65) and as a complication of percutaneous aortic balloon valvotomy. Progressive regurgitation may also occur in patients with myxomatous proliferation of the aortic valve. An increasingly common cause of valvular AR is structural deterioration of a bioprosthetic valve.

Less common causes of AR include various forms of congenital AR, such as unicommissural and quadricuspid valves, or rupture of a congenitally fenestrated valve, particularly in the presence of hypertension. Other less common causes of AR occur in association with systemic lupus erythematosus, rheumatoid arthritis, ankylosing spondylitis, Jaccoud arthropathy, Takayasu disease, Whipple disease, Crohn disease, and, in the past, the use of certain anorectic drugs. Isolated congenital AR is an uncommon lesion on necropsy studies but, when present, is usually associated with a bicuspid valve.

Aortic Root Disease

AR secondary to marked dilation of the ascending aorta is now more common than primary valve disease in patients undergoing AVR for isolated AR (see Chap. 60).[86] The conditions responsible for aortic root disease include age-related (degenerative) aortic dilation, cystic medial necrosis of the aorta (either isolated or associated with classic Marfan syndrome; see Fig. 15-81), aortic dilation related to bicuspid valves,[87] aortic dissection, osteogenesis imperfecta, syphilitic aortitis, ankylosing spondylitis, the Behçet syndrome, psoriatic arthritis, arthritis associated with ulcerative colitis, relapsing polychondritis, reactive arthritis, giant cell arteritis, and systemic hypertension, and exposure to some appetite suppressant drugs.[88]

When the aortic annulus becomes greatly dilated, the aortic leaflets separate and AR may ensue. Dissection of the diseased aortic wall may occur and aggravate the AR. Dilation of the aortic root may also have secondary effects on the aortic valve because dilation causes tension and bowing of the individual cusps, which may thicken, retract, and become too short to close the aortic orifice. This leads to intensification of the AR, further dilating the ascending aorta and thus leading to a vicious circle in which, as is the case for MR, regurgitation leads to regurgitation. AR, regardless of its cause, produces dilation and hypertrophy of the left ventricle, dilation of the mitral valve ring, and sometimes hypertrophy and dilation of the left atrium. Endocardial pockets frequently develop in the LV cavity at sites of impact of the regurgitant jet.

CHRONIC AORTIC REGURGITATION

Pathophysiology

In contrast to MR, in which a fraction of the LV stroke volume is ejected into the low-pressure left atrium, in AR the entire LV stroke volume is ejected into a high-pressure chamber (i.e., the aorta), although the low aortic diastolic pressure does facilitate ventricular emptying during early systole (**Fig. 66-9**). In MR, especially acute MR, the reduction of wall tension (i.e., reduced afterload) allows more complete systolic emptying; in AR the increase in LV end-diastolic volume (i.e., increased preload) provides hemodynamic compensation.[89,90]

Severe AR may occur with a normal effective forward stroke volume and a normal ejection fraction ([forward plus regurgitant stroke volume]/[end-diastolic volume]), together with an elevated LV end-diastolic volume, pressure, and stress (**Fig. 66-10**).[91] In accord with Laplace's law, which indicates that wall tension is related to the product of the intraventricular pressure and radius divided by wall thickness, LV dilation also increases the LV systolic tension required to develop any level of systolic pressure. Thus, in AR, there is an increase in preload and afterload. LV systolic function is maintained through the combination of chamber dilation and hypertrophy. This leads to eccentric hypertrophy, with replication of sarcomeres in series and elongation of myocytes and myocardial fibers. In compensated AR, there is sufficient wall thickening so that the ratio of ventricular wall thickness to cavity radius remains normal. This maintains or returns end-diastolic wall stress to normal levels. AR contrasts with AS, in which there is pressure overload (concentric) hypertrophy with replication of sarcomeres, largely in parallel, and an increased ratio of wall thickness to radius but, like AS, there is an increase in interstitial connective tissue. In AR, LV mass is usually greatly increased, often to levels even higher than in isolated AS. As AR persists and increases in severity over time, wall thickening fails to keep pace with the hemodynamic load and end-systolic wall stress rises. At this point, the afterload mismatch results in a decline in systolic function, and the ejection fraction falls.[90]

Patients with severe chronic AR have the largest end-diastolic volumes of those with any form of heart disease, resulting in so-called cor bovinum. However, end-diastolic pressure is not uniformly elevated

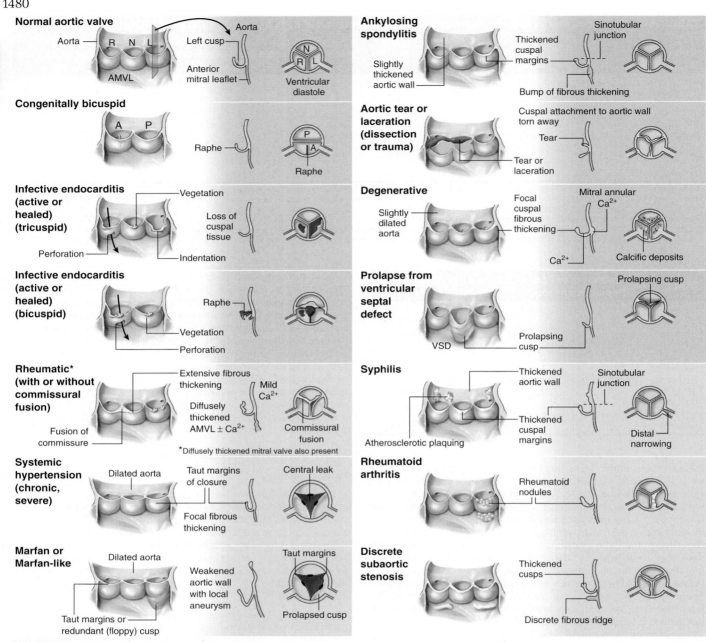

FIGURE 66-8 Diagram of various causes of pure aortic regurgitation. A = anterior; AMVL = anterior mitral valve leaflet; P = posterior; VSD = ventricular septal defect. *(From Waller BF: Rheumatic and nonrheumatic conditions producing valvular heart disease. Cardiovasc Clin 16:30, 1986.)*

(i.e., LV compliance is often increased; see Fig. 66-10). In more severe cases of AR, the regurgitant flow may exceed 20 liters/min, so the total LV output at rest approaches 25 liters/min, a level that can be achieved acutely only by a trained endurance runner during maximal exercise. Thus, the adaptive response to gradually increasing, chronic AR permits the ventricle to function as an effective high-compliance pump, handling a large stroke volume, often with little increase in filling pressure. During exercise, peripheral vascular resistance declines and, with an increase in heart rate, diastole shortens and the regurgitation per beat decreases, facilitating an increment in effective (forward) cardiac output without substantial increases in end-diastolic volume and pressure. The ejection fraction and related ejection phase indices are often within normal limits, both at rest and during exercise, even though myocardial function, as reflected in the slope of the end-systolic pressure-volume relationship, is depressed.

LEFT VENTRICULAR FUNCTION. As the left ventricle decompensates, interstitial fibrosis increases, compliance declines, and LV end-diastolic pressure and volume rise (see Fig. 66-10). In advanced stages of decompensation, left atrial, pulmonary artery wedge, pulmonary arterial, right

ventricular (RV), and right atrial pressures rise and the effective (forward) cardiac output falls, at first during exercise and then at rest. The normal decline in end-systolic volume or the rise in ejection fraction fails to occur during exercise. Symptoms of heart failure develop, particularly those secondary to pulmonary congestion.

MYOCARDIAL ISCHEMIA. When acute AR is induced experimentally, myocardial oxygen requirements rise substantially, secondary to an increase in wall tension. In patients with chronic severe AR, total myocardial oxygen requirements are also augmented by the increase in LV mass. Because the major portion of coronary blood flow occurs during diastole, when arterial pressure is lower than normal in AR, coronary perfusion pressure is reduced. Studies in experimentally induced AR have shown a reduction in coronary flow reserve, with a change in forward coronary flow from diastole to systole. The result—a combination of increased oxygen demands and reduced supply—sets the stage for the development of myocardial ischemia, especially during exercise. Thus, patients with severe AR exhibit a reduction of coronary reserve, which may be responsible for myocardial ischemia and which may in turn play a role in the deterioration of LV function.

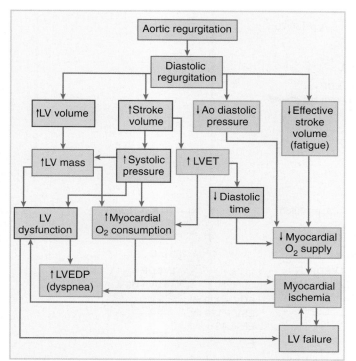

and femoral arteries than in the carotid arteries. A variety of auscultatory findings provide confirmation of a wide pulse pressure. The Traube sign (also known as pistol shot sounds) refers to booming systolic and diastolic sounds heard over the femoral artery, the Müller sign consists of systolic pulsations of the uvula, and the Duroziez sign consists of a systolic murmur heard over the femoral artery when it is compressed proximally and a diastolic murmur when it is compressed distally. Capillary pulsations (the Quincke sign) can be detected by transmitting a light through the patient's fingertips or exerting gentle pressure on the tip of a fingernail.

Systolic arterial pressure is elevated, and diastolic pressure is abnormally low. Korotkoff sounds often persist to zero even though the intra-arterial pressure rarely falls below 30 mm Hg. The point of change in Korotkoff sounds (i.e., the muffling of these sounds in phase IV) correlates with the diastolic pressure. As heart failure develops, peripheral vasoconstriction may occur and arterial diastolic pressure may rise, even though severe AR is present. The Hill sign (an exaggerated difference in systolic blood pressure between the upper and lower extremities) is an artifact of sphygmomanometric measurements and is no longer considered a sign of severe AR.

The apical impulse is diffuse and hyperdynamic and is displaced laterally and inferiorly; there may be systolic retraction over the parasternal region. A rapid ventricular filling wave is often palpable at the apex. The augmented stroke volume may create a systolic thrill at the base of the heart or suprasternal notch, and over the carotid arteries. In many patients, a carotid shudder is palpable.

AUSCULTATION. The aortic regurgitant murmur, the principal physical finding of AR, is high frequency and begins immediately after A_2. It may be distinguished from the murmur of pulmonic regurgitation by its earlier onset (i.e., immediately after A_2 rather than after P_2) and usually by the presence of a widened pulse pressure. The murmur is heard best with the diaphragm of the stethoscope while the patient is sitting up and leaning forward, with the breath held in deep exhalation. In severe AR, the murmur reaches an early peak and then has a dominant decrescendo pattern throughout diastole.

The severity of AR correlates better with the duration than with the intensity of the murmur. In mild AR, the murmur may be limited to early diastole and is typically high-pitched and blowing. In severe AR, the murmur is holodiastolic and may have a rough quality. When the murmur is musical (cooing dove murmur), it usually signifies eversion or perforation of an aortic cusp. In patients with severe AR and LV decompensation, equilibration of aortic and LV pressures in late diastole abolishes the late diastolic component of the regurgitant murmur. When regurgitation is caused by primary valvular disease, the diastolic murmur is heard best along the left sternal border in the third and fourth intercostal spaces. However, when it is caused mainly by dilation of the ascending aorta, the murmur is often more readily audible along the right sternal border.

Many patients with chronic AR have a harsh systolic outflow murmur caused by the increased total LV stroke volume and ejection rate, which often radiates to the carotid vessels. The systolic murmur is often more readily audible than the diastolic murmur. It may be higher pitched and less rasping than the murmur of AS but is often accompanied by a systolic thrill. Palpation of the carotid pulses will elucidate the cause of the systolic murmur and differentiate it from the murmur of AS.

A_2 may be normal or accentuated when AR is caused by disease of the aortic root but is soft or absent when the valve is causing AR. P_2 may be obscured by the early diastolic murmur. Thus, S_2 may be absent or single or exhibit narrow or paradoxical splitting. A systolic ejection sound, presumably related to abrupt distention of the aorta by the augmented stroke volume, is frequently audible. A third heart sound (S_3) correlates with an increased LV end-diastolic volume. Its development may be a sign of impaired LV function, which is useful in identifying patients with severe AR who are candidates for surgical treatment.

A mid-diastolic and late diastolic apical rumble, the Austin Flint murmur, is common in severe AR and may occur in the presence of a normal mitral valve. This murmur appears to be created by severe aortic reflux impinging on the anterior leaflet of the mitral valve or the free LV wall; there is no convincing evidence for obstruction to mitral inflow in these patients.

ECHOCARDIOGRAPHY. Echocardiography (see Chap. 15) is helpful in identifying the cause of AR (see Figs. 15-48 and 15-49) and may demonstrate a bicuspid valve, thickening of the valve cusps, other

FIGURE 66-9 Pathophysiology of aortic regurgitation. Aortic regurgitation results in an increased LV volume, increased stroke volume, increased aortic (Ao) systolic pressure, and decreased effective stroke volume. Increased LV volume results in an increased LV mass, which may lead to LV dysfunction and failure. Increased LV stroke volume increases systolic pressure and prolongation of LV ejection time (LVET). Increased LV systolic pressure results in a decrease in diastolic time. Decreased diastolic time (myocardial perfusion time), diastolic aortic pressure, and effective stroke volume reduce myocardial O_2 supply. Increased myocardial O_2 consumption and decreased myocardial O_2 supply produce myocardial ischemia, which further deteriorates LV function. LVEDP = LV end-diastolic pressure. (From Boudoulas H, Gravanis MB: Valvular heart disease. In Gravanis MB [ed]: Cardiovascular Disorders: Pathogenesis and Pathophysiology. St. Louis, CV Mosby, 1993, p 64.)

Clinical Presentation

SYMPTOMS. In patients with chronic severe AR, the left ventricle gradually enlarges while the patient remains asymptomatic.[83,91] Symptoms of reduced cardiac reserve or myocardial ischemia develop, most often in the fourth or fifth decade and usually only after considerable cardiomegaly and myocardial dysfunction have occurred. The principal complaints of exertional dyspnea, orthopnea, and paroxysmal nocturnal dyspnea usually develop gradually. Angina pectoris is prominent late in the course; nocturnal angina may be troublesome and is often accompanied by diaphoresis, which occurs when the heart rate slows and arterial diastolic pressure falls to extremely low levels. Patients with severe AR often complain of an uncomfortable awareness of the heartbeat, especially on lying down, and disagreeable thoracic pain caused by pounding of the heart against the chest wall. Tachycardia, occurring with emotional stress or exertion, may cause troubling palpitations and head pounding. Premature ventricular contractions are particularly distressing because of the great heave of the volume-loaded left ventricle during the postextrasystolic beat. These complaints may be present for many years before symptoms of overt LV dysfunction develop.

Physical Examination

In patients with chronic, severe AR, the head may bob with each heartbeat (de Musset sign), and there are water hammer pulses, with abrupt distention and quick collapse (Corrigan pulse). The arterial pulse is often prominent and can be best appreciated by palpation of the radial artery with the patient's arm elevated (see Chap. 12). A bisferiens pulse may be present and is more readily recognized in the brachial

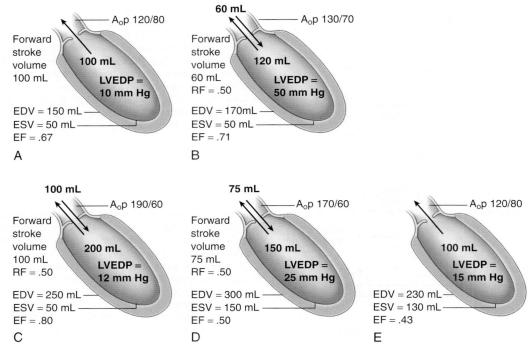

FIGURE 66-10 Hemodynamics of aortic regurgitation. **A,** Normal conditions. **B,** The hemodynamic changes that occur in severe acute aortic regurgitation. Although total stroke volume is increased, forward stroke volume is reduced. Left ventricular end-diastolic pressure (LVEDP) rises dramatically. **C,** Hemodynamic changes occurring in chronic compensated aortic regurgitation are shown. Eccentric hypertrophy produces increased end-diastolic volume (EDV), which permits an increase in total, as well as forward, stroke volume. The volume overload is accommodated, and left ventricular filling pressure is normalized. Ventricular emptying and end-systolic volume (ESV) remain normal. **D,** In chronic decompensated aortic regurgitation, impaired left ventricular emptying produces an increase in end-systolic volume and a fall in ejection fraction (EF), total stroke volume, and forward stroke volume. There is further cardiac dilation and reelevation of left ventricular filling pressure. **E,** Immediately following valve replacement, preload estimated by EDV decreases, as does filling pressure. ESV also is decreased, but to a lesser extent. The result is an initial fall in EF. Despite these changes, elimination of regurgitation leads to an increase in forward stroke volume, and with time ejection fraction increases. Aop = aortic pressure; RF = regurgitant fraction. *(From Carabello BA: Aortic regurgitation: Hemodynamic determinants of prognosis. In Cohn LH, DiSesa VJ [eds]: Aortic Regurgitation: Medical and Surgical Management. New York, Marcel Dekker, 1986, p 99-101.)*

congenital abnormalities, prolapse of the valve, a flail leaflet, or vegetation. In addition to leaflet anatomy and motion, the size and shape of the aortic root can be evaluated, although visualization of the ascending aorta is not always adequate and may require additional imaging procedures. Transthoracic imaging is usually satisfactory, but transesophageal echocardiography (TEE) often provides more detail, particularly of the aortic root.

Transthoracic echocardiography is useful for the measurement of LV end-diastolic and end-systolic dimensions and volumes, ejection fraction, and mass.[36] Two-dimensional guided M-mode measurements of LV dimensions are recommended when possible, because the high temporal resolution of this modality allows more accurate identification of endocardial borders. Care is needed to ensure that measurements are not oblique and are at the same site on subsequent studies. When the M-line is oblique, two-dimensional measurements are made in conjunction with the calculation of biplane ventricular end-diastolic and end-systolic volumes. Recent studies have suggested that end-systolic volume is a strong predictor of adverse clinical outcomes.[92,93] These measurements, when made serially, are of great value in selecting the optimal time for surgical intervention.

High-frequency fluttering of the anterior leaflet of the mitral valve during diastole may be seen in acute and chronic AR. However, it does not develop when the mitral valve is rigid, as occurs with rheumatic involvement. This sign, unlike the Austin Flint murmur, occurs even in mild AR and results from the movement imparted to the anterior leaflet of the mitral valve by the jet of blood regurgitating from the aorta.

Doppler echocardiography and color flow Doppler imaging are the most sensitive and accurate noninvasive techniques for the diagnosis

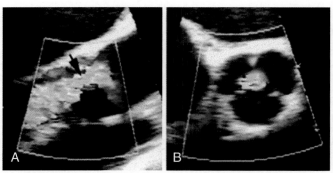

FIGURE 66-11 Transesophageal color Doppler imaging of the aortic regurgitant jet. **A,** Long-axis view. The black arrow indicates the vena contracta, the narrowest portion of the jet located at or just distal to its orifice. The width (in millimeters) of the vena contracta correlates well with volumetric measurement of regurgitant fraction and regurgitant volume. **B,** Short-axis view in the same patient. *(From Willett DL, Hall SA, Jessen ME, et al: Assessment of aortic regurgitation by transesophageal color Doppler imaging of the vena contracta: Validation against an intraoperative aortic flow probe. J Am Coll Cardiol 37:1450, 2001.)*

and evaluation of AR. They readily detect mild degrees of AR that may be inaudible on physical examination. Both the aortic regurgitant orifice size and aortic regurgitant flow can be estimated quantitatively (**Fig. 66-11;** see Figs. 15-48 and 15-49)[36,94] and are strongly recommended.[1] These quantitative data provide the basis for the definitions of mild, moderate, and severe AR (see Table 66-1). Serial studies permit determination of the progression of AR and its effect on the left ventricle.

OTHER DIAGNOSTIC EVALUATION MODALITIES

Electrocardiography. Chronic severe AR results in left axis deviation and a pattern of LV diastolic volume overload, characterized by an increase in initial forces (prominent Q waves in leads I, aVL, and V_3 through V_6) and a relatively small wave in lead V_1. With the passage of time, these initial forces diminish, but the total QRS amplitude increases. The T waves may be tall and upright in the left precordial leads early in the course, but more commonly they are inverted, with ST-segment depressions. An LV strain pattern correlates with the presence of dilation and hypertrophy (see Chap. 13). Intraventricular conduction defects occur late in the course and are usually associated with LV dysfunction. The electrocardiogram (ECG) is not an accurate predictor of the severity of AR or cardiac weight. When AR is caused by an inflammatory process, prolongation of the PR interval may be present.

Radiography. Cardiac size is a function of the duration and severity of regurgitation and the state of LV function (see Fig. 16-22). In acute AR, there may be minimal cardiac enlargement, but marked enlargement is a common finding in chronic AR. Typically, the left ventricle enlarges in an inferior and leftward direction, causing a significant increase in the long axis but sometimes causing little or no increase in the transverse diameter of the heart. Calcification of the aortic valve is uncommon in patients with isolated AR but is often present in patients with combined AS and AR. Distinct left atrial enlargement in the absence of heart failure suggests associated mitral valve disease. Aneurysmal dilation of the aorta suggests that aortic root disease (e.g., the Marfan syndrome, cystic medial necrosis, annuloaortic ectasia) is responsible for the AR. Linear calcifications in the wall of the ascending aorta are seen in syphilitic aortitis but are nonspecific and are also observed in degenerative disease.

Angiography. For angiographic assessment of AR, contrast material should be injected rapidly (i.e., 25 to 35 mL/sec) into the aortic root, and filming should be carried out in the right and left anterior oblique projections (see Chap. 20). Opacification may be improved by filming during a Valsalva maneuver. In acute AR, there is only a slight increase in LV end-diastolic volume but, with the passage of time, both the end-diastolic volume and thickness of the LV wall increase, usually in parallel.[87]

Cardiac Magnetic Resonance Imaging. CMR provides accurate measurements of regurgitant volumes and the regurgitant orifice in AR (see Fig. 18-20). It is the most accurate noninvasive technique for assessing LV end-systolic volume, diastolic volume, and mass (see Chap. 18). CMR accurately quantifies the severity of AR on the basis of the antegrade and retrograde flow volumes in the ascending aorta and is recommended when echocardiographic evaluation of regurgitation is suboptimal.[41,95]

Disease Course

NATURAL HISTORY OF CHRONIC AORTIC REGURGITATION. Moderately severe or even severe chronic AR often is associated with a generally favorable prognosis for many years. Quantitative measures of AR severity predict clinical outcome, and LV size and systolic function also are strong predictors of clinical outcome. In a study of 251 asymptomatic patients (mean age, 61 years), the 10-year survival was 94% ± 4% in those with mild AR, compared with 69% ± 9% in those with severe AR (**Fig. 66-12**).[94] In contrast, in series involving younger asymptomatic patients (mean age, 39 years) with severe AR and normal LV ejection fractions, the mortality rate was less than 1%/year[1,91] and more than 45% remained asymptomatic with normal LV function at 10 years. The average rate of developing symptoms or LV systolic dysfunction in these latter series was less than 6%/year (**Fig. 66-13** and **Table 66-5**).

However, as is the case for AS, once the patient becomes symptomatic, the downhill course becomes rapidly progressive. Congestive heart failure, punctuated by episodes of acute pulmonary edema, and sudden death may occur, usually in previously symptomatic patients who have considerable LV dilation. Data compiled in the presurgical

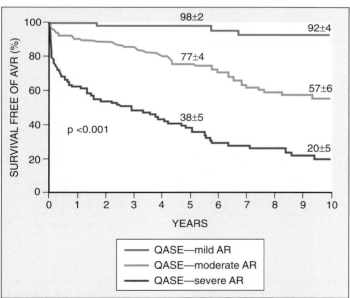

FIGURE 66-12 Composite end point of survival free of surgery for AR after diagnosis in asymptomatic patients. Patients are stratified according to quantitative criteria of the American Society of Echocardiography (QASE AR grading). The QASE-severe AR is defined as RV > 60 mL/beat or effective regurgitant orifice (ERO) > 30 mm² (red line). The QASE-mild AR is defined as RV < 30 mL/beat and ERO < 10 mm² (blue line) and QASE-moderate AR (yellow line) as larger than mild (RV, 30 mL/beat, or ERO, 10 mm²), but not reaching QASE-severe criteria. The 5- and 10-year rates of the endpoint ± standard error are indicated. Note the wide difference in outcome according to QASE grading at baseline. *(From Detaint D, Messika-Zeitoun D, Maalouf J, et al: Quantitative echocardiographic determinants of clinical outcome in asymptomatic patients with aortic regurgitation: A prospective study. J Am Coll Cardiol Img 1:1, 2008.)*

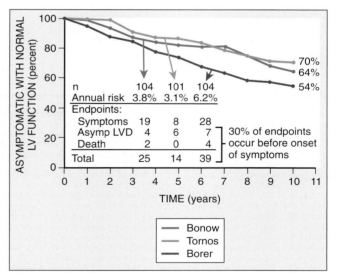

FIGURE 66-13 Natural history of chronic asymptomatic aortic regurgitation in patients with normal LV ejection fraction at rest in three series reported by Bonow and associates (blue line), Tornos and associates (yellow line), and Borer and colleagues (red line), each enrolling more than 100 patients. At 10 years, 54% to 70% of patients remained asymptomatic with normal LV function, such that the risk of developing symptoms, LV dysfunction (LVD), or death is approximately 3% to 6%/year. The endpoints encountered in these series are indicated. Most patients who deteriorated developed symptoms leading to aortic valve replacement. However, 25% to 30% of the endpoints, either asymptomatic LVD (Asymp LVD) or death, occurred without warning symptoms. *(Modified from Bonow RO, Lakatos E, Maron BJ, et al: Serial long-term assessment of the natural history of asymptomatic patients with chronic aortic regurgitation and normal left ventricular systolic function. Circulation 84:1625, 1991; Tornos MP, Olona M, Permanyer-Miralda G, et al: Clinical outcome of severe asymptomatic chronic aortic regurgitation: A long term prospective follow up study. Am Heart J 130:333, 1995; and Borer JS, Hochreiter C, Herrold EM, et al: Prediction of indications for valve replacement among asymptomatic and minimally symptomatic patients with chronic aortic regurgitation and normal left ventricular performance. Circulation 97:525, 1998.)*

TABLE 66-5 Studies of the Natural History of Asymptomatic Aortic Regurgitation

STUDY (YEAR)	Progression to Symptoms, Death, or LV Dysfunction			Progression to Asymptomatic LV Dysfunction		MORTALITY (NO. OF PATIENTS)	COMMENTS
	NO. OF PATIENTS	MEAN FOLLOW-UP (yr)	RATE/ yr (%)	NO. OF PATIENTS	RATE/ yr (%)		
Bonow et al (1983, 1991)	104	8.0	3.8	4	0.5	2	Outcome predicted by LV ESD, EDD, change in EF with exercise, rate of change in ESD and EF at rest with time
Scognamiglio et al (1986)*	30	4.7	2.1	3	2.1	0	Three patients developing asymptomatic LV dysfunction initially had lower PAP/ESV ratios and trend toward higher LV ESD and EDD and lower FS.
Siemienczuk et al (1989)	50	3.7	4.0	1	0.5	0	Patients included those receiving placebo and medical dropouts in a randomized drug trial; included some patients with NYHA FC II symptoms; outcome predicted by LV ESV, EDV, change in EF with exercise, and end-systolic wall stress
Scognamiglio et al (1994)*	74	6.0	5.7	15	3.4	0	All patients received digoxin as part of a randomized trial.
Tornos et al (1995)	101	4.6	3.0	6	1.3	0	Outcome predicted by pulse pressure, LV ESD, EDD, and EF at rest
Ishii et al (1996)	27	14.2	3.6	—	—	0	Development of symptoms predicted by systolic BP, LV ESD, EDD, mass index, and wall thickness; LV function not reported in all patients
Borer et al (1998)	104	7.3	6.2	7	0.9	4	20% of patients in NYHA FC II; outcome predicted by initial FC II symptoms, change in LV EF with exercise, LV ESD, and LV FS
Tarasoutchi et al (2003)	72	10	4.7	1	0.1	0	Development of symptoms predicted by LV ESD and EDD; LV function not reported in all patients
Evangelista et al (2005)	31	7	3.6	—	—	1	Placebo control group in 7-year vasodilator clinical trial
Detaint et al (2008)	251	8.0	5.0	17	2.1	33	10-year actuarial survival free of AVR: 92 ± 4% with mild AR (RV <30 mL and ERO < 0.1cm^2) 57 ± 5% with moderate AR 20 ± 5% with severe AR (RV ≥ 60 mL and ERO ≥ 0.3 cm^2)

*Two studies by same authors involved separate patient groups.

BP = blood pressure, EDD = end-diastolic dimension; EDV = end-diastolic volume; EF = ejection fraction; ESD = end-systolic dimension; ESV = end-systolic volume; FC = functional class; FS = fractional shortening; PAP = pulmonary artery pressure.

Modified from Bonow RO, Carabello BA, Chatterjee K, et al: ACC/AHA 2006 guidelines for the management of patients with valvular heart disease: A report of the American College of Cardiology/American Heart Association Task Force on Practice Guidelines (writing Committee to Revise the 1998 guidelines for the management of patients with valvular heart disease) developed in collaboration with the Society of Cardiovascular Anesthesiologists endorsed by the Society for Cardiovascular Angiography and Interventions and the Society of Thoracic Surgeons. J Am Coll Cardiol 48:e1, 2006

Data from Bonow RO, Rosing DR, McIntosh CL, et al: The natural history of asymptomatic patients with aortic regurgitation and normal left ventricular function. Circulation 68:509,1983; Bonow RO, Lakatos E, Maron BJ, Epstein SE: Serial long-term assessment of the natural history of asymptomatic patients with chronic aortic regurgitation and normal left ventricular systolic function. Circulation 84:1625, 1991; Scognamiglio R, Fasoli G, Dalla Volta S: Progression of myocardial dysfunction in asymptomatic patients with severe aortic insufficiency. Clin Cardiol 9:151, 1986; Siemienczuk D, Greenberg B, Morris C, et al: Chronic aortic insufficiency: Factors associated with progression to aortic valve replacement. Ann Intern Med 110:587, 1989; Scognamiglio R, Rahimtoola SH, Fasoli G, et al: Nifedipine in asymptomatic patients with severe aortic regurgitation and normal left ventricular function. N Engl J Med 331:689, 1994; Tornos MP, Olona M, Permanyer Miralda G, et al: Clinical outcome of severe asymptomatic chronic aortic regurgitation: A long-term prospective follow-up study. Am Heart J 130:333; 1995; Ishii K, Hirota Y, Suwa M, et al: Natural history and left ventricular response in chronic aortic regurgitation. Am J Cardiol 78:357, 1996; Borer JS, Hochreiter C, Herrold EM, et al: Prediction of indications for valve replacement among asymptomatic or minimally symptomatic patients with chronic aortic regurgitation and normal left ventricular performance. Circulation 97:525, 1998; Tarasoutchi F, Grinberg M, Spina GS, et al: Ten-year clinical laboratory follow-up after application of a symptom-based therapeutic strategy to patients with severe chronic aortic regurgitation of predominant rheumatic etiology. J Am Coll Cardiol 41:1316, 2003; Evangelista A, Tornos P, Sambola A, et al: Long-term vasodilator therapy in patients with severe aortic regurgitation. N Engl J Med 353:1342, 2005; Detaint D, Messika-Zeitoun D, Maalouf J, et al: Quantitative echocardiographic determinants of clinical outcome in asymptomatic patients with aortic regurgitation: a prospective study. J Am Coll Cardiol Img 1:1, 2008.

era indicated that without surgical treatment, death usually occurred within 4 years after the development of angina pectoris and within 2 years after the onset of heart failure. Even in the current era, 4-year survival without surgery in patients with NYHA Class III or IV symptoms is only approximately 30% (**Fig. 66-14**).

Gradual deterioration of LV function may occur even during the asymptomatic period, and some patients may develop significant impairment of systolic function before the onset of symptoms. Numerous surgical series over the past two decades have indicated that depressed LV ejection fraction is among the most important determinants of mortality after AVR, particularly when LV dysfunction is irreversible and does not improve after operation.[1,2] LV dysfunction is more likely to be reversible if detected early, before ejection fraction

becomes severely depressed, before the left ventricle becomes markedly dilated, and before significant symptoms develop. It is therefore important to intervene surgically before these changes have become irreversible.[30a,85,91]

Management

MEDICAL TREATMENT. There is no specific therapy to prevent disease progression in chronic AR. Patients with mild or moderate AR who are asymptomatic with normal or only minimally increased cardiac size require no therapy but should be followed clinically and by echocardiography every 12 or 24 months. Asymptomatic patients with chronic severe AR and normal LV function should be examined at intervals of approximately 6 months. In addition to clinical

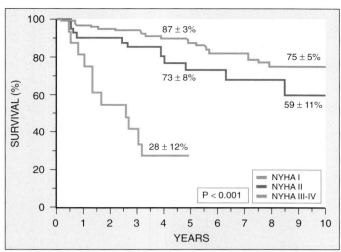

FIGURE 66-14 Survival without surgery in 242 patients with chronic aortic regurgitation, demonstrating the importance of symptoms in determining outcome. Patients with NYHA Class III or IV symptoms had a survival of only 28% at 4 years. In contrast, the 10-year survival in patients in Class I was 75%, which was identical to that of an age-matched normal population (75% at 10 years). *(From Dujardin KS, Enriquez-Sarano M, Schaff HV, et al: Mortality and morbidity of aortic regurgitation in clinical practice: A long-term follow-up study. Circulation 99:1851, 1999.)*

examination, serial echocardiographic assessments of LV size and ejection fraction should be made. CMR imaging is usually not necessary but may be useful for patients whose noninvasive test results are inconclusive or discordant with clinical findings or when further evaluation of aortic size is needed (see Fig 18-20). Patients with mild to moderate AR and those with severe AR with a normal ejection fraction and only mild ventricular dilation may engage in aerobic forms of exercise. However, patients with AR who have limitations of cardiac reserve and/or evidence of declining LV function should not engage in vigorous sports or heavy exertion.[54] Systemic arterial diastolic hypertension, if present, should be treated because it increases the regurgitant flow; vasodilating agents such as nifedipine or ACE inhibitors are preferred, and beta-blocking agents should be used with great caution. AF and bradyarrhythmias are poorly tolerated and should be prevented, if possible. If these arrhythmias occur, they must be treated promptly and vigorously. Recommendations for antibiotic prophylaxis for infective endocarditis have changed recently, and most patients with AR do not need prophylaxis (see Chap. 67).

Vasodilator Therapy. There is considerable uncertainty about whether patients with chronic AR and evidence of significant volume overload (increased end-diastolic dimension or volume) should be considered for vasodilator therapy.[96] Short-term studies spanning 6 months to 2 years have demonstrated beneficial hemodynamic effects of oral hydralazine, nifedipine, felodipine, and ACE inhibitors. One randomized study followed asymptomatic patients with severe AR for 6 years, comparing the effects of long-acting nifedipine (69 patients) and digoxin (74 patients) on LV function and symptoms. Nifedipine delayed the need for operation: at 6 years, 85% of patients receiving nifedipine remained asymptomatic, with a normal LV ejection fraction, compared with only 65% of patients receiving digoxin. However, a second randomized trial compared placebo, long-acting nifedipine, and enalapril in 95 consecutive patients who were followed for 7 years.[97] Neither nifedipine nor enalapril reduced the development of symptoms or LV dysfunction warranting AVR compared with placebo. Moreover, neither drug significantly altered LV dimension, ejection fraction, or mass over the course of time compared with placebo. In view of this equipoise, definitive recommendations regarding the indications for long-active nifedipine or ACE inhibitors are not possible.[1]

Symptomatic Patients

AVR is the treatment of choice for symptomatic patients. Chronic medical therapy may be necessary for some patients who refuse surgery or are considered to be inoperable because of comorbid conditions. These patients should receive an aggressive heart failure regimen (see Chap. 28) with ACE inhibitors (and perhaps other vasodilators), digoxin, diuretics, and salt restriction; beta blockers may also be beneficial.[98] Even though nitroglycerin and other nitrates are not as helpful in relieving anginal pain in patients with AR as they are in patients with coronary artery disease or AS, they are worth a try.

In patients who are candidates for surgery but who have severely decompensated LV dysfunction, vasodilator therapy may be particularly helpful in stabilizing patients while preparing for operation.

SURGICAL TREATMENT

Indications for Operation

Because of their excellent prognosis in the short and medium term, operative correction should be deferred in patients with chronic severe AR who are asymptomatic, have good exercise tolerance, and have an ejection fraction greater than 50% without severe LV dilation (i.e., end-diastolic diameter ≤75 mm; end-systolic diameter ≤55 mm) or progressive LV dilation on serial echocardiograms. In the absence of obvious contraindications or serious comorbidity, surgical treatment is advisable for symptomatic patients with severe AR and for asymptomatic patients with an ejection fraction of 50% or less, severe LV dilation (end-diastolic diameter > 75 mm or end-systolic diameter > 55 mm) or less severe dilation (end-diastolic diameter > 70 mm or end-systolic diameter > 50 mm), with evidence of progressive LV enlargement on serial echocardiograms.[1] Between these two ends of the clinical-hemodynamic spectrum are many patients in whom it may be difficult to balance the immediate risks of operation and the continuing risks of an implanted prosthetic valve, on the one hand, against the hazards of allowing a severe volume overload to damage the left ventricle, on the other.[85,90,91]

A proposed management strategy for patients with chronic severe AR is shown in **Figure 66-15**. Because severe symptoms (NYHA Class III or IV) and LV dysfunction with an ejection fraction less than 50% are independent risk factors for poor postoperative survival (**Fig. 66-16**), surgery should be carried out in NYHA Class II patients before severe LV dysfunction has developed.[1,2,83,92] Even after successful correction of AR, patients with severe LV dysfunction may have persistent cardiomegaly and depressed LV function. Such patients often exhibit persistent histologic changes in the left ventricle, including massive fiber hypertrophy and increased interstitial fibrous tissue. Therefore, it is highly desirable to operate on patients before irreversible LV changes have occurred.

Because AR has complex effects on preload and afterload, the selection of appropriate indices of ventricular contractility to identify patients for operation is challenging. The relationship between end-systolic wall stress and ejection fraction or percentage fractional shortening is a useful measurement,[35] as are more load-independent measures of LV contractility. However, in the absence of such complex measurements, serial changes in ventricular end-diastolic and end-systolic volumes or dimensions can be used to detect the relative deterioration of ventricular function.[90] Although LV end-diastolic volume and ejection phase indices (e.g., ejection fraction, ventricular fraction shortening) are strongly influenced by loading conditions, they are nonetheless useful empirical predictors of postoperative function.

Serial echocardiograms should be obtained to detect changes in LV size and function in asymptomatic patients with severe AR (see Fig. 66-15). Impaired LV function at rest is the basis for selecting patients for operation; normal LV function at rest with failure of the ejection fraction to rise normally with exercise is not considered an indication for surgery per se, but is an early warning sign that portends impaired function at rest. Echocardiographic measurements of LV size also are important, with M-mode LV end-diastolic and end-systolic dimensions, when possible, and with biplane apical calculations of the end-systolic volume index. Echocardiographic measurements should be made with side-by-side comparison of previous serial studies. A consistent change in dimensions or volumes, greater than measurement variability, must be ensured before recommending AVR for asymptomatic patients on the basis of these numbers alone.

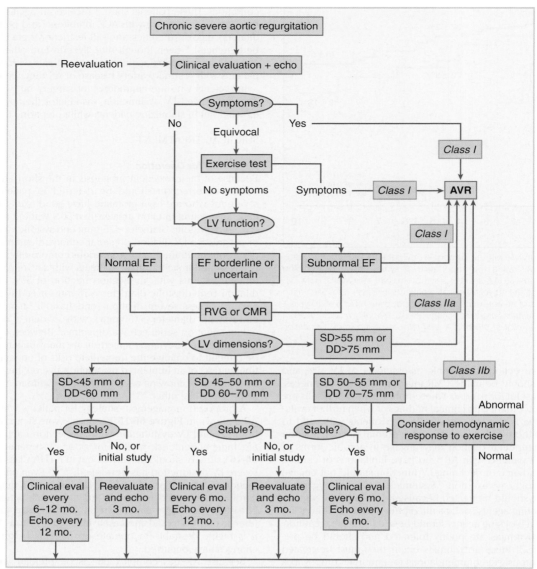

FIGURE 66-15 Management strategy for patients with chronic severe aortic regurgitation. Preoperative coronary angiography should be performed routinely as determined by age, symptoms, and coronary risk factors. Cardiac catheterization and angiography may also be helpful when there is discordance between clinical findings and echocardiography. "Stable" refers to stable echocardiographic measurements. In some centers, serial follow-up may be performed with radionuclide ventriculography (RVG) or CMR rather than echocardiography to assess LV volume and systolic function. DD = end-diastolic dimension; EF = ejection fraction; SD = end-systolic dimension. *(From Bonow RO, Carabello BA, Chatterjee K, et al: ACC/AHA 2006 guidelines for the management of patients with valvular heart disease: A report of the American College of Cardiology/American Heart Association Task Force on Practice Guidelines [writing committee to revise the 1998 Guidelines for the Management of Patients With Valvular Heart Disease]. Circulation 114:e84, 2006.)*

Asymptomatic patients with severe AR but normal LV function have an excellent prognosis and do not warrant prophylactic operation (see Table 66-5). On average, less than 6% of patients/year require operation because of the development of symptoms or of LV dysfunction (see Fig. 66-13), although the rate of symptom development is higher in patients older than 60 years.[94] The LV end-systolic dimension determined by echocardiography is valuable in predicting outcome in asymptomatic patients. Patients with severe AR and an end-systolic diameter less than 40 mm almost invariably remain stable and can be followed without immediate surgery. However, patients with an end-systolic diameter more than 50 mm have a 19% likelihood/year of developing symptoms of LV dysfunction, and those with an end-systolic diameter more than 55 mm have an increased risk of irreversible LV dysfunction if they are not operated on. Postoperative function and survival in this latter group is determined by the severity of symptoms, severity of LV dysfunction, and duration of LV dysfunction.[83,91] Indexed end-systolic dimension or volume (ESVI) may be a more robust indicator for timing of surgical intervention.[93,94] Patients with an ESVI ≥45 mL/m² are at higher risk of adverse outcomes.[94] Further data on the use of ESVI is needed before this approach becomes standard.

In summary, the following considerations apply to the selection of patients with chronic AR for surgical treatment.[1] Operation should be deferred in asymptomatic patients with normal and stable LV function and should be recommended for symptomatic patients (see Fig 66-15). In asymptomatic patients with LV dysfunction, a decision should be based not on a single abnormal measurement but rather on several observations of depressed performance and impaired exercise tolerance, carried out at intervals of 2 to 4 months. If evidence of LV dysfunction is borderline or inconsistent, continued close follow-up is indicated. If abnormalities are progressive and consistent (i.e., LV ejection fraction ≤ 50%, LV end-systolic diameter rises to >55 mm, or LV end-diastolic dimension rises to >75 mm), operation should be strongly considered, even in asymptomatic patients. It is also

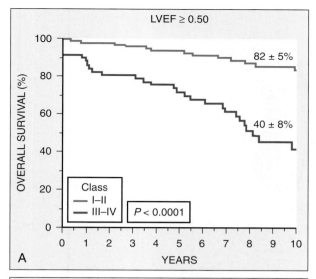

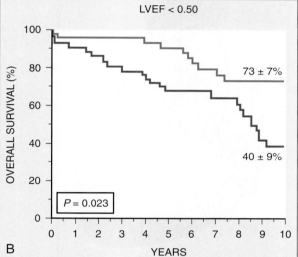

FIGURE 66-16 Long-term postoperative survival in patients with aortic regurgitation, stratified according to the severity of preoperative symptoms and preoperative left ventricular ejection fraction (LVEF). Patients with NYHA Class III or IV symptoms experienced significantly worse survival than those with Class I or II symptoms whether the echocardiographic LVEF was higher than 0.50 **(A)** or less than 0.50 **(B)** without associated coronary artery disease. *(From Klodas E, Enriquez-Sarano M, Tajik AJ, et al: Optimizing timing of surgical correction in patients with severe aortic regurgitation: Role of symptoms. J Am Coll Cardiol 30:746, 1997.)*

reasonable to consider AVR at lower levels of LV dilation (end-systolic dimension >50 mm; end-diastolic dimension >70 mm) in patients with progressive LV dilation on serial imaging studies. Symptomatic patients with severe AR who have normal, mildly depressed, or moderately depressed LV function should be operated on. Patients with severely impaired LV function (ejection fraction < 25%) are at high surgical risk and have a guarded prognosis, even after successful AVR. However, their outlook is also extremely poor when they receive medical therapy alone, and their management should be considered on an individual basis.

The indications for surgery for patients with severe AR secondary to aortic root disease are similar to those for patients with primary valvular disease. However, progressive expansion of the aortic root and/or a diameter more than 50 mm by echocardiography with any degree of regurgitation in patients with a bicuspid valve (or other connective tissue disorder) or with a diameter more than 55 mm in other patients is also an indication for aortic root replacement surgery.[1,98a]

As is the case for patients with other valvular lesions, adult surgical candidates who may have underlying coronary artery disease, based on symptoms, age, gender, and risk factors, should undergo preoperative coronary arteriography. Those with coronary artery stenoses should undergo revascularization at the time of AVR.

Operative Procedures

The standard surgical approach for chronic AR is valve replacement. Concurrent aortic root replacement is performed when aortic dilation is the cause or accompanies valve dysfunction. However, there is growing experience with surgical aortic valve repair, which is a viable option for selected patients in experienced centers.[99,100] Occasionally, when a leaflet has been torn from its attachments to the aortic annulus by trauma, surgical repair may be possible and, in patients with AR secondary to prolapse of an aortic leaflet, aortic cusp resuspension or cusp resection may be used. When AR is caused by leaflet perforation resulting from healed infective endocarditis, a pericardial patch can be used for repair. However, unlike patients with chronic MR, the large majority of patients with pure AR will require AVR rather than repair.

Because an increasing proportion of patients with severe isolated AR coming to operation now have primary aortic root rather than primary valvular disease, an increasing number can be treated surgically by correcting the dilated aortic root.[100,101] Aneurysmal dilation of the ascending aorta requires excision, replacement with a graft that includes a prosthetic valve, and reimplantation of the coronary arteries. In some patients with aortic root disease, the native valve can be spared when the aortic root is replaced or repaired (**Fig. 66-17**).

When AVR is performed in patients with severe AR, the aortic annulus often is larger than in patients with AS. Hence, a larger prosthetic valve can be inserted, and mild postoperative obstruction to LV outflow is less of a problem than it is in some patients with AS. In general, the risks and results of AVR in patients with AR are similar to those in patients with AS, with a large percentage of patients exhibiting striking improvement in symptoms. Reductions in heart size and in LV diastolic volume and mass occur in most patients.[90] Exceptions are patients who are in NYHA Class III or IV heart failure and/or patients who have severe LV dysfunction preoperatively. As is true for patients with AS, the operative risk of AVR for patients with AR depends on the general condition of the patient, state of LV function, and skill and experience of the surgical team. The mortality rate ranges from 3% to 8% in most medical centers (see Table 66-3). A late mortality of approximately 5% to 10%/year is observed in survivors who had marked cardiac enlargement and/or prolonged LV dysfunction preoperatively. Follow-up studies have shown both early rapid and then slower long-term reductions of LV mass, ejection fraction, myocyte hypertrophy, and ventricular fibrous content following relief of AR. By extending the indications for operation to symptomatic patients with normal LV function, as well as to asymptomatic patients with LV dysfunction, early and late results are improving. With the continued improvement of surgical techniques and results, it will likely become possible to extend the recommendation for operative treatment to asymptomatic patients with severe AR, normal LV systolic function, and only mild LV dilation. However, given the risks of operation and the long-term complications of presently available prosthetic valves, we do not believe that the time for such a policy has yet arrived.

ACUTE AORTIC REGURGITATION. Acute AR is caused most commonly by infective endocarditis, aortic dissection, or trauma (see Chaps. 60, 67, and 76).[102] The characteristic features of acute AR are tachycardia and an increase in LV diastolic pressures. In contrast to the pathophysiologic events in chronic AR just described, in which the left ventricle can adapt to the increased hemodynamic load, in acute AR the regurgitant volume fills a ventricle of normal size that cannot accommodate the combined large regurgitant volume and inflow from the left atrium. Because the ability of total stroke volume to rise acutely is limited, forward stroke volume declines. The sudden increase in LV filling causes the LV diastolic pressure to rise rapidly above left atrial pressure during early diastole (see Fig. 66-10), causing the mitral valve to close prematurely in diastole. Premature closure of the mitral valve, together with tachycardia that also shortens diastole, reduces the time interval during which the mitral valve is open. The tachycardia may compensate for the reduced forward stroke volume, and the LV and aortic systolic pressures may exhibit little change.

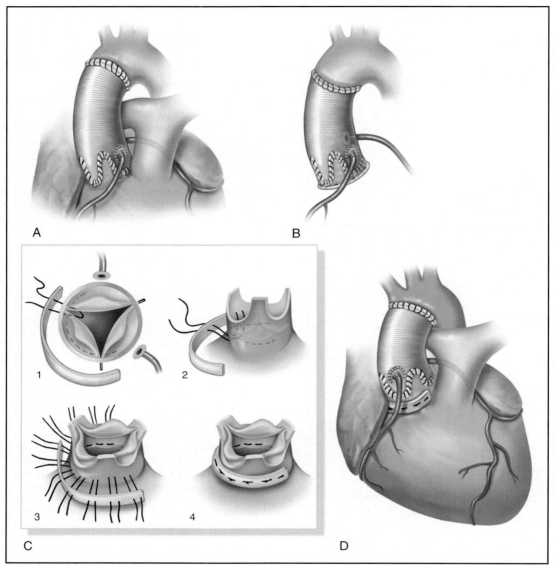

FIGURE 66-17 Repair of aortic regurgitation caused by aortic root dilation. **A,** Remodeling of the aortic root with replacement of all three aortic sinuses. **B,** Reimplantation of the aortic valve in patients with annuloaortic ectasia and aortic root aneurysm. **C, D,** Aortic annuloplasty in patients with annuloaortic ectasia. *(From David TE: Aortic root aneurysms: Remodeling or composite replacement? Ann Thorac Surg 64:1564, 1997.)*

However, acute severe AR may cause profound hypotension and cardiogenic shock. In light of the limited ability of the left ventricle to tolerate acute severe AR, patients with this valvular lesion often develop clinical manifestations of sudden cardiovascular collapse, including weakness, severe dyspnea, and profound hypotension secondary to the reduced stroke volume and elevated left atrial pressure. In some patients, the aortic diastolic pressure equilibrates with the elevated LV diastolic pressure.

PHYSICAL EXAMINATION. Patients with acute severe AR characteristically appear gravely ill, with tachycardia, severe peripheral vasoconstriction, and cyanosis, and sometimes pulmonary congestion and edema. The peripheral signs of AR are often not impressive and certainly not as dramatic as in patients with chronic AR. The normal or only slightly widened pulse pressure may lead to serious underestimation of the severity of the valvular lesion. The LV impulse is normal or almost normal, and the rocking motion of the chest characteristic of chronic AR is not apparent. S_1 may be soft or absent because of premature closure of the mitral valve, and the sound of mitral valve closure in mid or late diastole is occasionally audible. However, closure of the mitral valve may be incomplete, and diastolic MR may occur. Evidence of pulmonary hypertension, with an accentuated P_2, S_3, and S_4, is frequently present.

The early diastolic murmur of acute AR is lower pitched and shorter than that of chronic AR because as LV diastolic pressure rises, the (reverse) pressure gradient between the aorta and left ventricle is rapidly reduced. A systolic murmur is common, resulting in to and fro sounds. The Austin Flint murmur is often present, but is brief and ceases when LV pressure exceeds left atrial pressure in diastole. With premature diastolic closure of the mitral valve, the presystolic portion of the Austin Flint murmur is eliminated.

ECHOCARDIOGRAPHY. In acute AR the echocardiogram reveals a dense, diastolic Doppler signal with an end-diastolic velocity approaching zero and premature closure and delayed opening of the mitral valve. LV size and ejection fraction are normal. This contrasts with the findings in chronic AR, in which end-diastolic dimensions and wall motion are increased. Occasionally, with equilibration of aortic and LV pressures in diastole, premature opening of the aortic valve may be detected.

OTHER DIAGNOSTIC EVALUATION MODALITIES

Electrocardiography. In acute AR, the ECG may or may not show LV hypertrophy, depending on the severity and duration of the regurgitation. However, nonspecific ST-segment and T wave changes are common.

Radiography. In acute AR, there is often evidence of marked pulmonary venous hypertension and pulmonary edema. The cardiac silhouette is usually remarkably normal, although left atrial enlargement may be present and, depending on the cause of the AR, there may be enlargement of the ascending aorta.

MANAGEMENT OF ACUTE AORTIC REGURGITATION. Because early death caused by LV failure is frequent in patients with acute severe AR despite intensive medical management, prompt surgical intervention is indicated. Even a normal ventricle cannot sustain the burden of acute, severe volume overload. Therefore, the risk of acute AR is much greater than that of chronic AR.[1] While the patient is being prepared for surgery, treatment with an intravenous positive inotropic agent (dopamine or dobutamine) and/or a vasodilator (nitroprusside) is often necessary. The agent and dosage should be selected on the basis of arterial pressure (see Chap. 27). Beta-blocking agents and intra-aortic balloon counterpulsation are contraindicated, because either lowering the heart rate or augmenting peripheral resistance during diastole can lead to rapid hemodynamic decompensation. In hemodynamically stable patients with acute AR secondary to active infective endocarditis, operation may be deferred to allow 5 to 7 days of intensive antibiotic therapy (see Chap. 67). However, AVR should be undertaken at the earliest sign of hemodynamic instability or if echocardiographic evidence of diastolic closure of the mitral valve develops.

Bicuspid Aortic Valve Disease

EPIDEMIOLOGY. A congenital bicuspid aortic valve is present in about 1% to 2% of the population and is more prevalent in men, accounting for 70% to 80 % of cases. A subset of bicuspid aortic valve patients have familial clustering consistent with an autosomal dominant inheritance with incomplete penetrance.[4,6] In some families with bicuspid aortic valve and associated congenital anomalies, a mutation in the *NOTCH1* gene has been described.[103]

PATHOPHYSIOLOGY. The most prevalent anatomy for a bicuspid valve is two cusps with a right-left systolic opening, consistent with congenital fusion of the right and left coronary cusps, seen in 70% to 80% of patients. An anterior-posterior orientation, with fusion of the right and noncoronary cusps, is less common, seen in about 20% to 30% of cases.[104,105] Fusion of the left and noncoronary cusps is rarely seen. A prominent ridge of tissue or raphe may be present in the larger of the two cusps so that the closed valve in diastole may mimic a trileaflet valve. Echocardiographic diagnosis relies on imaging the systolic leaflet opening with only two aortic commissures. Unicuspid valves are distinguished from a bicuspid valve by having only one aortic commissure.

Bicuspid aortic valve disease is associated with an aortopathy, with dilation of the ascending aorta related to accelerated degeneration of the aortic media (see Chap. 60).[4-6,86,104] The presence, location, and severity of aortic dilation is related to valve morphology but does not appear to be related to the severity of valve dysfunction per se. The risk of aortic dissection in patients with a bicuspid aortic valve is five to nine times higher than the general population.[101,105a] Some studies have also suggested an association between bicuspid aortic valve disease (anterior-posterior leaflet opening) and mitral valve prolapse.[106]

CLINICAL PRESENTATION. Patients with a bicuspid valve may be diagnosed at any age based on the presence of an aortic ejection sound or a systolic or diastolic murmur. Some patients are initially diagnosed on echocardiography requested for other reasons. Often, the diagnosis is unknown until the patient develops valve dysfunction with physical examination findings and/or clinical symptoms.

DISEASE COURSE. Most bicuspid valves function normally until late in life, although a subset of patients present in childhood or adolescence with valve dysfunction. Overall, survival is not different than population estimates.[107,108] Risk factors for cardiac events are age older than 30 years, moderate or severe AR, and moderate or severe AS. Over a mean follow-up of 9 years, primary cardiac events occurred in 25% of 642 ambulatory adults with a bicuspid valve. Events included aortic valve or root replacement (22%), hospitalization for heart failure (2%), and cardiac death (3%; **Fig. 66-18**). Over their lifetime, approximately 20% of patients with bicuspid valves develop severe AR requiring AVR between 10 and 40 years of age. Patients with a bicuspid aortic valve also are at increased risk for endocarditis (0.4/100,000), accounting for about 1200 deaths/year in the United States. However, most patients with a bicuspid valve develop calcific valve stenosis later in life, typically presenting with severe AS after 50 years of age. Although the histopathology of calcific stenosis of a bicuspid aortic valve is no different than that of a trileaflet

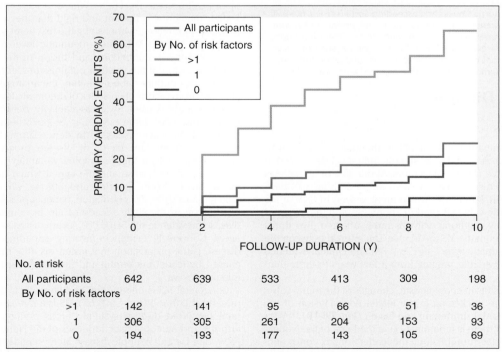

FIGURE 66-18 Outcome of patients with bicuspid aortic valves. The frequency of primary cardiac events in patients with more than one risk factor at baseline (*n* = 142) was 65% (standard deviation [SD] = 5%); in all participants (*N* = 642), 25% (SD = 2%); in patients with one risk factor at baseline (*n* = 306), 18% (SD = 3%); and in patients with no risk factors at baseline (*n* = 194), 6% (SD = 2%). The risk factors for primary cardiac events were age older than 30 years, moderate or severe aortic regurgitation, and moderate or severe aortic stenosis. (*From Tzemos N, Therrien J, Yip J, et al: Outcomes in adults with bicuspid aortic valves. JAMA 300:1317, 2008.*)

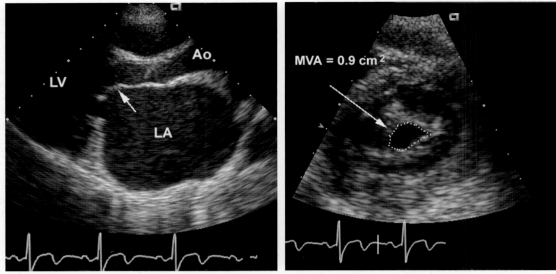

FIGURE 66-19 Parasternal long-axis **(left)** and short-axis **(right)** two-dimensional echocardiographic views showing the characteristic findings in rheumatic mitral stenosis. Note the commissural fusion that results in doming of the leaflets in the long-axis view and in a decrease in the width of the mitral orifice in the short-axis view. This patient has relatively thin, flexible leaflets with little subvalvular involvement. Ao = aorta; LA = left atrium; LV = left ventricle. *(From Otto CM: Valvular Heart Disease. Elsevier, Philadelphia, 2004.)*

valve, the turbulent flow and increased leaflet stress caused by the abnormal architecture is postulated to result in accelerated valve changes, providing an explanation for the earlier average age at presentation of patients with a bicuspid, compared with trileaflet, stenotic valve. Bicuspid valve disease accounts for over 50% of AVRs in the United States[3] and is a common cause of calcific AS, even in older individuals.

MANAGEMENT. The management of bicuspid aortic valve disease is directed toward the hemodynamic consequences of valve dysfunction—AS or AR—as discussed in these sections earlier. Currently, there are no effective medical therapies to prevent progressive valve deterioration when a bicuspid valve is diagnosed. In addition to appropriate follow-up for valve dysfunction, evaluation of the ascending aorta is needed, often with CT or CMR imaging to ensure adequate visualization and accurate measurement of the aortic sinuses and ascending aorta (see Fig. 60-4). If AVR is needed for stenosis or regurgitation, concurrent aortic root replacement is recommended if the maximum aortic dimension (measured at end-diastole) exceeds 45 mm. Even in the absence of aortic valve disease, aortic root replacement is recommended when the aortic dimension exceeds 50 mm in adults with a bicuspid aortic valve.[1,98a]

Mitral Valve Disease

Mitral Stenosis

CAUSE. The predominant cause of MS is rheumatic fever,[109] with rheumatic changes present in 99% of stenotic mitral valves excised at the time of mitral valve (MV) replacement. About 25% of all patients with rheumatic heart disease have isolated MS, and about 40% have combined MS and MR. Multivalve involvement is seen in 38% of MS patients, with the aortic valve affected in about 35% and the tricuspid valve in about 6%. The pulmonic valve is rarely affected. Two thirds of all patients with rheumatic MS are female. The interval between the initial episode of rheumatic fever (see Chap. 88) and clinical evidence of MV obstruction is variable, ranging from a few years to more than 20 years.[110]

Rheumatic fever results in characteristic changes of the mitral valve; diagnostic features are thickening at the leaflet edges, fusion of the commissures, and chordal shortening and fusion (**Fig. 66-19**).[111] With acute rheumatic fever, there is inflammation and edema of the leaflets, with small fibrin-platelet thrombi along the leaflet contact zones. Subsequent scarring leads to the characteristic valve deformity, with obliteration of the normal leaflet architecture by fibrosis, neovascularization and increased collagen and tissue cellularity. Aschoff bodies, the pathologic hallmark of rheumatic disease, are most frequently seen in

the myocardium, not the valve tissue, with Aschoff bodies identified in only 2% of autopsied patients with chronic valve disease.

These anatomic changes lead to a typical functional appearance of the rheumatic mitral valve. In earlier stages of the disease, the relatively flexible leaflets snap open in diastole into a curved shape because of restriction of motion at the leaflet tips. This diastolic doming is most evident in the motion of the anterior leaflet and becomes less prominent as the leaflets become more fibrotic and calcified. The symmetrical fusion of the commissures results in a small central oval orifice in diastole that on pathologic specimens is shaped like a fish mouth or buttonhole because the anterior leaflet is not in the physiological open position (see Fig. 66-19). With end-stage disease, the thickened leaflets may be so adherent and rigid that they cannot open or shut, reducing or, rarely, even abolishing the first heart sound and leading to combined MS and MR. When rheumatic fever results exclusively or predominantly in contraction and fusion of the chordae tendineae, with little fusion of the valvular commissures, dominant MR results.

A debate continues about whether the anatomic changes in severe MS result from recurrent episodes of rheumatic fever, a chronic autoimmune process caused by cross-reactivity between a streptococcal protein and valve tissue (see Chap. 88), or whether there is superimposed calcific valve disease.[112] Evidence supporting recurrent infection as an important factor in disease progression includes the correlation between the geographic variability in the prevalence of rheumatic heart disease and the age at which patients present with severe MS. In North America and Europe, where there is approximately 1 case/100,000 population, patients present with severe valve obstruction in the sixth decade of life. In contrast, in Africa, with a disease prevalence of 35/100,000, severe disease often is seen in teenagers. Conversely, evidence favoring superimposed calcific valve disease is the observation that restenosis after mitral valvuloplasty is caused by leaflet thickening and fibrosis rather than recurrent commissural fusion.[113]

Congenital MS is uncommon and typically is diagnosed in infancy or early childhood (see Chap. 65). MS is a rare complication of malignant carcinoid disease, systemic lupus erythematosus, rheumatoid arthritis, and mucopolysaccharidoses of the Hunter-Hurler phenotype, Fabry disease, and Whipple disease. Methysergide therapy is an unusual but documented cause of MS. The association of atrial septal defect with rheumatic MS is called Lutembacher syndrome.

Other conditions may result in obstruction to LV inflow, including a left atrial tumor, particularly myxoma (see Chap. 74), ball valve thrombus in the left atrium (usually associated with MS), infective endocarditis with large vegetations (see Chap. 67), or a congenital membrane in the left atrium (i.e., cor triatriatum; see Chap. 65). In older patients, extensive mitral annular calcification may result in restriction of the size and motion of the annulus and may extend onto the base of the mitral leaflets, resulting in functional MS, although obstruction rarely is severe.

PATHOPHYSIOLOGY. The most useful descriptor of the severity of mitral valve obstruction is the degree of valve opening in diastole, or the mitral valve orifice area. In normal adults, the cross-sectional area of the mitral valve orifice is 4 to 6 cm² (see Table 66-1). When the orifice is reduced to approximately 2 cm², which is considered to represent mild MS, blood can flow from the left atrium to the left ventricle only if propelled by a small, although abnormal, pressure gradient. When the mitral valve opening is reduced to 1 cm², which is considered to represent severe MS,[114] a left atrioventricular pressure gradient of approximately 20 mm Hg (and therefore, in the presence of a normal LV diastolic pressure, a mean left atrial pressure >25 mm Hg) is required to maintain normal cardiac output at rest (**Fig. 66-20**; see Fig. 20-14).

The transvalvular pressure gradient for any given valve area is a function of the square of the transvalvular flow rate.[114] Thus, a doubling of flow rate quadruples the pressure gradient. The elevated left atrial pressure, in turn, raises pulmonary venous and capillary pressures, resulting in exertional dyspnea. The first bouts of dyspnea in patients with MS are usually precipitated by tachycardia resulting from exercise, pregnancy, hyperthyroidism, anemia, infection, or AF. All these (1) increase the rate of blood flow across the mitral orifice, resulting in further elevation of the left atrial pressure, and (2) decrease the diastolic filling time, resulting in a reduction in forward cardiac output. Because diastole shortens proportionately more than systole as heart rate increases, the time available for flow across the mitral valve is reduced at higher heart rates. Therefore, at any given stroke volume, tachycardia results in a higher instantaneous volume flow rate and higher transmitral pressure gradient, which elevates left atrial pressures further. This higher transmitral gradient, often in combination with inadequate ventricular filling (because of the shortened diastolic filling time), explains the sudden occurrence of dyspnea and pulmonary edema in previously asymptomatic patients with MS who develop AF with a rapid ventricular rate. It also accounts for the equally rapid improvement in these patients when the ventricular rate is slowed.

Atrial contraction augments the presystolic transmitral valvular gradient by approximately 30% in patients with MS. AF is common in patients with MS, with an increasing prevalence with age. In patients with severe MS younger than 30 years, only about 10% are in AF compared with approximately 50% of those older than 50 years. Withdrawal of atrial transport when AF develops reduces cardiac output by approximately 20%, often resulting in symptom onset.

Obstruction at the mitral valve level has other hemodynamic consequences, which account for many of the adverse clinical outcomes associated with this disease. Elevated left atrial pressure results in pulmonary artery hypertension, with secondary effects on the pulmonary vasculature and right heart. In addition, left atrial enlargement and stasis of blood flow is associated with an increased risk of thrombus formation and systemic embolism. Typically, the left ventricle is relatively normal, unless there is coexisting MR, with the primary abnormalities of the left ventricle being a small underfilled chamber and paradoxical septal motion caused by RV enlargement and dysfunction.

HEMODYNAMIC CONSEQUENCES OF MITRAL STENOSIS

PULMONARY HYPERTENSION. In patients with MS and sinus rhythm, mean left atrial pressure is elevated (see Fig. 66-20), and the left atrial pressure curve shows a prominent atrial contraction (*a* wave), with a gradual pressure decline after mitral valve opening (*y* descent). In patients with mild to moderate MS without elevated pulmonary vascular resistance, pulmonary arterial pressure may be normal or only minimally elevated at rest but rises during exercise. However, in patients with severe MS and those in whom the pulmonary vascular resistance is significantly increased,

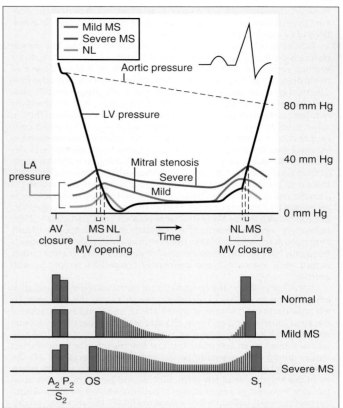

FIGURE 66-20 Schematic representation of LV, aortic, and left atrial (LA) pressures, showing normal relationships and alterations with mild and severe MS. Corresponding classic auscultatory signs of MS are shown at the bottom. The higher left atrial v wave of severe MS causes earlier pressure crossover and earlier MV opening, leading to a shorter time interval between aortic valve (AV) closure and the opening snap (OS). The higher left atrial end-diastolic pressure with severe MS also results in later closure of the mitral valve. With severe MS, the diastolic rumble becomes longer and there is accentuation of the pulmonic component (P₂) of the second heart sound (S₂) in relation to the aortic component (A₂).

pulmonary arterial pressure is elevated when the patient is at rest. Rarely, in patients with extremely elevated pulmonary vascular resistance, pulmonary arterial pressure may exceed systemic arterial pressure. Further elevations of left atrial and pulmonary vascular pressures occur during exercise and/or tachycardia.

Pulmonary hypertension in patients with MS results from the following: (1) passive backward transmission of the elevated left atrial pressure; (2) pulmonary arteriolar constriction, which presumably is triggered by left atrial and pulmonary venous hypertension (reactive pulmonary hypertension); and (3) organic obliterative changes in the pulmonary vascular bed, which may be considered to be a complication of long-standing and severe MS (see Chap. 78). With moderately elevated pulmonary arterial pressure (systolic pressure 30 to 60 mm Hg), RV performance is usually maintained. In time, severe pulmonary hypertension results in right-sided heart failure, with dilation of the right ventricle and its annulus, secondary tricuspid regurgitation (TR), and sometimes pulmonic regurgitation. These changes in the pulmonary vascular bed may also exert a protective effect; the elevated precapillary resistance makes the development of symptoms of pulmonary congestion less likely to occur by tending to prevent blood from surging into the pulmonary capillary bed and damming up behind the stenotic mitral valve. However, this protection occurs at the expense of a reduced cardiac output. In patients with severe MS, pulmonary vein–bronchial vein shunts occur. Their rupture may cause hemoptysis. Patients with severe MS manifest a reduction in pulmonary compliance, increase in the work of breathing, and redistribution of pulmonary blood flow from the base to the apex.

LEFT VENTRICULAR FUNCTION. The LV chamber typically is normal or small, with normal systolic function and normal LV end-diastolic pressure.

However, coexisting MR, aortic valve lesions, systemic hypertension, ischemic heart disease, and cardiomyopathy may all be responsible for elevations of LV diastolic pressure

EXERCISE HEMODYNAMICS. At any given severity of stenosis, the clinical picture is dictated largely by the levels of cardiac output and pulmonary vascular resistance with exertion. The response to a given degree of mitral obstruction may be characterized at one end of the hemodynamic spectrum by a normal cardiac output and high left atrioventricular pressure gradient or, at the opposite end of the spectrum, by a markedly reduced cardiac output and low transvalvular pressure gradient. Thus, in some patients with moderate MS (mitral valve area = 1.0 to 1.5 cm^2), cardiac output at rest may be normal and rises normally during exertion. However, the high transvalvular pressure gradient with exertion elevates left atrial and pulmonary capillary pressures, leading to pulmonary congestion during exertion. In contrast, in other patients with moderate MS, there is an inadequate rise in cardiac output during exertion, resulting in a smaller rise in pulmonary venous pressure. In these patients, symptoms are caused by a low cardiac output rather than by pulmonary congestion. In patients with severe MS (mitral valve area < 1 cm^2), particularly when pulmonary vascular resistance is elevated, cardiac output is usually depressed at rest and may fail to rise at all during exertion. These patients frequently have resting weakness and fatigue secondary to a low cardiac output, with low-output and pulmonary congestion symptoms with exercise.

LEFT ATRIAL CHANGES. The combination of mitral valve disease and atrial inflammation secondary to rheumatic carditis causes the following: (1) left atrial dilation; (2) fibrosis of the atrial wall; and (3) disorganization of the atrial muscle bundles. These changes lead to disparate conduction velocities and inhomogeneous refractory periods. Premature atrial activation, caused by an automatic focus or reentry, may stimulate the left atrium during the vulnerable period and thereby precipitate AF. The development of this arrhythmia correlates independently with the severity of the MS, degree of left atrial dilation, and height of the left atrial pressure. However, in a most studies of patients with severe MS undergoing percutaneous balloon mitral valvotomy (BMV), the strongest predictor of AF is older age. AF is often episodic at first but then becomes more persistent. AF per se causes diffuse atrophy of atrial muscle, further atrial enlargement, and further inhomogeneity of refractoriness and conduction. These changes, in turn, lead to irreversible AF.

CLINICAL PRESENTATION

Symptoms

DYSPNEA. The most common presenting symptoms of MS are dyspnea, fatigue, and decreased exercise tolerance.[115] Symptoms may be caused by a reduced ability to increase cardiac output normally with exercise or elevated pulmonary venous pressures and reduced pulmonary compliance. Dyspnea may be accompanied by cough and wheezing. Vital capacity is reduced, presumably because of the presence of engorged pulmonary vessels and interstitial edema. Patients who have critical obstruction to left atrial emptying and dyspnea with ordinary activity (NYHA functional Class III) generally have orthopnea as well and are at risk of experiencing attacks of frank pulmonary edema. The latter may be precipitated by effort, emotional stress, respiratory infection, fever pregnancy, or AF with a rapid ventricular rate or other tachyarrhythmia. Pulmonary edema may be caused by any condition that increases the flow rate across the stenotic mitral valve, either because of an increase in total cardiac output or a reduction in the time available for blood flow across the mitral orifice to occur. In patients with a markedly elevated pulmonary vascular resistance, RV function is often impaired and the presentation may also include symptoms and signs of right heart failure.

MS is a slowly progressive disease, and many patients remain seemingly asymptomatic merely by readjusting their lifestyles to a more sedentary level. Usually, symptom status can be accurately assessed by a directed history, asking the patient to compare current levels of maximum exertion to specific time points in the past. Exercise testing may be useful for selected patients to determine functional status in an objective manner and may be combined with Doppler echocardiography (see later) to assess exercise hemodynamics.

HEMOPTYSIS. Hemoptysis is rare in patients with a known diagnosis of MS because intervention is performed before severe obstruction becomes chronic. When hemoptysis does occur, it can be sudden and severe, caused by rupture of thin-walled, dilated bronchial veins, usually as a consequence of a sudden rise in left atrial pressure, or it may be milder, with only blood-stained sputum associated with attacks of paroxysmal nocturnal dyspnea. MS patients also may have pink frothy sputum characteristic of acute pulmonary edema with rupture of alveolar capillaries. Hemoptysis also may be caused by pulmonary infarction, a late complication of MS associated with heart failure.

CHEST PAIN. Chest pain is not a typical symptom of MS, but a small percentage, perhaps 15%, of patients with MS experience chest discomfort that is indistinguishable from that of angina pectoris. This symptom may be caused by severe RV hypertension secondary to the pulmonary vascular disease or by concomitant coronary atherosclerosis. Rarely, chest pain may be secondary to coronary obstruction caused by coronary embolization. In many patients, however, a satisfactory explanation for the chest pain cannot be uncovered, even after complete hemodynamic and angiographic studies.

PALPITATIONS AND EMBOLIC EVENTS. Patients with AF often are initially diagnosed when they present with AF or an embolic event.

OTHER SYMPTOMS. Compression of the left recurrent laryngeal nerve by a greatly dilated left atrium, enlarged tracheobronchial lymph nodes, and dilated pulmonary artery may cause hoarseness (Ortner syndrome). A history of repeated hemoptysis is common in patients with pulmonary hemosiderosis. Systemic venous hypertension, hepatomegaly, edema, ascites, and hydrothorax are all signs of severe MS with elevated pulmonary vascular resistance and right-sided heart failure.

PHYSICAL EXAMINATION. The most common findings on physical examination in patients with MS are an irregular pulse caused by AF and signs of left and right heart failure (see Chap. 12). The classic diastolic murmur and loud first heart sound are often difficult to appreciate. Patients with severe chronic MS, a low cardiac output, and systemic vasoconstriction may exhibit the so-called mitral facies, characterized by pinkish-purple patches on the cheeks. The arterial pulse is usually normal, but in patients with a reduced stroke volume, the pulse may be low in volume. The jugular venous pulse usually exhibits a prominent a wave in patients with sinus rhythm and elevated pulmonary vascular resistance. In patients with AF, the x descent of the jugular venous pulse disappears, and there is only one crest, a prominent v or c-v wave, per cardiac cycle. Palpation of the cardiac apex usually reveals an inconspicuous left ventricle; the presence of a palpable presystolic expansion wave or an early diastolic rapid filling wave speaks strongly against serious MS. A readily palpable, tapping S_1 suggests that the anterior mitral valve leaflet is pliable. When the patient is in the left lateral recumbent position, a diastolic thrill of MS may be palpable at the apex. Often, a RV lift is felt in the left parasternal region in patients with pulmonary hypertension. A markedly enlarged right ventricle may displace the left ventricle posteriorly and produce a prominent RV apex beat that can be confused with a LV lift. A loud P_2 may be palpable in the second left intercostal space in patients with MS and pulmonary hypertension.

AUSCULTATION. The auscultatory features of MS (see Fig. 66-20) include an accentuated S_1 with prolongation of the Q-S_1 interval, correlating with the level of the left atrial pressure. Accentuation of S_1 occurs when the mitral valve leaflets are flexible. It is caused, in part, by the rapidity with which LV pressure rises at the time of mitral valve closure, as well as by the wide closing excursion of the leaflets. Marked calcification and/or thickening of the mitral valve leaflets reduce the amplitude of S_1, probably because of diminished motion of the leaflets. As pulmonary arterial pressure rises, P_2 at first becomes accentuated and widely transmitted and can often be readily heard at both the mitral and the aortic areas. With further elevation of pulmonary arterial pressure, splitting of S_2 narrows because of reduced compliance of the pulmonary vascular bed, with earlier pulmonic valve closure. Finally, S_2 becomes single and accentuated. Other signs of severe pulmonary hypertension include a nonvalvular pulmonic ejection sound that diminishes during inspiration, because of dilation of the pulmonary artery, a systolic murmur of TR, a Graham Steell murmur of pulmonic regurgitation, and an S_4 originating from the right ventricle. An S_3 gallop originating from the left ventricle is absent in patients with MS unless significant MR or AR coexists.

The opening snap (OS) of the mitral valve is caused by a sudden tensing of the valve leaflets after the valve cusps have completed their opening excursion. The OS occurs when the movement of the mitral dome into the left ventricle suddenly stops. It is most readily audible at the apex, using the diaphragm of the stethoscope. The OS can usually be differentiated from P_2 because the OS occurs later, unless right bundle branch block is present. In addition, the OS usually is loudest at the apex, whereas S_2 is best heard at the cardiac base. The mitral valve cannot be totally rigid if it produces an OS, so an OS is usually accompanied by an accentuated S_1. Calcification confined to the tip of the mitral valve leaflets does not preclude an OS, although calcification of the body and tip does. The mitral OS follows A_2 by 0.04 to 0.12 second; this interval varies inversely with the left atrial pressure. A short A_2-OS interval is a reliable indicator of severe MS but accurate estimation of this time interval requires considerable experience.

The diastolic, low-pitched, rumbling murmur of MS is best heard at the apex, with the bell of the stethoscope (low-frequency mode on electronic stethoscopes) and with the patient in the left lateral recumbent position. When this murmur is soft, it is limited to the apex but, when louder, it may radiate to the left axilla or the lower left sternal area. Although the intensity of the diastolic murmur is not closely related to the severity of stenosis, the duration of the murmur is a guide to the severity of mitral valve narrowing. The murmur persists for as long as the left atrioventricular pressure gradient exceeds approximately 3 mm Hg. The murmur usually commences immediately after the OS. In mild MS, the early diastolic murmur is brief but, in the presence of sinus rhythm, it resumes in presystole. In severe MS, the murmur persists until end-diastole, with presystolic accentuation while sinus rhythm is maintained (see Figs. 66-20 and 12-8F).

OTHER AUSCULTATORY FINDINGS. A pansystolic murmur of TR and an S_3 originating from the right ventricle may be audible in the fourth intercostal space in the left parasternal region in patients with severe MS. These signs, which are secondary to pulmonary hypertension, may be confused with the findings of MR. However, the inspiratory augmentation of the murmur and of the S_3 and the prominent v wave in the jugular venous pulse aid in establishing that the murmur originates from the tricuspid valve. A high-pitched decrescendo diastolic murmur along the left sternal border in patients with MS and pulmonary hypertension may be audible pulmonic regurgitation (Graham Steell murmur), but more often is caused by concomitant AR.

DIAGNOSIS AND EVALUATION

DIFFERENTIAL DIAGNOSIS. MS is a rare diagnosis in developed countries and most apical diastolic murmurs have other causes. In older patients, an apical diastolic rumble most likely is caused by mitral annular calcification, and 90% of patients with a diastolic apical murmur have no evidence of MS on echocardiography. In severe MR—indeed, in any condition in which flow across a nonstenotic mitral valve is increased (e.g., a ventricular septal defect)—there may also be a short diastolic murmur following an S_3. Left atrial myxoma (see Chap. 74) may produce auscultatory findings similar to those in rheumatic valvular MS. A diastolic rumble may also be present in some patients with HCM, caused by early diastolic flow into the hypertrophied, nondistensible left ventricle (see Chap. 69).

Echocardiography

Echocardiography is the most accurate approach to the diagnosis and evaluation of MS (see Chap. 15).[36] It is recommended for all patients with MS at initial presentation, for reevaluation of changing symptoms or signs, and at regular intervals (depending on disease severity) for monitoring disease progression (see Table 66-1). Imaging shows the characteristic anatomy with leaflet thickening and restriction of opening caused by symmetric fusion of the commissures, resulting in "doming" of the leaflets in diastole (see Fig. 66-19 and Fig 15-46). As disease becomes more severe, thickening extends from the leaflet tips toward the base with further restriction of motion and less curvature of the leaflet in diastole. The mitral chords are variably thickening, fused, and shortened and there may be superimposed calcification of the valve apparatus (see Figs. 15-4C and 15-5C).

Mitral valve area is measured by direct planimetry from two-dimensional short-axis images and calculated by the Doppler pressure half-time method (see Figs. 15-39 and 15-47). The transmitral gradient is also calculated (see Fig. 15-36B) and any coexisting MR is quantitated

on the basis of the accepted guidelines.[30] Evaluation of the morphology of the valve is helpful for predicting the hemodynamic results and outcome of percutaneous BMV. A score of 0 to 4+ is given for leaflet thickness, mobility, calcification, and chordal involvement to provide an overall score that is favorable (low) or unfavorable (high) for valvuloplasty (see Table 15-11). Other important anatomic features of the valve are the degree of anterior leaflet doming, symmetry of commissural fusion, and distribution of leaflet calcification.[114]

Other key features on echocardiography are left atrial size, pulmonary artery pressures, LV size and systolic function, and RV size and systolic function. When pulmonary hypertension is present, the right ventricle is frequently dilated, with reduced systolic function. TR may be secondary to RV dysfunction and annular dilation or may be caused by rheumatic involvement of the tricuspid valve. Complete evaluation of aortic valve anatomy and function is also important because the aortic valve is affected in approximately one third of patients with MS. When transthoracic images are suboptimal, TEE is appropriate. TEE is also necessary to exclude left atrial thrombus and evaluate MR severity when percutaneous BMV is considered.

Exercise Testing with Doppler Echocardiography

Exercise testing is useful for many patients with MS to ascertain the level of physical conditioning and elicit covert cardiac symptoms. The exercise test can be combined with Doppler echocardiography to assess exercise pulmonary pressure,[70,114] usually with the Doppler examination performed at rest after termination of exercise. Exercise Doppler testing is recommended when there is a discrepancy between resting echocardiographic findings and the severity of clinical symptoms.[1] Useful parameters on exercise testing include the following: (1) exercise duration; (2) blood pressure and heart rate response; and (3) increase in pulmonary pressures with exercise, compared with the expected normal changes. An exercise pulmonary systolic pressure greater than 60 mm Hg is a key decision point in the management of these patients.

OTHER DIAGNOSTIC EVALUATION MODALITIES.

ELECTROCARDIOGRAPHY. The ECG is relatively insensitive for detecting mild MS, but it does show characteristic changes in moderate or severe obstruction (see Chap. 13). Left atrial enlargement (P wave duration in lead II >0.12 second and/or a P wave axis between +45 and −30 degrees) is a principal electrocardiographic feature of MS and is found in 90% of patients with significant MS and sinus rhythm. The electrocardiographic signs of left atrial enlargement correlate more closely with left atrial volume than with left atrial pressure and often regress following successful valvotomy. AF is common with long-standing MS, as noted.

Electrocardiographic evidence of RV hypertrophy correlates with RV systolic pressure. When RV systolic pressure is 70 to 100 mm Hg, approximately 50% of patients manifest ECG criteria for RV hypertrophy, including a mean QRS axis greater than 80 degrees in the frontal plane and an R:S ratio greater than 1 in lead V_1. Other patients with this degree of pulmonary hypertension have no frank evidence of RV hypertrophy, but the R:S ratio fails to increase from the right to the midprecordial leads. When RV systolic pressure is greater than 100 mm Hg in patients with isolated or predominant MS, electrocardiographic evidence of RV hypertrophy is consistently found.

RADIOGRAPHY. Patients with hemodynamically significant MS almost invariably have evidence of left atrial enlargement on the lateral and left anterior oblique views (see Chap. 16 and Figs. 16-10, 16-17, and 16-18), although the cardiac silhouette may be normal in the frontal projection. Extreme left atrial enlargement rarely occurs in isolated MS; when present, MR is usually severe (see Fig. 16-15). Enlargement of the pulmonary artery, right ventricle, and right atrium (as well as the left atrium) is commonly seen in patients with severe MS. Occasionally, calcification of the mitral valve is evident on the chest roentgenogram but, more commonly, fluoroscopy is required to detect valvular calcification.

Radiologic changes in the lung fields indirectly reflect the severity of MS. Interstitial edema, an indication of severe obstruction, is manifested as Kerley B lines (dense, short, horizontal lines most commonly seen in the costophrenic angles). This finding is present in 30% of patients with resting pulmonary arterial wedge pressures less than 20 mm Hg and in 70% of patients with pressures greater than 20 mm Hg. Severe long-standing mitral obstruction often results in Kerley A lines (straight, dense lines up to 4 cm in length, running toward the hilum), as well as the findings of pulmonary hemosiderosis and rarely of parenchymal ossification.

CARDIAC CATHETERIZATION. Catheter-based measurement of left atrial and LV pressures shows the expected hemodynamics (see Fig. 20-14) and allows measurement of the mean transmitral pressure gradient and, in conjunction with measurement of transmitral volume flow rate, calculation of the valve area using the Gorlin formula (see Chap. 20). Occasionally, diagnostic cardiac catheterization is necessary when echocardiography is nondiagnostic or results are discrepant with clinical findings.[116] More often, these measurements now are recorded for monitoring before, during, and after percutaneous BMV. Routine diagnostic cardiac catheterization is not recommended for the evaluation of MS.

DISEASE COURSE

Interval Between Acute Rheumatic Fever and Mitral Valve Obstruction

In temperate zones, such as the United States and Western Europe, patients who develop acute rheumatic fever have an asymptomatic period of approximately 15 to 20 years before symptoms of MS develop. It then takes approximately 5 to 10 years for most patients to progress from mild disability (i.e., early NYHA Class II) to severe disability (i.e., NYHA functional Class III or IV; **Fig. 66-21**). The progression is much more rapid in patients in tropical and subtropical areas, in Polynesians, and in Native Alaskans. In India, critical MS may be present in children as young as 6 to 12 years old. In North America and Western Europe, however, symptoms develop more slowly and occur most commonly between the ages of 45 and 65 years. The most likely causes for these differences are the relative prevalence of rheumatic fever and lack of primary and secondary prevention in developing countries, resulting in recurrent episodes of valve scarring (see Chap. 88).

Hemodynamic Progression

Serial echocardiographic data have described the rate of hemodynamic progression in patients with mild MS.[113-115] The two largest series followed a combined total of 153 adults, with a mean age of approximately 60 years, for an average of slightly more than 3 years. As in most series of MS patients, 75% to 80% were women. The initial valve area was $1.7 \pm 0.6 \ cm^2$ and the overall rate of progression was a decrease in valve area of $0.09 \ cm^2/yr$. Approximately one third of patients showed rapid progression, defined as a decrease in valve area greater than $0.1 \ cm^2/yr$. These data apply to the older MS patients seen in developed countries. There are little data on the rate of hemodynamic progression of rheumatic MS in underdeveloped countries in which the age of symptom onset is much younger.

Clinical Outcomes

Natural history data obtained in the presurgical era indicate that symptomatic patients with MS have a poor outlook, with 5-year survival rates of 62% among patients with MS in NYHA Class III but only 15% among those in Class IV. Data from unoperated patients in the surgical era still reported a 5-year survival rate of only 44% in patients with symptomatic MS who refused valvotomy (**Fig. 66-22**).

Overall clinical outcomes are greatly improved in patients who undergo surgical or percutaneous relief of valve obstruction on the basis of current guidelines. However, longevity is still shortened compared with that expected for age, largely because of complications of the disease process (AF, systemic embolism, pulmonary hypertension) and side effects of therapy (e.g., prosthetic valves, anticoagulation).

COMPLICATIONS

ATRIAL FIBRILLATION. The most common complication of MS is AF (see Chap. 40).[113,115] The prevalence of AF in patients with MS is related to the severity of valve obstruction and patient age. In historical series, AF was present in 17% of those 21 to 30 years, 45% of those 31 to 40 years, 60% of those 41 to 50 years, and 80% of those older than 51 years. Even when MS is severe, the prevalence of AF is related to age. In more recent BMV studies, the prevalence of AF ranged from 4% in a series of 600 patients from India, with a mean age of 27 years, and 27% in a series of 4832 patients from China, with a mean age of 37 years, to 40% in a series of 1024 patients from France, with a mean age of 49 years.

AF may precipitate or worsen symptoms caused by loss of the atrial contribution to filling and to a short diastolic filling period when the ventricular rate is not well controlled. In addition, AF predisposes to left

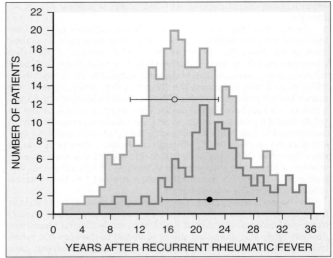

FIGURE 66-21 Interval between active rheumatic fever and clinical symptoms of valve disease in 177 patients with mitral stenosis (yellow bars) and 121 with aortic stenosis (blue bars). *(From Horstkotte D, Niehues R, Strauer BE: Pathomorphological aspects, aetiology, and natural history of acquired mitral valve stenosis. Eur Heart J 12[Suppl B]:55, 1991.)*

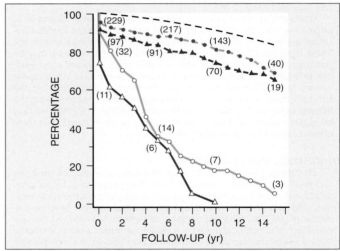

FIGURE 66-22 Natural history of 159 patients with isolated mitral stenosis (solid blue line) or mitral regurgitation (solid purple line) who were not operated on, even though the operation was indicated, compared with patients treated with valve replacement for mitral stenosis (dashed blue line) or mitral regurgitation (dashed purple line). The expected survival rate in the absence of mitral valve disease is indicated by the upper curve (dashed black line). *(From Horstkotte D, Niehues R, Strauer BE: Pathomorphological aspects, aetiology, and natural history of acquired mitral valve stenosis. Eur Heart J 12[Suppl B]:55, 1991.)*

atrial thrombus formation and systemic embolic events. AF conveys a worse overall prognosis in MS patients than in the general population. In patients with AF and MS, 5-year survival is only 64% compared with 85% in AF patients without MS.

SYSTEMIC EMBOLISM. Systemic embolism in patients with MS is caused by left atrial thrombus formation. Although systemic embolization most often occurs in patients with AF, 20% of patients with MS and a systemic embolic event are in sinus rhythm. When embolization occurs in patients in sinus rhythm, the possibility of transient AF or underlying infective endocarditis should be considered. However, up to 45% of patients with MS who are in normal sinus rhythm have prominent spontaneous left atrial contrast (a marker of embolic risk) seen by TEE (see Chap. 15). Atrial thrombi have been documented in a few MS patients in sinus rhythm, and many patients with new-onset AF have left atrial thrombi. It is postulated that the loss of atrial appendage contractile function, despite electrical evidence of sinus rhythm, leads to blood flow stasis and thrombus formation.

The risk of embolism correlates directly with patient age and left atrial size and inversely with the cardiac output. Before the advent of surgical treatment, this serious complication of MS developed in at least 20% of patients at some time during the course of their disease. Before the era of anticoagulant therapy and surgical treatment, approximately 25% of all fatalities in patients with mitral valve disease were secondary to systemic embolism.

Approximately half of all clinically apparent emboli are found in the cerebral vessels. Coronary embolism may lead to myocardial infarction and/or angina pectoris, and renal emboli may be responsible for the development of systemic hypertension. Emboli are recurrent and multiple in approximately 25% of patients who develop this complication. Rarely, massive thrombosis develops in the left atrium, resulting in a pedunculated ball valve thrombus, which may suddenly aggravate obstruction to left atrial outflow when a specific body position is assumed or may cause sudden death. Similar consequences occur in patients with free-floating thrombi in the left atrium. These two conditions are usually characterized by variability in the physical findings, often on a positional basis. They are very hazardous and require surgical treatment, often as an emergency.

INFECTIVE ENDOCARDITIS. MS is a predisposing factor for endocarditis (see Chap. 67) in less than 1% of cases in clinical series of bacterial endocarditis. The estimated risk of endocarditis in patients with MS is 0.17/1000 patient-years, which is much lower than the risk in patients with MR or aortic valve disease.

MANAGEMENT

Medical Treatment

The medical management of MS is primarily directed toward the following: (1) prevention of recurrent rheumatic fever; (2) prevention and treatment of complications of MS; and (3) monitoring disease progression to allow intervention at the optimal time point.[113,115] Patients with MS caused by rheumatic heart disease should receive penicillin prophylaxis for beta-hemolytic streptococcal infections to prevent recurrent rheumatic fever, per established guidelines (see Chap. 88). Prophylaxis for infective endocarditis is no longer recommended (see Chap. 67). Anemia and infections should be treated promptly and aggressively in patients with valvular heart disease. However, blood cultures should always be considered before beginning antibiotic therapy in patients with valve disease because the presentation of endocarditis often is mistaken for a noncardiac infection.

Anticoagulant therapy is indicated for prevention of systemic embolism in MS patients with AF (persistent or paroxysmal), any prior embolic events (even if in sinus rhythm), and documented left atrial thrombus. Anticoagulation also may be considered for patients with severe MS and sinus rhythm when there is severe left atrial enlargement (diameter >55 mm) or spontaneous contrast on echocardiography. Treatment with warfarin is used to maintain the international normalized ratio (INR) between 2 and 3.[117]

Asymptomatic patients with mild to moderate rheumatic mitral valve disease should have a history and physical examination annually, with echocardiography every 3 to 5 years for mild stenosis, every 1 to 2 years for moderate stenosis, and annually for severe stenosis. More frequent evaluation is appropriate for any change in signs or symptoms. All patients with significant MS should be advised to avoid occupations requiring strenuous exertion.

In patients with severe MS, with persistent symptoms after intervention or when intervention is not possible, medical therapy with oral diuretics and the restriction of sodium intake may improve symptoms. Digitalis glycosides do not alter the hemodynamics and usually do not benefit patients with MS and sinus rhythm, but these drugs are of value in slowing the ventricular rate in patients with AF and in treating patients with right-sided heart failure. Hemoptysis is managed by measures designed to reduce pulmonary venous pressure, including sedation, assumption of the upright position, and aggressive diuresis. Beta-blocking agents and rate-slowing calcium antagonists may increase exercise capacity by reducing heart rate in patients with sinus rhythm, especially in patients with AF.

TREATMENT OF ARRHYTHMIAS. AF is a frequent complication of severe MS. Management of AF for patients with MS is similar to management of AF of any cause (see Chap. 40). However, it typically is more difficult to restore and maintain sinus rhythm because of pressure overload of the left atrium in conjunction with effects of the rheumatic process on atrial tissue and the conducting system.

Immediate treatment of AF includes administration of intravenous heparin followed by oral warfarin. The ventricular rate should be slowed, as stated in the American College of Cardiology/American Heart Association (ACC/AHA) guidelines for the management of AF,[117] initially with an intravenous beta blocker or nondihydropyridine calcium channel antagonist, followed by long-term rate control with oral doses of these agents. When these medications are ineffective or when additional rate control is necessary, digoxin or amiodarone may be considered. Digoxin alone for long-term management of AF may be considered in patients with concurrent LV dysfunction or a sedentary lifestyle. An effort should be made to reestablish sinus rhythm by a combination of pharmacologic treatment and cardioversion. If cardioversion is planned in a patient who has had AF for more than 24 hours before the procedure, anticoagulation with warfarin for more than 3 weeks is indicated. Alternatively, if TEE results show no atrial thrombus, immediate cardioversion can be carried out provided the patient is effectively anticoagulated with intravenous heparin before and during the procedure, and with warfarin chronically thereafter. Paroxysmal AF and repeated conversions, spontaneous or induced, carry the risk of embolization. In patients who cannot be converted or maintained in sinus rhythm, digitalis should be used to maintain the ventricular rate at rest at approximately 60 beats/min. If this is not possible, small doses of a beta-blocking agent, such as atenolol (25 mg daily) or metoprolol (50 to 100 mg daily), may be added. Beta blockers are particularly helpful in preventing rapid ventricular responses that develop during exertion. Multiple repeat cardioversions are not indicated if the patient fails to sustain sinus rhythm while on adequate doses of an antiarrhythmic.

Patients with chronic AF who undergo surgical MV repair or MV replacement may undergo the maze procedure (atrial compartment operation).[118,119] More than 80% of patients undergoing this procedure can be maintained in sinus rhythm postoperatively and can regain normal atrial function, including a satisfactory success rate in those with significant left atrial enlargement. Early intervention with percutaneous valvotomy may prevent the development of AF.[120]

Mitral Valvotomy

PERCUTANEOUS BALLOON MITRAL VALVOTOMY. Patients with mild to moderate MS who are asymptomatic frequently remain so for years, and clinical outcomes are similar to age-matched normal patients. However, severe or symptomatic MS is associated with poor long-term outcomes if the stenosis is not relieved mechanically (see Fig. 66-22). Percutaneous BMV (see Chap. 59) is the procedure of choice for the treatment of MS so that surgical intervention is now reserved for patients who require intervention and are not candidates for a percutaneous procedure.[113]

BMV is recommended for symptomatic patients with moderate to severe MS (i.e., a mitral valve area < 1 cm²/m² body surface area [BSA] or <1.5 cm² in normal-sized adults) and with favorable valve morphology, no or mild MR, and no evidence of left atrial thrombus (**Fig. 66-23**). Even mild symptoms, such as a subtle decrease in exercise tolerance, are an indication for intervention because the procedure relieves symptoms and improves long-term outcome with a low procedural risk. In addition, BMV is recommended for asymptomatic patients with moderate to severe MS when mitral valve obstruction has resulted in pulmonary hypertension with a pulmonary systolic pressure greater than 50 mm Hg at rest or 60 mm Hg with exercise.

BMV also is reasonable for symptomatic patients who are at high risk for surgery, even when valve morphology is not ideal, including patients with restenosis after a previous BMV or previous commissurotomy who are unsuitable for surgery because of very high risk. These include very old frail patients, patients with associated severe ischemic heart disease, patients in whom MS is complicated by pulmonary, renal, or neoplastic disease, women of childbearing age

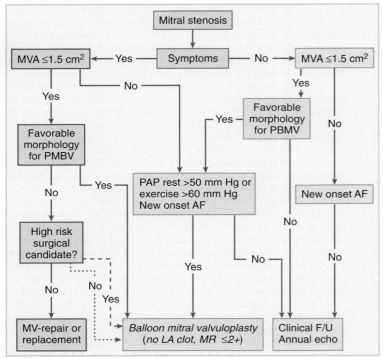

FIGURE 66-23 Management strategy for patients with mitral stenosis. F/U = follow-up; LA = left atrial; MVA = mitral valve area; PAP = pulmonary artery systolic pressure; PBMV = percutaneous balloon mitral valvotomy. *(Modified from Bonow RO, Carabello BA, Chatterjee K, et al: ACC/AHA 2006 guidelines for the management of patients with valvular heart disease: A report of the American College of Cardiology/American Heart Association Task Force on Practice Guidelines [writing committee to revise the 1998 Guidelines for the Management of Patients With Valvular Heart Disease]. Circulation 114:e84, 2006.)*

decreases in size in most. Rarely, the defect is large enough to cause right-sided heart failure; this complication most often is seen in conjunction with an unsuccessful mitral valvotomy.

The likelihood of hemodynamic benefit and the risk of complication with BMV are predicted by anatomic features of the stenosed valve. Rigid thickened valves with extensive subvalvular fibrosis and calcification lead to suboptimal results. One echocardiographic scoring system divides patients into three groups—those with a pliable, noncalcified anterior leaflet and little chordal disease (group 1); those with a pliable, noncalcified anterior leaflet but with chordal thickening and shortening (<10 mm long; group 2); and those with fluoroscopic evidence of calcification of any extent of the valve apparatus (group 3).[113] Event-free survival at 3 years is highest for group 1 (89%) compared with group 2 (78%) or group 3 (65%).[113,114] With an alternate echocardiographic scoring system, leaflet rigidity, leaflet thickening, valvular calcification, and subvalvular disease are each scored from 0 to 4 (see Table 15-11).[1,113] A score of 8 or lower is usually associated with an excellent immediate and long-term result, whereas scores exceeding 8 are associated with less impressive results (**Fig. 66-26**) including the risk of development of MR. Commissural calcification also is a predictor of poor outcomes.

TEE should be performed just prior to BMV to exclude left atrial thrombus and confirm that MR is not moderate or severe. TEE also is appropriate for the evaluation of MS severity and mitral valve morphology when transthoracic images are suboptimal, but the chordal apparatus is less well visualized compared with transthoracic imaging. During the procedure, transthoracic, transesophageal, or intracardiac echocardiography is used to monitor placement of the catheters and balloon, assess hemodynamic results after each inflation, and detect complications such as MR.

In patients with suitable anatomic findings, long-term results are favorable, with excellent survival rates without functional disability or need for surgery or repeat BMV.[113,115,121] A prospective randomized trial in which patients with severe MS were randomized to undergo BMV, closed surgical valvotomy, or open surgical valvotomy had similar clinical outcomes with BMV and the open surgical technique that were superior to the results of the closed surgical valvotomy. After 7 years, mitral valve area was equivalent in the BMV and open surgical groups, both significantly greater than in the closed valvotomy group (see Fig. 66-25). In another randomized study that included older patients with less favorable valve morphology, compared with open surgical commissurotomy, patients randomized to BMV had a smaller increase in valve area and higher likelihood of restenosis (28% versus 18% at 4 years). Excellent results have also been reported in children and adolescents in developing nations, where patients tend to be younger. These young patients usually have pliable valves, which are ideal for BMV.

in whom MV replacement is undesirable, and pregnant women with MS.

BMV may be considered for patients with moderate to severe MS and new-onset AF and those with mild MS when significant pulmonary hypertension is present (see Fig. 66-23). In this last group, it is likely that valve obstruction is the cause of pulmonary hypertension, even when stenosis severity does not meet the valve area criteria for severe obstruction.

This percutaneous technique consists of advancing a small balloon flotation catheter across the interatrial septum (after transseptal puncture), enlarging the opening, advancing a large (23- to 25-mm) hourglass-shaped balloon (the Inoue balloon), and inflating it within the orifice (**Fig. 66-24**).[121] Alternatively, two smaller (15- to 20-mm) side by side balloons across the mitral orifice may be used. A third technique involves retrograde, nontransseptal dilation of the mitral valve, in which the balloon is positioned across the mitral valve using a steerable guidewire.

Commissural separation and fracture of nodular calcium appear to be the mechanisms responsible for improvement in valvular function. In several series, the hemodynamic results of BMV have been favorable (**Fig. 66-25**), with reduction of the transmitral pressure gradient from an average of approximately 18 to 6 mm Hg (see Chap. 59), a small (average, 20%) increase in cardiac output, and an average doubling of the calculated mitral valve area, from 1 to 2 cm².[113-115] Results are especially impressive in younger patients without severe valvular thickening or calcification (see Fig. 66-19). Elevated pulmonary vascular resistance declines rapidly, although usually not completely. The reported mortality rate has ranged from 1% to 2%. Complications include cerebral emboli and cardiac perforation, each in approximately 1% of patients, and the development of MR severe enough to require operation in another 2% (approximately 15% develop lesser, but still undesirable, degrees of MR). Approximately 5% of patients are left with a small residual atrial septal defect, but this closes or

SURGICAL VALVOTOMY. Three operative approaches are available for the treatment of rheumatic MS: (1) closed mitral valvotomy using a transatrial or transventricular approach; (2) open valvotomy (i.e., valvotomy carried out under direct vision with the aid of cardiopulmonary bypass, which may be combined with other repair techniques, such as leaflet resection, chordal procedures, and annuloplasty when MR is present; and (3) MV replacement (**Table 66-6**). Surgical intervention for MS is recommended for patients with severe MS and significant symptoms (NYHA Class III or IV) when BMV is not available, BMV is contraindicated because of persistent left atrial thrombus or moderate to severe MR, or when the valve is calcified and surgical risk is acceptable.[122] The preferred surgical approach is valve repair (open valvotomy, with or without additional procedures) whenever possible. Surgery also is reasonable for patients with severe MS and severe pulmonary hypertension when BMV is not possible and may be considered for patients with moderate to severe MS with recurrent embolic events despite anticoagulation.

CLOSED MITRAL VALVOTOMY. Closed mitral valvotomy is rarely used in the United States today, having been replaced by BMV, which is more effective in patients who are candidates for closed mitral valvotomy. Closed mitral valvotomy is more popular in developing nations, where

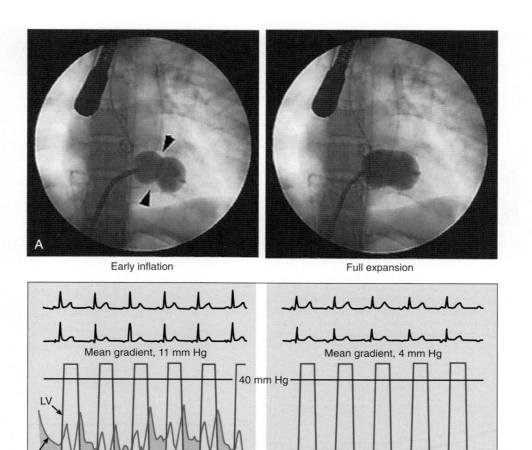

Early inflation   Full expansion

Before valvuloplasty   After valvuloplasty

FIGURE 66-24 Percutaneous balloon mitral valvotomy (BMV) for mitral stenosis using the Inoue technique (see Chap. 59). **A,** The catheter is advanced into the left atrium via the transseptal technique and guided antegrade across the mitral orifice. As the balloon is inflated, its distal portion expands first and is pulled back so that it fits snugly against the orifice. With further inflation, the proximal portion of the balloon expands to center the balloon within the stenotic orifice **(left).** Further inflation expands the central "waist" portion of the balloon **(right),** resulting in commissural splitting and enlargement of the orifice. **B,** Successful BMV results in significant increase in mitral valve area, as reflected by a reduction in the diastolic pressure gradient between left ventricle (magenta) and pulmonary capillary wedge (blue) pressure, as indicated by the shaded area. *(From Delabays A, Goy JJ: Images in clinical medicine: Percutaneous mitral valvuloplasty. N Engl J Med 345:e4, 2001.)*

the expense of open heart surgery and even of balloon catheters for BMV is an important factor and where patients with MS are younger and therefore have more pliable valves. However, even in these nations, closed mitral valvotomy is being replaced by BMV.

This procedure is performed without cardiopulmonary bypass but with the aid of a transventricular dilator. It is an effective operation, provided that MR, atrial thrombosis, or valvular calcification is not serious and that chordal fusion and shortening are not severe. Echocardiography is useful for selecting suitable candidates for this procedure by identifying patients without valvular calcification or dense fibrosis. If possible, closed mitral valvotomy should be carried out with pump standby; if the surgeon is unable to achieve a satisfactory result, the patient can be placed on cardiopulmonary bypass and the valvotomy carried out under direct vision or the valve replaced.

On average, the mitral valve area is increased by 1 cm², with only 20% to 30% of patients requiring MV replacement within 15 years. The hospital mortality rate is 1% to 2% in experienced centers. Marked symptomatic improvement occurs in most patients, and there is excellent long-term survival in patients selected with low echo scores.[122] Long-term follow-up has shown that the results are best if the operation is carried out before chronic AF and/or heart failure has occurred, and

complication rates are higher when valves are calcified and/or severely thickened.

OPEN VALVOTOMY. Most surgeons now prefer to carry out direct vision or open valvotomy. This operation is most frequently performed in patients with MS whose mitral valves are too distorted or calcified for BMV. Cardiopulmonary bypass is established and, to obtain a dry, quiet heart, body temperature is usually lowered, the heart is arrested, and the aorta is occluded intermittently. Thrombi are removed from the left atrium and its appendage, and the latter is often amputated to remove a potential source of postoperative emboli. The commissures are incised and, when necessary, fused chordae tendineae are separated, the underlying papillary muscle is split, and the valve leaflets are débrided of calcium. Mild or even moderate MR may be corrected using similar repair approaches as for primary MR. Left atrial and LV pressures are measured after bypass has been discontinued to confirm that the valvotomy has been effective. When it has not been effective, another attempt can be made. When repair is not possible—usually because of severe distortion and calcification of the valve and subvalvular apparatus, with accompanying MR that cannot be corrected—MV replacement should be carried out. In patients with AF, a left atrial maze or AF ablation procedure typically is done at the time of surgery to increase the likelihood of long-term

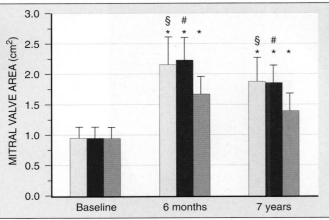

FIGURE 66-25 Mitral valve area before and 6 months and 7 years after valvotomy in a prospective, randomized trial of balloon mitral valvotomy (BMV, yellow bars), open surgical mitral commissurotomy (OMC, purple bars) and closed mitral commissurotomy (CMC, blue bars). At 6 months and 7 years, the results of BMV were equivalent to those of OMC and superior to those of CMC. §P<.001 for BMC versus CMC; #P<.001 for OMC versus CMC. *(From Farhat MB, Ayari M, Maatouk F, et al: Percutaneous balloon versus surgical closed and open mitral commissurotomy: Seven-year follow-up results of a randomized trial. Circulation 97:245, 1998.)*

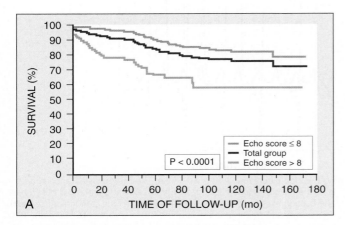

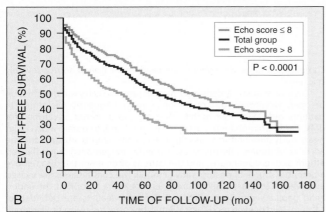

FIGURE 66-26 Long-term survival **(A)** and event-free survival **(B)** after balloon mitral valvotomy for 879 patients who were stratified by baseline echocardiographic morphology score, 8 or less (blue line) or more than 8 (gold line). Patients with the lower echo score had a significantly better outcome initially and over the next 12 to 13 years. *(From Palacios IF, Sanchez PL, Harrell LC, et al: Which patients benefit from percutaneous mitral balloon valvuloplasty? Prevalvuloplasty and postvalvuloplasty variables that predict long-term outcome. Circulation 105:1465, 2002.)*

TABLE 66-6	Approaches to Mechanical Relief of Mitral Stenosis	
APPROACH	**ADVANTAGES**	**DISADVANTAGES**
Closed surgical valvotomy	Inexpensive Relatively simple Good hemodynamic results in selected patients Good long-term outcome	No direct visualization of valve Only feasible with flexible, noncalcified valves Contraindicated if MR > 2+ Surgical procedure with general anesthesia
Open surgical valvotomy	Visualization of valve allows directed valvotomy Concurrent annuloplasty for MR is feasible	Best results with flexible, noncalcified valves Surgical procedure with general anesthesia
Valve replacement	Feasible in all patients regardless of extent of valve calcification or severity of MR	Surgical procedure with general anesthesia Effect of loss of annular-papillary muscle continuity on LV function Prosthetic valve Chronic anticoagulation
Balloon mitral valvotomy	Percutaneous approach Local anesthesia Good hemodynamic results in selected patients Good long-term outcome	No direct visualization of valve Only feasible with flexible noncalcified valves Contraindicated if MR > 2+

sinus rhythm. Open valvotomy is feasible and successful in more than 80% of patients referred for this procedure, with an operative mortality of 1%, rate of reoperation for MV replacement of 0% to 16% at 36 to 53 months, and 10-year actuarial survival rates of 81% to 100%.

RESTENOSIS AFTER VALVOTOMY. Mitral valvotomy, whether percutaneous or operative and open or closed, is palliative rather than curative and, even when successful, there is some degree of residual mitral valve dysfunction. Because the valve is not normal postoperatively, turbulent flow usually persists in the paravalvular region, and the resultant trauma may play a role in restenosis. These changes are analogous to the gradual development of obstruction in a congenitally bicuspid aortic valve and are not usually the result of recurrent rheumatic fever. It is likely that the process of superimposed leaflet calcification and increased stiffness superimposed on the rheumatic valve is similar to the calcific changes seen in aortic valve stenosis.

On clinical grounds alone, based on the reappearance of symptoms, the incidence of restenosis has been estimated to range widely, from 2% to 60%. Recurrence of symptoms is usually not caused by restenosis but may be caused by one or more of the following conditions: (1) an inadequate first operation with residual stenosis; (2) increased severity of MR, either at operation or as a consequence of infective endocarditis; (3) progression of aortic valve disease; or (4) development of coronary artery disease. True restenosis occurs in less than 20% of patients who are followed for 10 years.[113]

Thus, in properly selected patients, mitral valvotomy, however performed—percutaneous BMV, closed or open surgical valvotomy—is a low-risk procedure that results in a significant increase in the size of the mitral orifice and favorably alters the clinical course of an otherwise progressive disease. Pulmonary arterial pressure falls promptly and decisively when mitral obstruction is effectively relieved. Most patients maintain clinical improvement for 10 to 15 years of follow-up. When a second procedure is required because of symptomatic deterioration, the valve is usually calcified and more seriously deformed than at the time of the first operation, and adequate reconstruction may not be possible. Accordingly, MV replacement is often necessary at that time.

Mitral Valve Replacement

MV replacement is recommended for symptomatic patients with severe MR when BMV or surgical MV repair is not possible. Usually, MV replacement is required for patients with combined MS and moderate or severe MR, those with extensive commissural calcification, severe fibrosis, and subvalvular fusion, and those who have undergone previous valvotomy. The operative mortality rate for isolated MV replacement ranges from 3% to 8% in most centers and averaged 6.04% in the large data base of 16,105 such operations for patients with MS and/or MR reported in the Society of Thoracic Surgeons (STS) National Database (see Table 66-3). Prosthetic valves are associated with increased risk because of valve deterioration and chronic anticoagulation, so the threshold for operation should be higher in patients in whom preoperative evaluation suggests that MV replacement may be required than in patients in whom valvotomy alone appears to be indicated.

Generally, a mechanical valve is preferred when MV replacement for MS is necessary when AF is present because of the need for chronic anticoagulation. In patients younger than 65 years who are in sinus rhythm, a mechanical valve is reasonable because of the risk of tissue valve deterioration and likely need for a second operation in the future. However, some younger patients may choose a bioprosthetic valve for lifestyle considerations, despite the risk of valve deterioration. A bioprosthetic valve is appropriate in patients who cannot take warfarin and is reasonable in all patients older than 65 years.

MV replacement is indicated in two groups of patients with MS whose valves are not suitable for valvotomy: (1) those with a mitral valve area smaller than 1.5 cm^2 in NYHA Class III or IV; and (2) those with severe MS (mitral valve area ≤1 cm^2), NYHA Class II, and severe pulmonary hypertension (pulmonary artery systolic pressure >60 mm Hg). Because the operative mortality risk may be high (10% to 20%) in patients in NYHA Class IV, surgery should be carried out before patients reach this stage if possible. On the other hand, even such high-risk patients should not be denied this option unless they have comorbid conditions that preclude surgery or a satisfactory outcome.

Mitral Regurgitation

CAUSES AND PATHOLOGY. The mitral valve apparatus involves the mitral leaflets, chordae tendineae, papillary muscles, and mitral annulus (**Fig. 66-27**). Abnormalities of any of these structures may cause MR.[123] The major causes of MR include mitral valve prolapse (MVP), rheumatic heart disease, infective endocarditis, annular calcification, cardiomyopathy, and ischemic heart disease (**Table 66-7**). Specific aspects of the MVP syndrome, the most important cause of significant MR in the United States, are discussed later. Less common causes of MR include collagen vascular diseases, trauma, the hypereosinophilic syndrome, carcinoid, and exposure to certain drugs.

Abnormalities of Valve Leaflets

MR caused by involvement of the valve leaflets occurs in many situations.[124] MR in patients with chronic rheumatic heart disease, in contrast to MS, is more frequent in men than in women. It is a consequence of shortening, rigidity, deformity, and retraction of one or both mitral valve cusps and is associated with shortening and fusion of the chordae tendineae and papillary muscles. MVP involves both leaflets and chordae and is usually associated with annular dilation. Infective endocarditis can cause MR by perforating valve leaflets (see Chap. 67); vegetations can prevent leaflet coaptation, and valvular retraction during the healing phase of endocarditis can cause MR. Destruction of the mitral valve leaflets can also occur in patients with penetrating and nonpenetrating trauma (see Chap. 76). MR associated with drug exposure also results from anatomic changes in the valve leaflets.[125-127]

Abnormalities of the Mitral Annulus

DILATION. In a normal adult, the mitral annulus measures approximately 10 cm in circumference. It is soft and flexible, and contraction of the surrounding LV muscle during systole causes the annular constriction that contributes importantly to valve closure. MR secondary to dilation of the mitral annulus can occur in any form of heart disease characterized by dilation of the left ventricle, especially dilated cardiomyopathy. LV submitral aneurysm has been reported as a cause of

annular MR in sub-Saharan Africa and appears to be caused by a congenital defect in the posterior portion of the annulus. Diagnosis by TEE and surgical repair have been reported.

CALCIFICATION. Idiopathic (degenerative) calcification of the mitral annulus is one of the most common cardiac abnormalities found at autopsy; in most hearts, it is of little functional consequence. However, when severe (see Fig. 16-21), it may be an important cause of MR and, in contrast to MR secondary to rheumatic fever, is more common in women than in men. The development of degenerative calcification of the mitral annulus shares common risk factors with atherosclerosis, including systemic hypertension, hypercholesterolemia, and diabetes. Hence, mitral annular calcification is associated with coronary and carotid atherosclerosis and identifies patients at higher risk for cardiovascular morbidity and mortality.[128-130] Annular calcification may also be accelerated by an intrinsic defect in the fibrous skeleton of the heart, as in the Marfan and Hurler syndromes. In these two syndromes, the mitral annulus is not only calcified but dilated, further contributing to MR. The incidence of mitral annular calcification is also increased in patients who have chronic renal failure with secondary hyperparathyroidism. The annulus may also become thick, rigid, and calcified secondary to rheumatic involvement; when this process is severe, it also can interfere with valve closure.

With severe annular calcification, a rigid curved bar or ring of calcium encircles the mitral orifice, and calcific spurs may project into the adjacent LV myocardium. The calcification may immobilize the basal portion of the mitral leaflets, preventing their normal excursion in diastole and coaptation in systole, and aggravating the MR that results from loss of the normal sphincteric action of the mitral ring. Rarely, obstruction to LV filling may occur when severe calcification encroaches on or protrudes into the mitral orifice. In patients with severe calcification, the conduction system may be invaded by calcium, leading to atrioventricular and/or intraventricular conduction defects. Calcification of the aortic valve cusps is an associated finding in approximately 50% of patients with severe mitral annular calcification, but this rarely causes AS. Occasionally, calcific deposits extend into the coronary arteries.

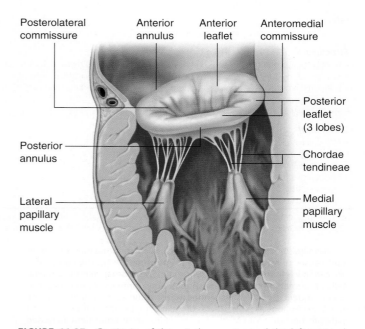

FIGURE 66-27 Continuity of the mitral apparatus and the left ventricular myocardium. MR may be caused by any condition that affects the leaflets or the structure and function of the left ventricle. Similarly, a surgical procedure that disrupts the mitral apparatus in an attempt to correct MR has adverse effects on left ventricular geometry, volume, and function. *(From Otto CM: Evaluation and management of chronic mitral regurgitation. N Engl J Med 345:740, 2001.)*

TABLE 66-7	**Causes of Acute and Chronic Mitral Regurgitation**

Acute

Mitral Annulus Disorders
- Infective endocarditis (abscess formation)
- Trauma (valvular heart surgery)
- Paravalvular leak caused by suture interruption (surgical technical problems or infective endocarditis)

Mitral Leaflet Disorders
- Infective endocarditis (perforation or interfering with valve closure by vegetation)
- Trauma (tear during percutaneous balloon mitral valvotomy or penetrating chest injury)
- Tumors (atrial myxoma)
- Myxomatous degeneration
- Systemic lupus erythematosus (Libman-Sacks lesion)

Rupture of Chordae Tendineae
- Idiopathic (e.g., spontaneous)
- Myxomatous degeneration (mitral valve prolapse, Marfan syndrome, Ehlers-Danlos syndrome)
- Infective endocarditis
- Acute rheumatic fever
- Trauma (percutaneous balloon valvotomy, blunt chest trauma)

Papillary Muscle Disorders
- Coronary artery disease (causing dysfunction and rarely rupture)
- Acute global left ventricular dysfunction
- Infiltrative diseases (amyloidosis, sarcoidosis)
- Trauma

Primary Mitral Valve Prosthetic Disorders
- Porcine cusp perforation (endocarditis)
- Porcine cusp degeneration
- Mechanical failure (strut fracture)
- Immobilized disc or ball of the mechanical prosthesis

Chronic

Inflammatory
- Rheumatic heart disease
- Systemic lupus erythematosus
- Scleroderma

Degenerative
- Myxomatous degeneration of mitral valve leaflets (Barlow click-murmur syndrome, prolapsing leaflet, mitral valve prolapse)
- Marfan syndrome
- Ehlers-Danlos syndrome
- Pseudoxanthoma elasticum
- Calcification of mitral valve annulus

Infective
- Infective endocarditis affecting normal, abnormal, or prosthetic mitral valves

Structural
- Ruptured chordae tendineae (spontaneous or secondary to myocardial infarction, trauma, mitral valve prolapse, endocarditis)
- Rupture or dysfunction of papillary muscle (ischemia or myocardial infarction)
- Dilation of mitral valve annulus and left ventricular cavity (congestive cardiomyopathies, aneurysmal dilation of the left ventricle)
- Hypertrophic cardiomyopathy
- Paravalvular prosthetic leak

Congenital
- Mitral valve clefts or fenestrations
- Parachute mitral valve abnormality in association with:
  Endocardial cushion defects
  Endocardial fibroelastosis
  Transposition of the great arteries
  Anomalous origin of the left coronary artery

Data from Jutzy KR, Al-Zaibag M: Acute mitral and aortic valve regurgitation. *In* Al-Zaibag M, Duran CMG (eds): Valvular Heart Disease. New York, Marcel Dekker, 1994, pp 345-362; and Haffajee CI: Chronic mitral regurgitation. In Dalen JE, Alpert JS (eds): Valvular Heart Disease. 2nd ed. Boston, Little, Brown, 1987, p 112.

ABNORMALITIES OF THE CHORDAE TENDINEAE. Such abnormalities are important causes of MR. Lengthening and rupture of the chordae tendineae are cardinal features of the MVP syndrome. The chordae may be congenitally abnormal; rupture may be spontaneous (primary) or may occur as a consequence of infective endocarditis, trauma, rheumatic fever or, rarely, osteogenesis imperfecta or relapsing polychondritis. In most patients, no cause for chordal rupture is apparent other than increased mechanical strain. Chordae to the posterior leaflet rupture more frequently than those to the anterior leaflet. Patients with idiopathic rupture of mitral chordae tendineae frequently exhibit pathologic fibrosis of the papillary muscles. It is possible that the dysfunction of the papillary muscles may cause stretching and ultimately rupture of the chordae tendineae. Chordal rupture may also result from acute LV dilation, regardless of the cause. Depending on the number of chordae involved in rupture and the rate at which rupture occurs, the resultant MR may be mild, moderate, or severe and acute, subacute, or chronic.

INVOLVEMENT OF THE PAPILLARY MUSCLES. Diseases of the LV papillary muscles are a frequent cause of MR. Because these muscles are perfused by the terminal portion of the coronary vascular bed, they are particularly vulnerable to ischemia, and any disturbance in coronary perfusion may result in papillary muscle dysfunction. When ischemia is transient, it results in temporary papillary muscle dysfunction and may cause transient episodes of MR that are sometimes associated with attacks of angina pectoris or pulmonary edema.[131] When ischemia of papillary muscles is severe and prolonged, it causes papillary muscle dysfunction and scarring, as well as chronic MR. The posterior papillary muscle, which is supplied by the posterior descending branch of the right coronary artery, becomes ischemic and infarcted more frequently than the antero-lateral papillary muscle; the latter is supplied by diagonal branches of the left anterior descending coronary artery and often by marginal branches from the left circumflex artery as well. Ischemia of the papillary muscles is usually caused by coronary atherosclerosis, but may also occur in patients with severe anemia, shock, coronary arteritis of any cause, or an anomalous left coronary artery. MR occurs frequently in patients with healed myocardial infarcts[132,133] and is most frequently caused by regional dysfunction of the LV myocardium at the base of a papillary muscle, resulting in tethering of the mitral leaflets and incomplete leaflet coaptation. Although necrosis of a papillary muscle is a frequent complication of myocardial infarction, frank rupture is far less common; the latter is usually fatal because of the extremely severe MR that it produces (see Chap. 55). However, rupture of one or two of the apical heads of a papillary muscle results in a lesser degree of MR and thus makes survival possible, usually following surgical therapy.

Various other disorders of the papillary muscles may also be responsible for the development of MR (see Chaps. 25, 57, and 68). These include congenital malposition of the muscles, absence of one papillary muscle, resulting in the so-called parachute mitral valve syndrome, and involvement or infiltration of the papillary muscles by a variety of processes, including abscesses, granulomas, neoplasms, amyloidosis, and sarcoidosis.

Left Ventricular Dysfunction

Ischemic LV dysfunction and dilated cardiomyopathy are important causative factors in the development of MR (see Fig. 66-27) and represent the second leading cause of MR after MVP in the United States. LV dilation of any cause including ischemia can alter the spatial relationships between the papillary muscles and chordae tendineae and thereby result in functional MR (see Fig. 66-27; see Fig 15-53).[133,134]

Some degree of MR is found in approximately 30% of patients with coronary artery disease who are being considered for coronary artery bypass surgery. In most of these patients, MR develops from tethering of the posterior leaflet because of regional LV dysfunction. The outlook for the patient with ischemic MR is substantially worse than that for MR from other causes because of the associated LV remodeling and systolic dysfunction. There may be additional ischemic damage to the papillary muscles, dilation of the mitral valve ring, and/or loss of systolic annular contraction contributing further to MR. In most of these patients, MR is mild; however, in the small percentage with severe MR (3% in one large series of patients with coronary artery disease proved by coronary arteriography), it is associated with a poor prognosis. The incidence and severity of regurgitation vary inversely with the LV ejection fraction and directly with the LV end-diastolic pressure. MR occurs in approximately 20% of patients following acute myocardial infarction and, even when mild, is associated with a higher risk of adverse outcomes.[135]

Other causes of MR, discussed in greater detail elsewhere, include obstructive HCM (see Chap. 69), the hypereosinophilic syndrome, endomyocardial fibrosis, trauma affecting the leaflets and/or papillary muscles, Kawasaki disease, left atrial myxoma, and various congenital anomalies, including cleft anterior leaflet and ostium secundum atrial septal defect (see Chaps. 65, 74, 76, and 89).

PATHOPHYSIOLOGY. Because the regurgitant mitral orifice is functionally in parallel with the aortic valve, the impedance to ventricular emptying is reduced in patients with MR. Consequently, MR enhances LV emptying. Almost 50% of the regurgitant volume is ejected into the left atrium before the aortic valve opens. The volume of MR flow depends on a combination of the instantaneous size of the regurgitant orifice and the (reverse) pressure gradient between the left ventricle and left atrium.[136] Both the orifice size and pressure gradient are labile. LV systolic pressure, and therefore the LV–left atrial gradient, depends on systemic vascular resistance and, in patients in whom the mitral annulus has normal flexibility, the cross-sectional area of the mitral annulus may be altered by many interventions. Thus,

increase of preload and afterload and depression of contractility increase LV size and enlarge the mitral annulus, and thereby the regurgitant orifice. When LV size is reduced by treatment with positive inotropic agents, diuretics, and particularly vasodilators, the regurgitant orifice size decreases, and the volume of regurgitant flow declines, as reflected in the height of the v wave in the left atrial pressure pulse and in the intensity and duration of the systolic murmur. Conversely, LV dilation, regardless of cause, may increase MR.[137]

Left Ventricular Compensation

The left ventricle initially compensates for the development of acute MR by emptying more completely and by increasing preload (i.e., by use of the Frank-Starling principle).[137] Because acute MR reduces late systolic LV pressure and radius, LV wall tension declines markedly (and proportionately to a greater extent than LV pressure), permitting a reciprocal increase in the extent and velocity of myocardial fiber shortening, leading to a reduced end-systolic volume (**Fig. 66-28**). Because regurgitation, particularly severe regurgitation, becomes chronic, the LV end-diastolic volume increases and the end-systolic volume returns to normal. By means of the Laplace principle, which states that myocardial wall tension is related to the product of intraventricular pressure and radius, the increased LV end-diastolic volume increases wall tension to normal or supranormal levels in the so-called chronic compensated stage of severe MR.[90] The resultant increase in LV end-diastolic volume and mitral annular diameter may create a vicious circle, in which MR leads to more MR. In patients with chronic MR, LV end-diastolic volume and mass are increased; that is, typical

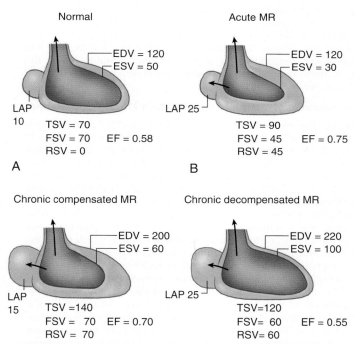

FIGURE 66-28 Three phases of MR are depicted and compared with normal physiology **(A). B,** In acute MR, an increase in preload and a decrease in afterload cause an increase in end-diastolic volume (EDV) and a decrease in end-systolic volume (ESV), producing an increase in total stroke volume (TSV). However, forward stroke volume (FSV) is diminished because 50% of the TSV regurgitates as the regurgitant stroke volume (RSV), resulting in an increase in left atrial pressure (LAP). **C,** In the chronic compensated phase, eccentric hypertrophy has developed and EDV is now increased substantially. Afterload has returned toward normal as the radius term of the Laplace relationship increases with the increase in EDV. Normal muscle function and a large increase in EDV permit a substantial increase in TSV from the acute phase. This, in turn, permits a normal FSV. Left atrial enlargement now accommodates the regurgitant volume at lower LAP. Ejection fraction (EF) remains greater than normal. **D,** In the chronic decompensated phase, muscle dysfunction has developed, impairing ejection fraction, diminishing both TSV and FSV. The EF, although still normal, has decreased to 0.55, and LAP is reelevated because less volume is ejected during systole, causing a higher ESV. (From Carabello BA: Progress in mitral and aortic regurgitation. Curr Probl Cardiol 28:553, 2003.)

volume overload (eccentric) hypertrophy develops. However, the degree of hypertrophy is often not proportional to the degree of LV dilation, so the ratio of LV mass to end-diastolic volume may be less than normal. Nonetheless, the reduced afterload permits maintenance of ejection fraction in the normal to supranormal range. The reduced LV afterload allows a greater proportion of the contractile energy of the myocardium to be expended in shortening than in tension development, and explains how the left ventricle can adapt to the load imposed by MR.

The eccentric ventricular hypertrophy that accompanies the elevated end-diastolic volume of chronic MR is secondary to new sarcomeres laid down in series. A shift to the right (greater volume at any pressure) occurs in the LV diastolic pressure-volume curve in patients with chronic MR. With decompensation, chamber stiffness increases, raising the diastolic pressure at any volume.

In most patients with severe primary MR, compensation is maintained for years, but in some patients the prolonged hemodynamic overload ultimately leads to myocardial decompensation.[137] End-systolic volume, preload, and afterload all increase, whereas ejection fraction and stroke volume decline. In such patients, there is evidence of neurohormonal activation and elevation of circulating proinflammatory cytokines. Plasma natriuretic peptide levels also increase in response to the volume load—more in patients with symptomatic decompensation.

Coronary flow rates may be increased in patients with severe MR, but the increases in myocardial oxygen consumption (MvO_2) are relatively modest compared with patients with AS and AR, because myocardial fiber shortening, which is elevated in patients with MR, is not one of the principal determinants of MvO_2 (see Chap. 24). One of these determinants, mean LV wall tension, may actually be reduced in patients with MR, whereas the other two, contractility and heart rate, may be little affected. Thus, patients with MR have a low incidence of clinical manifestations of myocardial ischemia compared with the much higher incidence in those with AS and AR, conditions in which MvO_2 is greatly augmented.

Assessment of Myocardial Contractility in Mitral Regurgitation

Because the ejection phase indices of myocardial contractility are inversely correlated with afterload, patients with early MR (with reduced LV afterload) often exhibit elevations in ejection phase indices of myocardial contractility, such as ejection fraction, fractional fiber shortening, and velocity of circumferential fiber shortening (VCF).[35,137] Many patients ultimately develop symptoms because of elevated left atrial and pulmonary venous pressures related to the regurgitant volume and with no change in these ejection phase indices, which remain elevated. However, in other patients, major symptoms reflect serious contractile dysfunction, at which time ejection fraction, fractional shortening, and mean VCF have declined to low-normal or below-normal levels (see Fig. 66-28). As MR persists, the reduction in afterload, which increases myocardial fiber shortening and the aforementioned ejection phase indices, is opposed by the impairment of myocardial function characteristic of severe chronic diastolic overload. However, even in patients with overt heart failure secondary to MR, the ejection fraction and fractional shortening may be only modestly reduced. Therefore, values in the low-normal range for the ejection phase indices of myocardial performance in patients with chronic MR may actually reflect impaired myocardial function, whereas moderately reduced values (e.g., ejection fraction 40% to 50%) generally signify severe, often irreversible, impairment of contractility, identifying patients who may do poorly after surgical correction of the MR (**Fig. 66-29**). An ejection fraction of less than 35% in patients with severe MR usually represents advanced myocardial dysfunction; such patients are high operative risks and may not experience satisfactory improvement following MV replacement.

End-Systolic Volume

Preoperative myocardial contractility is an important determinant of the risk of operative death, cardiac failure perioperatively, and postoperative level of LV function. Therefore, it is not surprising that the end-systolic pressure-volume (or stress-dimension) relationship

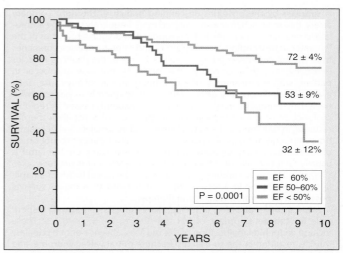

FIGURE 66-29 Late survival of patients after surgical correction of mitral regurgitation subdivided on the basis of the preoperative echocardiographic ejection fraction (EF). (From Enriquez-Sarano M, Tajik AJ, Schaff HV, et al: Echocardiographic prediction of survival after surgical correction of organic mitral regurgitation. Circulation 90:833, 1994.)

has emerged as a useful index for evaluating LV function in patients with MR. The simple measurement of end-systolic volume or diameter has been found to be a useful predictor of function and survival following mitral valve surgery.[136-138] A preoperative LV end-systolic diameter that exceeds 40 mm identifies a patient with a high likelihood of impaired LV systolic function following surgery.[1,139]

Hemodynamics

Effective (forward) cardiac output is usually depressed in severely symptomatic patients with MR, whereas total LV output (the sum of forward and regurgitant flow) is usually elevated until late in the patient's course. The cardiac output achieved during exercise, not the regurgitant volume, is the principal determinant of functional capacity. The atrial contraction a wave in the left atrial pressure pulse is usually not as prominent in MR as in MS, but the v wave is characteristically much taller (see Chap. 20) because it is inscribed during ventricular systole, when the left atrium is being filled with blood from the pulmonary veins and from the left ventricle. Occasionally, backward transmission of the tall v wave into the pulmonary arterial bed may result in an early diastolic pulmonary arterial v wave (**Fig. 66-30**). In patients with isolated MR, the y descent in the pulmonary capillary pressure pulse is particularly rapid because the distended left atrium empties rapidly during early diastole. However, in patients with combined MS and MR, the y descent is gradual. Although a left atrioventricular pressure gradient persisting throughout diastole signifies the presence of significant associated MS, a brief early diastolic gradient may occur in patients with isolated severe MR as a result of the rapid flow of blood across a normal-sized mitral orifice early in diastole, often accompanied by an early diastolic murmur at the apex.

LEFT ATRIAL COMPLIANCE. The compliance of the left atrium (and pulmonary venous bed) is an important determinant of the hemodynamic and clinical picture in patients with severe MR. Three major subgroups of patients with severe MR based on left atrial compliance have been identified and are characterized as follows.

NORMAL OR REDUCED COMPLIANCE. In this subgroup, there is little enlargement of the left atrium but marked elevation of the mean left atrial pressure, particularly of the v wave, and pulmonary congestion is a prominent symptom. Severe MR usually develops acutely, as occurs with rupture of the chordae tendineae, infarction of one of the heads of a papillary muscle, or perforation of a mitral leaflet as a consequence of trauma or endocarditis. In patients with acute MR, the left atrium initially operates on the steep portion of its pressure-volume curve, with a marked rise in pressure for a small increase in volume. Sinus rhythm is usually present; after the passage of weeks or a few months, the left atrial wall becomes hypertrophied, is capable of contracting vigorously, and

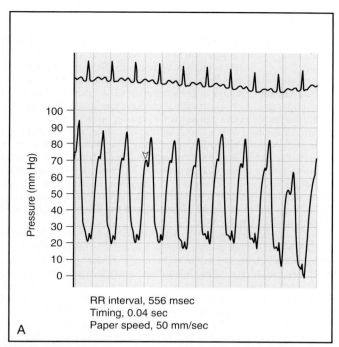

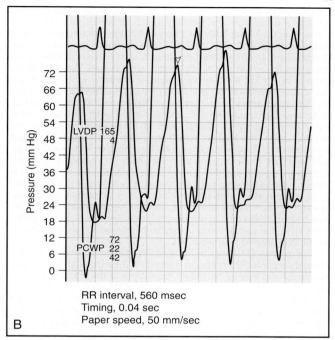

FIGURE 66-30 Hemodynamic tracings in a 45-year-old woman with acute mitral regurgitation from bacterial endocarditis. **A,** Pulmonary artery pressure. **B,** Simultaneous left ventricular diastolic pressure (LVDP) and pulmonary capillary wedge pressure (PCWP). The PCWP demonstrates a markedly elevated v wave (arrowhead, **B**) that transmits to the pulmonary artery pressure (arrowhead, **A**). *(Modified from Wisse B, Sniderman AD: Severe mitral regurgitation. N Engl J Med 343:1386, 2000.)*

facilitates LV filling. The thicker atrium is less compliant than normal, which further increases the height of the *v* wave. Thickening of the walls of the pulmonary veins and proliferative changes in the pulmonary arteries, as well as marked elevations of pulmonary vascular resistance and pulmonary artery pressure, usually develop over the course of 6 to 12 months after the onset of acute severe MR.

MARKEDLY INCREASED COMPLIANCE. At the opposite end of the spectrum from patients in the first group are those with severe long-standing MR with massive enlargement of the left atrium and normal or only slightly elevated left atrial pressure. The atrial wall contains only a small remnant of muscle surrounded by fibrous tissue. Long-standing MR in these patients has altered the physical properties of the left atrial wall and thereby displaced the atrial pressure-volume curve to the right, allowing a normal or almost normal pressure to exist in a greatly enlarged left atrium. Pulmonary arterial pressure and pulmonary vascular resistance may be normal or only slightly elevated at rest. AF and a low cardiac output are almost invariably present.

MODERATELY INCREASED COMPLIANCE. This most common subgroup consists of patients between the ends of the spectrum represented by the first and second groups. These patients have severe chronic MR and exhibit variable degrees of enlargement of the left atrium, associated with significant elevation of the left atrial pressure, and these two factors (in association with age) determine the likelihood that AF will ensue.

CLINICAL PRESENTATION

Symptoms

The nature and severity of symptoms in patients with chronic MR are functions of a combination of interrelated factors, including the severity of MR, rate of its progression, level of left atrial, pulmonary venous, and pulmonary arterial pressure, presence of episodic or chronic atrial tachyarrhythmias, and presence of associated valvular, myocardial, or coronary artery disease. Symptoms may occur with preserved LV contractile function in patients with chronic MR who have severely elevated pulmonary venous pressures or AF. In other patients, symptoms herald LV decompensation. In patients with rheumatic MR, the time interval between the initial attack of rheumatic fever and development of symptoms tends to be longer than in those with MS, and often exceeds two decades. Hemoptysis and systemic embolization are less common in patients with isolated or predominant MR than in those with MS. The development of AF affects the course adversely

but perhaps not as dramatically as in MS. Conversely, chronic weakness and fatigue secondary to a low cardiac output are more prominent features in MR.

Most patients with MR of rheumatic origin have only mild disability, unless regurgitation progresses as a result of chronic rheumatic activity, infective endocarditis, or rupture of the chordae tendineae. However, the indolent course of MR may be deceptive. By the time that symptoms secondary to a reduced cardiac output and/or pulmonary congestion become apparent, serious and sometimes even irreversible LV dysfunction may have developed.

In patients with severe chronic MR who have a greatly enlarged left atrium and relatively mild left atrial hypertension (patients with increased left atrial compliance), pulmonary vascular resistance does not usually rise markedly. Instead, the major symptoms, fatigue and exhaustion, are related to the depressed cardiac output. Right-sided heart failure, characterized by congestive hepatomegaly, edema, and ascites, may be prominent in patients with acute MR, elevated pulmonary vascular resistance, and pulmonary hypertension. Angina pectoris is rare unless coronary artery disease coexists.

PHYSICAL EXAMINATION. Palpation of the arterial pulse is helpful in differentiating AS from MR, both of which may produce a prominent systolic murmur at the base of the heart and apex (see Chap. 12). The carotid arterial upstroke is sharp in severe MR and delayed in AS; the volume of the pulse may be normal or reduced in the presence of heart failure. The cardiac impulse, like the arterial pulse, is brisk and hyperdynamic. It is displaced to the left, and a prominent LV filling wave is frequently palpable. Systolic expansion of the enlarged left atrium may result in a late systolic thrust in the parasternal region, which may be confused with RV enlargement.

AUSCULTATION. When chronic severe MR is caused by defective valve leaflets, S₁, produced by mitral valve closure, is usually diminished. Wide splitting of S₂ is common and results from the shortening of LV ejection and an earlier A₂ as a consequence of reduced resistance to LV ejection. In patients with MR who have severe pulmonary hypertension, P₂ is louder than A₂. The abnormal increase in the flow rate across the mitral orifice during the rapid filling phase is often associated with an S₃, which should not be interpreted as a feature of heart failure in these patients, and this may be accompanied by a brief diastolic rumble.

The systolic murmur is the most prominent physical finding; it must be differentiated from the systolic murmur of AS, TR, and ventricular septal defect. In most patients with severe MR, the systolic murmur commences immediately after the soft S_1 and continues beyond and may obscure the A_2 because of the persisting pressure difference between the left ventricle and left atrium after aortic valve closure. The holosystolic murmur of chronic MR is usually constant in intensity, blowing, high-pitched, and loudest at the apex, with frequent radiation to the left axilla and left infrascapular area. However, radiation toward the sternum or aortic area may occur with abnormalities of the posterior leaflet and is particularly common in patients with MVP involving this leaflet. The murmur shows little change, even in the presence of large beat to beat variations of LV stroke volume, as in AF. This contrasts with most midsystolic (ejection) murmurs, such as in AS, which vary greatly in intensity with stroke volume and therefore with the duration of diastole. There is little correlation between the intensity of the systolic murmur and severity of MR. In patients with severe MR caused by LV dilation, acute myocardial infarction, or paraprosthetic valvular regurgitation, or in those who have marked emphysema, obesity, chest deformity, or a prosthetic heart valve, the systolic murmur may be barely audible or even absent, a condition referred to as silent MR.

The murmur of MR may be holosystolic, late systolic, or early systolic. When the murmur is confined to late systole, the regurgitation is usually not severe and may be secondary to prolapse of the mitral valve or to papillary muscle dysfunction. These causes of MR are frequently associated with a normal S_1 because initial closure of the mitral valve cusps may be unimpaired. The late systolic murmur of papillary muscle dysfunction is particularly variable; it may become accentuated or holosystolic during acute myocardial ischemia and often disappears when ischemia is relieved. A midsystolic click preceding a mid to late systolic murmur, and the response of that murmur to a number of maneuvers, helps establish the diagnosis of MVP. Early systolic murmurs are typical of acute MR. When the left atrial v wave is markedly elevated in acute MR, the murmur may diminish or disappear in late systole as the reverse pressure gradient declines. As noted, a short, low-pitched diastolic murmur following S_3 may be audible in patients with severe MR, even without accompanying MS.

DYNAMIC AUSCULTATION. The holosystolic murmur of MR varies little during respiration. However, sudden standing usually diminishes the murmur, whereas squatting augments it. The late systolic murmur of MVP behaves in the opposite direction, decreasing in duration with squatting and increasing in duration with standing. The holosystolic MR murmur is reduced during the strain of the Valsalva maneuver and shows a left-sided response (i.e., a transient overshoot that occurs six to eight beats following release of the strain). The murmur of MR is usually intensified by isometric exercise, differentiating it from the systolic murmurs of valvular AS and obstructive HCM, both of which are reduced by this intervention. The murmur of MR caused by LV dilation decreases in intensity and duration following effective therapy with cardiac glycosides, diuretics, rest, and particularly vasodilators.

DIAGNOSIS AND EVALUATION

DIFFERENTIAL DIAGNOSIS. The holosystolic murmur of MR resembles that produced by a ventricular septal defect. However, the latter is usually loudest at the sternal border rather than the apex and is often accompanied by a parasternal, rather than an apical, thrill. The murmur of MR may also be confused with that of TR, but the latter is usually heard best along the left sternal border, is augmented during inspiration, and is accompanied by a prominent v wave and y descent in the jugular venous pulse.

When the chordae tendineae to the posterior leaflet of the mitral valve rupture, the regurgitant jet is often directed anteriorly, so that it impinges on the atrial septum adjacent to the aortic root and causes a systolic murmur that is most prominent at the base of the heart. This murmur can be confused with that of AS. On the other hand, when the chordae tendineae to the anterior leaflet rupture, the jet is usually directed to the posterior wall of the left atrium and the murmur may be transmitted to the spine or even the top of the head.

Patients with rheumatic disease of the mitral valve exhibit a spectrum of abnormalities, ranging from pure MS to pure MR. The presence of an S_3, a rapid LV filling wave and LV impulse on palpation, and a soft S_1 all favor predominant MR. In contrast, an accentuated S_1, a prominent OS with a short A_2-OS interval, and a soft, short systolic murmur all indicate predominant MS. Elucidation of the predominant valvular lesion may be complicated by the presence of a holosystolic murmur of TR in patients with pure MS and pulmonary hypertension; this murmur may sometimes be heard at the apex when the right ventricle is greatly enlarged and may therefore be mistaken for the murmur of MR.

Echocardiography

Echocardiography plays a central role in the diagnosis of MR, in determining its cause and potential for repair, and in quantifying its severity (see Chap. 15). In patients with severe MR, echocardiographic imaging shows enlargement of the left atrium and left ventricle, with increased systolic motion of both chambers. The underlying cause of the regurgitation, such as rupture of chordae tendineae, MVP (see Fig. 15-52), rheumatic mitral disease, a flail leaflet, vegetations (see Chap. 67), and LV dilation with leaflet tethering can often be determined on the transthoracic echocardiogram. It may also show calcification of the mitral annulus as a band of dense echoes between the mitral apparatus and posterior wall of the heart. This technique is also useful for estimating the hemodynamic consequences of MR on the left atrium and left ventricle; in patients with LV dysfunction, end-diastolic and end-systolic volumes are increased and the ejection fraction and shortening rate may decline.[138]

Doppler echocardiography in MR characteristically reveals a high-velocity jet in the left atrium during systole.[36,140] The severity of the regurgitation is reflected in the width of the jet across the valve (see Fig. 15-50) and the size of the left atrium. Qualitative assessment using color flow Doppler imaging or pulsed techniques correlates reasonably well with angiographic methods in estimating the severity of MR. However, color flow jet areas are significantly influenced by the cause of the regurgitation and jet eccentricity, thus limiting the accuracy of this approach. Quantitative methods to measure regurgitant fraction, regurgitant volume, and regurgitant orifice area have greater accuracy in comparison with angiography[141,142] (see Figs. 15-40, 15-41, 15-50, and 15-51), and these methods are strongly recommended (see Table 66-1).[1] The vena contracta, defined as the narrowest cross-sectional areas of the regurgitant jet as mapped by color flow Doppler echocardiography, also predicts the severity of MR (**Fig. 66-31**). The proximal isovelocity surface area (PISA) method estimates MR severity with isovelocity hemispheric shells as regurgitant flow accelerates toward the mitral orifice. Reversal of flow in the pulmonary veins during systole and a high peak mitral inflow velocity are also useful signs of severe MR.

Doppler echocardiography is also an important tool to estimate the pulmonary artery systolic pressure and to determine the presence and severity of associated AR or TR.

TEE (see Chap. 15) may be needed in addition to transthoracic echocardiography for assessment of the detailed anatomy of the regurgitant mitral valve (see Fig. 15-54) and the severity of MR in some patients. TEE is useful when the transthoracic images are suboptimal and also when determining whether MV repair is feasible or whether MV replacement is necessary. Three-dimensional transthoracic echocardiography and three-dimensional color Doppler[142] have also been reported to help elucidate the mechanism of MR.

Exercise echocardiography is helpful in determining severity of MR and hemodynamic abnormalities (e.g., pulmonary hypertension) during exercise.[70] This is a useful objective means to evaluate symptoms in patients who appear to have only mild MR at rest and, alternatively, to determine functional status and dynamic changes in hemodynamics in patients who otherwise appear stable and asymptomatic.

OTHER DIAGNOSTIC EVALUATION MODALITIES

ELECTROCARDIOGRAPHY. The principal electrocardiographic findings are left atrial enlargement and AF. Electrocardiographic evidence of LV enlargement occurs in about one third of patients with severe MR. Approximately 15% of patients exhibit electrocardiographic evidence of RV hypertrophy, a change that reflects the presence of pulmonary hypertension of sufficient severity to counterbalance the hypertrophied left ventricle of MR.

RADIOGRAPHY. Cardiomegaly with LV enlargement, and particularly with left atrial enlargement, is a common finding in patients with chronic severe MR (see Fig. 16-20). Although the left atrium may be severely enlarged, there is little correlation between left atrial size and pressure. Interstitial edema with Kerley B lines is frequently seen in patients with acute MR or with progressive LV failure.

In patients with combined MS and MR, overall cardiac enlargement and particularly left atrial dilation are prominent findings (see Fig. 16-15).

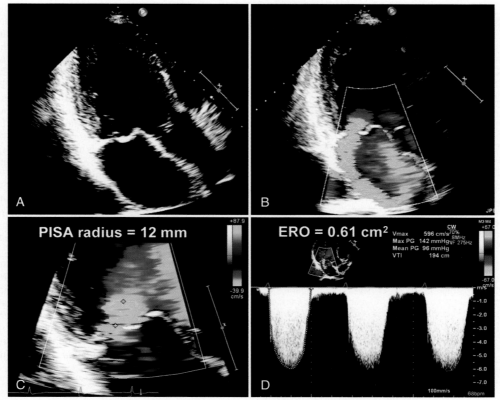

FIGURE 66-31 Severe MR caused by mitral valve prolapse with quantitative determination of effective regurgitant orifice area (ERO) on echocardiography. **A, B,** Severe prolapse of the mitral valve with severe MR was observed. **C, D,** ERO was calculated with the PISA radius and peak velocity of the MR jet. *(From Kang DH, Kim JH, Rim JH, et al: Comparison of early surgery versus conventional treatment in asymptomatic severe mitral regurgitation. Circulation 119:797, 2009.)*

Predominant MS is suggested by relatively mild cardiomegaly (principally straightening of the left cardiac border) and significant changes in the lung fields, whereas predominant MR is more likely when the heart is greatly enlarged and the changes in the lungs are relatively inconspicuous. Calcification of the mitral annulus, an important cause of MR in the elderly, is most prominent in the posterior third of the cardiac silhouette. The lesion is best visualized on chest films exposed in the lateral or right anterior oblique projections, in which it appears as a dense, coarse, C-shaped opacity (see Fig. 16-21).

CARDIAC MAGNETIC RESONANCE. CMR (see Chap. 18) provides accurate measurements of regurgitant flow that correlate well with quantitative Doppler imaging.[41,95] It is also the most accurate noninvasive technique for measuring LV end-diastolic volume, end-systolic volume, and mass. Although detailed visualization of mitral valve structure and function is obtained more reliably with echocardiography, CMR offers a promising approach for more accurate assessment of regurgitant severity.

LEFT VENTRICULAR ANGIOGRAPHY. The prompt appearance of contrast material in the left atrium following its injection into the left ventricle indicates the presence of MR. The injection should be rapid enough to permit LV opacification but slow enough to avoid the development of premature ventricular contractions, which can induce spurious regurgitation (see Chap. 20). The regurgitant volume can be determined from the difference between the total LV stroke volume, estimated by angiocardiography, and the simultaneous measurement of the effective forward stroke volume by the Fick method. In patients with severe MR, the regurgitant volume may approach, and even exceed, the effective forward stroke volume. Qualitative but clinically useful estimates of the severity of MR may be made by cineangiographic observation of the degree of opacification of the left atrium and pulmonary veins following the injection of contrast material into the left ventricle.

DISEASE COURSE

The natural history of MR is highly variable and depends on a combination of the volume of regurgitation, state of the myocardium, and cause of the underlying disorder. Asymptomatic patients with mild primary MR usually remain in a stable state for many years. Severe MR develops in only a small percentage of these patients, usually because of intervening infective endocarditis or rupture of the chordae tendineae. In patients with mild MR related to MVP, the rate of progression in severity of MR is highly variable; in most patients, progression is gradual unless a ruptured chordae or flail leaflet supervenes. Regurgitation tends to progress more rapidly in patients with connective tissue diseases, such as the Marfan syndrome, than in those with chronic MR of rheumatic origin. Acute rheumatic fever is a frequent cause of isolated severe MR in adolescents in developing nations, and these patients often have a rapidly progressive course.

AF is a common arrhythmia in patients with chronic MR, associated with age and left atrial dilation, and its onset is a marker for disease progression. Patients with AF have an adverse outcome compared with patients who remain in sinus rhythm,[143,144] and development of AF is considered an indication for operative intervention, especially in patients who are candidates for MV repair.[1]

Because the natural history of severe MR has been altered greatly by surgical intervention, it is difficult now to predict the course of patients who receive medical therapy alone. However, a 5-year survival of only 30% was reported in patients who were candidates for operation, presumably because of symptoms, but who declined (see Fig. 66-22). Among patients with severe MR resulting from flail leaflets, the annual mortality rate is as high as 6.3%,[145] and at 10 years 90% have died or undergone surgical correction (**Fig. 66-32**). This latter series included many patients who were initially symptomatic or had LV dysfunction or AF, and thus might be considered to be a higher risk.

Whether patients with severe MR who are asymptomatic, with normal LV function, are at risk of death is a subject of debate. One long-term retrospective study has demonstrated that patients with severe MR, defined quantitatively as an effective orifice area larger than 40 mm² (see Table 66-1), had a 4%/year risk of cardiac death.[141] In contrast, a second study reported the outcomes of 132 patients with

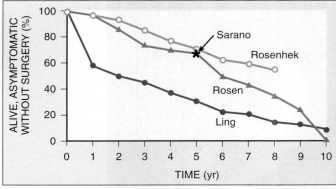

FIGURE 66-32 Four series examining the natural history of patients with severe MR, including a series of patients with flail mitral leaflets reported by Ling and associates (magenta), many of whom were symptomatic, had atrial fibrillation, or had evidence of left ventricular (LV) dysfunction, and three series reported by Rosen and colleagues (blue triangles), Sarano and coworkers (black asterisk), and Rosenhek and associates (gold open circles) in patients who initially were asymptomatic with normal LV function. Although the patients with flail leaflets had a steeper initial attrition rate, all series demonstrated that patients with severe MR have a high likelihood of developing symptoms or other indications for surgery over the course of 6 to 10 years. (*Modified from Ling LH, Enriquez-Sarano M, Seward JB, et al: Clinical outcome of mitral regurgitation due to flail leaflet. N Engl J Med 335:1417, 1996; Rosen SF, Borer JS, Hochreiter C, et al: Natural history of the asymptomatic patient with severe mitral regurgitation secondary to mitral valve prolapse and normal right and left ventricular performance. Am J Cardiol 74:374, 1994; Enriquez-Sarano M, Avierinos JF, Messika-Zeitoun D, et al: Quantitative determinants of the outcome of asymptomatic mitral regurgitation. N Engl J Med 352:875, 2005; and Rosenhek R, Rader F, Klaar U, et al: Outcome of watchful waiting in asymptomatic severe mitral regurgitation. Circulation 113:2238, 2006.*)

severe MR followed prospectively for 5 years,[146] during which the indications for surgery were symptoms or the development of LV dysfunction (ejection fraction < 0.60), LV end-systolic dimension larger than 45 mm, AF, or pulmonary hypertension. Only 2 patients in this latter study had cardiac death, both of whom met criteria for surgery but refused this intervention. A third study followed 286 asymptomatic patients with severe MR and normal LV function without surgery and reported an annual mortality less than 1% (5% mortality at 7 years); in 127 propensity score-matched patients in that study, the estimated actuarial 7 year survival was 99% ± 1% in those treated with early surgery compared with only 85% ± 4% for those treated according to current guidelines for watchful waiting.[147,148] However, mortality arguments aside, all studies uniformly indicated that among asymptomatic patients with initially normal LV ejection fractions, severe MR is associated with a high likelihood of requiring surgery over the next 6 to 10 years because of heart failure symptoms, LV dysfunction, or AF (see Fig. 66-32).

MANAGEMENT OF CHRONIC MITRAL REGURGITATION

Medical Treatment

DEGENERATIVE MITRAL REGURGITATION. The role of pharmacologic therapy for MR remains another subject of uncertainty and some debate.[137,145] Although there is no doubt that afterload reduction therapy is indicated, and may be lifesaving, in patients with acute MR, the indications for such therapy in patients with chronic MR are much less clear. Because afterload is not excessive in most patients with chronic MR, in whom systolic shortening is facilitated by the reduced systolic wall stress, systemic vasodilator therapy to reduce afterload further may not provide additional benefit. Acute administration of nitroprusside, nifedipine, and ACE inhibitors to severely symptomatic patients has been demonstrated to alter hemodynamics favorably in some studies, but these effects may not pertain to asymptomatic patients with preserved systolic function. Several small studies of chronic therapy with ACE inhibitors, ranging from 4 weeks to 6 months, have failed to provide evidence of hemodynamic benefit,

and there are no long-term studies and no randomized trials with which to make definitive recommendations. At present, there is a lack of convincing data that vasodilator therapy affects LV volumes or systolic function favorably in the absence of symptoms or hypertension, and current guidelines do not recommend the use of these agents for chronic therapy of primary degenerative MR. An exception would be those patients with severe chronic MR, with symptoms or LV dysfunction (or both) who are not candidates for surgery because of age or other comorbidities. These patients should receive standard, aggressive management for heart failure with ACE inhibitors and beta adrenergic blocking agents (see Chap. 28). Antibiotic prophylaxis to prevent infective endocarditis is no longer recommended routinely for patients with MR (see Chap. 67). All patients with AF, paroxysmal or chronic, should receive chronic anticoagulation.

FUNCTIONAL MITRAL REGURGITATION. Patients with secondary, functional MR stemming from LV dilation and dysfunction should undergo evidence-based aggressive medical management for LV systolic dysfunction (see Chap. 28). There is evidence that beneficial reverse remodeling with medical therapy will reduce the severity of MR in many patients.

RESYNCHRONIZATION THERAPY. In patients with a dilated or ischemic cardiomyopathy and secondary MR, resynchronization therapy with dual ventricular chamber pacing has been observed to decrease mitral regurgitant severity. The mechanism of this effect likely is similar to that achieved in some patients with medical management—LV remodeling with a reduction in ventricular size and associated improvement in alignment of the papillary muscles (see Chap. 29). This leads to improved leaflet coaptation and decreased backflow across the mitral valve.[145]

Surgical Treatment

Surgical treatment should be considered for patients with functional disability and/or for patients with no symptoms or only mild symptoms but with progressively deteriorating LV function or progressively increasing LV dimensions, as documented by noninvasive studies.[30a,136] In patients considered for surgery, two-dimensional transthoracic or TEE with Doppler evaluation and color flow Doppler imaging provide detailed assessment of mitral valve structure and function.[36,138] However, left heart catheterization, LV angiocardiography, and coronary arteriography are indicated for the following: (1) evaluating a discrepancy between echocardiographic findings and the clinical picture; (2) detecting and assessing the severity of any associated valvular lesions; and (3) determining the presence and assessing the extent of coronary artery disease.

Without surgical treatment, the prognosis for patients with MR and heart failure is poor (see Fig. 66-22), and hence MV repair or replacement is indicated for symptomatic patients. When operative treatment is being considered, the chronic and often slowly but relentlessly progressive nature of MR must be weighed against the immediate risks and long-term uncertainties attendant on surgery, especially if MV replacement is required. Surgical mortality depends on the following: patient's clinical and hemodynamic status (particularly the function of the left ventricle); patient's age (see Chap. 80)[149,150]; presence of comorbid conditions such as renal, hepatic, or pulmonary disease[82]; and the skill and experience of the surgical team.[151-153] The decision to replace or to repair the valve (**Fig. 66-33**) is of critical importance, and MV repair is strongly recommended whenever possible.[152-154] Replacement involves the operative risk, as well as the risks of thromboembolism and anticoagulation in patients receiving mechanical prostheses, of late structural valve deterioration in patients receiving bioprostheses, and of late mortality, especially in patients with associated coronary artery disease who require coronary artery bypass grafting (see Table 66-3). Surgical mortality in patients requiring MV replacement does not depend significantly on which of the currently used tissue or mechanical valve prostheses is selected.

Repair of the mitral valve is most often successful in the following: (1) children and adolescents with pliable valves; (2) adults with degenerative MR secondary to MVP; (3) annular dilation; (4) papillary muscle dysfunction secondary to ischemia or rupture; (5) chordal rupture; or (6) perforation of a mitral leaflet caused by infective endocarditis. This represents the vast majority of patients with MR in the United States and other developed countries. These procedures are less likely to be successful in older patients with the rigid, calcified, deformed valves of rheumatic heart disease or those with severe subvalvular chordal thickening and major loss of leaflet substance; many of these latter patients require MV replacement. Younger patients in developing countries who have severe rheumatic MR in the absence of active carditis may undergo successful repair.[152]

MV repair for degenerative MR consists of reconstruction of the valve, which is usually accompanied by a mitral annuloplasty using a rigid or flexible prosthetic ring (see Fig. 66-33). Prolapsed valves causing severe MR are usually treated with resection of the prolapsing segment(s) with plication and reinforcement of the annulus. Replacing, reimplanting, elongating, or shortening of the chordae tendineae, splitting the papillary muscles, and repairing the subvalvular apparatus have been successful in selected patients with pure or predominant MR in whom subvalvular pathology contributes to the MR.[152,155] Repair of anterior and posterior prolapsing leaflets has been successful in experienced centers.[153,156]

Ischemic MR secondary to regional LV dysfunction with annular dilation may be treated by annuloplasty (see Chap. 31). Annuloplasty is also successful in many patients with significant functional MR resulting from dilated cardiomyopathy. Episodic MR caused by transient ischemia is often eliminated by coronary revascularization, whereas moderate to severe chronic MR secondary to ischemic heart disease usually requires MV repair or replacement.[157,158] In patients undergoing coronary artery bypass surgery, some investigators recommend that concomitant MV repair be considered for even mild MR.[159]

Intraoperative TEE and Doppler is extremely useful for assessing the adequacy of MV repair.[160] In the minority of patients with persistent severe MR in whom the operative results are unsatisfactory, the problem can usually be corrected immediately or, if necessary, the valve can be replaced. LV outflow tract obstruction caused by systolic anterior motion of the mitral valve occurs in 5% to 10% of patients following MV repair for degenerative MR. The causes are not clear but may include excess valvular tissue with severe leaflet redundancy and/or an interventricular septum bulging into a small left ventricle. These complications may also be recognized intraoperatively by TEE. Treatment with volume loading and beta-blocking agents is often helpful. The obstruction usually disappears with time; if it does not, reoperation and rerepair or MV replacement may be necessary.

Preoperative AF is an independent predictor of reduced long-term survival after MV surgery for chronic MR.[144] The persistence of AF postoperatively requires long-term anticoagulation, thereby partially nullifying the advantages of MV repair. In patients who have developed AF, whether chronic or paroxysmal, outcomes are improved if a maze procedure is performed at the time of MV repair or replacement,[119,155] with reduced risk of postoperative stroke. The decision to perform a maze procedure should be based on surgical expertise as well as patient age and comorbidities, because this procedure may add to the length and complexity of the operation.

MITRAL VALVE REPAIR VERSUS REPLACEMENT. Although MV replacement has been used successfully in treating MR for almost four decades, there has been some dissatisfaction with the results of this operation. First, LV function often deteriorates following MV replacement, contributing to early and late mortality and late disability. The increase in afterload consequent to abolishing the low impedance leak was first believed to be responsible, but now it is clear that the loss of annular-chordal-papillary muscle continuity (see Fig. 66-27) interferes with LV geometry, volume, and function in patients who have undergone MV replacement. This does not occur after MV repair. Animal experiments have shown convincingly that the normal function of the MV apparatus primes the left ventricle for normal contraction that is prevented when surgery causes

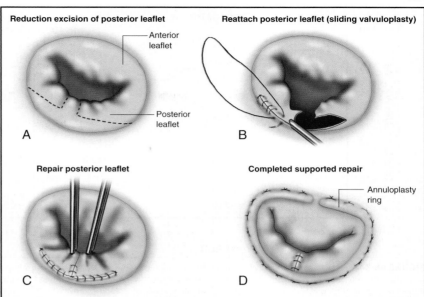

FIGURE 66-33 **A-D,** Mitral valve repair using reduction excision and reattachment of the posterior leaflet with implantation of an annuloplasty ring. *(From Doty DB [ed]: Cardiac Surgery: Operative Technique. St. Louis, Mosby Year Book, 1997, p 259.)*

discontinuity of this apparatus. There is evidence from animal experiments and from human patients that preservation of the papillary muscle and its chordal attachments to the mitral annulus is beneficial to postoperative LV function after MV reconstruction and replacement. Thus, preservation of these tissues, whenever possible, is now considered a critical feature of MV replacement.[145]

A second disadvantage of MV replacement is the prosthesis itself, including the risks of thromboembolism or hemorrhage associated with mechanical prostheses, late structural deterioration of bioprostheses, and infective endocarditis with all prostheses.

For these reasons, increasing efforts are being made to repair the mitral valve whenever possible in patients with isolated or predominant MR.[152-155] The STS National Database Committee reported an operative mortality rate of less than only 1.6% of 21,229 patients undergoing mitral valve repair from 2002 to 2006.[73] This compares favorably with the 5.7% operative mortality for the 12,238 patients undergoing isolated MV replacement. However, risk is high when concurrent CABG is necessary. Operative mortality for combining CABG and mitral valve replacement is 11.6% compared with 7.4% for mitral valve repair and CABG.[72] Long-term postoperative outcomes are also more favorable with MV repair versus MV replacement, whether or not concomitant CABG is required (**Fig. 66-34**).

With growing experience in MV repair for degenerative causes of MR, including MVP and rupture of chordae tendineae, as well as for ischemic MR, the number of patients in whom valve reconstruction is carried out is increasing on a yearly basis. In many centers in the United States, over two thirds of all patients requiring operation for pure or predominant MR now undergo MV repair. However, in 2003, only 42% of patients undergoing surgery for pure MR in the STS National Cardiac Surgery Database underwent repair and 58% underwent MV replacement. This percentage has steadily increased, and currently 69% of patients in the STS Database undergoing surgery for isolated MR undergo MV repair.[161] However, many patients who are candidates for repair continue to undergo MV replacement. MV repair is technically a more demanding procedure than MV replacement, with a distinct learning curve for the surgeon. In addition, MR recurs after MV repair in a subset of patient with degenerative valve disease that is predicted, in part, by the presence of residual MR immediately following repair. Hence, there is growing emphasis of referral of patients requiring surgery for pure MR to centers of excellence in performing MV repair.[1,152,162]

Minimally invasive surgical techniques using a small, low, asymmetrical sternotomy or anterior thoracotomy and percutaneous cardiopulmonary bypass[162,163] have been found to be less traumatic and can be used for MV repair and replacement. This approach has been reported to reduce cost, improve cosmetic results, and shorten the recovery time. However, it also is demanding technically and is successfully performed

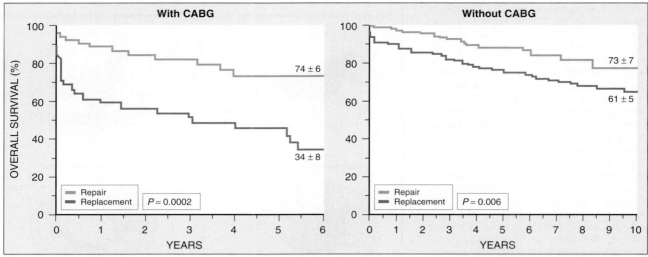

FIGURE 66-34 Plots of overall survival compared for mitral repair and replacement groups in patients who had **(left)** or did not have **(right)** associated CABG. Note that the outcome is better with repair than with replacement in both groups and that the outcome is worse in patients who underwent CABG and mitral valve replacement. *(From Enriquez-Sarano M, Schaff HV, Orszulak TA, et al: Valve repair improves the outcome of surgery for mitral regurgitation: A multivariate analysis. Circulation 91:1022, 1995.)*

by only a minority of cardiac surgeons. There is now growing interest in the development of percutaneous approaches to MV repair[164] using either the edge to edge technique[165] or the coronary sinus approach for percutaneous mitral annuloplasty.[166,167]

SURGICAL RESULTS. Operative mortality rates of 3% to 9% are now common in many centers for patients with pure or predominant MR (NYHA Class II or III) who undergo elective isolated MV replacement. The overall mortality rate was 5.7% in the STS National Database of more than 20,000 patients undergoing isolated MV replacement between 2002 and 2006 and 1.6% for the 21,000 patients undergoing MV repair.[72,73] In comparison, the operative mortality rate for isolated AVR during the same period was 3.2%. The combination of MV replacement with CABG, however, is associated with a mortality rate of 7% to 12% , and the mortality rate is higher (up to 25%) in patients with severe LV dysfunction, especially when MR is secondary to myocardial ischemia, when pulmonary or renal function is impaired, or when the operation must be carried out as an emergency.[82] Age per se is no barrier to successful surgery; MV repair or replacement can be performed in patients older than 75 years if their general health status is adequate[149-150a]; however, surgery in these patients has a higher risk than in younger patients (see Chap. 80). A review of Medicare data involving 684 U.S. hospitals and more than 61,000 patients has indicated that the average in-hospital mortality for isolated MV replacement in patients older than 65 years is 14.1% (20.5% in low-volume centers and 10.1% in high-volume centers).

Surgical treatment substantially improves survival in patients with symptomatic MR. Preoperative factors, such as age younger than 60 years, NYHA Class I or II, cardiac index exceeding 2.0 liters/min/m², LV end-diastolic pressure less than 12 mm Hg, and a normal ejection fraction and end-systolic volume, all correlate with excellent immediate and long-term survival rates. Both preoperative LV ejection fraction (see Fig. 66-29) and end-systolic diameter are important predictors of short- and long-term outcomes.[136,139] Excellent outcome is anticipated in patients with end-systolic diameters less than 40 mm and ejection fractions of 60% or more. Intermediate outcomes are observed in patients with end-systolic diameters between 40 and 50 mm and ejection fractions between 50% and 60%. Poor outcomes are associated with values beyond these limits.

A large proportion of operative survivors have improved clinical status, quality of life, and exercise tolerance following MV repair or replacement. Severe pulmonary hypertension is reduced, LV end-diastolic volume and mass decrease, and coronary flow reserve increases. Depressed contractile function improves, especially if the papillary muscles and chordal attachment to the annulus remain intact. However, patients with MR who have marked LV dysfunction preoperatively sometimes remain symptomatic, with depressed LV function, despite a technically satisfactory surgical procedure. Progressive LV dysfunction and death from heart failure may occur, presumably because LV dysfunction

may be advanced and largely irreversible by the time patients with pure MR develop serious symptoms. Thus, every effort should be made to operate on patients before they develop serious symptoms, and even asymptomatic patients with severe MR may be considered for surgery in an experienced center if there is a high likelihood (>90%) that the valve can be repaired successfully without residual MR.[1,2]

Even though surgical results are suboptimal in patients with MR who have developed severe symptoms or marked LV dysfunction,[145] operation is still indicated for most of these patients because conservative therapy has little to offer. Postoperative survival rates are lower in patients in AF than in those in sinus rhythm.[143,144] As with patients with MS, the arrhythmia by itself does not unfavorably influence outcome, but is a marker for older age and other clinical and hemodynamic features associated with less optimal results.

The cause of MR clearly plays an important role in determining outcome following surgical treatment.[152,156,158,168] In patients with primary degenerative disease of the mitral valve, MV repair or replacement has the potential to improve LV performance. However, in those with functional MR, the primary problem is disease of the LV myocardium, and prognosis is strongly influenced by the degree of LV dysfunction. MV repair or replacement in these latter patients has less beneficial effects on long-term outcome, particularly in those with ischemic MR, compared with patients with degenerative MR. Occlusive coronary artery disease coexisting with MR, but not the primary cause of MR, requires simultaneous coronary CABG and MV repair or replacement.[169] Coronary artery disease is associated with decreased perioperative and long-term postoperative survival (see Fig. 66-34).

INDICATIONS FOR OPERATION. A proposed management strategy for patients with chronic severe MR is shown in **Figure 66-35**.[1] The threshold for surgical treatment of MR is declining for several reasons. These include the reductions in operative mortality, the improvements in MV repair procedures, long-term results indicating stability of repair in experienced centers, and the recognition of the poor long-term results in many patients when MR is corrected only after a long history of symptoms, impaired LV function, AF, or pulmonary hypertension. A detailed echocardiographic examination should be carried out to assess the likelihood that MV repair, rather than MV replacement, is possible, and the difference in outcomes between these procedures should be weighed when deciding whether or not to proceed.

Asymptomatic Patients

Asymptomatic patients (NYHA Class I) should be considered for MV repair if they have LV systolic dysfunction (ejection fraction ≤60% and/ or LV end-systolic diameter ≥40 mm).[1,2] It is also reasonable to

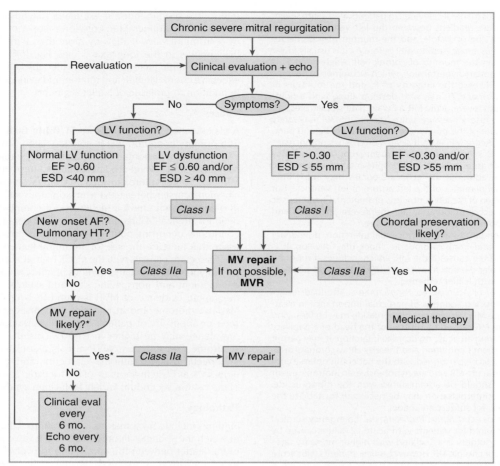

FIGURE 66-35 Management strategy for patients with chronic severe mitral regurgitation. EF = ejection fraction, ESD = end-systolic dimension, HT = hypertension; MVR = mitral valve replacement. *Mitral valve repair may be performed in asymptomatic patients with normal LV function if performed by an experienced surgical team and the likelihood of successful MV repair is greater than 90%. *(From Bonow RO, Carabello BA, Chatterjee K, et al: ACC/AHA 2006 guidelines for the management of patients with valvular heart disease: A report of the American College of Cardiology/American Heart Association Task Force on Practice Guidelines [writing committee to revise the 1998 Guidelines for the Management of Patients With Valvular Heart Disease]: Developed in collaboration with the Society of Cardiovascular Anesthesiologists: Endorsed by the Society for Cardiovascular Angiography and Interventions and the Society of Thoracic Surgeons. Circulation 114:e84, 2006.)*

consider MV repair in asymptomatic patients when AF or pulmonary hypertension is present.

A number of centers are moving toward a more aggressive surgical approach in which MV repair is recommended to all patients with severe MR, independent of symptoms or LV function. However, such a recommendation should be considered only for patients with severe MR (see Table 66-1) who are referred to centers in which the surgical experience indicates that the patient will undergo successful MV repair with a very high degree of certainty. Unfortunately, successful MV repair cannot be guaranteed and, even in the best of circumstances, some young asymptomatic patients may be subjected to the risks of prosthetic valves prematurely and unnecessarily with this approach.

When MV repair is not recommended, asymptomatic patients with normal LV function should be followed clinically and by echocardiography every 6 to 12 months. At times, a careful history and performance of an exercise test often reveal that these patients are not truly asymptomatic.

If MV replacement is likely to be necessary, a higher threshold for clinical and hemodynamic impairment should be used than if MV repair is contemplated, and there are few indications for MV replacement in asymptomatic patients other than LV systolic dysfunction (see Fig 66-35). Because of the higher operative mortality, older patients (>75 years) should, in general, undergo surgery only if they are symptomatic.

Symptomatic Patients

Patients with severe MR and moderate or severe symptoms (NYHA Classes II, III, and IV) should generally be considered for surgery. One exception is a patient in whom the LV ejection fraction is less than 30% and echocardiography suggests that MV replacement will be required and that the subvalvular apparatus cannot be preserved. Because of the high risk of operation and the poor long-term results in these patients, medical therapy is usually advised, but the outcome is poor in any event. However, when MV repair appears possible, even patients with serious LV dysfunction may be considered for operation (see Fig 66-35).

ACUTE MITRAL REGURGITATION. The causes of acute MR (see Table 66-7) are diverse and represent acute manifestations of disease processes that may, under other circumstances, cause chronic MR. Especially important causes of acute MR are spontaneous rupture of chordae tendineae, infective endocarditis with disruption of valve leaflets or chordal rupture, ischemic dysfunction or rupture of a papillary muscle, and malfunction of a prosthetic valve.[102]

Acute severe MR causes a marked reduction of forward stroke volume, slight reduction of end-systolic volume, and increase in end-diastolic volume. One major hemodynamic difference between acute and chronic MR derives from the differences in left atrial compliance. Patients who develop acute severe MR usually have a normal-sized left atrium, with normal or reduced left atrial compliance. The left atrial pressure rises abruptly, which often leads to pulmonary edema, marked elevation of pulmonary vascular resistance, and right-sided heart failure.

Because the *v* wave is markedly elevated in patients with acute severe MR, the reverse pressure gradient between the left ventricle and left atrium declines at the end of systole, and the murmur may be decrescendo rather than holosystolic, ending well before A$_2$. It is usually lower pitched and softer than the murmur of chronic MR. A left-sided S$_4$ is frequently found. Pulmonary hypertension, which is common in patients with acute MR, may increase the intensity of P$_2$ and the murmurs of pulmonary regurgitation and TR may also develop along with a right-sided S$_4$. In patients with severe, acute MR, a *v* wave (late systolic pressure rise) in the pulmonary artery pressure pulse (see Fig. 66-30) may rarely cause premature closure of the pulmonary valve, an early P$_2$, and paradoxical splitting of S$_2$. Acute MR, even if severe, often does not increase overall cardiac size, as seen on the chest roentgenogram, and may produce only mild left atrial enlargement despite marked elevation of left atrial pressure. In addition, the echocardiogram may show little increase in the internal diameter of the left atrium or left ventricle, but increased systolic motion of the left ventricle is prominent. Characteristic features on Doppler echocardiography are the severe jet of MR and elevation of the pulmonary artery systolic pressure.

In severe MR secondary to acute myocardial infarction, pulmonary edema, hypotension, and frank cardiogenic shock may develop. It is essential to determine the cause of the MR, which includes a ruptured papillary muscle, annular dilation from severe LV dilation, and papillary muscle displacement with leaflet tethering.

MEDICAL MANAGEMENT OF ACUTE MITRAL REGURGITATION. Afterload reduction with afterload-reducing agents is of particular importance in treating patients with acute MR. Intravenous nitroprusside may be lifesaving in patients with acute MR caused by rupture of the head of a papillary muscle that occurs during an acute myocardial infarction. It may permit stabilization of the patient's condition and thereby allow coronary arteriography and surgery to be performed with the patient in optimal condition. In patients with acute MR who are hypotensive, an inotropic agent such as dobutamine should be administered with the nitroprusside. Intra-aortic balloon counterpulsation may be necessary to stabilize the patient as preparations for surgery are made.

SURGICAL TREATMENT OF ACUTE MITRAL REGURGITATION. Emergency surgical treatment may be required for patients with acute LV failure caused by acute MR. Emergency surgery is associated with higher mortality rates than elective surgery for chronic MR. However, unless patients with acute severe MR and heart failure are treated aggressively, a fatal outcome is almost certain.

Acute papillary muscle rupture requires emergency surgery with MV repair or replacement. In patients with papillary muscle dysfunction, initial treatment should consist of hemodynamic stabilization, usually with the aid of an intra-aortic balloon pump, and surgery should be considered for those patients who do not improve with aggressive medical therapy. If patients with MR can be stabilized by medical treatment, it is preferable to defer operation until 4 to 6 weeks after the infarction. Vasodilator treatment may be useful during this period. However, medical management should not be prolonged if multisystem (renal and/or pulmonary) failure develops.[102]

Surgical mortality rates are also higher in patients with acute MR and refractory heart failure (NYHA Class IV), those with prosthetic valve dysfunction, and those with active infective endocarditis (of a native or prosthetic valve). Despite the higher surgical risks, the efficacy of early operation has been established in patients with infective endocarditis complicated by medically uncontrollable congestive heart failure and/or recurrent emboli (see Chap. 67).[170]

Mitral Valve Prolapse

CAUSES AND PATHOLOGY. MVP has been given many names, including the systolic click-murmur syndrome, Barlow syndrome, billowing mitral cusp syndrome, myxomatous mitral valve syndrome, floppy valve syndrome, and redundant cusp syndrome.[171,172] It is a variable clinical syndrome that results from diverse pathogenic mechanisms of one or more portions of the mitral valve apparatus, valve leaflets, chordae tendineae, papillary muscle, and valve annulus. MVP is one of the most prevalent cardiac valvular abnormalities. Using standardized echocardiographic diagnostic criteria, community-based studies have shown that MVP syndrome occurs in 2.4% of the population. MVP is twice as frequent in women as in men. However, serious MR occurs more frequently in older men (>50 years) with MVP than in young women with this disorder.

The clinical and echocardiographic criteria for the diagnosis of MVP have been well established. The characteristic systolic click and mid to late systolic murmur is a major diagnostic criterion. The most specific echocardiographic criterion is superior displacement of one or both mitral valve leaflets by more than 2 mm above the plane of the annulus in the long axis[171] (see Fig. 15-52). Other echocardiographic criteria include diffuse leaflet thickening and redundancy, excessive chordal length and motion, and evidence of ruptured chords, in addition to prolapse of leaflet segments.

Causes

A classification of MVP is shown in **Table 66-8**. Usually, MVP occurs as a primary condition that is not associated with other diseases and can be familial or nonfamilial. Familial MVP is transmitted as an autosomal trait and several chromosomal loci have been identified.[173] The MVP syndrome is more prevalent in young women, who generally have a benign course, whereas severe myxomatous disease is more common in older men, who have a higher risk of complications, including the need for surgical MV repair. MVP has also been associated with many conditions, occurring commonly in heritable disorders of connective tissue that increase the size of the mitral leaflets and apparatus.[171,172] MVP is seen in patients with the MASS (mitral, aortic, skin, and skeletal) phenotype, with associated findings of mild nonprogressive aortic root enlargement and nonspecific skin and skeletal changes.[174] Echocardiographic evidence of MVP is found in over 90% of patients with Marfan syndrome and in many of their first-degree relatives. MVP is seen in about 6% of patients with Ehlers-Danlos syndrome, but the prevalence may be higher in type IV (vascular type) Ehlers-Danlos syndrome (see Chap. 8). MVP also is associated with osteogenesis imperfecta, pseudoxanthoma elasticum, and congenital malformations such as Ebstein anomaly of the tricuspid valve, atrial septal defect of the ostium secundum variety, Holt-Oram syndrome, and HCM.

Pathology

Findings include myxomatous proliferation of the mitral valve leaflets, in which the spongiosa component of the valve (i.e., the middle layer of the leaflet between the atrialis and the ventricularis composed of loose, myxomatous material) is unusually prominent[111,171] and the quantity of acid mucopolysaccharide is increased. Electron microscopy shows a haphazard arrangement of cells with disruption and fragmentation of collagen fibrils. Secondary effects include fibrosis of the surface of the MV leaflets, thinning and/or elongation of the chordae tendineae, and ventricular friction lesions.

In mild cases, the valvular myxoid stroma is enlarged on histologic examination, but the leaflets are grossly normal. However, with increasing quantities of myxoid stroma, the leaflets become grossly abnormal, redundant, and prolapsed. There is interchordal hooding caused by leaflet redundancy that includes the rough and clear zones of the

---

TABLE 66-8   Classification of Mitral Valve Prolapse

Mitral Valve Prolapse Syndrome
- Younger age (20-50 yr)
- Predominantly female
- Click or click-murmur on physical examination
- Thin leaflets with systolic displacement on echocardiography
- Associated with low blood pressure, orthostatic hypotension, palpitations
- Benign long-term course

Myxomatous Mitral Valve Disease
- Older age (40-70 yr)
- Predominantly male
- Thickened, redundant valve leaflets
- Mitral regurgitation on physical exam and echocardiography
- High likelihood of progressive disease requiring mitral valve surgery

Secondary Mitral Valve Prolapse
- Marfan syndrome
- Hypertrophic cardiomyopathy
- Ehlers-Danlos syndrome
- Other connective tissue diseases

Modified from Otto CM: Valvular Heart Disease. 2nd ed. Philadelphia, WB Saunders, 2004, p 369.

involved leaflets. Regions of endothelial disruption are common and are possible sites of endocarditis or thrombus formation. The severity of MR depends on the extent of the prolapse. The cusps of the mitral valve, chordae tendineae, and annulus may all be affected by myxomatous proliferation. Degeneration of collagen and myxomatous changes within the central core of the chordae tendineae, with associated decreases in tensile strength,[124] are primarily responsible for chordal rupture, which often occurs and may intensify the severity of MR. Increased chordal tension resulting from the enlarged area of the valve cusps may play a contributory role. Myxomatous changes in the annulus may result in annular dilation and calcification, further contributing to the severity of MR.

Myxomatous proliferation, although most commonly affecting the mitral valve, has also been described in the tricuspid, aortic, and pulmonic valves, particularly in patients with the Marfan syndrome, and may lead to regurgitation of these valves and the mitral valve.

CLINICAL PRESENTATION. The clinical presentations of the MVP syndrome are diverse. The condition has been observed in patients of all ages and both genders. Despite the overestimation of prevalence in the population referred to earlier, MVP is the most common cause of isolated MR requiring surgical treatment in the United States and the most common cardiac condition predisposing patients to infective endocarditis (see Chap. 67).

Symptoms

The vast majority of patients with MVP are asymptomatic and remain so throughout their lives. Although early studies called attention to an MVP syndrome, with a characteristic systolic non-ejection click and various nonspecific symptoms, such as fatigability, palpitations, postural orthostasis, and anxiety and other neuropsychiatric symptoms, as well as symptoms of autonomic dysfunction, these associations have not been confirmed in carefully controlled studies.[171] How and even whether these symptoms relate to the presence of MVP is not clear.

Patients may complain of syncope, presyncope, palpitations, chest discomfort and, when MR is severe, symptoms of diminished cardiac reserve. Chest discomfort may be typical of angina pectoris but is more often atypical in that it is prolonged, not clearly related to exertion, and punctuated by brief attacks or severe stabbing pain at the apex. The discomfort may be secondary to abnormal tension on papillary muscles. In patients with MVP and severe MR, the symptoms of the latter (fatigue, dyspnea, and exercise limitation) may be present. Patients with MVP may also develop symptomatic arrhythmias (see later).

PHYSICAL EXAMINATION. The body weight is often low and the habitus may be asthenic (see Chap. 12). Blood pressure is usually normal or low; orthostatic hypotension may be present. As noted below, patients with MVP have a higher than expected prevalence of straight back syndrome, scoliosis, and pectus excavatum. MR ranges from absent to severe.

AUSCULTATION. The auscultatory findings unique to the MVP syndrome are best elicited with the diaphragm of the stethoscope. The patient should be examined in the supine, left decubitus, and sitting positions. The most important finding is a nonejection systolic click at least 0.14 second after S_1.[172] This can be differentiated from an aortic ejection click because it occurs after the beginning of the carotid pulse upstroke. Occasionally, multiple mid and late systolic clicks are audible, most readily along the lower left sternal border. The clicks are believed to be produced by sudden tensing of the elongated chordae tendineae and of the prolapsing leaflets. They are often, although not invariably, followed by a mid to late crescendo systolic murmur that continues to A_2. This murmur is similar to that produced by papillary muscle dysfunction, which is readily understandable because both result from mid to late systolic MR. In general, the duration of the murmur is a function of the severity of the MR. When the murmur is confined to the latter portion of systole, MR usually is not severe. However, as MR becomes more severe, the murmur commences earlier and ultimately becomes holosystolic.

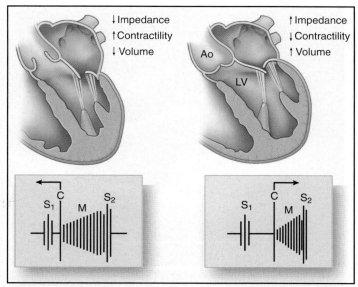

FIGURE 66-36 Dynamic auscultation in mitral valve prolapse. Any maneuver that decreases LV volume (e.g., decreased venous return, tachycardia, decreased outflow impedance, increased contractility) worsens the mismatch in size between the enlarged mitral valve and LV chamber, resulting in prolapse earlier in systole and movement of the click (C) and murmur (M) toward the first heart sound (S_1). Conversely, maneuvers that increase LV volume (e.g., increased venous return, bradycardia, increased outflow impedance, decreased contractility) delay the occurrence of prolapse, resulting in movement of the click and murmur toward the second heart sound (S_2). Ao = aorta. *(Modified from O'Rourke RA, Crawford MH: The systolic click-murmur syndrome: Clinical recognition and management. Curr Probl Cardiol 1:9, 1976.)*

There is considerable variability of the physical findings in the MVP syndrome. Some patients exhibit both a midsystolic click and a mid to late systolic murmur, others present with only one of these two findings, and still others have only a click on one occasion and only a murmur on another, both on a third examination, and no abnormality at all on a fourth. Conditions other than MVP that may cause midsystolic clicks include tricuspid valve prolapse, atrial septal aneurysms, and extracardiac factors.

DYNAMIC AUSCULTATION. The auscultatory findings are exquisitely sensitive to physiologic and pharmacologic interventions, and recognition of the changes induced by these interventions is of great value in the diagnosis of the MVP syndrome (**Fig. 66-36**). The mitral valve begins to prolapse when the reduction of LV volume during systole reaches a critical point at which the valve leaflets no longer coapt; at that instant, the click occurs and the murmur commences. Any maneuver that decreases LV volume, such as a reduction of impedance to LV outflow, reduction in venous return, tachycardia, or augmentation of myocardial contractility, results in an earlier occurrence of prolapse during systole. As a consequence, the click and onset of the murmur move closer to S_1. When prolapse is severe and/or LV size is markedly reduced, prolapse may begin with the onset of systole. As a consequence, the click may not be audible, and the murmur may be holosystolic. On the other hand, when LV volume is augmented by an increase in the impedance to LV emptying, an increase in venous return, reduction of myocardial contractility, or bradycardia, both the click and onset of the murmur will be delayed.

During the straining phase of the Valsalva maneuver and on sudden standing, cardiac size decreases, and the click and onset of the murmur occur earlier in systole. In contrast, a sudden change from the standing to the supine position, leg raising, squatting, maximal isometric exercise and, to a lesser extent, expiration will delay the click and the onset of the murmur. During the overshoot phase of the Valsalva maneuver (i.e., six to eight cycles following release), and with prolongation of the R-R interval, either following a premature contraction or in AF, the click and onset of the murmur are usually delayed, and the intensity of the murmur is reduced. Maneuvers that elevate arterial pressure, such as isometric exercise, increase the intensity of the click and murmur. In general, when the onset of the murmur is delayed, both its duration and intensity are diminished, reflecting a reduction in the severity of MR.

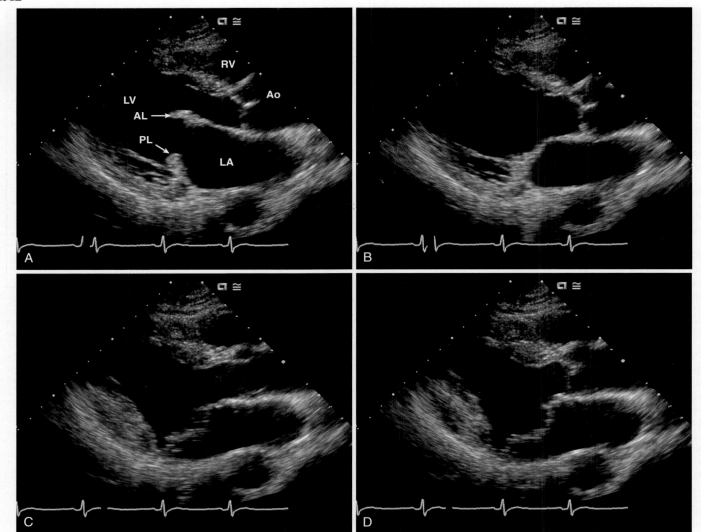

FIGURE 66-37 Parasternal long-axis two-dimensional echocardiographic images in a 41-year-old man with MVP and auscultatory findings of a midsystolic click and MR. **A,** End-diastolic image. The mitral valve leaflets are severely thickened, and the anterior leaflet (AL) is elongated. **B-D,** Serial images from early systole to midsystole demonstrating bileaflet prolapse. Color flow imaging in this patient demonstrated severe MR. Patients with these findings are at increased risk of complications, such as infective endocarditis, systemic emboli, and heart failure. Ao = aorta; LA = left atrium; LV = left ventricle; PL = posterior leaflet; RV = right ventricle.

The response to several interventions may be helpful in differentiating obstructive HCM from MVP (see Chap. 69). During the strain of the Valsalva maneuver, the murmur of HCM increases in intensity, whereas the murmur of MVP becomes longer but usually not louder. Following a premature beat, the murmur of HCM increases in intensity and duration, whereas that caused by MVP usually remains unchanged or decreases.

Echocardiography

Echocardiography (see Chap. 15) plays an essential role in the diagnosis of MVP and has been instrumental in the delineation of this syndrome (**Fig. 66-37**; see Fig. 15-52).[175] To establish the diagnosis, the two-dimensional echocardiogram must show that one or both mitral valve leaflets billow by at least 2 mm into the left atrium during systole in the long-axis view. Thickening of the involved leaflet to more than 5 mm supports the diagnosis. Findings of more severe myxomatous disease include increased leaflet area, leaflet redundancy, chordal elongation, and annular dilation. These findings are also helpful in identifying patients at significant risk for developing severe MR or infective endocarditis (**Table 66-9**). The mitral annular diameter is often abnormally increased. TEE provides additional details regarding

integrity of the mitral valve apparatus, such as rupture of the chordae tendineae. In MR secondary to MVP, the echocardiogram also provides valuable information regarding LV size and function.

The echocardiographic findings of MVP may be observed in patients without a click or murmur. Others have typical echocardiographic and auscultatory features. The echocardiographic findings of MVP have been reported to occur in a large number of first-degree relatives of patients with established MVP. Two-dimensional echocardiography has also revealed prolapse of the tricuspid and aortic valves in approximately 20% of patients with MVP. Conversely, however, prolapse of the tricuspid and aortic valves occurs uncommonly in patients without prolapse of the mitral valve.

Doppler echocardiography frequently reveals mild MR that is not always associated with an audible murmur. Moderate to severe MR is present in about two thirds of patients with posterior leaflet prolapse and in about 25% of patients with anterior leaflet prolapse. The severity of MR should be assessed quantitatively, as noted earlier (see Table 66-1).

OTHER DIAGNOSTIC EVALUATION MODALITIES
ELECTROCARDIOGRAPHY. The ECG is usually normal in asymptomatic patients with MVP. In a minority of asymptomatic patients and in many symptomatic patients, the ECG shows inverted or biphasic T waves and

TABLE 66–9	**Predictors of Clinical Outcome in Mitral Valve Prolapse**			
PREDICTOR	**SURVIVAL**	**VALVE SURGERY**	**ARRHYTHMIAS OR SUDDEN DEATH**	**ENDOCARDITIS**
Age	+++	+++	–	–
Gender	++	++	–	–
Leaflet thickness or redundancy	+++	+++	++++	++++
Severity of mitral regurgitation	++++	++++	++++	++++
Systolic click	+	–	–	–
Left ventricular dilation	+	++++	++	–
Left atrial dilation	–	++	+	

Symbols indicate the relative predictive value of each variable for the listed clinical outcomes on a scale of no predictive value (–) to strongly predictive (++++).

nonspecific ST-segment changes in leads II, III, and aVf and occasionally in the anterolateral leads as well.

ARRHYTHMIAS. A spectrum of arrhythmias has been observed in patients with MVP. These include atrial and ventricular premature contractions and supraventricular and ventricular tachyarrhythmias,[172] as well as bradyarrhythmias caused by sinus node dysfunction or varying degrees of atrioventricular block. The mechanism of the arrhythmias is not clear. Diastolic depolarization of muscle fibers in the anterior mitral leaflet in response to stretch has been demonstrated experimentally, and the abnormal stretch of the prolapsed leaflet may be of pathogenetic significance.

Paroxysmal supraventricular tachycardia is the most common sustained tachyarrhythmia in patients with MVP and may be related to an increased incidence of left atrioventricular bypass tracts. The incidence of MVP in patients with the Wolff-Parkinson-White syndrome is increased. There is also an increased association between MVP and prolongation of the QT interval, which may play a role in the pathogenesis of serious ventricular arrhythmias. Patients with MVP have an increased incidence of abnormal late potentials on signal-averaged ECGs, as well as reduced heart rate variability.

ANGIOGRAPHY. Angiography is not recommended for the diagnostic evaluation of MVP. However, if angiography is performed for other indications, there are features of the left ventriculogram that are characteristic of MVP. The right anterior oblique projection is most useful for defining the posterior leaflet of the mitral valve and the left anterior oblique projection is most useful for studying the anterior leaflet. The most helpful sign is extension of the mitral leaflet tissue inferiorly and posteriorly to the point of attachment of the mitral leaflets to the mitral annulus. Angiography may also reveal scalloped edges of the leaflets, reflecting redundancy of tissue. Other angiographic abnormalities in some patients with MVP include LV dilation, decreased systolic contraction (especially of the basal portion of the ventricle), and calcification of the mitral annulus.

MAGNETIC RESONANCE IMAGING AND CARDIAC COMPUTED TOMOGRAPHY. These advanced imaging techniques can help in determining the extent of MVP and LV function in patients with suboptimal echocardiographic examinations. CMR is also useful for evaluating the presence and severity of MR.

DISEASE COURSE. The outlook for patients with MVP in general is excellent; a large majority remain asymptomatic for many years without any change in clinical or laboratory findings.[171,172] Serious complications (need for cardiac surgery, acute infective endocarditis, or cerebral embolic events) occur at a rate of only 1/100 patient-years. In one study, 4% of patients died over an 8-year period. In contrast, another study reported a much more aggressive course in 833 patients with MVP, with a 19% mortality rate at 10 years and a 20% rate of MVP-related events, including heart failure, AF, cerebrovascular events, arterial thromboembolism, and endocarditis. The apparent explanation for these latter observations is that patients with MVP could be risk-stratified on the basis of several factors (**Fig. 66-38**). The primary risk factors were moderate to severe MR and/or LV ejection fraction less than 50%, and secondary risk factors included mild MR, left atrial dimension 40 mm or greater, flail leaflet, and age 50 years or older. Patients with a primary risk factor had excessive mortality and morbidity, as did those with two or more secondary risk factors. Other series have supported these observations, demonstrating greater risk of cardiac death or MVP-related complications in men, those older than

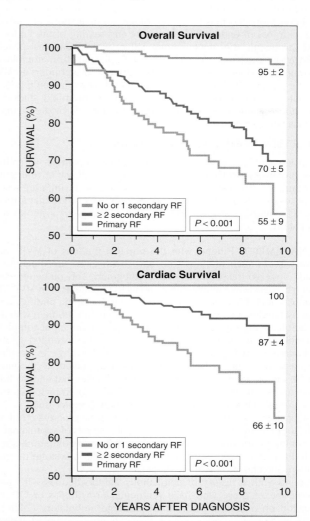

FIGURE 66-38 Survival in patients with mitral valve prolapse according to categories of baseline risk factors (RFs). Primary RFs were moderate to severe MR and ejection fraction <50%. Secondary RFs were mild MR, left atrium larger than 40 mm, flail leaflet, atrial fibrillation, and age older than 50 years. (*Modified from Avierinos JF, Gersh BJ, Melton LJ, et al: Natural history of asymptomatic mitral valve prolapse in the community. Circulation 106:1355, 2002.*)

45 years, those with holosystolic murmurs, those with severe MR, and those with left atrial dimension more than 40 mm. Those studies that reported a lower prevalence of adverse sequelae of MVP included relatively fewer patients with these risk factors. Variables associated with an adverse outcome are summarized in Table 66-9.

Progressive MR, with a gradual increase in left atrial and LV size, AF, pulmonary hypertension, and the development of congestive heart failure, is the most frequent serious complication, occurring in about

15% of patients over a 10- to 15-year period, with age and initial MR severity being the primary predictors of progression.[176] Patients with the MVP syndrome are also at risk of developing infective endocarditis. Both severe MR and endocarditis develop more frequently in patients with murmurs and clicks compared with those with an isolated click, patients with thickened (greater than 5 mm) and redundant mitral valve leaflets, and men older than 50 years (see Table 66-9). In many patients, rupture of the chordae tendineae is responsible for the precipitation and/or intensification of the MR. Infective endocarditis often aggravates the severity of MR and therefore precipitates the need for surgical treatment.

Acute hemiplegia, transient ischemic attacks, cerebellar infarcts, amaurosis fugax, and retinal arteriolar occlusions have been reported to occur more frequently in patients with the MVP syndrome, suggesting that cerebral emboli are unusually common in this condition. It has been proposed that these neurologic complications are associated with loss of endothelial continuity and tearing of the endocardium overlying the myxomatous valve, which initiates platelet aggregation and the formation of mural platelet-fibrin complexes. Although it has been proposed that embolization secondary to MVP may be a significant cause for unexplained strokes in young people without cerebrovascular disease, a large case-controlled study has show no association between MVP and ischemic neurologic events in persons younger than 45 years.[171]

Mitral Valve Prolapse and Sudden Death

The risk of sudden death is about twice normal in patients with mitral valve prolapse, most likely because of an increased risk of ventricular arrhythmias.[171] The risk of sudden death is increased with more severe MR or severe valvular deformity and with complex ventricular arrhythmias, QT interval prolongation, AF, and a history of syncope and palpitations.[158]

MANAGEMENT. Patients with the physical findings of MVP—and those without such findings who have been given the diagnosis—should undergo transthoracic echocardiography. This procedure also should be performed in first-degree relatives of patients with MVP.[1] The diagnosis of MVP requires definitive echocardiographic findings; overdiagnosis and incorrect labeling have been a major problem with this condition. Asymptomatic patients, or those whose principal complaint is anxiety, with no arrhythmias evident on a routine extended electrocardiographic tracing and without evidence of MR, have an excellent prognosis. They should be reassured about the favorable prognosis and be encouraged to engage in normal lifestyles, but should have follow-up examinations every 3 to 5 years. This should include a two-dimensional echocardiogram and a color flow Doppler study.

Patients with a long systolic murmur may show progression of MR and should be evaluated more frequently, at intervals of approximately 12 months. Endocarditis prophylaxis is no longer recommended routinely for patients with MVP, including those with a systolic murmur and typical echocardiographic findings (see Chap. 67).

Patients with a history of palpitations, lightheadedness, dizziness, or syncope, or those who have ventricular arrhythmias or QT prolongation on a routine ECG, should undergo ambulatory (24-hour) electrocardiographic monitoring and/or exercise electrocardiography to detect arrhythmias. Because of the risk, albeit very low, of sudden death, further electrophysiologic studies may be carried out to characterize arrhythmias, if they exist. Beta-adrenergic blockers are useful in the treatment of palpitations secondary to frequent premature ventricular contractions and for self-terminating episodes of supraventricular tachycardia. These drugs may also be useful in the treatment of chest discomfort, both for patients with associated coronary artery disease and those with normal coronary vessels in whom the symptoms may be caused by regional ischemia secondary to MVP. Radiofrequency ablation of atrioventricular bypass tracts is useful for frequent or prolonged episodes of supraventricular tachycardia.

Aspirin should be given to patients with MVP who have had a documented focal neurologic event and in whom no other cause, such as a left atrial thrombus or AF, is apparent.

Patients with MVP and severe MR should be treated similarly to other patients with severe MR and may require MV surgery. MV repair without replacement is possible in over 90% of patients (see Fig. 66-33). Therefore, the threshold for surgical treatment in these patients is lower than in patients with MR in whom MV replacement may be necessary, providing that patients are referred to a surgical team with established success in MV repair, as noted. Most of all MV repairs for MR are now carried out in patients with MVP. Resection of the most deformed leaflet segment, usually the middle scallop of the posterior leaflet, and insertion of an annuloplasty ring to reduce the dilated annulus is the most commonly used procedure. Repair of anterior leaflet prolapse is more challenging. Rupture of the chordae tendineae to the anterior leaflet can sometimes be treated by chordal transfer from the posterior leaflet. In other patients, shortening of the chordae tendineae and/or papillary muscle is necessary. The average operative mortality is 1.6%, and long-term studies demonstrate excellent durability of MV repair in most patients.[152-155] However, MR recurs in a subset of patients, at which point it may be necessary to perform repeat MV repair or replacement.

Although this discussion has focused attention on complications of MVP, it should not be forgotten that, on the whole, this is a benign condition. The vast majority of patients with this syndrome remain asymptomatic for their entire lives and require, at most, observation every few years and reassurance.

Tricuspid, Pulmonic, and Multivalvular Disease

Tricuspid Stenosis

CAUSES AND PATHOLOGY

Tricuspid stenosis (TS) is almost always rheumatic in origin.[177] Other causes of obstruction to right atrial emptying are unusual and include congenital tricuspid atresia (see Chap. 65), right atrial tumors, which may produce a clinical picture suggesting rapidly progressive TS (see Chap. 74), and the carcinoid syndrome (see Chap. 68), which more frequently produces TR. Rarely, obstruction to RV inflow can be caused by endomyocardial fibrosis, tricuspid valve vegetations, a pacemaker lead, or extracardiac tumors.

Most patients with rheumatic tricuspid valve disease present with TR or a combination of TS and TR. Isolated rheumatic TS is uncommon and almost never occurs as an isolated lesion but generally accompanies mitral valve disease. In many patients with TS, the aortic valve is also involved (i.e., trivalvular stenosis is present). TS is found at autopsy in about 15% of patients with rheumatic heart disease but is of clinical significance in only about 5%. Organic tricuspid valve disease is more common in India, Pakistan, and other developing nations near the equator than in North America or Western Europe. The anatomic changes of rheumatic TS resemble those of MS, with fusion and shortening of the chordae tendineae and fusion of the leaflets at their edges, producing a diaphragm with a fixed central aperture. However, valvular calcification is rare. As is the case with MS, TS is more common in women. The right atrium is often greatly dilated in TS, and its walls are thickened. There may be evidence of severe passive congestion, with enlargement of the liver and spleen.

PATHOPHYSIOLOGY. A diastolic pressure gradient between the right atrium and ventricle—the hemodynamic expression of TS—is augmented when the transvalvular blood flow increases during inspiration or exercise and is reduced when the blood flow declines during expiration. A relatively modest diastolic pressure gradient (i.e., a mean gradient of only 5 mm Hg) is usually sufficient to elevate the mean right atrial pressure to levels that result in systemic venous congestion and, unless sodium intake has been restricted or diuretics have been given, is associated with jugular venous distention, ascites, and edema.

In patients with sinus rhythm, the right atrial *a* wave may be very tall and may even approach the level of the RV systolic pressure. Resting

TABLE 66-10	Clinical and Laboratory Features of Rheumatic Tricuspid Stenosis

History
- Progressive fatigue, edema, anorexia
- Minimal orthopnea, paroxysmal nocturnal dyspnea
- Rheumatic fever in two thirds of patients
- Female preponderance
- Pulmonary edema and hemoptysis rare

Physical Findings
- Signs of multivalvular involvement
- Diastolic rumble at lower left sternal border, increasing in intensity with inspiration
- Often confused with mitral stenosis
- Peripheral cyanosis
- Neck vein distention, with prominent *a* waves and slow *y* descent
- Absent right ventricular lift
- Associated murmurs of mitral and aortic valve disease
- Hepatic pulsation
- Ascites, peripheral edema

Imaging Findings
- ECG—tall right atrial P waves and no right ventricular hypertrophy
- Chest roentgenogram—dilated right atrium without enlarged pulmonary artery segment
- Echocardiogram—diastolic doming of tricuspid valve leaflet

Modified from Ockene IS: Tricuspid valve disease. In Dalon JE, Alpert JS (eds): Valvular Heart Disease. 2nd ed. Boston, Little Brown, 1987, pp 356, 390.

cardiac output is usually markedly reduced and fails to rise during exercise. This accounts for the normal or only slightly elevated left atrial, pulmonary arterial, and RV systolic pressures, despite the presence of accompanying mitral valvular disease.

A mean diastolic pressure gradient across the tricuspid valve as low as 2 mm Hg is sufficient to establish the diagnosis of TS. However, exercise, deep inspiration, and the rapid infusion of fluids or the administration of atropine may greatly enhance a borderline pressure gradient in a patient with TS. Therefore, when this diagnosis is suspected, right atrial and ventricular pressures should be recorded simultaneously, using two catheters or a single catheter with a double lumen, with one lumen opening on either side of the tricuspid valve. The effects of respiration on any pressure difference should be examined.

CLINICAL PRESENTATION

Symptoms

The low cardiac output characteristic of TS causes fatigue, and patients often experience discomfort caused by hepatomegaly, ascites, and anasarca (**Table 66-10**). The severity of these symptoms, which are secondary to an elevated systemic venous pressure, is out of proportion to the degree of dyspnea. Some patients complain of a fluttering discomfort in the neck, caused by giant *a* waves in the jugular venous pulse. Despite the coexistence of MS, the symptoms characteristic of this valvular lesion (severe dyspnea, orthopnea, and paroxysmal nocturnal dyspnea) are usually mild or absent in the presence of severe TS because the latter prevents surges of blood into the pulmonary circulation behind the stenotic mitral valve. The absence of symptoms of pulmonary congestion in a patient with obvious MS should suggest the possibility of TS.

PHYSICAL EXAMINATION. Because of the high frequency with which MS occurs in patients with TS and the similarity in the physical findings between the two valvular lesions, the diagnosis of TS is commonly missed. The physical findings are mistakenly attributed to MS, which is more common and may be more obvious. Therefore, a high index of suspicion is required to detect the tricuspid valvular lesion. In the presence of sinus rhythm, the *a* wave in the jugular venous pulse is tall, and a presystolic hepatic pulsation is often palpable. The *y* descent is slow and barely appreciable. The lung fields are clear and, despite engorged neck veins and the presence of ascites and anasarca, the patient may be comfortable while lying flat. Thus, the diagnosis of TS may be suspected from inspection of the jugular venous pulse in a patient with MS but

without clinical evidence of pulmonary hypertension. This suspicion is strengthened when a diastolic thrill is palpable at the lower left sternal border, particularly if the thrill appears or becomes more prominent during inspiration.

The auscultatory findings of the accompanying MS are usually prominent and often overshadow the more subtle signs of TS. A tricuspid OS may be audible but is often difficult to distinguish from a mitral OS. However, the tricuspid OS usually follows the mitral OS and is localized to the lower left sternal border, whereas the mitral OS is usually most prominent at the apex and radiates more widely. The diastolic murmur of TS is also commonly heard best along the lower left parasternal border in the fourth intercostal space and is usually softer, higher pitched, and shorter in duration than the murmur of MS. The presystolic component of the TS murmur has a scratchy quality and a crescendo-decrescendo configuration that diminishes before S_1. The diastolic murmur and OS of TS are both augmented by maneuvers that increase transtricuspid valve flow, including inspiration, the Mueller maneuver (forced inspiration against a closed glottis), assumption of the right lateral decubitus position, leg raising, inhalation of amyl nitrite, squatting, and isotonic exercise. They are reduced during expiration or the strain of the Valsalva maneuver and return to control levels immediately (i.e., within two to three beats) after Valsalva release.

Echocardiography

The echocardiographic changes (see Chap. 15) of the tricuspid valve in TS resemble those observed in the mitral valve in MS.[177] Two-dimensional echocardiography characteristically shows diastolic doming of the leaflets (especially the anterior tricuspid valve leaflet), thickening and restricted motion of the other leaflets, reduced separation of the tips of the leaflets, and a reduction in diameter of the tricuspid orifice. TEE allows added delineation of the details of valve structure. Doppler echocardiography shows a prolonged slope of antegrade flow and compares well with cardiac catheterization in the quantification of TS and assessment of associated TR. Doppler evaluation of TS has largely replaced the need for catheterization to assess severity.

OTHER DIAGNOSTIC EVALUATION MODALITIES
ELECTROCARDIOGRAPHY. In the absence of AF in a patient with valvular heart disease, TS is suggested by the presence of electrocardiographic evidence of right atrial enlargement (see Chap. 13). The P wave amplitude in leads II and V_1 exceeds 0.25 mV. Because most patients with TS have mitral valvular disease, the electrocardiographic signs of biatrial enlargement are commonly found. The amplitude of the QRS complex in lead V_1 may be reduced by the dilated right atrium.

RADIOGRAPHY. The key radiologic finding is marked cardiomegaly with conspicuous enlargement of the right atrium (i.e., prominence of the right heart border), which extends into a dilated superior vena cava and azygos vein, but without conspicuous dilation of the pulmonary artery. The vascular changes in the lungs characteristic of mitral valvular disease may be masked, with little or no interstitial edema or vascular redistribution, but left atrial enlargement may be present.

Angiography following injection of contrast material into the right atrium and filming in the 30-degree right anterior oblique projection characteristically shows thickening and decreased mobility of the leaflets, a diastolic jet through the constricted orifice, and thickening of the normal atrial wall.

MANAGEMENT. Although the fundamental approach to the management of severe TS is surgical treatment, intensive sodium restriction and diuretic therapy may diminish the symptoms secondary to the accumulation of excess salt and water. A preparatory period of diuresis may diminish hepatic congestion and thereby improve hepatic function sufficiently to diminish the risks of subsequent operation.

Most patients with TS have coexisting valvular disease that requires surgery. In patients with combined TS and MS, the former must not be corrected alone because pulmonary congestion or edema may ensue. Surgical treatment of TS should be carried out at the time of MV repair or replacement in patients with TS in whom the mean diastolic pressure gradient exceeds 5 mm Hg and the tricuspid orifice is less than approximately 2.0 cm². The final decision concerning surgical treatment is often made at the operating table.

Because TS is almost always accompanied by some TR, simple finger fracture valvotomy may not result in significant hemodynamic

TABLE 66-11   Causes and Mechanisms of Pure Tricuspid Regurgitation

Causes
- Anatomically abnormal valve
  - Rheumatic
  - Nonrheumatic
    - Infective endocarditis
    - Ebstein anomaly
    - Floppy (prolapse)
    - Congenital (non-Ebstein)
    - Carcinoid
    - Papillary muscle dysfunction
    - Trauma
    - Connective tissue disorders (Marfan)
    - Rheumatoid arthritis
    - Radiation injury
- Anatomically normal valve (functional)
  - Elevated right ventricular systolic pressure (dilated annulus)

Mechanisms

CONDITION	LEAFLET AREA	ANNULAR CIRCUMFERENCE	LEAFLET INSERTION
Floppy	↑	↑	Normal
Ebstein anomaly	↑	↑	Abnormal
Pulmonary/right ventricular systolic hypertension	Normal	↑	Normal
Papillary muscle dysfunction	Normal	Normal	Normal
Carcinoid	↓/Normal	Normal	Normal
Rheumatic	↓/Normal	Normal	Normal
Infective endocarditis	↓/Normal	Normal	Normal

Modified from Waller BF: Rheumatic and nonrheumatic conditions producing valvular heart disease. In Frankl WS, Brest AN (eds): Cardiovascular Clinics: Valvular Heart Disease: Comprehensive Evaluation and Management. Philadelphia, FA Davis, 1989, pp 35, 95.

improvement but may merely substitute severe TR for TS. However, open valvotomy in which the stenotic tricuspid valve is converted into a functionally bicuspid valve may result in substantial improvement. The commissures between the anterior and septal leaflets and between the posterior and septal leaflets are opened. It is not advisable to open the commissure between the anterior and posterior leaflets for fear of producing severe TR. If open valvotomy does not restore reasonably normal valve function, the tricuspid valve may have to be replaced. A large bioprosthesis is preferred to a mechanical prosthesis in the tricuspid position because of the high risk of thrombosis of the latter and the longer durability of bioprostheses in the tricuspid than in the mitral or aortic positions. The feasibility of tricuspid balloon valvuloplasty has been demonstrated, and this procedure may be combined with mitral balloon valvuloplasty.

Tricuspid Regurgitation

CAUSES AND PATHOLOGY. The most common cause of TR is not intrinsic involvement of the valve itself (i.e., primary TR) but rather dilation of the right ventricle and of the tricuspid annulus causing secondary (functional) TR (**Table 66-11**).[177,178] This may be a complication of RV failure of any cause. It is observed in patients with RV hypertension secondary to any form of cardiac or pulmonary vascular disease, most commonly mitral valve disease.[179] In general, a RV systolic pressure greater than 55 mm Hg will cause functional TR. TR can also occur secondary to RV infarction, congenital heart disease (e.g., pulmonic stenosis and pulmonary hypertension secondary to Eisenmenger syndrome; see Chap. 65), primary pulmonary hypertension (see Chap. 78) and, rarely, cor pulmonale. In infants, TR may complicate RV failure secondary to neonatal pulmonary diseases and pulmonary hypertension with persistence of the fetal pulmonary circulation. In all these cases, TR reflects the presence of, and in turn aggravates, severe RV failure. Functional TR may diminish or disappear as the right ventricle decreases in size with the treatment of heart failure. TR can also occur as a consequence of dilation of the annulus in the Marfan syndrome, in which RV dilation secondary to pulmonary hypertension is not present.

A variety of disease processes can affect the tricuspid valve apparatus directly and lead to regurgitation (primary TR).[177] Thus, organic TR may occur on a congenital basis (see Chap. 65), as part of Ebstein anomaly, defects involving the atrioventricular canal, when the tricuspid valve is involved in the formation of an aneurysm of the ventricular septum, or in corrected transposition of the great arteries, or it may occur as an isolated congenital lesion. Rheumatic fever may involve the tricuspid valve directly. When this occurs, it usually causes scarring of the valve leaflets and/or chordae tendineae, leading to limited leaflet mobility and either isolated TR or a combination of TR and TS. Rheumatic involvement of the mitral, and often aortic, valves coexist.

TR or the combination of TR and TS is an important feature of the carcinoid syndrome (**Fig. 66-39**), which leads to focal or diffuse deposits of fibrous tissue on the endocardium of the valvular cusps and cardiac chambers and on the intima of the great veins and coronary sinus (see Chap. 68). The white, fibrous carcinoid plaques are most extensive on the right side of the heart, where they are usually deposited on the ventricular surfaces of the tricuspid valve and cause the cusps to adhere to the underlying RV wall, thereby producing TR. Endomyocardial fibrosis with shortening of the tricuspid leaflets and chordae tendineae is an important cause of TR in tropical Africa. TR may result from prolapse of the tricuspid valve caused by myxomatous changes in the valve and chordae tendineae (**Fig. 66-40**); prolapse of the mitral valve is usually present in these patients as well. Prolapse of the tricuspid valve occurs in about 20% of all patients with MVP. Tricuspid valve prolapse may also be associated with atrial septal defect. Other causes of TR include penetrating and nonpenetrating trauma, dilated cardiomyopathy, infective endocarditis (particularly staphylococcal endocarditis in IV drug users), and following surgical excision of the tricuspid valve in patients with infective endocarditis that is unresponsive to medical management. Less common causes of TR include cardiac tumors (particularly right atrial myxoma), transvenous pacemaker leads, repeated endomyocardial biopsy in a transplanted heart, endomyocardial fibrosis, methysergide-induced valvular disease, exposure to fenfluramine-phentermine, and systemic lupus erythematosus involving the tricuspid valve.

CLINICAL PRESENTATION

Symptoms

In the absence of pulmonary hypertension, TR is generally well tolerated. However, when pulmonary hypertension and TR coexist, cardiac output declines and the manifestations of right-sided heart failure become intensified. Thus, the symptoms of TR result from a reduced cardiac output and from ascites, painful congestive hepatomegaly, and massive edema. Occasionally, patients have throbbing pulsations in the neck, which intensify on effort and are caused by jugular venous distention, and systolic pulsations of the eyeballs have also been described. In the many patients with TR who have mitral valve disease, the symptoms of the latter usually predominate. Symptoms of pulmonary congestion may abate as TR develops but are replaced by weakness, fatigue, and other manifestations of a depressed cardiac output.

PHYSICAL EXAMINATION. Evidence of weight loss and cachexia, cyanosis, and jaundice are often present on inspection in patients with severe TR. AF is common. There is jugular venous distention, the normal x and x′ descents disappear, and a prominent systolic wave—a c-v wave (or s wave)—is apparent. The descent of this wave, the y descent, is sharp and becomes the most prominent feature of the venous pulse unless there is coexisting TS, in which case it is slowed. A venous systolic thrill and murmur in the neck may be present in patients with severe TR. The RV impulse is hyperdynamic and thrusting in quality. Systolic pulsations of an enlarged tender liver are commonly present initially. However, in patients with chronic TR and congestive cirrhosis, the liver may become firm and nontender. Ascites and edema are frequent.

Auscultation usually reveals an S₃ originating from the right ventricle, which is accentuated by inspiration. When TR is associated with and secondary to pulmonary hypertension, P₂ is accentuated as well. When TR occurs in the presence of pulmonary hypertension, the systolic murmur is usually high-pitched, pansystolic, and loudest in the fourth intercostal space in the parasternal region but occasionally is loudest in the subxiphoid area. When TR is mild, the murmur may be short. When TR occurs in the absence of pulmonary hypertension (e.g., in infective endocarditis or following trauma), the murmur is usually of low intensity and limited to the first half of systole. When the right ventricle is greatly dilated and occupies the anterior surface of the heart, the murmur may be prominent at the apex and difficult to distinguish from that produced by MR.

The response of the systolic murmur to respiration and other maneuvers is of considerable aid in establishing the diagnosis of TR. The murmur is characteristically augmented during inspiration (Carvallo sign). However, when the failing ventricle can no longer increase its stroke volume in the recumbent or sitting positions, the inspiratory augmentation may be elicited by standing. The murmur also increases during the Mueller maneuver (see earlier), exercise, leg raising, and hepatic compression. It demonstrates an immediate overshoot after release of the Valsalva strain but is reduced in intensity and duration in the standing position and during the strain of the Valsalva maneuver. Increased atrioventricular flow across the tricuspid orifice in diastole may cause a short early diastolic flow rumble in the left parasternal region following S₃. Tricuspid valve prolapse, like MVP, causes nonejection systolic clicks and late systolic murmurs. However, in tricuspid valve prolapse, these findings are more prominent at the lower left sternal border. With inspiration, the clicks occur later and the murmurs intensify and become shorter in duration

Echocardiography

The goal of echocardiography (see Figs. 15-55 and 15-56) is to detect TR, estimate its severity, and assess pulmonary arterial pressure and RV

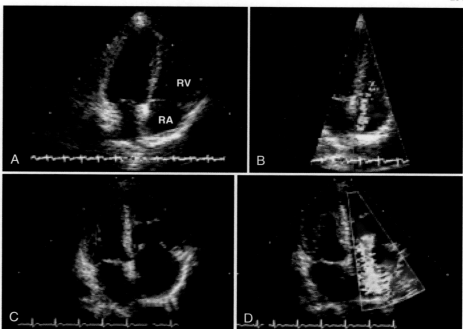

FIGURE 66-39 TR caused by carcinoid involvement of the tricuspid valve. Serial two-dimensional echocardiograms (**A** and **C**) and color Doppler studies (**B** and **D**), separated by 3 years are shown. **C,** After 3 years, there is severe thickening and fixation of the tricuspid leaflets, leading to severe TR and associated right ventricular (RV) and right atrial (RA) enlargement. *(From Møller JE, Connolly HM, Rubin J, et al: Factors associated with progression of carcinoid heart disease. N Engl J Med 348:1005, 2003.)*

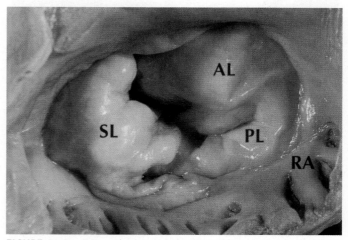

FIGURE 66-40 Tricuspid valve prolapse, viewed from the right atrium (RA). AL = anterior leaflet; PL = posterior leaflet; SL = septal leaflet. *(From Virmani R, Burke AP, Farb A: Pathology of valvular heart disease. In Rahimtoola SH [ed]: Valvular Heart Disease. In Braunwald E [series ed]: Atlas of Heart Diseases. Vol 11. Philadelphia, Current Medicine, 1997, p 1.17.)*

function. In patients with TR secondary to dilation of the tricuspid annulus, the right atrium, right ventricle, and tricuspid annulus are all usually greatly dilated on echocardiography. There is evidence of RV diastolic overload with paradoxical motion of the ventricular septum similar to that observed in atrial septal defect. Exaggerated motion and delayed closure of the tricuspid valve are evident in patients with Ebstein anomaly (see Fig. 15-93). Prolapse of the tricuspid valve caused by myxomatous degeneration may be evident on echocardiography. Echocardiographic indications of tricuspid valve abnormalities, especially TR by Doppler examination, can be detected in most patients with carcinoid heart disease (see Fig. 66-39). In patients with TR caused by endocarditis, echocardiography may reveal vegetations on the valve or a flail valve. TEE enhances detection of TR. Doppler

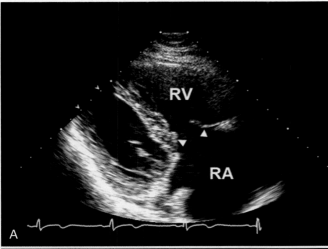

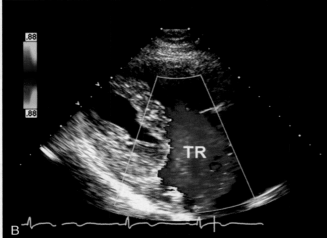

FIGURE 66-41 **A,** Two-dimensional echocardiographic systolic image (right ventricular inflow view) demonstrates thickened septal and anterior tricuspid valve leaflets (arrowheads) and enlargement of the right ventricle (RV) and right atrium (RA) in a patient with carcinoid heart disease. **B,** Color flow Doppler image demonstrates severe TR in the same patient. Note laminar color flow (blue) filling an enlarged right atrium. *(From Bruce CJ, Connolly HM: Right sided valve disease. In Otto CM, Bonow RO [eds]: Valvular Heart Disease: A Companion to Braunwald's Heart Disease. Philadelphia, Elsevier, 2009, pp 334-335.)*

echocardiography is a sensitive technique for visualizing the TR jet. The magnitude of TR can be quantified using techniques similar to those used to evaluation MR (**Fig. 66-41**).

OTHER DIAGNOSTIC EVALUATION MODALITIES

ELECTROCARDIOGRAPHY. The ECG is usually nonspecific and characteristic of the lesion causing TR. Incomplete right bundle branch block, Q waves in lead V_1, and AF are commonly found.

RADIOGRAPHY. In patients with functional TR, marked cardiomegaly is usually evident, and the right atrium is prominent. Evidence of elevated right atrial pressure may include distention of the azygos vein and the presence of a pleural effusion. Ascites with upward displacement of the diaphragm may be present. Systolic pulsations of the right atrium may be present on fluoroscopy.

HEMODYNAMIC FINDINGS. The right atrial and RV end-diastolic pressures are often elevated in TR whether the condition is caused by organic disease of the tricuspid valve or is secondary to RV systolic overload. The right atrial pressure tracing usually reveals absence of the *x* descent and a prominent *v* or *c-v* wave (ventricularization of the atrial pressure). Absence of these findings essentially excludes moderate or severe TR. As the severity of TR increases, the contour of the right atrial pressure pulse increasingly resembles that of the RV pressure pulse. A rise or no change in right atrial pressure on deep inspiration, rather than the usual fall, is a characteristic finding. Determination of the pulmonary arterial (or RV)

systolic pressure may be helpful in deciding whether the TR is primary (caused by disease of the valve or its supporting structures) or functional (secondary to RV dilation). A pulmonary arterial or RV systolic pressure less than 40 mm Hg favors a primary cause, whereas a pressure greater than 55 mm Hg suggests that TR is secondary.

MANAGEMENT. TR in the absence of pulmonary hypertension usually is well tolerated and may not require surgical treatment. Both human patients and experimental animals with normal pulmonary arterial pressure may tolerate total excision of the tricuspid valve as long as the RV systolic pressure is normal. Dilation of the right side of the heart usually occurs months or years after tricuspid valvectomy (usually carried out for acute infective endocarditis).

Surgical treatment of acquired TR secondary to annular dilation was greatly improved with the development of annuloplasty techniques, with or without an annuloplasty ring. At the time of mitral valve surgery in patients with TR secondary to pulmonary hypertension, the severity of the regurgitation should be assessed by palpation of the tricuspid valve. In addition, it should be determined whether the TR is secondary to pulmonary hypertension, in which case the valve is normal, or whether it is secondary to other disease processes. Patients with mild TR without annular dilation usually do not require surgical treatment; pulmonary vascular pressures decline following successful mitral valve surgery, and the mild TR tends to disappear. However, even mild TR should be repaired if there is dilation of the tricuspid annulus, because the TR is likely to progress in severity if left untreated.[180,181] Excellent results have been reported in patients with mild to moderate TR with the use of suture annuloplasty of the posterior (unsupported) portion of the annulus. Patients with severe TR, with or without annular dilation, require valvotomy and ring annuloplasty. A surgical mortality rate of 13.9% has been reported (see Table 66-3). Residual TR after tricuspid annuloplasty is determined principally by the degree of pre-operative tricuspid leaflet tethering.[182] If these procedures do not provide a good functional result at the operating table, as assessed by TEE, valve replacement using a large bioprosthesis may be required.

When organic disease of the tricuspid valve (Ebstein anomaly or carcinoid heart disease) causes TR severe enough to require surgery, valve replacement is usually needed. The risk of thrombosis of mechanical prostheses is greater in the tricuspid than in the mitral or aortic positions, presumably because pressure and flow rates are lower in the right side of the heart. For this reason, the artificial valve of choice for the tricuspid position in adults is a bioprosthesis. Anticoagulants are not required, and a graft durability of more than 10 years has been established.

In treating the difficult problem of tricuspid endocarditis in IV drug users (see Chap. 67), total excision of the tricuspid valve without immediate replacement can generally be tolerated by these patients, who usually do not have associated pulmonary hypertension. When antibiotic therapy is unsuccessful, valve replacement frequently results in reinfection or continued infection. Therefore, diseased valvular tissue should be excised to eradicate the endocarditis, and antibiotic treatment can then be continued. Initially, most patients tolerate loss of the tricuspid valve without great difficulty. However, RV dysfunction usually occurs subsequently. A bioprosthetic valve may therefore be inserted 6 to 9 months after valve excision and control of the infection.

Pulmonic Valve Disease

CAUSES AND PATHOLOGY

Pulmonic Stenosis

The congenital form is the most common cause of pulmonic stenosis (PS). Manifestations in children and adults are discussed in Chap. 65. Rheumatic inflammation of the pulmonic valve is very uncommon, is usually associated with involvement of other valves, and rarely leads to serious deformity. Carcinoid plaques, similar to those involving the tricuspid valve, are often present in the outflow tract of the right ventricle of patients with malignant carcinoid. The plaques result in constriction of the pulmonic valve ring, retraction and fusion of the valve cusps, and either PS or the combination of PS and pulmonic regurgitation. Obstruction in the region of the pulmonic valve may be extrinsic to the valve apparatus and may be produced by cardiac tumors or by aneurysm of the sinus of Valsalva (see Fig. 15-82). Management of congenital PS focuses on balloon dilation (see Chap. 59).

Pulmonic Regurgitation

Pulmonic regurgitation (PR) can result from dilation of the valve ring secondary to pulmonary hypertension (of any cause) or from dilation of the pulmonary artery. Infective endocarditis can involve the pulmonic valve, resulting in valve regurgitation. As more patients with congenital heart disease survive to adulthood, there is an increasing population of young adults with residual pulmonic regurgitation after surgical treatment of congenital PS or tetralogy of Fallot (**Fig. 66-42**). PR may also result from various lesions that directly affect the

pulmonic valve. These include congenital malformations, such as absent, malformed, fenestrated, or supernumerary leaflets. These anomalies may occur as isolated lesions but more often are associated with other congenital anomalies, particularly tetralogy of Fallot, ventricular septal defect, and pulmonic valvular stenosis. Less common causes include trauma, carcinoid syndrome, rheumatic involvement, injury produced by a pulmonary artery flow-directed catheter, syphilis, and chest trauma.

CLINICAL PRESENTATION. Like TR, isolated PR causes RV volume overload and may be tolerated for many years without difficulty unless it complicates, or is complicated by, pulmonary hypertension. In this case, PR is usually accompanied by and aggravates RV failure. Patients with PR caused by infective endocarditis who develop septic pulmonary emboli and pulmonary hypertension often exhibit severe RV

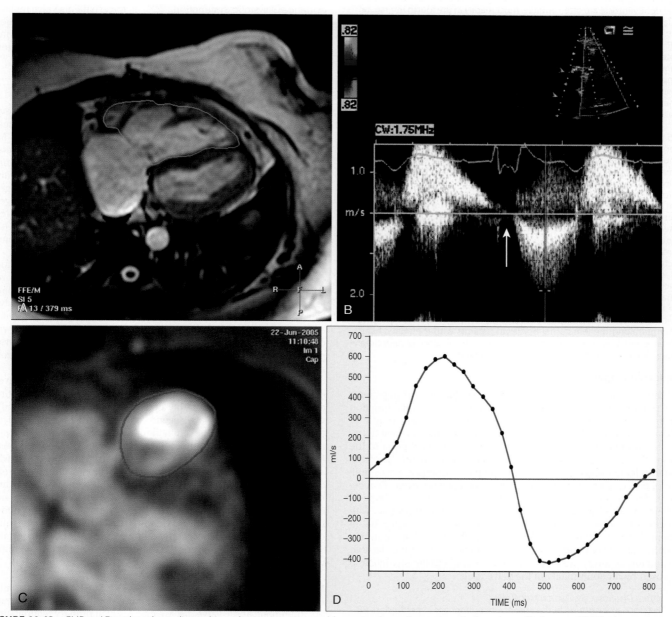

FIGURE 66-42 CMR and Doppler echocardiographic evaluation in a 40-year-old woman who underwent repair of tetralogy of Fallot as a child. She is asymptomatic but has significant right ventricular (RV) enlargement on echocardiography. **A,** RV dilation is confirmed in the CMR images, with a calculated RV end-diastolic volume of 444 mL. **B,** The Doppler tracing shows a dense signal in diastole with a steep deceleration slope that reaches the baseline before the end of diastole (arrow). **C,** Interrogation of pulmonary artery flow in the CMR phase-velocity images is performed by drawing a region of interest (red) around the pulmonary artery. **D,** Graph of the pulmonary artery flow within the region of interest indicated in **C** demonstrates both antegrade and retrograde flow. The total RV stroke volume was 245 mL, with antegrade flow of 98 mL, yielding a regurgitant fraction of 67%.

failure. In most patients, the clinical manifestations of the primary disease are severe and usually overshadow the PR, which often results only in incidental auscultatory findings.

PHYSICAL EXAMINATION. The right ventricle is hyperdynamic and produces palpable systolic pulsations in the left parasternal area, and an enlarged pulmonary artery often produces systolic pulsations in the second left intercostal space. Sometimes systolic and diastolic thrills are felt in the same area. A tap reflecting pulmonic valve closure is usually easily palpable in the second intercostal space in patients with pulmonary hypertension and secondary PR.

AUSCULTATION. P_2 is not audible in patients with congenital absence of the pulmonic valve; however, this sound is accentuated in patients with PR secondary to pulmonary hypertension. There may be wide splitting of S_2 caused by prolongation of RV ejection accompanying the augmented RV stroke volume. A nonvalvular systolic ejection click due to the sudden expansion of the pulmonary artery by the augmented RV stroke volume frequently initiates a midsystolic ejection murmur, most prominent in the second left intercostal space. An S_3 and S_4 originating from the right ventricle are often audible, most readily in the fourth intercostal space at the left parasternal area, and are augmented by inspiration.

In the absence of pulmonary hypertension, the diastolic murmur of PR is low-pitched and usually heard best at the third and fourth left intercostal spaces adjacent to the sternum. The murmur commences when pressures in the pulmonary artery and right ventricle diverge, approximately 0.04 second after P_2. It is diamond-shaped in configuration and brief, reaching a peak intensity when the gradient between these pressures is maximal, and ending with equilibration of the pressures. The murmur becomes louder during inspiration.

When systolic pulmonary arterial pressure exceeds approximately 55 mm Hg, dilation of the pulmonic annulus results in a high-velocity regurgitant jet resulting in the audible murmur of PR, or Graham Steell murmur. (Doppler ultrasonography reveals pulmonary regurgitation at much lower pulmonary arterial pressures.) This murmur is high-pitched, blowing, and decrescendo, beginning immediately after P_2 and is most prominent in the left parasternal region in the second to fourth intercostal spaces. Thus, although it resembles the murmur of AR, it is usually accompanied by severe pulmonary hypertension—that is, an accentuated P_2 or fused S_2, an ejection sound, and a systolic murmur of TR, and not by a widened arterial pulse pressure. Sometimes, a low-frequency presystolic murmur is present, originating from increased diastolic flow across the tricuspid valve.

The murmur of PR secondary to pulmonary hypertension usually increases in intensity with inspiration, is diminished during the Valsalva strain, and returns to baseline intensity almost immediately after release of the Valsalva strain. This PR murmur resembles and may be confused with the diastolic blowing murmur of AR. However, a diastolic blowing murmur along the left sternal border in patients with rheumatic heart disease and pulmonary hypertension (even in the absence of peripheral signs of AR) is usually caused by AR rather than PR.

Echocardiography

Two-dimensional echocardiography shows RV dilation and, in patients with pulmonary hypertension, RV hypertrophy as well. RV function can be evaluated. Abnormal motion of the septum characteristic of volume overload of the right ventricle in diastole and/or septal flutter may be evident. The motion of the pulmonic valve may point to the cause of the PR. Absence of a waves and systolic notching of the posterior leaflet suggest pulmonary hypertension; large a waves indicate pulmonic stenosis. Doppler echocardiography is extremely accurate in detecting PR and in helping estimate its severity (see Fig. 66-42 and Fig. 15-57). Abnormal Doppler signals in the RV outflow tract with velocity sustained throughout diastole are generally observed in patients in whom PR is caused by dilation of the valve ring secondary to pulmonary hypertension. When the velocity falls during diastole, the pulmonary artery pressure is usually normal, and the regurgitation is caused by an abnormality of the valve itself.

OTHER DIAGNOSTIC EVALUATION MODALITIES

ELECTROCARDIOGRAPHY. In the absence of pulmonary hypertension, PR often results in an ECG that reflects RV diastolic overload—an rSr (or rsR) configuration in the right precordial leads. PR secondary to pulmonary hypertension is usually associated with ECG evidence of RV hypertrophy.

RADIOGRAPHY. Both the pulmonary artery and right ventricle are usually enlarged, but these signs are nonspecific. Fluoroscopy may demonstrate pronounced pulsation of the main pulmonary artery. PR can be diagnosed by observing opacification of the right ventricle following injection of contrast material into the main pulmonary artery, but this diagnosis is made in almost all patients with echocardiography or cardiac magnetic resonance.

CARDIAC MAGNETIC RESONANCE. CMR plays an important role in assessing pulmonary artery dilation, imaging the regurgitant jet and quantifying PR severity (see Fig. 66-42). CMR also is useful in evaluating RV dilation and systolic function.[41,184]

MANAGEMENT. Except in patients with previous surgery for tetralogy of Fallot, PR alone is seldom severe enough to require specific treatment. Treatment of the primary condition, such as infective endocarditis, or the lesion responsible for the pulmonary hypertension, such as surgery for mitral valvular disease, often ameliorates the PR. The timing of surgery for severe PR after tetralogy of Fallot is controversial with current recommendations based on the degree of RV dilation and evidence of systolic dysfunction.[56,183,185] In these patients, valve replacement may be carried out, preferably with a pulmonary allograft. There is growing experience with catheter-based approaches to pulmonic valve replacement in native pulmonic valve disease and in PR following surgical correction of congenital heart defects (see Chap. 59).[186]

Multivalvular Disease

Multivalvular involvement is caused frequently by rheumatic fever and various clinical and hemodynamic syndromes can be produced by different combinations of valvular abnormalities. Myxomatous MR and associated pulmonary hypertension is a leading cause of concomitant TR, often with dilation of the tricuspid annulus. The Marfan syndrome and other connective tissue disorders may cause multivalve prolapse and dilation, resulting in multivalvular regurgitation. Degenerative calcification of the aortic valve may be associated with degenerative mitral annular calcification and cause AS and MR. Different pathologic conditions may affect two valves in the same patient (e.g., infective endocarditis on the aortic valve causing AR and ischemia causing MR).

In patients with multivalvular disease, the clinical manifestations depend on the relative severity of each of the lesions. When the valvular abnormalities are of approximately equal severity, clinical manifestations produced by the more proximal (upstream) of the two valvular lesions (i.e., the mitral valve in patients with combined mitral and aortic valvular disease and the tricuspid valve in patients with combined tricuspid and mitral valvular disease) are generally more prominent than those produced by the distal lesion. Thus, the proximal lesion tends to mask the distal lesion.

It is important to recognize multivalvular involvement preoperatively because failure to correct all significant valvular disease at the time of operation increases mortality considerably. In patients with multivalvular disease, the relative severity of each lesion may be difficult to estimate by clinical examination and noninvasive techniques because one lesion may mask the manifestations of the other. Therefore, patients suspected of having multivalvular involvement and who are being considered for surgical treatment should undergo careful clinical evaluation and full Doppler echocardiographic evaluation and right and left cardiac catheterization and angiography. If there is any question concerning the presence of significant AS in patients undergoing mitral valve surgery, the aortic valve should be inspected because overlooking this condition can lead to a high perioperative mortality. Similarly, it is useful to palpate the tricuspid valve at the time of mitral valve surgery.

MITRAL STENOSIS AND AORTIC VALVE DISEASE. Aortic valve involvement is present in about one third of patients with rheumatic MS. Rheumatic aortic valve disease may result in primary regurgitation, stenosis, or mixed stenosis and regurgitation. AR is evident on physical examination in about two thirds of patients with severe MS but only about 10% of patients with MS have severe rheumatic AR. On physical examination, a proximal lesion may mask signs of a distal lesion. For example, significant AR may be missed in patients with severe MS because the widened pulse pressure may be absent. On the other hand, MS may be missed or, conversely, may be falsely diagnosed on clinical examination of patients with obvious AR. An accentuated S_1 and an OS in a patient with AR should suggest the possibility of mitral valvular disease. AS is evident on physical examination based on the typical murmur, even when MS is present; however, cardiac output tends to be reduced more than in patients with isolated AS. On physical examination, an S_4 (which is common in patients with pure AS) is usually not present. The midsystolic murmur characteristic of AS may be reduced in intensity and duration because the stroke volume is reduced by the MS.

Echocardiography is of decisive value in the evaluation of patients with rheumatic disease and allows accurate diagnosis of the presence and severity of multivalve involvement, taking into consideration the altered flow conditions with serial lesions. For example, the gradient across the stenotic aortic valve may be relatively low when MS is present because of a low cardiac output; valve area calculations are especially helpful in this setting.

Because double-valve replacement is associated with increased short- and long-term risks, balloon mitral valvotomy can be the first procedure if MS is the predominant lesion, with subsequent AVR when needed. If percutaneous balloon valvotomy is not an option or concurrent AVR is needed, surgical valvotomy may be considered as an option.

It is vital to recognize the presence of hemodynamically significant aortic valvular disease (i.e., AS and/or AR) preoperatively in patients who are to undergo mitral valvotomy. This procedure may be hazardous because it can impose a sudden hemodynamic load on the left ventricle that had previously been protected by the MS and may lead to acute pulmonary edema.

AORTIC STENOSIS AND MITRAL REGURGITATION. AS is often accompanied by MR caused by mitral valve prolapse, annular calcification, rheumatic disease, or functional MR. The increased LV pressure secondary to LV outflow obstruction may augment the volume of MR flow, whereas the presence of MR may diminish the ventricular preload necessary for maintenance of the LV stroke volume in patients with AS. The result is a reduced forward cardiac output and marked left atrial and pulmonary venous hypertension. The development of AF (caused by left atrial enlargement) has an adverse hemodynamic effect in the presence of AS. Physical findings may be confusing because it may be difficult to recognize two distinct systolic murmurs. However, on echocardiography, the cause and severity of AS and MR can be accurately diagnosed. In most cases, MR is mild to moderate and it is appropriate to treat AS alone. When MR is severe or there is significant structural mitral valve disease, concurrent mitral repair (whenever possible) or valve replacement at the time of AVR should be considered.

AORTIC AND MITRAL REGURGITATION. This relatively infrequent combination of lesions may be caused by rheumatic heart disease, prolapse of both the aortic and the mitral valves because of myxomatous degeneration, or dilation of both annuli in patients with connective tissue disorders. The left ventricle is usually greatly dilated. The clinical features of AR usually predominate, and it is sometimes difficult to determine whether the MR is caused by organic involvement of this valve or dilation of the mitral valve ring secondary to LV enlargement. When both valvular leaks are severe, this combination of lesions is poorly tolerated. The normal mitral valve ordinarily serves as a backup to the aortic valve, and premature (diastolic) closure of the mitral valve limits the volume of reflux that occurs in patients with acute AR. With severe combined regurgitant lesions, regardless of the cause of the mitral lesion, blood may reflux from the aorta through both chambers of the left side of the heart into the pulmonary veins. Physical and laboratory examinations usually show evidence of both lesions. An S_3 and a brisk arterial pulse are frequently present. The relative severity of each lesion can be assessed best by Doppler echocardiography and contrast angiography. This combination of lesions leads to severe LV dilation. MR that occurs in patients with AR secondary to LV dilation often regresses following AVR alone. If severe, the

MR may be corrected by annuloplasty at the time of AVR. An intrinsically normal mitral valve that is regurgitant because of a dilated annulus should not be replaced.

SURGICAL TREATMENT OF MULTIVALVULAR DISEASE. Combined AVR and MV replacement is usually associated with a higher risk and poorer survival than replacement of either of the valves alone. The operative risk of double-valve replacement is about 70% higher than for single-valve replacement. The STS National Database Committee has reported an overall operative mortality rate of 9.6% for multiple (usually double) valve replacement in 3840 patients, compared with 3.2% and 5.7% for isolated AVR and MV replacement, respectively[72,73] (see Table 66-3). The long-term survival depends strongly on the preoperative functional status. Patients operated on for combined AR and MR have poorer outcomes than patients undergoing double-valve replacement for any of the other combinations of lesions, presumably because both AR and MR may produce irreversible LV damage. MV repair or balloon valvotomy in combination with AVR is preferable to double-valve replacement and should be carried out whenever possible. Risk factors that reduce long-term survival after double-valve replacement include advanced age, higher NYHA class, lower LV ejection fraction, greater LV enlargement, and accompanying ischemic heart disease requiring coronary artery bypass grafting.[73,82]

Given the higher risks, a higher threshold is required for multivalvular versus single-valve surgery. Thus, patients are generally advised not to undergo multivalvular surgery until they reach late NYHA Class II or Class III, unless there is evidence of declining LV function. Despite a detailed noninvasive and invasive workup, the decision to treat more than one valve is often made by palpation or by direct inspection at the operating table.

TRIPLE-VALVE DISEASE. Hemodynamically significant disease involving the mitral, aortic, and tricuspid valves is uncommon and typically is caused by rheumatic heart disease. Patients with trivalvular disease may present in advanced heart failure with marked cardiomegaly, and surgical correction of all three valvular lesions is imperative. However, triple-valve replacement is a long and complex operation. Early in the experience with this procedure, the mortality rate was 20% for patients in NYHA Class III and 40% for patients in Class IV. More recently, the mortality rate has declined, but nevertheless triple-valve replacement should be avoided if possible. In many patients with trivalvular disease, it is possible to replace the aortic valve, repair the mitral valve, and perform a tricuspid annuloplasty or valvuloplasty.

Patients who survive triple-valve replacement surgery usually show substantial clinical improvement during the early postoperative period, and postoperative catheterization studies show marked reductions in pulmonary arterial and capillary pressures. However, some patients die of arrhythmias or congestive heart failure in the late postoperative period despite three normally functioning prostheses. The cause of cardiac failure in this situation is unknown, but may be related to intraoperative myocardial ischemia, microemboli from the multiple prostheses, or continued subclinical episodes of rheumatic myocarditis.

When multiple prosthetic valves must be inserted, it is logical to select two bioprostheses or two mechanical prostheses for the left side of the heart. If the patient is to be exposed to the hazards of anticoagulants for one mechanical prosthesis, it seems unreasonable to add the potential risks of early failure of a bioprosthesis. However, if two mechanical prostheses are selected for the left side of the heart, the use of a bioprosthesis in the tricuspid position is suggested.

Prosthetic Cardiac Valves

The first successful human replacements of cardiac valves were accomplished in 1960 by Nina Braunwald and colleagues, Dwight Harken and coworkers, and Albert Starr and Lowell Edwards. Two major groups of prosthetic valves are currently available in models designed for the atrioventricular (mitral and tricuspid) and aortic positions, mechanical prostheses and bioprostheses (tissue valves; **Fig. 66-43**). The major differences are related to the risk of thromboembolism (higher with mechanical valves) and the risk of structural deterioration of the prosthesis (higher with bioprostheses).[187,188]

Mechanical Prostheses

Mechanical prosthetic valves are classified into three major groups—bileaflet, tilting disc, and ball cage. The bileaflet valves are the most

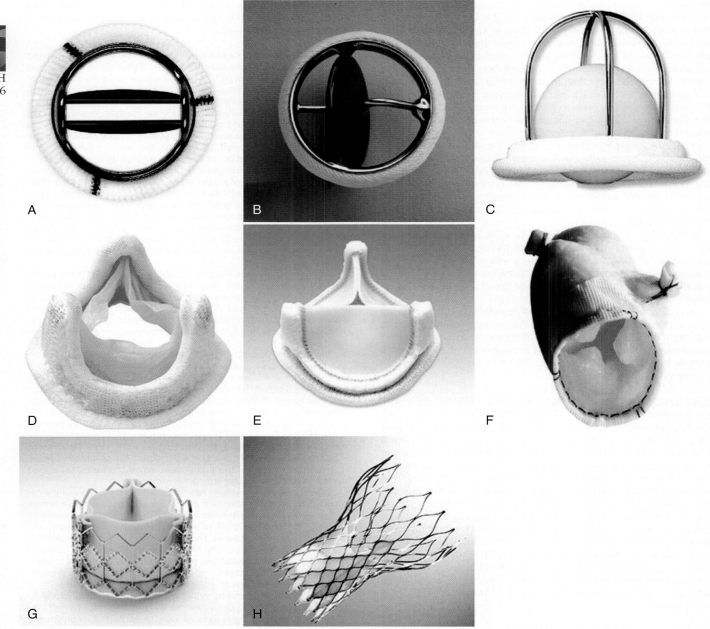

FIGURE 66-43 Different types of prosthetic valves. **A,** Bileaflet mechanical valve (St. Jude Medical, West Berlin, NJ). **B,** Monoleaflet mechanical valve (Medtronic-Hall, Medtronic, Minneapolis). **C,** Caged ball valve (Starr-Edwards,). **D,** Stented porcine bioprosthesis (Medtronic Mosaic). **E,** Stented pericardial bioprosthesis (Carpentier-Edwards Magna, Edwards Lifesciences, Irvine, Calif). **F,** Stentless porcine bioprosthesis (Medtronic Freestyle). **G,** Transcatheter bioprosthesis expanded over a balloon (Edwards SAPIEN). **H,** Self-expandable percutaneous bioprosthesis (CoreValve, Medtronic). *(From Pibarot P, Dumesnil JG: Prosthetic heart valves: Selection of the optimal prosthesis and long-term management. Circulation 119:1034, 2009.)*

commonly implanted mechanical valves because of their low bulk and flat profile and superior hemodynamics. Bileaflet valves are currently the most widely used mechanical prosthesis. The St. Jude bileaflet mechanical valve (St. Jude Medical, West Berlin, NJ) is coated with pyrolytic carbon and has two semicircular discs that pivot between open and closed positions without the need for supporting struts.[187-189] It has favorable flow characteristics and causes a lower transvalvular pressure gradient at any outer diameter and cardiac output than caged ball or tilting disc valves. Bileaflet valves appear to have particularly favorable hemodynamic characteristics in the smaller sizes. Thrombogenicity in the mitral position may be less than that associated with other prosthetic valves, although, as with other mechanical prostheses, lifelong anticoagulation is needed. A variation of the St. Jude valve, the CarboMedics prosthesis (Sorin group, Milan, Italy), is also a bileaflet valve composed of pyrolytic carbon with a titanium housing that can

be rotated to avoid interference with disc excursion by subvalvular tissue.

An example of a tilting disc valve in current use is the Medtronic-Hall valve (Medtronic, Minneapolis, Minn), which has a Teflon sewing ring and titanium housing; its thin, carbon-coated pivoting disc has a central perforation that allows improved hemodynamics. Thrombogenicity appears to be low (less than one episode/100 patient-years in the mitral position), and mechanical performance is excellent over the long term. Mechanical valves, both bileaflet and tilting disc, are associated with small (5 to 10 mL/beat) obligatory (normal) regurgitation. All have distinctive auscultatory features (**Fig. 66-44**).

Production of the Starr-Edwards caged-ball valve was discontinued in 2007, but patients in whom this valve was implanted are still encountered frequently in clinical practice. The poppet is made of silicone rubber, the cage of Stellite alloy, and the sewing ring

Type of Valve	Aortic Prosthesis		Mitral Prosthesis	
	Normal findings	Abnormal findings	Normal findings	Abnormal findings
Caged-Ball (Starr–Edwards)		Aortic diastolic murmur Decreased intensity of opening or closing click		Low-frequency apical diastolic murmur High-frequency holosystolic murmur
Single-Tilting-Disc (Björk–Shiley or Medtronic–Hall)		Decreased intensity of closing click		High-frequency holosystolic murmur Decreased intensity of closing click
Bileaflet-Tilting-Disc (St. Jude Medical)		Aortic diastolic murmur Decreased intensity of closing click		High-frequency holosystolic murmur Decreased intensity of closing click
Heterograft Bioprosthesis (Hancock or Carpentier–Edwards)		Aortic diastolic murmur		High-frequency holosystolic murmur

FIGURE 66-44 Auscultatory characteristics of various prosthetic valves in the aortic and mitral positions, with schematic diagrams of normal findings and descriptions of abnormal findings. AC = aortic closure; CC = closing click; DM = diastolic murmur; MC = mitral valve closure; MO = mitral opening; OC = opening click; SEM = systolic ejection murmur. *(From Vongpatanasin W, Hillis LD, Lange RA: Prosthetic heart valves. N Engl J Med 335:407, 1996.)*

of Teflon and polypropylene cloth. Because of the bulky cage design, the Starr-Edwards valve is not suitable for the mitral position in patients with a small LV cavity, for the aortic position in those with a small aortic annulus, or for those requiring a valve–aortic arch composite graft. In a small number of patients, this valve induces hemolysis, which may be greatly exaggerated and become clinically important if a perivalvular leak develops. When they are of small size, Starr-Edwards valves may cause mild obstruction, and the incidence of thromboembolism is slightly higher than with the tilting disc or bileaflet valve.

DURABILITY AND THROMBOGENICITY. All mechanical prosthetic valves have an excellent record of durability, up to 40 years for the Starr-Edwards valve and over 25 years for the St. Jude valve.[187,188] In the mitral position, perivalvular regurgitation appears to occur more frequently with mechanical than with tissue valves. Thrombosis and thromboembolism risks are greater with any mechanical valve in the mitral than in the aortic position, and higher doses of warfarin are generally recommended for mitral prostheses.[1] However, patients with any mechanical prosthesis, regardless of design or site of placement, require long-term anticoagulation and aspirin administration because of the hazard of thromboembolism, which is greatest in the first postoperative year. Without anticoagulants and aspirin, the incidence of thromboembolism is three- to sixfold higher than when proper doses of these medications are administered. Very rarely, thrombosis of the mechanical valve occurs. This may be a fatal event, but when nonfatal, it interferes with prosthetic valve function.

Warfarin should begin about 2 days after operation, and the INR should be in the range of 2.0 to 3.0 for patients with the bileaflet disc and the Medtronic-Hall valve in the aortic position. The INR should be between 2.5 and 3.5 for patients at higher risk for thrombosis (e.g., AF, previous thromboembolism) as well as for patients with other mechanical valves in the aortic position and for all valves in the mitral position (see Chap. 87).[1] This relatively conservative approach reduces the risk of anticoagulant hemorrhage but does not appear to be associated with a greater frequency of thromboembolism than an INR of 3.0 to 4.0. Antiplatelet agents without anticoagulants do not provide adequate protection. However, the addition of aspirin, 75 to 100 mg daily, together with warfarin may reduce the risk of thromboembolism and should be given to all patients with prosthetic valves.[1] Although this approach does increase the risk of bleeding slightly, there is a favorable risk-benefit profile.

Prosthetic valve thrombosis should be suspected by the sudden appearance of dyspnea and muffled sounds or new murmurs on auscultation. This serious complication is diagnosed by two-dimensional TEE and Doppler echocardiography (see Fig. 15-59). Unless surgical risk is high, the preferred treatment for left-sided valve thrombosis is emergency surgery when NYHA Class III-IV symptoms are present or there is a large clot burden. Fibrinolytic therapy is reasonable for right-sided valve thrombosis, left-sided valve thrombosis with a small clot burden, and only mild symptoms. Fibrinolytic therapy is followed by intravenous heparin and aspirin until the INR is therapeutic.[1,102,190]

The following must be recognized: (1) the administration of warfarin has an estimated mortality risk of 0.2/100 patient-years and serious hemorrhage of 2.2 episodes/100 patient-years; and (2) despite treatment with anticoagulants, the incidence of thromboembolic complications with the best mechanical prosthesis is still about 0.2 fatal complications and 1.0 to 2.0 nonfatal complications/100 patient-years for aortic valves and 2.0 to 3.0 nonfatal complications for mitral valves. Valve thrombosis, a particularly hazardous complication, occurs at an incidence of about 0.1%/year in the aortic position and 0.35%/year in the mitral position. Thrombosis of mechanical prostheses in the tricuspid position is high, and therefore bioprostheses are preferred at this site. The incidence of embolization in patients who have experienced repeated emboli from a prosthetic valve despite anticoagulants may be reduced by replacement with a tissue valve. Mechanical prostheses regularly cause mild hemolysis, but this is not severe enough to be of clinical importance unless the patient develops paraprosthetic regurgitation.

Bioprosthetic Valves

Tissue valves (bioprostheses) were developed primarily to overcome the risk of thromboembolism that is inherent in all mechanical prosthetic valves and the attendant hazards and inconvenience of permanent anticoagulant therapy.

STENTED BIOPROSTHETIC VALVES. A stented tissue valve consists of three tissue leaflets mounted on a ring with semirigid stents that facilitate implantation and maintain the three-dimensional relationship between the leaflets. Stented porcine aortic heterografts were developed for the mitral and aortic positions and have been in wide clinical use since 1965. Over the past 45 years, stented bioprosthetic valve design has improved to maximize orifice area by reconfiguration of the sewing ring and stents and improve durability by the use of other biologic tissues, improved fixation techniques, and anticalcification treatments. Bioprosthetic valves may be constructed from porcine valve tissue fixed and preserved in glutaraldehyde and mounted on a Dacron cloth–covered flexible polypropylene strut—for example the Hancock porcine bioprosthesis (Medtronic, Minneapolis, Minn), which was approved by the U.S. Food and Drug Administration (FDA) in 1989. Bioprosthetic valves also may be constructed using bovine pericardium—for example, the Carpentier-Edwards pericardial valve (Edwards Lifesciences, Irvine, Calif), which was FDA-approved in 1991. The Medtronic Mosaic valve, FDA-approved in 2000, is a porcine valve fixed at zero pressure to preserve leaflet function with an added anticalcification treatment.

During the first 3 postoperative months, while the sewing ring becomes endothelialized, there is a risk of thromboembolism so that warfarin anticoagulation is reasonable. Thereafter, anticoagulants are not required for porcine valves in the aortic position, and the thromboembolic rate is approximately one or two episodes/100 patient-years without these drugs.[1,187,188] When these valves have been placed in the mitral position in patients who are in sinus rhythm, do not have heart failure or thrombus in the left atrium or the left atrial appendage, and do not have a history of embolism preoperatively, anticoagulants are not needed after the first 3 postoperative months, and the thromboembolic rate is also approximately one or two episodes/100 patient-years. This rate is comparable to that observed in patients with the St. Jude or other mechanical valves who are receiving anticoagulants and are therefore subject to the risks of hemorrhage. It is unlikely that any MV replacement can be associated with a thromboembolic rate much below 0.5 episodes/100 patient-years because some of the emboli in patients with long-standing mitral disease are derived from the left atrium rather than from the valve itself. In patients undergoing MV replacement with a bioprosthesis who have experienced a previous embolism, in whom thrombus is found in the left atrium at operation, or who remain in AF postoperatively (approximately one third of all patients receiving MV replacement), the hazard of thromboembolism and the need for anticoagulants persist. This negates the principal advantage of the tissue valves and mechanical prostheses would appear to be preferable to bioprostheses in these patients.

The major problem with porcine bioprostheses is their limited durability (**Fig. 66-45**). Cuspal tears, degeneration, fibrin deposition, disruption of the fibrocollagenous structure, perforation, fibrosis, and calcification sufficiently severe to require reoperation begin to appear in some patients

in the fourth or fifth postoperative year, and by 10 years the rate of primary tissue failure averages 30%. It then accelerates and, by 15 years postoperatively, the actuarial freedom from bioprosthetic primary tissue failure has ranged from 30% to 60% in several series. In contrast, stented pericardial valves have a lower rate of primary tissue failure with 86% free of structural deterioration at 12 years. Prosthetic valve endocarditis is a serious, often grave, illness with the risk of endocarditis highest in the first few months after valve implantation (see Chap. 67).

Structural valve deterioration is more frequent in patients with bioprostheses in the mitral than in the aortic position, presumably because of the higher closing pressure. The rate of structural valve failure is age-dependent and is significantly lower in patients older than 65 years than in younger patients, especially in the aortic position (**Fig. 66-46**). In patients older than 65 years undergoing AVR with a porcine bioprosthesis, the rate of structural deterioration is less than 10% at 10 years. Valve failure is prohibitively rapid in children and in adults younger than 35 to 40 years. Therefore, bioprostheses are not advisable for these age groups. On the other hand, degeneration is rare when these valves are implanted into patients older than 70 years. Bioprostheses also have been reported to have extremely limited durability in patients with chronic renal failure, but recent studies have called this into question (see later). Other factors that increase the likelihood of bioprosthetic valve deterioration include abnormalities of calcium metabolism and, possibly, hypercholesterolemia and pregnancy. Fortunately, tissue valves usually do not fail suddenly, as is often the case for structural failure or thrombosis of mechanical prostheses. Rereplacement of a bioprosthetic valve should be carried out when significant and/or progressive structural deterioration is evident and standard criteria for intervention for native valve disease are present. The second operation, when carried out on an elective basis, may be associated with a surgical mortality rate that is two to three times higher than the initial valve replacement.

Echocardiographic evaluation is extremely helpful in the early detection of bioprosthetic valve malfunction. TEE is more sensitive than transthoracic imaging in detecting bioprosthetic mitral valve deterioration. A baseline echocardiographic study is recommended 2 to 4 weeks after hospital discharge for valve replacement. Annual cardiology follow-up is recommended with echocardiography during the first 5 years only if there are changes in symptoms or examination findings. After 5 years, annual echocardiography is reasonable, even in the absence of clinical findings, to evaluate for bioprosthetic valve deterioration.

STENTLESS BIOPROSTHETIC VALVES. Because the stent adds to the obstruction and thereby increases stress on the leaflets, stentless valves have been developed for the aortic position and are especially

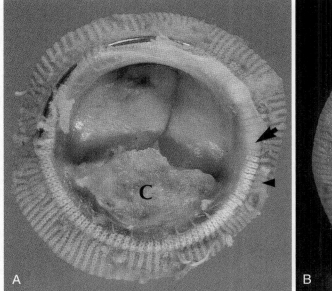
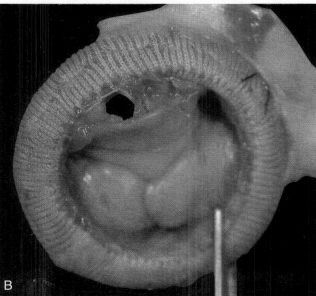

FIGURE 66-45 Structural deterioration of bioprosthetic valves. **A,** Valve failure related to mineralization and collagen degeneration. **B,** Cuspal tears and perforations. These processes may occur independently, or they may be synergistic. (**A,** From Virmani R, Burke AP, Farb A: Pathology of valvular heart disease. In Rahimtoola SH [ed]: Valvular Heart Disease. In Braunwald E [series ed]: Atlas of Heart Diseases. Vol 11. Philadelphia, Current Medicine, 1997, p 1.26; **B,** from Manabe H, Yutani C [eds]: Atlas of Valvular Heart Disease. Singapore, Churchill Livingstone, 1998, p 158.)

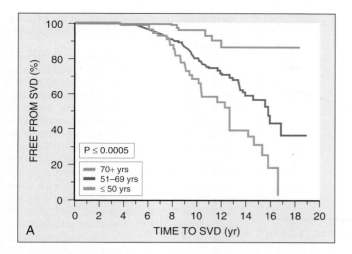

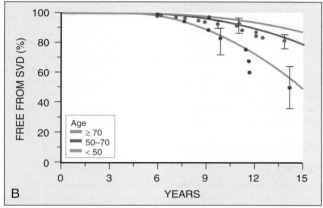

FIGURE 66-46 Estimates of freedom from structural valve deterioration (SVD) for patients undergoing porcine **(A)** and bovine pericardial **(B)** aortic valve replacement who are stratified according to age. (**A,** From Cohn LH, Collins JJ Jr, Rizzo RJ, et al: Twenty-year follow-up of the Hancock modified orifice porcine aortic valve. Ann Thorac Surg 66:S30, 1998; **B,** from Banbury MK, Cosgrove DM, White JA, et al: Age and valve size effect on the long-term durability of the Carpentier-Edwards aortic pericardial bioprosthesis. Ann Thorac Surg 72:753, 2001.)

useful for patients with small aortic roots. These include the Toronto SPV stentless valve (St. Jude Medical valve), Edwards stentless valve, and Medtronic Freestyle valve. These valves have been reported to have more physiologic flow and lower transvalvular gradients than stented porcine valves, with the potential for enhanced regression of LV hypertrophy and improved LV function. However, long-term outcome appears to be similar to that for other currently implanted tissue valves, in part because current generation stented bioprosthetic valves have better durability than older generation valves.[187,191,192]

TRANSCATHETER BIOPROSTHESES (see Chap. 59). Bioprosthetic valves that can be placed via a catheter in the aortic valve position are currently undergoing clinical trials in the United States and have been approved for use in Europe. These trileaflet bioprosthetic valves are mounted in a wire mesh stent that can be crimped to allow delivery of the valve over a catheter. Transcatheter aortic valve implantation (TAVI) may be performed using a catheter advanced from the femoral artery retrograde across the aortic valve, or from a small thoracotomy with the catheter positioned in the LV apex and passed antegrade across the aortic valve. This procedure is used for calcific AS with the native valve remaining in place, which helps anchor the valve stent. TAVI clinical trials have focused on adults with a high risk of cardiac surgery. In this subset of high-risk patients, procedural results and short-term outcomes are promising. The U.S. prospective randomized PARTNER trial, comparing TAVI with medical therapy (including balloon valvotomy) in patients considered to be at too high risk for conventional AVR, demonstrated substantial reduction in death and

hospitalization with TAVI, associated with significant improvement in symptoms.[64a] Long-term durability of these valves has not yet been evaluated in clinical trials.[61-64] Transcatheter valve implantation also holds promise for treating patients with failing bioprosthetic valves in the aortic and mitral positions, using a valve in valve approach.[193]

HOMOGRAFT (ALLOGRAFT) AORTIC VALVES. These are harvested from cadavers, usually within 24 hours of donor death. They are sterilized with antibiotics and cryopreserved for long periods at –196°C. They are inserted directly, usually in the aortic position, without being placed into a prosthetic stent. In the aortic position, the isolated valve is implanted in the subcoronary position or the valve and a portion of attached aorta are implanted as a root replacement, with reimplantation of the coronary arteries into the graft. Homograft hemodynamics are superior to those of stented porcine valves and similar to those of stentless porcine valves. Like porcine xenografts, their thrombogenicity is low, but cryopreserved valves appear to have similar issues with structural deterioration, with evidence that this rate is reduced with the use of freshly harvested valves, approximate matching of donor's and patient's ages, and use of the root replacement technique. The subcoronary technique is associated with a higher incidence of prosthetic AR and reoperation. In addition, the homograft valve and root are prone to severe calcification, making reoperation difficult. One possible advantage of homografts is in the avoidance of early endocarditis, and homografts are commonly used in the treatment of aortic valve endocarditis, particularly complex aortic root endocarditis, However, in randomized studies, there was no benefit of homografts compared with other tissue valves in outcome after endocarditis.[194]

PULMONARY AUTOGRAFTS. In this operation, the Ross procedure, the patient's own pulmonary valve and adjacent main pulmonary artery are removed and used to replace the diseased aortic valve and often the neighboring aorta, with reimplantation of the coronary arteries into the graft.[195] A human pulmonary or aortic homograft is then inserted into the pulmonary position. The autograft is nonthrombogenic. In children and adolescents, there is evidence that the autograft grows along with the patient.[196] The risk of endocarditis is very low, anticoagulants are not required, and, perhaps most importantly, the long-term durability appears to be excellent. A high incidence of pulmonary homograft stenosis has been reported in some series, which may represent a postoperative inflammatory reaction. The pulmonary artery tissue adapts to the aortic pressure and usually does not dilate. However, this procedure should not be performed in patients with bicuspid valves and dilated aortic roots, because the implanted pulmonary artery tissue exposed to the higher aortic pressures may also undergo degenerative changes, leading to significant dilation of the autograft. A subcoronary technique, in which the pulmonary autograft is inserted without a root replacement, may circumvent this problem, but late dilation of the autograft remains a concern.[197] The pulmonary autograft is the replacement valve of choice in children, adolescents, and younger adults who have a long (>20-year) life expectancy, particularly young women who wish to become pregnant. A prospective randomized clinical trial has demonstrated improved long-term survival in patients undergoing AVR who received a pulmonary autograft compared to those receiving a homograft.[197a] However, its use has been limited because the operation is technically much more demanding than a simple AVR. The procedure should be carried out only by highly experienced surgeons.

HEMODYNAMICS OF VALVE REPLACEMENTS. The most commonly used prosthetic valves—mechanical prostheses and stented porcine or pericardial xenografts—have an effective in vitro orifice size that is smaller than the normal valve at the same site.[187,189] Current generation tissue and mechanical valves have larger effective valve areas than older valves, particularly stented, valves, but still do not restore valve area or hemodynamics to normal. Although all prosthetic valves are inherently mildly stenotic, postoperative hemodynamic measurements show reasonably good function, with effective mitral valve orifice areas averaging 1.7 to 2.0 cm² and mitral valve gradients of 4 to 8 mm Hg at rest (see Tables 15-12 to 15-15). Aortic valve effective orifice areas and transvalvular gra-

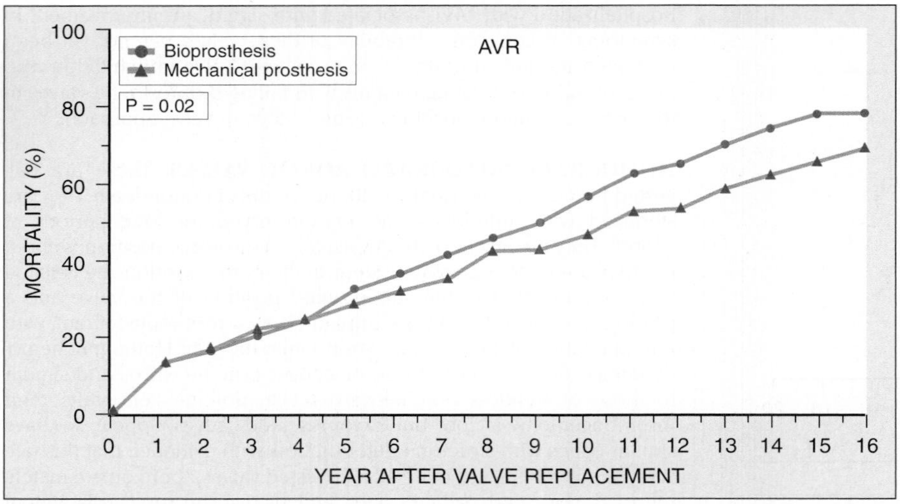

FIGURE 66-47 Mortality after AVR with the Björk-Shiley (Pfizer, New York) and porcine valves from the Department of Veterans Affairs trial. *(From Hammermeister KE, Sethi GK, Henderson WG, et al: Outcomes 15 years after valve replacement with a mechanical versus a bioprosthetic valve: Final report of the Veterans Affairs randomized trial. J Am Coll Cardiol 36:1152, 2000.)*

dients depend on valve size and type and have been detailed in published tables of normal values and guidelines.[187,188,198]

The degree of physiologic stenosis of a normally functioning prosthetic valve is considered significant (often called patient-prosthesis mismatch) when the effective valve orifice is 0.85 cm^2/m^2 or less and is severe when the effective orifice area is less than 0.65 cm^2/m^2. Patient prosthetic mismatch adversely affects short- and long-term survival after valve surgery.[199] Mismatch can be avoided by choosing a valve with an adequate orifice area for the patient's body size. In some cases, an annular enlarging procedure may be necessary. Rarely, reoperation to correct a malfunctioning prosthesis may be necessary.

Selection of an Artificial Valve

Most comparisons of mechanical and bioprosthetic valves indicate similar overall results in terms of early and late mortality, prosthetic valve endocarditis and other complications, and the need for reoperation, at least for the first 5 years postoperatively.[200] As indicated, there appear to be no significant differences when a valve size appropriate for the patient's body size is implanted.[187] Patients with a small aortic annulus may be better candidates for unstented homografts, heterografts, or pulmonary autografts. In general, patient outcome after valve surgery is related more to preoperative factors, such as age, LV function, associated coronary artery disease, and comorbid conditions, than to the prosthesis itself.

The major task when selecting an artificial valve is to weigh the advantage of durability and the disadvantages of the risks of thromboembolism and anticoagulant treatment inherent in mechanical prostheses on the one hand with the advantage of low thrombogenicity and the disadvantage of abbreviated durability of bioprostheses on the other.[200a] Overall survival after AVR is better with a mechanical compared with a bioprosthetic aortic valve (**Fig. 66-47**), principally because of the higher rate of structural deterioration of the bioprosthesis (especially in patients younger than 65 years). Much of the increased mortality in patients receiving a tissue valve is because of reoperation, which is associated with about twice the mortality of the initial procedure. With MV replacement, the prosthetic valve type does not influence survival nor the probability of developing other valve-related complications, including endocarditis, valve thrombosis, and systemic embolism, although anticoagulant-related bleeding is higher in patients receiving mechanical valves. Patients with mechanical valves also have a higher incidence of perivalvular regurgitation in the mitral position and a trend for this complication in the aortic position. The higher survival rates with mechanical compared with bioprosthetic valves have been confirmed in other studies as well. Therefore,

mechanical prostheses, usually of the bileaflet variety, are the valves of choice for most patients younger than 65 years.

However, the following groups of patients should receive bioprostheses: (1) patients with coexisting disease who are prone to hemorrhage and who therefore tolerate anticoagulants poorly, such as those with bleeding disorders, intestinal polyposis, and angiodysplasia; (2) patients who are likely to be noncompliant with permanent anticoagulant treatment, who are unwilling to take anticoagulants on a regular basis, or who live in developing nations and cannot be monitored; (3) patients older than 65 years in whom bioprosthetic valves deteriorate very slowly (see Fig. 66-46), who are unlikely to outlive their bioprostheses, and who because of their age may also be at greater risk of hemorrhage while taking anticoagulants; (4) patients with a small aortic annulus in whom an unstented (free) bioprosthetic graft may provide superior hemodynamics; and (5) younger women wishing to bear children, who require AVR. Patient preference plays an important role in determining the choice of a prosthetic valve. A bioprosthesis is reasonable for AVR in patients <65 years of age who elect to receive this valve for lifestyle considerations after detailed discussions of the risks of anticoagulation versus the likelihood that a second AVR may be necessary in the future.

SPECIAL CONSIDERATIONS

Pregnancy

Women with artificial valves can tolerate the hemodynamic burden of pregnancy well, but the hypercoagulable state of pregnancy increases the risk of thromboembolism in pregnant patients with mechanical prostheses (see Chap. 82).[201,202] Anticoagulation must not be interrupted, although an increased risk of fatal fetal hemorrhage occurs in women in whom anticoagulants are continued. There is also a risk of fetal malformation caused by the probable teratogenic effect of warfarin. Although these problems represent rationales for the use of tissue valves in all women of childbearing age, their limited durability in young adults makes their use unacceptable. Therefore, every effort should be made to defer valve replacement until after childbirth. In pregnant women with critical MS or AS, balloon valvuloplasty should be considered and, if at all possible, MV repair instead of replacement should be undertaken for patients with MR. Women of childbearing potential who have a mechanical prosthesis should be counseled against pregnancy.

When a woman who already has a mechanical prosthetic valve becomes pregnant, the risk of fetal defects with oral anticoagulants must be balanced against the risk of inadequate anticoagulation if oral therapy is interrupted. The management of anticoagulation in pregnant women with mechanical valves is controversial. All agree that the goal is continuous, effective, monitored anticoagulation and avoidance of fetal defects. In pregnant patients who receive warfarin, oral therapy is discontinued at week 36 of gestation and replaced with continuous intravenous unfractionated heparin. Heparin should be discontinued at the onset of labor but may be restarted, along with warfarin, several hours after delivery. Between weeks 1 to 36, the options include the following: (1) continued oral therapy with warfarin to maintain a therapeutic INR; (2) replacement of warfarin with dose-adjusted subcutaneous heparin or dose-adjusted subcutaneous low-molecular-weight heparin between weeks 6 and 12 (when the risk of fetal defects is highest); and (3) continuous intravenous or dose-adjusted subcutaneous heparin or dose-adjusted subcutaneous low-molecular-weight heparin for the duration of pregnancy.[1] The most important management principle is to ensure that anticoagulation is not interrupted and that the dose of anticoagulation is adequate based on frequent monitoring of the partial thromboplastin time (PTT; for intravenous or subcutaneous heparin), INR (for warfarin), or anti-Xa levels (for low-molecular-weight heparin).

Noncardiac Surgery

When noncardiac surgery is required for patients with prosthetic valves who are receiving anticoagulants, the risk depends on the valve type, location, and associated risk factors. In patients with an isolated AVR and no associated risk factors, the anticoagulant is stopped 1 to 3 days preoperatively and resumed as soon as possible postoperatively without the need for heparin therapy. However, when the risk of thromboembolism is higher, intravenous heparin is started when the INR falls below 2.0 and resumed postoperatively until the INR is again therapeutic. High-risk patients include those with a mechanical mitral valve prosthesis, AF, previous thromboembolism, LV dysfunction, hypercoagulable condition, older generation thrombotic valve, mechanical tricuspid valve, or more than one mechanical valve. The use of subcutaneous low-molecular-weight heparin in this situation has been advocated by some experts, but this topic represents another area of controversy.[1,203-205]

Children and Patients Receiving Chronic Hemodialysis

The high incidence of bioprosthetic valve failure in children and adolescents almost prohibits their use in these groups. In young adults between the ages of 25 and 35 years, the failure of bioprosthetic valves is somewhat higher than in older adults; this serves as a relative, but not an absolute, contraindication to their use in this age group.

In children, a mechanical prosthesis (generally the St. Jude valve), with its favorable hemodynamics and established durability, is preferred despite the disadvantages inherent in the need for anticoagulants in this age group. Alternatively, if an experienced surgical team is available and the patient requires an AVR, a pulmonary autograft is an excellent alternative.

Previous studies indicated a high rate of bioprosthetic structural deterioration in patients receiving chronic renal dialysis. However, several studies have reported no difference in survival of patients with a bioprosthesis or a mechanical valve, coupled with an unacceptably high rate of stroke and major bleeding in patients with the mechanical valves. Current guidelines no longer recommend mechanical valves for these patients, but this clearly is an area in which physician judgment is important for individual patients.

Tricuspid Position

The risk of thrombosis for all valves is highest in the tricuspid position because of the lower pressures and velocity of blood flow. This complication appears to be highest for tilting disc valves, intermediate for caged ball valves, and lowest for bioprostheses, which are the valves of choice as tricuspid replacements. Fortunately, bioprostheses exhibit a much slower rate of mechanical deterioration in the tricuspid position than in the mitral or aortic positions.

REFERENCES

1. Bonow RO, Carabello BA, Chatterjee K, et al: ACC/AHA 2006 guidelines for the management of patients with valvular heart disease: A report of the American College of Cardiology/American Heart Association Task Force on Practice Guidelines (Writing Committee to Revise the 1998 guidelines for the management of patients with valvular heart disease) developed in collaboration with the Society of Cardiovascular Anesthesiologists: Endorsed by the Society for Cardiovascular Angiography and Interventions and the Society of Thoracic Surgeons. J Am Coll Cardiol 48:e1, 2006.
2. Vahanian A, Baumgartner H, Bax J, et al: Guidelines on the management of valvular heart disease: The Task Force on the Management of Valvular Heart Disease of the European Society of Cardiology. Eur Heart J 28:230, 2007.

Aortic Stenosis

3. Roberts WC, Ko JM: Frequency by decades of unicuspid, bicuspid, and tricuspid aortic valves in adults having isolated aortic valve replacement for aortic stenosis, with or without associated aortic regurgitation. Circulation 111:920, 2005.
4. Braverman AC, Guven H, Beardslee MA, et al: The bicuspid aortic valve. Curr Probl Cardiol 30:470, 2005.
5. Lewin MB, Otto CM: The bicuspid aortic valve: Adverse outcomes from infancy to old age. Circulation 111:832, 2005.
6. Braverman AC: The bicuspid aortic valve. In Otto CM, Bonow RO (eds): Valvular Heart Disease: A Companion to Braunwald's Heart Disease. Philadelphia, Saunders/Elsevier, 2009, pp 169-186.
7. Stewart BF, Siscovick D, Lind BK, et al: Clinical factors associated with calcific aortic valve disease. J Am Coll Cardiol 29:630, 1997.
7a. Freeman RV, Otto CM: Spectrum of calcific aortic valve disease: Pathogenesis, disease progression, and treatment strategies. Circulation 111:3316, 2005.
8. Olsen MH, Wachtell K, Bella JN, et al: Aortic valve sclerosis relates to cardiovascular events in patients with hypertension (a LIFE substudy). Am J Cardiol 95:132, 2005.
9. Taylor HA Jr, Clark BL, Garrison RJ, et al: Relation of aortic valve sclerosis to risk of coronary heart disease in African-Americans. Am J Cardiol 95:401, 2005.
10. Owens DS, Otto CM: Is it time for a new paradigm in calcific aortic valve disease? J Am Coll Cardiol Img 2:928, 2009.
11. Rajamannan NM, Otto CM: Targeted therapy to prevent progression of calcific aortic stenosis. Circulation 110:1180, 2004.
12. Helske S, Otto CM: Lipid lowering in aortic stenosis: Still some light at the end of the tunnel? Circulation 119:2653, 2009.
13. O'Brien KD: Pathogenesis of calcific aortic valve disease: A disease process comes of age (and a good deal more). Arterioscler Thromb Vasc Biol 26:1721, 2006.
14. Miller JD, Chu Y, Brooks RM, et al: Dysregulation of antioxidant mechanisms contributes to increased oxidative stress in calcific aortic valvular stenosis in humans. J Am Coll Cardiol 52:843, 2008.
15. Rajamannan NM: Calcific aortic stenosis: Lessons learned from experimental and clinical studies. Arterioscler Thromb Vasc Biol 29:162, 2009.
16. Otto CM: Calcific aortic stenosis—time to look more closely at the valve. N Engl J Med 359:1395, 2008.
17. Bella JN, Tang W, Kraja A, et al: Genome-wide linkage mapping for valve calcification susceptibility loci in hypertensive sibships: The Hypertension Genetic Epidemiology Network Study. Hypertension 49:453, 2007.
18. Bosse Y, Mathieu P, Pibarot P: Genomics: The next step to elucidate the etiology of calcific aortic valve stenosis. J Am Coll Cardiol 51:1327, 2008.
19. Probst V, Le Scouarnec S, Legendre A, et al: Familial aggregation of calcific aortic valve stenosis in the western part of France. Circulation 113:856, 2006.
20. Ngo DTM, Sverdlov AL, Willoughby SR, et al: Determinants of occurrence of aortic sclerosis in an aging population. J Am Coll Cardiol Img 2:919, 2009.
21. Katz R, Wong ND, Kronmal R, et al: Features of the metabolic syndrome and diabetes mellitus as predictors of aortic valve calcification in the Multi-Ethnic Study of Atherosclerosis. Circulation 113:2113-2119, 2006.
22. Briand M, Dumesnil JG, Kadem L, et al: Reduced systemic arterial compliance impacts significantly on left ventricular afterload and function in aortic stenosis: Implications for diagnosis and treatment. J Am Coll Cardiol 46:291, 2005.
23. Rajamannan NM: Cellular, molecular and genetic mechanisms of valvular heart disease. In Otto CM, Bonow RO (eds): Valvular Heart Disease: A Companion to Braunwald's Heart Disease. Philadelphia, Saunders/Elsevier. 2009, pp 39-54.
24. Miller JD, Weiss RM, Serrano KM, et al: Lowering plasma cholesterol levels halts progression of aortic valve disease in mice. Circulation 119:2693, 2009.
25. Cowell SJ, Newby DE, Prescott RJ, et al: A randomized trial of intensive lipid-lowering therapy in calcific aortic stenosis. N Engl J Med 352:2389, 2005.
26. Moura LM, Ramos SF, Zamorano JL, et al: Rosuvastatin affecting aortic valve endothelium to slow the progression of aortic stenosis. J Am Coll Cardiol 49:554, 2007.
27. Rossebo AB, Pedersen TR, Boman K, et al: Intensive lipid lowering with simvastatin and ezetimibe in aortic stenosis. N Engl J Med 359:1343, 2008.
28. Chan KL, Teo K, Dumesnil JG, et al: Effect of lipid lowering with rosuvastatin on progression of aortic stenosis: Results of the Aortic Stenosis Progression Observation: Measuring Effects of Rosuvastatin (ASTRONOMER) Trial. Circulation 121:306, 2010.
29. Busseuil D, Shi Y, Mecteau M, et al: Regression of aortic valve stenosis by apo A-I mimetic peptide infusions in rabbits. Br J Pharmacol 154:765, 2008.
30. Baumgartner H, Hung J, Bermejo J, et al: Echocardiographic assessment of valve stenosis: EAE/ASE recommendations for clinical practice. Eur J Echocardiogr 10:1, 2009.
30a. Maganti K, Rigolin VH, Enriquez-Sarano M, Bonow RO. Heart valve disease: Diagnosis and management. Mayo Clin Proc 85:453, 2010.
31. Otto CM: Valvular aortic stenosis: Disease severity and timing of intervention. J Am Coll Cardiol 47:2141, 2006.
32. Monin JL, Lancellotti P, Monchi M, et al: Risk score for predicting outcome in patients with asymptomatic aortic stenosis. Circulation 120:69, 2009.
33. Coglianese EE, Davidoff R: Predicting outcome in patients with asymptomatic aortic stenosis. Circulation 120:9, 2009.
33a. Maréchaux S, Hachicha Z, Bellouin A, et al: Usefulness of exercise-stress echocardiography for risk stratification of true asymptomatic patients with aortic valve stenosis. Eur Heart J 31:1390, 2010.
34. Kadem L, Dumesnil JG, Rieu R, et al: Impact of systemic hypertension on the assessment of aortic stenosis. Heart 91:354, 2005.
35. Carabello BA, Paulus WJ: Aortic stenosis. Lancet 373:956, 2009.
36. Otto CM (ed): Textbook of Clinical Echocardiography. 4th ed. Philadelphia, Saunders/Elsevier, 2009.
37. Rosenhek R, Baumgartner H: Aortic stenosis. In Otto CM, Bonow RO (eds): Valvular Heart Disease: A Companion to Braunwald's Heart Disease. Philadelphia, Saunders/Elsevier, 2009, pp 127-154.
38. Rosenhek R: Aortic stenosis: Evaluation of disease severity, disease progression, and the role of echocardiography in clinical decision making. In Otto CM (ed): The Clinical Practice of Echocardiography. Philadelphia, Saunders/Elsevier, 2007, pp 516-551.
39. Baumgartner H: What influences the outcome of valve replacement in critical aortic stenosis? Heart 91:1254, 2005.
40. Chambers J, Bach D, Dumesnil J, et al: Crossing the aortic valve in severe aortic stenosis: No longer acceptable? J Heart Valve Dis 13:344, 2004.
41. Cawley PJ, Maki JH, Otto CM: Cardiovascular magnetic resonance imaging for valvular heart disease: Technique and validation. Circulation 119:468, 2009.
42. Otto CM: Calcific aortic valve disease: Outflow obstruction is the end stage of a systemic disease process. Eur Heart J 2009.
43. Dal-Bianco JP, Khandheria BK, Mookadam F, et al: Management of asymptomatic severe aortic stenosis. J Am Coll Cardiol 52:1279, 2008.
44. Varadarajan P, Kapoor N, Bansal RC, Pai RG: Clinical profile and natural history of 453 nonsurgically managed patients with severe aortic stenosis. Ann Thorac Surg 82:2111, 2006.

45. Rosenhek R, Klaar U, Schemper M, et al: Mild and moderate aortic stenosis. Natural history and risk stratification by echocardiography. Eur Heart J 25:199, 2004.
46. Pellikka PA, Sarano ME, Nishimura RA, et al: Outcome of 622 adults with asymptomatic, hemodynamically significant aortic stenosis during prolonged follow-up. Circulation 111:3290, 2005.
46a. Stewart RA, Kerr AJ, Walley GA, et al: Left ventricular systolic and diastolic function assessed by tissue Doppler imaging and outcome in asymptomatic aortic stenosis. Eur Heart J 31:2191, 2010.
47. Rosenhek R, Zilberszac R, Schemper M, et al: Natural history of very severe aortic stenosis. Circulation 121:151, 2010.
47a. Lancellotti P, Donal E, Magne J, et al: Risk stratification in asymptomatic moderate to severe aortic stenosis: The importance of the valvular, arterial and ventricular interplay. Heart 96:1364, 2010.
48. Bach DS, Siao D, Girard SE, et al: Evaluation of patients with severe symptomatic aortic stenosis who do not undergo aortic valve replacement: The potential role of subjectively overestimated operative risk. Circ Cardiovasc Qual Outcomes 2:533, 2009.
49 Das P, Rimington H, Chambers J: Exercise testing to stratify risk in aortic stenosis. Eur Heart J 26:1309, 2005.
50. Lancellotti P, Lebois F, Simon M, et al: Prognostic importance of quantitative exercise Doppler echocardiography in asymptomatic valvular aortic stenosis. Circulation 112:I377, 2005.
51. Bergler-Klein J, Klaar U, Heger M, et al: Natriuretic peptides predict symptom-free survival and postoperative outcome in severe aortic stenosis. Circulation 109:2302, 2004.
52. Lim P, Monin JL, Monchi M, et al: Predictors of outcome in patients with severe aortic stenosis and normal left ventricular function: Role of B-type natriuretic peptide. Eur Heart J 25:2048, 2004.
53. Gerber IL, Legget ME, West TM, et al: Usefulness of serial measurement of N-terminal pro-brain natriuretic peptide plasma levels in asymptomatic patients with aortic stenosis to predict symptomatic deterioration. Am J Cardiol 95:898, 2005.
53a. Monin JL, Lancellotti P, MD, Monchi M, et al: Risk score for predicting outcome in patients with asymptomatic aortic stenosis. Circulation 120:69, 2009.
54. Bonow RO, Cheitlin MD, Crawford MH, Douglas PS: Task Force 3: Valvular heart disease. J Am Coll Cardiol 45:1334, 2005.
55. Christ M, Sharkova Y, Geldner G, Maisch B: Preoperative and perioperative care for patients with suspected or established aortic stenosis facing noncardiac surgery. Chest 128:2944, 2005.
56. Warnes CA, Williams RG, Bashore TM, et al: ACC/AHA 2008 guidelines for the management of adults with congenital heart disease: A report of the American College of Cardiology/American Heart Association Task Force on Practice Guidelines (writing committee to develop guidelines on the management of adults with congenital heart disease). Circulation 118:e714, 2008.
57. Iung B, Cachier A, Baron G, et al: Decision-making in elderly patients with severe aortic stenosis: Why are so many denied surgery? Eur Heart J 26:2714, 2005.
58. Pereira JJ, Balaban K, Lauer MS, et al: Aortic valve replacement in patients with mild or moderate aortic stenosis and corbnary bypass surgery. Am J Med 118:735, 2005.
59. Gillinov AM, Garcia MJ: When is concomitant aortic valve replacement indicated in patients with mild to moderate stenosis undergoing coronary revascularization? Curr Cardiol Rep 7:101, 2005.
60. Munt B: Percutaneous aortic valve implantation. *In* Otto CM, Bonow RO (eds): Valvular Heart Disease: A Companion to Braunwald's Heart Disease. Philadelphia, Saunders/Elsevier, 2009, pp 209-220.
61. Rosengart TK, Feldman T, Borger MA, et al: Percutaneous and minimally invasive valve procedures: A scientific statement from the American Heart Association Council on Cardiovascular Surgery and Anesthesia, Council on Clinical Cardiology, Functional Genomics and Translational Biology Interdisciplinary Working Group, and Quality of Care and Outcomes Research Interdisciplinary Working Group. Circulation 117:1750, 2008.
62. Vahanian A, Alfieri O, Al-Attar N, et al: Transcatheter valve implantation for patients with aortic stenosis: A position statement from the European association of cardio-thoracic surgery (EACTS) and the European Society of Cardiology (ESC), in collaboration with the European Association of Percutaneous Cardiovascular Interventions (EAPCI). EuroIntervention 4:193, 2008.
63. Rodés-Cabau J, Webb JG, Cheung A, et al: Transcatheter aortic valve implantation for the treatment of severe symptomatic aortic stenosis in patients at very high or prohibitive surgical risk: Acute and late outcomes of the multicenter Canadian experience. J Am Coll Cardiol 55:1080, 2010.
64. Webb JG, Altwegg L, Boone RH, et al: Transcatheter aortic valve implantation: Impact on clinical and valve-related outcomes. Circulation 119:3009, 2009.
64a. Leon MB, Smith CR, Mack M, et al: Transcatheter aortic-valve implantation for aortic stenosis in patients who cannot undergo surgery. N Engl J Med 363:1667, 2010.
65. Chambers J: Low "gradient," low flow aortic stenosis. Heart 92:554, 2006.
66. Tribouilloy C, Levy F, Rusinaru D, et al: Outcome after aortic valve replacement for low-flow/low-gradient aortic stenosis without contractile reserve on dobutamine stress echocardiography. J Am Coll Cardiol 53:1865, 2009.
67. Levy F, Laurent M, Monin JL, et al: Aortic valve replacement for low-flow/low-gradient aortic stenosis operative risk stratification and long-term outcome: A European multicenter study. J Am Coll Cardiol 51:1466, 2008.
68. Quere JP, Monin JL, Levy F, et al: Influence of preoperative left ventricular contractile reserve on postoperative ejection fraction in low-gradient aortic stenosis. Circulation 113:1738, 2006.
69. Clavel MA, Fuchs C, Burwash IG, et al: Predictors of outcomes in low-flow, low-gradient aortic stenosis: Results of the multicenter TOPAS Study. Circulation 118:S234, 2008..
70. Picano E, Pibarot P, Lancellotti P, et al: The emerging role of exercise testing and stress echocardiography in valvular heart disease. J Am Coll Cardiol 54:2251, 2009.
71. Brown JM, O'Brien SM, Wu C, et al: Isolated aortic valve replacement in North America comprising 108,687 patients in 10 years: Changes in risks, valve types, and outcomes in the Society of Thoracic Surgeons National Database. J Thorac Cardiovasc Surg 137:82, 2009.
72. Shahian DM, O'Brien SM, Filardo G, et al: The Society of Thoracic Surgeons 2008 cardiac surgery risk models: Part 3—valve plus coronary artery bypass grafting surgery. Ann Thorac Surg 88:S43, 2009.
73. O'Brien SM, Shahian DM, Filardo G, et al: The Society of Thoracic Surgeons 2008 cardiac surgery risk models: Part 2—isolated valve surgery. Ann Thorac Surg 88:S23, 2009.
74. Goodney PP, O'Connor GT, Wennberg DE, Birkmeyer JE: Do hospitals with low mortality rates in coronary artery bypass also perform well in valve replacement? Ann Thorac Surg 76:1131, 2003.
75. Vahanian A, Otto CM: Risk stratification in aortic stenosis. Eur Heart J 31:416, 2010.
76. Dewey TM, Brown D, Ryan WH: Reliability of risk algorithms in predicting early and late operative outcomes in high-risk patients undergoing aortic valve replacement. J Thorac Cardiovasc Surg 135:180, 2008.
77. Wendt D, Osswald BR, Kayser K, et al: Society of Thoracic Surgeons score is superior to the EuroSCORE determining mortality in high risk patients undergoing isolated aortic valve replacement. Ann Thorac Surg 88:468, 2009.
78. Hannan EL, Wu C, Bennett EV, et al: Risk index for predicting in-hospital mortality for cardiac valve surgery. Ann Thorac Surg 83:921, 2008.
79. Pedrazzini GB, Masson S, Latini R, et al: Comparison of brain natriuretic peptide plasma levels versus logistic EuroSCORE in predicting in-hospital and late postoperative mortality in patients undergoing aortic valve replacement for symptomatic aortic stenosis. Am J Cardiol 102:749, 2008.
80. Kolh P, Kerzmann A, Honore C,et al: Aortic valve surgery in octogenarians: Predictive factors for operative and long-term results. Eur J Cardiothorac Surg 31:600, 2007.
81. Lung B: Management of the elderly patient with aortic stenosis. Heart 94:519, 2008.
81a. Malaisrie SC, McCarthy PM, McGee EC, et al: Contemporary perioperative results of isolated aortic valve replacement for aortic stenosis: Implications for referral of patients for valve replacement. Ann Thorac Surg 89:751, 2010.
82. Ambler G, Omar RZ, Royston P, et al: Generic, simple risk stratification model for heart valve surgery. Circulation 112:224, 2005.
82a. Maillet JM, Sommeb D, Hennel E, et al: Frailty after aortic valve replacement (AVR) in octogenarians. Arch Gerontol Geriatrics 48:391, 2009.

Aortic Regurgitation

83. Maurer G: Aortic regurgitation. Heart 92:994, 2006.
84. Bekeredjian R, Grayburn PA: Valvular heart disease: Aortic regurgitation. Circulation 112:125, 2005.
85. Enriquez-Sarano M, Tajik AJ: Clinical practice. Aortic regurgitation. N Engl J Med 351:1539, 2004.
86. Roberts WC, Ko JM, Moore TR, Jones WH III: Causes of pure aortic regurgitation in patients having isolated aortic valve replacement at a single U.S. tertiary hospital (1993 to 2005). Circulation 114:422, 2006.
87. Tadros TM, Klein MD, Shapira OM: Ascending aortic dilation associated with bicuspid aortic valve: Pathophysiology, molecular biology, and clinical implications. Circulation 119:880, 2009.
88. Palazzi C, D' AS, Lubrano E, Olivieri I: Aortic involvement in ankylosing spondylitis. Clin Exp Rheumatol 26:S13, 2008.
89. Bermudez EA, Gaasch WH: Regurgitant lesions of the aortic and mitral valves: Considerations in determining the ideal timing of surgical intervention. Heart Fail Clin 2:473, 2006.
90. Rigolin VH, Bonow RO: Hemodynamic characteristics and progression to heart failure in regurgitant lesions. Heart Fail Clin 2:453, 2006.
91. Tornos P, Bonow RO: Aortic regurgitation. *In* Otto CM, Bonow RO (eds): Valvular Heart Disease: A Companion to Braunwald's Heart Disease. Philadelphia, Saunders/Elsevier, 2009, pp 155-168.
92. Tornos P, Sambola A, Permanyer-Miralda G, et al: Long-term outcome of surgically treated aortic regurgitation: Influence of guideline adherence toward early surgery. J Am Coll Cardiol 47:1012, 2006.
93. Sambola A, Tornos P, Ferreira-Gonzalez I, Evangelista A: Prognostic value of preoperative indexed end-systolic left ventricle diameter in the outcome after surgery in patients with chronic aortic regurgitation. Am Heart J 155:1114, 2008.
94. Detaint D, Messika-Zeitoun D, Maalouf J, et al: Quantitative echocardiographic determinants of clinical outcome in asymptomatic patients with aortic regurgitation: A prospective study. J Am Coll Cardiol Img 1:1, 2008.
95. Gelfand EV, Hughes S, Hauser TH, et al: Severity of mitral and aortic regurgitation as assessed by cardiovascular magnetic resonance: optimizing correlation with Doppler echocardiography. J Cardiovasc Magn Reson 8:503, 2006.
96. Mahajerin A, Gurm HS, Tsai TT, et al: Vasodilator therapy in patients with aortic insufficiency: A systematic review. Am Heart J 153:454, 2007.
97. Evangelista A, Tornos P, Sambola A,et al: Long-term vasodilator therapy in patients with severe aortic regurgitation. N Engl J Med 353:1342, 2005.
98. Sampat U, Varadarajan P, Turk R, et al: Effect of beta-blocker therapy on survival in patients with severe aortic regurgitation: Results from a cohort of 756 patients. J Am Coll Cardiol 54;452, 2009.
98a. Hiratzka FD, Bakris GL, Beckman JA, et al: 2010 ACCF/AHA/AATS/ACR/ASA/SCA/SCAI/SIR/STS/SVM Guidelines for the diagnosis and management of patients with thoracic aortic disease: Executive summary. A Report of the American College of Cardiology Foundation/American Heart Association Task Force on Practice Guidelines, American Association for Thoracic Surgery, American College of Radiology, American Stroke Association, Society of Cardiovascular Anesthesiologists, Society for Cardiovascular Angiography and Interventions, Society of Interventional Radiology, Society of Thoracic Surgeons, and Society for Vascular Medicine. Circulation 121:1544, 2010.
99. Minakata K, Schaff HV, Zehr KJ, et al: Is repair of aortic valve regurgitation a safe alternative to valve replacement? J Thorac Cardiovasc Surg 127:645, 2004.
100. Stelzer P, Adams DH: The surgical approach to aortic valve disease. *In* Otto CM, Bonow RO (eds): Valvular Heart Disease: A Companion to Braunwald's Heart Disease. Philadelphia, Saunders/Elsevier, 2009, pp 187-208.
101. Borger MA, Preston M, Ivanov J, et al: Should the ascending aorta be replaced more frequently in patients with bicuspid aortic valve disease? J Thorac Cardiovasc Surg 128:677, 2004.
102. Stout KK, Verrier ED: Acute valvular regurgitation. Circulation 119:3232, 2009.

Bicuspid Aortic Valve

103. Garg V, Muth AN, Ransom JF, et al: Mutations in NOTCH1 cause aortic valve disease. Nature 437:270, 2005.
104. Schaefer BM, Lewin MB, Stout KK, et al: Usefulness of bicuspid aortic valve phenotype to predict elastic properties of the ascending aorta. Am J Cardiol 99:686, 2007.
105. Fernandez B, Duran AC, Fernandez-Gallego T, et al: Bicuspid aortic valves with different special orientations of the leaflets are distinct etiological entities. J Am Coll Cardiol 54:2312, 2009.
105a. Bonow RO: Bicuspid aortic valves and dilated aortas: A critical review of the critical review of the ACC/AHA guidelines recommendations. Am J Cardiol 102:111, 2008.

106. Schaefer BM, Lewin MB, Stout KK, et al: The bicuspid aortic valve: an integrated phenotypic classification of leaflet morphology and aortic root shape. Heart 94:1634, 2008.

107. Tzemos N, Therrien J, Yip J, et al: Outcomes in adults with bicuspid aortic valves. JAMA 300:1317, 2008.

108. Michelena HI, Desjardins VA, Avierinos JF, et al: Natural history of asymptomatic patients with normally functioning or minimally dysfunctional bicuspid aortic valve in the community. Circulation 117:2776, 2008.

Mitral Stenosis

109. Mensah GA: The burden of valvular heart disease. In Otto CM, Bonow RO (eds): Valvular Heart Disease: A Companion to Braunwald's Heart Disease. Philadelphia, Saunders/Elsevier, 2009, pp 1-18.

110. Essop MR, Nkomo VT: Rheumatic and nonrheumatic valvular heart disease: Epidemiology, management, and prevention in Africa. Circulation 112:3584, 2005.

111. Roberts WC, Ko JM: Clinical pathology of valvular heart disease. In Otto CM, Bonow RO (eds): Valvular Heart Disease: A Companion to Braunwald's Heart Disease. Philadelphia, Saunders/Elsevier, 2009, pp 19-38.

112. Rajamannan NM, Subramaniam M, Caira F, et al: Atorvastatin inhibits hypercholesterolemia-induced calcification in the aortic valves via the Lrp5 receptor pathway. Circulation 112 (suppl I):I-229, 2005.

113. Iung B, Vahanian A: Rheumatic mitral valve disease. In Otto CM, Bonow RO (eds): Valvular Heart Disease: A Companion to Braunwald's Heart Disease. Philadelphia, Saunders/Elsevier, 2009, pp 221-242.

114. Iung B, Vahanian A: Echocardiography in the patient undergoing catheter balloon mitral valvuloplasty: Patient selection, hemodynamic results, complications and long term outcome. In Otto CM (ed): The Clinical Practice of Echocardiography. Philadelphia, Saunders/Elsevier, 2007, pp 481-501.

115. Carabello BA: Modern management of mitral stenosis. Circulation 112:432, 2005.

116. Shavelle DM: Evaluation of valvular heart disease by cardiac catheterization and angiography. In Otto CM, Bonow RO (eds): Valvular Heart Disease: A Companion to Braunwald's Heart Disease. Philadelphia, Saunders/Elsevier, 2009, pp 85-100

117. Fuster V, Ryden LE, Cannom DS, et al: ACC/AHA/ESC 2006 guidelines for the management of patients with atrial fibrillation: A report of the American College of Cardiology/American Heart Association Task Force on Practice Guidelines and the European Society of Cardiology Committee for Practice Guidelines (Writing Committee to Revise the 2001 Guidelines for the Management of Patients With Atrial Fibrillation): Developed in collaboration with the European Heart Rhythm Association and the Heart Rhythm Society. Circulation 114:e257, 2006.

118. Abreu Filho CA, Lisboa LA, Dallan LA, et al: Effectiveness of the maze procedure using cooled-tip radiofrequency ablation in patients with permanent atrial fibrillation and rheumatic mitral valve disease. Circulation 112(Suppl I):I-20, 2005.

119. Doukas G, Samani NJ, Alexiou C, et al: Left atrial radiofrequency ablation during mitral valve surgery for continuous atrial fibrillation: A randomized controlled trial. JAMA 294:2357, 2005.

120. Krasuski RA, Assar MD, Wang A, et al: Usefulness of percutaneous balloon mitral commissurotomy in preventing the development of atrial fibrillation in patients with mitral stenosis. Am J Cardiol 93:936, 2004.

121. Song JK, Song JM, Kang DH, et al: Restenosis and adverse clinical events after successful percutaneous mitral valvuloplasty: Immediate post-procedural mitral valve area as an important prognosticator. Eur Heart J 30:1254, 2009.

122. Zakkar M, Amirak E, Chan KM, Punjabi PP: Rheumatic mitral valve disease: Current surgical status. Prog Cardiovasc Dis 51:478, 2009.

Mitral Regurgitation

123. Enriquez-Sarano M, Akins CW, Vahanian A: Mitral regurgitation. Lancet 373:1382, 2009.

124. Schoen FJ: Evolving concepts of cardiac valve dynamics: The continuum of development, functional structure, pathobiology, and tissue engineering. Circulation 118:1864, 2008.

125. Van CG, Flamez A, Cosyns B, et al: Treatment of Parkinson's disease with pergolide and relation to restrictive valvular heart disease. Lancet 363:1179, 2004.

126. Schade R, Andersohn F, Suissa S, et al: Dopamine agonists and the risk of cardiac-valve regurgitation. N Engl J Med 356:29-••, 2007.

127. Zanettini R, Antonini A, Gatto G, et al: Valvular heart disease and the use of dopamine agonists for Parkinson's disease. N Engl J Med 356:39, 2007.

128. Barasch E, Gottdiener JS, Larsen EK, et al: Clinical significance of calcification of the fibrous skeleton of the heart and aortosclerosis in community dwelling elderly: The Cardiovascular Health Study (CHS). Am Heart J 151:39, 2006.

129. Kizer JR, Wiebers DO, Whisnant JP, et al: Mitral annular calcification, aortic valve sclerosis, and incident stroke in adults free of clinical cardiovascular disease: The Strong Heart Study. Stroke 36:2533, 2005.

130. Allison MA, Cheung P, Criqui MH, et al: Mitral and aortic annular calcification are highly associated with systemic calcified atherosclerosis. Circulation 113:861, 2006.

131. Pierard LA, Lancellotti P: The role of ischemic mitral regurgitation in the pathogenesis of acute pulmonary edema. N Engl J Med 351:1627, 2004.

132. Levine RA: Dynamic mitral regurgitation—more than meets the eye. N Engl J Med 351:1681, 2004.

133. Levine RA, Schwammenthal E: Ischemic mitral regurgitation on the threshold of a solution: from paradoxes to unifying concepts. Circulation 112:745, 2005.

134. Agricola E, Galderisi M, Mele D, et al: Mechanical dyssynchrony and functional mitral regurgitation: Pathophysiology and clinical implications. J Cardiovasc Med (Hagerstown) 9:461, 2008.

135. Bursi F, Enriquez-Sarano M, Nkomo VT, et al: Heart failure and death after myocardial infarction in the community: The emerging role of mitral regurgitation. Circulation 111:295, 2005.

136. Nishimura RA, Schaff HV: Mitral regurgitation: timing of surgery. In Otto CM, Bonow RO (eds): Valvular Heart Disease: A Companion to Braunwald's Heart Disease. Philadelphia, Saunders/Elsevier, 2009, pp 274-290.

137. Gaasch WH, Meyer TE: Left ventricular response to mitral regurgitation: Implications for management. Circulation 118:2298, 2008.

138. Otto CM: Timing of intervention for chronic valve regurgitation: the role of echocardiography. In Otto CM (ed): The Clinical Practice of Echocardiography. Philadelphia, Saunders/Elsevier, 2007, pp 430-458.

139. Tribouilloy C, Grigioni F, Avierinos JF, et al: Survival implication of left ventricular end-systolic diameter in mitral regurgitation due to flail leaflets: A long-term follow-up multicenter study. J Am Coll Cardiol 54:1961, 2009.

140. Otto CM: Evaluation of valvular heart disease by echocardiography. In Otto CM, Bonow RO (eds): Valvular Heart Disease: A Companion to Braunwald's Heart Disease. Philadelphia, Saunders/Elsevier, 2009, pp 62-84.

141. Enriquez-Sarano M, Avierinos JF, Messika-Zeitoun D, et al: Quantitative determinants of the outcome of asymptomatic mitral regurgitation. N Engl J Med 352:875, 2005.

142. Hung J, Lang R, Flachskampf F, et al: 3D echocardiography: A review of the current status and future directions. J Am Soc Echocardiogr 20:213, 2007.

143. Bando K, Kasegawa H, Okada Y, et al: Impact of preoperative and postoperative atrial fibrillation on outcome after mitral valvuloplasty for nonischemic mitral regurgitation. J Thorac Cardiovasc Surg 129:1032, 2005.

144. Eguchi K, Ohtaki E, Matsumura T, et al: Pre-operative atrial fibrillation as the key determinant of outcome of mitral valve repair for degenerative mitral regurgitation. Eur Heart J 26:1866, 2005.

145. Carabello BA: The current therapy for mitral regurgitation. J Am Coll Cardiol 52:319, 2008.

146. Rosenhek R, Rader F, Klaar U, et al: Outcome of watchful waiting in asymptomatic severe mitral regurgitation. Circulation 113:2238, 2006.

147. Kang DH, Kim JH, Rim JH, et al: Comparison of early surgery versus conventional treatment in asymptomatic severe mitral regurgitation. Circulation 119:797, 2009.

148. Schaff HV: Asymptomatic severe mitral valve regurgitation: Observation or operation? Circulation 119:768, 2009.

149. DiGregorio V, Zehr KJ, Orszulak TA, et al: Results of mitral surgery in octogenarians with isolated nonrheumatic mitral regurgitation. Ann Thorac Surg 78:807, 2004.

150. Nagendran J, Norris C, Maitland A, et al: Is mitral valve surgery safe in octogenarians? Eur J Cardiothorac Surg 28:83, 2005.

150a. Chikwe J, Goldstone AB, Passage J, et al: A propensity score-adjusted retrospective comparison of early and mid-term results of mitral valve repair versus replacement in octogenarians. Eur Heart J. Published ahead of print doi:10.1093/eurheartj/ehq331.

151. Nowicki ER, Birkmeyer NJ, Weintraub RW, et al: Multivariable prediction of in-hospital mortality associated with aortic and mitral valve surgery in Northern New England. Ann Thorac Surg 77:1966, 2004.

152. Fedak PW, McCarthy PM, Bonow RO: Evolving concepts and technologies in mitral valve repair. Circulation 117:963, 2008.

153. Adams DH, Anyanwu AC: Seeking a higher standard for degenerative mitral valve repair: Begin with etiology. J Thorac Cardiovasc Surg 136:551, 2008.

154. Verma S, Mesana TG: Mitral-valve repair for mitral-valve prolapse. N Engl J Med 361:2261, 2009.

155. McCarthy PM, Malaisrie SC: Mitral valve repair and replacement, including associated atrial fibrillation and tricuspid regurgitation. In Otto CM, Bonow RO (eds): Valvular Heart Disease: A Companion to Braunwald's Heart Disease. Philadelphia, Saunders/Elsevier, 2009, pp. 291-306.

156. DeBonis M, Lorusso R, Lapenna E, et al: Similar long-term results of mitral valve repair for anterior compared with posterior leaflet prolapse. J Thorac Cardiovasc Surg 131:364, 2006.

157. Lam BK, Gillinov AM, Blackstone EH, et al: Importance of moderate ischemic mitral regurgitation. Ann Thorac Surg 79:462, 2005.

158. Bax JJ, Braun J, Somer ST, et al: Restrictive annuloplasty and coronary revascularization in ischemic mitral regurgitation results in reverse left ventricular remodeling. Circulation 110(Suppl II):II-103, 2004.

159. Schroder JN, Williams ML, Hata JA, et al: Impact of mitral valve regurgitation evaluated by intraoperative transesophageal echocardiography on long-term outcomes after coronary artery bypass grafting. Circulation 112:I293, 2005.

160. Shah PM: Intraoperative echocardiography for mitral valve disease. In Otto CM, Bonow RO (eds): Valvular Heart Disease: A Companion to Braunwald's Heart Disease. Philadelphia, Saunders/Elsevier, 2009, pp 322-333.

161. Gammie JS, Sheng S, Griffith BP, et al: Trends in mitral valve surgery in the United States: Results from the Society of Thoracic Surgeons Adult Cardiac Database. Ann Thorac Surg 87:1431, 2009.

162. Bridgewater B, Hooper T, Munsch C, et al: Mitral repair best practice: proposed standards. Heart 92:939, 2006.

163. Dogan S, Aybek T, Risteski PS, et al: Minimally invasive port access versus conventional mitral valve surgery: prospective randomized study. Ann Thorac Surg 79:492, 2005.

164. Vassiliades TA Jr, Block PC, Cohn LH, et al: The clinical development of percutaneous heart valve technology: A position statement of the Society of Thoracic Surgeons (STS), the American Association for Thoracic Surgery (AATS), and the Society for Cardiovascular Angiography and Interventions (SCAI) Endorsed by the American College of Cardiology Foundation (ACCF) and the American Heart Association (AHA). J Am Coll Cardiol 45:1554, 2005.

165. Feldman T, Wasserman HS, Herrmann HC, et al: Percutaneous mitral valve repair using the edge-to-edge technique: Six-month results of the EVEREST Phase I Clinical Trial. J Am Coll Cardiol 46:2134, 2005.

166. Webb JG, Harnek J, Munt BI, et al: Percutaneous transvenous mitral annuloplasty: initial human experience with device implantation in the coronary sinus. Circulation 113:851, 2006.

167. Block PC: Percutaneous transcatheter intervention for mitral regurgitation. In Otto CM, Bonow RO (eds): Valvular Heart Disease: A Companion to Braunwald's Heart Disease. Philadelphia, Saunders/Elsevier, 2009, pp 307-321.

168. Iung B, Rousseau-Paziaud J, Cormier B, et al: Contemporary results of mitral valve repair for infective endocarditis. J Am Coll Cardiol 43:386, 2004.

169. Beeri R, Otsuji Y, Schwammenthal E, Levine RA: Ischemic mitral regurgitation. In Otto CM, Bonow RO (eds): Valvular Heart Disease: A Companion to Braunwald's Heart Disease. Philadelphia, Saunders/Elsevier, 2009, pp 260-273.

170. Zegdi R, Debieche M, Latremouille C, et al: Long-term results of mitral valve repair in active endocarditis. Circulation 111:2532, 2005.

Mitral Valve Prolapse

171. Griffin BP: Myxomatous mitral valve disease. In Otto CM, Bonow RO (eds): Valvular Heart Disease: A Companion to Braunwald's Heart Disease. Philadelphia, Saunders/Elsevier, 2009, pp 243-259.

172. Hayek E, Gring CN, Griffin BP: Mitral valve prolapse. Lancet 365:507, 2005.
173. Nesta F, Leyne M, Yosefy C, et al: New locus for autosomal dominant mitral valve prolapse on chromosome 13: clinical insights from genetic studies. Circulation 112:2022, 2005.
174. Judge DP, Dietz HC: Marfan's syndrome. Lancet 366:1965, 2005.
175. Stewart WJ, Griffin BP: Intraoperative echocardiography in mitral valve repair. *In* Otto CM (ed): The Clinical Practice of Echocardiography. Philadelphia, Saunders/Elsevier, 2007, pp 459-480.
176. Avierinos JF, Detaint D, Messika-Zeitoun D, et al: Risk, determinants, and outcome implications of progression of mitral regurgitation after diagnosis of mitral valve prolapse in a single community. Am J Cardiol 101:662, 2008.

Tricuspid, Pulmonic, and Multivalve Disease

177. Bruce CJ, Connolly HM: Right-sided valve disease deserves a little more respect. Circulation 119:2726, 2009.
178. Rogers JH, Bolling SF: The tricuspid valve: Current perspective and evolving management of tricuspid regurgitation. Circulation 119:2718, 2009.
179. Forfia PR, Weigers SE: Echocardiographic findings in acute and chronic respiratory disease. *In* Otto CM (ed): The Clinical Practice of Echocardiography. Philadelphia, Saunders/Elsevier, 2007, pp 848-876.
180. McCarthy PM, Bhudia SK, Rajeswaran J, et al: Tricuspid valve repair: Durability and risk factors for failure. J Thorac Cardiovasc Surg 127:674, 2004.
181. Dreyfus GD, Corbi PJ, Chan KM, Bahrami T: Secondary tricuspid regurgitation or dilation: Which should be the criteria for surgical repair? Ann Thorac Surg 79:127, 2005.
182. Fukuda S, Song JM, Gillinov AM, et al: Tricuspid valve tethering predicts residual tricuspid regurgitation after tricuspid annuloplasty. Circulation 111:975, 2005.
183. Huehnergarth KV, Gurvitz M, Stout KK, Otto CM: Repaired tetralogy of Fallot in the adult: Monitoring and management. Heart 94:1663, 2008.
184. Therrien J, Siu SC, McLaughlin PR, et al: Pulmonary valve replacement in adults late after repair of tetralogy of fallot: Are we operating too late? J Am Coll Cardiol 36:1670, 2000.
185. Sommer RJ, Hijazi ZM, Rhodes JF: Pathophysiology of congenital heart disease in the adult: Part III: Complex congenital heart disease. Circulation 117:1340, 2008.
186. McElhinney DB, Hellenbrand WE, Zahn EM, et al: Short- and medium-term outcomes after transcatheter pulmonary valve placement in the expanded multicenter US melody valve trial. Circulation 122:507, 2010.

Prosthetic Cardiac Valves

187. Pibarot P, Dumesnil JG: Prosthetic heart valves: Selection of the optimal prosthesis and long-term management. Circulation 119:1034, 2009.
188. O'Gara PT, Bonow RO, Otto CM: Prosthetic heart valves. *In* Otto CM, Bonow RO (eds): Valvular Heart Disease: A Companion to Braunwald's Heart Disease. Philadelphia, Saunders/Elsevier, 2009, pp 383-398.
189. Yoganathan AP, Travis BR: Fluid dynamics of prosthetic valves. *In* Otto CM (ed): The Clinical Practice of Echocardiography. Philadelphia, Saunders/Elsevier, 2007, pp 552-576.

190. Tong AT, Roudaut R, Ozkan M, et al: Transesophageal echocardiography improves risk assessment of thrombolysis of prosthetic valve thrombosis: Results of the international PRO-TEE registry. J Am Coll Cardiol 43:77, 2004.
191. Schoen FJ, Levy RJ: Calcification of tissue heart valve substitutes: Progress toward understanding and prevention. Ann Thorac Surg 79:1072, 2005.
192. Ruel M, Kulik A, Rubens FD, et al: Late incidence and determinants of reoperation in patients with prosthetic heart valves. Eur J Cardiothorac Surg 25:364, 2004.
193. Webb JG, Wood DA, Ye J, et al: Transcatheter valve-in-valve implantation for failed bioprosthetic heart valves. Circulation 121:1848, 2010.
194. Leyh RG, Knobloch K, Hagl C, et al: Replacement of the aortic root for acute prosthetic valve endocarditis: Prosthetic composite versus aortic allograft root replacement. J Thorac Cardiovasc Surg 127:1416, 2004.
195. Takkenberg JJM, Klieverik LMA, Schoof PH, et al: The Ross procedure: A systematic review and meta-analysis. Circulation 119:222, 2009.
196. Raja SG, Pozzi M: Ross operation in children and young adults: The Alder Hey case series. BMC Cardiovasc Disord 4:3, 2004.
197. de Kerchove L, Rubay J, Pasquet A, et al: Ross operation in the adult: long-term outcomes after root replacement and inclusion techniques. Ann Thorac Surg 87:95, 2009.
197a. El-Hamamsy J, Eryigit A, Stevens LM, et al. Long-term outcomes after autograft versus homograft aortic root replacement in adults with aortic valve disease: A randomized controlled trial. Lancet 376:524, 2010.
198. Zabalgiotia M: Echocardiographic recognition and quantitation of prosthetic valve dysfunction. *In* Otto CM (ed): The Clinical Practice of Echocardiography. Philadelphia, Saunders/Elsevier, 2007, pp 577-604.
199. Pibarot P, Dumesnil JG: Prosthesis-patient mismatch: Definition, clinical impact, and prevention. Heart 92:1022, 2006.
200. Seiler C: Management and follow up of prosthetic heart valves. Heart 90:818, 2004.
200a. Rahimtoola SH: Choice of prosthetic heart valve in adults: An update. J Am Coll Cardiol 55:2413, 2010.
201. Elkayam U, Bitar F: Valvular heart disease and pregnancy part I: Native valves. J Am Coll Cardiol 46:223, 2005.
202. Stout KK: Valvular heart disease in pregnancy. *In* Otto CM, Bonow RO (eds): Valvular Heart Disease: A Companion to Braunwald's Heart Disease. Philadelphia, Saunders/Elsevier, 2009, pp 424-436.
203. Spyropoulos AC, Frost FJ, Hurley JS, Roberts M: Costs and clinical outcomes associated with low-molecular-weight heparin vs unfractionated heparin for perioperative bridging in patients receiving long-term oral anticoagulant therapy. Chest 125:1642, 2004.
204. Kovacs MJ, Kearon C, Rodger M, et al: Single-arm study of bridging therapy with low-molecular-weight heparin for patients at risk of arterial embolism who require temporary interruption of warfarin. Circulation 110:1658, 2004.
205. Salem DN, O'Gara PT, Madias C, Pauker SG, American College of Chest Physicians: Valvular and structural heart disease: American College of Chest Physicians Evidence-Based Clinical Practice Guidelines (8th Edition). Chest 133:593S, 2008.

GUIDELINES ROBERT O. BONOW AND CATHERINE M. OTTO*

Management of Valvular Heart Disease

The American College of Cardiology and the American Heart Association (ACC/AHA) first published guidelines for the management of patients with valvular heart disease in 1998.[1] These were revised in 2006[2] and updated in 2008.[3] Some material from the 2008 guidelines is presented elsewhere in other chapters. In addition to the guidelines tables and figures in Chap. 66, guidelines for the prevention and treatment of infective endocarditis are summarized in the appendix to Chap. 67 and guidelines for the management of anticoagulation in pregnancy are included in the appendix to Chap. 82. Other recommendations for valvular heart diseases are included in the ACC/AHA guidelines for the use of echocardiography,[4] appropriate use criteria for echocardiography from the ACC and other organizations,[5] ACC recommendations for assessment of athletes with cardiovascular abnormalities,[6] and AHA recommendations for cardiovascular assessment of athletes.[7]

The ACC/AHA guidelines emphasize that the clinical assessment should be based on the patient's symptomatic status and findings from the physical examination. Cardiac auscultation remains the most widely used method of screening for valvular heart disease. The chest radiograph and electrocardiogram (ECG), if normal, can often provide reassurance that a murmur is clinically insignificant. Echocardiography should be considered after assessment of these more routine data, and echocardiography is determined to be inappropriate for the evaluation of murmurs that experienced observers consider innocent or functional. In contrast, echocardiography is considered appropriate even in asymptomatic patients with murmurs suggesting significant valvular disease or with other signs or symptoms of cardiovascular disease (**Table 66G-1**), and there is emphasis on the use of Doppler echocardiography to quantify the severity of valvular

stenosis and regurgitation (see Table 66-1). In some cases, cardiac catheterization and angiography are appropriate, as is exercise stress testing.

As with other ACC/AHA guidelines, these use the standard ACC/AHA classification system for indications:

Class I: Conditions for which there is evidence and/or general agreement that the test is useful and effective

Class II: Conditions for which there is conflicting evidence and/or a divergence of opinion about the usefulness or efficacy of performing the test

Class IIa: Weight of evidence or opinion in favor of usefulness or efficacy

Class IIb: Usefulness or efficacy less well established by evidence or opinion

Class III: Conditions for which there is evidence and/or general agreement that the test is not useful or effective and in some cases may be harmful

Three levels are used to rate the evidence on which recommendations have been based. Level A recommendations are derived from data from multiple randomized clinical trials, level B recommendations are derived from a single randomized trial or nonrandomized studies, and level C recommendations are based on the consensus opinion of experts.

AORTIC STENOSIS

The guidelines indicate that Doppler echocardiography is a highly appropriate test for diagnosis and assessment of aortic stenosis (AS) and for evaluation of left ventricular (LV) function in patients with this condition. Yearly echocardiograms are helpful for the management of asymptomatic patients with severe AS, but intervals of 1 to 2 years are recommended for asymptomatic patients with moderate AS and 3 to 5 years for those with

---

*Dr. Thomas H. Lee contributed to this section in previous editions of this book.

TABLE 66G-1   ACC/AHA Guidelines for Echocardiography in Patients with a Cardiac Murmur

CLASS	INDICATION	LOE
I	Asymptomatic patients with diastolic, continuous, holosystolic, and late systolic murmurs, murmurs associated with ejection clicks, or those that radiate to the neck or back	C
	Patients with heart murmurs and symptoms or signs of heart failure, myocardial ischemia or infarction, syncope, thromboembolism, infective endocarditis, or other clinical evidence of structural heart disease	C
	Asymptomatic patients who have grade 3 or louder midpeaking systolic murmurs	C
IIa	Asymptomatic patients with murmurs associated with other abnormal cardiac physical findings or murmurs associated with an abnormal ECG or chest radiograph	C
	Patients whose symptoms and/or signs are likely noncardiac in origin but in whom a cardiac basis cannot be excluded by standard evaluation	C
III	Not recommended for patients with grade 2 or softer midsystolic murmurs identified as innocent or functional by an experienced observer	C

LOE = level of evidence.

TABLE 66G-2   ACC/AHA Guidelines for Management of Patients with Aortic Valve Stenosis

INDICATION	CLASS	RECOMMENDATION	LOE
Echocardiography	I	Diagnosis and assessment of AS severity	B
		Assessment of LV wall thickness, size, and function	B
		Diagnosis and assessment of AS severity	B
		Reevaluating patients with known AS and changing symptoms or signs	B
		Assessment changes in AS severity and LV function in patients with known AS during pregnancy	B
		Serial testing in asymptomatic patients—severe AS, every yr; moderate AS, every 1-2 yr; mild AS: every 3-5 yr	B
Exercise stress testing	IIb	Consider for asymptomatic patients to elicit exercise-induced symptoms and abnormal blood pressure responses	B
	III	Should not be performed in symptomatic patients with AS	B
Cardiac catheterization for hemodynamic assessment	I	Hemodynamic measurements for assessment of AS severity in symptomatic patients when noninvasive tests are inconclusive, or when there is a discrepancy between noninvasive tests and clinical findings regarding severity of AS	C
	III	Not recommended for assessment of AS severity when noninvasive tests are adequate and concordant with clinical findings	C
Coronary angiography	I	Indicated before AVR in patients at risk for CAD	B
		Indicated before AVR when pulmonary autograft (Ross procedure) is contemplated and origin of the coronary arteries is not identified by noninvasive techniques	C
Low-flow, low-gradient aortic stenosis	IIa	Dobutamine infusion during echocardiography or cardiac catheterization for evaluation of low-flow, low-gradient AS and LV dysfunction	B
Aortic valve replacement	I	Symptomatic patients with severe AS	B
		Patients with severe AS undergoing CABG or surgery on the aorta or other heart valves	C
		Patients with severe AS and LV systolic dysfunction (ejection fraction < 0.50)	B
	IIa	Patients with moderate AS undergoing CABG or surgery on the aorta or other heart valves	B
	IIb	Asymptomatic patients with severe AS and abnormal response to exercise	C
		Patients undergoing CABG who have mild AS and evidence that progression may be rapid	C
		Patients with severe asymptomatic AS if there is a high likelihood of rapid progression (age, calcification, and CAD) or if surgery might be delayed at the time of symptom onset	C
		Asymptomatic patients with extremely severe AS (aortic valve area < 0.6 cm^2, mean gradient > 60 mm Hg, and jet velocity > 5 m/sec) if expected operative mortality is ≤1%	C
	III	Not useful for the prevention of sudden death in asymptomatic patients with AS who have none of the findings listed under the Class IIa or IIb recommendations	B
Aortic balloon valvotomy	IIb	Bridge to surgery in hemodynamically unstable patients with AS who are at high risk for AVR	C
		Palliation in patients with AS in whom AVR cannot be performed because of serious comorbid conditions	C
	III	Not recommended as an alternative to AVR in adult patients with AS; certain younger adults without valve calcification may be exception	B

LOE = level of evidence.

mild AS (**Table 66G-2**). For patients with severe AS and low cardiac output (low-flow, low-gradient AS), dobutamine stress echocardiography may be a reasonable tool for evaluation.

Exercise testing of asymptomatic patients can be performed safely and may be a reasonable approach for eliciting symptoms, but it should not be performed in symptomatic patients. An experienced physician should supervise exercise tests for patients with AS and closely monitor blood pressure and the ECG. Physical activity should not be restricted in asymptomatic patients with mild AS. However, the 36th Bethesda Conference on Eligibility Recommendations for Competitive Athletes With Cardiovascular Abnormalities has recommended that patients with mild to moderate AS avoid competitive sports with high dynamic and static muscular demands.[6]

Cardiac Catheterization

The ACC/AHA guidelines indicate that coronary angiography is appropriate in patients with possible coronary artery disease (CAD), and catheterization may be necessary to assess the hemodynamic severity of AS in symptomatic patients when other data are not conclusive (see Table 66G-2). Catheterization is discouraged solely for the purposes of confirming information available from noninvasive tests or assessing LV function and severity of AS in asymptomatic patients. Cardiac catheterization with infusion of dobutamine may be useful for hemodynamic evaluation in patients with low-flow, low-gradient AS and LV dysfunction.

Aortic Valve Replacement

Surgery is recommended for almost all symptomatic patients with severe AS, and the ACC/AHA guidelines are generally supportive (Class IIa) of aortic valve replacement (AVR) for patients with moderate disease who are undergoing coronary artery bypass grafting (CABG) or surgery on the aorta or other heart valves. The guidelines are less supportive of AVR in patients who are asymptomatic despite severe AS (see Table 66G-2), although subgroups with a high likelihood of progressive disease are identified in whom this might be considered. Aortic balloon valvotomy was given qualified support as a bridge to surgery for hemodynamically unstable patients who cannot undergo immediate aortic valve replacement or

as palliation for those who cannot undergo valve replacement. It is not recommended as an alternative to AVR except in the case of some younger patients with congenital AS without valve calcification.

AORTIC REGURGITATION

Doppler echocardiography is a highly appropriate test for the diagnosis and serial assessment of patients with aortic regurgitation (AR; **Table 66G-3**). Serial echocardiography is indicated to evaluate LV size and function periodically in asymptomatic patients with severe AR and to reevaluate AR in patients with new or changing symptoms to ensure that rapid progression is not underway. Asymptomatic patients with mild AR, normal LV function, and little or no LV dilation can be seen on an annual basis, and echocardiography can be performed every 2 to 3 years in the absence of changes in symptoms. However, the guidelines support echocardiography every 6 to 12 months for patients with severe AR and significant LV dilation, such as end-diastolic dimension more than 60 mm. For patients with even more advanced LV dilation, echocardiography as often as every 3 months is endorsed.

TABLE 66G-3	ACC/AHA Guidelines for Management of Patients with Aortic Regurgitation		
INDICATION	**CLASS**	**RECOMMENDATION**	**LOE**
Echocardiography	I	Confirm presence and severity of acute or chronic AR.	B
		Assess cause of chronic AR (including valve morphology and aortic root size and morphology) and LV hypertrophy, LV dimension (or volume), and LV systolic function.	B
		Assess AR severity and severity of aortic dilation in patients with enlarged aortic root.	B
		Periodically reevaluate LV size and function in asymptomatic patients with severe AR.	B
		Reevaluate mild, moderate, or severe AR in patients with new or changing symptoms.	B
Exercise stress testing	IIa	Assess functional capacity and symptomatic response in patients with a history of equivocal symptoms.	B
		Evaluate symptoms and functional capacity before participation in athletic activities.	C
	IIb	Perform exercise testing with radionuclide angiography for assessment of LV function in asymptomatic or symptomatic patients with chronic AR.	B
Radionuclide imaging or CMR	I	Radionuclide angiography or CMR is indicated for the initial and serial assessment of LV volume and function at rest in patients with AR and suboptimal echocardiograms.	B
	IIa	Perform CMR for estimation of AR severity in patients with unsatisfactory echocardiograms	B
Vasodilator therapy	I	Chronic therapy in patients with severe AR who have symptoms or LV dysfunction when AVR is not recommended because of additional cardiac or noncardiac factors	B
	IIa	Short-term therapy to improve the hemodynamic profile of patients with severe heart failure symptoms and severe LV dysfunction before proceeding with AVR	C
	IIb	Long-term therapy for asymptomatic patients with severe AR and LV dilation but normal systolic function	B
	III	Not indicated for long-term therapy in asymptomatic, mild to moderate AR and normal LV systolic function	B
		Not indicated for long-term therapy in asymptomatic patients with LV systolic dysfunction who are otherwise candidates for AVR	C
		Not indicated for long-term therapy in symptomatic patients with either normal LV function or mild to moderate LV systolic dysfunction who are otherwise candidates for AVR	C
Cardiac catheterization for hemodynamic assessment and aortic root angiography	I	Assessment of AR severity, LV function, or aortic root size when noninvasive tests are inconclusive or discordant with clinical findings	B
	III	Not indicated for assessment of LV function, aortic root size, or AR severity before AVR when noninvasive tests are adequate and concordant with clinical findings	C
		Not indicated for assessment of LV function and severity of regurgitation in asymptomatic patients when noninvasive tests are adequate	C
Coronary angiography	I	Indicated before AVR in patients at risk for CAD	C
AVR or aortic valve repair	I	Symptomatic patients with severe AR irrespective of LV systolic function	B
		Asymptomatic patients with severe AR and LV systolic dysfunction (EF ≤ 0.50) at rest	B
		Patients with chronic severe AR undergoing CABG or surgery on the aorta or other heart valves	C
	IIa	Asymptomatic patients with severe AR and normal LV systolic function (EF > 0.50) but with severe LV dilation (EDD > 75 mm or ESD > 55 mm)*	B
	IIb	Patients with moderate AR while undergoing CABG or surgery on the ascending aorta	C
		Asymptomatic patients with severe AR and normal LV systolic function at rest (EF > 0.50) with LVEDD > 70 mm or LVESD >50 mm,* when there is evidence of progressive LV dilation, declining exercise tolerance, or abnormal hemodynamic response to exercise	C
	III	Not indicated for asymptomatic patients with mild, moderate, or severe AR and normal LV systolic function at rest (EF > 0.50) when LV dilation is not moderate or severe (EDD < 70 mm; ESD < 50 mm)*	B

*Consider lower thresholds for patients of small stature, regardless of gender.
EDD = end-diastolic dimension; EF = ejection fraction; ESD = end-systolic dimension; LOE = level of evidence.

Exercise testing is considered appropriate for the assessment of functional capacity in patients in whom the history is not definitive, but the impact of this test on management is not otherwise strongly supported. Cardiac magnetic resonance (CMR) is reasonable for estimating the severity of AR and LV volume and function in patients with equivocal echocardiograms. Radionuclide angiography is less positively endorsed as an alternative to echocardiography for the assessment of LV volume and function.

Medical Therapy

The ACC/AHA guidelines consider vasodilator therapy appropriate for patients with hypertension, with weak endorsement for those with severe AR, normal LV function, and evidence of LV dilation. However, there is no endorsement for long-term vasodilator therapy in normotensive patients with normal LV function and mild AR. Vasodilator therapy is not an alternative to surgery for patients who are appropriate candidates for valve replacement, including those with asymptomatic LV dysfunction.

Cardiac Catheterization

Cardiac catheterization is not routinely needed to confirm the diagnosis or assess the severity of AR when echocardiographic studies are adequate. The most common appropriate indication for cardiac catheterization is coronary angiography as a prelude to surgery.

Aortic Valve Replacement

The ACC/AHA guidelines deem AVR to be clearly appropriate for patients with symptoms (New York Heart Association [NYHA] Class II, III or IV), progressive LV dilation, mild to moderate LV systolic dysfunction, or declining exercise tolerance (see Table 66G-3). The guidelines were not supportive of surgery solely because of a decline in ejection fraction during exercise. Following AVR, close follow-up is necessary to evaluate both the function of the new valve and LV function. This usually includes an echocardiogram soon after surgery to be used as a baseline. Patients should be followed clinically at 6 months, 12, months, and then annually if the clinical course is uncomplicated. Serial postoperative echocardiograms after the initial early postoperative study are usually not indicated if the clinical course is uncomplicated. Patients with persistent LV dilation on the initial postoperative echocardiogram should be treated as any other patient with symptomatic or asymptomatic LV dysfunction, including treatment with angiotensin-converting enzyme (ACE) inhibitors and beta-adrenergic blocking agents.

BICUSPID AORTIC VALVE WITH DILATED ASCENDING AORTA

Transthoracic echocardiography should be used initially to evaluate patients with known bicuspid aortic valves (**Table 66G-4**). CMR or computed tomography (CT) should be used when echocardiography cannot adequately assess the aortic root or ascending aorta or to quantify the severity of dilation and involvement of the ascending aorta further. Surgical repair or replacement is indicated if the diameter of the aortic root or ascending aorta is more than 5 cm (or smaller in patients of small stature) or if the rate of increase in diameter is 0.5 cm/year or more.

MITRAL STENOSIS

Transthoracic echocardiography is endorsed in the ACC/AHA guidelines as the first-line test for the diagnosis and follow-up of patients with mitral stenosis (MS). Transesophageal echocardiography has a role for the detection of left atrial thrombus in patients being considered for percutaneous mitral balloon valvotomy or cardioversion (**Table 66G-5**) but not for routine evaluation of mitral valve morphology or hemodynamics, unless transthoracic echocardiography has been unsuccessful.

Medical Management

Patients with more than mild MS should be counseled to avoid unusual physical stresses. Anticoagulation is recommended for patients with MS if they have a history of atrial fibrillation, prior embolic event, or left atrial thrombus. The guidelines are not strongly supportive of anticoagulation on the basis of left atrial size alone.

Cardiac Catheterization

The guidelines support the use of cardiac catheterization for hemodynamic evaluation when noninvasive tests are not conclusive or yield discrepant results.

Percutaneous Mitral Balloon Valvotomy

In centers with skilled operators, the guidelines indicate that percutaneous mitral balloon valvotomy is the initial procedure of choice for symptomatic patients (NYHA functional Classes II to IV) with moderate or severe MS and favorable valve morphology, and for asymptomatic patients with pulmonary hypertension (see Table 66G-5). It is not indicated for patients with mild MS, left atrial thrombus, or moderate to severe mitral regurgitation (MR).

Surgical Options

When possible, mitral valve repair is indicated for patients with symptomatic (NYHA functional Classes II to IV) moderate or severe mitral valve stenosis when percutaneous mitral valve balloon valvotomy is not possible. Mitral valve repair may be considered for asymptomatic patients who experience recurrent embolic events despite adequate anticoagulation. Mitral valve replacement is an option when repair is not feasible.

MITRAL VALVE PROLAPSE

The diagnosis of mitral valve prolapse (MVP) should be made by physical examination; two-dimensional and Doppler echocardiography should be used primarily for evaluation of MR and ventricular compensation, as well as for excluding the diagnosis of MVP in patients who have been given the diagnosis inappropriately (**Table 66G-6**). Serial use of echocardiography in stable patients with mild or no regurgitation is discouraged.

Management

Reassurance is an important element of the management of patients with MVP. A normal lifestyle and regular exercise are encouraged, especially in patients with mild or no symptoms and mild MVP.

CH
66

VALVULAR HEART DISEASE

TABLE 66G-4 ACC/AHA Guidelines for Management of Patients with Bicuspid Aortic Valves and Dilated Ascending Aortas

INDICATION	CLASS	RECOMMENDATION	LOE
Echocardiography, CMR and cardiac CT	I	Initial transthoracic echo to assess the diameters of the aortic root and ascending aorta	B
		CMR or CT when morphology of the aortic root or ascending aorta cannot be assessed accurately by echo	C
		Serial evaluation of aortic root, ascending aorta size and morphology by echo, CMR, or cardiac CT annually when dilation of the aortic root or ascending aorta > 4 cm*	C
	IIa	CMR or cardiac CT in patients with bicuspid aortic valves when aortic root dilation is detected by echo to quantify severity of dilation and involvement of the ascending aorta further	B
Medical therapy	IIa	Beta-adrenergic blocking agents for patients with bicuspid valves and dilated aortic roots (diameter > 4 cm*) who are not candidates for surgical correction and who do not have moderate to severe AR	C
Surgery	I	Surgery to repair the aortic root or replace the ascending aorta indicated for patients with bicuspid aortic valves if the diameter of the aortic root or ascending aorta >5 cm* or rate of increase in diameter ≥ 0.5 cm/yr	C
		Repair of aortic root or replacement of ascending aorta if the diameter of the aortic root or ascending aorta > 4.5 cm* in patients with bicuspid valves undergoing AVR or repair because of severe AS or AR	C

*Consider lower thresholds for patients of small stature, regardless of gender .
Echo = echocardiography.

TABLE 66G-5 ACC/AHA Guidelines for Management of Patients with Mitral Stenosis

INDICATION	CLASS	RECOMMENDATION	LOE
Echocardiography	I	Diagnosis of MS, assessment of hemodynamic severity, assessment of concomitant valvular lesions, assessment of valve morphology (to determine suitability for PMBV)	B
		Reevaluation in patients with known MS and changing symptoms or signs	B
		Assess hemodynamic response of the mean gradient and PA pressure by exercise Doppler echo when there is a discrepancy among resting Doppler echo findings, clinical findings, symptoms, and signs.	C
		Transesophageal echo to assess presence or absence of left atrial thrombus and evaluate the severity of MR further in patients considered for PMBV	C
		Transesophageal echo to evaluate MV morphology and hemodynamics when transthoracic echo provides suboptimal data	C
	IIa	Reevaluation of asymptomatic patients with MS and stable clinical findings to assess PA pressure—severe MS, every yr; moderate MS, every 1-2 yr; mild MS, every 3-5 yr	C
	III	Transesophageal echo not indicated for routine evaluation of MV morphology and hemodynamics when complete transthoracic echo data are satisfactory	C
Anticoagulation therapy	I	Patients with MS and atrial fibrillation (paroxysmal, persistent, or permanent)	B
		Patients with MS and prior embolic event, even in sinus rhythm	B
		Patients with MS with left atrial thrombus	B
	IIb	Asymptomatic patients with severe MS and left atrial dimension ≥ 55 mm by echo	B
		Patients with severe MS, enlarged left atrium, and spontaneous contrast on echo	C
Cardiac catheterization for hemodynamic assessment	I	Assess severity of MS when noninvasive tests are inconclusive or when there is discrepancy between noninvasive tests and clinical findings.	C
		Hemodynamic evaluation (including left ventriculography to evaluate severity of MR) when there is a discrepancy between Doppler-derived mean gradient and valve area	C
	IIa	Assess PA and left atrial pressures during exercise when clinical symptoms and resting hemodynamics are discordant.	C
		Assess the cause of severe PA hypertension when out of proportion to severity of MS as determined by noninvasive testing.	C
	III	Not recommended when two-dimensional and Doppler echo data are concordant with clinical findings	C
PMBV	I	Indicated for symptomatic patients with moderate or severe MS and valve morphology favorable for PMBV in the absence of left atrial thrombus or moderate to severe MR	A
	IIa	Patients with moderate or severe MS who have a nonpliable calcified valve, are in NYHA functional Class III or IV, and are not candidates for surgery or are at high risk for surgery	C
	IIb	Asymptomatic patients with moderate or severe MS and valve morphology favorable for PMBV who have new-onset of atrial fibrillation in the absence of left atrial thrombus or moderate to severe MR	C
		Symptomatic patients with MV area >1.5 cm² if there is evidence of significant MS based on exercise PA systolic pressure > 60 mm Hg, exercise PA wedge pressure ≥ 25 mm Hg, or exercise mean MV gradient >15 mm Hg	C
		Alternative to surgery for patients with moderate or severe MS who have a nonpliable calcified valve and are in NYHA functional Class III or IV	C
	III	Not indicated for patients with mild MS	C
		Not indicated for patients with moderate to severe MR or left atrial thrombus	C
Surgery (repair if possible)	I	Indicated for symptomatic (NYHA functional Class III or IV) moderate or severe MS when PMBV is unavailable or contraindicated because of left atrial thrombus, despite anticoagulation or because concomitant moderate to severe MR is present	B
		Indicated for symptomatic (NYHA functional Class III or IV) moderate or severe MS when valve morphology is not favorable for PMBV in patients with acceptable operative risk	B
		Indicated for moderate to severe MS when there is moderate to severe MR	C
	IIa	MV replacement for severe MS and severe PA hypertension (PA systolic pressure > 60 mm Hg) with NYHA functional Class I or II symptoms in patients who are not candidates for PMBV or surgical MV repair	C
	IIb	MV replacement for symptomatic patients with moderate or severe MS who have had recurrent embolic events while receiving adequate anticoagulation and who have valve morphology favorable for repair	C
	III	Not indicated for patients with mild MS	C
		Closed commissurotomy should not be performed in patients undergoing MV repair; open commissurotomy is preferred approach	C

Echo = echocardiography; LOE = level of evidence; MV = mitral valve; PA = pulmonary artery; PMBV = percutaneous mitral balloon valvotomy.

In general, asymptomatic athletes with MVP need not have any restrictions, but recommendations from the ACC[6] and AHA[7] include restriction of patients to low-intensity competitive sports (e.g., golf and bowling) if any of the following are present: (1) history of syncope, judged probably arrhythmogenic in origin; (2) family history of sudden death caused by MVP; (3) repetitive supraventricular or complex ventricular tachyarrhythmias, particularly if exacerbated by exercise; (4) moderate to severe MR; and (5) prior embolic event.

Daily low-dose aspirin therapy is recommended for patients with MVP who have experienced transient ischemic attacks, as well as younger patients with atrial fibrillation but without MR, hypertension, or heart failure. Anticoagulation with warfarin is recommended for poststroke patients with MVP who have MR, atrial fibrillation, or left atrial thrombus. Warfarin is also recommended for poststroke patients with echocardiographic evidence of thickening or redundancy of the valve leaflets and those who experience recurrent transient ischemic attacks while taking aspirin.

Antibiotic prophylaxis is not considered appropriate for patients with the characteristic click-murmur complex or with echocardiographic evidence of MVP with MR (see summary of revised recommendations in Chap. 67 Guidelines).

TABLE 62G-6   ACC/AHA Guidelines for Management of Patients with Mitral Valve Prolapse

INDICATION	CLASS	RECOMMENDATION	LOE
Echocardiography	I	Diagnosis of MVP and assessment of MR, leaflet morphology, and LV compensation in asymptomatic patients with physical signs of MVP	B
	IIa	Exclude MVP in asymptomatic patients who have been diagnosed without clinical evidence to support the diagnosis.	C
		Risk stratification in asymptomatic patients with physical signs of MVP or known MVP	C
	III	Not indicated to exclude MVP in asymptomatic patients with ill-defined symptoms in the absence of a constellation of clinical symptoms or physical findings suggestive of MVP or a positive family history	B
		Not indicated for asymptomatic patients with MVP and no MR or with MVP and mild MR with no changes in clinical signs or symptoms	C
Antithrombotic therapy	I	Aspirin (75-325 mg/day) for patients with MVP who experience cerebral transient ischemic attacks	C
		Warfarin for patients with MVP and AF who are >65 yr or who have hypertension, MR murmur, or history of heart failure	C
		Aspirin (75-325 mg/day) for patients with MVP and AF < 65 yr and with no history of MR, hypertension, or heart failure	C
		Warfarin for patients with MVP and history of stroke who have MR, AF, or left atrial thrombus	C
	IIa	Warfarin for patients with MVP and history of stroke who do not have MR, AF, or left atrial thrombus when there is echo evidence of thickening (≥5 mm) and/or redundancy of the valve leaflets	C
		Aspirin (75-325 mg/day) for patients with MVP and history of stroke who do not have MR, AF, left atrial thrombus, or echo evidence of thickening (≥5 mm) or redundancy of the valve leaflets	C
	IIb	Aspirin (75-325 mg/day) for patients in sinus rhythm with echo evidence of high-risk MVP	C

AF = atrial fibrillation; echo = echocardiography; LOE= level of evidence.

MITRAL REGURGITATION

The ACC/AHA guidelines consider transthoracic echocardiography to be appropriate for the diagnosis of acute or chronic MR, as well as for annual or semiannual surveillance of LV function in patients with severe MR, even if asymptomatic (**Table 66G-7**). Serial use of chest radiographs and ECGs are considered to be of less value. In asymptomatic patients with mild MR and no evidence of LV dysfunction, the guidelines recommend annual evaluations to detect worsening symptomatic status but do not support annual echocardiography. Transesophageal echocardiography is considered most appropriate for intraoperative guidance and when transthoracic studies are inadequate.

Cardiac Catheterization

Catheterization is usually performed as a prelude to surgery in patients with MR, or when noninvasive tests yield discordant results or do not provide adequate information to guide management. The ACC/AHA guidelines do not consider catheterization routinely necessary in patients with MR when valve surgery is not planned.

Surgery

The guidelines consider mitral valve repair to be the operation of choice for patients with suitable valves when performed by an experienced operator. Surgery is deemed appropriate for acute symptomatic MR and for patients with chronic severe MR and symptoms of congestive heart failure, even if they have normal LV function (see Table 66G-7). Among asymptomatic patients, surgery is appropriate when there is evidence of mild or greater LV dysfunction (ejection fraction = 0.30 to 0.60 and/or end-systolic dimension >40 mm).

The 2006 and 2008 guidelines contained two important new recommendations regarding mitral valve repair. The first applies to asymptomatic patients with severe MR and normal LV function. The guidelines indicate that it is reasonable to consider mitral valve repair in such patients if they undergo surgery in experienced surgical centers in which the likelihood of successful repair without residual regurgitation is greater than 90% (Class IIa). A stronger recommendation (class I) indicates that mitral valve repair is recommended over mitral valve replacement for most patients who undergo surgery, and patients should be referred to surgical centers experienced in mitral valve repair.

OTHER VALVULAR DISEASE

Multiple Valve Disease

Given the large number of possible combinations and the slim evidence base for diagnosis and management, the ACC/AHA guidelines offer no specific recommendations for the management of mixed valve disease.

Tricuspid Valve Disease

Tricuspid valve repair is appropriate for correcting severe tricuspid regurgitation (TR) in patients with mitral valve disease requiring valve repair or replacement (**Table 66G-8**). Tricuspid valve replacement or annuloplasty is considered reasonable for patients with symptomatic severe primary TR. Annuloplasty may be considered for patients with mild to moderate TR who are undergoing surgery for mitral valve disease if they have pulmonary hypertension or dilation of the tricuspid annulus.

SURGICAL CONSIDERATIONS

Numerous options are available for the surgical management of valvular heart disease. The ACC/AHA guidelines generally favor mitral valve repair over replacement. The standard surgical approach usually entails a median sternotomy with cardiopulmonary bypass. However, numerous alternatives are gaining acceptance. These include minimally invasive approaches to valve repair such as ministernotomy, small right thoracotomy, or robotic surgery. Percutaneous approaches to mitral valve repair, pulmonary valve implantation, and aortic valve replacement have been conducted, with generally successful results,[8-10] and percutaneous devices are now approved for clinical use in Europe. Whether such catheter-based approaches gain widespread acceptance will depend on larger and longer-term clinical trial results and advances in device technology.

When replacement is necessary, several variables influence the selection of a bioprosthetic versus a mechanical valve (**Table 66G-9**). Patient preference plays an important role in determining the choice of a prosthetic valve. In the 1998 guidelines, bioprosthetic valves were considered appropriate only for patients older than 65 years for AVR and older than 70 years for mitral valve replacement. The 2006 and 2008 guidelines emphasize that a bioprosthesis is reasonable for patients younger than 65 years who elect to receive this valve for lifestyle considerations after detailed discussion of the risks of anticoagulation versus the likelihood that a second valve replacement may be necessary in the future.

The 1998 guidelines also considered bioprosthetic valves inappropriate for patients with end-stage renal failure, especially those undergoing chronic dialysis, because of concerns of accelerated calcification of bioprosthetic valves. Subsequent clinical studies have not demonstrated a difference in outcomes between mechanical and bioprosthetic valves in these patients, and this recommendation was removed in 2006.

Intraoperative Assessment

The ACC/AHA guidelines emphasize the importance of intraoperative transesophageal echocardiography by recommending its use during valve repair; valve replacement with a stentless xenograft, homograft, or autograft valve; or valve surgery for infective endocarditis. It may

TABLE 66G-7 ACC/AHA Guidelines for Management of Patients with Mitral Regurgitation

INDICATION	CLASS	RECOMMENDATION	LOE
Transthoracic echocardiography	I	Baseline evaluation of LV size and function, RV and LA size, PA pressure, and severity of MR in any patient suspected of having MR	C
		Delineation of the mechanism of MR	B
		Annual or semiannual surveillance of LV function (estimated by EF and ESD) in asymptomatic patients with moderate to severe MR	C
		Evaluate the MV apparatus and LV function after a change in signs or symptoms	C
		Initial evaluation of LV size and function and MV hemodynamics after MV replacement or repair	C
	IIa	Exercise Doppler echo in asymptomatic severe MR to assess exercise tolerance and effects of exercise on PA pressure and MR severity	C
	III	Not indicated for routine follow-up of asymptomatic mild MR with normal LV size and systolic function	C
Transesophageal echocardiography	I	Indicated when transthoracic echo provides nondiagnostic information regarding severity of MR, mechanism of MR, and/or status of LV function	B
		Preoperative or intraoperative assessment of the anatomic basis for severe MR to assess feasibility of repair and guide repair when surgery is recommended	B
	IIa	Preoperative assessment in asymptomatic patients with severe MR who are considered for surgery to assess feasibility of repair	C
	III	Not indicated for routine follow-up or surveillance of asymptomatic native valve MR	C
Cardiac catheterization for hemodynamic assessment and left ventriculography	I	Indicated when noninvasive tests are inconclusive regarding severity of MR, LV function, or need for surgery	C
		Indicated when PA pressure is out of proportion to the severity of MR as assessed by noninvasive testing	C
		Indicated when there is a discrepancy between clinical and noninvasive findings regarding severity of MR	C
	III	Not indicated in patients with MR in whom valve surgery is not contemplated	C
Coronary angiography	I	Indicated before MV repair or MV replacement in patients at risk for CAD	C
Surgery	I	Symptomatic patients with acute severe MR	B
		Patients with chronic severe MR and NYHA functional Class II, III, or IV symptoms in the absence of severe LV dysfunction (defined as EF < 0.30 and/or ESD > 55 mm)	B
		Asymptomatic patients with chronic severe MR and mild to moderate LV dysfunction, EF = 0.30 to 0.60, and/or ESD ≥ 40 mm	B
		MV repair recommended over MV replacement for most patients with severe chronic MR who require surgery; patients should be referred to surgical centers experienced in MV repair	C
	IIa	MV repair in experienced surgical centers for asymptomatic patients with chronic severe MR with preserved LV function (EF > 0.60 and ESD < 40 mm) in whom the likelihood of successful repair without residual MR is >90%	B
		Asymptomatic patients with chronic severe MR, preserved LV function, and new onset of atrial fibrillation or pulmonary hypertension (PA systolic pressure > 50 mm Hg at rest or > 60 mm Hg with exercise)	C
		Patients with chronic severe MR caused by primary abnormality of the mitral apparatus, NYHA functional Class III or IV symptoms, and severe LV dysfunction (EF < 0.30 and/or ESD > 55 mm) in whom MV repair is highly likely	C
	IIb	Patients with chronic severe secondary MR caused by severe LV dysfunction (EF < 0.30) who have persistent NYHA functional Class III or IV symptoms despite optimal therapy for heart failure, including biventricular pacing	C
	III	Not indicated for asymptomatic patients with MR and preserved LV function (EF > 0.60 and ESD < 40 mm) if there is significant doubt about the feasibility of repair	C
		Not indicated for patients with mild or moderate MR	C

Echo = echocardiography; EF = ejection fraction; ESD = end-systolic dimension; LA = left atrial; LOE = level of evidence; PA = pulmonary artery; RV = right ventricular.

TABLE 66G-8 ACC/AHA Guidelines for Management of Patients with Tricuspid Valve Disease

INDICATION	CLASS	RECOMMENDATION	LOE
Surgery	I	Severe TR in patients with MV disease requiring MV surgery	B
	IIa	Severe primary TR when symptomatic	C
		Tricuspid valve replacement for severe TR secondary to diseased or abnormal tricuspid valve leaflets not amenable to annuloplasty or repair	C
	IIb	Patients undergoing MV surgery when TR is not severe but there is pulmonary hypertension or tricuspid annular dilatation	C
	III	Not indicated in asymptomatic TR when PA systolic pressure < 60 mm Hg and MV is normal	C
		Not indicated in patients with mild primary TR	C

LOE= level of evidence.

also be reasonable for all patients undergoing cardiac valve surgery. The guidelines committee recommends that centers performing valve surgery establish consistent and credible intraoperative echocardiography programs capable of providing accurate anatomic and functional information relevant to valve operations. Given that even a generally safe procedure such as transesophageal echocardiography has risks, preoperative screening for risk factors and obtaining informed consent should be a routine part of each intraoperative transesophageal study.

Patients with Prosthetic Heart Valves

The ACC/AHA guidelines recommend warfarin therapy for patients with mechanical valves. For patients with aortic valve prostheses, those with bileaflet mechanical valves and Medtronic-Hall valves should maintain an international normalized ratio (INR) between 2 and 3, whereas those with Starr-Edwards valves or mechanical disc valves should maintain an INR between 2.5 and 3.5 (**Table 66G-10**). The same target is indicated following mitral valve replacement with a mechanical valve. Aspirin (75 to

TABLE 66G-9 ACC/AHA Major Criteria for the Selection of Replacement Valves for Individuals with Valvular Heart Disease

INDICATION	CLASS	RECOMMENDATION	LOE
Aortic valve replacement	I	Mechanical prosthesis in patients with a mechanical valve in the mitral or tricuspid position	C
		Bioprosthesis in patients of any age who will not take warfarin or who have major medical contraindications to warfarin therapy.	C
	IIa	Patient preference is a reasonable consideration in the selection of valve prosthesis. Mechanical prosthesis is reasonable for AVR in patients < 65 yr who do not have a contraindication to anticoagulation. A bioprosthesis is reasonable for AVR in patients < 65 yr who elect to receive this valve for lifestyle considerations after detailed discussions of the risks of anticoagulation versus the likelihood that a second AVR may be necessary in the future.	C
		Bioprosthesis is reasonable for patients ≥ 65 yr without risk factors for thromboembolism.	C
		Homograft is reasonable for patients undergoing repeat AVR with active prosthetic valve endocarditis.	
	IIb	Bioprosthesis might be considered for a woman of childbearing age.	C
Mitral valve replacement	I	Bioprosthesis in patients who will not take warfarin, is incapable of taking warfarin, or has a clear contraindication to warfarin therapy.	C
	IIa	Mechanical prosthesis reasonable for patients younger than 65 years of age with longstanding AF	C
		Bioprosthesis is reasonable in patients ≥ 65 yr	C
		Bioprosthesis is reasonable in patients < 65 yr in sinus rhythm who elect to receive this valve for life-style considerations after detailed discussions of the risks of anticoagulation versus the likelihood that a second MV replacement may be necessary in the future.	C

ACC/AHA = American College of Cardiology/American Heart Association; AF = atrial fibrillation; AVR = aortic valve replacement; LOE = level of evidence; MV = mitral valve.

TABLE 66G-10 Recommendations for Antithrombotic Therapy in Patients with Prosthetic Heart Valves*

PROSTHESIS	LOCATION	RISK*		ASPIRIN (75-100 mg)	WARFARIN (INR, 2-3)	WARFARIN (INR, 2.5-3.5)	NO WARFARIN
Mechanical prosthetic valves	AVR	Low	<3 mo	Class I	Class I	Class IIa	
			>3 mo	Class I	Class I		
		High		Class I		Class I	
	MVR			Class I		Class I	
Bioprosthetic valves	AVR	Low	<3 mo	Class I	Class IIa		Class IIb
			>3 mo	Class I			Class IIa
		High		Class I	Class I		
	MVR	Low	<3 mo	Class I	Class IIa		
			>3 mo	Class I			Class IIa
		High		Class I	Class I		

*Antithrombotic therapy must be individualized depending on a patient's clinical status. For patients receiving warfarin, aspirin is recommended in almost all situations. Risk factors include atrial fibrillation, left ventricular dysfunction, previous thromboembolism, and hypercoagulable condition. INR should be maintained between 2.5 and 3.5 for aortic disc valves and Starr-Edwards valves.

AVR = aortic valve replacement; INR = international normalized ratio; MVR = mitral valve replacement.

325 mg/day) is indicated for patients who are unable to take warfarin. Low-dose aspirin (75 to 100 mg/day) is recommended in addition to warfarin for all patients with mechanical heart valves and those with biologic valves who have risk factors such as atrial fibrillation, prior thromboembolism, LV dysfunction, or a hypercoagulable condition. Clopidogrel may be considered for those who cannot take aspirin.

Bridging Therapy
Antithrombotic medications must sometimes be interrupted in patients with mechanical valve prostheses for noncardiac surgery, invasive procedures, or dental care. In patients at low risk of thrombosis, warfarin should be stopped 48 to 72 hours before the procedure and started no more than 24 hours after the procedure (**Table 66G-11**). The ACC/AHA guidelines indicate that the use of heparin is usually unnecessary for patients at low risk of thrombosis, defined as those with a bileaflet mechanical aortic valve prosthesis with no risk factors. They recommend bridging anticoagulant therapy for higher risk individuals, including those with a mechanical mitral or tricuspid prosthesis or a mechanical aortic prosthesis who have risk factors such as atrial fibrillation, a recent thrombosis or embolus, LV dysfunction, or an older generation thrombogenic valve, and those with demonstrated thrombotic problems when previously off therapy. The recommended bridging therapy is intravenous unfractionated heparin (Class I), but subcutaneous doses of unfractionated heparin or low-molecular-weight heparin may also be considered (Class IIb). The use of low-molecular-weight heparin remains controversial for this indication.

Prosthetic Valve Thrombosis
Emergency surgery is reasonable for patients with a thrombosed left-sided prosthetic valve and moderate to severe symptoms (NYHA Class III or IV) or a large clot burden. Fibrinolytic therapy may be considered for patients with less severe symptoms, smaller clot burdens, or when surgery is high risk or unavailable (**Table 66G-12**).

Follow-up
After prosthetic valve implantation, asymptomatic patients should be seen 2 to 4 weeks after hospital discharge and then at 6-month or 1-year intervals (**Table 66G-13**). Routine annual echocardiography is not indicated in the absence of changes in clinical status. All patients should also receive primary and secondary prevention measures to reduce the risk of future cardiovascular events.

Patients who do not improve after receiving a prosthetic heart valve or who later show deterioration of functional capacity should undergo appropriate testing to determine the cause. Patients with postoperative LV systolic dysfunction, even if it is asymptomatic, should receive standard medical therapy for systolic heart failure indefinitely, even if systolic function or symptoms improve.

EVALUATION AND MANAGEMENT OF CORONARY ARTERY DISEASE IN PATIENTS WITH VALVULAR HEART DISEASE
Concomitant CAD is common in patients with valvular disease. Because of the impact of untreated CAD on perioperative and long-term

TABLE 66G-11 ACC/AHA Recommendations for Bridging Therapy in Patients with Mechanical Valves*

INDICATION	CLASS	RECOMMENDATION	LOE
Planned noncardiac invasive procedure	I	In patients at low risk of thrombosis,† warfarin should be stopped 48 to 72 hr before the procedure (so that the INR falls to <.5) and restarted within 24 hr after the procedure. Heparin is usually unnecessary.	B
	I	In patients at high risk of thrombosis,‡ start therapeutic doses of IV UFH when INR falls below 2 (typically 48 hr before surgery), stop 4 to 6 hr before the procedure, restart as early after surgery as bleeding stability allows, and continue until INR is again therapeutic with warfarin therapy.	B
	IIb	In patients at high risk of thrombosis,‡ therapeutic doses of subcutaneous UFH (15,000 U/12 hr) or LMWH (100 U/kg/12 hr) may be considered during the period of a subtherapeutic INR.	B
	III	High-dose vitamin K_1 should not be given routinely because this could create a hypercoagulable condition.	B
Emergency noncardiac surgery	IIa	Reasonable to give fresh-frozen plasma to patients with mechanical valves who require emergency interruption of warfarin therapy. Fresh frozen plasma is preferable to high-dose vitamin K_1.	B

*Who require interruption of warfarin therapy for noncardiac surgery, invasive procedures, or dental care.
†Low risk of thrombosis—bileaflet mechanical AVR with no risk factors (see below).
‡High risk of thrombosis—any mechanical MV replacement or mechanical AVR with any risk factor. Risk factors include atrial fibrillation, previous thromboembolism, LV dysfunction, hypercoagulable conditions, older generation thrombogenic valves, mechanical tricuspid valves, or more than one mechanical valve.
INR = international normalized ratio; IV = intravenous; LMWH = low-molecular-weight heparin; LOE = level of evidence; MV = mitral valve; UFH = unfractionated heparin.

TABLE 66G-12 ACC/AHA Guidelines for Management of Prosthetic Heart Valve Thrombosis

INDICATION	CLASS	RECOMMENDATION	LOE
Echocardiography	I	Indicated in patients with suspected prosthetic valve thrombosis to assess hemodynamic severity	B
	I	Transesophageal echo and/or fluoroscopy in patients with suspected valve thrombosis to assess valve motion and clot burden	B
Emergency operation	IIa	Reasonable for patients with thrombosed left-sided prosthetic valves and NYHA Class III or IV symptoms	C
	IIa	Reasonable for patients with thrombosed left-sided prosthetic valves and a large clot burden	C
Fibrinolytic therapy	IIa	Reasonable for patients with thrombosed right-sided prosthetic valves with NYHA Class III or IV symptoms or large clot burden	C
	IIb	May be considered as first-line therapy for patients with thrombosed left-sided prosthetic valves, NYHA Class I or II symptoms, and small clot burden	B
	IIb	May be considered as first-line therapy for patients with thrombosed left-sided prosthetic valves, NYHA Class III or IV symptoms, and a small clot burden if surgery is high risk or not available	B
	IIb	May be considered for patients with obstructed, thrombosed left-sided prosthetic valves, NYHA Class II or IV symptoms, and large clot burden if emergency surgery is high risk or not available	C
	IIb	May consider intravenous UFH as an alternative to fibrinolytic therapy for patients with thrombosed prosthetic valves, NYHA functional Class I or II, and small clot burden	C

Echo = echocardiography; LOE = level of evidence; UFH = unfractionated heparin.

TABLE 66G-13 ACC/AHA Guidelines for Patient Follow-up after Prosthetic Valve Implantation

INDICATION	CLASS	RECOMMENDATION	LOE
General patient follow-up	I	History, physical examination, and appropriate tests should be performed at the first postoperative outpatient evaluation, 2 to 4 wk after hospital discharge. This includes a transthoracic Doppler echo if a baseline echo was not obtained before hospital discharge.	C
		Routine annual follow-up visits, with earlier reevaluations (with echo) if there is a change in clinical status	C
	IIb	Consider annual echos after the first 5 yr in patients with bioprostheses in the absence of a change in clinical status.	C
	III	Routine annual echos not indicated in the absence of a change in clinical status in patients with mechanical valves or during the first 5 yr after valve replacement with a bioprosthesis	C
Follow-up of patients with complications	I	Patients with LV systolic dysfunction after valve surgery should receive standard medical therapy for systolic heart failure. This therapy should be continued even if there is improvement of LV dysfunction.	B

Echo = echocardiogram; LOE = level of evidence.

postoperative survival, preoperative identification of CAD is of great importance in patients with aortic or mitral valve disease. Thus, in symptomatic patients and/or those with LV dysfunction, the guidelines recommend preoperative coronary angiography in men 35 years and older, premenopausal women older than 35 years with coronary risk factors, and postmenopausal women.

The guidelines support the practice of bypassing all significant coronary artery stenoses when possible in patients undergoing AVR.

REFERENCES

1. Bonow RO, Carabello B, De Leon AC Jr, et al: ACC/AHA guidelines for the management of patients with valvular heart disease: A report of the American College of Cardiology/American Heart Association Task Force on Practice Guidelines (Committee on Management of Patients with Valvular Heart Disease). J Am Coll Cardiol 32:1486, 1998.
2. Bonow RO, Carabello BA, Chatterjee K, et al: ACC/AHA 2006 guidelines for the management of patients with valvular heart disease: A report

of the American College of Cardiology/American Heart Association Task Force on Practice Guidelines (writing committee to revise the 1998 guidelines for the management of patients with valvular heart disease) developed in collaboration with the Society of Cardiovascular Anesthesiologists and endorsed by the Society for Cardiovascular Angiography and Interventions and the Society of Thoracic Surgeons. J Am Coll Cardiol 48:e1, 2006.

3. Bonow RO, Carabello B, Chatterjee K, et al: 2008 focused update incorporated into the ACC/AHA 2006 Guidelines for the Management of Patients with Valvular Heart Disease. J Am Coll Cardiol 52:e1, 2008.

4. Cheitlin MD, Armstrong WF, Aurigemma GP, et al: ACC/AHA/ASE 2003 guideline update for the clinical application of echocardiography: A report of the American College of Cardiology/American Heart Association Task Force on Practice Guidelines (ACC/AHA/ASE Committee to Update the 1997 Guidelines for the Clinical Application of Echocardiography). J Am Coll Cardiol 42:954, 2003.

5. Douglas PS, Khandheria B, Stainback RF, et al: ACCF/ASE/ACEP/ASNC/SCAI/SCCT/SCMR 2007 Appropriateness criteria for transthoracic and transesophageal echocardiography: A report of the American College of Cardiology Foundation Quality Strategic Directions Committee Appropriateness Criteria Working Group, American Society of Echocardiography, American College of Emergency Physicians, American Society of Nuclear Cardiology, Society for Cardiovascular Angiography and Interventions, Society of Cardiovascular Computed Tomography, and the Society for Cardiovascular Magnetic Resonance Endorsed by the American College of Chest Physicians and the Society of Critical Care Medicine. J Am Coll Cardiol 50;187, 2007.

6. Bonow RO, Cheitlin MD, Crawford MH, Douglas PS: Task Force 3: Valvular heart disease. J Am Coll Cardiol 45:1334, 2005.

7. Maron BJ, Araujo CG, Thompson PD, et al: Recommendations for preparticipation screening and the assessment of cardiovascular disease in masters athletes: An advisory for healthcare professionals from the working groups of the World Heart Federation, the International Federation of Sports Medicine, and the American Heart Association Committee on Exercise, Cardiac Rehabilitation, and Prevention. Circulation 103:327, 2001.

8. Feldman T, Wasserman HS, Herrmann HC, et al: Percutaneous mitral valve repair using the edge-to-edge technique: Six-month results of the EVEREST Phase I Clinical Trial. J Am Coll Cardiol 46:2134, 2005.

9. Rosengart TK, Feldman T, Borger MA, et al: Percutaneous and minimally invasive valve procedures: A scientific statement from the American Heart Association Council on Cardiovascular Surgery and Anesthesia, Council on Clinical Cardiology, Functional Genomics and Translational Biology Interdisciplinary Working Group, and Quality of Care and Outcomes Research Interdisciplinary Working Group. Circulation 117:1750, 2008.

10. Webb JG, Altwegg L, Boone RH, et al: Transcatheter aortic valve implantation: Impact on clinical and valve-related outcomes. Circulation 119:3009, 2009.

VALVULAR HEART DISEASE

CHAPTER 67 Infective Endocarditis

Adolf W. Karchmer

The characteristic lesion of infective endocarditis (IE), the vegetation, is a variably sized amorphous mass of platelets and fibrin with abundant enmeshed microorganisms and moderate inflammatory cells. Infections involve heart valves most commonly but may occur at the site of a septal defect, on chordae tendineae, or on mural endocardium. Infections of arteriovenous shunts, arterioarterial shunts (patent ductus arteriosus), or coarctation of the aorta are clinically and pathologically similar to IE. Many species of bacteria cause IE; nevertheless, streptococci, staphylococci, enterococci, and fastidious gram-negative coccobacilli cause the majority of cases of IE.

IE is often called acute or subacute. Acute IE is caused typically by *Staphylococcus aureus*. It presents with marked toxicity and progresses during days to several weeks to valvular destruction and metastatic infection. Subacute IE, usually caused by viridans streptococci, enterococci, coagulase-negative staphylococci, or gram-negative coccobacilli, evolves during weeks to months with only modest toxicity and rarely causes metastatic infection.

Epidemiology

The incidence of IE remained relatively stable from 1950 through 2000 at about 3.6 to 7.0 cases per 100,000 patient-years.[1,2] In selected areas, the incidence may be increased because of the concentration of populations at uniquely high risk of infection, specifically intravenous (IV) drug users. For example, from 1988 to 1990, 11.6 episodes per 100,000 population were reported from metropolitan Philadelphia (Delaware Valley), with injection drug abuse accounting for approximately half of the cases. The stable incidence is illustrated in Olmsted County, Minnesota, where from 1970 to 2000 the 5-year interval IE incidence ranged from 5.0 to 7.0 per 100,000 person-years; and in France, the IE incidence in 1991 and 1999 was 3.1 and 2.6 per 100,000 population, respectively.[2] Risk factors in industrialized countries have shifted, however, from rheumatic and congenital heart disease to IV drug use, degenerative valve disease in the elderly, intracardiac devices, health care–associated infection, and hemodialysis. Endocarditis continues to occur more frequently in men than in women, with a 2:1 ratio, but the median age of patients has gradually increased and now is 57.9 years (interquartile range, 43.2 to 71.8 years).[3] The age-specific incidence of endocarditis increases from 5 cases per 100,000 person-years among persons younger than 50 years to 15 to 30 cases per 100,000 person-years in the sixth through eighth decades of life.[1] From 50% to 75% of patients with native valve endocarditis (NVE) have predisposing valve conditions. The nature of the predisposing conditions and, in part, the microbiology of IE correlate with the age of patients (**Table 67-1**). Recent case series from large tertiary care referral centers have illustrated not only the previously noted shift in risk factors but also concomitant changes in microbiology, in particular that *S. aureus* exceeds streptococci as a causative agent (**Fig. 67-1**).[3-5] In contrast, population-based series, particularly if they are not dominated by cases among drug abusers, illustrate the continued importance of rheumatic and congenital valvular disease as predispositions and the predominance of streptococci as causal agents.[2,6] Where NVE among adults is not skewed dramatically by IV drug abuse and nosocomial infection, the microbiology is as shown in Table 67-1.

Groups of Patients

CHILDREN. In the Netherlands, IE was noted in 1.7 and 1.2 per 100,000 male and female children younger than 10 years, respectively. IE among neonates often involves the tricuspid valve of structurally normal hearts and arises as a consequence of infected intravascular catheters or cardiac surgery. Most children with IE occurring after the neonatal period have identifiable structural cardiac abnormalities; congenital heart abnormalities are present in 75% to 90% of cases. In many cases, IE occurs at the site of surgical repair and reflects the persistent risk for infection after complex reconstructive surgery. Neither secundum atrial septal defect nor patent ductus arteriosus or pulmonic stenosis after repair is associated with IE. Mitral valve prolapse in association with a regurgitant murmur predisposes to IE in children. The clinical features and echocardiographic findings of IE in children are similar to those noted among adults with native or prosthetic valve endocarditis.

ADULTS. Mitral valve prolapse, a prominent predisposing structural cardiac abnormality in adults, accounts for 7% to 30% of NVE not related to drug abuse or nosocomial infection. The frequency of mitral valve prolapse in IE is not entirely a direct reflection of relative risk but rather a function of the frequency of the lesion in the general population. This increased risk of endocarditis is largely confined to patients with prolapse, thickened valve leaflets (>5 mm), and mitral regurgitation murmur, especially among men and patients older than 45 years (see Chap. 66). Among patients with mitral valve prolapse and a systolic murmur, the incidence of IE is 52 per 100,000 person-years, compared with a rate of 4.6 per 100,000 person-years among those with prolapse and no murmur or among the general population. The microbiology and morbidity of IE engrafted on mitral valve prolapse are similar to those of NVE that is not associated with drug abuse.

TABLE 67-1   Conditions Predisposing to and Microbiology of Native Valve Endocarditis

	Children (%)		Adults (%)	
CONDITIONS AND MICROBIOLOGY	**NEONATES**	**2 MONTHS-15 YEARS**	**15-60 YEARS**	**>60 YEARS**
Predisposing Conditions				
Rheumatic heart disease		2-10	25-30	8
Congenital heart disease	28	75-90*	10-20	2
Mitral valve prolapse		5-15	10-30	10
Degenerative heart disease			Rare	30
Parenteral drug abuse			15-35	10
Other			10-15	10
None	72†	2-5	25-45	25-40
Microbiology				
Streptococci	15-20	40-50	33-65‡	30-45‡
Enterococci		4	5-8	15
Staphylococcus aureus	40-50	25	30-40‡	25-30‡
Coagulase-negative staphylococci	10	5	3-10	5-10
Gram-negative bacteria§	10	5	4-8	5
Fungi	10	1	1	Rare
Polymicrobial	4		1	Rare
Other			1	2
Culture negative	4	0-15	3-10	5

*50% of cases follow surgery and may involve implanted devices and foreign material.
†Often tricuspid valve IE.
‡In recent large series from tertiary centers, the referral bias combined with health care–associated IE and prevalent IV drug abuse result in a reversal in the relative frequency of IE caused by S. aureus and streptococci (see text).
§Frequently *Haemophilus* species, *Aggregatibacter* species, *Cardiobacterium hominis* in cases after the neonatal period.

Rheumatic heart disease as a predisposing cardiac lesion for IE has become less prevalent in industrialized nations.[3] In patients with rheumatic heart disease, endocarditis occurs most frequently on the mitral valve, followed by the aortic valve.

Congenital heart disease is the substrate for IE in 10% to 20% of younger adults and 8% of older adults. Among adults, the common predisposing lesions are patent ductus arteriosus, ventricular septal defect, and bicuspid aortic valve, the last particularly found among older men (>60 years).

Infection with human immunodeficiency virus (HIV) is not a significant risk factor for IE (see Chap. 72). Among HIV-infected persons who are not IV drug abusers, organisms typical of NVE and those that are uniquely associated with AIDS, such as *Bartonella* species, *Salmonella* species, and *Streptococcus pneumoniae*, cause IE. In an urban cohort of HIV-infected patients, the incidence of first episodes of IE was 4.4 per 1000 patient-years. IE was associated with injection drug use, was caused commonly by *S. aureus*, recurred frequently, and resulted in high mortality rates.[7]

INTRAVENOUS DRUG ABUSERS. The risk for IE among IV drug abusers is several-fold greater than that for patients with rheumatic heart disease or prosthetic valves. From 65% to 80% of such cases of IE occur in men, aged 27 to 37 years. IE is located on the tricuspid valve in 46% to 78%, mitral valve in 24% to 32%, and aortic valve in 8% to 19%; as many as 16% of patients have infection at multiple sites. The valves were normal before infection in 75% to 93% of patients. IV drug abuse is a risk factor for recurrent NVE.

MICROBIOLOGY. *S. aureus* causes more than 50% of IE occurring in IV drug abusers overall and 60% to 70% of infections involving the tricuspid valve (**Table 67-2**).[3] The well-established predilection for *S. aureus* to infect normal heart valves is noted in addicts with frequent infection of normal tricuspid valves. Streptococci and enterococci infect previously abnormal mitral or aortic valves in addicts. Infection of right- and left-sided heart valves by *Pseudomonas aeruginosa* and other gram-negative bacilli and left-sided heart valves by fungi occurs with increased frequency among drug abusers. Unusual organisms related to injection of contaminated materials cause endocarditis in these patients (e.g., *Cory-*

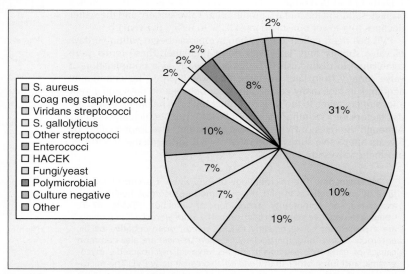

FIGURE 67-1   Microbiologic etiology of endocarditis in 1558 patients, 18 years old or older, admitted directly to 58 hospitals in 25 countries between June 2000 and September 2005. *(Data from Murdoch DR, Corey CR, Hoen B, et al: Clinical presentation, etiology, and outcome of infective endocarditis in the 21st century. Arch Intern Med 169:463, 2009.)*

nebacterium species, *Lactobacillus*, *Bacillus cereus*, and nonpathogenic *Neisseria* species). Polymicrobial endocarditis accounts for 3% to 5% of cases of IE.[3]

The clinical manifestations of IE in IV drug abusers depend on the valves involved and, to a lesser degree, on the infecting organism. Pleuritic chest pain, shortness of breath, cough, and hemoptysis occur with tricuspid valve endocarditis, particularly when it is caused by *S. aureus*. In 65% to 75% of patients, chest radiographs reveal abnormalities related to septic pulmonary emboli. Murmurs of tricuspid regurgitation are noted in less than half of these patients. Infection of the aortic or mitral valve in addicts clinically resembles IE seen in patients who are not drug abusers. HIV infection has been noted in 27% to 73% of IV drug abusers with IE (see Chap. 72).

TABLE 67-2   Microbiology of Endocarditis Associated with Intravenous Drug Abuse

ORGANISMS	Number of Cases (%) of Endocarditis in Drug Addicts*			
	RIGHT SIDED (N = 346)	LEFT SIDED (N = 204)	TOTAL (N = 675)	SPAIN, 1977-1993[†] (N = 1529)
Streptococci[‡]	17 (5)	31 (15)	80 (12)	131 (8.5)
Enterococci	7 (2)	49 (24)	59 (9)	21 (1)
Staphylococcus aureus	267 (77)	47 (23)	396 (57)	1138 (74)
Coagulase-negative staphylococci	—	—		44 (3)
Gram-negative bacilli[§]	7 (5)	26 (13)	45 (7)	23 (1.5)
Fungi (predominantly *Candida* species)	—	25 (12)	26 (4)	18 (1)
Polymicrobial/miscellaneous	28 (8)	20 (10)	49 (7)	48 (3)
Culture negative	10 (3)	6 (3)	20 (3)	106 (7)

*Ten patients with right- and left-sided infective endocarditis are counted twice.
[†]Data from Miro JM, del Rio A, Mestres CA: Infective endocarditis in intravenous drug abusers and HIV-1 infected patients. Infect Dis Clin North Am 16:273, 2002.
[‡]Includes viridans streptococci, *Streptococcus gallolyticus*, other non–group A groupable streptococci, *Abiotrophia* and *Granulicatella* species (nutritionally variant streptococci).
[§]*Pseudomonas aeruginosa, Serratia marcescens,* and Enterobacteriaceae.

Prosthetic Valve Endocarditis

Epidemiologic studies suggest that prosthetic valve endocarditis (PVE) constitutes 10% to 30% of all cases of IE in developed countries.[4,6,8,9] In patients undergoing valve surgery between 1965 and 1995, the cumulative incidence of PVE estimated actuarially ranged from 1.4% to 3.1% at 12 months and 3.0% to 5.7% at 5 years.[10] The frequency is greatest during the initial 6 months after valve surgery and thereafter declines to a lower but stable rate (0.2% to 0.35% per year).[10]

PVE has been called "early" when symptoms begin within 60 days of valve surgery and "late" with onset thereafter. These terms were established to distinguish PVE that arose early as a complication of valve surgery from later infection that was likely to be community acquired. In fact, many cases with onset between 60 days and 1 year after surgery relate to the surgical admission or to health care. Specific risk factors for PVE, other than prior IE, have not been clearly defined. Although the rates of PVE vary with time after valve implantation, by 5 years after valve surgery the rates of PVE for mechanical and bioprosthetic valves are similar.[10]

MICROBIOLOGY. The microbiology of PVE, when it is considered by time of onset, reflects in part the presumed nosocomial, health care–associated, or community acquisition of infection (**Table 67-3**). Coagulase-negative staphylococci, primarily *Staphylococcus epidermidis*, are a prominent cause of early PVE. *S. aureus,* gram-negative bacilli, enterococci, and fungi (particularly *Candida* species) are also common causes of early PVE. *Legionella* species, atypical mycobacteria, mycoplasma, and fungi other than *Candida* also cause early PVE. The microbiology of late PVE resembles that of community-acquired NVE; streptococci, *S. aureus,* enterococci, and coagulase-negative staphylococci are the major causes. Nosocomial and health care–associated late PVE has increased recently with attendant increases in infection caused by *S. aureus,* coagulase-negative staphylococci, and enterococci.[8,11]

PATHOLOGY. In contrast to the largely leaflet-confined pathology of NVE, infection on bioprostheses during the year after implantation or on mechanical prostheses commonly extends into the annulus and periannular tissue, causing dehiscence of the prosthesis with hemodynamically significant paravalvular regurgitation and conduction disturbances. Bulky vegetations can interfere with valve function at the mitral site and cause valve stenosis (**Fig. 67-2**).

Among 85 patients with mechanical valve PVE in whom the site of infection was examined at surgery or autopsy, annulus invasion was noted in 42%, myocardial abscess in 14%, valve obstruction in 4%, and pericarditis in 2%.[10] Among 49 patients with bioprosthetic PVE, 29 (59%) had later onset infection. Aortic site and clinical onset within a year of valve surgery correlate with an increased risk of invasive infection. Infected prosthetic valves can be distinguished from uninfected valves on histologic examination.

Signs and symptoms in patients developing PVE within 60 days of cardiac surgery may be obscured by surgery or postoperative complications. Peripheral signs of endocarditis (5% to 14%) and central nervous system emboli (10%) occur less frequently in these patients than in those

TABLE 67-3   Microbiology of Prosthetic Valve Endocarditis, 1970-2006

ORGANISMS	Number of Cases (%)* with Time of Onset After Valve Surgery	
	EARLY (N = 290) <12 MONTHS	LATE (N = 331) > 12 MONTHS
Streptococci[†]	7 (2)	93 (28)
Pneumococci	—	—
Enterococci	29 (10)	46 (14)
Staphylococcus aureus	72 (25)	57 (17)
Coagulase-negative staphylococci	85 (29)	41 (12)
Fastidious gram-negative coccobacilli (HACEK group)[‡]	—	13 (4)
Gram-negative bacilli	38 (13)	18 (5)
Fungi, *Candida* species	21 (7)	5 (2)
Polymicrobial/ miscellaneous	6 (2)	15 (5)
Diphtheroids	10 (3)	7 (2)
Coxiella burnetii	—	5 (2)
Culture negative	22 (8)	31 (9)

*Data from Karchner AW, Longworth DL: Infections of intracardiac devices. Infect Dis Clin North Am 16:477, 2002; Rivas P, Alonso J, Moya J, et al: The impact of hospital-acquired infections on the microbial etiology and prognosis of late-onset prosthetic valve endocarditis. Chest 128:764, 2005; Hill EE, Herregods MC, Vanderschueren S, et al: Management of prosthetic valve endocarditis. Am J Cardiol 101:1174, 2008; Wang A, Athan E, Pappas P, et al: Contemporary clinical profile and outcome of prosthetic valve endocarditis. JAMA 297:1354, 2007.
[†]Includes viridans streptococci, *Streptococcus gallolyticus*, other non–group A groupable streptococci, *Abiotrophia* and *Granulicatella* species (nutritionally variant streptococci).
[‡]Includes *Haemophilus* species, *Aggregatibacter* species, *Cardiobacterium hominis*, *Eikenella* species, and *Kingella* species.

with PVE occurring later. Among patients with later onset PVE, congestive heart failure (CHF) occurs in 40%, cerebrovascular complications in 26% to 28%, and peripheral signs in 15% to 28%.[10] Among patients with PVE treated since 1980, in-hospital mortality overall ranges from 14% to 41% and that for early and late infection from 30% to 46% and 19% to 34%, respectively.[9,11] Mortality for *S. aureus* PVE regardless of time of onset remains high, 36% to 47%.[8,12,13] Mortality is associated with age and complications of PVE, including CHF, stroke, intracardiac abscess, and persistent bacteremia.

Health Care–Associated Endocarditis

Health care–associated endocarditis includes nosocomial IE as well as IE arising in the community after a recent hospitalization or as a direct consequence of long-term indwelling devices, such as central venous lines and hemodialysis catheters. Health care–associated IE, unrelated to concurrent cardiac surgery, makes up 24% to 34% of cases in recent series and accounts for an even larger proportion of cases in the United States.[3,4,14] Infection may involve normal valves, including the tricuspid, as well as implanted intracardiac devices and valves.[3,5,6,10,11,14] Onset of health care–associated NVE is nosocomial or community based in 54% and 46%, respectively.[14]

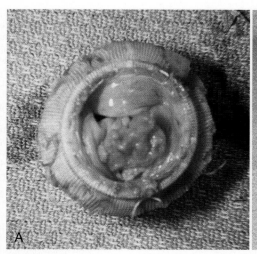 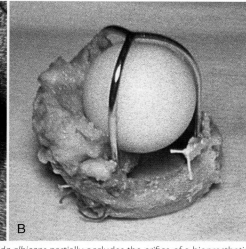

FIGURE 67-2 A, A large vegetation caused by *Candida albicans* partially occludes the orifice of a bioprosthetic valve removed from the mitral position. **B,** A Starr-Edwards prosthesis removed from the aortic position, where this large vegetation related to *Aspergillus* infection partially obstructed the outflow tract but also allowed regurgitation by preventing valve closure. (*A reproduced from Karchmer AW: Infections of prosthetic heart valves. In Korzeniowski OM [ed]: Cardiovascular Infection, vol X, Atlas of Infectious Diseases. Philadelphia, Churchill Livingstone, 1998, p 5.7.*)

The onset of health care–associated IE is usually acute, and although a changing murmur may be heard, other classic signs of endocarditis are infrequent. Mortality rates among these patients, many of whom are elderly and have serious underlying diseases, are high (27% to 38%).[6,14]

MICROBIOLOGY. Among 660 episodes of health care–associated IE from five series, *S. aureus* caused 305 (46%) infections (47% of *S. aureus* were methicillin resistant); coagulase-negative staphylococci, 94 (14%); enterococci, 105 (16%); streptococci, 72 (11%); *Candida* species, 18 (3%); gram-negative bacilli, 24 (4%); and other organisms, 6 (1%). Culture was negative in 36 cases (5%).

Catheter-associated and hemodialysis-associated *S. aureus* bacteremia occurs with sufficient frequency to be the predominant predisposing factor for health care–associated IE. Transesophageal echocardiography is recommended to exclude IE in patients with catheter-related *S. aureus* bacteremia (see Chap. 15). Patients with *S. aureus* catheter-related bacteremia who have abnormal heart valves, prosthetic valves, or persisting fever or bacteremia for 3 or 4 days after catheter removal and initiation of therapy should be treated for presumed IE.

Etiologic Microorganisms

Viridans Streptococci

These streptococci, which in developed countries cause 18% to 30% of NVE cases unrelated to drug abuse and health care, are normal inhabitants of the oropharynx, characteristically produce alpha-hemolysis when grown on sheep blood agar, and are usually nontypable by the Lancefield system.[2,6] By earlier taxonomy, the non–beta-hemolytic streptococci causing NVE were distributed as follows: *Streptococcus mitior,* 31% of cases; *Streptococcus sanguis,* 24%; *Streptococcus bovis,* 27%; *Streptococcus mutans,* 7%; *Streptococcus milleri* (now called *Streptococcus anginosus* group and includes *Streptococcus intermedius, anginosus,* and *constellatus*), 4%; *Streptococcus faecalis* (now *Enterococcus faecalis*), 7%; and *Streptococcus salivarius* and other species, 2%. Nutritional variant organisms that require media supplemented with either pyridoxal hydrochloride or L-cysteine for growth, previously speciated as *Streptococcus adjacens* or *Streptococcus defectivus,* cause 5% of cases of streptococcal NVE. These organisms have been reclassified as *Granulicatella* species and *Abiotrophia defectiva* species, respectively. *Gemella morbillorum,* previously called *Streptococcus morbillorum,* shares some characteristics with nutritionally variant organisms and should be treated with similar antibiotic therapy.[15]

The viridans streptococci causing IE have been, in general, highly susceptible to penicillin; 5% to 8% of these have penicillin minimum inhibitory concentrations (MICs) >0.1 μg/mL. These streptococci are killed in a synergistic manner by penicillin plus gentamicin.

Streptococcus bovis and Other Streptococci

Streptococcus gallolyticus (formerly *S. bovis*), part of the gastrointestinal tract normal flora, causes 20% to 40% of the episodes of streptococcal NVE. Although it superficially resembles the enterococci, the distinction is important because *S. gallolyticus* is highly penicillin susceptible, in contrast to the relative penicillin resistance of enterococci. *S. gallolyticus* type I endocarditis is frequently associated with coexistent polyps or malignant disease in the colon; accordingly, colonoscopy is warranted in these patients.

Group A streptococci cause rare episodes of endocarditis. Among IV drug abusers, group A streptococci have caused tricuspid valve IE similar to that noted with *S. aureus*. Group B organisms (*Streptococcus agalactiae,* part of the normal flora of the mouth, genital tract, and gastrointestinal tract) infect normal and abnormal valves and cause a morbid NVE syndrome with a high incidence of systemic emboli and septic musculoskeletal complications (arthritis, discitis, osteomyelitis). The *S. anginosus* group cause destructive extracardiac infections and IE with intracardiac complications. Beta-hemolytic (groups A, B, C, and G) streptococcal IE often occurs in the absence of valvular disease and causes frequent intracardiac or extracardiac complications. Surgical intervention is often necessary in treatment of beta-hemolytic streptococcal and *S. anginosus* IE.

Streptococcus pneumoniae

S. pneumoniae accounts for only 1% to 3% of NVE cases. Pneumococcal IE frequently involves a normal aortic valve and progresses rapidly with valve destruction, myocardial abscess formation, and acute CHF. The diagnosis of IE is often delayed until intracardiac complications or systemic emboli are evident. The clinical presentation, complications, and outcome of endocarditis caused by penicillin-susceptible and penicillin-resistant *S. pneumoniae* are similar. Patients commonly require cardiac surgery because of valve dysfunction, CHF, or persisting fever. Mortality (35%) is related to left-sided heart failure and not to the penicillin susceptibility of the infecting strain.

Enterococci

E. faecalis and *Enterococcus faecium* cause 85% and 10% of cases of enterococcal IE, respectively. Enterococci, which are part of the normal gastrointestinal flora and cause genitourinary tract infection, account for 5% to 15% of cases of both NVE and PVE (see Tables 67-2 and 67-3).[2,4,6,14,16] Disease typically occurs with equal frequency in older men (often from a urinary tract portal of entry) and women, and 15% to 25% of cases are nosocomial.[16] Enterococci infect abnormal valves and prosthetic valves. IE may be acute or subacute. Mortality rates are comparable to those noted with viridans streptococcal IE.

Enterococci are resistant to cephalosporins, semisynthetic penicillinase-resistant penicillins (oxacillin and nafcillin), and therapeutic concentrations of aminoglycosides. Most enterococci are inhibited by modest concentrations of the cell wall–active antibiotics: penicillin, ampicillin, vancomycin, teicoplanin (not licensed in the United States), daptomycin, and linezolid. Bactericidal antienterococcal activity can be achieved by combining an inhibitory cell wall–active agent and streptomycin or gentamicin. This bactericidal activity, called synergy, is essential for optimal treatment of enterococcal IE. Strains of enterococci that are resistant to penicillin and ampicillin, resistant to vancomycin, or highly resistant to streptomycin or gentamicin have been identified as causes of IE. These resistant strains of enterococci may be unresponsive to standard antienterococcal regimens and defy development of synergistic bactericidal therapy.[17] The antibiotic susceptibility of any enterococcus causing IE must be thoroughly evaluated if optimal therapy is to be ensured.

Staphylococci

The coagulase-positive staphylococci are a single species: *S. aureus*. Of the 13 species of coagulase-negative staphylococci that colonize humans, *S. epidermidis* has emerged as an important pathogen in the setting of implanted devices and health care–associated infection.

S. aureus

This organism is a major cause of IE in all population groups (see Fig. 67-1 and Tables 67-1 to 67-3). *S. aureus* is the most common cause of IE noted in large international series from tertiary care centers.[3,4,18] In general, 25% to 30% of isolates are methicillin resistant; however, among nosocomial and health care–associated cases, rates of methicillin resistance are 57% and 40%, respectively.[14] *S. aureus* IE is characterized by a highly toxic febrile illness, frequent focal metastatic infection, 30% to 50% rate of CHF, and central nervous system complications.[4] A cerebrospinal fluid polymorphonuclear pleocytosis, with or without *S. aureus* cultured from the cerebrospinal fluid, is common. Heart murmurs as a consequence of intracardiac damage are ultimately heard in 75% to 85%. The mortality rate in nonaddicts with left-sided *S. aureus* endocarditis ranges from 16% to 65% overall and is increased with age, with significant underlying diseases, or when IE is complicated by a major neurologic event, perivalvular abscess and valve dysfunction, or CHF.[4,18] Among addicts, left-sided *S. aureus* IE resembles that in nonaddicts. With *S. aureus* IE limited to the tricuspid valve (see Fig. 15-e21 on website), systemic complications are rare and mortality rates are only 2% to 4%, although occasional patients suffer overwhelming septic pulmonary emboli, pyopneumothorax, and severe respiratory insufficiency.

Coagulase-Negative Staphylococci

These organisms, particularly *S. epidermidis*, are a major cause of PVE, an important cause of nosocomial IE, and the cause of 8% to 10% of NVE, usually in the setting of prior valve abnormalities (see Fig. 67-1).[3,14,19] Non-*epidermidis* species cause NVE that is not associated with health care. Coagulase-negative staphylococcal NVE is often complicated and fatal.[19] *Staphylococcus lugdunensis*, a community-acquired, antibiotic-susceptible coagulase-negative species, causes valve damage and frequently requires surgical intervention.

Gram-Negative Bacteria

The HACEK organisms (*Haemophilus parainfluenzae*, *Aggregatibacter* [previously *Haemophilus*] *aphrophilus*, *Aggregatibacter* [previously *Actinobacillus*] *actinomycetemcomitans*, *Cardiobacterium hominis*, *Eikenella corrodens*, and *Kingella kingae*), which are part of the upper respiratory tract and oropharyngeal flora, infect abnormal cardiac valves, causing subacute NVE and PVE that occurs a year or more after valve surgery.

Although fastidious and slow growing, HACEK organisms are usually detected in blood cultures within 5 days of incubation; more prolonged incubation is occasionally required. HACEK NVE has been associated with large vegetations and a high incidence of systemic emboli.

Gram-negative bacilli, despite causing frequent episodes of bacteremia, are implicated in only sporadic cases of IE. *Escherichia coli* and *P. aeruginosa* are the most commonly implicated species.[20] Mortality rates are high (25% to 50%).

Neisseria gonorrhoeae, a rare cause of endocarditis today, causes acute IE with valve destruction and intracardiac abscesses. Antibiotic resistance is widespread among *N. gonorrhoeae*; accordingly, treatment must be based on the susceptibility of the implicated isolate. Other *Neisseria* species (nongonococcal, nonmeningococcal) cause rare episodes of subacute IE, usually in the setting of preexisting valvulopathy.

Other Organisms

Corynebacterium species, called diphtheroids, although often contaminants in blood cultures, cannot be ignored when they are isolated from multiple blood cultures. They are an important cause of PVE and cause endocarditis involving abnormal valves. *Listeria monocytogenes* occasionally infects abnormal left-sided heart valves and prosthetic devices. *Tropheryma whipplei*, the cause of Whipple disease, causes a cryptic afebrile form of IE with associated arthralgias but without diarrhea as well as valvular disease as part of typical Whipple disease. The diagnosis has been established by identification of the organism on excised valves by periodic acid–Schiff stain or by polymerase chain reaction (PCR). IE caused by *T. whipplei* often does not fulfill the Duke criteria for diagnosis (**Table 67-4**); thus, detection requires a high index of suspicion.

The rickettsia *Coxiella burnetii*, an uncommon cause of IE in the United States, is a prominent cause of IE in other parts of the world. IE follows acute infection by *C. burnetii* (Q fever) in persons with abnormal mitral or aortic valves and particularly those with prosthetic valves. Patients with acute Q fever and echocardiographically confirmed valvulopathy should receive prolonged antibiotic treatment with doxycycline plus hydroxychloroquine to prevent IE.[21] IE commonly is manifested with low-grade fever, fatigue, weight loss, hepatosplenomegaly, digital clubbing, and an immune complex vasculitis-induced purpuric rash. Vegetations are small, have smooth surfaces, and are not uniformly visible on the echocardiogram. The diagnosis is typically based on high immunoglobulin G antibody titers to phase I *C. burnetii* antigens plus immunoglobulin A antibody or demonstration of the organism in excised cardiac valves by immunohistologic or Gimenez staining or by PCR testing.

Bartonella quintana and *Bartonella henselae* together may cause 3% of NVE. In the absence of special blood culturing efforts, PCR detection of genetic material in excised vegetations, or serologic testing, many cases would have been "culture negative." *B. henselae*, the etiologic agent of cat-scratch disease, causes IE in patients with prior valve injury and cat exposure. *B. quintana*, the agent of trench fever, causes IE on normal valves largely in homeless people who are exposed to infected body lice. *Bartonella* IE arises insidiously; diagnosis is often delayed, and CHF and systemic emboli frequently complicate infection. Treatment commonly requires valve surgery.

Fungi

Candida species, *Histoplasma*, and *Aspergillus* species are the most common of the many fungal organisms identified as causing IE. Unusual so-called emerging fungi and molds account for 25% of cases. Risk factors include previous valve surgery, antibiotic use, injection drug abuse, intravascular catheters, surgery other than cardiac, and immunocompromised state. Fever, murmurs, embolization including major limb artery occlusion, neurologic abnormalities, and CHF are common. Blood cultures are positive commonly when IE is caused by *Candida* species but rarely when it is caused by molds. Culture and histologic examination of vegetations and peripheral emboli yield a microbiologic diagnosis in 75% to 95% of cases.

Pathogenesis

The interactions between the human host and selected microorganisms that culminate in IE involve the vascular endothelium, hemostatic mechanisms, host immune system, gross anatomic abnormalities in the heart, surface properties of microorganisms, enzyme and toxin production by microorganisms, and peripheral events that initiate bacteremia. Each component is in itself complex, influenced by many factors. On occasion, these interactions result in a pathogenetic sequence wherein microorganisms gain access to the bloodstream, rapidly adhere to valve surfaces, become persistent at the site of adherence, proliferate

TABLE 67-4 Diagnosis of Infective Endocarditis (Modified Duke Criteria)

Definite Infective Endocarditis

Pathologic criteria
　Microorganisms: demonstrated by culture or histology in a vegetation, or in a vegetation that has embolized, or in an intracardiac abscess, or
　Pathologic lesions: vegetation or intracardiac abscess present, confirmed by histology showing active endocarditis
Clinical criteria, using specific definitions listed below
　Two major criteria, or
　One major criterion and three minor criteria, or
　Five minor criteria

Possible Infective Endocarditis

One major criterion and one minor criterion or three minor criteria

Rejected

Firm alternative diagnosis for manifestations of endocarditis, or
Sustained resolution of manifestations of endocarditis, with antibiotic therapy for 4 days or less, or
No pathologic evidence of infective endocarditis at surgery or autopsy, after antibiotic therapy for 4 days or less

Criteria for Diagnosis of Infective Endocarditis
Major Criteria

Positive blood culture
　Typical microorganism for infective endocarditis from two separate blood cultures
　　Viridans streptococci, *Streptococcus bovis*, HACEK group or *Staphylococcus aureus* or community-acquired enterococci in the absence of a primary focus, or
　Persistently positive blood culture, defined as recovery of a microorganism consistent with infective endocarditis from:
　　Blood cultures (≥2) drawn more than 12 hr apart, or
　　All of three or a majority of four or more separate blood cultures, with first and last drawn at least 1 hr apart
　Single positive blood culture for *Coxiella burnetii* or anti–phase I IgG antibody titer >1:800
Evidence of endocardial involvement
　Positive echocardiogram (TEE advised for PVE or complicated infective endocarditis)
　　Oscillating intracardiac mass, on valve or supporting structures, or in the path of regurgitant jets, or on implanted material, in the absence of an alternative anatomic explanation, or
　　Abscess, or
　　New partial dehiscence of prosthetic valve, or
　New valvular regurgitation (increase or change in preexisting murmur not sufficient)

Minor Criteria

Predisposition: predisposing heart condition or intravenous drug use
Fever ≥38.0°C (100.4°F)
Vascular phenomena: major arterial emboli, septic pulmonary infarcts, mycotic aneurysm, intracranial hemorrhage, conjunctival hemorrhages, Janeway lesions
Immunologic phenomena: glomerulonephritis, Osler nodes, Roth spots, rheumatoid factor
Microbiologic evidence: positive blood culture but not meeting major criterion as noted previously* or serologic evidence of active infection with organism consistent with infective endocarditis

*Excluding single positive cultures for coagulase-negative staphylococci and organisms that do not cause endocarditis commonly.
IgG = immunoglobulin G; PVE = prosthetic valve endocarditis; TEE = transesophageal echocardiography.
Modified from Durack DT, Lukes AS, Bright DK: New criteria for diagnosis of infective endocarditis: Utilization of specific echocardiographic findings. Am J Med 96:200, 1994; modified per Li JS, Sexton DJ, Mick N, et al: Proposed modifications to the Duke criteria for the diagnosis of infective endocarditis. Clin Infect Dis 30:633, 2000.

to cause local damage and vegetation growth, and ultimately disseminate hematogenously with or without emboli. Studies have begun to elucidate the pathogenesis of IE caused by viridans streptococci and *S. aureus*.[1] The rarity of endocarditis in spite of frequent bacteremia indicates that the intact endothelium is relatively resistant to infection. It is hypothesized that platelet-fibrin deposition occurs spontaneously on abnormal valves and at sites of cardiac endothelium injury or inflammation and that these deposits, called nonbacterial thrombotic endocarditis (NBTE), are the sites at which microorganisms adhere during bacteremia to initiate IE.[1]

Development of Nonbacterial Thrombotic Endocarditis

Two major mechanisms appear pivotal in the formation of NBTE: endothelial injury and a hypercoagulable state. Marantic NBTE, thought to be a result of hypercoagulability, has been found in 1.3% of patients at autopsy and is more common with increasing age and in patients with malignant disease, disseminated intravascular coagulation, uremia, burns, systemic lupus erythematosus (see Fig. 15-62), valvular heart disease, and intracardiac catheters. NBTE occurs at the valve closure contact line on the atrial surfaces of the mitral and tricuspid valves and on the ventricular surfaces of the aortic and pulmonic valves. Three hemodynamic circumstances may injure the endothelium, initiating NBTE: (1) a high-velocity jet striking endothelium; (2) flow from a high-pressure to a low-pressure chamber; and (3) flow across a narrow orifice at high velocity.

During bacteremia, blood flow through a narrowed orifice deposits bacteria maximally at the low-pressure sink immediately beyond an orifice as a consequence of the Venturi effect or at the site where a jet stream strikes a surface. These are the same sites where NBTE forms as a result of endothelial injury or hypercoagulability. The superimposition of NBTE formation and preferential deposition of bacteria helps explain the distribution of infected vegetations.

Conversion of Nonbacterial Thrombotic Endocarditis to Infective Endocarditis

Bacteremia is the event that converts NBTE to IE. The frequency and magnitude of bacteremia associated with daily activities and health care procedures appear related to the specific mucosal surfaces and skin, the density of colonizing bacteria, the disease state of the surface, and the extent of the local trauma. Bacteremia rates are highest for events that traumatize the oral mucosa, particularly the gingiva, and progressively decrease with procedures involving the genitourinary tract and the gastrointestinal tract. For viable circulating microorganisms to reach NBTE, they must be resistant to the complement-mediated bactericidal activity of serum.

The adherence of microorganisms to the NBTE or to apparently intact valve endothelium, a pivotal early event in the development of IE, is mediated by bacterial surface molecules (adhesins). Collectively, these adhesins are known as microbial surface components recognizing adhesive matrix molecules (MSCRAMMs). Streptococci that produce surface polysaccharides called glucans or dextran cause endocarditis more frequently than strains that do not. Surface dextran mediates the adherence of streptococci to platelet-fibrin lattices and injured valves and facilitates the development of endocarditis in experimental models.[1] Dextran production, however, is not universal among the major microbial causes of IE; thus, other mechanisms of adherence are likely. FimA protein of *Streptococcus parasanguis* facilitates adherence to fibrin and development of experimental endocarditis. Collagen adhesins and biofilm-associated pili on the surface of *E. faecalis* and *E. faecium* similarly facilitate development of endocarditis in experimental models.[22,23]

Fibronectin, an important factor in the pathogenesis of IE, has been identified in lesions on heart valves and is produced by endothelial cells, platelets, and fibroblasts in response to vascular injury; a soluble form binds with fibrinogen and fibrin to exposed subendothelial collagen. Receptors for fibronectin, MSCRAMMs, are present on the surface of *S. aureus;* viridans streptococci; groups A, C, and G streptococci; enterococci; *S. pneumoniae;* and *C. albicans*. Fibronectin has numerous binding domains and thus can bind simultaneously to fibrin, collagen, cells, and microorganisms and facilitate adherence of bacteria to the valve at the site of injury or NBTE. Fibronectin-binding proteins A and B in *S. aureus* are critical in the induction of experimental endocarditis. Clumping factor (or fibrinogen-binding surface protein) of *S. aureus* also mediates the binding of these organisms to platelet-fibrin thrombi and to aortic valves in models of endocarditis.[1] The glycocalyx or slime on the surface of *S. epidermidis* does not appear to function as an adhesin but may render organisms more virulent by enhancing their ability to avoid eradication by host defenses.

The mechanism by which virulent organisms colonize and infect intact valvular endothelium is less clearly understood. Degenerative valve sclerosis may be associated with local inflammation that in turn may promote endothelial cell expression of integrins that bind fibronectin and other extracellular matrix molecules. Particulate material injected during IV drug abuse might stimulate similar endothelial events. These endothelial changes could allow *S. aureus* adherence through MSCRAMMs to apparently normal valves.[1] Adherent *S. aureus* triggers its own internalization by intact endothelial cells. Multiplication of the organism intracellularly results in cell death, which in turn disrupts the endothelial surface and initiates formation of platelet-fibrin deposits and additional sites for bacterial adherence and subsequently IE.

After adherence to NBTE or the endothelium, bacteria must persist and multiply if IE is to develop. Resistance of viridans streptococci and *S. aureus* to platelet antimicrobial proteins is associated with increased ability to cause experimental endocarditis.[1] Persistence and multiplication result in a complex dynamic process during which the infected vegetation increases in size by platelet-fibrin aggregation, microorganisms multiply and are shed into the blood, and vegetation fragments embolize. Staphylococcal and streptococcal surface proteins bind to platelets and promote aggregation and growth of the vegetation. Organisms that bind and aggregate platelets are more virulent in experimental models. Streptococci and staphylococci increase local procoagulant activity by inducing fibrin-adherent monocytes to elaborate tissue factor (a tissue thromboplastin that binds to activated factor VII to initiate clotting). Also, *S. aureus* can induce tissue factor production by endothelial cells, which would facilitate endocarditis development on normal valves. Multiple replications of this cycle from adherence to multiplication and platelet-fibrin deposition result in clinical IE.

Pathophysiology

Aside from the constitutional symptoms of infection, which are probably mediated by cytokines, the clinical manifestations of IE result from (1) the local destructive effects of intracardiac infection; (2) the embolization of bland or septic fragments of vegetations to distant sites, resulting in infarction or infection; (3) the hematogenous seeding of remote sites during continuous bacteremia; and (4) an antibody response to the infecting organism with subsequent tissue injury caused by deposition of preformed immune complexes or antibody-complement interaction with antigens deposited in tissues.

The intracardiac consequences of IE range from an infected vegetation with no attendant tissue damage to destruction of valves and adjacent structures. Distortion or perforation of valve leaflets, rupture of chordae tendineae, and fistulas between major vessels and cardiac chambers or between chambers themselves may result in CHF that is progressive (**Fig. 67-3**). Infection may extend into paravalvular tissue and result in abscesses and consequent persistent fever, disruption of the conduction system with electrocardiographic conduction abnormalities and arrhythmias, or purulent pericarditis. Large vegetations, particularly at the mitral valve, can result in functional valvular stenosis. In general, intracardiac complications involving the aortic valve evolve more rapidly than those associated with the mitral valve; nevertheless, the progression is highly variable and unpredictable in individual patients.

Clinically apparent emboli, half of which cause strokes, occur in 11% to 43% of patients.[24,25] Pathologic evidence of emboli at autopsy is more frequent (45% to 65%). Pulmonary emboli, which are often septic, occur in 66% to 75% of IV drug abusers with tricuspid valve IE. IE caused by virulent organisms, particularly *S. aureus,* beta-hemolytic streptococci, or other pyogenic organisms, is complicated more

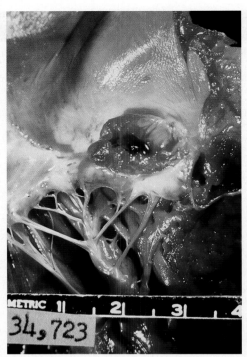

FIGURE 67-3 A normal valve with a large, bulky vegetation caused by *S. aureus* infection. Clot is present centrally in the vegetation, obscuring a valve fenestration.

frequently by metastatic infection, often with local signs and symptoms or persistent fever during therapy, than IE due to avirulent bacteria (e.g., viridans streptococci). Metastatic infection assumes particular importance when the required therapy is more than the antibiotics indicated for IE (e.g., when abscesses require drainage or meningitis requires antibiotics penetrating into the cerebrospinal fluid).

Clinical Features

The interval between the presumed initiating bacteremia and the onset of symptoms of IE is estimated to be less than 2 weeks in more than 80% of patients with NVE. Interestingly, in some patients with candidemia causing IE or with intraoperative or perioperative infection of prosthetic valves, the incubation period may be prolonged (5 months or more).

Fever is almost universal (**Table 67-5**). However, it may be absent or minimal in those with CHF, severe debility, or chronic renal failure. Heart murmurs are usually emblematic of the lesion predisposing to IE. Murmurs are commonly not audible in patients with tricuspid valve IE. The new or changing regurgitant murmurs indicative of valve damage are relatively infrequent in subacute NVE and are more prevalent in acute IE and PVE (e.g., that due to *S. aureus*). They are frequently harbingers of CHF. Enlargement of the spleen is more common in subacute IE of long duration.

The classic peripheral manifestations of IE are encountered infrequently today and are virtually absent in IE restricted to the tricuspid valve. Petechiae, the most common of these manifestations, are found on the palpebral conjunctiva, the buccal and palatal mucosa, and the extremities. Splinter or subungual hemorrhages are dark red, linear, or occasionally flame-shaped streaks in the proximal nailbed. Distal lesions at the nail tip are probably caused by trauma. Osler nodes are small, tender subcutaneous nodules in the pulp of the digits, or occasionally more proximal, that persist for hours to several days. Janeway lesions are small erythematous or hemorrhagic macular nontender lesions on the palms and soles and are the consequence of septic embolic events. Embolic infarcts in the digits (**Fig. 67-4**) are common in left-sided *S. aureus* IE. Roth spots, oval retinal hemorrhages with pale

TABLE 67-5	Clinical Features of Infective Endocarditis		
SYMPTOMS	PERCENTAGE OF PATIENTS	SIGNS	PERCENTAGE OF PATIENTS
Fever	80-85	Fever	80-96
Chills	42-75	Murmur	80-85
Sweats	25	Changing or new murmur	10-40
Anorexia	25-55	Neurologic abnormalities†	30-40
Weight loss	25-35	Embolic event	20-40
Malaise	25-40	Splenomegaly	15-50
Dyspnea	20-40	Clubbing	10-20
Cough	25	Peripheral manifestations	
Stroke	13-20	Osler nodes	7-10
Headache	15-40	Splinter hemorrhage	5-15
Nausea or vomiting	15-20	Petechiae	10-40
Myalgia arthralgia	15-30	Janeway lesion	6-10
Chest pain*	8-35	Retinal lesion or Roth spots	4-10
Abdominal pain	5-15		
Back pain	7-10		
Confusion	10-20		

*More common in intravenous drug abusers with right-sided infective endocarditis.
†Central nervous system.

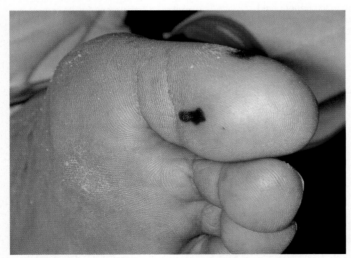

FIGURE 67-4 Digit infarcts in a patient with infective endocarditis due to *S. aureus*. *(Courtesy of Alan J. Lesse, MD.)*

centers, are infrequent findings in IE. Neither these nor Osler nodes nor conjunctival petechiae are pathognomonic for IE.

Musculoskeletal symptoms, unrelated to focal infection, are relatively common in patients with IE. These include arthralgias and myalgias, occasional true arthritis with nondiagnostic but inflammatory synovial fluid findings, and prominent back pain without demonstrable infection of vertebrae, disc space, epidural space, or sacroiliac joint. In patients with arthritis or back pain, focal infection must be excluded because additional therapy may be required.

Symptomatic systemic emboli frequently antedate or coincide with the diagnosis of IE; the incidence decreases promptly during administration of effective antibiotic therapy. Embolic events are infrequent after 2 weeks of therapy.[25] The risks of emboli generally increase with large vegetations (>10 mm), mitral vegetations, *S. aureus* IE, and increasing vegetation size during therapy.[4,24,25] Embolic stroke syndromes (clinically evident), predominantly involving the middle cerebral artery territory, occur in 15% to 35% of patients with NVE and PVE. A similar additional frequency of asymptomatic embolic infarcts may be detected with careful routine imaging. Coronary artery emboli, common findings at autopsy, rarely cause transmural infarction. Emboli to the extremities may produce pain and overt ischemia, and emboli to mesenteric arteries may cause abdominal pain, ileus, and guaiac-positive stools.

Neurologic symptoms and signs are caused most commonly by embolic strokes, are more frequent when IE is caused by *S. aureus*, and are associated with increased mortality rates.[24-26] Intracranial hemorrhage, which occurs in 5% of patients, results from rupture of a mycotic aneurysm, rupture of an artery related to septic arteritis at the site of embolic occlusion, or hemorrhage into an infarct. Cerebritis with microabscesses complicates IE caused by invasive pathogens such as *S. aureus*, but large brain abscesses are rare. Purulent meningitis complicates some episodes of IE caused by *S. aureus* or *S. pneumoniae*, but more typically the cerebrospinal fluid, if abnormal, has an aseptic profile. Other neurologic manifestations include severe headache (a potential clue to a mycotic aneurysm), seizures, and encephalopathy.

CHF primarily results from valve destruction or distortion or rupture of chordae tendineae. Intracardiac fistulas, myocarditis, or coronary artery embolization may occasionally contribute to the genesis of CHF, as obviously can underlying cardiac disease.

Renal insufficiency as a result of immune complex–mediated glomerulonephritis occurs in less than 15% of patients with IE. Azotemia as a result of this process may develop or progress during initial therapy but usually improves with continued administration of effective antibiotic therapy. Focal glomerulonephritis and embolic renal infarcts cause hematuria but rarely result in azotemia. The most common cause of renal dysfunction in patients with IE is impaired hemodynamics or antimicrobial toxicities (interstitial nephritis or aminoglycoside toxicity).

Diagnosis

The symptoms and signs of endocarditis are often constitutional and, when localized, may result from a remote complication rather than reflect the intracardiac infection itself (see Table 67-5). Consequently, to avoid overlooking the diagnosis of IE, a high index of suspicion must be maintained. The diagnosis must be investigated when patients with fever present with one or more of the cardinal elements of IE: predisposing cardiac lesion or behavior pattern, bacteremia, embolic phenomenon, and evidence of an active endocardial process or new prosthetic valve dysfunction. Among patients with a predisposition to IE, unexplained weight loss, malaise, azotemia, and anemia should prompt consideration of IE even in the absence of fever. Even when the illness seems typical of endocarditis, the definitive diagnosis requires positive blood cultures or positive cultures (or histology or PCR recovery of the DNA of a microorganism) from the vegetation or an embolus. There are many mimics of IE: atrial myxoma (see Chap. 74), acute rheumatic fever (see Chap. 88), systemic lupus erythematosus or other collagen-vascular disease (see Chap. 89), marantic endocarditis, antiphospholipid syndrome, carcinoid syndrome, renal cell carcinoma with increased cardiac output, and thrombotic thrombocytopenic purpura.

The modified Duke criteria provide a schema that facilitates evaluation of patients for endocarditis (see Table 67-4).[27] Clinical and laboratory data, including echocardiography, should be collected to assess the presence or absence of the listed major and minor criteria. Finding evidence of two major criteria or one major criterion plus three minor criteria or five minor criteria establishes a clinical diagnosis of "definite endocarditis," whereas finding one major criterion plus one minor criterion or three minor criteria indicates "possible endocarditis." When used judiciously over the entire evaluation (i.e., not limited to initial findings), these criteria are sensitive and specific for the diagnosis of IE.[27] Erroneous rejection of the diagnosis of endocarditis is unlikely. When the criteria are used to guide therapy, patients who are categorized with possible endocarditis should be treated as if they have IE. Requiring at least one major criterion plus one minor criterion or three minor criteria to designate possible endocarditis reduces the potential for overdiagnosis (failure to reject the diagnosis).[27] Nevertheless, because the echocardiogram cannot fully distinguish healed vegetations and other valvular masses from actively infected vegetations, these guidelines are vulnerable to misidentification of patients as having culture-negative IE when vegetations that complicate marasmus, malignant disease, cryptic collagen-vascular disease, antiphospholipid antibody syndrome, or previously treated IE are detected. To use bacteremia caused by coagulase-negative staphylococci or diphtheroids (organisms that may cause IE but more often contaminate blood cultures) to support the diagnosis of endocarditis, blood cultures must be persistently positive or the organisms recovered in several sporadically positive cultures must be proved to represent a single clone.[27]

Echocardiography

Inclusion of echocardiographic evidence of endocardial infection in these criteria recognizes the high sensitivity of two-dimensional echocardiography with color Doppler study, especially if biplane or multiplanar transesophageal echocardiography (TEE) and transthoracic echocardiography (TTE) are combined (see Chap. 15), and the relative infrequency of false-positive studies when experienced operators use specific definitions for vegetations.[28] TEE provides improved resolution and allows visualization of smaller vegetations compared with TTE (see Fig. 15-60). The sensitivity of TTE for the detection of vegetations, even with the use of harmonic imaging and other modern techniques, in patients with NVE is approximately 45% to 65%, whereas that of TEE in these patients is 85% to 95%. The likelihood of a false-negative study can be reduced to 5% to 10% if TEE is repeated.[15] TEE is the preferred approach in patients in whom TTE is technically suboptimal and is the

procedure of choice for imaging of the pulmonic valve and patients with suspected PVE.[28,29] Among patients with PVE, the diagnostic sensitivity of TTE is 15% to 45%. In contrast, the sensitivity of TEE for detection of signs of PVE ranges from 82% to 96% with mechanical or bioprosthetic devices in the aortic or mitral position. Thus, the highly sensitive TEE helps preclude the diagnosis of IE when the clinical suspicion is low; when the clinical suspicion is high, even these studies cannot exclude the diagnosis or need for treatment.[28] When initial TEE is normal and the clinical suspicion of IE remains, repeating TEE in 7 to 10 days is advocated.[15,30]

The American Heart Association (AHA) and the American College of Cardiology (ACC) guidelines recommend echocardiographic evaluation in all patients with suspected IE (see Table 67G-2).[15,30a] Echocardiography should not be used as a screening test for IE in unselected patients with positive blood cultures or in evaluating patients with fevers of unknown origin when the clinical probability of IE is low.[28,29] A decision analysis evaluation assessed the use of echocardiography to make the diagnosis and to initiate treatment of NVE in patients with bacteremia; the study suggests that, assuming the diagnostic enhancement of TEE over TTE is 15%, the most cost-effective strategies are as follows: (1) if prior probability of IE is less than 2%, treat for bacteremia without echocardiography; (2) if prior probability is 2% to 4%, use TTE; and (3) if prior probability is 5% to 45%, use TEE initially in lieu of TTE. If the prior probability of IE is greater than 45%, therapy for IE without echocardiography is cost-effective, although imaging is preferred to evaluate for complications and other risks. The approach for use of echocardiography advocated by the AHA is outlined in **Figure 67-5**. The ACC 2007 appropriateness criteria for transthoracic and transesophageal echocardiography also endorse TEE as a highly appropriate initial study to aid in the management of patients with a moderate or high pretest probability of IE.[31]

Studies suggest that among patients with a high prior probability of NVE, data derived from TEE rarely alter the decisions to treat for endocarditis based on the clinical presentation and TTE. Exceptions to this, when TEE provides pivotal information, include when TTE is technically inadequate, when PVE is suspected, and when there is S. aureus or enterococcal bacteremia. In patients with clinically uncomplicated catheter-associated S. aureus bacteremia, in whom the risk of IE ranges from 6% to 23%, use of TEE to seek vegetations and to determine the duration of antibiotic therapy (4 to 6 weeks versus 2 weeks, i.e., treatment for IE or not) is more cost-effective and less morbid than empiric selection of either treatment duration.

Despite the sensitivity of TEE in detecting vegetations in patients with proven IE, echocardiography does not itself provide a definite diagnosis. Vegetations and valve dysfunction may be demonstrated, but determination of causality requires clinical or direct anatomic and microbiologic confirmation. In addition to noninfected vegetations, thickened valves, ruptured chordae or valves, valve calcification, and nodules may be mistaken for infected vegetations.

Establishing the Microbial Cause

A microbial cause of IE is established by recovering the infecting agent from the blood or by identifying it in vegetations or embolic material. In detecting the continuous bacteremia of IE, there is no advantage to obtaining blood cultures in relation to fever or from arterial blood. In patients who have not received prior antibiotics and who will ultimately have blood culture–positive IE, it is likely that 95% to 100% of all cultures obtained will be positive and that one of the first two cultures will be positive in at least 95% of patients. Prior antibiotic therapy is a major cause of blood culture–negative IE, particularly when the causative microorganism is highly antibiotic susceptible. After

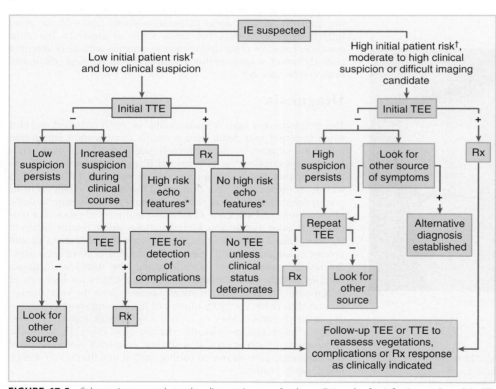

FIGURE 67-5 Schematic approach to the diagnostic use of echocardiography for infective endocarditis (IE). *High-risk echocardiographic features include large vegetations, valve insufficiency, suggestion of perivalvular extension, and ventricular dysfunction. †Patients with high initial risk include those with prosthetic heart valves, complex congenital heart disease, prior IE, new murmur, and heart failure. Rx indicates initiation of antibiotic therapy for IE. TEE = transesophageal echocardiography; TTE = transthoracic echocardiography. *(Reproduced from Bayer AS, Bolger AF, Taubert KA, et al: Diagnosis and management of infective endocarditis and its complications. Circulation 98:2936, 1998.)*

subtherapeutic antibiotic exposure, the time required for reversion to positive cultures is directly related to the duration of antimicrobial therapy and the susceptibility of the causative agent; days to a week or more may be required.

Obtaining Blood Culture Specimens

Three separate sets of blood cultures, each from a separate venipuncture, obtained during 24 hours, are recommended to evaluate patients with suspected endocarditis.[28] Each set should include a bottle containing an aerobic medium and one containing thioglycollate broth (anaerobic medium); at least 10 mL of blood should be placed into each bottle. If a clinically stable patient has received an antimicrobial agent during the past several weeks, it is prudent to delay therapy so that repeated cultures can be performed on successive days without further confounding by antibiotics. If endocarditis caused by fungi or unusual bacteria (*Legionella* species or *Bartonella* species) is suspected, the laboratory should be consulted for guidance regarding optimal culture techniques. Serologic tests can be used to make the presumptive diagnosis of endocarditis caused by *Brucella* species, *Legionella* species, *Bartonella* species, *C. burnetii*, *Aspergillus* species, or *Chlamydia* species. By use of special techniques, including PCR and antigen detection, these agents and others that are difficult to recover in blood culture can be identified in blood or vegetations.[28,32]

In evaluation of positive blood cultures, sustained bacteremia, which is typical of IE, should be distinguished from transient bacteremia. When several blood culture samples obtained during 24 hours or more are positive, the diagnosis of IE must be considered. The identity of the organism is also helpful in determining the intensity with which the diagnosis is entertained. Organisms can be divided into those that commonly or rarely cause IE and the intermediate-behaving organisms, such as enterococci and *S. aureus*, which, when in the blood, may or may not indicate IE. Finally, the presence or absence of alternative sources for the bacteremia aids in the assessment of bacteremia.

Laboratory Tests

Anemia, with normochromic normocytic red blood cell indices, low serum iron level, and low serum iron-binding capacity, is found in 70% to 90% of patients. Anemia worsens with increased duration of illness and thus in acute IE may be absent. In subacute IE, the white blood cell count is usually normal; in contrast, a leukocytosis with increased segmented granulocytes is common in acute IE. Thrombocytopenia occurs only rarely. The erythrocyte sedimentation rate is elevated (average approximately 55 mm/hr) in almost all patients with IE; the exceptions are those with CHF, renal failure, or disseminated intravascular coagulation. The C-reactive protein is elevated with mean concentrations ranging from 67 to 179 mg/liter, depending on the causative organism. The rheumatoid factor is increased in 50% of patients. Proteinuria and microscopic hematuria are noted in 50% of patients even when renal function remains normal. In patients with diffuse immune complex glomerulonephritis, circulating immune complexes are detectable and complement is depressed.

Imaging

ECHOCARDIOGRAPHY. In addition to its role in diagnosis, echocardiography (see Chap. 15) may identify complications or a need for surgery and provide information central to the management of IE. Valve dysfunction, obstructing vegetations, or evidence of decompensated CHF can be visualized and quantitated by echocardiography with Doppler study. Some degree of regurgitation by Doppler evaluation is almost universal early in the course of NVE and PVE and does not necessarily predict progressive hemodynamic deterioration. Extension of infection beyond the valve leaflet results in abscesses in the annulus or adjacent structures, mycotic aneurysms of the sinus of Valsalva or mitral valve, intracardiac fistulas, and purulent pericarditis. Myocardial abscesses are more readily detected by TEE than by TTE in patients with NVE or PVE (see Fig. 15-61). The sensitivity and specificity for abscess detection are 28% and 98% for TTE, compared with 87% and 95% for TEE. TEE is also more sensitive and accurate than TTE for recognizing subaortic invasive disease and valve perforations. Progressive CHF, new electrocardiographic conduction changes, changes in heart murmurs, and evidence of pericarditis warrant

prompt evaluation by TEE to plan care. To facilitate long-term care, valve morphology and function, vegetation size, and ventricular function should be determined by TTE at the conclusion of treatment.

OTHER IMAGING. Scintigraphy is insufficiently sensitive to be clinically useful. Magnetic resonance imaging and multislice computed tomography (CT) can define cardiac anatomy and supplement TEE evaluation (see Chaps. 18 and 19). Multislice CT with contrast media may be comparable to TEE in the diagnosis of IE and provide better paravalvular anatomic detail (see Fig. 19-22), as well as visualization of the coronary arteries.[33]

Treatment

Two major objectives must be achieved to treat IE effectively. The infecting microorganism in the vegetation must be eradicated. Failure to accomplish this results in relapse of infection. Also, invasive, destructive intracardiac and focal extracardiac complications of infection must be resolved if morbidity and mortality are to be minimized. The second objective often exceeds the capacity of effective antimicrobial therapy and requires cardiac or other surgical intervention.

Bacteria in vegetations multiply to population densities approaching 10^9 to 10^{10} organisms per gram of tissue, become metabolically dormant, and are difficult to eradicate. Clinical experience and animal model experiments suggest that optimal therapy requires bactericidal antibiotics or antibiotic combinations rather than bacteriostatic agents. To reach effective antibiotic concentrations in avascular vegetations by passive diffusion, high serum concentrations must be achieved. Parenteral antimicrobial therapy is used whenever feasible to achieve suitable serum antibiotic concentrations and to avoid the potentially erratic absorption of orally administered therapy. Treatment is continued for prolonged periods to ensure eradication of dormant microorganisms.

In selecting antimicrobial therapy for patients with IE, one must consider the MIC and the ability of potential agents to kill the causative organism. The MIC is the lowest concentration that inhibits growth, and the minimum bactericidal concentration (MBC) is the lowest concentration that decreases a standard inoculum of organisms 99.9% during 24 hours. For most streptococci and staphylococci, the MIC and MBC of penicillins, cephalosporins, or vancomycin are the same or differ by only a factor of 2 to 4. Organisms for which the MBC for these antibiotics is 10-fold or greater than the MIC are occasionally encountered. This phenomenon has been termed tolerance. Most of the tolerant strains are simply killed more slowly than nontolerant strains, and with prolonged incubation (48 hours) their MICs and MBCs are similar. Enterococci exhibit what superficially appears to be tolerance when tested against penicillins and vancomycin; however, these organisms are, in fact, not killed by these agents but are merely inhibited even after longer incubation times. Enterococci can be killed by the synergistic activity of selected penicillins or vancomycin and an aminoglycoside. A similar effect can be seen with these combinations against streptococci and staphylococci.

A synergistic bactericidal effect is required for optimal therapy for enterococcal endocarditis and has been used to achieve more effective therapy or effective short-course therapy for IE caused by other organisms. Tolerance in streptococci or staphylococci has not been correlated with decreased cure rates or delayed responses to treatment with penicillins, cephalosporins, or vancomycin and is not an indication for combination therapy. In fact, regimens are designed using the MICs of these organisms.[15]

The regimens recommended for the treatment of IE caused by specific organisms are designed to provide concentrations of antibiotics in serum and deep in vegetations that exceed the organism's MIC throughout most of the interval between doses. Although antibiotic concentrations in vegetations of patients with IE have been measured infrequently, the success of the recommended regimens suggests that this goal is achieved. Accordingly, for optimal therapy, it is important that the recommended regimens be followed carefully.

Antimicrobial Therapy for Specific Organisms

Optimal antimicrobial therapy, which is based on the susceptibility of the causative organism, should sterilize the vegetation while causing little or no toxicity. Antibiotic modifications may be needed to accommodate end-organ dysfunction, allergies, or anticipated toxicities. In anticipation of the possible need to modify therapy, the organism causing endocarditis should be saved until successful therapy has been completed. With the exception of staphylococcal endocarditis, the antimicrobial regimens recommended for the treatment of NVE and PVE are similar, although more prolonged treatment is often advised for PVE.[10,15]

Penicillin-Susceptible Viridans Streptococci or *Streptococcus gallolyticus (bovis)*

Multiple regimens provide highly effective, comparable therapy for patients with uncomplicated NVE caused by penicillin-susceptible streptococci and *S. gallolyticus* (**Table 67-6**). The 4-week regimens yield bacteriologic cure rates of 98%. The synergistic combination of penicillin or ceftriaxone plus gentamicin for 2 weeks is as effective in selected cases as treatment with the 4-week regimens.[15] The short-course combination regimens are recommended for patients who have uncomplicated NVE and who are not at increased risk for aminoglycoside toxicity. Patients with endocarditis caused by nutritionally variant organisms (*Granulicatella* species, *Abiotrophia defectiva, G. morbillorum*) and patients with PVE or endocarditis complicated by a mycotic aneurysm, myocardial abscess, perivalvular infection, or an extracardiac focus of infection should not be treated with a short-course regimen.

From 2% to 8% of viridans streptococci and *S. gallolyticus* causing endocarditis are highly resistant to streptomycin (MIC >2000 µg/mL) and are not killed synergistically by penicillin plus streptomycin but are killed synergistically by penicillin plus gentamicin. Consequently, gentamicin is recommended for use in the short-course combination regimen. Ceftriaxone 2 g once daily plus either gentamicin (3 mg/kg) or netilmicin (4 mg/kg) given as a single daily dose for 14 days has effectively treated endocarditis caused by penicillin-susceptible streptococci. The nutritionally variant organisms are generally more

resistant to penicillin than viridans streptococci are; thus, IE caused by these organisms is treated with regimens recommended for enterococcal endocarditis (see later); however, outcome remains unsatisfactory.

For the treatment of streptococcal endocarditis in patients with a history of urticarial or anaphylactic reactions to a penicillin or cephalosporin, vancomycin is recommended (see Table 67-6). Patients with other forms of penicillin allergy (delayed maculopapular rash) may be treated cautiously with the ceftriaxone regimens (see Table 67-6). For patients with PVE caused by penicillin-susceptible streptococci, treatment with 6 weeks of penicillin is recommended, with or without gentamicin 3 mg/kg/day in three divided doses given during the initial 2 weeks.[10,15]

RELATIVELY PENICILLIN RESISTANT STREPTOCOCCI. Treatment with 4 weeks of high-dose parenteral penicillin or ceftriaxone plus an aminoglycoside (primarily gentamicin for the reasons noted previously) during the initial 2 weeks is recommended for endocarditis caused by streptococci with MICs for penicillin between >0.1 and 0.5 µg/mL (**Table 67-7**). Patients who cannot tolerate penicillin because of immediate hypersensitivity reactions can be treated with vancomycin alone. For those with non-immediate penicillin hypersensitivity, effective treatment can be accomplished either with vancomycin alone or with the ceftriaxone-gentamicin regimen (see Table 67-7). NVE caused by streptococci that are "fully" resistant to penicillin (MIC >0.5 µg/mL; *Granulicatella* species, *Abiotrophia defectiva,* and *G. morbillorum*) or PVE caused by relatively or fully penicillin-resistant organisms should be treated for 6 weeks with penicillin or ceftriaxone plus gentamicin (doses per Table 67-7 or Table 67-8) or vancomycin alone.[15,34]

STREPTOCOCCUS PYOGENES, STREPTOCOCCUS PNEUMONIAE, AND GROUP B, C, AND G STREPTOCOCCI. Endocarditis caused by these streptococci has been either refractory to antibiotic therapy or associated with extensive valvular damage. Penicillin G in a dose of 3 million units intravenously every 4 hours for 4 weeks is recommended for the treatment of group A streptococcal endocarditis. Ceftriaxone and vancomycin, depending on the degree of penicillin allergy, are treatment alternatives (see Table 67-7).

IE caused by group G, C, or B streptococci is more difficult to treat than that caused by penicillin-susceptible viridans streptococci. Consequently, the addition of gentamicin to the first 2 weeks of a 4-week regimen using high doses of penicillin is often advocated (see Table 67-7). Early cardiac surgery to correct intracardiac complications is needed in almost half of these cases and may improve outcome.

In selecting treatment for pneumococcal IE, both antibiotic resistance in the infecting strain and coexisting meningitis are important considerations.[15] The treatment of IE caused by penicillin-susceptible pneumococci (MIC ≤0.1 µg/mL) with or without concomitant meningitis is penicillin G 4 million units intravenously every 4 hours, ceftriaxone 2 g

TABLE 67-6	Treatment of Native Valve Endocarditis Caused by Penicillin-Susceptible Viridans Streptococci and *Streptococcus gallolyticus (bovis)* (MIC <0.1 µg/mL)*	
ANTIBIOTIC	**DOSAGE AND ROUTE†**	**DURATION**
Aqueous penicillin G	12-18 million units/24 hr IV either continuously or every 4 hr in six equally divided doses	4 weeks
or		
Ceftriaxone	2 g once daily IV or IM	4 weeks
Aqueous penicillin G	12-18 million units/24 hr IV either continuously or every 4 hr in six equally divided doses	2 weeks
or		
Ceftriaxone	2 g once daily IV or IM	2 weeks
plus		
Gentamicin	3 mg/kg/day IM or IV as a single daily dose or divided in equal doses every 8 hr	2 weeks
Vancomycin	30 mg/kg/24 hr IV in two equally divided doses, not to exceed 2 g/24 hr unless serum levels are monitored	4 weeks

Three treatment options are recommended.

*For nutritionally variant organisms (*Granulicatella* species, *Gemella morbillorum, Abiotrophia defectiva*), see text and Table 67-8.

†Dosages given are for patients with normal renal function. Vancomycin and gentamicin doses must be reduced for treatment of patients with renal dysfunction. Gentamicin doses are calculated by ideal body weight (men = 50 kg + 2.3 kg per inch over 5 feet; women = 45.5 kg + 2.3 kg per inch over 5 feet). Vancomycin doses are based on actual body weight. Vancomycin doses are adjusted to yield 1-hour postinfusion serum concentration of 30 to 45 µg/mL and trough of 15 µg/mL. Gentamicin administered every 8 hours should be adjusted to achieve a 1-hour peak concentration of 3 to 3.5 µg/mL and a trough of <1.0 µg/mL. Lengthening of the dose-to-dose interval may be required to achieve these parameters in patients with renal dysfunction.

Modified from Baddour LM, Wilson WR, Bayer AS, et al: Infective endocarditis: Diagnosis, antimicrobial therapy, and management of complications. Circulation 111:3167, 2005.

TABLE 67-7	Treatment of Native Valve Endocarditis Caused by Strains of Viridans Streptococci and *Streptococcus gallolyticus (bovis)* Relatively Resistant to Penicillin G (MIC >0.1 µg/mL and <0.5 µg/mL)*	
ANTIBIOTIC	**DOSAGE AND ROUTE†**	**DURATION**
Aqueous penicillin G	24 million units/24 hr IV either continuously or every 4 hr in six equally divided doses	4 weeks
or		
Ceftriaxone	2 g once daily IV or IM	
plus		
Gentamicin	3 mg/kg/day IM or IV as a single daily dose or divided in equal doses every 8 hr	2 weeks
Vancomycin	30 mg/kg/24 hr IV in two equally divided doses, not to exceed 2 g/24 hr unless serum levels are monitored	4 weeks

Two treatment options are recommended.

*For streptococci with penicillin MIC > 0.5 µg/mL, see text and Table 67-8.

†Dosages are for patients with normal renal function; see Table 67-6 footnote.

Modified from Baddour LM, Wilson WR, Bayer AS, et al: Infective endocarditis: Diagnosis, antimicrobial therapy, and management of complications. Circulation 111:3167, 2005.

intravenously every 12 hours, or cefotaxime 4 g intravenously every 6 hours. In the absence of meningitis, these regimens are effective for IE caused by pneumococci that are relatively penicillin resistant (MIC 0.1 to 1.0 µg/mL). If IE, including that caused by relatively penicillin resistant isolates when complicated by meningitis, is caused by a penicillin-resistant (MIC = 2.0 µg/mL) or cefotaxime-resistant (MIC = 2.0 µg/mL) pneumococcus, therapy with ceftriaxone 2 g intravenously every 12 hours or cefotaxime 4 g intravenously every 6 hours plus vancomycin 15 mg/kg intravenously every 12 hours and rifampin is preferred. CHF rather than penicillin resistance is associated with mortality; thus, intervention early with cardiac surgery may be essential for an optimal outcome.

Enterococci

Optimal therapy for enterococcal endocarditis requires synergistic bactericidal interaction of an antimicrobial targeted against the bacterial cell wall (penicillin, ampicillin, or vancomycin) and an aminoglycoside that is able to exert a lethal effect (streptomycin or gentamicin). High-level resistance, defined as the inability of high concentrations of streptomycin (1000 or 2000 µg/mL) or gentamicin (500 to 2000 µg/mL) to inhibit the growth of an enterococcus, predicts the agent's inability to exert this lethal effect and to participate in the bactericidal synergistic interaction. Similarly, resistance to the cell wall–targeted agents indicates their inability to contribute to synergistic killing. The standard regimens recommended for the treatment of enterococcal endocarditis (**Table 67-8**) are designed to achieve bactericidal synergy and to result in cure rates of approximately 85%, compared with 40% with single-agent, nonbactericidal treatment. Isolates with high-level gentamicin resistance are not routinely high-level streptomycin resistant. In the absence of high-level resistance to streptomycin in a causative strain, streptomycin, 7.5 mg/kg intramuscularly or intravenously every 12 hours to achieve a 1-hour peak serum concentration of approximately 20 to 35 µg/mL and a trough of <10 µg/mL, can be substituted for gentamicin in the standard regimens. The streptomycin dose must be reduced if renal function is decreased. The vancomycin-aminoglycoside regimen (see Table 67-8) is recommended only for

patients allergic to penicillin. Desensitization to penicillin may be desirable when preexisting renal dysfunction favors avoidance of the potentially more nephrotoxic vancomycin-aminoglycoside combination. Therapy is administered for 4 to 6 weeks, with the longer course used to treat patients with PVE or IE that was symptomatic for more than 3 months or is complicated. Careful monitoring of patients clinically and of serum creatinine and aminoglycoside levels is required to prevent nephrotoxicity and ototoxicity.

Favorable outcomes with regimens using shortened courses of aminoglycosides suggest that the aminoglycoside component of combination therapy can be abbreviated if toxicity becomes significant. Of 93 patients treated for enterococcal IE (66 with NVE, 27 with PVE), 75 (81%) were cured, 15 (16%) died, and 3 (3%) relapsed. Cure was achieved with a median duration of cell wall–active antimicrobial therapy and aminoglycoside therapy of 42 and 15 days, respectively. In 39 of the patients who were cured, aminoglycosides were administered for 21 days or less. Experimental data and limited clinical data suggest that double beta-lactam antibiotic therapy (ceftriaxone or cefotaxime plus ampicillin) may be bactericidal and provide a nonnephrotoxic alternative for treatment of E. faecalis infection.[15,35]

Enterococci causing endocarditis must be tested for high-level resistance to both streptomycin and gentamicin and susceptibility to penicillin, ampicillin, and vancomycin (**Table 67-9**). High-level resistance to gentamicin predicts resistance to all other aminoglycosides except streptomycin. With use of these data, an attempt should be made to design a regimen containing a cell wall–active agent to which the isolate is susceptible plus gentamicin or streptomycin, depending on the absence of high-level resistance. If a bactericidal synergistic regimen is not feasible, an alternative treatment plus possible surgery should be considered (see Table 67-9).[15,17]

TABLE 67-8	Standard Therapy for Endocarditis Caused by Enterococci*	
ANTIBIOTIC	**DOSAGE AND ROUTE†**	**DURATION**
Aqueous penicillin G	18-30 million units/24 hr IV given continuously or every 4 hr in six equally divided doses	4-6 weeks
plus		
Gentamicin	1 mg/kg IM or IV every 8 hr	4-6 weeks
Ampicillin	12 g/24 hr IV given continuously or every 4 hr in six equally divided doses	4-6 weeks
plus		
Gentamicin	1 mg/kg IM or IV every 8 hr	4-6 weeks
Vancomycin‡	30 mg/kg/24 hr IV in two equally divided doses not to exceed 2 g/24 hr unless serum levels are monitored	4-6 weeks
plus		
Gentamicin	1 mg/kg IM or IV every 8 hr	4-6 weeks

Three treatment options are recommended.
*All enterococci causing endocarditis must be tested for antimicrobial susceptibility for selection of optimal therapy. These regimens are for treatment of endocarditis caused by enterococci that are susceptible to penicillin, ampicillin, or vancomycin and not highly resistant to gentamicin. These may also be used for treatment of endocarditis caused by penicillin-resistant (MIC > 0.5 µg/mL) viridans streptococci and nutritionally variant organisms or enterococcal prosthetic valve endocarditis.
†Dosages are for patients with normal renal function; see Table 67-6 footnote.
‡For patients allergic to penicillin or ampicillin. Alternatively, desensitize to penicillin. For enterococcal IE, cephalosporins are not alternatives to penicillin or ampicillin in penicillin-allergic patients.
Modified from Baddour LM, Wilson WR, Bayer AS, et al: Infective endocarditis: Diagnosis, antimicrobial therapy, and management of complications. Circulation 111:3167, 2005.

TABLE 67-9	Strategy to Select Therapy for Enterococcal Endocarditis Caused by Strains Resistant to Components of the Standard Regimen

I. Ideal therapy includes a cell wall–active agent plus an effective aminoglycoside to achieve bactericidal synergy (see text)
II. Cell wall–active antimicrobial
  A. Determine MIC for ampicillin and vancomycin; test for beta-lactamase production (nitrocefin test)
  B. If ampicillin and vancomycin susceptible, use ampicillin
  C. If ampicillin resistant (MIC ≥16 µg/mL) and vancomycin susceptible, use vancomycin
  D. If beta-lactamase produced, use vancomycin or consider ampicillin-sulbactam
  E. If ampicillin resistant and resistant to vancomycin (MIC > 8 µg/mL) and teicoplanin* (MIC ≥ 8 µg/mL), see IV C, D†
III. Aminoglycoside to be used with cell wall–active antimicrobial
  A. If no high-level resistance to streptomycin (MIC < 1000 or 2000 µg/mL) or gentamicin (MIC < 500-2000 µg/mL), use gentamicin or streptomycin
  B. If high-level resistance to gentamicin (MIC > 500-2000 µg/mL), test streptomycin; if no high-level resistance to streptomycin, use streptomycin (see IV B)
  C. If high-level resistance to gentamicin and streptomycin, omit aminoglycoside therapy; use prolonged therapy (8-12 wk) with cell wall–active antimicrobial if the organism is susceptible (see II A-E) or alternative therapy (see IV C, D, E)†
IV. Alternative regimens and approaches (use with consultative assistance of infectious disease specialist)
  A. Single-drug therapy (see III C) and possible surgical intervention
  B. Consider ampicillin, vancomycin (or teicoplanin), streptomycin based on absence of high-level resistance
  C. Consider quinupristin-dalfopristin therapy for infective endocarditis caused by susceptible Enterococcus faecium and surgical intervention
  D. Consider linezolid therapy for E. faecalis or E. faecium with or without surgical intervention
  E. Daptomycin active in vitro against vancomycin-resistant enterococci but few clinical data for this treatment

*Not approved by the Food and Drug Administration for use in the United States.
†See Stevens MP, Edmond MB: Endocarditis due to vancomycin-resistant enterococci: Case report and review of the literature. Clin Infect Dis 41:1134, 2005.
MIC = minimum inhibitory concentration.

Staphylococci

ANTIBIOTIC RESISTANCE. In excess of 90% of *S. aureus* and coagulase-negative staphylococci, whether acquired in the hospital or community, produce beta-lactamase and thus are resistant to penicillin, ampicillin, and the ureidopenicillins. Penicillin-resistant *S. aureus* can be further subdivided into isolates that are either methicillin susceptible, that is, susceptible to penicillinase-resistant beta-lactam antibiotics (nafcillin, oxacillin, cloxacillin, and cefazolin), or methicillin-resistant, that is, resistant to all beta-lactam antibiotics but susceptible, with rare exceptions, to vancomycin, teicoplanin (not approved for use in the United States), and daptomycin. Previously, the majority of *S. aureus* infections were caused by methicillin-susceptible isolates. Currently, methicillin-resistant *S. aureus* (MRSA) have become a common cause of staphylococcal infections that are nosocomial or community acquired (both health care associated and not health care associated). Accordingly, empiric therapy for suspected *S. aureus* IE should be effective against MRSA. Coagulase-negative staphylococci causing community-acquired infections are frequently methicillin susceptible, whereas those causing nosocomial IE are commonly methicillin resistant. Methicillin-resistant coagulase-negative staphylococci may not always phenotypically express this resistance (a property called heteroresistance) and require special testing. Most methicillin-resistant strains of *S. aureus* and coagulase-negative staphylococci remain susceptible to vancomycin, teicoplanin, and daptomycin. *S. aureus* and coagulase-negative staphylococci with reduced susceptibility (and occasionally overt resistance) to vancomycin, teicoplanin, and daptomycin have emerged as pathogens.[36] Reduced susceptibility to vancomycin among MRSA is manifested as vancomycin intermediate *S. aureus* (VISA, MIC 4 to 16 µg/mL) or heteroresistant vancomycin intermediate *S. aureus* (hVISA). In hVISA, although the MIC suggests that the isolate is vancomycin susceptible (MIC ≤2.0 µg/mL), there are subpopulations that require higher concentrations for inhibition and killing.[37] VISA and hVISA may emerge during vancomycin treatment and result in failure.[38] MRSA that develop reduced susceptibility to vancomycin may be nonsusceptible to daptomycin. Thus, the antibiotic susceptibility of MRSA recovered from patients who have failed vancomycin therapy must be carefully reassessed.

Among staphylococci killed by beta-lactam antibiotics or vancomycin, the bactericidal effects of these agents can be enhanced by aminoglycosides. Combinations of semisynthetic penicillinase-resistant penicillins or vancomycin with rifampin do not result in predictable bactericidal synergism; nevertheless, rifampin has unique activity against staphylococcal infections that involve foreign material and is included in regimens for staphylococcal PVE.[39]

STAPHYLOCOCCAL NATIVE VALVE ENDOCARDITIS. The semisynthetic penicillinase-resistant penicillins are the preferred treatment of endocarditis caused by methicillin-susceptible staphylococci. When patients have a non-immediate penicillin allergy, a first-generation cephalosporin can be used. Treatment with beta-lactam antibiotics plus gentamicin has not increased the cure rates for staphylococcal endocarditis, although this combination has modestly accelerated the eradication of staphylococci in vegetations and in the blood.[39] The potential benefit from adding gentamicin to beta-lactam therapy for *S. aureus* IE, even when it is limited to the initial 3 to 5 days of therapy, however, is offset by nephrotoxicity. Thus, routine use of this combination is not advised.[36,40] The role for combination therapy is less well defined in NVE caused by coagulase-negative staphylococci.

In IV drug addicts, methicillin-susceptible *S. aureus* endocarditis that is uncomplicated and limited to the right-sided heart valves has been effectively treated with 2 weeks of semisynthetic penicillinase-resistant penicillin (but not vancomycin) given alone or in combination with gentamicin 1 mg/kg intravenously or intramuscularly every 8 hours (normal renal function). Patients with right-sided *S. aureus* who develop peripheral signs suggesting left-sided infection or with other localized infection are not candidates for abbreviated therapy. Vancomycin or daptomycin (6 mg/kg once daily) for 4 weeks is recommended when right-sided IE is caused by MRSA.[15,36]

Left-sided NVE caused by MRSA requires treatment with vancomycin (**Table 67-10**) or daptomycin. Vancomycin doses to achieve trough serum concentrations of 15 to 20 µg/mL are recommended even though this may be associated with nephrotoxicity.[41] Vancomycin killing of MRSA with a vancomycin MIC of 1.5 to 2.0 µg/mL may be suboptimal even with aggressive dosing. Accordingly, in this setting, some experts prefer treatment with daptomycin (doses from 6 to 10 mg/kg daily, normal renal function) even though this indication is not approved by the Food and Drug Administration. Bacteremia in MRSA IE often persists for 5 to 7 days in spite of treatment.[36,38] With vancomycin therapy, persistent bacteremia or later relapse may be accompanied by emergence of reduced susceptibility (see earlier) and requires infectious disease consultation. Experience in treating MRSA IE with linezolid, although the isolates are usually susceptible, is limited. Teicoplanin (not available in the United States) is a possible alternative, but its efficacy is potentially less than that of vancomycin. Combining gentamicin with vancomycin to enhance activity against MRSA is associated with nephrotoxicity and is not recommended routinely.[15] The addition of rifampin to vancomycin for treatment of methicillin-resistant *S. aureus* NVE has not been beneficial.

STAPHYLOCOCCAL PROSTHETIC VALVE ENDOCARDITIS. *S. aureus* and coagulase-negative staphylococcal PVE should be treated with three antibiotics in combination (**Table 67-11**).[15,39] Rifampin provides unique antistaphylococcal activity when infection involves foreign bodies. However, rifampin-resistant staphylococci rapidly emerge when rifampin is used alone or in combination with only vancomycin or a beta-lactam antibiotic. Consequently, staphylococcal PVE is treated with two antimicrobials plus rifampin.[10,15,39]

For PVE caused by methicillin-resistant staphylococci, start treatment with vancomycin plus gentamicin and add rifampin after 2 or 3 days if the organism is susceptible to gentamicin. If the organism is resistant to gentamicin, an effective alternative antibiotic, such as another aminoglycoside or a quinolone, should be used in lieu of gentamicin.[10,15] Trimethoprim-sulfamethoxazole or linezolid could be considered also. For treatment of PVE caused by methicillin-susceptible staphylococci, a semisynthetic penicillinase-resistant penicillin should be substituted for vancomycin in the combination regimen (see Table 67-11). Because heteroresistance may confound detection of methicillin resistance in coagulase-negative staphylococci, these organisms should be considered methicillin resistant, particularly when PVE occurs during the initial postoperative year, until susceptibility is conclusively established.

Coagulase-negative staphylococcal PVE that occurs within the initial year after valve placement and *S. aureus* PVE are often complicated by perivalvular extension of infection. Their outcome is improved if early surgical intervention is combined with appropriate combination antimicrobial therapy.[12,13,15]

TABLE 67-10	**Treatment of Staphylococcal Endocarditis in the Absence of Prosthetic Material**	
ANTIBIOTIC	**DOSAGE AND ROUTE***	**DURATION**
Methicillin-susceptible staphylococci†		
Nafcillin or oxacillin	2 g IV every 4 hr	4-6 weeks
or		
Cefazolin	2 g IV every 8 hr	4-6 weeks
or		
Vancomycin	15 to 20 mg/kg actual body weight, IV every 8 to 12 hr	4-6 weeks
Methicillin-resistant staphylococci‡		
Vancomycin§	15 to 20 mg/kg actual body weight, IV every 8 to 12 hr	4-6 weeks

*Dosages are for patients with normal renal function; see Table 67-6 footnote.
†For treatment of endocarditis caused by penicillin-susceptible staphylococci (MIC ≤ 0.1 µg/mL), aqueous penicillin G 18-24 million units/24 hr) can be used for 4 to 6 weeks instead of nafcillin or oxacillin. Cefazolin or vancomycin may be used in selected penicillin-allergic patients contingent on degree of allergic response.
‡For staphylococcal infection, vancomycin target trough serum concentration is 15 to 20 µg/mL.
§If vancomycin MIC > 1.5 µg/mL, see text for daptomycin use.
Modified from Baddour LM, Wilson WR, Bayer AS, et al: Infective endocarditis: Diagnosis, antimicrobial therapy, and management of complications. Circulation 111:3167, 2005.

TABLE 67-11	Treatment of Staphylococcal Endocarditis in the Presence of a Prosthetic Valve or Other Prosthetic Material	
ANTIBIOTIC	**DOSAGE AND ROUTE***	**DURATION**
Regimen for methicillin-resistant staphylococci†		
Vancomycin‡	15 to 20 mg/kg actual body weight, IV every 8 to 12 hr	≥6 weeks
plus		
Rifampin	300 mg PO every 8 hr	≥6 weeks
and		
Gentamicin§	1.0 mg/kg IM or IV every 8 hr	2 weeks
Regimen for methicillin-susceptible staphylococci		
Nafcillin or oxacillin¶	2 g IV every 4 hr	≥6 weeks
plus		
Rifampin	300 mg PO every 8 hr	≥6 6weeks
and		
Gentamicin§	1.0 mg/kg IM or IV every 8 hr	2 weeks

*Dosages are for patients with normal renal function. See Table 67-6 footnote for gentamicin dosing.
†If vancomycin MIC >1.5 μg/mL, see text for daptomycin use.
‡For staphylococcal infection, vancomycin trough serum concentration is 15 to 20 μg/mL.
§Use during initial 2 weeks of treatment. If strain is gentamicin resistant, see text for alternatives.
¶Cefazolin 2 g IV every 8 hours can be used in lieu of these agents in patients with non–immediate-type penicillin allergy. Vancomycin is used with immediate-type allergy.
Modified from Baddour LM, Wilson WR, Bayer AS, et al: Infective endocarditis: Diagnosis, antimicrobial therapy, and management of complications. Circulation 111:3167, 2005.

TABLE 67-12	Treatment of Endocarditis Caused by HACEK Microorganisms*	
ANTIBIOTIC	**DOSAGE AND ROUTE†**	**DURATION**
Ceftriaxone‡	2 g once daily IV or IM	4 weeks
or		
Ampicillin-sulbactam	12 g/24 hr IV given every 4 hr in six equally divided doses	4 weeks

*HACEK microorganisms are Haemophilus species, Aggregatibacter aphrophilus or actinomycetemcomitans, Cardiobacterium hominis, Eikenella corrodens, and Kingella species.
†Dosages are for those with normal renal function; see Table 67-6 footnote.
‡Cefotaxime or another third- or fourth-generation cephalosporin in comparable doses may be substituted for ceftriaxone. See text for treatment of patients unable to take beta-lactam antibiotics.
Modified from Baddour LM, Wilson WR, Bayer AS, et al: Infective endocarditis: Diagnosis, antimicrobial therapy, and management of complications. Circulation 111:3167, 2005.

Haemophilus species, *Aggregatibacter* (previously *Actinobacillus*) *actinomycetemcomitans, Cardiobacterium hominis, Eikenella corrodens,* and *Kingella* species (HACEK organisms)

HACEK organisms may produce beta-lactamase, resulting in ampicillin resistance. HACEK organisms are highly susceptible to third-generation cephalosporins; accordingly, these agents are recommended for treatment of NVE or PVE (**Table 67-12**).[15] Treatment with a fluoroquinolone has been recommended for patients who cannot tolerate a beta-lactam antibiotic.[15]

Other Pathogens

Recommendations for therapy of IE caused by unusual organisms are contained in the AHA Scientific Statement and the guidelines of the European Society of Cardiology.[15,42] Amphotericin desoxycholate or a less toxic liposomal amphotericin formulation, at full doses, often combined with 5-fluorocytosine, is recommended for treatment of *Candida* endocarditis. Although it is not of proven benefit, surgical intervention shortly after beginning of medical treatment is advised. Sporadic cases of *Candida* NVE and PVE have been successfully treated with caspofungin, a fungicidal echinocandin agent. Prolonged or indefinite oral azole therapy has been advocated for patients treated either medically or surgically.[15]

Many corynebacteria (diphtheroids) causing IE remain susceptible to penicillin, vancomycin, and aminoglycosides. Strains susceptible

to aminoglycosides are killed synergistically by penicillin in combination with an aminoglycoside. *Corynebacterium jeikeium,* although often resistant to penicillin and aminoglycosides, is killed by vancomycin. NVE or PVE caused by *Corynebacterium* species can be treated with the combination of penicillin plus an aminoglycoside or vancomycin, contingent on the susceptibilities of the causative strain.

The antibiotic susceptibility of Enterobacteriaceae (*Escherichia coli, Klebsiella, Enterobacter, Serratia, Salmonella,* and *Proteus* species) and *P. aeruginosa* is unpredictable. IE caused by these organisms is treated with high doses of a highly active beta-lactam plus full doses of an aminoglycoside (i.e., gentamicin 1.7 mg/kg every 8 hours).[15] If *P. aeruginosa* is susceptible, the preferred treatment of IE is tobramycin (8 mg/kg/day intravenously once daily with peak and trough serum concentrations of 15 to 20 μg/mL and <2 μg/mL, respectively) plus piperacillin, ceftazidime, or cefipime.[15]

C. burnetii IE is difficult to eradicate. Treatment for at least 4 years using doxycycline (100 mg twice daily) combined with a quinolone has been advocated. Treatment with doxycycline combined with hydroxychloroquine for 18 to 48 months (mean, 31 months; median, 26 months) may be more effective than longer courses of doxycycline plus a quinolone. Surgery is important in effective treatment.

CULTURE-NEGATIVE ENDOCARDITIS. Special studies must be performed to diagnose IE caused by fastidious bacteria and other organisms (see Obtaining Blood Culture Specimens) and to distinguish these from noninfectious mimics of IE (marantic endocarditis, atrial myxoma, antiphospholipid antibody syndrome, acute rheumatic fever, hypernephroma, carcinoid syndrome, and so on). Clinical and epidemiologic clues, such as acute versus subacute presentation, partial response to prior antibiotics, or presence and duration of prosthetic valve, are important in designing therapy. Recommended therapy for patients with suspected NVE who received confounding antibiotic therapy is either ampicillin-sulbactam plus gentamicin (3 mg/kg/day) or vancomycin plus gentamicin and ciprofloxacin; for those with suspected PVE, it is vancomycin plus gentamicin, cefepime, and rifampin.[15] For patients with suspected IE in whom negative cultures are not confounded by prior antibiotics, fastidious organisms must be considered. *Bartonella* species and *C. burnetii* may be the most common of these causes. Suspected *Bartonella* IE is treated with 6 weeks of ceftriaxone plus gentamicin (1 mg/kg every 8 hours for at least 2 weeks) with an additional 6 weeks of doxycycline (100 mg intravenously or orally every 12 hours) if diagnostic studies are confirmatory (see Diagnosis).[43] For those who do not fully respond to empiric antimicrobial therapy, surgical intervention both as therapy and to obtain vegetations for a detailed microbiologic, PCR, and pathologic examination is recommended (see Diagnosis).

Timing the Initiation of Antimicrobial Therapy

Cost-containment pressures frequently result in initiation of antimicrobial therapy for suspected endocarditis immediately after blood culture specimens have been obtained. This practice is appropriate for patients with acute IE that is highly destructive and rapidly progressive and for those presenting with hemodynamic decompensation requiring urgent surgical intervention. Precipitous initiation of therapy in hemodynamically stable patients with suspected subacute endocarditis does not prevent early complications and may, by compromising subsequent blood cultures, obscure the etiologic diagnosis. In the latter patients, particularly in those who have received antibiotics recently, delay of antibiotic therapy briefly pending the results of the initial blood cultures is prudent. If these cultures are not immediately positive, this delay provides an important opportunity to perform additional blood cultures without the confounding effect of empiric treatment.

MONITORING THERAPY FOR ENDOCARDITIS. Patients must be carefully monitored during therapy and for several months thereafter. Failure of antimicrobial therapy, myocardial or metastatic abscess, emboli, hypersensitivity to antimicrobial agents, and other complications of therapy (catheter-related infection, thrombophlebitis) or intercurrent illness may be manifested by persistent or recurrent fever. Adverse reactions (fever, rash, neutropenia, and hepatic or renal toxicity) occur in 33% of patients treated for IE with beta-lactam antimicrobials. The serum concentration of vancomycin or aminoglycosides should be measured periodically and doses adjusted to ensure optimal therapy and to avoid adverse events.

Renal function should be monitored in patients receiving these two anti-microbials, and the complete blood count should be monitored in patients receiving high-dose beta-lactam antibiotics or vancomycin. Repeated blood cultures should be performed during the initial days of therapy or if fever persists or recurs to determine whether the bacteremia has been controlled and to detect relapse or new infections.

OUTPATIENT ANTIMICROBIAL THERAPY. Technical advances allowing safe administration of complex antimicrobial regimens combined with well-developed home care systems that provide supplies and monitor treatment make outpatient treatment feasible. However, only patients who have responded to initial therapy and are free of fever, who are not experiencing threatening complications, who will be compliant with therapy, and who have a home situation that is physically suitable should be considered for outpatient treatment. Because most threatening complications of IE occur during the initial 2 weeks of therapy, some clinicians have suggested that treatment during this period be administered in the inpatient setting or an outpatient setting that provides daily physician oversight. Patients must be instructed to seek advice promptly on encountering unexpected or untoward clinical events and to have regular physician supervision and laboratory monitoring. Outpatient therapy must not result in compromises leading to suboptimal treatment.

Surgical Treatment of Intracardiac Complications

INDICATIONS FOR SURGICAL INTERVENTION. Cardiac surgical intervention has an important role in the treatment of infection that is unresponsive to antibiotics as well as the intracardiac complications of endocarditis (see Table 67G-3). Retrospective data suggest that mortality is unacceptably high when these aspects of IE are treated medically, whereas mortality is reduced when treatment combines antibiotics and surgical intervention.[44,45] The indications for cardiac surgery evolve from these experiences (see Table 67G-3). Surgical intervention for these indications has not been evaluated in randomized prospective trials. However, most retrospective studies of patients with left-sided IE, particularly NVE, wherein the analysis of outcome of surgical versus medical treatment is adjusted for predictors of mortality and the presence of surgical indications, demonstrate improved survival rates with surgery. Benefit of surgery measured at hospital discharge is apparent in those with the most urgent need for intervention and among all patients if the cohort is observed for at least 6 months.[45-49]

Congestive Heart Failure

Medical therapy for NVE that is complicated by moderate to severe (New York Heart Association [NYHA] Class III and IV) CHF related to new or worsening valvular dysfunction results in mortality rates of 50% to 90% versus 20% to 40% for a similar group of patients treated with antibiotics and cardiac surgery.[44] In an analysis controlled for bias against operating on severely ill patients with NVE, surgery on those with moderate to severe CHF was associated with a significantly improved 6-month survival compared with medical treatment.[45] Survival rates among surgically treated patients with PVE complicated by valvular dysfunction and CHF are 45% to 85%; in contrast, few patients with these complications are alive at 6 months when they are treated with antibiotics alone.[10] Patients with aortic valve dysfunction require surgery on a more urgent basis when CHF supervenes. Severe mitral valve insufficiency, nevertheless, results in inexorable CHF and ultimately requires surgical intervention. Echocardiography indicating significant valvular regurgitation during the initial week of endocarditis treatment does not reliably predict the patients who require valve replacement during active endocarditis. Alternatively, despite the absence of significant valvular regurgitation on early echocardiography, marked CHF may still develop. Thus, decisions about surgical intervention should be based on careful serial monitoring.

Unstable Prostheses

Dehiscence of an infected prosthetic valve is a manifestation of paravalvular infection and often results in hemodynamically significant valvular dysfunction. Surgical intervention is recommended for PVE patients with these complications. The risk of invasive infection is increased among patients with onset of PVE within the year after valve implantation and in those with infection of aortic valve prostheses, endocarditis, and PVE caused by invasive antimicrobial-resistant organisms. Clinically stable patients who have overtly unstable and hypermobile prostheses, a finding indicative of dehiscence in excess of 40% of the circumference, are likely to experience progressive valve instability and warrant urgent surgery. Occasional patients with PVE caused by noninvasive, highly antibiotic-susceptible organisms (e.g., streptococci), despite a favorable clinical course, experience minor valve dehiscence without prosthesis instability or hemodynamic deterioration. Surgical treatment of these patients can be deferred unless clear indications arise.

Uncontrolled Infection or Unavailable Effective Antimicrobial Therapy

Surgical intervention has improved the outcome of IE when maximal antibiotic therapy fails to eradicate infection. Surgical intervention is recommended for fungal PVE or NVE, particularly with intracardiac complications; endocarditis caused by some gram-negative bacilli (e.g., *P. aeruginosa*, *Burkholderia cepacia*, *Brucella* species); and enterococcal endocarditis caused by a strain resistant to synergistic bactericidal therapy when antibiotic therapy is failing. Perivalvular invasive infection is in some instances a form of ineradicable infection. Relapse of PVE after optimal antimicrobial therapy reflects invasive disease or the difficulty in eradicating infection involving foreign devices and merits surgical intervention. In contrast, patients with uncomplicated NVE who relapse, unless infected with a highly resistant microorganism, are often treated again with intensified, prolonged antimicrobial therapy.

S. AUREUS PROSTHETIC VALVE ENDOCARDITIS. Crude mortality rates for *S. aureus* PVE treated medically range from 48% to 73% as contrasted to 28% to 48% for treatment with antibiotics plus surgery.[9,12,13] Assessment of management strategy is undoubtedly distorted by selection bias, the most ill patients often being denied surgery. Among 33 cases of *S. aureus* PVE analyzed in a multivariate model to adjust for confounding variables, the presence of intracardiac complications was associated with a 13.7-fold increased risk of death, and surgical intervention during active disease was accompanied by a 20-fold reduction in mortality. Data suggest that early surgical treatment can improve outcome of patients with *S. aureus* PVE and intracardiac complications.[9,12] Some patients younger than 50 years, with an American Society of Anesthesiologists score of 3 and neither intracardiac nor central nervous system complications, may do well with medical therapy.[13]

PERIVALVULAR INVASIVE INFECTION. Perivalvular abscess or intracardiac fistula formation occurs in 10% to 14% of patients with NVE and 45% to 60% of those with PVE. Persistent, otherwise unexplained fever despite appropriate antimicrobial therapy or pericarditis in patients with aortic valve endocarditis suggests infection extending beyond the valve leaflet. New-onset and persistent electrocardiographic conduction abnormalities, although not a sensitive indicator of perivalvular infection (28% to 53%), are relatively specific (85% to 90%). TEE is superior to TTE for detection of invasive infection in patients with NVE and PVE. Abscesses suspected but not detected by initial and repeated TEE may be detected by cardiac magnetic resonance imaging or multislice CT scans. Cardiac catheterization adds little to these imaging studies and is not recommended unless coronary angiography is needed.

Cardiac surgery should be considered to débride abscesses, allowing eradication of uncontrolled infection, and to reconstruct cardiac structures, restoring hemodynamics and alleviating CHF. Sporadic patients with small, structurally insignificant abscesses in which the cavity is open to the circulatory stream have been treated medically.[15]

LEFT-SIDED S. AUREUS ENDOCARDITIS. Because this infection is difficult to control, highly destructive, and associated with high mortality (25% to 47%), some investigators have suggested that these patients should be considered for surgical treatment when the response to antimicrobial therapy is not prompt and complete. Patients with *S. aureus* left-sided NVE and vegetations that are visible by TTE (versus requiring TEE) are at increased risk for arterial emboli and death and thus should be considered for surgery. IV drug abusers with *S. aureus* endocarditis limited to the tricuspid or pulmonary valves often experience prolonged fever during antimicrobial therapy; nevertheless, most respond to antimicrobial therapy and do not require surgery.

UNRESPONSIVE CULTURE-NEGATIVE ENDOCARDITIS. Patients who have culture-negative endocarditis and do not respond to empiric anti-microbial therapy, particularly those with PVE, should be considered for surgical intervention. If endocarditis is not marantic, persistent fever likely represents either unrecognized perivalvular infection or ineffective antimicrobial therapy. Surgery may help clarify the cause as well as facilitate treatment.

LARGE VEGETATIONS (>10 MM) AND THE PREVENTION OF SYSTEMIC EMBOLI. Systemic embolization is increased in patients with vegetations larger than 10 mm versus those with smaller or undetectable vegetations (33% to 37% versus 19%). In addition, mitral valve location and *S. aureus* infection increase the risk of an embolic event.[25] Although a relation may exist between vegetation characteristics—including size, mobility, and extent (number of leaflets involved)—and embolic complications, the implications for surgical intervention are not clear. The recommendation for valve surgery to prevent arterial emboli based on vegetation characteristics or after two major arterial emboli can be questioned.[15,17,42]

In deciding to intervene with cardiac surgery to prevent arterial emboli, many factors must be considered carefully. The rate of systemic or cerebral emboli in patients with NVE and PVE decreases rapidly during the course of effective antibiotic therapy. Thus, maximum benefit requires early surgery.[25,42] Also, it is not clear that valve replacement reduces the frequency of systemic emboli. The morbidity and mortality caused by cerebral and coronary emboli, the major events to be prevented, must be compared with the immediate and long-term risks of valve replacement or, if feasible, vegetectomy and valve repair. The sum of the clinical findings, risk of embolization, and other surgically correctable intracardiac complications may be sufficient to justify surgery in spite of these immediate and remote hazards. However, only on rare occasions is vegetation size alone or a prior systemic embolus a sufficient independent indication for surgical intervention.[15,28,42]

REPAIR OF INTRACARDIAC DEFECTS

Timing of Surgical Intervention

When endocarditis is complicated by valvular regurgitation and significant CHF, surgical intervention before the development of severe intractable hemodynamic dysfunction is recommended, regardless of the duration of antimicrobial therapy.[15,44,45,50] Postoperative mortality correlates with the severity of preoperative hemodynamic dysfunction; consequently, this approach is justified.[15] In patients who have valvular dysfunction and in whom infection is controlled and cardiac function is compensated, surgery may be delayed until antimicrobial therapy has been completed.

More specific recommendations for timing of surgery have been presented.[44] Strong clinical evidence suggests emergent (same day) surgery for acute aortic regurgitation with mitral valve preclosure, acute severe mitral or aortic valve regurgitation with pulmonary edema or cardiogenic shock, sinus of Valsalva rupture into the right side of the heart, and fistula to the pericardial sac; urgent (1 to 2 days) surgery for valve obstruction, unstable prosthesis, acute aortic or mitral regurgitation with CHF (NYHA Class III to IV), septal perforation, perivalvular extension of infection, and no effective antimicrobial therapy; and early elective surgery for progressive paravalvular regurgitation, valve dysfunction and persistent fever, and fungal IE.[42,44]

It may be desirable to delay surgical intervention to avoid worsening of neurologic status or death in patients who have sustained recent neurologic injury. Among patients who have had a nonhemorrhagic embolic stroke, exacerbation of cerebral dysfunction occurs during cardiac surgery in 44% of cases when the interval between the stroke and surgery is 7 days or less but decreases progressively with time to 10% or less when more than 2 weeks has elapsed. After hemorrhagic intracerebral events, the risk for neurologic worsening or death with cardiac surgery persists at 20% even after 1 month.[51] Thus, when the response of IE to antimicrobial therapy and hemodynamic status permit, delay of cardiac surgery for 2 to 3 weeks after a significant embolic infarct and at least a month after intracerebral hemorrhage (with prior repair of a mycotic aneurysm) has been recommended.[42,51] Alternatively, in patients at immediate risk of death in the absence of cardiac surgery, operation during the early days after cerebral infarction has been advocated as lifesaving in spite of potential neurologic risk.[42] Urgent surgery should not be delayed by the fortuitous discovery of an asymptomatic cerebral infarct, nor is routine screening for asymptomatic infarcts recommended as a guide for timing surgery.

Duration of Antimicrobial Therapy After Surgical Intervention

Inflammatory changes and bacteria visible with Gram stain have been found in vegetations removed from patients who had successfully completed standard recommended antibiotic therapy for IE: 29 of 53 (55%) still taking antibiotics; 7 of 15 (47%) without antibiotics for less than a month; and 4 of 18 (22%) without antibiotics for 1 to 6 months. Cultures of these vegetations yielded bacteria in 5, 0, and 1 instances, respectively. If vegetation cultures are negative, neither visible bacteria nor PCR detection of bacterial DNA indicates that antimicrobial therapy has failed or that a full course of antibiotic therapy is needed postoperatively. The duration of antimicrobial therapy after surgery depends on the length of preoperative therapy, the antibiotic susceptibility of the causative organism, the presence of paravalvular invasive infection, and the culture status of the vegetation. In general, for uncomplicated NVE caused by relatively antibiotic-responsive organisms with negative cultures of operative specimens, the duration of preoperative plus postoperative therapy should at least equal a full course of recommended therapy with perhaps 2 weeks or less of therapy postoperatively.[52] For patients with prostheses sewn into a débrided abscess cavity or with positive intraoperative cultures, a full course of therapy should be given postoperatively.[15] Patients with PVE should receive a full course of antimicrobial therapy postoperatively when the causative organism is seen or cultured in resected material.

Treatment of Extracardiac Complications

SPLENIC ABSCESS. Three percent to 5% of patients with IE develop a splenic abscess.[15] Although splenic defects can be identified by ultrasonography and computed tomography, these tests in isolation usually cannot reliably discriminate between abscess and the far more common infarct. Persistent fever and progressive enlargement of the lesion during antimicrobial therapy suggest that it is an abscess. Successful therapy for splenic abscesses requires drainage percutaneously or a splenectomy.[15,28,42] If possible, abscesses in the spleen should be treated effectively before valve replacement surgery; alternatively, splenectomy should be performed as soon thereafter as surgical risks permit.[28,42]

MYCOTIC ANEURYSMS AND SEPTIC ARTERITIS. Two percent to 10% of patients with IE have mycotic aneurysms, and half of these involve cerebral vessels. Cerebral mycotic aneurysms occur at the branch points in cerebral vessels and are generally located distally over the cerebral cortex, particularly in branches of the middle cerebral artery. Aneurysms arise either from occlusion of vessels by septic emboli with secondary arteritis and vessel wall destruction or from injury caused by bacteremia seeding the vessel wall through the vasa vasorum. *S. aureus* is commonly implicated in the former mechanism and viridans streptococci in the latter. Devastating intracranial hemorrhage is the initial clinical event in many patients with mycotic aneurysms. Focal deficits from embolic events, persistent focal headache, unexplained neurologic deterioration, or cerebrospinal fluid with erythrocytes and xanthochromia may be premonitory. Magnetic resonance or spiral computed tomographic angiography, each of which has a 90% to 95% sensitivity for aneurysms >5 mm, has been recommended for patients experiencing premonitory symptoms, especially if cardiac surgery or anticoagulant therapy is planned.[28] Cerebral angiography is required to evaluate patients with suspected small (≤2 mm) aneurysms or intracerebral hemorrhage. Rupture or leakage may occur at any point before or during early antibiotic therapy or rarely later. Mortality is 80% with aneurysm rupture.

Unruptured mycotic aneurysms should be observed during antimicrobial therapy. Half of these may resolve.[28] If it is feasible anatomically, aneurysms that have ruptured should be repaired.[53] Surgery should be considered for a single aneurysm that enlarges during or after antimicrobial therapy. Anticoagulant therapy should be avoided in patients with a persisting mycotic aneurysm. There is no accurate estimation of risk for late rupture of persisting aneurysms. Prevailing opinion favors the resection of single aneurysms, particularly those larger than 7 mm, that persist after therapy whenever possible without serious neurologic injury.[53] The potential existence of occult aneurysms in patients without neurologic symptoms or in those who have had a nondiagnostic angiographic evaluation is not considered a contraindication to anticoagulant therapy after completion of antimicrobial therapy.

Extracranial mycotic aneurysms should be managed as outlined for cerebral aneurysms. Those that leak, that are expanding during therapy, or that persist after therapy should be repaired. Particular attention

CH
67

should be given to aneurysms that involve intra-abdominal arteries, rupture of which could result in life-threatening hemorrhage.[28]

ANTICOAGULANT THERAPY. Patients with PVE involving devices that would usually warrant maintenance anticoagulation are continued on careful anticoagulant therapy with either warfarin or heparin. Some investigators advise that anticoagulant therapy be withdrawn from patients with *S. aureus* PVE during the initial 2 weeks of treatment.[15] In the absence of an accepted indication, anticoagulation is not initiated as prophylaxis against IE-related thromboembolism in patients with PVE involving devices that do not usually require this therapy. Anticoagulant therapy in patients with NVE is limited to patients for whom there is a clear indication and no increased risk for intracranial hemorrhage. If central nervous system complications occur in patients who are receiving anticoagulant therapy, anticoagulation should be reversed immediately. In a randomized blinded trial, initiation of aspirin, 325 mg daily, did not reduce the risk of emboli and was likely associated with increased bleeding.[54] Data are inconclusive about the benefits or risks of continued aspirin in patients who were using this medication before having IE diagnosed.

Response to Therapy

Within a week after initiation of effective antimicrobial therapy, almost 70% of patients with NVE or PVE are afebrile, and 90% have defervesced by the end of the second week of treatment. Fever persists longer in patients with *S. aureus, P. aeruginosa,* or culture-negative IE as well as IE characterized by microvascular phenomena and major embolic complications. Persistence (or recurrence) of fever or a low percentage decline in C-reactive protein more than 10 days after initiation of antibiotic therapy identifies patients with increased mortality rates and with complications of infection or therapy.[55] These patients should be evaluated for intracardiac complications, focal extracardiac septic complications, intercurrent nosocomial infections, recurrent pulmonary emboli (patients with right-sided IE), drug-associated fever, additional underlying illnesses, and, if appropriate, in-hospital substance abuse. Blood cultures should be repeated and the antimicrobial susceptibility of the causative organism should be reevaluated. Fever attributed to the antimicrobial therapy may warrant revision of treatment if a suitable alternative is available. In the absence of effective alternative therapy, treatment can be continued despite drug fever if there is no significant end-organ toxicity. The increased erythrocyte sedimentation rate and anemia may not correct until after therapy has been completed.

Mortality rates for large series of patients with NVE treated since 1980 ranged from 13% to 20%.[3,6,18] Death from IE has been associated with increased age (>65 to 70 years), underlying diseases, infection involving the aortic valve, development of CHF, nosocomial origin, *S. aureus* infection, renal failure, and central nervous system complications.[6,26] Early surgical treatment of CHF due to valve dysfunction has decreased the mortality associated with CHF. As a result, neurologic events, uncontrolled infection, and myocardial abscess have accounted for a larger proportion of deaths in recent series.

Mortality rates among patients with IE caused by viridans streptococci, enterococci, and *S. gallolyticus* have ranged from 4% to 16%. Mortality rates are higher with left-sided NVE caused by other organisms: *S. aureus,* 25% to 47%; non-viridans streptococci (groups B, C, and G), 13% to 50%; *C. burnetii,* 5% to 37%; *P. aeruginosa,* Enterobacteriaceae, and fungi, >50%.

Outcome for patients with PVE, as contrasted with NVE, has been less favorable. Before 1980, mortality rates for PVE with onset less than 60 days after surgery and PVE with later onset averaged 70% and 45%, respectively. With the recognition that PVE outcome would benefit from surgical intervention, mortality rates have decreased to 14% to 36%.[9,11] Among patients with PVE treated surgically, survival rates at 4 to 6 years ranged from 50% to 82%. Long-term survival was adversely affected by the presence of moderate or severe CHF at discharge. Survival rates are not related to time of onset after cardiac surgery.

Among patients with NVE (nonaddicts) discharged after medical or medical-surgical therapy, survival was 71% to 88% at 5 years and 61% to 81% at 10 years. Among patients treated surgically for NVE, survival at 5 years ranged from 70% to 80%.

RELAPSE AND RECURRENCE. Relapse of IE usually occurs within 2 months of discontinuation of antibiotic treatment. Patients who have NVE caused by penicillin-susceptible viridans streptococci and who receive a recommended course of therapy experience less than 2% relapse. From 8% to 20% of patients with enterococcal IE relapse after standard therapy. Patients with IE caused by *S. aureus,* Enterobacteriaceae, or fungi are more likely to experience overt failure of therapy rather than relapse; nevertheless, 4% of patients with *S. aureus* IE suffer relapse. Relapse of fungal endocarditis, which occurs in at least 17% to 30% of cases, may be seen at long intervals after treatment. Relapse occurs in 10% of patients with PVE overall and in 6% to 15% of those treated surgically.

Among nonaddicts with an initial episode of NVE or PVE, 4.5% to 7% experience one or more additional episodes. Recurrent IE episodes share the clinical and microbiologic features and response to therapy noted in primary episodes. IV drug abuse is now the most common predisposing factor for recurrent IE.

Prevention

The AHA has dramatically restricted its recommendations for the chemoprophylaxis for IE.[56] These recommendations reflect an evaluation of data documenting procedure-related bacteremia, the antibiotic susceptibility of procedure-related bacteremic organisms that cause endocarditis most commonly, the results of prophylaxis studies in animal models of endocarditis, population-based studies of endocarditis and the prevalence of valvulopathy at risk for endocarditis, the association of excess morbidity with specific forms of endocarditis, and retrospective and prospective studies of endocarditis prophylaxis. The committee recommends that prophylactic antibiotics be used in conjunction with dental and oral procedures only in those patients with underlying cardiac conditions at the highest risk for a severe morbid outcome as a consequence of endocarditis. The recommendations are acknowledged to be "less well established by evidence" and to represent the consensus opinion of experts. The committee's reasoning is summarized here.

GENERAL METHODS. The incidence of IE can be significantly reduced by total surgical correction of some congenital lesions, such as patent ductus arteriosus, ventricular septal defect, and pulmonary stenosis. Maintaining good oral hygiene, which decreases the frequency of bacteremia that accompanies daily activities, is an important preventive measure. Oral hygiene and dental health should be addressed before prosthetic valves are placed electively. Some activities or procedures likely to induce bacteremia should be avoided. Oral irrigating devices are not recommended. The use of central intravascular catheters and urinary catheters should be minimized. Infections associated with bacteremia must be treated promptly and, if possible, eradicated before the involved tissues are incised or manipulated.

CHEMOPROPHYLAXIS. Transient bacteremia occurs commonly after manipulation of the teeth and periodontal tissues and various dental procedures. In addition, transient bacteremia frequently develops during routine daily activities involving the oral cavity: brushing and flossing teeth, using water irrigation devices, and chewing. Considering the relative infrequency of dental visits or oral surgery, the cumulative exposure of cardiac structures to bacteremia is dramatically greater from routine daily activities than from dental procedures. It has been estimated that brushing teeth twice daily for a year results in 154,000 times greater bacteremia exposure than extraction of a single tooth, the dental procedure that induces the greatest risk of bacteremia. Thus, the risk of seeding cardiac structures is far greater from routine daily activities than from dental manipulations. Furthermore, the ability of antibiotics or topical antiseptics to prevent or to reduce bacteremia precipitated by dental procedures is not established and is impaired even further by the gradual increase in the frequency of resistance of viridans streptococci to antibiotics advocated for prophylaxis.

The causal association of dental manipulations with endocarditis is not established, and in fact, the often implied association may result from biased observations. Population-based studies in the Netherlands concluded that dental procedures caused at best only a small fraction of IE cases and that prophylaxis, even if totally effective, would prevent only a small number of cases. Strom and associates did not find that premorbid dental procedures increased in patients with endocarditis compared with uninfected controls.[57] In France, the estimate of IE related to unprotected procedures was 1 per 10,700 and 1 per 54,300, with prosthetic and native valve predispositions, respectively.[58] Thus, a huge prophylaxis effort may be required to prevent one case of IE.

The committee recognized the absence of data documenting that antibiotic prophylaxis prevents endocarditis as a result of procedure-induced bacteremia; however, it could not exclude that a small number of IE cases could be prevented by antibiotic prophylaxis. Nevertheless, in weighing the benefits, potential adverse events, and cost associated with antibiotic prophylaxis, the committee considered that prophylaxis is not warranted on the basis of a lifetime increased risk of IE related to cardiac disease but rather that prophylaxis should be restricted to those patients whose cardiac abnormality places them at the highest risk for a morbid outcome from IE (see Table 67G-1). Notably, prophylaxis is no longer recommended for patients with mitral valve prolapse or for cardiac conditions other than those noted (see Table 67G-1).

The new guidelines advise that prophylaxis be used in the high-risk group before any dental procedures that involve gingival tissue or the periapical region of a tooth or that perforate oral mucosa. Procedures and events not warranting prophylaxis include routine intraoral anesthetic injection through uninfected tissue, taking of dental radiographs, placement or adjustment of removable prosthodontic or orthodontic brackets or appliances, shedding of deciduous teeth, or bleeding due to lip or oral mucosa trauma.[56] The regimens recommended are single-dose modifications of those previously advocated (**Table 67-13**). These same regimens are considered appropriate for at-risk patients (see Table 67G-1) who will undergo incision or biopsy of the respiratory mucosa, such as tonsillectomy, adenoidectomy, or bronchoscopy.

The causal relationship between gastrointestinal and genitourinary tract procedures and IE is less well defined than that for dental procedures. Consequently, antibiotics are not recommended to prevent endocarditis when at-risk patients undergo these procedures.[56] When at-risk patients with gastrointestinal or genitourinary tract infection are to receive antibiotic therapy to prevent wound infections or procedure-induced sepsis, it is reasonable to include an agent active against enterococci. Eradication of genitourinary tract infection, especially that caused by enterococci, before manipulation is advised. Similarly, in at-risk patients undergoing surgery on infected skin or musculoskeletal tissue, antibiotic therapy should include an agent active against anticipated or documented *S. aureus* (including methicillin-resistant strains) and beta-hemolytic streptococci.

TABLE 67-13	Regimens for Prophylaxis Against Endocarditis: Use with Dental, Oral, and Upper Respiratory Tract Procedures	
SETTING PROCEDURE	**REGIMEN ADMINISTERED 30-60 MINUTES BEFORE***
Standard regimen†	Amoxicillin 2.0 g PO
Amoxicillin- or penicillin-allergic patients	Cephalexin 2 g PO† *or* Azithromycin or clarithromycin 500 mg PO *or* Clindamycin 600 mg PO
Patients unable to take oral medications	Ampicillin 2.0 g IM or IV *or* Cefazolin or ceftriaxone 1 g IV†
Ampicillin-, amoxicillin-, or penicillin-allergic patients unable to take oral medications	Clindamycin 300 mg IV 30 min before procedure, then 150 mg 6 hr after initial dose

*Dosages for adults. Initial pediatric dosages are as follows: ampicillin or amoxicillin, 50 mg/kg; clindamycin, 20 mg/kg; azithromycin or clarithromycin, 15 mg/kg.
†Cephalosporins are not used in patients with history of anaphylaxis, angioedema, or urticaria associated with penicillin, ampicillin, or cephalosporins.
Modified from Wilson W, Taubert KA, Gewitz M, et al: Prevention of infective endocarditis: Guidelines from the American Heart Association. Circulation 116:1736, 2007.

Patients with at-risk cardiac lesions should be given written material about their predisposing lesion and the recommended antibiotic prophylaxis.

Future Perspectives

The continued significant mortality and morbidity associated with IE stimulate ongoing efforts to improve diagnostic, preventive, and therapeutic strategies. Molecular detection of nonviable, nonculturable, and even routine causative organisms is likely and will provide more rapid, efficient, and sensitive diagnostic tests. The increasing prominence of *S. aureus* as a cause of IE and its increasing resistance to antibiotics have stimulated efforts to develop staphylococcal vaccines. If it is proven to be efficacious, a vaccine could protect patients at continuous high risk for *S. aureus* IE (e.g., patients with chronic health care exposure [hemodialysis] and implanted cardiac devices). New antibiotics are under development for treatment of resistant gram-positive bacteria, including MRSA. Groups of investigators are collaborating to develop large prospectively collected endocarditis data bases. Using sophisticated analytic techniques, these investigators will address therapeutic questions that are not amenable to randomized clinical trials and thus provide data for evidenced-based decision making in difficult areas of treatment, such as surgical indications for and treatment of unusual causes of IE.

REFERENCES

Epidemiology

1. Moreillon P, Que YA: Infective endocarditis. Lancet 363:139, 2004.
2. Tleyjeh IM, Steckelberg JM, Murad HS, et al: Temporal trends in infective endocarditis: A population-based study in Olmsted County, Minnesota. JAMA 293:3022, 2005.
3. Murdoch DR, Corey GR, Hoen B, et al: Clinical presentation, etiology, and outcome of infective endocarditis in the 21st century. Arch Intern Med 169:463, 2009.
4. Fowler VG Jr, Miro JM, Hoen B, et al: *Staphylococcus aureus* endocarditis: A consequence of medical progress. JAMA 293:3012, 2005.
5. Hill EE, Herijgers P, Claus P, et al: Infective endocarditis: Changing epidemiology and predictors of 6-month mortality: A prospective cohort study. Eur Heart J 28:196, 2007.
6. Martin-Davila P, Fortun J, Navas E, et al: Nosocomial endocarditis in a tertiary hospital: An increasing trend in native valve cases. Chest 128:772, 2005.
7. Gebo KA, Burkey MD, Lucas GM, et al: Incidence of, risk factors for, clinical presentation, and 1-year outcomes of infective endocarditis in an urban HIV cohort. J AIDS 43:426, 2006.

Etiologic Microorganisms

8. Wang A, Athan E, Pappas PA, et al: Contemporary clinical profile and outcome of prosthetic valve endocarditis. JAMA 297:1354, 2007.
9. Habib G, Tribouilloy C, Thuny F, et al: Prosthetic valve endocarditis: Who needs surgery? A multicentre study of 104 cases. Heart 91:954, 2005.
10. Karchmer AW, Longworth DL: Infections of intracardiac devices. Cardiol Clin 21:253, 2003.
11. Rivas P, Alonso J, Moya J, et al: The impact of hospital-acquired infections on the microbial etiology and prognosis of late-onset prosthetic valve endocarditis. Chest 128:764, 2005.
12. Chirouze C, Cabell CH, Fowler VG Jr, et al: Prognostic factors in 61 cases of *Staphylococcus aureus* prosthetic valve infective endocarditis from the International Collaboration on Endocarditis merged database. Clin Infect Dis 38:1323, 2004.
13. Sohail MR, Martin KR, Wilson WR, et al: Medical versus surgical management of *Staphylococcus aureus* prosthetic valve endocarditis. Am J Med 119:147, 2006.
14. Benito N, Miro JM, de Lazzari E, et al: Health care–associated native valve endocarditis: Importance of non-nosocomial acquisition. Ann Intern Med 150:586, 2009.
15. Baddour LM, Wilson WR, Bayer AS, et al: Diagnosis, antimicrobial therapy, and management of complications. A statement for healthcare professionals from the Committee on Rheumatic Fever, Endocarditis, and Kawasaki Disease, Council on Cardiovascular Disease in the Young, and the Councils on Clinical Cardiology, Stroke, and Cardiovascular Surgery and Anesthesia, American Heart Association. Circulation 111:e394, 2005.
16. McDonald JR, Olaison L, Anderson DJ, et al: Enterococcal endocarditis: 107 cases from the international collaboration on endocarditis merged database. Am J Med 118:759, 2005.
17. Stevens MP, Edmond MB: Endocarditis due to vancomycin-resistant enterococci: Case report and review of the literature. Clin Infect Dis 41:1134, 2005.
18. Miro JM, Anguera I, Cabell CH, et al: *Staphylococcus aureus* native valve infective endocarditis: Report of 566 episodes from the International Collaboration on Endocarditis merged database. Clin Infect Dis 41:507, 2005.
19. Chu VH, Woods CW, Miro JM, et al: Emergence of coagulase-negative staphylococci as a cause of native valve endocarditis. Clin Infect Dis 46:232, 2008.
20. Morpeth S, Murdoch D, Cabell CH, et al: Non-HACEK gram-negative bacillus endocarditis. Ann Intern Med 147:829, 2007.
21. Fenollar F, Thuny F, Xeridat B, et al: Endocarditis after acute Q fever in patients with previously undiagnosed valvulopathies. Clin Infect Dis 42:818, 2006.

Pathogenesis, Clinical Features, Diagnosis

22. Nallapareddy SR, Singh KV, Sillanpaa J, et al: Endocarditis and biofilm-associated pili of *Enterococcus faecalis*. J Clin Invest 116:2799, 2006.
23. Nallapareddy SR, Singh KV, Murray BE: Contribution of the collagen adhesin Acm to pathogenesis of *Enterococcus faecium* in experimental endocarditis. Infect Immun 76:4120, 2010.

24. Thuny F, DiSalvo G, Belliard O, et al: Risk of embolism and death in infective endocarditis: Prognostic value of echocardiography. A prospective multicenter study. Circulation 112:69, 2005.

25. Dickerman SA, Abrutyn E, Barsic B, et al: The relationship between the initiation of antimicrobial therapy and the incidence of stroke in infective endocarditis: An analysis from the ICE prospective cohort study (ICE-PCS). Am Heart J 154:1086, 2007.

26. Hasbun R, Vikram HR, Barakat LA, et al: Complicated left-sided native valve endocarditis in adults: Risk classification for mortality. JAMA 289:1933, 2003.

27. Li JS, Sexton DJ, Mick N, et al: Proposed modifications to the Duke criteria for the diagnosis of infective endocarditis. Clin Infect Dis 30:633, 2000.

28. Bayer AS, Bolger AF, Taubert KA, et al: Diagnosis and management of infective endocarditis and its complications. Circulation 98:2936, 1998.

29. Kini V, Logani S, Ky B, et al: Transthoracic and transesophageal echocardiography for the indication of suspected infective endocarditis: Vegetations, blood cultures and imaging. J Am Soc Echocardiograph 23:396, 2010.

30. Vieira MLC, Grinberg M, Pomerantzeff PM, et al: Repeated echocardiographic examinations of patients with suspected infective endocarditis. Heart 90:1020, 2004.

30a. Bonow RO, Carabello B, Chatterjee K, et al: 2008 focused update incorporated into the ACC/AHA 2006 guidelines for the management of patients with valvular heart disease. Circulation 118:e523, 2008.

31. Douglas PS, Khandheria B, Stainback RF, et al: ACCF/ASE,ACEP/ASNC/SCAI/ SCCT/SCMR 2007 appropriateness criteria for transthoracic and transesophageal echocardiography. J Am Coll Cardiol 50:187, 2007.

32. Grijalva M, Horvath R, Dendis M, et al: Molecular diagnosis of culture negative infective endocarditis: Clinical validation in a group of surgically treated patients. Heart 89:263, 2003.

33. Feuchtner GM, Stolzmann P, Dichtl W, et al: Multislice computed tomography in infective endocarditis. J Am Coll Cardiol 53:436, 2009.

Treatment

34. Knoll B, Tleyjeh IM, Steckelberg JM, et al: Infective endocarditis due to penicillin-resistant viridans group streptococci. Clin Infect Dis 44:1585, 2007.

35. Gavalda J, Len O, Miro JM, et al: Treatment of *Enterococcus faecalis* endocarditis with ampicillin plus ceftriaxone. Ann Intern Med 146:574, 2007.

36. Fowler VG Jr, Boucher HW, Corey GR, et al: Daptomycin versus standard therapy for bacteremia and endocarditis caused by *Staphylococcus aureus*. N Engl J Med 355:653, 2006.

37. Tenover FC, Moellering RC Jr: The rationale for revising the Clinical and Laboratory Standards Institute vancomycin minimal inhibitory concentration interpretive criteria for *Staphylococcus aureus*. Clin Infect Dis 44:1208, 2007.

38. Hawkins C, Huang J, Jin N, et al: Persistent *Staphylococcus aureus* bacteremia. Arch Intern Med 167:1861, 2007.

39. Drinkovic D, Morris AJ, Pottumarthy S, et al: Bacteriological outcome of combination versus single-agent treatment for staphylococcal endocarditis. J Antimicrob Chemother 52:820, 2003.

40. Cosgrove SE, Vigliani GA, Campion M, et al: Initial low-dose gentamicin for *Staphylococcus aureus* bacteremia and endocarditis is nephrotoxic. Clin Infect Dis 48:713, 2009.

41. Rybak MJ, Lomaestro BM, Rotschafer JC, et al: Vancomycin therapeutic guidelines. A summary of consensus recommendations from the Infectious Diseases Society of America, the American Society of Health-System Pharmacists and the Society of Infectious Disease Pharmacists. Clin Infect Dis 49:325, 2009.

42. Habib G, Hoen B, Tornos P, et al: Guidelines on the prevention, diagnosis, and treatment of infective endocarditis (new version 2009). Eur Heart J 30:2369, 2009.

43. Rolain JM, Brouqui P, Koehler JE, et al: Recommendations for treatment of human infections caused by *Bartonella* species. Antimicrob Agents Chemother 48:1921, 2004.

44. Olaison L, Pettersson G: Current best practices and guidelines indications for surgical intervention in infective endocarditis. Cardiol Clin 21:235, 2003.

45. Vikram HR, Buenconsejo J, Hasbun R, et al: Impact of valve surgery on 6-month mortality in adults with complicated, left-sided native valve endocarditis: A propensity analysis. JAMA 290:3207, 2003.

46. Bannay A, Hoen B, Duval X, et al: The impact of valve surgery on short- and long-term mortality in left-sided infective endocarditis: Do differences in methodological approaches explain previous conflicting results? Eur Heart J doi:10.1093/eurheartj/ehp008:2009.

47. Aksoy O, Sexton DJ, Wang A, et al: Early surgery in patients with infective endocarditis: A propensity score analysis. Clin Infect Dis 44:364, 2007.

48. Nadji G, Goissen T, Brahim A, et al: Impact of early surgery on 6-month outcome in acute infective endocarditis. Int J Cardiol 129:227, 2009.

49. Cabell CH, Abrutyn E, Fowler VG Jr, et al: Use of surgery in patients with native valve infective endocarditis: Results from the International Collaboration on Endocarditis merged database. Am Heart J 150:1092, 2005.

50. Thuny F, Beurtheret S, Mancini J, et al: The timing of surgery influences mortality and morbidity in adults with severe complicated infective endocarditis: A propensity analysis. Eur Heart J doi:10.1093/eurheartj/ehp089:2009.

51. Eishi K, Kawazoe K, Kuriyama Y, et al: Surgical management of infective endocarditis associated with cerebral complications: Multicenter retrospective study in Japan. J Thorac Cardiovasc Surg 110:1745, 1995.

52. Morris AJ, Drinkovic D, Pottumarthy S, et al: Bacteriological outcome after valve surgery for active infective endocarditis: Implications for duration of treatment after surgery [abstract]. Clin Infect Dis 41:187, 2005.

53. Phuong LK, Link M, Wijdicks E: Management of intracranial infectious aneurysms: A series of 16 cases. Neurosurgery 51:1145, 2002.

54. Chan KL, Dumesnil JG, Cujec B, et al: A randomized trial of aspirin on the risk of embolic events in patients with infective endocarditis. J Am Coll Cardiol 42:775, 2003.

55. Verhagen DWM, Hermanides J, Korevaar JC, et al: Prognostic value of serial C-reactive protein measurements in left-sided native valve endocarditis. Arch Intern Med 168:302, 2008.

Prevention

56. Wilson W, Taubert KA, Gewitz M, et al: Prevention of infective endocarditis. Guidelines from the American Heart Association. Circulation 116:1736, 2007.

57. Strom BL, Abrutyn E, Berlin JA, et al: Dental and cardiac risk factors for infective endocarditis: A population-based, case-control study. Ann Intern Med 129:761, 1998.

58. Duval X, Alla F, Hoen B, et al: Estimated risk of endocarditis in adults with predisposing cardiac conditions undergoing dental procedures with or without antibiotic prophylaxis. Clin Infect Dis 42:e102, 2006.

 GUIDELINES ROBERT O. BONOW

Infective Endocarditis

The American Heart Association (AHA) guidelines for prevention of infective endocarditis have been evolving for the last 50 years, with the most recent key updates providing recommendations for antibiotic prophylaxis published in 2007.[1] The AHA scientific statement regarding the recommendations for diagnosis and management of this condition were published in 1997.[2] Other guidelines with recommendations relevant to this condition include the American College of Cardiology/American Heart Association (ACC/AHA) guidelines for management of patients with valvular heart disease, updated most recently in 2008.[3]

PREVENTION

The 2007 AHA guidelines represent a marked departure from prior recommendations, previously published in 1997,[4] and greatly reduce the patient population for which prophylactic antibiotics are recommended. These new guidelines note that prior recommendations were based on research showing that antimicrobial prophylaxis is effective for prevention of experimental infective endocarditis in animal models but also acknowledge the lack of evidence that antimicrobial prophylaxis is effective in humans for prevention of endocarditis after dental, gastrointestinal, or genitourinary procedures. The expert committee also considered the complexity of prior guidelines, which required stratification of patients and procedures on their risk for infective endocarditis.

The 2007 AHA guidelines committee concluded that only an extremely small number of cases of infective endocarditis might be prevented by antibiotic prophylaxis for dental procedures even if such prophylaxis was 100% effective. Accordingly, the revised guidelines recommend infective endocarditis prophylaxis for dental procedures only for patients with underlying cardiac conditions associated with the highest risk of adverse outcomes from infective endocarditis (**Table 67G-1**). These new recommendations were incorporated in the 2008 ACC/AHA guidelines update for management of patients with valvular heart disease.[3] That guidelines update, however, also included the following statement regarding individualization of preventive strategies based on physician and patient preference:

> The committee recognizes that decades of previous recommendations for patients with most forms of valvular heart disease and other conditions have been abruptly changed by the new AHA guidelines. Because this may cause consternation among patients, clinicians should be available to discuss the rationale for these new changes with their patients, including the lack of scientific evidence to demonstrate a proven benefit for infective endocarditis prophylaxis. In select circumstances, the committee also understands that some clinicians and some patients may still feel more comfortable continuing with prophylaxis for infective endocarditis, particularly for those with bicuspid aortic valve or coarctation of the aorta, severe mitral valve prolapse, or hypertrophic obstructive cardiomyopathy. In those settings, the clinician should determine that the risks associated with antibiotics are low before continuing a prophylaxis regimen. Over time, and with continuing education, the committee anticipates increasing acceptance of the new guidelines among both provider and patient communities.

For patients with the conditions in which antibiotic prophylaxis is recommended, the antibiotics are intended for dental procedures that involve manipulation of gingival tissue or the periapical region of teeth or

TABLE 67G-1	Cardiac Conditions and Dental Procedures for Which Antibiotic Prophylaxis Is Recommended

Cardiac Conditions Associated with the Highest Risk of Adverse Outcome from Endocarditis for which Prophylaxis with Dental Procedures is Recommended

Prosthetic cardiac valve

Previous infective endocarditis

Congenital heart disease (CHD)

    Unrepaired cyanotic CHD, including those with palliative shunts and conduits

    Completely repaired CHD with prosthetic material or device either by surgery or by catheter intervention during the first 6 months after the procedure

    Repaired CHD with residual defects at the site or adjacent to the site of a prosthetic patch or prosthetic device (which inhibit endothelialization)

    Except for the conditions listed above, antibiotic prophylaxis is no longer recommended for any other form of CHD

Cardiac transplantation recipients who develop cardiac valvulopathy

Dental Procedures for which Endocarditis Prophylaxis is Recommended for High-Risk Patients (see above)

All dental procedures and events that involve manipulation of gingival tissue or the periapical region of teeth or perforation of the oral mucosa **except** the following:

Routine anesthetic injections through noninfected tissue

Taking dental radiographs

Placement of removable prosthodontic or orthodontic appliances

Adjustment of orthodontic appliances

Placement of orthodontic brackets

Shedding of deciduous teeth and bleeding from trauma to the lips or oral mucosa

From Wilson W, Taubert KA, Gewitz M, et al: Prevention of infective endocarditis. Recommendations by the American Heart Association. Circulation 116:1736, 2007.

perforation of the oral mucosa. The guidelines recommend a single dose of amoxicillin or ampicillin as the preferred prophylactic agent for individuals who do not have a history of type I hypersensitive reactions to a penicillin. For individuals who are allergic to penicillins or amoxicillin, alternative recommendations include first-generation oral cephalosporins, clindamycin, azithromycin, or clarithromycin.

Antibiotic administration is not recommended for patients undergoing genitourinary or gastrointestinal tract procedures solely for the purpose of preventing endocarditis. This recommendation is in contrast with previous guidelines that recommended endocarditis antibiotic prophylaxis before some procedures and not others. Antibiotic prophylaxis for bronchoscopy is not recommended unless the procedure involves incision of the respiratory tract mucosa.

INDICATIONS FOR ECHOCARDIOGRAPHY

Echocardiography is strongly supported in virtually all patients with suspected or known infective endocarditis (**Table 67G-2**).[3] The guidelines urge use of transesophageal echocardiography (TEE) when specific questions are not adequately addressed by an initial transthoracic echocardiographic evaluation, such as when the transthoracic study is of poor quality, if the transthoracic echocardiogram is negative despite a high clinical suspicion of endocarditis, if a prosthetic valve is involved, and if there is a high suspicion such as in a patient with staphylococcal bacteremia or in an elderly patient with valvular abnormalities that make diagnosis by transthoracic imaging difficult.

Diagnosis of prosthetic valve endocarditis with transthoracic echocardiography is more difficult than diagnosis of endocarditis of native valves. Thus, the ACC/AHA guidelines suggest a lower threshold for performance of TEE in patients with prosthetic valves and suspected endocarditis (see Table 67G-2).[3]

SURGERY FOR ACTIVE ENDOCARDITIS

The ACC/AHA guidelines for valvular heart disease support performance of surgery for patients with life-threatening congestive heart failure or cardiogenic shock related to active endocarditis.[3] Indications for surgery for patients with stable endocarditis are considered less clear (**Table 67G-3**).

ACKNOWLEDGMENT

Thomas H. Lee, MD, contributed to this section in previous editions of this book.

TABLE 67G-2	ACC/AHA Guidelines for Echocardiography in Endocarditis		
INDICATION	**CLASS**	**RECOMMENDATION**	**LOE**
Transthoracic echocardiography	Class I	Detection and characterization of valvular lesions, their hemodynamic severity, and/or ventricular compensation	B
		Detection of vegetations and characterization of lesions in patients in whom IE is suspected	B
		Detection of associated complications (e.g., abscesses, shunts)	B
		Reevaluation in complex IE (e.g., virulent organism, severe hemodynamic lesion, aortic valve involvement, new murmur, persistent or recurrent fever or bacteremia, clinical change, or symptomatic deterioration)	C
	Class IIa	Persistent fever without bacteremia or a new murmur in patients with prosthetic heart valves	C
	Class IIb	Reevaluation of prosthetic valve IE during antibiotic therapy in the absence of clinical deterioration	C
	Class III	Not indicated to reevaluate uncomplicated (including no regurgitation on baseline echocardiogram) native valve IE during antibiotic treatment in the absence of clinical deterioration, new physical findings, or persistent fever	C
Transesophageal echocardiography	Class I	Assess severity of valvular lesions in symptomatic patients with IE, if transthoracic echocardiography is nondiagnostic	C
		Diagnose IE in patients with valvular heart disease and positive blood cultures, if transthoracic echocardiography is nondiagnostic	C
		Assess complications of IE with potential impact on prognosis and management (e.g., abscesses, perforation, and shunts)	C
		First-line diagnostic study to diagnose prosthetic valve IE and assess for complications	C
		Preoperative evaluation in patients with known IE, unless the need for surgery is evident on transthoracic imaging and unless preoperative imaging will delay surgery in urgent cases	C
		Intraoperative monitoring of patients undergoing valve surgery for IE	C
	Class IIa	Diagnose possible IE in patients with persistent staphylococcal bacteremia without a known source	C
	Class IIb	Detection of IE in patients with nosocomial staphylococcal bacteremia	C

IE = infective endocarditis; LOE = level of evidence.

From Bonow RO, Carabello B, Chatterjee K, et al: 2008 focused update incorporated into the ACC/AHA 2006 guidelines for the management of patients with valvular heart disease. Circulation 118:e1, 2008.

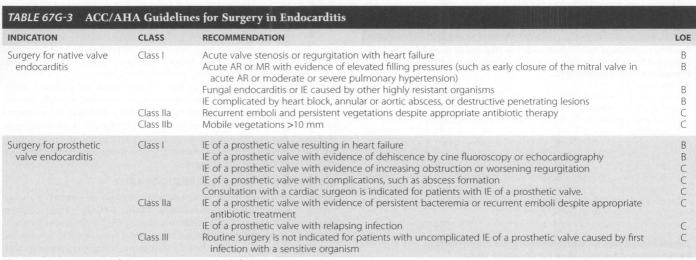

TABLE 67G-3 ACC/AHA Guidelines for Surgery in Endocarditis

INDICATION	CLASS	RECOMMENDATION	LOE
Surgery for native valve endocarditis	Class I	Acute valve stenosis or regurgitation with heart failure	B
		Acute AR or MR with evidence of elevated filling pressures (such as early closure of the mitral valve in acute AR or moderate or severe pulmonary hypertension)	B
		Fungal endocarditis or IE caused by other highly resistant organisms	B
		IE complicated by heart block, annular or aortic abscess, or destructive penetrating lesions	B
	Class IIa	Recurrent emboli and persistent vegetations despite appropriate antibiotic therapy	C
	Class IIb	Mobile vegetations >10 mm	C
Surgery for prosthetic valve endocarditis	Class I	IE of a prosthetic valve resulting in heart failure	B
		IE of a prosthetic valve with evidence of dehiscence by cine fluoroscopy or echocardiography	B
		IE of a prosthetic valve with evidence of increasing obstruction or worsening regurgitation	C
		IE of a prosthetic valve with complications, such as abscess formation	C
		Consultation with a cardiac surgeon is indicated for patients with IE of a prosthetic valve.	C
	Class IIa	IE of a prosthetic valve with evidence of persistent bacteremia or recurrent emboli despite appropriate antibiotic treatment	C
		IE of a prosthetic valve with relapsing infection	C
	Class III	Routine surgery is not indicated for patients with uncomplicated IE of a prosthetic valve caused by first infection with a sensitive organism	C

AR = aortic regurgitation; IE = infective endocarditis; LOE = level of evidence; MR = mitral regurgitation.
From Bonow RO, Carabello B, Chatterjee K, et al: 2008 focused update incorporated into the ACC/AHA 2006 guidelines for the management of patients with valvular heart disease. Circulation 118:e1, 2008.

REFERENCES

1. Wilson W, Taubert KA, Gewitz M, et al: Prevention of infective endocarditis. Recommendations by the American Heart Association. Circulation 116:1736, 2007.
2. Bayer AS, Bolger AF, Taubert KA, et al: Diagnosis and management of infective endocarditis and its complications. Circulation 98:2936, 1998.
3. Bonow RO, Carabello B, Chatterjee K, et al: 2008 focused update incorporated into the ACC/AHA 2006 guidelines for the management of patients with valvular heart disease. Circulation 118:e1, 2008.
4. Dajani AS, Taubert KA, Wilson W, et al: Prevention of bacterial endocarditis: Recommendations by the American Heart Association. Circulation 96:363, 1997.

CHAPTER 68   The Dilated, Restrictive, and Infiltrative Cardiomyopathies

Joshua M. Hare

Cardiomyopathies are diseases of heart muscle that result from myriad insults, such as genetic defects, cardiac myocyte injury, and infiltration of myocardial tissues. Thus, cardiomyopathies result from both insults to cellular elements of the heart, notably the cardiac myocyte, and processes that are external to cells, such as deposition of abnormal substances into the extracellular matrix. Cardiomyopathies are traditionally defined on the basis of structural and functional phenotypes (**Tables 68-1 and 68-2**), notably dilated (characterized primarily by an enlarged ventricular chamber and reduced cardiac performance),[1] hypertrophic (characterized primarily by thickened, hypertrophic ventricular walls and enhanced cardiac performance), and restrictive (characterized primarily by thickened, stiff ventricular walls that impede diastolic filling of the ventricle; cardiac systolic performance is typically close to normal).[2] A fourth and increasingly appreciated structural and functional phenotype is a cardiomyopathy that primarily involves the right ventricle—arrhythmogenic right ventricular dysplasia/cardiomyopathy. The dilated cardiomyopathy phenotype is often viewed as a "final common pathway" of numerous types of cardiac injuries and is the most common cardiomyopathic phenotype.[3]

The use of the term *cardiomyopathy* was previously reserved for primary diseases of the heart, not including processes affecting valvular structures, coronary vasculature, or pericardium. Because of the recognition of the final common pathway phenomenon, the term *cardiomyopathy* has entered into common use to denote specific cardiomyopathies, such as ischemic cardiomyopathy[4] or valvular cardiomyopathy (see Table 68-1). There is biologic support for this because there is substantial (but clearly not complete[5]) overlap in the altered signaling pathways and compensatory mechanisms in the failing heart, regardless of underlying cause.[3]

SPECIFIC CAUSES. Classification of the causes of cardiomyopathy continues to be a challenge, and a satisfactory and uniformly agreed on classification system remains in evolution.[6] Classification schemes are plagued by the fact that as the causal basis of heart muscle disease becomes increasingly understood, it is also appreciated that for a given etiology, there may be a spectrum of phenotypes that can overlap or evolve. For example, both myocarditis and amyloidosis can have a spectrum of phenotypes ranging from restrictive to dilated. Recently, a new classification of cardiomyopathies that incorporates molecular insights was proposed by an American Heart Association Scientific Statement panel.[6] This classification divides cardiomyopathy into primary and secondary causes, in a manner similar to traditional classification schemes, but adds important subcharacterization of the primary cardiomyopathies into genetic, mixed, and acquired groups (**Fig. 68-1**). From the clinical perspective, where the objective is diagnosis and delivery of effective therapy that may be cause-specific, there is major overlap with the concept of an acquired primary cardiomyopathy and a secondary cardiomyopathy. An important new addition to the genetic subgroup is that of ion channel disorders, which often are not accompanied by structural heart disease but clearly can be considered a primary disorder of the heart (see Chap. 9 for further discussion). Ischemic heart disease can also lead to a cardiomyopathy and is discussed in Chaps. 25, 52, and 54. The hypertrophic cardiomyopathies are discussed in Chaps. 8 and 69.

Operationally, disagreement about classification of cardiomyopathies does not necessarily impede patient management. Rather, the disagreement reinforces the key principle in patient evaluation—there are many primary, secondary, and systemic disorders that manifest with cardiac dysfunction or congestive heart failure. Accordingly, the patient with an abnormality in cardiac structure or function requires comprehensive evaluation for a broad array of disorders. The main goal of this approach is to identify disorders that cause reversible cardiac dysfunction, capable of significant improvement with treatment of the underlying cause of the heart failure.[7,8] Thus, a key principle for management of the cardiomyopathy patient is an exhaustive evaluation to determine the underlying etiologic diagnosis. Throughout this chapter, the issue of reversibility will be addressed (see Chap. 25). In contrast to the principle that the underlying etiologic basis of cardiomyopathy is broad is the therapeutic concept that therapies for heart failure are somewhat similar. A common approach of addressing the patient's volume status and use of neurohormonal blockade is appropriate management regardless of etiology (see Chap. 28). Only now are specific etiology-based therapies entering into clinical testing.

TABLE 68-1 Classification of the Cardiomyopathies

DISORDER	DESCRIPTION
Dilated cardiomyopathy	Dilation and impaired contraction of the left ventricle or both ventricles
	Caused by familial-genetic, viral, immune, alcoholic-toxic, or unknown factors or is associated with recognized cardiovascular disease
Hypertrophic cardiomyopathy	Left and/or right ventricular hypertrophy, often asymmetric, which usually involves the interventricular septum
	Mutations in sarcoplasmic proteins cause the disease in many patients
Restrictive cardiomyopathy	Restricted filling and reduced diastolic size of either ventricle or both ventricles with normal or near-normal systolic function
	Idiopathic or associated with other disease (e.g., amyloidosis, endomyocardial disease)
Arrhythmogenic right ventricular cardiomyopathy	Progressive fibrofatty replacement of the right, and to some degree the left, ventricular myocardium
	Familial disease is common
Unclassified cardiomyopathy	Diseases that do not fit readily into any category; examples include systolic dysfunction with minimal dilation, mitochondrial disease, and fibroelastosis
Specific Cardiomyopathies	
Ischemic cardiomyopathy	Arises as dilated cardiomyopathy with depressed ventricular function not explained by the extent of coronary artery obstructions or ischemic damage
Valvular cardiomyopathy	Arises as ventricular dysfunction that is out of proportion to the abnormal loading conditions produced by the valvular stenosis and/or regurgitation
Hypertensive cardiomyopathy	Arises with left ventricular hypertrophy with features of cardiac failure related to systolic or diastolic dysfunction
Inflammatory cardiomyopathy	Cardiac dysfunction as a consequence of myocarditis
Metabolic cardiomyopathy	Includes a wide variety of causes, including endocrine abnormalities, glycogen storage disease, deficiencies (such as hypokalemia), and nutritional disorders
General systemic disease	Includes connective tissue disorders and infiltrative diseases such as sarcoidosis and leukemia
Muscular dystrophies	Includes Duchenne, Becker-type, and myotonic dystrophies
Neuromuscular disorders	Includes Friedreich ataxia, Noonan syndrome, and lentiginosis
Sensitivity and toxic reactions	Includes reactions to alcohol, catecholamines, anthracyclines, irradiation, and others
Peripartum cardiomyopathy	First becomes manifested in the peripartum period, but it is probably a heterogeneous group

Derived from Richardson P, McKenna W, Bristow M, et al: Report of the 1995 World Health Organization/International Society and Federation of Cardiology Task Force on the Definition and Classification of Cardiomyopathies. Circulation 93:841, 1996. Copyright 1996, American Heart Association.

TABLE 68-2 Functional Classification of the Cardiomyopathies

DILATED	RESTRICTIVE	HYPERTROPHIC
Symptoms		
Congestive heart failure, particularly left sided	Dyspnea, fatigue	Dyspnea, angina pectoris
Fatigue and weakness	Right-sided congestive heart failure	Fatigue, syncope, palpitations
Systemic or pulmonary emboli	Signs and symptoms of systemic disease, e.g., amyloidosis, iron storage disease	
Physical Examination		
Moderate to severe cardiomegaly; S_3, S_4	Mild to moderate cardiomegaly; S_3 or S_4	Mild cardiomegaly
Atrioventricular valve regurgitation, especially mitral	Atrioventricular valve regurgitation; inspiratory increase in venous pressure (Kussmaul sign)	Apical systolic thrill and heave; brisk carotid upstroke
		S_4 common
		Systolic murmur that increases with Valsalva maneuver
Chest Radiography		
Moderate to marked cardiac enlargement, especially left ventricular	Mild cardiac enlargement	Mild to moderate cardiac enlargement
Pulmonary venous hypertension	Pulmonary venous hypertension	Left atrial enlargement
Electrocardiography		
Sinus tachycardia	Low voltage	Left ventricular hypertrophy
Atrial and ventricular arrhythmias	Intraventricular conduction defects	ST-segment and T wave abnormalities
ST-segment and T wave abnormalities	Atrioventricular conduction defects	Abnormal Q waves
Intraventricular conduction defects		Atrial and ventricular arrhythmias
Echocardiography		
Left ventricular dilation and dysfunction	Increased left ventricular wall thickness and mass	Asymmetric septal hypertrophy
Abnormal diastolic mitral valve motion secondary to abnormal compliance and filling pressures	Small or normal-size left ventricular cavity	Narrow left ventricular outflow tract
	Normal systolic function	Systolic anterior motion of the mitral valve
	Pericardial effusion	Small or normal-sized left ventricle
Radionuclide Studies		
Left ventricular dilation and dysfunction (RVG)	Infiltration of myocardium (^{201}Tl)	Small or normal-sized left ventricle (RVG)
	Small or normal-sized left ventricle (RVG)	Vigorous systolic function (RVG)
	Normal systolic function (RVG)	Asymmetric septal hypertrophy (RVG or ^{201}Tl)
Cardiac Catheterization		
Left ventricular enlargement and dysfunction	Diminished left ventricular compliance	Diminished left ventricular compliance
Mitral and/or tricuspid regurgitation	"Square root" sign in ventricular pressure recordings	Mitral regurgitation
Elevated left- and often right-sided filling pressures	Preserved systolic function	Vigorous systolic function
Diminished cardiac output	Elevated left- and right-sided filling pressures	Dynamic left ventricular outflow gradient

RVG = radionuclide ventriculogram; ^{201}Tl = thallium-201.

Dilated Cardiomyopathy

The hallmarks of dilated cardiomyopathy (DCM), the most common cardiomyopathy, are enlargement of one or both of the ventricles and systolic dysfunction (**Fig. 68-2**; see Fig. 68-e1 on website). It is not uncommon for chamber enlargement to precede signs and symptoms of congestive heart failure. Recent classification revision attempts recognize that chamber dilation is part of the spectrum of genetic and environmental disorders affecting the heart; thus, a patient presenting with DCM may have a broad array of cardiac or systemic conditions. Nevertheless, DCM is an important and frequent clinical presentation. In 50% or more of patients with a DCM, an etiologic basis will not be identified, in which case the patient is referred to as having an idiopathic DCM.[1,7]

Natural History

The natural history of DCM remains incompletely understood. This is because this diagnosis clearly contains a variety of causes and patients have highly variable presentations. The presentations of patients can range from asymptomatic left ventricular dysfunction to mild, moderate, or severe congestive heart failure. Different studies report wide-ranging estimates of annual mortality that are between 10% and 50%.[9] Traditionally, it is held that symptomatic heart failure is invariably progressive. However, several factors suggest that this concept should be reexamined and that biologic factors may determine favorable or unfavorable long-term outcomes.[10] First, there has been an impact of therapy on the natural history of patients. Whereas the 1-year mortality in the placebo arm was approximately 50% in the Cooperative North Scandinavian Enalapril Survival Study (CONSENSUS) conducted in the 1980s, similar patients experienced ~20% annual mortality in the Carvedilol Prospective Randomized Cumulative Survival (COPERNICUS) trial conducted in the 1990s, and this dropped further in the 2000s to ~10% (see Chap. 28). There is also growing awareness that treatment with pharmacologic therapies that antagonize the neurohormonal system can lead to myocardial recovery or "reverse left ventricular remodeling" in some patients with DCM (see Chap. 25). Finally, it is reported that between

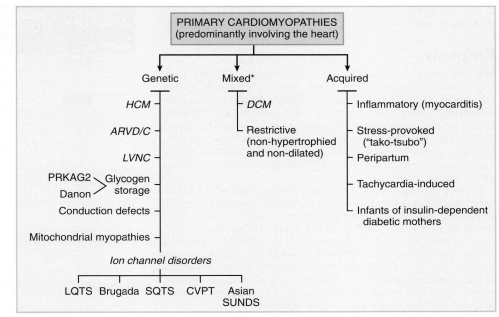

FIGURE 68-1 Primary and specific cardiomyopathies that are primarily manifested with cardiac involvement. *The mixed group comprises predominantly nongenetic causes; however, within this group, familial disease with a genetic origin has been reported in a minority of cases. ARVD/C = arrhythmogenic right ventricular dysplasia/cardiomyopathy; CVPT = catecholaminergic polymorphic ventricular tachycardia; DCM = dilated cardiomyopathy; HCM = hypertrophic cardiomyopathy; LQTS = long-QT syndrome; LVNC = left ventricular noncompaction; PRKAG2 = gene encoding the γ_2 regulatory subunit of the AMP-activated protein kinase; SQTS = short-QT syndrome; SUNDS = sudden unexplained nocturnal death syndrome. *(From Maron BJ, Towbin JA, Thiene G, et al: Contemporary definitions and classification of the cardiomyopathies: An American Heart Association Scientific Statement from the Council on Clinical Cardiology, Heart Failure and Transplantation Committee; Quality of Care and Outcomes Research and Functional Genomics and Translational Biology Interdisciplinary Working Groups; and Council on Epidemiology and Prevention. Circulation 113:1807, 2006.)*

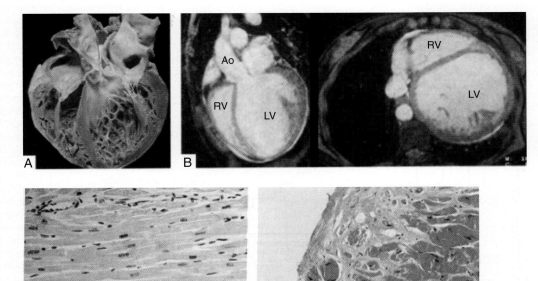

FIGURE 68-2 Dilated cardiomyopathy, gross and microscopic appearance. Affected hearts exhibit four-chamber enlargement as shown by gross cardiac specimen **(A)** and with cardiac magnetic resonance imaging **(B)**. Cardiac myocytes are hypertrophied **(D)** with variable size and enlarged nuclei compared with normally aligned myocytes **(C)**. In addition, there is significant interstitial deposition of fibrotic tissue **(D)**. Ao = aorta; LV = left ventricle; RV = right ventricle. *(From Hare JM: Etiologic basis of congestive heart failure. In Colucci WS [ed]: Atlas of Heart Failure. 5th ed. Philadelphia, Springer, Current Medicine Group, 2008, pp 29-56. Copyright 2008, Current Medicine LLC.)*

25% and 33% of patients presenting with new-onset DCM experience meaningful cardiac recovery.[11]

Prognosis

The prognosis of DCM may be much more variable than previously appreciated.[9,10] Several features of the clinical presentation may be valuable in predicting patient outcome (**Table 68-3**). In addition, the underlying etiology of the cardiomyopathy clearly has a substantial impact on the natural history, thus warranting an exhaustive search for causes (**Fig. 68-3**). Some cardiomyopathies have excellent long-term survival, whereas others, particularly amyloidosis and human immunodeficiency virus (HIV)–related disease, carry grave prognoses.[7]

In terms of idiopathic DCM, the natural history may not be inextricably progressive, and patients may experience variable courses. In some cases, patients may enter into periods of stability during which symptoms completely stabilize; such periods can last years or even decades. Associated but not clearly linked with periods of stability is reverse remodeling, a phenomenon appreciated only in the last decade (see Chap. 25). Reverse remodeling may be spontaneous or in response to pharmacologic or device therapy. A study using microarray analysis to measure gene expression in endomyocardial tissue obtained from patients suggested that patients who have favorable long-term outcomes accompanied by reverse remodeling can be detected at the time of clinical presentation[10] (**Fig. 68-4**). Alternatively, it is clear that some patients may experience sudden deterioration after a period of stability or never experience a quiescent time.[12] It is also critical to appreciate that certain patients may have severe and life-threatening hemodynamic embarrassment at initial presentation. For these patients, a diagnostic evaluation including endomyocardial biopsy should be rapidly performed[13]; these patients are critically ill and frequently require inotropic or mechanical support as a lifesaving therapy.

The determinants of the natural history are not entirely clear, but several studies suggest that biomarkers or panels of laboratory values may have prognostic value.[9,10] As discussed subsequently, there is growing appreciation for the genetic component of DCM, and it is likely that inherited predisposition plays a major role in the natural history of this disorder.

TABLE 68-3 Factors Associated with an Adverse Outcome in Dilated Cardiomyopathy

CLINICAL	NONINVASIVE	INVASIVE
NYHA Class III/IV	Low LV ejection fraction	High LV filling pressures
Increasing age	Marked LV dilation	
Low exercise peak oxygen consumption	Low LV mass	
Marked intraventricular conduction delay	≥Moderate mitral regurgitation	
Complex ventricular arrhythmias	Abnormal diastolic function	
Abnormal signal-averaged ECG	Abnormal contractile reserve	
Evidence of excessive sympathetic stimulation	Right ventricular dilation or dysfunction	
Protodiastolic gallop (S₃)		
Elevated serum BNP		
Elevated uric acid		
Decreased serum sodium		

BNP = brain natriuretic peptide; ECG = electrocardiogram; LV = left ventricular; NYHA = New York Heart Association.

Pathology

MACROSCOPIC EXAMINATION. Gross inspection of the heart demonstrates four-chamber enlargement (see Fig. 68-2). Most often, the ventricular walls are increased in thickness consistent with the myocyte hypertrophy that accompanies this disorder. Increasing chamber thickness is attributed to a compensatory mechanism aimed at reducing wall stress and is thus thought to play a beneficial role, averting further chamber remodeling.[3] The valvular structures themselves are normal, although chamber enlargement frequently leads to a dilation of the valvular orifice. Intracavitary thrombi are often noted and are preferentially located in the ventricular apices. The coronary circulation is most commonly normal, although the presence of nonocclusive epicardial disease can raise a diagnostic conundrum wherein the degree of cardiomyopathy is "out of proportion to the underlying coronary artery disease." A definition for ischemic cardiomyopathy has been arbitrarily set at a requirement for a greater than 70% stenosis in a major epicardial coronary artery, although pathologic studies have reported greater degrees of disease.[4] Preferential involvement of the right ventricle should suggest the diagnoses of arrhythmogenic right ventricular dysplasia/cardiomyopathy (ARVD/C)[14] or cor pulmonale (secondary to pulmonary hypertension).

HISTOLOGIC EXAMINATION. Histologic evaluation of the myocardium reveals varying degrees of myocyte hypertrophy and interstitial fibrosis (see Fig. 68-2).[4] Fibrosis most often affects the left ventricular subendocardium or throughout the myocardium in interstitial or perivascular patterns. A finding

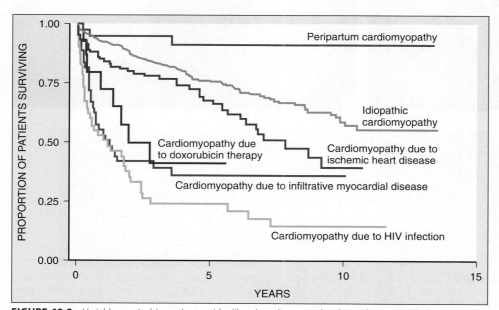

FIGURE 68-3 Variable survival in patients with dilated cardiomyopathy depending on underlying etiologic basis. HIV = human immunodeficiency virus. *(From Felker GM, Thompson RE, Hare JM, et al: Underlying causes and long-term survival in patients with initially unexplained cardiomyopathy. N Engl J Med 342:1077, 2000.)*

of replacement fibrosis, an island of fibrotic tissue, often signifies a small area of tissue necrosis and suggests an ischemic etiology. It has been difficult to identify characteristic immunologic or infectious findings; however, progress is being made, particularly with regard to viral persistence within the heart (see later). Scattered cells considered to be lymphocytes are a frequent observation and may lead to a diagnosis of borderline myocarditis. This does not appear to affect prognosis.[15]

Etiology

DCM accounts for approximately 25% of the cases of congestive heart failure in the United States.[16] The majority of the additional cases are due to specific cardiomyopathies, most notably ischemic or hypertensive cardiomyopathies,[16] or nonsystolic heart failure.[17] The DCM phenotype can be manifested from specific systemic diseases or primary acquired processes, and intensive diagnostic evaluations in referral centers can reveal a specific associated cause of cardiomyopathy in ~50% of patients; the remaining 50% are assigned the diagnosis of exclusion, idiopathic DCM.[7,8] It is increasingly being appreciated that many of the so-called cases of idiopathic DCM result from underlying genetic abnormalities or previous environmental insults that are difficult to detect at the time of clinical presentation. With the advent of sophisticated molecular and imaging technologies in clinical medicine, it is likely in the future that an increasing number of the idiopathic cases will have a specific diagnosis assigned.

Specific Cardiomyopathies with a Dilated Phenotype

Clinically, there are a host of important causes of secondary DCM (see Table 68-1) that include alcohol and cocaine abuse (see Chap. 73), HIV infection (see Chap. 72), and metabolic abnormalities as well as the cardiotoxicity of anticancer drugs (see Chap. 90), most notably doxorubicin and newly introduced drugs that inhibit tyrosine kinases (e.g., herceptin and imitinab). The following four specific disorders are particularly important to recognize in that correct diagnosis has a major impact on patient management and chance for recovery.

STRESS (TAKO-TSUBO OR BROKEN HEART SYNDROME).[18] An acute cardiomyopathy can be provoked by a stressful or emotional situation or exposure to high doses of catecholamines (sympathomimetic drugs)[18,19] (see Chap. 28). This cardiomyopathy is most common among middle-aged women, appears to be related to catecholamine release, and in most cases is fully reversible with supportive care (**Fig. 68-5**; see Fig. 15-32). Electrocardiographic findings of myocardial infarction in the presence of left ventricular dysfunction and absence of epicardial coronary stenoses should prompt the diagnosis. Endomyocardial biopsy is of value to exclude myocarditis, which can also mimic acute myocardial infarction, and demonstrates contraction band necrosis.

PERIPARTUM CARDIOMYOPATHY. Peripartum cardiomyopathy[20,21] is defined as a cardiomyopathy manifesting between the last month of pregnancy and 6 months post partum. The etiology is unclear, but inflammatory factors are highly implicated, and some studies reveal a high incidence of lymphocytic inflammation. Peripartum cardiomyopathy is common in Africa but also is manifested in the developed world; it has an excellent long-term natural history if patients survive the initial period (see Fig. 68-4), during which time hemodynamic compromise may be severe.[22] Prognosis is worse in the developing world and among indigent patients in the United States.[23] It is important to differentiate peripartum cardiomyopathy from a chronic cardiomyopathy exacerbated by the volume load occurring during pregnancy.[20] Women who recover are at increased risk of recurrences with subsequent pregnancies; women with full recovery are more likely to tolerate a subsequent pregnancy than are those with residual left ventricular dysfunction.[21]

TACHYCARDIA-INDUCED CARDIOMYOPATHY. Patients may develop a DCM with congestive heart failure in the face of recurrent or persistent tachycardias. The most common association is with atrial fibrillation or supraventricular tachycardia. There is a high rate of full recovery with control of the arrhythmia.[24] This cardiomyopathy is notable for the degree to which it resembles idiopathic DCM phenotypically, yet it is characterized by a remarkable degree of recovery in left ventricular function once the arrhythmia is controlled. Patients presenting with an atrial

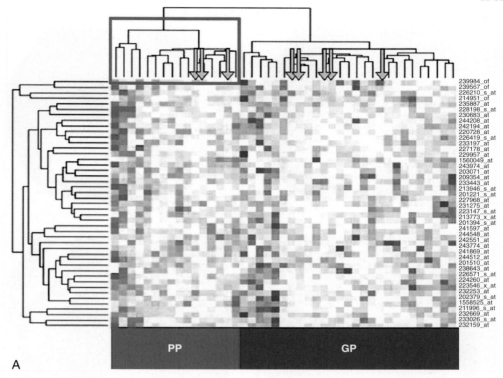

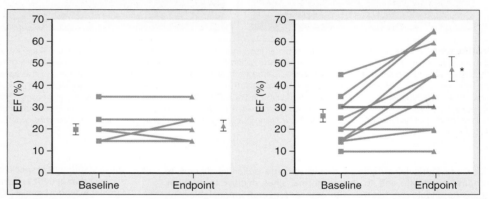

FIGURE 68-4 Inherent biologic processes affect long-term survival in patients with idiopathic dilated cardiomyopathy. **A,** Microarray transcriptomic analysis revealed a gene signature that predicted long-term event-free survival compared with poor prognosis manifesting as death or need for heart transplantation within 2 years. The dendograms depict individual signatures in specific columns and specific genes in rows. **B,** Patients with gene signature predicting favorable outcome undergo reverse remodeling and improvement in ejection fraction (EF). Yellow arrows in **A** and green line in **B** (at right) denote misclassified samples. GP = good prognosis; PP = poor prognosis. *(From Heidecker B, Kasper EK, Wittstein IS, et al: Transcriptomic biomarkers for individual risk assessment in new-onset heart failure. Circulation 118:238, 2008.)*

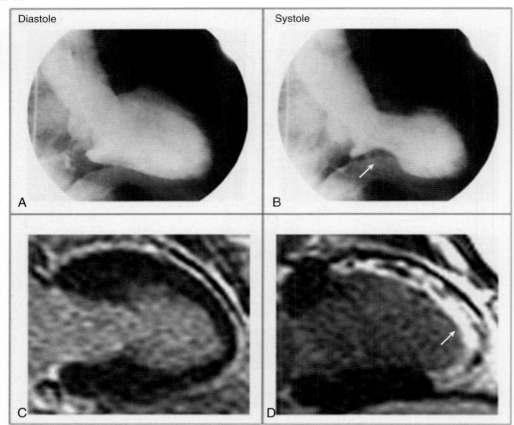

Diastole	Systole
A	B
C	D

FIGURE 68-5 Ventriculographic assessment of cardiac function and cardiac magnetic resonance (CMR) assessment of myocardial viability at admission in a patient with stress cardiomyopathy. Contrast-enhanced ventriculography during diastole, in **A,** and systole, in **B,** demonstrates apical and midventricular akinesis, with relative sparing of the base of the heart (arrow). **C,** CMR in the long-axis view reveals that the akinetic regions seen on ventriculography are dark and hypoenhanced, consistent with the presence of viable myocardium. **D,** presented for purposes of comparison, shows hyperenhancement (arrow), indicative of necrosis and decreased viability, after an acute anterior myocardial infarction. *(From Wittstein IS, Thiemann DR, Lima JA, et al: Neurohumoral features of myocardial stunning due to sudden emotional stress. N Engl J Med 352:539, 2005.)*

conditions, particularly muscular dystrophies, had cardiomyopathy as a component.[25,29] There are now abundant gene linkage studies with multiple genes identified; autosomal dominant and recessive as well as X-linked modes of inheritance exist (see Chap. 8).[25]

Most of the genes encode structural elements of the cell, notably members of the dystrophin-associated glycoprotein complex, or components of the sarcomeric contractile machinery. A mutation in the gene encoding phospholamban[30] implicates abnormalities in the excitation-contraction cascade as a cause of cardiomyopathy and supports attempts to treat cardiomyopathy with other elements of the calcium cycling machinery (i.e., delivery of the gene encoding the sarcoplasmic reticulum calcium pump [SERCA]).[31]

The fact that genetic abnormalities play a role offers insights into the phenotype in general. Clearly, genetic predisposition may be a central factor in the development of primary and secondary DCMs. Genetic defects may be primary causes of DCM, or they may act as predisposing factors in the setting of an environmental stressor-host-environment interaction. Primary examples of the latter are viral infections and hypertension, wherein exposure may lead to DCM only in subpopulations of exposed individuals. Genetic predisposition may be of fundamental importance in the variable natural history of DCM and may contribute to responsiveness to therapy.[32]

Knowledge of the genetics of DCM has led to the entry of genetic screening into the clinical arena and the development of specialty clinics at referral centers. Recent guidelines suggest that genetic screening and counseling should be considered in families in whom familial DCM is suspected, as a means of early detection of cardiomyopathy in family members.[25]

INFLAMMATORY AND INFECTIOUS MYOCARDITIS. The diagnosis and management of infectious myocarditis are discussed in Chap. 70 and reviewed here only briefly. Myocarditis may result from viral (or other pathogen) infection, autoimmune disease, or a combination (autoimmune reaction stimulated by a viral infection).[33] It is also increasingly possible that genetic factors increase the risk for development of cardiac disease after viral infection.

It has long been postulated that viral infection in susceptible hosts may be a proximate cause of cardiomyopathy and may serve as a precursor to the development of DCM. This hypothesis has been difficult to prove because of challenges in confirming viral infection in affected individuals coupled with the fact that common viruses are implicated in viral cardiomyopathy, leading to concerns of a high false-positive rate when viruses are detected in patients with heart failure. Lymphocytic myocarditis with or without myocyte necrosis has been considered the hallmark diagnostic finding necessary for a diagnosis, and criteria established for the histologic evaluation are termed the Dallas criteria.[33] The link between myocarditis and viral heart disease is problematic because true inflammatory myocarditis can occur in the absence of an infectious agent (see later). As discussed in Chap. 70, the application of the polymerase chain reaction (PCR) to detect viral particles in myocardial samples taken from patients with DCM has provided important insights into the role played by viruses in heart muscle disease.

Two general mechanisms for postviral cardiac injury have been invoked: autoimmune reactions and direct tissue injury resulting from viral infection of the heart (see Chap. 70). Both of these mechanisms are incompletely proved and remain controversial. The presence or absence

or supraventricular arrhythmia should undergo definitive therapy to control heart rate and to restore normal sinus rhythm. In addition, patients should be treated with standard neurohormonal blocking agents and carefully monitored with echocardiography in the weeks to months after presentation for signs of recovery.

ALCOHOLIC CARDIOMYOPATHY. Alcoholic cardiomyopathy is a common cause of DCM and the most common secondary cardiomyopathy. Phenotypically and clinically, it closely resembles idiopathic DCM (see also Chap. 73). The disorder is linked to ongoing excessive alcohol consumption and appears to be both dose related and responsive to cessation of alcohol exposure. Alcohol exposure also increases risk for comorbidities that can contribute to cardiovascular disease, such as hypertension, stroke, arrhythmias, and sudden death. Alcoholic cardiomyopathy is discussed in Chap. 73.

Etiologic Basis for Idiopathic Dilated Cardiomyopathy

Rapidly advancing knowledge in four areas is shedding light on pathophysiologic mechanisms that may contribute to DCM and may in turn lead to new therapeutic approaches. These areas include (1) familial and genetic factors,[25] (2) inflammatory and infectious factors, particularly viral infection,[26] (3) cytotoxicity, and (4) cell loss and abnormalities in endogenous repair mechanisms.[27,28]

GENETIC AND FAMILIAL FACTORS. Studies of the genetics of DCM offer major insights into the etiology of the disease. Two general lines of evidence initially suggested a genetic component to DCM.[25] Familial studies indicated that in excess of 20% of patients with DCM had other family members with the condition, and conversely, certain inherited

of inflammation on endomyocardial biopsy, which varies greatly from study to study, is used to substantiate immunologic injury. However, other studies have suggested different criteria (e.g., complement or immunoglobulin deposition). The postviral hypothesis has increasing support, and viral material has been detected on the basis of elevated viral titers, presence of viral genomic material by PCR, and detection of viral particles.

AUTOIMMUNITY. Studies support abnormalities of humoral and cellular immunity in DCM. Two general theories are proposed for an autoimmune cause of DCM: (1) viral components incorporate into the cardiac myocyte membrane, stimulating an antigenic response; and (2) anti–heart antibodies are generated as a result of myocardial damage as opposed to being the proximate cause. Certain specific human leukocyte antigen (HLA) class II antigens (particularly DR4) are associated with DCM. In addition, numerous circulating antimyocardial antibodies have been measured in DCM patients that react with a variety of antigens, including the myosin heavy chain, the beta adrenoceptor, the muscarinic receptor, sarcolemmal sodium-potassium adenosine triphosphatase, laminin, and mitochondrial proteins. Whether anti-inflammatory therapies have efficacy in treating DCM has been difficult to prove; corticosteroid trials performed in the 1980s have been neutral, but there are ongoing attempts to test the value of immunoabsorption strategies. A regimen of prednisone and azathioprine has recently been shown to improve ejection fraction in patients with virus-negative myocarditis.[34]

CYTOTOXICITY AND DERANGED INTRACELLULAR SIGNALING. The direct action of various circulating factors is implicated in the pathophysiology of myocyte dysfunction. For example, tumor necrosis factor and endothelin levels are elevated in DCM. The exact role of these factors remains incompletely understood, and therapies to antagonize their effects have not been definitively established.

An additional molecular mechanism gaining increased experimental and clinical support is that of nitroso-redox imbalance, an intracellular phenomenon characterized by dysregulation of nitric oxide production coupled with increased production of reactive oxygen species.[35] This imbalance is described in experimental animal models and in humans with DCM and causes cellular dysfunction and possibly cytotoxicity. Although not definitively proved, one mechanism postulated to explain the response of DCM patients to hydralazine–isosorbide dinitrate is a restoration of nitroso-redox balance (see Chap. 25).

INJURY, CELL LOSS, AND ENDOGENOUS REPAIR. A variety of other causes related to damage to cellular constituents of the heart are proposed as etiologic factors. Although none is accepted as the absolute cause, the variety of mechanisms highlights the notion of a final common pathway, with various insults converging on a set of mechanisms that all result in a common phenotypic response to injury. Many of the mechanisms, such as endocrine disturbances and toxic exposures, derive from the existence of specific examples of secondary cardiomyopathies. The appearance of DCM in only a small fraction of subjects with a common disorder is supportive of the idea that specific host (gene)–environment interactions lead to the cardiac manifestations of the exposure.

Ischemia due to hyperreactivity or spasm of the microvasculature may contribute to diffuse myocyte necrosis and replacement fibrosis. The classic disorder in which this is manifested is scleroderma heart disease. Increased myocyte apoptosis is described in DCM and ARVD/C, leading to the suggestion that augmented cell loss may contribute to the development of left ventricular remodeling in DCM processes. Although there are an increasing number of experimental studies supporting cardiac recovery when antiapoptotic agents are administered in animal models,[36] the exact role of apoptosis in these conditions is not known. Further, the role of cell loss in DCM has become more interesting in light of recent accumulating data supporting the idea that endogenous cardiac stem cells repopulate cardiac myocytes throughout life,[28] thereby serving a homeostatic balancing mechanism for ongoing cell loss and cell replacement after tissue injury (see Chap. 11). Indeed, studies already support the idea of cardiac stem cell senescence contributing to the development of human cardiomyopathy.[27] Thus, depletion or dysfunction of endogenous cells with capacity to divide and to differentiate in cardiac cellular constituents may be a central pathophysiologic contributor to cardiomyopathic processes.[27]

Clinical Evaluation of the Dilated Cardiomyopathies

HISTORY. DCM affects individuals of all ages, including neonates and children.[37,38] In adults, the incidence of DCM is estimated to be between 5 and 8 per 100,000 persons per year. DCM is most frequent in middle age and affects men to a greater degree than women. Although the incidence of ischemic cardiomyopathy is higher than that of DCM, these two diagnoses account for an equal number of heart transplantations performed.

The clinical presentation of patients with heart failure is discussed in Chap. 26. In the case of DCM, the clinical presentation of patients can vary substantially. In some patients, symptoms develop very gradually and diagnosis can result from the detection of cardiomegaly on routine chest radiography. Patients presenting with clear-cut symptoms of congestive heart failure report the development of progressive symptoms for periods varying from weeks to months. Intercurrent illnesses frequently precipitate congestive heart failure in individuals with DCM. A significant minority of patients with DCM present with aggressive, life-threatening congestive heart failure (fulminant heart failure) that can require the most intensive forms of mechanical intervention.[15] The causes of the fulminant presentation vary from idiopathic cardiomyopathy to fulminant lymphocytic myocarditis to giant cell myocarditis (see Chap. 70).[13,16] The determinants of these various forms of clinical presentation are poorly understood.

EVALUATION FOR SECONDARY CARDIOMYOPATHIES. An initial history must focus on identifying etiologic factors[7] (see Table 68-1). A past or associated history of rheumatologic, endocrine, or infectious diseases or of previous neoplasia should be sought.[7] In patients with a history of cancer, treatment with anthracyclines, tyrosine kinase inhibitors, or irradiation is particularly relevant. The family history can often reveal heritable forms of cardiomyopathy. Patients should be questioned about the consumption of alcohol, tobacco, and illicit drugs. Travel history can reveal exposure to geographically related infectious pathogens.

The most typical symptoms are those of congestive heart failure and include dyspnea, fatigue, and volume gain. A minority of patients report chest pain, which can signify epicardial coronary disease, subendocardial disease, or pulmonary embolism. A report of abdominal discomfort or anorexia is frequent in late stages of the disease and suggests hepatomegaly or bowel edema, respectively.

Common late complications include thromboembolic events, which may be systemic, originating from dislodgment of left atrial and ventricular intracardiac or pulmonary thrombi from the lower extremity venous system.

PHYSICAL EXAMINATION. The physical examination for patients with heart failure is discussed in Chaps. 12 and 26. Particular attention should be paid in the physical examination to excluding findings of valvular heart disease. S_3 and S_4 gallops are invariably present in DCM. The S_3 must be differentiated from a pericardial knock or an opening snap of mitral stenosis, both of which are higher pitched sounds than the S_3. Patients with fulminant heart failure of new onset will frequently be tachycardic and will develop a gallop rhythm in which S_3 and S_4 fuse. Attention should be paid to differentiation of right-sided gallops and murmurs to consider the possibility of right-sided involvement.

NONINVASIVE EVALUATION. The diagnostic evaluation of patients with heart failure is discussed in Chap. 26. For patients presenting with DCM, the initial evaluation should focus on identification of reversible and secondary causes. Even though the presentation of the patient with a dilated ventricle and heart failure may be fairly uniform, a wide array of specific and secondary cardiomyopathies may cause a clinical presentation of a DCM. The first step in the diagnostic evaluation involves screening biochemical testing, including serum electrolytes, phosphorus, calcium, and markers of renal function (serum creatinine and urea).[7] Endocrine function should be screened, notably thyroid function (hyperthyroidism and hypothyroidism) and possibly urinary evaluation of catecholamine levels to exclude pheochromocytoma. To screen for rheumatologic conditions, an antinuclear antibody and erythrocyte sedimentation rate should be obtained. When suspected, rarer causes of cardiomyopathy can be excluded with blood testing. For example, Lyme titers can be a useful screen for

Lyme carditis. Iron studies may assist in evaluating hemochromatosis, and HIV testing is valuable.

The use of biomarkers (such as troponin) to assess myocardial necrosis and the use of circulating brain natriuretic peptide (BNP or pro-BNP) levels may serve as useful adjunctive strategies to help determine diagnosis or prognosis (see Chap. 26). Further, there is increasing support for the use of serum uric acid levels as a prognostic marker.[9,39] A chest radiograph offers supporting evidence for the diagnosis and in some cases is the initial mode of detection. Cardiomegaly may be appreciated, as may evidence of pulmonary vascular redistribution. Rarely, interstitial and alveolar edema are present on initial presentation. With advancing heart failure, pleural effusions are present, and dilated azygos veins and superior vena cava indicate right-sided volume overload.

ELECTROCARDIOGRAPHY. There are no specific electrocardiographic findings signifying DCM. Sinus tachycardia is often present in proportion to the degree of heart failure. Typical changes in the QRS complex include poor R wave progression, intraventricular conduction delays, and left bundle branch block. A wide QRS complex portends a worse prognosis and has now emerged as a clinical indicator of responsiveness to cardiac resynchronization therapy (see Chaps. 28 and 29). Patients with substantial left ventricular fibrosis may exhibit anterior Q waves even in the absence of a discrete scar or epicardial coronary artery obstructions. A broad array of abnormalities may be manifested, such as nonspecific ST-segment and T wave abnormalities as well as P wave alterations, notably left atrial abnormality. Nonsustained ventricular tachycardia is extremely common on 24-hour ambulatory monitoring and represents a predictor of all-cause mortality. Persistent supraventricular or ventricular tachyarrhythmias represent an important etiologic factor for ventricular dysfunction,[24] and restoration of sinus rhythm or heart rate control may lead to recovery of ventricular function. Control of atrial fibrillation is also important because of atrial transport issues contributing to cardiac output. In addition, atrial fibrillation should prompt consideration of tachycardia-induced cardiomyopathy.

ECHOCARDIOGRAPHY. Echocardiography is a cornerstone in the evaluation and management of patients with DCM (see Chaps. 15 and 26). Two-dimensional echocardiography is a highly useful and readily available technique to assess ventricular size and performance and to exclude associated valvular or pericardial abnormalities. Doppler echocardiography permits the evaluation of valvular regurgitation or stenosis and the quantification of cardiac output (see Figs. 15-53 and 15-63). Doppler detection of restrictive filling patterns may indicate disease of greater severity (see Fig. 15-64). Pericardial effusion may be present. Performing echocardiography during dobutamine stimulation may identify occult coronary artery disease by provoking regional wall motion abnormalities, differentiating these patients from those with idiopathic DCM. Moreover, significant contractile reserve during dobutamine infusion represents a positive prognostic finding. Three-dimensional echocardiography may be of additional value in assessing mitral valve orifice remodeling and determining ventricular dyssynchrony.

RADIONUCLIDE IMAGING. Nuclear imaging protocols for myocardial perfusion stress imaging may be useful to exclude an ischemic cause of dilated heart failure. Radionuclide ventriculography also provides evidence of cardiac structure and function, showing increased chamber volumes at end diastole and end systole; it provides quantification of reduced ejection fraction in either or both ventricles, and it can elucidate the regional nature of wall motion abnormalities (see Chap. 17). Not always necessary, this technique can be of particular value if echocardiography is technically suboptimal.

CARDIAC MAGNETIC RESONANCE IMAGING AND MULTIDETECTOR COMPUTED TOMOGRAPHY (see Fig. 68-2). Cardiac magnetic resonance imaging (CMR) and multidetector computed tomography are relatively new imaging modalities that are likely to become increasingly useful to evaluate patients with

cardiomyopathies (see Chap. 18).[40] Specific cardiomyopathic disorders in which CMR has proved particularly valuable include ARVD/C,[41] endocardial fibroelastosis, myocarditis,[42] amyloidosis,[43] and sarcoidosis. CMR evaluation is also emerging as a critical tool to understand DCM pathophysiology and may contribute to identification of patients at particular risk for complications, such as sudden cardiac death (e.g., within DCM subsets, those with or without areas of replacement fibrosis that may predispose to electrical instability and sudden cardiac death).[44] CMR is also emerging as an important tool in the delineation of infiltrative and inflammatory cardiomyopathies.

INVASIVE EVALUATION INCLUDING ENDOMYOCARDIAL BIOPSY. Catheterization for the exclusion of epicardial coronary disease is essential in the management of the patient presenting with DCM. Because DCM and heart failure increase the false-positive and false-negative rates of noninvasive nuclear assessment for myocardial ischemia, performance of coronary angiography is often necessary to exclude epicardial coronary obstructive disease.[4] It is increasingly relevant to obtain hemodynamic assessments in individuals presenting with acute or worsening heart failure. Use of these diagnostic tests is currently nonuniform.[45] Catheterization usually reveals elevated left ventricular end-diastolic and pulmonary artery wedge pressures. Pulmonary arterial hypertension may be of variable degrees, ranging from mild to severe. The right ventricle is frequently involved and enlarged, hemodynamically manifesting with increased right ventricular end-diastolic, right atrial, and central venous pressures.

Left ventriculography demonstrates varying degrees of ventricular dilation and diffuse chamber hypokinesis. There may be a degree of regionality to the decreased function resembling ischemic heart disease, although a diffuse pattern is frequently present. Filling defects may be present because of left ventricular thrombi, and mild mitral regurgitation is not unusual. It is not always possible to distinguish between left ventricular dilation due to severe mitral regurgitation associated with primary mitral valve disease and DCM with secondary mitral regurgitation.

Coronary arteriography is particularly important to exclude coronary obstructive disease. In patients with DCM, the arterial circulation is typically normal although vasodilator function may be abnormal.

BIOPSY. The role of endomyocardial biopsy to evaluate the myocardium histologically has been historically controversial in the evaluation of the patient presenting with structural heart disease or symptoms of heart failure.[8,46] Recently, however, expert guidelines have been published that offer significant guidance as to the indications for endomyocardial biopsy (see Table 70-4).[13] This procedure, which is routine in the management of heart transplant recipients, allows the acquisition of small pieces of myocardium by use of a flexible bioptome. Currently available bioptomes are advanced transvenously, most commonly by a right internal jugular venous approach, to the right ventricular septum. If it is required, the left ventricular septum may be sampled by a transarterial approach. This procedure is currently performed with either fluoroscopic or echocardiographic guidance. Although not reported in the literature, the widespread use of disposable bioptomes, which have replaced reusable Stanford-Caves devices, has led to a reduction of complications, particularly right ventricle perforation.

Perhaps the most compelling reason in favor of routine biopsy is the detection of a few relatively rare diseases in which accurate diagnosis yields a life-threatening disease with specific management.[15,47] For example, lymphocytic and giant cell myocarditis must be detected early in the course of the presentation for patients to survive and can be separated from each other only by histologic evaluation.[34,48] Biopsy is also an established method for grading the severity of anthracycline cardiomyopathy and has potential similar value for cardiac amyloidosis. A biopsy finding that is negative for inflammation is also valuable in patients with rapidly progressive severe decompensated heart failure, insofar as it may prompt advancement to aggressive mechanical support earlier in the patient's clinical course. Whereas widespread use of the myocardial biopsy is no longer routinely recommended, recent guidelines and treatment trials continue to add clarity around appropriate selection of patients. As reflected in the guidelines, the determination of whether to perform the procedure remains a balance between exposing a patient to a low-yield procedure in the entire population versus the lifesaving potential in a relatively fewer number of patients. In patients with fulminant heart failure, particularly those with new-onset cardiomyopathy, the risk-benefit assessment is more clearly in favor of performing a biopsy to more rationally allocate patients for emergent heart transplantation listing or for insertion of a mechanical assist device. Patients who have fulminant lymphocytic myocarditis have excellent long-term prognosis after short-term hemodynamic support[15]; those with giant cell myocarditis should be aggressively immunosuppressed or listed for heart transplantation[48]; and those with idiopathic cardiomyopathy (suggested by the absence of myocardial inflammation on biopsy) should be aggressively supported and converted to conventional therapy once stabilized. Not infrequently, the endomyocardial biopsy reveals an unsuspected cause of cardiomyopathy.

Management

PHARMACOLOGIC AND DEVICE THERAPY. Whereas the concept of specific etiology-based therapies represents an ongoing quest for patients with DCM, the general treatment of these patients should follow the practice guidelines for all patients with heart failure (see Guidelines: Management of Heart Failure[49] and Chaps. 27, 28, and 30). Indeed, treatment with neurohormonal antagonists to prevent disease progression and the use of diuretics to maintain the volume balance are the therapeutic cornerstones for the management of patients with DCM.[49] Similarly, the use of prophylactic implantable cardiac defibrillators and biventricular pacemakers is indicated in appropriate patients with nonischemic and ischemic DCM (see Chaps. 28, 29, and 38).[49,50]

SURGERY. The surgical management for patients with heart failure is discussed in Chap. 31. Patients with valvular heart disease, coronary artery disease, pericardial disease, or congenital heart defects should have these conditions corrected surgically, when appropriate. Other specific operations geared toward the cardiomyopathic heart include approaches motivated by the concept of restoring chamber geometry or interventions to provide mechanical support. Approaches to achievement of reverse remodeling surgically include left ventricular reconstruction and implantation of external restraint devices (see Chap. 31). Left ventricular assist devices provide aggressive mechanical support to patients with advanced decompensated heart failure (see Chap. 32).

EMERGING SPECIFIC THERAPIES. Only recently are specific etiology-based therapies being evaluated. These include agents to eradicate persistent viral infections and immunomodulatory agents (see Chap. 70). Stem cells for cardiac regeneration and gene therapy approaches are in clinical trials (see Chaps. 11 and 33).

Restrictive and Infiltrative Cardiomyopathy

Relative to the dilated and hypertrophic cardiomyopathies, restrictive cardiomyopathy occurs with lower frequency in the developed world. Specific forms of restrictive cardiomyopathy, such as endomyocardial disease (**Table 68-4**), are important causes of morbidity and mortality common in specific geographic locales, especially in underdeveloped countries.[51-53] The pathophysiologic feature that defines restrictive cardiomyopathy is the increase in stiffness of the ventricular walls, which causes heart failure because of impaired diastolic filling of the ventricle (see also Chaps. 24 and 26).[16] In early stages of the syndrome, systolic function may be normal, although deterioration in systolic function is usually observed as the disease progresses.[2]

Restrictive cardiomyopathy must be distinguished from constrictive pericarditis, which is also characterized by normal or nearly normal

TABLE 68-4	**Classification of Types of Restrictive Cardiomyopathy According to Cause**

Myocardial
Noninfiltrative
Idiopathic cardiomyopathy*
Familial cardiomyopathy
Hypertrophic cardiomyopathy
Scleroderma
Pseudoxanthoma elasticum
Diabetic cardiomyopathy

Infiltrative
Amyloidosis*
Sarcoidosis*
Gaucher disease
Hurler disease
Fatty infiltration

Storage Disease
Hemochromatosis
Fabry disease
Glycogen storage disease

Endomyocardial
Endomyocardial fibrosis*
Hypereosinophilic syndrome
Carcinoid heart disease
Metastatic cancers
Radiation*
Toxic effects of anthracycline*
Drugs causing fibrous endocarditis (serotonin, methysergide, ergotamine, mercurial agents, busulfan)

*These conditions are more likely than the others to be encountered in clinical practice.
From Kushwaha S, Fallon JT, Fuster V: Restrictive cardiomyopathy. N Engl J Med 336:267, 1997. Copyright 1997, Massachusetts Medical Society.

systolic function but abnormal ventricular filling (see Chap. 75).[2] Differentiation of these two conditions represents a classic diagnostic challenge and is one of significant clinical importance because pericardial constriction may be treated successfully with pericardiectomy.

Approximately 50% of cases of restrictive cardiomyopathy result from specific clinical disorders, whereas the remainder represents an idiopathic process. The most common specific cause of restrictive cardiomyopathy is infiltration caused by amyloidosis; there are both acquired and genetic causes of amyloid.[54] Although there are other specific pathologic presentations associated with restrictive cardiomyopathy, their precise etiology often remains obscure. Like DCM, there are inflammatory and genetic factors important in the etiology of restrictive cardiomyopathy. The identification of specific infiltrative processes may have prognostic and therapeutic implications (**Fig. 68-6**).[7] The abnormal diastolic properties of the ventricle are attributable to myocardial fibrosis, infiltration, or scarring of the endomyocardial surface. Myocyte hypertrophy is common, particularly in idiopathic restrictive cardiomyopathy (**Fig. 68-7**).

Clinical Evaluation

CARDIAC CATHETERIZATION AND ENDOMYOCARDIAL BIOPSY. A classic diagnostic challenge is to differentiate restrictive cardiomyopathy from constrictive pericarditis, which is manifested with similar clinical and hemodynamic features. Cardiac catheterization is a key step in this evaluation (see Chaps. 20 and 75). Whereas there is equalization of diastolic pressures in constrictive pericarditis (pressures differ by no more than 5 mm Hg), they may vary to a greater extent in restrictive cardiomyopathy (see Fig. 20-15). Pulmonary hypertension is worse in restrictive cardiomyopathy, with systolic pulmonary pressures often exceeding 50 mm Hg. In constrictive pericarditis, the plateau of right ventricular diastolic pressure is usually at least one third of peak systolic pressure; in restrictive cardiomyopathy, this is most often lower. Hemodynamically, both conditions have a rapid early diastolic pressure decline followed by a rapid rise and plateau

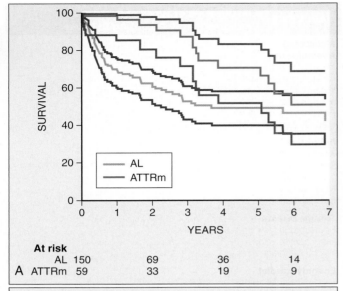

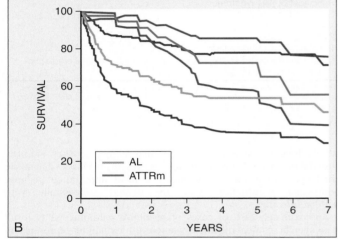

FIGURE 68-6 Variable prognosis in patients with cardiac amyloidosis based on the specific etiology. Overall survival (with 95% confidence intervals) of patients with transthyretin-related (ATTRm) and light chain (AL) amyloidosis before **(A)** and after **(B)** adjustment for renal involvement or insufficiency. *(From Rapezzi C, Merlini G, Quarta CC, et al: Systemic cardiac amyloidoses. Disease profiles and clinical courses of the 3 main types. Circulation 120:1203, 2009.)*

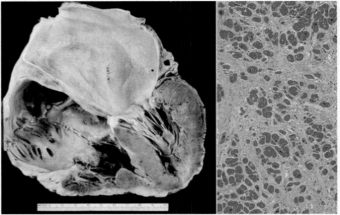

FIGURE 68-7 Pathology of idiopathic restrictive cardiomyopathy in a 63-year-old woman. **Left,** Gross cardiac specimen, shown in four-chamber format, demonstrating prominent biatrial enlargement, with normal-sized ventricles. **Right,** Light microscopy showing marked interstitial fibrosis (light pink areas). Hematoxylin and eosin; magnification ×120. *(From Ammash NM, Seward JB, Bailey KR, et al: Clinical profile and outcome of idiopathic restrictive cardiomyopathy. Circulation 101:2490, 2000.)*

in early diastole, the so-called square root sign. The atrial pressure tracing is manifested as either a classic square root pattern or an M or W waveform when the x descent is also rapid. Both a and v waves are prominent and frequently have the same amplitude. Right- and left-sided atrial filling pressures are elevated, although in the case of restrictive cardiomyopathy, the left ventricular filling pressure typically is 5 mm Hg, or more, greater than the right ventricular diastolic pressure. This difference may be accentuated by Valsalva maneuver, exercise, or a fluid challenge.

Endomyocardial biopsy can also be valuable in the evaluation of these patients to exclude an infiltrative process or cardiomyopathic-appearing myocytes and received a Class IIa recommendation in the guidelines.[13] A normal-appearing biopsy specimen supports the diagnosis of a pericardial process. Surgical exploration is needed far less often, given the availability of biopsy and imaging technology (see later).

Prognosis

Restrictive cardiomyopathy carries a variable prognosis dependent on etiology (see Fig. 68-e2 on website). Most often, especially in the case

of amyloidosis, it is invariably progressive with an accelerated mortality.[55] A longitudinal study of 233 patients revealed the importance of the underlying type of amyloidosis in outcome; patients fared better with the transthyretin-related form of amyloid than with immunoglobulin associated (see Fig. 68-6).[54] There is no specific therapy for the idiopathic form of restrictive cardiomyopathy, but intensive fluid and supportive management are required to maintain a patient with a reasonable quality of life. There are ongoing aggressive attempts to devise therapies for secondary forms of restrictive cardiomyopathy tailored to the etiology (e.g., iron removal in hemochromatosis or enzyme replacement therapy in Fabry disease).

Clinical Manifestations

Patients with restrictive cardiomyopathy frequently present with exercise intolerance that results from an impaired ability to augment cardiac output during increasing heart rate because of the restriction of diastolic filling. Other notable symptoms are weakness, dyspnea, and edema, and exertional chest pain is reported by some but not all patients. With advancing disease, profound edema occurs that includes peripheral edema, hepatomegaly, ascites, and anasarca. These patients represent the most difficult volume management because of the balance between volume status and hypotension that can result during diuresis by reduced preload filling of the ventricles. Physical examination is notable for an elevated jugular venous pulse, often with the Kussmaul sign, a rising jugular pressure during inspiration (because of the restriction to filling). Both S3 and S4 gallops are common, and the apical pulse is palpable (in contrast to constrictive pericarditis). Patients with restrictive cardiomyopathy are highly prone to development of atrial fibrillation.[2]

Laboratory Studies

Computed tomography and CMR are valuable for differentiation of constrictive and restrictive disease.(see Chaps. 18 and 19). A thickened pericardium supports the diagnosis of pericardial constriction. Other ancillary tests also may be helpful. For example, chest radiography may detect pericardial calcification. The electrocardiogram may disclose atrial fibrillation. Echocardiography (see Fig. 15-68) should be routinely performed in patients suspected of restrictive cardiomyopathy or constriction and may reveal biatrial dilation and increasing wall thickness associated with myocardial infiltration as well as alterations in the appearance of the myocardium (e.g., speckling). Doppler echocardiography supplemented with tissue Doppler reveals evidence of impaired myocardial relaxation with increased early left ventricular filling velocity, decreased atrial filling velocity, and decreased isovolumetric relaxation time (see Figs. 15-69 and 15-70); these findings are additionally useful for the discrimination from constrictive disease.[2,56] BNP levels may be used to discriminate between restrictive cardiomyopathy and constrictive disease, with concentrations approximately five times greater in the former compared with the latter.[57]

Amyloidosis

Etiology and Types

Amyloidosis is a unique disease process that results from tissue deposition of proteins that have a unique secondary structure (twisted beta-pleated sheet fibrils; **Fig. 68-8**). Amyloid may be found in almost any organ but does not produce clinically evident disease unless tissue infiltration is extensive. Several classification systems have been used to characterize the different clinical presentations of amyloidosis. Primary (acquired) amyloidosis results from the deposition of portions of immunoglobulin light chains (designated AL amyloid) within tissues. In most cases, the excess production of this protein results from a monoclonal expansion of plasma cells in the setting of multiple myeloma. Rarely, a patient with a plasma cell dyscrasia may develop restrictive cardiomyopathy due to deposition of light chains in a non-amyloid manner. Importantly, the latter form of disease may be reversible. Historically, primary amyloidosis occurred from other chronic untreated inflammatory conditions. Secondary amyloidosis (also known as reactive systemic amyloidosis) results from the excess production of a nonimmunoglobulin protein known as AA.

FAMILIAL (HEREDITARY) AMYLOIDOSIS. In the past decade, there has been growing recognition that various familial diseases can lead to amyloid deposition in the heart. An autosomal dominant form results from the deposition of a variant form of prealbumin serum carrier termed transthyretin in tissues. Multiple (>100) point mutations in the transthyretin gene are associated with amyloidosis.[54] Transthyretin amyloidosis usually produces one of three different clinical scenarios—nephropathy, neuropathy, or cardiomyopathy. Isolated cardiomyopathy occurring with older age, associated with the Ile 122 variant, is more common in individuals of African American descent.[58] Given that transthyretin is produced within the liver, liver transplantation may be contemplated in affected individuals who are detected early.

SENILE SYSTEMIC AMYLOIDOSIS. This form of amyloidosis results from amyloid deposition of proteins that are like either atrial natriuretic peptide or transthyretin.[59] This form of amyloidosis is increasing in incidence as the population ages, with a predilection for elderly men. Although it affects individuals of older age, the prognosis is better than that of AL disease.[59] Deposition of amyloid in the atria and pulmonary vessels is often found at autopsy in octogenarians and may be a risk factor for atrial fibrillation.

CARDIAC AMYLOIDOSIS. Cardiac amyloidosis is an invariably progressive infiltrative cardiomyopathy that carries a grave prognosis.[55] Cardiac involvement may be present in up to one third of patients with primary amyloidosis resulting from plasma cell dyscrasias. When the heart is studied pathologically, AL protein deposits are present invariably at necropsy even if clinically silent in life. Myocardial infiltration tends to be less with secondary amyloidosis, in which the AA protein deposits tend to be smaller and more perivascular in location, where they are less likely to produce myocardial dysfunction.

Approximately one quarter of patients with transthyretin-induced (familial) amyloidosis experience clinically significant cardiac involvement that is often marked by involvement of the conduction system. Neurologic or renal involvement may also predominate in this form of amyloidosis. Patients will typically present with clinical symptoms after the age of 35 years. In half of the cases involving deposition of transthyretin, the mode of death is cardiac, from either heart failure or sudden cardiac death. In senile amyloidosis, deposits vary from isolated atrial involvement to extensive ventricular infiltration causing severe restrictive cardiomyopathy. Cardiac amyloidosis is observed more frequently in men than in women and is rare before the age of 40 years.

Pathology

The term *amyloidosis* was coined by Virchow and means "starch-like." The heart infiltrated with amyloid appears tan and waxy and is rubbery in consistency. The atria are also significantly enlarged (see Fig. 68-8). On histologic examination, amyloid deposits can be detected with Congo red or Sirius red staining and are present between cardiac myocytes.[16,55] Amyloidosis may cause focal thickening of the cardiac valves but infrequently leads to valvular dysfunction. In addition, amyloid may deposit within the media and adventitia of intramural coronary arteries and may cause impairment in coronary perfusion.

Clinical Manifestations

There are four overlapping cardiovascular syndromes that may occur with cardiovascular involvement of amyloidosis, including restrictive cardiomyopathy, systolic heart failure, orthostatic hypotension, and presentation with conduction system disease.

RESTRICTIVE CARDIOMYOPATHY. Amyloid infiltration and circulating immunoglobulins produce classic restrictive physiology leading to increased diastolic chamber stiffness with a resultant impairment of left ventricular filling. The impairment of chamber filling leads to fluid retention and peripheral edema, hepatomegaly, and elevated jugular venous pressure. Hemodynamic measurements reveal the classic dip and plateau square root sign. One feature differentiating amyloidosis from constrictive pericarditis is the rate of early diastolic filling, which is accelerated in pericardial disease but is diminished in amyloidosis.

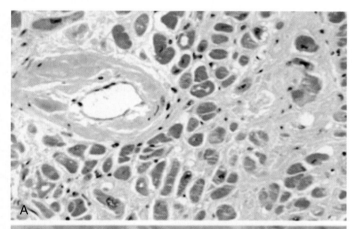
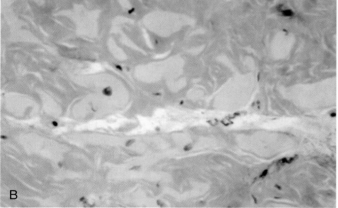

FIGURE 68-8 Histologic phenotype of cardiac amyloidosis. **A,** Endomyocardial biopsy specimen, stained with hematoxylin and eosin, from a patient with cardiac amyloidosis. The amyloid stains light pinkish red and is seen as an amorphous material that separates the darker-staining myocytes. **B,** Staining of the tissue from the same patient with sulfated Alcian blue. The amyloid stains turquoise green and the myocytes stain yellow, characteristic of amyloid. *(From Falk RH: Diagnosis and management of the cardiac amyloidoses. Circulation 112:2047, 2005.)*

SYSTOLIC HEART FAILURE. Although systolic function may be normal early in the disease, it frequently deteriorates late in the disease as the degree of amyloid deposition increases. Deposition of amyloid in the atrium can also lead to atrial arrest, even though the sinus node is fully functional. The loss of atrial transport function may contribute to worsening heart failure, particularly in the face of restrictive cardiac physiology. Patients may also exhibit angina pectoris, although epicardial coronary arteries are normal angiographically. This form of the disease is usually relentlessly progressive.

ORTHOSTATIC HYPOTENSION. Approximately 10% of affected individuals will exhibit orthostasis caused by amyloid infiltration of the autonomic nervous system, blood vessels, or both.[60] Infiltration of the heart and adrenal glands may contribute to the pathogenesis of this variant. Renal failure resulting in the nephrotic syndrome and volume retention can worsen the postural hypotension. Patients with amyloidosis frequently experience frank syncope often associated with emotional or physical stress, a phenomenon that may be associated with left ventricular outflow obstruction. Syncope during exertion represents an extremely poor prognosis, with demise likely within 3 months.

CONDUCTION SYSTEM DISEASE. Abnormal propagation of cardiac electrical signals is the least common form of amyloidosis and may result in arrhythmias and conduction disturbances. Sudden cardiac death, caused by malignant arrhythmias or conduction block, is an important mode of death. Episodes of syncope may herald more severe events, such as sudden cardiac death.

Physical Examination

Most commonly, patients with cardiac amyloidosis present with signs of congestive heart failure. The jugular venous pulse is elevated, often massively, and there are signs of systemic edema with hepatomegaly, ascites, and edema. On auscultation, apical systolic murmurs due to mitral regurgitation and S_3 gallops are frequently present, although the S_4 is typically absent when there is atrial infiltration with amyloid that leads to impaired atrial contraction. The blood pressure is normal to reduced, and the pulse pressure may be quite narrow, consistent with low cardiac output.

Noninvasive Testing

Cardiomegaly is present on chest radiography in patients with systolic dysfunction but not in those with restrictive presentations. Pulmonary congestion will be detected if heart failure is present. The electrocardiogram most often reveals low QRS voltage, and bundle branch block and abnormal axis are also common. A pattern of old anterior myocardial infarction may be simulated by diminutive or absent R waves in the right precordial leads or by inferior Q waves. Amyloid infiltration of the atrium predisposes to atrial fibrillation, and ventricular arrhythmias are also common. Signal-averaged electrocardiography has proved valuable in predicting increased risk for sudden cardiac death. Atrioventricular conduction defects are common, are particularly prominent in familial amyloidosis with polyneuropathy, and may portend a poor prognosis. Electrophysiologic testing is usually necessary to detect significant intrahisian block. Sinus node dysfunction is also common, and the electrocardiogram may show sick sinus syndrome.

ECHOCARDIOGRAPHY. Echocardiography is valuable and reveals increased ventricular wall thickness with small intracavitary chambers, enlarged atria, and a thickened interatrial septum (see Fig. 15-78). As noted, systolic function is normal early in the course of the disease, but progressive left ventricular dysfunction ensues with advancing amyloid deposition. The walls of the ventricles often reveal a distinctive appearance with a sparkling and granular texture, most likely resulting from the amyloid deposition itself. The cardiac valves may have a thickened appearance but typically have normal excursion. Pericardial effusions may be present but do not advance to tamponade. Patterns of chamber hypertrophy are, on occasion, regional, leading to a pattern reminiscent of hypertrophic cardiomyopathy. The echocardiographic appearance of thickened left ventricular walls associated with low voltage on electrocardiography is valuable for differentiation from pericardial disease. Both Doppler echocardiography and radionuclide

ventriculography are valuable to evaluate diastolic dysfunction (see Fig. 15-79), the degree of which offers prognostic information.

RADIONUCLIDE AND MAGNETIC RESONANCE CARDIAC IMAGING. Technetium-99m pyrophosphate scintigraphy and other agents that bind to calcium may be valuable for amyloid detection. This tool is frequently strongly positive when amyloidosis is extensive and correlates with the degree of cardiac infiltration; however, false-negative results may occur. Both CMR and indium-labeled antimyosin antibody imaging are useful for the detection of cardiac amyloid involvement. CMR has a very high sensitivity for the detection of cardiac amyloid (see Fig. 18-14) and may also be valuable in measuring the extent of amyloid deposition in the heart, which may be of significant prognostic importance.[43] There are specialized agents that may detect sympathetic denervation in patients with cardiac amyloidosis.

Diagnosis

In the past, systemic amyloidosis was frequently diagnosed at autopsy. However, the increasing awareness and the availability of endomyocardial biopsy now allow antemortem diagnosis in the majority of patients. Biopsy of alternative tissue locations, such as the abdominal fat pad, rectum, gingiva, bone marrow, liver, and kidney, is also useful for the detection of systemic amyloidosis. For the diagnosis of cardiac amyloidosis, endomyocardial biopsy performed by an experienced operator is safe and definitive and allows evaluation of the extent of tissue infiltration, which may offer prognostic information.[61] Tissue may be examined by immunohistochemistry to identify specific amyloid proteins, which is increasingly important for targeted therapy. Measurement of circulating serum proteins may also be diagnostically valuable. The importance of seeking the identity of the specific amyloidogenic protein is underscored by a study showing that unsuspected hereditary amyloidosis was detected in nearly 10% of patients initially thought to have primary (AL) amyloidosis. In addition, the specific type of transthyretin amyloidosis has prognostic implications.[54]

Management

Patients with cardiac amyloidosis have few treatment options, although there are ongoing attempts to modify the severe natural history of this disorder (**Fig. 68-9**).[62] Approaches for patients with AL amyloidosis involve chemotherapy with alkylating agents alone or in combination with autologous bone marrow stem cell transplantation. Heart transplantation with concomitant autologous bone marrow transplants has been reported with variable degrees of success with a 39% 4-year survival in one study and 30% 5-year survival in another, although amyloid is likely to recur in the transplanted heart.[63] Nevertheless, survival rates may exceed those if the patient is left untreated. Moreover, combination bone marrow and cardiac transplantation may offer better survival rates in the future. For patients with transthyretin amyloid, liver transplantation may remove the source of the abnormal amyloidogenic protein.[64] No form of therapy is effective in the senile form of amyloidosis, although the clinical course is more benign than in primary amyloidosis.

In terms of conventional cardiac medications, the use of digitalis glycosides requires additional vigilance because patients with cardiac amyloidosis have increased sensitivity to digitalis preparations. In spite of this, digitalis glycosides are sometimes useful for successful control of the ventricular rate in atrial fibrillation. Calcium channel antagonists also require caution because their negative inotropic effect has the potential to exacerbate heart failure. Pacemakers are frequently indicated for conduction system disturbances, and implantable cardioverter-defibrillators (ICDs) should be considered for appropriate patients. Perhaps the mainstay of symptom relief in volume overloaded patients is the judicious use of diuretics, which requires very careful titration, in combination with rigorous fluid restriction. Vasodilator agents may also afford symptom relief and enhance diuresis but must be used cautiously to avoid systemic hypotension.

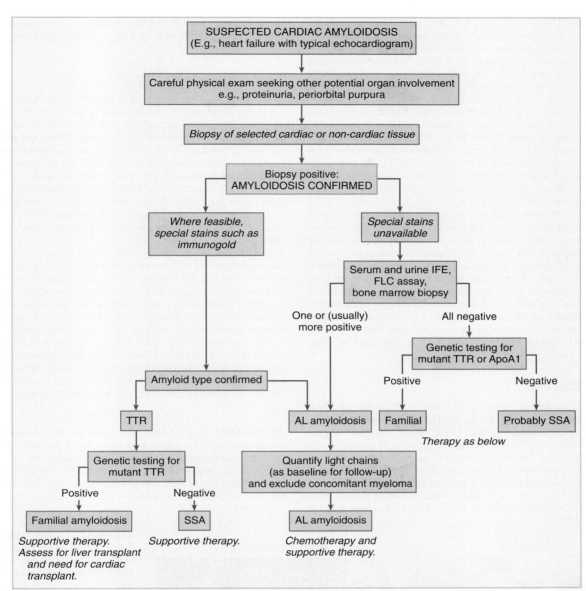

FIGURE 68-9 Flow diagram outlining the evaluation of a patient with suspected cardiac amyloidosis. Clinical evaluation may reveal clues that strengthen the likelihood of amyloidosis, but a tissue diagnosis is mandatory. Although special staining of the biopsy specimen may confirm the type of amyloid, further workup of amyloid (AL) is required to exclude myeloma and to quantify free light chains. If the biopsy specimen stains positive for transthyretin, further testing is needed to determine whether this is a wild-type or mutant transthyretin. ApoA1 = apoprotein type A1; FLC = free light chain; IFE = immunofixation electrophoresis; SSA = senile systemic amyloidosis; TTR = transthyretin. *(From Falk RH: Diagnosis and management of the cardiac amyloidoses. Circulation 112:2047, 2005.)*

Anticoagulation should be considered in the case of atrial standstill or atrial fibrillation.

Inherited and Acquired Infiltrative Disorders Causing Restrictive Cardiomyopathy

The heritable metabolic disorders resulting from the myocardial accumulation or infiltration of abnormal metabolic products represent an important cause of restrictive cardiomyopathy. These disorders produce classic restrictive cardiomyopathy with diastolic impairment and variable degrees of systolic dysfunction. The heritable metabolic disorders include Fabry disease, Gaucher disease, the glycogenoses, and the mucopolysaccharidoses. Early diagnosis is increasingly important because of the availability, in some cases, of effective enzyme replacement therapy.

Fabry Disease

Fabry disease, also referred to as angiokeratoma corporis diffusum universale, is an X-linked recessive disorder that results in deficiency of alpha-galactosidase A, a lysosomal enzyme, and the resultant accumulation of glycosphingolipids (most notably globotriaosylceramide) in lysosomes.[65,66] The major clinical features result from the accumulation of glycolipid substrate in the endothelium. More than 160 different mutations are described that have varying impact, ranging from absence of alpha-galactosidase activity to an attenuated level of activity of this enzyme. Patients with absent alpha-galactosidase activity exhibit widespread systemic manifestations with prominent kidney and cutaneous manifestations, whereas those with an attenuated level of enzyme activity have atypical variants of Fabry disease that may cause isolated myocardial disease. Histologic evaluation of the heart demonstrates diffuse involvement of the myocardium, vascular endothelium, conduction system, and valves, most notably the mitral valve (see Fig. 68-e3 on website).

CARDIAC FINDINGS. Patients with Fabry disease often experience angina pectoris and myocardial infarction caused by the accumulation of lipid species in the coronary endothelium, although epicardial coronary arteries are angiographically normal. The ventricular walls are thickened and have mildly diminished diastolic compliance with normal systolic function. Mild mitral regurgitation may be present. Diastolic abnormalities detected by Doppler echocardiography may be one of the earlier manifestations preceding cardiac hypertrophy. Males almost always present with symptomatic cardiovascular involvement, whereas female carriers may be completely asymptomatic or have only minimal symptoms.[67] Other common features of the disorder include systemic hypertension, congestive heart failure, and mitral valve prolapse. Echocardiography demonstrates increased ventricular wall thickness, which may mimic hypertrophic cardiomyopathy.[65] Whereas echocardiography may not be sufficient to do so, CMR may be able to differentiate Fabry disease from other infiltrative processes such as amyloidosis (see Fig. 68-e4 on website).[68] The surface electrocardiogram may reveal a short PR interval, atrioventricular block, and ST-segment and T wave abnormalities. The endomyocardial biopsy and low plasma alpha-galactosidase A activity offer a definitive diagnosis, which has therapeutic implications because enzyme replacement therapy for Fabry disease is safe and effective; moreover, heart biopsy may be used to monitor response to therapy.[69] Administration of recombinant alpha-galactosidase A can ameliorate the stores of globotriaosylceramide from the heart and other tissues, leading to symptomatic, clinical, and echocardiographic improvement (**Fig. 68-10**).[69]

Gaucher Disease

Gaucher disease results from a heritable deficiency of beta-glucosidase, which leads to an accumulation of cerebrosides in diffuse organs including spleen, liver, bone marrow, lymph nodes, brain, and heart. Cardiac disease is manifested as a stiffened ventricle caused by reduced chamber compliance, leading to impaired cardiac performance. Other manifestations include left ventricular failure and enlargement, hemorrhagic pericardial effusion, and sclerotic, calcified left-sided valves. Gaucher disease is responsive to enzyme replacement therapy or, in more extreme cases, hepatic transplantation; both therapies contribute to reducing tissue infiltration by cerebrosides and can lead to varying degrees of clinical improvement.[70]

Hemochromatosis

Hemochromatosis results from excessive deposition of iron in a variety of parenchymal tissues, notably the heart, liver, gonads, and pancreas. The classic pentad is a symptom complex of heart failure, cirrhosis, impotence, diabetes, and arthritis. The most frequent form of hemochromatosis is inherited as an autosomal recessive disorder (see Chap. 8) that arises from a mutation in the *HFE* gene, which codes for a transmembrane protein that is responsible for regulating iron uptake in the intestine and liver. Hemochromatosis may also arise from ineffective erythropoiesis secondary to a defect in hemoglobin synthesis as well as from chronic liver disease, or it may be acquired as a result of chronic and excessive oral or parenteral intake of iron (or blood transfusions).[71]

Iron deposition in the heart is almost always accompanied by varying degrees of infiltration of the liver, spleen, pancreas, and bone marrow, although the degrees of different organ system involvement may not parallel each other. Cardiac involvement produces a mixed pattern of systolic and diastolic dysfunction that is often accompanied by arrhythmias. The severity of hemochromatosis is less and age at onset is later in women because of the menstrual loss of iron. Cardiac toxicity results directly from the free iron moiety in addition to adverse effects of tissue infiltration. Death results most frequently from cirrhosis and hepatocellular carcinoma, whereas cardiac mortality accounts for an additional one third of the mortality and is particularly important in the group of male patients who present at relatively younger ages.

PATHOLOGY. In gross appearance, the hearts are dilated and ventricular walls are thickened. Iron deposits locate preferentially in the myocyte sarcoplasmic reticulum, more frequently in ventricular versus atrial cardiomyocytes. Frequently, the conduction system is involved, and loss of myocytes with fibrosis is often present. The degree of iron deposition correlates with the extent of myocardial dysfunction.

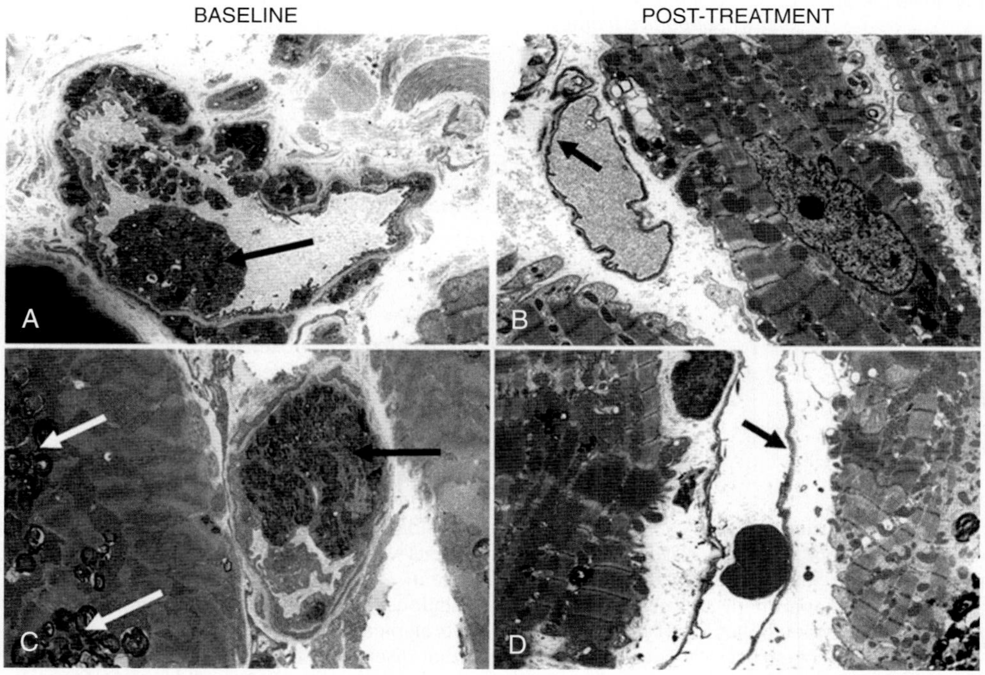

CLINICAL MANIFESTATIONS. Symptoms at presentation vary widely, and some patients are asymptomatic although evidence exists for myocardial involvement. Echocardiography reveals increased left ventricular wall thickness, ventricular dilation, and ventricular dysfunction. Both computed tomography and CMR are useful to detect early subclinical myocardial involvement at a time when therapy is most effective.[72] Electrocardiographic manifestations occur with advancing cardiac involvement and include ST-segment and T wave abnormalities and supraventricular arrhythmias.

Clinical and echocardiographic features usually are diagnostic, and endomyocardial biopsy is confirmatory but because of false negativity cannot definitively rule out the diagnosis. Evaluation of iron metabolism may aid in the diagnosis. Plasma iron levels are elevated, total iron-binding capacity is low or normal, and serum ferritin, urinary iron, liver iron, and especially saturation of transferrin are markedly elevated. Management should include repeated phlebotomies or treatment with chelating agents such as deferox-

FIGURE 68-10 Electron microscopy demonstrates clearance of GL-3 from cardiac capillaries. *(From Thurberg BL, Fallon JT, Mitchell R, et al: Cardiac microvascular pathology in Fabry disease: Evaluation of endomyocardial biopsies before and after enzyme replacement therapy. Circulation 119:2561, 2009.)*

BASELINE

POST-TREATMENT

amine. For advanced disease, cardiac transplantation carries acceptable 5- and 10-year survival rates.[73]

Glycogen Storage Disease

Patients with type II, III, IV, and V glycogen storage diseases may have cardiac involvement. However, survival to adulthood is rare with the exception of patients with type III disease (glycogen debranching enzyme deficiency). The most typical cardiac involvement is left ventricular hypertrophy, with electrocardiographic and echocardiographic findings, often with the absence of symptoms. A subset of patients may present with overt cardiac dysfunction, arrhythmias, and presentation of a DCM.

Inflammatory Causes of Infiltrative Cardiomyopathy

SARCOIDOSIS

Sarcoidosis is a systemic inflammatory condition characterized by the formation of noncaseating granulomas, most commonly involving the lungs, reticuloendothelial system, and skin. Sarcoid has been reported to involve essentially all tissues including the heart, which is recognized in 20% to 30% of autopsies of affected patients. Cardiac impairment may also arise secondary to pulmonary sarcoidosis, in which case extensive pulmonary fibrosis leads to advancing right-sided heart failure. The main clinical manifestations of sarcoid heart disease result from infiltration of the conduction system and myocardium, producing heart block, malignant arrhythmias, heart failure, and sudden cardiac death. Patients with cardiac sarcoidosis may also present with a restrictive cardiomyopathy caused by increased ventricular chamber stiffness.[47]

PATHOLOGY. Noncaseating granulomas surrounded by multinucleated giant cells are the diagnostic feature of the disorder and are found in multiple organs. In the heart, they infiltrate the myocardium and lead to the formation of fibrotic scars. The condition must be separated from two other inflammatory conditions of the heart—chronic active myocarditis and giant cell myocarditis (see Chap. 70). Giant cell myocarditis, which is characterized by diffuse giant cell inflammation in the absence of discrete granulomas, has a much more fulminant course than cardiac sarcoid (**Fig. 68-11**).[13,48] In sarcoidosis, the granulomas may involve discrete areas of the ventricular walls in a patchy fashion, increasing the likelihood of a false-negative endomyocardial biopsy result. Granulomas are most commonly observed in the interventricular septum and left ventricular free wall, and patients with conduction system disease typically have involvement of the basal portion of the interventricular septum. Left ventricular aneurysm formation may occur with extensive transmural free wall involvement. In terms of the coronary anatomy, the large conductance vessels are usually spared, but small coronary artery branches may be involved.

CLINICAL MANIFESTATIONS.

The clinical manifestations result from infiltration of the conduction system and myocardium. The most devastating presentation is that of sudden death due to malignant ventricular arrhythmia. Patients may also present with heart block, congestive heart failure, and syncope. Both atrial and ventricular arrhythmias are common.[74] Patients may be asymptomatic despite significant cardiac involvement. Heart failure may result from direct myocardial involvement or cor pulmonale due to extensive pulmonary fibrosis. Survival may

range from months to years, with a positive endomyocardial biopsy finding heralding a grave outcome.[75] Excellent long-term outcome may be achieved with aggressive immunosuppression. Isolated cardiac sarcoid has been reported.

The initial detection of cardiac sarcoidosis often results from the presence of bilateral hilar lymphadenopathy on chest radiographs in individuals with clinical or electrocardiographic findings suggesting myocardial disease. Endomyocardial biopsy should be performed if it is available because of the importance of positive findings, but it has a high false-negative rate.[13,75] Multiple imaging modalities assist in assessing diagnosis and prognosis. Echocardiography may demonstrate either global or regional left ventricular dysfunction and rarely may reveal aneurysm formation. Echocardiography is also valuable to evaluate right ventricular hypertrophy and to estimate pulmonary artery systolic pressures. CMR is emerging as a highly sensitive and specific test (see Fig. 18-13).[76] Other modalities include myocardial nuclear imaging with thallium-201 or technetium-99m, which can reveal segmental perfusion defects due to granulomatous inflammation, and [^{18}F]-fluorodeoxyglucose positron emission tomography, which can reveal focal uptake consistent with sarcoid. Uptake of technetium pyrophosphate, gallium, or labeled antimyosin antibody may also contribute to making the diagnosis.

The physical examination may show evidence of extracardiac sarcoid or may be totally normal. An apical systolic murmur due to mitral regurgitation is frequently present, often arising from cardiac chamber dilation as opposed to direct papillary muscle infiltration. Murmurs of tricuspid regurgitation, pulmonic regurgitation, and right-sided third heart sounds suggest pulmonary hypertension and cor pulmonale. Both S_3 and S_4 are frequently appreciated.

Electrocardiography typically demonstrates nonspecific findings suggestive of myocardial involvement, with T wave abnormalities commonly present. The electrocardiogram is highly valuable to assess the degree of conduction system involvement in terms of intraventricular delays and atrioventricular block (see Fig. 68-e5 on website). Q waves may be present, indicating severe and extensive myocardial replacement and fibrosis. Typical findings on echocardiography include left ventricular dilation with global or regional hypokinesis, right-sided enlargement and hypertrophy, possible left ventricular aneurysm formation, and, not infrequently, pericardial effusion. On occasion, increased echogenicity suggests an infiltrative process.

MANAGEMENT. Sarcoidosis is generally treated with immunosuppression.[13,47] Conduction disturbance, arrhythmias, and myocardial dysfunction may all respond to corticosteroids. Steroids effectively halt the progression of inflammation, and some studies suggest that therapy may offer improved survival. Other drugs that may be of benefit in sarcoidosis include hydroxychloroquine, methotrexate, and cyclophosphamide. It is important to distinguish cardiac sarcoidosis from giant cell myocarditis, a much more aggressive disorder that requires intensive immunosuppression and frequently mechanical support or heart transplantation (see Chap. 70). Whereas antiarrhythmic therapy is often ineffective for control of malignant arrhythmias,

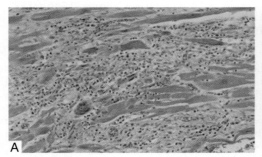 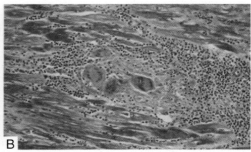

FIGURE 68-11 Sarcoid versus giant cell myocarditis. Giant cell myocarditis (**A**) is characterized by lymphocytic infiltration, myocyte necrosis, and giant cells. Sarcoidosis (**B**) is characterized by the presence of true noncaseating granulomas. *(From Hare JM: Etiologic basis of congestive heart failure. In Colucci WS [ed]: Atlas of Heart Failure. 5th ed. Philadelphia, Springer, Current Medicine Group, 2008, pp 29-56. Copyright 2008, Current Medicine LLC.)*

ICD therapy is appropriate for patients at risk for sudden cardiac death. Implantation of a permanent pacemaker is often required in the case of conduction system disease. Heart or heart-lung transplantation should be considered in the case of intractable heart failure, although sarcoid may recur in the grafted organ.

Endomyocardial Disease

DEFINITION AND PATHOGENESIS. A common form of restrictive cardiomyopathy found in a geographic location close to the equator is known as endomyocardial disease. Endomyocardial disease is common in equatorial Africa and is manifested less frequently in South America, Asia, and nontropical countries, including the United States. Two variants are described that, despite similar phenotypes, are likely unique processes, both manifesting as aggressive endocardial scarring obliterating the ventricular apices and subvalvular regions. Endomyocardial fibrosis or Davies disease is the first variant and occurs primarily in tropical regions; the second, Löffler endocarditis parietalis fibroplastica, or the hypereosinophilic syndrome, is encountered in more temperate zones. Although the pathologic appearance of these two disorders is similar, there are sufficient differences between the two disorders to suggest that they indeed are two distinct entities. Löffler endocarditis is more aggressive and rapidly progresses, affects mainly males, and is associated with hypereosinophilia, thromboemboli, and systemic arteritis; endomyocardial fibrosis occurs in a younger distribution, affects young children, and is only variably associated with eosinophilia.

DIFFERENCES BETWEEN LÖFFLER ENDOCARDITIS AND ENDOMYOCARDIAL FIBROSIS. Overlap between Löffler endocarditis and endomyocardial fibrosis is suggested by the observation that both diseases are attributable to the direct toxic effects of eosinophils in the myocardium. It is suggested that hypereosinophilia (regardless of cause) produces the first phase of endomyocardial disease, which is characterized by necrosis, intense myocarditis, and arteritis (i.e., Löffler endocarditis). This phase lasts for a period of months and is then followed by a thrombotic stage a year after the initial presentation, in which nonspecific thickening of the myocardium with a layer of thrombus replaces the inflammatory portion of myocardium. In the late phase, final healing is achieved by the formation of fibrosis, at which point the clinical features of endomyocardial fibrosis are present. Most of the support for this three-stage pathophysiologic process, namely, necrotic, thrombotic, and fibrotic, comes from autopsy studies. Nonetheless, definitive evidence that each patient passes sequentially through these stages is lacking.

ROLE OF EOSINOPHILS. The mechanism by which eosinophils participate in the development of cardiac disease remains incompletely understood. These cells have the capacity to directly infiltrate tissues or to release factors that may exert toxicity. The observation that patients with Löffler endocarditis have degranulated eosinophils in their peripheral blood supports the idea that these granules contain cardiotoxic substances, capable of causing the necrotic phase of endomyocardial disease, which leads to the thrombotic and fibrotic phases once the eosinophilia resolves. It is conceivable that this effect may occur only in temperate zones of the world, as the link between eosinophilia and endomyocardial fibrosis is less clear (although parasitic diseases have increased incidence), suggesting that endomyocardial fibrosis may result from a different mechanism in tropical countries. Factors implicated include elevated cerium levels and hypomagnesemia.

Löffler Endocarditis: The Hypereosinophilic Syndrome

In temperate climates, endomyocardial disease is closely associated with significant hypereosinophilia, which can have several different causes. Hypereosinophilia associated with Löffler endocarditis usually is characterized by eosinophil counts exceeding 1500/mm³ for at least 6 months. Most patients with this degree of hypereosinophilia will have cardiac involvement. The eosinophilia may be secondary to leukemia, reactive disorders such as parasite infection, allergies, granulomatous syndromes, hypersensitivity, or neoplastic disorders. In addition, patients with Churg-Strauss syndrome, characterized by asthma or allergic rhinitis and a necrotizing vasculitis, often have cardiac involvement.[77]

PATHOLOGY. The hypereosinophilic syndrome involves several organ systems beyond the heart, including the lungs, brain, and bone marrow. Both chambers of the heart are involved and show endocardial thickening of the inflow regions and ventricular apices. On histologic examination, there are variable degrees of eosinophilic myocarditis of the myocardium and subendocardium, thrombosis and inflammation of small intramural coronary vessels, mural thrombosis containing eosinophils, and endocardial fibrotic thickening of several millimeters.

CLINICAL MANIFESTATIONS. Patients with hypereosinophilic syndrome exhibit weight loss, fever, cough, rash, and congestive heart failure. Early in the course of cardiac involvement, patients may be asymptomatic; but with progression, in excess of 50% of patients will have overt congestive heart failure or cardiomegaly. Murmurs of mitral regurgitation are common. Systemic emboli occur frequently, resulting in neurologic and renal sequelae. Death results from heart failure associated with renal, hepatic, or pulmonary involvement. Sudden cardiac death and syndromes mimicking acute myocardial infarction are described.

LABORATORY EXAMINATION. Chest radiography may demonstrate an enlarged cardiac silhouette accompanied by evidence of pulmonary congestion or, less frequently, pulmonary infiltrates. Changes on the electrocardiogram are nonspecific and include ST-segment and T wave abnormalities. Atrial fibrillation and conduction defects, most notably right bundle branch block, are often noted. The echocardiogram often shows regional thickening of the posterobasal portion of the left ventricular wall, with substantial impairment in the motion of the posterior leaflet of the mitral valve. The apex may be obliterated by thrombus (see Fig. 15-80). The atria are often dilated, and there is Doppler ultrasound evidence of atrioventricular regurgitation. As is typical for restrictive cardiomyopathy, systolic function is often normal. Hemodynamic measurements support a restrictive cardiomyopathic appearance with abnormal diastolic filling, secondary to the dense endocardial scarring and reduced size of the ventricular cavity from the organized thrombus. Regurgitation through atrioventricular valves results from involvement of their respective supporting structures. Cardiac catheterization reveals markedly elevated ventricular filling pressures, and there may be evidence of tricuspid or mitral regurgitation. A characteristic feature on angiocardiography is largely preserved systolic function with obliteration of the apex of the ventricles. Endomyocardial biopsy can provide diagnostic confirmation but is not always positive.

MANAGEMENT. There is a role for both medical and surgical therapy in improving quality and quantity of life in patients with Löffler endocarditis. There is evidence that both corticosteroids and cytotoxic drugs such as hydroxyurea may have an important favorable effect on survival. In refractory patients, treatment with interferon may offer a valuable adjunctive therapy. Routine supportive cardiac therapy with diuretics, neurohormonal blockade, and anticoagulation as indicated is appropriate for management of these patients. Surgical therapy consisting of endocardiectomy and valve replacement or repair appears to provide significant symptomatic palliation once the fibrotic stage of the disease is manifested.

Endomyocardial Fibrosis

Endomyocardial fibrosis is a disorder found typically in tropical and subtropical Africa, notably in Uganda, Nigeria, and Mozambique, and is a major cause of morbidity and mortality, accounting for 25% of cases of congestive heart failure and death in equatorial Africa.[53,78,79] A population-based study in rural Mozambique revealed a prevalence of the disorder affecting 19.8% of the population.[53] In this study, only 48 of 211 patients were symptomatic at time of detection, and familial occurrence was high.

The disease is increasingly recognized in other tropical and subtropical regions within 15 degrees of the equator, including India, Brazil, Colombia, and Sri Lanka.[52] Importantly, it is also recognized in the Middle East, particularly Saudi Arabia.[79] Cardiac dysfunction occurs because of fibrous lesions that affect the inflow of the right and left ventricles and that may also involve the atrioventricular valves, thereby producing regurgitant lesions. Endomyocardial fibrosis has increased incidence among the Rwanda tribe of Uganda and in individuals of low socioeconomic status.[51] It has a slight male preponderance, is most common in children[78] and young adults,[53] but has been described in individuals into the sixth decade of life (see Fig. 68-e6 on website). Although most cases occur in black individuals, there are occasional presentations in white subjects residing in temperate climates. There are rare reports of endomyocardial fibrosis in individuals who have not resided in tropical areas.

PATHOLOGY. Endomyocardial fibrosis affects both the right and left ventricles in approximately 50% of patients, purely the left in 40%, and the right ventricle alone in the remaining 10%.[52,79] The typical gross appearance is that of a normal to slightly enlarged heart. The right atrium may be dilated in proportion to the severity of right ventricular involvement. There is often a pericardial effusion, which may be large. The right-sided heart border may be indented because of apical scarring. The hallmark feature of the disorder is fibrotic obliteration of the apex of the affected ventricles (**Fig. 68-12**). The fibrosis involves the papillary muscles and chordae tendineae, leading to atrioventricular valve distortion and regurgitation. In the left ventricle, the fibrosis extends from the apex to the posterior mitral valve leaflet, usually sparing the anterior mitral leaflet and the ventricular outflow tract. Endocardial calcific deposits can be present involving diffuse areas of the ventricle. The fibrotic tissue often creates a nidus for thrombus formation, which can be extensive. Atrial thrombi also occur. The process usually does not involve the epicardium, and the coronary artery obstruction is distinctly uncommon.

HISTOLOGIC FINDINGS. Endomyocardial fibrosis is clearly apparent histologically, presenting as a thick layer of collagen overlying loosely arranged connective tissue.[79] In addition, there are fibrous and granular septations extending into the underlying myocardial tissue. Myocyte hypertrophy is common.[52] Whereas cellular infiltration is uncommon, interstitial edema is frequently present. Fibroelastosis that is found in the ventricular outflow tracts beneath the semilunar valves often represents a secondary process caused by local trauma. Examination of intramural coronary arteries may show involvement with medial degeneration, the deposition of fibrin, and fibrosis.

CLINICAL MANIFESTATIONS. The symptomatic status of patients at presentation relates to which ventricles are involved. Pulmonary congestion signals left-sided involvement, whereas predominantly right-sided disease may mimic restrictive cardiomyopathy or constrictive pericarditis. Atrioventricular valve regurgitation is common. The disease may be heralded by an acute febrile illness or may be simply insidious. Endomyocardial fibrosis is a relentless and progressive process, although the time course of decline may vary considerably, with some patients appearing to have periods of stability. Modes of death include progressive heart failure, infection, infarction, sudden cardiac death, and complications of surgery. Atrial fibrillation and ascites are reported to be poor prognostic indicators.[80,81]

RIGHT VENTRICULAR ENDOMYOCARDIAL FIBROSIS. In pure or predominant right ventricular involvement, the right ventricular apex is characterized by fibrous obliteration, which may extend to involve the supporting structures of the tricuspid valve, with ensuing tricuspid regurgitation. Patients exhibit an elevated jugular venous pressure, a prominent *v* wave with rapid *y* descent, and a right-sided S_3 gallop. There is prominent hepatomegaly with a pulsatile liver, ascites, splenomegaly, and peripheral edema, but pulmonary congestion is typically absent

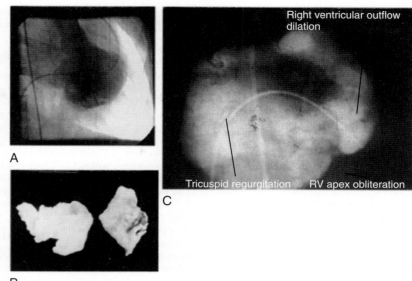

FIGURE 68-12 Right- and left-sided endomyocardial fibrosis. **A,** Left-sided endomyocardial fibrosis is characterized by apical obliteration, patchy filling defects, and severe mitral regurgitation. **B,** The management of endomyocardial fibrosis often requires surgical excision of the endocardial fibrosis. Depicted are pieces of excised endocardial fibrosis. **C,** Right ventricular (RV) angiogram of a patient with RV endomyocardial fibrosis showing RV outflow tract dilation, RV apex obliteration, and tricuspid regurgitation. (**A** and **B** from Joshi R, Abraham S, Kumar AS: New approach for complete endocardiectomy in left ventricular endomyocardial fibrosis. J Thorac Cardiovasc Surg 125:40, 2003. **C** from Seth S, Thatai D, Sharma S, et al: Clinico-pathological evaluation of restrictive cardiomyopathy [endomyocardial fibrosis and idiopathic restrictive cardiomyopathy] in India. Eur J Heart Fail 6:723, 2004.)

because of the lack of left-sided involvement. In this regard, pulmonary artery and pulmonary capillary wedge pressures are normal. A large pericardial effusion is often present. The right atrium may be enormously dilated. The electrocardiogram often has findings consistent with right-sided enlargement, especially a qR pattern in lead V_1, and supraventricular arrhythmias are common. The chest radiograph often demonstrates obvious right atrial prominence, a pericardial effusion, and calcification in the walls of the right and, less frequently, the left ventricle. Echocardiography demonstrates thickening of the right ventricle with obliteration of the apex, a dilated atrium, hyperechoic endocardial surfaces, and abnormal septal motion in patients with tricuspid regurgitation. On angiography, the right ventricular apex is typically not visualized because of fibrous obliteration; tricuspid regurgitation, right atrial enlargement, and filling defects in the right atrium caused by thrombi may be present.

LEFT VENTRICULAR ENDOMYOCARDIAL FIBROSIS. In cases of predominant left-sided disease, fibrosis involves the ventricular apex and often the chordae tendineae or the posterior mitral valve leaflet, producing mitral regurgitation. The associated murmur may be late systolic, characteristic of a papillary muscle dysfunction murmur, or pansystolic. Findings of pulmonary hypertension may be prominent, and an S_3 protodiastolic gallop is frequently present. The electrocardiogram usually shows ST-segment and T wave abnormalities, low-voltage QRS complexes if a pericardial effusion is present, or left ventricular hypertrophy. Left atrial abnormality is often noted. As with right-sided involvement, atrial fibrillation is often present and portends a poor prognosis. Echocardiography reveals increased endocardial echoreflectivity, preserved systolic function, apical obliteration, enlarged atrium, pericardial effusion of varying size, and Doppler ultrasound evidence of mitral regurgitation. Pulmonary hypertension is typically observed during cardiac catheterization, as well as left atrial hypertension and a reduced cardiac index. Left ventriculography shows mitral regurgitation, and ventricular filling defects caused by intracavitary thrombi may be present. Coronary arteriography usually excludes obstructive epicardial vessel stenoses.

BIVENTRICULAR ENDOMYOCARDIAL FIBROSIS. Biventricular endomyocardial fibrosis is more common then either isolated right- or left-sided disease. The typical clinical presentation of endomyocardial fibrosis resembles right ventricular endomyocardial fibrosis; however, a murmur of mitral regurgitation is indicative of left-sided involvement. Unless left ventricular involvement is extensive, severe pulmonary hypertension is absent and the right-sided findings are the predominant mode of presentation. Approximately 15% of patients will experience systemic embolization, and only 2% will have infective endocarditis.

DIAGNOSIS. Detection of endomyocardial fibrosis in individuals from the appropriate geographic area requires typical clinical and laboratory findings as well as angiography. Eosinophilia is variably present and may result from parasitic infection.[51] Endomyocardial biopsy is diagnostic, but false negatives can occur because of the patchy nature of the disease. Insofar as myocardial biopsy may be complicated by systemic emboli, left-sided myocardial biopsy is contraindicated.

MANAGEMENT. The medical management of endomyocardial fibrosis remains challenging. One third to one half of patients with advanced disease die within 2 years, whereas those who are less symptomatic fare better. The development of atrial fibrillation is a poor prognostic indicator, although symptomatic relief can be achieved with rate control.[80] Heart failure is difficult to control, and diuretics are effective only in early stages of disease, losing efficacy with advanced ascites. Once endomyocardial fibrosis progresses to severe endocardial fibrosis, surgical resection with atrioventricular valve replacement on affected sides is the treatment of choice.[82] Surgical therapy consisting of endocardiectomy and valve replacement or repair usually results in hemodynamic improvement with reductions in ventricular filling pressures, increased cardiac output, and normalized angiographic appearance (see Fig. 68-12). Operative mortality is high, between 15% and 25%, and may be lower if valve replacement is not necessary.[83] Fibrosis may recur, although there are case reports of excellent long-term survival.[84]

Endocardial Fibroelastosis

Endocardial fibroelastosis is a disorder of fetuses and infants of unclear etiology that is characterized by deposition of collagen and elastin, leading to ventricular hypertrophy and diffuse endocardial thickening (see Fig. 68-e7 on website). Causes are incompletely understood, and there are reports of associations with viral infections (especially mumps), metabolic disorders, autoimmune disease, and congenital left-sided obstructive lesions. Two recent reports implicate mitochondrial disorders and placental insufficiency.[85,86] Like DCM, endocardial fibroelastosis usually progresses to severe congestive heart failure and subsequent death. The echocardiographic finding of a highly reflective endocardial surface of the ventricular myocardium suggests endocardial fibroelastosis.

Neoplastic Infiltrative Cardiomyopathy—Carcinoid Heart Disease

The carcinoid syndrome results from the metastasis of carcinoid tumors from the gut to the heart.[87] The symptoms include marked cutaneous flushing, diarrhea, bronchoconstriction, and endocardial plaques composed of a unique type of fibrous tissue. The symptom complex is caused in large part by the release of serotonin and other circulating substances secreted by the tumor. Essentially all patients experience diarrhea and flushing, 50% have cardiac lesions detected echocardiographically, and about 25% of the patients have severe right-sided involvement.

Carcinoid tumors originate largely from the gut, with 60% to 90% being found in the small bowel and appendix and the remainder arising from other regions of the gastrointestinal tract or the bronchi. Carcinoid tumors arising in the ileum pose the greatest risk of metastasis, most likely affecting regional lymph nodes and the liver. The carcinoid tumors arising in the liver affect the heart. The severity of the cardiac lesions is related to the circulating concentrations of serotonin and 5-hydroxyindoleacetic acid (its primary metabolite), which are produced primarily by the carcinoid tumors in the liver. The observation that the right side of the heart is preferentially affected in the carcinoid syndrome reflects inactivation of the circulating toxic substances in the lung; the 5% to 10% of individuals presenting with

left-sided lesions are likely to have right-to-left shunts or tumor involvement of the lungs.

Pathology

The characteristic lesions are fibrous plaques involving locations "downstream" of the tricuspid and pulmonic valves, the endocardium, and the intima of the venae cavae, pulmonary artery, and coronary sinus. Both stenotic and regurgitant valvular lesions result from fibrotic distortion originating in the plaques.[87] The plaque material appears as a layer of fibrous tissue composed of smooth muscle cells, collagen, and mucopolysaccharides overlying the endocardium and in some cases extending into the underlying regions. Interestingly, identical pathology results from exposure to the anorectic drugs fenfluramine and dexfenfluramine. On occasion, there is actual metastasis of the tumor to one or both of the ventricles.

Clinical Manifestations

Cardiac murmurs indicating right-sided valve involvement are widely appreciated. A systolic murmur of tricuspid regurgitation along the left sternal border is almost always present, and pulmonic valve murmurs of either stenosis or regurgitation may also be present (see Chap. 66). The chest radiograph may be normal or may show cardiac enlargement and pleural effusions or nodules. The pulmonary artery trunk is most often not enlarged, and poststenotic dilation is also absent, differentiating pulmonic involvement from congenital pulmonic stenosis. Although there are no specific changes on the electrocardiogram diagnostic of carcinoid heart disease, it is not uncommon to encounter right atrial enlargement without other findings of right ventricular hypertrophy, nonspecific ST-segment and T wave abnormalities, and sinus tachycardia. Patients with advanced disease are likely to have low QRS voltage. Echocardiography often reveals tricuspid or pulmonary valve thickening and enlargement of the right atrium and ventricle (see Figs. 66-39 and 66-41); a minority of patients may have a small pericardial effusion. CMR may offer additional value in evaluating the right side of the heart that may be difficult to image with echocardiography.[88]

Management

For mild congestive heart failure, standard therapy with diuretics and neurohormonal antagonists is appropriate. Both somatostatin analogues and chemotherapy can lead to improved symptoms and possibly enhanced survival, but neither is effective at amelioration of progressive cardiac disease in patients with carcinoid syndrome. A key element of management is relief of stenotic lesions of the tricuspid and pulmonary valves. This may be achieved with either balloon valvuloplasty or surgery, both of which can achieve symptomatic relief. Operative mortality is traditionally high, but it has improved significantly in experienced centers.[87]

Arrhythmogenic Right Ventricular Dysplasia/Cardiomyopathy

Arrhythmogenic right ventricular dysplasia/cardiomyopathy (ARVD/C), first described in 1977 by Fontaine and coworkers, is a genetic form of cardiomyopathy characterized prototypically by fibrofatty infiltration of the right ventricle (**Figs. 68-13** and **68-14**). ARVD/C accounts for 20% of cases of sudden cardiac death, and importantly, among young athletes dying suddenly, the prevalence of this condition is higher.[89,90]

Presenting Symptoms and Natural History

Patients typically present between the teenage years and the forties, with only 10% falling outside of this age range. The natural history of the disorder is characterized by four phases: a concealed phase in which patients are asymptomatic, a phase characterized by an overt clinical manifestation of an electrical system disturbance, progression

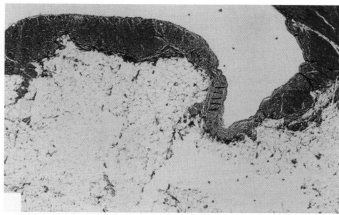

FIGURE 68-13 Arrhythmogenic right ventricular dysplasia/cardiomyopathy (ARVD/C). Histologic appearance of ARVD/C showing fibrosis, adipose infiltration, and myocardial thinning. *(From Hare JM: Etiologic basis of congestive heart failure.* In *Colucci WS [ed]: Atlas of Heart Failure. 5th ed. Philadelphia, Springer, Current Medicine Group, 2008, pp 29-56. Copyright 2008, Current Medicine LLC.)*

present at younger ages and are more likely to have malignant arrhythmias.[89] This finding suggests the prognostic importance of genetic testing for ARVD/C. In addition, immunohistochemical detection of plakoglobin is proposed to be of value in diagnosis.[91]

Diagnosis

A task force has set diagnostic criteria to aid in the study and characterization of ARVD/C. The diagnostic criteria involve features obtained from imaging, electrocardiography, signal-averaged electrocardiography, and histologic evaluation as well as a positive family history and a history of arrhythmias.[14] Early diagnosis of ARVD/C remains challenging. Whereas endomyocardial biopsy may offer valuable diagnostic information, CMR is emerging as a more definitive diagnostic tool.[41] The main limitation of endomyocardial biopsy is a high false-negative rate because of sampling error and the fact that the right ventricle septum may lack the characteristic histologic changes; however, immunohistochemical detection of plakoglobin may enhance the value of tissue diagnosis.[91] Tandri and colleagues[41] have reported that characterization of the ventricular wall morphology with delayed enhancement gadolinium CMR correlated well with

to signs and symptoms of right ventricular failure, and finally frank biventricular congestive heart failure. Accordingly, presenting symptoms range from palpitations to syncope and sudden cardiac death. A majority of patients who subsequently experience sudden cardiac death have a history of syncope, which thus represents an important prognostic event.[90] Progression to heart failure occurs in the minority of patients but is the predominant mode of death in individuals who are protected from sudden cardiac death by ICD implantation.

Pathology

Characteristically, a heart affected with ARVD/C exhibits fatty or fibrofatty replacement of the myocardium predominantly affecting the right ventricle. Rarely, the process extends to the left ventricle (see Fig. 18-11).

Genetics

Several genes and gene loci are associated with ARVD/C, and both autosomal dominant and recessive modes of inheritance are described. Most but not all genes encode desmosomal proteins.[91] Implicated genes include desmoplakin, junctional plakoglobin (*JUP*), the cardiac ryanodine receptor plakophilin 2 (*PKP2*), and transforming growth factor-β3. *JUP* mutations are causally implicated in Naxos disease, a syndrome characterized by ARVD/C, wooly hair, and palmoplantar keratoderma. Individuals with mutations in *PKP2*

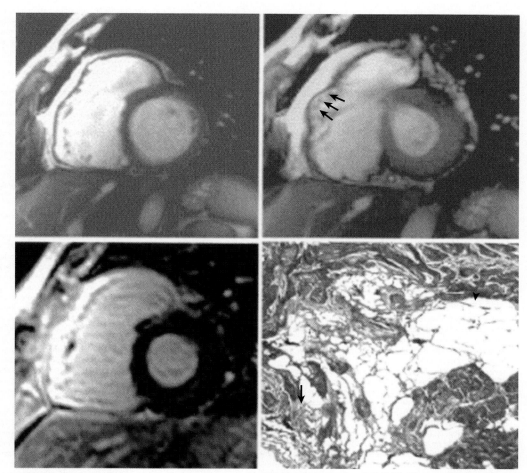

FIGURE 68-14 Arrhythmogenic right ventricular dysplasia/cardiomyopathy (ARVD/C). The **top left and right panels** represent the end-diastolic and end-systolic frames of a short-axis cine magnetic resonance image showing an area of dyskinesia on right ventricular free wall characterizing a focal ventricular aneurysm (arrows). The **bottom left panel** displays the delayed-enhanced magnetic resonance image with increased signal intensity within the right ventricular myocardium (arrows), at the location of right ventricular aneurysms. The **bottom right panel** shows the corresponding endomyocardial biopsy. Trichrome stain of the right ventricle at high magnification shows marked replacement of the ventricular muscle by adipose tissue. The adipose tissue cells (arrowhead) are irregular in size and infiltrate the ventricular muscle. There is also abundant replacement fibrosis (arrow). There is no evidence of inflammation. *(From Tandri H, Saranathan M, Rodriguez ER, et al: Noninvasive detection of myocardial fibrosis in arrhythmogenic right ventricular cardiomyopathy using delayed-enhancement magnetic resonance imaging. J Am Coll Cardiol 45:98, 2005.)*

histologic findings as well as with inducibility of ventricular tachycardia during electrophysiologic testing.

Management

Patients diagnosed with ARVD/C should receive an ICD. Antiarrhythmic therapy is appropriate before ICD insertion and in some cases after, in patients who have recurrent ICD firings. Use of an ICD can have an enormous clinical impact on reducing the major cause of mortality in affected individuals. It is also recommended that patients receive neurohormonal blockade with angiotensin-converting enzyme inhibitors and beta adrenoreceptor antagonists. In individuals progressing to overt heart failure, management involves the same principles for the treatment of other forms of cardiomyopathy. Consideration of heart transplantation is indicated for patients with overt biventricular failure.

Summary and Future Perspectives

Our current understanding of cardiomyopathic processes is still fairly rudimentary as evidenced by the large percentage of patients who are assigned as having idiopathic disease. Continual advances are being made with respect to genetics and cellular biology (stem cells) that are revealing important insights into the etiology, natural history, and potentially the management of dilated, restrictive, and right ventricular cardiomyopathy. The strong genetic basis of several cardiomyopathic disorders coupled with new high-throughput technologies will allow the possibility of widespread genetic testing of affected individuals and their family members. Genetic testing will also facilitate understanding of which patients have a genetic cause of their disease as opposed to a genetic predisposition to an environmental insult. In addition to genetics, measurement of expressed genes (transcriptomics), microRNA abnormalities,[92] and proteins (proteomics) has the potential to aid in understanding etiology, prognosis, and individualized responses to therapy (personalized medicine). A key example of the last is the attempt to identify patients with a viral cause of cardiomyopathy and to treat those patients with appropriate antiviral therapy, on the one hand, and those without viral infection with immunosuppressive therapy, on the other hand. The most recent advance with significant future implications is the observation that the body, including the bone marrow and the heart, possesses reservoirs of endogenous stem cells regulated in stem cell niches; the discovery of these cells and their niches offers new insights into the causes of cardiomyopathy and may, in the future, provide a new therapeutic avenue.

REFERENCES

Dilated Cardiomyopathy

1. Dec GW, Fuster V: Idiopathic dilated cardiomyopathy. N Engl J Med 331:1564, 1994.
2. Ammash NM, Seward JB, Bailey KR, et al: Clinical profile and outcome of idiopathic restrictive cardiomyopathy. Circulation 101:2490, 2000.
3. Mann DL, Bristow MR: Mechanisms and models in heart failure: The biomechanical model and beyond. Circulation 111:2837, 2005.
4. Hare JM, Walford GD, Hruban RH, et al: Ischemic cardiomyopathy: Endomyocardial biopsy and ventriculographic evaluation of patients with congestive heart failure, dilated cardiomyopathy and coronary artery disease. J Am Coll Cardiol 20:1318, 1992.
5. Kittleson MM, Minhas KM, Irizarry RA, et al: Gene expression analysis of ischemic and nonischemic cardiomyopathy: Shared and distinct genes in the development of heart failure. Physiol Genomics 21:299, 2005.
6. Maron BJ, Towbin JA, Thiene G, et al: Contemporary definitions and classification of the cardiomyopathies: An American Heart Association Scientific Statement from the Council on Clinical Cardiology, Heart Failure and Transplantation Committee; Quality of Care and Outcomes Research and Functional Genomics and Translational Biology Interdisciplinary Working Groups; and Council on Epidemiology and Prevention. Circulation 113:1807, 2006.
7. Felker GM, Thompson RE, Hare JM, et al: Underlying causes and long-term survival in patients with initially unexplained cardiomyopathy. N Engl J Med 342:1077, 2000.
8. Ardehali H, Qasim A, Cappola T, et al: Endomyocardial biopsy plays a role in diagnosing patients with unexplained cardiomyopathy. Am Heart J 147:919, 2004.
9. Levy WC, Mozaffarian D, Linker DT, et al: The Seattle Heart Failure Model: Prediction of survival in heart failure. Circulation 113:1424, 2006.
10. Heidecker B, Kasper EK, Wittstein IS, et al: Transcriptomic biomarkers for individual risk assessment in new-onset heart failure. Circulation 118:238, 2008.
11. McNamara DM, Holubkov R, Starling RC, et al: Controlled trial of intravenous immune globulin in recent-onset dilated cardiomyopathy. Circulation 103:2254, 2001.
12. Teuteberg JJ, Lewis EF, Nohria A, et al: Characteristics of patients who die with heart failure and a low ejection fraction in the new millennium. J Card Fail 12:47, 2006.
13. Cooper LT, Baughman KL, Feldman AM, et al: The role of endomyocardial biopsy in the management of cardiovascular disease: A scientific statement from the American Heart Association, the American College of Cardiology, and the European Society of Cardiology. Circulation 116:2216, 2007.
14. Marcus FI, Zareba W, Calkins H, et al: Arrhythmogenic right ventricular cardiomyopathy/dysplasia clinical presentation and diagnostic evaluation: Results from the North American Multidisciplinary Study. Heart Rhythm 6:984, 2009.
15. McCarthy RE, Boehmer JP, Hruban RH, et al: Long-term outcome of fulminant myocarditis as compared with acute (nonfulminant) myocarditis. N Engl J Med 342:690, 2000.
16. Hare JM: The etiologic basis of congestive heart failure. In Colucci WS (ed): Atlas of Heart Failure. 5th ed. Philadelphia, Springer, Current Medicine Group, 2008, pp 29-56.
17. Owan TE, Hodge DO, Herges RM, et al: Trends in prevalence and outcome of heart failure with preserved ejection fraction. N Engl J Med 355:251, 2006.
18. Wittstein IS, Thiemann DR, Lima JA: Neurohumoral features of myocardial stunning due to sudden emotional stress. N Engl J Med 352:539, 2005.
19. Abraham J, Mudd JO, Kapur NK, et al: Stress cardiomyopathy after intravenous administration of catecholamines and beta-receptor agonists. J Am Coll Cardiol 53:1320, 2009.
20. Elkayam U, Akhter MW, Singh H, et al: Pregnancy-associated cardiomyopathy: Clinical characteristics and a comparison between early and late presentation. Circulation 111:2050, 2005.
21. Elkayam U, Tummala PP, Rao K, et al: Maternal and fetal outcomes of subsequent pregnancies in women with peripartum cardiomyopathy. N Engl J Med 344:1567, 2001.
22. Felker GM, Jaeger CJ, Klodas E, et al: Myocarditis and long-term survival in peripartum cardiomyopathy. Am Heart J 140:785, 2000.
23. Modi KA, Illum S, Jariatul K, et al: Poor outcome of indigent patients with peripartum cardiomyopathy in the United States. Am J Obstet Gynecol 201:171, 2009.
24. Redfield MM, Kay GN, Jenkins LS, et al: Tachycardia-related cardiomyopathy: A common cause of ventricular dysfunction in patients with atrial fibrillation referred for atrioventricular ablation. Mayo Clinic Proc 75:790, 2000.
25. Hershberger RE, Lindenfeld J, Mestroni L, et al: Genetic evaluation of cardiomyopathy—a Heart Failure Society of America practice guideline. J Card Fail 15:83, 2009.
26. Poller W, Kuhl U, Tschoepe C, et al: Genome-environment interactions in the molecular pathogenesis of dilated cardiomyopathy. J Mol Med 83:579, 2005.
27. Chimenti C, Kajstura J, Torella D, et al: Senescence and death of primitive cells and myocytes lead to premature cardiac aging and heart failure. Circ Res 93:604, 2003.
28. Kajstura J, Urbanek K, Perl S, et al: Cardiomyogenesis in the adult human heart. Circ Res 107:305, 2010.
29. Lee DS, Pencina MJ, Benjamin EJ, et al: Association of parental heart failure with risk of heart failure in offspring. N Engl J Med 355:138, 2006.
30. Schmitt JP, Kamisago M, Asahi M, et al: Dilated cardiomyopathy and heart failure caused by a mutation in phospholamban. Science 299:1410, 2003.
31. Lyon AR, Sato M, Hajjar RJ, et al: Gene therapy: Targeting the myocardium. Heart 94:89, 2008.
32. McNamara DM, Tam SW, Sabolinski ML, et al: Aldosterone synthase promoter polymorphism modulates outcome in black patients with heart failure: Results from the A-HeFT trial. J Am Coll Cardiol 48:1277, 2006.
33. Cooper LT Jr: Myocarditis. N Engl J Med 360:1526, 2009.
34. Frustaci A, Russo MA, Chimenti C: Randomized study on the efficacy of immunosuppressive therapy in patients with virus-negative inflammatory cardiomyopathy: The TIMIC study. Eur Heart J 30:1995, 2009.
35. Zimmet JM, Hare JM: Nitroso-redox interactions in the cardiovascular system. Circulation 114:1531, 2006.
36. Dorn GW: Apoptotic and non-apoptotic programmed cardiomyocyte death in ventricular remodelling. Cardiovasc Res 81:465, 2009.
37. Towbin JA, Lowe AM, Colan SD, et al: Incidence, causes, and outcomes of dilated cardiomyopathy in children. JAMA 296:1867, 2006.
38. Cox GF, Sleeper LA, Lowe AM, et al: Factors associated with establishing a causal diagnosis for children with cardiomyopathy. Pediatrics 118:1519, 2006.
39. Hare JM, Mangal B, Brown J, et al: Impact of oxypurinol in patients with symptomatic heart failure. Results of the OPT-CHF study. J Am Coll Cardiol 51:2301, 2008.
40. Williams TJ, Manghat NE, Kay-Ferguson A, et al: Cardiomyopathy: Appearances on ECG-gated 64-detector row computed tomography. Clin Radiol 63:464, 2008.
41. Tandri H, Saranathan M, Rodriguez ER, et al: Noninvasive detection of myocardial fibrosis in arrhythmogenic right ventricular cardiomyopathy using delayed-enhancement magnetic resonance imaging. J Am Coll Cardiol 45:98, 2005.
42. Friedrich MG, Sechtem U, Schulz-Menger J, et al: Cardiovascular magnetic resonance in myocarditis: A JACC White Paper. J Am Coll Cardiol 53:1475, 2009.
43. Maceira AM, Joshi J, Prasad SK, et al: Cardiovascular magnetic resonance in cardiac amyloidosis. Circulation 111:186, 2005.
44. Nazarian S, Bluemke DA, Lardo AC, et al: Magnetic resonance assessment of the substrate for inducible ventricular tachycardia in nonischemic cardiomyopathy. Circulation 112:2821, 2005.
45. Kurtz CE, Gerber Y, Weston SA, et al: Use of ejection fraction tests and coronary angiography in patients with heart failure. Mayo Clinic Proc 81:906, 2006.
46. Ardehali H, Kasper EK, Baughman KL: Diagnostic approach to the patient with cardiomyopathy: Whom to biopsy. Am Heart J 149:7, 2005.
47. Okura Y, Dec GW, Hare JM, et al: A clinical and histopathologic comparison of cardiac sarcoidosis and idiopathic giant cell myocarditis. J Am Coll Cardiol 41:322, 2003.
48. Cooper LT Jr, Hare JM, Tazelaar HD, et al: Usefulness of immunosuppression for giant cell myocarditis. Am J Cardiol 102:1535, 2008.
49. Jessup M, Abraham WT, Casey DE, et al: 2009 focused update: ACCF/AHA Guidelines for the Diagnosis and Management of Heart Failure in Adults: A report of the American College of Cardiology Foundation/American Heart Association Task Force on Practice Guidelines: Developed in collaboration with the International Society for Heart and Lung Transplantation. Circulation 119:1977, 2009.
50. Cleland JG, Daubert JC, Erdmann E, et al: The effect of cardiac resynchronization on morbidity and mortality in heart failure. N Engl J Med 352:1539, 2005.

Restrictive and Infiltrative Cardiomyopathy

51. Rutakingirwa M, Ziegler JL, Newton R, et al: Poverty and eosinophilia are risk factors for endomyocardial fibrosis (EMF) in Uganda. Trop Med Int Health 4:229, 1999.
52. Seth S, Thatai D, Sharma S, et al: Clinico-pathological evaluation of restrictive cardiomyopathy (endomyocardial fibrosis and idiopathic restrictive cardiomyopathy) in India. Eur J Heart Fail 6:723, 2004.
53. Mocumbi AO, Ferreira MB, Sidi D, et al: A population study of endomyocardial fibrosis in a rural area of Mozambique. N Engl J Med 359:43, 2008.

Amyloidosis

54. Rapezzi C, Merlini G, Quarta CC, et al: Systemic cardiac amyloidoses. Disease profiles and clinical courses of the 3 main types. Circulation 120:1203, 2009.
55. Falk RH: Diagnosis and management of the cardiac amyloidoses. Circulation 112:2047, 2005.
56. Ha JW, Ommen SR, Tajik AJ, et al: Differentiation of constrictive pericarditis from restrictive cardiomyopathy using mitral annular velocity by tissue Doppler echocardiography. Am J Cardiol 94:316, 2004.
57. Leya FS, Arab D, Joyal D, et al: The efficacy of brain natriuretic peptide levels in differentiating constrictive pericarditis from restrictive cardiomyopathy. J Am Coll Cardiol 45:1900, 2005.
58. Jacobson DR, Pastore RD, Yaghoubian R, et al: Variant-sequence transthyretin (isoleucine 122) in late-onset cardiac amyloidosis in black Americans. N Engl J Med 336:466, 1997.
59. Ng B, Connors LH, Davidoff R, et al: Senile systemic amyloidosis presenting with heart failure: A comparison with light chain–associated amyloidosis. Arch Int Med 165:1425, 2005.
60. Wang AK, Fealey RD, Gehrking TL, et al: Patterns of neuropathy and autonomic failure in patients with amyloidosis. Mayo Clin Proc 83:1226, 2008.
61. Rahman JE, Helou EF, Gelzer-Bell R, et al: Noninvasive diagnosis of biopsy-proven cardiac amyloidosis. J Am Coll Cardiol 43:410, 2004.
62. Palladini G, Merlini G: Current treatment of AL amyloidosis. Haematologica 94:1044, 2009.
63. Sack FU, Kristen A, Goldschmidt H, et al: Treatment options for severe cardiac amyloidosis: Heart transplantation combined with chemotherapy and stem cell transplantation for patients with AL-amyloidosis and heart and liver transplantation for patients with ATTR-amyloidosis. Eur J Cardiothorac Surg 33:257, 2008.
64. Delahaye N, Rouzet F, Sarda L, et al: Impact of liver transplantation on cardiac autonomic denervation in familial amyloid polyneuropathy. Medicine (Baltimore) 85:229, 2006.

Inherited and Acquired Infiltrative Disorders Causing Restrictive Cardiomyopathy

65. Pieroni M, Chimenti C, de Cobelli F, et al: Fabry's disease cardiomyopathy: Echocardiographic detection of endomyocardial glycosphingolipid compartmentalization. J Am Coll Cardiol 47:1663, 2006.
66. Sheppard MN, Cane P, Florio R, et al: A detailed pathologic examination of heart tissue from three older patients with Anderson-Fabry disease on enzyme replacement therapy. Cardiovasc Pathol 19:293, 2010.
67. Glass RBJ, Astrin KH, Norton KI, et al: Fabry disease: Renal sonographic and magnetic resonance imaging findings in affected males and carrier females with the classic and cardiac variant phenotypes. J Comput Assist Tomogr 28:158, 2004.
68. Imbriaco M, Pisani A, Spinelli L, et al: Effects of enzyme-replacement therapy in patients with Anderson-Fabry disease: A prospective long-term cardiac magnetic resonance imaging study. Heart 95:1103, 2009.
69. Thurberg BL, Fallon JT, Mitchell R, et al: Cardiac microvascular pathology in Fabry disease: Evaluation of endomyocardial biopsies before and after enzyme replacement therapy. Circulation 119:2561, 2009.
70. Elstein D, Zimran A: Review of the safety and efficacy of imiglucerase treatment of Gaucher disease. Biologics 3:407, 2009.
71. Hoffbrand AV: Diagnosing myocardial iron overload. Eur Heart J 22:2140, 2001.
72. Ptaszek LM, Price ET, Hu MY, et al: Early diagnosis of hemochromatosis-related cardiomyopathy with magnetic resonance imaging. J Cardiovasc Magn Reson 7:689, 2005.
73. Caines AE, Kpodonu J, Massad MG, et al: Cardiac transplantation in patients with iron overload cardiomyopathy. J Heart Lung Transplant 24:486, 2005.
74. Koplan BA, Soejima K, Baughman K, et al: Refractory ventricular tachycardia secondary to cardiac sarcoid: Electrophysiologic characteristics, mapping, and ablation. Heart Rhythm 3:924, 2006.
75. Ardehali H, Howard DL, Hariri A, et al: A positive endomyocardial biopsy result for sarcoid is associated with poor prognosis in patients with initially unexplained cardiomyopathy. Am Heart J 150:459, 2005.
76. Smedema JP, Snoep G, van Kroonenburgh MP, et al: Evaluation of the accuracy of gadolinium-enhanced cardiovascular magnetic resonance in the diagnosis of cardiac sarcoidosis. J Am Coll Cardiol 45:1683, 2005.
77. Pela G, Tirabassi G, Pattoneri P, et al: Cardiac involvement in the Churg-Strauss syndrome. Am J Cardiol 97:1519, 2006.
78. Marijon E, Ou P: What do we know about endomyocardial fibrosis in children of Africa? Pediatr Cardiol 27:523, 2006.
79. Hassan WM, Fawzy ME, Al Helaly S, et al: Pitfalls in diagnosis and clinical, echocardiographic, and hemodynamic findings in endomyocardial fibrosis: A 25-year experience. Chest 128:3985, 2005.
80. Barretto ACP, Mady C, Nussbacher A, et al: Atrial fibrillation in endomyocardial fibrosis is a marker of worse prognosis. Int J Cardiol 67:19, 1998.
81. Barretto AC, Mady C, Oliveira SA, et al: Clinical meaning of ascites in patients with endomyocardial fibrosis. Arq Bras Cardiol 78:196, 2002.
82. Joshi R, Abraham S, Kumar AS: New approach for complete endocardiectomy in left ventricular endomyocardial fibrosis. J Thorac Cardiovasc Surg 125:40, 2003.
83. Moraes F, Lapa C, Hazin S, et al: Surgery for endomyocardial fibrosis revisited. Eur J Cardiothorac Surg 15:309, 1999.
84. Cherian SM, Jagannath BR, Nayar S, et al: Successful reoperation after 17 years in a case of endomyocardial fibrosis. Ann Thorac Surg 82:1115, 2006.
85. Corradi D, Tchana B, Miller D, et al: Dilated form of endocardial fibroelastosis as a result of deficiency in respiratory-chain complexes I and IV. Circulation 120:e38, 2009.
86. Perez MH, Boulos T, Stucki P, et al: Placental immaturity, endocardial fibroelastosis and fetal hypoxia. Fetal Diagn Ther 26:107, 2009.

Carcinoid Heart Disease and Arrhythmogenic Right Ventricular Dysplasia/Cardiomyopathy

87. Moller JE, Pellikka PA, Bernheim AM, et al: Prognosis of carcinoid heart disease: Analysis of 200 cases over two decades. Circulation 112:3320, 2005.
88. Bastarrika G, Cao MG, Cano D, et al: Magnetic resonance imaging diagnosis of carcinoid heart disease. J Comput Assist Tomogr 29:756, 2005.
89. Dalal D, Molin LH, Piccini J, et al: Clinical features of arrhythmogenic right ventricular dysplasia/cardiomyopathy associated with mutations in plakophilin-2. Circulation 113:1641, 2006.
90. Dalal D, Nasir K, Bomma C, et al: Arrhythmogenic right ventricular dysplasia: A United States experience. Circulation 112:3823, 2005.
91. Asimaki A, Tandri H, Huang H, et al: A new diagnostic test for arrhythmogenic right ventricular cardiomyopathy. N Engl J Med 360:1075, 2009.
92. Matkovich SJ, Van Booven DJ, Youker KA, et al: Reciprocal regulation of myocardial microRNAs and messenger RNA in human cardiomyopathy and reversal of the microRNA signature by biomechanical support. Circulation 119:1263, 2009.

THE DILATED, RESTRICTIVE, AND INFILTRATIVE CARDIOMYOPATHIES

CHAPTER 69 **Hypertrophic Cardiomyopathy**

Barry J. Maron

Hypertrophic cardiomyopathy (HCM), the most common of the genetic cardiovascular diseases, is caused by a multitude of mutations in genes encoding proteins of the cardiac sarcomere.[1-5] HCM is characterized by heterogeneous clinical expression, unique pathophysiology, and diverse natural history.[6-13] This condition is the most common cause of sudden death in the young, including competitive athletes,[14] and it is responsible for heart failure–related disability at virtually any age.[1,7] Since the modern description of HCM more than 50 years ago, our understanding of the clinical complexity and spectrum of this disease has evolved dramatically. This chapter represents a contemporary summary of HCM with respect to diagnosis, natural history, and management.

Definition, Prevalence, and Nomenclature

HCM is characterized by a thickened but nondilated left ventricle in the absence of other cardiac or systemic conditions (e.g., aortic valve stenosis, systemic hypertension, and some expressions of physiologic athlete's heart) capable of producing the magnitude of left ventricular (LV) hypertrophy evident (**Figs. 69-1 and 69-2**).[1,3,5,7] Several epidemiologic studies have reported a similar prevalence of the HCM phenotype in the general population (e.g., about 0.2%; 1 : 500), equivalent to 600,000 people in the United States with this disease.[15] This estimated frequency in the general population far exceeds the relatively uncommon occurrence of HCM in cardiology practice, inferring that most affected individuals may remain unidentified and in most cases probably without symptoms or shortened life expectancy.[1,7] HCM is a global disease[16] reported in more than 50 countries from all continents, although most cases have come from the United States and Canada, western Europe, Israel, and Asia (Japan and China).

The first contemporary reports of HCM in 1958 are from Brock in the cardiac catheterization laboratory and from Teare, who described at autopsy "asymmetrical hypertrophy of the heart" as responsible for sudden cardiac death in a small group of young people. The disease rapidly acquired a confusing array of names,[5] with most emphasizing the highly visible feature of LV outflow obstruction.[13,17] However, since obstruction to LV outflow is not invariable and about 30% of patients have the nonobstructive form,[13] names once in common use, such as idiopathic hypertrophic subaortic stenosis, hypertrophic obstructive cardiomyopathy, and muscular subaortic stenosis (as well as their acronyms, IHSS, HOCM, and MSS) have been largely abandoned.[1,5,7] Hence, the preferred and generally accepted name for this condition is now hypertrophic cardiomyopathy (HCM).[1,5,7]

Genetic Basis (see Chap. 8)

HCM is transmitted as a mendelian trait with an autosomal dominant pattern of inheritance.[1,5,7] Molecular studies, conducted intensively during almost two decades, have provided access to definitive laboratory-based diagnosis by identification of pathologic disease-causing mutations (even in patients without obvious clinical evidence of the disease), in the process affording important insights into the broad clinical expression of HCM and genetic counseling, as well as promoting recognition of greater numbers of affected individuals.

Eleven mutated genes encoding proteins of the cardiac sarcomere are presently associated with HCM, accounting for about 50% of patients, most commonly beta-myosin heavy chain (the first identified) and myosin-binding protein C (see Fig. 8-1).[2,4,5] Each of the other nine genes appears to account for far fewer cases; these include troponin T and I, alpha-tropomyosin, regulatory and essential myosin light chains, titin, alpha-actin, alpha-myosin heavy chain, and muscle LIM protein (MLP). This diversity is compounded by considerable intragenetic heterogeneity, with myriad individual mutations identified (total >1000). The characteristic diversity of the HCM phenotype (even among closely related family members) is likely to be attributable to the disease-causing mutations as well as the influence of modifier genes and environmental factors. Neither the complete number of genes nor the number of HCM-causing mutations is known, and many others remain to be identified. Genetic testing is now commercially available, translating genomics into the clinical arena.[4]

Non-sarcomeric protein mutations cause storage diseases that are phenocopies of sarcomeric HCM and require molecular diagnosis, namely, Fabry disease, γ_2 regulatory subunit of adenosine monophosphate–activated protein kinase (PRKAG2), and lysosome-associated membrane protein 2 (LAMP2; Danon disease; **Fig. 69-3**).[18,19] Clinical presentation is often indistinguishable from sarcomeric HCM, although PRKAG2 and LAMP2 are frequently associated with ventricular preexcitation. LAMP2 cardiomyopathy, which is characterized by massive LV hypertrophy (see Fig. 69-3) and profound clinical course refractory to defibrillator therapy (with survival beyond 25 years unusual), necessitates consideration for early heart transplantation.[19]

Morphology

Left Ventricular Hypertrophy (see Chaps. 15 and 18)

Clinical diagnosis of HCM is usually made with two-dimensional echocardiography (see Fig. 69-1; see Figs. 15-65, 15-66, and 15-67),[1] although more recently cardiovascular magnetic resonance imaging (CMR) has emerged with an expanding role in noninvasive diagnosis by virtue of its high-resolution tomographic imaging capability (see Fig. 69-2; see

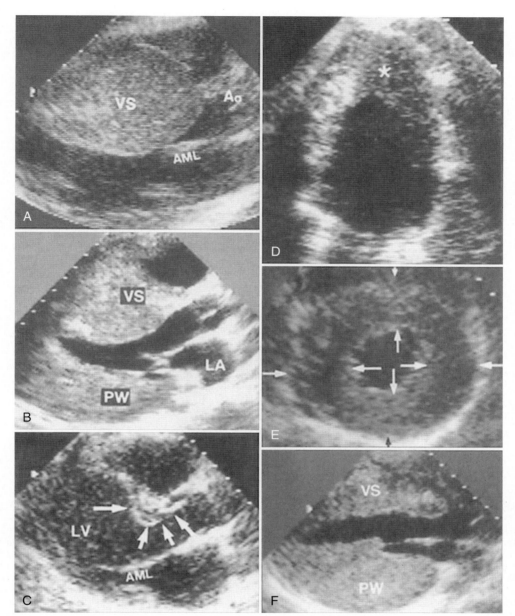

FIGURE 69-1 Patterns of LV hypertrophy in HCM. Heterogeneous distribution and extent of LV wall thickening by echocardiography. **A,** Massive asymmetric hypertrophy of ventricular septum (VS) with thickness >50 mm. **B,** Septal hypertrophy with distal portion considerably thicker than proximal region. **C,** Hypertrophy confined to proximal septum just below aortic valve (arrows). **D,** Hypertrophy localized to LV apex (asterisk), that is, apical HCM. **E,** Relatively mild hypertrophy in symmetric pattern showing similar or identical thicknesses within each segment (paired arrows). **F,** Inverted pattern with posterior free wall (PW) thicker (40 mm) than anterior VS. Calibration marks = 1 cm. Ao = aorta; AML = anterior mitral leaflet; LA = left atrium. *(From Maron BJ: Hypertrophic cardiomyopathy: A systematic review. JAMA 287:1308, 2002. Reproduced with permission of the American Medical Association.)*

Fig. 18-10).[8,9] CMR is complementary to echocardiography by clarifying technically ambiguous LV wall thicknesses, by visualizing abnormalities often not identifiable with echocardiography (e.g., areas of segmental hypertrophy in the anterolateral free wall[8,9]; see Fig. 69-2), or by depicting pathologic changes in the apical region including hypertrophy[9] and aneurysm formation[12] (**Fig. 69-4**) that may clarify diagnosis or in some patients alter management strategies (see Fig. 69-2).

Diverse patterns of asymmetric LV hypertrophy are characteristic of HCM, including dissimilar phenotypes in relatives (with the exception of identical twins; see Fig. 69-1). Typically, one or more regions of the LV wall are of greater thickness than other areas, frequently with sharp transitions in thickness between adjacent areas or noncontiguous patterns of segmental hypertrophy, as well as extension into the right ventricle.[20] However, there is not a single "classic" morphologic form,

and virtually all possible patterns of LV hypertrophy have been reported in HCM, including genetically affected children and adults with normal LV wall thicknesses (see Fig. 69-1).[1,7,9] There is no evidence that specific patterns of LV hypertrophy are consistently related to outcome.[1,7]

Hypertrophy is frequently diffuse, involving portions of both ventricular septum and LV free wall, including some patients with the greatest magnitude of LV hypertrophy observed in any cardiac disease with wall thicknesses ranging to 50 to 60 mm (see Fig. 69-1).[9] However, in about 50% of patients, LV hypertrophy is nondiffuse, including a sizeable minority with wall thickening confined to segmental areas of the LV chamber. Wall thickening limited to the most distal portion of the LV chamber (apical HCM) represents a morphologic form characterized by a "spade" deformity of the distal left ventricle and marked T

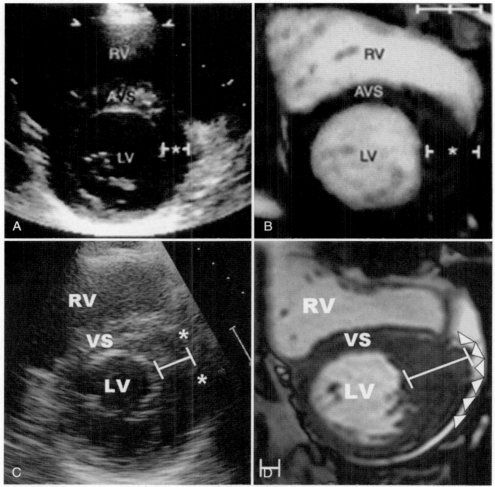

FIGURE 69-2 Cardiovascular magnetic resonance (CMR) identification of segmental LV wall thickening in HCM. Diagnosis: two-dimensional echocardiogram **(A)** and comparative CMR image **(B)** acquired in short-axis plane at end diastole at same level from 13-year-old asymptomatic identical twin. **A,** Echocardiogram shows normal anterolateral free wall thickness (asterisk). **B,** CMR shows segmental area of hypertrophy confined to anterolateral LV free wall (20 mm) and small portion of contiguous anterior septum (asterisk). Calibration marks are 1 cm apart. *(From Rickers C, Wilke NM, Jerosch-Herold M, et al: Utility of cardiac magnetic resonance imaging in the diagnosis of hypertrophic cardiomyopathy. Circulation 112:855, 2005. Reproduced with permission of the American Heart Association.)* Management implications: echocardiogram **(C)** and comparative CMR image **(D)** from 46-year-old man with HCM. **C,** Echocardiographic short-axis image shows anterolateral free wall thickness of 18 mm. **D,** CMR shows focal area of massive LV hypertrophy (wall thickness, 35 mm) in the same region of LV, significantly underestimated by two-dimensional echocardiography. This finding defined high-risk status, prompting altered management strategy with an ICD recommendation for primary prevention of sudden death. Calibration markers are 1 cm apart. AVS = anterior ventricular septum. LV = left ventricle; RV = right ventricle; VS = ventricular septum. *(From Maron MS, Lesser JR, Maron BJ: Management implications of massive left ventricular hypertrophy in hypertrophic cardiomyopathy significantly underestimated by echocardiography but identified by cardiovascular magnetic resonance. Am J Cardiol 105:1842, 2010.)*

wave negativity on electrocardiography that may be due to mutations in proteins of the cardiac sarcomere (see Fig. 69-1; see Fig. 15-67). Increased LV mass (calculated by CMR) is not invariable in HCM and is normal or nearly normal in 20% of patients when hypertrophy is localized and segmental.[10]

LV hypertrophy commonly develops dynamically after a variable period of latency (**Fig. 69-5**). Typically, the HCM phenotype is incomplete until adolescence, when accelerated growth and maturation are often accompanied by spontaneous and striking increases in LV wall thickness (i.e., average 100% change) and more extensive distribution of hypertrophy.[1,7] These structural changes, which occasionally may be delayed until later in midlife, are part of a genetically predetermined remodeling process not usually associated with development of symptoms or arrhythmia-related events. In genetically affected individuals, 12-lead electrocardiographic abnormalities or subtle preclinical evidence of diastolic dysfunction (usually diminished E′ velocity) detectable by tissue Doppler imaging may precede the appearance of LV hypertrophy,[21] including the possibility that some athletes with marked repolarization abnormalities on electrocardiogram may later manifest clinical and phenotypic evidence of HCM.[22]

Mitral Valve Apparatus

Structural abnormalities of the mitral valve apparatus that are responsible for LV outflow obstruction include diverse alterations in valvular size and shape and represent a primary morphologic abnormality in HCM, most frequently evident in younger patients.[1,7] The mitral valve may be as much as twice normal size from elongation of both leaflets or segmental enlargement of only the anterior leaflet or the midportion of the posterior leaflet. In a small subset of patients, congenital and anomalous anterolateral papillary muscle insertion into the anterior mitral leaflet (without the interposition of chordae tendineae) produces muscular midcavity outflow obstruction.[7]

Histopathology

In HCM, cardiac muscle cells (myocytes) in both ventricular septum and LV free wall show increased transverse diameter and bizarre shapes, often maintaining intercellular connections with several adjacent cells.[7] Many myocytes (and myofilaments) are arranged in chaotic, disorganized patterns at oblique and perpendicular angles

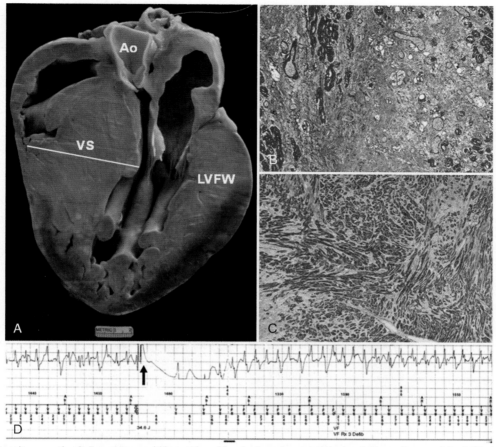

FIGURE 69-3 *LAMP2* cardiomyopathy. **A,** From 14-year-old boy with sudden death and septal thickness of 65 mm (heart weight, 1425 g). Ao = aorta; LVFW = left ventricular free wall; VS = ventricular septum. **B,** Clusters of myocytes with vacuolated sarcoplasm (stained red) embedded in area of scar (stained blue; Masson trichrome). **C,** Disorganized arrangement of myocytes most typical of sarcomeric HCM. **D,** Intracardiac electrogram. ICD elicited five defibrillation shocks that failed to interrupt ventricular fibrillation (280 beats/min). *(From Maron BJ, Roberts WC, Arad M, et al: Clinical outcome and phenotypic expression in LAMP2 cardiomyopathy. JAMA 301:1253, 2009. Reproduced with permission of the American Medical Association.)*

(**Fig. 69-6**). Areas of disorganized architecture are evident in 95% of HCM patients at autopsy, usually occupying substantial portions of hypertrophied (as well as nonhypertrophied) LV myocardium (33% of septum and 25% of free wall).[7]

Abnormal intramural coronary arteries with thickened walls (composed of increased intimal and medial components) and narrowed lumen are present in 80% of patients at necropsy, most frequently within or close to areas of replacement fibrosis[1,7,23] (see Fig. 69-6). This microvascular small-vessel disease[23] is responsible for clinically silent myocardial ischemia[23] and myocyte death, leading to a repair process in the form of replacement (often transmural) with fibrosis[7,11,23,24] (see Fig. 69-6). Also, the volume of the interstitial (matrix) collagen compartment, constituting the structural LV framework, is greatly expanded.

It is likely that the disorganized cellular architecture and replacement fibrosis evident in HCM impair transmission of electrophysiologic impulses and predispose to disordered patterns and increased dispersion of electrical depolarization and repolarization, in turn serving as an electrically unstable substrate and nidus for reentry ventricular tachyarrhythmias and sudden death.

Pathophysiology

Left Ventricular Outflow Obstruction

Longstanding LV outflow tract obstruction (basal gradient, ≥30 mm Hg) is a strong determinant of HCM-related progressive heart failure symptoms and cardiovascular death[17,25] (**Fig. 69-7**). However, only a weak relationship is evident between outflow obstruction and specifically the risk for sudden cardiac death (usually in patients without significant heart failure symptoms).[17,25]

Subaortic obstruction in HCM represents true mechanical impedance to LV outflow, producing markedly increased intraventricular pressures that may be detrimental to LV function, probably by increasing myocardial wall stress and oxygen demand.[17,25] In most patients, obstruction is produced in the proximal left ventricle by systolic anterior motion (SAM) of mitral valve and midsystolic ventricular septal contact. Characteristic of SAM, particularly in young patients, is abrupt anterior motion of the mitral valve in which elongated leaflets move toward the septum with a sharp-angled 90-degree bend. SAM appears to be generated largely by a drag effect, that is, hydrodynamic pushing force of flow directly on the leaflets. Magnitude of the outflow gradient, reliably estimated with continuous-wave Doppler, is directly related to duration of mitral valve–septal contact. Mitral regurgitation is a secondary consequence of SAM, with the jet (usually mild to moderate in degree) directed posteriorly.[1] Severe mitral regurgitation suggests an intrinsic valve abnormality, such as myxomatous degeneration.

Subaortic gradients (and systolic ejection murmurs) in HCM are often dynamic, with spontaneous variability,[1] or reduced or abolished by interventions that decrease myocardial contractility (e.g., beta-adrenergic blocking drugs) or increase ventricular volume or arterial pressure (e.g., squatting, isometric handgrip, phenylephrine).[6] Alternatively, gradients can be augmented by circumstances in which arterial pressure or ventricular volume is reduced (e.g., Valsalva maneuver, nitroglycerin or amyl nitrite administration, blood loss, dehydration) or

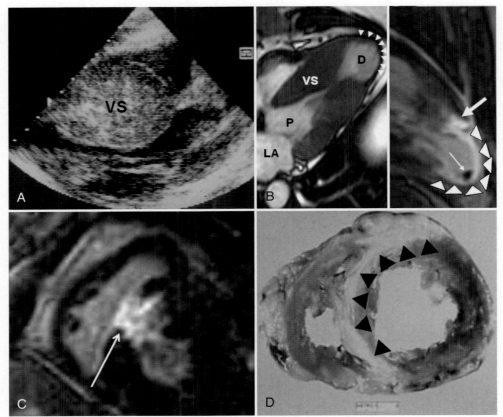

FIGURE 69-4 LV morphology associated with risk for sustained ventricular tachyarrhythmias and sudden death. **A,** Massive hypertrophy with ventricular septal (VS) thickness of 55 mm. **B, left,** Akinetic thin-walled LV apical aneurysm, associated with midcavity muscular apposition; contrast-enhanced CMR images demonstrated substantial, transmural delayed enhancement contiguous with the aneurysm. D = distal (cavity); LA = left atrium; P = proximal (cavity). **B, right,** Contrast-enhanced CMR image showing delayed enhancement (i.e., scar) involving thin aneurysm rim (arrowheads) and contiguous myocardium (large arrow); small apical thrombus is evident (small arrow). **C,** Large transmural ventricular septal scar (arrow), resulting from alcohol septal ablation procedure. *(From Valeti US, Nishimura RA, Holmes DR, et al: Comparison of surgical septal myectomy and alcohol septal ablation by cardiac magnetic resonance imaging in patients with hypertrophic obstructive cardiomyopathy. J Am Coll Cardiol 49:350, 2007. Reproduced with permission of the American College of Cardiology.)* **D,** End-stage heart showing extensive, transmural scarring involving the septum and extending into anterior free wall (arrowheads).

contractility is increased, such as with premature ventricular contractions, infusion of isoproterenol or dobutamine, or exercise.[6]

Consumption of a heavy meal or small amounts of alcohol can also transiently increase subaortic gradient and produce dyspnea. Furthermore, a large proportion of HCM patients without outflow obstruction (or SAM) at rest may generate outflow gradients with physiologic exercise, sometimes associated with severe heart failure symptoms.[13] Fully 70% of a hospital-based HCM cohort have the propensity to develop an outflow gradient ≥30 mm Hg, either at rest or during exercise.[13]

Microvascular

Myocardial ischemia due to microvascular dysfunction occurs in HCM and is an important pathophysiologic component of the disease process, promoting LV myocardial scarring and remodeling and affecting clinical course.[23] Active ischemia, demonstrable with positron emission tomography, is a determinant of progressive heart failure and cardiovascular mortality.[23] However, the relationship between chest pain commonly encountered in HCM and active myocardial ischemia is unresolved.

Diastolic Dysfunction

Evidence of impaired LV relaxation and filling, by mitral inflow pulsed Doppler and tissue Doppler imaging (see Chap. 15), is present in as many as 80% of HCM patients, probably contributing to heart failure symptoms of exertional dyspnea, although not directly related to severity of LV hypertrophy.[1] The rapid filling phase is usually prolonged, associated with decreased rate and volume of LV filling and (in sinus rhythm) a compensatory increase in the contribution of atrial systole to overall filling.[1,21] Parameters of diastolic function have limited applicability to patient management and do not accurately predict prognosis, symptoms, or filling pressures, although restrictive LV filling patterns may be linked to adverse outcome in some HCM patients.

Reduced ventricular compliance in HCM probably results largely from those factors determining passive elastic properties of the LV chamber, such as hypertrophy, replacement scarring and interstitial fibrosis, and disorganized cellular architecture. Diastolic dysfunction is likely to be the fundamental mechanism by which heart failure occurs in nonobstructive HCM with preserved LV systolic function (see Chap. 30).

FAMILY SCREENING STRATEGIES

Clinical screening of relatives in HCM families (in the absence of genetic testing) is performed with two-dimensional echocardiography and 12-lead electrocardiography (also CMR) as well as by history taking and physical examination. Screening evaluations are usually performed on a 12- to 18-month basis, beginning at the age of 12 years.[26] If these studies do not show LV hypertrophy by the time full growth is achieved (18 to 21 years), it is usually reasonable to conclude that an HCM-causing mutation is likely absent. However, morphologic conversions to HCM phenotypes (i.e., LV hypertrophy) can be delayed into adulthood, and it is not possible to provide unequivocal reassurance that a normal echocardiogram at maturity defines a genetically unaffected relative.[1,2,7,26] In such circumstances, it may be prudent to pursue genetic testing[4] or to extend echocardiographic surveillance into adulthood at 5-year intervals.[26]

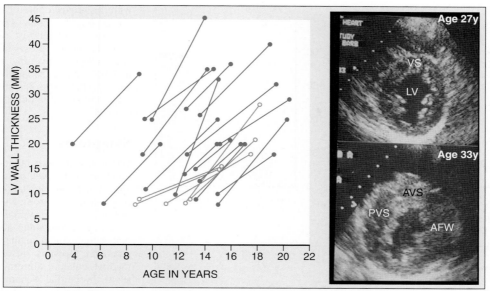

FIGURE 69-5 LV remodeling with development or progression of HCM phenotype. **Left,** Childhood/adolescence. Increased echocardiographic LV wall thickness in patients with familial HCM, unassociated with changes in clinical course. Open symbols denote those without initial evidence of hypertrophy in any LV segment. *(From Maron BJ, Spirito P, Wesley Y, Arce J: Development and progression of left ventricular hypertrophy in children with hypertrophic cardiomyopathy. N Engl J Med 315:610, 1986. Reproduced with permission of the Massachusetts Medical Society.)* **Right,** Adulthood. Woman with myosin-binding protein C mutation at age 27 years, with normal LV thickness (≤12 mm) in all segments of the wall **(top)**; 6 years later, at age 33 years, wall thickness has increased to 20 mm in both anterior ventricular septum and posterior septum as well as anterolateral free wall **(bottom)**. LV wall thickness eventually increased to >30 mm, and the patient was prophylactically implanted with a defibrillator for primary prevention of sudden death. Calibration marks are 10 mm apart. *(From Maron BJ, Niimura H, Casey SA, et al: Development of left ventricular hypertrophy in adults in hypertrophic cardiomyopathy caused by cardiac myosin-binding protein C gene mutations. J Am Coll Cardiol 38:315, 2001. Reproduced with permission of the American College of Cardiology.)*

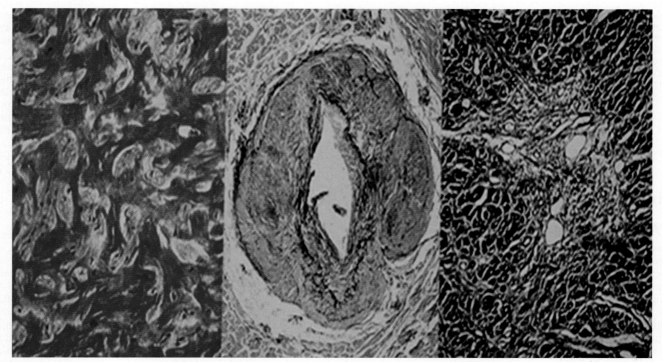

FIGURE 69-6 Arrhythmogenic myocardial substrate. **Left,** Disorganized LV architecture with myocyte disarray. **Center,** Small-vessel disease; remodeled intramural coronary arteriole with thickened media and narrowed lumen. **Right,** Repair process with replacement fibrosis, the consequence of silent myocardial ischemia and myocyte death.

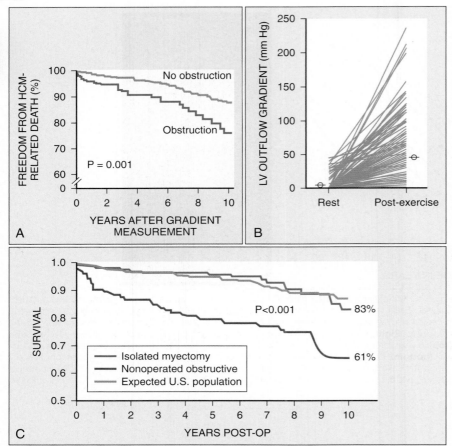

FIGURE 69-7 Left ventricular outflow tract obstruction. **A,** Probability of severe progressive heart failure (NYHA Class III or IV), heart failure death, or stroke in patients with LV outflow obstruction significantly exceeds that in patients without obstruction (relative risk, 4.4; P < 0.001). *(From Maron MS, Olivotto I, Betocchi S, et al: Effect of left ventricular outflow tract obstruction on clinical outcome in hypertrophic cardiomyopathy. N Engl J Med 348:295, 2003. Reproduced with permission of the Massachusetts Medical Society.)* **B,** Changes in LV outflow tract gradient from resting (basal) conditions to immediately after termination of treadmill exercise. Each patient is depicted by a line connecting the two gradient measurements. θ indicates the mean. *(From Maron MS, Olivotto I, Zenovich AG, et al: Hypertrophic cardiomyopathy is predominantly a disease of left ventricular outflow tract obstruction. Circulation 114:216, 2006. Reproduced with permission of the American Heart Association.)* **C,** After myectomy with relief of LV outflow obstruction, survival free from all-cause mortality compared with age- and gender-matched U.S. population and also patients with nonoperated obstruction (P < 0.001). *(From Ommen SR, Maron BJ, Olivotto I, et al: Long-term effects of surgical septal myectomy on survival in patients with obstructive hypertrophic cardiomyopathy. J Am Coll Cardiol 46:470, 2005. Reproduced with permission of the American College of Cardiology.)*

Clinical Features

Physical Examination

Physical examination findings in patients with HCM are variable and related in large measure to hemodynamic state (see Chap. 12). Initial clinical suspicion of HCM may be triggered by recognition of a heart murmur on routine examination or before sports participation, although the majority of patients are still identified by virtue of clinically overt symptom onset or cardiac events.[27] Patients with outflow obstruction characteristically have a medium-pitch systolic ejection murmur at the lower left sternal border and apex that varies in intensity with the magnitude of the subaortic gradient, increasing with the Valsalva maneuver, during or immediately after exercise, or on standing. Most patients with loud murmurs of at least grade 3/6 are likely to have LV outflow gradients >30 mm Hg; arterial pulses usually rise rapidly

with bisferiens contour, and double or triple apical impulses may be palpable, reflecting outward systolic thrust caused by ventricular contraction and presystolic accentuated atrial contraction. Conversely, physical findings in patients without subaortic gradients are more subtle, with no or soft systolic murmur, although a forceful apical impulse may arouse suspicion of HCM.

Symptoms

Symptoms of heart failure (with preserved LV function) may develop unpredictably at any age, with functional limitation due to exertional dyspnea or fatigue, and in advanced stages by orthopnea or paroxysmal nocturnal dyspnea.[1,7] Disability is frequently accompanied by chest pain, either typical angina pectoris or atypical in character, possibly resulting from structural microvasculature abnormalities responsible for silent myocardial ischemia. HCM patients may also experience impaired consciousness with syncope (or near-syncope) and lightheadedness potentially explained by several mechanisms, including arrhythmias and outflow obstruction. Severity of symptoms in HCM may be similar, independent of whether obstruction to LV outflow is present.[1]

Electrocardiographic Findings

The 12-lead electrocardiogram (ECG) is abnormal in more than 90% of probands with HCM and in about 75% of asymptomatic relatives.[1,3] ECGs show a wide variety of abnormal patterns, some of which are distinctly altered or even bizarre, although none is typical or characteristic of the disease. Most common abnormalities include increased voltages consistent with LV hypertrophy, ST-T changes including marked T wave inversion in the lateral precordial leads, left atrial enlargement, deep and narrow Q waves, and diminished R waves in the lateral precordial leads.[28] Normal electrocardiographic patterns (present in about 5% of patients) are associated with less severe phenotype and favorable cardiovascular course[29] but are not predictive of future sudden death events or appropriate defibrillator interventions.[28] Increased voltages (tall R waves or deep S waves) are only weakly correlated with the magnitude of LV hypertrophy evident on echocardiography and do not reliably distinguish the obstructive and nonobstructive forms.[28]

Gender and Race

HCM occurs with equal frequency in men and women.[2] The predominance of men in the literature reflects underdiagnosis in women, who achieve clinical recognition less frequently, at older ages, and with more pronounced symptoms than in men.[30] Furthermore, women have greater risk than men do for progression to advanced heart failure (usually associated with outflow obstruction), although there is no relation between gender and sudden death or overall mortality.[30] HCM has been reported in many races[1] but is underrecognized in African Americans, with most competitive athletes who die suddenly of HCM previously undiagnosed black men.[31] Phenotypic expression of HCM is similar throughout the world, with the possible exception of the morphologic form characterized by hypertrophy confined to the LV apex, most common in Japan.[7,16]

Athletes

Athlete's Heart and Hypertrophic Cardiomyopathy

Long-term athletic training can increase LV diastolic cavity dimension, wall thickness, and calculated mass, known as the athlete's heart.[31] Physiologically induced increases in absolute LV wall thickness are usually modest, are more substantial in some elite and highly trained individuals participating in rowing and cycling, but are not associated with purely isometric sports such as weightlifting.[31] A diagnostic dilemma may arise in distinguishing clinically benign and physiologic LV hypertrophy (as a consequence of athletic training) from pathologic conditions such as HCM. Clinical parameters that favor the diagnosis of HCM in trained athletes in the ambiguous "gray zone" of overlap between the two conditions (maximum LV wall thicknesses, 13 to 15 mm) include identification of a disease-causing sarcomeric protein mutation or recognition of HCM in a relative, transmitral Doppler waveform consistent with altered LV relaxation and filling, and LV end-diastolic cavity dimension <45 mm (**Fig. 69-8**). Parameters favoring physiologic athlete's heart include regression of wall thickness after a short (4- to 6-week) period of deconditioning assessed with CMR and enlarged LV cavity size exceeding 55 mm.

Preparticipation Screening

Detection of cardiovascular abnormalities having the potential for sudden death associated with intense physical training and competition is a major objective of preparticipation screening for high-school and college-aged sports participants.[31,32] In the United States, customary screening practice dictates a personal and family history and physical examination. Although HCM can be suspected and identified by this process, in other instances the disease remains undetected, given that many affected individuals do not have a heart murmur or historical clues (e.g., syncope or family history of HCM). Mandatory incorporation of noninvasive testing (such as with ECGs) into a national screening program for competitive athletes is not practical or feasible within the current U.S. health care system for several reasons, including limited physician resources.[32] The frequency of borderline and false-positive test results (and the uncertainty that accompanies these circumstances), the variations in ECG patterns with respect to race,[33] and the possibility that HCM phenotypes are not always detectable in early adolescence represent other limitations to mass ECG screening. Broad-based screening of athletes with echocardiography would not appear to be cost-effective.[34]

Clinical Course

Natural History

HCM is perhaps unique among cardiovascular diseases with the potential for clinical presentation during all phases of life, from infancy to old age (birth to >90 years).[1,7,35] Affected patients at either extreme of this age range appear to have the same basic disease process, although not necessarily with the same clinical course. During the last decade, greater clarity and general understanding have emerged regarding the natural history of HCM. Community-based patient populations, uncontaminated by tertiary center referral bias (and most representative of the true disease state), have reported overall HCM-related mortality rates of about 1%/year (**Fig. 69-9**), although somewhat higher in children (i.e., 2%/year).[1,7,14] This characterization of HCM contrasts with the older literature. Previously reported annual mortality rates of 4% to 6% were derived from highly selected cohorts at major referral centers incorporating substantial patient referral bias and skewed toward high-risk patients. This extreme perception of the natural history of HCM patients has been rendered obsolete with respect to the contemporary population.

Although clinical course is typically variable, patients with HCM may remain stable during long periods.[1,7,35] Notably, HCM is compatible with normal life expectancy with little or no disability and without the necessity for major therapeutic interventions to achieve this outcome (see Fig. 69-9).[1,7,29,35] Indeed, adults with HCM have the same overall life expectancy as that of an age- and sex-matched general population, underscoring the important principle that many patients with this disease deserve a large measure of reassurance regarding prognosis.

Nevertheless, subgroups at higher risk for important disease complications and premature death reside within an HCM population. Such patients proceed along specific adverse pathways, punctuated by clinical events that ultimately dictate targeted treatment strategies[1,7,11,14,17,35-40]: (1) sudden and unexpected death; (2) progressive heart failure with exertional dyspnea and functional limitation (often accompanied by chest pain) in the presence of preserved LV systolic function; and (3) atrial fibrillation (AF), with the risk for embolic stroke and heart failure. However, prediction of clinical course and outcome for individual patients with HCM remains encumbered by the markedly diverse disease expression and the long period of potential risk for young patients.[1,7,38,39]

Heart Failure

Whereas some degree of heart failure with exertional dyspnea is common in HCM, progression to severe functional limitation with preserved LV systolic function (i.e., New York Heart Association [NYHA] Class III or IV) is infrequent, occurring in probably 10% to 15% of the overall patient population.[1,7] The principal determinants of progressive heart failure and heart failure–related death appear to be LV outflow obstruction, AF, and diastolic dysfunction.[13,17,20,21,23,25,35] Also, microvascular dysfunction[23] has been advanced as a predictor of long-term outcome and heart failure death. In contrast to the risk specifically for sudden death (which bears a linear relationship to magnitude of LV hypertrophy) greater degrees of LV wall thickness are

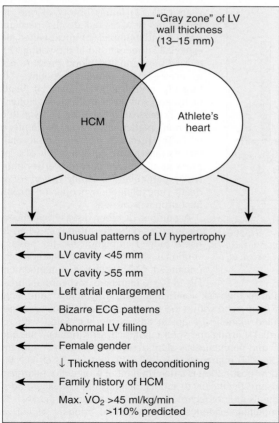

FIGURE 69-8 Differential diagnosis of HCM versus physiologic athlete's heart. Clinical criteria used to distinguish nonobstructive HCM from athlete's heart when maximal LV wall thickness is within the shaded gray area of overlap, consistent with both diagnoses. ↓ = decreased. (*Modified from Maron BJ, Pelliccia A: The heart of trained athletes: Cardiac remodeling and the risks of sports including sudden death. Circulation 114;1633, 2006. Reproduced with permission of the American Heart Association.*)

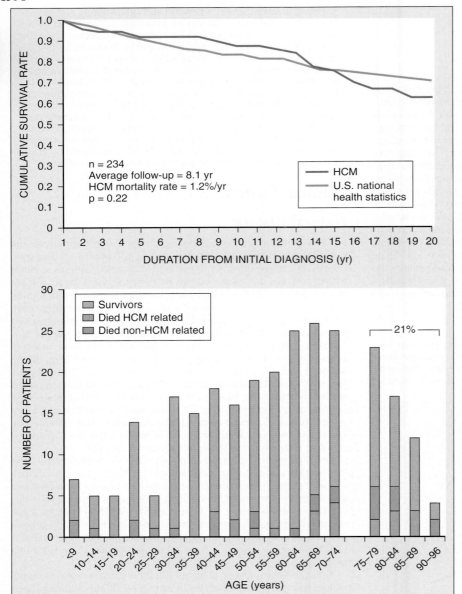

FIGURE 69-9 Clinical course of HCM patients. **Top,** Cumulative survival in a community-based adult HCM population. Total mortality of 1%/year does not differ significantly from that expected in the general U.S. population after adjustment for age, gender, and race. **Bottom,** Age at initial presentation with >20% of patients achieving normal life expectancy (≥75 years). *(From Maron BJ, Casey SA, Poliac LC, et al: Clinical course of hypertrophic cardiomyopathy in a regional United States cohort. JAMA 281:650, 1999. Reproduced with permission of the American Medical Association.)*

Risk Stratification and Sudden Death

Sudden death in HCM may occur at a wide range of ages but most commonly in adolescents and young adults <30 to 35 years of age (**Fig. 69-10**).[1,7,14,31,36,38] These events are arrhythmia based, caused by primary ventricular tachycardia and ventricular fibrillation.[38,39] Sudden death is often the initial clinical manifestation of HCM, occurring commonly in asymptomatic individuals, many of whom are undiagnosed during life. Whereas most sudden deaths occur while sedentary or during modest physical activity, such events are also frequently associated with vigorous exertion, consistent with the observation that HCM is the most common cardiovascular cause of athletic field deaths (see Fig. 69-10).[14] Association of HCM with vigorous exercise and sudden death constitutes the basis for prudent recommendations by the 36th Bethesda Conference to disqualify young athletes with HCM from intense competitive sports to reduce sudden death risk.[41]

The greatest risk for sudden death is associated with specific clinical markers (**Fig. 69-11**). For secondary prevention, these are prior cardiac arrest and sustained ventricular tachycardia. For primary prevention, risk markers include one or more of the following, which assume greater weight in younger patients (<50 years old): (1) family history of one or more premature HCM-related deaths, particularly if sudden and multiple; (2) unexplained syncope, especially if recent and in the young; (3) hypotensive or attenuated blood pressure response to exercise; (4) multiple, repetitive (or prolonged) nonsustained bursts of ventricular tachycardia on serial ambulatory (Holter) ECGs; and (5) massive LV hypertrophy (wall thickness, ≥30 mm), particularly in young patients (see Fig. 69-4). The presence of one or more major risk factors may justify consideration of a primary prevention implantable cardioverter-defibrillator (ICD), particularly if family history of sudden death, unexplained syncope, or massive LV hypertrophy is present.

A number of other disease features can be regarded as potential arbitrators when level of risk is judged ambiguous on the basis of conventional markers. These include contrast-enhanced CMR[24] delayed enhancement (see Fig. 18-10) (a marker for myocardial fibrosis with a relation to high-risk ventricular tachyarrhythmia)[42] and subgroups that have emerged within the heterogeneous HCM disease spectrum: thin-walled akinetic LV apical aneurysms associated with regional myocardial scarring and ventricular tachyarrhythmias,[12] the end-stage phase,[11] and percutaneous alcohol septal ablation[38,43-45] with transmural myocardial infarction in select patients (see Fig. 69-4).[46] Whereas LV outflow obstruction is a determinant of progressive heart failure, its relationship specifically to sudden death is much weaker, and subaortic gradients are not regarded per se as a major risk marker.[17] There is no compelling evidence that myocardial bridging of left anterior descending coronary artery is a sudden death risk factor in HCM.[47]

At present, there is very limited prognostic significance that can be attributed to specific HCM-causing mutations for stratification of risk and clinical decision-making in individual patients.[1] Moreover, prognosis appears to be benign in gene carriers without LV hypertrophy, with little evidence[48] to justify disqualification from most competitive sports or employment opportunities.[41]

not associated with higher likelihood for development of progressive heart failure symptoms.[40] HCM is a rare cause of heart failure in infants and young children, and this presentation is regarded as an unfavorable prognostic sign.[1,3]

About 3% of HCM patients manifest the end stage characterized by systolic dysfunction (ejection fraction <50%; see Fig. 69-4).[11] This profound form of progressive heart failure (often associated with AF) may be expressed by various patterns of LV remodeling, including wall thinning and cavity dilation, associated with diffuse transmural scarring that can be identified in vivo by CMR[11,23,24] (the consequence of small-vessel mediated myocardial ischemia). Clinical course is unpredictable, but progression to refractory heart failure or sudden death is frequent (10%/year). The most reliable risk marker for evolution to the end stage is a family history of the end stage.[11]

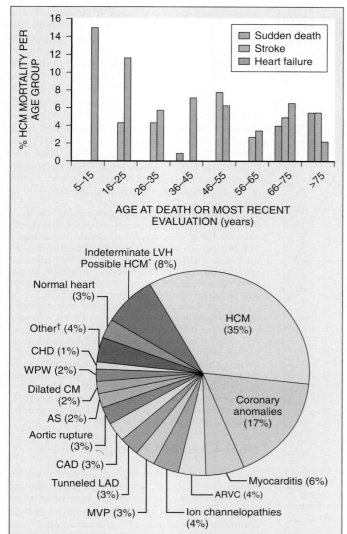

FIGURE 69-10 Clinical profile of sudden death. **Top,** Sudden death is most common in children and young adults before about 25 years of age, whereas heart failure and stroke generally occur later in life. *(From Maron BJ, Olivotto I, Spirito P, et al: Epidemiology of hypertrophic cardiomyopathy–related death: Revisited in a large non-referral-based patient population. Circulation 102:858, 2000. Reproduced with permission of the American Heart Association.)* **Bottom,** HCM is the single most common cause of sudden death in young competitive athletes in the United States. ARVC = arrhythmogenic right ventricular cardiomyopathy; AS = aortic valve stenosis; CAD = coronary artery disease; CHD = congenital heart disease; CM = cardiomyopathy; LAD = left anterior descending; LVH = left ventricular hypertrophy; MVP = mitral valve prolapse; WPW = Wolff-Parkinson-White. *Regarded as possible (but not definitive) evidence for HCM at autopsy with mildly increased LV wall thicknesses (18 ± 4 mm) and heart weight (447 ± 76 g). †Includes most commonly Kawasaki disease, sickle cell trait, and sarcoidosis. *(From Maron BJ, Doerer JJ, Haas TS, et al: Sudden deaths in young competitive athletes: Analysis of 1866 deaths in the U.S., 1980-2006. Circulation 119:1085, 2009. Reproduced with permission of the American Heart Association.)*

Management

Prevention of Sudden Death

The ICD has altered the natural history of HCM for many patients by virtue of effectively and reliably aborting potentially lethal ventricular tachyarrhythmias (see Chap. 38),[38,39,49-52] for both secondary prevention after cardiac arrest (11%/year) and primary prevention for risk factors (4%/year) (see Fig. 69-e1 on website).[38,49] Noteworthy is the extended time (i.e., 5 to 10 years) that may elapse between the clinical decision to implant an ICD and the time at which the device is required to

terminate ventricular tachyarrhythmias (**Fig. 69-12**). The unpredictability of arrhythmic events in HCM is underscored by the absence of a distinct circadian pattern, the occurrence of a substantial proportion during sleep,[39] and the long periods that may elapse after cardiac arrest without a recurrent event.[38,49,51] Notably, development of heart failure symptoms appears to be uncommon in the years after an appropriate ICD intervention.[51]

Age may alter the threshold for prophylactic ICD implants; elderly patients are less often targeted for devices, given that HCM-related sudden death is uncommon in this age group and survival to advanced age itself generally declares lower risk status. Whereas it appears that current risk stratification strategy for HCM reliably identifies most high-risk patients, nevertheless this algorithm is probably incomplete, and a small minority of patients without any of the traditional primary prevention risk factors may be susceptible to sudden death.[52] Prophylactic, empiric pharmacologic treatment with amiodarone for asymptomatic high-risk patients to reduce sudden death risk is an obsolete strategy that has been abandoned, given the lack of proven efficacy and the likelihood for important side effects during the long risk period of young HCM patients.[1,7]

Medical Treatment of Heart Failure (see Fig. 69-12)

Symptoms of heart failure, that is, exertional dyspnea (sometimes fatigue) and chest pain, are attributable to diastolic dysfunction, outflow tract obstruction, or microvascular myocardial ischemia or combinations of these pathophysiologic variables. Symptom relief due to medical treatment can be highly variable, and drug administration is often empirically tailored to requirements of individual patients. Since the mid-1960s, beta-adrenergic receptor blocking drugs have been used extensively to relieve symptoms of heart failure in obstructive or nonobstructive HCM by slowing heart rate and reducing force of LV contraction, thus augmenting ventricular filling and relaxation and decreasing myocardial oxygen consumption. Long-acting preparations of propranolol, atenolol, metoprolol, or nadolol are now commonly used. By inhibiting sympathetic stimulation of the heart, beta blockers also have the potential to blunt LV outflow gradient triggered by physiologic exercise.[6]

Verapamil improves symptoms and exercise capacity, largely in patients without marked obstruction to LV outflow, probably because of its beneficial effect on ventricular relaxation and filling. Some investigators favor disopyramide as a third option (in combination with a beta blocker) to ameliorate symptoms when other drugs fail to achieve symptom control.[53] Diuretic agents may be judiciously administered, in conjunction with beta blockers or verapamil, to reduce pulmonary congestion and LV filling pressures. Either beta blockers or verapamil can be administered initially, although there is no evidence that combining these drugs is advantageous, and together they may excessively lower heart rate or blood pressure.

Therapeutic strategies for patients with systolic dysfunction in the end stage are similar to those employed for congestive heart failure in other cardiac diseases, including the administration of beta blockers, angiotensin-converting enzyme inhibitors or angiotensin receptor blockers, and diuretics or possibly spironolactone as well as warfarin.[11] End stage with widespread LV scarring also represents a sudden death risk factor with consideration for ICD as a bridge to heart transplantation.[1,7,11]

Atrial Fibrillation (see Fig. 69-12)

AF is the most common sustained arrhythmia in HCM, frequently accounting for unexpected hospital admissions and lost productivity and on occasion requiring aggressive therapeutic intervention (see Chap. 40).[1,7] AF, either paroxysmal or chronic, occurs in about 20% of HCM patients, increasing in incidence with age and linked to enlargement of the left atrium (a finding that has also been associated with overall adverse outcome in HCM, even independent of AF).[54] AF is well tolerated by about one third of patients but not uncommonly associated with adverse consequences, including embolic stroke (incidence, 1%/year; prevalence, 6%), and progressive heart failure, particularly

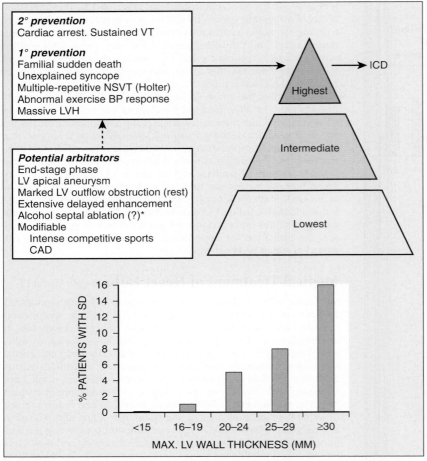

2° prevention
Cardiac arrest. Sustained VT

1° prevention
Familial sudden death
Unexplained syncope
Multiple-repetitive NSVT (Holter)
Abnormal exercise BP response
Massive LVH

ICD

Highest

Intermediate

Lowest

Potential arbitrators
End-stage phase
LV apical aneurysm
Marked LV outflow obstruction (rest)
Extensive delayed enhancement
Alcohol septal ablation (?)*
Modifiable
  Intense competitive sports
  CAD

FIGURE 69-11 Sudden death risk stratification. **Top,** Risk pyramid currently used to identify the most likely candidates for prevention of sudden death with ICDs. BP = blood pressure; CAD = coronary artery disease; ICD = implantable cardiac defibrillator; LV = left ventricle. LVH = left ventricular hypertrophy; NSVT = nonsustained ventricular tachycardia; VT = ventricular tachycardia. **Bottom,** Relation between magnitude of LV hypertrophy (maximum [max] wall thickness by echocardiography) and sudden death risk in an unselected HCM cohort. Mild hypertrophy conveys generally lower risk and extreme hypertrophy (wall thickness ≥30 mm) the highest risk. *(From Spirito P, Bellone P, Harris KM, et al: Magnitude of left ventricular hypertrophy and risk of sudden death in hypertrophic cardiomyopathy. N Engl J Med 342:1778-85, 2000. Reproduced with permission of the Massachusetts Medical Society.)* *Sustained ventricular tachyarrhythmias have been reported in a significant minority of patients (10%) short term after the alcohol septal ablation procedure.[43-46,59,60]

when it is associated with outflow obstruction or onset before the age of 50 years.

Because of potential for clot formation and embolization, a low threshold for initiation of anticoagulant therapy with warfarin is prudent, although such decisions should be tailored to individual patients after consideration of lifestyle modifications, hemorrhagic risk, and expectations for compliance. Although data specifically in HCM are limited, amiodarone is considered the most effective drug in reducing AF recurrences. Beta blockers and verapamil are usually administered to control heart rate in chronic AF. Some success in treatment of refractory AF complicating HCM with radiofrequency catheter ablation has been reported in relatively small numbers of patients, but long-term outcome is largely unresolved.[56,58,59]

Surgery (see Fig. 69-12)

On the basis of the extensive worldwide experience during more than 45 years, surgical septal myectomy remains the preferred treatment option for patients with severe drug-refractory heart failure symptoms and marked functional disability (i.e., NYHA Classes III and IV in adults, but less limitation in children) associated with obstruction to LV outflow under basal conditions or with physiologic exercise (i.e., gradient ≥50 mm Hg).[1,7,56-59] Inducing gradients with nonphysiologic

maneuvers, such as the infusion of inotropic and catecholamine inducing drugs (e.g., dobutamine and isoproterenol), is not advisable in selecting patients for septal myectomy (or alcohol ablation).

Patients with obstructive HCM have mechanical impedance to LV outflow and a form of heart failure that is reversible by surgery.[1,7,17,25,56-59] Transaortic ventricular septal myectomy (Morrow procedure) involves resection of a small portion of muscle (usually 3 to 10 g) from the basal septum.[57] Some surgeons now perform a more aggressive myectomy, extended in the septum for about 7 cm distal from the aortic valve.[56,58,59] Operative mortality has steadily decreased and is now <1% during the last 15 years at the most experienced myectomy centers.[58,59]

The primary objective of surgical myectomy is reduction in heart failure symptoms and improved quality of life, by virtue of relieving outflow obstruction. Indeed, 95% of patients undergoing myectomy experience permanent abolition of the basal outflow gradient, without compromise of global LV function.[56-59] As a result, long-term follow-up studies reported relief of symptoms in 85% of patients during periods of up to 25 years.[56-59]

Myectomy also beneficially alters the clinical course of HCM; surgical patients achieve long-term survival equivalent to that expected in the general population and superior to that of nonsurgical HCM patients with outflow obstruction[56] (see Fig. 69-6). At present, surgical myectomy is not recommended for asymptomatic (or mildly symptomatic) patients, as conclusive evidence is lacking that prophylactic relief of obstruction is of benefit long term. There is no evidence that myectomy predisposes patients to the end-stage phase with systolic dysfunction and LV remodeling.[11,58,59]

Dual-Chamber Pacing (see Fig. 69-12)

About 20 years ago, permanent dual-chamber pacing was promoted as an alternative to myectomy for obstructive HCM patients with refractory heart failure symptoms. Although modest reduction in subaortic gradient may result from pacing in some patients, this benefit is inconsistent, particularly compared with that achieved by myectomy or alcohol ablation.[1] Several randomized studies demonstrated that the subjectively perceived symptomatic benefit from pacing was not accompanied by objective evidence of improved exercise capacity and appeared to be largely a placebo effect.[1,7] The overall role for pacing in HCM has become particularly limited during the last decade.

Alcohol Septal Ablation (see Chap. 59)

Percutaneous alcohol septal ablation, an alternative to myectomy only in selected patients (see Fig. 69-12; see Fig. 59-5),[1] involves introduction of 1 to 3 mL of 95% alcohol into a major septal perforator coronary artery to create necrosis and a permanent transmural myocardial infarction in the proximal ventricular septum (see Fig. 69-4).[43-46] This scar leads to progressive thinning and restricted septal excursion, outflow tract enlargement, and reduction in LV outflow tract gradient and mitral regurgitation in most patients.

Alcohol ablation resolves heart failure symptoms in many patients, although follow-up is short compared with myectomy, and even in expert centers, it may be associated with procedural mortality and complication rates exceeding those of myectomy.[44,45,59] Nonrandomized, comparative data show that gradient reduction after alcohol ablation is similar to myectomy, although less consistent or complete, and patients ≤65 years experience better symptom resolution with myectomy than with ablation.[45] About 20% of patients require repeated ablations because of unsatisfactory hemodynamic and symptomatic results or permanent pacing for complete heart block.[44]

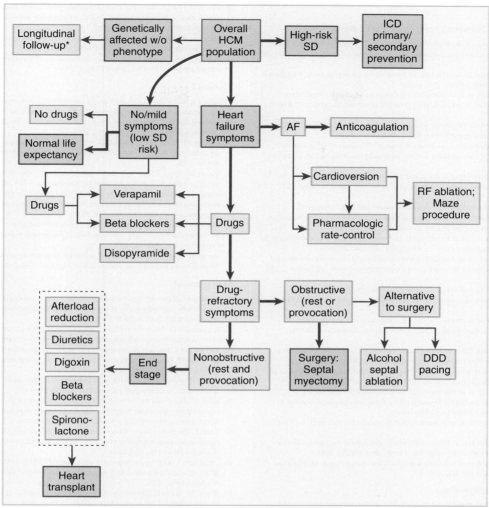

FIGURE 69-12 Management strategies for subgroups of patients within the broad HCM clinical spectrum. *Generally no specific treatment or intervention indicated. AF = atrial fibrillation; DDD = dual-chamber; ICD = implanted cardioverter-defibrillator; RF= radiofrequency; SD = sudden death.

An American College of Cardiology/European Society of Cardiology expert consensus panel[1] recommended surgical myectomy as the preferred and primary management option for patients with severe refractory symptoms and marked outflow obstruction. Alcohol ablation is regarded as an alternative treatment strategy for patients not considered optimal operative candidates (e.g., advanced age, significant comorbidity and increased operative risk, or strongly adverse to surgery personally).

Long-term issues remain unresolved, most importantly the clinical significance of the alcohol-induced transmural scar (occupying about 10% of the LV wall; see Fig. 69-4),[46] which represents a potentially unstable arrhythmogenic substrate that in some patients has triggered potentially lethal ventricular tachyarrhythmias and could raise sudden death risk in some susceptible patients.[43-46,59,60] Indeed, there is a recognized risk for life-threatening sustained ventricular tachyarrhythmias largely during the short term[43-46,59,60] (with postprocedural annual event rates of 3% to 5% involving approximately 10% of reported patients).[43,60] On the basis of this consideration, some practitioners have prudently implanted ICDs prophylactically in selected patients with alcohol septal ablation.[60] It is, however, unlikely that a randomized myectomy versus ablation trial will be carried out to resolve the level of risk conveyed long term by alcohol ablation.[61]

Other Management Issues

There is no evidence that HCM patients are generally at increased risk during pregnancy and delivery. Maternal mortality appears confined to the very small subset of symptomatic women with high-risk clinical profiles, such as severe heart failure, ventricular tachyarrhythmias, or possibly marked LV outflow obstruction, who should be afforded specialized and preventive obstetric care. Otherwise, most women with HCM can undergo normal vaginal delivery, without the necessity for cesarean section.

Bacterial endocarditis is an uncommon complication of HCM (prevalence <1%), virtually confined to patients with LV outflow obstruction. Vegetations most commonly involve anterior mitral leaflet or septal endocardium at the site of mitral valve contact. Prevention of bacterial endocarditis by antimicrobial prophylaxis remains a prudent strategy before dental or surgical procedures for this patient group.[62]

Future Directions

The last decade has witnessed a substantially increased understanding of the diagnosis, clinical profile, and natural history of HCM as well as substantial advances in management. Future clinical directions will include the development of more precise risk stratification strategies to more reliably identify those patients at unacceptably high risk for sudden death and deserving of consideration for ICD therapy. Also, there will be a continuing effort to define the proper role of alcohol septal ablation relative to surgical septal myectomy in the management of severely symptomatic drug-refractory patients with outflow obstruction, as well as the role of commercial genetic testing.

REFERENCES

Definition, Prevalence, Nomenclature, and Genetic Basis

1. Maron BJ, McKenna WJ, Danielson GK, et al: American College of Cardiology/European Society of Cardiology Clinical Expert Consensus Document on Hypertrophic Cardiomyopathy. J Am Coll Cardiol 42:1687, 2003.
2. Alcalai R, Seidman JG, Seidman CE: Genetic basis of hypertrophic cardiomyopathy: From bench to the clinics. J Cardiovasc Electrophysiol 19:104, 2008.
3. Maron BJ, Towbin JA, Thiene G, et al: Contemporary definitions and classification of the cardiomyopathies. An American Heart Association Scientific Statement. Circulation 113:1807, 2006.
4. Bos JM, Towbin JA, Ackerman MJ: Diagnostic, prognostic, and therapeutic implications of gene testing for hypertrophic cardiomyopathy. J Am Coll Cardiol 54:201, 2009.
5. Maron BJ, Seidman CE, Ackerman MJ, et al: What's in a name? Dilemmas in nomenclature characterizing hypertrophic cardiomyopathy and left ventricular hypertrophy. Circ Cardiovasc Genet 2:8, 2009.
6. Braunwald E, Lambrew C, Rockoff D, et al: Idiopathic hypertrophic subaortic stenosis. I. Description of the disease based on the analysis of 64 patients. Circulation 30(Suppl IV):1, 1964.
7. Maron BJ: Hypertrophic cardiomyopathy: A systematic review. JAMA 287:1308, 2002.
8. Rickers C, Wilke NM, Jerosch-Herold M, et al: Utility of cardiac magnetic resonance imaging in the diagnosis of hypertrophic cardiomyopathy. Circulation 112:855, 2005.
9. Maron MS, Maron BJ, Harrigan C, et al: Hypertrophic cardiomyopathy phenotype revisited at 50 years with cardiovascular magnetic resonance. J Am Coll Cardiol 54:220, 2009.
10. Olivotto I, Maron MS, Autore C, et al: Assessment and significance of left ventricular mass by cardiovascular magnetic resonance in hypertrophic cardiomyopathy. J Am Coll Cardiol 52:559, 2008.
11. Harris KM, Spirito P, Maron MS, et al: Prevalence, clinical profile and significance of left ventricular remodeling in the end-stage phase of hypertrophic cardiomyopathy. Circulation 114;216, 2006.
12. Maron MS, Finley JJ, Bos JM, et al: Prevalence, clinical significance and natural history of left ventricular apical aneurysms in hypertrophic cardiomyopathy. Circulation 118:1541, 2008.
13. Maron MS, Olivotto I, Zenovich AG, et al: Hypertrophic cardiomyopathy is predominantly a disease of left ventricular outflow tract obstruction. Circulation 114:216, 2006.
14. Maron BJ, Doerer JJ, Haas TS, et al: Sudden deaths in young competitive athletes: Analysis of 1866 deaths in the U.S., 1980-2006. Circulation 119:1085, 2009.
15. Maron BJ, Gardin JM, Flack JM, et al: Assessment of the prevalence of hypertrophic cardiomyopathy in a general population of young adults: Echocardiographic analysis of 4111 subjects in the CARDIA Study. Circulation 92:785, 1995.
16. Maron BJ: Hypertrophic cardiomyopathy: An important global disease [editorial]. Am J Med 116:63, 2004.
17. Maron MS, Olivotto I, Betocchi S, et al: Effect of left ventricular outflow tract obstruction on clinical outcome in hypertrophic cardiomyopathy. N Engl J Med 348:295, 2003.
18. Arad M, Maron BJ, Gorham JM, et al: Glycogen storage diseases presenting as hypertrophic cardiomyopathy. N Engl J Med 352:362, 2005.

Morphology and Pathophysiology

19. Maron BJ, Roberts WC, Arad M, et al: Clinical outcome and phenotypic expression in LAMP2 cardiomyopathy. JAMA 301:1253, 2009.
20. Maron MS, Hauser TH, Dubrow E, et al: Right ventricular involvement in hypertrophic cardiomyopathy. Am J Cardiol 100:1293, 2007.
21. Ho CY, Carlsen C, Thune JJ, et al: Echocardiographic strain imaging to assess early and late consequences of sarcomere mutations in hypertrophic cardiomyopathy. Circ Cardiovasc Genet 2:14, 2009.
22. Pelliccia A, DiPaolo FM, Quattrini FM, et al: Outcomes in athletes with marked ECG repolarization abnormalities. N Engl J Med 358:152, 2008.
23. Maron MS, Olivotto I, Maron BJ, et al: The case for myocardial ischemia in hypertrophic cardiomyopathy: An emerging but under-recognized pathophysiologic mechanism. J Am Coll Cardiol 54:866, 2009.
24. Maron MS, Appelbaum E, Harrigan C, et al: Clinical profile and significance of delayed enhancement in hypertrophic cardiomyopathy. Circ Heart Fail 1:184, 2008.
25. Maron BJ, Maron MS, Wigle ED, Braunwald E: 50 year history of left ventricular outflow tract obstruction in hypertrophic cardiomyopathy: From idiopathic hypertrophic subaortic stenosis to hypertrophic cardiomyopathy. J Am Coll Cardiol 54:191, 2009.

Family Screening, Clinical Features, and Athletes

26. Maron BJ, Seidman JG, Seidman CE: Proposal for contemporary screening strategies in families with hypertrophic cardiomyopathy. J Am Coll Cardiol 44:2125, 2004.
27. Adabag AS, Kuskowski MA, Maron BJ: Determinants for clinical diagnosis of hypertrophic cardiomyopathy. Am J Cardiol 98:1507, 2006.
28. Montgomery JV, Harris KM, Casey SA, et al: Relation of electrocardiographic patterns to phenotypic expression and clinical outcome in hypertrophic cardiomyopathy. Am J Cardiol 96:270, 2005.
29. McLeod CJ, Ackerman MJ, Nishimura RA, et al: Outcome of patients with hypertrophic cardiomyopathy and a normal electrocardiogram. J Am Coll Cardiol 54:229, 2009.
30. Olivotto I, Maron MS, Adabag AS, et al: Gender-related differences in the clinical presentation and outcome of hypertrophic cardiomyopathy. J Am Coll Cardiol 46:480, 2005.
31. Maron BJ, Pelliccia A: The heart of trained athletes: Cardiac remodeling and the risks of sports including sudden death. Circulation 114:1633, 2006.

32. Maron BJ, Haas TS, Doerer JJ, et al: Comparison of U.S. and Italian experiences with sudden cardiac deaths in young competitive athletes and implications for preparticipation screening strategies. Am J Cardiol 104:276, 2009.
33. Magalski A, Maron BJ, Main ML, et al: Relation of race to electrocardiographic patterns in elite American football players. J Am Coll Cardiol 51:2250, 2008.
34. Basavarajaiah S, Wilson M, Whyte G, et al: Prevalence of hypertrophic cardiomyopathy in highly trained athletes. J Am Coll Cardiol 51:1033, 2008.

Clinical Course

35. Sorajja P, Nishimura RA, Gersh BJ, et al: Outcome of mildly symptomatic or asymptomatic obstructive hypertrophic cardiomyopathy. J Am Coll Cardiol 54:234, 2009.
36. Spirito P, Autore C, Rapezzi C, et al: Syncope and risk of sudden death in hypertrophic cardiomyopathy. Circulation 119:1703, 2009.
37. Adabag AS, Casey SA, Kuskowski MA, et al: Spectrum and prognostic significance of arrhythmias on ambulatory Holter electrocardiogram in hypertrophic cardiomyopathy. J Am Coll Cardiol 45:697, 2005.
38. Maron BJ, Spirito P, Shen W-K, et al: Implantable cardioverter-defibrillators and prevention of sudden cardiac death in hypertrophic cardiomyopathy. JAMA 298:405, 2007.
39. Maron BJ, Semsarian C, Shen W-K, et al: Circadian patterns in the occurrence of malignant ventricular tachyarrhythmias triggering defibrillator interventions in patients with hypertrophic cardiomyopathy. Heart Rhythm 6:603, 2009.
40. Maron MS, Zenovich AG, Casey SA, et al: Significance and relationship between magnitude of left ventricular hypertrophy and heart failure symptoms in hypertrophic cardiomyopathy. Am J Cardiol 95:1329, 2005.
41. Maron BJ, Zipes DP: 36th Bethesda Conference: Eligibility Recommendations for Competitive Athletes with Cardiovascular Abnormalities. J Am Coll Cardiol 45:1312, 2005.

Management

42. Adabag AS, Maron BJ, Appelbaum E, et al: Occurrence and frequency of arrhythmias in hypertrophic cardiomyopathy in relation to delayed enhancement on cardiovascular magnetic resonance. J Am Coll Cardiol 51:1369, 2008.
43. Noseworthy PA, Rosenberg MA, Fifer MA, et al: Ventricular arrhythmia following alcohol septal ablation for obstructive hypertrophic cardiomyopathy. Am J Cardiol 104:128, 2009.
44. van der Lee C, ten Cate FJ, Geleijnse ML, et al: Percutaneous versus surgical treatment for patients with hypertrophic obstructive cardiomyopathy and enlarged anterior mitral valve leaflets. Circulation 112:482, 2005.
45. Sorajja P, Valeti U, Nishimura RA, et al: Outcome of alcohol septal ablation for obstructive hypertrophic cardiomyopathy. Circulation 118:131, 2008.
46. Valeti US, Nishimura RA, Holmes DR, et al: Comparison of surgical septal myectomy and alcohol septal ablation by cardiac magnetic resonance imaging in patients with hypertrophic obstructive cardiomyopathy. J Am Coll Cardiol 49:350, 2007.
47. Basso C, Thiene G, Mackey-Bojack S, et al: Myocardial bridging: A frequent component of the hypertrophic cardiomyopathy phenotype lacks systematic association with sudden cardiac death. Eur Heart J 30:1627, 2009.
48. Christiaans I, Lekanne dit Deprez RH, van Langen IM, Wilde AAM: Ventricular fibrillation in MYH7-related hypertrophic cardiomyopathy before onset of ventricular hypertrophy. Heart Rhythm 6:1366, 2009.
49. Maron BJ, Spirito P: Implantable defibrillators and prevention of sudden death in hypertrophic cardiomyopathy. J Cardiovasc Electrophysiol 19:1118, 2008.
50. Woo A, Monakier D, Harris L, et al: Determinants of implantable defibrillator discharges in high-risk patients with hypertrophic cardiomyopathy. Heart 93:1044, 2007.
51. Maron BJ, Haas TS, Shannon KM, et al: Long-term survival after cardiac arrest in hypertrophic cardiomyopathy. Heart Rhythm 6:993, 2009.
52. Maron BJ, Maron MS, Lesser JR, et al: Sudden cardiac arrest in hypertrophic cardiomyopathy in the absence of conventional criteria for high risk status. Am J Cardiol 101:544, 2008.
53. Sherrid MV, Barac I, McKenna WJ, et al: Multicenter study of the efficacy and safety of disopyramide in obstructive hypertrophic cardiomyopathy. J Am Coll Cardiol 45:1251, 2005.
54. Nistri S, Olivotto I, Betocchi S, et al: Prognostic significance of left atrial size in patients with hypertrophic cardiomyopathy (from the Italian Registry for Hypertrophic Cardiomyopathy). Am J Cardiol 98:960, 2006.
55. Kilicaslan F, Verma A, Saad E, et al: Efficacy of catheter ablation of atrial fibrillation in patients with hypertrophic obstructive cardiomyopathy. Heart Rhythm 3:275, 2006.
56. Ommen SR, Maron BJ, Olivotto I, et al: Long-term effects of surgical septal myectomy on survival in patients with obstructive hypertrophic cardiomyopathy. J Am Coll Cardiol 46:470, 2005.
57. Woo A, Williams WG, Choi R, et al: Clinical and echocardiographic determinants of long-term survival following surgical myectomy in obstructive hypertrophic cardiomyopathy. Circulation 111:2033, 2005.
58. Maron BJ, Dearani JA, Ommen SR, et al: The case for surgery in obstructive hypertrophic cardiomyopathy. J Am Coll Cardiol 44:2044, 2004.
59. Maron BJ: Controversies in cardiovascular medicine. Surgical myectomy remains the primary treatment option for severely symptomatic patients with obstructive hypertrophic cardiomyopathy. Circulation 116:196, 2007.
60. Cuoco FA, Spencer WH III, Fernandes VL, et al: Implantable cardioverter-defibrillator therapy for primary prevention of sudden death after alcohol septal ablation of hypertrophic cardiomyopathy. J Am Coll Cardiol 52:1718, 2008.
61. Olivotto I, Ommen SR, Maron MS, et al: Surgical myectomy versus percutaneous alcohol septal ablation for obstructive hypertrophic cardiomyopathy: Will there ever be a randomized trial? J Am Coll Cardiol 50:831, 2007.
62. Maron BJ, Lever H: In defense of antimicrobial prophylaxis for prevention of infective endocarditis in patients with hypertrophic cardiomyopathy. J Am Coll Cardiol 54:2339, 2009.

CHAPTER **70**   # Myocarditis

Peter Liu and Kenneth L. Baughman

Myocarditis is defined as inflammation of the heart muscle. The most common causes today are infectious agents such as viruses or parasites and autoimmune conditions. True viral myocarditis is probably more common than currently diagnosed, largely because of its protean manifestations and the reliance on myocardial biopsies for pathologic confirmation. The availability of new diagnostic modalities, such as cardiac magnetic resonance imaging, helps increase the appropriate identification of suspected cases. New molecular tools to identify the viral genome from cardiac tissues also help in defining the appropriate etiology.

The pathogenesis of myocarditis is a classic paradigm of cardiac injury followed by immunologic response from the host as cardiac inflammation. The relative incidence of viral causes is continually evolving as new diagnostic tools based on molecular epidemiology become available. Just as important, if the host immune response is overwhelming or inappropriate, the inflammation may destroy the heart tissue acutely or lingers on and produces cardiac remodeling, leading to dilated cardiomyopathy, heart failure, or death. For the appropriate diagnosis of myocarditis, a heightened clinical suspicion is required. A composite diagnostic criterion is also evolving. Fortunately for the majority of patients, clinical myocarditis is often self-limited if proper support and follow-up are available. The role of endomyocardial biopsy has been evaluated in a recently published consensus report. Ventricular function after myocarditis may recover without residual damage, result in some degree of dysfunction, or progress rapidly to life-threatening cardiac compromise. Because of the high incidence of ultimate recovery, aggressive therapy including ventricular assist is indicated for patients with severe hemodynamic compromise. With the evolution of new understanding of pathophysiology and new therapies for this condition, the outlook for myocarditis is continuing to improve.

Definition and Incidence

Myocarditis

Myocarditis broadly refers to inflammation of the heart muscle. Inflammation can be found after any form of injury to the heart, including ischemic damage, mechanical trauma, and genetic cardiomyopathies. However, classic myocarditis refers to inflammation of the heart muscle as a result of exposure to either discrete external antigens (such as viruses, bacteria, parasites, toxins, or drugs) or internal triggers, such as autoimmune activation against self antigens.[1] The classic Dallas criteria for the pathologic diagnosis of myocarditis require the presence of inflammatory cells simultaneous with evidence of myocyte necrosis on the same microscopic section on examination of a myocardial biopsy specimen. Borderline myocarditis is characterized by inflammatory cell infiltrate without myocardial necrosis (**Fig. 70-1**).[2] However, the Dallas criteria have been criticized as too restrictive. These concerns include sampling error, intraobserver variability of interpretation, and failure of the criteria to be associated with demonstrated viral infection by molecular techniques and clinical outcomes. A broader definition including the presence of viral genome or molecular markers of immune activation has since evolved, but consensus has not yet been achieved on these additional measures.[3]

It is not surprising, then, that the precise incidence of myocarditis is difficult to ascertain, depending on inclusion and diagnostic criteria applied. One estimate has been about 8 to 10 per 100,000 population. However, because of failure to make the appropriate diagnosis or failure to detect subclinical cases, many deaths due to myocarditis may go unrecognized. Therefore, the prevalence of myocarditis among unselected autopsy series is as high as 1 to 5 per 100. Recent pathologic series examining young adults who had suffered sudden deaths suggested an even higher incidence of myocarditis around 8.6%.[4] When patients with idiopathic dilated cardiomyopathy only are considered, myocarditis accounts for 10% to 40% of the cases overall.[5] This suggests that myocarditis is not clinically suspected in a large number of cases, leading to death or severe heart failure.

Dilated Cardiomyopathy (see Chap. 68)

Cardiomyopathy with systolic dysfunction refers to disorders of the heart muscle with decreased contractility and usually increased internal diastolic dimensions of the left ventricular chamber. This generally includes cardiac dysfunction *not* associated with overt ischemic heart disease. About one third of dilated cardiomyopathy cases can be attributed to single-gene mutations involving defects of cytoskeletal proteins, such as actin, dystrophin complex, plakoglobin, or laminin. Myocarditis may also be an antecedent event leading to dilated

Supported in part by grants from the Heart and Stroke Foundation, the Canadian Institutes of Health Research; and National Heart, Lung and Blood Institute, National Institutes of Health.

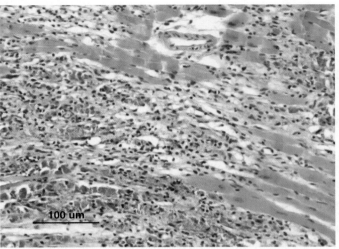

FIGURE 70-1 Myocardial biopsy section under high power (hematoxylin and eosin stain). This section is diagnostic of myocarditis by the Dallas criteria. The Dallas criteria require the presence of a lymphocyte-rich inflammatory infiltrate associated with myocyte degeneration or necrosis in the same view. However, the Dallas criteria are viewed as overly conservative, in view of the patchy nature of the inflammatory foci and less than ideal reproducibility.

cardiomyopathy, with ventricular dilation a consequence of inflammation-induced myocyte loss and interstitial fibrosis. In one pediatric series of patients with dilated cardiomyopathy, 46% of the cases could be attributed to antecedent myocarditis.[6]

In that 50% of patients with new-onset cardiomyopathy or heart failure submitted to endomyocardial biopsy who have no cause of their dysfunction identified, it is conceivable that viral myocarditis or postviral autoimmune activation may cause a large proportion of these cases. Therefore, understanding of myocarditis may allow improved diagnosis of and therapy for patients otherwise destined to the natural history of cardiomyopathy with systolic dysfunction.

Viruses such as coxsackievirus can also elaborate proteases that directly modify the cytoskeleton components, such as the dystrophin complex in the heart, leading to ventricular dilation.[7] Dilated cardiomyopathy is associated with relatively poor prognosis and is one of the most common indications for cardiac transplantation worldwide.

Acute Pericarditis (see Chap. 75)

Acute pericarditis is characterized by typical pericardial chest pain, pericardial friction rub, diffuse ST elevation by standard electrocardiography, and usually an associated pericardial effusion on transthoracic echocardiography. In approximately 15% of patients with pericarditis, myocardial involvement (myopericarditis) is diagnosed when, in addition, there is elevation of cardiac enzymes and diffuse or focal wall motion abnormalities by echocardiography. Patients may have associated supraventricular or ventricular arrhythmias and, less frequently, atrial ventricular block. Most patients respond to treatment with aspirin or nonsteroidal anti-inflammatory agents; however, approximately 15% report recurrence of pain, with or without evidence of myopericarditis. By 12 months after the acute event, virtually all patients will have resolved their symptoms and electrocardiographic and echocardiographic abnormalities. Those who fail to respond to aspirin or nonsteroidal anti-inflammatory drugs and require corticosteroids for relief of pain may have a higher rate of complications.[8]

Epidemiology

Myocarditis has been more often a diagnosis of exclusion rather than a specific diagnosis. However, the incidence of myocarditis is increasing with the advent of newer molecular diagnostic techniques in place of the absolute requirement of inflammatory cell infiltrates on myocardial biopsy. Multiple investigators evaluating heart biopsy samples in patients with clinical myocarditis or new-onset cardiomyopathy have demonstrated cardiotropic viral agents with no evidence of myocardial inflammation or myocyte destruction compatible with myocarditis as required by the Dallas criteria. Other investigators have demonstrated upregulation of immune markers in these populations, suggesting that a postviral autoimmune response is responsible.[9,10]

Meanwhile, the increasing prevalence of human immunodeficiency virus (HIV) infection with the improved survival of patients with acquired immunodeficiency syndromes (AIDS) introduced the new condition of HIV-associated myocarditis (see Chap. 72). This condition is associated with very poor prognosis and is probably related to both the HIV infection and multiple comorbidities in these patients.

CHANGING ETIOLOGY AND DIVERGENT GEOGRAPHIC DISTRIBUTION. The etiologic agents accounting for myocarditis have changed not only temporally but also geographically around the globe. Previously, the most common etiologic agents globally have been enteroviruses, with coxsackieviruses predominating. However, more recent series have indicated that the traditional dominance of coxsackieviruses has been replaced by a broader spectrum of viral causes, including adenoviruses, parvoviruses, and cytomegaloviruses. There is also an evolving distinct viral profile in different regions of the globe.

In Europe, Kuhl and colleagues' recent series of biopsies from 245 patients with dilated cardiomyopathy found that 51.4% of the biopsy samples tested positively for parvovirus B19, 21.6% for human herpesvirus 6, but only 9.4% for enterovirus and 1.6% for adenovirus.[11] Interestingly, 27.3% had evidence of multiple infections.

In contrast, Bowles and coworkers analyzed biopsy specimens from 624 patients with polymerase chain reaction (PCR) and found that overall viral positivity was 38% (or 239/624).[12] On analysis, 22.8% tested positive for adenovirus, 13.6% for enterovirus, but only 1.0% for parvovirus. This group of patients was younger, resided mainly in North America, and certainly showed a distinct viral etiologic profile (see Fig. 70-e1 on website). Meanwhile, in Japan, hepatitis C virus infection of the heart, particularly related to a hypertrophic cardiomyopathy, dominated the etiologic profile. Both hepatitis C virus antibodies and genome have been detected in the serum and myocardial biopsy specimens of patients with myocarditis.[13]

Whereas PCR has expanded our ability to identify viral pathogens, there are limitations to this technology. PCR is performed to identify specific viral pathogens predetermined by the investigator. At this time, there is no proven methodology to screen heart tissue for all viral agents. Doing so may further enhance our ability to associate cardiomyopathy with viral causes.

Globally, a common cause of dilated cardiomyopathy in the Third World is still Chagas' disease, an inflammatory myocarditis caused by the parasite *Trypanosoma cruzi*. Therefore, there are major regional differences in etiologic profile of myocarditis, showing the footprints of genetic and environmental interaction. Some of these differences may be due to the differences in the prevalence of these viruses in the local population, but others may be due to differences of definition and inclusion criteria.

Specific Etiologic Agents

Myocarditis most commonly results from an external inflammatory trigger, such as a virus, inducing host immune response, which may range from a minimally transient response to fulminant overwhelming inflammation. Characterization of the etiologic triggers has benefited significantly from molecular tools such as PCR amplification and in situ hybridization to detect external agents such as viral genome. These techniques have shown that the viral genome may persist in the myocardium for variable periods, with or without the accompaniment of an inflammatory cell infiltrate.

Recent series of molecular analysis in patients with suspected myocarditis have confirmed that indeed viruses are the most common etiologic agents associated with the condition (**Table 70-1**). Meta-analysis of PCR studies in patients who had heart biopsies with clinically suspected myocarditis or cardiomyopathy demonstrated an odds ratio of 3.8 for viral presence compared with control patients. The persistence of viral genome in the myocardium is also associated

TABLE 70-1 Etiologic Agents of Myocarditis

Viral (Most Common)
Adenovirus
Coxsackievirus, enterovirus
Cytomegalovirus
Parvovirus B19
Hepatitis C virus
Influenza virus
Human immunodeficiency virus
Herpesvirus
Epstein-Barr virus
Mixed infections

Bacterial
Mycobacterial species
Chlamydia pneumoniae
Streptococcal species
Mycoplasma pneumoniae
Treponema pallidum

Fungal
Aspergillus
Candida
Coccidioides
Cryptococcus
Histoplasma

Protozoal
Trypanosoma cruzi

Parasitic
Schistosomiasis
Larva migrans

Toxins
Anthracyclines
Cocaine

Hypersensitivity
Clozapine
Sulfonamides
Cephalosporins
Penicillins
Tricyclic antidepressants

Autoimmune Activation
Smallpox vaccination
Giant cell myocarditis
Churg-Strauss syndrome
Sjögren syndrome
Inflammatory bowel disease
Celiac disease
Sarcoidosis
Systemic lupus erythematosus
Takayasu arteritis
Wegener granulomatosis

with progressive ventricular dysfunction and worse outcome during follow-up.[11]

Viruses

ENTEROVIRUSES INCLUDING COXSACKIEVIRUSES. The most common etiologic agent of viral myocarditis has traditionally been the enteroviruses, single-stranded RNA viruses that include the coxsackieviruses and echoviruses. Because coxsackieviruses can also infect susceptible strains of mice, they are the model system on which the current understanding of the pathophysiology of viral myocarditis in humans is based.

Current evidence suggests that coxsackieviruses enter the host gastrointestinal or respiratory system by the coxsackie-adenoviral receptor (CAR), a junctional protein important for cell-cell communication and critical for internalization of the virus.[14,15] CAR localization is particularly concentrated in the cardiovascular, immune, and neurologic systems. Use of the CAR for viral entry also triggers host immune activation through its associated receptor tyrosine kinases, leading to the subsequent inflammatory response. The virus is usually cleared from the host by the immune system in 1 to 2 weeks; however, in some instances, the virus genome can persist in the host myocardium for 6 months or longer, constituting a nidus for chronic inflammatory response and a known risk factor for worse prognosis. There is also evidence to suggest that coxsackieviral infection may contribute to sudden cardiac death in those with acute coronary thrombosis.[16]

More recent series of myocarditic patients have demonstrated a decrease in the prevalence of enteroviruses as an etiologic agent, particularly in western Europe. This could be related to the development of herd immunity after a period of prolonged exposure, leading to temporary decrease in the prevalence of infections in the community.

ADENOVIRUS. Adenovirus is a DNA virus that commonly infects the human mucosal surface, particularly in the pediatric population. Adenoviruses also use the CAR (shared with coxsackievirus) as well as the integrin receptor to gain entry into cells. Adenoviral infections can be much more virulent than coxsackievirus infections and can cause extensive cell death without comparable inflammatory response. The immunologic profile associated with adenovirus is very different from that found with enterovirus, with markedly decreased CD2, CD3, and CD45RO T-lymphocyte counts in those with adenoviral genome present in the myocardium.

PARVOVIRUS. A new entry in the epidemiology of myocarditis is the parvovirus B19 family of viruses. Parvoviruses are single-stranded DNA viruses that cause common childhood infections, such as the fever and exanthem seen in pediatric populations known as fifth disease. However, in recent biopsy series from Europe, parvovirus B19 genome has been found in more than 51% of the patients with dilated cardiomyopathy.[10] Questions have been raised as to whether this is mere association, contamination, or truly causal. By autopsy myocardial analysis, even in those without cardiac dysfunction, parvovirus B19 may persist in most patients who are seropositive for this pathogen. Demonstration of immunoglobulin M parvovirus B19 antibody response may help determine those with an acute as opposed to a chronic inflammation.[17] There have been cases of myocarditis or heart failure reported after clinical fifth disease, and this can be accompanied by persistent detection of parvovirus B19 in the circulation. Patients with parvovirus myocarditis are frequently symptomatic with nonspecific chest pain, and, interestingly, parvovirus is mainly resident and trophic in the endothelial cells of the vasculature. Persistent viral infection, particularly with parvovirus B19, in patients with myocarditis has been associated with decreased flow-mediated vasodilation.[18] There is recent evidence that endothelial dysfunction from the parvovirus infection may contribute to local inflammation and vasospasm, producing the symptoms of chest pain and ventricular dysfunction.[19] This may also be consistent with the high prevalence of parvovirus infection in patients with diastolic dysfunction and myocarditis.[9]

HEPATITIS C VIRUS. In contrast to the high prevalence of parvovirus in Europe, hepatitis C virus appears to be a new etiologic agent mainly seen in Asian countries such as Japan.[13] Myocardial biopsy samples have demonstrated the hepatitis C viral genome; serum samples show confirmatory antibody rise in those patients affected. Hepatitis C infection is also overall much more prevalent in Asia than in other parts of the world and may account for the higher detection rates. The phenotype of myocarditis also appears to be different; many of the patients exhibit a hypertrophic cardiomyopathy phenotype rather than a dilated heart. This may suggest that hepatitis C directly alters the growth and hypertrophy program within the myocardium. Symptomatic myocarditis is generally observed in the first to third week of illness. Patients may have dyspnea, palpitations, and anginal chest pain; fatalities have been reported. Once the virus clears, the heart has been reported to return to normal function and morphology.

HUMAN IMMUNODEFICIENCY VIRUS. With improved survival in patients with HIV infection, the prevalence of ventricular dysfunction and associated myocarditis is also increasing (see Chap. 72). From histologic analysis of postmortem cases infected with HIV, 14 of 21 patients (67%) had criteria for myocarditis, and this increases to 83% in another study when one concentrates only on high-risk patients. In asymptomatic patients with HIV infection, the annual incidence of progression to dilated cardiomyopathy has been estimated to be around 15.9 cases per 1000 individuals. It is often impossible to determine the precise cause of the ventricular dysfunction in a given patient as it may be attributable to the HIV infection itself, immunologic dysregulation, side effects of antiretroviral treatment, opportunistic coinfection or comorbid conditions, or a combination of any of these factors.

INFLUENZA. During epidemics, 5% to 10% of infected patients may experience cardiac symptoms. The presence of pre-existing cardiovascular disease greatly increases the risk of morbidity and mortality. Cardiac involvement typically occurs within 4 days to 2 weeks of the onset of the illness. Death may be associated with massive hemorrhagic pulmonary edema due to viral or bacterial involvement of the lungs.

Mixed Viral Infections. Another interesting new finding is the detection of mixed or multiple etiologic agents from a single myocardial biopsy specimen by multiplexed molecular detection tools. It appears that multiple viruses can enhance each other's virulence in a given host by cooperating as coinfections. This may occur for both coxsackieviruses and adenoviruses as they share the same receptor CAR, which can be upregulated in the presence of cardiomyopathy.[20] Conversely, this may also be an indication that the host's immune system is incapable of clearing multiple types of viruses as a result of a likely genetic defect, which then leads to worse ventricular function and outcome.[11]

Bacteria

Virtually any bacterial agent can cause myocardial dysfunction. This occurs because of activation of inflammatory mediators (see Chap. 25) through specific interactions with toll-like receptors 2 and 4, bacterial invasion, microabscess formation, and toxins elaborated by the pathogen. Other clinical manifestations of the infection mask or delay the appreciation of myocardial involvement. Accordingly, the clinician must always be alert for cardiac involvement during systemic bacterial infections.

Clostridial Infection. Cardiac involvement is common in patients with clostridial infections with multiple organ involvement. The myocardial damage results from the toxin elaborated by the bacteria, with gas bubbles present in the myocardium. An inflammatory infiltrate is usually absent. *Clostridium perfringens* may cause myocardial abscess formation with myocardial perforation and resultant purulent pericarditis.

Diphtheria. Myocardial involvement is a serious complication of diphtheria and occurs in up to half of cases. Indeed, myocardial involvement is the most common cause of death in this infection, and half of the fatal cases demonstrate cardiac involvement. Cardiac damage is due to the liberation of a toxin that inhibits protein synthesis by interfering with the transfer of amino acids from soluble RNA to polypeptide chains under construction. The toxin appears to have a particular affinity for the cardiac conducting system. Antitoxin should be administered as rapidly as possible. Antibiotic therapy is of less urgency. The development of complete atrioventricular block is an ominous complication, and mortality is high despite insertion of a transvenous pacemaker.

Streptococcal Infection. The most commonly detected cardiac finding after beta-hemolytic streptococcal infection is acute rheumatic fever. Involvement of the heart by the streptococcus may produce a myocarditis that is distinct from acute rheumatic carditis. It is characterized by an interstitial infiltrate composed of mononuclear cells with occasional polymorphonuclear leukocytes, and the infiltrate may be focal or diffuse. Electrocardiographic abnormalities, including prolongation of the PR and QT intervals, occur frequently. Rarely, this may result in sudden death, conduction disturbances, and arrhythmias.

Tuberculosis. Involvement of the myocardium by *Mycobacterium tuberculosis* (not tuberculous pericarditis) is rare. Tuberculous involvement of the myocardium occurs by means of hematogenous or lymphatic spread or directly from contiguous structures and may cause nodular, miliary, or diffuse infiltrative disease. On occasion, it may lead to arrhythmias, including atrial fibrillation and ventricular tachycardia, complete atrioventricular block, heart failure, left ventricular aneurysms, and sudden death.

Whipple Disease. Although overt involvement is rare, intestinal lipodystrophy, or Whipple disease, is not uncommonly associated with cardiac involvement, and periodic acid–Schiff–positive macrophages can be found in the myocardium, pericardium, coronary arteries, and heart valves of patients with this disorder. Electron microscopy has demonstrated rod-shaped structures in the myocardium similar to those found in the small intestine, representing the causative agent of the disease, *Tropheryma whipplei*, a gram-negative bacillus related to the actinomycetes. There may be an associated inflammatory infiltrate and foci of fibrosis. The valvular fibrosis may be severe enough to result in aortic regurgitation and mitral stenosis. Although it is usually asymptomatic, nonspecific electrocardiographic changes are most common; systolic murmurs, pericarditis, complete heart block, and even overt congestive heart failure may occur. Antibiotic therapy appears to be effective in treatment of the basic disease, but relapses can occur, often more than 2 years after initial diagnosis.

Spirochetal Infections: Lyme Carditis. Lyme disease is caused by a tick-borne spirochete *(Borrelia burgdorferi)*. It usually begins during the summer months with a characteristic rash (erythema chronicum migrans), followed by acute neurologic, joint, or cardiac involvement and usually few long-term sequelae.[21] About 10% of patients with Lyme disease develop evidence of transient cardiac involvement, the most common manifestation being variable degrees of atrioventricular block. Syncope due to complete heart block is frequent with cardiac involvement because often there is an associated depression of ventricular escape rhythms. Diffuse ST-segment and T wave abnormalities are transient and usually asymptomatic. An abnormal gallium scan is compatible with cardiac involvement, and the demonstration of spirochetes in myocardial biopsy specimens of patients with Lyme carditis suggests a direct cardiac effect. Patients with second-degree or complete heart block should be hospitalized and undergo continuous electrocardiographic monitoring. Temporary transvenous pacing may be required for a week or longer in patients with high-grade block. Although the efficacy of antibiotics is not established, they are used routinely in patients with Lyme carditis. Intravenous antibiotics are suggested, although oral antibiotics can be used when there is only mild cardiac involvement. Corticosteroids may reduce myocardial inflammation and edema, which in turn can shorten the duration of heart block. It is thought that treatment of the early manifestations of the disease will prevent development of late complications.

Protozoal Infections

CHAGAS' DISEASE (see Chap. 71). Chagas' disease is still one of the most common causes of dilated cardiomyopathy worldwide. The World Health Organization estimates that currently there are 18 million infected cases worldwide, and 5 million will develop symptomatic disease.[22] The causative organism is the protozoan *Trypanosoma cruzi*, spread by arthropods as the vector in endemic regions in the world, most notably in South America. Organs other than the heart may also be involved. The parasite incites an intense acquired T lymphocyte–mediated inflammatory response in the host, akin to viral myocarditis, leading to extensive scarring and remodeling of the myocardium, resulting in chagasic cardiomyopathy. Treatment is most effective during the acute phase of the disease. Ultimately, prevention through public health measures will be most cost-effective.

Metazoal Myocardial Diseases

Echinococcosis (Hydatid Cyst). Echinococcosis is endemic in many sheep-raising areas of the world, particularly Argentina, New Zealand, Greece, North Africa, and Iceland; however, cardiac involvement in patients with hydatid disease is uncommon (<2%). The usual host of *Echinococcus granulosus* is the dog, but humans may serve as intermediate hosts if they accidentally ingest ova from contaminated dog feces. When cardiac involvement is present, the cysts usually are intramyocardial in the interventricular septum or left ventricular free wall. A myocardial cyst can degenerate and calcify, develop daughter cysts, or rupture. Rupture of the cyst is the most dreaded complication; rupture into the pericardium can result in acute pericarditis, which may progress to chronic constrictive pericarditis. Rupture into the cardiac chambers can result in systemic or pulmonary emboli. Rapidly progressive pulmonary hypertension can occur with rupture of right-sided cysts, with subsequent embolization of hundreds of scolices into the pulmonary circulation. The liberation of hydatid fluid into the circulation can produce profound, fatal circulatory collapse due to an anaphylactic reaction to the protein constituents of the fluid. It is estimated that only about 10% of patients with cardiac hydatid cysts have clinical symptoms. The electrocardiogram may reflect the location of the cyst. Chest pain is usually due to rupture of the cyst into the pericardial space with resultant pericarditis. Large cystic masses sometimes produce right-sided obstruction. The chest radiograph may show an abnormal cardiac silhouette or a calcified lobular mass adjacent to the left ventricle. Two-dimensional echocardiography, computed tomography, or magnetic resonance imaging may aid in the detection and localization of heart cysts. Eosinophilia, when present, is a useful adjunctive finding. The Casoni skin test, or serologic evaluations for echinococcus, have a limited role in cardiac diagnosis. In terms of therapy, despite the availability of effective drugs such as mebendazole and albendazole, surgical excision is generally recommended, even for asymptomatic patients. This is because of the significant risk of rupture of the cyst and its attendant serious and sometimes fatal consequences.

Trichinosis. Infestation with *Trichinella spiralis* is common, but clinically detectable cardiac involvement occurs in only a minority of patients. Symptomatic involvement is uncommon and may be responsible for the fatalities. Less frequently, death is due to pulmonary embolism secondary to venous thrombosis or neurologic complications. Although the parasite can invade the heart, it does not usually encyst there, and it is rare to find larvae or larval fragments in the myocardium. The heart may be dilated and flabby, and a pericardial effusion may be present. A prominent focal infiltrate composed of lymphocytes and eosinophils can be found, with occasional microthrombi in the intramural arterioles. Areas of muscle degeneration and necrosis are present. The clinical myocarditis in trichinosis is usually mild and goes unnoticed, but in occasional cases it is manifested by heart failure and chest pain, usually appearing around the third week of the disease. Electrocardiographic abnormalities are detected in about 10% of patients with trichinosis and parallel the time course of clinical cardiac involvement, initially appearing in the second or third week and usually resolving by the seventh week of the illness. The most common electrocardiographic abnormalities are repolarization abnormalities and ventricular premature complexes. The diagnosis is usually based on the demonstration of indirect immunofluorescent antibody in a patient with the clinical features of trichinosis. Eosinophilia, when present, is a supportive finding. The skin test result is usually but not invariably positive. Treatment is with anthelmintics and corticosteroids; dramatic improvement in cardiac function has been reported after their use.

Hypersensitivity Reactions: Vaccines and Drugs

Drug-induced hypersensitivity syndrome may involve the heart and be associated with myocarditis. The syndrome usually occurs within 8 weeks of the initiation of a new drug but can occur at any time after drug consumption. Common agents include antiepileptics, antimicrobials, allopurinol, and sulfa-based drugs. Dobutamine, often used as hemodynamic support in patients with failing hearts, may be associated with eosinophilic myocarditis, and the drug should be stopped when eosinophilia appears or there is an unexpected decline in left ventricular function. Presenting characteristics usually include a rash (unless the patient is immunologically compromised), fever, and multiorgan dysfunction (including hepatitis, nephritis, and myocarditis). Diffuse myocardial involvement may result in systemic hypotension and thromboembolic events. Magnetic resonance imaging and cardiac biomarkers may help identify patients with cardiac involvement. Endomyocardial biopsy may demonstrate eosinophils, histiocytes, lymphocytes, myocardial necrosis, and occasionally granuloma and vasculitis. Myocardial involvement is patchy and therefore definitively diagnosed only when the biopsy finding is positive. Corticosteroids and drug withdrawal usually resolve this syndrome; however, some patients may display a prolonged and relapsing course (see Chap. 70 Online Supplement for further details about physical agents).[23]

Physical Agents

A wide variety of substances other than infectious agents can act on the heart and damage the myocardium. In some cases, the damage is acute, transient, and associated with evidence of an inflammatory myocardial infiltrate with myocyte necrosis (e.g., with the arsenicals and lithium). Other agents that damage the myocardium can lead to chronic changes with resulting histologic evidence of fibrosis and a clinical picture of a dilated or restrictive cardiomyopathy. Numerous chemicals and drugs (both industrial and therapeutic) can lead to cardiac damage and

dysfunction. Several physical agents (e.g., radiation and excessive heat) can also contribute directly to myocardial damage (see Chap. 70 Online Supplement for further details about physical agents).

Pathophysiology

Our current understanding of the pathogenesis of viral myocarditis is derived mostly from enteroviral models of myocarditis in the mouse, and the principles have been generalized to other types of myocarditis.[1,24] The disease represents a delicate interaction between the virus and the host. Myocarditis can be considered to have three phases in its pathophysiology (**Fig. 70-2**). The first is the viral phase, followed by the immunologic response phase (including innate and acquired immunity components), followed by the cardiac remodeling phase (**Fig. 70-3**).

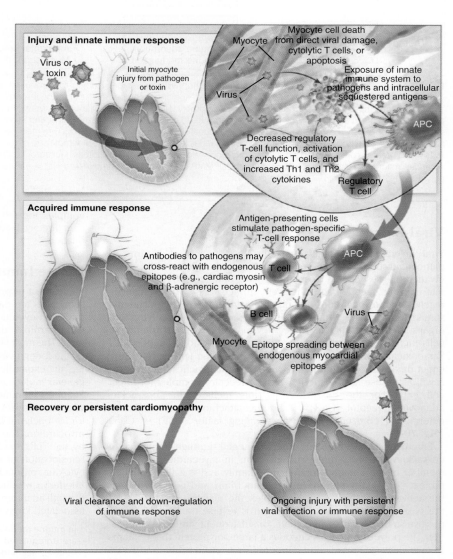

FIGURE 70-2 Pathogenesis of myocarditis. The current understanding of the cellular and molecular pathogenesis of postviral and autoimmune myocarditis is based solely on animal models. In these models, the progression from acute injury to chronic dilated cardiomyopathy may be simplified into a three-stage process. Acute injury leads to cardiac damage, exposure of intracellular antigens such as cardiac myosin, and activation of the innate immune system. During weeks, specific immunity that is mediated by T lymphocytes and antibodies directed against pathogens and similar endogenous heart epitopes causes robust inflammation. In most patients, the pathogen is cleared and the immune reaction is downregulated with few sequelae. However, in other patients, the virus is not cleared and causes persistent myocyte damage, and heart-specific inflammation may persist because of mistaken recognition of endogenous heart antigens as pathogenic entities. APC = antigen-presenting cell. *(From Cooper LT Jr: Myocarditis. N Engl J Med 360:1526, 2009. Copyright © 2009 Massachusetts Medical Society. All rights reserved.)*

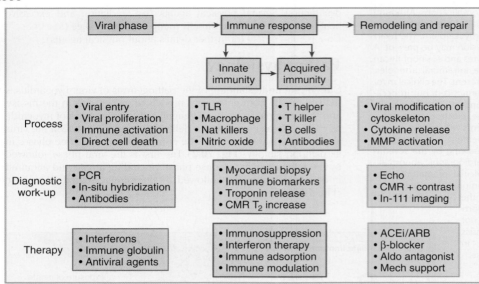

FIGURE 70-3 Conceptual framework of the three pathophysiologic stages leading to chronic myocarditis, including viral phase, immune response phase, and remodeling and repair phase. The immune response can be subdivided into the innate and acquired immune responses, with significant collaboration between the two processes. Both the viral and immune processes contribute to cell death, cardiac remodeling, and inflammatory response by the host. The therapeutic efficacy unfortunately has not been as well documented because of heterogeneity of the population, high rates of spontaneous improvement, and small sample size of the studies. ACEi = angiotensin-converting enzyme inhibitors; Aldo = aldosterone; ARB = angiotensin receptor blocker; CMR = cardiac magnetic resonance; Mech = mechanical; MMP = matrix metalloproteinases; Nat = natural; PCR = polymerase chain reaction; TLR = toll-like receptors.

Viral Entry

Viral myocarditis is initiated by the introduction of a virus of pathogenic strain (e.g., enterovirus such as coxsackievirus B3), which invades the susceptible host through a portal of entry by a virus internalizing receptor on the cell surface. The virus ultimately reaches the myocardium through hematogenous or lymphangitic spread. Many of the viruses are initially processed in the lymphoid organs, such as the spleen, where the virus will proliferate in immune cells themselves, including macrophages and T and B lymphocytes. Paradoxically, through host immune activation, the viruses reach the target organs, such as the heart. Once the virus reaches the myocyte, it will again use its specific receptor or receptor complex for target cell entry. For the coxsackievirus, this includes the coxsackie-adenoviral receptor (CAR)[14,20] and the attachment and virulence-determining coreceptor decay-accelerating factor (DAF) or CD55 (**Fig. 70-4**).

Enteroviruses use the CAR complex, hence the high frequency of coxsackievirus and adenovirus infection in myocarditis. CAR is a member of the immunoglobulin superfamily and is a tight junction protein particularly present in the heart, brain, and gut.[14,24] Through the activation of this receptor complex, the negative strand RNA of the coxsackievirus enters the cell and is reverse transcribed into a positive strand to act as a template for subsequent viral RNA duplication. The polycistronic RNA encodes a large polyprotein that contains its own cleavage enzyme and important viral capsid subunits VP1-VP4. Exuberant viral replication in a susceptible host lacking suitable immunity defenses can cause acute myocardial damage and early death of the host.

Entry of the virus through the receptor also activates its signaling system, including tyrosine kinase p56lck, Fyn, and Abl.[14,15] Activation of these signals modifies the host cell cytoskeleton to permit more viral entry. At the same time, these signals also mediate the activation of T cells, which are critically dependent on p56lck and Fyn. Interestingly, heart tissue damage and inflammation upregulate the CAR receptor and increase the susceptibility of the host to coxsackieviral infection.[20]

Immune Activation and Viral Persistence (see Fig. 70-2)

Whereas viral entry triggers the immune activation, the immune system has a dual role. On one hand, it is activated to eliminate as many virus-infected cells as possible to control the infection. On the other hand, the response needs to be modulated by negative controls; otherwise, there will be excessive tissue damage from the inflammatory response with organ dysfunction. The virus has an elaborate system in place to escape host immunologic surveillance, including molecular mimicry, proliferation in immunocytes, and upregulation of its own receptors, and it can persist in the myocyte for months to years.

Viral persistence can expose the host to persistent antigenic trigger and chronic immune activation and the potential of chronic myocarditis. Persistence of the viral genome, such as coxsackievirus in the myocyte, has been directly linked to the development of dilated cardiomyopathy through cytoskeleton remodeling. Knowlton and colleagues have identified that the enteroviral protease 2A can directly cleave the dystrophin-sarcoglycan complex located at the myocyte–extracellular matrix junction.[7] This can directly lead to myocyte remodeling and subsequent cardiac dilation.[24]

Innate Immunity (see Fig. 70-2)

The earliest responses of the host to the presence of foreign genome sequences are members of the innate immune system. Innate immunity is an evolutionarily ancient host protective system that provides early warnings for the cells to deal with an adverse external environment. The most common pathway for innate immunity to be triggered by the foreign virus is the ubiquitous toll-like receptors (TLRs), which are an expanding family of cell surface receptors that recognize general molecular patterns without the high specificity conferred by acquired immune players, such as T and B cells. For example, TLR3, which recognizes double-stranded RNA, and TLR4, which is the receptor for bacterial lipopolysaccharide, are present in abundance in the myocardium. The presence of foreign genetic material can be detected by the TLRs, leading to signaling activation that ultimately leads to translocation of transcription factors such as NF-κB, with amplified cytokine production, and interferon regulatory factors, leading to interferon production (see Fig. 70-4). The activation of TLRs signals through adaptors and kinases such as MyD88 and interleukin receptor–associated kinases (IRAKs).

In murine models of myocarditis, many components of innate immunity are upregulated immediately on viral exposure, including MyD88 and IRAK-4,[25] leading to NF-κB activation. In turn, the activation of NF-κB appears to be modulated by the interferon production pathways, including interferon regulatory factors such as IRF3.[24,25] Downregulation of MyD88 and in turn of NF-κB and activation of acquired immunity are accompanied by the upregulation of type I interferons (IFN-α and IFN-β). Interferon is critical for host protection and survival, and its absence leads to excessive viral proliferation and direct cardiac damage.[26] Type I interferon thus may have an ideal dual role of control of viral proliferation and downregulation of acquired immune pathways of T-cell activation and clonal expansion. Besides these positive regulators of host defense responses, there are also systems of negative modulators that will counteract the excessive cytokine activation. One system, the intracellular suppressors of cytokine signaling (SOCS), negatively regulates innate immune response.[27] The SOCS system particularly downregulates cytokine signals going through the gp130 receptor on the myocytes. Normal signals through the gp130 receptor serve to stabilize the dystrophin complex and confer protection for the host. This appears to be a SOCS3-dependent phenomenon, as cardiac-restricted overexpression of SOCS3 in a transgenic model led to gp130 instability and worse outcome.

Acquired Immunity

Acquired immunity refers to the ability of the immune system to recognize and to respond specifically to a single viral or tissue antigen through T and B cells that recognize very specific peptide sequences. This system is triggered by the recognition of a precise "foreign" molecular pattern by the variable region of the T-cell receptor. The T cell is then stimulated to clonally expand to attack the source of "antigen," which could be from the viral coat protein or sometimes from parts of the myocardium (such as myosin), which may resemble the pattern of the virus (molecular mimicry), triggering autoimmunity. However, this process is very much dependent on costimulation from inflammatory signals, often linked to innate immunity signaling activated earlier in the injury process.

The result of acquired immune activation is the production of T killer cells that can directly attack the virus and virally infected cells. The activation of T cells also leads to B-cell activation and the production of specific antibodies to neutralize the antigen. This results in subacute and chronic inflammation observed in myocarditis and contributes to the subsequent myocyte necrosis, fibrosis, and remodeling. The critical contributory role of the signals through the acquired immune pathways has been examined in mouse models of myocarditis. A common downstream signaling pathway from the T-cell receptor is the tyrosine kinase p56lck. Interestingly, p56lck is the same tyrosine kinase signal attached to the CAR-DAF receptor complex for viral entry. When p56lck is genetically removed from the mouse by transgenic knockout techniques, the mouse is no longer susceptible to the inflammation seen in typical myocarditis, and the mortality is almost completely eliminated.[15] T cells, when present, will attempt to seek out the infected cells and destroy them by mechanisms such as cytokine-mediated signaling[28] or perforin-mediated cell death. This confirms that the T-cell receptor activation sequence ultimately does lead to the detrimental phenotype of the disease and supports the concept that decreasing inflammation from acquired immunity, while finding ways to control the virus through innate immunity, will lead to the most beneficial outcomes of the disease.

A more recently recognized counterregulatory system in acquired immunity is the small population of T-regulatory cells (or Tregs). These cells also derive from part of the T-cell activation process but are present in small numbers to act as a counterbalancing population to T killer cells. This population of cells were known earlier as T helper CD4+ cells. Currently, Tregs are more precisely defined as

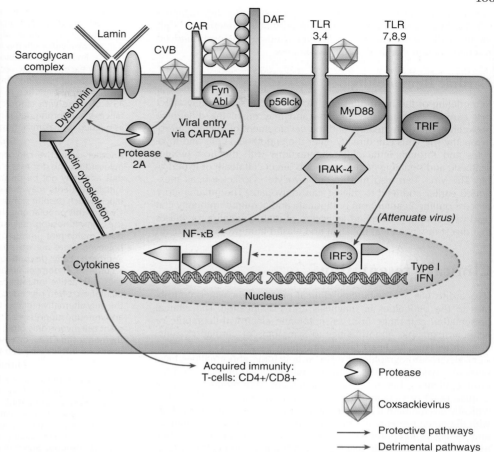

FIGURE 70-4 The pathogenesis of viral myocarditis, such as that caused by coxsackievirus. The virus enters the cell membrane through internalization receptors of coxsackie-adenoviral receptor (CAR), which in turn can trigger receptor-associated kinases such as p56lck, Fyn, and Abl to alter host myocyte cytoskeleton to facilitate viral entry. Viruses such as the coxsackievirus (CVB) can directly produce enzymes such as protease 2A that can disassemble the important cytoskeletal components such as dystrophin-sarcoglycan complex, leading to myocyte remodeling and destruction. Engagement of the receptor also activates tyrosine kinases, which are important for T-cell clonal expansion and linking between the innate and the acquired immune systems. The virus also activates innate immunity by engaging toll-like receptors (TLR) through adaptors such as MyD88 and TRIF. Activation and translocation of NF-κB, on the one hand, will produce cytokines and trigger acquired immunity such as CD4/CD8 T-cell mobilization. On the other hand, this can be attenuated by the activation of IRF3 and type I interferon (IFN) production. The latter may be protective through multiple mechanisms, including attenuation of the virus. DAF = decay-accelerating factor, CVB coreceptor; IRAK = interleukin receptor–associated kinase, a signaling protein in innate immune pathway; IRF = interferon regulatory factor.

CD4+CD25+Foxp3+ T cells. Enhanced levels of Tregs in models of myocarditis appear to be protective by reducing inflammatory cytokine response and inducing tolerance to self antigens. Therefore, Tregs may one day have a therapeutic potential in viral myocarditis.

To understand why certain individuals develop overwhelming myocarditis after exposure to the virus and rapidly die of the disease and others do not even show inflammation, we have been methodically mapping the major determinants of the host immune system by molecular targeting strategies in knockout mice. Earlier work identified that components of innate immunity, such as interferon and IRF3, are critical for host survival, yet T-cell signaling and activation are injurious to the host. Through CD4−/CD8− knockout mice, we have established that both CD4 and CD8 T cells contribute to the host autoimmune inflammatory disease, accompanied by a shift of cytokine profile from Th1 to Th2 response. More recently, we have identified that p56lck triggers downstream ERK activation in the host target cell and appears to be critical for the determinant of host susceptibility.[28] To validate these observations, we have also investigated the function of the associated tyrosine phosphatase CD45 linked in function to the p56lck kinase and confirmed that CD45−/− animals are also resistant to viral myocarditis. After careful dissection, it was apparent that CD45 is an important Src as well as JAK/STAT phosphatase, and virally triggered CD45 activation shuts down interferon production. Interferon levels are markedly increased once CD45 is removed, and the host is indeed rescued through this dual protective process.

Cardiac Remodeling (see Chap. 25)

Remodeling of the heart after cardiac injury can significantly affect that cardiac structure and function and may mean the difference between appropriate healing and the development of dilated cardiomyopathy. The virus can directly enter the endothelial cells and myocytes and through intracellular interactions with the host protein synthetic and signaling pathways lead to direct cell death or hypertrophy. The virus can also modify the myocyte cytoskeleton, as mentioned earlier, and lead to dilated cardiomyopathy. The inflammatory process outlined earlier from both innate and acquired immunity can lead to cytokine release and activation of matrix metalloproteinases that digest the interstitial collagen and elastin framework of the heart (see Chap. 25).

Clinical Presentation

Myocarditis has a wide-ranging clinical presentation, which contributes to the difficulties in diagnosis and classification. The clinical presentation can range from asymptomatic electrocardiographic or echocardiographic abnormalities to symptoms of cardiac dysfunction, arrhythmias or heart failure, and hemodynamic collapse. Transient electrocardiographic or echocardiographic abnormalities have been observed frequently during community viral outbreaks or influenza epidemics, but most patients remain asymptomatic from a cardiac point of view and have few long-term sequelae. Myocarditis typically has a bimodal distribution in terms of age in the population, with the acute presentation more commonly seen in young children and teenagers. In contrast, the presenting symptoms are more subtle and insidious, often with dilated cardiomyopathy and heart failure, in the older adult population. Felker and colleagues have observed earlier in consecutive cases of new-onset dilated cardiomyopathy in adults that 9% to 16% have classic myocarditis on biopsy by the Dallas criteria.[29] The difference in presentation is probably related to the maturity of the immune system, whereby the young tend to have an exuberant response to the initial exposure of a provocative antigen. On the other hand, the older individual would have developed a greater degree of tolerance and show a chronic inflammatory response only to the chronic presence of a foreign antigen or a dysregulated immune system that predisposes to autoimmunity.

Acute Myocarditis

Classically, patients with myocarditis present with nonspecific symptoms related to the heart. In a recent series of 245 patients with clinically suspected myocarditis, the most common symptoms included fatigue (82%), dyspnea on exertion (81%), arrhythmias (55%, both supraventricular and ventricular), palpitations (49%), and chest pain at rest (26%).[10] These can be difficult to distinguish from acute ischemic syndromes because they result in release of troponin, ST-segment elevation on electrocardiography, and segmental wall motion abnormalities on echocardiography. Therefore, the symptoms can be quite nonspecific, although some symptoms indicate cardiac involvement. The viral prodrome of fever, chills, myalgias, and constitutional symptoms occurs in between 20% and 80% of the cases, can be readily missed by the patient, and thus cannot be relied on for diagnosis.

Many cases of myocarditis present with de novo onset of heart failure, particularly when the patient is middle aged or older. When the health care team fails to identify other causes of heart failure, viral myocarditis along with idiopathic dilated cardiomyopathy becomes the diagnosis of exclusion. To distinguish myocarditis from idiopathic dilated cardiomyopathy, almost one third of the cases of viral myocarditis will recover to normal cardiac function with appropriate supportive therapy, which is less frequent in genetic dilated cardiomyopathy.

Fulminant Myocarditis

Approximately 10% of patients with biopsy-proven myocarditis display fulminant myocarditis. This entity is characterized by an abrupt onset, usually within 2 weeks of a viral illness. Patients have hemodynamic compromise and hypotension, often requiring pressors or mechanical support. The echocardiogram reveals diffuse global hypofunction, rarely cardiac dilation, and typically thickening of the ventricular wall probably due to myocardial edema from myocardial inflammation and cytokine release. Endomyocardial biopsy reveals typical and diffuse myocarditis in virtually each histologic section, making endomyocardial biopsy confirmation straightforward. On follow-up, 93% of the original cohort were alive and transplant free 11 years after initial biopsy, compared with only 45% of those with chronic myocarditis.[30] This underscores the importance of supporting patients with fulminant myocarditis as aggressively as needed to maximize time for recovery.

Giant Cell Myocarditis

Another distinctive clinicopathologic form of myocarditis is giant cell myocarditis. This disorder is more subtle in onset than fulminant myocarditis and may not be distinguishable from other forms of myocarditis initially. Patients may present with heart failure, arrhythmia, or heart block, which despite standard medical therapy fails to improve. The survival for this population is less than 6 months and is improved with the use of immunosuppressive therapy.[31] Preliminary data suggest that high-dose multiagent immunosuppression may improve the prognosis; however, there are no prospective randomized trials to confirm this approach. Early discontinuation of immunosuppression may lead to recurrence. Endomyocardial biopsy reveals a distinctive pattern of giant cells with active inflammation and scar tissue. Currently, cardiac transplantation, often preceded by mechanical circulatory support, remains the only alternative for most patients with this disorder. Early recognition and immunosuppressive therapy may alter this approach. Patients with giant cell myocarditis often have other autoimmune disorders including thymoma and Crohn disease. The pathophysiologic mechanism remains unknown but is suspected to be autoimmune in nature.

Chronic Active Myocarditis

This group represents most older adult patients with myocarditis, and the onset is often insidious and difficult to pinpoint. The patient presents with symptoms compatible with moderate ventricular dysfunction, such as fatigue and dyspnea. Pathologic examination of a myocardial biopsy specimen may show active myocarditis, but more frequently it is only borderline or generalized chronic myopathic changes with fibrosis and myocyte dropout. Some may progress to diastolic dysfunction with predominantly fibrosis, resembling ultimately a restrictive cardiomyopathy.

This category encompasses 60% to 70% of patients with active or borderline myocarditis who present with dilated cardiomyopathy of unknown etiology. Use of newer imaging approaches such as magnetic resonance imaging with gadolinium enhancement and positron emission tomography–computed tomography (PET-CT), molecular diagnosis by immunohistopathologic analysis, assessment of upregulation of immune markers, and molecular testing, including PCR and in situ hybridization, may expand this population significantly.

Eosinophilic Myocarditis

The eosinophil may be associated with myocardial inflammation in three distinct forms of myocardial inflammation. Allergic eosinophilic myocarditis is caused by a hypersensitivity reaction to a foreign antigen, almost always a drug. This form of myocarditis requires a high degree of suspicion (related to the initiation of new agents) and subtle declines in left ventricular function. Withdrawal of the offending agent and administration of corticosteroids usually result in resolution. The heart may be inflamed in association with systemic eosinophilic disorders, resulting in myocardial, endocardial, and valvular involvement (Löffler endocarditis). The outcome is dependent on control of the underlying condition. Finally, fulminant necrotic myocarditis presents in a fashion similar to fulminant myocarditis, has no clear etiology, and requires aggressive medical immunosuppression and occasional mechanical support.

Peripartum Cardiomyopathy

Peripartum cardiomyopathy is characterized by the onset of left ventricular dysfunction in the last month of pregnancy or within 5 months of delivery, with no pre-existing cardiac dysfunction and no recognized cause of the cardiomyopathy. There is evidence that patients submitted to endomyocardial biopsy early after presentation have a high frequency of myocarditis.[29] As most patients with this disorder recover with standard therapy, biopsy is recommended only for those with persistent left ventricular dysfunction and symptoms despite heart failure management.

Diagnostic Approaches

The diagnosis of myocarditis has traditionally required a histologic diagnosis according to the classic Dallas criteria.[2] However, because

TABLE 70-2	Expanded Criteria for Diagnosis of Myocarditis
Suggestive of myocarditis:	2 positive categories
Compatible with myocarditis:	3 positive categories
High probability of being myocarditis:	all 4 categories positive

(Any matching feature in category = positive for category)

Category I: Clinical Symptoms
Clinical heart failure
Fever
Viral prodrome
Fatigue
Dyspnea on exertion
Chest pain
Palpitations
Presyncope or syncope

Category II: Evidence of Cardiac Structural or Functional Perturbation *in the absence* of Regional Coronary Ischemia
Echocardiography evidence
    Regional wall motion abnormalities
    Cardiac dilation
    Regional cardiac hypertrophy
Troponin release
    High sensitivity (>0.1 ng/mL)
Positive indium In 111 antimyosin scintigraphy
and
Normal coronary angiography *or*
Absence of reversible ischemia by coronary distribution on perfusion scan

Category III: Cardiac Magnetic Resonance Imaging
Increased myocardial T2 signal on inversion recovery sequence
Delayed contrast enhancement after gadolinium-DTPA infusion

Category IV: Myocardial biopsy—Pathologic or Molecular Analysis
Pathology findings compatible with Dallas criteria
Presence of viral genome by polymerase chain reaction or in situ hybridization

DTPA = diethylenetriamine penta-acetic acid.

TABLE 70-3	Comparison of Efficacy of Various Diagnostic Modalities for Myocarditis		
DIAGNOSTIC MODALITY		**SENSITIVITY RANGE (%)**	**SPECIFICITY RANGE (%)**
Electrocardiographic changes (AV block; Q wave, ST changes)		47	?
Troponin (lower threshold of >0.1 ng/mL)		34-53	89-94
Creatine kinase MB isoform		6	?
Antibodies to virus or myosin		25-32	40
Indium 111 antimyosin scintigraphy		85-91	34-53
Echocardiography (ventricular dysfunction)		69	?
Cardiac magnetic resonance		86	95
Myocardial biopsy (Dallas criteria of pathology)		35-50	78-89
Myocardial biopsy (viral genome by PCR)		38-65	80-100

? = indeterminate or poor; AV = atrioventricular; PCR = polymerase chain reaction.

of low sensitivity due to the patchy nature of the inflammatory infiltrates in the myocardium and the reluctance of clinicians to perform an invasive diagnostic procedure, myocarditis is severely underdiagnosed. Because the incidence of the disease is likely to be much higher than is appreciated, a high level of clinical suspicion, together with hybrid clinical and laboratory criteria and new imaging modalities, may help secure the diagnosis without necessarily resorting to biopsy in all cases.

With the advent of a number of new diagnostic strategies for myocarditis, one may now *strongly suspect myocarditis* if two of the following criteria are present, and the diagnosis is *highly probable as myocarditis* if three or more criteria are present: (1) compatible clinical symptoms; (2) evidence of cardiac structural or functional defect or myocardial damage in the absence of active regional coronary ischemia; (3) regional delayed contrast enhancement or increased T2 signal on cardiac magnetic resonance imaging; and (4) presence of inflammatory cell infiltrate or positive viral genome signals on myocardial biopsy or pathologic examination (**Table 70-2**). Of course, myocardial biopsy still provides the most specific diagnosis for myocarditis.

For example, myocarditis as a diagnosis should be suspected when a young patient presents with unexplained symptoms of heart failure or chest pain but the coronary arteries are found to be normal on angiography. When young patients such as this present with minimal risk factors for coronary disease with acute chest pain or ischemic electrocardiographic abnormalities, 32% will have biopsy evidence of acute myocarditis according to the Dallas criteria. An even higher proportion will also be viral genome positive on molecular analysis. A major limitation to the accurate diagnosis of myocarditis is the lack of a highly sensitive and specific tool that is noninvasive and widely applicable. The common diagnostic modalities and their reported sensitivities and specificities are outlined in **Table 70-3**.

Clinical Symptoms

The clinical symptoms of myocarditis are not specific and very much depend on the mode of presentation as outlined before. Younger patients most often complain of chest pain and fatigue. Patient with cardiac dysfunction may present with new-onset heart failure, dyspnea, or fatigue. Some patients are also symptomatic of the supraventricular or ventricular arrhythmias, including palpitations, presyncope, and syncope. In most severe cases, such as those with fulminant myocarditis, patients may present with cardiogenic shock and intractable arrhythmias. Some patients may present with constitutional symptoms, such as fever and viral prodrome. However, these are infrequent and unreliable for diagnosis.

Laboratory Testing

Severe myocarditis will lead to myocardial damage secondary to the presence of inflammatory cell infiltrates and cytokine activation as well as some contribution directly from virus-mediated cell death. These processes can severely depress cardiac function and produce evidence of cardiac damage. This can be detected as leakage of cardiac enzymes such as creatine kinase and troponin when the damage is severe or chronic (see Table 70-2). However, in most cases, the leakage of enzymes is relatively minor, and standard laboratory testing for creatine kinase or its isoform MB is too insensitive (overall sensitivity for myocarditis is only 8%). Enzyme biomarkers such as troponin are more useful when high sensitivity thresholds are used. For example, when a serum troponin T threshold of >0.1 ng/mL is used as a cutoff, the sensitivity can be increased from 34% to 53% without compromising specificity. Similar findings have been noted for troponin I. Other biomarkers, such as cytokines, complement, and antiviral or anti–heart antibodies, are either too insensitive or inadequately standardized to make them generally useful clinically.

The cardiac damage can also be manifested as electrocardiographic abnormalities (see Chap. 13) that range from T wave inversions to frank ST-segment elevation and bundle branch block, depending on the region and extent of inflammatory damage. Kuhl and associates have noted that arrhythmias may be present in 55% of the patients, including both supraventricular and ventricular arrhythmias.

Imaging techniques such as two-dimensional echocardiography (see Chap. 15) are useful for initial diagnostic evaluation of the patient to detect the regional ventricular dysfunction that often accompanies the condition. Parameters of ventricular remodeling, including chamber dilation, regional hypertrophy, and regional wall motion abnormalities, are often seen with myocarditis, but these changes may be indistinguishable from those of myocardial ischemia or infarction at the outset. The absence of matching regional coronary disease and evidence of rapid recovery of ventricular dysfunction during follow-up are general clues to the diagnosis of myocarditis. Retrospective analysis of echocardiograms from 42 patients with biopsy-proven myocarditis identified ventricular dysfunction in 69% of the patients, but the presence of cardiac dilation is much more variable. Newer techniques such as tissue characterization and tissue Doppler imaging may permit better diagnostic accuracy in the future. Additional validation studies will be needed to determine their ultimate clinical role. However, echocardiography is certainly useful as a follow-up imaging modality to monitor the natural history of the patient's ventricular function or response to treatment. Two-dimensional echocardiography may also help distinguish fulminant from more classic forms of myocarditis; fulminant myocarditis shows less diastolic dimensional increase but increased septal thickness, whereas the more classic forms of myocarditis show a much greater degree of ventricular dilation.

Newer imaging techniques, such as PET-CT, may reveal inflammation of the myocardium and associated mediastinal and thoracic structures. This technique is particularly beneficial in conditions such as sarcoidosis.

Cardiac Magnetic Resonance Imaging

(see Chap. 18)

A new approach to the diagnosis of myocarditis is cardiac magnetic resonance (CMR). CMR imaging is attractive for the detection of myocarditis because of its ability to characterize tissue according to water content and changes in contrast kinetics. CMR also allows visualization of the entire myocardium and is thus well suited to detect the local patchy nature of the myocarditic lesions.[32] The local inflammatory process in myocarditis leads to cytokine release and mobilization of inflammatory cells to the infected foci. This in turn produces local changes in membrane permeability, tissue edema, and ultimately tissue fibrosis. These changes directly affect the T2 relaxation parameters of the tissues, which are dependent on water content. Furthermore, extracellular contrast agents such as gadolinium-DTPA will also distribute and clear very differently in inflamed or scarred tissue compared with normal tissue, leading to changes in T1 relaxation and thus contrast changes or delayed enhancement on T1 weighted images (**Fig. 70-5**; see Fig. 18-12).

Evaluation of the relative accuracy of the CMR technique in the detection of myocarditis has demonstrated the relative merit of using a T2-weighted imaging strategy, such as the inversion recovery sequence. This approach to detection of myocarditic lesions showed a sensitivity of 84% and specificity of 74% based on biopsy or natural history evidence of myocarditis.[33] The addition of the T2-weighted imaging to the more commonly used gadolinium-DTPA–based extracellular T1-altering contrast agent and the inclusion of local delayed enhancement further increased the diagnostic accuracy to more than 90% by collation of all of the current studies.[32] The delayed contrast enhancement phenomenon is often associated with recent cardiac necrosis or healing of the myocardium after myocardial infarction; but in the setting of myocarditis, it also further increases the sensitivity and specificity of diagnosis. The mechanism is not clear but may be related to the deposition of local collagen bundles during the healing process that can also temporarily bind the gadolinium-DTPA to delay its clearance.

The ability to localize areas of tissue signature abnormality together with regional wall motion abnormality visualized by CMR has permitted contrast-enhanced CMR to also guide subsequent myocardial biopsy. Mahrholdt and coworkers used this CMR-guided cardiac biopsy in 32 patients with suspected myocarditis. Biopsy in these abnormal regions showed remarkable positive and negative predictive values of 71% and 100%, respectively.[34] Interestingly, CMR suggested that the lateral wall may actually be the most common location

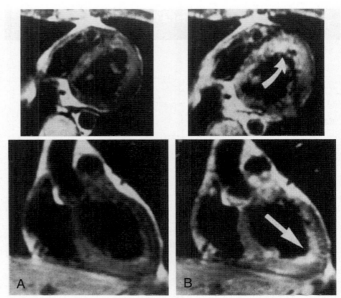

FIGURE 70-5   A, Precontrast T1-weighted transaxial **(upper)** and coronal **(lower)** magnetic resonance images through the left ventricle in a patient with myocarditis. **B,** Postcontrast magnetic resonance images at the same levels after injection of contrast material. Note enhancement of the myocardial signal in the septum and apical region (arrows). *(From Matsouka H, Hamada M, Honda T, et al: Evaluation of acute myocarditis and pericarditis by Gd-DTPA enhanced magnetic resonance imaging. Eur Heart J 15:283, 1994.)*

for lesion development, not the septum, from which most of the biopsy samples have been taken previously.

A consensus document on the role of CMR in myocarditis was published in 2009.[35] The recommended indications for CMR in suspected myocarditis include a combination of (1) new-onset or persisting symptoms suggestive of myocarditis, (2) evidence of recent or ongoing myocardial injury or dysfunction, and (3) suspected viral or nonischemic etiology. The generally agreed on CMR criteria of myocarditis include at least two of the following indicators of inflammation: (1) regional or global myocardial signaling intensity increase in T2-weighted images; (2) increased global myocardial early gadolinium enhancement ratio between myocardium and skeletal muscle in gadolinium-enhanced T1-weighted images; and (3) at least one focal lesion with nonischemic regional distribution in inversion recovery prepared gadolinium-enhanced T1-weighted images (late gadolinium enhancement).

Myocardial Biopsy

HISTOLOGIC EVALUATION. The Dallas criteria for the diagnosis of myocarditis represented the first attempt to standardize the pathologic definition of myocarditis. The Dallas criteria require an inflammatory infiltrate and associated myocyte necrosis or damage not characteristic of an ischemic event. Borderline myocarditis requires a less intense inflammatory infiltrate and no light microscopic evidence of myocyte destruction. Despite insensitivity for detection of myocarditis, the Dallas criteria remain the gold standard for unequivocal diagnosis.

The reasons for the insensitivity of the Dallas criteria are many, and some of them are outlined here. Because of the patchy nature of the myocarditic lesions in the myocardium, standard biopsy sampling of myocardial tissue of about 30 mg in mass is very much a "hit or miss" phenomenon. Chow and McManus first demonstrated this insensitivity by biopsy of postmortem hearts from patients with myocarditis. They demonstrated that with a single endomyocardial biopsy sample, histologic myocarditis could be demonstrated in only 25% of cases. Even with five random biopsy samples, correct diagnosis of myocarditis by the classic Dallas criteria could be reached in only about two thirds of subjects. This is further compounded by a recent magnetic resonance imaging study showing that the earliest myocardial inflammatory abnormalities in myocarditis are located commonly in the lateral wall of the left ventricle, a site difficult to reach with a standard bioptome.[34] Therefore, there is considerable built-in sampling error and insensitivity with the standard diagnosis of myocarditis with endomyocardial biopsies. To compound the situation further, there are also variations in the interpretation of histologic samples by expert pathologists experienced in reading cardiac biopsies. For example, of the 111 patients recruited in the original National Institutes of Health (NIH) Myocarditis Treatment Trial diagnosed with myocarditis by heart biopsy, only 64% had that diagnosis confirmed by the expert pathology panel during consensus reading of the same biopsy samples later.[36]

INDICATIONS FOR ENDOMYOCARDIAL BIOPSY. The AHA/ACC/ESC/HFSA guidelines for endomyocardial biopsy in the analysis of patients with new-onset cardiomyopathy or heart failure provide guidance to the clinician in the determination of the appropriateness of endomyocardial biopsy based on the patient's clinicopathologic presentation (**Table 70-4**). Whereas these guidelines are evidence based, there are very few prospective randomized trials to guide management, and most recommendations are the result of expert opinions. Nonetheless, patients presenting with a clinicopathologic picture compatible with fulminant, giant cell, or eosinophilic myocarditis or who are thought to have cardiac sarcoidosis should undergo endomyocardial biopsy. As the diagnosis of cardiomyopathy from a viral pathogen is enhanced by additional molecular techniques, these categories in which biopsy must or should be performed may be expanded in the future.[37]

RISKS OF ENDOMYOCARDIAL BIOPSY. Studies suggest that the complication rate of myocardial biopsy in patients with dilated cardiomyopathy is approximately 2% to 5%. Approximately half of these complications are related to venous access and the remainder to the biopsy procedure itself. Complications related to venous access include inadvertent arterial puncture, pneumothorax, vasovagal reaction, and bleeding after sheath removal. The use of ultrasonographically guided techniques to identify the internal jugular vein or to guide vein cannulation improves the success rate and decreases the complication rate and access time. Complications associated with the procedure include arrhythmias, cardiac conduction abnormalities, and cardiac perforation, which can lead to pericardial tamponade and rarely death. Patients with perforation report pain, which otherwise should not be experienced during the procedure. These patients may deteriorate rapidly because of the rapid accumulation of blood in the pericardial space and underlying left ventricular dysfunction. The rapid accumulation of blood in the pericardial space can form a clot acutely, which may interfere with percutaneous pericardial evacuation of blood. Patients who cannot be immediately resuscitated by percutaneous pericardiocentesis should have open chest evacuation of the hematoma. This requires coordination with cardiovascular surgery and preparation in the laboratory for the occurrence of these rare but expected complications. The complication rate with biopsies through the femoral vein is at least equivalent to that experienced with a jugular venous procedure. Performance of left ventricular biopsies shares similar perforation complication rates, despite the greater wall thickness of the left ventricle. In addition, left ventricular endomyocardial biopsy may be complicated by arterial embolization. Some operators use antiplatelet agents to diminish this complication. If noninvasive techniques continue to reveal evidence of left rather than right ventricular septal involvement, it is likely that more left ventricular biopsy procedures will be done in the future.

IMAGE-GUIDED BIOPSIES. Patients with arrhythmogenic right ventricular dysplasia may at times represent underlying chronic active myocarditis, with positive viral signals on molecular analysis of biopsy specimens[38] or contrast enhancement on magnetic resonance imaging. To clarify the diagnosis, patients with suspected arrhythmogenic right ventricular cardiomyopathy are sometimes submitted to endomyocardial biopsy.[39] Image-guided biopsy, usually in the triangle of dysplasia, provides the most useful histology. Whereas fat and fibrosis are

TABLE 70-4	The Role of Endomyocardial Biopsy in 14 Clinical Scenarios		
SCENARIO NUMBER	CLINICAL SCENARIO	CLASS OF RECOMMENDATION (I, IIa, IIb, III)	LEVEL OF EVIDENCE (A, B, C)
1	New-onset heart failure of <2 weeks' duration associated with a normal-sized or dilated left ventricle and hemodynamic compromise	I	B
2	New-onset heart failure of 2 weeks' to 3 months' duration associated with a dilated left ventricle and new ventricular arrhythmias, second- or third-degree heart block, or failure to respond to usual care within 1 to 2 weeks	I	B
3	Heart failure of >3 months' duration associated with a dilated left ventricle and new ventricular arrhythmias, second- or third-degree heart block, or failure to respond to usual care within 1 to 2 weeks	IIa	C
4	Heart failure associated with a DCM of any duration associated with suspected allergic reaction and/or eosinophilia	IIa	C
5	Heart failure associated with suspected anthracycline cardiomyopathy	IIa	C
6	Heart failure associated with unexplained restrictive cardiomyopathy	IIa	C
7	Suspected cardiac tumors	IIa	C
8	Unexplained cardiomyopathy in children	IIa	C
9	New-onset heart failure of 2 weeks' to 3 months' duration associated with a dilated left ventricle, without new ventricular arrhythmias or second- or third-degree heart block, that responds to usual care within 1 to 2 weeks	IIb	B
10	Heart failure of >3 months' duration associated with a dilated left ventricle, without new ventricular arrhythmias or second- or third-degree heart block, that responds to usual care within 1 to 2 weeks	IIb	C
11	Heart failure associated with unexplained HCM	IIb	C
12	Suspected ARVD/C	IIb	C
13	Unexplained ventricular arrhythmias	IIb	C
14	Unexplained atrial fibrillation	III	C

ARVD/C = arrhythmogenic right ventricular dysplasia/cardiomyopathy; DCM = dilated cardiomyopathy; HCM = hypertrophic cardiomyopathy.
From Cooper LT, Baughman KL, Feldman AM, et al: The role of endomyocardial biopsy in the management of cardiovascular disease: A scientific statement from the American Heart Association, the American College of Cardiology, and the European Society of Cardiology. Circulation 116:2216, 2007.

considered "diagnostic," PET-CT imaging may reveal inflammation of the myocardium and associated mediastinal and thoracic structures. This technique is particularly beneficial in conditions such as sarcoidosis.

MOLECULAR EVALUATION. Whereas the traditional Dallas criteria based on standard pathologic analysis of myocardial biopsy specimens have limitations, advances in molecular techniques in detecting the viral genome and inflammatory activation within the same biopsy sample have expanded our ability to detect viral myocarditis significantly, to delineate the potential viral etiology, and to improve the sensitivity of the biopsy as a diagnostic technique.

Molecular detection techniques for viral genome, such as in situ hybridization seeking the presence of viral genetic signatures in a pathologic sample and multiplexed PCR amplification of the RNA from the biopsy specimen itself, have increased the sensitivity of detecting virus signatures in the heart. These techniques have demonstrated that viral RNA can be significantly associated with symptoms and prognosis. However, the surprise was that the presence of viral genome is entirely independent of the presence or absence of inflammatory cells on the same biopsy specimen. Thus, a tissue sample can be Dallas positive only, molecularly positive only, both, or neither. This underscores that myocarditis is truly a disease of both the molecular trigger by the virus and the immunologic response by the host; either alone will be able to produce the disease syndrome.

PCR is limited by the requirement that the viral pathogen to be searched for must be declared in advance of the analysis, which is usually based on historical demonstration of pathogens in other series of patients. Techniques capable of demonstrating any viral pathogen would greatly enhance the recognition of viral causes of cardiomyopathy and may allow correlation of specific pathogens with clinical pathologic entities.

Analysis of immunologic activation on the biopsy tissues may also provide additional information. The tissues can be analyzed for inflammatory cell infiltration subtypes or signal activation, such as cytokine and complement signals. The tissues can also be analyzed for the upregulation of major histocompatibility complex (MHC) antigens. Whereas the sensitivity and specificity of MHC antigen upregulation have been shown to be 80% and 85%, respectively, from studies of very small sample size, this has not been replicated in larger series. Nevertheless, MHC expression has been used to guide therapy for patients with myocarditis and inflammatory cardiomyopathy in one study evaluating immunosuppressive therapy.

Prognosis

Patients with acute myocarditis and mild cardiac involvement generally will recover in the majority of cases without long-term sequelae. However, patients with more advanced cardiac dysfunction accompanying myocarditis may have a more varied outlook. Paradoxically, patients with severe hemodynamic collapse at presentation (fulminant myocarditis) have a surprisingly good prognosis, with one series documenting transplant-free survival of 93% in 11 years.[30] Those with chronic myocarditis may recover (30%), maintain some degree of left ventricular compromise, or progress to dilated cardiomyopathy and require intensive medical therapy, mechanical support, or cardiac transplantation.[40] Patients with giant cell myocarditis have extremely poor prognosis, with median survival of less than 6 months, and most will require transplantation to avoid succumbing to the disease (**Fig. 70-6**). On the other hand, patients with chronic active myocarditis with dilated cardiomyopathy, like those recruited into the NIH Myocarditis Treatment Trial, still have a relatively poor prognosis. These patients all had the diagnosis of myocarditis based on the Dallas biopsy criteria and showed a mortality of 20% at 1 year and 56% at 4.3 years, with many cases of chronic heart failure despite optimal medical management (**Fig. 70-7**).[36]

Several studies have attempted to identify clinical variables that can predict adverse outcomes in viral myocarditis. Although many of these variables cannot be replicated from study to study, several factors do appear to predict death or transplantation, including presentation with syncope, bundle branch block on electrocardiography, and ejection fraction of less than 40%. Additional predictors of poor outcome included New York Heart Association Class III or IV, pulmonary capillary wedge pressure greater than 15 mm Hg, immunopathologic evidence of myocardial inflammation, failure to use beta-blocking

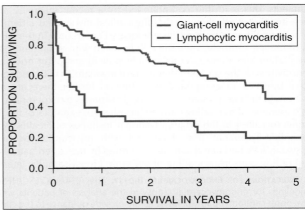

FIGURE 70-6 Prognosis in patients with giant cell myocarditis. Patients with giant cell myocarditis have much worse survival compared with patients with lymphocytic myocarditis, particularly in the acute phase soon after presentation.

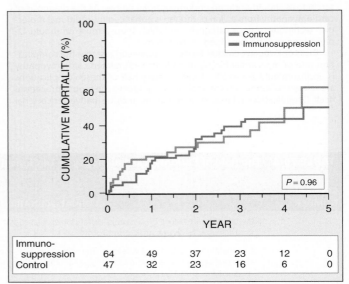

| Immuno-suppression | 64 | 49 | 37 | 23 | 12 | 0 |
| Control | 47 | 32 | 23 | 16 | 6 | 0 |

FIGURE 70-7 The cumulative mortality data from the NIH-sponsored Myocarditis Treatment Trial. The mortality curve confirms the general poor prognosis of patients with myocarditis, who unfortunately did not demonstrate that the immunosuppressive treatment conferred any mortality benefit over standard medical therapy (control). Overall, 20% of the patients were dead in 1 year, and 54% died during 4.3 years of follow-up. There was a temporary improvement in the immunosuppressive arm that was not sustained. *(Modified from Mason JW, O'Connell JB, Herskowitz A, et al: A clinical trial of immunosuppressive therapy for myocarditis. N Engl J Med 333:269, 1995.)*

therapy,[41] biventricular failure, and giant cell or viral genome on biopsy.[42] On the other hand, two-dimensional echocardiographic evidence of a small left atrial and left ventricular size was predictive of myocardial recovery from a small study of 15 patients. Whereas general pathologic features of the biopsy specimen did not predict prognosis in more recent series, the resolution of myocarditis on follow-up biopsy and the absence of azan-Mallory staining of cardiac myocytes (a marker of cellular edema or myocytolysis) do appear to herald functional ventricular recovery.[41,43]

Why and associates reported that of 120 patients with dilated cardiomyopathy, the group (34%) who were positive for enteroviral minus strand RNA had a significantly worse outcome during 2 years (68% versus 92%; $P = 0.02$) compared with those who were enteroviral genome negative.[44] More recent studies have also demonstrated that viral genome persistence on myocardial biopsy predicted more rapid deterioration of ventricular function during follow-up.[11,42] Interestingly, molecular markers of cell apoptosis may turn out to be good prognosticators. Fuse and colleagues from Japan found that serum levels of soluble Fas and Fas ligand were significantly higher in patients with fatal myocarditis than in survivors. Sheppard more recently examined the patients who participated in the Intervention in Myocarditis and Acute Cardiomyopathy (IMAC II) trial. Patients with myocardial expression of Fas ligand or tumor necrosis factor receptor 1 (TNFR1) showed minimal recovery, suggesting again that excessive apoptosis is a poor prognosticator in patients with acute myocarditis. Because of the diversity of outcomes in patients with myocarditis and the general lack of dramatic response to treatment, meticulous follow-up of patients to determine their natural history is very important. This will also help determine the need for continuation or additional therapy and ongoing risk.

Therapeutic Approaches

Supportive Therapy

The first-line therapy for all patients with myocarditis and heart failure is supportive care (see Chap. 28). A very small proportion of patients will require hemodynamic support (**Fig. 70-8**) that ranges from vasopressors (see Chap. 27) to intra-aortic balloon pump and ventricular assist devices (see Chap. 32). These patients should be treated like any patient with clinical heart failure, including initial diuretics to remove excessive volume overload if present. Patients may also benefit from intravenous vasodilators such as nitroglycerin and nesiritide in appropriate doses with appropriate monitoring to improve cardiac output and to lower filling pressures (see Chap. 27). The recommended therapy for heart failure, such as angiotensin modulators (angiotensin-converting enzyme [ACE] inhibitors or angiotensin receptor blockers) and beta blockers, should then be initiated as soon as the patient is

clinically stable and able to tolerate these medications (see Chap. 28). The current ACC/AHA/ESC/CCS guidelines for heart failure care should be followed.[45]

There is usually an urgent discussion of whether immunosuppressive therapies should be used for patients with myocarditis, but what is not well recognized is that the traditional heart failure therapies may already have significant anti-inflammatory effect. ACE inhibitors together with beta blockers represent the cornerstones of modern heart failure therapy. It has been previously well documented that angiotensin is a potent proinflammatory and pro-oxidative agent. ACE inhibitors have been shown to decrease the expression of adhesion molecules on the surface of the endothelium. ACE inhibitors also have general anti-inflammatory properties in terms of attenuating inflammatory cell mobilization and cytokine release. The effect of ACE inhibition observed to date in heart failure and atherosclerosis is consistent with its effect on inflammation. Even though beta blockers have traditionally been associated mainly with blockade of the adrenergic system, more recently there is appreciation that they may also have an impact on inflammatory cytokine signaling. In a canine model of heart failure, the effective use of beta blockade in this setting can significantly reduce cytokine gene expression in the myocardium. This is accompanied by improvements in ventricular function and reverses remodeling of the left ventricle.

Immunosuppression

Because inflammatory cell infiltrates have consistently been found on myocardial biopsy or autopsy of patients who have myocarditis, the general belief has been that immunosuppression should be beneficial for myocarditis. However, this is very much an unproven hypothesis, as our current understanding of inflammation suggests that the immune response can be as much protective as harmful and that broad immunosuppressive regimens may produce as much harm as benefit. To date, there is no shortage of small trials evaluating a variety of immunosuppressive regimens. However, all of them are fraught with significant limitations, including (1) the high degree of spontaneous improvement in the control and treatment arms, (2) the small sample size with a heterogeneous collection of recruited patients, (3) the patchy nature of myocardial biopsy detection of myocarditis, and (4) the lack of relationship between pathologic abnormalities and clinical prognosis.

The first systematic approach to evaluate immune modulatory therapy in heart disease is the NIH-sponsored Myocarditis Treatment Trial (see Fig. 70-8). In this trial, patients with biopsy-proven myocarditis according to the Dallas criteria were randomized to receive either conventional therapy, including ACE inhibitors and standard anti–heart failure regimen, or the addition of immunosuppressive therapy. The immunosuppressive therapy regimen consisted of steroids, azathioprine, or cyclosporine. The results showed that there was a significant improvement in ejection fraction in both arms of the randomized trial, such that at the end of the follow-up period at 4.3 years, there was no significant difference between the two arms.[36] The overall outcome of patients with myocarditis and dilated cardiomyopathy is still poor in the trial. Predictors of improvement included high initial left ventricular ejection fraction (LVEF), less intensive conventional therapy, and short duration of symptoms. When the survival was examined in more detail, there was a trend for improvement in the immunosuppressed arm while the treatment was actively being administered. However, because the immunosuppression was given for only 6 months and was discontinued thereafter, the effect was not sustained. In retrospect, during the time in which the Myocarditis Treatment Trial was conducted, the clinical approach was focused on the overly simplified notion of immune activation in myocarditis and heart failure. The immunosuppressive regimen used was nonspecific for the innate or acquired arms of immunity. In addition, there was no delineation of the viral etiology in the trial itself. Finally, the patients entered in the trial were at various stages of development of cardiomyopathy, and the sample size was not adequate in retrospect to detect a transient albeit potentially important benefit during the short term.[1] A series from Italy examined 112 patients with active biopsy-proven

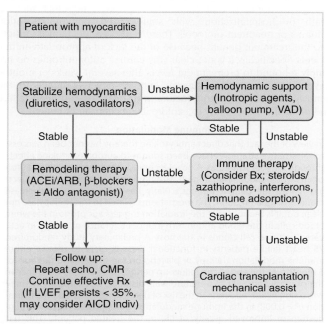

FIGURE 70-8 Treatment algorithms for patients with myocarditis, depending on hemodynamic stability and response to general supportive and remodeling treatment regimen at each step. All patients should have aggressive support and appropriate follow-up. Immune therapy at present is still mainly to support those who have failed to improve spontaneously. ACEi = angiotensin-converting enzyme inhibitors; AICD = automatic implantable cardioverter-defibrillator; Aldo = aldosterone; ARB = angiotensin receptor blockers; Bx = biopsy; CMR = cardiac magnetic resonance; indiv = based on individual assessment of risk versus benefit; LVEF = left ventricular ejection fraction; VAD = ventricular assist device.

myocarditis, of whom 41 were treated with prednisone and azathio-prine because of failure of conventional therapy. The responders to the immunosuppressive regimen were 90% positive for cardiac autoanti-bodies, and there was no evidence of persisting viral genome. Polish investigators demonstrated improved ejection fraction and subjective symptoms in patients with myocarditis defined by alternative endo-myocardial biopsy markers of immunologic activation, as opposed to standard Dallas criteria. This suggested that there may evolve to be predictors of response to immunosuppression.

On the basis of the results of the foregoing studies, immunosuppres-sion should not be routinely considered for patients with myocarditis. However, patients with giant cell myocarditis, myocarditis due to auto-immune or hypersensitivity reactions, or severe hemodynamic com-promise and deteriorating conditions may benefit from a trial of immunosuppressive therapy in the hope of stabilizing the hemody-namic condition of the patient. The best responders may be those with active autoimmune response without persisting viral genome. We need to be aware that this is unlikely to influence the ultimate mortal-ity of the patient, but it may improve the short-term natural history.

Interferon

Type I interferons (IFN-α and IFN-β) exert antiviral activity by virtue of their ability to phosphorylate interferon-stimulated genes (ISGs) in the host innate immune system. These ISGs together can lead to deg-radation of foreign viral RNA, and the small GTPase Mx (a component of the ISG) can interfere with the accumulation of viral RNA and coat protein. IFN-β has been shown to be most effective in animal models of viral myocarditis, and we have demonstrated recently that IFN-β knockout animals (IFN-β[−/−]) have a higher viral titer, increased inflam-matory cell infiltrate, increased mortality, and worse cardiac function.[26]

To determine if this strategy can be applied to patients, Kuhl and associates have evaluated 22 patients with dilated cardiomyopathy and biopsy evidence of viral persistence.[46] The patients were treated with subcutaneous IFN-β for a period of 24 weeks. The interferon treat-ment was able to eliminate the viral genome from all of the patients, and ventricular function improved in 15 of 22 patients. The mean LVEF improved from 44.6% to 53.1% ($P < 0.001$). Overall, the patients also improved in clinical status. These encouraging phase II results have paved the way for a phase IIb trial of IFN-β in patients with dilated cardiomyopathy. Preliminary data in this trial suggested that there was a reduction in viral load from myocardial biopsy samples in the interferon-treated group.[47] There was also improvement in New York Heart Association functional class and quality of life indices in the IFN-β–treated group. However, this is an encouraging and intriguing result. This will need to be replicated to represent a true advancement for the treatment of myocarditis.

Intravenous Immune Globulin

Many causes of acute-onset dilated cardiomyopathy, including peri-partum cardiomyopathy, are likely to represent an autoimmune inflammatory process in the myocardium that is triggered by a tran-sient viral infection. Instead of anticytokine therapy or active immune suppression, a possible strategy is passive immunization through the infusion of immune globulins. In cases of pediatric heart failure, par-ticularly myocarditis, uncontrolled studies suggested a potential benefit with intravenous immune globulins.

Retrospective analysis suggested that in patients with peripartum cardiomyopathy, many of whom also had concurrent myocarditis, those who received intravenous immune globulin appear to have better ventricular function during follow-up.[48] To test this hypothesis more thoroughly and prospectively in adults, McNamara and associ-ates conducted a randomized double-blinded trial involving 62 patients with acute heart failure and randomized the patients with 2 g/kg intravenous immune globulin or placebo, followed up for changes in LVEF from the baseline to 6 months and 12 months (IMAC II trial).[40] Overall, there was impressive improvement of LVEF from 25% to 41% at 6 months and to 42% at 12 months; however, the improvement was

identical in both the intravenous immune globulin treatment arm and in the placebo arm. The transplant-free survival was 92% at 1 year. In IMAC, the patients spontaneously improved left ventricular ejection significantly with or without immune globulin treatment. The rapid improvement in LVEF in the control precluded any possibility of dem-onstrating a treatment effect. In retrospect, the evaluation of this agent in a more advanced chronic cardiomyopathy population with evi-dence of inflammation in the heart may have produced a more defini-tive result. Accordingly, at present, there is no primary indication for immune globulins in myocarditis, except perhaps in pediatric popula-tions and those refractory to immunosuppressive therapy.

Immune Adsorption Therapy

A physical approach to removal of potential cardiac depressant factors is immune adsorption therapy through plasmapheresis of peripheral blood. There have been previous suggestions that in addi-tion to cytokines, circulating antibodies may target against specific components of the myocyte under stress, such as the beta-adrenergic receptor, the adenosine triphospate (ATP) carrier, or even the myosin molecule, leading to eventual cell dysfunction and cell death. Various strategies have been developed to capture these cardiodepressant factors or antibodies by use of immune adsorption columns.

In one earlier randomized trial using immune adsorption therapy, 34 patients were randomized to standard therapy or immune adsorp-tion therapy aimed at removal of antibodies against the beta-adrenergic receptor. After 1 year of treatment, the treated group demonstrated a change of LVEF from a mean of 22% to 38%, whereas the placebo or standard treatment arm did not show any significant improvement. There was also accompanying improvement in patients' symptomatic status. More recently, other groups have demonstrated further specific-ity by identifying the IgG3 subclass of antibodies to be particularly responsible for cardiac depression.[49,50] Patients who had effective removal of the IgG3 class of antibodies are particularly the patients who demonstrated improvement in ejection fraction.

However, these innovative approaches have not been subjected to a large randomized trial examining objective endpoints, such as death or hospitalization, with standardized immunoadsorption columns or treatment protocols. There is also no mechanistic insight into the treatment benefit because of the lack of appropriate animal models. Specifically, it is not clear why cardiac autoantibodies do not simply rebound to pretreatment levels after several weeks or months. Nevertheless, this does represent another novel approach to the removal of proinflammatory factors in myocarditis and heart failure and offers the opportunity to explore its mechanism of benefit.

Immune Modulation

In view of the fact that direct anticytokine therapy has not been success-ful, alternative strategies have been sought to abrogate cytokine effects through indirect strategies. A novel technique that involves taking autol-ogous whole blood, irradiating it with ultraviolet radiation, and reinject-ing it into the patient intramuscularly has been shown to decrease markers of inflammation. The mechanisms related to this therapy are not clear, but it is thought that the irradiation triggers apoptosis in the white blood cells in the blood and in turn induces tolerance or anergy in acti-vated immune cell clones in the host. A preliminary study randomized 75 heart failure patients in functional Class III or IV to receive either immune modulation therapy or placebo on top of standard therapy for 6 months. At the end of the follow-up period, there was no difference in the primary endpoint of 6-minute walk distance, but surprisingly there was a significant reduction in the risk of death ($P = 0.022$) and hospitaliza-tion ($P = 0.008$) in the immune modulation group. There was also a sug-gestion of improved quality of life in the treated patients. This has resulted in a large follow-up mortality and morbidity trial involving more than 2400 patients (the ACCLAIM trial).[51] During 10.2 months of follow-up, there was no overall difference in the composite endpoints of time to death or transplantation for cardiovascular reasons. Nonetheless, two prespecified subgroups, those with no history of myocardial infarction and those with Class II New York Heart Association heart failure, dis-played significant reductions in the primary endpoint. The failure of immunomodulation therapy to improve left ventricular compromise relates to redundancy of the immune system and alternative effects of TNFR1 and TNFR2 on NF-κB, inflammation, apoptosis, and hypertrophy.

Hemodynamic Support (see Chap. 32)

Whereas there has been no universally applicable specific therapy for patients with myocarditis, general supportive measures, even for those patients with hemodynamic compromise, have been effective because a significant portion of patients recover spontaneously. Patients with myocarditis presenting with profound hemodynamic compromise secondary to fulminant myocarditis or cardiogenic shock can be supported effectively with devices ranging from intra-aortic balloon pumps to full ventricular assist devices (VAD). Indeed, many of the cases of spontaneous recovery after VAD support without the need for transplantation, or so-called bridge to recovery, are in patients with the primary diagnosis of myocarditis. For example, Simon and colleagues reported a single-center series of 154 patients receiving VAD therapy, of whom 10 had successful recovery without transplantation.[52] The majority of cases were nonischemic cardiomyopathy, including myocarditis in three patients and peripartum cardiomyopathy in four patients.

Vaccination

If viruses continue as the most common cause of myocarditis and dilated cardiomyopathy, one may consider in the future the possibility of targeted vaccination. Patients who may be genetically susceptible to myocarditis may receive vaccination against the most common causative agents, thus obviating the risk for development of the disease. One example is the disappearance of endocardial fibroelastosis causing dilated cardiomyopathy in children associated with the mumps vaccination program. If vaccination is effective, this could lead to an effective prevention program of myocarditis and dilated cardiomyopathy, with attendant reduction in cost and improvement in morbidity and mortality.

Future Perspectives

Myocarditis serves as an excellent model for the study of host injury and repair. The outcome is critically dependent on the virulence of the causative agent, the ability of the host immune system to mount an appropriate response, and the ability of the host to repair the injury effectively and efficiently. Future determination of the genetic risk factors leading to the phenotype of myocarditis and its potential interactions with the environment and the ability to predict who will or will not recover will be beneficial in identifying those at particular high risk for development of long-term sequelae of the condition.

Meanwhile, the diagnostic techniques are evolving to identify novel blood-based biomarkers reflecting cardiac inflammation through microarray and proteomic analysis of tissues of both laboratory models and patient samples. The goal in the near future is to develop a blood-based diagnostic tool or panel with sufficient sensitivity and specificity to obviate the need for myocardial biopsies. The combination of blood samples of biomarkers together with imaging techniques such as cardiac magnetic resonance imaging may help properly diagnose and stage the disease and avoid the current problem of severe underdiagnosis due to dependence on the Dallas criteria by biopsy.

With the understanding of new pathophysiologic mechanisms, new therapies are also being developed and evaluated in clinical trials. Ongoing interferon and immune-modifying strategies may become more refined as data determining their relative efficacies compared with traditional therapies become available. This may help develop more evidence-based guidelines for treatment of these very ill patients. In addition, the increased refinement of ventricular assist strategies to support patients and ultimately to wean them from support without necessary transplantation represents another unique opportunity to improve outcomes for the patients presenting with dramatic hemodynamic collapse. One long-term goal would be to identify individuals at risk for myocarditis and to evaluate the opportunity and cost-effectiveness of developing a combination vaccine to prevent the development of disease in these individuals despite exposure to the causative agents.

In Memoriam

Kenneth L. Baughman's scientific contributions to the study of myocarditis, the subject of this chapter, were legion. He was also a consummate clinician, a caring and dedicated physician, a generous mentor, a valued colleague, and a trusted and loyal friend. He was an avid athlete who regularly competed in triathlons. He was also a loving and devoted husband, father, and grandfather. His untimely death while attending the American Heart Association meeting in Orlando, Florida, in November 2009 has had a lasting impact on the editors and his colleagues at the Brigham and Women's Hospital. He is sorely missed, and the editors dedicate this chapter to his memory.

REFERENCES

Definition, Incidence, and Epidemiology

1. Cooper LT Jr: Myocarditis. N Engl J Med 360:1526, 2009.
2. Aretz HT, Billingham ME, Edwards WD, et al: Myocarditis, a histopathologic definition and classification. Am J Cardiovasc Pathol 1:3, 1987.
3. Baughman KL: Diagnosis of myocarditis: Death of Dallas criteria. Circulation 113:593, 2006.
4. Fabre A, Sheppard MN: Sudden adult death syndrome and other non-ischaemic causes of sudden cardiac death. Heart 92:316, 2006.
5. Nugent AW, Daubeney PE, Chondros P, et al: The epidemiology of childhood cardiomyopathy in Australia. N Engl J Med 348:1639, 2003.
6. Towbin JA, Lowe AM, Colan SD, et al: Incidence, causes, and outcomes of dilated cardiomyopathy in children. JAMA 296:1867, 2006.
7. Xiong D, Yajima T, Lim BK, et al: Inducible cardiac-restricted expression of enteroviral protease 2A is sufficient to induce dilated cardiomyopathy. Circulation 115:94, 2007.
8. Imazio M, Cecchi E, Demichelis B, et al: Myopericarditis versus viral or idiopathic acute pericarditis. Heart 94:498, 2008.
9. Tschope C, Bock CT, Kasner M, et al: High prevalence of cardiac parvovirus B19 infection in patients with isolated left ventricular diastolic dysfunction. Circulation 111:879, 2005.
10. Kuhl U, Pauschinger M, Noutsias M, et al: High prevalence of viral genomes and multiple viral infections in the myocardium of adults with "idiopathic" left ventricular dysfunction. Circulation 111:887, 2005.
11. Kuhl U, Pauschinger M, Seeberg B, et al: Viral persistence in the myocardium is associated with progressive cardiac dysfunction. Circulation 112:1965, 2005.
12. Bowles NE, Ni J, Kearney DL, et al: Detection of viruses in myocardial tissues by polymerase chain reaction: Evidence of adenovirus as a common cause of myocarditis in children and adults. J Am Coll Cardiol 42:466, 2003.

Etiologic Agents

13. Matsumori A: Hepatitis C virus infection and cardiomyopathies. Circ Res 96:144, 2005.
14. Coyne CB, Bergelson JM: Virus-induced Abl and Fyn kinase signals permit coxsackievirus entry through epithelial tight junctions. Cell 124:119, 2006.
15. Liu P, Aitken K, Kong YY, et al: Essential role for the tyrosine kinase p56lck in coxsackievirus B3 mediated heart disease. Nat Med 6:429, 2000.
16. Andreoletti L, Venteo L, Douche-Aourik F, et al: Active coxsackieviral B infection is associated with disruption of dystrophin in endomyocardial tissue of patients who died suddenly of acute myocardial infarction. J Am Coll Cardiol 50:2207, 2007.
17. Schenk T, Enders M, Pollak S, et al: High prevalence of human parvovirus B19 DNA in myocardial autopsy samples from subjects without myocarditis or dilative cardiomyopathy. J Clin Microbiol 47:106, 2009.
18. Vallbracht KB, Schwimmbeck PL, Kuhl U, et al: Endothelium-dependent flow-mediated vasodilation of systemic arteries is impaired in patients with myocardial virus persistence. Circulation 110:2938, 2004.
19. Yilmaz A, Mahrholdt H, Athanasiadis A, et al: Coronary vasospasm as the underlying cause for chest pain in patients with PVB19 myocarditis. Heart 94:1456, 2008.
20. Noutsias M, Fechner H, de Jonge H, et al: Human coxsackie-adenovirus receptor is colocalized with integrins αvβ3 and αvβ5 on the cardiomyocyte sarcolemma and upregulated in dilated cardiomyopathy: Implications for cardiotropic viral infections. Circulation 104:275, 2001.
21. Nowakowski J, Nadelman RB, Sell R, et al: Long-term follow-up of patients with culture-confirmed Lyme disease. Am J Med 115:91, 2003.
22. Barrett MP, Burchmore RJ, Stich A, et al: The trypanosomiases. Lancet 362:1469, 2003.
23. Ben m'rad M, Leclerc-Mercier S, Blanche P, et al: Drug-induced hypersensitivity syndrome: Clinical and biologic disease patterns in 24 patients. Medicine (Baltimore) 88:131, 2009.

Pathophysiology

24. Maekawa Y, Ouzounian M, Opavsky MA, Liu PP: Connecting the missing link between dilated cardiomyopathy and viral myocarditis: Virus, cytoskeleton, and innate immunity. Circulation 115:5, 2007.
25. Fuse K, Chan G, Liu Y, et al: Myeloid differentiation factor-88 plays a crucial role in the pathogenesis of coxsackievirus B3 induced myocarditis and influences type I interferon production. Circulation 112:2276, 2005.
26. Deonarain R, Cerullo D, Fuse K, et al: Protective role for interferon-β in coxsackievirus B3 infection. Circulation 110:3540, 2004.

27. Yajima T, Yasukawa H, Jeon ES, et al: Innate defense mechanism against virus infection within the cardiac myocyte requiring gp130-STAT3 signaling. Circulation 114:2364, 2006.

28. Opavsky MA, Martino T, Rabinovitch M, et al: Enhanced ERK-1/2 activation in mice susceptible to coxsackievirus-induced myocarditis. J Clin Invest 109:1561, 2002.

Clinical Presentation and Diagnosis

29. Felker GM, Thompson RE, Hare JM, et al: Underlying causes and long-term survival in patients with initially unexplained cardiomyopathy. N Engl J Med 342:1077, 2000.

30. McCarthy RE 3rd, Boehmer JP, Hruban RH, et al: Long-term outcome of fulminant myocarditis as compared with acute (nonfulminant) myocarditis. N Engl J Med 342:690, 2000.

31. Cooper LT Jr, Hare JM, Tazelaar HD, et al: Usefulness of immunosuppression for giant cell myocarditis. Am J Cardiol 102:1535, 2008.

32. Liu PP, Yan AT: Cardiovascular magnetic resonance for the diagnosis of acute myocarditis: Prospects for detecting myocardial inflammation. J Am Coll Cardiol 45:1823, 2005.

33. Abdel-Aty H, Boye P, Zagrosek A, et al: Diagnostic performance of cardiovascular magnetic resonance in patients with suspected acute myocarditis: Comparison of different approaches. J Am Coll Cardiol 45:1815, 2005.

34. Mahrholdt H, Goedecke C, Wagner A, et al: Cardiovascular magnetic resonance assessment of human myocarditis: A comparison to histology and molecular pathology. Circulation 109:1250, 2004.

35. Friedrich MG, Sechtem U, Schulz-Menger J, et al: Cardiovascular magnetic resonance in myocarditis: A JACC White Paper. J Am Coll Cardiol 53:1475, 2009.

36. Mason JW, O'Connell JB, Herskowitz A, et al: A clinical trial of immunosuppressive therapy for myocarditis. N Engl J Med 333:269, 1995.

37. Cooper LT, Baughman KL, Feldman AM, et al: The role of endomyocardial biopsy in the management of cardiovascular disease: A scientific statement from the American Heart Association, the American College of Cardiology, and the European Society of Cardiology. Circulation 116:2216, 2007.

38. Bowles NE, Ni J, Marcus F, Towbin JA: The detection of cardiotropic viruses in the myocardium of patients with arrhythmogenic right ventricular dysplasia/cardiomyopathy. J Am Coll Cardiol 39:892, 2002.

39. Pieroni M, Dello Russo A, Marzo F, et al: High prevalence of myocarditis mimicking arrhythmogenic right ventricular cardiomyopathy: Differential diagnosis by electroanatomic mapping–guided endomyocardial biopsy. J Am Coll Cardiol 53:681, 2009.

40. McNamara DM, Holubkov R, Starling RC, et al: Controlled trial of intravenous immune globulin in recent-onset dilated cardiomyopathy. Circulation 103:2254, 2001.

41. Kindermann I, Kindermann M, Kandolf R, et al: Predictors of outcome in patients with suspected myocarditis. Circulation 118:639, 2008.

42. Caforio AL, Calabrese F, Angelini A, et al: A prospective study of biopsy-proven myocarditis: Prognostic relevance of clinical and aetiopathogenetic features at diagnosis. Eur Heart J 28:1326, 2007.

43. Mann DL: Determinants of myocardial recovery in myocarditis has the time come for molecular fingerprinting? J Am Coll Cardiol 46:1043, 2005.

44. Why HJ, Meany BT, Richardson PJ, et al: Clinical and prognostic significance of detection of enteroviral RNA in the myocardium of patients with myocarditis or dilated cardiomyopathy. Circulation 89:2582, 1994.

45. Hunt SA, Abraham WT, Chin MH, et al: ACC/AHA 2005 Guideline Update for the Diagnosis and Management of Chronic Heart Failure in the Adult: A report of the American College of Cardiology/American Heart Association Task Force on Practice Guidelines (Writing Committee to Update the 2001 Guidelines for the Evaluation and Management of Heart Failure). Circulation 112:1825, 2005.

46. Kuhl U, Pauschinger M, Schwimmbeck PL, et al: Interferon-β treatment eliminates cardiotropic viruses and improves left ventricular function in patients with myocardial persistence of viral genomes and left ventricular dysfunction. Circulation 107:2793, 2003.

47. Schultheiss HP, Poller W, Kuhl U, et al: Interferon β-1b in patients with chronic viral cardiomyopathy. American Heart Association meeting; New Orleans, La; November 2008.

48. Bozkurt B, Villaneuva FS, Holubkov R, et al: Intravenous immune globulin in the therapy of peripartum cardiomyopathy. J Am Coll Cardiol 34:177, 1999.

49. Staudt A, Schaper F, Stangl V, et al: Immunohistological changes in dilated cardiomyopathy induced by immunoadsorption therapy and subsequent immunoglobulin substitution. Circulation 103:2681, 2001.

50. Staudt A, Bohm M, Knebel F, et al: Potential role of autoantibodies belonging to the immunoglobulin G-3 subclass in cardiac dysfunction among patients with dilated cardiomyopathy. Circulation 106:2448, 2002.

51. Torre-Amione G, Anker SD, Bourge RC, et al: Results of a non-specific immunomodulation therapy in chronic heart failure (ACCLAIM trial): A placebo-controlled randomised trial. Lancet 371:228, 2008.

52. Simon MA, Kormos RL, Murali S, et al: Myocardial recovery using ventricular assist devices: Prevalence, clinical characteristics, and outcomes. Circulation 112:I32, 2005.

CHAPTER 71   # Chagas' Disease

José A.F. Ramires, Andrei C. Sposito, Edécio Cunha-Neto, and
Maria de Lourdes Higuchi

Chagas' disease, or American trypanosomiasis, is an infection caused by the protozoan *Trypanosoma cruzi* (*T. cruzi*), originally transmitted by hematophagous triatomine insects.[1,2] Triatominae infected by *T. cruzi* inhabit 18 countries in North and South America, ranging from the southern United States to southern Argentina, and the prevalence of the disease relates to the proximity between infected triatomines and humans. The infection can also result from maternal-fetal transmission, from food contaminated with feces or urine from infected Triatominae, from laboratory accidents, and from blood transfusion or organs transplanted from infected donors. Some 20,000 people die annually from Chagas' disease, 16 to 18 million people are infected, and 100 million people are at risk of contracting the infection. During its life cycle, *T. cruzi* can assume three forms (**Fig. 71-1**).

Pathologic Findings

Manifestations of Chagas' disease vary during the course of infection. In the acute phase, at the site of inoculation, local swelling occurs (called a chagoma). The histology typically shows amastigote forms of *T. cruzi* in macrophages, adipose cells, and muscle fibers in the subcutaneous tissue, associated with lymphohystiocytic inflammatory infiltrate, vascular proliferation, edema, and congestion.[3] Some metastatic chagomas (cutaneous nodes showing inflammation without parasites) may occur. The parasites entering the bloodstream (**Fig. 71-2A**) reach almost all organs and infect different types of cells, including macrophages, endothelial cells, smooth and skeletal muscle cells, cardiac myocytes, and fibroblasts.

The most common cause of death in this phase is an acute myocarditis characterized macroscopically by a flabby congested dilated heart, with normal or moderately increased volume, and microscopically by moderate to severe mononuclear inflammatory infiltration with some neutrophils, edema, myocytolysis, and many intramyocyte nests of amastigotes, with no inflammation when cells remain intact (see Fig. 71-2B). An inflammatory infiltrate injures nerves and parasympathetic ganglia. Parasites and mononuclear inflammatory infiltrate can also affect skeletal muscles (see Fig. 71-2C) and smooth muscle of the esophagus and large intestine, destroying myenteric plexus. Meningoencephalitis can also cause death in this phase.[3]

Reactivation of the disease during the chronic phase may occur because of immunosuppression, as in AIDS or neoplasia or after heart transplantation.[4,5] *T. cruzi* may be detected in peripheral blood or bone marrow or in subcutaneous nodes, resembling primary chagomas (see Fig. 71-2D and E). An asymptomatic period called the indeterminate phase follows the acute phase of infection with *T. cruzi*. Endomyocardial biopsies of 15% of patients in this phase show mild lymphocytic myocarditis without substantial structural alterations such as fibrosis, hypertrophy, or myocytolysis.[6]

Several years after initial infection, an estimated 30% of infected people will develop clinical Chagas' cardiomyopathy. In necropsy

studies,[3,7] patients who died because of Chagas' cardiomyopathy presented with rounded globe-shaped hearts; severe chamber dilation, mainly on the right side; myocardial hypertrophy; congested epicardial veins; and intracavitary thrombosis, usually in the left ventricular apex and right atrial appendage (**Fig. 71-3A**). Microscopy shows a variable degree of lymphocytic inflammatory infiltrate surrounding nonparasitized myocytes, severe myofiber hypertrophy (see Fig. 71-3B), and fibrosis (see Fig. 71-3C). In this phase, nests of *T. cruzi* are rare. Immunohistochemistry and polymerase chain reaction (PCR) techniques have demonstrated antigens and DNA of the parasite at sites of inflammation (see Fig. 71-3D), but their quantity does not relate to the intensity of myocarditis, suggesting involvement of other factors.[8,9]

Segmental fibrotic lesions often occur in the myocardium of patients with chronic Chagas' disease.[3,8,10] One is the so-called apex lesion, characterized by a thinning of the left ventricular apex, with total or partial disappearance of the myocardium (replaced by fibrosis), a pathognomonic sign of Chagas' disease. In necropsy studies, other segmental thinning of the myocardial wall is usually found at the inferolateral wall of the left ventricle. These lesions are accompanied by mural thrombosis and aneurysm dilatation (**Fig. 71-4**). In patients, myocardial delayed enhancement by contrast cardiac magnetic resonance (CMR)[11] has also demonstrated fibrosis in the inferolateral wall associated with clinical manifestation of sustained ventricular tachycardia. Segmental fibrotic lesions often occur in the watershed zone of coronary circulation (**Fig. 71-5**), and may correspond to healed ischemic injury, explaining also the segmental fibrosis in the conduction system (see Fig. 71-4D).

The apex lesion might result from conduction system fibrosis, which would delay the electric stimulus to the apex,[12] parasympathetic denervation. Altered myocardial perfusion occurs in patients with Chagas' disease who manifest myocardial ischemia in the absence of epicardial coronary stenosis; the imbalance between the sympathetic and parasympathetic nervous systems may account for this coronary flow disturbance.[13-15]

Pathophysiology

Chagas' cardiomyopathy is essentially a myocarditis.[3,8,16,17] The inflammatory process, although more intense in the acute phase, is clinically silent but incessant in patients in the indeterminate and chronic phases of the disease. The T-cell rich mononuclear cell inflammatory infiltrate seems to play a major pathogenic role in the disease.[18,19] Various observations support this view: (1) the worse prognosis of Chagas' disease compared with cardiomyopathies of noninflammatory cause; (2) the relationship between the frequency of myocarditis and the severity of cardiomyopathy; and (3) the correlation between ventricular dilation and the intensity of myocarditis in Syrian hamsters chronically infected by *T. cruzi*.[20] The scarcity of *T. cruzi* parasites in the

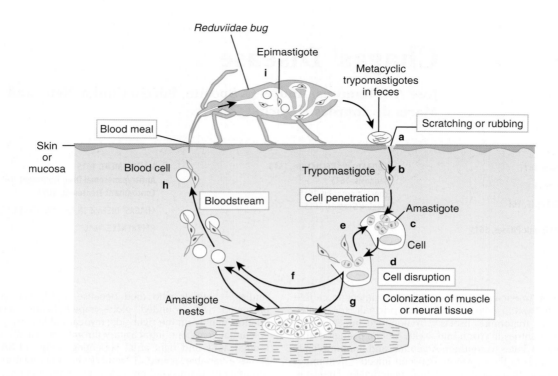

FIGURE 71-1 The life cycle of *Trypanosoma cruzi*. Reduvid bugs transmit *T. cruzi*. While partaking of a blood meal (a), the insect defecates on the host's skin, releasing the infective trypomastigote form of the parasite. The trypomastigotes penetrate the host's skin or mucous membrane through abrasion caused by scratching or rubbing the bitten area (b). Trypomastigotes can infect host cardiac, skeletal, smooth muscle, or neural cells, and give rise to the round amastigote form that can replicate intracellularly (c). Amastigotes can give rise to trypomastigotes that can lyse cells (d). Amastigotes and trypomastigotes released from dying cells can propagate the infection or reenter the circulation (e-g). Insects can pick up the parasite when consuming a blood meal (h), and develop the epimastigote form that replicates in the insect gut (i). *(From Macedo AM, Oliveira RP, Pena SD: Chagas' disease: Role of parasite genetic variation in pathogenesis. Expert Rev Mil Med 4:1, 2002.)*

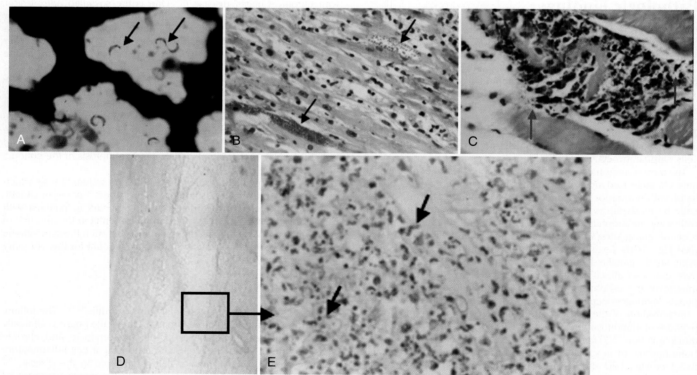

FIGURE 71-2 Microscopic features of acute or reactivation of Chagas' disease. **A,** Diagnosis of the disease is made during the second or third week by microscopic detection of *T. cruzi* organisms in the blood or tissues, appearing in peripheral blood stains as long, slender, C- or S-shaped flagellates, 15 to 20 μm in length (arrows). **B,** Myocardium presenting intracellular nests of amastigotes, which are ovoid, aflagellate forms 2 to 5 μm in length (arrows), and inflammatory mononuclear infiltrate with occasional neutrophils. **C,** Infected ruptured skeletal muscle fiber infiltrated by lymphocytic inflammatory cells, exhibiting many free amastigotes (arrows). **D,** Chagoma-like subcutaneous inflammatory lesion in a reactivation episode of Chagas' disease after heart transplantation. **E,** Close-up view of the lesion in **D,** showing many *T. cruzi* amastigotes in macrophages and endothelial cells stained brown by immunostaining (arrows).

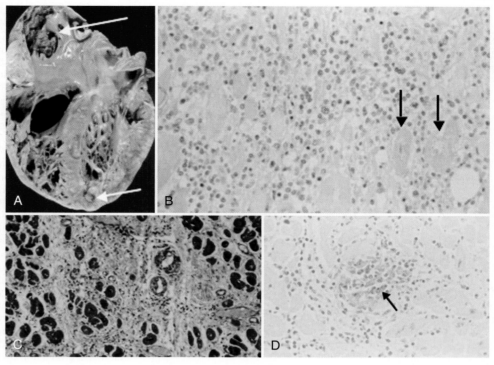

FIGURE 71-3 Macroscopic and microscopic aspects of chronic cardiac Chagas' disease with heart failure. **A,** A dilated globular heart with the most frequent sites of intracavitary thrombosis at the left ventricle apex and right atrial appendage (arrows). **B,** Lymphocytic myocarditis destroying nonparasitized myocardial fibers, suggesting an autoimmune myocarditis. The myofibers exhibit severe hypertrophy with aberrant nuclei (arrows) (H&E stain, ×40). **C,** Ischemic-like fibrotic areas and thin diffuse fibrosis surrounding small groups or individual myocytes (Masson trichrome stain, ×20). **D,** Scarce *T. cruzi* antigens (arrow; immunoperoxidase stain, ×40) surrounded by intense lymphomononuclear inflammatory infiltrate.

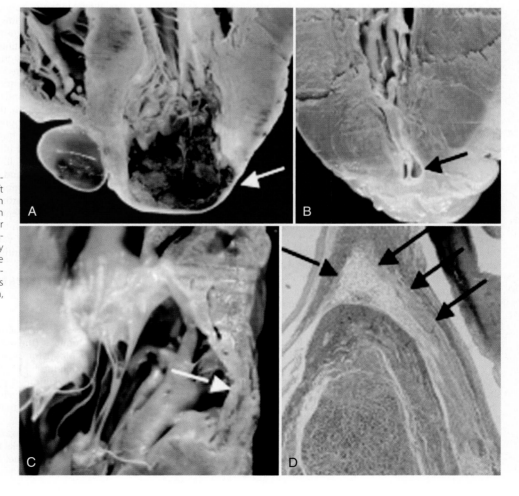

FIGURE 71-4 Necropsy findings of segmental fibrotic chagasic lesions (arrows). **A,** The left ventricle apex lesion shows aneurysm dilation and thrombosis in a patient who died from heart failure. **B,** Focal small apex left ventricular lesion in a sudden death patient. **C,** Lateroposterior basal subvalvar lesion characterized by myocardial wall thinning. **D,** Histology of the conduction system at the His bundle bifurcation, almost completely replaced by fibrosis and adipose tissue (Masson trichrome stain, ×2.5).

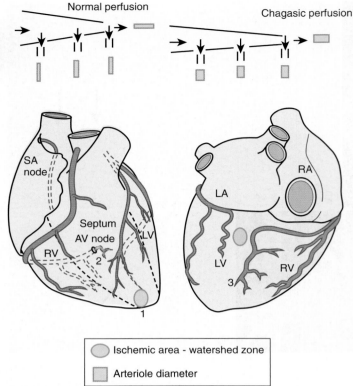

FIGURE 71-5 Schematic representation of three regions that frequently have segmental replacement by fibrosis or adipose tissue in dilated chagasic hearts, and that correspond to watershed regions in the coronary circulation. These lesions may have been caused by ischemia resulting from imbalanced blood flow distribution in the presence of arteriolar vessel dilation. Watershed regions: apex of the left ventricle, irrigated by the anterior and posterior descending interventricular arteries (1); His bundle, irrigated by the crux cordis branch originated from the right coronary artery and septal branch originated from the anterior descending interventricular branch of the left coronary artery (2); lateroposterior basal wall of left ventricle (LV), irrigated by posterior descending right and circumflex coronary arteries. AV = atrioventricular; LA = left atrium; RA = right atrium; RV = right ventricle; SA = sinoatrial.

intensely inflamed heart tissue of patients with Chagas' cardiomyopathy has cast doubt on whether *T. cruzi* antigens trigger myocardial inflammation. The autoimmune hypothesis of pathogenesis has predicted that T cells infiltrating the myocardium should recognize heart proteins as a result of chronic *T. cruzi* infection.[21] Numerous reports have documented autoimmune recognition of neuroantigens, cardiovascular receptors, highly conserved proteins, and cardiac myosin by sera or T cells from patients with Chagas' disease and experimentally infected animals.[22,23] Both *T. cruzi*–specific and autoimmune CD4+ T cells that cross-reactively recognize cardiac myosin and *T. cruzi* proteins populate the myocardium of patients with Chagas' cardiomyopathy, indicating that both antigenic stimuli contribute to sustained inflammation-induced myocardial damage.

Animal studies have shown that inflammatory cytokines play a central part in acute *T. cruzi* infection. Shortly after the acute infection starts, *T. cruzi* components, including DNA and membrane glycoconjugates, trigger innate immunity via Toll-like receptors 2, 4, and 9 in macrophages and dendritic cells.[24] On activation, these cells secrete proinflammatory cytokines and chemokines, express costimulatory receptors, and increase endocytosis and intracellular killing of parasites through the release of reactive oxygen and nitrogen species. The release of proinflammatory cytokines, such as interleukin-1 (IL-1), IL-6, IL-12, IL-18, IL-27, and tumor necrosis factor-α (TNF-α), amplifies and propagates the local inflammatory response. Macrophages and dendritic cells that have endocytosed the parasite subsequently elicit a strong T-cell and antibody response against *T. cruzi*. The resultant *T. cruzi*–specific T cells produce the signature T-helper 1 (Th1) cytokine

interferon-γ (IFN-γ)[25] which, together with other inflammatory cells, migrate to sites of *T. cruzi*-induced inflammation in response to chemokines such as CCL2, CCL3, CCL4, CCL5, CXCL9, and CXCL10.[26] This inflammatory T-cell and antibody response leads to control of, but not complete elimination of, tissue and blood parasitism. Immunologic changes found in the indeterminate and chronic phases of Chagas' disease are consistent with low-grade persistent infection by *T. cruzi*. These changes include moderate to high-titer anti–*T. cruzi* immunoglobulin G (IgG) serum antibodies, increased plasma TNF-α levels, IFN-γ–producing *T. cruzi*–specific CD4+ and CD8+ T cells, and suppressed production of the Th2 cytokine IL-4.

The subset of patients that develops Chagas' cardiomyopathy manifest an array of immunologic alterations consistent with an exacerbated Th1 immune response. They display an increased number of peripheral blood IFN-γ–producing T cells,[25] with reduced numbers of IL-10–producing and FoxP3+ regulatory T cells[19] as compared with patients with indeterminant-phase Chagas' disease. Among patients showing ventricular dysfunction, circulating levels of both TNF-α and CCL2 exceed those in indeterminant-phase patients, or those displaying electrocardiographic alterations but no ventricular dysfunction.[25] The exacerbated Th1 response observed in the peripheral blood reflects the nature of the inflammatory infiltrate found in the myocardium of patients with Chagas' cardiomyopathy.[16] The mononuclear cell inflammatory infiltrate contains macrophages, CCR5+, CXCR3+, and IFN-γ–producing T cells, granzyme-expressing cytotoxic CD8+ T cells, and CD4+ T cells. The chemokines CCL2, CXCL9 and CXCL10, also expressed in Chagas' disease myocardium, attract the cell types found in the infiltrate. Local production of cytokines such as IFN-γ, TNF-α, IL-4, IL-6, IL-7, and IL-15 indicates ongoing T-cell or macrophage activation. Enhanced transforming growth factor-β (TGF-β) signaling may contribute to the pronounced fibrosis found in heart lesions.[19] Increased myocardial expression of adhesion molecules and human leukocyte antigen (HLA) classes I and II result from exposure to cytokines such as IFN-γ and facilitate inflammatory-cell influx and antigen presentation. In vitro experiments have shown that IFN-γ can change the cardiomyocyte gene expression program, inducing the hypertrophic gene expression program and modulating energy metabolism pathways.[22] Together, these observations suggest that IFN-γ–producing T cells migrate to the heart, where IFN-γ–mediated chronic myocardial inflammation could sustain inflammation and act directly on cardiomyocyte function.

The reasons why only one third of infected patients develop Chagas' cardiomyopathy are poorly understood. Familial aggregation of cases suggests a genetic component to risk. Single nucleotide polymorphisms (SNPs) in DNA in immune or inflammatory genes (e.g., *MAL/TIRAP*) involved in signal transduction of Toll-like receptors, the proinflammatory cytokines IL-1β, TNF-α, lymphotoxin-α (LTα), and IL-12β, chemokine CCL2, and chemokine receptor CCR5 are all associated with the development of Chagas' cardiomyopathy. Among patients with Chagas' cardiomyopathy who also have overt heart failure, particular TNF-α genotypes are associated with a significantly shortened survival.[25] Given the important role played by such inflammatory molecules in the various stages of pathogenesis, functional genotypic variants likely influence the course of Chagas' disease.

Clinical Manifestations

Acute Phase

Chagas disease is usually acquired after contact between humans and infected triatomines (the vectors). However, the disease can also be acquired by blood transfusion, contaminated food, across the placenta or through the birth canal, laboratory accidents, or organ transplantation.[1] In addition, in patients in the indeterminate or chronic phases of Chagas' disease, HIV infection may induce the elevation of the parasitemia or the manifestation of symptoms of the acute phase.[27,28]

The acute phase of Chagas' disease is frequently asymptomatic and lasts for the first few weeks or months of the infection.[29] Symptoms may include fever, fatigue, body pain, headache, cutaneous rash, diarrhea, and vomiting. Physical examination shows slight hepatosplenomegaly, lymphadenopathy, and the chagoma. The classic chagoma, or swelling of the eyelid on the side of the face nearest the bite wound, is called the Romaña sign. Even in individuals who manifest symptoms in the acute phase, 90% of these symptoms abate spontaneously within 2 to 12 weeks, but the infection persists, leading to the indeterminate phase of the disease.

Indeterminate and Chronic Phases

The indeterminate phase is asymptomatic and may last indefinitely. The appearance of clinical manifestations[20] defines the onset of the chronic phase and may become apparent through the gradual onset of dementia (3%), cardiomyopathy (30%), or dilation of the digestive tract (6%).

Chagas' cardiomyopathy can cause arrhythmias, heart failure, and sudden death.[11,30] Arrythmias occur in about 50% of patients, and constitute the most frequent clinical manifestation in the chronic phase. Extensive myocardial fibrosis creates a substrate for reentry and for delays in cardiac conduction, including the sinus-atrial node, atrioventricular node, His bundle, His bundle branches, and Purkinje fibers.[20] Polymorphic ventricular extrasystoles are a common finding, followed by complete right bundle branch block, left anterior hemiblock, various degrees of atrioventricular block, and changes in ventricular repolarization. These arrhythmias are generally well tolerated or even unapparent. However, depending on its severity, the atrioventricular block can cause fainting, syncope, and seizures caused by reduced cardiac output and cerebral blood flow.

Myocardial fibrosis can also cause malignant ventricular tachyarrhythmias, a major cause of sudden death in patients with chronic Chagas' disease. Structural abnormalities of the myocardium, such as foci of inflammation and fibrosis, can lead to areas of unidirectional block or slow conduction in circumscribed ventricular regions, and to the formation of reentrant circuits. Such reentrant circuits can occur in various regions in both ventricles, but are more often found in regions of fibrotic thinning of the inferolateral wall of the left ventricle. Accordingly, ventricular arrhythmias typically affect individuals with systolic dysfunction, and rarely those with a normal electrocardiogram (ECG) and cardiac anatomy.

The progressive nature of chronic Chagas' myocarditis promotes a slow replacement of myocardial fibers by fibrosis, leading to systolic dysfunction. The onset of heart failure usually follows the development of ventricular arrhythmias late in the course of chagasic myocardial injury. Once present, heart failure generally leads to death in 5 years or less.

In general, systolic dysfunction in Chagas' disease is biventricular, but the initial clinical manifestation with predominantly right ventricular failure characterizes Chagas' cardiomyopathy. These patients often present with elevated jugular venous pressure, painful hepatomegaly, and pedal edema, without signs of pulmonary congestion or orthopnea. Patients at this stage usually have cardiomegaly, electrocardiographic changes, and diffuse and segmental hypokinesis of both ventricles. Several schemes classify the stages of Chagasic cardiomyopathy.[31]

Carlos Chagas recognized the high prevalence of sudden death in the chronic phase in his original description of the disease in 1912. Sustained ventricular tachycardia progressing to ventricular fibrillation most commonly causes sudden death.[32,33] Less commonly, sudden death can result from ventricular asystole, ventricular failure, or systemic embolism. Near-syncope or syncope, systolic dysfunction, ventricular arrhythmias (sustained or unsustained), sinus node dysfunction, and advanced atrioventricular block may predict sudden death.

Laboratory Evaluation

Diagnosis

For decades, the diagnosis of Chagas' disease has been based on the presence of parasites in the blood or tissues. These techniques are especially useful for monitoring drug therapy for T. cruzi. In the acute phase, parasites can be easily found through microscopic examination of fresh blood. When parasitemia is low, procedures for parasite concentration (e.g., microhematocrit, Strout) or amplification by indirect methods (e.g., xenodiagnosis, blood culture) can aid in the diagnosis.

In the microhematocrit, blood is centrifuged and the parasite sought in the buffy coat. In the Strout preparation, blood cells are removed by precipitation and centrifugation and the parasites are sought microscopically. The xenodiagnostic method consists of feeding uninfected Triatominae with blood from the patient under examination and searching for T. cruzi in the intestinal contents of the insects 30, 60, and 90 days later.[34] In addition to these methods, amplification of T. cruzi DNA by PCR assay recently has become feasible and is the method of choice for the detection of parasites in blood and tissues. Although it is more sensitive than xenodiagnosis and blood culture, the sensitivity of PCR also depends on the parasite burden.

Antibodies against T. cruzi can also support the diagnosis of Chagas' disease—IgM in the early phase, and IgG after the acute phase. Three methods can be used for the indirect diagnosis—hemagglutination, immunofluorescence, and enzyme-linked immunosorbent assay (ELISA). Despite the possibility of false-positive test results for cross reactions with other pathogens or autoimmune diseases, these tests have high sensitivity, and a positive result in two of these tests is sufficient to diagnose the disease. In conjunction with PCR to estimate parasitemia, serologic tests can be used to monitor patients undergoing causative treatment.

Echocardiography (see Chap. 15)

In the early stages of the disease, diastolic dysfunction commonly occurs, resulting from the presence of myocarditis foci on the ventricular wall that reduces its compliance. With the progression of the disease, these foci eventually become hypokinetic, akinetic, or dyskinetic areas. As noted, the involvement of the right ventricle often precedes, and can occur even in the absence of, any anomaly detectable in the left ventricle. Because echocardiography has a low accuracy for detecting right ventricular dysfunction, CMR or radionuclide angiography is preferred for this evaluation. Initially, global systolic dysfunction may be apparent only during stress induced by dobutamine or phenylephrine, indicating reduced systolic reserve. In advanced stages, the region of myocarditis at the apex becomes an aneurysm, and the global systolic function of the left and right ventricles deteriorates.[11,17]

Imaging Studies

RADIONUCLIDE IMAGING (see Chap. 17). Myocardial ischemia in the absence of coronary obstruction often occurs in patients with Chagas' disease and probably relates to autonomic denervation and inflammatory damage in the coronary endothelium. Transient or permanent perfusion defects are often observed, particularly in the apex and inferolateral segments of the left ventricle. Similar changes in coronary endothelium-dependent or -independent vasodilation may also accompany idiopathic dilated cardiomyopathy, suggesting that microvascular dysfunction is unlikely to be pathogen-dependent, but rather is an early sign of ventricular disease.[13,15]

CARDIAC MAGNETIC RESONANCE (see Chap. 18). CMR with delayed hyperenhancement can demonstrate areas of myocardial fibrosis, even in individuals in the indeterminate phase. Early detection of areas of fibrosis may be useful for the characterization and treatment of arrhythmogenic foci and estimation of the severity of myocardial damage.[11,30]

Management

Antitrypanosomal Drug Treatment

Nitrofuran and nitroimidazole derivatives (nifurtimox and benznidazole, respectively) remain the treatment of choice for Chagas' disease.

These compounds exert their trypanosomicidal action by the generation of superoxide anions, causing oxidative stress and cell death in the parasites.[35] In the acute phase or congenital infection, both compounds significantly reduce the parasite load and improve serologic test results. In the indeterminate phase, however, the results are less promising. Although treatment with nitroimidazole derivatives, especially benznidazole, can reduce the blood parasite load and titers of specific antibodies, their effectiveness in delaying or preventing the onset of chronic symptomatic disease is unknown.

In individuals in the chronic phase of Chagas' disease, the benefit of this type of treatment is even less clear. In these subjects, the disappearance of specific antibodies is not common and can take as long as 10 to 20 years. The DNA of the parasite is present in various tissues, and parasite antigens can induce an immune response during treatment and perhaps even disease progression. Current evidence does not demonstrate substantial clinical benefit in the antiparasitic treatment of patients in the chronic phase of Chagas' disease. Recommendations for antitrypanosomal drug treatment vary among different patient categories.[31]

Concomitant Treatment

In the acute phase of the disease, symptoms disappear spontaneously within 2 months. In rare cases of severe acute myocarditis, concomitant treatment with corticosteroids or immunosuppressants has been attempted empirically, with inconsistent results. Studies are too scarce in this small group of patients to validate this treatment strategy. In the chronic phase, mortality from Chagas' disease is caused primarily by heart failure and life-threatening arrhythmias. The treatment of heart failure should resemble that for other cardiomyopathies (see Chap. 28).[36]

In patients with severe heart failure, cardiac transplantation is feasible. Although immunosuppression may cause some complications in patients with Chagas' disease, including reactivation of the disease[37] or the development of cancer,[38] the clinical complications are well known and preventive strategies are well established. Current strategies for changing the degree of immunosuppression, especially the substitution of mycophenolate mofetil for azathioprine or low doses of mycophenolate mofetil, have proven effective in reducing Chagas' disease reactivation.[39] Monitoring for parasitemia is required and reactivation warrants causative treatment.

Prevention of sudden death is of high priority in patients with heart failure secondary to Chagas' disease. As in other patients with heart failure, treatment with amiodarone reduces the incidence of complex ventricular arrhythmias and sudden death. Its effectiveness, however, is further attenuated in patients with severe systolic dysfunction. Thus, ablation by catheter or surgical procedures and implantation of an implantable cardioverter-defibrillator (ICD) is frequently required (see Chaps. 38 and 41). Reentry is the primary arrhythmogenic substrate for ventricular tachyarrhythmias in Chagas' disease, and the circuits typically localize in the perianeurysmal zone or in focal areas of fibrosis in the inferolateral segment of the left ventricle. Surgical aneurysmectomy associated with myocardial or endocardial resection and/or isolation of reentry sites by endocardectomy or cryoablation guided by electrophysiologic mapping has been a treatment of choice.[32,33] Nevertheless, because the mortality of the procedure is high, surgical ablation should be considered in the absence of severe systolic dysfunction and when other surgical procedures, such as aneurysmectomy, are indicated.

Simultaneous percutaneous ablation of endocardial and epicardial sites is an alternative approach for the treatment of patients with Chagas' disease and recurrent ventricular tachycardia who are unfit for surgery. The sites of reentry could be endocardial, intramural, or epicardial, so this combined approach is essential for the treatment of recurrent ventricular tachycardia in these patients. In addition, in patients with severe systolic dysfunction, especially those with left ventricular ejection fraction below 30%, the implantation of an ICD is recommended.

Symptomatic or high-risk bradycardia is often manifested in these patients and limits antiarrhythmic treatment. Thus, concomitant pacemaker and ICD implantation is often indicated. ICDs can prevent death caused by ventricular tachyarrhythmias, but frequent shocks triggered by tachycardia, whether life-threatening or not, may reduce quality of life. Therefore, a combination of ICD, antiarrhythmic therapy, and catheter ablation is the ideal approach for these patients.[32,33]

Chagas' Disease in the United States

An estimated 100,000 individuals infected with *T. cruzi* are in the United States, placing this nation in the top 10 countries with regard to the prevalence of Chagas' disease. Most infected individuals acquired the infection in endemic areas and then migrated to North America, resulting in many unrecognized chronic infections in the United States. There is a small risk of vector-borne infection; approximately six species of insect vectors inhabit the United States. Many common animal species can provide reservoirs for infections, including rodents, dogs, ungulates, squirrels, and skunks. The major cause of new *T. cruzi* infections in North America is transfusion or aquisition from transplanted organs. Screening of donated blood in the United States using a U.S. Food and Drug Administration (FDA)–approved ELISA for *T. cruzi* was instituted in 2007. This program has identified those with unrecognized infection.

The antitrypanosomal drugs benznidazole and nifurtimox are available from the Centers for Disease Control and Prevention (CDC), through the CDC drug service (http://www.cdc.gov/). An excellent recent review provides details regarding the evaluation and treatment of Chagas' disease in the United States, including an algorithm for evaluation of the patient with newly diagnosed *T. cruzi* infection.[31]

REFERENCES

Background

1. Coura JR: Chagas disease: What is known and what is needed—a background article. Mem Inst Oswaldo Cruz 102(Suppl 1):113, 2007.
2. Moncayo A, Silveira AC: Current epidemiological trends for Chagas disease in Latin America and future challenges in epidemiology, surveillance and health policy. Mem Inst Oswaldo Cruz 104 Suppl 1:17, 2007.
3. Andrade Z, Andrade S: Patologia. *In* Brener Z, Andrade Z (eds): Trypanosoma cruzi e doença de Chagas. Guanabara, Brazil, Koogan, 1979, pp 199-248.
4. Bocchi EA, Bellotti G, Mocelin AO, et al: Heart transplantation for chronic Chagas' heart disease. Ann Thorac Surg 61:1727, 1996.

Pathophysiology

5. Cunningham DS, Grogl M, Kuhn RE: Suppression of antibody responses in humans infected with Trypanosoma cruzi. Infect Immun 30:496, 1980.
6. Pereira Barretto AC, Mady C, Arteaga-Fernandez E, et al: Right ventricular endomyocardial biopsy in chronic Chagas' disease. Am Heart J 111:307, 1986.
7. Rossi MA: Fibrosis and inflammatory cells in human chronic chagasic myocarditis: Scanning electron microscopy and immunohistochemical observations. Int J Cardiol 66:183, 1998.
8. Higuchi Mde L, Benvenuti LA, Martins Reis M, Metzger M: Pathophysiology of the heart in Chagas' disease: Current status and new developments. Cardiovasc Res 60:96, 2003.
9. Jones EM, Colley DG, Tostes S, et al: Amplification of a Trypanosoma cruzi DNA sequence from inflammatory lesions in human chagasic cardiomyopathy. Am J Trop Med Hyg 48:348, 1993.
10. Lopes E, Chapadeiro E, Almeida H, Rocha A: Contribuição ao estudo da anatomia patológica dos corações de chagásicos falecidos subitamente. Rev Soc Bras Med Trop 9:269, 1975.
11. Rochitte CE, Oliveira PF, Andrade JM, et al: Myocardial delayed enhancement by magnetic resonance imaging in patients with Chagas' disease: A marker of disease severity. J Am Coll Cardiol 246:1553, 2005.
12. Andrade ZA, Andrade SG, Oliveira GB, Alonso DR: Histopathology of the conducting tissue of the heart in Chagas' myocarditis. Am Heart J 95:316, 1978.
13. Marin-Neto JA, Marzullo P, Marcassa C, et al: Myocardial perfusion abnormalities in chronic Chagas' disease as detected by thallium-201 scintigraphy. Am J Cardiol 69:780, 1992.
14. Higuchi ML, Fukasawa S, De Brito T, et al: Different microcirculatory and interstitial matrix patterns in idiopathic dilated cardiomyopathy and Chagas' disease: A three-dimensional confocal microscopy study. Heart 82:279, 1999.
15. Torres FW, Acquatella H, Condado JA, et al: Coronary vascular reactivity is abnormal in patients with Chagas' heart disease. Am Heart J 129:995, 1995.
16. Higuchi M de L, Gutierrez PS, Aiello VD, et al: Immunohistochemical characterization of infiltrating cells in human chronic chagasic myocarditis: comparison with myocardial rejection process. Virchows Arch A Pathol Anat Histopathol 423:157, 1993.
17. Higuchi M de L, de Morais CF, Pereira Barreto AC, et al: The role of active myocarditis in the development of heart failure in chronic Chagas' disease: A study based on endomyocardial biopsies. Clin Cardiol 10:665, 1987.
18. Araujo FF, Gomes JA, Rocha MO, et al: Potential role of CD4+CD25HIGH regulatory T cells in morbidity in Chagas' disease. Front Biosci 12:2797, 2007.
19. Araujo-Jorge TC, Waghabi MC, Soeiro M de N, et al: Pivotal role for TGF-beta in infectious heart disease: The case of Trypanosoma cruzi infection and consequent Chagasic myocardiopathy. Cytokine Growth Factor Rev 19:405, 2008.

20. Marin-Neto JA, Cunha-Neto E, Maciel BC, Simoes MV: Pathogenesis of chronic Chagas' heart disease. Circulation 115:1109, 2007.

21. Cunha-Neto E, Coelho V, Guilherme L, et al: Autoimmunity in Chagas' disease. Identification of cardiac myosin-B13 Trypanosoma cruzi protein crossreactive T cell clones in heart lesions of a chronic Chagas' cardiomyopathy patient. J Clin Invest 98:1709, 1996.

22. Cunha-Neto E, Dzau VJ, Allen PD, et al: Cardiac gene expression profiling provides evidence for cytokinopathy as a molecular mechanism in Chagas' disease cardiomyopathy. Am J Pathol 167:305, 2005.

23. Fonseca SG, Moins-Teisserenc H, Clave E, et al: Identification of multiple HLA-A*0201-restricted cruzipain and FL-160 CD8+ epitopes recognized by T cells from chronically Trypanosoma cruzi-infected patients. Microbes Infect 7:688, 2005.

24. Bafica A, Santiago HC, Goldszmid R, et al: Cutting edge: TLR9 and TLR2 signaling together account for MyD88-dependent control of parasitemia in Trypanosoma cruzi infection. J Immunol 177:3515, 2006.

25. Bilate AM, Cunha-Neto E: Chagas disease cardiomyopathy: Current concepts of an old disease. Rev Inst Med Trop Sao Paulo 50:67, 2008.

26. Teixeira MM, Gazzinelli RT, Silva JS: Chemokines, inflammation and Trypanosoma cruzi infection. Trends Parasitol 18:262, 2002.

Clinical Manifestations and Management

27. Rosemberg S, Chaves CJ, Higuchi ML, et al: Fatal meningoencephalitis caused by reactivation of Trypanosoma cruzi infection in a patient with AIDS. Neurology 42(Pt 1):640, 1992.

28. Sartori AM, Ibrahim KY, Nunes Westphalen EV, et al: Manifestations of Chagas' disease (American trypanosomiasis) in patients with HIV/AIDS. Ann Trop Med Parasitol 101:31, 2007.

29. Acquatella H, Perez JE, Condado JA, Sanchez I: Limited myocardial contractile reserve and chronotropic incompetence in patients with chronic Chagas' disease: Assessment by dobutamine stress echocardiography. J Am Coll Cardiol 33:522, 1999.

30. Bocchi EA, Kalil R, Bacal F, et al: Magnetic resonance imaging in chronic Chagas' disease: Correlation with endomyocardial biopsy findings and gallium-67 cardiac uptake. Echocardiography 15:279, 1998.

31. Bern C, Montgomery SP, Herwaldt BL, et al: Evaluation and treatment of Chagas' disease in the United States: A systematic review. JAMA 298:2171, 2007.

32. d'Avila A, Splinter R, Svenson RH, et al: New perspectives on catheter-based ablation of ventricular tachycardia complicating Chagas' disease: Experimental evidence of the efficacy of near infrared lasers for catheter ablation of Chagas' VT. J Interv Card Electrophysiol 7:23, 2002.

33. Sosa E, Scanavacca M, D'Avila A, et al: Radiofrequency catheter ablation of ventricular tachycardia guided by nonsurgical epicardial mapping in chronic Chagasic heart disease. Pacing Clin Electrophysiol 22(Pt 1):128, 1999.

34. Schenone H: Xenodiagnosis. Mem Inst Oswaldo Cruz 94(Suppl 1):289, 1999.

35. Villar JC, Marin-Neto JA, Ebrahim S, Yusuf S: Trypanocidal drugs for chronic asymptomatic Trypanosoma cruzi infection. Cochrane Database Syst Rev (1):CD003463, 2002.

36. Ramires FJ, Salemi VM, Ianni BM, et al: Aldosterone antagonism in an inflammatory state: Evidence for myocardial protection. J Renin Angiotensin Aldosterone Syst 7:162, 2006.

37. Bacal F, Silva CP, Bocchi EA, et al: Mycophenylate mofetil increased Chagas' disease reactivation in heart transplanted patients: Comparison between two different protocols. Am J Transplant 5:2017, 2005.

38. Bocchi EA, Higuchi ML, Vieira ML, et al: Higher incidence of malignant neoplasms after heart transplantation for treatment of chronic Chagas' heart disease. J Heart Lung Transplant 17:399, 1998.

39. Bacal F, Silva CP, Pires PV, et al: Transplantation for Chagas' disease: an overview of immunosuppression and reactivation in the last two decades. Clin Transplant 24:E29, 2010.

CHAPTER 72

Cardiovascular Abnormalities in HIV-Infected Individuals

Stacy D. Fisher and Steven E. Lipshultz

Background

Infection with the human immunodeficiency virus (HIV) is one of the leading causes of acquired heart disease and specifically of symptomatic heart failure and pulmonary arterial hypertension (**Table 72-1**). Cardiac complications of HIV infection tend to occur late in the disease or are associated with related therapies and are therefore becoming more prevalent as therapy and longevity improve.[1-6] Complicated drug therapies for HIV infection have sustained life but may increase cardiovascular risk and accelerate atherosclerotic disease and events.[7]

Approximately 33 million adults and children were living with HIV infection at the end of 2007. Two million deaths and 2.7 million new infections were reported that year. In the United States, approximately 10% of those infected are older than 50 years and more than 85% of HIV-infected individuals survive more than 10 years.[8,9] The 2- to 5-year incidence of symptomatic heart failure ranges from 4% to 28%,[1,10] suggesting a prevalence of symptomatic HIV-related heart failure of between 4 and 5 million cases worldwide. Among HIV-infected children, up to 10 years of age, 25% die with chronic cardiac disease, and 28% experience serious cardiac events after an AIDS-defining illness.[11] Antiretroviral therapy clearly increases survival, and goals now involve balancing survival and toxicities with therapy. As survival improves, atherosclerotic cardiovascular disease has become an increasingly important cause of morbidity and mortality among patients with HIV infection (**Fig. 72-1**).

A range of cardiac abnormalities (see Table 72-1) associated with HIV infection has been suggested by autopsy studies; the conditions, in order of frequency, are pericardial effusion, lymphocytic interstitial myocarditis, dilated cardiomyopathy (frequently with myocarditis), infective endocarditis, and malignancy (myocardial Kaposi sarcoma and B-cell immunoblastic lymphoma).[3,4] Even more prevalent are drug effects and interactions, which directly challenge the cardiovascular system.

Left Ventricular Dysfunction

Left Ventricular Systolic Dysfunction

CLINICAL PRESENTATION. In HIV-infected patients, concurrent pulmonary infections, pulmonary hypertension, anemia, portal hypertension, malnutrition, or malignancy can alter or confuse the characteristic signs that define heart failure in other populations. Thus, patients with left ventricular systolic dysfunction can be asymptomatic or can present with New York Heart Association Class III or IV heart failure.

Echocardiography (see Chap. 15) is useful for assessing left ventricular systolic function in this population and, in addition to diagnosing left ventricular dysfunction, often reveals low to normal wall thickness or left ventricular hypertrophy and a dilated left ventricle.[5,12] Echocardiography should be performed in any patient at elevated cardiovascular risk, with any clinical manifestations of cardiovascular disease, or with unexplained or persistent pulmonary symptoms or viral coinfections at baseline and every 1 to 2 years thereafter, or as clinically indicated.[11]

Electrocardiography (see Chap. 13) can reveal nonspecific conduction defects or repolarization changes. The chest radiograph has low sensitivity and specificity for congestive heart failure in patients with HIV infection.[13] In small studies of HIV-infected patients and large populations of patients without HIV infection, brain natriuretic peptide levels have been inversely correlated with left ventricular ejection fraction and can be useful in the differential diagnosis of congestive cardiomyopathy in HIV-infected patients.[14]

Patients with encephalopathy are more likely to die of congestive heart failure than those without encephalopathy (hazard ratio, 3.4).[15] HIV persists in reservoir cells in the myocardium and the cerebral cortex, even after antiretroviral therapy. These cells seem to be important in the development and progression of cardiomyopathy and encephalopathy. Reservoir cells may hold HIV on their surfaces for extended periods of time and cause progressive tissue damage by chronic release of cytotoxic cytokines.

INCIDENCE. A 4-year observational study of 296 patients with a spectrum of HIV-related disease before highly active antiretroviral therapy (HAART) found 44 (15%) with dilated cardiomyopathy (fractional shortening < 28%, with global left ventricular hypokinesis), 13 (4%) with isolated right ventricular dysfunction (right ventricle larger than left ventricle on standard two-dimensional views), and 12 (4%) with borderline left ventricular dysfunction (left ventricular end-systolic diameter > 58 mm but fractional shortening > 28%, or global dysfunction reported by one or two but not all three observers).[1] Dilated cardiomyopathy was strongly associated with a CD4 count lower than 100 cells/mL.[5]

Left ventricular (LV) dysfunction is a common consequence of HIV infection in children. In a study of 205 children infected with HIV by maternal-fetal transmission (enrolled at a median age of 22 months and observed with echocardiography every 4 to 6 months and with electrocardiography, Holter monitoring, and chest radiography every year), the prevalence of decreased left ventricular function (fractional shortening < 28%) was 5.7%. The 2-year cumulative incidence was 15.3%.[4] The cumulative incidence of symptomatic congestive heart failure, the use of cardiac medications, or both was 10% over 2 years.[16] Progressive LV dilation is common in HIV-infected children, may be a harbinger of congestive heart failure (CHF; 5-year cumulative incidence, 12.3%), and is associated with inadequate LV hypertrophy, elevated afterload, and reduced LV function.

PATHOGENESIS. A wide variety of possible causative agents has been postulated for HIV-related cardiomyopathy (see Table 72-1), including myocardial infection with HIV itself, opportunistic infections,

TABLE 72-1 Summary of HIV-Associated Cardiovascular Diseases

TYPE OF DISEASE	POSSIBLE CAUSES	INCIDENCE, PREVALENCE	DIAGNOSIS	TREATMENT
Dilated cardiomyopathy	Drug-related: Cocaine, AZT, IL-2, doxorubicin, interferon. Infectious: HIV, toxo-plasma, coxsackievirus group B, EBV, CMV, adenovirus. Metabolic or endocrine: selenium or carnitine deficiency, anemia, hypocalcemia, hypophosphatemia, hyponatremia, hypokalemia, hypoalbuminemia, hypothyroidism, growth hormone deficiency, adrenal insufficiency, hyperinsulinemia, hemochromatosis, pheochromocytoma, sarcoidosis, amyloidosis. Cytokines: TNF-α, nitric oxide, TGF-β, endothelin-I, interleukins. Immunodeficiency: CD4 < 100 cells/mm^3. Autoimmune factors	≤8% of asymptomatic patients; ≤25% of autopsy cases; systolic > diastolic	Chest radiograph findings: Nonspecific conduction abnormalities, PVCs, PACs. Echocardiographic findings: Low-normal LV wall thickness, increased LV mass, dilated LV, systolic LV dysfunction. Possible laboratory studies: Troponin T, brain natriuretic peptide, CD4 count, viral load, viral PCR, Toxoplasma serology, thyroid-stimulating hormone, cortisol, carnitine, selenium, serum ACE, vanillylmandelic acid, amyloid, urinanalysis, stress testing, myocardial biopsy, cardiac catheterization	Diuretics, digoxin, ACE inhibitors, beta blockers. Adjunctive treatment in HIV patients: Treatment of infection, nutritional replacement, IVIg. Intensify antiretroviral therapy. Follow-up: Serial echocardiograms
Pericardial	Bacteria: Staphylococcus, Streptococcus, Proteus, Klebsiella, Enterococcus, Listeria, Nocardia, Mycobacterium. Viral pathogens: HIV, HSV, CMV, adenovirus, echovirus. Other pathogens: Cryptococcus, Toxoplasma, Histoplasma. Malignancy: Kaposi sarcoma, lymphoma, capillary leak, wasting, malnutrition. Hypothyroidism. Immunodeficiency. Uremia	11%/yr; spontaneous resolution in 42% of affected patients; ≈30% increase in 6-mo mortality	Pericardial rub on examination. Echocardiogram. Fluid analysis for gram stain, and culture, cytology. ECG: Low voltage, PR depression. Associated pleural and peritoneal fluid analysis. Pericardial biopsy	Treat the cause. Follow-up: Serial echocardiograms. Intensify antiretroviral therapy. Pericardiocentesis or window
Infective endocarditis	Autoimmune factors. Bacteria: Staphylococcus aureus or Staphylococcus epidermidis, Salmonella, Streptococcus, Haemophilus parainfluenzae, Pseudallescheria boydii, HACEK (see Chap. 67). Fungal: Aspergillus fumigatus, Candida, Cryptococcus neoformans	6% increased incidence in IVDA, regardless of HIV status	Blood cultures; echocardiogram	IV antibiotics, valve replacements
Nonbacterial thrombotic endocarditis	Valvular damage, vitamin C deficiency, malnutrition, wasting, DIC, hypercoagulable state, prolonged acquired immunodeficiency	Rare but clinically relevant emboli in 42% of cases	Echocardiogram	Anticoagulation, treat vasculitis or underlying illness
Malignancy	Kaposi sarcoma, non-Hodgkin lymphoma, leiomyosarcoma, low CD4 count, prolonged immunodeficiency, HHV-8, EBV	Approximately 1% incidence; usually metastatic in HIV-positive patients	Echocardiogram, biopsy	Chemotherapy possible
Right ventricular and pulmonary disease	Recurrent pulmonary infections, pulmonary arteritis, microvascular pulmonary emboli		ECG, echocardiogram, right heart catheterization	Diuretics, treat underlying lung infection or disease, anticoagulation
Primary pulmonary hypertension	Plexogenic pulmonary arteriopathy	0.5%	ECG, echocardiogram, right heart catheterization	Anticoagulation, vasodilators, prostacyclin analogues
Vasculitis	Drug therapy with antibiotics and antivirals	Increasing incidence	Clinical diagnosis	Systemic corticosteroids, withdrawal of drug
Accelerated atherosclerosis	Protease inhibitors, atherogenesis with virus-infected macrophages, chronic inflammation, glucose intolerance, dyslipidemia	≤8% prevalence	Stress testing, echocardiogram, lipid profile, CT angiogram, calcium scoring	Minimize risk factors, exercise, controversial statin use
Autonomic dysfunction	CNS disease, drug therapy, prolonged immunodeficiency, malnutrition	Increased in patients with CNS disease	Tilt-table test, Holter monitoring	Procedural precautions
Arrhythmias	Drug therapy, pentamidine, autonomic dysfunction, acidosis electrolyte abnormalities		ECG: Long-QT, Holter monitoring, exercise stress testing	Discontinue drug, procedural precautions
Lipodystrophy	Drug therapy: Protease inhibitors		Echocardiogram, lipid profile, cardiac catheterization, coronary calcium score	Lipid therapy (beware of drug interactions), aerobic exercise, altered antiretroviral therapy, cosmetic surgery, fat implantation

CMV = cytomegalovirus; DIC = disseminated intravascular coagulation; EBV = Epstein-Barr virus; ECG = electrocardiogram; HSV = herpes simplex virus; HTN = hypertension; IVDA = intravenous drug abuse; IVIg = intravenous immunoglobulin; PAC = premature atrial complex; PCR = polymerase chain reaction; PVC = premature ventricular complex.

CH 72 CARDIOVASCULAR ABNORMALITIES IN HIV-INFECTED INDIVIDUALS

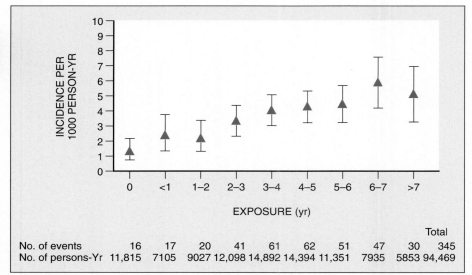

									Total
No. of events	16	17	20	41	61	62	51	47	30 345
No. of persons-Yr	11,815	7105	9027	12,098	14,892	14,394	11,351	7935	5853 94,469

FIGURE 72-1 Risk of myocardial infarction according to exposure to combination antiretroviral therapy. The crude incidence of primary events was assessed beginning at baseline according to the cumulative duration of combination antiretroviral therapy since the initiation of therapy, stratified in 1-year intervals from the initiation of therapy to more than 7 years of exposure. The adjusted relative rate of myocardial infarction according to cumulative exposure to combination antiretroviral therapy was 1.16/year of exposure (95% confidence interval [CI], 1.09 to 1.23). The I bars denote the 95% CIs. *(From DAD Study Group: Class of antiretroviral drugs and the risk of myocardial infarction. N Engl J Med 356:1723, 2007.)*

viral infections, autoimmune response to viral infection, cardiotoxicity or direct mitochondrial injury from therapeutic or illicit drugs, nutritional deficiencies, and cytokine overexpression.

Myocarditis is perhaps the best studied of the possible causes (see Chap. 70). Dilated cardiomyopathy can be related to a direct action of HIV on the myocardial tissue or to proteolytic enzymes or cytokine mediators induced by HIV alone or in conjunction with coinfecting viruses.[16-18] *Toxoplasma gondii,* coxsackievirus group B, Epstein-Barr virus, cytomegalovirus, adenovirus, and HIV in myocytes have been found in biopsy specimens.

Autopsy and biopsy results have revealed only scant and patchy inflammatory cell infiltrates in the myocardium.[11,17] HIV can clearly infect myocardial interstitial cells but not the cardiac myocyte. Increased numbers of infected interstitial cells have been found in patients with confirmed myocarditis in which proteolytic enzymes or increased levels of tumor necrosis factor-α (TNF-α) or interleukin may injure the myocytes. Increased levels of TNF-α, inducible nitric oxide synthase, and interleukin-6 in affected patients and experimental models have been reported.

Notably, HIV-related cardiomyopathy is often not associated with any specific opportunistic infection, and approximately 40% of patients have not experienced any opportunistic infection before the onset of cardiac symptoms.[11]

Pathogenesis in Children

In children with vertically transmitted HIV infection, two mechanisms of pathogenesis have been described. One is dilation of the left ventricle with a reduction in the ratio of thickness to end-systolic dimension of the ventricle. The other is concentric hypertrophy of the muscle; with dilation, the ratio of thickness to end-systolic dimension remains normal or is increased.[5]

CYTOKINE ALTERATIONS. HIV infection increases the production of TNF-α, which alters intracellular calcium homeostasis and increases nitric oxide production, transforming growth factor-β, and endothelin-1 upregulation.[15] High levels of nitric oxide induced experimentally had a negative inotropic effect and were cytotoxic to myocytes.

In one study, HIV-infected individuals with dilated cardiomyopathy were much more likely to have myocarditis and had a broader spectrum of viral infections than HIV-negative patients with idiopathic dilated cardiomyopathy. Also, levels of TNF-α and induced nitric oxide synthase were higher in myocytes from the HIV-infected patients with dilated cardiomyopathy, particularly those with viral coinfections, and levels varied inversely with the CD4 count. Immunodeficiency may favor the selection of those viral variants with increased pathogenicity or enhance the cardiovirulence of viral strains.[15,17]

NUTRITIONAL DEFICIENCIES. Nutritional deficiencies are common in HIV infection, particularly in those with late-stage disease. Poor absorption and diarrhea both lead to electrolyte imbalances and deficiencies in elemental nutrients. Deficiencies of trace elements have been associated with cardiomyopathy. For example, selenium deficiency increases the virulence of coxsackie virus to cardiac tissue.[11] Selenium replacement reverses cardiomyopathy and restores LV function in nutritionally depleted patients. Levels of vitamin B_{12}, carnitine, and growth and thyroid hormone can also be altered in HIV disease; all have been associated with LV dysfunction.

COURSE OF DISEASE. Patients with asymptomatic LV dysfunction (fractional shortening < 28%, with global left ventricular hypokinesis) may have transient disease by echocardiographic criteria. In one serial echocardiographic study, three of six patients with abnormal fractional shortening had normal readings after a mean of 9 months. The three with persistently depressed LV function died within 1 year of baseline.[11]

PROGNOSIS. Mortality in HIV-infected patients with cardiomyopathy is increased, independently of CD4 count, age, gender, and HIV risk group. The median survival to AIDS-related death was 101 days in patients with LV dysfunction and 472 days in patients with a normal heart at a similar stage of infection before HAART (see Fig. 72-1).[1,11] Isolated right ventricular dysfunction or borderline LV dysfunction did not place patients at risk.

In the Pediatric Pulmonary and Cardiovascular Complications of Vertically Transmitted HIV Infection (P2C2 HIV) study of children with vertically transmitted HIV infection (median age, 2.1 years), 5-year cumulative survival was 64%.[10] Mortality was higher in children with baseline measurements showing depressed left ventricular fractional shortening or increased LV dimension, thickness, mass, wall stress, heart rate, or blood pressure. Decreased LV fractional shortening and increased wall thickness also predicted survival after adjustment for age, height, CD4 count, HIV RNA copy number, clinical center, and encephalopathy[3,4] (**Fig. 72-2**).

Fractional shortening was abnormal for up to 3 years before death, whereas wall thickness identified a population at risk only 18 to 24 months before death. Thus, in children, fractional shortening may be a useful long-term predictor, and wall thickness may be a useful short-term predictor of mortality.[19]

Postmortem cardiomegaly was associated with echocardiographic evidence of increased LV mass and documented chronically increased heart rate before death but not with anemia, encephalopathy, or HIV viral load.[12] In HIV-infected children, mild persistent depression of LV function and elevated LV mass were associated with higher all-cause mortality.[19] A 2-SD decrease in LV fractional shortening from 34% to 30% in a 10-year old, levels that most cardiologists would not consider to be action values, is associated with an increase in 5-year mortality from 15% to 55%.

Rapid-onset congestive heart failure has a grim prognosis in HIV-infected adults and children, with more than half of patients dying

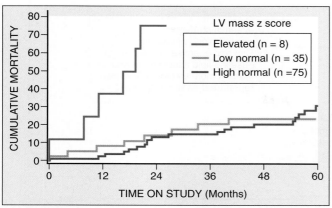

FIGURE 72-2 Mildly increased LV mass is a risk marker for early HIV mortality, even though it is still inadequate for LV dimension. This National Heart, Lung and Blood Institute study shows cumulative mortality in 113 HIV-infected children by degree of LV mass abnormality. *(From Fisher SD, Easley KA, Orav EJ, et al: Mild dilated cardiomyopathy and increased LV mass predict mortality: The prospective P2C2 HIV Multicenter Study. Am Heart J 150:439, 2005.)*

from primary cardiac failure within 12 months of presentation.[10,11] Chronic-onset heart failure may respond better to medical therapy in these patients.

THERAPY. Therapy for dilated cardiomyopathy associated with HIV infection is generally similar to therapy for nonischemic cardiomyopathy. It includes diuretics, digoxin, beta blockers, aldosterone antagonists, and angiotension-converting enzyme (ACE) inhibitors, as tolerated (see Chap. 28). No studies have investigated the efficacy of specific cardiac therapeutic regimens other than intravenous immunoglobulin.[2] A suggested evaluation of cardiac dysfunction is presented in **Figure 72-3**.

Opportunistic or other infections should be sought aggressively and treated to improve or resolve the cardiomyopathy. Right ventricular biopsy may be useful for identifying infectious causes of failure and to suggest targeted therapy.[11,13] However, right ventricular biopsy is probably underused.

After medical therapy is begun, serial echocardiographic studies should be performed at 4-month intervals (see Fig. 72-3).[13] Monitoring recommendations for testing and timing of follow-up are based on studies relating impairment of fractional shortening to a worse prognosis. If function continues to worsen or the clinical course deteriorates, a biopsy should be considered. Patients with congestive heart failure who have not responded to 2 weeks of medical therapy may benefit from cardiac catheterization and endomyocardial biopsy, which may reveal lymphocytic infiltrates suggesting myocarditis or treatable opportunistic infections (by special stains), permitting aggressive therapy of an underlying pathogen. Tissue should be evaluated for the presence of abnormal mitochondria that could benefit from an antiretroviral drug holiday. Angiography should be performed selectively if there are risk factors for atherosclerotic disease or suggestive clinical symptoms.

Intravenous immunoglobulins have had some success in treating acute congestive cardiomyopathy and nonspecific myocarditis in patients who are not infected with HIV. Monthly immunoglobulin infusions in HIV-infected children have minimized LV dysfunction, increased LV wall thickness, and reduced peak LV wall stress, suggesting that both impaired myocardial growth and LV dysfunction can be immunologically mediated.[2]

Patients should be evaluated for nutritional status, and any patients with deficiencies should receive supplements. Supplementation with selenium, carnitine, multivitamins, or all three can be helpful, especially for anorexic patients or those with wasting or diarrhea syndromes.

Heart transplantation has been reported, including one HIV-infected man believed to have anthracycline-related cardiomyopathy. At 24 months of follow-up, his course was complicated by more frequent and higher grade episodes of rejection than average, but otherwise was relatively uneventful and productive.[20] Transplantation therapy is not currently widely available but is an area of active consideration and discussion.

ANIMAL MODELS. Chronic pathogenic simian immunodeficiency virus (SIV) infection in rhesus macaques has resulted in marked depression of LV ejection fraction and extensive coronary arteriopathy suggestive of a cell-mediated immune response.[21] Notably, 9 of 15 chronically infected macaques who died of SIV had myocardial pathology with lymphocytic myocarditis, and 9 had coronary arteriopathy (6 alone and 3 in combination with myocarditis). Coronary arteriopathy was associated with evidence of vessel occlusion and recanalization, with associated areas of myocardial necrosis in four animals. Two animals had marantic endocarditis, and one had a LV mural thrombus. Animals with cardiac pathology were emaciated to a greater extent than those with SIV and similar periods of infection who did not experience cardiac pathology.

Transgenic mouse models with cardiac pathologic changes have been studied and may help evaluate the impact of environmental factors, therapeutic or illicit drugs, or drug combinations in both the cause and treatment of HIV-associated myocarditis.[22]

Left Ventricular Diastolic Dysfunction

Clinical and echocardiographic findings suggest that diastolic dysfunction (see Chaps. 25 and 27) is relatively common in long-term survivors of HIV infection. LV diastolic dysfunction may precede systolic dysfunction.[7,16,18]

Pericardial Effusion (see Chap. 75)

CLINICAL PRESENTATION. HIV-infected patients with pericardial effusions generally have a lower CD4 count than those without effusions, indicating more advanced disease.[7,18] Effusions are generally small and asymptomatic.

INCIDENCE. Asymptomatic pericardial effusions are common in HIV-infected patients. The 5-year Prospective Evaluation of Cardiac Involvement in AIDS (PRECIA) study found that 16 of 231 patients (59 patients with asymptomatic HIV, 62 with AIDS-related complex, and 74 with AIDS) had pericardial effusions.[18] Three had an effusion on enrollment and 13 experienced effusions during follow-up (12 had AIDS). Pericardial effusions were small (maximum pericardial space < 10 mm at end-diastole) in 13 and asymptomatic in 14 patients. The incidence of pericardial effusion in those with AIDS was 11%/year. The prevalence of effusion in AIDS patients increases over time, reaching a mean in asymptomatic patients of about 22% after 25 months of follow-up.

HIV infection should be suspected whenever young patients have pericardial effusion or tamponade. In a retrospective series of cardiac tamponade cases in a city hospital, 13 of 37 patients (35%) had HIV infection.[11]

PATHOGENESIS. Pericardial effusion may be related to an opportunistic infection, metabolic abnormality, or malignancy (see Table 72-1), but usually the cause is not clear. The effusion is often part of a generalized serous effusive process also involving pleural and peritoneal surfaces. This capillary leak syndrome may be related to enhanced cytokine production in the later stages of HIV disease. Other causes can include uremia from HIV-associated nephropathy or drug nephrotoxicity. Fibrinous pericarditis with or without effusion is also well described, constituting 9% of cardiac lesions found in AIDS patients in one autopsy series.[18]

COURSE OF DISEASE AND PROGNOSIS. Effusion markedly increases mortality. For example, in the PRECIA study, it almost tripled the risk of death among AIDS patients.[17] Also, 2 of 16 patients with effusions experienced pericardial tamponade. Pericardial effusion may, however, resolve spontaneously in up to 42% of patients.[11]

MONITORING AND THERAPY. Screening echocardiography is recommended for HIV-infected individuals, regardless of the stage of disease.[13] All HIV-infected patients with evidence of heart failure, Kaposi sarcoma, tuberculosis, or other pulmonary infections should undergo baseline echocardiography and electrocardiographic testing.

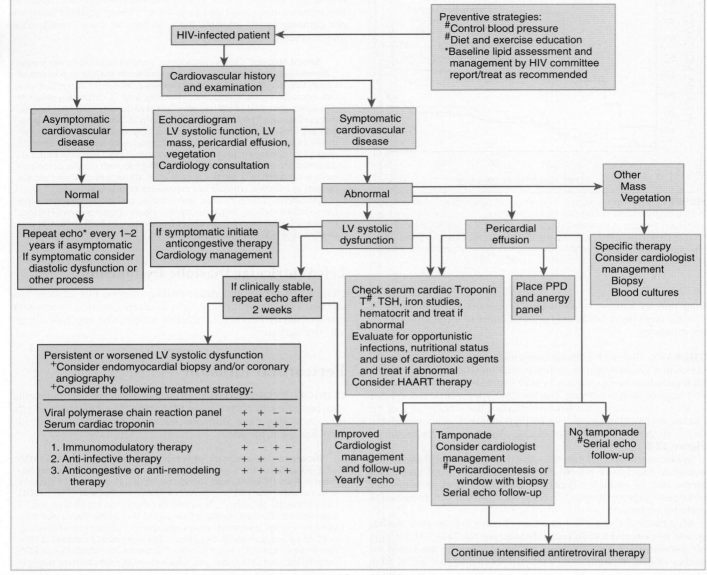

FIGURE 72-3 Cardiac dysfunction in HIV-infected patients. *Evidence-based; #non-HIV standard of care data; +considered for future research. PPD = purified protein derivative; TSH = thyroid-stimulating hormone. *(From Dolin R, Masur H, Saag MS [eds]: AIDS Therapy. 2nd ed. New York, Churchill Livingstone, 2003, p 817.)*

Patients should undergo pericardiocentesis if they have pericardial effusion and clinical signs of tamponade (e.g., elevated jugular venous pressure, dyspnea, hypotension, persistent tachycardia, pulsus paradoxus) or echocardiographic signs of tamponade (e.g., continuous-wave Doppler evidence of respiratory variation in valvular inflow, septal bounce, right ventricular diastolic collapse, a large effusion).

Patients with pericardial effusion without tamponade should be evaluated for treatable opportunistic infections, such as tuberculosis, and for malignancy. Highly active antiretroviral therapy (HAART) should be considered if therapy has not already been instituted. Repeated echocardiography is recommended after 1 month, or sooner if clinical symptoms direct (see Fig. 72-3).

Other Disorders

Infective Endocarditis

Injection drug users are at greater risk than the general population for infective endocarditis, chiefly of right-sided heart valves (see Chap. 67). Surprisingly, HIV-infected patients may not have a higher incidence of endocarditis than people with similar risk behaviors.[7]

Because the autoimmune response to bacterial endocarditis is often largely responsible for the valvular destruction associated with endocarditis, the course of the disease in HIV-infected patients may vary. For example, HIV-infected patients have a higher risk of salmonella endocarditis than immunocompetent patients because they are more likely to experience salmonella bacteremia during salmonella infection. However, they respond better to antibiotic therapy and may be less likely to sustain valvular damage because of their impaired immune response.[11,18,23]

Common organisms associated with endocarditis in HIV-infected patients include *Staphylococcus aureus* and *Salmonella* species. Fungal endocarditis with organisms such as *Aspergillus fumigatus*, *Candida* species, and *Cryptococcus neoformans* are more common in intravenous drug users with HIV than in those without it, and again may be responsive to therapy (see Table 72-1).[11]

Fulminant courses of infective endocarditis with high mortality can occur in late-stage AIDS patients with poor nutritional status and severely compromised immune systems, but several patients have been successfully treated with antibiotic therapy. Operative indications in HIV-infected patients with endocarditis include hemodynamic instability, failure to sterilize blood cultures after appropriate intravenous antibiotics, and severe valvular destruction in patients with a reasonable life expectancy after recovery from surgery.

Nonbacterial Thrombotic Endocarditis

Nonbacterial thrombotic endocarditis (or marantic endocarditis) involves large, friable, sterile vegetations that form on the cardiac valves. These lesions have been associated with disseminated intravascular coagulation and systemic embolization. Lesions are rarely diagnosed ante mortem; among patients who do receive the diagnosis, clinically relevant emboli occur in a high percentage of cases.[11] In the early HIV epidemic, several case series suggested a high incidence of this uncommon disorder; however, few cases have since been reported, and almost none have been found in prospective series. Marantic endocarditis should be suspected in any patient with systemic embolization, but should be considered rare in AIDS patients.

Treatment of nonbacterial thrombotic endocarditis should focus on reducing the underlying disease causing coagulation abnormalities, valvular endothelial damage, or both. An anticoagulation risk-benefit assessment must be made on an individual basis.

Cardiovascular Malignancy

Malignancy affects many AIDS patients, generally in the later stages of disease (see Chap. 74). Cardiac malignancy is usually metastatic disease.

Kaposi sarcoma (angiosarcoma) is associated with human herpesvirus 8 and affects up to 35% of AIDS patients, particularly homosexuals, with an incidence inversely related to the CD4 count. Autopsy studies have found that 28% of HIV-infected patients with widespread Kaposi sarcoma had cardiac involvement and rarely described it as a primary cardiac tumor.[3] Kaposi sarcoma has not been found invading the coronary arteries but is often an endothelial cell neoplasm, with a predilection in the heart for subpericardial fat around the coronary arteries.

Kaposi sarcoma involving the heart is generally an incidental finding at autopsy and rarely causes cardiac symptoms. Specific symptoms can be related to pericardial effusion associated with the epicardial location of the tumor. Pericardial fluid in patients with cardiac Kaposi sarcoma is typically serosanguineous, without malignant cells or infection.[3]

Kaposi sarcoma is difficult to treat, although most affected patients die from opportunistic infections related to the advanced stage of immunodeficiency rather than from the malignancy. Protease inhibitors have significantly decreased the incidence of Kaposi sarcoma from the reported incidence in the pre-HAART era.[24]

Primary cardiac malignancy associated with HIV infection is generally caused by cardiac lymphoma. Non-Hodgkin lymphomas are 25 to 60 times more common in HIV-infected individuals. They are the first manifestation of AIDS in up to 4% of new cases.[3] Patients with primary cardiac lymphoma can present with dyspnea, right-sided heart failure, biventricular failure, chest pain, or arrhythmias. Cardiac lymphoma is associated with rapid progression to cardiac tamponade, symptoms of congestive heart failure, myocardial infarction (MI), tachyarrhythmias, conduction abnormalities, or superior vena cava syndrome. Pericardial fluid typically reveals malignant cells but can be histologically normal. Systemic multiagent chemotherapy with and without concomitant radiation or surgery has been beneficial for some patients, but overall the prognosis is poor (**Fig. 72-4**). HAART has not substantially affected the incidence of HIV-related non-Hodgkin lymphomas, but cumulative viremia has been associated, even during HAART therapy.[25] An intracardiac mass in late-stage HIV infection is associated with a uniformly poor prognosis.

Isolated Right Ventricular Disease

Isolated right ventricular hypertrophy, with or without right ventricular dilation, is relatively uncommon in HIV-infected individuals and is generally related to pulmonary disease that increases

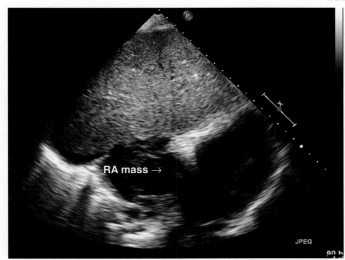

FIGURE 72-4 Burkitt's lymphoma in an AIDS patient. This four-chamber apical echocardiogram view shows near obliteration of the right atrial (RA) cavity, with tumor invading through hepatic veins directly into the right atrium.

pulmonary vascular resistance. Possible causes include multiple bronchopulmonary infections, pulmonary arteritis from the immunologic effects of HIV disease, or microvascular pulmonary emboli caused by thrombus or contaminants in injected drugs.

Pulmonary Hypertension

Primary pulmonary arterial hypertension (see Chap. 78) has been described in a disproportionate number of HIV-infected individuals, estimated to occur in about 0.5% of hospitalized AIDS patients.[4,7] Histologic analysis often reveals plexogenic pulmonary arteriopathy characterized by remodeling of the pulmonary vasculature, with intimal fibrosis and replacement of normal endothelial structure. All these patients had clear lung fields on examination and chest radiography and normal perfusion scans.

Primary pulmonary arterial hypertension (PAH) has been reported in HIV-infected patients without a history of thromboembolic disease, intravenous drug use, or pulmonary infections associated with HIV.[4] One autopsy and one biopsy specimen revealed precapillary muscular pulmonary artery and arteriole medial hypertrophy, fibroelastosis, and eccentric intimal fibrosis, without direct viral infection of pulmonary artery cells. This finding suggests mediator release from infected cells elsewhere. Primary PAH has also been found in hemophiliacs receiving lyophilized factor VIII, intravenous drug users, and patients with LV dysfunction, obscuring any relationship with HIV. A controversial association is present between human herpesvirus 8 (HHV-8) and PAH. It may be that HIV or a coinfection causes endothelial damage and mediator-related vasoconstriction of the pulmonary arteries.

The CD4 count has been independently associated with survival in HIV PAH patients, and pulmonary hypertension was the direct cause of death in 72% of those affected. Survival rates at 1, 2, and 3 years were 73%, 60%, and 47%, respectively. Survival rates in New York Heart Association functional Class III and IV patients at the time of diagnosis were 60%, 45%, and 28%.[26,27]

A high rate or response has been reported to vasodilator testing (37%) in HIV PAH patients.[27,28] Standard treatments for PAH including prostaglandin E5 (PGE5) inhibitors, endothelin antagonists, and prostacyclin analogues have all been shown effective in the HIV infected population. Therapy also includes anticoagulation (on the basis of individual risk-benefit analysis). HAART has been continued in affected patients. Notably, in HIV PAH patients, the PAH is the immediate threat to life and should be aggressively approached. Best current practice is to follow guidelines set for PAH patients because the morbidity and mortality reflect the PAH more than the HIV infection and respond to current strategies.

Vasculitis

Clinically, suspicion occurs in the setting of fever of unknown origin, unexplained multisystem disease, unexplained arthritis or myositis, glomerulonephritis, peripheral neuropathy, especially mononeuritis multiplex, or unexplained gastrointestinal, cardiac, or central nervous system (CNS) ischemia. Many types of vasculitis (see Chap. 89) have been described in HIV-infected patients, including systemic necrotizing vasculitis, hypersensitivity vasculitis, Henoch-Schönlein purpura, lymphomatoid granulomatosis, and primary angiitis of the CNS. Successful immunomodulatory therapy, chiefly with systemic corticosteroid therapy, has been described.

HIV protein transactivator of transcription (tat) has been implicated in the pathogenesis of vasculitis, where transduction of this gene into a monocyte cell line led to TNF-α and TNF-β production.

Accelerated Atherosclerosis

Accelerated atherosclerosis (see Chap. 43) has been observed in young HIV-infected adults and children without traditional coronary risk factors.[29,30] Pronounced coronary lesions were discovered at autopsy in several HIV-positive patients 23 to 32 years of age who died unexpectedly. Endothelial dysfunction is possibly the most plausible link between HIV infection and atherosclerosis. Increased expression of adhesion molecules such as intercellular adhesion molecule-1 (ICAM)-1 and endothelial adhesion molecule (E-selectin) and inflammatory cytokines such as TNF)-α and interleukin-6 (IL-6) have been reported in HIV-positive patients. Higher plasma TNF-α, IL-6, and von Willebrand factor levels also correlate with viral load, supporting the presence of endothelial response to injury.[31,32] Clinically, this also may manifest after percutaneous coronary interventions; restenosis may be higher in these patients than in other populations.

Premature cerebrovascular disease is common in AIDS patients. The prevalence of stroke in AIDS patients was estimated to be 8% on review of autopsy records between 1983 and 1987. Of the patients with stroke, 4 of 13 had evidence of cerebral emboli, and in 3 of those 4, the embolus had a clear cardiac source.[31]

Protease inhibitor therapy markedly alters lipid metabolism and can be associated with premature atherosclerotic disease. Chronic inflammatory states have also been associated with premature atherosclerotic vascular disease. Atherosclerotic disease in the HIV-infected individual is believed to be multifactorial in cause and prone to plaque rupture, possibly related to the host environment.[32] In a large, prospective observational study, the adjusted risk of MI was 16%/year of protease inhibitor exposure, an approximate doubling over 5 years. The adjusted risk with non-nucleotide reverse transcriptase inhibitors (NNRTIs) increased by 5%/year, but this was not statistically significant. The risk of MI associated with the use of protease inhibitors was attenuated when traditional risk factors were added to the model, suggesting that some but not all of the protease inhibitor–associated MI risk can be attributed to metabolic changes.[32]

Overall, however, protease inhibitor therapy, specifically HAART, have clearly improved morbidity and mortality, with no short-term evidence of increased cardiovascular mortality.[32] Lipodystrophy, including fat redistribution with increased truncal obesity, temporal wasting, increased triglyceride levels, elevated levels of small, dense low-density lipoproteins, and glucose intolerance, should be recognized and treated because of an elevated 10-year cardiovascular risk.[7,31] Risk stratification based on traditional risk factors, plus diet, alcohol intake, physical exercise, hypertriglyceridemia, cocaine use, heroin use, thyroid disease, renal disease, and hypogonadism, should be considered for long-term cardiac preventive care.[13,30]

Fat redistribution is seen in 42% of children after more than 5 years of antiretroviral therapy.[29] Routine physical and laboratory assessment should be part of routine follow-up to balance cardiovascular risk and necessary HIV therapies. Diet and exercise modification are recommended to reduce cardiovascular risk.

Autonomic Dysfunction

Early clinical signs of autonomic dysfunction (see Chap. 94) in HIV-infected patients include syncope and presyncope, diminished sweating, diarrhea, bladder dysfunction, and impotence. In one study, heart rate variability; Valsalva ratio; cold pressor testing; and hemodynamic responses to isometric exercise, tilt-table testing, and standing showed that autonomic dysfunction occurred in patients with HIV and was pronounced in AIDS patients. AIDS patients receiving HAART were relatively protected. Patients with HIV-associated nervous system disease had the most abnormalities in autonomic function (**Fig. 72-5**).[33] Screening and augmented procedural precautions in patients with clinical symptoms need to be applied.

Long-QT Interval

HIV infection is associated with QT prolongation and torsades de pointes ventricular tachycardia; the incidence increases with progression to AIDS (see Chaps. 36 and 39).[34] Hepatitis C is independently associated with increased QT duration, and coinfection with HIV almost doubles the risk of clinically important QT prolongation (i.e., QT_c values of 470 milliseconds or longer). The risk of QT prolongation was 16% with HIV alone and 30% with both HIV and hepatitis C infections.[35]

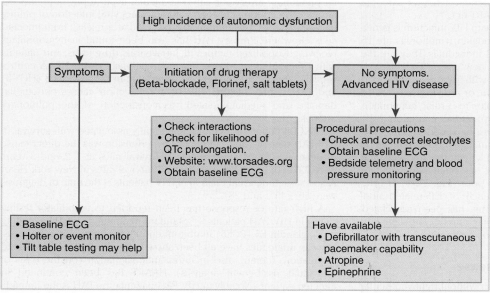

FIGURE 72-5 Evaluation and management of dysautonomia. ECG = electrocardiogram. *(From Dolin R, Masur H, Saag MS [eds]: AIDS Therapy. 2nd ed. New York, Churchill Livingstone, 2003, p 817.)*

Complications of Therapy for HIV

Complications in Adults

Potent antiretroviral medications and HAART, which generally combines three or more agents and usually includes a protease inhibitor, have clearly increased the life span and quality of life of HIV-infected patients.[9] However, protease inhibitors, particularly when used in combination therapy or in HAART, are associated with lipodystrophy, fat wasting and redistribution, metabolic abnormalities, hyperlipidemia, insulin resistance, and increased atherosclerotic risk (**Fig. 72-6**). HIV-infected patients treated with protease inhibitors have reported substantial decreases in total body fat with peripheral lipodystrophy (fat wasting of the face, limbs, and buttocks) and relative conservation or enhancement of central adiposity (truncal obesity, breast enlargement, and buffalo hump) compared with patients who have not received protease inhibitors. Lipid alterations associated with protease inhibitors include higher triglyceride, total cholesterol, insulin, lipoprotein (a), and C-reactive protein levels and lower high-density lipoprotein levels, all promoting an atherogenic profile.[29]

Lipid abnormalities vary with different protease inhibitors. Ritonavir has the most adverse effects on lipids, with a mean increase in total cholesterol of 2.0 mmol/L and a mean increase in triglyceride level of 1.83 mmol/L. More modest increases of total cholesterol without marked triglyceride increases were found in patients taking indinavir and nelfinavir. Combination with saquinavir did not further elevate total cholesterol. Protease inhibitor therapy increased lipoprotein(a) by 48% in patients with elevated pretreatment values (>20 mg/dL).[36] In some cases, switching protease inhibitors may reverse elevations in triglyceride levels and abnormal fat deposition. Low-level aerobic exercise may also help reverse lipid abnormalities.[7,37]

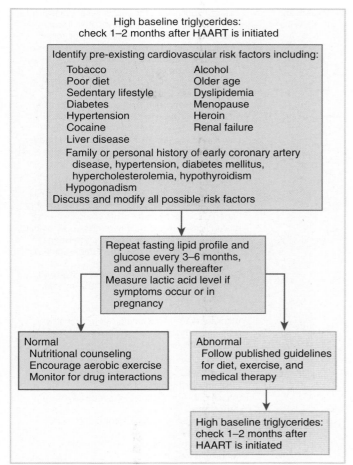

FIGURE 72-6 Cardiovascular considerations when initiating HAART.

Zidovudine (azidothymidine, AZT) has been implicated in skeletal muscle myopathies. In culture, AZT causes a dose-dependent destruction of human myotubes. Human cultured cardiac muscle cells treated with AZT have developed mitochondrial abnormalities, and NNRTIs in general have been associated with altered mitochondrial DNA replication.[38] However, cardiac myopathies have not been evident in clinical data. Rarely, patients with LV dysfunction have improved with cessation of AZT therapy.

Intravenous pentamidine, used to treat *Pneumocystis jiroveci* pneumonia in patients intolerant of trimethoprim-sulfamethoxazole, has been associated with cases of torsades de pointes and refractory ventricular tachycardia.[11,38] Pentamidine should be reserved for patients whose QTc interval is 48 milliseconds or less. Multiple medication reactions and interactions have occurred during the treatment of HIV infection and are a major cause of cardiac emergencies in HIV-infected patients. Common cardiac drug interactions are outlined in **Table 72-2**.

Perinatal Transmission and Vertically Transmitted HIV Infection

Most children with HIV are infected in the perinatal period, but HIV transmission can be minimized if mothers are given antiretroviral therapy in the second and third trimesters or short courses before parturition.[39] The incidence of vertical transmission can be limited to less than 2% with current therapies, some including up to 6 months of neonatal AZT.

Rates of congenital cardiovascular malformations in cohorts of HIV-uninfected and HIV-infected children born to HIV-infected mothers have ranged from 5.6% to 8.9%. These rates were 5 to 10 times higher than those reported in population-based epidemiologic studies but are not higher than in normal populations similarly screened.[11]

In the same cohorts, serial echocardiograms obtained at 4- to 6-month intervals have shown subclinical cardiac abnormalities to be common, persistent, and often progressive.[5] Some dilated cardiomyopathy (LV contractility ≥ 2 SDs below the normal mean; LV end-diastolic dimension ≥2 SDs above the mean) and some had mildly increased cardiac mass for height and weight. Depressed LV function correlated with immune dysfunction at baseline but not longitudinally, suggesting that the CD4 cell count may not be a useful surrogate marker of HIV-associated LV dysfunction. The development of encephalopathy was highly correlated with a decline in fractional shortening.

In children with vertically transmitted HIV-1 infection, disease can progress rapidly or slowly.[10] Rapid progressors have higher heart rates, higher respiratory rates, and lower fractional shortening on serial examinations than nonrapid progressors and HIV-uninfected children who are similarly screened. Rapid progressors have higher 5-year cumulative mortality, higher HIV-1 viral loads, and lower CD8+ (cytotoxic) T-cell counts than nonrapid progressors. Knowing the patterns of disease allows more aggressive therapy to be initiated earlier in rapid progressors.

Evaluating non-HIV infected infants born to HIV infected mothers has shown that fetal exposure to HAART is associated with reduced LV mass, LV dimension, and septal wall thickness and higher LV fractional shortening and contractility during the first 2 years of life. In utero exposure to HAART may impair myocardial growth while initially improving LV function, although LV function was less than normal. These effects are more pronounced in girls. Long-term monitoring of these infants is still needed to define the mechanism of these effects better and to evaluate their long-term clinical importance.[5,40]

Monitoring Recommendations

Routine, systematic cardiac evaluation, including a comprehensive history and thorough cardiac examination, is essential for the care of HIV-infected adults and children. The history should include traditional risk factors, environmental exposures, and therapeutic and illicit drug use. Routine blood pressure monitoring is important because HIV-infected individuals have been reported to experience

TABLE 72-2 Cardiovascular Actions and Interactions of Drugs Commonly Used in HIV Therapy*

CLASS	CARDIAC DRUG INTERACTIONS	CARDIAC SIDE EFFECTS
Antiretroviral		
Nucleotide reverse transcriptase inhibitors	Zidovudine, dipyridamole	Rare—lactic acidosis, hypotension Accelerated risk with cardiopulmonary bypass Zidovudine—skeletal muscle myopathy, myocarditis
Non-nucleotide reverse transcriptase inhibitors	Calcium channel blockers, warfarin, beta blockers, nifedipine, quinidine, steroids, theophylline Delavirdine—can cause serious toxic effects if given with antiarrhythmic drugs and calcium channel blockers	
Protease inhibitors	Metabolized by cytochrome P-450 and interact with other drugs metabolized through this pathway, such as selected antimicrobials, antidepressant, and antihistamine agents; cisapride, HMG-CoA reductase inhibitors (lovastatin, simvastatin), sildenafil Potentially dangerous interactions that require close monitoring or dose adjustment; can occur with amiodarone, disopyramide, flecainide, lidocaine, mexiletine, propafenone, quinidine Ritonavir—most potent cytochrome activator (CYP3A) and P-glycoprotein inhibitor; most likely to interact Indinavir, amprenavir, and nelfinavir—moderate Saquinavir—lowest probability to interact Calcium channel blockers, prednisone, quinine, beta blockers (1.5- to 3-fold increase) Decrease theophylline concentrations	Implicated in premature atherosclerosis, dyslipidemia, insulin resistance, diabetes mellitus, fat wasting and redistribution
Anti-infective		
Antibiotics	Rifampin—reduces therapeutic effect of digoxin by inducing intestinal P-glycoprotein, reduces protease inhibitor concentration and effect Erythromycin—cytochrome P-450 metabolism and drug interactions Trimethoprim-sulfamethoxazole (Bactrim)—increases warfarin effects	Erythromycin—orthostatic hypotension, ventricular tachycardia, bradycardia, torsades (with drug interactions) Clarithromycin—QT prolongation and torsades de pointes Trimethoprim-sulfamethoxazole—orthostatic hypotension, anaphylaxis, QT prolongation, torsades de pointes, hypokalemia Sparfloxacin (fluoroquinolones)— QT prolongation
Antifungal agents	Amphotericin B—digoxin toxicity Ketoconazole or itraconazole—cytochrome P-450 metabolism and drug interactions; increases levels of sildenafil, warfarin, HMG-CoA reductase inhibitors, nifedipine, digoxin	Amphotericin B—hypertension, arrhythmia, renal failure, hypokalemia, thrombophlebitis, bradycardia, angioedema, dilated cardiomyopathy; liposomal formulations still have potential for electrolyte imbalance and QT prolongation Ketoconazole, fluconazole, itraconazole—QT prolongation, torsades de pointes
Antiviral	Ganciclovir—zidovudine	Foscarnet—reversible cardiac failure, electrolyte abnormalities Ganciclovir—ventricular tachycardia, hypotension
Antiparasitic		Pentamidine—hypotension, QT prolongation, arrhythmias (torsades de pointes), ventricular tachycardia, hyperglycemia, hypoglycemia, sudden death; these effects enhanced by hypomagnesemia and hypokalemia
Chemotherapeutic	Vincristine, doxorubicin—decrease digoxin level	Vincristine—arrhythmia, MI, cardiomyopathy, autonomic neuropathy Recombinant human interferon-alfa—hypertension, hypotension, tachycardia, acute coronary events, dilated cardiomyopathy, arrhythmias, sudden death, atrioventricular block, peripheral vasodilation Contraindicated in patients with unstable angina or recent MI IL-2—hypotension, arrhythmia, sudden death, MI, dilated cardiomyopathy, capillary leak, thyroid alterations Anthracyclines (doxorubicin, daunorubicin, mitoxantrone)—myocarditis, cardiomyopathy Liposomal anthracyclines—as above for doxorubicin and vasculitis
Other		
Systemic corticosteroids	Corticosteroids—decrease salicylate levels, increase gastric ulceration in combination with salicylates	Corticosteroids—ventricular hypertrophy, cardiomyopathy, hyperglycemia
Pentoxifylline		Pentoxifylline—decreased triglyceride levels, arrhythmias, chest pain Megestrol acetate—edema, thrombophlebitis, hyperglycemia
Megestrol acetate (Megace)		Epoetin alfa (erythropoietin)—hypertension, ventricular dysfunction
Methadone		Prolonged QT interval
Amphetamines		Increased heart rate and blood pressure

*See Piscitelli SC, Gallicano KD: Interactions among drugs for HIV and opportunistic infections. N Engl J Med 344:984, 2001, for cytochrome P-450 isoforms and selected drugs used in the care of HIV-infected patients.
HMG-CoA = 3-hydroxy-3-methylglutaryl coenzyme A.

hypertension at a younger age and more frequently than in the general population.[11,13,18]

Routine electrocardiographic and Holter monitoring are not warranted unless patients have symptoms such as palpitations, syncope, stroke, or dysautonomia. These tests can also be useful for baseline and monitoring before, during, and after therapies, such as pentamidine, methadone, or antibiotics, that may prolong the QT interval.[13,18]

Asymptomatic cardiac disease related to HIV can be fatal, and cardiac symptoms are often disguised by secondary effects of HIV infection, so systematic echocardiographic monitoring is warranted. We recommend an echocardiogram at the time of HIV diagnosis and every 1 to 2 years thereafter (see Fig. 72-3). Symptomatic patients with HIV infection without cardiovascular abnormalities should have annual echocardiographic follow-up. Echocardiography should also be considered for patients with unexplained or persistent pulmonary symptoms and those with viral coinfection at risk for myocarditis.[13]

An international consensus panel has recommended slightly less aggressive echocardiographic monitoring, with a baseline, for any patient at high risk or with any clinical manifestation of cardiovascular disease, and serial studies repeated every 1 to 2 years or as clinically indicated. Patients with cardiac symptoms should have a formal cardiac assessment, including baseline echocardiography, electrocardiography, and Holter monitoring, and should begin directed therapy.[13] Brain natriuretic peptide levels may be helpful for diagnosing ventricular dysfunction.

In patients with LV dysfunction, serum troponin assays are indicated. Serum troponin level elevations warrant consideration of cardiac catheterization and endomyocardial biopsy. Myocarditis proven by biopsy warrants considering therapy with intravenous immunoglobulin.[2] Cytomegalovirus inclusions on the biopsy specimen support the use of antiviral therapy, and abnormal mitochondria should encourage consideration of a drug holiday from zidovudine. Echocardiography should be repeated after 2 weeks of therapy to allow a more aggressive approach if LV dysfunction persists or worsens and to encourage continued therapy if improvement has occurred.[13]

Because HIV has become a chronic disease, cardiovascular disease will predominate as a cause of mortality and will surface as a vital area of research. Research may translate to other populations if HIV can be used as a model of chronic immunosuppression in a large population. Understanding genetic predispositions to QT prolongation may guide therapy, and determining the causes of cardiomyopathy may benefit diverse research efforts, such as the effects of cytokines, mitochondria, and neurohormonal pathways. Observations such as increased mortality related to LV mass and very mild LV dysfunction may enhance diagnostic testing in at-risk populations affected by other poorly understood cardiomyopathies.

REFERENCES

History

1. Currie PF, Jacob AJ, Foreman AR, et al: Heart muscle disease related to HIV infection: Prognostic implications. BMJ 309:1605, 1994.
2. Lipshultz SE, Orav EJ, Sanders SP, Colan SD: Immunoglobulins and LV structure and function in pediatric HIV infection. Circulation 92:2220, 1995.
3. Jenson HB, Pollock BH: Cardiac cancers in HIV-infected patients. In Lipshultz SE (ed): Cardiology in AIDS. New York, Chapman & Hall, 1998, pp 255-263.
4. Saidi A, Bricker JT: Pulmonary hypertension in patients infected with HIV. In Lipshultz SE (ed): Cardiology in AIDS. New York, Chapman & Hall, 1998, pp 187-194.
5. Lipshultz SE, Easley KA, Orav EJ, et al: Cardiac dysfunction and mortality in HIV-infected children: The Prospective P2C2 HIV Multicenter Study. Circulation 102:1542, 2000.
6. Felker GM, Thompson RE, Hare JM, et al: Underlying causes and long-term survival in patients with initially unexplained cardiomyopathy. N Engl J Med 342:1077-1084, 2000.

Background

7. Morse CG, Kovacs JA: Metabolic and skeletal complications of HIV infection: The price of success. JAMA 296:844, 2006.
8. UNAIDS (Joint United Nations Programme on HIV/AIDS): 2008 Report on the Global AIDS Epidemic (http://www.unaids.org/en/KnowledgeCentre/HIVData/GlobalReport/2008).
9. Stein JH: Managing cardiovascular risk in patients with HIV infection. J Acquir Immune Defic Syndr 38:115, 2005.
10. Ho JE, Hsue PY: Cardiovascular manifestations of HIV infection. Heart 95:1193, 2009.
11. Al-Attar I, Orav EJ, Exil V, et al: Predictors of cardiac morbidity and related mortality in children with acquired immunodeficiency syndrome. J Am Coll Cardiol 41:1598, 2003.

LV Systolic and Diastolic Dysfunction

12. Kearney DL, Perez-Atayde AR, Easley KA, et al: Postmortem cardiomegaly and echocardiographic measurements of LV size and function in children infected with the human immunodeficiency virus. The Prospective P2C2 HIV Multicenter Study. Cardiovasc Pathol 12:140, 2003.
13. Lipshultz SE, Fisher SD, Lai WW, Miller TL: Cardiovascular risk factors, monitoring, and therapy for HIV-infected patients. AIDS 17:S96, 2003.
14. Mansoor A, Althoff K, Gange S, et al: Elevated NT-pro-BNP levels are associated with comorbidities among HIV-infected women. AIDS Res Hum Retroviruses 25:997, 2009.
15. Fisher SD, Bowles NE, Towbin JA, Lipshultz SE: Mediators in HIV-associated cardiovascular disease: A focus on cytokines and genes. AIDS 17:S29, 2003.
16. Starc TJ, Lipshultz SE, Easley KA, et al: Incidence of cardiac abnormalities in children with human immunodeficiency virus infection: The prospective P2C2 HIV study. J Pediatr 141:327, 2002.
17. Currie PF, Boon NA: Immunopathogenesis of HIV-related heart muscle disease: Current perspectives. AIDS 17:S21, 2003.
18. Sudano I, Spieker LE, Noll G, et al: Cardiovascular disease in HIV infection. Am Heart J 151:1147, 2006.
19. Fisher SD, Easley KA, Orav EJ, et al: Mild dilated cardiomyopathy and increased LV mass predict mortality: The prospective P2C2 HIV Multicenter Study. Am Heart J 150:439, 2005.
20. Calabrese LH, Albrecht M, Young J, et al: Successful cardiac transplantation in an HIV-1–infected patient with advanced disease. N Engl J Med 348:2323, 2003.

Animal Models

21. Yearley JH, Mansfield KG, Carville AA, et al: Antigenic stimulation in the simian model of HIV infection yields dilated cardiomyopathy through effects of TNFalpha. AIDS 22:585, 2008.
22. Kohler JJ, Cucoranu I, Fields E, et al: Transgenic mitochondrial superoxide dismutase and mitochondrially targeted catalase prevent antiretroviral-induced oxidative stress and cardiomyopathy. Lab Invest 89:782, 2009.

Infective Endocarditis

23. Martin-Davila P, Navas E, Fortun J, et al: Analysis of mortality and risk factors associated with native valve endocarditis in drug users: The importance of vegetation size. Am Heart J 150:1099, 2005.

Cardiovascular Malignancy

24. Bruno R, Sacchi P, Filice G: Overview on the incidence and the characteristics of HIV-related opportunistic infections and neoplasms of the heart: Impact of highly active antiretroviral therapy. AIDS 17:S83, 2003.
25. Zoufaly A, Stellbrink HJ, Heiden MA: Cumulative HIV viremia during highly active antiretroviral therapy is a strong predictor of AIDS-related lymphoma. J Infect Dis 200:8, 2009.

Right Ventricular Dysfunction and Pulmonary Hypertension

26. Degano B, Guillaume M, Savale L, et al: HIV-associated pulmonary arterial hypertension: survival and prognostic factors in the modern therapeutic era. AIDS 24:67, 2010.
27. Opravil M, Sereni D: Natural history of HIV-associated pulmonary arterial hypertension: trends in the HAART era. AIDS 22 Suppl 3:S35-S40, 2008.
28. McLaughlin VV, Archer SL, Badesch DB, et al: ACCF/AHA 2009 expert consensus document on pulmonary hypertension: A report of the American College of Cardiology Foundation Task Force on Expert Consensus Documents and the American Heart Association: Developed in collaboration with the American College of Chest Physicians, American Thoracic Society, Inc., and the Pulmonary Hypertension Association. Circulation 119:2250, 2009.

Accelerated Atherosclerosis

29. Grinspoon S, Carr A: Cardiovascular risk and body-fat abnormalities in HIV-infected adults. N Engl J Med 352:48, 2005.
30. Boccara F, Teiger E, Cohen A, et al: Percutaneous coronary intervention in HIV infected patients: Immediate results and long term prognosis. Heart 92:543, 2006.
31. Kotler DP: HIV and antiretroviral therapy: lipid abnormalities and associated cardiovascular risk in HIV-infected patients. J Acquir Immune Defic Syndr 49(Suppl 2):S79, 2008.
32. DAD Study Group, Friis-Møller N, Reiss P, Sabin CA, et al: Class of antiretroviral drugs and the risk of myocardial infarction. N Engl J Med 356:1723, 2007.

Autonomic Dysfunction

33. Correia D, Rodrigues De Resende LA, Molina RJ, et al: Power spectral analysis of heart rate variability in HIV-infected and AIDS patients. Pacing Clin Electrophysiol 29:53, 2006.

Long-QT Interval

34. Sani MU, Okeahialam BN: QTc interval prolongation in patients with HIV and AIDS. J Natl Med Assoc 97:1657, 2005.
35. Nordin C, Kohli A, Beca S, et al: Importance of hepatitis C coinfection in the development of QT prolongation in HIV-infected patients. J Electrocardiol 39:199, 2006.

Complications of Therapy for HIV

36. Fisher SD, Miller TL, Lipshultz SE: Impact of HIV and highly active antiretroviral therapy on leukocyte adhesion molecules, arterial inflammation, dyslipidemia, and atherosclerosis. Atherosclerosis 185:1, 2006.
37. Nanavati KA, Fisher SD, Miller TL, Lipshultz SE: HIV-related cardiovascular disease and drug interactions. Am J Cardiovasc Drugs 4:315, 2004.
38. Zareba KM, Miller TL, Lipshultz SE: Cardiovascular disease and toxicities related to HIV infection and its therapies. Expert Opin Drug Saf 4:1017, 2005.

Perinatal Transmission and Vertically Transmitted HIV Infection

39. Mofenson LM, Brady MT, Danner SP, et al: Guidelines for the Prevention and Treatment of Opportunistic Infections among HIV-exposed and HIV-infected children: Recommendations from CDC, the National Institutes of Health, the HIV Medicine Association of the Infectious Diseases Society of America, the Pediatric Infectious Diseases Society, and the American Academy of Pediatrics. MMWR Recomm Rep 58(RR-11):1, 2009.
40. Lavigne JE, Shearer WT, Thompson B: Cardiovascular outcomes of pediatric seroreverters perinatally exposed to HAART: Design of a longitudinal clinical study. Cardiovasc Toxicol 4:187, 2004.

CH 72

CARDIOVASCULAR ABNORMALITIES IN HIV-INFECTED INDIVIDUALS

CHAPTER **73** **Toxins and the Heart**

Richard A. Lange and L. David Hillis

Because many toxins, some used by a substantial portion of the population, may affect the heart adversely, it is important to understand the myriad of ways in which these substances may influence the cardiovascular system. This chapter focuses on environmental exposures and commonly prescribed pharmacologic agents, as well as frequently used illicit drugs, including cocaine and amphetamines. Chap. 90 discusses the toxicities of various chemotherapeutic agents in greater detail.

Ethanol

An estimated two thirds of Americans occasionally consume ethanol, and approximately 10% are considered to be heavy consumers. Although the ingestion of a moderate amount of ethanol (usually defined as three to nine drinks/week) is associated with a reduced risk of cardiovascular disease, the consumption of excessive amounts has the opposite effect. When ingested in substantial amounts, ethanol may cause ventricular systolic and/or diastolic dysfunction, systemic arterial hypertension, angina pectoris, arrhythmias, and even sudden cardiac death.

Effects of Ethanol on Cardiac Myocyte Structure and Function

Ethanol may cause myocardial damage via several mechanisms (**Table 73-1**).[1] First, ethanol and its metabolites, acetaldehyde and acetate, may exert a direct toxic effect on the myocardium. Second, deficiencies of certain vitamins (e.g., thiamine), minerals (e.g., selenium), or electrolytes (e.g., magnesium, phosphorus, potassium) that sometimes occur in heavy ethanol consumers may adversely affect myocardial function. Third, certain substances that sometimes contaminate alcoholic beverages, such as lead (often found in moonshine) or cobalt, may damage the myocardium.

Ethanol impairs excitation-contraction, mitochondrial oxidative phosphorylation, and cardiac contractility by adversely affecting the function of the sarcolemmal membrane, the sarcoplasmic reticulum, mitochondria, and contractile proteins. Electron microscopic studies of the hearts of experimental animals in close temporal proximity to heavy ethanol ingestion have demonstrated dilated sarcoplasmic reticula and swollen mitochondria, with fragmented cristae and glycogen-filled vacuoles. With sustained exposure to ethanol, myofibrillar degeneration and replacement fibrosis appear. In addition to

the effects of ethanol on the myocardial contractile apparatus, acute or chronic consumption may adversely influence myofibrillar protein synthesis. Microscopically, the hearts of chronic heavy consumers of ethanol manifest an increased accumulation of collagen in the extracellular matrix, as well as increased intermolecular cross links.

Effects of Ethanol on Organ Function

Chronic heavy ethanol ingestion may induce left ventricular diastolic and/or systolic dysfunction. Diastolic dysfunction, which is caused at least in part by interstitial fibrosis of the myocardium, is often demonstrable in heavy consumers of ethanol, even in the absence of symptoms or obvious signs. About 50% of asymptomatic chronic alcoholics have echocardiographic evidence of left ventricular hypertrophy with preserved systolic performance. By Doppler echocardiography, the left ventricular relaxation time is often prolonged, the peak early diastolic velocity is reduced, and the acceleration of early diastolic flow is slowed—all manifestations of left ventricular diastolic dysfunction. Abnormal increases in left ventricular filling pressure during volume or pressure loading may be observed.

Ethanol may induce asymptomatic left ventricular systolic dysfunction, even when it is ingested by healthy individuals in relatively small quantities, as occurs in subjects who are considered social drinkers. As many as 30% of asymptomatic chronic alcoholics have echocardiographic evidence of left ventricular systolic dysfunction. With continued heavy ethanol ingestion, these subjects often develop symptoms and signs of congestive heart failure, which is caused by a dilated cardiomyopathy (see Chap. 68). In fact, ethanol abuse is the leading cause of nonischemic dilated cardiomyopathy in industrialized countries, accounting for approximately half of those who carry this diagnosis. The likelihood of developing an ethanol-induced dilated cardiomyopathy correlates with the amount of ethanol that is consumed in a lifetime. Most men who develop an ethanol-induced dilated cardiomyopathy have consumed more than 80 g of ethanol/day (i.e., 1 liter of wine, 8 standard-sized beers, or 0.5 pint of hard liquor) for at least 5 years. Women appear to be even more susceptible to ethanol's cardiotoxic effects, in that they may develop a dilated cardiomyopathy following the consumption of a smaller amount of ethanol daily and over their lifetime when compared with their male counterparts.

Although the heavy intake of ethanol is associated with nonischemic dilated cardiomyopathy, individuals with light to moderate ethanol consumption actually have a lower incidence of congestive

TABLE 73-1	Mechanisms of Ethanol-Induced Myocardial Injury

Direct Toxic Effects
Uncoupling of the excitation-contraction system
Reduced calcium sequestration in sarcoplasmic reticulum
Inhibition of sarcolemmal ATP-dependent Na+/K+ pump
Reduction in mitochondrial respiratory ratio
Altered substrate uptake
Increased interstitial-extracellular protein synthesis

Toxic Effect of Metabolites
Acetaldehyde
Ethyl esters

Nutritional or Trace Metal Deficiencies
Thiamine
Selenium

Electrolyte Disturbances
Hypomagnesemia
Hypokalemia
Hypophosphatemia

Toxic Additives
Cobalt
Lead

TABLE 73-2	Qualitative Effects of Light to Moderate and Heavier Alcohol Intake on Cardiovascular (CV) Risk Factors and Outcomes	
CV RISK FACTORS AND OUTCOMES	**LIGHT TO MODERATE ALCOHOL INTAKE***	**HEAVIER ALCOHOL INTAKE†**
Blood pressure	↔	↑↑
HDL-C	↑↑	↑↑↑
Triglycerides	↑	↑↑
LDL-C	↔ or ↓	↑
Platelet aggregability or coagulability	↓	↓↓
Systemic inflammation	↓	↑
CHF	↓	↑↑
CAD (angina, non-fatal MI)	↓↓	↓
Atrial fibrillation	↔	↑↑
Stroke	↓	↑↑
SCD	↓↓	↑

*Less than two drinks/day.
†More than two drinks/day.
↔ = Indicates no or equivocal effect; ↑ = indicates mild effect; ↑↑ = indicates modest effect; ↑↑↑ = indicates substantial effect.

heart failure when compared with those who do not drink at all.[2] In patients with left ventricular dysfunction, light to moderate ethanol ingestion does not exacerbate heart failure. In subjects with an ischemic cardiomyopathy, light to moderate ethanol consumption may reduce mortality.[3]

Subjects with markedly symptomatic ethanol-induced dilated cardiomyopathy may manifest a substantial improvement in left ventricular systolic function and symptoms of heart failure with complete abstinence or a dramatic reduction in ethanol consumption (i.e., to less than 60 g of ethanol/day or the equivalent of four standard drinks). Although most of this improvement occurs in the first 6 months of abstinence, it often continues for as long as 2 years of observation.

Ethanol and Systemic Arterial Hypertension

Experts estimate that ethanol is a causative factor in up to 11% of men with hypertension (see Chap. 45). Individuals who consume more than two drinks daily are 1.5 to 2 times more likely to have hypertension when compared with age- and sex-matched nondrinkers. This effect is dose-related and is most prominent when the daily ethanol intake exceeds five drinks (i.e., 30 g of ethanol).[3,4] Social ethanol consumption is associated with a modest rise in systolic arterial pressure, whereas heavy consumption and binge drinking may lead to a substantial increase. Although the mechanism whereby ethanol induces a rise in systemic arterial pressure is poorly understood, studies have demonstrated that ethanol consumption increases plasma levels of catecholamines, renin, and aldosterone, each of which may cause systemic arterial vasoconstriction. In individuals with ethanol-induced hypertension, abstinence often normalizes systemic arterial pressure.

Ethanol and Lipid Metabolism

Ethanol consumption inhibits the oxidation of free fatty acids by the liver, which stimulates hepatic triglyceride synthesis and the secretion of very low-density lipoprotein (LDL) cholesterol. Most commonly, therefore, ethanol consumption causes hypertriglyceridemia. In addition, heavy ingestion may cause an increase in the serum concentrations of total and LDL cholesterol. Regular ethanol consumption increases the serum concentration of high-density lipoprotein (HDL) cholesterol. Subjects with hyperlipidemia should be encouraged to limit their ethanol intake.

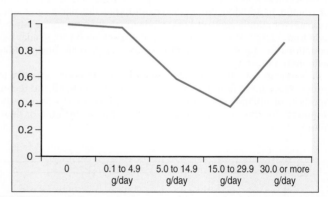

FIGURE 73-1 Relative risk of MI according to daily alcohol intake in men already at low risk for cardiovascular disease on the basis of body mass index, physical activity, smoking, and diet. Moderate alcohol intake is associated with a lower risk of MI.

Coronary Artery Disease

Heavy ethanol use is associated with an increased incidence of atherosclerotic coronary artery disease and resultant cardiovascular morbidity and mortality (see Chaps. 44 and 49). This rise may result at least in part, from the increased likelihood that heavy ethanol consumers (compared with nondrinkers) have systemic arterial hypertension, an increased left ventricular muscle mass (with concomitant diastolic and/or systolic dysfunction), and hypertriglyceridemia (**Table 73-2**). Conversely, light to moderate ethanol intake (two to seven drinks/week) is associated with a decreased risk of cardiovascular morbidity and mortality in men and women.[3-5] Even in men already at low risk for cardiovascular disease on the basis of body mass index, physical activity, smoking, and diet, moderate alcohol intake is associated with a reduced risk of myocardial infarction (MI) (**Fig 73-1**).[6] This lower risk of cardiovascular morbidity and mortality among consumers of moderate amounts of ethanol—when compared with nondrinkers or heavy consumers—is supported by numerous retrospectively and prospectively conducted studies. The French were noted to have a reduced incidence of coronary artery disease when compared with inhabitants of other countries, despite high smoking rates and a diet that is high in fat (the so-called French paradox). Although this diminished incidence initially was attributed to the antioxidant and hemostatic properties of red wine, similar findings subsequently were reported in mild to moderate consumers of other alcoholic beverages and in other study populations.[7] Several prospectively performed cohort studies have demonstrated that drinkers of moderate amounts of ethanol are 40% to 70% less likely to manifest coronary artery disease or ischemic stroke when compared with non-drinkers or heavy consumers.[7] Some studies have suggested that the consumption of all alcoholic beverages exerts such an effect, whereas others have reported that this so-called cardioprotection is strongest with the consumption of wine.[8] The mechanism(s) whereby the consumption of moderate amounts of ethanol reduces cardiovascular risk appear to be multifactorial, in that moderate consumption exerts several beneficial effects, including the following: (1) an increase in the serum concentrations of HDL cholesterol and apolipoprotein A-I; (2) inhibition of platelet aggregation; (3) a decreased serum fibrinogen concentration; (4) increased antioxidant activity (from the phenolic compounds and flavonoids contained in red wine); (5) anti-inflammatory effects (with lower concentrations of white blood cells and C-reactive protein); and (6) improved fibrinolysis resulting from increased concentrations of endogenous tissue plasminogen activator and a concomitant decrease in endogenous plasminogen activator inhibitor activity (**Fig. 73-2**).[5,8]

Men and women manifest a difference in the cardioprotective effect of alcohol (**Fig. 73-3**). The maximal beneficial effect of ethanol occurs at lower doses for women than for men, and the range of alcohol consumption with which it is protective is wider for men than for women. In addition, the relative cardioprotective effect of ethanol is greater for middle-aged and older individuals than for young adults.[8] Light to moderate ethanol consumption is associated with similar risk reductions in coronary artery disease among diabetic and nondiabetic men and women.[9]

In survivors of MI, moderate ethanol consumption appears to reduce subsequent mortality. In the setting of an acute MI, the recent ingestion of ethanol does not appear to reduce infarct size or the propensity for the subsequent appearance of an arrhythmia or heart failure.

Arrhythmias

Ethanol consumption is associated with a variety of atrial and ventricular arrhythmias, most commonly the following: (1) atrial or ventricular premature beats; (2) supraventricular tachycardia; (3) atrial flutter; (4) atrial fibrillation; (5) ventricular tachycardia; or (6) ventricular fibrillation (see Chap. 40). The most common ethanol-induced arrhythmia is atrial fibrillation. Ethanol is a causative factor in about one third of subjects with new-onset atrial fibrillation; in those younger than 65 years of age, it may be responsible in as many as two thirds. Most episodes occur after binge drinking, usually on weekends or holidays—hence, the term *holiday heart*. Electrophysiologic testing in humans without cardiac disease has shown that ethanol enhances vulnerability to the induction of atrial flutter and fibrillation. The treatment of these ethanol-induced arrhythmias is abstinence.

Ethanol may be arrhythmogenic via several mechanisms. In many ethanol consumers, concomitant factors may predispose to arrhythmias, including cigarette smoking, electrolyte disturbances, metabolic abnormalities, hypertension, or sleep apnea. Acute ethanol ingestion

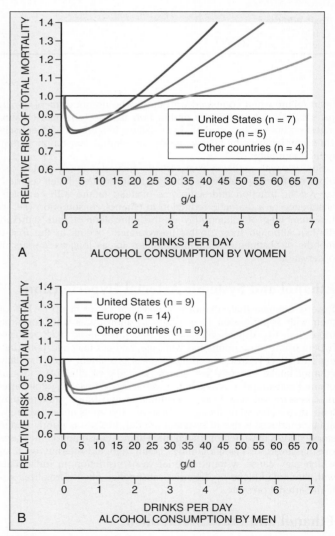

FIGURE 73-3 Relative risk of total mortality and alcohol intake in women **(A)** and men **(B)** in the United States, Europe, and other countries (Australia, Japan, and China). A J-shaped relationship between alcohol consumption and total mortality is observed in men and women. Consumption of alcohol, up to four drinks/day in men and two drinks/day in women, is inversely associated with total mortality. Higher doses of alcohol were associated with increased mortality. The inverse association in women disappears at lower doses than in men. *(From Di Castelnuovo A, Constanzo S, Bagnardi V, et al: Alcohol dosing and total mortality in men and women. An updated meta-analysis of 34 prospective studies. Arch Intern Med 166:2437, 2006.)*

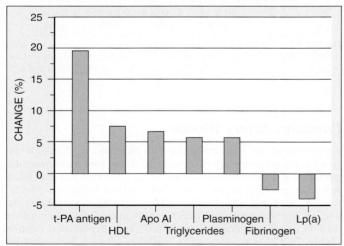

FIGURE 73-2 Percentage change in various serologic variables caused by ethanol ingestion. The ingestion of ethanol, 30 g daily for 1 to 9 weeks, was associated with increased serum concentrations of tissue type plasminogen activator (t-PA) antigen, HDL cholesterol, apolipoprotein A-I (Apo AI), serum triglycerides, and serum plasminogen, as well as decreased concentrations of serum fibrinogen and lipoprotein(a) [Lp(a)]. The reduced risk of cardiovascular events seen in subjects who consume moderate amounts of ethanol may be caused, at least in part, by these beneficial changes in serologic variables. *(From Rimm EB, Williams P, Fosher K, et al: Moderate alcohol intake and lower risk of coronary heart disease: meta-analysis of effects on lipids and haemostatic factors. BMJ 319:1523, 1999.)*

induces a diuresis, which is accompanied by the concomitant urinary loss of sodium, potassium, and magnesium. The presence of myocardial interstitial fibrosis, ventricular hypertrophy, cardiomyopathy, and autonomic dysfunction also may enhance the likelihood of dysrhythmias.

Sudden Death

In subjects without known cardiac disease, the decrease in cardiovascular mortality associated with moderate ethanol intake results largely from a reduction in the incidence of sudden death (**Fig. 73-4**). Of the more than 21,000 men in the Physicians Health Study, those who consumed two to four drinks/week or five to six drinks/week had a significantly reduced risk of sudden death (relative risks, 0.40 and 0.21, respectively) when compared with those who rarely or never drank.[10] In contrast, heavy ethanol consumption (i.e., six or more drinks/day) or binge drinking was associated with an increased risk of sudden death. Heavy ethanol consumption is associated with an increased incidence of sudden death independent of the presence of coronary artery disease (see Chap. 41). The incidence of ethanol-induced sudden death increases with age and the amount of ethanol that is ingested. For example, the daily ingestion of more than 80 g of ethanol

is associated with a threefold increased incidence of mortality when compared with a daily consumption of a lesser amount.

Cocaine

Cocaine is currently the most commonly used illicit drug among subjects seeking care in hospital emergency departments, and is the most frequent cause of drug-related deaths reported by medical examiners in the United States.[11] Its widespread use is attributable to the following: (1) its ease of administration; (2) the ready availability of relatively pure drug; (3) its relatively low cost; and (4) the misperception that its recreational use is safe. As cocaine abuse has increased in frequency, the number of cocaine-related cardiovascular complications, including angina pectoris, MI, cardiomyopathy, and sudden death, has increased (**Table 73-3**).

Pharmacology and Mechanisms of Action

Cocaine (benzoylmethylecgonine) is an alkaloid extracted from the leaf of the *Erythroxylon coca* bush, which grows primarily in South America. It is available in two forms, the hydrochloride salt and the freebase. Cocaine hydrochloride is prepared by dissolving the alkaloid in hydrochloric acid to form a water-soluble powder or granule, which can be taken orally, intravenously, or intranasally (so-called chewing, mainlining, or snorting, respectively). The freebase form is manufactured by processing the cocaine with ammonia or sodium bicarbonate (baking soda). Unlike the hydrochloride form, freebase cocaine is heat-stable so that it can be smoked. It is known as crack because of the popping sound that it makes when heated.

Cocaine hydrochloride is well absorbed through all mucous membranes; therefore, users may achieve a high blood concentration with intranasal, sublingual, vaginal, or rectal administration. The route of administration determines the rapidity of onset and duration of action (**Table 73-4**). The euphoria associated with smoking crack cocaine occurs within seconds and is short-lived. Crack cocaine is considered the most potent and addictive form of the drug. Cocaine is metabolized by serum and liver cholinesterases to water-soluble metabolites, primarily benzoylecgonine and ecgonine methyl ester, which are excreted in the urine. Because cocaine's serum half-life is only 45 to 90 minutes, it is detectable in blood or urine only for several hours after its use. However, its metabolites persist in blood or urine for 24 to 36 hours after its administration.

When applied locally, cocaine acts as an anesthetic by virtue of its inhibition of membrane permeability to sodium during depolarization, thereby blocking the initiation and transmission of electrical signals. When given systemically, it blocks the presynaptic reuptake of norepinephrine and dopamine, thereby producing an excess of these neurotransmitters at the site of the postsynaptic receptor (**Fig. 73-5**). In short, cocaine acts as a powerful sympathomimetic agent.

Cocaine-Related Myocardial Ischemia and Infarction

Since 1982, numerous reports have associated cocaine use with myocardial ischemia and infarction. In one survey of 10,085 adults 18 to 45 years of age, 25% of nonfatal MIs were attributed to cocaine use.[12] Cocaine-related myocardial ischemia or infarction may result from the following: (1) increased myocardial oxygen demand in the setting of a limited or fixed oxygen supply; (2) marked coronary arterial vasoconstriction; and (3) enhanced platelet aggregation and thrombus formation (**Fig. 73-6**).

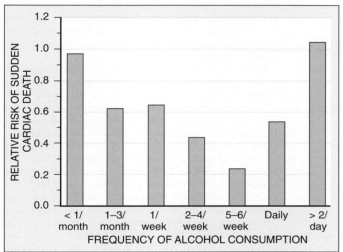

FIGURE 73-4 Ethanol consumption and the risk of sudden cardiac death in U.S. male physicians. In comparison to those who had less than one drink/month (far left bar), those who consumed small or moderate amounts of ethanol (middle bars) had a reduced risk of sudden cardiac death. In contrast, those who consumed at least two drinks/day (far right bar) had an increased risk.

TABLE 73-3 Cardiovascular Complications of Cocaine Use

- Myocardial ischemia
- Angina pectoris
- Myocardial infarction
- Sudden death
- Arrhythmias
- Pulmonary edema
- Myocarditis
- Endocarditis
- Aortic dissection

TABLE 73-4 Pharmacokinetics of Cocaine According to Route of Administration

ROUTE OF ADMINISTRATION	ONSET OF ACTION	PEAK EFFECT	DURATION OF ACTION
Inhalation (smoking)	3-5 sec	1-3 min	5-15 min
Intravenous	10-60 sec	3-5 min	20-60 min
Intranasal or other mucosal	1-5 min	15-20 min	60-90 min

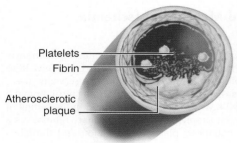

FIGURE 73-5 *Mechanism whereby cocaine alters sympathetic tone. Cocaine blocks the reuptake of norepinephrine by the preganglionic neuron, resulting in excess amounts of this neurotransmitter at postganglionic receptor sites.*

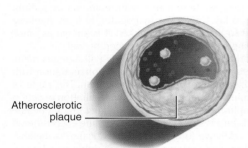

Increased myocardial oxygen demand with limited oxygen supply

Increased heart rate
Increased blood pressure
Increased myocardial contractility

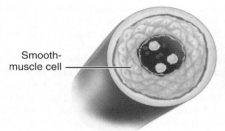

Vasoconstriction

Increased α-adrenergic stimulation
Increased endothelin production
Decreased nitric oxide production

Accelerated atherosclerosis and thrombosis

Increased plasminogen-activator inhibitor
Increased platelet activation and aggregability
Increased endothelial permeability

FIGURE 73-6 *Mechanisms whereby cocaine may induce myocardial ischemia or infarction. Cocaine may increase the determinants of myocardial oxygen demand in the setting of limited oxygen supply (top), cause intense coronary arterial vasoconstriction (middle), or induce accelerated atherosclerosis and thrombosis (bottom). (From Lange RA, Hills LD: Cardiovascular complications of cocaine use. N Engl J Med 345:351, 2001.)*

By virtue of its sympathomimetic effects, cocaine increases the three major determinants of myocardial oxygen demand—heart rate, left ventricular wall tension, and left ventricular contractility. At the same time, the ingestion of even small amounts of the drug causes vasoconstriction of the epicardial coronary arteries (so-called inappropriate vasoconstriction), in that myocardial oxygen supply decreases as demand increases. Cocaine induces vasoconstriction in normal coronary arteries but exerts a particularly marked vasoconstrictive effect in diseased segments. As a result, cocaine users with atherosclerotic coronary artery disease probably have an especially high risk for an ischemic event after cocaine use. Cocaine-induced coronary arterial vasoconstriction results primarily from the stimulation of coronary arterial alpha-adrenergic receptors, because it is reversed by phentolamine (an alpha-adrenergic antagonist) and exacerbated by propranolol (a beta-adrenergic antagonist). In addition, cocaine causes increased endothelin production of endothelin (a potent vasoconstrictor) and decreased production of nitric oxide (a potent vasodilator), which also may promote vasoconstriction.

Cocaine use may enhance platelet activation and aggregability, as well as increase concentrations of plasminogen activator inhibitor, which may promote thrombus accumulation. The presence of premature atherosclerotic coronary artery disease, as observed in postmortem studies of long-term cocaine users, may provide a nidus for thrombosis. In vitro studies have shown that cocaine causes structural abnormalities in the endothelial cell barrier, increasing its permeability to low-density lipoprotein and enhancing the expression of endothelial adhesion molecules, thereby favoring leukocyte migration, all of which are associated with atherogenesis.

Chest pain is the most common cardiovascular complaint of patients seeking medical assistance following cocaine use. Approximately 6% of those who come to the emergency department with cocaine-associated chest pain have enzymatic evidence of myocardial necrosis. Most subjects with cocaine-related MI are young, nonwhite, male cigarette smokers, without other risk factors for atherosclerosis, who have a history of repeated cocaine use (**Table 73-5**). Similar to cocaine, cigarette smoking induces coronary arterial vasoconstriction through an alpha-adrenergic mechanism. The deleterious effects of cocaine on myocardial oxygen supply and demand are exacerbated substantially by concomitant cigarette smoking. Following concomitant cocaine use and smoking, heart rate and systemic arterial pressure increase markedly, and coronary arterial vasoconstriction is more intense than with either alone.

In subjects who are considered otherwise to be at low risk for MI, the risk of infarction increases 24-fold during the first 60 minutes after cocaine use. The occurrence of MI after cocaine use appears to be unrelated to the amount ingested, its route of administration, and the frequency of its use; cocaine-related infarction has been reported with doses ranging from 200 to 2000 mg, after ingestion by all routes, and in habitual and first-time users. About 50% of patients with cocaine-related MI have no angiographic evidence of atherosclerotic coronary artery disease. Therefore, when subjects with no or few risk factors for atherosclerosis, particularly those who are young or have a history of substance abuse, present with acute MI, urine and blood samples should be analyzed for cocaine and its metabolites.

Cardiovascular complications resulting from cocaine-related MI are relatively uncommon, with ventricular arrhythmias occurring in 4% to 17%, congestive heart failure in 5% to 7%, and death in less than 2%. This low incidence of complications is caused, at least in part, by the young age and absence of extensive multivessel coronary artery disease of most patients with cocaine-related infarction. If complications develop, most occur within 12 hours of presentation to the hospital.[13]

TABLE 73-5	Characteristics of Patients with Cocaine-Induced Myocardial Infarction

Dose of Cocaine
Five or six lines (150 mg), up to 2 g
Serum concentration, 0.01-1.02 mg/liter

Frequency of Use
Reported in chronic, recreational, and first-time users

Route of Administration
Occurs with all routes of administration
75% of reported MIs occurred after intranasal use

Age
Mean, 34 yr (range, 17-71 yr)
20% younger than 25 yr

Sex
80%-90% male

Timing
Often within minutes of cocaine use
Reported as late as 5-15 hr after use

TABLE 73-6	Cardiac Dysrhythmias and Conduction Disturbances Reported with Cocaine Use

Sinus tachycardia
Sinus bradycardia
Supraventricular tachycardia
Bundle branch block
Complete heart block
Accelerated idioventricular rhythm
Ventricular tachycardia
Ventricular fibrillation
Asystole
Torsades de pointes
Brugada pattern (right bundle branch block with ST-segment elevation in leads V_1, V_2, and V_3)

Following hospital discharge, continued cocaine use and recurrent chest pain are common. Occasionally, a patient has recurrent nonfatal or fatal MI.

Most subjects with cocaine-related myocardial ischemia or infarction have chest pain within an hour of cocaine use, when the blood cocaine concentration is highest. Occasionally some individuals note the onset of symptoms several hours after the administration of the drug, when the blood cocaine concentration is low or even undetectable. With cocaine ingestion, the diameter of the coronary arteries decreases as the drug concentration increases. Then, as the drug concentration declines, the vasoconstriction resolves. Thereafter, as the concentrations of cocaine's major metabolites (benzoylecgonine and ecgonine methyl ester) rise, delayed (i.e., recurrent) coronary arterial vasoconstriction occurs, thereby explaining why myocardial ischemia or infarction has been reported to occur several hours after drug use.

Cocaethylene

In individuals who use cocaine in temporal proximity to the ingestion of ethanol, hepatic transesterification leads to the production of a unique metabolite, cocaethylene. Cocaethylene is often detected postmortem in subjects who are presumed to have died of cocaine and ethanol toxicity. Similar to cocaine, cocaethylene blocks the reuptake of dopamine at the synaptic cleft, thereby possibly potentiating the systemic toxic effects of cocaine. In experimental animals, in fact, cocaethylene is more lethal than cocaine. In humans, the combination of cocaine and ethanol causes a substantial increase in myocardial oxygen demand. The concomitant use of cocaine and ethanol is associated with a higher incidence of disability and death than either agent alone. Individuals presumably dying of a combined cocaine-ethanol overdose have much lower blood cocaine concentrations than those presumably dying of a cocaine overdose alone, thereby suggesting an additive or synergistic effect of ethanol on the catastrophic cardiovascular events that are induced by cocaine.

Cocaine-Induced Myocardial Dysfunction

Long-term cocaine abuse has been associated with left ventricular hypertrophy, as well as with left ventricular diastolic and/or systolic dysfunction. Several reports have described dilated cardiomyopathy in long-term cocaine abusers, and others have described profound but reversible myocardial depression after binge cocaine use. Approximately 7% of long-term chronic users without cardiac symptoms have radionuclide ventriculographic evidence of left ventricular systolic dysfunction.

Cocaine may adversely affect left ventricular systolic function by several mechanisms. First, as noted, cocaine may induce myocardial ischemia or infarction. Second, the profound repetitive sympathetic stimulation induced by cocaine is similar to that observed in patients with pheochromocytoma; either may induce a cardiomyopathy and characteristic microscopic changes of subendocardial contraction band necrosis. Third, the concomitant administration of adulterants or infectious agents may cause myocarditis, which has been seen on occasion in intravenous cocaine users studied post mortem. Fourth, studies in experimental animals have shown that cocaine increases the production of reactive oxygen species, alters cytokine production in the endothelium and in circulating leukocytes, induces the transcription of genes responsible for changes in the composition of myocardial collagen and myosin, and induces myocyte apoptosis.

Aside from the effects of long-term cocaine use on myocardial performance, it may cause an acute deterioration of left ventricular systolic and/or diastolic function or transient apical ballooning (also called takotsubo cardiomyopathy, or broken heart syndrome). In some subjects, this deterioration results from neurohormonal, metabolic, and/or acid-base disturbances that accompany cocaine intoxication, whereas in others it may be caused by a direct toxic effect of the drug. The intracoronary infusion of cocaine, in an amount sufficient to produce a concentration in coronary sinus blood similar in magnitude to the peripheral blood concentration found in abusers presumably dying of cocaine intoxication, exerts a deleterious effect on left ventricular systolic and diastolic function.

Arrhythmias

Cardiac dysrhythmias may occur with cocaine (**Table 73-6**), but the precise arrhythmogenic potential of the drug is poorly defined. In many cases, the dysrhythmias ascribed to cocaine occur in the setting of profound hemodynamic or metabolic derangements, such as hypotension, hypoxemia, seizures, or MI. Nonetheless, because of cocaine's sodium and potassium channel–blocking properties and its ability to enhance sympathetic activation, it is considered a likely cause of cardiac arrhythmias.[14] The development of lethal arrhythmias with cocaine use may require an underlying substrate of abnormal myocardium. Studies in experimental animals have shown that cocaine precipitates ventricular arrhythmias only in the presence of myocardial ischemia or infarction. In humans, life-threatening arrhythmias and sudden death associated with cocaine use occur most often in those with myocardial ischemia or infarction, or in those with nonischemic myocellular damage. Long-term cocaine use is associated with increased left ventricular mass and wall thickness, which are known risk factors for ventricular dysrhythmias. In some cocaine users, such an increased mass may provide the substrate for arrhythmias.

Cocaine may affect the generation and conduction of cardiac impulses by several mechanisms. First, its sympathomimetic properties may increase ventricular irritability and lower the threshold for fibrillation. Second, it inhibits action potential generation and conduction (i.e., it prolongs the QRS and QT intervals) as a result of its sodium channel–blocking effects. In so doing, it acts in a manner similar to that of a Class I antiarrhythmic agent. Accordingly, Brugada-type electrocardiographic features and torsades de pointes have been observed following cocaine use. Third, cocaine increases the intracellular calcium concentration, which may result in afterdepolarizations and triggered ventricular arrhythmias. Fourth, it reduces vagal activity, thereby potentiating its sympathomimetic effects.

Endocarditis

Although the intravenous administration of any illicit drug associates with an increased risk of bacterial endocarditis, the intravenous use of cocaine appears to be accompanied by a greater risk of endocarditis than the intravenous administration of other drugs. The reason for this enhanced risk of endocarditis in intravenous cocaine users is unknown, but several hypotheses have been proposed. The increases in heart rate and systemic arterial pressure that accompany cocaine use may induce valvular injury that predisposes to bacterial invasion. Cocaine's immunosuppressive effects may increase the risk of infection. The manner in which cocaine is manufactured, as well as the adulterants that are often present in it, may increase the risk of endocarditis. In contradistinction to the endocarditis associated with other drugs, the endocarditis of cocaine users more often involves the left-sided cardiac valves.

Aortic Dissection

Because aortic dissection or rupture has been temporally related to cocaine use, it should be considered as a possible cause of chest pain in cocaine users. In one study of 38 patients with acute aortic dissection, 14 (37%) were related to cocaine use, with an average interval from cocaine use to the onset of symptoms of 12 hours (range, 0 to 24 hours).[15] Dissection probably results from a cocaine-induced increase in systemic arterial pressure. In addition to aortic rupture, the cocaine-related rupture of mycotic and intracerebral aneurysms has been reported.

Amphetamines

Amphetamines were previously prescribed for the treatment of obesity, attention deficit disorder, and narcolepsy; at present, their use is strictly limited. The most frequently abused amphetamines are dextroamphetamine, methcathinone, methamphetamine, methylphenidate, ephedrine, propylhexedrine, phenmetrazine, and 3,4-methylenedioxymethamphetamine (MDMA, also known as ecstasy). Ice is a freebase form of methamphetamine that can be inhaled, smoked, or injected. Because amphetamines are sympathomimetic agents, their use has been associated with systemic arterial hypertension, premature coronary artery disease, acute coronary syndromes, MI, myocardial damage consistent with catecholamine excess, aortic dissection, and lethal arrhythmias.[16,17] Similar to cocaine, amphetamines may induce intense coronary arterial vasoconstriction, with or without thrombus formation.[18] Finally, dilated cardiomyopathy following repetitive amphetamine can occur, with recovery of cardiovascular function after drug discontinuation.[17]

Catecholamines and Beta-Adrenergic Receptor Agonists

Catecholamines, administered exogenously or secreted by a neuroendocrine tumor (e.g., pheochromocytoma or neuroblastoma), may produce acute myocarditis (with focal myocardial necrosis and inflammation), cardiomyopathy, tachycardia, and arrhythmias. Similar abnormalities have been described with the excessive use of beta-adrenergic receptor agonist inhalants and methylxanthines in patients with severe pulmonary disease. The administration of beta receptor agonists or catecholamines (i.e., dobutamine or epinephrine, respectively) has been associated with the appearance of transient left ventricular apical dyskinesis and anterior electrocardiographic T wave inversions. This entity, known as takotsubo or stress cardiomyopathy, is more likely to occur in women than in men. It resolves spontaneously when catecholamine secretion abates.[19,20]

Several mechanisms may be responsible for the acute and chronic myocardial damage associated with catecholamines. They may exert a direct toxic effect on the myocardium through changes in autonomic tone, enhanced lipid mobility, calcium overload, free radical production, or increased sarcolemmal permeability. Alternatively, myocardial damage may be secondary to a sustained increase in myocardial oxygen demands and/or decrease in myocardial oxygen supply—the latter caused by catecholamine-induced coronary arterial vasoconstriction or platelet aggregation.

Inhalants

Inhalants may be classified as organic solvents, organic nitrites (e.g., amyl nitrite or amyl butyl), and nitrous oxide. The organic solvents include toluene (airplane glue, rubber cement, paint thinner), Freon, kerosene, gasoline, carbon tetrachloride, acrylic paint sprays, shoe polish, degreasers, nail polish remover, typewriter correction fluid, adhesives, permanent markers, room freshener, deodorants, dry-cleaning agents, and lighter fluid. These solvents are most often inhaled by children or young adolescents. Acute or chronic inhalant use occasionally has been reported to induce cardiac abnormalities, most commonly dysrhythmias; rarely, inhalant use has been associated with myocarditis, MI, and sudden death. The inhalation of Freon, for example, can sensitize the myocardium to catecholamines; in these individuals, fatal arrhythmias have been reported to occur when the user is startled during inhalation.

Pharmaceuticals

Antiretroviral Agents

Subjects treated with highly active antiretroviral therapy (HAART; see Chap. 72) have been observed to have severe hypertriglyceridemia (serum triglyceride levels >1000 mg/dL), marked elevations in lipoprotein(a), hypercholesterolemia, increased LDL and decreased HDL cholesterol levels, and insulin resistance.[21] Not surprisingly, therefore, patients who are maintained on these agents have an increased risk of atherosclerosis.[22] Dilated cardiomyopathy in association with HIV antiretroviral therapy has been reported.[23-25] In mice, zidovudine produces a cardiomyopathy, with pathologic changes demonstrable in the mitochondria, and similar ultrastructural mitochondrial changes have been observed in myocardial biopsy specimens from HIV-infected patients treated with this agent.[25] In one individual, discontinuation of zidovudine resulted in a reversal of cardiac dysfunction.

Serotonin Agonists

The medicinal use of serotonin agonists, such as ergotamine and methysergide (migraine therapy); bromocriptine, cabergoline, and pergolide (Parkinson's disease therapy); and fenfluramine and dexfenfluramine (appetite suppressants) has been associated with left- and right-sided valvular disease.[26-29] Echocardiographic and histopathologic findings resemble those described in patients with carcinoid syndrome. Grossly, the valve leaflets and chordae tendineae are thickened and have a glistening white appearance. Histologically, leaflet architecture is intact, but a plaque-like encasement of the leaflets and chordal structures occurs, and proliferative myofibroblasts surround an abundant extracellular matrix.

Two medications used to treat subjects with migraine headaches, ergotamine and sumatriptan, have been associated with acute MI. Ergotamine causes vasoconstriction of intracerebral and extracranial arteries; rarely, its use has been associated with coronary arterial vasospasm and acute MI. Its vasoconstrictor effects are exaggerated by concomitant caffeine ingestion or beta-adrenergic blocker use. Sumatriptan, a selective 5-hydroxytryptamine agonist, also exerts its therapeutic effects by inducing cerebral arterial vasoconstriction. There have been several reports of patients in whom coronary vasospasm and acute MI occurred following the administration of therapeutic doses of sumatriptan, some of which were complicated by ventricular tachycardia or fibrillation and sudden cardiac death.

Chemotherapeutic Agents

Several chemotherapeutic agents may adversely affect cardiac function (see Chap. 90). Some of these substances have been reported to induce hypertension, acute cardiomyopathy, myocardial ischemia or infarction, dysrhythmias, QT prolongation, and/or sudden death (**Table 73-7**; see Table 90-2).[30,31] Among the agents that cause cardiotoxicity, the anthracyclines are known to induce acute myocarditis and long-standing cardiomyopathy. Tyrosine kinase inhibitors may cause a decrease in left ventricular ejection fraction, which is especially likely to occur if administered in conjunction with paclitaxel or anthracyclines. In contrast to anthracycline cardiotoxicity, however, the cardiotoxicity associated with a tyrosine kinase inhibitor is not cumulative or dose-dependent, and cardiac function often returns to normal after the agent is discontinued. As a result, its repeat administration is acceptable once cardiac function has normalized.

Up to 31% of patients who receive paclitaxel as a chemotherapeutic agent develop transient asymptomatic bradycardia. More substantial cardiac disturbances, including atrioventricular block, left bundle branch block, ventricular tachycardia, and myocardial ischemia, occur in up to 5% of subjects. Finally, 5-fluorouracil and capecitabine may cause myocardial ischemia or infarction by inducing coronary vasospasm.

Environmental Exposures

Cobalt

In the mid-1960s, an acute and fulminant form of dilated cardiomyopathy was described in heavy beer drinkers. It was suggested that the cobalt chloride that was added to the beer as a foam stabilizer was the causative agent; therefore, its addition was discontinued. Subsequently, this acute and severe form of cardiomyopathy disappeared. More recently, several reports of dilated cardiomyopathy after occupational exposure to cobalt have appeared; in these individuals, high concentrations of cobalt were demonstrated in endomyocardial biopsy specimens.

Lead

Patients with lead poisoning typically have complaints that are referable to the gastrointestinal and central nervous systems. On occasion, subjects with lead poisoning have electrocardiographic abnormalities, atrioventricular conduction defects, and overt congestive heart failure. Rarely, myocardial involvement may contribute to or be the principal cause of death.

Mercury

Occupational exposure to metallic mercuric vapors may cause systemic arterial hypertension and myocardial failure. Although some studies have suggested that a high mercury content of fish may counteract the beneficial effects of its omega-3 fatty acids, thereby increasing the risk of atherosclerotic cardiovascular disease, more recent assessments have not supported an association between total mercury exposure and the risk of coronary artery disease.

Antimony

Various antimony compounds have been used in the treatment of patients with schistosomiasis. Their use is often associated with electrocardiographic abnormalities, including prolongation of the QT interval and T wave flattening or inversion. Rarely, chest pain,

TABLE 73-7	Cardiotoxic Effects of Chemotherapeutic Agents
AGENT	**INCIDENCE (%)**
Chemotherapy Associated with Left Ventricular Dysfunction	
Anthracyclines	
Doxorubicin (Adriamycin)*	3-26*
Epirubicin (Ellence)	0.9-3.3
Idarubicin (Idamycin)	5-18
Alkylating Agents	
Cyclophosphamide (Cytoxan)	7-28
Ifosfamide (Ifex)	17
Antimetabolites	
Clofarabine (Clolar)	27
Antimicrotubule Agents	
Docetaxel (Taxotere)	2.3-8
Monoclonal Antibody–Based Tyrosine Kinase Inhibitors	
Bevacizumab (Avastin)	1.7-3
Trastuzumab (Herceptin)	2-28
Proteasome Inhibitors	
Bortezomib (Velcade)	2-5
Small-Molecule Tyrosine Kinase Inhibitors	
Dasatinib (Sprycel)	2-4
Imatinib mesylate (Gleevec)	0.5-1.7
Lapatinib (Tykerb)	1.5-2.2
Sunitinib (Sutent)	2.7-11
Chemotherapy Associated with Ischemia	
Antimetabolites	
Capecitabine (Xeloda)	3-9
Fluorouracil (Adrucil)	1-68
Antimicrotubule Agents	
Paclitaxel (Taxol)	<1-5
Docetaxel (Taxotere)	1.7
Monoclonal Antibody–Based Tyrosine Kinase Inhibitors	
Bevacizumab (Avastin)	0.6-1.5
Small-Molecule Tyrosine Kinase Inhibitors	
Erlotinib (Tarceva)	2.3
Sorafenib (Nexavar)	2.7-3
Chemotherapy Associated with Bradycardia	
Angiogenesis Inhibitors	
Thalidomide (Thalomid)	0.12-55
Antimicrotubule Agents	
Paclitaxel (Taxol)	<0.1-31
Chemotherapy Associated with QT Prolongation	
Histone Deacetylase Inhibitors	
Vorinostat (Zolinza)	3.5-6
Miscellaneous	
Arsenic trioxide (Trisenox)	26-93
Small-Molecule Tyrosine Kinase Inhibitors	
Dasatinib (Sprycel)	<1-3
Lapatinib (Tykerb)	16
Nilotinib (Tasigna)	1-10

* At a cumulative dose of 550 mg/m².

bradycardia, hypotension, ventricular arrhythmias, and sudden death have been reported.

Arsenic

Arsenic exposure typically occurs from pesticide poisoning. Its cardiac manifestations include pericardial effusion, myocarditis, and various electrocardiographic abnormalities, including QT interval prolongation with T wave inversion.

Carbon Monoxide

Carbon monoxide has a higher affinity for hemoglobin than oxygen; as a result, elevated blood concentrations of carbon monoxide lead to reduced tissue oxygen delivery. Although central nervous system symptoms are the predominant manifestations of carbon monoxide poisoning, cardiac toxicity may occur because of myocardial hypoxia or a direct toxic effect of the gas on myocardial mitochondria. Such cardiac involvement may appear promptly after carbon monoxide exposure or may be delayed for several days. Sinus tachycardia and various arrhythmias, including ventricular extrasystoles and atrial fibrillation, are common; bradycardia and atrioventricular block may occur in more severe cases. Angina pectoris or MI may be precipitated by carbon monoxide exposure in patients with or without underlying coronary artery disease. Electrocardiographic ST-segment and T wave abnormalities occur commonly, and transient ventricular dysfunction may occur. The administration of 100% oxygen or treatment in a hyperbaric oxygen chamber usually results in rapid resolution of the cardiac abnormalities.

Thallium

Thallium salts are toxic when inhaled, ingested, or absorbed through the skin. Gastrointestinal and neurologic symptoms of poisoning occur within 12 to 24 hours of a single toxic dose (>1 g in adults). Several weeks after acute exposure, individuals are predisposed to cardiac arrhythmias and sudden death.

Cardenolides

Cardenolides are naturally occurring plant toxins that act primarily on the heart, causing serious dysrhythmias—including second- or third-degree heart block—and cardiac arrest. Poisoning with the digitalis cardenolides (digoxin and digitoxin) is reported worldwide. Cardiotoxicity from other cardenolides, such as the yellow, pink, or white oleander and sea mango tree, is a major problem in South Asia. In India and Sri Lanka, yellow oleander has become a popular means of self-injury, with tens of thousands of ingestions annually and a case fatality ratio of 5% to 10%.[32] Prolonged hospitalization and observation is recommended, because the occurrence of dangerous dysrhythmias may be delayed up to 72 hours after ingestion.

"Mad Honey"

Honey produced from the nectar of rhododendrons growing on the mountains of the eastern Black Sea region of Turkey may contain grayanotoxins, which bind to voltage-dependent sodium channels in the heart and lead to bradycardia and atrioventricular block.[33] Symptoms of "mad honey" poisoning (e.g., nausea, vomiting, hypotension, syncope) occur a few minutes to several hours after honey ingestion, with the severity of the poisoning dependent on the amount ingested. Grayanotoxins are metabolized and excreted rapidly, so the toxic effects of honey poisoning are rarely fatal and typically resolve in 2 to 9 hours.

Scombroid

Acute severe myocardial dysfunction caused by histamine poisoning has been reported within 1 hour of the ingestion of spoiled scombroid fish, such as tuna or bonito.[34] The flesh of these fish is rich in histidine, which is metabolized by gastrointestinal flora to histamine. The diagnosis is mainly based on clinical findings, but can be documented by the determination of histamine concentrations in the ingested fish or increased plasma histamine levels in the patient within 4 hours of fish ingestion.

Envenomations

Black widow spider, bee, wasp, jellyfish, cobra, and scorpion envenomation have been associated with cardiac complications, including MI, acute cardiac failure, myocarditis, bradyarrhythmias, heart block, ventricular tachyarrhythmias, and sudden death.[35,36] The mechanisms whereby these adverse outcomes occur include the systemic release of catecholamines, cardiac ion channel modulation, coronary arterial vasoconstriction, and direct myotoxic effects.

REFERENCES

Ethanol

1. Lucas DL, Brown RA, Wassef M, Giles TD: Alcohol and the cardiovascular system: Research challenges and opportunities. J Am Coll Cardiol 45:1916, 2005.
2. Djousse L, Gaziano JM: Alcohol consumption and heart failure: A systematic review. Curr Atheroscler Rep 10:117, 2008.
3. Kloner RA, Rezkalla SH: To drink or not to drink? That is the question. Circulation 116:1306, 2007.
4. di Castelnuovo A, Constanza S, Bagnardi V, et al: Alcohol dosing and total mortality in men and women. An updated meta-analysis of 34 prospective studies. Arch Intern Med 166:2437, 2006.
5. Mukanal KJ, Rimm EB: Alcohol consumption: risks and benefits. Curr Atheroscler Rep 10:536, 2008.
6. Mukamal KJ, Chiuve SE, Rimm EB: Alcohol consumption and risk for coronary heart disease in men with healthy lifestyles. Arch Intern Med 166:2145, 2006.
7. Mukamal KJ, Conigrave KM, Mittleman MA, et al: Roles of drinking pattern and type of alcohol consumed in coronary heart disease in men. N Engl J Med 348:109, 2003.
8. Tolstrup J, Gronbaek M: Alcohol and atherosclerosis: Recent insights. Curr Atheroscler Rep 9:116, 2007.
9. Koppes LL, Dekker JM, Hendriks HF, et al: Meta-analysis of the relationship between alcohol consumption and coronary heart disease and mortality in type 2 diabetic patients. Diabetologia 49:648, 2006.
10. Albert CM, Manson JE, Cook NR, et al: Moderate alcohol consumption and the risk of sudden cardiac death among US male physicians. Circulation 31:944, 1999.

Cocaine

11. Drug Abuse Warning Network (DAWN): National Estimates of Drug-Related Emergency Department Visits, 2006. DHHS Publication No. 08-4339. Substance Abuse and Mental Health Services Administration, Office of Applied Studies. Rockville, MD, 2008.
12. Qureshi AI, Suri MF, Guterman LR, et al: Cocaine use and the likelihood of nonfatal myocardial infarction and stroke: Data from the Third National Health and Nutrition Examination Survey. Circulation 103:502, 2001.
13. Weber JE, Shofer FS, Larkin GL, et al: Validation of a brief observation period for patients with cocaine-associated chest pain. N Engl J Med 348:510, 2003.
14. Bauman JL, DiDomenico RJ: Cocaine-induced channelopathies: Emerging evidence on the multiple mechanisms of sudden death. J Cardiovasc Pharmacol Ther 7:195, 2002.
15. Hsue PY, Salinas CL, Bolger AF, et al: Acute aortic dissection related to crack cocaine. Circulation 105:1592, 2002.

Amphetamines and Methamphetamines

16. Jacobs W: Fatal amphetamine-associated cardiotoxicity and its medicolegal implications. Am J Forens Med Pathol 27:156, 2006.
17. Kaye S, McKEtin R, Duflou J, Darke S: Methamphetamine and cardiovascular pathology. Addiction 102:1204, 2007.
18. Costa G, Pizzi C, Bresciani B, et al: Acute myocardial infarction caused by amphetamines: A case report and review of the literature. Ital Heart J 2:478, 2001.

Catecholamines and Beta-Adrenergic Receptor Agonists

19. Abraham J, Mudd JO, Kapur N, et al: Stress cardiomyopathy after intravenous administration of catecholamines and beta-receptor agonists. J Am Coll Cardiol 53:1320, 2009.
20. Akashi YJ, Nakazawa K, Sakakibara M, et al: Reversible left ventricular dysfunction "takotsubo" cardiomyopathy related to catecholamine cardiotoxicity. J Electrocardiol 35: 351, 2002.

Antiretroviral Agents (Protease Inhibitors)

21. Calza L, Manfredi R, Pocaterra D, Chiodo R: Risk of premature atherosclerosis and ischemic heart disease associated with HIV infection and antiretroviral therapy. J Infect 57:16, 2008.
22. Kulasekaram R, Peters BS, Wiersbicki AS: Dyslipidemia and cardiovascular risk in HIV infection. Curr Med Res Opin 21:1717, 2005.
23. Sudano I, Spieker LE, Noll G, et al: Cardiovascular disease in HIV infection. Am Heart J 151: 1147, 2006.
24. Zareba KM, Lavigne JE, Lipshultz SE: Cardiovascular effects of HAART in infants and children of HIV-infected mothers. Cardiovasc Toxicol 4:271, 2004.
25. Lewis W: Mitochondrial DNA replication, nucleoside reverse-transcriptase inhibitors, and AIDS cardiomyopathy. Prog Cardiovasc Dis 45:305, 2003.

Serotonin Agonists

26. Connolly Antonini A, Poewe W: Fibrotic heart-valve reactions to dopamine-agonist treatment in Parkinson's disease. Lancet Neurol 6:826, 2007.
27. Zanettini R, Antonini A, Gatto G, et al: Valvular heart disease and the use of dopamine agonists for Parkinson's disease. N Engl J Med 356:39, 2007.
28. Schade R, Andersohn F, Suissa S, et al: Dopamine agonists and the risk of cardiac-valve regurgitation. N Engl J Med 356:29, 2007.
29. Weissman NJ, Panza JA, Tighe JF, et al: Natural history of valvular regurgitation 1 year after discontinuation of dexfenfluramine therapy. A randomized, double-blind, placebo-controlled trial. Ann Intern Med 134:267, 2001.

Chemotherapeutic Agents

30. Force T, Kerkela R: Cardiotoxicity of the new cancer therapeutics— mechanisms of, and approaches to, the problem. Drug Disc Today 13:778, 2008.
31. Yeh ET: Cardiotoxicity induced by chemotherapy and antibody therapy. Ann Rev Med 57:485, 2006.

Environmental Exposures

32. Roberts DM, Buckley N: Antidotes for acute cardenolide (cardiac glycoside) poisoning. Cochrane Database Syst Rev (4):CD005490, 2006.

33. Gunduz A, Turedi S, Uzun H, Topbas M: Mad honey poisoning. Am J Emerg Med 24:595, 2006.
34. Grinda J-m, Bellenfant F, Bribet FG, et al: Biventricular assist device for scombroid poisoning with refractory myocardial dysfunction: A bridge to recovery. Crit Care Med 32:1957, 2004.
35. Valkanas MA, Bowman S, Dailey M: Electrocardiographic myocardial infarction without structural lesion in the setting of acute hymenoptera envenomation. Am J Emerg Med 25:1082, 2007.
36. Tibbals J: Australian venomous jellyfish, envenomation syndromes, toxins, and therapy. Toxicon 48:830, 2006.

CHAPTER 74 # Primary Tumors of the Heart

Bruce McManus

Primary tumors of the heart are rare across all age groups, with a reported prevalence of 0.001% to 0.03% in autopsy series.[1] Secondary involvement of the heart by extracardiac tumors is 20 to 40 times more common than by primary cardiac tumors.[1-3] Despite rarity, multiple histologic types of primary cardiac tumors are recognized. Excluding tumors that are primarily based in the pericardium, like mesotheliomas and teratomas (see Chap. 75), the overwhelming majority of primary cardiac tumors are mesenchymal tumors that display the full spectrum of differentiation as those in the soft tissue do. Non-neoplastic hamartomatous lesions represent the majority of pediatric tumors; in the fetus, there is a higher proportion of germ cell tumors.[4] About 75% of all primary cardiac tumors are regarded as benign neoplasms; cardiac myxoma accounts for at least half of them. However, the oncologic designation of benignity understates the potentially devastating effect any benign primary cardiac tumor may impose on the patient. By virtue of their anatomic locations, primary cardiac tumors are capable of producing myriad cardiac, embolic, and systemic symptoms, sometimes with fatal consequences. Of the remaining 25% of primary cardiac tumors that are considered to be malignant neoplasms, the majority are sarcomas; lymphomas are the next most common. Because many symptoms of malignant primary cardiac tumors occur relatively late in the disease course, findings of locally infiltrative or systemically widespread disease at initial presentation are not uncommon.

The diagnosis of primary cardiac tumors is frequently challenging. The symptoms associated with most primary cardiac tumors are nonspecific, and they often mimic far more commonly encountered disease entities. Furthermore, many tumors are manifested with mild and vague symptoms such that most routine workups will fail to identify the underlying abnormality. This elusiveness often results in a delay in the diagnosis of disease. Fortunately, the more widespread use of noninvasive and relatively sensitive imaging modalities such as echocardiography, computed tomography (CT), cardiac magnetic resonance (CMR), and positron emission tomography (PET) (see Chaps. 15, 17, 18, and 19) should facilitate the identification of cardiac lesions. However, the consideration of primary cardiac tumor in the differential diagnosis combined with a high index of suspicion is also paramount in arriving at the correct diagnosis. In addition to the diagnostic challenges, the management of some primary cardiac tumors is also not straightforward even when the histologic diagnosis has been made. Many benign primary cardiac tumors are now found incidentally in asymptomatic individuals. Therefore, the treatment decision requires a thorough analysis of the potential benefits and harms of surgery versus conservative management. Because of our limited experience with the natural clinical course of many primary cardiac tumors, this treatment decision may be difficult to reach.

Clinical Presentations

Primary cardiac tumors are great masqueraders of many commonly encountered cardiac and systemic diseases. Depending on the location, size, mobility, friability, and histologic type of the lesions, cardiac tumors can produce a variety of symptoms and clinical findings. The clinical manifestations that are produced by primary cardiac tumors overall can be divided into four general mechanistic categories: systemic manifestations, embolic manifestations, cardiac manifestations, and phenomena secondary to metastatic diseases.

Systemic Manifestations

Primary cardiac tumors, whether benign or malignant, are capable of producing a multitude of systemic symptoms that can add to the challenge of reaching the proper diagnosis. Patients with primary cardiac tumors may experience constitutional symptoms of fever, chills, fatigue, malaise, and weight loss. In addition, these symptoms mimic those of several connective tissue diseases and vasculitides such as myalgia, arthralgia, muscle weakness, and Raynaud phenomenon.[5,6] Routine laboratory tests may reveal evidence of leukocytosis, polycythemia, anemia, thrombocytosis, thrombocytopenia, hypergammaglobulinemia, and increased erythrocyte sedimentation rate. These systemic manifestations are believed to be produced by secretory products released by the tumor or by tumor necrosis. Among the benign primary cardiac tumors, cardiac myxomas are the most notorious for causing systemic symptoms, and an elevated serum interleukin-6 (IL-6) frequently found in these patients is believed to mediate such symptoms.[7,8] Malignant primary cardiac tumors, similar to their counterparts from extracardiac sites, are also frequently associated with constitutional findings.

Embolic Phenomena

Primary cardiac tumors can cause systemic or pulmonary embolism by way of tumor emboli or thromboemboli that are released from or formed on the surface of the tumor, respectively. The propensity for cardiac tumors to cause embolic phenomena depends largely on the predominant origin of the tumor (intramural or intracavitary), the type of the tumor, and the friability of the intraluminal tumor surface.[9] Among the benign primary cardiac neoplasms, cardiac myxomas are most frequently associated with embolic findings, especially when the tumor possesses a villous surface.[9] Other benign primary cardiac neoplasms that are known to produce emboli include papillary fibroelastomas, hemangiomas, and lymphangiomas.[10-12] Embolism related to malignant primary cardiac tumors is not uncommon because many malignant tumors have a friable and sometimes necrotic luminal surface. However, systemic and pulmonary metastases from the malignant tumor must be excluded because they can produce similar manifestations. Primary cardiac tumors can embolize to almost any organ, resulting in ischemia, infarction, and even delayed aneurysm formation in the organs or the body sites involved.[1,6,13,14] The brain is the most common site of involvement for systemic emboli produced by primary cardiac tumors, and the involvement of both hemispheres and multiple regions is seen more than 40% of the time.[13] The multifocal nature of cerebral involvement should therefore prompt a search for embolic origin with echocardiography and carotid Doppler ultrasound in these instances. Cerebral embolism most commonly results in a transient ischemic attack or an ischemic stroke, but intracranial hemorrhage may occur as well. Depending on the region of the brain involved, patients may experience a variety of psychiatric and neurologic disturbances that range in severity from mild vertigo to seizure and even coma. Delayed aneurysm formation presumably at the site of previous cerebral tumor emboli represents another dreadful complication of the disease.[14] In addition to the brain, the tumor emboli or tumor-associated thromboemboli can occur in almost any organ or tissue. This includes tumor emboli to a coronary artery that result in clinical findings of myocardial infarction, which can further conceal the underlying abnormality. Careful examination of embolectomy specimens is therefore important because it may reveal evidence of tumor emboli. Pulmonary embolization is typically caused by a right-sided tumor, although emboli from a left-sided tumor located proximal to the site of a left-to-right intracardiac shunt can also result in pulmonary embolism in rare instances. Consideration should be given to the possibility of a primary cardiac tumor in patients presenting with findings of pulmonary embolism when no identifiable source of emboli surfaces after conventional assessment.

Cardiac Manifestations

The cardiac manifestations of primary cardiac tumors can result from direct mechanical interference with myocardial or valvular function, interruption of coronary blood flow, interference with electrophysiologic conduction, and accumulation of pericardial fluid. The propensity for various cardiac manifestations depends primarily on the location of the tumor (pericardial, intramural, or intracavitary), the chamber involved, the size, and the infiltrative nature. Pericardial tumors are not addressed in this chapter because they are dealt with elsewhere (see Chap. 75).

Primary cardiac tumors that are completely or predominantly intramural or myocardial are typically asymptomatic, especially if the sizes are small. Large intramural tumors that are within or pressing on major cardiac conduction pathways may, however, cause a wide variety of arrhythmias, including complete heart block and asystole in more severe cases.[5] In addition, large intramural tumors may also compress the cardiac cavities, obstruct the ventricular outflow tract, or contribute to insufficiency of the mitral valve.

In contrast to intramural tumors, primary cardiac tumors with a significant intracavitary component tend to cause more symptoms for patients. Furthermore, intracavitary tumors that are pedunculated and mobile can be especially problematic because of their tendency to interfere with valvular and myocardial function. The precise cardiac manifestations depend also on the locale of a tumor in the heart. For left atrial tumors, intracavitary lesions that are pedunculated and mobile can interfere with the mitral valve and produce clinical findings typical of mitral regurgitation that include fatigue, dyspnea, orthopnea, paroxysmal nocturnal dyspnea, cough, hemoptysis, chest pain, pulmonary edema, and peripheral edema. However, findings atypical for mitral regurgitation, such as the aforementioned systemic and constitutional symptoms, should prompt further investigation. These symptoms can be sudden in onset, intermittent, and positional. Physical examination may reveal signs of pulmonary congestion with an S_3 and loud and widely split S_1, a holosystolic murmur most prominent at the apex with radiation to the axilla, a diastolic murmur from turbulent blood flow through the mitral orifice, and a tumor "plop." Such tumor plop is thought to result from the tumor's striking the endocardial wall or the abrupt halt of tumor excursions. It occurs later

than an opening snap but earlier than an S_3. For intracavitary tumors located in the right atrium, findings of right-sided heart failure that include fatigue, peripheral edema, ascites, hepatosplenomegaly, and elevated jugular venous pressure with a prominent a wave are the most common cardiac presentations.

Because of the right atrial location, the diagnosis is often delayed, with an average time interval from presentation to the correct diagnosis of 3 years. Patients frequently present with rapidly progressive right-sided heart failure and also new-onset heart murmurs because of mechanical interference with the tricuspid valve. In patients with a patent foramen ovale, the buildup of right atrial pressure can produce right-to-left intracardiac shunting with resulting systemic hypoxia, cyanosis, clubbing, and polycythemia. On occasion, patients may also present with superior vena cava syndrome caused by a large right atrial tumor. Physical examination may reveal findings of peripheral edema, hepatosplenomegaly, ascites, elevated jugular venous pressure with prominent a wave and steep y descent, and an early diastolic murmur or holosystolic murmur that exhibits significant respiratory or positional variation.

Right ventricular tumors with a significant intracavitary component may obstruct the filling or the outflow of the right ventricle and as such can produce right-sided heart failure that includes dyspnea, peripheral edema, ascites, and hepatosplenomegaly. Precordial auscultation may reveal a systolic ejection murmur at the left sternal border, an S_3, and a delayed P_2. An elevated jugular venous pressure and Kussmaul sign may also be present. These findings may vary significantly, depending on the position of the patient. In addition, left ventricular tumors with a significant intracavitary component can obstruct the left ventricular outflow tract and produce findings of left-sided heart failure and syncope as well as atypical chest pain from obstruction of a coronary artery by either direct tumor involvement or tumor emboli. Physical examination may reveal evidence of pulmonary edema, low blood pressure, and systolic murmurs that mimic the findings of aortic or subaortic stenosis. The murmurs and blood pressure may display considerable positional variation. In the case of malignant primary cardiac tumors, such as angiosarcomas and primary cardiac lymphomas, malignant hemorrhagic pericardial effusion may be present. Life-threatening cardiac tamponade and cardiac rupture leading to sudden death may also occur.[15-17]

Metastatic Diseases

Truly metastatic diseases are by definition features of malignant primary cardiac tumors. Most malignant primary cardiac tumors are detected at a late stage with systemic dissemination present. In some cases, symptoms secondary to the metastatic disease may represent the initial clinical manifestation of the malignant primary cardiac tumor.[18] Common sites of metastases for most primary cardiac sarcomas like angiosarcomas and rhabdomyosarcomas include lung, brain, and bone,[15,19,20] although metastases to the liver, lymph node, adrenal gland, spleen, and skin have also been reported.

DIAGNOSTIC APPROACH

Primary cardiac tumors are among the most challenging disease entities to diagnose because of their rarity and their highly variable and usually nonspecific clinical presentations. Therefore, it is understandable that clinicians who first encounter a patient with a primary cardiac tumor generally attribute the findings to other, more commonly encountered disease entities and proceed with the investigation accordingly. Thus, the key to proper and timely diagnosis of a primary cardiac tumor lies not necessarily in its immediate diagnostic recognition but rather in the consideration of primary cardiac tumor in the differential diagnosis. In addition, clinicians need to maintain a high index of suspicion for rare entities like primary cardiac tumors, especially when atypical features are present. A thorough clinical evaluation including a complete history and physical examination coupled with appropriate laboratory tests is necessary because pertinent information may be present to help support a possible diagnosis of primary cardiac tumor (see Table 74-e1 on website) or secondary cardiac tumor. When cardiac tumor is considered in the differential diagnosis, the most ideal initial method of evaluation is echocardiography (see Chap. 15), either transthoracic or transesophageal, depending on the clinical circumstances. The sensitivities of transthoracic and transesophageal echocardiography for detection of a cardiac mass are 93% and 97%, respectively.[21] Thus, transesophageal echocardiography is more comprehensive and accurate in assessment compared with transthoracic echocardiography, and transesophageal echocardiography is especially advantageous in evaluating right atrial tumors. Three-dimensional echocardiography can assess the size of cardiac masses and describe complex anatomy of the heart.[22] If a cardiac lesion is identified, chest CT with contrast enhancement and CMR with contrast are superior modalities for characterization of the lesions and delineation of the extent of tumor involvement (see Chaps. 18 and 19). They can also help exclude the possibility of direct cardiac extension of a tumor that originates from adjacent mediastinal structures. CT and CMR are particularly good at depicting the pericardium and great vessels and evaluating the extent of disease, and CT can also detect calcification, which is important in the differential diagnosis.[23] Features suggestive of malignant cardiac tumors include a large broad-based lesion occupying most of the affected cardiac chamber, hilar lymphadenopathy, extensive pericardial involvement, and hemorrhagic pericardial effusions. However, the diagnosis of a cardiac tumor, whether benign or malignant, cannot be made with imaging studies alone, and histologic evaluation is necessary for definitive diagnosis. Depending on the clinical settings, tissue diagnosis may be made with less invasive methods such as cytologic evaluation of pericardial or pleural fluids, echocardiographically guided percutaneous cardiac biopsy, or echocardiographically guided transvenous cardiac biopsy.[15,24,25] However, a negative finding on biopsy performed through these less invasive methods does not rule out a diagnosis of malignancy because the false-negative rate of these methods can be significant. Therefore, more invasive methods of tumor biopsy through mediastinoscopy or even thoracotomy may be necessary to obtain a definitive diagnosis. In the scenarios in which the presence of a malignant cardiac tumor is confirmed through tissue diagnosis or strongly suspected on the basis of clinical and imaging findings, a full metastatic workup should be performed if it is clinically feasible. Of note, the great majority of malignant cardiac tumors represent local or distant metastases by an extracardiac tumor, and most malignant primary cardiac tumors are diagnosed at an advanced stage with distant metastases already present. Therefore, a thorough physical examination and a complete series of imaging may help locate probable extracardiac origin of the primary tumor or identify potential metastatic lesions from the primary cardiac tumor. This information will help in the disease staging and prognostication as well as in the planning of a treatment course.

Benign Tumors

Myxomas

Myxoma, the most common type of primary cardiac tumor, accounts for 30% to 50% of all primary tumors of the heart.[1] It has an annual incidence of 0.5 per million population and most commonly presents in adults 30 to 50 years of age, although it can occur in nearly all age groups ranging from 1 to 83 years.[8] Sixty-five percent of cardiac myxomas occur in women, and 4.5% to 10% of cardiac myxomas are familial[8]; thus, routine screening of first-degree relatives of myxoma patients is recommended.[22] Although there was debate in the past about whether cardiac myxoma was, indeed, a neoplastic entity or an organized thrombus, recent gene expression and immunohistochemical studies have shown that cardiac myxoma is a neoplasm with tumor cells arising most likely from multipotent mesenchymal cells.[26-32] Other features suggestive of its being a neoplastic process include its ability to recur, occurrence in multiple sites, and occurrence in families. Despite several documented reports of metastases to various anatomic sites, the typical cardiac myxoma is regarded as a benign neoplasm in a conventional sense, and the reported metastases most likely represent tumor growth from embolic tumor fragments that are deposited along the arterial circulation in different remote sites. Thus, although histopathologically benign, cardiac myxomas can cause chronic systemic inflammation, embolism, or intracardiac obstructions, leading to increased morbidity.[33]

The pathogenesis of cardiac myxoma is poorly understood, especially for those tumors that occur sporadically. Studies have, however, shed more light on the pathogenesis of familial cases of cardiac myxomas. Carney syndrome accounts for the majority of familial cases of cardiac myxoma and for 7% of all cardiac myxomas.[27]

Carney syndrome or complex is an autosomal dominant syndrome characterized by myxoma formation in cardiac and several extracardiac locations, spotty skin pigmentation, endocrine hyperactivity, and other tumors (such as testicular Sertoli cell tumor, psammomatous melanotic schwannoma, pituitary adenoma, and thyroid tumors).[27] The cardiac myxomas occurring in the setting of Carney syndrome and sporadic cases are histologically indistinguishable. However, cardiac myxomas associated with Carney syndrome show no age or gender predilection, can be single or multiple, can occur in any intracardiac location, and tend to recur with a rate of 20% despite adequate surgical excision. In contrast, sporadic cases of cardiac myxoma tend to occur in women of middle age and as isolated lesions in the left atrial aspect of interatrial septum. Sporadic cases have a lower recurrence rate (roughly 3%) than those mentioned previously. Mutations in *PRKAR1A*, a regulatory subunit 1A of cAMP-dependent protein kinase A (PKA), and in *MYH8*, a non-PKA phosphorylated perinatal myosin isoform, are believed to be responsible for cardiac myxoma formation in most individuals with Carney syndrome. The precise mechanism of tumorigenesis involving these mutations is unknown. However, there may be a role for genetic testing for these mutations in asymptomatic kindreds of individuals with myxomas to guide further investigation and management.[34]

Clinically, patients with symptomatic cardiac myxoma can have a variety of nonspecific findings, depending on its size, location, and mobility. However, the majority of the patients will present with at least one of the classic triad of obstructive cardiac, embolic, and constitutional or systemic signs.[1,5] The obstructive cardiac findings including dizziness, dyspnea, cough, pulmonary edema, and heart failure are the result of mechanical interference with the mitral valve by the tumor and account for the most common presenting findings in the triad. Tumor embolism is another common basis for clinical presentation and can affect the systemic or pulmonary circulation, depending on the location of the tumor and the patency of the foramen ovale. Cardiac myxoma is the most common primary cardiac tumor to produce tumor emboli, and it has been reported to embolize to virtually any organ or tissue. Constitutional and nonembolic systemic findings secondary to cardiac myxoma include several nonspecific symptoms, such as fever, weight loss, fatigue, myalgia, arthralgia, muscle weakness, and Raynaud syndrome. These nonspecific symptoms often create the most confusion and difficulty in the diagnosis because they may mimic immunologic diseases.[6,7,35] They are believed to be related to IL-6 release by the myxoma tumor cells. A significant subset (approximately two thirds) of patients with cardiac myxoma have abnormal electrocardiograms (ECGs), commonly showing evidence of left atrial enlargement, although a variety of abnormalities can be seen.[6,9,36] However, atrial arrhythmias or conduction disturbances are rare. On chest radiography, about one third of patients have normal findings. Evidence of elevated left atrial pressure, such as left atrial enlargement, vascular redistribution, prominent pulmonary trunk, and pulmonary edema, is found in 53% of patients with left atrial myxoma.[5] Cardiomegaly is seen in 37% and 50% of left and right atrial myxomas, respectively. Intracardiac tumor calcification is a rare finding in left atrial myxomas but is found in 56% of patients with right atrial myxoma. The typical imaging modalities used for diagnostic and preoperative assessment purposes include CT, CMR, and echocardiography. Most cardiac myxomas appear as spherical or ovoid masses with lobular contour on CT and CMR scans.[5] Two thirds of myxomas are heterogeneous, whereas one third appear homogeneous on CT.

Contrast-enhanced CT reveals that most myxomas have an overall attenuation lower than that of myocardium; few such tumors have equivalent attenuation, but in no instance have the tumors shown higher attenuation. CMR shows heterogeneous signal intensity in 90% of cardiac myxomas; the T1-weighted images show isointense signal in 79% and hyperintense signal in 14% of the cases (see Chap. 18). Cine gradient-echo CMR appears to be superior to other imaging modalities in the assessment of cardiac tumors because it allows better visualization of the size, location, and point of attachment of the tumor.[5] Echocardiography is the most commonly used modality for diagnostic purposes, and transesophageal echocardiography is the recommended method for initial assessment of suspected cardiac lesions.[3]

Cardiac myxoma most commonly occurs in the left atrium (**Fig. 74-1**). A recent meta-analysis showed that 83% of cardiac myxomas occur in the left atrium (see Fig. 15-86), 12.7% occur in the right atrium, and 1.3% are biatrial.[8] Occurrence in the ventricles is uncommon; only 1.7% and 0.6% of myxomas occur in the left ventricle and the right ventricle, respectively.[1] The majority (>90%) of myxomas are solitary, although multiple synchronous cardiac myxomas can occur, especially in the setting of Carney syndrome. Cardiac myxomas are generally pedunculated tumors with a fibrovascular stalk attaching to the subendothelial base. The usual site of attachment is the interatrial septum in the region of the fossa ovalis.[6,37] Rarely, cardiac myxoma can involve heart valves directly. Most have sizes ranging from 4 to 8 cm in diameter, although they can reach a size of 16 cm.[4,5,8] The mean weight is 37 g, with a range of 15 to 180 g. Approximately half of the cardiac myxomas have a smooth compact surface, whereas the remaining half have a villous surface. Evidence suggests that myxomas with a villous surface are more likely to embolize.[9] On cross section, cardiac myxomas have a gelatinous appearance, although foci of hemorrhage, calcification (see Fig. 74-e1 on website), ossification, and cystic change can also be present.[5] On histologic examination, the myxoma contains sparsely distributed uniform spindle- and stellate-shaped cells within an extensive myxoid stroma. Although generally hypocellular, the degree of cellularity can vary from tumor to tumor. Tumor spindle- and stellate-shaped cells typically possess round or oval nuclei, with indistinct nucleoli and indistinct cell borders. Binucleate or multinucleate cells may be seen. Mitotic figures are rarely present. The myxoid stroma is composed of acid mucopolysaccharides that are hyaluronidase sensitive. The stroma typically contains prominent thin-walled vessels. Necrosis, calcification, and Gamna bodies (calcified elastic fibers) can be seen in a small subset of cardiac myxomas.[4,5] Smooth muscle cells and fibroblasts are occasionally present in the stroma.[32] A mixed inflammatory infiltrate is also commonly seen. Although infrequent, cardiac myxomas may contain epithelial or glandular, hematopoietic, chondroid, and thymic elements.[32,38,39] Experts suspect that these heterotopic elements represent a form of choristoma. Even more rarely, malignant transformation of these heterotopic elements can occur, giving rise to various malignant neoplasms.[38] On histochemical evaluation, both the stroma and the tumor cells stain positive with periodic acid–Schiff, whereas only the stroma shows positive staining with alcian blue. On immunohistochemical evaluation, the stromal tumor cells show vimentin positivity and variable S100 and NSE positivity, but never keratin positivity.[32] When embolic myxoma is suspected in embolectomy specimens, calretinin and IL-6 may be useful in differentiating between embolic myxoma and myxoid thrombus.[9,40]

The treatment of symptomatic cardiac myxoma is prompt surgical resection of the tumor with the patient placed on cardiopulmonary bypass.[41] Complete excision is the goal, although this may not be possible in all instances.[42] Immediate postoperative mortality in most series ranges from 0% to 7.5%.[6,37,43] Other common postoperative complications include arrhythmias, which may require long-term medication.[37] Recurrence develops in about 3% of tumors, although the rate is higher with familial cardiac myxomas and can occur anywhere from 3 months up to 14 years postoperatively.[5,23-25] Recurrences can be local or in extracardiac locations, such as the brain, lung, skeletal muscle, bone, kidney, gastrointestinal tract, skin, and other soft tissue sites. Recurrence of myxoma in the brain, which probably represents growth of the embolized tumor fragments, can be difficult to manage, but chemotherapy is not recommended because embolic myxomas do not truly represent metastatic diseases.[44] A particularly rare but potentially life-threatening complication is the development of cerebral aneurysm secondary to embolic tumor fragments.[14]

Lipomas and Lipomatous Hypertrophy of the Atrial Septum

Benign lipomatous tumor is the second most common primary neoplasm of the heart and can be divided into two major groups primarily on the basis of the degree of encapsulation—lipoma and lipomatous hypertrophy of the atrial septum (LHAS). Cardiac lipomas (**Fig. 74-2**) can occur sporadically at all ages with equal frequency in both sexes.[45]

Although lipomas from other body sites, such as skin, frequently show cytogenetic abnormalities involving chromosome 12 in q15,[46] the molecular and genetic basis of cardiac lipomas is not elucidated. Clinically, most cardiac lipomas are asymptomatic and typically are incidental findings. However, the tumor can produce a variety of symptoms, depending on its size and location. Cardiac lipomas can occur at any atrial or ventricular surface.[1] They originate most commonly in the subepicardial and subendocardial locations, although intramyocardial lesions have also been reported. Subendocardial lipomas with a prominent intracavitary component can interfere with mechanical function of the heart, resulting in symptoms of heart failure.[47] Subepicardial tumors are usually asymptomatic, but large lesions may cause compression of the heart and produce pericardial effusion.[1] Intramyocardial lipoma may interfere with electrical conduction in the heart and cause arrhythmias. Diagnostically, even though transesophageal echocardiography can be used to assess the location, size, and mobility of these cardiac lesions, it may not be possible to accurately determine the tissue type because typical cardiac lipomas have a nonspecific appearance on ultrasound examination.[45,48] CT can provide better tissue characterization because cardiac lipomas display a low attenuation signal similar to subcutaneous or mediastinal fat.[45] In gross appearance, cardiac lipomas usually are single well-encapsulated masses, although multiple lesions can occur, especially in patients with tuberous sclerosis.[45] Size typically ranges from 1 to 8 cm in diameter. Similar to lipomas found in other sites, cardiac lipoma is histopathologically composed of mature fat cells with occasional fibrous connective tissue (fibrolipoma) and vacuolated brown fat (hibernoma-like). Areas of degeneration and extensive radiographically apparent calcification may be present.[49] The treatment of symptomatic cardiac lipomas is surgical resection, and the postoperative prognosis is excellent.[1,47]

In contrast to lipoma, LHAS (**Fig. 74-3**), also known as massive fatty deposits of the atrial septum, is a nonencapsulated excessive accumulation of fat in the atrial septum at the level of the fossa ovalis that is more than 2 cm in thickness and typically occurs in elderly, obese patients; the mean age at diagnosis in most series is about 70 years.[48] A study revealed that this disease as diagnosed by CT scan may have an incidence as high as 2.2%, which is considerably higher than previously estimated.[48] The cause of LHAS is unknown, and there is controversy about whether the condition truly represents a neoplasm in most instances.[1,48,50] Its apparent association with advanced age and obesity has led to the suggestion that it may represent a metabolic process. However, the observed occurrence in nonobese patients suggests otherwise.[1] Clinically, the great majority of LHAS does not cause any symptoms. On occasion, it can result in a variety of rhythm disturbances and even sudden death.[45] These rhythm disturbances are speculated to involve fatty tissue infiltration into atrial myocyte tissue, which alters the architecture and function of the myocytes.[51] In rare instances in which the tumor protrudes into the right atrium and the superior vena cava, patients can present with symptoms related to blood flow obstruction.[52] CT and CMR are the most desirable modalities for the diagnosis of LHAS because they are superior to echocardiography in differentiating between fat and connective tissue. Multislice CT is the most advantageous method of diagnosis because it has greater coverage, has a decreased number of motion artifacts, and provides sharper images (see Fig. 15-90).[51] On imaging, the atrial septum is thickened to up to 7 cm, whereas normally it is less than 1 cm,[48,53] but this thickening always avoids the fossa ovalis, giving the atrial septum a dumbbell or hourglass shape.[51] The lipomatous hypertrophy appears macroscopically as circumscribed, nonencapsulated, slightly firm adipose tissue and cannot be differentiated from epicardial fat.[51] Accumulation of the fat beneath the atrial septal endocardium may bulge into the right atrium. On histologic examination, LHAS contains an infiltrating mixture of mature fat and vacuolated adipose cells resembling brown fat with enlarged cardiac myocytes. There is a focal excess of fibrous tissue. No mitotic activity is observed in the fat cells in contrast to liposarcoma.[1] Occasional mononuclear cells are present, and mast cells are also not uncommon in association with the adipose cells. LHAS with symptomatic arrhythmias can be managed medically; surgical excision should be restricted to the rare cases in which the disease causes symptomatic hemodynamic obstruction.[48,54]

Papillary Tumors of the Heart Valves

Papillary fibroelastoma is the third most common primary cardiac tumor with an incidence of up to 0.33% in autopsy series.[55] It is believed to be an acquired lesion of fibroblastic origin with a slow growth rate that is distinct from Lambl excrescences.[12,56] It does not spontaneously regress. It also may have focal calcification and occasionally cystic degeneration.[33] Clinically, most patients with papillary fibroelastoma are asymptomatic. However, a review of the literature shows that nearly half of

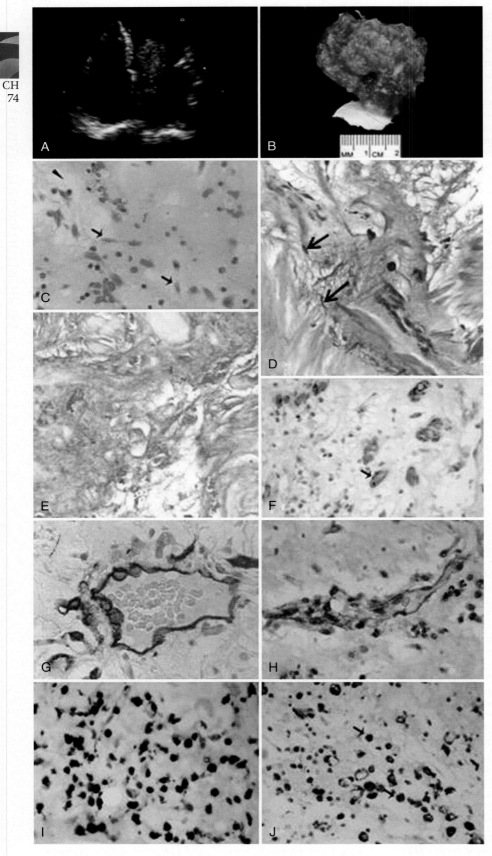

FIGURE 74-1 **A,** Four-chamber echocardiogram of a left atrial myxoma in a 71-year-old woman showing a mass on the left side of the heart projecting from the atrial septum through the mitral valve into the left ventricle. **B,** Gross photograph of the left atrial myxoma that was surgically excised from the same woman. The tumor is a pedunculated, variegated mass with a friable, gelatinous texture. **C,** Hematoxylin and eosin staining of the loose, proteoglycan-rich tumor (×200). The tumor is highly vascular, with vessels containing red blood cells admixed with lipidic cells present in a network throughout the tumor matrix (arrows). **D,** Movat pentachrome staining aids in defining the composition of a myxoma (×400). A variably loose (bubbly turquoise appearance) glycosaminoglycan-rich connective tissue is interspersed with collagen (yellow), rare mononuclear cells, and lipidic mesenchymal cells (arrows, magenta). **E,** Immunohistochemical staining indicates prominent expression of versican (golden brown), a major proteoglycan in myxomas (×400). **F, G,** and **H,** Immunohistochemical staining for vessels was positive for alpha smooth muscle actin (arrow), CD34, and CD31, respectively (×400). **I,** Staining for leukocyte common antigen is positive for mononuclear cells (×400). **J,** Staining for CD68 shows several macrophages (arrows), some of which are hemosiderin laden, reflecting previous hemorrhage, a common occurrence in myxomas (×400).

patients can be symptomatic[55] with transient ischemic attacks, stroke, angina, myocardial infarction, and dyspnea. Cerebral embolic symptoms are present in more than half of the symptomatic patients.[55] Rarely, patients present with subacute bacterial endocarditis–like findings, and pulmonary embolism and sudden death have also been reported. Cardiac papillary fibroelastomas are usually firmly attached to the valvular or mural endocardium. In contrast to other cardiac neoplasms like cardiac myxoma, the embolic material from papillary fibroelastoma is believed to be fibrin or a thrombus originating from the fragile papillary fronds of the tumor surface because fragments of tumor have only rarely been found in the vessels involved.[57] Transesophageal echocardiography is the recommended imaging modality for the diagnosis and characterization of papillary fibroelastoma (see Fig. 15-88), with a sensitivity and specificity of 89% and 88%, respectively, for lesions measuring 2 cm or more.[58] A papillary fibroelastoma generally appears as a round, oval, or irregular lesion that is well demarcated and homogeneous on echocardiography. A diagnosis is supported by the echodensity of the tumor's central collagen core. CMR can differentiate between a tumor and a thrombus by the delayed enhancement after the administration of extracellular contrast media. With multislice scanners, CT is just as effective as echocardiography in depicting small moving structures. Cine CMR can also assess myocardial and valvular function, but the spatial resolution is reduced.[33] Even though papillary fibroelastoma can be found anywhere in the heart, 80% to 90% are found on the valvular endocardium.[58] The aortic valve is the most common site (37% to 45%), although fibroelastomas can also originate on the mitral, tricuspid, or pulmonary valves and less commonly on the left atrial and left ventricular endocardium.[55,58-60] The lesions are single in 91% of the cases,[58] although multiple papillary fibroelastomas from different sites can be found in a small subset of patients.[61,62] The average size of a reported papillary fibroelastoma is about 1 cm in diameter, and it can range from 0.2 to 4.6 cm. In gross appearance, the papillary fibroelastoma has often been compared with the sea anemone because of the numerous and delicate papillary fronds. The tumor is soft, white to tan, and often friable with adherent thrombus, which likely represents the source of the emboli. Forty-four percent of papillary fibroelastomas have a 1- to 3-mm stalk, and this mobile type of papillary fibroelastoma appears more likely to give rise to embolism.[55,58,63] Papillary

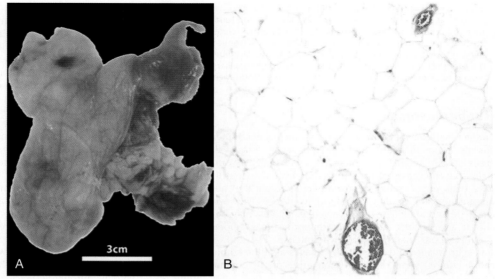

FIGURE 74-2   A, Gross photograph of a pericardial lipoma from a 71-year-old man. **B,** Hematoxylin and eosin staining depicts mature adipocytes in the tumor with associated vascular supply (×200).

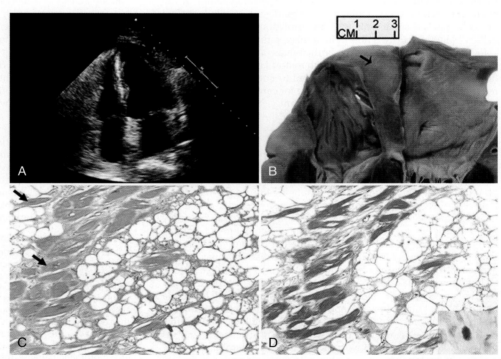

FIGURE 74-3   A, Four-chamber echocardiogram demonstrating lipomatous hypertrophy of the atrial septum in a 72-year-old woman. **B,** Lipomatous hypertrophy of the atrial septum in a heart from a 62-year-old man. The atrial septum superior to the fossa ovale was measured to have a thickness greater than 3 cm (arrow). **C,** Hematoxylin and eosin staining depicts variably hypertrophied and atrophied cardiac myocytes (arrows), with associated fibrous tissue and an admix of mature (larger) and immature (smaller and granular) adipocytes (×200). **D,** Movat pentachrome staining highlights the myocytes (red) and associated excess collagen (yellow) as well as the unusual adipose tissue (×200). **D, inset,** Chloracetate esterase staining shows the presence of mast cells (×400). (**A** and **B** courtesy of Dr. Kenneth Gin, University of British Columbia, Division of Cardiology.)

fibroelastoma has a distinct histologic appearance with multiple narrow, elongated, avascular papillary villous fronds radiating from a central stalk. Each frond has a surface that is covered by a single hyperplastic layer of endothelial cells frequently with attached fibrin thrombi, and the matrix of the papillary fronds consists of variable amounts of mucopolysaccharides, collagen, elastic fibers, and rare spindle cells resembling smooth muscle cells or fibroblasts. The treatment of papillary fibroelastoma is surgical excision or tumor shaving from the valvular leaflets with

either reconstitution or, less commonly, replacement of the valve.[33,50,58] In prospective studies involving 45 patients with suspected papillary fibroelastomas based on transesophageal echocardiography, 6.6% of the patients went on to develop embolic-type symptoms in a 1-year follow-up period.[58] However, the risk of papillary fibroelastoma–related complication must be weighed against the risk of surgery from patient to patient. Asymptomatic patients with small, left-sided, nonmobile-type papillary fibroelastomas can be cautiously observed, whereas excision should be considered for patients with larger (≥1 cm) or mobile-type papillary fibroelastomas .[50,53,58] Aortic valve location and tumor mobility are good predictors for cardiac papillary fibroelastoma–related deaths.[33] No data are currently available to support the use of systemic anticoagulation to prevent the embolic complications of papillary fibroelastoma. The prognosis for patients with surgically resectable papillary fibroelastoma is excellent, and there is no reported case of recurrence to date.[58]

Rhabdomyomas

Cardiac rhabdomyomas are the most frequently encountered primary cardiac tumor in infants and children. Nearly 80% of the reported cases of cardiac rhabdomyomas occur in patients younger than 1 year,[29] but rare cases of cardiac rhabdomyomas occurring in adults have been encountered.[64] Arrhythmias represent the most common presentation for adult-type rhabdomyomas.[64,65] However, for both fetal-type and adult-type rhabdomyomas, patients may be asymptomatic if the lesions are small. Rhabdomyomas appear as well-circumscribed masses with hyperintense T1- and T2-weighted spin-echo images and hypointense images after the administration of gadolinium. Cardiac rhabdomyoma arises more commonly in the ventricles, although up to 30% of cases can involve either atrium.[1,66] On histologic examination, cardiac rhabdomyoma is a well-demarcated lesion composed of enlarged cells with clear cytoplasm and occasional "spider cells."[1] Adult-type cardiac rhabdomyoma histologically resembles the extracardiac rhabdomyoma found in the head and neck region of adults, with a high degree of cellularity, foci of tightly packed small cells, and inconspicuous vacuolated spider cells.[59,61] Mitotic activity is absent in adult-type rhabdomyoma.

In symptomatic patients with arrhythmias, antiarrhythmic drugs may be used, and surgical excision with removal of the culprit portion of the lesion is indicated if the drugs fail to control symptoms.[4] No recurrence has been documented to date for cardiac rhabdomyomas, and the prognosis of this disease is excellent.

Fibromas and Hamartomas

Cardiac fibroma is the second most common primary cardiac neoplasm in infants and children after rhabdomyomas.[1] About 90% of the reported cases occur in children before the age of 1 year, although fibromas can occur in any age group ranging from a few days to 83 years. Some cases of cardiac fibroma have also been diagnosed prenatally by ultrasound.[67] There is no sex predilection, and the majority of cases appear to be nonfamilial.[1] The exact nature of cardiac fibroma is unknown, and it is unclear whether it represents a hamartoma or a true neoplasm. The majority of cardiac fibromas behave like hamartomas with no tendency to recur or to grow aggressively.[1] Of note, hamartomas usually cause arrhythmogenic disorders such as ventricular tachycardia, atrial fibrillation, and right or left bundle branch block.[4] They typically appear as subendocardial yellow-tan nodules or plaques. Histologic findings show multifocal hamartomatous proliferation of cardiac cells with oncocytic features, such as nests of foamy-appearing myocytes resembling macrophages.[4] The first line of treatment is antiarrhythmic drugs, allowing the regression of lesions. Other treatments include surgical excision, electrophysiologic mapping and cryoablation, or direct-vision cryoablation of nodular tumors. The survival rate is approximately 80%.[4] Some cardiac fibromas behave like benign neoplasms with the ability to recur but never metastasize. Although most cardiac fibromas appear to occur sporadically, some appear to develop as part of the Gorlin syndrome (nevoid basal cell carcinoma syndrome), which is a result of germline mutations in the *PTC* gene that maps to chromosome 9q22.3 and is homologous to the Drosophila *patched* gene.[4,68]

Clinically, heart failure, heart murmurs, arrhythmias, and syncope are the more common presenting findings in patients with cardiac fibroma.[1] Less common presenting findings include sudden death and atypical chest pain. However, up to one third of patients with cardiac fibroma can remain asymptomatic. The ECG can show a number of abnormalities, including evidence of left ventricular hypertrophy, right ventricular hypertrophy, bundle branch block, and

atrioventricular (AV) block as well as ventricular tachycardia.[69] Chest radiography may reveal cardiomegaly with or without a focal bulge, and calcification is visible in 15% of cases. Because of its tendency to occur in children, cardiac fibroma must be considered in the differential diagnosis for children with unexplained heart failure, arrhythmias, cardiomegaly, murmur, and pericardial effusion. On echocardiography, cardiac fibroma usually appears as a solitary homogeneous echogenic lesion (see Fig. 15-87).[67] For preoperative assessment, CT and CMR are more desirable for evaluating the "resectability" of the lesion. CT can delineate the heterogeneity of the mural mass, the degree of calcification, and its three-dimensional characteristics.[23] In gadolinium-enhanced CMR and first-pass perfusion imaging, fibromas demonstrate a hypoperfused tumor core that is readily distinguishable from the surrounding myocardium.[4] Cardiac fibromas typically appear grossly as solitary, rounded, intramural masses with a fibrous, whorled cut surface.[1] The mass can be grossly circumscribed or infiltrative with a pushing margin. The average size of the tumor is 5 cm, although lesions up to 10 cm have been reported.[1] Cardiac fibromas are generally single lesions, and they are commonly found in the ventricular septum or the left ventricular free wall, with occurrence in the right ventricle or the atria in less than 10% of cases. On histologic examination, cardiac fibroma shows a proliferation of monomorphic fibroblasts with little or no cellular atypia and resembles fibromatoses with infiltrating margins. The degree of cellularity decreases with age, whereas the amount of collagen deposition increases with age.[1]

Mitotic activity is usually absent but can be present in infants who are only a few months old.[1] A variable amount of elastic fibers and lymphocytic and histiocytic infiltrates may exist. Immunohistochemical examination may demonstrate some degree of smooth muscle actin positivity, but staining for desmin, CD34, and S100 should be negative.[70] The differential diagnosis, especially in the more cellular cases, includes low-grade fibrosarcoma and inflammatory myofibroblastic tumors. The differential feature favoring fibroma over rhabdomyoma is calcification, which occurs in fibromas but not in rhabdomyomas.[4] Because of the potential for cardiac fibroma to cause arrhythmias and occasionally to recur, complete surgical resection in symptomatic cases is recommended. The postoperative prognosis is typically good, although some surgical attempts in infants younger than 4 months have resulted in death.[1] If complete resection is not feasible, palliative partial resection may be considered. Periodic echocardiography may be necessary to monitor for recurrence of the tumor. For large, unresectable tumors, cardiac transplantation may be considered if symptoms such as arrhythmias persist.

Hemangiomas and Lymphangiomas

Primary benign vascular tumors of the heart include hemangiomas, lymphangiomas, and hemangioendotheliomas. Lymphangiomas and hemangioendotheliomas are extremely rare, with only a few reported cases in the literature.[1] In comparison, cardiac hemangioma is more frequent but accounts for less than 2% of primary cardiac neoplasms.[10] Hemangioma can occur in any age group ranging from a few months to the seventh decade of life.[1] Cardiac hemangiomas are considered to be benign neoplasms with potential for recurrence, but the etiology is not defined. Patients with cardiac hemangioma may remain asymptomatic. In symptomatic patients, the clinical presentation of cardiac hemangioma is variable. Depending on the nature and location of the tumor, patients can present with palpitations,[71] arrhythmias,[1,10] heart failure,[1,10] pericardial effusion, ventricular outflow tract obstruction, pseudoangina,[11] cerebral embolism,[9,10] and, in more extreme cases, sudden death. In some instances, giant cardiac hemangioma can result in Kasabach-Merritt syndrome, characterized by thrombosis, consumptive thrombocytopenia, and coagulopathy. Cardiac hemangioma can occasionally be associated with hemangioma in extracardiac sites, such as the gastrointestinal tract and on the skin or face. Echocardiography is a sensitive, noninvasive method for detection of the tumor, with cardiac hemangioma appearing typically as a hyperechoic lesion.[3] Coronary angiography can sometimes demonstrate blood supply to the tumor, with the presence of "tumor blush."[3,10] On chest CT, cardiac hemangioma is characterized by heterogeneous signal with intense enhancement in most cases after contrast material administration.[3,68] On CMR, cardiac hemangiomas appear as masses with intermediate signal intensity on T1-weighted images and hypointense signal on T2-weighted images, and there may be rapid enhancement during infusion of the contrast agent.[72] In gross appearance, cardiac hemangiomas can range from less than 1 cm to 8 cm in size and can occur as intracavitary, intramural, epicardial, or pericardial lesions. They can occur in any chamber, although occurrences in the ventricles are more frequent than in the atria. Multiple tumors are seen in about 30% of cases.[73] Although usually well demarcated, some cardiac hemangiomas can have an infiltrative border, which makes complete surgical resection difficult.[1] The histologic appearance of cardiac hemangiomas is similar to that of hemangiomas arising in other sites. Three main histologic subtypes exist: (1) the cavernous hemangioma, which is composed of multiple thin- or thick-walled dilated vessels; (2) the capillary hemangioma, which is composed of lobules of endothelial cells forming small, capillary-like vessels; and (3) the arteriovenous hemangioma, which is composed of dysplastic thick-walled arterioles, venous-like vessels, and capillaries. The cavernous type of cardiac hemangioma tends not to show a rapid signal enhancement with administration of contrast material on imaging because of the slow blood flow.[3] In contrast to angiosarcoma, necrosis, marked nuclear atypia, and mitotic activity are not seen in hemangioma. In symptomatic patients, radical resection of the tumor is recommended because of the potential for recurrence, especially if the resection is incomplete.[11] The postoperative prognosis is excellent in patients with resectable tumors.[74] Because cardiac hemangiomas may regress spontaneously, conservative management may be considered in asymptomatic patients, particularly if complex and potentially hazardous excision is required.[3] In instances in which surgical resection is high risk, treatment of a congenital pericardial hemangioma next to the coronary artery with high-dose corticosteroid therapy may lead to regression of the tumor.[75] Notably, a single case of cardiac angiosarcoma developing 7 years after surgical excision of a cardiac hemangioma has been reported.[76] As such, in all cases of cardiac hemangioma, periodic echocardiography is recommended to examine for recurrence of tumor growth.

Malignant Tumors

Approximately one fourth of all cardiac tumors are considered malignant, and about one half to three quarters of all malignant primary cardiac tumors are sarcomas; primary cardiac lymphomas are the next most common group.[1,77] Of note is that metastatic tumors to the heart are 20 to 40 times more common (see Chap. 90). Most common malignant neoplasms that involve the heart or pericardium include lung and breast cancer. However, Hodgkin disease, non-Hodgkin lymphomas, malignant melanoma (see Fig. 18-18), numerous primary gastrointestinal malignant neoplasms, and various types of sarcomas arising from extracardiac locations can also secondarily involve the heart. Therefore, it is important as well as logical to consider the possibility that a cardiac lesion confirmed histologically to be a sarcoma may actually be a metastasis from a sarcoma in another anatomic location. A thorough clinical examination combined with a series of imaging studies should help rule out this possibility. The more common malignant primary tumors of the heart (excluding malignant mesothelioma that arises from the pericardium) include angiosarcomas, leiomyosarcomas, rhabdomyosarcomas, malignant fibrous histiocytomas, undifferentiated sarcomas, fibrosarcomas, and malignant lymphomas. Other rarely encountered primary cardiac sarcomas include liposarcomas, synovial sarcomas, and malignant peripheral nerve sheath tumors. In general, the individual histologic subtypes of primary cardiac sarcomas do not appear to influence the outcome as significantly as the histologic grade of the sarcomas, which is evaluated on the basis of a combination of mitotic activity, amount of necrosis, and degree of cellular differentiation. Sarcomas showing high mitotic activity (>5 mitotic figures/10 high-power fields), extensive tumor necrosis, and poor cellular differentiation have a worse prognosis than sarcomas without these features.[1] The presence of metastases also confers a poorer prognosis. In terms of imaging studies, nearly all sarcomas occurring in the heart are aggressive tumors that show a highly infiltrative pattern of growth. They often appear on CT or CMR as large, heterogeneous, broad-based masses that frequently occupy most of the affected cardiac chambers.[3] CMR is usually the method of choice for imaging of sarcomas because it provides excellent tissue characterization and local extent of the tumor.[23] The tumors may also show evidence of extension into other cardiac chambers and the

pericardium, and there may also be associated pericardial effusions and hilar lymphadenopathy.

Angiosarcomas

Primary cardiac angiosarcoma is the most common primary cardiac sarcoma in adults, accounting for 30% to 37% of the cases.[1,2,78] Other malignant vascular tumors, such as Kaposi sarcoma and malignant epithelioid hemangioendothelioma, are even rarer by comparison. Cardiac angiosarcomas typically occur in adults 30 to 50 years old but can occur in almost any age group from 2 to 80 years. A slight male predilection exists.[2,18] With the exception of a single report of familial occurrence of cardiac angiosarcomas, all others appear to occur sporadically.[79] Little is known about the oncogenesis of angiosarcoma. Complex cytogenetic changes and mutations in p53 have been identified in some angiosarcomas.[79,80] Clinically, patients with primary cardiac angiosarcomas typically present with advanced disease, with 66% to 89% of patients already demonstrating evidence of metastatic disease at initial presentation.[2] Initial findings may include dyspnea, chest pain, heart murmur, constitutional symptoms, arrhythmias, superior vena cava syndrome, and evidence of heart failure.[1,2,15,81,82] Because of the propensity for cardiac angiosarcoma to involve pericardium, pericardial effusion and cardiac tamponade may also be the presentation.[14,15,72] Hemorrhagic pericardial tamponade usually indicates tumor infiltration through the myocardium.[23] Less commonly, symptoms related to the metastatic disease, such as stroke-like neurologic symptoms secondary to cerebral metastases, are the initial presentation in patients with cardiac angiosarcoma.[2,83] The ECG may reveal nonspecific ST changes, arrhythmias, and AV block. The chest radiograph may show nonspecific changes like cardiomegaly, widened mediastinum, hilar lymphadenopathy, and pleural effusion.[78] Transesophageal echocardiography is the initial imaging modality of choice[14,73] for detection of the lesion, but echocardiography has limited ability to demonstrate tumor infiltration and cannot depict mediastinal and extracardiac involvement. CT and CMR are therefore required[78] for a better characterization of the tumor growth and involvement (**Fig. 74-4**). Angiosarcomas typically appear as low-attenuation, invasive, irregular nodular masses showing heterogeneous enhancement with the administration of contrast media on CT and heterogeneous mass on CMR. They frequently show extensive pericardial involvement and hemorrhagic pericardial effusions.[3] For histologic diagnosis, invasive methods like echocardiographically guided transvenous cardiac biopsy may provide diagnostic material, but a negative biopsy finding does not rule out the possibility of angiosarcoma.[14,21] Alternatively, biopsy of the metastatic lesion in a more accessible location or cytology examination on pericardiocentesis fluid may also assist in the diagnosis.[15] In gross appearance, angiosarcomas are typically large, multilobular, dark brown intramural masses that may protrude into or replace most of the atrial cavity.[1] About 90% of angiosarcomas arise in the right atrium, and this is thought to contribute to the late onset of symptoms. Involvement of adjacent structures such as the tricuspid valve, pulmonary valve, and vena cava as well as extension into the pericardium may occur. On histologic examination, cardiac angiosarcomas usually exhibit evidence of endothelial differentiation with formation of vascular channels or papillary structures.[1] In contrast to benign vascular lesions, the lining cells are atypical and form irregular anastomosing sinusoid structures. Moderate nuclear and mitotic pleomorphisms are also observed. In some cases, the tumor is composed primarily of anaplastic or spindle cells with little evidence of endothelial derivation, and the identification of poorly formed vascular channels or intracytoplasmic vacuoles containing red blood cells can aid in the diagnosis. Immunohistochemical study can be used to further support evidence of endothelial differentiation by demonstrating CD31, CD34, and von Willebrand factor positive immunophenotype in the tumor cells.[84] Novel lymphatic endothelial markers including D2-40 and LYVE-1 can further identify tumors showing more lymphatic endothelial differentiation than vascular endothelial differentiation.[85-87]

Cardiac angiosarcomas are aggressive-behaving neoplasms that are associated with a poor prognosis and mean survival of 9 to 10 months.[82]

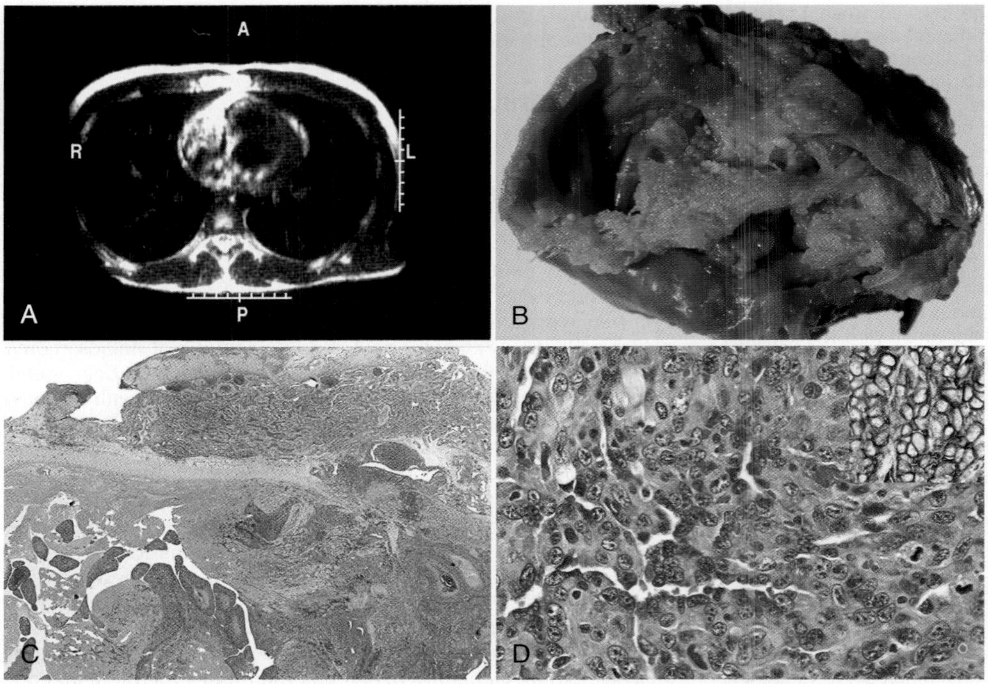

FIGURE 74-4 **A,** CMR imaging of the heart of a 20-year-old man with an angiosarcoma in the right atrium. CMR confirmed findings from a transesophageal echocardiogram that showed a 3 × 3 × 3.5-cm intra-arterial mass with extension toward the inferior vena cava. **B,** Angiosarcoma tumor resected from the right atrium of a 20-year-old man. This tumor was surgically resected from the superior vena cava down to the annulus of the tricuspid valve. The surgical resected specimen shows a tan-red, multilobulated tumor mass. **C** and **D,** Section of angiosarcoma (hematoxylin and eosin; **D** ×400). **D, inset,** Brightly positive staining for CD31 in tumor cells. (**A** and **C** courtesy of Drs. Gerald Berry and Kizhake Kurian, Department of Pathology, Stanford University, Calif., and Department of Cardiovascular Medicine, UFSHC at Jacksonville, Fla., respectively. **B** and **D** from Kurian KC, Weisshaar D, Parekh H, et al: Primary cardiac angiosarcoma: Case report and review of the literature. Cardiovasc Pathol 15:110, 2006.)

This is partially because of the late detection of the disease; most patients present with advanced-stage disease. Common sites of metastases include lung, liver, brain, and bone, although metastases to lymph nodes, adrenal glands, spleen, and skin have also been reported.[14,18] Even though no consistent, effective treatment has been identified for cardiac angiosarcoma to date,[82] a multidisciplinary approach to the treatment of cardiac angiosarcoma is advocated.[15,18] Such an integrated approach includes a combination of surgery, irradiation, adjuvant or neoadjuvant chemotherapy, and immunotherapy with interleukin-12 (IL-12). Chemotherapy with doxorubicin, an anthracycline antibiotic with antineoplastic activity, has been shown to improve the survival of patients.[88] The aim of the surgery is still complete tumor resection.[89] Neoadjuvant chemotherapy may be administered to reduce the tumor mass and to facilitate surgical excision.[90] However, the prognosis for patients with angiosarcomas is still poor. The use of heart transplantation remains controversial in this setting.[2] For patients with advanced-stage unresectable disease, palliative treatment including the use of metallic stents for superior vena cava syndrome and for severe right ventricular outflow tract obstruction may help improve the patient's short-term quality of life.[2,90] It has been shown that the MDM2 protein binds to and inhibits p53 activity. The *MDM2* gene is often overexpressed in angiosarcomas even when the p53 expression is normal. MDM2 directly induces cellular transformation and is associated with vascular endothelial growth factor overproduction and angiogenesis. Thus, inhibition of angiogenesis through MDM2 may potentially be a therapeutic target used to treat angiosarcomas.[91]

Rhabdomyosarcomas

Cardiac rhabdomyosarcomas are the most common primary sarcoma of the heart in children. The average age at disease presentation is in the second decade of life, but it can also occur in young adults. A slight male predominance, especially in the pediatric population,

exists.[1] Because of its rarity, the etiology of primary cardiac rhabdomyosarcomas remains elusive. Heart failure, arrhythmias, cardiac murmurs, and constitutional symptoms are common manifestations of the disease.[1] Occasional cases are also associated with hypereosinophilia, hypertrophic osteoarthropathy, and polyarthritis.[92,93] Nonspecific electrocardiography and chest radiography findings are often present. As with other cardiac sarcomas, transthoracic echocardiography and transesophageal echocardiography are reasonable imaging modalities in the initial workup of the patient thought to have a cardiac lesion.[20,93] Chest CT or CMR is necessary for better delineation of the nature, origin, and extent of the lesion, especially if a malignant lesion is suspected.[20,93] Although echocardiographically guided transvenous cardiac biopsy may be attempted for tissue diagnosis, a negative result cannot be relied on because there is a high rate of false negatives. In contrast to angiosarcomas, cardiac rhabdomyosarcomas show no predilection for a specific cavity, and multiple lesions are frequently present (60%).[20,93] The histologic features of cardiac rhabdomyosarcomas are similar to those of their extracardiac counterparts. The embryonal type and pleomorphic type of rhabdomyosarcomas are more commonly seen as primary tumors in the heart, whereas the alveolar type of rhabdomyosarcomas is typically found as a metastatic disease to the heart.[1] Cardiac rhabdomyosarcomas are aggressive neoplasms with a tendency to produce local and distant metastases, most commonly to the lung and lymph nodes, although spread to various other organs has also been documented previously.[20] Cardiac rhabdomyosarcomas have a dismal prognosis, and survival is usually less than 1 year. Tumors demonstrating a high mitotic activity, extensive tumor necrosis, lack of cellular differentiation, and extensive myocardial and pericardial extension are associated with the worst prognosis.[1,93] The primary aim of treatment is complete surgical resection, but the highly infiltrative nature of tumor often precludes this. Furthermore, the tumor has a poor response to radiation therapy and chemotherapy.[94] In selected cases, heart transplantation may be considered if no obvious distant metastases are present.[93]

Leiomyosarcomas

Leiomyosarcomas are malignant mesenchymal tumors that demonstrate histologic and immunophenotypic evidence of smooth muscle differentiation. The mean age at presentation is in the fourth decade, and there is no apparent sex predilection.[1] The exact oncogenesis of leiomyosarcomas is not known. The common clinical presentations include dyspnea, pericardial effusions, chest pain, atrial arrhythmias, and heart failure.[1,95,96] Approximately 70% to 80% of leiomyosarcomas arise from the left atrium, and they tend to extend into the pulmonary trunk.[95] The tumor is typically solitary but can be multiple in 30% of patients.[1,96] Echocardiography can help identify the cardiac lesion, and contrast-enhanced CT or CMR can help to further characterize the nature and extent of tumor growth.[96,97] On histologic examination, typical leiomyosarcomas show intersecting fascicles of spindle cells with blunt-ended nuclei and well-defined eosinophilic cytoplasm with longitudinal striations. Some leiomyosarcomas contain a large number of highly atypical pleomorphic cells. Immunohistochemical demonstration of smooth muscle differentiation in the form of smooth muscle actin and desmin positivity is required to confirm the diagnosis of leiomyosarcoma, especially for pleomorphic tumors.

Cardiac leiomyosarcomas are rapidly growing tumors with a high rate of local recurrence and distant metastases; the prognosis is poor, with a mean survival of 6 months after diagnosis.[95] Because of the tendency of leiomyosarcomas to recur, cardiac transplantation is not a realistic option. Effective treatment of this progressively lethal disease is unknown. Palliative surgery may be considered in severely symptomatic patients to improve their quality of life.

Other Sarcomas

Besides rhabdomyosarcomas, other nonvascular sarcomas include malignant fibrous histiocytomas, undifferentiated sarcomas, osteosarcomas, fibrosarcomas, myxosarcomas, synovial sarcomas, and malignant peripheral nerve sheath tumors.[1] Inflammatory myofibroblastic tumors are often diagnosed as sarcomas, especially in the pediatric population. They vary in appearance from inflammatory, reactive-appearing proliferations to low-grade sarcomas.[4] Inflammatory myofibroblastic tumors are thought to originate from the endocardium, but the precise nature of their origin is still undetermined. On histologic examination, they are variably cellular with abundant myxoid matrix and surface fibrin and a general background of lymphocytic infiltrate.[4] With the exception of malignant fibrous histiocytomas, the remaining types of sarcomas occur extremely rarely as primary tumors of the heart. The majority of these sarcomas arise in the left atrium, and they can produce symptoms and signs of chest pain, heart failure, valvular insufficiency, arrhythmias, and systemic embolism.[1,3] Constitutional symptoms and those secondary to tumor metastases are also frequently encountered. Like angiosarcomas, rhabdomyosarcomas, and leiomyosarcomas, the other primary cardiac sarcomas are all highly aggressive tumors that show little or no response to chemotherapy and radiation therapy. Complete surgical excision is often attempted in resectable cases, but local recurrences and metastatic disease are common even after apparently complete surgical excision. Furthermore, for tumors extending from the posterior to the anterior wall of the heart, a major obstacle to complete surgical excision is the difficulty in exposing the posterior aspect of the heart. An extreme method of treatment suggested is to excise the heart, to resect the tumor ex vivo, and then to reimplant the heart into the patient, but this is not highly recommended.[91] The mean survival is typically less than 1 year for the different histologic types of primary cardiac sarcomas,[3] and palliative surgery may help improve patients' quality of life.

Lymphomas

Primary cardiac lymphomas are rare neoplasms that account for 1.3% to 2% of all primary cardiac tumors.[16,22] They can arise in both immunocompetent and immunocompromised individuals, with occurrences in immunocompromised individuals being more common.[98] In recent years, there have been increasing reports of primary cardiac lymphomas, particularly in association with human immunodeficiency virus (HIV) infections (see Chap. 72). In the scenarios of solid organ transplantation, posttransplantation lymphoproliferative disease (PTLD) is another setting in which primary cardiac lymphoma can occur,[99] in this case caused by chronic immunosuppression and Epstein-Barr virus infection. Lymphomas associated with HIV infection and PTLD usually have extracardiac involvement at presentation, and isolated cardiac involvement is rare. The average age at diagnosis of primary cardiac lymphomas is 62 to 67 years, with a range of 13 to 90 years,[17,25] and there is a slight male predominance. The common clinical presentations of primary cardiac lymphomas include chest pain, heart failure, pericardial effusion, palpitation, and arrhythmias.[17,25,98] Constitutional symptoms may be present in a subset of patients.[25] Less common presentations of primary cardiac lymphomas are cardiac tamponade, pulmonary and systemic embolism,[100,101] superior vena cava syndrome, and sudden death.[17] Routine chemistry shows elevation of lactate dehydrogenase in 16% to 23% of patients and elevation of sedimentation rate in 20%.[17] Electrocardiographic findings are nonspecific and not uncommonly reveal evidence of AV block and supraventricular arrhythmias.[25,102,103] Chest radiography is typically not helpful, but echocardiography, especially transesophageal, is excellent for initial visualization of such cardiac lesions. CT and CMR are superior at delineating the infiltrative nature of the tumor, and CMR has the highest sensitivity for detection of primary cardiac lymphomas.[25] However, the CT and CMR signals of primary cardiac lymphomas are not specific, and histopathologic examination is required for definitive diagnosis. Cytology of pericardial effusion has proved to be diagnostic in 60% of cases.[25] Transesophageal echocardiography–guided transvenous biopsy and percutaneous intracardiac biopsy may provide diagnostic tissue samples. However, if all else fails, biopsy performed through mediastinoscopy or thoracotomy may be necessary in some cases for diagnosis. Primary cardiac lymphoma involves the right side of the heart in 69% to 72% of the cases.[17,25] It appears as a single lesion in 66% and as multiple lesions in 34% of the cases.[17] Pericardial effusion is present in 49% of the cases, and in some cases, only the pericardial effusion may be evident. Primary cardiac lymphomas range from 3 to 12 cm in size with a mean of 7 cm.[17] On histologic examination, about 80% of primary cardiac lymphomas found in immunocompetent individuals are of the diffuse large B-cell lymphoma type, although cases of small cell lymphomas, Burkitt lymphomas, and T-cell lymphomas have also been reported.[17,104] In immunocompromised patients, small noncleaved or immunoblastic lymphomas are more commonly seen. Flow cytometry and immunohistochemistry can aid in the diagnosis and determination of specific subtypes of cardiac lymphomas. Therapeutically, primary cardiac lymphomas are similar to any aggressive lymphomas arising from other sites in that they are all sensitive to chemotherapy. Early implementation of anthracycline-based chemotherapy with or without radiation therapy has become the mainstay for treatment of primary cardiac lymphomas,[25] and radical surgical excision is generally discouraged.[105] More recently, the use of rituximab, a monoclonal antibody targeted against CD20, in combination with conventional chemotherapy, has shown some promise in improving survival of patients.[106,107] Overall, because of the aggressive nature of most primary cardiac lymphomas, the current prognosis of primary cardiac lymphoma remains relatively poor regardless of the treatment given, and about 60% of patients die of the disease within 2 months after the initial diagnosis.[17] In contrast, the prognosis of patients with primary cardiac PTLD is better, and a trial of reduced immunosuppression is the recommended initial approach in all cases.[41]

Management of Primary Cardiac Tumors

Management of primary cardiac tumors is discussed briefly and in detail in earlier sections.[41] Because of the rarity of primary cardiac neoplasms, no prospective randomized controlled trials have been performed to date. The treatment of benign primary cardiac tumors is mostly surgical, and the urgency of surgical intervention depends primarily on the patient's symptoms and the type of tumor, although consideration should also be given to the general medical status of the patient. For most benign cardiac tumors, no clinical data will allow clinicians to prospectively assess the annual risks of the patient for tumor-related complications. This can sometimes create therapeutic dilemmas, especially if the patient is a poor surgical candidate and minimally symptomatic. For cardiac myxomas, prompt complete surgical excision after diagnosis, regardless of whether the patient is currently symptomatic, is strongly recommended because of the risk of significant morbidity or mortality from tumor embolism or severe hemodynamic compromise. Similarly, because of the risk of embolism, prompt surgical excision is also recommended for patients with papillary fibroelastomas if they are large (≥1 cm) or of the mobile type, although conservative management for patients with small, left-sided, and nonmobile-type papillary fibroelastoma may also be considered.[55,58,63] In contrast, surgical intervention for patients with cardiac lipomas or LHAS should be restricted to those with significant hemodynamic dysfunction.[41] For patients with cardiac fibromas, hemangiomas, or lymphangiomas, complete surgical resection in symptomatic cases is recommended because of the potential for tumor recurrence if the resection is incomplete. Surgery is generally curative for benign primary cardiac tumors like myxomas, and the prognosis of the surgically resectable tumors is generally excellent.

The treatment of malignant primary cardiac tumors like sarcomas and lymphomas is guided primarily by experiences derived from the treatment of their extracardiac pathologic counterparts. For primary cardiac sarcomas, surgery is the mainstay for therapy and offers the only chance for curative therapy, although it is usually limited by early metastases and local spread or recurrence. Most operations are palliative and are performed to relieve cardiac compression or hemodynamic obstruction with partial resection or placement of stents.[41] Neoadjuvant chemotherapy may be administered to reduce the tumor mass and to facilitate surgical excision in some cases.[90] For cardiac angiosarcomas, an integrated approach that includes a combination of surgery, irradiation, adjuvant or neoadjuvant chemotherapy, and immunotherapy with IL-12 is currently advocated for clinically suitable candidates. For other primary cardiac sarcomas, chemotherapy is the treatment of first choice for sarcomas that are unresectable or that present with extracardiac metastases, and combinations of several agents are more effective than single-agent therapy. Radiation therapy may play an adjunct role in these cases. Despite the use of these conventional systemic therapies, the mean survival of patients with most primary cardiac sarcomas is typically less than 1 year regardless of the histologic types,[3] and palliative surgery may offer the only means to improve patients' quality of life. Orthotopic heart transplantation remains controversial but has been employed for treatment of malignant primary cardiac tumors. It has shown success in the context of complex disease and in treating recurrent disease.[22]

As reviewed in detail earlier,[41] primary cardiac lymphomas are generally sensitive to systemic chemotherapy. Prompt implementation of conventional chemotherapy with or without radiation therapy has become the mainstay for treatment of primary cardiac lymphomas,[25] and radical surgical excision is generally discouraged.[105] The use of rituximab may also be considered in some cases.[106,107] For PTLD, early diagnosis is essential to its successful management, and a trial of reduced immunosuppression is the recommended initial approach in all cases.

FUTURE OUTLOOK

The diagnosis and treatment of primary cardiac tumors can be an unexpected challenge for clinicians and surgeons because of their rarity and the lack of clearly defined guidelines in their management. For the initial evaluation of a suspected cardiac mass, echocardiography will likely remain the preferred modality in the years and perhaps decades to come. Although CT and CMR are superior to echocardiography at identification and characterization of cardiac lesions, emerging imaging modalities such as combined PET-CT with the use of novel radiopharmaceutical agents may eventually prove to be more sensitive and specific for diagnosis and characterization of the lesions.[108,109] Furthermore, although not yet demonstrated, it is highly probable that PET-CT will become a more valuable tool for detection of recurrent primary cardiac tumors and metastases of primary cardiac tumors.[108] Recent developments in multidetector CT have further improved diagnostic evaluation of heart tumors with incredible detail.[23] Such approaches further improve diagnostic capabilities for cardiac tumors by delineating tumors, assessing their impact on cardiac function, and planning for surgical intervention.[23]

Genetic analysis with associated gene therapy is an evolving therapeutic option for patients with cardiac tumors. Investigation of the different apoptotic pathways in the heart may lead to safer use of new anticancer drugs. Induction of apoptosis in cancer cells can be achieved by targeting mRNA with antisense oligonucleotides, leading to downregulation of protein expression.[91] Apoptosis in rhabdomyosarcoma cells has been shown to be modifiable by antisense oligonucleotides directed at the oncoprotein mRNA.[91] Other malignant changes in cells and resistance to apoptosis are made possible by the production of chimeric genes that code for fusion proteins. These genes are products of translocations, which occur between chromosomes 12 and 15 [t(12;15) (p13q25)], and the resultant fusion protein is a transcription factor fused to a tyrosine kinase receptor. This fusion protein is a tyrosine kinase that has oncogenic potential.[91] New tyrosine kinase inhibitors may be therapeutically beneficial. Other fusion proteins that have been found in rhabdomyosarcomas have the effect of increasing the production of the antiapoptotic protein Bcl-xL.[91]

With the more widespread use of various imaging modalities and the aging population, it is conceivable that more cases of primary cardiac tumors, especially of benign varieties, will be uncovered incidentally in patients who are not experiencing any clinical symptoms. The management of these patients may become a clinical dilemma, especially for the tumor types for which the conventional treatment is radical tumor excision. Therefore, it is crucial for us to gain a better appreciation of the natural history of many of these benign primary cardiac tumors when they present as small, asymptomatic lesions. For instance, understanding the annual risk of embolism for small papillary fibroelastomas or small,

nonpedunculated myxomas with smooth surfaces will allow proper assessment of the risks and benefits of surgical intervention. Given the rarity of these diseases, an international consortium or network may be required to accumulate the treatment and follow-up data of patients with primary cardiac tumors. Such a source of information will undoubtedly provide valuable data for the clinicians and patients in determining the most appropriate management plan. A similar collective effort is also necessary for primary cardiac sarcomas. Despite our best intentions and effort thus far, primary cardiac sarcomas are incurable diseases with dismal prognoses in most cases.

Studies using high-throughput gene array technology to examine gene expression level or copy number changes in tumors may be a reasonable initial step for identification of genes of interest in the different subtypes of primary cardiac sarcomas.[110] Again, an international network or tumor registry can assist in collecting tissues from surgical specimens of patients undergoing curative or palliative surgical excision for their primary cardiac sarcomas. Furthermore, because of our lack of understanding of primary cardiac sarcomas and sarcomas in general, the classification of sarcomas is in a constant state of evolution.[111] One of the more noteworthy changes stems from our recognition that many sarcomas once considered to be malignant fibrous histiocytomas actually represent poorly differentiated types of other sarcomas like leiomyosarcomas and myxofibrosarcomas.[112] A new term, undifferentiated pleomorphic sarcoma, has now replaced malignant fibrous histiocytoma, reflecting the fact that this tumor truly lacks evidence of specific mesenchymal differentiation.

ACKNOWLEDGMENT

The author is deeply indebted to Dr. Cheng Han Lee, Ms. Lise Matzke, and Ms. Crystal Leung for their incredible assistance with all aspects of this chapter. I also appreciate the generosity and expertise of Dr. Gerald J. Berry, Stanford University, Stanford, Calif.; Dr. Kizhake C. Kurian, University of Florida Health Science Center, Jacksonville; Dr. Glenn Taylor, The Hospital for Sick Children, Toronto; Dr. Kenneth Gin, Vancouver General Hospital, Vancouver; and Dr. Suzanne Chan, British Columbia Children's Hospital, Vancouver. Without their contributions, this work would not have been possible.

REFERENCES

1. Burke A, Virmani R: Tumors of the Heart and Great Vessels. Atlas of Tumor Pathology. 3rd Series, Fascicle 16. Washington, DC, Armed Forces Institute of Pathology, 1996.
2. Best AK, Dobson RL, Ahmad AR: Best cases from the AFIP: Cardiac angiosarcoma. Radiographics 23(Spec No):S141, 2003.
3. Grebenc ML, Rosado-de-Christenson ML, Burke AP, et al: Primary cardiac and pericardial neoplasms: Radiologic-pathologic correlation. Radiographics 20:1073, 2000.
4. Burke A, Virmani R: Pediatric heart tumors. Cardiovasc Pathol 17:193, 2008.

Clinical Presentation

5. Grebenc ML, Rosado-de-Christenson ML, Green CE, et al: Cardiac myxoma: Imaging features in 83 patients. Radiographics 22:673, 2002.
6. Pinede L, Duhaut P, Loire R: Clinical presentation of left atrial cardiac myxoma. A series of 112 consecutive cases. Medicine (Baltimore) 80:159, 2001.
7. Mendoza CE, Rosado MF, Bernal L: The role of interleukin-6 in cases of cardiac myxoma. Clinical features, immunologic abnormalities, and a possible role in recurrence. Tex Heart Inst J 28:3, 2001.
8. Kuon E, Kreplin M, Weiss W, et al: The challenge presented by right atrial myxoma. Herz 29:702, 2004.
9. Acebo E, Val-Bernal JF, Gomez-Roman JJ, et al: Clinicopathologic study and DNA analysis of 37 cardiac myxomas: A 28-year experience. Chest 123:1379, 2003.
10. Kocak H, Ozyazicioglu A, Gundogdu C, et al: Cardiac hemangioma complicated with cerebral and coronary embolization. Heart Vessels 20:296, 2005.
11. Kipfer B, Englberger L, Stauffer E, et al: Rare presentation of cardiac hemangiomas. Ann Thorac Surg 70:977, 2000.
12. Fox E, Brunson C, Campbell W, et al: Cardiac papillary fibroelastoma presents as an acute embolic stroke in a 35-year-old African American male. Am J Med Sci 331:91, 2006.
13. Ekinci EI, Donnan GA: Neurological manifestations of cardiac myxoma: A review of the literature and report of cases. Intern Med J 34:243, 2004.
14. Sabolek M, Bachus-Banaschak K, Bachus R, et al: Multiple cerebral aneurysms as delayed complication of left cardiac myxoma: A case report and review. Acta Neurol Scand 111:345, 2005.
15. Brandt RR, Arnold R, Bohle RM, et al: Cardiac angiosarcoma: Case report and review of the literature. Z Kardiol 94:824, 2005.
16. Sakaguchi M, Minato Y, Katayama Y, et al: Cardiac angiosarcoma with right atrial perforation and cardiac tamponade. Ann Thorac Cardiovasc Surg 12:145, 2006.
17. Chalabreysse L, Berger F, Loire R, et al: Primary cardiac lymphoma in immunocompetent patients: A report of three cases and review of the literature. Virchows Arch 441:456, 2002.
18. Pomper GJ, Gianani R, Johnston RJ, et al: Cardiac angiosarcoma: An unusual presentation with cutaneous metastases. Arch Pathol Lab Med 122:273, 1998.
19. Sinatra R, Brancaccio G, di Gioia CR, et al: Integrated approach for cardiac angiosarcoma. Int J Cardiol 88:301, 2003.
20. Villacampa VM, Villarreal M, Ros LH, et al: Cardiac rhabdomyosarcoma: Diagnosis by MR imaging. Eur Radiol 9:634, 1999.

Diagnostic Approach

21. Meng Q, Lai H, Lima J, et al: Echocardiographic and pathologic characteristics of primary cardiac tumors: A study of 149 cases. Int J Cardiol 84:69, 2002.
22. Ekmektzoglou KA, Samelis GF, Xanthos T: Heart and tumors: Location, metastasis, clinical manifestations, diagnostic approaches and therapeutic considerations. J Cardiovasc Med (Hagerstown) 9:769, 2008.
23. van Beek EJ, Stolpen AH, Khanna G, et al: CT and MRI of pericardial and cardiac neoplastic disease. Cancer Imaging 7:19, 2007.
24. Nitta R, Sakomura Y, Tanimoto K, et al: Primary cardiac angiosarcoma of the right atrium undiagnosed by transvenous endocardial tumor biopsy. Intern Med 37:1023, 1998.
25. Anghel G, Zoli V, Petti N, et al: Primary cardiac lymphoma: Report of two cases occurring in immunocompetent subjects. Leuk Lymphoma 45:781, 2004.

Benign Tumors

26. Terracciano LM, Mhawech P, Suess K, et al: Calretinin as a marker for cardiac myxoma. Diagnostic and histogenetic considerations. Am J Clin Pathol 114:754, 2000.
27. Wilkes D, Charitakis K, Basson CT: Inherited disposition to cardiac myxoma development. Nat Rev Cancer 6:157, 2006.
28. Orlandi A, Ciucci A, Ferlosio A, et al: Cardiac myxoma cells exhibit embryonic endocardial stem cell features. J Pathol 209:231, 2006.
29. Amano J, Kono T, Wada Y, et al: Cardiac myxoma: Its origin and tumor characteristics. Ann Thorac Cardiovasc Surg 9:215, 2003.
30. Kodama H, Hirotani T, Suzuki Y, et al: Cardiomyogenic differentiation in cardiac myxoma expressing lineage-specific transcription factors. Am J Pathol 161:381, 2002.
31. Kono T, Koide N, Hama Y, et al: Expression of vascular endothelial growth factor and angiogenesis in cardiac myxoma: A study of fifteen patients. J Thorac Cardiovasc Surg 119:101, 2000.
32. Pucci A, Gagliardotto P, Zanini C, et al: Histopathologic and clinical characterization of cardiac myxoma: Review of 53 cases from a single institution. Am Heart J 140:134, 2000.
33. Sydow K, Willems S, Reichenspurner H, et al: Papillary fibroelastomas of the heart. Thorac Cardiovasc Surg 56:9, 2008.
34. Aspres N, Bleasel NR, Stapleton KM: Genetic testing of the family with a Carney-complex member leads to successful early removal of an asymptomatic atrial myxoma in the mother of the patient. Australas J Dermatol 44:121, 2003.
35. Mochizuki Y, Okamura Y, Iida H, et al: Interleukin-6 and "complex" cardiac myxoma. Ann Thorac Surg 66:931, 1998.
36. Komiya N, Isomoto S, Hayano M, et al: The influence of tumor size on the electrocardiographic changes in patients with left atrial myxoma. J Electrocardiol 35:53, 2002.
37. Ipek G, Erentug V, Bozbuga N, et al: Surgical management of cardiac myxoma. J Card Surg 20:300, 2005.
38. Miller DV, Tazelaar HD, Handy JR, et al: Thymoma arising within cardiac myxoma. Am J Surg Pathol 29:1208, 2005.
39. Pucci A, Bartoloni G, Tessitore E, et al: Cytokeratin profile and neuroendocrine cells in the glandular component of cardiac myxoma. Virchows Arch 443:618, 2003.
40. Val-Bernal JF, Acebo E, Gomez-Roman JJ, et al: Anticipated diagnosis of left atrial myxoma following histological investigation of limb embolectomy specimens: A report of two cases. Pathol Int 53:489, 2003.
41. Rosenberg FM, Chan A, Lichtenstein SV, et al: Cardiac neoplasms. Curr Treat Options Cardiovasc Med 1:243, 1999.
42. Bjessmo S, Ivert T: Cardiac myxoma: 40 years' experience in 63 patients. Ann Thorac Surg 63:697, 1997.
43. Selkane C, Amahzoune B, Chavanis N, et al: Changing management of cardiac myxoma based on a series of 40 cases with long-term follow-up. Ann Thorac Surg 76:1935, 2003.
44. Altundag MB, Ertas G, Ucer AR, et al: Brain metastasis of cardiac myxoma: Case report and review of the literature. J Neurooncol 75:181, 2005.
45. Salanitri JC, Pereles FS: Cardiac lipoma and lipomatous hypertrophy of the interatrial septum: Cardiac magnetic resonance imaging findings. J Comput Assist Tomogr 28:852, 2004.
46. Mitelman F: Catalog of Chromosome Aberrations in Cancer. New York, Wiley-Liss, 1998.
47. Akram K, Hill C, Neelagaru N, Parker M: A left ventricular lipoma presenting as heart failure in a septuagenarian: A first case report. Int J Cardiol 114:386, 2007 .
48. Heyer CM, Kagel T, Lemburg SP, et al: Lipomatous hypertrophy of the interatrial septum: A prospective study of incidence, imaging findings, and clinical symptoms. Chest 124:2068, 2003.
49. Nova M, Steiner I: A rationale for a stone on the heart—subepicardial lipoma. Cardiovasc Pathol 15:176, 2006.
50. Meaney JF, Kazerooni EA, Jamadar DA, et al: CT appearance of lipomatous hypertrophy of the interatrial septum. AJR Am J Roentgenol 168:1081, 1997.
51. Xanthos T, Giannakopoulos N, Papadimitriou L: Lipomatous hypertrophy of the interatrial septum: A pathological and clinical approach. Int J Cardiol 121:4, 2007.
52. Christiansen S, Stypmann J, Baba HA, et al: Surgical management of extensive lipomatous hypertrophy of the right atrium. Cardiovasc Surg 8:88, 2000.
53. Roberts WC: Primary and secondary neoplasms of the heart. Am J Cardiol 80:671, 1997.
54. Nadra I, Dawson D, Schmitz SA, et al: Lipomatous hypertrophy of the interatrial septum: A commonly misdiagnosed mass often leading to unnecessary cardiac surgery. Heart 90:e66, 2004.
55. Howard RA, Aldea GS, Shapira OM, et al: Papillary fibroelastoma: Increasing recognition of a surgical disease. Ann Thorac Surg 68:1881, 1999.
56. Sumino S, Paterson HS: No regrowth after incomplete papillary fibroelastoma excision. Ann Thorac Surg 79:e3, 2005.
57. Roberts WC: Papillary fibroelastomas of the heart. Am J Cardiol 80:973, 1997.
58. Sun JP, Asher CR, Yang XS, et al: Clinical and echocardiographic characteristics of papillary fibroelastomas: A retrospective and prospective study in 162 patients. Circulation 103:2687, 2001.
59. Saad RS, Galvis CO, Bshara W, et al: Pulmonary valve papillary fibroelastoma. A case report and review of the literature. Arch Pathol Lab Med 125:933, 2001.
60. Georghiou GP, Erez E, Vidne BA, et al: Tricuspid valve papillary fibroelastoma: An unusual cause of intermittent dyspnea. Eur J Cardiothorac Surg 23:429, 2003.

61. Davoli G, Bizzarri F, Enrico T, et al: Double papillary fibroelastoma of the aortic valve. Tex Heart Inst J 31:448, 2004.
62. Eslami-Varzaneh F, Brun EA, Sears-Rogan P: An unusual case of multiple papillary fibroelastoma, review of literature. Cardiovasc Pathol 12:170, 2003.
63. Nawaz MZ, Lander AR, Schussler JM, et al: Tumor excision versus valve replacement for papillary fibroelastoma involving the mitral valve. Am J Cardiol 97:759, 2006.
64. Burke AP, Gatto-Weis C, Griego JE, et al: Adult cellular rhabdomyoma of the heart: A report of 3 cases. Hum Pathol 33:1092, 2002.
65. Krasuski RA, Hesselson AB, Landolfo KP, et al: Cardiac rhabdomyoma in an adult patient presenting with ventricular arrhythmia. Chest 118:1217, 2000.
66. Chen X, Hoda SA, Edgar MA: Cardiac rhabdomyoma. Arch Pathol Lab Med 126:1559, 2002.
67. Kim TH, Kim YM, Han MY, et al: Perinatal sonographic diagnosis of cardiac fibroma with MR imaging correlation. AJR Am J Roentgenol 178:727, 2002.
68. Bossert T, Walther T, Vondrys D, et al: Cardiac fibroma as an inherited manifestation of nevoid basal-cell carcinoma syndrome. Tex Heart Inst J 33:88, 2006.
69. Wong JA, Fishbein MC: Cardiac fibroma resulting in fatal ventricular arrhythmia. Circulation 101:E168, 2000.
70. de Montpreville VT, Serraf A, Aznag H, et al: Fibroma and inflammatory myofibroblastic tumor of the heart. Ann Diagn Pathol 5:335, 2001.
71. Eftychiou C, Antoniades L: Cardiac hemangioma in the left ventricle and brief review of the literature. J Cardiovasc Med (Hagerstown) 10:565, 2009.
72. Oshima H, Hara M, Kono T, et al: Cardiac hemangioma of the left atrial appendage: CT and MR findings. J Thorac Imaging 18:204, 2003.
73. Moniotte S, Geva T, Perez-Atayde A, et al: Images in cardiovascular medicine. Cardiac hemangioma. Circulation 112:e103, 2005.
74. Kojima S, Sumiyoshi M, Suwa S, et al: Cardiac hemangioma: A report of two cases and review of the literature. Heart Vessels 18:153, 2003.
75. Wu G, Jones J, Sequeira IB, et al: Congenital pericardial hemangioma responding to high-dose corticosteroid therapy. Can J Cardiol 25:e139, 2009.
76. Chalet Y, Mace L, Franc B, et al: Angiosarcoma 7 years after surgical excision of histiocytoid haemangioma in left atrium. Lancet 341:1217, 1993.

Malignant Tumors

77. Farah HH, Jacob M, Aragam J: Images in cardiology: A case of cardiac angiosarcoma presenting as pericardial tamponade. Heart 86:665, 2001.
78. Deetjen AG, Conradi G, Mollmann S, et al: Cardiac angiosarcoma diagnosed and characterized by cardiac magnetic resonance imaging. Cardiol Rev 14:101, 2006.
79. Casha AR, Davidson LA, Roberts P, et al: Familial angiosarcoma of the heart. J Thorac Cardiovasc Surg 124:392, 2002.
80. Zu Y, Perle MA, Yan Z, et al: Chromosomal abnormalities and p53 gene mutation in a cardiac angiosarcoma. Appl Immunohistochem Mol Morphol 9:24, 2001.
81. Amonkar GP, Deshpande JR: Cardiac angiosarcoma. Cardiovasc Pathol 15:57, 2006.
82. Kurian KC, Weisshaar D, Parekh H, et al: Primary cardiac angiosarcoma: Case report and review of the literature. Cardiovasc Pathol 15:110, 2006.
83. Liassides C, Katsamaga M, Deretzi G, et al: Cerebral metastasis from heart angiosarcoma presenting as multiple hematomas. J Neuroimaging 14:71, 2004.
84. Weiss SW, Goldblum J: Enzinger and Weiss's Soft Tissue Tumors. 4th ed. St. Louis, Mosby, 2001.
85. Arai E, Kuramochi A, Tsuchida T, et al: Usefulness of D2-40 immunohistochemistry for differentiation between kaposiform hemangioendothelioma and tufted angioma. J Cutan Pathol 33:492, 2006.
86. Khan MA, Mujahed MA: Atrial myxoma producing a saddle embolus in a child. Thorax 25:634, 1970.
87. Xu H, Edwards JR, Espinosa O, et al: Expression of a lymphatic endothelial cell marker in benign and malignant vascular tumors. Hum Pathol 35:857, 2004.
88. Pigott C, Welker M, Khosla P, et al: Improved outcome with multimodality therapy in primary cardiac angiosarcoma. Nat Clin Pract Oncol 5:112, 2008.
89. Hoffmeier A, Scheld HH, Tjan TD, et al: Ex situ resection of primary cardiac tumors. Thorac Cardiovasc Surg 51:99, 2003.
90. Totaro M, Miraldi F, Ghiribelli C, et al: Cardiac angiosarcoma arising from pulmonary artery: Endovascular treatment. Ann Thorac Surg 78:1468, 2004.
91. Neragi-Miandoab S, Kim J, Vlahakes GJ: Malignant tumours of the heart: A review of tumour type, diagnosis and therapy. Clin Oncol (R Coll Radiol) 19:748, 2007.
92. Lo Re V 3rd, Fox KR, Ferrari VA, et al: Hypereosinophilia associated with cardiac rhabdomyosarcoma. Am J Hematol 74:64, 2003.
93. Grandmougin D, Fayad G, Decoene C, et al: Total orthotopic heart transplantation for primary cardiac rhabdomyosarcoma: Factors influencing long-term survival. Ann Thorac Surg 71:1438, 2001.
94. Aksoylar S, Kansoy S, Bakiler AR, et al: Primary cardiac rhabdomyosarcoma. Med Pediatr Oncol 38:146, 2002.
95. Ishikawa K, Takanashi S, Mihara W, et al: Surgical treatment for primary cardiac leiomyosarcoma causing right ventricular outflow obstruction. Circ J 69:121, 2005.
96. Clarke NR, Mohiaddin RH, Westaby S, et al: Multifocal cardiac leiomyosarcoma. Diagnosis and surveillance by transoesophageal echocardiography and contrast enhanced cardiovascular magnetic resonance. Postgrad Med J 78:492, 2002.
97. Ogimoto A, Hamada M, Ohtsuka T, et al: Rapid progression of primary cardiac leiomyosarcoma with obstruction of the left ventricular outflow tract and mitral stenosis. Intern Med 42:827, 2003.
98. Rockwell L, Hetzel P, Freeman JK, et al: Cardiac involvement in malignancies. Case 3. Primary cardiac lymphoma. J Clin Oncol 22:2744, 2004.
99. Nart D, Nalbantgil S, Yagdi T, et al: Primary cardiac lymphoma in a heart transplant recipient. Transplant Proc 37:1362, 2005.
100. Binder J, Pfleger S, Schwarz S: Images in cardiovascular medicine. Right atrial primary cardiac lymphoma presenting with stroke. Circulation 110:e451, 2004.
101. Quigley MM, Schwartzman E, Boswell PD, et al: A unique atrial primary cardiac lymphoma mimicking myxoma presenting with embolic stroke: A case report. Blood 101:4708, 2003.

102. Engelen MA, Juergens KU, Breithardt G, et al: Interatrial conduction delay and atrioventricular block due to primary cardiac lymphoma. J Cardiovasc Electrophysiol 16:926, 2005.

103. Fujisaki J, Tanaka T, Kato J, et al: Primary cardiac lymphoma presenting clinically as restrictive cardiomyopathy. Circ J 69:249, 2005.

104. Giunta R, Cravero RG, Granata G, et al: Primary cardiac T-cell lymphoma. Ann Hematol 83:450, 2004.

105. Rolla G, Bertero MT, Pastena G, et al: Primary lymphoma of the heart. A case report and review of the literature. Leuk Res 26:117, 2002.

106. Dawson MA, Mariani J, Taylor A, et al: The successful treatment of primary cardiac lymphoma with a dose-dense schedule of rituximab plus CHOP. Ann Oncol 17:176, 2006.

107. Nakagawa Y, Ikeda U, Hirose M, et al: Successful treatment of primary cardiac lymphoma with monoclonal CD20 antibody (rituximab). Circ J 68:172, 2004.

Management of Primary Cardiac Tumors

108. Messa C, Di Muzio N, Picchio M, et al: PET/CT and radiotherapy. Q J Nucl Med Mol Imaging 50:4, 2006.

109. von Schulthess GK, Steinert HC, Hany TF: Integrated PET/CT: Current applications and future directions. Radiology 238:405, 2006.

110. Nielsen TO, West RB, Linn SC, et al: Molecular characterisation of soft tissue tumours: A gene expression study. Lancet 359:1301, 2002.

111. Fletcher CD: The evolving classification of soft tissue tumours: An update based on the new WHO classification. Histopathology 48:3, 2006.

112. Fletcher CD, Gustafson P, Rydholm A, et al: Clinicopathologic re-evaluation of 100 malignant fibrous histiocytomas: Prognostic relevance of subclassification. J Clin Oncol 19:3045, 2001.

CHAPTER 75 Pericardial Diseases

Martin M. LeWinter and Marc D. Tischler

Anatomy and Physiology of the Pericardium

The pericardium is composed of two layers,[1,2] the visceral pericardium, a monolayer membrane of mesothelial cells and associated collagen and elastin fibers that is adherent to the epicardial surface of the heart, and the fibrous parietal layer, which is about 2 mm thick in normal humans and surrounds most of the heart. The parietal pericardium is largely acellular and also contains both collagen and elastin fibers. Collagen is the major structural component and appears as wavy bundles at low levels of stretch. With further stretch, the bundles straighten, resulting in increased stiffness. The visceral pericardium reflects back near the origins of the great vessels, becoming continuous with and forming the inner layer of the parietal pericardium. The pericardial space or sac is contained within these two layers and normally contains up to 50 mL of serous fluid. The reflection of the visceral pericardium is a few centimeters proximal to the junctions of the caval vessels with the right atrium; portions of these vessels lie within the pericardial sac (**Fig. 75-1**). Posterior to the left atrium, the reflection occurs at the oblique sinus of the pericardium. The left atrium is largely extrapericardial. The parietal pericardium has ligamentous attachments to the diaphragm, sternum, and other structures. These ensure that the heart occupies a fixed position within the thoracic cavity regardless of respiration and body position. The only noncardiovascular macrostructures associated with the pericardium are the phrenic nerves enveloped by the parietal pericardium.

Although pericardiectomy does not result in obvious negative consequences, the normal pericardium does have functions. As noted before, it maintains the position of the heart relatively constant. It may also be a barrier to infection and provides lubrication between visceral and parietal layers. The pericardium is well innervated with mechanoreceptors and chemoreceptors and phrenic afferents. The roles of these receptors are incompletely understood, but they probably participate in reflexes arising from the pericardium and epicardium (e.g., the Bezold-Jarisch reflex) as well as in transmission of pericardial pain. The pericardium also secretes prostaglandins and related substances that may modulate neural traffic and coronary tone by effects on coronary receptors.

The best-characterized mechanical function of the pericardium is its restraining effect on cardiac volume. This reflects the mechanical properties of the pericardial tissue. The parietal pericardium has a tensile strength similar to that of rubber. At low applied stresses similar to those at physiologic or subphysiologic cardiac volumes, it is very elastic (see Fig. 75-e1, top, on website). As stretch increases, the tissue fairly abruptly becomes stiff and resistant to further stretch. The point on the pericardial stress-strain relation (see Fig. 75-e1, top, on website) where this transition occurs probably corresponds to stresses present around the upper range of physiologic cardiac volumes and is likely related to straightening of collagen bundles.

The pressure-volume relation of the parietal pericardial sac parallels the properties of the isolated tissue (see Fig. 75-e1, bottom, left curve, on website), that is, a relatively flat, compliant segment transitioning relatively abruptly to a noncompliant segment, with the transition in the range of the upper limit of normal total cardiac volume. Thus, the pericardial sac has a relatively small reserve volume. When it is exceeded, the pressure within the sac operating on the surface of the heart increases rapidly and is transmitted to the inside of the cardiac chambers. The shape of the pericardial pressure-volume relation accounts for the fact that once a critical level of effusion is reached, relatively small amounts of additional fluid cause large increases in intrapericardial pressure and have marked effects on cardiac function. Conversely, removal of small amounts of fluid can result in striking benefit.

The shape of the pericardial pressure-volume relation suggests that it can normally restrain cardiac volume, that is, the force it exerts on the surface of the heart can limit filling, with a component of intracavitary filling pressure representing transmission of the pericardial pressure. This has been examined with flattened balloons designed to measure surface contact pressures. These studies demonstrate a substantial pericardial contact pressure, especially when the upper limit of normal cardiac volume is exceeded. This pressure is proportionally more important for the right side of the heart, whose filling pressures are normally lower than the left.

Pericardial contact pressure has also been estimated by quantifying the change in the right- and left-sided heart diastolic pressure-volume relation before and after pericardiectomy. A decrease in pressure at a given volume is the effective pericardial pressure at that volume. Studies in canine hearts using this approach indicate negligible pericardial restraint at low normal filling volumes, with contact pressures in the range of 2 to 4 mm Hg at the upper end of the normal range. With additional filling, contact pressure rapidly increases. At left-sided filling pressure of ~25 mm Hg, estimated contact pressure is ~10 mm Hg, accounting for most of the right-sided heart pressure at this level of filling. Thus, the normal pericardium can acutely restrain cardiac volume and influences intracavitary filling pressure. Moreover, patients with normal preoperative cardiac volumes undergoing pericardiotomy in conjunction with heart surgery develop mild postoperative increases in cardiac mass and volume (similar to chronic volume overload), consistent

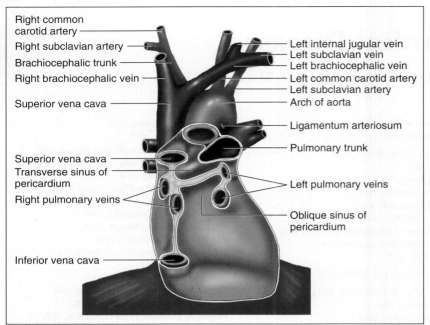

Right common carotid artery
Right subclavian artery
Brachiocephalic trunk
Right brachiocephalic vein
Superior vena cava

Superior vena cava
Transverse sinus of pericardium
Right pulmonary veins

Inferior vena cava

Left internal jugular vein
Left subclavian vein
Left brachiocephalic vein
Left common carotid artery
Left subclavian artery
Arch of aorta
Ligamentum arteriosum
Pulmonary trunk

Left pulmonary veins

Oblique sinus of pericardium

FIGURE 75-1 The pericardial reflections near the origins of the great vessels shown after removal of the heart. Note that portions of the caval vessels are within the pericardial space. *(From Johnson D: The pericardium. In Standring S, et al [eds]: Gray's Anatomy. New York, Elsevier Churchill Livingstone, 2005, pp 995-996.)*

with relief of underlying, normally occurring restraint to filling by the pericardium. It has recently been shown that the visceral pericardium also restrains cardiac volume.[2]

The normal pericardium also contributes to diastolic interaction, the transmission of intracavitary filling pressure to adjoining chambers. Thus, for example, a portion of right ventricular diastolic pressure is transmitted to the left ventricle across the interventricular septum and contributes to left ventricular diastolic pressure. Because its presence increases right ventricular intracavitary pressure, the normal pericardium amplifies diastolic interaction. Thus, as cardiac volume increases above the physiologic range, the pericardium contributes increasingly to intracavitary filling pressures, directly because of the external contact pressure and indirectly because of increased diastolic interaction.

The Passive Role of the Normal Pericardium in Heart Disease

When the cardiac chambers dilate rapidly, the restraining effect of the pericardium and its contribution to diastolic interaction become markedly augmented, resulting in a hemodynamic picture with features of both cardiac tamponade and constrictive pericarditis. The most common example is right ventricular myocardial infarction (MI),[3] usually in conjunction with inferior left ventricular MI. Here, the right side of the heart dilates markedly and rapidly such that total heart volume exceeds the pericardial reserve volume. As a result of increased pericardial constraint and augmented interaction, left- and right-sided filling pressures equilibrate at elevated levels, and a paradoxical pulse and inspiratory increase in systemic venous pressure (Kussmaul sign) may be observed (see Chap. 12). Other conditions with similar effects include acute pulmonary embolus and subacute mitral regurgitation.

Chronic cardiac dilation due to dilated cardiomyopathy or regurgitant valvular disease can result in cardiac volumes well in excess of the normal pericardial reserve volume. Despite this, exaggerated restraining effects are not ordinarily encountered. This implies that the pericardium undergoes chronic adaptation to accommodate marked increases in cardiac volume. In experimental chronic volume overload, the pericardial pressure-volume relation shifts to the right and its slope decreases (see Fig. 75-e1, bottom, right curve, on website), that is,

it becomes more compliant in association with increased pericardial area and mass and a decreased effect on the left ventricular diastolic pressure-volume relation. Thus, apparent growth of pericardial tissue occurs in response to chronic stretch. A similar effect presumably occurs with very large, slowly accumulating effusions.

Acute Pericarditis

Etiology, Epidemiology, and Pathophysiology

Table 75-1 is a partial list of diseases that can involve the pericardium. Acute pericarditis, defined as symptoms or signs resulting from pericardial inflammation of no more than 1 to 2 weeks in duration, can occur in a variety of these diseases (denoted by asterisks in Table 75-1), but the majority of cases are idiopathic.[4,5] The term *idiopathic* is used to denote acute pericarditis for which no specific cause can be found with routine diagnostic testing as outlined later. Most cases of acute idiopathic pericarditis are presumed to be viral in etiology, but testing for specific viruses is not routine because of cost and the fact that this knowledge rarely alters management.

The incidence of acute pericarditis is difficult to quantify because there are undoubtedly many undiagnosed cases. At autopsy, the frequency is ~1%.[6] Pericarditis is common in patients presenting to the emergency department, accounting for up to 5% of those with nonischemic chest pain. The fraction of all acute cases accounted for by idiopathic pericarditis is also uncertain and is influenced by population demographics and regional and seasonal variation in viral infections. However, 80% to 90% seems a reasonable estimate.[4-6] This percentage is lower in patients with pericarditis who require hospitalization and higher in young, previously healthy patients. Tuberculous pericarditis is included in Table 75-1 as a cause of acute pericarditis, but it usually presents with more chronic symptoms. Bacterial pericarditis is also included because it can present with signs and symptoms of acute pericardial inflammation, but these patients are usually critically ill, and other components of their illness, including pericardial effusions, sepsis, and pneumonias, typically dominate the picture. Pericarditis occurring 24 to 72 hours after transmural MI caused by local inflammation and the delayed pericarditis of Dressler syndrome used to be common (see Chap. 54). Their incidence has markedly declined during the era of early reperfusion. Other than this, the etiologic distribution of acute pericarditis has changed little over time. In contrast, the epidemiology of pericardial effusion and constriction has changed considerably.

The pathophysiology of uncomplicated acute pericarditis is straightforward, that is, symptoms and signs result from inflammation of pericardial tissue. A minority of cases are complicated, as discussed later, and some are associated with myocarditis.[4-6] Coexistent myocarditis is usually manifested solely by modest release of biomarkers such as troponin I (see Chap. 70). Rarely, however, myocardial dysfunction occurs in conjunction with clinically manifested pericarditis.

History and Differential Diagnosis

Acute pericarditis almost always presents with chest pain.[4] A few cases are diagnosed during evaluation of symptoms, such as dyspnea and fever, or incidentally in conjunction with noncardiac manifestations of systemic diseases, such as systemic lupus erythematosus (SLE). The pain of pericarditis can be quite severe. It is variable in quality but almost always pleuritic. It usually does not have the viselike, constricting or oppressive features of myocardial ischemia. Pericardial pain typically has a relatively rapid onset and sometimes begins remarkably abruptly. It is most commonly substernal but can be

TABLE 75-1 Categories of Pericardial Disease and Selected Specific Causes

Idiopathic*
Infectious
    Viral* (echovirus, coxsackievirus, adenovirus, cytomegalovirus, hepatitis B, infectious mononucleosis, HIV/AIDS)
    Bacterial* (pneumococcus, staphylococcus, streptococcus, mycoplasma, Lyme disease, *Haemophilus influenzae, Neisseria meningitidis,* and others)
    Mycobacterial* (*Mycobacterium tuberculosis, Mycobacterium avium-intracellulare*)
    Fungal (histoplasmosis, coccidioidomycosis)
    Protozoal
Immune-inflammatory
    Connective tissue disease* (systemic lupus erythematosus, rheumatoid arthritis, scleroderma, mixed)
    Arteritis (polyarteritis nodosa, temporal arteritis)
    Inflammatory bowel disease
    Early post–myocardial infarction
    Late post–myocardial infarction (Dressler syndrome),* late post-cardiotomy/thoracotomy*
    Late post-trauma*
    Drug induced* (procainamide, hydralazine, isoniazid, cyclosporine, others)
Neoplastic disease
    Primary: mesothelioma, fibrosarcoma, lipoma, others
    Secondary*: breast and lung carcinoma, lymphomas, Kaposi sarcoma
Radiation induced*
Early post–cardiac surgery and post–orthotopic heart transplantation
Hemopericardium
    Trauma
    Post–myocardial infarction free wall rupture
    Device and procedure related: percutaneous coronary procedures, implantable defibrillators, pacemakers, post–arrhythmia ablation, post–atrial septal defect closure, post–valve repair or replacement
    Dissecting aortic aneurysm
Trauma
    Blunt and penetrating,* post–cardiopulmonary resuscitation*
Congenital
    Cysts, congenital absence
Miscellaneous
    Cholesterol ("gold paint" pericarditis)
    Chronic renal failure, dialysis related
    Chylopericardium
    Hypothyroidism and hyperthyroidism
    Amyloidosis
    Aortic dissection

*Causes that can present as acute pericarditis.

centered in the left anterior chest or epigastrium. Left arm radiation is not unusual. The most characteristic radiation is to the trapezius ridge, which is highly specific for pericarditis. Pericardial pain is almost always relieved by sitting forward and worsened by lying down. Associated symptoms can include dyspnea, cough, and occasionally hiccoughs. An antecedent history of symptoms suggesting a viral syndrome is common. It is important to review the past medical history for clues to specific etiologic diagnoses. A history of cancer or an autoimmune disorder, high fevers with shaking chills, rash, or weight loss should alert the physician to specific diseases that can cause pericarditis.

The differential diagnosis of chest pain is extensive (see Chaps. 12 and 53). Diagnoses most easily confused with pericarditis include pneumonia or pneumonitis with pleurisy (which may coexist with pericarditis), pulmonary embolus or infarction, costochondritis, and gastroesophageal reflux disease. Acute pericarditis is usually relatively easily distinguished from myocardial ischemia or infarction, but coronary angiography is occasionally required to resolve this issue. Other considerations include aortic dissection, intra-abdominal processes, pneumothorax, and herpes zoster pain before skin lesions appear. Finally, acute pericarditis is occasionally the presenting manifestation of a preceding, silent MI.

Physical Examination

Patients with uncomplicated acute pericarditis often appear uncomfortable and anxious and may have low-grade fever and sinus tachycardia. Otherwise, the only abnormal physical finding is the friction rub caused by contact between visceral and parietal pericardium. The classic rub is easily recognized and pathognomonic of pericarditis. It consists of three components corresponding to ventricular systole, early diastolic filling, and atrial contraction and is similar to the sound made when walking on crunchy snow. The rub is usually loudest at the lower left sternal border and is best heard with the patient leaning forward. It is often dynamic, disappearing and returning during short periods. Thus, it is often rewarding to listen frequently to a patient with suspected pericarditis who does not have an audible rub initially. Sometimes what is considered a pericardial rub has only two components or even one component. Such findings should be labeled rubs with caution because the sound may actually represent a murmur. It is important to perform a careful, complete physical examination in a patient with acute pericarditis and to look for clues to specific etiologic diagnoses. The examiner must also be alert to findings indicating significant pericardial effusion, as discussed subsequently.

Laboratory Testing

ELECTROCARDIOGRAPHY. The electrocardiogram (ECG) is the most important laboratory test for diagnosis of acute pericarditis (see Chap. 13). The classic finding is diffuse ST-segment elevation (**Fig. 75-2**; see Fig. 13-45).[4-6] The ST-segment vector typically points leftward, anterior, and inferior, with ST-segment elevation in all leads except aVR and often V$_1$. The ST segment is usually coved upward and resembles the current of injury of acute, transmural ischemia. However, the distinction between acute pericarditis and transmural ischemia is usually not difficult because of more extensive lead involvement in pericarditis and the presence of much more prominent reciprocal ST-segment depression in ischemia. However, ST elevation in pericarditis sometimes involves a smaller number of leads, in which case the distinction is more difficult. In other cases, the ST segment more closely resembles early repolarization. Here again, pericarditis usually involves more leads than typical early repolarization. As with the rub, electrocardiographic changes can be dynamic. Frequent recordings can yield a diagnosis in patients with suspected pericarditis who present initially with neither rub nor ST elevation. PR-segment depression is also common (see Fig. 75-2). PR depression can occur without ST elevation and be the initial or sole electrocardiographic manifestation of acute pericarditis. Electrocardiographic abnormalities other than ST elevation and PR depression are unusual in patients presenting soon after the onset of symptoms of acute pericarditis. Subsequent electrocardiographic changes are variable.[4-6] In some, the ECG reverts to normal during days or weeks. In others, the elevated ST segment passes through the isoelectric point and progresses to ST-segment depression and T wave inversions in leads with upright QRS complexes. These changes can persist for weeks or even months but have no known significance in patients who have otherwise recovered. In patients presenting late after the onset of symptoms, these electrocardiographic changes can be difficult to distinguish from ischemia.

Electrocardiographic abnormalities other than these should be considered carefully because they suggest diagnoses other than idiopathic pericarditis or the presence of complications. As examples, atrioventricular block may indicate Lyme disease, pathologic Q waves can signify a previous silent MI with pericardial pain as its first manifestation, and low voltage or electrical alternans points toward significant effusion.

HEMOGRAM. Modest elevations of the white blood cell count with mild lymphocytosis are common in acute idiopathic pericarditis. Higher counts are an alert for the presence of other causes, as is anemia.

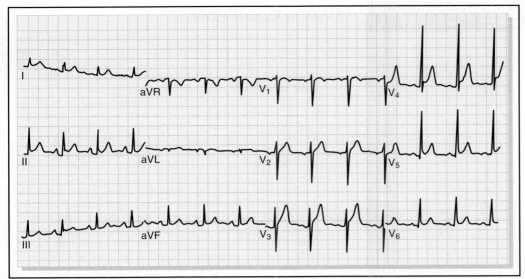

FIGURE 75-2 The electrocardiogram in acute pericarditis. Note both diffuse ST-segment elevation and PR-segment depression.

Initial management should be focused on screening for specific causes that would alter management, detection of effusion and other echocardiographic abnormalities, alleviation of symptoms, and appropriate treatment if a specific cause is discovered. Initially, we recommend obtaining the laboratory data discussed before, that is, ECG, hemogram, chest radiograph, serum creatine kinase and troponin I, and echocardiogram. In young women, it is not unreasonable to test for SLE. However, low antinuclear antibody (ANA) titers appear to be common in patients with recurrent idiopathic pericarditis who do not meet other criteria for SLE.[7] Thus, the significance of low ANA titers in the setting of an initial presentation is somewhat uncertain. **Table 75-2** summarizes our recommendations for initial assessment and treatment of patients with definite or suspected acute pericarditis.

Acute idiopathic pericarditis is a self-limited disease without significant complications or recurrence in 70% to 90% of patients.[4,6,8,9] If laboratory data support the clinical diagnosis, symptomatic treatment with nonsteroidal anti-inflammatory drugs (NSAIDs) should be initiated.[4,6] Because of its excellent safety profile, we prefer ibuprofen (600 to 800 mg orally three times daily) with discontinuation if pain is no longer present after 2 weeks. Many patients have very gratifying responses to the first dose or two of the NSAID, and most respond fully and need no additional treatment. Reliable patients with no more than small effusions who respond well to NSAIDs need not be admitted to the hospital.[10] Patients who do not respond well initially, have larger effusions, or have a suspected cause other than idiopathic pericarditis should be hospitalized for additional observation, diagnostic testing, and treatment as necessary.

Patients who respond slowly or inadequately to NSAIDs may require supplementary narcotic analgesics to allow time for a full response or a course of colchicine. Colchicine is administered as a 2- to 3-mg oral loading dose followed by 1 mg daily for 10 to 14 days.[5,11,12] It is unusual not to achieve a satisfactory response to a regimen of an NSAID, with colchicine added if necessary. On the basis of two randomized trials,[11,12] colchicine has been proposed as a standard adjuvant to NSAIDs for initial treatment. However, these trials have uncertain applicability as they were open label, and the treatment arms consisted of aspirin versus aspirin plus colchicine for either 3 or 6 months, much longer than the usual recommendation for acute pericarditis. Poorly

CARDIAC ENZYMES AND TROPONIN MEASUREMENTS. A significant fraction of patients with a diagnosis of acute pericarditis without other evidence of myocarditis (see Chap. 70) or MI (see Chap. 54) have elevated creatine kinase MB fraction or troponin I values. This suggests a significant incidence of concomitant, otherwise silent myocarditis. Pericarditis patients with elevated biomarkers of myocardial injury almost always have ST-segment elevation. Another concern in patients with elevated biomarkers is silent MI presenting with subsequent pericarditis. Post-MI pericarditis usually (but not always) occurs after MIs with transmural electrocardiographic changes.

CHEST RADIOGRAPHY (see Chap. 16). The chest radiograph is usually normal in uncomplicated acute idiopathic pericarditis. On occasion, small pulmonary infiltrates or pleural effusions are present, presumably due to viral or possibly mycoplasmal infections. Other than this, pulmonary parenchymal or other abnormalities suggest diagnoses other than idiopathic pericarditis. Thus, bacterial pericarditis often occurs in conjunction with severe pneumonia. Tuberculous pericarditis can occur with or without associated pulmonary disease. Mass lesions and enlarged lymph nodes suggestive of neoplastic disease also have great significance. Small to even moderate effusions may not cause an abnormal cardiac silhouette; thus, even modest enlargement is a cause for concern.

ECHOCARDIOGRAPHY (see Chap. 15). The echocardiogram is normal in most patients with acute idiopathic pericarditis. The main reason for its performance is to exclude an otherwise silent effusion. There are no modern data delineating the incidence of effusions. Most patients do not have effusions, but small ones are fairly common and not a cause for concern. Moderate or larger effusions are unusual and may signal a diagnosis other than idiopathic pericarditis. Echocardiography is also useful in delineating whether associated myocarditis is severe enough to alter ventricular function as well as in detection of MI.

Natural History and Management

The European Society of Cardiology has published guidelines for the diagnosis and management of pericardial diseases.[5] Although these are useful, there have been few randomized clinical trials devoted to the diagnosis or management of pericardial disease. It is therefore important to keep in mind that objective data to support the following recommendations for management of acute pericarditis as well as other pericardial diseases are limited.

TABLE 75-2	**Initial Approach to the Patient with Definite or Suspected Acute Pericarditis**

If the diagnosis is suspected but not certain, listen frequently for pericardial rub and obtain frequent ECGs to look for diagnostic findings.

If the diagnosis is suspected or certain, obtain the following tests to determine if a specific etiologic diagnosis is likely or significant associated conditions or complications are present:
- Chest radiograph
- Hemogram
- Echocardiogram
- Creatine kinase with MB fraction, troponin I
- Echocardiogram
- Consider serum antinuclear antibody if patient is young woman

If diagnosis is certain, initiate therapy with a nonsteroidal anti-inflammatory drug.

responding patients have typically been treated with short courses of corticosteroids. However, corticosteroids should be avoided as they appear to encourage recurrences.[5,6,13] If they simply cannot be avoided to manage an initial episode, we recommend prednisone 60 mg orally daily for 2 days with tapering to zero during a week.

Complications of acute pericarditis include effusion, tamponade, and constriction (myocarditis is best considered an associated condition rather than a complication). As noted earlier, small effusions are common. Relatively little is known about the incidence of more significant complications. In the largest modern report on this topic,[9] a specific cause was identified in 17% of patients with acute pericarditis. During an average 31-month follow-up period, 3.1% developed tamponade and 1.5% developed constriction. Most complications occurred in patients with identified causes. Thus, in patients without an identified cause, the incidence of complications (including larger effusions) is extremely low during the acute episode and for the longer term.

Relapsing and Recurrent Pericarditis

Perhaps 15% to 30% of patients with acute, apparently idiopathic pericarditis who respond satisfactorily to treatment as outlined before suffer a relapse.[4-6,9] Women and patients in whom initial therapy with NSAIDs fails are at increased risk.[9] A minority develop recurrent bouts of pericardial pain, which can be chronic and debilitating. Recurrent pain is often not associated with objective signs of pericardial inflammation. Evidence of a specific cause is manifested in some patients with what is initially thought to be idiopathic pericarditis as they develop recurrences. Accordingly, repeated evaluation for specific causes, especially autoimmune disorders, is appropriate. A pericardial biopsy to look for a specific cause in patients with recurrent pain *without effusion* is rarely indicated because it is unlikely that a diagnosis will actually result or that the information obtained will alter management. The complication rate, including constrictive pericarditis, is very low in patients with recurrent pericarditis, and the long-term prognosis is good; most patients eventually have a full remission.[14,15]

Treatment of recurrent pain is empiric. For an initial relapse, a second 2-week course of an NSAID is often effective. A course of colchicine may be at least as effective.[11] For bouts of recurrent pain beyond an initial relapse, we recommend colchicine prophylaxis.[11,16] There is now a substantial experience with colchicine as prophylaxis for recurrent pericardial pain due to idiopathic pericarditis and other causes (e.g., after thoracotomy, SLE). This experience indicates that colchicine is at least as effective as corticosteroid therapy and has a much more favorable side effect profile. The usual dose is a 2- to 3-mg oral load followed by 1 mg orally daily. Initiation of prophylactic therapy does not preclude simultaneous use of NSAIDs. The most common difficulty in using colchicine is nausea or diarrhea, which results in dose reduction or termination in 10% to 15% of patients.

Patients with recurrent pericardial pain despite NSAIDs and colchicine (or who cannot tolerate colchicine) are a challenging problem. One option is a brief course of prednisone as outlined before whenever symptoms first appear. Maintenance corticosteroid therapy should be avoided if at all possible. If prednisone therapy must be continued for longer periods, lower doses appear to be preferable. In a retrospective study,[17] 0.2 to 0.5 mg/kg of oral prednisone daily was associated with a lower recurrence and hospitalization rate than an average of 1.0 mg/kg daily; only the higher dose range was associated with severe side effects. Nonsteroidal immunosuppressive therapy with drugs such as azathioprine and cyclophosphamide is another alternative, but there has been no systematic, published experience. Pericardiectomy has occasionally been employed for recurrent pericarditis but appears to be effective in only a minority of patients.[4-6]

Pericardial Effusion and Tamponade

Etiology

Idiopathic pericarditis and any infection, neoplasm, and autoimmune or inflammatory process that can cause pericarditis can cause an effusion (see Table 75-1).[5,6,18] Effusions are common early after both routine cardiac surgery and orthotopic heart transplantation,[19] but tamponade is unusual, and they almost always resolve within several weeks to a few months. A lengthy list of miscellaneous, noninflammatory diseases can cause effusion (see Table 75-1). Patients with severe circulatory congestion can have small to moderate transudative effusions. Bleeding into the pericardial sac occurs after blunt and penetrating trauma (see Chap. 76), following post-MI rupture of the free wall of the left ventricle, and as a complication of percutaneous cardiac procedures and device implantation. Retrograde bleeding is an important cause of death due to aortic dissection (see Chap. 60). Last, occasional patients are encountered with large, silent pericardial effusion.[20] These are generally stable, but instances of tamponade do occur over time.

Those causes of effusion with a high incidence of progression to tamponade include bacterial (including mycobacterial) infections, fungal infections, human immunodeficiency virus (HIV)–associated infections (see Chap. 72), bleeding, and neoplastic involvement. Whereas large effusions due to acute idiopathic pericarditis are unusual, this form of pericarditis accounts for a significant percentage of tamponade cases because of its high frequency. About 20% of large, symptomatic effusions without an obvious cause after routine evaluation constitute the initial presentation of a previously unrecognized cancer.[21] Details of pericardial effusion pertinent to specific disease entities are discussed later.

Pathophysiology and Hemodynamics

Formation of an effusion is a component of the inflammatory response when there is an inflammatory or infectious process affecting the pericardium. This is also the likely mechanism with pericardial tumor implants (see Chap. 74). Lymphomas occasionally cause effusion in association with enlarged mediastinal lymph nodes by obstructing pericardial lymph drainage. The pathophysiologic mechanism of effusions in situations in which there is no obvious inflammation (e.g., uremia) is very poorly understood.

Cardiac tamponade represents a continuum from an effusion causing minimal effects to full-blown circulatory collapse. Clinically, the most critical point occurs when an effusion reduces the volume of the cardiac chambers such that cardiac output begins to decline. Determinants of the hemodynamic consequences of an effusion are the pressure in the pericardial sac and the ability of the heart to compensate for elevated pressure. The pressure in turn depends on the amount of fluid and the pericardial pressure-volume relation. As discussed earlier, the pericardium normally has little reserve volume. As a result, relatively modest amounts of rapidly accumulating fluid can have major effects on cardiac function. Large, slowly accumulating effusions are often well tolerated, presumably because of chronic changes in the pericardial pressure-volume relation described earlier. The compensatory response to a significant pericardial effusion includes increased adrenergic stimulation and parasympathetic withdrawal, which cause tachycardia and increased contractility[22] and can maintain cardiac output and blood pressure for a time. Eventually, however, cardiac output and blood pressure progressively decline. Patients who cannot mount a normal adrenergic response (e.g., those receiving beta-adrenergic blocking drugs) are more susceptible to the effects of an effusion. In terminal tamponade, a depressor reflex with paradoxical bradycardia can supervene.

The hemodynamic consequences of pericardial effusion have fascinated physiologists and physicians for years.[18,22] Non–steady-state responses to an abrupt increase in pericardial pressure provide insights into the mechanisms of these derangements. **Figure 75-3** shows an experiment in a dog in which aortic and pulmonary arterial flow (stroke volume) were measured beat to beat before and after a large amount of fluid was abruptly introduced into the pericardial sac, indicated by the arrow. This causes an immediate decrease in pulmonary arterial stroke volume but no change in aortic stroke volume. Two beats later, aortic stroke volume decreases, and eventually a new steady state is achieved with equivalent decreases in aortic and pulmonary arterial stroke volume. During the time required to achieve a new steady state, pulmonary stroke volume is less than aortic stroke volume. The transient inequality in left- and

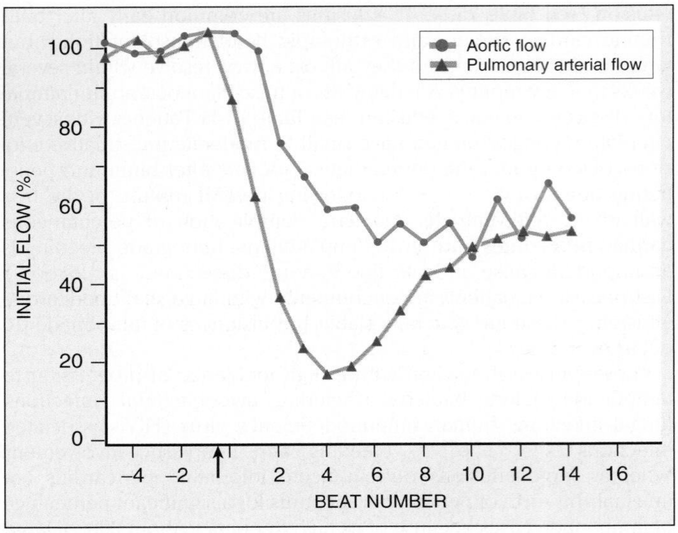

FIGURE 75-3 Beat-to-beat changes in pulmonary arterial and aortic stroke volume (as percentage of control) after abrupt production of cardiac tamponade (at arrow). Note that pulmonary arterial stroke volume decreases immediately, but there is a brief lag before aortic stroke volume decreases. Pulmonary arterial stroke volume is lower than aortic stroke volume until new steady state is reached. (*From Ditchey R, Engler R, LeWinter M, et al: The role of the right heart in acute cardiac tamponade in dogs. Circ Res 48:701, 1981.*)

right-sided heart output results in transfer of blood out of the pulmonary and into the systemic circulation and may explain the decrease in pulmonary vascularity on the chest radiograph in tamponade. In parallel studies, right-sided heart volume was shown to decrease more than left-sided heart volume in response to a given increase in pericardial pressure. These results indicate that high pericardial pressure exerts its effect mainly by impeding right-sided heart filling, with much of the effect on the left side of the heart due to secondary underfilling.

As fluid accumulates, left- and right-sided atrial and ventricular diastolic pressures rise and in severe tamponade equalize at a pressure similar to that in the pericardial sac, typically 15 to 20 mm Hg (**Fig. 75-4**). Equalization is closest during inspiration. Thus, the pericardial pressure dictates the intracavitary pressure, and the transmural filling pressures of the cardiac chambers are very low. Correspondingly, cardiac volumes progressively decline. The small end-diastolic ventricular volume (decreased preload) mainly accounts for the small stroke volume. Because of compensatory increases in contractility, end-systolic volume also decreases, but not enough to normalize stroke volume (hence, the importance of tachycardia in maintaining cardiac output). Because transmural right-sided heart filling pressure is normally lower than left-sided heart filling pressure (upper limit of right atrial pressure ~7 mm Hg, left atrial pressure ~12 mm Hg), as fluid accumulates, filling pressure increases more rapidly in the right side than in the left side of the heart.

In addition to elevated and equal intracavitary filling pressures, low transmural filling pressures, and small cardiac volumes, two other hemodynamic abnormalities are characteristic of tamponade. One is loss of the *y* descent of the right atrial or systemic venous pressure (see Fig. 75-4). The *x* and *y* descents of the venous pressure waveform correspond to periods when flow is increasing. Loss of the *y* descent has been explained on the basis of the concept that total heart volume is fixed in severe tamponade.[18,22] Thus, blood can enter the heart only when blood is simultaneously leaving. The right atrial *y* descent begins when the tricuspid valve opens, that is, when blood is not leaving the heart. Thus, no blood can enter, and the *y* descent is lost. In contrast, the *x* descent occurs during ventricular ejection. Because blood is leaving the heart, venous inflow can increase and the *x* descent is retained. Loss of the *y* descent can be difficult to discern at the bedside but is easily appreciated in recordings of systemic venous or right atrial pressure and provides a useful clue to the presence of very significant tamponade.

The second characteristic hemodynamic finding is the paradoxical pulse (**Fig. 75-5**), an abnormally large decline in systemic arterial pressure during inspiration (usually defined as a drop of >10 mm Hg in systolic pressure). Other causes of pulsus paradoxus include constrictive pericarditis, pulmonary embolus, and pulmonary disease with large

variations in intrathoracic pressure. In severe tamponade, the arterial pulse is impalpable during inspiration. The mechanism of the paradoxical pulse is multifactorial, but respiratory changes in systemic venous return are certainly important.[18,22] In tamponade, in contrast to constriction, the normal inspiratory increase in systemic venous return is retained. Therefore, the normal decline in systemic venous pressure on inspiration is present (and Kussmaul sign is absent). The increase in right-sided heart filling occurs, once again, under conditions in which total heart volume is fixed and left-sided heart volume is markedly reduced to start. The interventricular septum shifts to the left in exaggerated fashion on inspiration, encroaching on the left ventricle such that its stroke volume and pressure generation are further reduced (see Fig. 75-5). Although the inspiratory increase in right-sided heart volume (preload) causes an increase in right ventricular stroke volume, this requires several cardiac cycles to increase left ventricular filling and stroke volume and to counteract the septal shift. Other factors that may contribute to the paradoxical pulse include increased afterload caused by transmission of negative intrathoracic pressure to the aorta and traction on the pericardium caused by descent of the diaphragm, which increases pericardial pressure. Associated with these mechanisms are the striking findings that left- and right-sided heart pressure and stroke volume variations are exaggerated and 180 degrees out of phase (see Fig. 75-5). **Table 75-3** lists the major hemodynamic findings of tamponade in comparison with constrictive pericarditis.

When there are pre-existing elevations in diastolic pressures or volume, tamponade can occur without a paradoxical pulse.[18,22] Examples are patients with left ventricular dysfunction, aortic regurgitation, and atrial septal defect. In patients with retrograde bleeding into the pericardial sac due to aortic dissection, tamponade can occur without a paradoxical pulse because of aortic valve disruption and regurgitation.

Although left- and right-sided filling pressures are usually 15 to 20 mm Hg in severe tamponade, tamponade can occur at lower levels of filling pressure, which is termed low-pressure tamponade.[18,22,23] Low-pressure tamponade occurs when there is a decrease in blood volume in the setting of a pre-existing effusion that would not otherwise cause significant hemodynamic consequences. A relatively modestly elevated pericardial pressure can then lower transmural filling pressure to levels at which stroke volume is compromised. Because the venous pressure is only modestly elevated or even normal, the diagnosis may not be suspected. Low-pressure tamponade is typically observed during hemodialysis, when it may be signaled by hypotension; in patients with blood loss and dehydration; and when diuretics are administered to patients with effusions (see Chap. 93). In the only large published experience with this entity,[23] about 20% of patients undergoing combined cardiac catheterization and closed pericardiocentesis met criteria for low-pressure tamponade. Compared with high-pressure tamponade, low-pressure tamponade patients were less often critically ill and signs of tamponade were less prominent. Echocardiographic findings were similar to those of high-pressure tamponade, and substantial hemodynamic benefit was derived from pericardiocentesis.

Pericardial effusions can be loculated or localized, resulting in regional tamponade, which is most commonly encountered after cardiac surgery.[22] Regional tamponade can cause atypical hemodynamic findings, that is, reduced cardiac output with unilateral filling pressure elevation. However, reports of hemodynamics are scarce, and it is difficult to generalize about this entity. Regional tamponade should be considered whenever there is hypotension in a setting in which a loculated effusion is present or suspected. Large pleural effusions can also compress the heart and even cause clinical cardiac tamponade.[24]

Clinical Presentation

Obviously, in patients with pericardial effusions, a history pertinent to a specific cause can often be elicited. On occasion, large, asymptomatic chronic effusions are discovered when a chest imaging study is performed for an unrelated reason.[20] As discussed earlier, specific causes are usually not found in these cases. Effusions do not cause symptoms unless tamponade is present, although many patients with effusions have pericardial pain because of associated pericarditis. Patients with tamponade may complain of true dyspnea, whose mechanism is uncertain because there is no pulmonary congestion. They almost always are more comfortable sitting forward. Other symptoms reflect the severity of cardiac output and blood pressure reduction. Pericardial pain or a nonspecific sense of discomfort may dominate the clinical picture.

A complete physical examination of patients with pericardial effusion can provide clues to a specific cause (see Chap. 12). In pericardial effusion without tamponade, the cardiovascular examination findings are normal except that if the effusion is large, the cardiac impulse can be difficult to palpate and the heart sounds muffled. A friction rub can of course also be present. Tubular breath sounds may be heard in the left axilla or left base due to bronchial compression. The Beck triad of hypotension, muffled heart sounds, and elevated jugular venous pressure remains a useful clue to the presence of severe tamponade. Patients with tamponade almost always appear uncomfortable, with signs reflecting varying degrees of reduced cardiac output and shock, including tachypnea, diaphoresis, cool extremities, peripheral cyanosis, depressed sensorium, and, rarely, yawning.[25] Hypotension with reduced pulse pressure is usually present, although compensatory mechanisms maintain the blood pressure in early stages. A paradoxical pulse is the rule, but it is important to be alert to those situations in which it may not be present. It is quantified by cuff sphygmomanometry by noting the difference between the pressure at which Korotkoff sounds first appear and that at which they are present with each heart beat. In severe tamponade, the inspiratory decrease in arterial pressure is palpable and most obvious in arteries distant from the heart. Tachycardia is also the rule unless heart rate–lowering drugs have been administered, conduction system disease coexists, or a preterminal bradycardic reflex has supervened. The jugular venous pressure is markedly elevated except in low-pressure tamponade, and the y descent is absent (see Fig. 75-4). The normal decrease in venous pressure on inspiration is retained. Examination of the heart itself is simply consistent with an effusion, as outlined before. Tamponade can be confused with anything that causes hypotension, shock, and elevated jugular venous pressure, including myocardial failure, right-sided heart failure due to pulmonary embolus or other causes of pulmonary hypertension, and right ventricular MI.

Laboratory Testing

ELECTROCARDIOGRAPHY. Electrocardiographic abnormalities characteristic of pericardial effusion and tamponade are reduced voltage and electrical alternans[22] (**Fig. 75-6**; see Fig. 13-51). Reduced voltage is nonspecific and can be caused by several other conditions (e.g., emphysema, infiltrative myocardial disease, pneumothorax). Electrical alternans is specific but relatively insensitive for large effusions. It is caused by anterior-posterior swinging of the heart with each heart beat. When pericarditis coexists, the usual electrocardiographic findings may be present (see Chap. 13).

CHEST RADIOGRAPHY (see Chap. 16). The cardiac silhouette is normal until effusions are at least moderate in size. With moderate and larger effusions, the anteroposterior cardiac silhouette assumes a rounded, flasklike

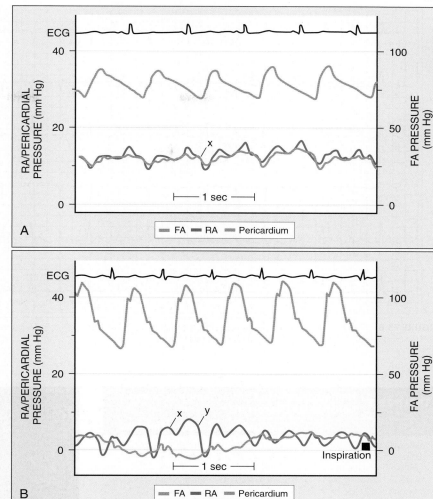

FIGURE 75-4 Femoral arterial (FA), right atrial (RA), and pericardial pressure before **(A)** and after **(B)** pericardiocentesis in a patient with cardiac tamponade. Both right atrial and pericardial pressures are about 15 mm Hg before pericardiocentesis. In this case, there was a negligible paradoxical pulse. Note presence of x descent but absence of y descent before pericardiocentesis. Pericardiocentesis results in marked increase in femoral arterial pressure and marked decrease in right atrial pressure. During inspiration, pericardial pressure becomes negative, there is clear separation between right atrial and pericardial pressures, and y descent is now prominent, suggesting the possibility of an effusive-constrictive picture. *(Modified from Lorell BH, Grossman W: Profiles in constrictive pericarditis, restrictive cardiomyopathy and cardiac tamponade.* In *Baim DS, Grossman W [eds]: Grossman's Cardiac Catheterization, Angiography, and Intervention. Philadelphia, Lippincott Williams & Wilkins, 2000, p 840.)*

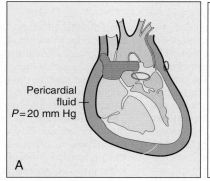

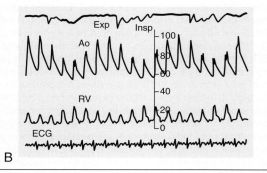

FIGURE 75-5 A, Schematic illustration of leftward septal shift with encroachment of left ventricular volume during inspiration in cardiac tamponade. **B,** Respiration marker and aortic and right ventricular pressure tracings in cardiac tamponade. Note paradoxical pulse and marked, 180-degree out-of-phase respiratory variation in right- and left-sided pressures. *(From Shabetai R: The Pericardium. New York, Grune & Stratton, 1981, p 266.)*

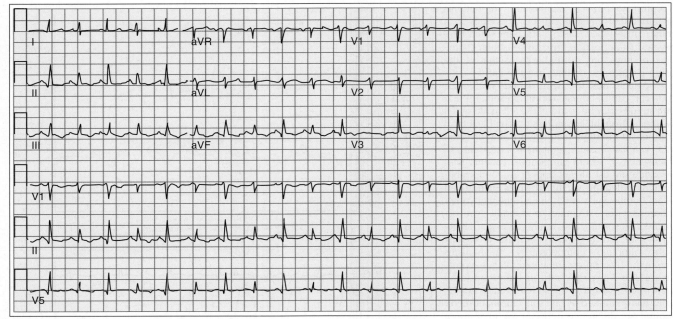

FIGURE 75-6 ECG in cardiac tamponade showing electrical alternans. *(From Lau TK, Civitello AB, Hernandez A, Coulter SA: Cardiac tamponade and electrical alternans. Tex Heart Inst J 48:67, 2002. Copyright 2002 Texas Heart Institute.)*

TABLE 75-3	**Hemodynamics in Cardiac Tamponade and Constrictive Pericarditis**	
	TAMPONADE	**CONSTRICTION**
Paradoxical pulse	Usually present	Present in ~⅓
Equal left- and right-sided filling pressures	Present	Present
Systemic venous wave morphology	Absent *y* descent	Prominent *y* descent (M or W shape)
Inspiratory change in systemic venous pressure	Decrease (normal)	Increase or no change (Kussmaul sign)
"Square root" sign in ventricular pressure	Absent	Present

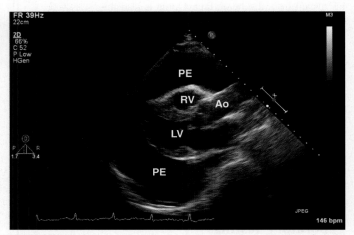

FIGURE 75-7 Two-dimensional echocardiogram of a large, circumferential pericardial effusion (PE). Ao = aorta; LV = left ventricle; RV = right ventricle. *(From Kabbani SS, LeWinter M: Cardiac constriction and restriction. In Crawford MH, DiMarco JP [eds]: Cardiology. St. Louis, Mosby, 2001, p 5, 15.5.)*

appearance (see Fig. 75-e2 on website). Lateral views may reveal the pericardial fat pad sign, a linear lucency between the chest wall and the anterior surface of the heart representing separation of parietal pericardial fat from epicardium. The lungs appear oligemic.

ECHOCARDIOGRAPHY (see Chap. 15). Because of their convenience, M-mode and two-dimensional Doppler echocardiography remain the standard noninvasive diagnostic methods for detection of pericardial effusion and tamponade. A pericardial effusion appears as a lucent separation between parietal and visceral pericardium (**Fig. 75-7**; see Fig. 15-72). With a true effusion, separation is present for the entire cardiac cycle. Small effusions are first evident over the posterobasal left ventricle. As the fluid increases, it spreads anteriorly, laterally, and behind the left atrium, where its limit is demarcated by the visceral pericardial reflection. Ultimately, the separation becomes circumferential. Video 75-1 on the website shows a cine image of an echocardiogram demonstrating a large, circumferential effusion in a patient with tamponade. Ordinarily, tamponade does not occur without a circumferential effusion, and the diagnosis should be viewed with skepticism if this is not the case. However, as discussed earlier, loculated effusions can cause regional tamponade. Computed tomography (CT) scanning and cardiac magnetic resonance (CMR) are more precise than echocardiography for imaging of the pericardium itself (see Chaps. 18 and

19). Frondlike or shaggy-appearing structures in the pericardial space detected by echocardiography suggest clots or chronic inflammatory or neoplastic pericardial processes.

As discussed before, tamponade is best considered a spectrum of severity of cardiac compression. Several findings indicate that tamponade is severe enough to cause at least some degree of hemodynamic compromise. Early diastolic collapse of the right ventricle (**Fig. 75-8**; see also Video 75-1 on website) and right atrium (which occurs during *ventricular* diastole; **Fig. 75-9**) are sensitive and specific signs that appear relatively early during tamponade.[18,22] Both occur when the pericardial pressure transiently exceeds intracavitary pressure. Right atrial collapse is more sensitive and right ventricular collapse more specific for tamponade.[18] As noted earlier, a large pleural effusion can also cause right-sided chamber collapse. Rarely, left ventricular collapse and left atrial collapse occur with loculated effusions after cardiac surgery.[18] The cardiac chambers are small in tamponade, and as discussed before, the heart may swing anteroposteriorly within the effusion. Distention of the caval vessels that does not diminish with inspiration is also a useful sign.

Reflecting the hemodynamic abnormalities discussed earlier, Doppler velocity recordings demonstrate exaggerated respiratory variation in right- and left-sided venous and valvular flow, with inspiratory increases on the right and decreases on the left (see Fig. 15-73).[18,22] As a result of reduced systemic venous inflow during early diastole with loss of the y descent, most caval and pulmonary venous inflow occurs during ventricular systole. These flow patterns were found to have good sensitivity and high specificity for diagnosis of tamponade. The absence of chamber collapse is especially useful in excluding tamponade in patients with effusions, but its presence is less well correlated with tamponade than abnormal venous flow patterns are. Newer techniques such as tissue Doppler do not as yet have a well-defined, additive role in cardiac tamponade. In most cases of pericardial effusion, transthoracic echocardiography provides sufficient diagnostic information for informed management decisions to be made. Transesophageal studies provide better quality images but are often impractical in sick patients unless they are intubated.

OTHER IMAGING MODALITIES. Fluoroscopy is useful in the cardiac catheterization laboratory for detection of procedure-related effusions because they may cause damping or abolition of cardiac pulsation.

CT (see Chap. 19) and CMR (see Chap. 18) are useful adjuncts to echocardiography in the characterization of effusion and tamponade.[26,27] Neither is ordinarily required or advisable in sick patients who require prompt management and treatment decisions. They have an important ancillary role in situations in which hemodynamics are atypical, other conditions complicate interpretation, and the presence and severity of tamponade are less certain. They are of course invaluable when

echocardiography is technically inadequate. Video 75-2 on the website shows a CMR cine image revealing a large, circumferential pericardial effusion and a small, underfilled left ventricle. In this case, the right ventricle is not compressed because of longstanding pulmonary hypertension as evidenced by significant right ventricular hypertrophy.

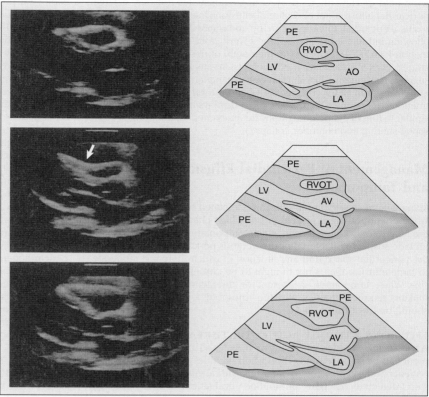

FIGURE 75-8 Two-dimensional echocardiogram illustrating diastolic collapse or indentation of the right ventricle in cardiac tamponade. **Top,** Systole. **Middle,** Early diastole with indentation indicated by arrow. **Bottom,** Late diastole with return of normal configuration. AO = aorta; AV = aortic valve; LA = left atrium; LV = left ventricle; PE = pericardial effusion; RVOT = right ventricular outflow tract. *(From Weyman AE: Principles and Practice of Echocardiography. Philadelphia, Lea & Febiger, 1994, p 1119.)*

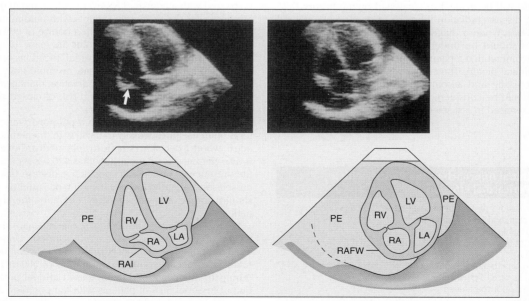

FIGURE 75-9 Two-dimensional echocardiogram illustrating right atrial collapse or indentation in cardiac tamponade. LA = left atrium; LV = left ventricle; PE = pericardial effusion; RA = right atrium; RAFW = right atrial free wall; RAI = right atrial inversion; RV = right ventricle. *(From Gillam LD, Guyer DE, Gibson TC, et al: Hemodynamic compression of the right atrium: A new echocardiographic sign of cardiac tamponade. Circulation 68:294, 1983.)*

It is important to recognize this constellation of findings because coexistent pulmonary hypertension reduces the accuracy of echocardiographic signs of cardiac tamponade. CT and CMR provide more detailed quantitation and regional localization than echocardiography does and are especially useful for loculated effusions and in the presence of coexistent pleural effusions. In Video 75-3 on the website, the wide field of view afforded by CMR demonstrates not only a large pericardial effusion but also pleural effusions in a patient with polyserositis. Pericardial thickness can be measured with both methods, allowing indirect assessment of the severity and chronicity of inflammation (see Fig. 18-17). Clues to the nature of pericardial fluid can be gained from CT attenuation coefficients. Attenuation similar to water suggests transudative; higher than water, malignant, bloody, or purulent; and lower than water, chylous. CMR can be used to make similar distinctions. Real-time CT or CMR cine displays provide information similar to that of echocardiography for assessment of tamponade (e.g., septal shifting and chamber collapse).

Management of Pericardial Effusion and Tamponade

Management of pericardial effusion is dictated first and foremost by whether tamponade is present or has a high chance of developing in the near term.[18,22] Situations in which tamponade is a near-term threat include suspected bacterial or tuberculous pericarditis, bleeding into the pericardial space, and any situation in which there is a moderate to large effusion that is not thought to be chronic or is increasing in size. When tamponade is present or threatened, clinical decision making requires urgency, and the threshold for pericardiocentesis should be low (**Table 75-4**).

EFFUSIONS WITHOUT ACTUAL OR THREATENED TAMPONADE. In the absence of actual or threatened tamponade, management can be more leisurely. This cohort includes several categories of patients. Some have acute pericarditis with a small to moderate effusion detected as part of routine evaluation. Others undergo echocardiography because of diseases known to involve the pericardium. The rest are asymptomatic and have effusions detected when diagnostic tests are performed for reasons other than suspected pericardial disease, such as when echocardiography is performed to evaluate an enlarged cardiac silhouette on the chest radiograph or CT or CMR is used to investigate thoracic disease.

In many cases of effusion when tamponade is neither present nor threatened, a cause will be evident or suggested by the history (e.g., known neoplastic disease, radiation therapy) or previously obtained diagnostic test results. When a diagnosis is not clear, an assessment of specific causes should be undertaken. This should include the diagnostic tests recommended for acute pericarditis and anything else dictated by the clinical picture. Thus, skin testing for tuberculosis and screening for neoplastic and autoimmune diseases, infections, and hypothyroidism should be considered. At the same time, careful judgment should be exercised in test selection. Thus, a patient with severe

heart failure and circulatory congestion with a small, asymptomatic effusion does not need testing. In contrast, patients with evidence of a systemic disease deserve very careful attention. Titers of serum antibodies to viruses usually are not helpful in these cases because results may be nonspecific or negative despite a viral etiology. However, situations occasionally arise in which evidence of a viral etiology, if present, is helpful in clarifying diagnostic dilemmas, providing reassurance, and avoiding unnecessary diagnostic testing or treatments. Thus, it may be useful to save serum obtained at presentation should there be a need to measure viral titers at a later date.

In most of these patients, pericardiocentesis (closed or open with biopsy) needs to be undertaken only for diagnostic purposes and is usually not required. As discussed before, in many cases, a diagnosis will either be obvious when the effusion is first noted or become evident as part of initial investigations. Moreover, in this setting, analysis of pericardial fluid alone in general has a low yield for providing a specific diagnosis.[18] In occasional situations in which pericardiocentesis is thought to be necessary for diagnostic purposes, consideration should be given to open drainage with biopsy.

Occasional patients with large, asymptomatic effusions and no evidence of tamponade or a specific cause are a special category.[20] The effusions are by definition chronic because tamponade would be present if this were not the case. They are in general stable, and specific causes usually are not evident. However, a minority develop tamponade unpredictably. After closed pericardiocentesis, the effusions typically do not reaccumulate.[20] Thus, there is a rationale for pericardiocentesis after routine evaluation for specific causes as outlined before. This decision can be individualized, however, as little is lost by conservative management in reliable patients. Before pericardiocentesis is undertaken, a course of NSAID or colchicine should be considered because this will shrink some of these effusions. A course of corticosteroids may have the same effect, but this is controversial because of the possibility of an increased likelihood of recurrence.

EFFUSIONS WITH ACTUAL OR THREATENED TAMPONADE. These patients should be considered a true or potential medical emergency. With the exception of those who do not wish prolongation of life (mainly those with metastatic cancer), hospital admission and hemodynamic and echocardiographic monitoring are mandatory. Most patients require pericardiocentesis to treat or to prevent tamponade. Treatment should be individualized, and thoughtful clinical judgment is critical. Thus, for example, patients with acute, apparently idiopathic pericarditis who have no more than mild tamponade can be treated with a course of NSAID or colchicine in the hope that their effusions will shrink rapidly. Patients with autoimmune diseases can be treated in the same way or with a course of corticosteroids (there is no evidence that corticosteroids increase recurrence in these patients). Those with possible bacterial infections or bleeding into the pericardial sac whose effusions are no more than moderate in size may be suitable for initial conservative management and careful monitoring, especially because the risk of closed pericardiocentesis is increased with smaller effusions.

Hemodynamic monitoring with a pulmonary artery balloon catheter is often useful, especially in those with threatened or mild tamponade in whom a decision is made to defer pericardiocentesis. Monitoring is also helpful after pericardiocentesis to assess reaccumulation and the presence of underlying constrictive disease (see Fig. 75-4), as discussed subsequently. However, insertion of a pulmonary artery catheter should not be allowed to delay definitive therapy in critically ill patients.

For most patients in this category, management should be oriented toward urgent or emergent pericardiocentesis. Once actual or threatened tamponade is diagnosed, intravenous hydration should be instituted. In a recent report, administration of 500 mL of normal saline during 10 minutes modestly increased arterial pressure and cardiac output in about 50% of patients with tamponade.[28] Positive inotropes can also be employed but are of limited efficacy. Hydration and positive inotropes are temporizing measures and should not be allowed to substitute for or to delay pericardiocentesis.

TABLE 75-4	Initial Approach to the Patient with a Pericardial Effusion

Determine if tamponade is present or threatened on the basis of history, physical examination, and echocardiogram.
If tamponade is not present or threatened:
- If the cause is not apparent, consider diagnostic tests as for acute pericarditis.
- If the effusion is large, consider course of NSAID or corticosteroid; if no response, consider closed pericardiocentesis.
If tamponade is present or threatened:
- Urgent or emergent closed pericardiocentesis or careful monitoring is indicated if a trial of medical treatment to reduce effusion is considered appropriate.

In most circumstances, closed pericardiocentesis is the treatment of choice. Before proceeding, it is important to be confident that there is an effusion large enough to cause tamponade, especially if hemodynamics are atypical. Loculated effusions or effusions containing clots or fibrinous material are also of concern because the risk and difficulty of closed pericardiocentesis are increased. In these situations, if removal of fluid is thought to be necessary, an open approach should be considered for safety and to obtain pericardial tissue and to create a window. One of the more difficult management decisions is whether to perform closed versus open pericardiocentesis in patients with known or suspected bleeding into the pericardial space. The danger of a closed approach is that lowering the intrapericardial pressure will simply encourage more bleeding without affording an opportunity to correct its source. In cases of trauma or rupture of the wall of the left ventricle after MI, closed pericardiocentesis should in general be avoided. However, if bleeding is slower (e.g., due to a procedural coronary perforation or puncture of a cardiac chamber), closed pericardiocentesis is often appropriate because bleeding may stop spontaneously or the procedure can provide temporary relief before definitive repair.

The most commonly employed approach to closed pericardiocentesis is subxiphoid needle insertion with echocardiographic guidance to minimize the risk of myocardial puncture and to assess completeness of fluid removal. Once the needle has entered the pericardial space, a modest amount of fluid should be immediately removed (perhaps 50 to 150 mL) in an effort to produce immediate hemodynamic improvement. A guidewire is then inserted, and the needle is replaced with a pigtail catheter. The catheter is manipulated with continuing echocardiographic guidance to maximize fluid removal. In a large series from the Mayo Clinic,[29] procedural success rate was 97% and complication rate 4.7% (major, 1.2%; minor, 3.5%). Whenever possible, the procedure should be performed in the cardiac catheterization laboratory with experienced personnel in attendance. If echocardiographic guidance is unavailable, the needle should be directed toward the left shoulder and then replaced with a catheter for subsequent fluid removal. Fluoroscopy-guided drainage is an alternative when echocardiography cannot be used.

If a pulmonary artery catheter has been inserted, pulmonary capillary wedge and systemic arterial pressures and cardiac output should be monitored before, during, and after the procedure. Ideally, pericardial fluid pressure should also be measured. As discussed before, removal of relatively small amounts of fluid can result in substantial hemodynamic improvement. Hemodynamic monitoring before and after pericardiocentesis is useful for several reasons. Initial measurements confirm and document the severity of tamponade. Assessment after completion establishes a baseline to assess reaccumulation. As discussed later, some patients presenting with tamponade have a coexisting component of constriction (i.e., effusive-constrictive pericarditis),[30] which is difficult to detect when an effusion dominates the picture. Filling pressures that remain elevated after pericardiocentesis and the appearance of venous waveforms typical of constriction (rapid x and y descents) indicate coexistent constriction.

After pericardiocentesis, repeated echocardiography and in many cases continued hemodynamic monitoring are useful to assess reaccumulation. The duration of monitoring is a matter of judgment, but 24 hours is typically sufficient. A follow-up echocardiogram should be obtained immediately before hemodynamic monitoring is discontinued. We recommend consideration of leaving intrapericardial catheters in place for several days to allow continued fluid removal. This has been shown to minimize recurrences[5,18] and facilitates delivery of intrapericardial drugs if indicated.

Open pericardiocentesis is occasionally preferred for initial removal of pericardial fluid. Bleeding due to trauma and rupture of the left ventricular free wall has been mentioned previously in this regard. Loculated effusions or effusions that are borderline in size are drained more safely in the operating room. Recurring effusions, especially those causing tamponade, may initially be drained by a closed approach because of logistical considerations. However, open pericardiocentesis with biopsy and establishment of a pericardial window are preferred for most recurrences that are severe enough to cause tamponade. Creation of a window reliably eliminates future tamponade and provides pericardial tissue to assist in diagnosis. The surgeon should inspect the pericardium carefully and obtain multiple biopsy specimens.

More recently, percutaneous balloon techniques have been used for drainage. These methods are safe and effective for producing pericardial windows but are available at relatively few centers. Balloon pericardiotomy appears to be particularly useful in patients with malignant effusions,[31] in whom the incidence of recurrence is high and a definitive approach without a surgical procedure is desirable.

ANALYSIS OF PERICARDIAL FLUID. Normal pericardial fluid in general has the features of a plasma ultrafiltrate.[32] However, the lactate dehydrogenase level is 2.4 times and the mean protein level is 0.6 times that of plasma. Lymphocytes are the predominant cell type.

Although analysis of pericardial fluid does not have a high yield in identifying the cause of pericardial disease, careful analysis can be rewarding. Assuming that a diagnosis is not known before fluid removal, routine pericardial fluid measurements should include specific gravity, white blood cell count and differential, hematocrit, and protein content.[5,18,32] Although most effusions are exudates, detection of a transudate reduces the diagnostic possibilities considerably. Sanguinous fluid is nonspecific and does not necessarily indicate bleeding. Chylous effusions can occur after traumatic or surgical injury to the thoracic duct or obstruction by a neoplastic process. On occasion, they are idiopathic. Cholesterol-rich ("gold paint") effusions occur in severe hypothyroidism.

Pericardial fluid should routinely be stained and cultured for detection of bacteria, including tuberculosis, and fungi. As much fluid as possible should be submitted for detection of malignant cells as there is a reasonably high diagnostic yield. In tuberculous pericardial disease, several tests other than culture of fluid and examination of biopsy specimens are useful.[5,18,32-35] These include adenosine deaminase (ADA), interferon-γ, and the polymerase chain reaction (PCR), discussed in more detail later. Unless some other cause is evident, we believe that some relatively rapid test for tuberculosis (ADA, PCR) should be routine because of the difficulty in diagnosis of tuberculous pericarditis and the delays involved in making a diagnosis by culture. There may also be a role for routine measurement of selected tumor markers as a general screen for malignant effusion and an adjunct to direct detection of malignant cells.[5]

PERICARDIOSCOPY AND PERCUTANEOUS BIOPSY. Some experts advocate the routine use of pericardioscopy-guided biopsy in patients with pericardial effusion without an etiologic diagnosis. Seferovic and colleagues[35] compared the diagnostic yield of percutaneous, fluoroscopy-guided parietal biopsy (3 to 6 samples) with that of targeted, pericardioscopy-guided biopsy with either limited (3 to 6 samples) or extended (18 to 20 samples) sampling. Tissue was examined by routine histology. Pericardioscopic biopsy was found to have a higher sampling efficiency than fluoroscopic guidance and a much higher diagnostic yield. Extended sampling performed best, leading to a new diagnosis in 41% and a specific etiology in 53% of cases. The technique was especially useful in detecting malignant involvement, and few complications occurred. However, pericardioscopy is technically challenging, and few individuals have significant experience. Moreover, in earlier reports, major complications were occasionally encountered, and it is as yet uncertain whether its use will significantly improve long-term outcomes. Thus, this procedure should be undertaken only by individuals with appropriate training and experience.

Constrictive Pericarditis

Etiology

Constrictive pericarditis is the end stage of an inflammatory process involving the pericardium. Virtually any process listed in Table 75-1 can cause constriction. In the developed world, the etiology is most commonly idiopathic, postsurgical, or radiation injury[6,18] (**Table 75-5**). Tuberculosis was the most common cause in the developed world before the advent of effective drug therapy and remains important in developing countries. Although constriction can follow an initial insult by as little as several months, it usually takes years to develop. The end result is dense fibrosis, often calcification, and adhesions of the parietal and visceral pericardium. Scarring is usually more or less symmetric and impedes filling of all heart chambers. In a subset of patients, the process develops relatively rapidly and is reversible. This variant is seen most commonly after cardiac surgery.[36]

Pathophysiology

The pathophysiologic consequence of pericardial scarring is markedly restricted filling of the heart.[18] This results in elevation and equilibration of filling pressures in all chambers and the systemic and pulmonary veins. In early diastole, the ventricles fill abnormally rapidly because of markedly elevated atrial pressures and accentuated early diastolic ventricular suction, the latter related to small end-systolic volumes. During early to mid diastole, ventricular filling abruptly ceases when intracardiac volume reaches the limit set by the stiff pericardium. As a result, almost all ventricular filling occurs early in diastole. Systemic venous congestion results in hepatic congestion, peripheral edema, ascites and sometimes anasarca, and cardiac cirrhosis. Reduced cardiac output is a consequence of impaired ventricular filling and causes fatigue, muscle wasting, and weight loss. In "pure" constriction, contractile function is preserved, although ejection fraction can be reduced because of reduced preload. The myocardium is occasionally involved in the chronic inflammation and fibrosis, leading to true contractile dysfunction that can at times be quite severe and predicts a poor response to pericardiectomy.

Failure of transmission of intrathoracic respiratory pressure changes to the cardiac chambers is an important contributor to the pathophysiologic process of constrictive pericarditis (**Fig. 75-10**). These pressure changes continue to be transmitted to the pulmonary circulation. Thus, on inspiration, the drop in intrathoracic pressure (and therefore pulmonary venous pressure) is not transmitted to the left side of the heart.[18]

TABLE 75-5 Causes of Constrictive Pericarditis
Idiopathic
Irradiation
Postsurgical
Infectious
Neoplastic
Autoimmune (connective tissue) disorders
Uremia
Post-trauma
Sarcoid
Methysergide therapy
Implantable defibrillator patches

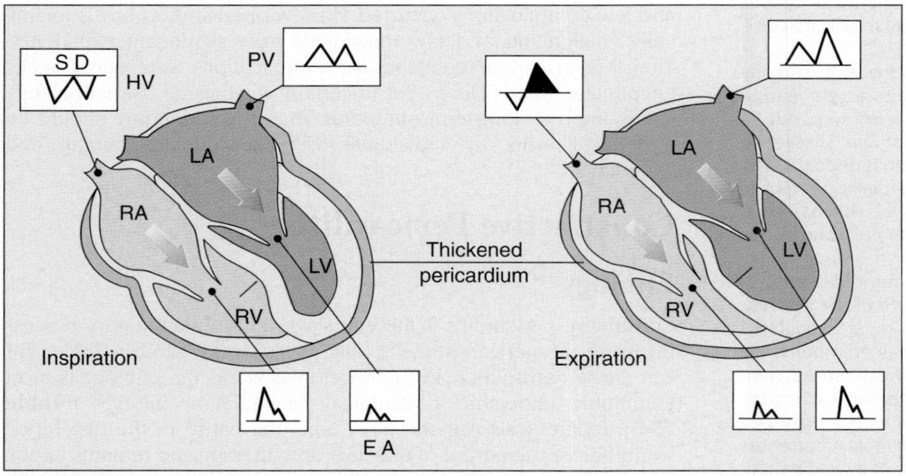

FIGURE 75-10 Schematic representation of transvalvular and central venous flow velocities in constrictive pericarditis. During inspiration, the decrease in left ventricular filling results in a leftward septal shift, allowing augmented flow into the right ventricle. The opposite occurs during expiration. D = diastole; EA = mitral inflow; HV = hepatic vein; LA = left atrium; LV = left ventricle; PV = pulmonary venous flow; RA = right atrium; RV = right ventricle; S = systole.

Consequently, the small pulmonary venous to left atrial pressure gradient that normally drives left-sided heart filling is reduced, resulting in decreased transmitral inflow. The inspiratory decrease in left ventricular filling allows an increase in right ventricular filling and an interventricular septal shift to the left. The opposite sequence occurs with expiration.

High systemic venous pressure and reduced cardiac output result in compensatory retention of sodium and water by the kidneys. Inhibition of natriuretic peptides also may contribute to renal sodium retention, further exacerbating increased filling pressures.[37]

Clinical Presentation

The usual presentation consists of signs and symptoms of right-sided heart failure. At a relatively early stage, these include lower extremity edema, vague abdominal complaints, and passive hepatic congestion. As the disease progresses, hepatic congestion worsens and can progress to ascites, anasarca, and jaundice due to cardiac cirrhosis. Signs and symptoms ascribable to elevated pulmonary venous pressures, such as exertional dyspnea, cough, and orthopnea, may also appear with progressive disease. Atrial fibrillation and tricuspid regurgitation, which further exacerbate venous pressure elevation, may also appear at this stage. In end-stage constrictive pericarditis, the effects of a chronically low cardiac output are prominent, including severe fatigue, muscle wasting, and cachexia. Other findings include recurrent pleural effusions and syncope. Constrictive pericarditis can be mistaken for any cause of right-sided heart failure as well as end-stage primary hepatic disease. Of course, venous pressure is not elevated in the latter circumstance.

Physical Examination

Physical findings include markedly elevated jugular venous pressure with a prominent, rapidly collapsing *y* descent. This, combined with a normal *x* descent, results in an M- or W-shaped venous pressure contour. At the bedside, this is best appreciated as two prominent descents with each cardiac cycle. In patients in atrial fibrillation, the *x* descent is lost, leaving only the prominent *y* descent (see Fig. 12-3). The latter is very difficult to distinguish from tricuspid regurgitation, which, as noted before, may itself be due to constrictive pericarditis. Kussmaul sign, an inspiratory increase in systemic venous pressure, is usually present,[18] or the venous pressure may simply fail to decrease on inspiration. Kussmaul sign reflects loss of the normal increase in right-sided heart venous return on inspiration, even though tricuspid flow increases. These characteristic abnormalities of the venous waveform contrast with tamponade. A paradoxical pulse occurs in perhaps one third of patients with constriction, especially when there is an effusive-constrictive picture (see later). It is best explained by the aforementioned lack of transmission of decreased intrathoracic pressure to the left-sided heart chambers. Table 75-3 is a comparison of hemodynamic findings in tamponade and constrictive pericarditis.

In cases with extensive calcification and adhesion of the heart to adjacent structures, the position of the cardiac point of maximal impulse may fail to change with changes in body position. However, the most notable cardiac finding is the pericardial knock, an early diastolic sound best heard at the left sternal border or the cardiac apex (see Fig. 12-3). It occurs slightly earlier and has a higher frequency content than a typical third heart sound. The knock corresponds to the early, abrupt cessation of ventricular filling. Widening of second heart sound splitting may also be present. As noted, patients may have secondary tricuspid regurgitation with its characteristic murmur.

Abdominal examination reveals hepatomegaly, often with palpable venous pulsations, with or without ascites. Other signs of hepatic congestion or cardiac cirrhosis include jaundice, spider angiomas, and palmar erythema. Lower extremity edema is the rule. As noted before, with end-stage constriction, muscle wasting, cachexia, and massive ascites and anasarca may appear.

Laboratory Testing

ELECTROCARDIOGRAPHY. There are no specific electrocardiographic findings. Nonspecific T wave abnormalities, reduced voltage, and left atrial abnormality may be present. Atrial fibrillation is also common.

CHEST RADIOGRAPHY (see Chap. 16). The cardiac silhouette can be enlarged secondary to a coexisting pericardial effusion. Pericardial calcification is seen in a minority of patients and suggests tuberculosis (**Fig. 75-11**; see Fig. 16-11), but calcification per se is not diagnostic of constrictive physiology. The lateral view may reveal pericardial calcification along the right-sided heart border and in the atrioventricular groove. Isolated calcification of the left ventricular apex or posterior wall suggests ventricular aneurysm rather than pericardial calcification. Pleural effusions are occasionally noted and can be a presenting sign of constrictive pericarditis. When left-sided heart filling pressures are markedly elevated, pulmonary vascular congestion and redistribution can be present.

ECHOCARDIOGRAPHY (see Chap. 15). M-mode and two-dimensional transthoracic echocardiographic findings include pericardial thickening, abrupt displacement of the interventricular septum during early diastole (septal "bounce"),[5,18] and signs of systemic venous congestion such as dilation of hepatic veins and distention of the inferior vena cava with blunted respiratory fluctuation. Premature pulmonic valve opening as a result of elevated right ventricular early diastolic pressure may also be observed. Exaggerated septal shifting during respiration is often present.

Lack of transmission of intrathoracic pressure to the cardiac chambers and resulting mitral and tricuspid inflow patterns have been discussed earlier. In accordance with these patterns, Doppler measurements often reveal exaggerated respiratory variation in both mitral inflow velocity

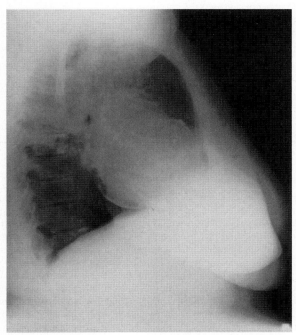

FIGURE 75-11 Chest radiograph showing marked pericardial calcification in a patient with constrictive pericarditis.

and tricuspid-mitral inflow velocity, with the latter 180 degrees out of phase (see Fig. 15-73). Although there is some overlap with tamponade, these inflow patterns have good sensitivity and specificity for diagnosis of constrictive pericarditis and also help distinguish restrictive cardiomyopathy from constriction.[5,18] Typically, patients with constriction demonstrate a ≥25% increase in mitral E velocity during expiration compared with inspiration and increased diastolic flow reversal with expiration in the hepatic veins. Mitral E wave deceleration time is usually but not always <160 milliseconds. However, up to 20% of patients with constriction do not exhibit typical respiratory changes, most likely because of markedly increased left atrial pressure or possibly a mixed constrictive-restrictive pattern due to myocardial involvement by the constrictive process. In patients without typical respiratory mitral-tricuspid flow findings, examination after maneuvers that decrease preload (head-up tilt, sitting) can unmask characteristic respiratory variation in mitral E velocity.[18] Tissue Doppler examination reveals increased E′ velocity of the mitral annulus as well as septal abnormalities corresponding to the bounce.[38,39] Tissue Doppler appears to be at least as sensitive as mitral-tricuspid inflow Doppler for diagnosis of constriction.

Similar patterns of respiratory variation in mitral inflow velocity can be observed in chronic obstructive lung disease, right ventricular infarction, pulmonary embolism, and pleural effusion. These conditions have other clinical and echocardiographic features that differentiate them from constrictive pericarditis. Superior vena caval flow velocities are helpful in distinguishing constrictive pericarditis from chronic obstructive pulmonary disease. Patients with pulmonary disease display a marked increase in inspiratory superior vena caval systolic forward flow velocity, which is not seen in constriction.

Transesophageal echocardiography is superior to transthoracic echocardiography for measuring pericardial thickness and has an excellent correlation with CT. When mitral inflow velocities by transthoracic echocardiography are technically inadequate or equivocal, measurement of transesophageal pulmonary venous Doppler velocity demonstrates pronounced respiratory variation, larger than that observed across the mitral valve.

CARDIAC CATHETERIZATION AND ANGIOGRAPHY (see Chap. 20). Cardiac catheterization in patients with suspected constriction provides documentation of the hemodynamics of constrictive physiology and assists in discriminating between constrictive pericarditis and restrictive cardiomyopathy.[5,18] Whereas there is limited need for contrast ventriculography, coronary angiography should ordinarily be performed in patients being considered for pericardiectomy. On rare occasions, external pinching or compression of the coronary arteries by the constricting pericardium is detected.

Right atrial, right ventricular diastolic, pulmonary capillary wedge, and pre–a wave left ventricular diastolic pressures are elevated and equal, or nearly so, at around 20 mm Hg. Differences of more than 3 to 5 mm Hg between left- and right-sided heart filling pressures are rarely encountered. The right atrial pressure tracing shows a preserved x descent, a prominent y descent, and roughly equal a and v wave height, with the resultant M or W configuration. Both right and left ventricular pressures reveal an early, marked diastolic dip followed by a plateau ("dip and plateau" or "square root" sign; **Fig. 75-12**). Pulmonary artery and right ventricular systolic pressures are often modestly elevated, in the range of 35 to 45 mm Hg. Greater elevation of the pulmonary artery systolic pressure is not a feature of constrictive pericarditis and casts doubt on the diagnosis. Hypovolemia (e.g., secondary to diuretic therapy) can mask typical hemodynamic findings. Rapid volume challenge of 1000 mL of normal saline during 6 to 8 minutes may reveal typical hemodynamic features. Stroke volume is almost always reduced, but resting cardiac output can be preserved because of tachycardia. Depression of stroke volume is primarily caused by reduced diastolic filling. In the absence of extensive coexisting myocardial involvement, left ventricular ejection fraction is normal or slightly reduced.

COMPUTED TOMOGRAPHY AND CARDIAC MAGNETIC RESONANCE. CT (see Chap. 19) provides detailed pericardial images and is helpful in detecting even minute amounts of pericardial calcification[26,27] (see Fig. 75-e3 on website). Its major disadvantage is the frequent need for iodinated contrast medium to best display pericardial disease. The thickness of the normal pericardium measured by CT is <2 mm. CMR[26,27] (see Chap. 18) provides a detailed and comprehensive examination of the pericardium without the need for contrast material

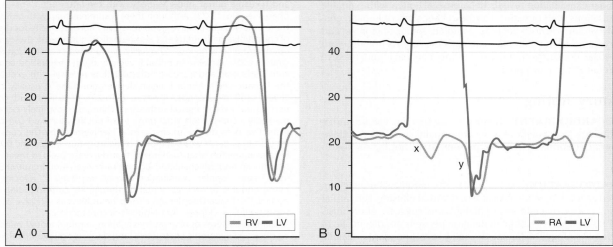

FIGURE 75-12 Pressure recordings in a patient with constrictive pericarditis. **A,** Simultaneous right ventricular (RV) and left ventricular (LV) pressure tracings with equalization of diastolic pressure as well as "dip and plateau" morphology. **B,** Simultaneous right atrial (RA) and LV pressure tracings with equalization of RA and LV diastolic pressure. Note the prominent y descent. *(From Vaitkus PT, Cooper KA, Shuman WP, Hardin NJ: Images in cardiovascular medicine: Constrictive pericarditis. Circulation 93:834, 1996.)*

or ionizing radiation. It is somewhat less sensitive than CT for detection of calcification. The "normal" pericardium visualized by CMR is up to 3 to 4 mm in thickness. This measurement most likely reflects the entire pericardial "complex," with physiologic fluid representing a component of the measured thickness.

Demonstration of a thickened pericardium indicates acute or chronic pericarditis. If there is clinical evidence of impaired diastolic filling, pericardial thickening, especially with calcification, is virtually diagnostic of constriction. Absence of pericardial thickening argues against the diagnosis of constriction but does not completely rule it out. The pericardium can be globally or focally thickened. Localized compression of the heart caused by focal thickening is reported and is much more common on the right than on the left side. In patients being considered for pericardiectomy, delineation of the location and severity of thickening and calcification aids the surgeon with respect to both risk stratification and planning of surgery. Additional findings include distorted ventricular contours, hepatic venous congestion, ascites, pleural effusions, and occasionally pericardial effusion. Cine acquisition (CMR or CT) shows abnormal motion of the interventricular septum (septal bounce) in early diastole (see Video 75-4 on website). Finally, enhanced uptake of gadolinium appears useful for detection of pericardial inflammation.[40]

There is a cohort of patients with well-documented constriction who have no pericardial thickening on the basis of measurements in pathologic specimens despite histologic evidence of inflammation and calcification. These patients constituted 18% of those with constrictive pericarditis in a Mayo Clinic series.[41] Almost all had normal pericardial thickness by CT. Calcification and distorted ventricular contours occurred in a majority, providing clues to the diagnosis despite normal thickness.

TABLE 75-6	Hemodynamic and Echocardiographic Features of Constrictive Pericarditis Compared with Restrictive Cardiomyopathy	
	CONSTRICTION	**RESTRICTION**
Prominent y descent in venous pressure	Present	Variable
Paradoxical pulse	~⅓ of cases	Absent
Pericardial knock	Present	Absent
Equal right- and left-sided filling pressures	Present	Left at least 3-5 mm Hg > right
Filling pressures >25 mm Hg	Rare	Common
Pulmonary artery systolic pressure >60 mm Hg	No	Common
"Square root" sign	Present	Variable
Respiratory variation in left- and right-sided pressures or flows	Exaggerated	Normal
Ventricular wall thickness	Normal	Usually increased
Atrial size	Possible left atrial enlargement	Biatrial enlargement
Septal bounce	Present	Absent
Tissue Doppler E' velocity	Increased	Reduced
Pericardial thickness	Increased	Normal

Differentiation of Constrictive Pericarditis from Restrictive Cardiomyopathy

Because their treatment is radically different, distinguishing constrictive pericarditis from restrictive cardiomyopathy is extremely important (**Table 75-6**). Their presentation and course overlap in many respects. A pericardial knock points to constriction, but prominent third heart sounds in restrictive disease can be confusing. Electrocardiographic and chest radiographic findings are mostly nonspecific. However, a calcified pericardium indicates constriction, whereas low QRS voltage suggests amyloidosis. There are some useful echocardiographic distinctions. Patients with restrictive cardiomyopathy usually have thick-walled ventricles due to infiltrative processes such

as amyloidosis (see Fig. 15-77). Marked biatrial enlargement is also common in restriction (see Fig. 68-7). In constriction, the most distinctive finding is the septal bounce. As discussed before, the pericardium is usually thickened in constriction, but this may be difficult to assess with transthoracic echocardiography. As noted, transesophageal echocardiographic measurements of pericardial thickness correlate well with CT, although they are limited by their narrow field of view. With use of two-dimensional speckle tracking, differences in contraction mechanics that are useful in distinguishing constriction from restriction have been described.[42] In constriction, deformation of the left ventricle and early diastolic recoil velocity were attenuated in the circumferential direction, whereas in restriction, they were attenuated in the longitudinal direction.

Doppler measurements are also useful in differentiating constrictive from restrictive physiology.[18,38,39] Enhanced respiratory variation in mitral inflow velocity (>25%) is seen in constriction; in restriction, velocity varies by <10% (see Fig. 75-10; see Fig. 15-75). In restriction, pulmonary venous systolic flow is markedly blunted and diastolic flow is increased. This is not observed in constriction. Hepatic veins demonstrate enhanced expiratory flow reversal with constriction, in contrast to increased inspiratory flow reversal in restriction (see Figs. 15-70 and 15-76). Tissue Doppler echocardiography and color M-mode flow propagation are complementary to mitral Doppler respiratory variation in distinguishing constriction from restrictive cardiomyopathy. Higher tissue Doppler mitral annulus E' values in constriction versus restrictive cardiomyopathy (see Figs. 15-69 and 15-77) are reported to have a higher sensitivity than mitral inflow parameters for making the distinction.[38,39]

Hemodynamic differentiation between constrictive pericarditis and restrictive cardiomyopathy in the cardiac catheterization laboratory can be difficult. However, careful attention to the hemodynamic profile usually allows successful distinction (see Table 75-6). In both conditions, right and left ventricular diastolic pressures are markedly elevated. In restrictive cardiomyopathy, diastolic pressure in the left ventricle is usually higher than in the right ventricle by at least 3 to 5 mm Hg; in constrictive pericarditis, left- and right-sided diastolic pressures typically track closely and rarely differ by more than 3 to 5 mm Hg. Pulmonary hypertension is common with restrictive cardiomyopathy but rare in constriction. The absolute level of atrial or ventricular diastolic pressure elevation is also sometimes useful in distinguishing the two conditions, with extremely high pressures (>25 mm Hg) much more common in restrictive cardiomyopathy.[5,18] Finally, the ratio of right ventricular to left ventricular systolic pressure-time area during inspiration versus expiration[43] is greater in constriction versus restriction (reflecting exaggerated ventricular interaction) and is reported to have a high sensitivity and specificity for distinguishing between them (see Fig. 20-15).

CT and CMR, because of their ability to provide detailed assessment of pericardial thickness and calcification, are useful in differentiating constriction from restriction.[26,27] Occasional patients with constriction and normal pericardial thickness have been discussed before. Pericardial calcification or distorted ventricular contour is helpful in making the correct diagnosis in these patients. Endomyocardial or abdominal fat pad biopsy establishes the diagnosis of restrictive cardiomyopathy due to amyloidosis. Brain natriuretic peptide (BNP) levels may be useful in distinguishing constriction from restriction. BNP is reported to be elevated in restrictive cardiomyopathy and normal in constriction.[37] More recent data[43] indicate that this difference is more useful in secondary constriction (e.g., postoperative, irradiation) than in idiopathic cases.

Availability of the multiple diagnostic modalities discussed before has made it very rare to have to resort to exploratory thoracotomy to distinguish constriction from restriction.

Management

Constrictive pericarditis is a progressive disease but has a variable course. With the exception of patients with transient constriction, surgical pericardiectomy is the definitive treatment. Transient constriction should be suspected in patients presenting relatively earlier after cardiac surgery or with relatively rapid development of symptoms. Such patients can be monitored for several months to look for spontaneous improvement. They may respond to a course of corticosteroids, and there is little to lose by managing them in this way. Patients with major comorbidities or severe debilitation are often at too high risk to undergo pericardiectomy. Radiation-induced disease is also considered a relative contraindication to pericardiectomy. Healthy older patients with very mild constriction may also be managed nonsurgically, with pericardiectomy held in reserve until there is disease progression. Otherwise, surgery should not be delayed once the diagnosis is made. Medical management with diuretics and salt restriction is useful for relief of fluid overload and edema, but patients ultimately become refractory. Because sinus tachycardia is a compensatory mechanism, beta-adrenergic blockers and calcium antagonists that slow the heart rate should be avoided. In patients with atrial fibrillation and a rapid ventricular response, digoxin is recommended as initial treatment to slow the ventricular rate before resorting to beta blockers or calcium antagonists. In general, the rate should not be allowed to drop below 80 to 90 beats/min.

Pericardiectomy can be performed through either a median sternotomy or a left fifth interspace thoracotomy and involves radical excision of as much of the parietal pericardium as possible.[5] The visceral pericardium is then inspected and resection considered if it is involved in the disease process. Most surgeons initially attempt to perform pericardiectomy without cardiopulmonary bypass. Cardiopulmonary bypass is available as backup and is frequently required to facilitate access to the lateral and diaphragmatic surfaces of the left ventricle and to allow safe removal of a maximal amount of pericardial tissue. Ultrasonic or laser débridement[5,44] is useful as an adjunct to conventional surgical débridement or as the sole technique in high-risk patients with extensive, calcified adhesions between pericardium and epicardium. Occasional patients may be candidates for video-assisted thoracoscopic pericardiectomy in centers with appropriate expertise.

Hemodynamic and symptomatic improvement is achieved in some patients immediately after operation. In others, improvement may be delayed for weeks to months. Videos 75-5 and 75-6 on the website show cine CMR images before and after successful pericardial stripping, demonstrating relief of exaggerated variations in right- and left-sided heart volume. After pericardiectomy, 70% to 80% of patients remain free from adverse cardiovascular outcomes at 5 years and 40% to 50% at 10 years.[45] Long-term results are worse in patients with radiation-induced disease, impaired renal function, relatively high pulmonary artery systolic pressure, reduced left ventricular ejection fraction, moderate or severe tricuspid regurgitation, low serum sodium, and advanced age.[45,46] Left ventricular diastolic function based on echocardiography returns to normal in about 40% of patients early and in nearly 60% late after pericardiectomy. Persistence of abnormal filling was correlated with postoperative symptoms. Delayed or inadequate responses to pericardiectomy have been attributed to longstanding disease with myocardial atrophy or fibrosis, incomplete pericardial resection, and development of recurrent cardiac compression by mediastinal inflammation and fibrosis. Lack of improvement after pericardiectomy may also be due to inadequate resection of visceral pericardium. Tricuspid regurgitation usually does not improve after surgery[47] and can cause postoperative hemodynamic deterioration.

Pericardiectomy has a 5% to 15% perioperative mortality in patients with constriction. In a Cleveland Clinic series,[45] 63% of patients were alive after a median follow-up of 6.9 years, but long-term results were variable. Early mortality results primarily from low cardiac output, often in debilitated patients with prolonged cardiopulmonary bypass and difficult dissections. Sepsis, uncontrolled hemorrhage, and renal and respiratory insufficiency also contribute to early mortality.[45,46] The highest mortality occurs in patients with Class III or IV symptoms, supporting the recommendation of early pericardiectomy.

Effusive-Constrictive Pericarditis

A number of patients with pericardial disease present with a syndrome combining elements of effusion or tamponade and constriction. They often have a subacute course initially. An inflammatory effusion may dominate early, with constriction more prominent later. As noted previously, these patients are often identified when hemodynamics fail to normalize after pericardiocentesis. Sagrista-Sauleda and coworkers[30] defined effusive-constrictive pericarditis as a failure of the right atrial pressure to decline by at least 50% to a level below 10 mm Hg when the pericardial pressure is reduced to near 0 mm Hg by pericardiocentesis. In their series at a referral center, 8% of those undergoing pericardiocentesis met these criteria. Causes are diverse. The most common are idiopathic, malignant disease, radiation, and tuberculosis. Physical, hemodynamic, and echocardiographic findings are often mixtures of those associated with effusion and constriction and may vary with time as the syndrome progresses. Diagnosis may require acquisition of pericardial fluid and biopsy specimens if the cause is not obvious and tamponade does not mandate pericardiocentesis. It is important to be cautious in performing closed pericardiocentesis in patients without large effusions. Management is tailored to the specific cause, if it is known. Pericardiectomy is often ultimately required.

Specific Causes of Pericardial Disease

The pericardium is involved in a wide variety of diseases. Some are relatively common, but pericardial involvement is rare (e.g., inflammatory bowel disease). Conversely, there are a number of very rare diseases in which pericardial involvement is often common. Following is a discussion of the most significant categories of diseases affecting the pericardium.

Viral Pericarditis

ETIOLOGY AND PATHOPHYSIOLOGY. Viral pericarditis is the most common form of pericardial infection.[5,6,48] It is caused by either direct damage resulting from viral replication or immune responses. Numerous viruses have been implicated (HIV is discussed separately later). Echoviruses and coxsackieviruses are the most common. Cytomegalovirus has a predilection for immunocompromised patients. Other than identification of specific viral particles, the most definitive way to diagnose viral pericarditis is by detection of DNA by PCR or in situ hybridization in pericardial fluid or tissue. As discussed earlier, this is rarely necessary.

CLINICAL FEATURES AND MANAGEMENT. These have been discussed earlier in conjunction with the syndrome of acute pericarditis.

Bacterial Pericarditis

ETIOLOGY AND PATHOPHYSIOLOGY. Bacterial pericarditis is usually characterized by a purulent effusion. A wide variety of organisms can be causative.[5,6,48,49] Direct extension from pneumonia or empyema accounts for a majority of cases. The most common agents are staphylococci, pneumococci, and streptococci. Hematogenous spread during bacteremia and contiguous spread after thoracic surgery or trauma are also important. Hospital-acquired, post–thoracic surgery methicillin-resistant staphylococcal pericarditis has been increasing. Anaerobic organisms have also been increasing in frequency,[49] usually in association with concomitant infection in the mediastinum, head, or neck.

Bacterial pericarditis can also result from rupture of perivalvular abscesses into the pericardial space (see Chap. 67). Rarely, pericardial invasion spreads along fascial planes from the oral cavity (e.g., periodontal and peritonsillar abscesses). The pericardium can become infected in the course of meningococcal sepsis with or without concurrent meningitis. In contrast to the usual purulent fluid, *Neisseria* can evoke a sterile effusion accompanied by systemic reactions such as arthritis, pleuritis, and ophthalmitis. This responds to anti-inflammatory drugs.

CLINICAL FEATURES. The clinical presentation of bacterial pericarditis is usually high-grade fever with shaking chills, but these may be absent in debilitated patients. Patients may complain of dyspnea and chest pain. A pericardial friction rub is present in the majority. Bacterial pericarditis can take a fulminant course with rapid development of tamponade and may be unsuspected because associated illnesses dominate the clinical picture. Laboratory findings include leukocytosis with marked left shift. Pericardial fluid shows polymorphonuclear leukocytosis and low glucose, high protein, and elevated lactate dehydrogenase levels. Frank pus is occasionally drained. The chest radiograph shows widening of the cardiac silhouette if the effusion is large. With gas-producing organisms, an air-fluid interface may be observed. The ECG shows typical ST-T wave changes of acute pericarditis along with low voltage if there is a large effusion. Echocardiography almost always demonstrates a significant pericardial effusion with or without adhesions.

MANAGEMENT. Suspected or proven bacterial pericarditis should be considered a medical emergency and prompt closed pericardiocentesis or surgical drainage performed.[5,6,48] We recommend at least 3 to 4 days of subsequent catheter drainage. Fluid should be Gram stained and cultured for aerobic and anaerobic bacteria with appropriate antibiotic sensitivity testing. Fungal and tuberculosis staining and cultures should also be performed. Blood, sputum, urine, and surgical wounds should all be cultured. Broad-spectrum antibiotics should be started promptly and modified according to culture results. Anaerobic coverage is critical when pericarditis associated with head and neck infections is suspected.

Purulent pericardial effusions are likely to recur. Thus, surgical drainage with construction of a window is often needed. In patients with thick, purulent effusions and dense adhesions, extensive pericardiectomy may be required to achieve adequate drainage and to prevent the development of constriction. Early surgical drainage may also help prevent late constriction. Intrapericardial streptokinase has been administered to selected patients with purulent or loculated effusions and may obviate the need for a window.[50] The prognosis of bacterial pericarditis is poor,[6] with survival in the range of 30% even in modern series.

Pericardial Disease and Human Immunodeficiency Virus (see Chap. 72)

ETIOLOGY AND PATHOPHYSIOLOGY. A wide variety of pericardial diseases have been reported in patients infected with HIV. About 20% of HIV-infected patients have pericardial involvement at some time. Pericardial disease is the most common cardiac manifestation, and the most common abnormality is an effusion.[51,52] Most are small, asymptomatic, and, in the developed world, idiopathic. Effusions may also be part of a generalized seroeffusive process. This "capillary leak" syndrome is likely related to enhanced cytokine expression in the later stages of HIV disease. Moderate to large effusions are more frequent with more advanced stages of infection. Congestive heart failure, Kaposi sarcoma, tuberculosis, and other pulmonary infections are independently associated with moderate to large effusions, but most remain idiopathic. In some cases, the virus itself appears to be the cause. Tuberculosis is the most common etiology of pericardial effusion in African HIV-infected patients.[34,53] Other, less frequent forms of pericardial disease include involvement by various neoplasms, classic acute pericarditis, and myopericarditis. Constrictive pericarditis is rare; when present, it is usually due to *Mycobacterium tuberculosis*.

CLINICAL FEATURES. Symptomatic patients with pericardial disease usually present with dyspnea or chest pain secondary to pericardial inflammation or a large effusion. Large effusions are often caused by infection or neoplasm. The most common agents identified in symptomatic effusions are *M. tuberculosis* and *M. avium-intracellulare*. However, a wide variety of organisms, often unusual, have been implicated. Lymphomas and Kaposi sarcoma are the most common neoplasms associated with effusion (see Chap. 74).

MANAGEMENT. Asymptomatic patients with small to moderate pericardial effusions do not require treatment. Most are idiopathic and usually remain asymptomatic or resolve spontaneously. Symptomatic, large effusions should be drained and an identifiable cause sought. Even though it is often small and asymptomatic, effusion in HIV disease often occurs in the context of or heralds the onset of full-blown acquired immunodeficiency syndrome and is strongly associated with a shortened survival.[51] Importantly, highly active antiretroviral therapy has substantially reduced the incidence and severity of the myopericardial complications of HIV disease.[52,53]

Tuberculous Pericarditis

ETIOLOGY AND PATHOPHYSIOLOGY. The incidence of pericardial tuberculosis has decreased markedly in the developed world. Of patients with pulmonary tuberculosis, 1% to 8% develop pericardial involvement.[5,34,54] In a modern series of acute to subacute pericardial disease, tuberculosis was diagnosed in only 4% overall and 7% of patients who developed cardiac tamponade. Similarly, tuberculosis is now a rare cause of constrictive pericarditis. However, pericardial tuberculosis remains a major problem in immunocompromised hosts and the Third World. It is estimated to account for 70% of large pericardial effusions and most cases of constrictive pericarditis in developing countries.[34,54] Mortality is estimated to be 17% to 40%, with a similar proportion going on to constriction after development of an effusion.[34] Tuberculous pericarditis is by far the most common cause of pericardial disease in African HIV-infected patients. Evidence of pericardial involvement in patients with HIV infection in African countries where tuberculosis and HIV infection are endemic is sufficient to prompt antituberculous therapy.[54] Pericardial involvement is usually secondary to retrograde spread from peribronchial, peritracheal, or mediastinal lymph nodes or hematogenous spread from the primary focus. Less commonly, the pericardium is involved by breakdown and contiguous spread of a necrotic lesion in the lung.

CLINICAL FEATURES. The clinical presentation of tuberculous pericarditis is usually subacute to chronic, with fever, malaise, and dyspnea in association with an effusion. Cough, night sweats, orthopnea, weight loss, and ankle edema are also common. The most frequent findings are radiographic cardiomegaly, pericardial rub, fever, and tachycardia. Evidence of cardiac tamponade with severe hemodynamic compromise, paradoxical pulse, increased venous pressure, pleural effusion, and distant heart sounds is common. Many patients have a subacute, effusive-constrictive syndrome.[30] Late constrictive pericarditis may develop despite antituberculous treatment.[30,34,54] Clinical evidence of pulmonary tuberculosis may be absent or subtle, a chief reason that the diagnosis is sometimes unsuspected.

Diagnosis of tuberculous pericardial disease has been notoriously difficult.[5,34,48] A definitive diagnosis is made by isolating the organism from pericardial fluid or a biopsy specimen or identifying it histologically. However, the yield for isolation from pericardial fluid is low.[54] The probability of making a diagnosis is increased if both pericardial fluid and biopsy specimens are examined early in the effusive stage of the disease. Thus, there is a definite role for pericardial biopsy. Pericardial tissue reveals either granulomas or organisms in 80% to 90% of cases. The optimal diagnostic workup (as well as management) of suspected tuberculous pericarditis includes a pericardial window with fluid and tissue sent for culture and histopathologic examination. The presence of granulomas without bacilli in biopsy tissue is helpful but not diagnostic of tuberculous pericarditis because granulomas can be found in rheumatoid and sarcoid disease. A positive skin test response increases suspicion, but a negative test response does not exclude the diagnosis, especially in immunocompromised hosts. A positive skin test response is also less helpful in populations with a high endemic incidence of tuberculosis. Unexplained pericarditis in a patient with proven tuberculosis elsewhere makes the diagnosis highly likely.

Measurement of ADA, an enzyme produced by white blood cells in pericardial fluid, was the first modern test to markedly improve the accuracy and speed of diagnosis of tuberculous pericarditis.[5,34,55] A recent systematic review[55] indicates that ADA >40 units/liter in pericardial fluid has a sensitivity of 88% and a specificity of 83%. Increased interferon-γ in pericardial fluid is an additional marker. Combined with ADA, it provides even greater diagnostic accuracy. Most recently, PCR to detect *M. tuberculosis* DNA has been used and can be performed in minute amounts of fluid or tissue, even in patients with constriction.[56] Use of one or more of these modern tests should be routine whenever tuberculous pericarditis is suspected.

MANAGEMENT. The goals of therapy are to treat symptoms as well as tamponade and to prevent progression to constriction. Multidrug antimycobacterial treatment is mandatory and has greatly decreased mortality.[55] The role of corticosteroids and the issue of open surgical drainage versus closed pericardiocentesis have been debated for some time. In studies performed in the 1980s in South Africa,[34,54] patients were randomly allocated to open biopsy and complete surgical drainage of fluid or percutaneous pericardiocentesis and further randomized to receive or not to receive prednisolone. All patients

were treated with isoniazid, streptomycin, rifampin, and pyrazinamide. The outcomes suggested that patients who undergo open drainage are less likely to require repeated pericardiocentesis, and there was a trend in the open drainage group toward reduced constriction. Corticosteroids did not influence the risk of death or progression to constriction but did speed the resolution of symptoms and decrease fluid reaccumulation. Subsequent meta-analyses[5] tend to support these conclusions, but individual studies have been inconclusive, and there are no modern, appropriately powered, controlled trials of corticosteroids. In contrast, a recent prospectively performed trial[57] in patients with large effusions concluded that there is no benefit from the use of systemic or intrapericardial triamcinolone, but the total number of patients was only 57. No studies have specifically addressed the use of corticosteroids in HIV-positive patients with tuberculous pericarditis, in whom outcomes could be different. If corticosteroids are administered, high doses (1 to 2 mg/kg/day with tapering during 6 to 8 weeks) are recommended[5,54] because rifampin induces their hepatic metabolism. Because data are inconclusive, selection of closed versus open drainage and corticosteroid use are necessarily based on clinical judgment. There is no rationale for corticosteroids once established constriction is present.

Fungal Pericarditis

ETIOLOGY AND PATHOPHYSIOLOGY. Fungal infections can rarely cause pericarditis. They are mainly due to locally endemic organisms such as *Histoplasma* and *Coccidioides* or opportunistic fungi such as *Candida* and *Aspergillus*,[5,48] although a number of other organisms have been reported. Histoplasmosis is the most common. It is endemic in Ohio, the Mississippi River valley, and the western Appalachians; it is acquired by inhalation and can infect otherwise healthy patients living in endemic areas. Coccidioidomycosis is endemic in the Southwest. The organism is acquired by inhalation.[58] Immunocompromised patients, those taking corticosteroids or broad-spectrum antibiotics, and drug addicts are at increased risk.

CLINICAL FEATURES AND MANAGEMENT. Pericardial histoplasmosis usually occurs in a previously healthy patient and is thought to represent an inflammatory process in response to infection of adjacent mediastinal lymph nodes.[5,48] Accordingly, isolation of organisms from pericardial fluid is unusual. The fluid is serous, xanthochromic, or hemorrhagic. The disease usually begins with respiratory symptoms followed by pericardial pain. Effusion leading to tamponade occurs in almost half the cases. The diagnosis must be considered in endemic zones and is aided by rising complement fixation titers. Provided effusions are drained as needed, pericardial involvement eventually resolves with or without anti-inflammatory drugs. Antifungal agents are indicated only for disseminated histoplasmosis.

Coccidioidomycosis pericarditis occurs as a complication of progressive, disseminated infection[5,48,58] in chronically ill, debilitated patients. Pericardial involvement does not occur in the self-limited influenza-like form of the infection. Physical findings suggestive of cardiac compression may be the first clues to the diagnosis. Treatment is directed at the disseminated infection with intravenous amphotericin B. Pericardiocentesis is of course indicated when tamponade occurs.

Pericarditis due to opportunistic fungi such as *Candida* and *Aspergillus* usually occurs in patients who are immune suppressed or receiving broad-spectrum antibiotics as well as in patients recovering from open heart surgery,[5,48] typically in the setting of disseminated infection. The prognosis is poor, and the diagnosis is often made at autopsy.

Pericarditis in Patients with Renal Disease

(see Chap. 93)

ETIOLOGY AND PATHOPHYSIOLOGY. The incidence of classic uremic pericarditis has decreased markedly since the advent of widespread dialysis. Its pathophysiology was never fully elucidated, but it is correlated with levels of blood urea nitrogen and creatinine. Toxic metabolites, hypercalcemia, hyperuricemia, and hemorrhagic, viral, and autoimmune mechanisms have all been proposed as etiologic factors.[5,59] The acute or subacute phase is characterized by shaggy, hemorrhagic, fibrinous exudates on both parietal and visceral surfaces with minimal inflammatory reaction. Subacute or chronic constriction may develop with organization of the effusion and formation of thick adhesions within the pericardial space. Large, gradually accumulating effusions are typical.

What we term *dialysis-associated pericardial disease* is now much more common than classic uremic pericarditis.[5,59] It is characterized by de novo appearance of pericardial disease in patients undergoing chronic dialysis, despite normal or mildly elevated blood urea nitrogen and creatinine. Its mechanisms and relation to classic uremic pericarditis are unclear. Small pericardial effusions are often caused by volume overload.

An increased incidence of asymptomatic pericardial effusion has been found in patients with autosomal dominant polycystic kidney disease.[60] About half are moderate to large. They do not appear to cause tamponade and are not correlated with renal function.

CLINICAL FEATURES. In modern populations of dialysis patients, the clinical presentation is sometimes that of acute pericarditis with chest pain, fever, leukocytosis, and pericardial friction rub. Small, asymptomatic effusions are common. Alternatively, patients can present with a pericardial effusion causing hypotension during or after ultrafiltration (low-pressure tamponade). Although conventional cardiac tamponade with acute or subacute hemodynamic compromise can occur, the extremely large, asymptomatic effusions typical of classic uremic pericarditis are unusual today.

The ECG most often is not markedly affected and reflects a high incidence of associated abnormalities (left ventricular hypertrophy, previous MI, electrolyte abnormalities). The chest radiograph may demonstrate cardiac enlargement related to myocardial dysfunction, volume overload, or pericardial effusion.

MANAGEMENT. The management of classic uremic pericarditis is intensive hemodialysis and drainage in patients with effusions causing hemodynamic compromise.[5,48,59] Patients with symptomatic pericarditis almost always respond. Heparin should be used cautiously during hemodialysis because of the possibility of causing hemorrhagic pericarditis. Pericardial effusions without hemodynamic compromise usually resolve after several weeks of intensive hemodialysis.

Treatment of pericardial disease appearing de novo in patients on chronic dialysis is empiric.[5,48,59] Tamponade of course requires drainage. In our experience, intensification of dialysis is variably beneficial, presumably because these patients are already receiving most of its benefits. Use of NSAIDs for pericardial pain is appropriate. Corticosteroids are probably ineffective. There is little experience with colchicine, but its use is not unreasonable. A pericardial window may be required and is usually the most effective approach in patients with recurring effusions. For patients requiring drainage, instillation of a nonabsorbable corticosteroid in the pericardial space was found beneficial in small series of patients.

Early Post—Myocardial Infarction Pericarditis and Dressler Syndrome (see Chap. 54)

ETIOLOGY AND PATHOPHYSIOLOGY. Early post-MI pericarditis occurs during the first 1 to 3 days and no more than a week after the index event.[5] It is due to transmural necrosis with inflammation affecting the adjacent visceral and parietal pericardium. Pericardial involvement is correlated with infarct size. At autopsy, around 40% of patients with large, Q-wave MIs have pericarditis. Thrombolysis and mechanical revascularization have markedly reduced the incidence of this form of pericarditis. Thus, in a recent report,[61] only 4% of patients undergoing primary percutaneous intervention for acute MI had clinical evidence of early post-MI pericarditis.

Late pericarditis is characterized by polyserositis with pericardial or pleural effusions.[5,48] The syndrome was initially described by Dressler and had an estimated incidence of 3% to 4%. Its incidence has also markedly diminished since the onset of early revascularization and was only 0.1% in the same recent report.[61] Dressler syndrome is believed to have an autoimmune etiology due to sensitization to myocardial cells at the time of MI. Antimyocardial antibodies have been

demonstrated. In contrast to early post-MI pericarditis, inflammation is diffuse and not localized to the myocardial injury site.

CLINICAL FEATURES. Most commonly, early post-MI pericarditis is asymptomatic and identified by auscultation of a rub, usually within 1 to 3 days after presentation. Many are monophasic (usually systolic) and can be confused with murmurs of mitral regurgitation or ventricular septal defect. Early post-MI pericarditis virtually never causes tamponade by itself. However, tamponade does occur with left ventricular free wall rupture. Because of its association with large MIs, early post-MI pericarditis should alert the clinician to this possibility, especially if an effusion is present. Symptomatic patients develop pleuritic chest pain within the above time frame. It is important to distinguish pericardial pain from recurrent ischemic discomfort. Ordinarily, this is not difficult on clinical grounds. However, typical electrocardiographic changes of acute pericarditis are uncommon after MI. Pericardial inflammation is localized to the infarcted area; hence, electrocardiographic changes usually involve subtle re-elevation of the ST segment in originally involved leads. An atypical T wave evolution consisting of persistent upright T waves or early normalization of inverted T waves may occur and appears to be highly sensitive for early post-MI pericarditis.

Dressler syndrome occurs as early as 1 week to a few months after acute MI. Symptoms include fever and pleuritic chest pain. The physical examination may reveal pleural or pericardial friction rubs. The chest radiograph may show a pleural effusion or enlargement of the cardiac silhouette, and the ECG often demonstrates ST elevation and T wave changes typical of acute pericarditis. Although pericardial effusions are common, tamponade is unusual.

MANAGEMENT. Although it is associated with large, transmural MIs, early post-MI pericarditis per se is almost invariably a benign process that does not *independently* affect in-hospital mortality. Treatment is therefore based on symptoms. Augmentation of usual post-MI aspirin doses (650 mg orally three or four times per day for 2 to 5 days) or acetaminophen is usually effective.[5,48] Corticosteroids and perhaps some nonaspirin NSAIDs interfere with conversion of MI into a scar, resulting in greater wall thinning and a higher incidence of post-MI rupture.[5,18] Thus, these drugs should be avoided. Because significant hemopericardium is extremely rare with early post-MI pericarditis and there is no evidence that heparin or other antithrombotic drugs increase its risk, their administration need not be modified.

Although Dressler syndrome is a self-limited disorder, admission to the hospital for observation and monitoring should be considered if there is a substantial pericardial effusion or other conditions (e.g., pulmonary infarction) are also being considered. Aspirin or other NSAIDs are effective for symptomatic relief.[5,48] Colchicine is also likely effective. A short course of prednisone, 40 to 60 mg orally per day with a 7- to 10-day taper, can be used in patients not responding to treatment or for recurrent symptoms.

Post-Pericardiotomy and Post–Cardiac Injury Pericarditis
(see Chap. 76)

Blunt or penetrating injury of the chest and heart with myocardial contusion can cause acute pericarditis. The pericarditis is rarely of clinical significance compared with other effects of the trauma. However, pericarditis can develop days to months after cardiac surgery, thoracotomy, or chest trauma. The pathogenesis of this syndrome is thought to involve production of anti-heart antibodies in response to myocardial injury.[5] A systemic inflammatory response occurs and is characterized by low-grade fever, mild leukocytosis, and pleuropericardial inflammation with associated chest discomfort. The chest radiograph typically shows pleural effusions. A few patients demonstrate pulmonary infiltrates. The ECG reveals changes consistent with acute pericarditis in about 50% of cases. The echocardiogram usually shows a small to moderate pericardial effusion, but tamponade is rare. NSAIDs are first-line treatment, with an excellent response usually occurring within 48 hours. Colchicine is also likely effective. Treatment should be maintained for 2 to 3 weeks. Corticosteroid therapy is reserved for patients with unresponsive, severe, or recurrent symptoms.

Radiation-Induced Pericarditis
Mediastinal and thoracic radiation therapy remains standard treatment of a variety of thoracic neoplasms. Hodgkin disease, non-Hodgkin

lymphoma, and breast carcinoma are most commonly associated with radiation pericarditis (see Chap. 90). Factors that influence pericardial injury include the total dose, the amount of cardiac silhouette exposed, the nature of the radiation source, and the duration and fractionation of therapy. There is about a 2% incidence of clinically evident pericarditis in conjunction with modern radiation delivery.[5,48] However, the incidence can be as high as 20% when the entire pericardium is exposed.

Radiation pericarditis takes one of two forms, an acute illness with chest pain and fever and a delayed form that can occur years after treatment. Self-limited, asymptomatic effusions are common soon after radiation therapy, but tamponade is unusual. Late manifestations of radiation injury occur from about a year to up to 20 years after exposure. Patients can present with symptomatic pericarditis and effusion with or without cardiac compression or circulatory congestion due to constrictive pericarditis. Effusions can evolve into constriction (i.e., an effusive-constrictive syndrome).[30]

Radiation-induced pericarditis and effusion can be confused with malignant effusions. The malignant effusions are usually associated with other evidence of disease recurrence. Hypothyroidism induced by mediastinal irradiation can also contribute to pericardial effusion. Pericardiocentesis with fluid analysis for malignant cells and thyroid function tests differentiate radiation-induced effusion from other causes. Large, symptomatic pericardial effusions may be drained either percutaneously or surgically. Recurrent pericardial effusions are usually best treated surgically with either a window or pericardiectomy. Pericardiectomy is the treatment of choice for patients with constriction. However, perioperative mortality is higher than with idiopathic constrictive pericarditis.

Metastatic Pericardial Disease (see Chaps. 74 and 90)

Pericardial tumor implants are the usual cause of effusion in patients with known malignant neoplasms, although as noted earlier, obstruction of lymphatic drainage by enlarged mediastinal nodes is occasionally observed.[5,21,48,62] Malignant disease is a leading cause of cardiac tamponade in developed countries. Lung carcinoma is the most common, accounting for about 40% of malignant effusions; breast carcinoma and lymphomas are responsible for about another 40%. Gastrointestinal carcinoma, melanoma, sarcomas, and other cancers are less common. With the advent of HIV disease, the incidence of Kaposi sarcoma and lymphomatous involvement of the pericardium increased, but highly active antiretroviral therapy has reduced their incidence (see Chap. 72).

Pericardial tumor implants can cause pericardial pain. However, the dominant feature is usually an effusion. Effusive-constrictive patterns are common. An asymptomatic, incidentally discovered pericardial effusion can be the presenting sign of a malignant neoplasm. However, most patients present with symptomatic effusions or tamponade. In a recent series,[63] 18% of large, symptomatic effusions represented the first presentation of a malignant neoplasm after exclusion of those with an easily identifiable cause. The ECG in malignant effusions is variable but usually shows nonspecific T wave abnormalities with low-voltage QRS. ST-segment elevation is somewhat unusual but can occur. In addition to echocardiography, CT and CMR are useful in evaluating the extent of metastatic disease to the pericardium and adjacent structures.

In most cancer patients with effusions, it is important that metastatic involvement of the pericardium be confirmed by identification of malignant cells or tumor markers in pericardial fluid. This is because of occasional patients with obstructed lymphatic drainage, the possibility of confusion with radiation-induced disease, and the fact that other forms of pericardial disease can occur in patients who have cancer. However, there are many exceptions when clinical judgment dictates that pericardial fluid need not be obtained, especially when effusions are not large and specific treatment (e.g., instillation of drugs in the pericardial space) is not being contemplated.

It is essential to evaluate the life expectancy of patients before performing pericardiocentesis and choosing treatment modalities. In terminally ill patients, drainage should be performed only to aid in relief of symptoms. However, patients with better prognoses deserve a more aggressive approach, which can be gratifying in a surprisingly large number. In many cases, a single drainage will provide prolonged relief as well as fluid for analysis, although it is likely that the only factor to ultimately influence survival is successful treatment of the underlying cancer. For this reason, pericardiocentesis should be the initial step in most patients, with several days of drainage and careful attention to detection of reaccumulation. For recurrences and perhaps in some cases of a first effusion, intrapericardial instillation of tetracycline or chemotherapeutic agents has a reasonable record.[5] Cisplatin appears effective in treating pericardial involvement by lung adenocarcinoma[64]; bleomycin is useful for non–small cell lung cancer.[65] Thiotepa[66] has a good record with a variety of malignant neoplasms. External beam radiation therapy

is an option in patients with radiation-sensitive tumors. A pericardial window or even complete surgical pericardiectomy should be considered in unusual patients with unresponsive, recurrent effusions who continue to have a good prognosis otherwise.

Primary Pericardial Tumors

A number of primary pericardial neoplasms, all exceedingly rare, have been reported. They include malignant mesotheliomas, fibrosarcomas, lymphangiomas, hemangiomas, teratomas, neurofibromas, and lipomas.[5,67] Because of their rarity, it is difficult to generalize about their clinical presentation and course. They are usually either locally invasive or compress cardiac structures or are detected because of an abnormal cardiac silhouette on the chest radiograph. Mesotheliomas and fibrosarcomas are lethal. Others, such as lipomas, are benign. CT and CMR are helpful in delineating the anatomy of these tumors, but surgery is usually required for diagnosis and treatment.

Autoimmune and Drug-Induced Pericardial Disease

Pericardial involvement can occur in virtually any autoimmune disease, but the bulk of cases occur in rheumatoid arthritis, SLE, and progressive systemic sclerosis (scleroderma).[5,48] In addition, many drugs have been reported to cause pericarditis as part of an autoimmune process. Maisch and colleagues[68] coined the general term *autoreactive pericarditis* when an autoimmune mechanism is thought to be involved as the cause of pericarditis. Assignment to this group is not dependent on establishment of a specific diagnosis (e.g., SLE); rather, evaluation includes analysis of pericardial fluid that is designed to systematically exclude nonautoimmune causes. In a selected cohort, 32% of patients with pericardial effusion were found to have autoreactive pericarditis. Maisch and colleagues[68] advocate treatment of these patients with intrapericardial instillation of triamcinolone. However, theirs was not a controlled study, follow-up was relatively short, and a significant number of patients suffered transient Cushing syndrome. Thus, the overall effectiveness of this approach is uncertain.

RHEUMATOID ARTHRITIS. Pericardial involvement is common in rheumatoid arthritis[5,48] (see Chap. 89). Older autopsy studies revealed pericardial inflammation in about 50% of patients. There are no contemporary pathologic or clinical studies addressing the incidence of pericardial involvement. Clinically evident pericardial involvement is reported in up to 25% of patients. Patients can present with chest pain, fever, and dyspnea due to acute pericarditis, which usually occurs in conjunction with exacerbation of underlying disease. Asymptomatic pericardial effusion and cardiac tamponade can also be presenting manifestations. Pericardial fluid is characterized by low glucose concentration, neutrophilic leukocytosis, elevated titers of rheumatoid factor, low complement levels, and, rarely, high cholesterol levels. Constrictive pericarditis also can occur as the result of longstanding pericardial inflammation. In patients with joint exacerbations, management of acute pericarditis or asymptomatic effusion is first and foremost effective treatment of the exacerbation. Pericardial manifestations seem to respond well to high-dose aspirin or NSAIDs. Effusions causing tamponade should be drained both to treat tamponade and to establish with confidence that there is no other cause (e.g., infection) in patients who may be receiving immunosuppressive drugs. In general, the response to treatment of underlying disease exacerbations is too slow and uncertain to advocate a period of watchful waiting in the hope that large effusions will shrink. Recurrent tamponade and large effusions are good indications for a pericardial window. Therapy with colchicine has also been shown to be effective for recurrences.[5] In some patients receiving anti–tumor necrosis factor therapy, pericardial effusion may be drug rather than disease related.[69]

SYSTEMIC LUPUS ERYTHEMATOSUS. Pericarditis is the most common cardiovascular manifestation of SLE (see Chap. 89).[5,48] Acute pericarditis can be the first manifestation of the disease. About 40% of patients with SLE develop pericarditis at some time, usually in conjunction with a flare and involvement of other serosal surfaces. Typical patients present with pleuritic chest pain and low-grade fever. Large effusions can occur but are unusual. The ECG often shows typical findings of acute pericarditis. The chest radiograph may show enlargement of the cardiac silhouette if effusion is present, along with pleural effusions and often parenchymal infiltrates. Pericardial effusions have high protein and low glucose contents and a white blood cell count below 10,000/mL³. As with rheumatoid arthritis, it is important to exclude purulent, fungal, or tuberculous pericarditis because many patients are immunosuppressed. Most patients respond to corticosteroids or immunosuppressive therapy used to treat disease flares. Hemodynamic compromise secondary to cardiac tamponade may occur in as many as 10% to 20% of patients with SLE.[70] Accordingly, we recommend hospitalization to monitor for hemodynamic complications until stability is ensured. Closed drainage combined with corticosteroids is reported to have a good outcome in these patients.[6,70] However, a significant proportion of patients with tamponade may require a window despite high-dose corticosteroids.

PROGRESSIVE SYSTEMIC SCLEROSIS (SCLERODERMA) (see Chap. 89). There is about a 10% incidence of acute pericarditis with chest pain and pericardial rub in progressive systemic sclerosis.[5,48] Pericardial involvement is found at autopsy in about 50% of patients. Pericardial effusion is detected by echocardiography in up to 40%. Most are small and asymptomatic, but there are occasional instances of large effusions. Late constrictive pericarditis has been described. Treatment of acute pericarditis in scleroderma patients is often unrewarding, with an unpredictable response to aspirin and NSAIDs. Although there is no published experience, colchicine should be considered. Right-heart catheterization is useful in patients presenting with dyspnea or right-sided heart failure to evaluate pulmonary vascular disease, which is relatively common and can be confused with pericardial involvement. Moreover, various pericardial CT scan abnormalities are associated with pulmonary hypertension due to systemic sclerosis.[71]

DRUG-INDUCED PERICARDITIS. The great majority of cases of drug-induced pericardial disease occur as a component of drug-induced SLE syndromes.[5] There are no recent studies of the epidemiology or etiology of drug-induced SLE, and the list of offending agents is long. Isoniazid and hydralazine are probably the most common current offenders. Large effusions, tamponade, and even constriction have been reported but are rare in drug-induced SLE pericarditis. In addition to drug cessation, management is dictated by the specific elements of the SLE syndrome present as well as usual efforts aimed at detection and treatment of effusions. Rarely, drug-induced pericarditis due to agents such as penicillin and cromolyn involves eosinophilic hypersensitivity reactions without an SLE picture.

Hemopericardium

Any form of chest trauma can cause hemopericardium[5,48] (see Chap. 76). Post-MI free wall rupture with hemopericardium occurs within several days of transmural MI and is discussed in Chap. 54. Hemopericardium due to retrograde bleeding into the pericardial sac is an important complication and frequent cause of death in type I dissecting aortic aneurysm (see Chap. 60). These patients may also have the combination of acute volume overload due to disruption of the aortic valve and tamponade without a paradoxical pulse.

Puncture of atrial or ventricular walls can occur during mitral valvuloplasty and is signaled by abrupt chest pain.[5,48] Tamponade commonly ensues and can occur rapidly or with a delayed course. It is usually managed with percutaneous drainage. Small pericardial effusions are occasionally observed after device closure of atrial septal defects, but tamponade appears to be rare.[72]

Pericardial effusion with tamponade is a rare but important complication of percutaneous coronary intervention[73] (see Chap. 58). The incidence is 0.1% to 0.6% and may have increased in the 1990s in relation to aggressive treatment of complex lesions with atherectomy and debulking devices and stiff or hydrophilic guidewires. With more modern equipment and experience, the incidence may be decreasing or at least stabilizing. Cardiac tamponade during percutaneous coronary intervention is almost always a result of coronary perforation. The clinical presentation is usually rapidly progressive cardiac decompensation and severe hypotension, although it can occasionally be delayed and more insidious. The diagnosis of perforation is usually made by detection of extravasation of dye from the coronary circulation into the pericardial space. Loss of cardiac pulsation on fluoroscopy indicates that a significant pericardial effusion is present. Management of tamponade requires sealing of the perforation, pericardiocentesis, and reversal of anticoagulation.[5,73] If perforation cannot be managed percutaneously, emergency surgery is indicated.

Pericardial effusion and tamponade can also occur as a complication of catheter-based arrhythmia procedures, especially atrial fibrillation ablations. In a large, prospective series,[74] 0.8% of patients had pericardial effusions that did not require pericardiocentesis and 0.6% had cardiac tamponade, which was successfully drained in all. Reduction of energy appears to reduce the incidence. Management is similar to that for coronary perforations. Right ventricular perforation is an occasional immediate complication of pacemaker and implantable defibrillator lead insertion but rarely causes tamponade. The risk of delayed right ventricular perforation (>5 days after implantation) by small-diameter active fixation pacing and implantable defibrillator leads has recently been emphasized.[75] The clinical presentation is variable, but cardiac tamponade occurs in a significant number of cases.

Last, right ventricular perforation remains an occasional complication of right ventricular endomyocardial biopsy but very rarely causes tamponade.[76]

Thyroid-Associated Pericardial Disease (see Chap. 86)

Of patients with severe hypothyroidism, 25% to 35% develop pericardial effusions.[5] These can be large but rarely if ever cause tamponade. Effusions occasionally occur in subclinical hypothyroidism. Hypothyroid effusions often have high concentrations of cholesterol. The effusions gradually resolve with thyroid replacement. Rarely, effusion can occur in hyperthyroidism.

Pericardial Disease in Pregnancy (see Chap. 82)

Small, clinically insignificant pericardial effusions are observed in about 40% of healthy pregnant women.[5] There is no evidence that pregnancy per se influences the incidence, etiology, or course of pericardial disease, and it is in general managed no differently than in nonpregnant patients. However, colchicine is contraindicated, and pericardiocentesis should be performed only for effusions causing tamponade or if a treatable infectious cause is suspected. Early during pregnancy, fluoroscopically guided pericardiocentesis should be avoided.

Congenital Anomalies of the Pericardium

PERICARDIAL CYSTS. Pericardial cysts are rare, benign congenital malformations.[5,67] They are usually fluid filled, located at the right costophrenic angle, and identified as an incidental finding on a chest radiograph. The diagnosis is usually confirmed by echocardiography. Management is conservative.

CONGENITAL ABSENCE OF THE PERICARDIUM. Congenital absence of the pericardium is rare (see Chap. 65). Usually part or all of the left parietal pericardium is absent, but partial absence of the right side has also been reported.[5] Partial absence of the left pericardium is associated with other anomalies, including atrial septal defect, bicuspid aortic valve, and pulmonary malformations. It is often symptomatic and may allow herniation of portions of the heart through the defect or torsion of the great vessels, with potentially life-threatening consequences. Recurrent pulmonary infections are occasionally seen. Patients can present with chest pain, syncope, or even sudden death. The ECG typically reveals incomplete right bundle branch block. Absence of all or most of the left pericardium results in a characteristic chest radiograph with a leftward shift of the cardiac silhouette, elongated left-sided heart border, and radiolucent bands between the aortic knob and the main pulmonary artery and the left diaphragm and the base of the heart. Echocardiography reveals paradoxical septal motion and right ventricular enlargement. CT or CMR can be employed to establish a definitive diagnosis. Pericardiectomy should be advised to ameliorate symptoms and to prevent herniation.

REFERENCES

Classic Reading List

Ditchey R, Engler R, LeWinter M, et al: The role of the right heart in acute cardiac tamponade in dogs. Circ Res 48:701, 1981.

Hatle LK, Appleton CP, Popp RL: Differentiation of constrictive pericarditis and restrictive cardiomyopathy by Doppler echocardiography. Circulation 79:357,1989.

LeWinter MM, Myhre EESP, Slinker BK: Influence of the pericardium and ventricular interaction on diastolic function. In Gaasch WH, LeWinter MM (eds): Heart Failure and Left Ventricular Diastolic Function. Philadelphia, Lea & Febiger, 1993, pp 103-117.

Shabetai R: The Pericardium. New York, Grune & Stratton, 1981.

Singh S, Wann LS, Schuchard GH, et al: Right ventricular and right atrial collapse in patients with cardiac tamponade—a combined echocardiographic and hemodynamic study. Circulation 70:966, 1984.

Anatomy and Physiology of the Pericardium

1. Johnson D: The pericardium. In Standring S, et al (eds): Gray's Anatomy. New York, Elsevier Churchill Livingstone, 2005, pp 995-996.
2. Jöbsis PD, Ashikaga H, Wen H, et al: The visceral pericardium: Macromolecular structure and contribution to passive mechanical properties of the left ventricle. Am J Physiol 293:H3379, 2007.

The Passive Role of the Normal Pericardium in Heart Disease

3. O'Rourke RA, Dell'Italia LJ: Diagnosis and management of right ventricular myocardial infarction. Curr Probl Cardiol 29:6, 2004.

Acute Pericarditis

4. Lange RA, Hillis LD: Clinical practice. Acute pericarditis. N Engl J Med 351:2195, 2004.
5. Maisch B, Seferovic PM, Ristic AD, et al: Guidelines on the diagnosis and management of pericardial diseases executive summary; the Task force on the diagnosis and management of pericardial diseases of the European Society of Cardiology. Eur Heart J 25:587, 2004.
6. Troughton RW, Asher CR, Klein AL: Pericarditis. Lancet 363:717, 2004.
7. Imazio M, Brucato A, Doria A, et al: Antinuclear antibodies in recurrent idiopathic pericarditis: Prevalence and clinical significance. Int J Cardiol 136:289, 2009. Epub 2008 Jul 31.
8. Imazio M, Demichelis B, Parrini I, et al: Management, risk factors, and outcomes in recurrent pericarditis. Am J Cardiol 96:736, 2005.
9. Imazio M, Cecchi E, Demichelis B, et al: Indicators of poor prognosis of acute pericarditis. Circulation 115:2739, 2007.
10. Imazio M, Demichelis B, Parrini I, et al: Day-hospital treatment of acute pericarditis: A management program for outpatient therapy. J Am Coll Cardiol 43:1042, 2004.

11. Imazio M, Bobbio M, Cecchi E, et al: Colchicine as first-choice therapy for recurrent pericarditis: Results of the CORE (COlchicine for REcurrent pericarditis) trial. Arch Intern Med 165:1987, 2005.
12. Imazio M, Bobbio M, Cecchi E, et al: Colchicine in addition to conventional therapy for acute pericarditis: Results of the COlchicine for acute PEricarditis (COPE) trial. Circulation 112:2012, 2005.
13. Artom G, Koren-Morag N, Spodick DH, et al: Pretreatment with corticosteroids attenuates the efficacy of colchicine in preventing recurrent pericarditis: A multi-centre all-case analysis. Eur Heart J 26:723, 2005.
14. Brucato A, Brambilla G, Moreo A, et al: Long-term outcomes in difficult-to-treat patients with recurrent pericarditis. Am J Cardiol 98:267, 2006.
15. Imazio M, Brucato A, Adler Y, et al: Prognosis of idiopathic recurrent pericarditis as determined from previously published reports. Am J Cardiol 100:1026, 2007.
16. Imazio M, Brucato A, Trinchero R, et al: Colchicine for pericarditis: Hype or hope? Eur Heart J 30:532, 2009.
17. Imazio M, Brucato A, Cumetti D, et al: Corticosteroids for recurrent pericarditis: High versus low doses: A nonrandomized observation. Circulation 118:667, 2008.

Pericardial Effusion and Tamponade

18. Little WC, Freeman GL: Pericardial disease. Circulation 113:1622, 2006.
19. Al-Dadah AS, Guthrie TJ, Pasque MK, et al: Clinical course and predictors of pericardial effusion following cardiac transplantation. Transplant Proc 39:1589, 2007.
20. Goland S, Caspi A, Malnick S, et al: Idiopathic chronic pericardial effusion. N Engl J Med 342:1449, 2000.
21. Ben-Horin S, Bank I, Guetta V, Livneh A: Large symptomatic pericardial effusion as the presentation of unrecognized cancer: A study in 173 consecutive patients undergoing pericardiocentesis. Medicine (Baltimore) 85:49, 2006.
22. Spodick DM: Acute cardiac tamponade. N Engl J Med 349:684, 2003.
23. Sagristà-Sauleda J, Angel J, Sambola A, et al: Low-pressure cardiac tamponade: Clinical and hemodynamic profile. Circulation 114:945, 2006.
24. Kopterides P, Lignos M, Papanikolaou S, et al: Pleural effusion causing cardiac tamponade: Report of two cases and review of the literature. Heart Lung 35:66, 2006.
25. Krantz MJ, Lee JK, Spodick DH: Repetitive yawning associated with cardiac tamponade. Am J Cardiol 94:701, 2004.
26. Wang ZJ, Reddy GP, Gotway MB, et al: CT and MR imaging of pericardial disease. Radiographics 23:S167, 2003.
27. Oyama N, Oyama N, Komuro K, et al: Computed tomography and magnetic resonance imaging of the pericardium: Anatomy and pathology. Magn Res Med Sci 3:145, 2004.
28. Sagristà-Sauleda J, Angel J, Sambola A, Permanyer-Miralda G: Hemodynamic effects of volume expansion in patients with cardiac tamponade. Circulation 117:1545, 2008.
29. Tsang TS, Enriquez-Sarano M, Freeman WK, et al: 1127 consecutive therapeutic echocardiographically guided pericardiocenteses: Clinical profile, practice patterns, and outcomes spanning 21 years. Mayo Clin Proc 77:429, 2002.
30. Sagristà-Sauleda J, Angel J, Sanchez A, et al: Effusive-constrictive pericarditis. N Engl J Med 350:469, 2004.
31. Swanson N, Mirza I, Wijesinghe N, Devlin G: Primary percutaneous balloon pericardiotomy for malignant pericardial effusion. Catheter Cardiovasc Interv 71:504, 2008.
32. Ben-Horin S, Shinfeld A, Kachel E, et al: The composition of normal pericardial fluid and its implications for diagnosing pericardial effusions. Am J Med 118:636, 2005.
33. Permanyer-Miralda G: Acute pericardial disease: Approach to the aetiologic diagnosis. Heart 90:252, 2004.
34. Mayosi BM, Burgess LJ, Doubell AF: Tuberculous pericarditis. Circulation 112:3608, 2005.
35. Seferovic PM, Ristic AD, Maksimovic R, et al: Diagnostic value of pericardial biopsy: Improvement with extensive sampling enabled by pericardioscopy. Circulation 107:978, 2003.

Constrictive Pericarditis

36. Haley JH, Tajik AJ, Danielson GK, et al: Transient constrictive pericarditis: Causes and natural history. J Am Coll Cardiol 43:271, 2004.
37. Leya FS, Arab D, Joyal D, et al: The efficacy of brain natriuretic peptide levels in differentiating constrictive pericarditis from restrictive cardiomyopathy. J Am Coll Cardiol 45:1900, 2005.
38. Ha JW, Ommen SR, Tajik AJ, et al: Differentiation of constrictive pericarditis from restrictive cardiomyopathy using mitral annular velocity by tissue Doppler echocardiography. Am J Cardiol 94:316, 2004.
39. Sengupta PP, Mohan JC, Mehta V, et al: Doppler tissue imaging improves assessment of abnormal interventricular septal and posterior wall motion in constrictive pericarditis. J Am Soc Echocardiogr 18:226, 2005.
40. Taylor AM, Dymarkowski S, Verbeken EK, Bogaert J: Detection of pericardial inflammation with late-enhancement cardiac magnetic resonance imaging: Initial results. Eur Radiol 16:569, 2006.
41. Talreja DR, Edwards WD, Danielson GK, et al: Constrictive pericarditis in 26 patients with histologically normal pericardial thickness. Circulation 108:1852, 2003.
42. Sengupta PP, Krishnamoorthy VK, Abhayaratna WP, et al: Disparate patterns of left ventricular mechanics differentiate constrictive pericarditis from restrictive cardiomyopathy. JACC Cardiovasc Imaging 1:29, 2008.
43. Talreja DR, Nishimura RA, Oh JK, Holmes DR: Constrictive pericarditis in the modern era: Novel criteria for diagnosis in the cardiac catheterization laboratory. J Am Coll Cardiol 22:315, 2008.

44. Hirai S, Hamanaka Y, Mitsui N, et al: Surgical treatment of chronic constrictive pericarditis using an ultrasonic scalpel. Ann Thorac Cardiovasc Surg 11:204, 2005.
45. Ling LH, Oh JK, Schaff HV, et al: Constrictive pericarditis in the modern era: Evolving clinical spectrum and impact on outcome after pericardiectomy. Circulation 100:1380, 1999.
46. Bertog SC, Thambidorai SK, Parakh K, et al: Constrictive pericarditis: Etiology and cause-specific survival after pericardiectomy. J Am Coll Cardiol 43:1445, 2004.
47. Góngora E, Dearani JA, Orszulak TA: Tricuspid regurgitation in patients undergoing pericardiectomy for constrictive pericarditis. Ann Thorac Surg 85:163, 2008.

Specific Causes of Pericardial Disease

48. Maisch B, Ristic AD: Practical aspects of the management of pericardial disease. Heart 89:1096, 2003.
49. Brook I: Pericarditis caused by anaerobic bacteria. Int J Antimicrob Agents 33:297, 2009.
50. Tomkowski WZ, Gralec R, Kuca P, et al: Effectiveness of intrapericardial administration of streptokinase in purulent pericarditis. Herz 29:802, 2004.
51. Barbaro G: Pathogenesis of HIV-associated cardiovascular disease. Adv Cardiol 40:49, 2003.
52. Ntsekhe M, Hakim J: Impact of human immunodeficiency virus infection on cardiovascular disease in Africa. Circulation 112:3602, 2005.
53. Sudano I, Spieker LE, Noll G, et al: Cardiovascular disease in HIV infection. Am Heart J 151:1147, 2006.
54. Syed FF, Mayosi BM: A modern approach to tuberculous pericarditis. Prog Cardiovasc Dis 50:218, 2007.
55. Tuon FF, Litvoc MN, Lopes MI: Adenosine deaminase and tuberculous pericarditis—a systematic review with meta-analysis. Acta Trop 99:67, 2006.
56. Zamirian M, Mokhtarian M, Motazedian MH, et al: Constrictive pericarditis: Detection of Mycobacterium tuberculosis in paraffin-embedded pericardial tissues by polymerase chain reaction. Clin Biochem 40:355, 2007.
57. Reuter H, Burgess LJ, Louw VJ, Doubell AF: Experience with adjunctive corticosteroids in managing tuberculous pericarditis. Cardiovasc J S Afr 17:233, 2006.
58. Arsura EL, Bobba RK, Reddy CM: Coccidioidal pericarditis. Int J Infect Dis 10:86, 2006.
59. Alpert MA, Ravenscraft MD: Pericardial involvement in end-stage renal disease. Am J Med Sci 325:228, 2003.
60. Qian Q, Hartman RP, King BF, Torres VE: Increased occurrence of pericardial effusion in patients with autosomal dominant polycystic kidney disease. Clin J Am Soc Nephrol 2:1223, 2007.
61. Imazio M, Negro A, Belli R, et al: Frequency and prognostic significance of pericarditis following acute myocardial infarction treated by primary percutaneous coronary intervention. Am J Cardiol 103:1525, 2009.
62. Imazio M, Demichelis B, Parrini I, et al: Relation of acute pericardial disease to malignancy. Am J Cardiol 95:1393, 2005.
63. Ben-Horin S, Bank I, Guetta V, Livneh A: Large symptomatic pericardial effusion as the presentation of unrecognized cancer: A study in 173 consecutive patients undergoing pericardiocentesis. Medicine (Baltimore) 85:49, 2006.
64. Bischiniotis TS, Lafaras CT, Platogiannis DN, et al: Intrapericardial cisplatin administration after pericardiocentesis in patients with lung adenocarcinoma and malignant cardiac tamponade. Hellenic J Cardiol 46:324, 2005.
65. Maruyama R, Yokoyama H, Seto T, et al: Catheter drainage followed by the instillation of bleomycin to manage malignant pericardial effusion in non–small cell lung cancer: A multi-institutional phase II trial. J Thorac Oncol 2:65, 2007.
66. Martinoni A, Cipolla CM, Cardinale D, et al: Long-term results of intrapericardial chemotherapeutic treatment of malignant pericardial effusions with thiotepa. Chest 126:1412, 2004.
67. Duwe BV, Sterman DH, Musani AI: Tumors of the mediastinum. Chest 128:2893, 2005.
68. Maisch B, Ristic AD, Pankuweit S: Intrapericardial treatment of autoreactive pericardial effusion with triamcinolone; the way to avoid side effects of systemic corticosteroid therapy. Eur Heart J 23:1503, 2002.
69. Edwards MH, Leak AM: Pericardial effusions on anti-TNF therapy for rheumatoid arthritis—a drug side effect or uncontrolled systemic disease? Rheumatology (Oxford) 48:316, 2009.
70. Rosenbaum E, Krebs E, Cohen M, et al: The spectrum of clinical manifestations, outcome and treatment of pericardial tamponade in patients with systemic lupus erythematosus: A retrospective study and literature review. Lupus 16:608, 2009.
71. Fischer A, Misumi S, Curran-Everett D, et al: Pericardial abnormalities predict the presence of echocardiographically defined pulmonary arterial hypertension in systemic sclerosis–related interstitial lung disease. Chest 131:988, 2007.
72. Elshershari H, Cao QL, Hijazi ZM: Transcatheter device closure of atrial septal defects in patients older than 60 years of age: Immediate and follow-up results. J Invasive Cardiol 20:177, 2008.
73. Fasseas P, Orford JL, Panetta CJ, et al: Incidence, correlates, management, and clinical outcome of coronary perforation: Analysis of 16,298 procedures. Am Heart J 147:140, 2004.
74. Bertaglia E, Zoppo F, Tondo C, et al: Early complications of pulmonary vein catheter ablation for atrial fibrillation: A multicenter prospective registry on procedural safety. Heart Rhythm 4:1265, 2007.
75. Laborderie J, Barandon L, Ploux S, et al: Management of subacute and delayed right ventricular perforation with a pacing or an implantable cardioverter-defibrillator lead. Am J Cardiol 102:1352, 2008.
76. Holzmann M, Nicko A, Kühl U, et al: Complication rate of right ventricular endomyocardial biopsy via the femoral approach: A retrospective and prospective study analyzing 3048 diagnostic procedures over an 11-year period. Circulation 118:1722, 2008.

CHAPTER 76 Traumatic Heart Disease

Matthew J. Wall, Jr., Peter I. Tsai, and Kenneth L. Mattox

Incidence

Thoracic trauma is responsible for 25% of the deaths from vehicular accidents. These can be comprised of six lethal injuries—airway obstruction, tension pneumothorax, cardiac tamponade, open pneumothorax, massive hemothorax, and flail chest. There are six hidden injuries, which can be potentially lethal; these should be detected during secondary survey and include thoracic aortic disruption, tracheobronchial disruption, blunt cardiac injury, traumatic diaphragmatic tear, esophageal disruption, and pulmonary contusion.[1] Of motor vehicle fatalities, 10% to 70% may have been the result of blunt cardiac rupture. Penetrating cardiac trauma is a highly lethal injury, with relatively few victims surviving long enough to reach the hospital. In a series of 1198 patients with penetrating cardiac injuries in South Africa, only 6% of patients reached the hospital with any signs of life.[2] With improvements in organized emergency medical transport systems, up to 45% of those who sustain significant heart injury may reach the emergency department with signs of life. Transport times shorter than 5 minutes and successful endotracheal intubation are positive factors for survival when the patient suffers a pulseless cardiac injury.[3] However, the overall mortality for penetrating cardiac trauma has not changed significantly, even in the major trauma centers.[4]

Traumatic heart disease can be categorized on the basis of the mechanism of injury (**Table 76-1**). Knowledge of the various types of cardiac injuries, methods available to facilitate rapid diagnosis, and familiarity of the techniques for surgical repair are no longer an academic exercise but a lifesaving necessity.[5] This chapter deals primarily with the presentation, evaluation, and treatment of penetrating, nonpenetrating, and miscellaneous cardiac injuries.

Penetrating Cardiac Injury

Causes

Penetrating trauma is the most common cause of significant cardiac injury seen in the hospital setting, with the predominant cause being firearms and knives.[6,7] Other mechanisms, such as shotguns, ice picks, and fence post impalement, have also been reported.

The location of injury to the heart often correlates with the location of injury on the chest wall. Because of their anterior location, the anatomic chambers at greatest risk for injury are the right and left ventricles. A review of 711 patients with penetrating cardiac trauma has reported 54% sustained stab wounds and 42% gunshot wounds. The right ventricle was injured in 40% of cases, the left ventricle in 40%, the right atrium in 24%, and the left atrium in 3%.[6]

In one study, one third of cardiac injuries involved multiple cardiac structures.[6] Significant complex cardiac injuries involved the coronary arteries ($n = 39$), valvular apparatus (mitral; $n = 2$), intracardiac fistulas (i.e., ventricular septal defects [VSDs]; $n = 14$), and unusual injuries ($n = 10$). Only 2% of patients surviving the initial injury and undergoing an operation required reoperation for a residual defect, and most of these repairs were performed on a semielective basis.

Thus, most injuries are to the myocardium. These are readily managed by the general, trauma, or acute care surgeon.

Clinical Presentation and Pathophysiology

Wounds involving the epigastrium and precordium should raise suspicion for cardiac injury. Stab wounds present a more predictable path of injury than gunshot wounds. Patients with cardiac injury can present with a clinical spectrum from full cardiac arrest with no vital signs to asymptomatic with normal vital signs. Up to 80% of stab wounds that injure the heart eventually manifest tamponade. The weapon injures the pericardium and heart but as the weapon is removed, the pericardium may not allow the blood to escape. Rapid bleeding into the pericardium favors clotting rather than defibrination.[8] As pericardial fluid accumulates, a decrease in ventricular filling occurs, leading to a decrease in stroke volume. A compensatory rise in catecholamine levels leads to tachycardia and increased right heart filling pressures. The limits of distensibility are reached as the pericardium is filled with blood and the septum shifts toward the left side, further compromising left ventricular function. If this cycle persists, ventricular output can continue to deteriorate, leading to irreversible shock. As little as 60 to 100 mL of blood in the pericardial sac can produce the clinical picture of tamponade.

The rate of accumulation depends on the location of the wound. Because it has a thicker wall, wounds to the right ventricle seal themselves more readily than wounds to the right atrium. Patients with penetrating injuries to the coronary arteries present with rapid onset of tamponade combined with cardiac ischemia.

The classic findings of Beck's triad (muffled heart sounds, hypotension, and distended neck veins) are seen in only 10% of trauma patients. Pulsus paradoxus (a substantial fall in systolic blood pressure during inspiration) and Kussmaul's sign (increase in jugular venous distention on inspiration) may be present but are not reliable signs.[9] A valuable and reproducible sign of pericardial tamponade is a narrowing of the pulse pressure. An elevation of the central venous pressure often accompanies rapid and cyclic hyperresuscitation with crystalloid solutions, but in such cases a widening of the pulse pressure occurs.

In contrast to stab wounds, gunshot wounds to the heart are more frequently associated with hemorrhage than with tamponade. Of gunshot wounds to the heart, 20% manifest as tamponade. With firearms, the kinetic energy is greater and the wounds to the heart and pericardium are frequently larger. Thus, these patients present with exsanguination into a pleural cavity and arrest more often.[9]

TABLE 76-1 Causes of Traumatic Heart Diseases

I. Penetrating
  A. Stab wounds—knives, swords, ice picks, fence posts, wire, sports
  B. Gunshot wounds—handguns, rifles, nail guns, lawnmower projectiles
  C. Shotgun wounds—pellets, close versus distant range
II. Nonpenetrating (blunt)
  A. Motor vehicle accident
    1. Seat belt
    2. Air bag
    3. Dashboard, steering wheel
  B. Vehicle-pedestrian accident
  C. Falls from height
  D. Crushing—industrial accident
  E. Blasts—improvised explosive devices, grenades, fragments (combined blunt and penetrating)
  F. Assault
  G. Sternal or rib fractures
  H. Recreational—sporting events, rodeo, baseball
III. Iatrogenic
  A. Catheter-induced
  B. Pericardiocentesis-induced
  C. Percutaneous
IV. Metabolic
  A. Traumatic response to injury
  B. "Stunning"
  C. Systemic inflammatory response syndrome
V. Other
  A. Burn
  B. Electrical
  C. Factitious—needles, foreign bodies
  D. Embolic—missiles

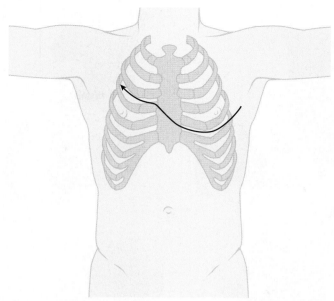

FIGURE 76-1 Left anterior thoracotomy (extension across the sternum if required). See text for details. *(Redrawn from Baylor College of Medicine, 2005.)*

Evaluation

The evaluation of suspected heart injury differs, depending on whether the presenting patient is clinically stable or in extremis. The diagnosis of heart injury requires a high index of suspicion. On initial presentation to the emergency center, airway, breathing, and circulation (ABCs) under the Advanced Trauma Life Support protocol are evaluated and established.[10] Intravenous access is obtained and blood is typed and cross-matched. The patient undergoes chest radiography[11] followed by focused abdominal sonography for trauma (FAST)[12] and can be examined for Beck's triad of muffled heart sounds, hypotension, and distended neck veins, as well as for pulsus paradoxus and Kussmaul's sign. These findings suggest cardiac injury but are present in only 10% of patients with cardiac tamponade. If the FAST results demonstrates pericardial fluid in an unstable patient (systemic blood pressure < 90 mm Hg), transfer of the patient to the operating room to address the injury is recommended.

Patients in extremis often require emergency thoracotomy for resuscitation. The clear indications for emergency department thoracotomy by surgical personnel include the following[13,14]:

1. Salvageable postinjury cardiac arrest (e.g., patients who have experienced cardiac arrest with a high likelihood of intrathoracic injury, particularly penetrating cardiac wounds)
2. Severe postinjury hypotension (i.e., systolic blood pressure < 60 mm Hg) caused by cardiac tamponade, air embolism, or thoracic hemorrhage

If vital signs are regained after resuscitative thoracotomy, the patient can be transferred to the operating room for definitive repair. The patient with confirmed pericardial fluid by FAST, with normal vital signs (systemic blood pressure > 90 mm Hg), may undergo a thorough evaluation to identify associated injuries. If other injuries are excluded, open exploration may then proceed to exclude cardiac injury. In the absence of known causes of the presence of pericardial fluid (e.g., malignant pericardial effusion), a missed cardiac injury can lead to delayed bleeding, deterioration, or death.

Surgeons are increasingly performing ultrasonography for thoracic trauma, paralleling the use of ultrasonography for blunt abdominal trauma. The FAST examination evaluates four anatomic windows for the presence of intra-abdominal or pericardial fluid.[12] Ultrasonography in this setting is not intended to reach the precision of studies performed in the radiology or cardiology suite but is merely intended to determine the presence of abnormal fluid collections, which aids in surgical decision making. Ultrasonography is safe, portable, and expeditious and can be repeated as indicated. If performed by a trained surgeon, the FAST examination has a sensitivity of almost 100% and a specificity of 97.3%. As the use of FAST evolves, the most universally agreed indication is evaluation for pericardial blood.

Chest radiography is nonspecific, but can identify hemothorax or pneumothorax. Other possibly indicated examinations include ultrasonography, central venous pressure measurements, computed tomography (CT) scan for trajectory, thoracoscopy, and laparoscopy.

Treatment

Definitive treatment involves surgical exposure through an anterior thoracotomy or median sternotomy. The goals of treatment are relief of tamponade and hemorrhagic control. Concomitantly, correction of acidosis and hypothermia and reestablishment of effective coronary perfusion are addressed by appropriate resuscitation.

Exposure of the heart is accomplished via a left anterolateral thoracotomy (**Fig. 76-1**), which allows access to the pericardium and heart and exposure for aortic cross-clamping if necessary. This incision can be extended across the sternum to gain access to the right side of the chest and for better exposure of the right atrium or right ventricle. Once the left pleural space is entered, the lung is retracted to expose the descending thoracic aorta for cross-clamping. The amount of blood present in the left chest indicates whether one is dealing with hemorrhage or tamponade. The pericardium anterior to the phrenic nerve is opened, injuries are rapidly identified, and repair is performed. In selected cases, particularly stab wounds to the precordium, median sternotomy can be used. This incision allows excellent exposure to the anterior structures of the heart, but difficulty with access to the posterior mediastinal structures and descending thoracic aorta for cross-clamping may be encountered.

Cardiorrhaphy should be carefully performed. Poor technique can result in enlargement of the lacerations or injury to the coronary arteries. If the initial treating physician is uncomfortable with the suturing technique, digital pressure can be applied until a more experienced surgeon arrives. Other techniques that have been described include

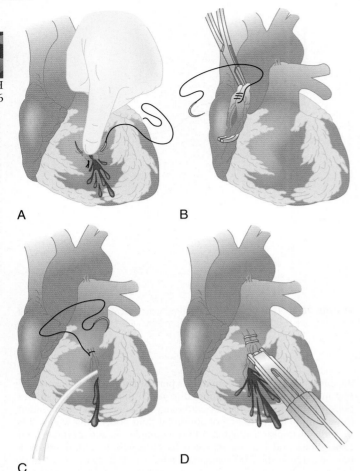

FIGURE 76-2 Temporary techniques to control bleeding. **A,** Finger occlusion. **B,** Partial occluding clamp. **C,** Foley balloon catheter. **D,** Skin staples. *(Redrawn from Baylor College of Medicine, 2005.)*

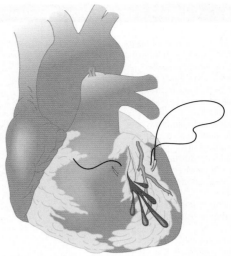

FIGURE 76-3 Injuries adjacent to coronary arteries can be addressed by placing sutures deep, avoiding injury to the artery. *(Redrawn from Baylor College of Medicine, 2005.)*

Intracardiac fistulas include VSDs, atrial septal defects, and atrioventricular fistulas, with an incidence of 1.9% among cardiac injuries. Management depends on symptoms and degree of cardiac dysfunction, with only a minority of these patients requiring repair. These injuries are often identified after primary repair is carried out, and they can be repaired after the patient has recovered from the original and associated injuries. Cardiac catheterization and detailed echocardiography should be performed before repair so that specific anatomic sites of injury and incision planning can be addressed.

The overall hospital survival rate for patients with penetrating heart injuries ranges from 30% to 90%. The survival rate for patients with stab wounds is 70% to 80%, whereas survival after gunshot wounds is 30% to 40%.[4]

Blunt Cardiac Injury

Causes

The term *nonpenetrating* or *blunt cardiac trauma* has replaced the term *cardiac contusion* and describes injury ranging from minor bruises of the myocardium to cardiac rupture. It can be caused by direct energy transfer to the heart or compression of the heart between the sternum and vertebral column at the time of the accident. It can even include cardiac contusion and cardiac rupture during external cardiac massage as part of cardiopulmonary resuscitation (CPR).[15,16] Within this spectrum, blunt cardiac injuries can manifest as septal rupture, free wall rupture, coronary artery thrombosis, cardiac failure, complex and simple dysrhythmias, and/or rupture of chordae tendineae or papillary muscles.[17-19] The incidence can be as high as 75% of patients with severe bodily trauma. Mechanisms include motor vehicle accidents, vehicle-pedestrian accidents, falls, crush injuries, blasts, assaults, CPR, and recreational events. Such injuries can be associated with sternal or rib fractures. A fatal cardiac dysrhythmia can occur when the sternum is struck by a ball,[20] which may be a form of commotio cordis.[21,22]

Cardiac rupture carries a significant risk of mortality. The biomechanics of cardiac rupture include the following: (1) direct transmission of increased intrathoracic pressure to the chambers of the heart; (2) hydraulic effect from a large force applied to the abdominal or extremity veins, causing force to be transmitted to the right atrium; (3) decelerating force between fixed and mobile areas, explaining atriocaval tears; (4) direct force causing myocardial contusion, necrosis, and delayed rupture; and (5) penetration from a broken rib or fractured sternum.[8,23]

Blunt rupture of the cardiac septum occurs most frequently near the apex of the heart when the injury occurs in late diastole or early

the use of a Foley balloon catheter and a skin stapler (**Fig. 76-2**). Injuries adjacent to coronary arteries can be managed by placing the sutures deep to the artery (**Fig. 76-3**).

Complex cardiac injuries include coronary artery injury, valvular apparatus injury (annulus, papillary muscles, and chordae tendineae), intracardiac fistulas, arrhythmias, and delayed tamponade. These delayed sequelae have been reported to have a broad incidence (4% to 56%), depending on the definition.

Coronary artery injury is a rare injury, occurring in 5% to 9% of patients with cardiac injuries, with a 69% mortality rate.[6] A coronary artery injury is most often controlled by simple ligation, but bypass grafting using a saphenous vein may be required for proximal left anterior descending injuries (with cardiopulmonary bypass). With a resurrection of the old concept of coronary artery bypass grafting without cardiopulmonary bypass (off-pump bypass), this technique can theoretically be used for these injuries in the highly unlikely event that the patient is hemodynamically stable.

Valvular apparatus dysfunction is rare (0.2% to 9%) and can occur with blunt and penetrating trauma. The aortic valve is most frequently injured, followed by the mitral and tricuspid valves, although many victims of aortic valve injuries die at the scene. Often, these injuries are identified after the initial cardiorrhaphy and resuscitation have been performed. Timing of repair depends on the patient's condition. If severe cardiac dysfunction exists at the time of the initial operation, immediate valve repair or replacement may be required; otherwise, delayed repair is usually advised.[6]

systole. Multiple ruptures as well as disruption of the conduction system have been reported.[19] From autopsy data, blunt cardiac trauma with ventricular rupture most often involves the left ventricle, followed by the right ventricle. In contrast, in patients who arrive alive to the hospital, right atrial disruption is more common.[24] This is seen at the superior vena cava–atrial junction, inferior vena cava–atrial junction, or the appendage. VSDs can occur, with the most common tear involving the membranous and muscular portions of the septum. Injury to only the membranous portion of the septum is the least common type of blunt VSD. Traumatic rupture of the thoracic aorta is associated with lethal cardiac rupture in almost 25% of cases.[25] Blunt pericardial rupture results from pericardial tears secondary to increased intra-abdominal pressure or lateral decelerative forces. Tears can occur on the left side, most often parallel to the phrenic nerve, to the right of the pleuropericardium, to the diaphragmatic surface of the pericardium, and finally to the mediastinum. Cardiac herniation with cardiac dysfunction can occur in conjunction with these tears.[26] The heart can be displaced into either pleural cavity or even into the abdomen. In the case of right pericardial rupture, the heart can become twisted, leading to the surprising discovery of an empty pericardial cavity at resuscitative left anterolateral thoracotomy. With a left-sided cardiac herniation through a pericardial tear, a trapped distending heart prevents the heart from returning to the pericardium, and the term *strangulated heart* has been applied. Venous filling is impaired and, unless the cardiac herniation is reduced, hypotension and cardiac arrest can occur.[27] One clue to the presence of cardiac herniation is sudden loss of pulse when the patient is repositioned, such as when moved to a stretcher.

Clinical Presentation and Pathophysiology

As in penetrating cardiac trauma, clinically severe blunt cardiac trauma (e.g., cardiac rupture) manifests as tamponade or hemorrhage into the pleural cavity, depending on the status of the pericardium. If the pericardium is intact, tamponade develops; if it is not intact, extrapericardial bleeding occurs and hypovolemic shock ensues. Tamponade is sometimes combined with hypovolemia, thus complicating the clinical presentation.

Blunt cardiac injury can be divided into clinically significant and insignificant injuries. Clinically significant injuries include cardiac rupture (ventricular or atrial), septal rupture, valvular dysfunction, coronary thrombosis, and caval avulsion. These injuries manifest as tamponade, hemorrhage, or severe cardiac dysfunction. Septal rupture and valvular dysfunction (e.g., leaflet tear, papillary muscle, chordal rupture) can initially appear without symptoms but later demonstrate the delayed sequelae of heart failure.[8,17] Blunt cardiac injury can also appear as a dysrhythmia, most commonly premature ventricular contractions, the precise mechanism of which is unknown. Ventricular tachycardia can occur and degenerate into ventricular fibrillation. Supraventricular tachyarrhythmias can also occur. These symptoms commonly occur within the first 24 to 48 hours after injury.

A major difficulty in managing blunt cardiac injury relates to definitions. *Cardiac contusion* is a nonspecific term that should likely be abandoned. It is best to describe these injuries as "blunt cardiac trauma with ..." followed by the clinical manifestation, such as dysrhythmia or heart failure.[28]

Evaluation

Blunt cardiac injury can often present like a penetrating injury, especially if there is tear and laceration to the heart resulting in pericardial tamponade. The routine ABCs and FAST used for penetrating cardiac injury apply here as well. A high suspicion of the mechanism of injury leads to monitoring for blunt cardiac injury.[29-31]

ELECTROCARDIOGRAPHY. In cases of blunt cardiac injury, conduction disturbances are common.[29,30] Thus, a screening 12-lead electrocardiogram (ECG) can be helpful for evaluation. Sinus tachycardia is the most common rhythm disturbance seen.

Other common disturbances include T wave and ST-segment changes, sinus bradycardia, first- and second-degree atrioventricular block, right bundle branch block, right bundle branch block with hemiblock, third-degree block, atrial fibrillation, premature ventricular contractions, ventricular tachycardia, and ventricular fibrillation.[29,30]

CARDIAC ENZYMES. Much has been written previously about the use of cardiac enzyme level determinations in evaluating blunt cardiac injury. However, no correlation among serum assays (e.g., creatine phosphokinase–myocardial band, cardiac troponin T, cardiac troponin I) and identification and prognosis of injury have been demonstrated with blunt cardiac injury. Therefore, cardiac enzyme level assays are not helpful unless one is evaluating concomitant coronary artery disease, or are considered with other diagnostic modalities (e.g., 12-lead ECG, echocardiography) to improve the diagnosis.[29-32]

ECHOCARDIOGRAPHY. Transthoracic echocardiography (TTE) has limited use in evaluating blunt cardiac trauma because most patients also have significant chest wall injury, thus rendering the test suboptimal. Its major use is in diagnosing intrapericardial blood, suggesting an injury or chamber rupture. To evaluate more subtle findings of blunt cardiac injury, such as wall motion, valvular, or septal abnormalities in the stable patient, transesophageal echocardiography (TEE) is a more sensitive test for evaluating blunt cardiac injury.[29,30] Cardiac septal defects and valvular insufficiency are readily diagnosed with TEE. Because echocardiography is operator-dependent, the approach is often based on the local expertise available.

Ventricular dysfunction can often mimic cardiac tamponade in its clinical presentation. Echocardiography is particularly useful for older patients with preexisting ventricular dysfunction. However, most blunt cardiac injuries identified by echocardiography in stable patients rarely require acute treatment.[33]

Treatment

Much debate and discussion has occurred about the clinical relevance of cardiac contusion. Most trauma surgeons conclude that this diagnosis should be eliminated because it does not affect how these injuries are treated. Thus, a normotensive patient with a normal initial ECG and suspected blunt cardiac injury is managed in observation units, with no expected clinical significance. Patients with an abnormal ECG are admitted for monitoring and treated accordingly. Patients who present in cardiogenic shock are evaluated for a structural injury, which is then repaired.[28]

Dysrhythmias can occur as a result of blunt injury, ischemia, or electrolyte abnormalities and are addressed according to the injury (**Table 76-2**). Complex cardiac injuries from blunt trauma remain rare, and treatment is similar to that for penetrating cardiac injuries of the valvular, septal, and atrial-ventricular apparatus. Cardiac rupture has a worse prognosis than penetrating injuries to the heart, with a survival rate of approximately 20%.

Miscellaneous Cardiac Trauma

Iatrogenic Cardiac Injury

Iatrogenic cardiac injury can occur with central venous line insertion, cardiac catheterization procedures, endovascular interventions, percutaneous pericardiocentesis, or while creating an open pericardial window.[34] Cardiac injuries caused by central venous lines usually occur with placement from the left subclavian or left internal jugular vein.

Perforation causing tamponade has also been reported with a right internal jugular introducer sheath for transjugular intrahepatic portocaval shunts. Vigorous insertion of left-sided central lines, especially during dilation of the line tract, can lead to cardiac perforations.

Even appropriate technique carries a discrete rate of iatrogenic injury secondary to central venous catheterization. Common sites of

TABLE 76-2 Dysrhythmias Associated with Cardiac Injury

Penetrating Cardiac Injury
Sinus tachycardia
ST-segment changes associated with ischemia
Supraventricular tachycardia
Ventricular tachycardia, fibrillation

Blunt Cardiac Injury
Sinus tachycardia
ST-segment, T wave abnormalities
Atrioventricular conduction alterations, bradycardia
Ventricular tachycardia, fibrillation

Electrical Injury
Sinus tachycardia
ST-segment, T wave abnormalities
Bundle branch blocks
Axis deviation
Prolonged QT
Paroxysmal supraventricular tachycardia
Atrial fibrillation
Ventricular tachycardia, fibrillation (alternating current)
Asystole (lightning strike)

cardiac injury include the superior vena cava–atrium junction and superior vena cava–innominate junction. These small perforations often lead to a compensated cardiac tamponade. Drainage by pericardiocentesis is often unsuccessful, and evacuation via a subxiphoid pericardial window or full median sternotomy is sometimes required. Once access to the pericardial space is gained, the site of injury has sometimes sealed and may be difficult to find.

Complications from cardiac catheterization are fortunately relatively rare, but include perforation of the coronary arteries, cardiac perforation, and aortic dissection. These can be catastrophic and require emergency surgical intervention. Other potential iatrogenic causes of cardiac injury include external and internal cardiac massage, endovascular interventions, transthoracic percutaneous interventions, right ventricular injury during pericardiocentesis, and intracardiac injections.[35]

Intracardiac Foreign Bodies and Missiles

Intrapericardial and intracardiac foreign bodies can cause complications of acute suppurative pericarditis, chronic constrictive pericarditis, foreign body reaction, and hemopericardium.[36] Intrapericardial foreign bodies that have been reported to result in complications include bullets,[37] explosive device and missile fragments, knitting needles, and hypodermic needles. Needles and similar foreign bodies have been noted after deliberate insertion by patients, usually those with psychiatric diagnoses. A report by LeMaire and colleagues[36] has advocated removal of those intrapericardial foreign bodies that are larger than 1 cm, contaminated, or produce symptoms.

Intracardiac missiles are foreign bodies that are embedded in the myocardium, retained in the trabeculations of the endocardial surface, or free in a cardiac chamber. These are the result of direct penetrating thoracic injury or injury to a peripheral venous structure, with embolization to the heart. Location and other conditions determine the type of complications that can occur and the treatment required. Observation might be considered when the missile is small, right-sided, embedded completely in the wall, contained within a fibrous covering, not contaminated, and/or producing no symptoms. Right-sided missiles can embolize to the lung, at which point they can be removed if large. In rare cases they can embolize paradoxically through a patent foramen ovale or atrial septal defect. Left-sided missiles can manifest as systemic embolization shortly after the initial injury. Diagnosis is pursued with radiography in two projections, fluoroscopy, echocardiography, or angiography. More recently, rapid CT scanning can be used to diagnose and locate these fragments.

The full body topogram can help identify all missiles and then the cross-sectional images can locate them precisely. Treatment of retained missiles is individualized. Removal is recommended for missiles that are left-sided, larger than 1 to 2 cm, rough in shape, or produce symptoms. Although a direct approach, with or without cardiopulmonary bypass, has been advocated in the past, a large percentage of right-sided foreign bodies can now be removed by endovascular techniques.

Metabolic Cardiac Injury and Burns

Metabolic cardiac injury refers to cardiac dysfunction in response to injury and may be associated with injuries caused by burns, electrical injury, sepsis, the systemic inflammatory response syndrome, and multisystem trauma.[38,39] Intraoperatively, myocardial depression can occur shortly after restoring blood flow to an ischemic extremity. The exact mechanism responsible for this dysfunction is unclear, but responses to trauma can induce a release of cytokines that may have a direct effect on the myocardium, with gender differences in response.[40] Endotoxin, tumor necrosis factor-α, tumor necrosis factor-β, interleukin-1, interleukin-6, interleukin-10, catecholamines (epinephrine, norepinephrine), cell adhesion molecules, and nitric oxide are all possible mediators.[41-43]

Metabolic cardiac injury can manifest clinically as conduction disturbances or decreased contractility leading to decreased output. Myocardial depression can occur in response to the mediator storm and can alter calcium uptake and depression of the myocyte responsiveness to beta-adrenergic stimulation.[44]

Myocytes have altered calcium uptake in patients with injuries from burns. The activation of constitutive nitric oxide synthase can modulate cardiac responsiveness to cholinergic and adrenergic stimulation, and production of inducible nitric oxide synthase can depress myocyte contractile responsiveness to beta-adrenergic agonists. The myocardial depressive effects appear to be reversible.[39]

Treatment of metabolic cardiac injury has been supportive, with correction of the initiating insults, but some practitioners have attempted to address the involved mediators using intravenous phosphodiesterase inhibitors, corticosteroids, arginine, granulocyte-macrophage colony-stimulating factor, and glutamate.[44,45] Use of an intra-aortic counterpulsation balloon pump can be considered to treat such myocardial depression, but no controlled series have tested this hypothesis.

Cardiac complications in the early postburn period are a major cause of death. The initial cardiovascular effect of burn injury is attributable to the profound reduction in cardiac output that can occur within minutes of injury. The overall cardiac response has been described as an ebb and flow pattern, with the initial ebb phase lasting between 1 and 3 days, marked by hypovolemia and myocardial depression, and the flow phase characterized by a prolonged period of increased metabolic demand, with increased cardiac output and peripheral blood flow. The reduction in cardiac output observed in the initial period of burn injury is the result of a dramatic and rapid decrease in intravascular volume and of direct myocardial depression.

Hypovolemia results from the capillary leak caused by endothelial injury and may be mediated by platelet-activating factor, complement, cytokines, arachidonic acid, or oxygen free radicals. Myocardial depression manifested by a decrease in myocardial contractility and abnormalities in ventricular compliance becomes apparent with a total body surface area burn of 20% to 25%. Myocardial depressant factor, tumor necrosis factor-α, vasopressin, oxygen free radicals, and interleukins may be responsible for the depression.[46-48]

Electrical Injury

Cardiac complications are a common cause of death after electrical injury. An estimated 1100 to 1300 deaths occur annually in the United States from electrical injury, including lightning strikes.

The cardiac complications after electrical injury include immediate cardiac arrest, acute myocardial necrosis with or without ventricular failure, myocardial ischemia, dysrhythmias, conduction abnormalities, acute hypertension with peripheral vasospasm, and asymptomatic nonspecific abnormalities evident on the ECG. Damage from electrical injury is caused by direct effects on the excitable tissues, heat generated from the electrical current, and accompanying associated injuries (e.g., falls, explosions, fires).[49] Thus, electrical injuries can result in later complications and algorithms have been developed for monitoring after the event.[50,51]

Pericardial Injury

Small isolated tears in the pericardium can lead to cardiac herniation. This is a rare complication of pericardial rupture and depends on the size of the pericardial tear. If large enough, cardiac herniation can occur, leading to acute cardiac dysfunction.[8,27,52] Traumatic pericardial rupture is rare. Most patients with pericardial rupture do not survive transport to the hospital because of other significant associated injuries. The overall mortality of those who are treated at trauma centers with such injury remains as high as 64%.[53] Motor vehicle accidents are is the most common causes of pericardial rupture. Sixty percent of pericardial ruptures occur along the left pleuropericardial surface.[53] Most of these cases are diagnosed intraoperatively or on autopsy.[27] The clinical presentation of pericardial rupture can mimic that of pericardial tamponade with associated cardiac electrical-mechanical dissociation caused by impaired venous return. When the heart returns to its normal position in the pericardium, venous return resumes.

Positional hypotension is a manifestation of cardiac herniation caused by pericardial rupture,[27] whereas pericardial tamponade is associated with persistent hypotension until the pericardium is decompressed. Therefore, a high index of suspicion should be maintained when evaluating polytrauma patients with unexplained positional hypotension.

Late Sequelae

Secondary sequelae in survivors of cardiac trauma include valvular abnormalities and intracardiac fistulas.[6,54,55] These abnormalities can be identified intraoperatively by gross palpation of a thrill[5] or with the use of TEE. TEE may not be feasible, however, in the acutely injured patient. Early postoperative clinical examination and electrocardiographic findings are unreliable. Thus, echocardiography is recommended during the initial hospitalization to identify occult injury and establish a baseline study. Because the incidence of late sequelae can be as high as 56%, follow-up echocardiography 3 to 4 weeks after injury has been recommended by some.

Summary

The approach to the injured patient follows a well-defined plan. Patients with penetrating trauma who arrive alive at a trauma center can have hemopericardium diagnosed by FAST. Urgent operation performed in the trauma resuscitation area or the operating room can result in survival. Blunt cardiac trauma can produce a range of presentation, from minor electrocardiographic changes to frank rupture of the septum, free wall, or cardiac valves. Associated injuries are common. Stable patients can undergo more extensive evaluation, but unstable patients require rapid imaging and urgent operation. Late sequelae of fistula, valve dysfunction, coronary occlusion, and heart failure are rare and are most often detected by echocardiography or catheterization within the first year after injury.

REFERENCES

Incidence

1. Yamamoto L, Schroeder C, Morley D, Beliveau C: Thoracic trauma: The deadly dozen. Crit Care Nurs Q 28:22, 2005.
2. Campbell NC, Thomsen SR, Murkart DJ, et al: Review of 1198 cases of penetrating cardiac trauma. Br J Surg 84:1737, 1997.
3. Durham LA, Richardson R, Wall MJ, et al: Emergency center thoracotomy: Impact of prehospital resuscitation. J Trauma 32:779, 1992.
4. Thourani VH, Feliciano DV, Cooper WA, et al: Penetrating cardiac trauma at an urban trauma center: A 22-year perspective. Am Surg 65: 811, 1999.
5. Embrey R: Cardiac trauma. Thorac Surg Clin 17:87, 2007.

Penetrating Cardiac Injury

6. Wall MJ Jr, Mattox KL, Chen CD, Baldwin JC: Acute management of complex cardiac injuries. J Trauma 42:905, 1997.
7. Degiannis E, Loogna P, Doll D, et al: Penetrating cardiac injuries: Recent experience in South Africa. World J Surg 30:1258, 2006.
8. Ivatury RR: The injured heart. In Moore ES, Feliciano DV, Mattox KL (eds): Trauma. 5th Ed. New York, McGraw Hill, 2004, pp 555-568.
9. Brown J, Grover FL: Trauma to the heart. Chest Surg Clin North Am 7:325, 1997.
10. American College of Surgeons, Committee on Trauma: Advanced Trauma Life Support. Chicago, American College of Surgeons, 2008.
11. Ho ML, Gutierrez FR: Chest radiography in thoracic polytrauma. AJR Am J Roentgenol 192:599, 2009.
12. Rozycki GS, Schmidt JA, Oschner MG, et al: The role of surgeon-performed ultrasound in patients with possible penetrating wounds: A prospective multicenter study. J Trauma 45:190, 1998.
13. Biffl WD, Moore EE, Johnson JL: Emergency department thoracotomy. In Moore EE, Feliciano DV, Mattox KL (eds): Trauma. 5th ed. New York, McGraw-Hill, 2004, pp 239-252.
14. Working Group, Ad Hoc Subcommittee on Outcomes, American College of Surgeons-Committee on Trauma: Practice management guidelines for emergency department thoracotomy. J Am Coll Surg 193:303, 2001.

Blunt Cardiac Injury

15. Hashimoto Y, Moriya F, Furumiya J: Forensic aspects of complications resulting from cardiopulmonary resuscitation. Leg Med (Tokyo) 9:94, 2007.
16. Bansal MK, Maraj S, Chewaproug D, Amanullah A: Myocardial contusion injury: Redefining the diagnostic algorithm. Emerg Med J 22:465, 2005.
17. Choi JS, Kim EJ: Simultaneous rupture of the mitral and tricuspid valves with left ventricular rupture caused by blunt trauma. Ann Thorac Surg 86:1371, 2008.
18. Varahan SL, Farah GM, Caldeira CC, et al: The double jeopardy of blunt chest trauma: A case report and review. Echocardiography 23:235, 2006.
19. Schaffer RB, Berdat PA, Seiler C, Carrel TP: Isolated rupture of the ventricular septum after blunt chest trauma. Ann Thorac Surg 67:853, 1999.
20. Wahl P, Schreyer N, Yersin B: Injury pattern of the Flash-Ball, a less-lethal weapon used for law enforcement: Report of two cases and review of the literature. J Emerg Med 31:325, 2006.
21. Maron BJ, Link MS, Wang PJ, et al: Clinical profile of commotio cordis: An underappreciated cause of sudden death in young during sports and other activities. J Cardiovasc Electrophysiol 10:114, 1999.
22. Hsing DD, Madikians A: True-true, unrelated: A case report. Pediatr Emerg Care 21:755, 2005.
23. Bakaeen FG, Wall MJ Jr, Mattox KL: Successful repair of an avulsion of the superior vena cava from the right atrium inflicted by blunt trauma. J Trauma 59:1486, 2005.
24. Vougiouklakis T, Peschos D, Doulis A, et al: Sudden death from contusion of the right atrium after blunt chest trauma: Case report and review of the literature. Injury 36:213, 2005.
25. Howanitz EP, Buckley D, Galbraith TA, et al: Combined blunt traumatic rupture of the heart and aorta: Two case reports and review of the literature. J Trauma 30:506, 1990.
26. Nassiri N, Yu A, Statkus N, Gosselin M: Imaging of cardiac herniation in traumatic pericardial rupture. J Thorac Imaging 24:69, 2009.
27. Wall MJ Jr, Mattox KL, Wolf DA: The cardiac pendulum—blunt rupture of the pericardium with strangulation of the heart. J Trauma 59:136, 2005.
28. Mattox KL, Flint LM, Carrico CJ, et al: Blunt cardiac injury (formerly termed "myocardial contusion") [editorial]." J Trauma 31:653, 1992.
29. Holanda MS, Domínguez MJ, López-Espadas F, et al: Cardiac contusion following blunt chest trauma. Eur J Emerg Med 13:373, 2006.
30. Elie MC: Blunt cardiac injury. Mt Sinai J Med 73:542, 2006.
31. Jackson L, Stewart A: Best evidence topic report. Use of troponin for the diagnosis of myocardial contusion after blunt chest trauma. Emerg Med J 22:193, 2005.
32. Bertinchant JP, Polge A, Mohty D, et al: Evaluation of incidence, clinical significance and prognostic value of circulating cardiac troponin I and T elevation in hemodynamically stable patients with suspected myocardial contusion after blunt chest trauma. J Trauma 48:924, 2000.
33. Karalis DG, Victor MF, Davis GA, et al: The role of echocardiography in blunt chest trauma: A transthoracic and transesophageal echocardiographic study. J Trauma 36:53, 1994.

Iatrogenic Cardiac Injury

34. Barleben A, Huerta S, Mendoza R, et al: Left ventricle injury with a normal pericardial window: Case report and review of the literature. J Trauma. 63:414, 2007.
35. Ivatury RR, Simon RJ, Rohman M: Cardiac complications. In Mattox KL (ed): Complications of Trauma. New York, Churchill Livingstone, 1994, pp 409-428.

Intracardiac Foreign Bodies and Missiles

36. LeMaire SA, Wall MJ Jr, Mattox KL: Needle embolus causing cardiac puncture and chronic constrictive pericarditis. Ann Thorac Surg 65:1786, 1998.
37. Davis RE, Bruno AD 2nd, Larsen WB, et al: Mobile intrapericardial bullet: Case report and review of the literature. J Trauma 58:378, 2005.

Metabolic Cardiac Injury and Burns

38. Huang YS, Yang ZC, Tan BG, et al: Pathogenesis of early cardiac myocyte damage after sear burns. J Trauma 46:428, 1999.
39. Sharkey SW, Shear W, Hodges M, Herzog CA: Reversible myocardial contraction abnormalities in patients with an acute non-cardiac illness. Chest 114:98, 1998.
40. Kher A, Wang M, Tsai BM, et al: Sex differences in the myocardial inflammatory response to acute injury. Shock 23:1, 2005.
41. Kumar A, Thota V, Dee L, et al: TNF-alpha and IL-1 are regulators for depression of in vitro myocardial cell contractility induced by serum from humans with septic shock. J Exp Med 183:949, 1996.
42. Meldrum DR, Shenkar R, Sheridan BC, et al: Hemorrhage activates myocardial NF-kappa and increases TNF-alpha in the heart. J Mol Cell Cardiol 29:2849, 1997.

43. Horton JW, Lin C, Maass D: Burn trauma and tumor necrosis factor alpha alter calcium handling by cardiomyocytes. Shock 10:270, 1998.

44. Heinz G, Geppert A, Delle Karth G, et al: IV milrinone for cardiac output increase and maintenance: Comparison in nonhyperdynamic SIRS/sepsis and congestive heart failure. Intensive Care Med 25:620, 1999.

45. Flohe S, Borgermann J, Dominquez FE, et al: Influence of granulocyte-macrophage colony-stimulating factor (GM-CSF) on whole blood endotoxin responsiveness following trauma, cardiopulmonary bypass, and severe sepsis. Shock 12:17, 1999.

46. Maass DL, White J, Horton JW: IL-1beta and IL-6 act synergistically with TNF-alpha to alter cardiac contractile function after burn trauma. Shock 18:360, 2002.

47. Horton JW: Oxygen free radicals contribute to post-burn cardiac cell membrane dysfunction. J Surg Res 61:97, 1996.

48. Horton JW: Cellular basis for burn-mediated cardiac dysfunction in adult rabbits. Am J Physiol 271:H2615, 1996.

49. Lee RC: Injury by electrical forces: Pathophysiology, manifestations, and therapy. Curr Probl Surg 34:677, 1997.

50. Chen EH: Do children require ECG evaluation and inpatient telemetry after household electrical exposures? Ann Emerg Med 49:64, 2007.

51. Arnoldo B, Klein M, Gibran NS: Practice guidelines for the management of electrical injuries. J Burn Care Res 27:439, 2006.

Pericardial Injury

52. Nassiri N, Yu A, Statkus N, Gosselin M: Imaging of cardiac herniation in traumatic pericardial rupture. J Thorac Imaging 24:69, 2009.

53. Galindo Gallego M, Lopez-Cambra MJ, Fernandez-Acenero MJ, et al: Traumatic rupture of the pericardium. Case report and literature review. J Cardiovasc Surg (Torino) 37:187, 1996.

Late Sequelae

54. Meyer DM, Jessen ME, Grayburn PA: Use of echocardiography to detect occult cardiac injury after penetrating thoracic trauma: A prospective study. J Trauma 39:902, 1995.

55. Mattox KL, Limacher MC, Feliciano DV, et al: Cardiac evaluation following heart injury. J Trauma 25:758, 1985.

CHAPTER **77** # Pulmonary Embolism

Samuel Z. Goldhaber

Pulmonary embolism (PE) and deep venous thrombosis (DVT) constitute one of the "big three" cardiovascular killers, along with myocardial infarction and stroke. Known collectively as venous thromboembolism (VTE), PE and DVT account for several hundred thousand deaths annually in the United States and afflict millions of individuals worldwide. The case fatality rate for PE, approximately 15%, exceeds the mortality rate for acute myocardial infarction. PE survivors may have to deal with an impaired quality of life because of chronic thromboembolic pulmonary hypertension or chronic venous insufficiency (also called post-thrombotic syndrome) of the legs. During the past decade, VTE has become integrated into the curriculum for cardiovascular medicine training. The American Heart Association, the American College of Cardiology, and the European Society of Cardiology have targeted PE as an area requiring special guidelines[1] and professional education. The U.S. government has created VTE policies both with a "big stick" (exacting penalties on hospitals that do not optimize prophylaxis) and simultaneously with a "carrot" (increasing federal funding for basic and clinical VTE research projects as well as educational outreach programs for health care professionals and the public). The U.S. Surgeon General has issued a call to action to prevent DVT and PE in which he describes VTE as the most preventable cause of death among hospitalized patients.[2] New nonprofit organizations have formed and include patient advocacy as part of their core mission to improve public education and awareness of VTE and to support innovative research on VTE prevention and treatment.[3] Momentum from these activities is beginning to reap rewards because the case fatality rate for PE is decreasing in the United States.[4]

VTE is a common problem, yet it is often difficult to diagnose. It strikes a wide range of individuals, from teenagers to nonagenarians. Its onset is usually unpredictable. The likelihood of recurrence after completion of a time-limited course of anticoagulation is high, especially when surgery, trauma, or estrogens do not precipitate the initial event. VTE exacts a psychological toll on patients, who wonder whether they will suffer a recurrent event, whether it will affect their family members, and whether it will diminish their quality of life and shorten their life span.

No diagnostic test for PE has utility unless PE is considered in the differential diagnosis. Therefore, clinicians must remain vigilant to detect PE, which has been known for generations as the great masquerader because it mimics other illnesses such as pneumonia and congestive heart failure. For imaging of PE, chest computed tomography (CT) scanning has virtually replaced ventilation-perfusion lung scanning. When the clinical likelihood of PE is low and the result of a screening blood test, the plasma D-dimer assay, is negative, the exclusion of PE is usually straightforward and accurate. The principal challenge now is to confront runaway technology that has led to overuse of CT scanning, with too little attention paid to history, physical examination, and clinical likelihood scoring systems. This trend toward relying on advanced imaging technology, typical of many

aspects of contemporary medicine, has led to excessive exposure to radiation and to intravenous contrast material, with its attendant complications of renal dysfunction, anaphylaxis, and exponential increases in cost.

As soon as the diagnosis of acute PE is established, rapid and precise risk stratification is of paramount importance. Effective anticoagulation serves as the foundation of therapy. High-risk patients may also benefit from thrombolysis, catheter embolectomy, surgical embolectomy, or placement of an inferior vena caval filter. Accurate prognostication relies on classic clinical assessment of general appearance, heart rate, blood pressure, and respiratory rate, as well as a new array of poor prognosis indicators that include elevation of cardiac biomarkers, right ventricular hypokinesis assessed by echocardiography, and right ventricular enlargement detected by chest CT. These risk stratification variables can predict the development of clinical deterioration and adverse outcomes that occur several days after admission to the hospital, despite an initial presentation of hemodynamic stability.

The selection of immediately active parenteral anticoagulant drugs has expanded beyond unfractionated heparin (UFH). Low-molecular-weight heparins (LMWH) and fondaparinux provide convenient fixed-dose, weight-based therapy as an alternative to an adjusted-dose continuous intravenous infusion of UFH monitored by the activated partial thromboplastin time (aPTT). Three direct thrombin inhibitors—argatroban, lepirudin, and bivalirudin—are available for use in patients with suspected or proven heparin-induced thrombocytopenia. Although warfarin is the only oral anticoagulant approved for the treatment of acute PE, its effectiveness and safety are improving with a combination of centralized anticoagulation management services (often run by pharmacists or nurses), more widespread use of self-testing fingerstick machines for rapid turnaround of coagulation results, development of computer-driven dosing nomograms that factor clinical variables and response to prior warfarin doses into the algorithm, and use of rapid turnaround genetic testing during warfarin dose initiation.[5] Meanwhile, novel oral anticoagulants have immediate action and fixed-dose administration and do not require routine coagulation monitoring.[6] Two are approved in Canada and Europe for VTE prevention after orthopedic surgery—the anti-Xa agent rivaroxaban[7,8] and the direct thrombin inhibitor dabigatran[9] (see Chap. 87). In a primary prevention trial of cardiovascular disease, rosuvastatin 20 mg daily reduced the symptomatic VTE rate by 43% within 2 years compared with placebo.[10] This finding points to emerging pharmacologic approaches to VTE prevention other than standard anticoagulation.

A key to reducing VTE incidence will be the implementation of prophylaxis measures that have proven safe and effective in rigorously executed trials.[11] Currently, a wide gap exists between extensive evidence-based knowledge of VTE prevention and meager prescription of anticoagulants or mechanical measures. At-risk

TABLE 77-1	Modifiable Risk Factors for Venous Thromboembolism

Obesity
Metabolic syndrome
Cigarette smoking
Hypertension
Abnormal lipid profile
High consumption of red meat and low consumption of fish, fruits, and vegetables

TABLE 77-2	Major Risk Factors for Venous Thromboembolism That Are Not Readily Modifiable

Advancing age
Arterial disease, including carotid and coronary disease
Personal or family history of venous thromboembolism
Recent surgery, trauma, or immobility, including stroke
Congestive heart failure
Chronic obstructive pulmonary disease
Acute infection
Air pollution
Long-haul air travel
Pregnancy, oral contraceptive pills, or postmenopausal hormone replacement therapy
Pacemaker, implantable cardiac defibrillator leads, or indwelling central venous catheter
Hypercoagulable states
    Factor V Leiden resulting in activated protein C resistance
    Prothrombin gene mutation 20210
    Antithrombin deficiency
    Protein C deficiency
    Protein S deficiency
    Antiphospholipid antibody syndrome

patients hospitalized[12] on medical services[13] and medical subspecialty services, including cardiology and heart failure patients,[14] less often receive guideline-approved prophylaxis[15] than surgical service patients do.[16] Yet, prevention is much easier than diagnosis and treatment of PE or DVT and is far more cost-effective.[17] Failure to prevent VTE has important ramifications after hospital discharge because hospitalized patients receiving inadequate prophylaxis contribute to the burden of out-of-hospital PE and DVT, where three of every four VTE events occur.[18] Universal VTE prophylaxis among at-risk hospitalized patients will bring us toward the goal of near eradication of PE, both in the hospital setting and in the community after hospital discharge of high-risk patients. Strategies to improve implementation of prophylaxis include enhanced education, performance-based incentives, financial penalties if VTE occurs, electronic computerized alerts,[19] and "human alerts" from a hospital staff member to the responsible physicians[20] whose high-risk patients are not receiving prophylaxis.

Epidemiology

The incidence of VTE is about 1.5 per 1000 person-years. There are approximately twice as many DVT as PE cases. Although children and adolescents are susceptible,[21] incidence rises with age[22] and is similar in men and women. About half the cases are idiopathic and occur without antecedent trauma, surgery, immobilization, or the diagnosis of cancer.[23] Several gene polymorphisms associate independently with an increased risk of VTE apart from those with widely known prothrombotic effects, such as factor V Leiden. These include polymorphisms in the beta$_2$-adrenergic receptor and lipoprotein lipase genes.[24] Clinical predictors for fatal PE include anatomically massive PE, neurologic disease, age older than 75 years, and cancer.[25]

A major breakthrough in epidemiology is the discovery that VTE and arterial thrombosis share many identical risk factors, including increasing age, obesity, cigarette smoking, diabetes mellitus, and unfavorable lipid profile.[26] In a cohort of 5451 patients with ultrasound-confirmed DVT from 183 U.S. hospitals, the five most frequent comorbidities were hypertension (50%), surgery within 3 months (38%), immobility within 30 days (34%), cancer (32%), and obesity (27%).[27] Patients with newly diagnosed VTE have an increased long-term risk for development of myocardial infarction or stroke.[28] A meta-analysis of 63,552 patients with VTE and control subjects found that the relative risk for VTE was 2.3 for obesity, 1.5 for hypertension, 1.4 for diabetes mellitus, 1.2 for cigarette smoking, and 1.2 for hypercholesterolemia. High-density lipoprotein (HDL) cholesterol levels were lower in VTE patients.[29] The metabolic syndrome is a risk factor for VTE.[30] Persistent stress also predisposes to VTE.[31] Eating less red meat and more fish, fruit, and vegetables is associated with a lower incidence of VTE.[32] An especially problematic VTE risk factor is obesity, which has become pandemic in the United States. Obesity doubles or triples the likelihood of VTE.[33] The overlap between venous and arterial thrombosis means that the cardiovascular medicine practitioner can counsel patients on steps to reduce VTE and coronary heart disease risk simultaneously. **Table 77-1** lists modifiable VTE risk factors.

Many risk factors for VTE are not readily modifiable (**Table 77-2**). Acute urinary tract infection or respiratory infection may precipitate VTE.[34] Heart failure is a common problem in patients with VTE. The combination of higher medical acuity, increased frequency of VTE

risk factors, and low rate of VTE prophylaxis constitutes a "triple threat" to patients with heart failure.[14] As patients survive longer with cancer, the frequency of VTE is increasing because cancer patients have twice the incidence of VTE (see Chap. 90).[35] This increased risk of VTE not only accompanies adenocarcinomas of the pancreas, stomach, lung, esophagus, prostate, and colon, but also threatens patients with "liquid tumors" such as myeloproliferative disease, lymphoma, and leukemia. In patients with a first VTE and without the diagnosis of cancer, the risk for detection of a subsequent new cancer is 1% to 2% per year and is higher in patients with unprovoked VTE and in those with advanced age.[36]

Pregnancy,[37] hormonal contraception,[38] and postmenopausal hormonal therapy[39] each contribute to increased risk. Less well known risk factors include chronic obstructive pulmonary disease,[40] nephrotic syndrome,[41] and air pollution.[42]

Perhaps the most frequently discussed acquired risk factor is long-haul air travel. The risk of fatal PE in this setting is less than 1 in 1 million. However, when death occurs, it is dramatic and especially tragic because the victim is often an otherwise healthy young person. It appears that among some individuals, there is activation of the coagulation system during air travel.[43] For each 2-hour increase in travel duration, there appears to be an 18% higher risk of VTE.[44]

Hospitalized patients with medical illnesses[13] such as pneumonia and congestive heart failure have a high risk for development of VTE. The stasis and immobilization associated with postoperative venous thrombosis may paradoxically increase after hospital discharge because with short hospital lengths of stay, patients may be too weak and debilitated at home to ambulate after surgery. Vigilance is required to ensure that appropriate patients receive extended VTE prophylaxis at the time of hospital discharge.

Upper extremity DVT is an increasingly important clinical entity because of more frequent placement of pacemakers and internal cardiac defibrillators, as well as more frequent use of chronic indwelling catheters for chemotherapy and nutrition. Patients with upper extremity DVT are at risk for PE, superior vena caval syndrome, and loss of vascular access.[45]

Risk factors for VTE in the community include advancing age, cancer, prior VTE, venous insufficiency, pregnancy, trauma, frailty, and immobility. Of those suffering VTE in the community in the Worcester Venous Thromboembolism Study, 23% had undergone surgery and 36% had been hospitalized within the preceding 3 months. Among those patients, fewer than half had received anticoagulant prophylaxis.[18] More than half of VTE events occurred in subjects 65 years of age or older.[46]

Pathophysiology

Hypercoagulable States (see Chap. 90)

In 1856, Rudolf Virchow postulated a triad of factors that predispose to intravascular coagulation: local trauma to the vessel wall, hypercoagulability, and stasis. Classically, the pathogenesis of PE has been dichotomized as caused by either inherited (primary) or acquired (secondary) risk factors. It appears likely, however, that a combination of thrombophilia and acquired risk factors (see Table 77-2) often precipitates overt thrombosis.

The two most common genetic causes of thrombophilia are factor V Leiden and the prothrombin gene mutation. Normally, a specified amount of activated protein C (aPC) can be added to plasma to prolong the aPTT. Patients with "aPC resistance" have a blunted aPTT prolongation and a predisposition to development of PE and DVT. The phenotype of aPC resistance is associated with a single point mutation, designated factor V Leiden, in the factor V gene. Factor V Leiden triples the risk for development of VTE. This genetic mutation is also a risk factor for recurrent pregnancy loss, possibly caused by placental vein thrombosis. Use of oral contraceptives by patients with factor V Leiden increases the risk of VTE by at least 10-fold. A single point mutation in the 3′ untranslated region of the prothrombin gene (G-to-A transition at nucleotide position 20210) is associated with increased levels of prothrombin. In the Physicians' Health Study, the prevalence of the prothrombin gene mutation was 3.9%, and this mutation doubled the risk of venous thrombosis. The Agency for Healthcare Research and Quality concluded that there is no direct evidence that testing for these mutations leads to improved clinical outcomes in adults with a history of VTE or their adult family members. The test results have variable clinical validity for predicting VTE in these populations and have only weak clinical utility.[47]

The most common acquired thrombophilia is the antiphospholipid syndrome.[48] It can cause venous or arterial thrombosis, thrombocytopenia, recurrent fetal loss, or acute ischemic encephalopathy.[49] A careful family history remains the most rapid and cost-effective method of identifying a predisposition to venous thrombosis. Investigation with blood tests can be misleading. For example, consumption coagulopathy caused by venous thrombosis may be misdiagnosed as deficiency of antithrombin, protein C, or protein S. Heparin administration can depress antithrombin levels. Use of warfarin ordinarily causes a mild deficiency of protein C or protein S. Both oral contraceptives and pregnancy depress protein S levels.

Relationship Between Deep Venous Thrombosis and Pulmonary Embolism

When venous thrombi detach from their sites of formation, they flow through the venous system toward the vena cava. They pass through the right atrium and right ventricle and then enter the pulmonary arterial circulation. An extremely large embolus may lodge at the bifurcation of the pulmonary artery, forming a saddle embolus (**Fig. 77-1**). More commonly, a major pulmonary vessel is occluded. Many patients with large PEs do not have ultrasonographic evidence of DVT, probably because the clot has already embolized to the lungs.

RIGHT VENTRICULAR DYSFUNCTION. The extent of pulmonary vascular obstruction and the presence of underlying cardiopulmonary disease are probably the most important factors determining whether right ventricular dysfunction ensues.[50] As obstruction increases, pulmonary artery pressure rises. Further increases in pulmonary vascular resistance and pulmonary hypertension are caused by secretion of vasoconstricting compounds such as serotonin, reflex pulmonary artery vasoconstriction, and hypoxemia.[51] The overloaded right ventricle[51] releases cardiac biomarkers such as pro–brain natriuretic peptide (pro-BNP), brain natriuretic peptide (BNP), and troponin, all of which predict an increased likelihood of an adverse clinical outcome.

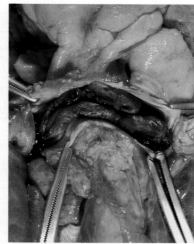

FIGURE 77-1 A 41-year-old woman with poorly controlled hypertension suffered an intracerebral hemorrhage, complicated 6 days later by acute pulmonary embolism. Emergency catheter embolectomy was unsuccessful, and she suffered cardiac arrest. At autopsy, a large saddle embolus extended from the root of the pulmonary artery into the left and right lungs.

VENTRICULAR INTERDEPENDENCY. The sudden rise in pulmonary artery pressure abruptly increases right ventricular afterload, with consequent elevation of right ventricular wall tension followed by right ventricular dilation and dysfunction (**Fig. 77-2**). As the right ventricle dilates, the interventricular septum shifts toward the left, with resultant underfilling and decreased left ventricular diastolic distensibility. With underfilling of the left ventricle, systemic cardiac output and systolic arterial pressure both decline, potentially impairing coronary perfusion and producing myocardial ischemia. Elevated right ventricular wall tension after massive PE[52] reduces right coronary artery flow, increases right ventricular myocardial oxygen demand, and causes ischemia. Perpetuation of this cycle can lead to right ventricular infarction, circulatory collapse, and death.[53]

Summary of Pathophysiology

PE can have the following pathophysiologic effects: increased pulmonary vascular resistance caused by vascular obstruction, neurohumoral agents, or pulmonary artery baroreceptors; impaired gas exchange caused by increased alveolar dead space from vascular obstruction and hypoxemia from alveolar hypoventilation, low ventilation-perfusion units, and right-to-left shunting as well as impaired carbon monoxide transfer caused by loss of gas exchange surface; alveolar hyperventilation caused by reflex stimulation of irritant receptors; increased airway resistance due to bronchoconstriction; and decreased pulmonary compliance due to lung edema, lung hemorrhage, and loss of surfactant.

Diagnosis

Diagnosis of PE is more difficult than treatment or prevention. Fortunately, noninvasive diagnostic approaches have become increasingly reliable and streamlined. The greatest challenge is to remember to consider the possible diagnosis of PE and to realize that it can masquerade as many other illnesses, such as asthma, pneumonia, and congestive heart failure. PE can occur concomitantly with other illnesses, thereby confounding the diagnostic workup. The most useful approach is the clinical assessment of likelihood, based on presenting symptoms and signs, in conjunction with judicious diagnostic testing. When PE is not highly suspected, a normal plasma D-dimer enzyme-linked immunosorbent assay (ELISA) usually suffices to rule out this condition. When PE is highly suspected, especially with an elevated D-dimer ELISA, chest CT scanning is the best imaging test. Another problem is that patients often delay seeking medical attention.[54] Among 1152 patients with confirmed DVT or PE at 70 North American

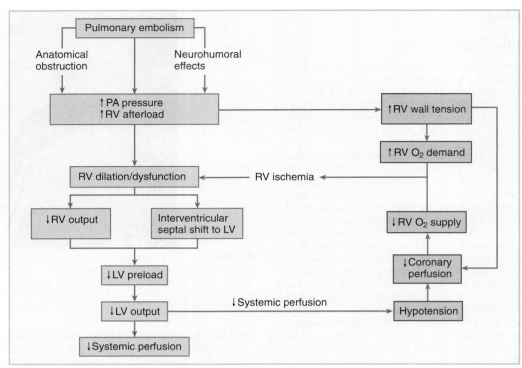

FIGURE 77-2 Pathophysiology of right ventricular dysfunction. LV = left ventricular; PA = pulmonary artery; RV = right ventricular.

TABLE 77-3	Most Common Symptoms and Signs of Pulmonary Embolism

Symptoms
Otherwise unexplained dyspnea
Chest pain, either pleuritic or "atypical"
Anxiety
Cough

Signs
Tachypnea
Tachycardia
Low-grade fever
Left parasternal lift
Tricuspid regurgitant murmur
Accentuated P_2
Hemoptysis
Leg edema, erythema, tenderness

medical centers, 21% of DVT patients and 17% of PE patients received diagnoses more than 1 week after symptom onset.

CLINICAL PRESENTATION. Symptoms and signs of PE are nonspecific. Hence, clinical suspicion of PE is of paramount importance in guiding diagnostic testing. Clinical gestalt and clinical experience are helpful, but the incremental gain in diagnostic accuracy is small when comparing attending physicians with interns.[55] Dyspnea is the most frequent symptom and tachypnea is the most frequent sign of PE (**Table 77-3**). In general, severe dyspnea, syncope, or cyanosis portends a major life-threatening PE, which is often devoid of chest pain. Paradoxically, severe pleuritic pain often signifies that the embolism is small and located in the distal pulmonary arterial system, near the pleural lining.

PE should be suspected in hypotensive patients when (1) there is evidence of venous thrombosis or predisposing factors for it and (2) there is clinical evidence of acute cor pulmonale (acute right ventricular failure), such as distended neck veins, right-sided S_3 gallop, right ventricular heave, tachycardia, or tachypnea, especially if (3) there are echocardiographic findings of right ventricular dilation and hypokinesis or electrocardiographic evidence of acute cor pulmonale

manifested by a new $S_1Q_3T_3$ pattern, new right bundle branch block, or right ventricular ischemia (**Fig. 77-3** and see Fig. 13-21).

A reliable set of clinical decision rules can stratify patients into high clinical likelihood or non–high clinical likelihood of PE with a set of seven bedside assessment questions (**Table 77-4**). This approach was validated in a large Dutch study in which almost half of the patients could be categorized as "PE unlikely." In this low-risk group, only about 5% of patients were subsequently diagnosed with PE.[56] But the problem with this scoring system, known as the Wells criteria, is that it appears at first glance to be time-consuming and, therefore, has not been adopted into everyday use. Simplified Wells criteria have been developed and validated[57] (**Table 77-5**).

DIFFERENTIAL DIAGNOSIS. The differential diagnosis of PE is broad and covers a wide spectrum from life-threatening disease such as acute myocardial infarction to innocuous anxiety states (**Table 77-6**). Some patients have concomitant PE and other illnesses. For example, if pneumonia or heart failure does not respond to appropriate therapy, the possibility of coexisting PE should be considered. Idiopathic pulmonary hypertension may present with sudden exacerbations that mimic acute PE.

Clinical Syndromes of Pulmonary Embolism

Classification of acute PE (**Table 77-7**) can assist with prognostication and clinical management. Massive PE occurs rarely in most hospitals. Submassive PE is more common, and small to moderate PE is most common.

MASSIVE PULMONARY EMBOLISM. Patients with massive PE are susceptible to cardiogenic shock and multisystem organ failure. Renal insufficiency, hepatic dysfunction, and altered mentation are common findings. Thrombosis is widespread, affecting at least half of the pulmonary arterial vasculature. Clot is typically present bilaterally. Dyspnea is usually the most noticeable symptom; chest pain is unusual, transient cyanosis is common, and systemic arterial hypotension requiring pressor support is frequent. Excessive fluid boluses may worsen right-sided heart failure and render therapy more difficult.

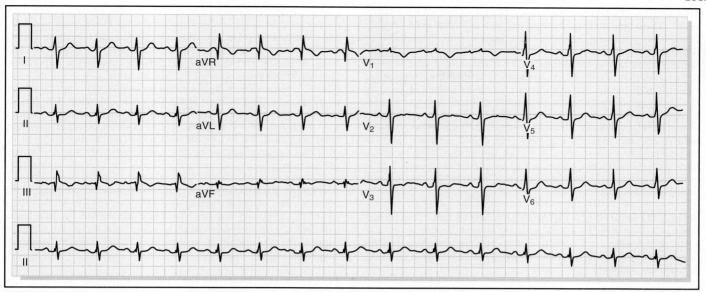

FIGURE 77-3 Electrocardiogram from a 33-year-old man who presented with a left main pulmonary artery embolism on chest CT scan. He was hemodynamically stable and had normal right ventricular function on echocardiography. His troponin and brain natriuretic peptide levels were normal. He was managed with anticoagulation alone. On the initial electrocardiogram, he has a heart rate of 90/min, $S_1Q_3T_3$, and incomplete right bundle branch block, with inverted or flattened T waves in leads V_1 through V_4.

TABLE 77-4	Classic Wells Criteria to Assess Clinical Likelihood of Pulmonary Embolism

>4 score points = high probability

≤4 score points = non–high probability

	SCORE POINTS
DVT symptoms or signs	3
An alternative diagnosis is less likely than PE	3
Heart rate >100/min	1.5
Immobilization or surgery within 4 weeks	1.5
Prior DVT or PE	1.5
Hemoptysis	1
Cancer treated within 6 months or metastatic	1

TABLE 77-5	Simplified Wells Criteria to Assess Clinical Likelihood of Pulmonary Embolism

>1 score point = high probability

≤1 score point = non–high probability

	SCORE POINTS
DVT symptoms or signs	1
An alternative diagnosis is less likely than PE	1
Heart rate >100/min	1
Immobilization or surgery within 4 weeks	1
Prior DVT or PE	1
Hemoptysis	1
Cancer treated within 6 months or metastatic	1

TABLE 77-6	Differential Diagnosis of Pulmonary Embolism

Anxiety, pleurisy, costochondritis
Pneumonia, bronchitis
Myocardial infarction
Pericarditis
Congestive heart failure
Idiopathic pulmonary hypertension

TABLE 77-7	Classification of Acute Pulmonary Embolism	
CLASSIFICATION	**PRESENTATION**	**THERAPY**
Massive PE	Systolic blood pressure <90 mm Hg or poor tissue perfusion or multisystem organ failure plus right or left main pulmonary artery thrombus or "high clot burden"	Thrombolysis or embolectomy or inferior vena caval filter plus anticoagulation
Submassive PE	Hemodynamically stable but moderate or severe right ventricular dysfunction or enlargement	Addition of thrombolysis, embolectomy, or filter remains controversial
Small to moderate PE	Normal hemodynamics and normal right ventricular size and function	Anticoagulation

MODERATE TO LARGE (SUBMASSIVE) PULMONARY EMBOLISM. These patients frequently present with moderate or severe right ventricular hypokinesis as well as elevations in troponin, pro-BNP, or BNP, but they maintain normal systemic arterial pressure. Usually, one third or more of the pulmonary artery vasculature is obstructed. If there is no prior history of cardiopulmonary disease, they may appear clinically well, but this initial impression is often misleading. They are at risk for recurrent PE, even with adequate anticoagulation. Most survive, but they may require escalation of therapy with pressor support or mechanical ventilation. Therefore, especially if moderate or severe right ventricular dysfunction persists, one should consider thrombolytic therapy or embolectomy. If neither thrombolysis nor embolectomy appears warranted, placement of an inferior vena caval filter is controversial but may be employed as a "back-up" in case heparin anticoagulation fails.

SMALL TO MODERATE PULMONARY EMBOLISM. This presentation is characterized by normal systemic arterial pressure, no cardiac biomarker release, and normal right ventricular function. Patients appear clinically stable. Adequate anticoagulation results in an excellent clinical outcome.

PULMONARY INFARCTION. This syndrome (**Table 77-8**) is characterized by pleuritic chest pain that may be unremitting or may wax and wane. The pleurisy is occasionally accompanied by hemoptysis. The embolus usually lodges in the peripheral pulmonary arterial tree, near the pleura. Tissue infarction usually occurs 3 to 7 days after embolism. The syndrome often includes fever, leukocytosis, elevated erythrocyte sedimentation rate, and radiologic evidence of infarction.

PARADOXICAL EMBOLISM. This syndrome may present with a sudden stroke. The cause is a small DVT that embolizes to the arterial system, usually through a patent foramen ovale. VTE is rarely detected in patients who suffer paradoxical embolism; the DVT is small and breaks away from a tiny leg vein completely, leaving no residual evidence of thrombosis that can be imaged on venous ultrasound examination. After a "cryptogenic stroke," echocardiography with bubble study may diagnose a patent foramen ovale. Contemporary management requires choosing between indefinite duration of anticoagulation and closure of the patent foramen ovale, usually percutaneously.

NONTHROMBOTIC PULMONARY EMBOLISM. Sources of embolism other than thrombus are uncommon. They include fat, tumor, air, and amniotic fluid. Fat embolism syndrome is most often observed after blunt trauma complicated by long bone fractures. Air embolus can occur during placement or removal of a central venous catheter. Amniotic fluid embolism may be catastrophic and is characterized by respiratory failure, cardiogenic shock, and disseminated intravascular coagulation. Intravenous drug abusers sometimes self-inject hair, talc, and cotton that contaminate the drug they have acquired. These patients also have susceptibility to septic PE, which can cause endocarditis of the tricuspid or pulmonic valves.

Nonimaging Diagnostic Methods

PLASMA D-DIMER ASSAY. This blood screening test relies on the principle that most patients with PE have ongoing endogenous fibrinolysis that is not effective enough to prevent PE but that does break down some of the fibrin clot to D-dimers. Although elevated plasma concentrations of D-dimers are sensitive for the presence of PE, they are not specific. Levels are elevated for at least 1 week postoperatively and are increased in patients with myocardial infarction, sepsis, cancer, or almost any other systemic illness. Therefore, the plasma D-dimer assay is ideally suited for outpatients or emergency department patients who have suspected PE but no coexisting acute systemic illness. This test is generally not useful for acutely ill hospitalized inpatients because their D-dimer levels are usually elevated. A normal D-dimer assay appears to be as diagnostically useful as a normal lung scan to exclude PE.[58] A randomized trial at seven Canadian university hospitals found that in patients with a low clinical probability of PE who had negative D-dimer results, additional diagnostic testing was not necessary.[59]

ARTERIAL BLOOD GASES. Arterial blood gases are not part of the contemporary diagnostic algorithm for PE. They used to be the principal blood screening test but have been supplanted by the plasma D-dimer assay. Noninvasive oximetry meters placed on the finger or earlobe are now usually used instead of blood gases to determine oxygen saturation.

ELECTROCARDIOGRAM. The electrocardiogram (ECG) helps exclude acute myocardial infarction and may raise suspicion or help confirm the diagnosis of PE among patients with electrocardiographic manifestations of right-sided heart strain (**Table 77-9**), which is an ominous prognostic finding.[60] Right-sided heart strain is not specific, however, and may be observed in patients with asthma or idiopathic pulmonary hypertension. Patients with massive PE may have sinus tachycardia, slight ST and T wave abnormalities, or even entirely normal ECGs. Other abnormalities include incomplete or complete right bundle branch block or an $S_1Q_3T_3$ complex (see Fig. 77-3). T wave inversion in leads V_1 to V_4 has the greatest accuracy for identification of right ventricular dysfunction in patients with acute PE.

Imaging Methods

CHEST RADIOGRAPHY. The chest radiograph is usually the first imaging study obtained in patients with suspected PE. A near-normal radiograph in the setting of severe respiratory compromise is highly suggestive of massive PE. Major chest radiographic abnormalities are uncommon. Focal oligemia (Westermark sign) indicates massive central embolic occlusion. A peripheral wedge-shaped density above the diaphragm (Hampton hump) usually indicates pulmonary infarction. Subtle abnormalities suggestive of PE include enlargement of the descending right pulmonary artery. The vessel often tapers rapidly after the enlarged portion. The chest radiograph can also help identify patients with diseases that can mimic PE, such as lobar pneumonia and pneumothorax, but patients with these illnesses can also have concomitant PE.

CHEST COMPUTED TOMOGRAPHY. Chest CT has supplanted pulmonary radionuclide perfusion scintigraphy as the initial imaging test in most patients with suspected PE (**Fig. 77-4**, Fig. 19-23C).[61] Lung scans have caused consternation because most are nondiagnostic. An unequivocal normal or high probability scan is the exception, not the rule. Lung scans depend on expert interpretation, and there is a great deal of interobserver variability even among experts. Therefore, the medical community has welcomed the advent of chest CT to provide definitive diagnosis or exclusion of PE. Only three indications to obtain

TABLE 77-8 Pulmonary Infarction Syndrome
Caused by a tiny peripheral pulmonary embolism
Pleuritic chest pain, often not responsive to narcotics
Low-grade fever
Pleural rub
Occasional scant hemoptysis
Leukocytosis

TABLE 77-9 Electrocardiographic Signs of Pulmonary Embolism
Sinus tachycardia
Incomplete or complete right bundle branch block
Right-axis deviation
T wave inversions in leads III and aVF or in leads V_1-V_4
S wave in lead I and a Q wave and T wave inversion in lead III ($S_1Q_3T_3$)
QRS axis greater than 90 degrees or an indeterminate axis
Atrial fibrillation or atrial flutter

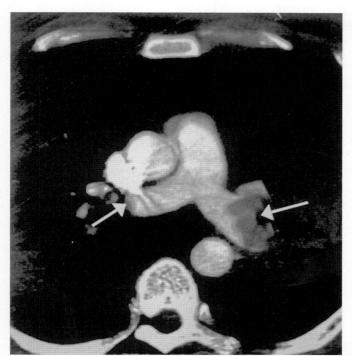

FIGURE 77-4 A 62-year-old physician suffered a massive pulmonary embolism 2 weeks after prostatectomy. Spiral chest CT with contrast enhancement provided a definitive diagnosis, with a large thrombus burden apparent in the right and left main pulmonary arteries (arrows).

TABLE 77-10	Chest Computed Tomography

When reviewing results, the clinician should *learn* the following:
The type of scanner used (single-slice versus multislice) and the resolution for visualizing thrombus
Whether the bolus of injected contrast material was technically adequate
Whether a CT protocol specific for PE was used, versus an aortic dissection protocol or a cancer staging protocol
Whether the images extend to the pelvic and deep leg veins

When reviewing results, the clinician should *look for* the following:
Size, location, and extent of thrombus
Other diagnoses that may coexist with PE or explain PE symptoms:
   Pneumonia
   Atelectasis
   Pericardial effusion
   Pneumothorax
   Left ventricular enlargement
Pulmonary artery enlargement, suggestive of pulmonary hypertension
Age of thrombus: acute, subacute, chronic
Location of thrombus: pulmonary arteries, pelvic veins, deep leg veins, upper extremity veins
Right ventricular enlargement
Contour of the interventricular septum: whether it bulges toward the left ventricle, thus indicating right ventricular pressure overload
Incidental masses or nodules in lung

TABLE 77-11	Echocardiographic Signs of Pulmonary Embolism

Right ventricular enlargement or hypokinesis, especially free wall hypokinesis, with sparing of the apex (the McConnell sign)
Interventricular septal flattening and paradoxical motion toward the left ventricle, resulting in a D-shaped left ventricle in cross section
Tricuspid regurgitation
Pulmonary hypertension with a tricuspid regurgitant jet velocity >2.6 m/sec
Loss of respiratory-phasic collapse of the inferior vena cava with inspiration
Dilated inferior vena cava without physiologic inspiratory collapse
Direct visualization of thrombus (more likely with transesophageal echocardiography)

a lung scan exist: (1) renal insufficiency, (2) anaphylaxis to intravenous contrast agent that cannot be suppressed with high-dose corticosteroids, and (3) pregnancy (lower radiation exposure to the fetus).

CT scanners are technologic marvels for patients with suspected PE.[62] Multiple generations of CT scanners exist. Even first-generation "single-slice" machines provide images that are clear, rapidly acquired, and accurate in delineating the proximal pulmonary arterial tree. Massive PE can easily be visualized and can confirm surgical or catheter accessibility to the centrally located thrombus. Multidetector-row CT scanners can rapidly image the entire chest with submillimeter resolution. The latest generation of scanners can image thrombus in sixth-order vessels. These thrombi are so tiny that their clinical significance is uncertain.

A meta-analysis of chest CT for suspected PE comprised 3500 patients. All patients were followed for at least 3 months. The overall negative predictive value of a chest CT scan was 99.4%.[63] A validated outcome strategy is D-dimer testing followed by multidetector-row chest CT for patients with abnormally elevated D-dimer levels. With use of this strategy, only 1.5% of patients in whom PE was ruled out developed DVT or PE during 3-month follow-up.[64] For patients with PE, the CT scan serves as a prognostic and diagnostic test. Right ventricular enlargement on CT portends a complicated hospital course. Thus, the CT scan can serve as a "one-stop shop" for diagnosis, detection of source of thrombus, and prognosis. The chest CT scan can also detect other pulmonary diseases that are present in conjunction with PE or that explain a clinical presentation that mimics PE. These include pneumonia, atelectasis, pneumothorax, and pleural effusion that might not be well visualized on the chest radiograph. At times, the chest CT scan detects an incidental but critical finding, such as a small lung carcinoma.

When ordering a CT scan, it is of paramount importance to know what generation of scanners is available (**Table 77-10**). Routine use of CT leg venography increases radiation exposure and rarely changes clinical management.[65] The CT scan reports should always comment on the size of the right ventricle compared with the left ventricle. Three-dimensional images can be reconstructed, and color can be added electronically to enhance details of thrombus localization.[66] Clinical outcome studies differ from studies testing the accuracy of a particular diagnostic modality. The Prospective Investigation of Pulmonary Embolism Diagnosis II (PIOPED II) trial found that the accuracy of CT plummeted on the rare occasions when the imaging results and clinical probability assessment were discordant.[67]

ECHOCARDIOGRAPHY. Echocardiography (**Table 77-11**) is normal in about half of unselected patients with acute PE. Therefore, echocardiography is not recommended as a routine diagnostic test for PE. However, it is a rapid, practical, and sensitive technique for detection of right ventricular overload among patients with established and large PE. Moderate or severe right ventricular hypokinesis, persistent pulmonary hypertension, patent foramen ovale, and free-floating thrombus in the right atrium or right ventricle help identify patients at high risk of death or recurrent thromboembolism. Echocardiography can also help identify illnesses that may mimic PE, such as myocardial infarction and pericardial disease. For those patients in whom transthoracic imaging is unsatisfactory, transesophageal echocardiography can be carried out.

VENOUS ULTRASONOGRAPHY. The primary diagnostic criterion for DVT is loss of vein compressibility. Normally, the vein collapses completely when gentle pressure is applied to the skin overlying it. Upper extremity DVT can be more difficult to diagnose than leg DVT because the clavicle can hinder attempts to compress the subclavian vein. When PE is suspected, venous ultrasonography is useful if it demonstrates DVT, because DVT can be considered a surrogate for PE. But at least half of patients with PE have no imaging evidence of DVT. *Therefore, if clinical suspicion of PE is moderate or high, patients without evidence of DVT should undergo further investigation for PE.*

LUNG SCANNING. Pulmonary radionuclide perfusion scintigraphy (lung scanning) uses radiolabeled aggregates of albumin or microspheres that lodge in the pulmonary microvasculature. Patients with large PE often have multiple perfusion defects. If ventilation scanning is performed on a patient with PE but no intrinsic lung disease, a normal

CH
77

ventilation study is expected, yielding a ventilation-perfusion mismatch and a lung scan interpreted as high probability for PE. However, many patients with low-probability scans but high clinical suspicion for PE do, in fact, have PE proven by invasive pulmonary angiography. Therefore, the term *low-probability scan* is a potentially lethal misnomer.

MAGNETIC RESONANCE IMAGING. Gadolinium-enhanced magnetic resonance angiography (MRA) is far less sensitive than CT for the detection of PE. However, unlike chest CT or catheter-based pulmonary angiography, MRA does not require ionizing radiation or injection of iodinated contrast agent. In addition, magnetic resonance pulmonary angiography can assess right ventricular size and function. Three-dimensional MRA can be carried out during a single breath-hold and may provide high resolution from the main pulmonary artery through the segmental pulmonary artery branches.[68]

PULMONARY ANGIOGRAPHY. Invasive pulmonary angiography was formerly the reference standard for diagnosis of PE, but it is now rarely performed. It is an uncomfortable and potentially risky procedure. However, pulmonary angiography is required when interventions are planned, such as suction catheter embolectomy, mechanical clot fragmentation, or catheter-directed thrombolysis. In cases of chronic thromboembolic PE, pulmonary arteries appear pouched. The thrombus usually organizes with a concave edge. Bandlike defects called webs may be present, in addition to intimal irregularities and abrupt narrowing or occlusion of lobar vessels.

CONTRAST VENOGRAPHY. Although contrast phlebography was once the reference standard for DVT diagnosis, venograms are now rarely obtained. Venography is costly, invasive, and potentially harmful. It can cause contrast-induced renal failure, anaphylaxis, or chemical phlebitis. Furthermore, difficulty in interpretation of contrast venograms causes considerable disagreement among experienced readers. Invasive contrast phlebography is required, of course, for interventional procedures such as catheter-directed thrombolysis, suction embolectomy, angioplasty, stenting, and placement of an inferior vena caval filter. In patients undergoing total hip or knee replacement, contrast venography is more sensitive than venous ultrasonography for the diagnosis of acute DVT. In one large study of orthopedic surgery patients, sensitivity of venous ultrasound compared with contrast venography was about 30%.[69]

Overall Strategy: An Integrated Diagnostic Approach

A wide array of diagnostic tests is available for the investigation of suspected PE (**Table 77-12**). Familiarity with each test's strengths and weaknesses will enable a concise and streamlined workup. The key to success is to consider PE a possible diagnosis in assessing symptoms, signs, and associated clinical circumstances and comorbidities (**Fig. 77-5**). The first step in an integrated diagnostic strategy is a directed history and physical examination to assess the clinical likelihood of acute PE. An assessment of non–high clinical probability is followed by D-dimer testing. A normal D-dimer assay usually concludes the workup for PE. If the D-dimer is elevated, chest CT usually provides the definitive diagnosis or exclusion of PE. If the CT scan is normal, there is no need to obtain venous ultrasonography of the leg to exclude the diagnosis of PE.[70] For patients in whom the clinical likelihood of PE is high, skip the D-dimer testing and proceed directly to chest CT scanning. For the rare equivocal CT result, venous ultrasonography of the legs may help. Diagnostic pulmonary angiography may be useful if PE is strongly suspected and both the chest CT and the venous ultrasound study of the legs are normal.

Management

Risk Stratification

PE presents with a wide spectrum of illness ranging from mild to severe. Therefore, rapid and accurate risk stratification is of paramount importance. Appropriate care can range from prevention of recurrent PE with anticoagulation alone in low-risk patients to thrombolysis or embolectomy in high-risk patients. High-risk patients may require intensive hemodynamic and respiratory support with pressors or mechanical ventilation while the PE itself is managed with aggressive medical, percutaneous interventional, or surgical therapy (**Fig. 77-6**). The three key components for risk stratification are (1) clinical

TABLE 77-12	Diagnostic Tests for Suspected Pulmonary Embolism
TEST	**COMMENTS**
Oxygen saturation	Nonspecific, but suspect PE if there is a sudden, otherwise unexplained decrement
D-dimer	An excellent "rule-out" test if normal, especially if accompanied by non–high clinical probability
Electrocardiography	May suggest an alternative diagnosis, such as myocardial infarction or pericarditis
Lung scanning	Usually provides ambiguous result; used in lieu of chest CT for patients with anaphylaxis to contrast agent, renal insufficiency, or pregnancy
Chest CT	The most accurate diagnostic imaging test for PE (see Table 77-10); beware if CT result and clinical likelihood probability are discordant
Pulmonary angiography	Invasive, costly, uncomfortable; used primarily when local catheter intervention is planned
Echocardiography	Best used as a prognostic test in patients with established PE rather than as a diagnostic test (see Table 77-11); many patients with large PE will have normal echocardiograms
Venous ultrasonography	Excellent for diagnosis of acute symptomatic proximal DVT; a normal study does not rule out PE because a recent leg DVT may have embolized completely; calf vein imaging is operator dependent
Magnetic resonance	Reliable only for imaging of proximal segmental pulmonary arteries; requires gadolinium but does not require iodinated contrast agent

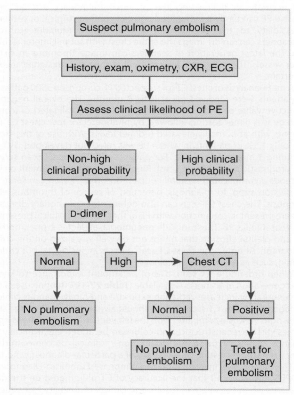

FIGURE 77-5 Integrated diagnostic approach. CXR = Chest x-ray.

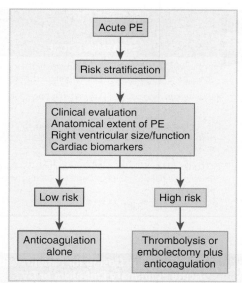

FIGURE 77-6 Management strategy for acute PE, based on risk stratification.

TABLE 77-13	The Pulmonary Embolism Severity Index: Predictors of Low Prognostic Risk
PREDICTOR	**SCORE POINTS**
Age, per year	Age, in years
Male sex	10
History of cancer	30
History of heart failure	10
History of chronic lung disease	10
Pulse ≥110/min	20
Systolic blood pressure <100 mm Hg	30
Respiratory rate ≥30/min	20
Temperature <36°C	20
Altered mental status	60
Arterial oxygen saturation <90%	20

Low prognostic risk is defined as ≤85 points.

evaluation, (2) assessment of right ventricular size and function, and (3) analysis of cardiac biomarkers such as troponin, pro-BNP, and BNP (even though troponin-based risk stratification has been challenged).[71]

Clinical evaluation is straightforward if the patient looks and feels well and has no evidence of right ventricular dysfunction. The Pulmonary Embolism Severity Index has identified 11 features from demographics, history, and clinical findings that can be weighted and scored to predict good prognosis and to identify low-risk patients[72] (**Table 77-13**). The practitioner can detect right ventricular dysfunction on physical examination by seeking distended jugular veins, a systolic murmur of tricuspid regurgitation, or an accentuated P₂. Obese necks may make jugular vein assessment difficult. Noisy emergency departments can obscure the subtle auscultatory findings of right ventricular dysfunction. Clinical assessment should be supplemented by electrocardiography to look for a right ventricular strain pattern (right bundle branch block, $S_1Q_3T_3$, negative T waves in V_1 through V_4),[60] echocardiography,[73] or chest CT[74] for evidence of right ventricular enlargement, which predicts increased 30-day mortality, and elevated cardiac biomarkers, which indicate right ventricular microinfarction or right ventricular pressure overload and a potentially

TABLE 77-14	Predictors of Increased Mortality

Hemodynamic instability
Right ventricular hypokinesis on echocardiogram
Right ventricular enlargement on echocardiogram or chest CT scan
Right ventricular strain on electrocardiogram
Elevated cardiac biomarkers

TABLE 77-15	Intravenous Unfractionated Heparin "Raschke Nomogram"	
VARIABLE	**ACTION**	
Initial heparin bolus	80 units/kg bolus, then 18 units/kg/hr	
aPTT <35 seconds (<1.2 times control)	80 units/kg bolus, then increase by 4 units/kg/hr	
aPTT 35 to 45 seconds (1.2 to 1.5 times control)	40 units/kg bolus, then increase by 2 units/kg/hr	
aPTT 46 to 70 seconds (1.5 to 2.3 times control)	No change	
aPTT 71 to 90 seconds (2.3 to 3 times control)	Decrease infusion rate by 2 units/kg/hr	
aPTT >90 seconds (>3 times control)	Hold infusion 1 hr, then decrease infusion rate by 3 units/kg/hr	

From Raschke RA, Reilly BM, Guidry JR, et al: The weight-based heparin dosing nomogram compared with a "standard care" nomogram: A randomized controlled trial. Ann Intern Med 119:874, 1993.

ominous prognosis[75] (**Table 77-14**). The combination of right ventricular hypokinesis and elevated cardiac biomarkers identifies the highest-risk group of PE patients.[76]

Certain hospital, patient, and socioeconomic factors portend high risk and poor outcome. Patients with PE admitted on weekends have a higher short-term mortality than those admitted on weekdays.[77] Those with a very short length of stay had a greater postdischarge mortality compared with those with a typical length of stay.[78] In a study of 14,426 PE patients discharged from 186 hospitals in Pennsylvania, early readmission after PE occurred in 14% and was associated with black race, Medicaid insurance, and high baseline PE Severity Index (see Table 77-13).[79]

Anticoagulation (see Chap. 87)

UNFRACTIONATED HEPARIN. Heparin is the cornerstone for treatment of acute PE. For patients with average bleeding risk, begin with an intravenous UFH bolus of 80 units/kg, followed by a continuous infusion at 18 units/kg per hour. Target the aPTT between 1.5 and 2.5 times the control value.[80] Commonly, the therapeutic range is 60 to 80 seconds. A nomogram may be helpful for heparin dose adjustment (**Table 77-15**). Although there is a trend toward the use of LMWH for patients who present with acute PE, the shorter half-life of UFH is advantageous for patients who might require insertion of an inferior vena caval filter, thrombolysis, or embolectomy. In patients with active major bleeding, withhold heparin and consider nonpharmacologic treatment with insertion of an inferior vena caval filter. Alternative UFH dosing regimens, used rarely, employ fixed-dose weight-adjusted subcutaneous UFH[81] or adjusted-dose subcutaneous UFH.[82]

UFH is a highly sulfated glycosaminoglycan that is partially purified, most often from porcine intestinal mucosa. Heparin acts primarily by binding to antithrombin, a protein that inhibits the coagulation factors thrombin (factor IIa), Xa, IXa, XIa, and XIIa. Heparin subsequently promotes a conformational change in antithrombin that accelerates its activity approximately 100- to 1000-fold. This prevents additional thrombus formation and permits endogenous fibrinolytic mechanisms

TABLE 77-16 Low-Molecular-Weight Heparins

NAME	STATUS	MOLECULAR WEIGHT	ANTI-Xa/ANTI-IIa RATIO	TREATMENT DOSE
Enoxaparin	FDA approved for DVT treatment	4800	3.9	1 mg/kg twice daily (approved as an inpatient or outpatient dose), or 1.5 mg/kg once daily (inpatient dose only)
Dalteparin	FDA approved for cancer-associated DVT	5000	2.2	100 units/kg twice daily, or 200 units/kg once daily
Nadroparin	Not available in the United States	4500	3.5	4100 units twice daily for patients weighing <50 kg, 6150 units twice daily for 50-70 kg, and 9200 units twice daily for >70 kg
Reviparin	Not available in the United States	3900	3.3	3500 units twice daily for patients weighing 35-45 kg, 4200 units twice daily for 46-60 kg, and 6300 units twice daily for >60 kg
Tinzaparin	FDA approved for DVT treatment	4500	1.5	175 units/kg once daily

to lyse clot that has already formed. Heparin does *not* directly dissolve thrombus that already exists. The world's heparin supplies were temporarily contaminated by oversulfated chondroitin sulfate, which caused severe anaphylactoid reactions in some patients.[83,84] Contamination ended after closer factory inspection and additional analytic testing were instituted.

LOW-MOLECULAR-WEIGHT HEPARIN. LMWH consists of fragments of UFH that exhibit less binding than UFH to plasma proteins and endothelial cells. Therefore, LMWH has greater bioavailability, a more predictable dose response, and a longer half-life than UFH. These features permit weight-based LMWH dosing without laboratory tests for dose adjustment in most instances. Consequently, LMWHs have revolutionized the management of DVT and converted the treatment from a mandatory minimum 5-day hospitalization to either an overnight stay or outpatient therapy for most patients (**Table 77-16**). Whereas this approach has been shown to be feasible, safe, and cost-effective in DVT treatment, further data are needed before the strategy of shortened hospital stay can be endorsed for the management of PE.[85]

In 2007, the Food and Drug Administration (FDA) approved the LMWH dalteparin as monotherapy without warfarin in cancer patients with acute VTE. In a trial of 672 patients with VTE and cancer, those randomized to dalteparin monotherapy had a much lower VTE recurrence rate than did patients receiving dalteparin as a "bridge" to warfarin: 8.8% versus 17.4%.[86] At times, LMWH is used off label as monotherapy without warfarin to treat VTE patients without cancer who cannot tolerate warfarin or who suffer recurrent VTE despite warfarin.[87]

LMWH is usually dosed according to weight. However, if a quantitative assay is desired, an anti-Xa level can be obtained. Whether use of anti-Xa levels improves efficacy and safety remains controversial. The plasma anti-Xa level may be useful in five situations: (1) UFH anticoagulation with baseline elevated aPTT caused by a lupus anticoagulant or anticardiolipin antibodies, (2) LMWH dosing in obese patients, (3) LMWH dosing in patients with renal dysfunction, (4) pregnancy, and (5) determination of the origin of an unexpected bleeding or clotting problem in patients receiving what appeared to be appropriate anticoagulant dosing.

FONDAPARINUX. Fondaparinux is an anticoagulant pentasaccharide that specifically inhibits activated factor X. By selectively binding to antithrombin, fondaparinux potentiates (about 300 times) the neutralization of factor Xa by antithrombin. Its predictable and sustained pharmacokinetic properties allow a fixed-dose, once-daily subcutaneous injection, without the need for coagulation laboratory monitoring or dose adjustment. Fondaparinux does not cross-react with heparin-induced antibodies. The FDA has approved fondaparinux for initial treatment of acute PE and acute DVT as a bridge to oral anticoagulation with warfarin.[88] The subcutaneous dosing regimen to treat VTE is straightforward (**Table 77-17**). Fondaparinux is often used off label for the management of suspected or proven heparin-induced thrombocytopenia[89] (see later). At times, fondaparinux is used off label as monotherapy without warfarin to treat VTE patients without cancer who cannot tolerate warfarin or who suffer recurrent VTE despite warfarin.[90] The dose for VTE prophylaxis is a fixed low dose of 2.5 mg once daily, regardless of body weight. However, fondaparinux elimination is prolonged in patients with renal impairment.

TABLE 77-17 Fondaparinux Dosing for Patients with Acute Pulmonary Embolism or DVT

Patient weight	<50 kg	50-100 kg	>100 kg
Daily dose of fondaparinux*	5 mg	7.5 mg	10 mg

*Assumes normal renal function.

HEPARIN-INDUCED THROMBOCYTOPENIA. Heparin-induced thrombocytopenia is a serious,[91] costly,[92] and perhaps increasingly frequent immune-mediated complication.[93] It occurs about 10 times more often with UFH than with LMWH. Immunoglobulin G antibodies bind to a heparin–platelet factor 4 complex and activate platelets, causing release of prothrombotic microparticles, platelet consumption, and thrombocytopenia. The microparticles promote excessive thrombin generation, which can result in paradoxical thrombosis. The thrombosis is usually extensive DVT or PE but can be manifested as myocardial infarction, stroke, or unusual arterial thrombosis such as mesenteric arterial thrombosis. Suspect heparin-induced thrombocytopenia when the platelet count decreases to less than 100,000 or to less than 50% of baseline. Typically, heparin-induced thrombocytopenia occurs after 5 to 10 days of heparin exposure. UFH or LMWH should be immediately discontinued, and platelets should not be transfused. A direct thrombin inhibitor[94] such as argatroban, bivalirudin, or lepirudin should be used.

WARFARIN. Warfarin is a vitamin K antagonist that prevents gamma-carboxylation activation of coagulation factors II, VII, IX, and X. The full anticoagulant effect of warfarin may not be apparent for 5 to 7 days, even if the prothrombin time, used to monitor warfarin's effect, becomes elevated more rapidly. Elevation in the prothrombin time, used to adjust the dose of warfarin, may initially reflect depletion of coagulation factor VII, which has a short half-life of about 6 hours, whereas factor II has a long half-life of about 5 days. The prothrombin time should be standardized and reported according to the international normalized ratio (INR), not the prothrombin time ratio or the prothrombin time expressed in seconds. For VTE patients, the usual target INR range is between 2.0 and 3.0.

WARFARIN OVERLAP WITH HEPARIN. Initiation of warfarin as monotherapy to treat acute VTE without UFH, LMWH, or fondaparinux may paradoxically exacerbate hypercoagulability, increasing the likelihood of recurrent thrombosis. Warfarin monotherapy decreases the levels of two endogenous anticoagulants, proteins C and S, thus increasing thrombogenic potential. Overlapping warfarin for at least 5 days with an immediately effective parenteral anticoagulant counteracts the procoagulant effect of unopposed warfarin.

DOSING AND MONITORING OF WARFARIN. Dosing of warfarin is both an art and a science. Warfarin is traditionally dosed by an "educated guess" coupled with trial and error. Controversy exists over the optimal initial warfarin dose, and whether it should be 5 mg or 10 mg. One open-label, randomized trial compared two warfarin initiation nomograms (5 mg versus 10 mg) in 50 patients with acute VTE.[95] The median time to two consecutive target INRs was 5 days in both groups ($P = 0.69$), whether the initial dose was 5 mg or 10 mg. Nevertheless, most practitioners begin with warfarin 5 mg daily. A new and promising approach is to use computer-assisted warfarin dosing,[96] which appears to be at least as accurate and cost-effective as conventional dosing.[97]

Some patients have unexplained variability in their INR response to warfarin. Large body stores of phylloquinone allow steady clotting factor activation and stable control of anticoagulation. Therefore, although it seems paradoxical and counterintuitive, administration of vitamin K supplementation can improve anticoagulation control in patients with unexplained instability of response to warfarin.[98]

Monitoring of warfarin requires walking a tightrope. High INRs predispose to bleeding complications,[99] but subtherapeutic dosing makes patients vulnerable to recurrent VTE. An overview of more than 22,000 warfarin-treated patients found that their time within the therapeutic INR range was only about 50%.[100] All patients taking warfarin should wear a medical alert bracelet or necklace. This allows emergency medical personnel to reverse warfarin quickly if major trauma causes catastrophic bleeding.

Warfarin is plagued by multiple drug-drug and drug-food interactions. Most antibiotics increase the INR, but some, like rifampin, lower the INR. Even benign-sounding drugs such as acetaminophen increase the INR in a dose-dependent manner. The warfarin dose should be reduced in the management of debilitated or elderly patients. On the other hand, green leafy vegetables have vitamin K and lower the INR. Concomitant medications with antiplatelet effects may increase the bleeding risk without increasing the INR. These include fish oil supplements, vitamin E, and alcohol.

Centralized anticoagulation clinics, staffed by nurses or pharmacists, have eased the administrative burden of prescribing warfarin and have facilitated safer and more effective anticoagulation. In a report encompassing 50,208 patients from 67 studies, patients managed by anticoagulation clinics or clinical trials remained in the therapeutic INR range 66% of the time. However, patients managed by community practices were therapeutic for only 57% of the study period.[101] "Point-of-care" devices provide the INR result within 2 minutes by use of a drop of whole blood obtained from a fingertip puncture. Appropriately selected patients can be taught to obtain their own INRs and to self-manage their warfarin dosing at home. In a meta-analysis of self-monitoring and self-adjustment of oral anticoagulation among 3049 patients in 14 trials, self-monitoring of INR was associated with a 55% reduction in thromboembolic events and a 39% reduction in all-cause mortality compared with conventional management. Those patients capable of both self-monitoring and self-adjustment of therapy had fewer thromboembolic events (73% less) and 63% lower mortality compared with those who undertook self-monitoring alone compared with, conventional management.[102]

WARFARIN PHARMACOGENOMICS. (See Chap. 10.) Genetic determinants of warfarin dose response include CYP2C9 variant alleles, which impair the hydroxylation of S-warfarin, resulting in extremely low warfarin dose requirements, and variants in the gene encoding vitamin K epoxide reductase complex 1 (VKORC1). Variability in the INR response to warfarin appears more strongly associated with VKORC1 than with CYP2C9.[103] A multiple regression model using the predictors of CYP2C9, VKORC1, age, sex, and drug interactions explains about half of the variance in warfarin dose.[104] Use of a pharmacogenetic algorithm for initiation of warfarin dosing appears to be of greatest benefit among those patients requiring very high or very low doses of warfarin.[5] This approach may be cost-effective when warfarin is initiated in patients at high risk for hemorrhage.[105] The largest randomized trial to date studied 206 patients who received either pharmacogenetic-guided or standard warfarin dosing. The primary endpoint, reduction in out-of-range INRs, was not achieved in the group undergoing rapid turnaround genetic testing.[106] The National Heart, Lung and Blood Institute (NHLBI) is sponsoring a larger trial (NCT00839657) with more than 1200 patients who will be randomized to a genotype-guided versus clinical-guided warfarin dosing algorithm. The primary endpoint is the percentage of time that participants spend within the therapeutic INR range. Results should be available in 2012.

COMPLICATIONS OF ANTICOAGULATION. The most important adverse effect of anticoagulation is hemorrhage. Major bleeding

during anticoagulation may unmask a previously silent lesion, such as bladder or colon cancer. Resumption of anticoagulation at a lower dose or implementation of alternative therapy depends on the severity of the bleeding, the risk of recurrent thromboembolism, and the extent to which bleeding may have resulted from excessive anticoagulation. For management of bleeding caused by heparin, cessation of UFH or LMWH will usually suffice. However, the anticoagulation effect will persist longer with LMWH than with UFH. With life-threatening or intracranial hemorrhage, protamine sulfate can be administered at the time heparin is discontinued. With warfarin, the risk of bleeding increases as the INR increases. The dose of warfarin should be adjusted downward when an "intranormal rise" in the INR occurs, such as an increase from 2.2 to 2.8 in patients whose target INR range is 2 to 3. Ironically, for patients who develop warfarin-associated intracerebral hemorrhage, the INR is often less than 3 at the time of diagnosis.[107] Be aware that an INR specimen that is not assayed promptly after blood collection can be spuriously high. In addition, point-of-care machines generally have higher INRs than central laboratories when the INR value exceeds 4. These abnormally high INR results should be verified with standard central laboratory instrumentation.[108] Life-threatening bleeding caused by warfarin can be managed with enough cryoprecipitate or fresh frozen plasma to normalize the INR and to achieve immediate hemostasis. Recombinant human factor VIIa concentrate can also be used to achieve rapid warfarin reversal.

NOVEL ANTICOAGULANTS. Novel oral anticoagulants[6] promise immediate onset of action and administration in fixed doses without routine laboratory coagulation monitoring. They will compete against warfarin, the only oral anticoagulant licensed in the United States since 1954. These drugs have few drug-drug or drug-food interactions, making them more "user friendly" than warfarin for patients and for health care providers. The onset of action of these new drugs is rapid, and the half-life is short. Therefore, when they must be stopped for a diagnostic or surgical procedure, no "bridging" is needed with a parenteral anticoagulant. Dabigatran is a direct thrombin inhibitor. It has proven noninferior to enoxaparin in three major orthopedic surgery trials of total knee or hip arthroplasty.[9,109] In a large-scale trial of acute VTE, dabigatran was noninferior to warfarin. Rivaroxaban is a factor Xa inhibitor with 80% bioavailability and a 5- to 9-hour half-life. Its efficacy has proven superior to enoxaparin to prevent VTE after total knee[8] and hip[7] arthroplasty. Both dabigatran and rivaroxaban are approved in Canada and Europe for VTE prevention after knee or hip arthroplasty.

OPTIMAL DURATION OF ANTICOAGULATION.

Provoked VTE (Including Cancer)

Management is more straightforward and less controversial for provoked rather than unprovoked VTE (**Table 77-18**). For patients with first-time PE or proximal leg DVT provoked by surgery, trauma, oral contraceptives, pregnancy, or hormone replacement, the optimal

TABLE 77-18	Optimal Duration of Anticoagulation
CLINICAL SETTING	RECOMMENDATION
First provoked PE/proximal leg DVT	3 to 6 months
First provoked upper extremity DVT or isolated calf DVT	3 months
Second provoked VTE	Uncertain
Third VTE	Indefinite duration
Cancer and VTE	Consider indefinite duration or until cancer is resolved
Unprovoked PE/proximal leg DVT	Consider indefinite duration
First unprovoked calf DVT	3 months
Second unprovoked calf DVT	Uncertain

duration of anticoagulation is 3 to 6 months, with a target INR between 2.0 and 3.0. For patients with a first-time isolated calf or upper extremity DVT, with any of the same provoking factors, the optimal duration of anticoagulation is 3 months, with a target INR between 2.0 and 3.0. For a second VTE with the same provoking factors, many clinicians double the duration of anticoagulation, and a few favor indefinite-duration anticoagulation. For a third VTE, a broad and strong consensus supports lifelong anticoagulation.

For patients with cancer and a first episode of DVT, there is now a consensus from the American College of Chest Physicians,[110] the National Comprehensive Cancer Network,[111] and the American Society of Clinical Oncology[112] to manage the first 3 to 6 months of treatment with LMWH as monotherapy without warfarin. Consider continuation of anticoagulation indefinitely or until the cancer has resolved. There is uncertainty as to whether subsequent anticoagulation should be continued with LMWH as monotherapy or whether cancer patients should be switched to warfarin.

Unprovoked VTE

No area of VTE management is more hotly debated than the optimal duration of anticoagulation for idiopathic and unprovoked VTE, which accounts for about half of all PE and DVT cases. Unprovoked VTE includes patients who develop VTE during long-haul air travel or "out of the blue." Recurrent VTE develops more often after discontinuation of anticoagulant therapy among patients with unprovoked events than among those who had provoked VTE. The emerging concept is that VTE is a chronic illness, with latent periods between flares of acute PE or DVT. Those who favor a population-based approach anticoagulate unprovoked VTE patients indefinitely, whereas those who favor a personalized approach consider each patient's clinical profile—including age, sex, comorbid conditions, and thrombophilia workup—to devise an individualized plan for the duration of anticoagulation.[113] Debate also surrounds the intensity of anticoagulation after the first 6 months of therapy. Whereas many continue to use standard-intensity warfarin, with a target INR range between 2.0 and 3.0, a low-intensity anticoagulant regimen with a target INR range between 1.5 and 2.0 is effective and safe.[114]

Recurrent VTE has a high fatality rate, especially when it occurs despite ongoing anticoagulation within the first week of diagnosis.[115] Even after completion of a 6-month course of anticoagulation, the case fatality rate for recurrent PE remains high.[116] Risk factors for recurrent VTE can be subdivided into variables that increase the likelihood of recurrence either while anticoagulants are being taken or after anticoagulants are discontinued (**Table 77-19**). Persistent right ventricular dysfunction on echocardiography after acute PE is an independent risk factor for recurrent VTE.[117] However, it is surprising and counterintuitive that most thrombophilias do not appear to increase the risk of recurrent VTE.[118] Risk factors for recurrent VTE after anticoagulants are discontinued include male sex,[119,120] overweight,[121] initial presentation with symptomatic PE rather than symptomatic DVT,[122] low levels of HDL-cholesterol,[123] and residual DVT with failure to recanalize the deep veins on subsequent venous ultrasonography.[124] Persistent thrombus imaged on chest CT does not predict recurrent PE.

TABLE 77-19	Risk Factors for Recurrent Venous Thromboembolism

While anticoagulants are being taken
Increasing age
Immobilization
Cancer
Chronic obstructive pulmonary disease
Right ventricular enlargement or right ventricular dyskinesis

After anticoagulants are discontinued
Male sex
Overweight
Presenting symptoms of PE rather than DVT
Low levels of HDL-cholesterol
Lack of leg vein recanalization on venous ultrasound examination

About half of PE patients have persistent imaging defects on chest CT 6 months after the initial event.[125]

Persistent abnormally elevated D-dimer levels after withdrawal of anticoagulation may reflect an ongoing hypercoagulable state. In the placebo group of the PREVENT trial, patients with unprovoked VTE received only 6 months of anticoagulation. D-dimer was measured 7 weeks after discontinuation of warfarin.[126] The subsequent recurrence rate was twice as high in those with elevated D-dimer levels. Thus, D-dimer might be useful to identify patients at particularly high risk of recurrence if warfarin is withdrawn after an initial 6 months of anticoagulation. However, an overview of 1888 patients who had unprovoked VTE showed that they had a high 3.5% annual risk of recurrence despite normal D-dimer levels after stopping of anticoagulation.[127] In a separate meta-analysis of patients with idiopathic VTE, those with normal D-dimer levels measured 1 month after discontinuation of oral anticoagulation had a clinically important 7.2% recurrence rate.[128] No guideline committee has endorsed the use of D-dimer levels to direct the optimal duration of anticoagulation.

INFERIOR VENA CAVAL FILTERS. The two major indications for placement of an inferior vena caval filter are major hemorrhage that precludes anticoagulation, and recurrent PE despite well-documented anticoagulation. Eight-year follow-up of a randomized controlled trial of filters shows that filters reduce the risk of PE, increase the risk of DVT, and have no long-term impact on survival.[129] Nevertheless, insertion of filters has markedly increased, with a 25-fold increase in use in the United States during the past two decades.[130] In a prospective DVT registry of 5451 patients at 183 U.S. sites, 14% underwent insertion of filters.[131] Some patients have a temporary contraindication to anticoagulation. Under these circumstances, placement of a nonpermanent, retrievable filter may be appropriate. Retrievable filters can be left in place for weeks to months or can remain permanently, if necessary, because of a trapped large clot or a persistent contraindication to anticoagulation.[132]

FIBRINOLYSIS. When it is successfully used, thrombolysis will reverse right-sided heart failure by physical dissolution of anatomically obstructing pulmonary arterial thrombus, thereby reducing right ventricular pressure overload; prevent the continued release of serotonin and other neurohumoral factors that can worsen pulmonary hypertension; and dissolve thrombus in the pelvic or deep leg veins, thereby at least theoretically decreasing the likelihood of recurrent PE. Thrombolysis may also improve pulmonary capillary blood flow and reduce the likelihood for development of chronic thromboembolic pulmonary hypertension. The American College of Chest Physicians advises: "For patients with evidence of hemodynamic compromise, we recommend use of thrombolytic therapy unless there are major contraindications owing to bleeding risk (Grade 1B)…. In selected high-risk patients without hypotension who are judged to have a low risk of bleeding, we suggest administration of thrombolytic therapy (Grade 2B)."[110]

The FDA has approved alteplase for massive PE, in a dose of 100 mg as a continuous infusion during 2 hours, without concomitant heparin. Unlike patients receiving myocardial infarction thrombolysis, patients with PE have a wide "window" for effective use of thrombolysis. Those who receive thrombolysis up to 14 days after new symptoms or signs maintain an effective response, probably because of the bronchial collateral circulation. Guidelines for heparin before and after alteplase are provided in **Table 77-20**.

Thrombolysis in normotensive high-risk PE patients remains controversial.[133] The fear is that the risk of bleeding complications, especially intracranial hemorrhage, outweighs any potential benefit. Women may not gain as much benefit from PE thrombolysis as men do. In a German multicenter PE registry, thrombolysis was associated with a 79% reduction in 30-day mortality in men but no statistically significant reduction in women. Women had a 27% rate of major bleeding compared with 15% in men.[134] The rationale in favor of thrombolysis is that improved survival will ensue. However, a study of patients who received thrombolysis within a cohort of 15,116 PE patients from Pennsylvania does not support this concept.[135] In the International

TABLE 77-20	Use of Heparin Before and After Thrombolysis

1. Discontinue the continuous infusion of intravenous UFH as soon as the decision has been made to administer thrombolysis.
2. Proceed to order thrombolysis. Use the U.S. Food and Drug Administration–approved regimen of alteplase 100 mg as a continuous infusion during 2 hours.
3. Do not delay the thrombolysis infusion by obtaining an activated partial thromboplastin time (aPTT).
4. Infuse thrombolysis as soon as it becomes available.
5. At the conclusion of the 2-hour infusion, obtain a stat aPTT.
6. If the aPTT is 80 seconds or less (which is almost always the case), resume UFH as a continuous infusion without a bolus.
7. If the aPTT exceeds 80 seconds, hold off from resuming heparin for 4 hours and repeat the aPTT. At this time, the aPTT has virtually always declined to <80 seconds. If this is the case, resume continuous infusion of intravenous UFH without a bolus.

Cooperative Pulmonary Embolism Registry, 108 patients presented with massive PE and hypotension. Counterintuitively, among those with massive PE who received thrombolysis, mortality was not reduced.[136]

Thrombolysis is being tested in high-risk normotensive PE patients in an ambitious multicentered European randomized trial that plans to enroll about 1000 patients (NCT00639743). The primary clinical composite endpoint is all-cause mortality or hemodynamic collapse. At Brigham and Women's Hospital, we tend to prescribe thrombolysis when patients have elevation in cardiac biomarkers as well as moderate or severe right ventricular hypokinesis. Despite more than two decades of experience with thrombolysis for acute PE, review of our alteplase-treated patients revealed a major bleeding rate of 19%.[137]

DEEP VENOUS THROMBOSIS INTERVENTIONS. Indications for catheter-directed DVT thrombolysis remain controversial because no convincing reduction in post-thrombotic syndrome has yet been demonstrated. Common indications for thrombolysis include extensive iliofemoral or upper extremity venous thrombosis. Totally occlusive venous thrombosis usually does not improve if the agent is infused through a peripheral vein. Therefore, DVT thrombolysis is almost always administered locally through a catheter. This intervention frequently accompanies catheter-directed suction embolectomy, venous angioplasty, or venous stenting. The American College of Chest Physicians guidelines endorse catheter-directed thrombolysis in selected patients with extensive acute proximal DVT (e.g., iliofemoral DVT, symptoms for <14 days, good functional status, life expectancy ≥1 year) who have a low risk of bleeding.[110] The NHLBI is funding a randomized trial of pharmacomechanical catheter-directed thrombolysis versus conventional anticoagulation in approximately 700 patients with iliac or femoral vein DVT (NCT00790335). The primary endpoint is the incidence of post-thrombotic syndrome in each group. Results are expected in 2014.

CATHETER EMBOLECTOMY. Interventional catheterization techniques[138] for massive PE include mechanical fragmentation of thrombus with a standard pulmonary artery catheter, clot pulverization with a rotating basket catheter, percutaneous rheolytic thrombectomy,[139] and pigtail rotational catheter embolectomy. Another approach is mechanical clot fragmentation and aspiration,[140] which can be combined if necessary with pharmacologic thrombolysis[141] (**Fig. 77-7**). Pulmonary artery balloon dilation and stenting can also be considered. Successful catheter embolectomy rapidly restores normal blood pressure and decreases hypoxemia. Catheter techniques have been limited by poor maneuverability, mechanical hemolysis, macroembolization, and microembolization.

SURGICAL EMBOLECTOMY. Emergency surgical embolectomy with cardiopulmonary bypass has reemerged as an effective strategy for management of patients with massive PE and systemic arterial hypotension or submassive PE with right ventricular dysfunction[142] in whom contraindications preclude thrombolysis (**Fig. 77-8**). This operation is also suited for acute PE patients who require surgical excision of a right atrial thrombus or closure of a patent foramen ovale. Surgical embolectomy can also rescue patients refractory to thrombolysis.[143] The results of embolectomy will be optimized if patients are referred before the onset of cardiogenic shock. In one study, 47 patients underwent surgical embolectomy in a 4-year period, with a 96% survival rate.[144] We perform the

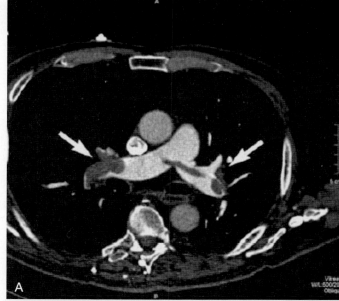

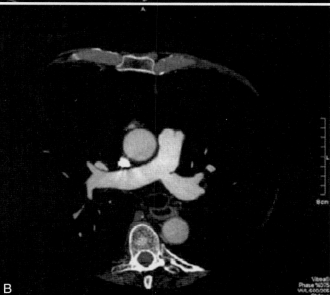

FIGURE 77-7 **A,** Chest CT demonstrates thrombus in the right and left main stem pulmonary arteries, with clot extending into lobar and segmental branches (arrows). **B,** One month after catheter-directed intrapulmonary administration of tissue plasminogen activator and rheolytic thrombectomy, the thrombus has resolved.

procedure off bypass, with normothermia, without aortic cross-clamping or cardioplegic or fibrillatory arrest. Avoidance of blind instrumentation of the fragile pulmonary arteries is imperative. Extraction is limited to directly visible clot, which can be accomplished through the segmental pulmonary arteries.

EMOTIONAL SUPPORT. Patients find PE to be emotionally draining. They and their families seek constant reassurance that most patients have good outcomes once the diagnosis has been established. They must confront PE-related issues such as genetic predisposition, potential long-term disability, changes in lifestyle related to anticoagulation, and the possibility of suffering a recurrent event. By discussing the implications of PE with patients and their families, we can help allay the emotional burden. A Pulmonary Embolism Support Group for patients can fill this need. Our group meets at the hospital once monthly in the evening. We discuss the anxieties and day-to-day difficulties that occur in the aftermath of PE.

MASSIVE PULMONARY EMBOLISM. Hospitals should establish written protocols and rehearse interdisciplinary management for patients with

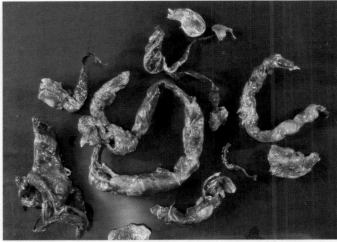

FIGURE 77-8 This 72-year-old woman presented with presyncope, hypotension, and hypoxia. She was diagnosed with massive pulmonary embolism by chest CT scan and underwent emergency pulmonary embolectomy.

TABLE 77-22	Regimens for Venous Thromboembolism Prevention
CONDITION	**PROPHYLAXIS**
Hospitalization with medical illness	Unfractionated heparin 5000 units SC bid or tid *or* Enoxaparin 40 mg SC qd *or* Dalteparin 5000 units SC qd *or* Fondaparinux 2.5 mg SC qd (in patients with a heparin allergy such as heparin-induced thrombocytopenia) *or* Graduated compression stockings or intermittent pneumatic compression for patients with contraindications to anticoagulation Consider combination pharmacologic and mechanical prophylaxis for high-risk patients Consider surveillance lower extremity ultrasonography for intensive care unit patients
General surgery	Unfractionated heparin 5000 units SC bid or tid *or* Enoxaparin 40 mg SC qd *or* Dalteparin 2500 or 5000 units SC qd
Major orthopedic surgery	Warfarin (target INR 2 to 3) *or* Enoxaparin 30 mg SC bid *or* Enoxaparin 40 mg SC qd *or* Dalteparin 2500 or 5000 units SC qd *or* Fondaparinux 2.5 mg SC qd Rivaroxaban 10 mg qd (in Canada and Europe) Dabigatran 220 mg bid (in Canada and Europe)
Neurosurgery	Unfractionated heparin 5000 units SC bid *or* Enoxaparin 40 mg SC qd *and* Graduated compression stockings or intermittent pneumatic compression Consider surveillance lower extremity ultrasonography
Oncologic surgery	Enoxaparin 40 mg SC qd
Thoracic surgery	Unfractionated heparin 5000 units SC tid *and* Graduated compression stockings or intermittent pneumatic compression

INR = international normalized ratio; qd = daily; SC = subcutaneous; bid = twice daily; tid = three times daily.

TABLE 77-21	Massive Pulmonary Embolism

- Begin bolus high-dose intravenous unfractionated heparin as soon as massive pulmonary embolism is suspected.
- Begin continuous infusion of unfractionated heparin to achieve a target aPTT of at least 80 seconds.
- Try volume resuscitation with no more than 500 to 1000 mL of fluid.
- Excessive volume resuscitation will worsen right ventricular failure.
- Have a low threshold for administration of vasopressors and inotropes.
- Decide whether thrombolysis can be safely administered, without a high risk of major hemorrhage.
- If thrombolysis is too risky, consider placement of an inferior vena caval filter, catheter embolectomy, or surgical embolectomy.
- Do not use a combination of thrombolysis and vena caval filter insertion. The prongs of the filter insert into the caval wall. Concomitant thrombolysis predisposes to caval wall hemorrhage.
- Consider immediate referral to a tertiary care hospital specializing in massive pulmonary embolism.

massive PE.[52] The policies and procedures to treat massive PE should become as firmly established and enforced as those for acute ST-segment elevation myocardial infarction. **Table 77-21** presents some management tips. Rapid integration of historical information, physical findings, and laboratory data and coordination with a team composed of cardiologists, cardiac surgeons, emergency department physicians, radiologists, and other specialists are crucial to maximize success. Immediate patient referral to hospitals specializing in massive PE should be considered.

POST-THROMBOTIC SYNDROME AND CHRONIC VENOUS INSUFFICIENCY. Dysfunction of the valves of the deep venous system often results from damage due to prior DVT.[145] Obstruction of the deep veins may limit the outflow of blood, causing increased venous pressure with muscle contraction. Abnormal hemodynamics in the large veins of the leg are transmitted into the microcirculation. The eventual result is venous microangiopathy. Physical findings may include varicose veins, abnormal pigmentation of the medial malleolus, and skin ulceration. The economic impact is high because of time lost from work and the expense of medical diagnosis and treatment. Chronic venous disease is associated with a reduced quality of life due to pain, decreased physical function, and decreased mobility. A mainstay of therapy is vascular compression stockings, below knee, 30 to 40 mm Hg. Compression stockings improve venous hemodynamics, reduce edema, and minimize skin discoloration. By alleviation of calf discomfort, stockings improve the quality of life. Risk factors for development of post-thrombotic syndrome include proximal (rather than calf) DVT, male sex, and high D-dimer levels after completion of a course of anticoagulation.[146]

CHRONIC THROMBOEMBOLIC PULMONARY HYPERTENSION. Chronic thromboembolic pulmonary hypertension occurs much more frequently after acute PE than previously believed.[147] The old teaching was that chronic thromboembolic pulmonary hypertension had a prevalence of 1 in 500 or 1 in 1000 cases of acute PE. New data indicate that the frequency is between 1% and 4%. Although acute PE is the initiating event, pulmonary vascular remodeling may cause severe pulmonary hypertension out of proportion to the pulmonary vascular obliteration observed on pulmonary angiography.[148] Primary therapy is pulmonary thromboendarterectomy, which, if successful, can reduce and at times even cure pulmonary hypertension.[149] The operation involves a median sternotomy, institution of cardiopulmonary bypass, and deep hypothermia with circulatory arrest periods. Incisions are made in both pulmonary arteries into the lower lobe branches. Sildenafil[150] and bosentan,[151] which are established therapies for idiopathic pulmonary hypertension, also appear promising for the treatment of chronic thromboembolic pulmonary hypertension.

Prevention

PE is the most preventable cause of in-hospital death. However, once it occurs, PE is difficult to diagnose, expensive to treat, and potentially lethal despite therapy. Therefore, VTE prevention is of paramount importance. Low fixed-dose anticoagulant prophylaxis is effective.[152] Fortunately, numerous prophylaxis options are available (**Table 77-22**). North American[15] and European[153] consensus conferences have recommended detailed guidelines using various mechanical measures and pharmacologic agents. Often, multiple options are available for each category of risk. Computer-generated alerts to physicians whose hospitalized patients are not receiving prophylaxis can reduce the frequency of symptomatic PE and DVT[19] and maintain effectiveness over time.[154]

There appears to be a failure-to-use-prophylaxis phenomenon. The problem is more widespread among medical service patients than among surgical service patients. For example, 227 American hospitals were surveyed for medical patients 40 years of age or older and requiring at least 6 days of hospitalization without contraindications to anticoagulation.[155] Almost 200,000 patients were identified, all of whom should have received VTE prophylaxis. However, only 62% received any preventive measures, and only 38% received prophylaxis administered in accordance with the American College of Chest Physicians 8th Edition guidelines (2008).

Failure to use prophylaxis during hospitalization has adverse effects that continue after hospital discharge.[18] In a survey of 1897 patients with VTE in the Worcester, Massachusetts, area, 74% developed DVT or PE in the outpatient setting. Of the 516 who had been hospitalized within the prior 3 months and subsequently developed VTE, 67% developed VTE within 1 month after the hospitalization. These findings indicate the need to consider extension of VTE prophylaxis after hospital discharge.

Medicare will not pay the incremental cost to manage a "never event," defined as a medical complication that should never happen. Rather, the hospital bears the additional financial burden. In 2008, Medicare selected the occurrence of VTE after total knee or hip replacement to be listed as a never event.[156] It is now clear that the fiercely independent practitioner, who used to be free to accept or to reject VTE prophylaxis without oversight, is a fading memory destined to become a footnote in the history of medicine.

Mechanical Measures

Mechanical measures consist of intermittent pneumatic compression devices, which enhance endogenous fibrinolysis and increase venous blood flow, and graduated compression stockings. Mechanical measures are prescribed for patients who have an absolute contraindication to anticoagulation. A meta-analysis of intermittent pneumatic compression devices was undertaken in 2270 postoperative patients from 15 studies. In comparison to no prophylaxis, intermittent pneumatic compression devices reduced the risk of DVT by 60%.[157] They also appear to be cost-effective.[158] However, in a large study of stroke patients, thigh-high graduated compression did not confer protection.[159] Pharmacologic prophylaxis appears to be more effective.[160]

Pharmacologic Agents

Pharmacologic prophylaxis options include low fixed-dose UFH, LMWH, fondaparinux, and full-dose warfarin. The American College of Chest Physicians does not consider aspirin to confer meaningful prophylaxis against VTE.

Unconventional Approaches

VITAMIN E. The Women's Health Study randomized 39,876 women to receive 600 units of vitamin E or placebo.[161] After a median follow-up of 10 years, there was a 21% reduction in VTE among women assigned to vitamin E. The reduction was most striking among women with VTE before randomization (44% reduction) and in women with either the factor V Leiden mutation or the prothrombin gene mutation (49% reduction). These data suggest that supplementation with vitamin E may reduce VTE risk in women, especially those with a prior history of VTE or with a genetic predisposition.

STATINS. Observational studies suggest that statins as a class reduce VTE. In the JUPITER study, 17,802 apparently healthy men and women with both low-density lipoprotein cholesterol levels of less than 130 mg/dL and high-sensitivity C-reactive protein levels of 2.0 mg/dL or higher were randomized to receive rosuvastatin, 20 mg/day, or placebo.[10] During a median follow-up period of 1.9 years, the prespecified endpoint of symptomatic VTE was reduced by 43% in the rosuvastatin group ($P = 0.007$). Thus, rosuvastatin appears to prevent VTE. Notably, statins do not increase bleeding risk, in contrast to most other pharmacologic approaches to VTE prevention.

Future Perspectives

PE and DVT are major cardiovascular illnesses that cause suffering and death. VTE has much in common with coronary heart disease—risk factors are similar, prevention has not received adequate emphasis, and drug therapy has not been adequately integrated with lifestyle modification. During the next several years, we will witness widespread institution of electronic decision support to prevent in-hospital VTE. Hospitalized patients will subsequently be observed closely after discharge to ensure that preventive efforts are maintained in the community. Public and professional education and awareness of PE and DVT will increase. These trends should reduce the delay in seeking medical assistance and will lead to more rapid diagnosis, risk stratification, and effective therapy. For the minority of patients requiring advanced therapy for massive PE, specialized hospitals modeled after trauma centers will offer catheter-directed thrombolysis, pharmacomechanical thrombectomy, and surgical embolectomy. Novel anticoagulants will be introduced into clinical medicine and will provide increased convenience for the patient and practitioner, and perhaps superior efficacy. Translational and clinical research in VTE will intensify and flourish.

REFERENCES

1. Torbicki A, Perrier A, Konstantinides S, et al: Guidelines on the diagnosis and management of acute pulmonary embolism: The Task Force for the Diagnosis and Management of Acute Pulmonary Embolism of the European Society of Cardiology (ESC). Eur Heart J 29:2276, 2008.
2. Galson S: The Surgeon General's Call to Action to Prevent Deep Vein Thrombosis and Pulmonary Embolism. Available at: http://www.surgeongeneral.gov/topics/deepvein/.
3. North American Thrombosis Forum (www.natfonline.org).
4. Park B, Messina L, Dargon P, et al: Recent trends in clinical outcomes and resource utilization for pulmonary embolism in the United States: Findings from the nationwide inpatient sample. Chest 136:983, 2009.
5. Klein TE, Altman RB, Eriksson N, et al: Estimation of the warfarin dose with clinical and pharmacogenetic data. N Engl J Med 360:753, 2009.
6. Gross PL, Weitz JI: New anticoagulants for treatment of venous thromboembolism. Arterioscler Thromb Vasc Biol 28:380, 2008.
7. Eriksson BI, Borris LC, Friedman RJ, et al: Rivaroxaban versus enoxaparin for thromboprophylaxis after hip arthroplasty. N Engl J Med 358:2765, 2008.
8. Lassen MR, Ageno W, Borris LC, et al: Rivaroxaban versus enoxaparin for thromboprophylaxis after total knee arthroplasty. N Engl J Med 358:2776, 2008.
9. Wolowacz SE, Roskell NS, Plumb JM, et al: Efficacy and safety of dabigatran etexilate for the prevention of venous thromboembolism following total hip or knee arthroplasty. A meta-analysis. Thromb Haemost 101:77, 2009.
10. Glynn RJ, Danielson E, Fonseca FA, et al: A randomized trial of rosuvastatin in the prevention of venous thromboembolism. N Engl J Med 360:1851, 2009.
11. Dentali F, Douketis JD, Gianni M, et al: Meta-analysis: Anticoagulant prophylaxis to prevent symptomatic venous thromboembolism in hospitalized medical patients. Ann Intern Med 146:278, 2007.
12. Anderson FA Jr, Zayaruzny M, Heit JA, et al: Estimated annual numbers of US acute-care hospital patients at risk for venous thromboembolism. Am J Hematol 82:777, 2007.
13. Piazza G, Seddighzadeh A, Goldhaber SZ: Double trouble for 2,609 hospitalized medical patients who developed deep vein thrombosis: Prophylaxis omitted more often and pulmonary embolism more frequent. Chest 132:554, 2007.
14. Piazza G, Seddighzadeh A, Goldhaber SZ: Heart failure in patients with deep vein thrombosis. Am J Cardiol 101:1056, 2008.
15. Geerts WH, Bergqvist D, Pineo GF, et al: Prevention of venous thromboembolism: American College of Chest Physicians Evidence-Based Clinical Practice Guidelines (8th Edition). Chest 133:381S, 2008.
16. Cohen AT, Tapson VF, Bergmann JF, et al: Venous thromboembolism risk and prophylaxis in the acute hospital care setting (ENDORSE study): A multinational cross-sectional study. Lancet 371:387, 2008.
17. Deitelzweig SB, Becker R, Lin J, et al: Comparison of the two-year outcomes and costs of prophylaxis in medical patients at risk of venous thromboembolism. Thromb Haemost 100:810, 2008.
18. Spencer FA, Lessard D, Emery C, et al: Venous thromboembolism in the outpatient setting. Arch Intern Med 167:1471, 2007.
19. Kucher N, Koo S, Quiroz R, et al: Electronic alerts to prevent venous thromboembolism among hospitalized patients. N Engl J Med 352:969, 2005.
20. Piazza G, Rosenbaum EJ, Pendergast W, et al: Physician alerts to prevent symptomatic venous thromboembolism in hospitalized patients. Circulation 119:2196, 2009.

Epidemiology

21. Parasuraman S, Goldhaber SZ: Venous thromboembolism in children. Circulation 113:e12, 2006.
22. Naess IA, Christiansen SC, Romundstad P, et al: Incidence and mortality of venous thrombosis: A population-based study. J Thromb Haemost 5:692, 2007.
23. Cushman M, Tsai AW, White RH, et al: Deep vein thrombosis and pulmonary embolism in two cohorts: The longitudinal investigation of thromboembolism etiology. Am J Med 117:19, 2004.
24. Zee RY, Cook NR, Cheng S, et al: Polymorphism in the beta$_2$-adrenergic receptor and lipoprotein lipase genes as risk determinants for idiopathic venous thromboembolism: A multilocus, population-based, prospective genetic analysis. Circulation 113:2193, 2006.

25. Laporte S, Mismetti P, Decousus H, et al: Clinical predictors for fatal pulmonary embolism in 15,520 patients with venous thromboembolism: Findings from the Registro Informatizado de la Enfermedad TromboEmbolica venosa (RIETE) Registry. Circulation 117:1711, 2008.

26. Zhu T, Martinez I, Emmerich J: Venous thromboembolism: Risk factors for recurrence. Arterioscler Thromb Vasc Biol 29:298, 2009.

27. Goldhaber SZ, Tapson VF: A prospective registry of 5,451 patients with ultrasound-confirmed deep vein thrombosis. Am J Cardiol 93:259, 2004.

28. Sorensen HT, Horvath-Puho E, Pedersen L, et al: Venous thromboembolism and subsequent hospitalisation due to acute arterial cardiovascular events: A 20-year cohort study. Lancet 370:1773, 2007.

29. Ageno W, Becattini C, Brighton T, et al: Cardiovascular risk factors and venous thromboembolism: A meta-analysis. Circulation 117:93, 2008.

30. Borch KH, Braekkan SK, Mathiesen EB, et al: Abdominal obesity is essential for the risk of venous thromboembolism in the metabolic syndrome: The Tromsø study. J Thromb Haemost 7:739, 2009.

31. Rosengren A, Freden M, Hansson PO, et al: Psychosocial factors and venous thromboembolism: A long-term follow-up study of Swedish men. J Thromb Haemost 6:558, 2008.

32. Steffen LM, Folsom AR, Cushman M, et al: Greater fish, fruit, and vegetable intakes are related to lower incidence of venous thromboembolism: The Longitudinal Investigation of Thromboembolism Etiology. Circulation 115:188, 2007.

33. Stein PD, Beemath A, Olson RE: Obesity as a risk factor in venous thromboembolism. Am J Med 118:978, 2005.

34. Smeeth L, Cook C, Thomas S, et al: Risk of deep vein thrombosis and pulmonary embolism after acute infection in a community setting. Lancet 367:1075, 2006.

35. Stein PD, Beemath A, Meyers FA, et al: Incidence of venous thromboembolism in patients hospitalized with cancer. Am J Med 119:60, 2006.

36. Douketis JD, Gu C, Piccioli A, et al: The long-term risk of cancer in patients with a first episode of venous thromboembolism. J Thromb Haemost 7:546, 2009.

37. Marik PE, Plante LA: Venous thromboembolic disease and pregnancy. N Engl J Med 359:2025, 2008.

38. Blanco-Molina A, Trujillo-Santos J, Tirado R, et al: Venous thromboembolism in women using hormonal contraceptives. Findings from the RIETE Registry. Thromb Haemost 101:478, 2009.

39. Cushman M, Kuller LH, Prentice R, et al: Estrogen plus progestin and risk of venous thrombosis. JAMA 292:1573, 2004.

40. Rizkallah J, Man SF, Sin DD: Prevalence of pulmonary embolism in acute exacerbations of COPD: A systematic review and metaanalysis. Chest 135:786, 2009.

41. Mahmoodi BK, ten Kate MK, Waanders F, et al: High absolute risks and predictors of venous and arterial thromboembolic events in patients with nephrotic syndrome: Results from a large retrospective cohort study. Circulation 117:224, 2008.

42. Baccarelli A, Martinelli I, Pegoraro V, et al: Living near major traffic roads and risk of deep vein thrombosis. Circulation 119:3118, 2009.

43. Schreijer AJ, Cannegieter SC, Meijers JC, et al: Activation of coagulation system during air travel: A crossover study. Lancet 367:832, 2006.

44. Chandra D, Parisini E, Mozaffarian D: Travel and risk for venous thromboembolism. Ann Intern Med 151:1, 2009.

45. Rooden CJ, Tesselaar ME, Osanto S, et al: Deep vein thrombosis associated with central venous catheters—a review. J Thromb Haemost 3:2409, 2005.

46. Spencer FA, Gore JM, Lessard D, et al: Venous thromboembolism in the elderly. A community-based perspective. Thromb Haemost 100:780, 2008.

Pathophysiology

47. Segal JB, Brotman DJ, Necochea AJ, et al: Predictive value of factor V Leiden and prothrombin G20210A in adults with venous thromboembolism and in family members of those with a mutation: a systematic review. JAMA 301:2472, 2009.

48. Dalen JE: Should patients with venous thromboembolism be screened for thrombophilia? Am J Med 121:458, 2008.

49. Lim W, Crowther MA, Eikelboom JW: Management of antiphospholipid antibody syndrome: A systematic review. JAMA 295:1050, 2006.

50. Konstantinides S: Pulmonary embolism: Impact of right ventricular dysfunction. Curr Opin Cardiol 20:496, 2005.

51. Piazza G, Goldhaber SZ: The acutely decompensated right ventricle: Pathways for diagnosis and management. Chest 128:1836, 2005.

52. Kucher N, Goldhaber SZ: Management of massive pulmonary embolism. Circulation 112:e28, 2005.

53. Tapson VF: Acute pulmonary embolism. N Engl J Med 358:1037, 2008.

Diagnosis

54. Elliott CG, Goldhaber SZ, Jensen RL: Delays in diagnosis of deep vein thrombosis and pulmonary embolism. Chest 128:3372, 2005.

55. Kabrhel C, Camargo CA Jr, Goldhaber SZ: Clinical gestalt and the diagnosis of pulmonary embolism: Does experience matter? Chest 127:1627, 2005.

56. van Belle A, Buller HR, Huisman MV, et al: Effectiveness of managing suspected pulmonary embolism using an algorithm combining clinical probability, D-dimer testing, and computed tomography. JAMA 295:172, 2006.

57. Douma RA, Gibson NS, Gerdes VE, et al: Validity and clinical utility of the simplified Wells rule for assessing clinical probability for the exclusion of pulmonary embolism. Thromb Haemost 101:197, 2009.

58. Stein PD, Hull RD, Patel KC, et al: D-dimer for the exclusion of acute venous thrombosis and pulmonary embolism: A systematic review. Ann Intern Med 140:589, 2004.

59. Kearon C, Ginsberg JS, Douketis J, et al: An evaluation of D-dimer in the diagnosis of pulmonary embolism: A randomized trial. Ann Intern Med 144:812, 2006.

60. Vanni S, Polidori G, Vergara R, et al: Prognostic value of ECG among patients with acute pulmonary embolism and normal blood pressure. Am J Med 122:257, 2009.

61. Stein PD, Kayali F, Olson RE: Trends in the use of diagnostic imaging in patients hospitalized with acute pulmonary embolism. Am J Cardiol 93:1316, 2004.

62. Goldhaber SZ: Multislice computed tomography for pulmonary embolism—a technological marvel. N Engl J Med 352:1812, 2005.

63. Quiroz R, Kucher N, Zou KH, et al: Clinical validity of a negative computed tomography scan in patients with suspected pulmonary embolism: A systematic review. JAMA 293:2012, 2005.

64. Perrier A, Roy PM, Sanchez O, et al: Multidetector-row computed tomography in suspected pulmonary embolism. N Engl J Med 352:1760, 2005.

65. Hunsaker AR, Zou KH, Poh AC, et al: Routine pelvic and lower extremity CT venography in patients undergoing pulmonary CT angiography. AJR Am J Roentgenol 190:322, 2008.

66. Schoepf UJ, Goldhaber SZ, Costello P: Spiral computed tomography for acute pulmonary embolism. Circulation 109:2160, 2004.

67. Stein PD, Fowler SE, Goodman LR, et al: Multidetector computed tomography for acute pulmonary embolism. N Engl J Med 354:2317, 2006.

68. Stein PD, Chenevert TL, Fowler SE, et al: Gadolinium-enhanced magnetic resonance angiography for pulmonary embolism: a multicenter prospective study (PIOPED III). Ann Intern Med 152:434, 2010.

69. Schellong SM, Beyer J, Kakkar AK, et al: Ultrasound screening for asymptomatic deep vein thrombosis after major orthopaedic surgery: The VENUS study. J Thromb Haemost 5:1431, 2007.

70. Righini M, Le Gal G, Aujesky D, et al: Diagnosis of pulmonary embolism by multidetector CT alone or combined with venous ultrasonography of the leg: A randomised non-inferiority trial. Lancet 371:1343, 2008.

Management

71. Jimenez D, Uresandi F, Otero R, et al: Troponin-based risk stratification of patients with acute nonmassive pulmonary embolism: Systematic review and metaanalysis. Chest 136:974, 2009.

72. Donze J, Le Gal G, Fine MJ, et al: Prospective validation of the Pulmonary Embolism Severity Index. A clinical prognostic model for pulmonary embolism. Thromb Haemost 100:943, 2008.

73. Fremont B, Pacouret G, Jacobi D, et al: Prognostic value of echocardiographic right/left ventricular end-diastolic diameter ratio in patients with acute pulmonary embolism: Results from a monocenter registry of 1,416 patients. Chest 133:358, 2008.

74. Schoepf UJ, Kucher N, Kipfmueller F, et al: Right ventricular enlargement on chest computed tomography: A predictor of early death in acute pulmonary embolism. Circulation 110:3276, 2004.

75. Becattini C, Vedovati MC, Agnelli G: Prognostic value of troponins in acute pulmonary embolism: A meta-analysis. Circulation 116:427, 2007.

76. Scridon T, Scridon C, Skali H, et al: Prognostic significance of troponin elevation and right ventricular enlargement in acute pulmonary embolism. Am J Cardiol 96:303, 2005.

77. Aujesky D, Jimenez D, Mor MK, et al: Weekend versus weekday admission and mortality after acute pulmonary embolism. Circulation 119:962, 2009.

78. Aujesky D, Stone RA, Kim S, et al: Length of hospital stay and postdischarge mortality in patients with pulmonary embolism: A statewide perspective. Arch Intern Med 168:706, 2008.

79. Aujesky D, Mor MK, Geng M, et al: Predictors of early hospital readmission after acute pulmonary embolism. Arch Intern Med 169:287, 2009.

80. Konstantinides S: Clinical practice. Acute pulmonary embolism. N Engl J Med 359:2804, 2008.

81. Kearon C, Ginsberg JS, Julian JA, et al: Comparison of fixed-dose weight-adjusted unfractionated heparin and low-molecular-weight heparin for acute treatment of venous thromboembolism. JAMA 296:935, 2006.

82. Prandoni P, Carnovali M, Marchiori A: Subcutaneous adjusted-dose unfractionated heparin vs fixed-dose low-molecular-weight heparin in the initial treatment of venous thromboembolism. Arch Intern Med 164:1077, 2004.

83. Blossom DB, Kallen AJ, Patel PR, et al: Outbreak of adverse reactions associated with contaminated heparin. N Engl J Med 359:2674, 2008.

84. Kishimoto TK, Viswanathan K, Ganguly T, et al: Contaminated heparin associated with adverse clinical events and activation of the contact system. N Engl J Med 358:2457, 2008.

85. Hull RD: Treatment of pulmonary embolism: The use of low-molecular-weight heparin in the inpatient and outpatient settings. Thromb Haemost 99:502, 2008.

86. Lee AY, Levine MN, Baker RI, et al: Low-molecular-weight heparin versus a coumarin for the prevention of recurrent venous thromboembolism in patients with cancer. N Engl J Med 349:146, 2003.

87. Kucher N, Quiroz R, McKean S, et al: Extended enoxaparin monotherapy for acute symptomatic pulmonary embolism. Vasc Med 10:251, 2005.

88. Buller HR, Davidson BL, Decousus H, et al: Fondaparinux or enoxaparin for the initial treatment of symptomatic deep venous thrombosis: A randomized trial. Ann Intern Med 140:867, 2004.

89. Baroletti S, Labreche M, Niles M, et al: Prescription of fondaparinux in hospitalised patients. Thromb Haemost 101:1091, 2009.

90. Shetty R, Seddighzadeh A, Parasuraman S, et al: Once-daily fondaparinux monotherapy without warfarin for long-term treatment of venous thromboembolism. Thromb Haemost 98:1384, 2007.

91. Oliveira GB, Crespo EM, Becker RC, et al: Incidence and prognostic significance of thrombocytopenia in patients treated with prolonged heparin therapy. Arch Intern Med 168:94, 2008.

92. Baroletti S, Piovella C, Fanikos J, et al: Heparin-induced thrombocytopenia (HIT): Clinical and economic outcomes. Thromb Haemost 100:1130, 2008.

93. Arepally GM, Ortel TL: Clinical practice. Heparin-induced thrombocytopenia. N Engl J Med 355:809, 2006.

94. Di Nisio M, Middeldorp S, Buller HR: Direct thrombin inhibitors. N Engl J Med 353:1028, 2005.

95. Quiroz R, Gerhard-Herman M, Kosowsky JM, et al: Comparison of a single end point to determine optimal initial warfarin dosing (5 mg versus 10 mg) for venous thromboembolism. Am J Cardiol 98:535, 2006.

96. Poller L, Keown M, Ibrahim S, et al: A multicentre randomised assessment of the DAWN AC computer-assisted oral anticoagulant dosage program. Thromb Haemost 101:487, 2009.

97. Jowett S, Bryan S, Poller L, et al: The cost-effectiveness of computer-assisted anticoagulant dosage: Results from the European Action on Anticoagulation (EAA) multicentre study. J Thromb Haemost 7:1482, 2009.

98. Sconce E, Avery P, Wynne H, et al: Vitamin K supplementation can improve stability of anticoagulation for patients with unexplained variability in response to warfarin. Blood 109:2419, 2007.

99. Koo S, Kucher N, Nguyen PL, et al: The effect of excessive anticoagulation on mortality and morbidity in hospitalized patients with anticoagulant-related major hemorrhage. Arch Intern Med 164:1557, 2004.

100. Baker WL, Cios DA, Sander SD, et al: Meta-analysis to assess the quality of warfarin control in atrial fibrillation patients in the United States. J Manag Care Pharm 15:244, 2009.

101. van Walraven C, Jennings A, Oake N, et al: Effect of study setting on anticoagulation control: A systematic review and metaregression. Chest 129:1155, 2006.

102. Heneghan C, Alonso-Coello P, Garcia-Alamino JM, et al: Self-monitoring of oral anticoagulation: A systematic review and meta-analysis. Lancet 367:404, 2006.

103. Schwarz UI, Ritchie MD, Bradford Y, et al: Genetic determinants of response to warfarin during initial anticoagulation. N Engl J Med 358:999, 2008.

104. Wadelius M, Chen LY, Lindh JD, et al: The largest prospective warfarin-treated cohort supports genetic forecasting. Blood 113:784, 2009.

105. Eckman MH, Rosand J, Greenberg SM, et al: Cost-effectiveness of using pharmacogenetic information in warfarin dosing for patients with nonvalvular atrial fibrillation. Ann Intern Med 150:73, 2009.

106. Anderson JL, Horne BD, Stevens SM, et al: Randomized trial of genotype-guided versus standard warfarin dosing in patients initiating oral anticoagulation. Circulation 116:2563, 2007.

107. Rosand J, Eckman MH, Knudsen KA, et al: The effect of warfarin and intensity of anticoagulation on outcome of intracerebral hemorrhage. Arch Intern Med 164:880, 2004.

108. Dorfman DM, Goonan EM, Boutilier MK, et al: Point-of-care (POC) versus central laboratory instrumentation for monitoring oral anticoagulation. Vasc Med 10:23, 2005.

109. Eikelboom JE, Weitz JI: Dabigatran etexilate for prevention of venous thromboembolism. Thromb Haemost 101:2, 2009.

110. Kearon C, Kahn SR, Agnelli G, et al: Antithrombotic therapy for venous thromboembolic disease: American College of Chest Physicians Evidence-Based Clinical Practice Guidelines (8th Edition). Chest 133:454S, 2008.

111. Wagman LD, Baird MF, Bennett CL, et al: Venous thromboembolic disease. Clinical practice guidelines in oncology. J Natl Compr Canc Netw 4:838, 2006.

112. Lyman GH, Khorana AA, Falanga A, et al: American Society of Clinical Oncology guideline: Recommendations for venous thromboembolism prophylaxis and treatment in patients with cancer. J Clin Oncol 25:5490, 2007.

113. Goldhaber SZ: Optimal duration of anticoagulation after venous thromboembolism: Fixed and evidence-based, or flexible and personalized? Ann Intern Med 150:644, 2009.

114. Ridker PM: Long-term low-dose warfarin use is effective in the prevention of recurrent venous thromboembolism: Yes. J Thromb Haemost 2:1034, 2004.

115. Nijkeuter M, Sohne M, Tick LW, et al: The natural course of hemodynamically stable pulmonary embolism: Clinical outcome and risk factors in a large prospective cohort study. Chest 131:517, 2007.

116. Douketis JD, Gu CS, Schulman S, et al: The risk for fatal pulmonary embolism after discontinuing anticoagulant therapy for venous thromboembolism. Ann Intern Med 147:766, 2007.

117. Grifoni S, Vanni S, Magazzini S, et al: Association of persistent right ventricular dysfunction at hospital discharge after acute pulmonary embolism with recurrent thromboembolic events. Arch Intern Med 166:2151, 2006.

118. Christiansen SC, Cannegieter SC, Koster T, et al: Thrombophilia, clinical factors, and recurrent venous thrombotic events. JAMA 293:2352, 2005.

119. Cushman M, Glynn RJ, Goldhaber SZ, et al: Hormonal factors and risk of recurrent venous thrombosis: The prevention of recurrent venous thromboembolism trial. J Thromb Haemost 4:2199, 2006.

120. Kyrle PA, Minar E, Bialonczyk C, et al: The risk of recurrent venous thromboembolism in men and women. N Engl J Med 350:2558, 2004.

121. Eichinger S, Hron G, Bialonczyk C, et al: Overweight, obesity, and the risk of recurrent venous thromboembolism. Arch Intern Med 168:1678, 2008.

122. Eichinger S, Weltermann A, Minar E, et al: Symptomatic pulmonary embolism and the risk of recurrent venous thromboembolism. Arch Intern Med 164:92, 2004.

123. Eichinger S, Pecheniuk NM, Hron G, et al: High-density lipoprotein and the risk of recurrent venous thromboembolism. Circulation 115:1609, 2007.

124. Prandoni P, Prins MH, Lensing AW, et al: Residual thrombosis on ultrasonography to guide the duration of anticoagulation in patients with deep venous thrombosis: A randomized trial. Ann Intern Med 150:577, 2009.

125. Nijkeuter M, Hovens MM, Davidson BL, et al: Resolution of thromboemboli in patients with acute pulmonary embolism: A systematic review. Chest 129:192, 2006.

126. Shrivastava S, Ridker PM, Glynn RJ, et al: D-dimer, factor VIII coagulant activity, low-intensity warfarin and the risk of recurrent venous thromboembolism. J Thromb Haemost 4:1208, 2006.

127. Verhovsek M, Douketis JD, Yi Q, et al: Systematic review: D-dimer to predict recurrent disease after stopping anticoagulant therapy for unprovoked venous thromboembolism. Ann Intern Med 149:481, W494, 2008.

128. Bruinstroop E, Klok FA, Van De Ree MA, et al: Elevated D-dimer levels predict recurrence in patients with idiopathic venous thromboembolism: A meta-analysis. J Thromb Haemost 7:611, 2009.

129. The PREPIC Study Group: Eight-year follow-up of patients with permanent vena cava filters in the prevention of pulmonary embolism: The PREPIC (Prevention du Risque d'Embolie Pulmonaire par Interruption Cave) randomized study. Circulation 112:416, 2005.

130. Stein PD, Kayali F, Olson RE: Twenty-one-year trends in the use of inferior vena cava filters. Arch Intern Med 164:1541, 2004.

131. Jaff MR, Goldhaber SZ, Tapson VF: High utilization rate of vena cava filters in deep vein thrombosis. Thromb Haemost 93:1117, 2005.

132. Stein PD, Alnas M, Skaf E, et al: Outcome and complications of retrievable inferior vena cava filters. Am J Cardiol 94:1090, 2004.

133. Todd JL, Tapson VF: Thrombolytic therapy for acute pulmonary embolism: A critical appraisal. Chest 135:1321, 2009.

134. Geibel A, Olschewski M, Zehender M, et al: Possible gender-related differences in the risk-to-benefit ratio of thrombolysis for acute submassive pulmonary embolism. Am J Cardiol 99:103, 2007.

135. Ibrahim SA, Stone RA, Obrosky DS, et al: Thrombolytic therapy and mortality in patients with acute pulmonary embolism. Arch Intern Med 168:2183; discussion 2191, 2008.

136. Kucher N, Rossi E, De Rosa M, et al: Massive pulmonary embolism. Circulation 113:577, 2006.

137. Fiumara K, Kucher N, Fanikos J, et al: Predictors of major hemorrhage following fibrinolysis for acute pulmonary embolism. Am J Cardiol 97:127, 2006.

138. Kucher N: Catheter embolectomy for acute pulmonary embolism. Chest 132:657, 2007.

139. Margheri M, Vittori G, Vecchio S, et al: Early and long-term clinical results of AngioJet rheolytic thrombectomy in patients with acute pulmonary embolism. Am J Cardiol 101:252, 2008.

140. Eid-Lidt G, Gaspar J, Sandoval J, et al: Combined clot fragmentation and aspiration in patients with acute pulmonary embolism. Chest 134:54, 2008.

141. Kuo WT, van den Bosch MA, Hofmann LV, et al: Catheter-directed embolectomy, fragmentation, and thrombolysis for the treatment of massive pulmonary embolism after failure of systemic thrombolysis. Chest 134:250, 2008.

142. Sukhija R, Aronow WS, Lee J, et al: Association of right ventricular dysfunction with in-hospital mortality in patients with acute pulmonary embolism and reduction in mortality in patients with right ventricular dysfunction by pulmonary embolectomy. Am J Cardiol 95:695, 2005.

143. Meneveau N, Seronde MF, Blonde MC, et al: Management of unsuccessful thrombolysis in acute massive pulmonary embolism. Chest 129:1043, 2006.

144. Leacche M, Unic D, Goldhaber SZ, et al: Modern surgical treatment of massive pulmonary embolism: Results in 47 consecutive patients after rapid diagnosis and aggressive surgical approach. J Thorac Cardiovasc Surg 129:1018, 2005.

145. Bergan JJ, Schmid-Schonbein GW, Smith PD, et al: Chronic venous disease. N Engl J Med 355:488, 2006.

146. Stain M, Schonauer V, Minar E, et al: The post-thrombotic syndrome: Risk factors and impact on the course of thrombotic disease. J Thromb Haemost 3:2671, 2005.

147. McLaughlin VV, Archer SL, Badesch DB, et al: ACCF/AHA 2009 expert consensus document on pulmonary hypertension: A report of the American College of Cardiology Foundation Task Force on Expert Consensus Documents and the American Heart Association: Developed in collaboration with the American College of Chest Physicians, American Thoracic Society, Inc., and the Pulmonary Hypertension Association. Circulation 119:2250, 2009.

148. Hoeper MM, Mayer E, Simonneau G, et al: Chronic thromboembolic pulmonary hypertension. Circulation 113:2011, 2006.

149. Corsico AG, D'Armini AM, Cerveri I, et al: Long-term outcome after pulmonary endarterectomy. Am J Respir Crit Care Med 178:419, 2008.

150. Suntharalingam J, Treacy CM, Doughty NJ, et al: Long-term use of sildenafil in inoperable chronic thromboembolic pulmonary hypertension. Chest 134:229, 2008.

151. Jais X, D'Armini AM, Jansa P, et al: Bosentan for treatment of inoperable chronic thromboembolic pulmonary hypertension: BENEFiT (Bosentan Effects in iNopErable Forms of chronIc Thromboembolic pulmonary hypertension), a randomized, placebo-controlled trial. J Am Coll Cardiol 52:2127, 2008.

Prevention

152. Wein L, Wein S, Haas SJ, et al: Pharmacological venous thromboembolism prophylaxis in hospitalized medical patients: A meta-analysis of randomized controlled trials. Arch Intern Med 167:1476, 2007.

153. Nicolaides AN, Breddin HK, Carpenter P, et al: Thrombophilia and venous thromboembolism. International consensus statement. Guidelines according to scientific evidence. Int Angiol 24:1, 2005.

154. Lecumberri R, Marques M, Diaz-Navarlaz MT, et al: Maintained effectiveness of an electronic alert system to prevent venous thromboembolism among hospitalized patients. Thromb Haemost 100:699, 2008.

155. Amin A, Stemkowski S, Lin J, et al: Thromboprophylaxis rates in US medical centers: Success or failure? J Thromb Haemost 5:1610, 2007.

156. Streiff MB, Haut ER: The CMS ruling on venous thromboembolism after total knee or hip arthroplasty: Weighing risks and benefits. JAMA 301:1063, 2009.

157. Urbankova J, Quiroz R, Kucher N, et al: Intermittent pneumatic compression and deep vein thrombosis prevention. A meta-analysis in postoperative patients. Thromb Haemost 94:1181, 2005.

158. Nicolaides A, Goldhaber SZ, Maxwell GL, et al: Cost benefit of intermittent pneumatic compression for venous thromboembolism prophylaxis in general surgery. Int Angiol 27:500, 2008.

159. Dennis M, Sandercock PA, Reid J, et al: Effectiveness of thigh-length graduated compression stockings to reduce the risk of deep vein thrombosis after stroke (CLOTS trial 1): A multicentre, randomised controlled trial. Lancet 373:1958, 2009.

160. Turpie AG, Bauer KA, Caprini JA, et al: Fondaparinux combined with intermittent pneumatic compression vs. intermittent pneumatic compression alone for prevention of venous thromboembolism after abdominal surgery: A randomized, double-blind comparison. J Thromb Haemost 5:1854, 2007.

161. Glynn RJ, Ridker PM, Goldhaber SZ, et al: Effects of random allocation to vitamin E supplementation on the occurrence of venous thromboembolism: Report from the Women's Health Study. Circulation 116:1497, 2007.

CHAPTER **78** # Pulmonary Hypertension

Stuart Rich

Normal Pulmonary Circulation

The lung has a unique double arterial blood supply from the pulmonary and bronchial arteries, as well as double venous drainage into the pulmonary and azygos veins.[1] Each pulmonary artery accompanies the appropriate-generation bronchus and divides with it down to the level of the respiratory bronchiole. The pulmonary arteries are classified as elastic or muscular. The elastic arteries are conducting vessels, highly distensible at low transmural pressure. As the arteries decrease in size, the number of elastic laminae decreases and smooth muscle increases. Eventually, in vessels between 100 and 500 μm, elastic tissue is lost from the media and the arteries become muscular. The intima of the pulmonary arteries consists of a single layer of endothelial cells and their basement membrane. The adventitia is composed of dense connective tissue in direct continuity with the peribronchial connective tissue sheath. The muscular arteries are 500 μm in diameter or smaller and are characterized by a muscular media bounded by internal and external elastic laminae. Arterioles are precapillary arteries smaller than 100 μm in outer diameter and composed solely of a thin intima and single elastic lamina. The alveolar capillaries are lined with a continuous layer of endothelium resting on a continuous basement membrane and focally connected to scattered pericytes located beneath the basement membrane. Within the respiratory units, the pulmonary arteries and arterioles are centrally located and give rise to precapillary arterioles, from which a network of capillaries radiates into the alveolar walls. The alveolar capillaries collect at the periphery of the acini and then drain into venules located in the interlobular and interlobar septa.

The bronchial circulation provides nutrition to the airways. The bronchial arteries ramify into a capillary network drained by bronchial veins; some empty into the pulmonary veins, and the remainder empty into the systemic venous bed. The bronchial circulation therefore constitutes a physiologic right-to-left shunt. Normally, blood flow through this system amounts to approximately 1% of the cardiac output; the resulting desaturation of left atrial blood is usually trivial. However, in some forms of pulmonary disease (e.g., severe bronchiectasis) and in the presence of many congenital cardiovascular malformations that cause cyanosis, blood flow through the bronchial circulation can increase to as much as 30% of left ventricular output and produce a significant right-to-left shunt.

The pulmonary circulation is characterized by high flow and by low pressure and low resistance (**Table 78-1**) The normal pulmonary vascular bed offers less than 10% of the resistance to flow offered by the systemic bed and can be approximated as the ratio of pressure drop (ΔP, in mm Hg) to mean flow (Q, in liters per minute). The ratio can be multiplied by 80 to express the results in dyne-sec · cm^{-5}, or

expressed in mm Hg/liter/min, which is referred to as a Wood unit. The calculated pulmonary vascular resistance in normal adults is 67 ± 23 (standard deviation, SD) dyne-sec · cm^{-5}, or 1 Wood unit.

FETAL AND NEONATAL CIRCULATION. In the fetus, oxygenated blood enters the heart from the inferior vena cava and streams across the foramen ovale to the left atrium (see Chap. 65). Desaturated blood returns from the superior vena cava and into the right ventricle and pulmonary artery. Because the resistance of the pulmonary vascular bed in the collapsed fetal lung is extremely high, only 10% to 30% of the right ventricular output passes through the lungs, with the remainder being shunted across the ductus arteriosus to the descending aorta and then back to the placenta. An abrupt change in the pulmonary circulation occurs at birth. With the first breath, expansion of the lungs and the abrupt rise in the partial pressure of oxygen (PO_2) of blood lead to a reversal of pulmonary arteriolar vasoconstriction and stretching and dilation of muscular pulmonary arteries and arterioles, with a marked drop in vascular resistance. This decreased resistance facilitates a large increase in pulmonary blood flow and raises left atrial volume and pressure. The latter closes the flap valve of the foramen ovale, and interatrial right-to-left shunting ordinarily ceases within the first hour of life. Normally, the ductus arteriosus closes over the next 10 hours as a result of contraction of the thick smooth muscle bundles within its wall in response to rising arterial oxygen tension and a change in the prostaglandin milieu. Following the initial dramatic fall in pulmonary vascular resistance at birth, a continuous decline occurs over the first few months of life, associated with thinning of the media of muscular pulmonary arteries and arterioles until the normal adult pattern is achieved.

AGING. In older adults, the main pulmonary artery becomes mildly dilated, and shallow atheromas may develop in the elastic pulmonary arteries. Mild medial thickening and eccentric intimal fibrosis may occur in the muscular pulmonary arteries; the capillaries become slightly thicker and the veins are frequently involved by intimal hyalinization, with mild luminal narrowing. Pulmonary artery pressure and pulmonary vascular resistance increase with advanced age. Changes in the pulmonary arteries are also affected by the reduced compliance of left ventricular filling with age that is reflected back in the pulmonary vascular bed.

EXERCISE. With moderate exercise, a large increase in pulmonary blood flow is normally accompanied by only a small increase in pulmonary artery pressure. Exercise results in an increase in left atrial pressure that is progressive with exercise intensity and accounts for most of the increase in observed pulmonary arterial pressure. This

TABLE 78-1	Hemodynamic Comparison of the Pulmonary and Systemic Circulations			
	Pulmonary Circulation		Systemic Circulation	
PARAMETER	RANGE	MEAN	RANGE	MEAN
Arterial pressure, mm Hg	25/10	15	120/80	90
Capillary pressure, mm Hg	6-9	7	10-30	17
Venous pressure, mm Hg	1-4	2	0-10	6
Arterial M/D ratio, %*	3-7	5	15-25	20
Venous M/D ratio, %*	2-5	3	3-6	5
Vascular resistance, units	1-4	3	10-25	15
Blood flow, liter/min	4-6	5	4-6	5

*M/D ratio = ratio of the medial thickness to the external diameter of the vessel.

marked effect of downstream pressure on upstream pressure is unique to the lung circulation. Because of the high vascular compliance in the normal lung microcirculation, an increase in left atrial pressure that results from the increased flow will act to distend the small vessels, contributing to the fall in pulmonary vascular resistance during exercise.

ALTITUDE. Life at high altitudes is associated with pulmonary hypertension of variable severity, reflecting the range of susceptibilities of different persons to the pulmonary vasoconstrictive effect of chronic hypoxia. Altitude decreases the inspired PO_2 because of a decrease in barometric pressure. At sea level, PO_2 is on average 150 mm Hg. At high altitudes (3000 to 5500 m), PO_2 decreases to 80 to 100 mm Hg and, and at extreme altitudes (5500 to 8840 m), PO_2 decreases to 40 to 80 mm Hg. Corresponding alveolar PO_2 (PAO_2) and arterial PO_2 (PaO_2) depend on the hypoxic ventilatory response and associated respiratory alkalosis. Mild pulmonary hypertension in adults living at high altitudes occurs at rest and may increase substantially with exercise.[2] It is not immediately reversed by breathing of oxygen, does not seem to limit exercise capacity, and is rarely the cause of right ventricular failure. Severe pulmonary hypertension may occur with high-altitude pulmonary edema, subacute mountain sickness, and chronic mountain sickness. Transient right ventricular dysfunction has also been described with strenuous exercise at high altitudes.

Regulation of Pulmonary Vascular Tone and Blood Flow

ALVEOLAR OXYGENATION. Changes in alveolar oxygenation affect the small pulmonary arteries and arterioles by direct gaseous diffusion from the alveoli, respiratory bronchioles, and alveolar ducts in the pulmonary arterioles, even though the latter are upstream in relation to the alveoli. This fact, taken together with evidence for a reduction in pulmonary arterial blood volume during hypoxia, supports the view that the small pulmonary arteries and arterioles are the main sites of vasoconstriction and increased resistance in the pulmonary circulation during hypoxia. Although alveolar oxygen tension is a major physiologic determinant of pulmonary arteriolar tone, a reduction in oxygen tension in the mixed venous blood flowing through the small pulmonary arteries and arterioles may also contribute to pulmonary arterial vasoconstriction.[3]

The effect of oxygen on the pulmonary vasculature is the most distinctive characteristic by which it differs from the systemic vasculature. The hypoxic pulmonary vasoconstrictor response is an important adaptive mechanism in human physiology. Alveolar hypoxia results in local vasoconstriction so that blood flow is shunted away from hypoxic regions toward better ventilated areas of the lung, improving the ventilation-perfusion matching in the lung. Although the acute effects of this response are beneficial, chronic hypoxemia can result in sustained elevation of pulmonary artery pressure, vascular remodeling,

and development of pulmonary arterial hypertension (PAH). The response of smooth muscle cells in the pulmonary arteries to hypoxia begins within seconds. Hypoxia causes pulmonary vascular smooth muscle membrane depolarization and inhibition of potassium currents (Kv 1.5 channels) as a result of changes in the membrane redox status. Increased calcium ion (Ca^{2+}) entry into the vascular smooth muscle cells via Ca^{2+} (L-type) channels also mediates hypoxic pulmonary vasoconstriction. Within the cell, Ca^{2+} can be mobilized from the sarcoplasmic reticulum and mitochondrial membrane, or the inner aspect of the cell membrane. Pulmonary vascular tone is also modulated by the balance between local kinase and phosphatase activities.

Whereas acute hypoxia causes reversible changes in vascular tone, chronic hypoxia induces structural remodeling and is mediated by a number of growth factors. The endothelial cell manifests marked changes in permeability, coagulant, inflammatory, and protein synthetic capabilities in response to chronic hypoxic exposure. Distinct smooth muscle cell populations with membrane-bound receptors sensitive to hypoxic activation engage specific intracellular signaling pathways, conferring unique hypoxic proliferative responses. Vascular endothelial growth factor (VEGF), an endothelial cell-specific mitogen, is upregulated during exposure to chronic hypoxia; this is thought to be a protective mechanism. Hypoxia-inducible factor-1α (HIF-1α) has been identified as a nuclear factor that is induced by hypoxia and bound to a site in the erythropoietin response element. HIF-1α represents a vital link between oxygen sensing, gene transcription, and the physiologic adaptation to chronic hypoxia in vivo. Expression of HIF-1α is tightly regulated by cellular oxygen tension. Acidosis increases pulmonary vascular resistance and acts synergistically with hypoxia. In contrast, an increase in arterial PCO_2 seems to exert no direct effect but rather operates by way of the induced increase in hydrogen ion concentration. Hypoxia and acidemia frequently coexist and their interaction, which is clinically important, follows a predictable pattern.

NITRIC OXIDE. Nitric oxide (NO) relaxes vascular smooth muscle by raising levels of cyclic guanosine monophosphate (cGMP).[4] Endothelial NO synthase is found in the vascular endothelium of the normal pulmonary vasculature, where it generates NO to regulate vascular tone. Release of NO occurs in response to a multitude of physiologic stimuli, including thrombin and shear stress. In addition to its direct hemodynamic effects, NO inhibits platelet activation and confers an important antithrombotic property on the endothelial surface. NO also inhibits the growth of vascular smooth muscle cells and is probably involved in vascular remodeling in response to injury. NO is also important in the signal transduction of angiogenesis in that VEGF receptor activation results in increased NO production.

ADRENERGIC CONTROL. The pulmonary vasculature expresses both alpha and beta adrenoreceptors, which help regulate pulmonary vascular tone by producing vasoconstriction or vasodilation, respectively. Alpha$_1$ adrenoreceptors in the pulmonary arteries have increased affinity and responsiveness to their agonists when compared with other vessels. The downstream signaling events in alpha$_1$-adrenergic stimulation are an increase in Ca^{2+} levels and activation of protein kinase, which mediate vascular contractile and proliferative responses. The increased sensitivity of alpha$_1$ adrenoreceptors to norepinephrine in the pulmonary arteries may facilitate local regulation of vascular tone in response to acute changes in oxygen concentrations, thereby adjusting regional perfusion. Excessive stimulation of alpha$_1$-adrenergic receptors produces smooth muscle contraction, proliferation, and growth.

Pathobiology of Pulmonary Arterial Hypertension

By definition, the precise cause of idiopathic pulmonary arterial hypertension (IPAH) is unknown, but it likely represents the clinical expression of PAH as the final common pathway from multiple biologic abnormalities in the pulmonary circulation.[5] Our understanding of the underlying pathobiology of pulmonary hypertension associated with clinical disease states has become increasingly complex as a multitude of genetic and molecular pathways have been identified.[6] Overall, it appears that varying degrees of thrombosis, vasoconstriction, vascular proliferation, and inflammation underlie chronic PAH. The initiating cell line remains unclear, but abnormalities in pulmonary endothelial cell (EC) function and pulmonary artery smooth muscle cells (PASMCs) may cause or contribute to the development of pulmonary hypertension in humans.[7] Disease progression is invariably accompanied by worsening of cellular function, which itself can further promote disease progression.

THROMBOSIS. The observation that chronic warfarin anticoagulation has been associated with a marked survival advantage in several longitudinal studies lends support to the important role of thrombosis in PAH.[8] Several lines of evidence point to the widespread development of in situ thrombosis of the small pulmonary arteries, with intraluminal thrombin deposition as an important causative feature of PAH. In studies of pulmonary vascular histopathology in IPAH, the prevalence rates of thrombotic lesions were more than 50%.[9] The promotion of PAH through the coagulation and fibrinolytic systems is likely a result of endothelial dysfunction. Thrombin appears to play a key role. Receptors for thrombin are present on ECs and PASMCs. Thrombin activation directly upregulates angiogenesis-related genes, including VEGF, VEGF receptors, tissue factor (TF), basic fibroblast growth factor (bFGF), and matrix metalloproteinase-2, all of which have been reported to be increased in PAH.[10,11] Thrombin indirectly upregulates the transcription of VEGF by inducing the production of reactive oxygen species (ROS) and the expression of the HIF-1α transcription factor. Thrombin also activates platelets.

There is increased expression of TF in the vasculature of patients with severe PAH. TF activation leads to rapid initiation of coagulation when a vessel is damaged and is involved in the migration and proliferation of PASMCs (**Fig. 78-1**). TF can induce angiogenesis by clotting-dependent mechanisms via thrombin generation and fibrin deposition.[12] Plasma levels of fibrinopeptide A, a byproduct and marker of fibrin generation, are elevated in PAH patients.

Abnormalities in platelet activation and function also occur in PAH. In addition to promoting thrombosis, platelet activation leads to the release of granules that contain mitogenic and vasoconstrictive substances, including VEGF, bFGF, platelet-derived growth factor (PDGF), and serotonin, which contribute to increased endothelial cell proliferation and migration.

VASOCONSTRICTION. The initial report of a patient with IPAH demonstrated a reversible fall in PA pressure in response to intravenous vasodilators. As a result, PAH has traditionally been thought of as a disease of inappropriate pulmonary vasoconstriction. However, clinical experiences from multiple registries and large referral centers have documented that reversible vasoconstriction plays an important role in less than 20% of patients with PAH.[13] Although it has not been possible to relate the presence of vasoreactivity specifically to the vascular changes noted on histology, one study reported a qualitative relationship in patients, showing that those with more advanced lesions had a reduced likelihood to respond to acute vasodilator testing.

An important concept in the pathobiology of PAH is that the disease develops in patients with an underlying genetic predisposition following exposure to specific stimuli, which serve as triggers. The finding of increased pulmonary vascular reactivity and vasoconstriction in patients with IPAH suggests that a vasoconstrictive tendency underlies the development of IPAH in predisposed individuals. Voltage-dependent and calcium-dependent potassium channels found throughout the pulmonary vascular bed (see Chap. 52) modulate pulmonary vascular tone. Inhibition of the voltage-regulated potassium channel by hypoxia or drugs can produce vasoconstriction and has been described in PASMCs harvested from patients with IPAH.[14] It has been suggested that abnormalities in the potassium channel of PASMCs are involved in the initiation or progression of pulmonary hypertension[15] (**Fig. 78-2**).

VASCULAR PROLIFERATION. A striking feature of the pulmonary vasculature in patients with PAH is intimal proliferation, which in some vessels causes complete vascular occlusion. Several growth factors have been implicated in the development of this type of vascular pathology. Enhanced growth factor release, activation, and intracellular signaling may lead to PASMC proliferation and migration, as well as extracellular matrix synthesis.[16] Even advanced lesions show evidence of in situ activity of ongoing synthesis of connective tissue proteins such as elastin, collagen, and fibronectin. In PAH, PASMCs have abnormalities that favor decreased apoptosis and enhanced proliferation. The impaired apoptosis appears to be multifactorial, related to abnormal mitochondrial hyperpolarization, activation of transcription factors such as HIF-1α[17] and the nuclear factor of activated T cells (NFAT),[18] and de novo expression of the antiapoptotic protein survivin.[19] The PASMCs in PAH also display excessive proliferation in response to transforming growth factor-β (TGF-β), which is exacerbated by impaired smooth muscle cell apoptosis.[20] Other processes,

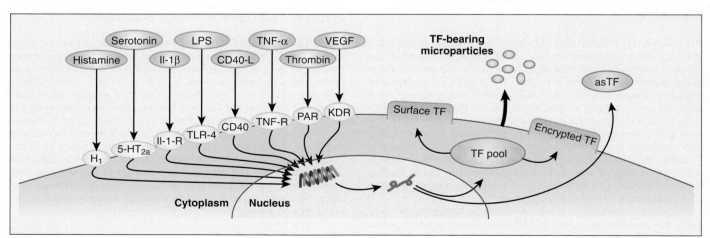

FIGURE 78-1 Molecular mechanisms of thrombosis-mediated remodeling. Induction of tissue factor (TF) is exemplified in an endothelial cell. Various mediators induce TF expression through activation of their receptors. Induction of TF primarily occurs at the transcriptional level, resulting in an increase in TF mRNA and, eventually, in TF protein expression. TF is distributed in three cellular pools as cytoplasmic TF, surface TF, and encrypted TF. Moreover, TF-containing microparticles are released from the cell. Alternative splicing results in a soluble secreted form of TF (asTF). CD40-L = CD40-ligand; H$_1$ = histamine H1 receptor; 5-HT$_{2a}$ = 5-hydroxytryptamine 2a receptor; IL-1-R = interleukin-1 receptor; KDR = VEGF receptor 2; LPS = lipopolysaccharide; PAR = protease-activated receptor; TLR-4 = Toll-like receptor 4; TNF-R = tumor necrosis factor receptor. *(From Steffel J, Lüscher TF, Tanner FC: Tissue factor in cardiovascular diseases: Molecular mechanisms and clinical implications. Circulation 113:722, 2006.)*

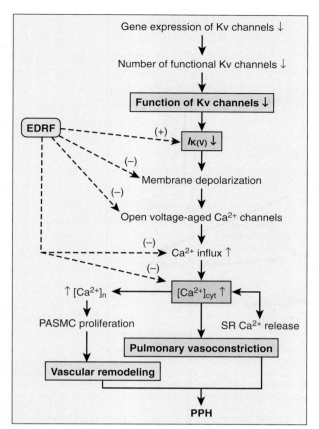

FIGURE 78-2 Molecular mechanisms of vasoconstriction-mediated remodeling. The process may be initiated by abnormal gene transcription and expression of Kv channels. Resultant reduction of Kv currents [$I_{K(v)}$] causes membrane depolarization and opens voltage-gated Ca^{2+} channels. Increased Ca^{2+} influx through sarcolemmal Ca^{2+} channels and Ca^{2+}-induced Ca^{2+} release from intracellular Ca^{2+} stores (mainly sarcoplasmic reticulum [SR]) raise cytoplasmic Ca^{2+} concentrations ([Ca^{2+}]$_{cyt}$), which triggers pulmonary vasoconstriction. An increase in [Ca^{2+}]$_{cyt}$ would also increase nuclear Ca^{2+} concentration ([Ca^{2+}]$_n$) and stimulate cell proliferation, which causes pulmonary vascular remodeling. Endothelium-derived relaxing factors (EDRFs) may participate in regulating Em and [Ca^{2+}]$_{cyt}$ through activation of K^+ (KCa and Kv) channels and/or inhibition of voltage-gated Ca^{2+} channels in PASMCs. (+) = increase (or enhance); (−) = decrease (or inhibit). *(From Yuan J, Aldinger A, Juhaszova M, et al: Dysfunctional voltage-gated K+ channels in pulmonary artery smooth muscle cells of patients with primary pulmonary hypertension. Circulation 98:1400, 1998.)*

such as mitochondrial and ion channel dysregulation, seem to convey a state of cellular resistance to apoptosis; this has recently emerged as a necessary event in the pathogenesis of pulmonary vascular remodeling.

Animal and human data point to a key role for serotonin in PAH (**Fig. 78-3**). Serotonin is an important constituent of platelet-dense granules and is released on activation. It is a vasoconstrictor that promotes smooth muscle cell hypertrophy and hyperplasia by exerting mitogenic effects on PASMCs.[21] Elevated plasma levels of serotonin and reduced platelet serotonin concentration have been described in IPAH patients. One series reported increased serotonin levels in patients with PAH associated with the use of fenfluramine and with connective tissue disease. Data indicate that the serotonin transporter (SERT) in the lung is a key determinant of pulmonary vessel remodeling because of its effects on PASMC growth.[22,23] The SERT is abundantly expressed in the lung and appears specific to PASMCs, because no similar effect has been reported with other SMC types. Mutations in the SERT and 5-hydroxytryptamine 2B receptor have now been reported in patients with IPAH.[24]

INFLAMMATION. The frequent association of PAH in well-defined inflammatory conditions, as well as the presence of PAH associated

with connective tissue diseases (CTDs; see Chap. 89), indicate a role for vascular inflammation leading remodeling of the vessel in PAH[25,26] (**Fig. 78-4**). Macrophages and both T and B lymphocytes are present in the vascular lesions of IPAH and PAH related to CTD and human immunodeficiency virus (HIV; see Chap. 72). Inflammatory infiltrates have been identified in plexiform lesions in the lungs of patients with severe IPAH and mononuclear inflammatory cells surround vascular sites of plexiform growth in patients with scleroderma-related PAH. Autoantibodies from patients with CTD have been shown to induce upregulation of immunoactive molecules, such as intercellular adhesion molecule-1, endothelial leukocyte adhesion molecule-1, and major histocompatibility complex class II, on human pulmonary ECs. The nuclear factor of activated T-cells (NFAT) increases the transcription of multiple inflammatory mediators and activating T and B cells.[18] NFAT activation causes myocardial downregulation of Kv1.5, and NFATc2-activated circulating inflammatory cells are found in the blood and pulmonary arterial wall in PAH patients. Several interleukins and tumor necrosis factor-α are increased in patients with PAH,[27] and many of these cytokines are regulated by NFAT.

Inflammation has been observed in affected vessels in HIV patients with PAH, although development of severe PAH seems to be unrelated to the degree of immune deficiency. HIV patients with PAH also had significantly higher autoantibody levels than a matched HIV non-PAH control group. Similarly, the presence of circulating chemokines and cytokines, viral protein components (e.g., HIV-1 Nef), and increased expression of growth factors (e.g., VEGF, PDGF) in these patients are thought to contribute directly to further recruitment of inflammatory cells.[28] Many IPAH patients without immunodeficiency or other associated systemic diseases have evidence of autoimmunity and/or active inflammation. These include detectable levels of antinuclear antibodies, elevated serum levels of the proinflammatory cytokines interleukin-1 (IL-1) and IL-6, and increased pulmonary expression of PDGF or macrophage inflammatory protein-1. Clinically, there is also an association of IPAH with autoimmune thyroid disease

Cellular Pathology of Pulmonary Arterial Hypertension

Morphologic abnormalities in each cell line of the pulmonary vasculature have been described in PAH[29] (**Fig. 78-5**). Although endothelial dysfunction has been described in PAH, it is not known at what stage during the evolution of PAH that EC proliferation occurs. It has been proposed, however, that a somatic mutation rather than nonselective cell proliferation in response to injury accounts for the growth advantage of ECs in patients with IPAH. Heterogeneity in the PASMC and fibroblast populations also contributes to discordance between phenotype and function. Interconversion between cell types (fibroblast to smooth muscle cell, or endothelium to smooth muscle cell), in addition to neovascularization, may occur. PASMC hypertrophy and increased connective tissue and extracellular matrix are found in the large muscular and elastic arteries. In the subendothelial layer, increased thickness may be the result of recruitment and/or proliferation of smooth muscle-like cells. It is possible that precursor smooth muscle cells are in a continuous layer in the subendothelial layer along the entire pulmonary artery. These cells are similar to the pericytes responsible for the appearance of muscle in normally nonmuscular arteries and that contribute to intimal thickening in larger arteries. Alterations in the extracellular matrix secondary to proteolytic enzymes also play a role in the pathology of PAH. Matrix-degrading enzymes can release mitogenically active growth factors that stimulate PASMC proliferation. In addition, elastase and matrix metalloproteinases contribute to the upregulation of proliferation. Degradation of elastin has also been shown to stimulate upregulation of the glycoprotein fibronectin, which in turn stimulates smooth muscle cell migration.

The most common vascular changes in PAH are characterized as a hypertensive pulmonary arteriopathy, which is present in 85% of cases (**Table 78-2**). These changes involve medial hypertrophy of the arteries and arterioles, often in conjunction with other vascular changes. Isolated medial hypertrophy is uncommon and, when present, has

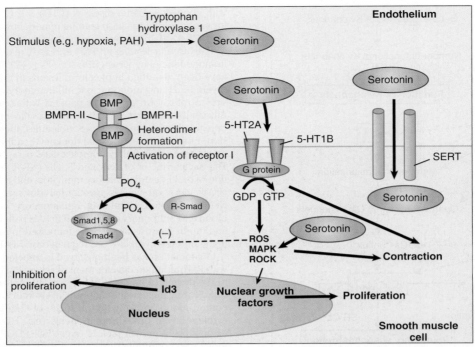

FIGURE 78-3 Molecular mechanisms of cellular proliferation–mediated remodeling. Serotonin synthesis via tryptophan hydroxylase 1 acts in a paracrine fashion on underlying PASMCs. Serotonin enters PASMC via SERT and signal transduction is initiated involving SERT-dependent generation of reactive oxygen species (ROS), rho kinase (ROCK), and mitogen-activated protein kinases (MAPK). This may contribute to contraction or, via nuclear translocation of pERK1/2, increase the expression of nuclear growth factors such as GATA 4, leading to proliferation. Serotonin may also stimulate 5-hydroxytryptamine (5-HT) 1A and 2B receptors to induce contraction and ROS, ROCK, and MAPK activation. Signaling by wild-type BMPRII involves heterodimerization with the transmembrane serine-threonine kinases type I BMPR-IA and BMPR-IB receptors at the cell membrane. On ligand binding, the constitutively active BMPR-II phosphorylates the type I receptor. Activated type I receptors phosphorylate the cytoplasmic signaling proteins known as receptor-mediated Smads (R-Smads) 1, 5, and 8. These complex with Smad4 and translocate to the nucleus, where they activate downstream target genes such as the inhibitors of DNA binding 3 (Ids), which inhibit proliferation. Serotonin may antagonize the antiproliferative BMPR-II/Smad 1, 5, 8 pathway, inhibit Id3 activation, and facilitate proliferation. (−) = inhibitory effect. *(From MacLean MR, Dempsie Y: Serotonin and pulmonary hypertension—from bench to bedside? Curr Opin Pharmacol 9:281, 2009.)*

been assumed to represent an early stage of the disease. The intimal proliferation may appear as concentric laminar intimal fibrosis, eccentric intimal fibrosis, or concentric nonlaminar intimal fibrosis. The frequency of these findings differs from case to case and within regions of the same lung in the same patient. In addition, plexiform and dilation lesions, as well as a necrotizing arteritis, may be seen throughout the lungs. The fundamental nature of the plexiform lesion remains a mystery. Morphologically, it represents a mass of disorganized vessels with proliferating ECs, PASMCs, myofibroblasts, and macrophages. Whether the plexiform lesion represents impaired proliferation or angiogenesis remains unclear (**Fig. 78-6**).

The other major pattern of vascular changes in PAH is that of a thrombotic pulmonary arteriopathy. Typical features include medial hypertrophy of the arteries and arterioles, with both eccentric and concentric nonlaminar intimal fibrosis. The presence of colander lesions, which represent recanalized thrombi, is also typical. These lesions are believed to arise as a result of primary in situ thrombosis of the small vascular arteries and not from recurrent pulmonary embolism. Many patients have characteristics of both patterns of arteriopathy in varying degrees. This suggests that the vascular changes from PAH occur across a spectrum and are likely influenced by genetic and environmental factors.

Role of Genetics in Pulmonary Arterial Hypertension

An important concept in the development of PAH is that the disease develops in patients with an underlying genetic predisposition following exposure to specific stimuli, which serve as triggers.[30] Predisposition to the development of pulmonary hypertension has been noted by the marked heterogeneity in responses of the pulmonary

vasculature in various disease states. Examples include the considerable variability among individuals to vasoconstrictive stimuli such as hypoxia or acidosis, which can produce marked pulmonary hypertension in one person and be essentially without effect in another. Also, the severity of pulmonary hypertension and level of pulmonary vascular resistance vary considerably among individuals with congenital heart disease and comparably sized ventricular septal defects.

Using linkage analysis, the locus designated PPH-1 on chromosome 2q33 led to the discovery of the PPH-1 gene.[31] The bone morphogenetic protein receptor type II gene (*BMPR-II*) codes for a receptor member of the TGF-β family (**Fig. 78-7**). *BMPR-II* modulates vascular cell growth by activating the intracellular pathways of Smad and LIM kinase. The mutations ascribed to the locus interrupt the BMP-mediated signaling pathway, resulting in a predisposition to proliferation rather than apoptosis of cells in small pulmonary arteries.[32] These molecular studies have suggested that the target cells within the pulmonary arterial wall are sensitive to *BMPR-II* gene dosage and that the TGF-β pathway mediated through *BMPR-II* is critical for the maintenance and/or normal response to injury of the pulmonary vasculature. It is clear, however, that additional factors, environmental or genetic, are required in the pathogenesis of the disease.[33] Recent data have supported the hypothesis that the dominant genetic mechanism underlying PAH is haploinsufficiency for *BMPR-II*.[34] How defects in BMPR-II contribute to EC proliferation, PASMC hypertrophy, and fibroblast deposition in patients with PAH remains unclear. It is interesting to note that about one in four cases of IPAH actually have germline mutations in the gene encoding the *BMPR-II* receptor.[35] Patients with hereditary hemorrhagic telangiectasia and IPAH have been described and found to have mutations of the *ALK1* gene, also within the TGF-β superfamily.

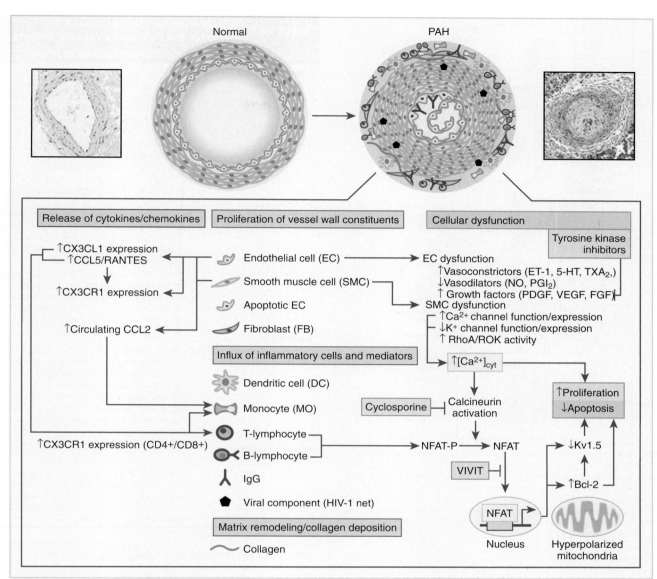

FIGURE 78-4 Molecular mechanisms of inflammation-mediated remodeling. This schematic features inflammatory mediators, cells, and mechanisms involved in pulmonary vascular remodeling as well as potential therapeutic targets. Release of cytokines and chemokines in remodeled vessels (e.g., plexiform lesions) or in the circulation, from activated ECs and smooth muscle cells (SMCs), mediate the influx of inflammatory cells (e.g., monocytes, T and B lymphocytes). Cellular dysfunction (particularly involving ECs and SMCs) contributes to the release of vasomotor and growth mediators, activation of transcriptional factors (e.g., nuclear factor of activated T lymphocytes [NFAT]), influx of calcium, and mitochondrial dysfunction. The net effect is a shift of balance in favor of cell proliferation and decreased apoptosis, leading to remodeling and narrowing of the pulmonary vascular lumen. Potential therapeutic target sites include inhibition of growth factors with tyrosine kinase inhibitors, calcineurin with cyclosporine, and prevention of NFAT activation with VIVIT polypeptide, a competitive peptide that inhibits the docking of NFAT to calcineurin. Specific mechanisms are detailed further in the text. bcl2 = B-cell lymphoma 2; CCL2 = chemokine (C-C motif) ligand 2; CCL5 = chemokine (C-C motif) ligand 5 or RANTES (**r**egulated upon **a**ctivation, **n**ormal **T** cell **e**xpressed and **s**ecreted); CX3CL1 = chemokine (C-X3-C motif) ligand 1 (fractalkine); CX3CR1 = chemokine (C-X3-C motif) receptor 1; DC = dendritic cells; FB = fibroblasts; FGF = fibroblast growth factor; 5-HT = serotonin; HIV-1 = human immunodeficiency virus 1; IgG = immunoglobulin G; MO = monocyte; PGI2 = prostacyclin; ROK = rho kinase. *(From Hassoun PM, Mouthon L, Barbera JA, et al: Inflammation, growth factors, and pulmonary vascular remodeling. J Am Coll Cardiol 54:S10, 2009.)*

Other genetic factors that have been associated with PAH suggest that polymorphisms in other genes could contribute to the development of PAH. The overexpression of SERT in pulmonary arteries and platelets from patients with PAH has been reported, with the increased activity of SERT responsible for the associated PASMC hyperplasia.[36] In addition, increased PASMC proliferation is related to SERT expression and activity in cultured PASMCs from patients with PAH. SERT is encoded by a single gene on chromosome 17q11.2, and a variant in the upstream promotor region of the SERT gene has been described. This polymorphism, with long (L) and short (S) forms, affects SERT expression and function, with the L allele inducing a greater rate of SERT gene transcription than the S allele. One study has shown that the L-allelic variant is found to be present in homozygous form in 65% of IPAH patients but in only 27% of control subjects.

Clinical Assessment of Patients with Suspected Pulmonary Hypertension

History

A careful and detailed history of the patient with suspected pulmonary hypertension is often revealing. Because the earliest symptoms in patients with pulmonary hypertension are manifest with exercise,

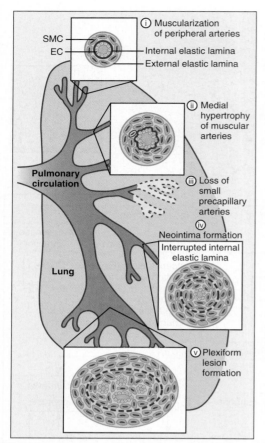

i Muscularization
of peripheral arteries

SMC
EC
Internal elastic lamina
External elastic lamina

ii Medial
hypertrophy
of muscular
arteries

**Pulmonary
circulation**

iii Loss of
small
precapillary
arteries

iv Neointima formation
Interrupted internal
elastic lamina

Lung

v Plexiform
lesion
formation

FIGURE 78-5 Vascular abnormalities associated with pulmonary hypertension. Shown are the abnormalities throughout the pulmonary circulation, including abnormal muscularization of distal precapillary arteries (i), medial hypertrophy (thickening) of large pulmonary muscular arteries (ii), loss of precapillary arteries (iii), neointima formation that is particularly occlusive in vessels 100 to 500 μM in size (iv), and formation of plexiform lesions in these vessels (v). (*From Rabinovitch M: Molecular pathogenesis of pulmonary arterial hypertension. J Clin Invest 118:2372, 2008.*)

TABLE 78-2	Histopathologic Classification of Hypertensive Pulmonary Vascular Disease
CLASSIFICATION	**CHARACTERISTIC FEATURES**
Arteriopathy	
Isolated medial hypertrophy*	Medial hypertrophy—increase of medial muscle in muscular arteries, muscularization of nonmuscularized arterioles; no appreciable intimal or luminal obstructive lesions; no plexiform lesions
Plexogenic	Plexiform and dilation lesions; medial hypertrophy; pulmonary eccentric or concentric laminar and nonlaminar arteriopathy, arteriopathy, intimal thickening; fibrinoid necrosis, arteritis, and thrombotic lesions
Thrombotic	Thrombi (fresh, organizing, or organized and pulmonary colander lesions); eccentric and concentric nonlaminar arteriopathy, intimal thickening, varying degrees of medial hypertrophy; no plexiform lesions
Isolated pulmonary arteritis	Active or healed arteritis, limited to pulmonary arteries; varying pulmonary degrees of medial hypertrophy, intimal fibrosis, and thrombotic arteritis lesions; no plexiform lesions; no systemic arteritis
Venopathy	
Pulmonary venoocclusive disease	Eccentric intimal fibrosis and recanalized thrombi in diseased pulmonary veins and venules; arterialized veins, capillary congestion, alveolar edema and siderophages, dilated lymphatics, pleural and septal edema, and arterial medial hypertrophy; intimal thickening and thrombotic lesions
Microangiopathy	
Pulmonary capillary hemangiomatosis	Infiltrating thin-walled blood vessels throughout pulmonary parenchyma, pleura, bronchi, and walls of pulmonary veins and arteries; medial hypertrophy and intimal thickening of muscular pulmonary arteries and arterioles

*Medial hypertrophy includes muscularization of arterioles.
From Pietra GG: Pathology of primary pulmonary hypertension. *In* Rubin LJ, Rich S (eds): Primary Pulmonary Hypertension. New York, Marcel Dekker, 1997, pp 19-61.

pulmonary hypertension can have an insidious onset. With the onset of right ventricular failure, lower extremity edema from venous congestion is characteristic. Angina is also common, likely reflecting reduced coronary blood flow to a markedly hypertrophied right ventricle.[37] As the cardiac output becomes fixed and eventually falls, patients may have episodes of syncope or near-syncope. Patients with pulmonary hypertension related to left ventricular diastolic dysfunction will characteristically have orthopnea and paroxysmal nocturnal dyspnea. Patients with underlying lung disease may also report episodes of coughing. Hemoptysis is relatively uncommon in patients with pulmonary hypertension and may be associated with underlying thromboembolism and pulmonary infarction. Some patients with advanced mitral stenosis also present with hemoptysis (see Chap. 66).

Physical Examination

Cardiovascular findings consistent with pulmonary hypertension and right ventricular pressure overload include a large a wave in the jugular venous pulse, low-volume carotid arterial pulse with a normal upstroke, left parasternal (right ventricular) heave, systolic pulsation produced by a dilated pulmonary artery in the second left interspace, ejection click and flow murmur in the same area, narrowly split second heart sound with a loud pulmonic component, and fourth heart sound of right ventricular origin. Late in the course, signs of

right ventricular failure (e.g., hepatomegaly, peripheral edema, ascites) may be present. Patients with severe pulmonary hypertension may also have prominent v waves in the jugular venous pulse as a result of tricuspid regurgitation, third heart sound of right ventricular origin, a high-pitched early diastolic murmur of pulmonic regurgitation, and holosystolic murmur of tricuspid regurgitation. Tricuspid regurgitation is a reflection of right ventricular dilation. Cyanosis is a late finding and, unless the patient has associated lung disease, is usually attributable to a markedly reduced cardiac output, with systemic vasoconstriction and ventilation-perfusion mismatch in the lung. Uncommonly, the left laryngeal nerve becomes paralyzed as a consequence of compression by a dilated pulmonary artery (Ortner syndrome).

Diagnostic Tests

LABORATORY TESTS. The results of these studies (**Table 78-3**) are usually normal in patients with pulmonary hypertension. If chronic arterial oxygen desaturation exists, polycythemia should be present. Hypercoagulable states, abnormal platelet function, defects in fibrinolysis, and other abnormalities of coagulation are found in some patients with PAH. Brain natriuretic peptide (BNP) levels are elevated in patients with pulmonary hypertension and correlate with the pulmonary artery pressure.[38] Uric acid levels are elevated in patients with

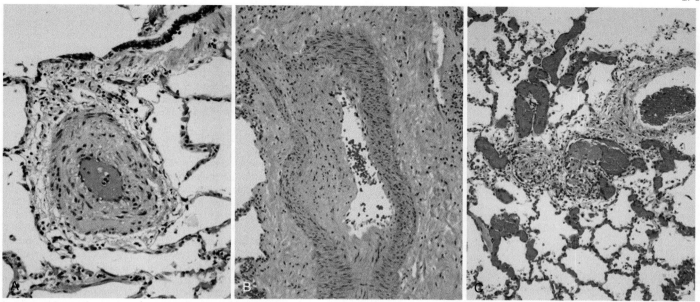

FIGURE 78-6 Photomicrographs of PA histologic lesions seen in cases of clinically unexplained pulmonary hypertension. **A,** Medical hypertrophy with intimal proliferation. The vascular lumen is markedly reduced, contributing to the elevated resistance. **B,** Eccentric intimal fibrosis. These are believed to be related to local thrombin deposition. **C,** Plexiform lesion demonstrating obstruction in the arterial lumen, aneurysmal dilation, and proliferation of anastomosing vascular channels. Hematoxolyn and cosin stains. **A** and **B,** magnification ×20; **C,** magnification ×4.

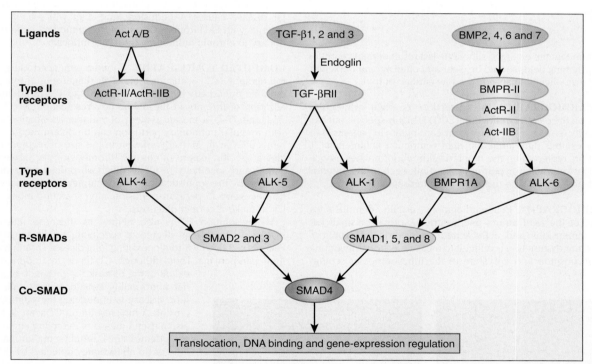

FIGURE 78-7 Transforming growth factor-β (TGF-β) signaling pathway. TGF ligands bind to a range of type II receptors to form complexes that interact with type I receptors. The receptors then form heterotetramers, which result in the phosphorylation and activation of receptor-regulated SMADs (R-SMADs) that subsequently form complexes with the common SMAD (Co-SMAD) SMAD4. This complex translocates to the nucleus, where it regulates gene transcription directly or indirectly. Endoglin is a coreceptor for both TGF-1 and TGF-3. Act = activin; ActR = activin receptor; ALK = activin-like kinase; TGF-R = TGF receptor. *(From Waite KA, Eng C: Developmental disorder to heritable cancer: It's all in the BMP/TGF family. Nat Rev Genet 4:763, 2003.)*

pulmonary hypertension and correlate with hemodynamics. Although the mechanism is uncertain, it may relate to overproduction and impaired uric acid excretion caused by the low cardiac output and tissue hypoxia. There is an increased incidence of thyroid disease in patients with PAH (see Chap. 86), which can mimic the symptoms of right ventricular failure.[39] Consequently, it is advised that thyroid function tests be monitored serially in all patients.

CHEST RADIOGRAPHY. A chest radiograph (see Chap. 16) shows enlargement of the main pulmonary artery and its major branches, with marked tapering of peripheral arteries. The right ventricle and atrium may also be enlarged. Dilation of the right ventricle gives the heart a globular appearance, but right ventricular hypertrophy or dilation is not easily discernible on a plain chest radiograph. Encroachment of the retrosternal air space on the lateral film may be a helpful

TABLE 78-3	Clues for Interpretation of Diagnostic Tests for Pulmonary Hypertension
TEST	**NOTABLE FINDINGS**
Chest x-ray	Enlargement of central pulmonary arteries reflects level of PA pressure and duration
Electrocardiography	Right axis deviation and precordial T wave abnormalities are early signs.
Pulmonary function tests	Elevated pulmonary artery pressure causes restrictive physiology.
Perfusion lung scan	Nonsegmental perfusion abnormalities can occur from severe pulmonary vascular disease.
Chest computed scan	Minor interstitial changes may reflect diffuse disease; mosaic tomography perfusion pattern indicates thromboembolism and/or left heart failure.
Echocardiography	Right ventricular enlargement will parallel the severity of the pulmonary hypertension.
Contrast echocardiography	Minor right to left shunting rarely produces hypoxemia.
Doppler echocardiography	This is too unreliable for following serial measurements to monitor therapy
Exercise testing	This is very helpful to assess the efficacy of therapy. Severe exercise-induced hypoxemia should cause consideration of a right-to-left shunt.

sign to confirm that the enlarged silhouette is a result of right ventricular dilation. The lung fields should be clear and often appear darkened from the relative oligemia caused by a low cardiac output.

ELECTROCARDIOGRAPHY. The detection of right ventricular hypertrophy on the electrocardiogram (ECG) is highly specific but has a low sensitivity (see Chap. 13). The electrocardiogram in patients with PAH usually exhibits right atrial and right ventricular enlargement. T wave inversion, representing the repolarization abnormalities associated with right ventricular hypertrophy, is usually seen in the anterior precordial leads and may be mistaken for anteroseptal ischemia.

ECHOCARDIOGRAPHY. Echocardiography usually demonstrates enlargement of the right atrium and ventricle, normal or small left ventricular dimensions, and a thickened interventricular septum.[40] Right ventricular dysfunction is difficult to measure echocardiographically, but the position and curvature of the intraventricular septum

provide an indication of right ventricular afterload. Echocardiographic findings that portend a poor prognosis include pericardial effusion and a markedly diminished left ventricular cavity. Doppler echocardiographic estimates of right ventricular systolic pressures can be obtained by measuring the velocity of the tricuspid regurgitant jet and by using the Bernoulli formula (see Chap. 15). Although Doppler measurements correlate with right ventricular systolic pressure, they are relatively imprecise (±20 mm Hg) and are not a substitute for catheterization if a correct measurement of pulmonary pressure is needed.[41]

PULMONARY FUNCTION TESTS. Although pulmonary function in patients with PAH is often completely normal, reductions in lung volumes of 20% are common, making the differentiation from interstitial lung disease on the basis of pulmonary function tests (PFTs) difficult.[40] A significant obstructive pattern is not characteristic and should suggest obstructive airways disease. In patients with PAH, the diffusing lung capacity for carbon monoxide (DLCO) is reduced to approximately 60% to 80% of that predicted. The presence of mild to moderate arterial hypoxemia is caused by ventilation-perfusion mismatch and/or reduced mixed venous oxygen saturations resulting from low cardiac output. A severe reduction of both pulmonary arterial and systemic arterial oxygen saturations can be caused by right-to-left intracardiac or extracardiac shunts and/or intrapulmonary shunts. Consequently, PaO_2 and SaO_2 may vary markedly among patients with different constellations of associated abnormalities.

LUNG SCINTIGRAPHY. Patients with PAH may reveal a relatively normal perfusion pattern or diffuse, patchy perfusion abnormalities (**Fig. 78-8**). The latter is associated with a variety of pulmonary vascular disease causes. A perfusion lung scan will reliably distinguish patients with PAH from those who have pulmonary hypertension secondary to chronic pulmonary thromboembolism

COMPUTED TOMOGRAPHY. Contrast enhanced chest computed tomography (CT) scans are helpful in diagnosing chronic thromboembolic pulmonary hypertension (see Chap. 19). In addition to visualization of thrombi in the pulmonary vasculature (see Figs. 19-23C, 77-4, and 77-7), a mosaic pattern of variable attenuation compatible with irregular pulmonary perfusion can be determined in the nonenhanced CT scan. Marked variation in the size of segmental vessels is also a specific feature of chronic thromboembolic disease. The sensitivity and specificity of CT to diagnose pulmonary embolism are affected by the sophistication of the scanner. In some patients, it may be necessary to perform perfusion lung scanning along with chest CT to make a correct diagnosis.

High-resolution CT is also helpful to diagnose interstitial lung disease. It has a high degree of specificity, but its sensitivity is low. Patients with PAH without coexisting lung disease should have normal lung parenchyma. Thus, although CT tends to underrepresent the extent of the disease, the presence of any interstitial abnormality should suggest that interstitial lung disease is underlying the pulmonary hypertension. A high-resolution CT scan of the chest is also a useful means of detecting emphysema and may demonstrate emphysema in patients with little or no abnormality detected by PFTs.

CARDIAC MAGNETIC RESONANCE IMAGING. Advances in magnetic resonance imaging technology (see Chap. 18) have led to the development of techniques for the assessment of hemodynamics in the pulmonary circulation and identification of right ventricular morphologic changes. Cardiovascular magnetic resonance (CMR) is now regarded as the reference standard for the assessment of right ventricular structure and function via the measurement of right ventricular volumes and ejection fraction, which makes CMR an attractive modality for serial follow-up in PAH management to determine

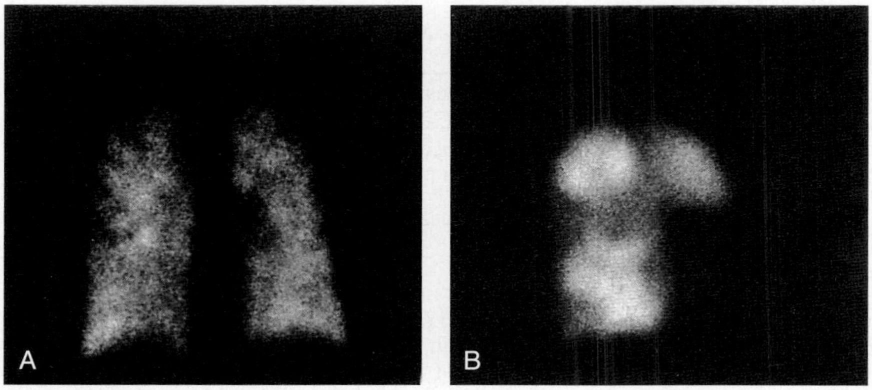

FIGURE 78-8 Perfusion lung scans in patients with pulmonary hypertension. **A,** Patient with IPAH. **B,** Patient with CTEPH. Both perfusion scans are abnormal. The scan in **A** shows a mottled distribution in a nonsegmental nonanatomic manner. The scan in **B** reveals lobar, segmental, and subsegmental defects, highly suggestive of an anatomic obstruction to pulmonary blood flow.

treatment response.[42] One study that used CMR to assess the response to continuous intravenous epoprostenol in IPAH patients over 1 year showed a significant increase in right ventricular stroke volume and reduction in pulmonary vascular resistance.

EXERCISE TESTING. The use of a symptom-limited exercise test (see Chap. 14) can be very helpful in the evaluation of patients with pulmonary hypertension. The 6-minute walk test is commonly used in clinical trials as an endpoint for the efficacy of therapy in patients with pulmonary hypertension.[43] It has been correlated with workload, heart rate, oxygen saturation, and dyspnea response. Its drawbacks include the fact that anthropometric factors such as gait speed, age, weight, muscle mass, and length of stride can affect the test results. Treadmill testing using the Naughton-Balke protocol, which creates increases in work of 1-MET (metabolic equivalent) increments at 2-minute stages has also been used and compares with the 6-minute walk test in reflecting drug efficacy. Cardiopulmonary exercise testing using an upright bicycle and measurements of gas exchange have the potential to grade the severity of exercise limitation in patients with pulmonary hypertension noninvasively.[44]

CARDIAC CATHETERIZATION. In addition to confirming the diagnosis and allowing the exclusion of other causes, cardiac catheterization (see Chap. 20) also establishes the severity of disease and allows an assessment of prognosis. By definition, patients with PAH should have a low or normal pulmonary capillary wedge pressure. Because this is a critical measurement in distinguishing a patient with PAH from one with pulmonary venous hypertension, quality measures must be established in the catheterization laboratory to ensure that correct values are obtained.[45] The transducers must be carefully adjusted to reflect the height of the midchest of every patient. Pressures should never be determined by the electronically integrated mean pressure from the laboratory's computer, because these measurements ignore respiratory influences.[46] Instead, measurements of all pressures are properly made at end-expiration to avoid incorporating negative intrathoracic pressures. When a reproducible wedge pressure cannot be obtained, direct measurement of left ventricular end-diastolic pressure is advised. If the wedge pressure is increased, it should be correlated with left ventricular end-diastolic pressure and not attributed to a falsely elevated reading.

It can be difficult to pass a catheter into the pulmonary artery in patients with pulmonary hypertension because of the tricuspid regurgitation, dilated right atrium and ventricle, and low cardiac output. A specific flow-directed thermodilution balloon catheter has been developed for patients with pulmonary hypertension (American Edwards Laboratories, Irvine, Calif); it has an extra port for the placement of a 0.25-inch guidewire to provide better stiffness to the catheter, which greatly facilitates the procedure.

VASODILATOR TESTING. Several vasodilators are of value in the assessment of pulmonary vasoreactivity in patients with PAH (**Table 78-4**). All appear to have similar efficacy in identifying patients who are vasoreactive. Adenosine and epoprostenol are vasodilators at low doses but they possess potent inotropic properties which become manifest at higher doses, whereas NO has little effect on cardiac output at any dose. An increase in cardiac output with no change in pulmonary arterial pressure will result in a reduction in calculated pulmonary vascular resistance, and may be erroneously interpreted as a vasodilator response[45] (**Table 78-5**). Changes in pulmonary capillary wedge pressure can also have important influences on the

TABLE 78-4	Agents Used for Determination of Acute Pulmonary Vasoreactivity				
AGENT	**MODE OF ADMINISTRATION**	**DOSAGE**	**ADVANTAGES**	**DISADVANTAGES**
Prostacyclin	Intravenous	2 ng/kg/min (stepwise increase every 10-15 min); maximum dose, 10 ng/kg/min	Affects PA pressure, cardiac output; can be used as chronic therapy	Systemic hypotension; dramatic side effects
Adenosine	Intravenous	50 µg/kg/min increased by 50 µg/kg/min every 2 min; maximum dose, 250 µg/kg/min	Affects PA pressure, cardiac output; rapid onset, rapid washout	Bradycardia
Nitric oxide	Inhaled	5-80 ppm for 10 min	Affects PA pressure alone; rapid onset, rapid washout	Rebound pulmonary hypertension in a few cases
Iloprost	Inhaled	2.5-5.0 µg/inhaled dose	Affects PA pressure selectively with minimal effects on cardiac output; can be used as chronic therapy	Potential dosing variabilities depending on investigator experience, inhalation device, and breathing pattern of patient

TABLE 78-5	Hemodynamic Assessment of Vasodilators in Pulmonary Hypertension	
PARAMETER MEASURED	**DESIRED ACUTE CHANGES**	**COMMENTS**
Mean pulmonary artery pressure (PAP)	>10-mm Hg decrease; ideally, mean PAP < 30 mm Hg	Must not be associated with significant fall in systemic blood pressure
Pulmonary vascular resistance (PVR)	>33% decrease; ideally PVR < 6 units	Cardiac output unchanged or increased
Pulmonary capillary wedge pressure	No change	Increase in wedge pressure suggests pulmonary venoocclusive disease or coexisting left ventricular dysfunction
Cardiac output	Increase	Increase should be from increased stroke volume rather than increased heart rate
Heart rate	No significant change	Chronic increased heart rate will result in RV failure; watch for bradycardia if using high doses of diltiazem
Systemic arterial oxygen saturation	Increase if reduced on room air, little change if normal	Decrease in systemic arterial oxygen saturation suggests lung disease or right-to-left shunt; prohibits chronic use
Pulmonary artery (mixed venous) oxygen saturation	Increase; should parallel increase in cardiac output and reflect improved tissue oxygenation	

calculation of pulmonary vascular resistance. A rising capillary wedge pressure secondary to increased cardiac output may be the first sign of impending left ventricular failure and an adverse effect of a drug, whereas the calculated pulmonary vascular resistance may be lower and suggest a beneficial effect. The resting heart rate is a physiologic parameter of marked importance in patients with congestive heart failure, and treatments that cause an increased heart rate are likely to yield deleterious long-term results. Finally, the systemic arterial oxygen content should be evaluated in patients with pulmonary hypertension. Vasodilator drugs can result in vasodilation of blood vessels supplying poorly ventilated areas of the lung and can worsen hypoxemia. This effect is particularly noticeable in patients with underlying chronic lung disease.

CLASSIFICATION OF PULMONARY HYPERTENSION

Pulmonary hypertension, in its simplest sense, refers to any elevation in the pulmonary arterial pressure above normal. The presence of pulmonary hypertension may reflect a serious underlying pulmonary vascular disease or a manifestation of high cardiac output from thyrotoxicosis. Consequently, an accurate diagnosis of the cause of pulmonary hypertension in a patient is essential to establish an effective treatment plan. In addition, therapies that may be beneficial for patients with some types of pulmonary hypertension may be harmful for patients with other types.

The diagnosis of pulmonary hypertension relies on establishing an elevation in pulmonary artery pressure above normal. The upper limit of normal for pulmonary artery mean pressure is 19 mm Hg. However, this assumes that there are no abnormalities in downstream pressures of the left atrium or left ventricle, or an increased cardiac output. That is why a patient can have pulmonary hypertension from the standpoint of an elevated pulmonary artery pressure, but normal pulmonary vascular resistance. Parameters for normal pulmonary arterial systolic pressure derived by echocardiographic Doppler studies have suggested that the upper limit of normal of pulmonary arterial systolic pressure in the general population may be higher than previously appreciated.

In 1998, a new clinical classification for pulmonary hypertension was developed. This classification catalogued clinical conditions based on common causative features to serve as a guide in the clinical assessment and treatment of these patients (**Table 78-6**). Several modifications to this classification have since been proposed.[47] In addition, a functional classification, similar to the New York Heart Association (NYHA) functional classification for heart disease, has been developed to allow comparisons of patients with respect to the clinical severity of their symptoms. Because heart and lung diseases commonly coexist in these patients, a worsening functional class may not necessarily reflect worsening pulmonary hypertension.

PAH refers to pulmonary vascular disease originating from the arterioles that results in an elevation in pressure and vascular resistance and a normal pulmonary capillary wedge pressure. Although IPAH (formerly referred to as primary pulmonary hypertension, or PPH) is relatively rare, with an estimated incidence of 1 to 2/million, severe PAH associated with other conditions such as connective tissue CTDs and congenital heart defects is considerably more common. The Centers for Disease Control and Prevention has surveyed the number of hospitalizations of persons with pulmonary hypertension from any cause in the United States from 1980 to 2002 and found a dramatic increase since 1990, with 260,000 hospitalizations and 15,668 deaths reported annually since 2000.[48]

Pulmonary Arterial Hypertension

IDIOPATHIC PULMONARY ARTERIAL HYPERTENSION. IPAH is the diagnosis given to patients with pulmonary hypertension of unexplained cause. However, the clinical features, usual age of onset, progression of the disease, and autopsy findings make IPAH a distinct clinical entity. There are sporadic and familial forms. The prevalence of familial PAH (FPAH) is uncertain, but it occurs in at least 6% of IPAH cases, and the incidence is likely higher. Many unique features are associated with the transmission and development of FPAH. The age of onset is variable and the low penetrance of the gene confers only about a 10% to 20% likelihood of development of the disease. Many individuals in families with PAH inherit the gene and have progeny in whom PAH never develops. Patients with FPAH have a similar female-to-male ratio, age of onset, and natural history of the disease as those with IPAH.

Documentation of FPAH can be difficult because remote common ancestry occurs in patients with PAH and skip generations caused by

TABLE 78-6	Clinical Classification of Pulmonary Hypertension

Category 1: Pulmonary Arterial Hypertension

Key feature: Elevation in PAP with normal pulmonary capillary wedge pressure (PCWP)

Includes the following:

Idiopathic (IPAH)
- Sporadic
- Familial
- From exposure to drugs or toxins
- From exposure to HIV infection
- Persistent pulmonary hypertension of the newborn

Associated with other active conditions:
- Congenital systemic to pulmonary shunts
- Collagen vascular disease
- Portal hypertension

Pulmonary capillary hemangiomatosis (PCH)

Category 2: Pulmonary Venous Hypertension

Key feature: Elevation in PAP with elevation in PCWP

Includes the following:
- Left-sided atrial or ventricular heart disease
- Left-sided valvular heart disease
- Pulmonary venous obstruction
- Pulmonary venoocclusive disease (PVOD)

Category 3: Pulmonary Hypertension Associated with Hypoxemic Lung Disease

Key feature: Chronic hypoxia with mild elevation of PA pressure

Includes the following:
- Chronic obstructive lung disease
- Interstitial lung disease
- Sleep-disordered breathing
- Alveolar hypoventilation disorders
- Chronic exposure to high altitude
- Developmental abnormalities

Category 4: Pulmonary Hypertension Caused by Chronic Thromboembolic Disease

Key feature: Elevation of PAP with documentation of PA obstruction for >3 mo

Includes the following:
- Chronic pulmonary thromboembolism
- Nonthrombotic pulmonary embolism (tumor, foreign material)

Category 5: Pulmonary Hypertension from Conditions with Uncertain Mechanisms

Key feature: Elevation in PAP pressure in association with systemic disease where a causal relationship is possible but not clearly understood

Includes the following:
- Sarcoidosis
- Chronic anemias
- Schistosomiasis
- Histiocytosis X
- Lymphangiomatosis

incomplete penetrance or by variable expression can mimic sporadic disease. Vertical transmission has been demonstrated in as many as five generations in one family and is indicative of a single autosomal dominant gene for PAH. Genetic anticipation has been described in FPAH since the early reports. Most cases of FPAH can be attributed to the mutation of *BMPR-2*. On clinical grounds, FPAH and IPAH appear identical.

Natural History and Symptoms

The most extensive study on the natural history of IPAH was reported from the National Institutes of Health (NIH) Registry on Primary Pulmonary Hypertension from 1981 to 1987. Of the patients, 63% were female, and the mean age was 36 ± 15 years (range, 1 to 81 years) at the time of diagnosis. The mean interval from the onset of symptoms to diagnosis was 2 years, and the most common initial symptoms were dyspnea (80%), fatigue (19%), and syncope or near-syncope (13%). No ethnic or racial differentiation was observed, with 12.3% of patients being black and 2.3% being Hispanic.

RIGHT VENTRICULAR FUNCTION. Right ventricular failure from pulmonary hypertension is a result of chronic pressure overload and associated volume overload, with the development of tricuspid regurgitation. The mechanism of right ventricular failure in patients with pulmonary hypertension is complex. The chronic pressure overload that induces right ventricular hypertrophy and reduced contractility has been shown to cause a reduction in coronary blood flow to the right ventricular myocardium, which can produce right ventricular ischemia acutely and chronically.[37] Such right ventricular dysfunction appears to be a result of a reduction in right ventricular coronary artery driving pressure. In animals, acute right ventricular failure secondary to right ventricular hypertension was overcome by increasing aortic pressure, which resulted in an increase in right ventricular coronary driving pressure.

LEFT VENTRICULAR FUNCTION. On occasion, patients with pulmonary hypertension have a reduced left ventricular ejection fraction and even regional wall motion abnormalities of the left ventricle. These findings had been attributed to mechanisms related to interventricular dependence, which suggests that in some way a dysfunctional right ventricle can lead to a dysfunctional left ventricle. More recently, extrinsic compression of the left main coronary artery by the pulmonary artery in patients with chronic pulmonary hypertension has been described and may be associated with classic angina-like symptoms. It is advisable to look for extrinsic compression of the left main coronary artery with coronary angiography in patients with long-standing pulmonary hypertension who have abnormal left ventricular function.

Clinical Course

The clinical course of patients with IPAH can be highly variable. The NIH registry demonstrated that the mean right atrial pressure, mean pulmonary artery pressure, and cardiac index were significantly related to mortality. The NYHA functional classification was also strongly related to survival. However, with the onset of overt right ventricular failure manifested by worsening symptoms and systemic venous congestion, patient survival is generally limited to approximately 6 months. The most common cause of death in patients with IPAH in the NIH registry was progressive right-sided heart failure. Sudden cardiac death was limited to patients who were in NYHA functional Class IV, suggesting that it is a manifestation of end-stage disease rather than a phenomenon that occurs early or unpredictably in the clinical course of the disease. The remainder of the patients died of other medical complications, such as pneumonia or bleeding, which suggests that patients with IPAH do not tolerate coexistent medical conditions well.

Management

With the current classification system, patients within a category of pulmonary hypertension are commonly treated alike. Differences in the efficacy and safety of therapies for pulmonary hypertension associated with other conditions are discussed later. However, the general principles surrounding the management of pulmonary hypertension patients are usually consistent.

LIFESTYLE CHANGES. The diagnosis of PAH does not necessarily imply total disability for the patient. However, marked increases in pulmonary artery have been documented to occur early in the onset of increased physical activity. For that reason, graded exercise activities, such as bicycle riding or swimming, in which patients can gradually increase their workload and easily limit the extent of their work, are thought to be safer than isometric activities. Isometric activities such as lifting weights or stair climbing can be associated with syncopal events and should be limited or avoided. One recent study has reported an improvement in exercise capacity in patients who underwent a training program that far exceeded the effects of vasodilator treatments.[49]

PREGNANCY. Pregnancy should be discussed with women of childbearing age. The physiologic changes that occur in pregnancy can potentially activate the disease and result in death of the mother and/or fetus. In addition to the increased circulating blood volume and oxygen consumption that will increase right ventricular work,

circulating procoagulant factors and the risk of pulmonary embolism from deep vein thrombosis and amniotic fluid are serious concerns. Syncope and cardiac arrest have also been reported to occur during active labor and delivery, and a syndrome of postpartum circulatory collapse has been described. For these reasons, surgical sterilization should be given strong consideration by women with PAH or their husbands, and pregnancy should be strongly discouraged.

MEDICAL THERAPY. The mainstay of therapy has focused on the use of vasodilators. However, these patients suffer from right heart failure; thus, measures that have been shown to be effective for the treatment of heart failure are often used.

Digoxin

Animal studies of right ventricular systolic overload have shown that prior administration of digoxin helps prevent the reduction in contractility of the right ventricle. Clinically, digoxin can increase cardiac output by approximately 10% when given acutely to patients with right ventricular failure from pulmonary hypertension, which is similar to observations made in patients with left ventricular systolic failure. In addition, digoxin caused a reduction in circulating norepinephrine, which is markedly increased.

Diuretics

These drugs appear to be of marked benefit in symptom relief of patients with PAH. Their traditional role has been limited to patients manifesting right ventricular failure and systemic venous congestion. However, patients with advanced PAH can have increased left ventricular filling pressures that contribute to the symptoms of dyspnea and orthopnea, which can be relieved with diuretics. Diuretics may also serve to reduce right ventricular wall stress in patients with concomitant tricuspid regurgitation and volume overload. The fear that diuretics will induce systemic hypotension is unfounded, because the main factor limiting cardiac output is pulmonary vascular resistance and not pulmonary blood volume. Patients with severe venous congestion may require high doses of loop diuretics or the use of combined diuretics. In these cases, electrolyte levels need to be carefully monitored to avoid hyponatremia and hypokalemia. Elevated plasma aldosterone concentrations are associated with endothelial dysfunction, left ventricular hypertrophy, and cardiac death in left heart failure. Given the similarities between left and right heart failure in regard to activation of the renin-angiotensin-aldosterone system, it seems reasonable to use aldosterone antagonists in patients with PAH.

Supplemental Oxygen

Hypoxic pulmonary vasoconstriction can contribute to pulmonary vascular disease. Patients with PAH who exhibit resting hypoxemia or arterial oxygen desaturation with activity may benefit from supplemental oxygen because increased oxygen extraction occurs with fixed oxygen delivery. Patients with severe right-sided heart failure and resting hypoxemia resulting from markedly increased oxygen extraction at rest should be treated with continuous oxygen therapy to maintain their arterial oxygen saturation above 90%. Patients with hypoxemia caused by a right-to-left shunt may not improve their level of oxygenation to an appreciable degree with supplemental oxygen.

Anticoagulants

Oral anticoagulant therapy is widely recommended for patients with PAH, supported by the numerous studies implicating thrombin as contributing to disease progression.[50] A number of retrospective and prospective observational studies have shown a significant survival advantage in patients with PAH treated with warfarin. The current recommendation is to use warfarin in relatively low doses, as has been recommended for the prophylaxis of venous thromboembolism, with the international normalized ratio (INR) maintained at 2.0 to 3.0 times that of controls.

PRINCIPLES OF VASODILATOR DRUG TREATMENT OF PULMONARY ARTERIAL HYPERTENSION

- Establish a correct diagnosis. The symptoms of pulmonary hypertension attributable to PAH can be indistinguishable from pulmonary hypertension of other causes. In addition, treatments that may be helpful in PAH can often be harmful or dangerous in other conditions. For these reasons, it is essential that a correct diagnosis of the cause be made in every case. Lack of an obvious history should not be relied on as adequate, because patients with congenital heart disease may never have been told of a heart murmur, and patients with chronic thromboembolic pulmonary hypertension often have no antecedent history of pulmonary embolism. Given the poor survival of pulmonary hypertension of any cause, every patient should undergo thorough testing, including cardiac catheterization, prior to initiating therapy.

- Obtain baseline assessments of the disease. To determine whether a treatment of PAH is effective, it is important to evaluate the patient's response objectively. Regardless of which test or tests are used (e.g., exercise testing, catheterization), an adequate baseline assessment of the patient's disease must be obtained to monitor the patient's response to therapy.

- Test vasoreactivity. Because of the dramatic effect that calcium blockers have on improving survival in patients who are vasoreactive, patients should be tested at the time of diagnosis so that potentially reactive patients are not missed.

- Vasoreactive patients should undergo a trial of calcium channel blockers. Calcium blockers are the drugs of choice for those patients who demonstrate vasoreactivity at the time of testing. There is no evidence to suggest that these patients would have a similarly beneficial response with other therapies. Some patients who demonstrate reactivity may not respond to calcium blockers or may respond for only a limited period. It is essential that the drugs are used in the high doses that have been described to realize full benefit for the patient.

  Nonreactive patients should be offered other therapies. Currently, there are no comparative trials regarding the efficacy of the various approved therapies, so no specific treatment can or should be considered first-line treatment. However, foremost should be consideration of which treatment the physician believes will offer the patient the best chance for improved symptoms and long-term survival. This will often depend on personal opinion, because there are no long-term controlled trials of any therapies for pulmonary hypertension.

- Follow-up assessment of drug efficacy is essential. In all the clinical trials for pulmonary hypertension, the full treatment effect was reached within 1 month of the patient receiving the active drug at full dose. There are no data to suggest that patients who do not respond initially might respond over time with longer exposure. Thus, it is recommended that a repeat measure of drug efficacy be performed within 2 months of starting any new drug treatment.

- Treatments that are ineffective should be replaced. All approved therapies for PAH have inherent risks and are expensive. If a treatment is deemed ineffective by an assessment of efficacy, a different treatment should be substituted rather than added. Patients who clinically fail all treatments should be considered for lung transplantation.

- Benefits and risks of combination therapies are largely unknown. The use of these treatments in combination is becoming popular. However, the only randomized controlled trial of combination therapy demonstrating efficacy has been the addition of oral sildenafil to stable patients with PAH on intravenous epoprostenol.[51] Trials evaluating the combination of bosentan with epoprostenol and bosentan with tadalafil have failed to demonstrate increased efficacy.

- Repeated measures of efficacy should be adhered to. Evidence suggests that some therapies may lose efficacy over time. Thus, even in patients in whom it has been shown that drug therapy has been helpful initially, serial assessments of drug efficacy should be performed periodically to check for loss of efficacy over time.

VASODILATOR THERAPIES. All the approved therapies for pulmonary hypertension are considered to be pulmonary vasodilators. Current practice guidelines recommend that calcium channel blockers be used in vasoreactive patients, which is not an U.S. Food and Drug Administration (FDA)-approved use.[8] The approved vasodilators are recommended for patients who are shown to be nonresponsive to acute vasodilator testing. Regulatory approval has been based on the demonstration that they improve exercise tolerance over 12 to 16 weeks and is not based on a fall in pulmonary artery pressure. Although there is a presumption that they also lower pulmonary arterial pressure, the usual decrease in pulmonary artery pressure is less than 10%.

Calcium Channel Blockers

It has been reported that up to 20% of patients with IPAH are vasoreactive and will respond to high doses of calcium channel blockers, with a dramatic reduction in pulmonary artery pressure and pulmonary vascular resistance; on serial catheterization, this has been maintained for more than 20 years.[52] It appears essential that high doses (e.g., amlodipine, 20 to 30 mg/day; nifedipine, 180 to 240 mg/day; diltiazem, 720 to 960 mg/day) must be used to realize full benefit. When patients respond favorably, quality of life is restored, with improved functional class, and survival (94% at 5 years) is improved when compared with nonresponders and historical control subjects. This experience suggests that a select subset of patients with IPAH have the ability to have their pulmonary hypertension reversed and their quality of life and length of survival enhanced. It is unknown whether the response to calcium channel blockers identifies two subsets of patients with IPAH, different stages of IPAH, or a combination of both. However, patients who do not exhibit a dramatic hemodynamic response to calcium channel blockers do not appear to benefit from their long-term administration.

Prostacyclins

Prostacyclin is produced by vascular endothelial cells and has vasodilatory and antiproliferative activities. It is also a potent inhibitor of platelet aggregation. Abnormalities in prostacyclin production and metabolism have been described in PAH. Continuous intravenous infusion of epoprostenol (synthetic prostacyclin) has been shown in randomized clinical trials to improve symptoms related to IPAH, exercise tolerance, hemodynamics, and short-term survival.[53] It appears effective when given chronically, even if it does not seem effective acutely. Epoprostenol is administered through a central venous catheter that is surgically implanted and delivered by an ambulatory infusion system. The delivery system is complex and requires patients to learn the techniques of sterile drug preparation, operation of the pump, and care of the intravenous catheter. Most serious complications that have occurred with epoprostenol therapy have been attributable to the delivery system; these include catheter-related infections and temporary interruption of the infusion because of pump malfunction. The short half-life (6 minutes) of epoprostenol is believed to contribute to the hemodynamic collapse that has occurred when the infusion is abruptly interrupted. Side effects related to epoprostenol include flushing, headache, diarrhea, and a unique type of jaw discomfort that occurs with eating. In most patients, these symptoms are minimal and well tolerated. Chronic foot pain and a diffuse rash develop in some patients. To date, epoprostenol has been given to patients with PAH for more than 15 years with sustained effectiveness. In some patients (NYHA Class IV) who are critically ill, it serves as a bridge to lung transplantation by stabilizing the patient to a more favorable preoperative state. Patients who are less critically ill may do so well with epoprostenol therapy that the need to consider transplantation may be delayed, perhaps indefinitely.

The optimal dose of epoprostenol has never been determined, but doses between 25 and 40 ng/kg/min are typical. A high cardiac output state has been reported in a series of patients with IPAH receiving chronic epoprostenol therapy and is consistent with the drug having positive inotropic effects. The development of a chronic high-output state could have long-term detrimental effects on underlying cardiac function and should be avoided. The follow-up assessment of patients receiving intravenous epoprostenol is variable among medical centers, but it does appear important to determine the cardiac output response to therapy periodically to optimize dosing. The experience

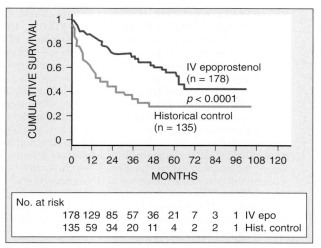

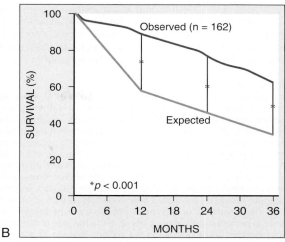

A

B

FIGURE 78-9 Kaplan-Meier survival estimates in patients with IPAH treated with epoprostenol therapy. **A,** Patient survival is compared with patients with IPAH matched for NYHA functional class who never received epoprostenol therapy. **B,** Patient survival compared with untreated patients with IPAH from the NIH registry survival prediction equation. The observed survival with epoprostenol therapy from both studies was remarkably similar and considerably better than what would have been expected. (**A** from Sitbon O, Humbert M, Nunes H, et al: Long-term intravenous epoprostenol infusion in primary pulmonary hypertension. J Am Coll Cardiol 40:780, 2002; **B** from McLaughlin V, Shillington A, Rich S: Survival in primary pulmonary hypertension: The impact of epoprostenol therapy. Circulation 106:1477, 2002.)

with epoprostenol in patients with IPAH for more than 10 years has been reported by two large centers (**Fig. 78-9**). Survival rates longer than 5 years were improved compared with survival in historical control subjects and the natural history predicted by the NIH Registry. Predictors of survival included NYHA functional class, exercise tolerance, and acute vasodilator responsiveness. Both studies provided important data for identifying patients who would do well over the long term, versus those in whom transplantation should be considered.

Treprostinil is a stable prostacyclin analogue that has pharmacologic actions similar to those of epoprostenol, but differs in that it is chemically stable at room temperature and has a longer half-life (4 hours). This allows it to be administered through continuous subcutaneous infusion, although infusion site pain is common. In a large, randomized clinical trial in patients with PAH, treprostinil was effective in reducing symptoms of dyspnea associated with exercise.[54] Treprostinil has also been approved for intravenous administration. The optimal dose of treprostinil has never been determined, but doses of 75 to 150 ng/kg/min are typical. Because there is no difference in bioavailability between the subcutaneous and intravenous routes, patients can be transitioned from one route of administration to the other without the need for adjusting the dosage. It has been reported that the use of intravenous treprostinil is associated with a higher incidence of gram-negative sepsis than intravenous epoprostenol.

A key element of the long-term efficacy of the parenteral prostacyclins appears to be related to the strategy of upward dose titration of the drug over time. It is important to increase the dose to tolerated side effects in patients who remain symptomatic because there is a direct relationship between the dose of drug and improvement in exercise testing and hemodynamics. Once an optimal dose has been achieved, the dose is kept constant thereafter. Patients who deteriorate after a long period of stability usually do not respond to further dose increases.

Iloprost, an analogue of prostacyclin, has been approved for use via inhalation. Because of the short half-life of iloprost, however, it requires frequent (up to 12/day) inhalations. Iloprost is given by 2.5- or 5.0-μg ampules via a dedicated nebulizer that limits the dose of drug that can be delivered. Beraprost is an orally active prostacyclin analogue that improved exercise capacity and symptoms over a 12-week period in a European trial. A similar trial conducted in the United States, however, showed similar efficacy at 12 weeks, only to document the loss of effectiveness over 1 year. This is the only randomized clinical trial to follow patients for a period of 1 year and underscores how initial improvements with therapies might not be

sustained for longer periods. At present, beraprost is only approved for use in Japan.

Phosphodiesterase Type 5 Inhibitors

Inhibition of the phosphodiesterase type 5 (PDE5) enzyme produces pulmonary vasodilation by promoting an enhanced and sustained level of cGMP, an identical effect to that of inhaled NO. Sildenafil is a PDE5 inhibitor that has been shown to be a selective pulmonary vasodilator with similar efficacy to that of inhaled NO in lowering pulmonary artery pressure. Sildenafil has a preferential effect on the pulmonary circulation because of the high expression of the PDE5 isoform in the lung. Recent studies have also suggested that PDE5 inhibitors may improve cardiac function by direct effects on the myocardium.[55] In a large, randomized clinical trial sildenafil caused significant improvements in 6-minute walk distance and hemodynamics in patients with PAH.[56] The recommended dosage is 20 mg three times daily, but dosages as high as 80 mg three times daily have been used safely, and in some patients may be more effective. Side effects are generally mild and mainly related to vasodilation (headache, flushing, and nasal congestion). Tadalafil is a long-acting selective PDE5 inhibitor that has been recently approved for PAH.[57] In the pivotal clinical trial, it was similarly well tolerated and improved exercise tolerance and quality of life measures. The effective dose was 40 mg once daily.

Endothelin Receptor Blockers

Endothelin (ET)-1 exerts vasoconstrictor and mitogenic effects and is activated in PAH. Three endothelin receptor blockers have been approved for PAH. Although there have never been direct comparative trials, all three appear to have similar efficacy.[58] Bosentan, a nonselective ET receptor blocker, has produced an improvement in 6-minute walk distance after 16 weeks as compared with placebo in several clinical trials. It also has been shown to lengthen a composite endpoint of time to clinical worsening. The approved dosage of bosentan is 125 mg twice daily. Ambrisentan is an ET$_A$-selective endothelin receptor blocker that can be given once daily at a 5-mg dose, which can be increased to 10 mg if the drug is well tolerated. Sitaxsentan is an ET$_A$-selective endothelin receptor blocker that can be given once daily at a 100 mg dose. Sitaxsentan is currently approved only in the European Union, Canada, and Australia.

These drugs have similar side effects, which include peripheral edema. They also have a potential of causing liver toxicity requiring monthly monitoring of liver enzyme levels, and have interactions with warfarin that require careful monitoring of the INR and dose adjustments when used together. This is particularly important with sitaxsentan. Pregnancy monitoring (when indicated), as well as quarterly hematocrit testing, is also advised. Caution should also be used when they are coadministered with cyclosporine, strong CYP3A4 inhibitors (ketoconazole), or CYP2C19 inhibitors (omeprazole).

SURGICAL THERAPY

Atrial Septostomy. The rationale for the creation of an atrial septostomy in patients with PAH is based on experimental and clinical observations suggesting that an intra-atrial defect allowing right-to-left shunting in the setting of severe pulmonary hypertension might be of benefit. Indications for the procedure include recurrent syncope and/or right ventricular failure despite maximum medical therapy, as a bridge to transplantation if deterioration occurs in the face of maximum medical therapy, or when no other option exists.[59] The rate of procedure-related mortality with atrial septostomy in patients with PAH is high, and thus the procedure should be attempted only in centers with an established record for the treatment of advanced pulmonary hypertension and experience in performing atrial septostomy with a low rate of morbidity. The recommended technique is graded balloon dilation of the fosse ovalis, which can be achieved in stages over several weeks in unstable patients. It should not be performed in a patient with impending death and severe right ventricular failure. Predictors of procedure-related failure or death include a mean right atrial pressure higher than 20 mm Hg, a pulmonary vascular resistance index higher than 55 units/m², or a predicted 1-year survival rate of less than 40%. The mechanisms responsible for the beneficial effects of atrial septostomy remain unclear. Possibilities include increased oxygen delivery at rest and/or with exercise, reduced right ventricular end-diastolic pressure or wall stress, improvement in right ventricular function, or relief of right ventricular ischemia.

Heart-Lung and Lung Transplantation. Heart-lung transplantation (see Chap. 31) has been performed successfully in patients with PAH since 1981. Currently, bilateral lung transplantation has become the procedure of choice, allowing the donor heart to be given to another patient.[60] Hemodynamic studies have shown an immediate reduction in pulmonary artery pressure and pulmonary vascular resistance associated with an improvement in right ventricular function. The 1-year survival rate is 70% to 75%, the 2-year survival rate is 55% to 60%, and the 5-year survival rate is between 40% to 45%. The major long-term complications in patients are the high incidence of bronchiolitis obliterans in the transplanted lungs, acute organ rejection, and opportunistic infection.

Transplantation should be reserved for patients with pulmonary hypertension that has progressed despite optimal medical management. It is generally accepted that patients should be considered for transplantation when they are in NYHA functional Class III or IV despite therapy with a parenteral prostacyclin. However, the recent adoption of a lung allocation score system for candidates has made it increasingly difficult for these patients to become transplanted. The scoring system was developed to reduce the mortality of patients on the waiting list, prioritize candidates on the basis of urgency, and avoid futile transplants. Because patients with pulmonary hypertension have a higher postoperative mortality than patients with lung disease, they receive a lower score. However, their long-term survival is comparable.

PULMONARY ARTERIAL HYPERTENSION FROM EXPOSURE TO ANOREXIGENS.

Several anorexigens have been demonstrated to cause pulmonary hypertension in humans. The first observation was made in 1967, when an epidemic of PAH in Europe was associated with the use of aminorex, which has similarities to adrenaline and ephedrine in its chemical structure. The clinical features of pulmonary hypertension were identical to those attributed to IPAH. The association between the use of fenfluramine appetite suppressants and the development of PAH was established in a case-control study conducted in Europe in 1992 to 1994. Anorexigens such as amphetamines were also implicated. Ultimately, the marked increase in the number of cases of PAH and cardiac valvulopathy ascribed to the use of fenfluramine drugs in the United States led to their withdrawal in 1997. In most patients, the development of pulmonary hypertension was progressive, despite withdrawal of the anorexigen. In addition, many of the patients did not develop clinical symptoms of PAH for more than 5 years after their last ingestion. Animal models have suggested that the fenfluramines produce pulmonary hypertension via the SERT by allowing for serotonin to stimulate PASMC proliferation by some type of permissive effect.[61]

PULMONARY ARTERIAL HYPERTENSION FROM EXPOSURE TO HUMAN IMMUNODEFICIENCY VIRUS INFECTION.

Although well documented, it remains unclear how HIV infection results in an increased incidence of PAH in HIV-infected patients (see Chap. 72). A direct pathogenic role of HIV seems unlikely inasmuch as no viral constituents have been detected in the vascular endothelium of these patients. On the other hand, reports of pulmonary arteriopathy with intimal proliferation in monkeys experimentally infected with the simian immunodeficiency virus and in a murine model of acquired immunodeficiency syndrome have suggested a pathogenetic link between infection with an immunodeficiency virus and the development of PAH, possibly mediated by the release of inflammatory mediators or by autoimmune mechanisms.[28] The Swiss HIV Cohort Study reported the cumulative incidence of HIV-associated PAH to be 1/200 patients in the HIV-infected population. PAH was diagnosed in patients in all stages of HIV infection; it was unrelated to the CD4 cell counts. The clinical and hemodynamic features of these patients were similar to those of patients with IPAH.

PERSISTENT PULMONARY HYPERTENSION OF THE NEWBORN.

Three forms of persistent pulmonary hypertension of the newborn (PPHN) have been described. In the hypertrophic type, the muscular tissue of the pulmonary arteries is hypertrophied and extends peripherally to the acini, which causes narrowing of the arteries, an increase in pulmonary pressure, and a reduction in pulmonary blood flow. It is believed to be the result of sustained fetal hypertension from vasoconstriction caused by chronic fetal distress. In the hypoplastic type, the lungs and pulmonary arteries are underdeveloped, usually as the result of a congenital diaphragmatic hernia or prolonged leakage of amniotic fluid. The cross-sectional area of the pulmonary vascular bed is inadequate for normal neonatal pulmonary blood flow. In the reactive type, lung histology is presumably normal but vasoconstriction causes pulmonary hypertension. High levels of vasoconstrictive mediators such as thromboxane, norepinephrine, and leukotrienes may be responsible and may result from streptococcal infection or acute asphyxia at birth. Although PPHN can vary in severity, severe cases are life-threatening. It is commonly associated with severe hypoxemia and the need for mechanical ventilation. Right-to-left shunting at the level of the ductus arteriosus or foramen ovale is common. Inhaled nitric oxide has provided encouraging results through improvement in oxygenation in these patients. Intravenous epoprostenol has also been used and may even have effects additive to those of inhaled NO.

Alveolar capillary dysplasia is a very rare cause of pulmonary hypertension in neonates and is characterized by a developmental abnormality in the pulmonary vasculature. The antemortem diagnosis can be made only with open lung biopsy. Despite aggressive treatment with NO, epoprostenol, and even extracorporeal membrane oxygenation, survival in the setting of alveolar capillary dysplasia is rare.

PULMONARY ARTERIAL HYPERTENSION ASSOCIATED WITH CONGENITAL HEART DISEASE.

Pulmonary hypertension can develop from any congenital heart defect that increases pulmonary blood flow (see Chap. 65).[62] If a congenital defect causes pulmonary hypertension from the time of birth, the small muscular arteries of the fetal lung may undergo delayed or only partial involution, with subsequent persistently high levels of pulmonary vascular resistance. This is especially true in lesions in which a left-to-right shunt enters the right ventricle or pulmonary artery directly (i.e., a post-tricuspid shunt, such as ventricular septal defect or patent ductus arteriosus). These patients experience a higher incidence of severe and irreversible pulmonary vascular damage than those in whom the shunt is proximal to the tricuspid valve (pretricuspid shunts, as in atrial septal defect and partial anomalous pulmonary venous drainage). An important feature of PAH in congenital heart disease is the right ventricular adaptive response to elevated pulmonary arterial pressure. When the onset is early in life, there is marked hypertrophy and preservation of a fetal-like phenotype. As a result, these patients can sustain an increased afterload for many years or decades as compared with patients in whom the pulmonary hypertension occurs later in life.

The vascular changes that occur in pulmonary hypertension associated with congenital heart disease are identical to those seen in IPAH. It is believed that ECs release mediators that induce PASMC growth in response to changes in pulmonary blood flow or pressure. Experimental data have suggested that medial hypertrophy can be converted to a neointimal pattern when pulmonary vascular injury is coupled with increased pulmonary blood flow. Early changes, characterized by hypertrophy of the media and intimal proliferation of the muscular pulmonary arteries and arterioles, are believed to be reversible. Advanced disease, characterized by the presence of concentric laminar fibrosis, with obliteration of many arterioles and small arteries, and plexiform lesions are considered irreversible.

Eisenmenger Syndrome

Eisenmenger syndrome refers to any anomalous circulatory communication that leads to obliterative pulmonary vascular disease. The long-term prognosis of patients with Eisenmenger syndrome is better than that of patients with IPAH, with survival reported to be 80% at 10 years, 77% at 15 years, and 42% at 25 years. A major distinction between Eisenmenger syndrome and other forms of PAH is the presence of cyanosis. Pulse oximetry at rest and with exercise is a useful way to monitor the progress of these patients and their response to therapy. Patients with bidirectional shunting may have normal resting pulse oximetry that will fall during exercise, reflecting shunt reversal. The magnitude of the fall may be helpful in deciding how to intervene. Patients with advanced pulmonary vascular disease will have hypoxemia at rest that worsens significantly with any level of exercise activity. Although this can have deleterious effects on organ function, these patients commonly have significant secondary erythrocytosis, which can effectively improve tissue oxygenation. Because erythrocytosis provides an important compensatory mechanism, patients should take supplemental iron to maintain their hematocrit. The use of anticoagulants is somewhat controversial, because these patients generally have thrombosis of the pulmonary vasculature but an increased risk of hemoptysis. It is recommended that warfarin anticoagulation be prescribed unless there is a history of bleeding.

All the approved vasodilators for PAH have been used in congenital heart disease to improve exercise tolerance, but the only randomized clinical trial conducted specifically in these patients (BREATHE-5) was with bosentan.[63] Intravenous epoprostenol therapy has also been reported to be effective, but the presence of an underlying right-to-left shunt presents a risk for systemic embolization from the indwelling venous catheter, which needs to be monitored closely.

PULMONARY ARTERIAL HYPERTENSION ASSOCIATED WITH CONNECTIVE TISSUE DISEASES. All the CTDs have been associated with the development of PAH, which is the leading cause of death in patients with scleroderma (see Chap. 89). Advanced pulmonary hypertension has also been described in patients with systemic lupus erythematosus, mixed CTDs, polymyositis, dermatomyositis, rheumatoid arthritis, and Sjögren syndrome. Patients with severe pulmonary hypertension usually have a pulmonary vasculature with histologic features that resemble those of IPAH, but coexisting interstitial fibrosis is extremely common and likely contributes to hypoxemia. Because CTDs may have an insidious onset and slowly progressive course, early recognition of the symptoms of pulmonary hypertension may be difficult. Dyspnea is the most common initial symptom. A reduced DLCO on pulmonary function tests has been shown to be predictive of the presence of pulmonary vascular disease. Scleroderma is associated with mild pulmonary hypertension in as many as one third of patients, which would make periodic screening with echocardiography in these patients reasonable.

The prognosis for patients with CTD in whom pulmonary hypertension develops is poor. Conventional therapy with digitalis, diuretics, and anticoagulation has been recommended to provide a clinical benefit similar to the practice in IPAH. Because hypoxemia is so common, patients should be tested with pulse oximetry during exercise, and supplemental oxygen used whenever indicated. All the approved therapies for PAH apply to the CTDs. The principles of drug selection and management for IPAH are similar, but their long-term

efficacy is considerably less.[64] Patients with coexisting lung disease must be watched carefully for worsening oxygenation from the vasodilators.

PULMONARY ARTERIAL HYPERTENSION ASSOCIATED WITH PORTAL HYPERTENSION. Pulmonary abnormalities are commonly associated with the development of hepatic cirrhosis and include hepatopulmonary syndrome (HPS), and portopulmonary hypertension (POPH). HPS is characterized by vascular dilation that produces severe arterial hypoxemia from intrapulmonary shunting in the setting of normal hemodynamics. No proven medical therapy exists for HPS, except for supplemental oxygen.

POPH hypertension is progressive and is unrelated to the severity of hepatic dysfunction, with no reports of spontaneous resolution.[65] There is a strong association between portal hypertension and pulmonary hypertension, regardless of whether liver disease is present. The prevalence of pulmonary hypertension in patients with portal hypertension is estimated as 2% to 6%, with an estimated 5-year survival of 10% to 30%. Patients with POPH are similar to patients with PAH without cirrhosis, with the exception that they tend to have higher cardiac output and consequently lower systemic and pulmonary vascular resistance, which is characteristic of the cirrhotic state. Treatment of POPH generally follows the guidelines developed for treating patients with IPAH, but many of these drugs pose a risk of liver toxicity and should not be used. Although severe pulmonary hypertension is considered a contraindication to liver transplantation because of the risk of irreversible right-sided heart failure, successful liver transplantation has been reported in patients with mild pulmonary hypertension treated successfully with intravenous epoprostenol.

Pulmonary Capillary Hemangiomatosis

Pulmonary capillary hemangiomatosis (PCH) was first described in 1978 as a very rare cause of pulmonary hypertension. The typical chest radiographic appearance is a diffuse, bilateral, reticular nodular pattern associated with enlarged central pulmonary arteries. The most characteristic finding on high-resolution CT scan is diffuse bilateral thickening of the interlobular septa and small centrilobular, poorly circumscribed, nodular opacities. Diffuse ground-glass opacities have also been described. Histologic findings often include irregular small nodular foci of thin-walled capillary-sized vessels that diffusely invade the lung parenchyma, bronchiolar walls, and adventitia of large vessels.[66] These nodular lesions are often associated with alveolar hemorrhage. Most patients appear to be young adults and present with dyspnea and/or hemoptysis. A hereditary form with probable autosomal recessive transmission has been reported. It can be difficult to distinguish PCH from IPAH clinically. The clinical course of patients with this condition is usually one of progressive deterioration, leading to severe pulmonary hypertension, right-sided heart failure, and death. The only definitive treatment for these patients is lung transplantation.

Pulmonary Venous Hypertension

Patients with pulmonary venous hypertension have elevated pulmonary venous pressure (as reflected in the pulmonary capillary wedge pressure) as a consequence of left ventricular dysfunction (see Chap. 25), mitral and aortic valve disease (see Chap. 66), cardiomyopathy (see Chap. 68), cor triatriatum (see Chap. 65), and pericardial disease (see Chap. 75). Although mitral stenosis was the most common cause of this disorder decades ago, left ventricular diastolic dysfunction is the most common cause of pulmonary venous hypertension seen in the Western world today. It is presumed that the mechanism of both is similar. Specifically, a chronic elevation in the diastolic filling pressure of the left heart causes a backward transmission of the pressure to the pulmonary venous system, which appears to trigger vasoconstriction in the pulmonary arterial bed.

PATHOLOGY. Histologically, abnormal thickening of the pulmonary veins and formation of a neointima are seen. The latter can be extensive. There is medial hypertrophy and thickening of the neointima on the arterial side of the pulmonary circulation as well. Patients with chronic severe pulmonary venous hypertension may show distention of pulmonary capillaries, thickening and rupture of the basement membranes of endothelial cells, and transudation of erythrocytes through these ruptured membranes into the alveolar spaces, which contain fragments of disintegrating erythrocytes. Pulmonary hemosiderosis is commonly observed and may progress to extensive fibrosis. In the late stages of pulmonary venous hypertension, areas of hemorrhage may be scattered throughout the lungs, edema fluid, coagulum may collect in the alveolar spaces, and widespread organization and fibrosis of pulmonary alveoli may be present. Pulmonary lymphatics may become markedly distended and give the appearance of lymphangiectasis, particularly when the pulmonary venous pressure exceeds 30 mm Hg.

PATHOPHYSIOLOGY. Increased resistance to pulmonary venous drainage will force the PA pressure to increase. The severity of pulmonary hypertension depends, in part, on the contractility of the right ventricle. In the presence of a normal right ventricle, an increase in left atrial pressure initially results in a decrease in pulmonary vascular resistance and the pressure gradient across the lungs, reflecting distention of compliant small vessels, recruitment of additional vascular channels, or both. With further increases in left atrial pressure, PA pressure rises along with pulmonary venous pressure, so that at a constant pulmonary blood flow, the pressure gradient between the pulmonary artery and veins and pulmonary vascular resistance remains constant. When pulmonary venous pressure approaches or exceeds 25 mm Hg on a chronic basis, a disproportionate elevation in pulmonary artery pressure occurs, so that the pressure gradient between the pulmonary artery and veins rises while pulmonary blood flow remains constant or falls. This is indicative of an elevation in pulmonary vascular resistance caused in part by pulmonary arterial vasoconstriction. Some patients may have a genetic predisposition, allowing the chronically elevated pulmonary venous pressures to serve as a trigger for the development of structural changes similar to those found in IPAH. Marked reactive pulmonary hypertension with PA systolic pressures in excess of 80 mm Hg occurs in less than one third of patients whose pulmonary venous pressures are elevated more than 25 mm Hg, which suggests a broad spectrum of pulmonary vascular reactivity to chronic increases in pulmonary venous pressure. The molecular mechanisms involved in elevating pulmonary vascular resistance are unclear.

CLINICAL IMPLICATIONS. Pulmonary hypertension is a common and well-recognized complication of left ventricular systolic dysfunction and is an independent predictor of survival in these patients. Patients with a high pulmonary artery pressure and a low right ventricular ejection fraction have a sevenfold higher risk of death compared with heart failure patients with a normal pulmonary artery pressure and right ventricular ejection fraction. Treatment of pulmonary venous hypertension as caused by left ventricular systolic dysfunction should include traditional therapy for the underlying disease. Both epoprostenol and endothelin receptor antagonists have been studied in these patients and have been demonstrated to increase mortality or have no benefit, respectively. Recently, sildenafil has been used with some success.

Pulmonary venous hypertension related to left ventricular diastolic dysfunction, now referred to as heart failure with preserved ejection fraction (HFpEF), is less appreciated than that related to systolic dysfunction, and is commonly mistaken for IPAH (see Chap. 30). The features of pulmonary hypertension in patients with HFpEF have recently been characterized.[67] Patients tend to be older than IPAH patients and often have other conditions that may contribute to pulmonary hypertension, including obesity and obstructive sleep apnea. However, important and distinctive symptoms are orthopnea and paroxysmal nocturnal dyspnea, which is not a feature of PAH. Atrial fibrillation and absence of right axis deviation on the ECG should increase the suspicion for pulmonary venous hypertension. The chest x-ray will often show pulmonary vascular congestion, pleural effusions and, on occasion, pulmonary edema. A high-resolution chest CT scan can be particularly helpful because it will often reveal ground-glass opacities consistent with chronic pulmonary edema and a mosaic perfusion pattern. Left atrial enlargement on the echocardiogram also

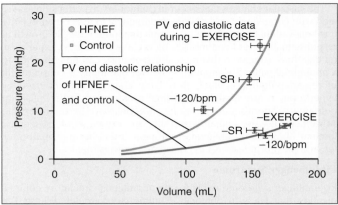

FIGURE 78-10 End-diastolic pressure-volume relationships from patients with heart failure with normal ejection fraction (HFNEF) and control subjects (arrows indicate curve for HFNEF and control subjects, respectively). Yellow circles indicate mean end-diastolic volume (EDV, with horizontal error bars indicating the standard error of the mean [SEM]) and pressure (with vertical error bars indicating SEM) during sinus rhythm (SR), during pacing with 120 bpm (beats/min), or during exercise of the HFNEF group. Blue squares indicate mean EDV and pressure (with vertical and horizontal error bars indicating SEM) of control subjects. The abnormal curve illustrates why patients with elevated left ventricular EDV or pulmonary wedge pressures experience such severe dyspnea with exercise, because any increase in stroke volume causes the pressure to rise. Conversely, a reduction in left ventricular filling pressure may relieve the symptoms of orthopnea and dyspnea and obscure the clinical picture of heart failure with a normal ejection fraction. *(From Westermann D, Kasner M, Steendijk P, et al: Role of left ventricular stiffness in heart failure with normal ejection fraction. Circulation 117:2051, 2008.)*

suggests pulmonary venous hypertension rather than PAH. Although echocardiographic techniques for the assessment of left ventricular diastolic function are advancing, heart catheterization is required to document left heart filling pressures in those with pulmonary hypertension. To make the diagnosis of PAH, the pulmonary capillary wedge pressure or left ventricular end-diastolic pressure must be less than 16 mm Hg. If an ideal wedge pressure tracing cannot be obtained, left ventricular end diastolic pressure should be directly measured. The reduction in diastolic filling time that occurs with an increased heart rate during exercise may further increase left heart filling pressures and, as a result, pulmonary artery (PA) pressures (**Fig. 78-10**).

Two hemodynamic profiles have been described that are common in these patients. Some patients will have an elevation in pulmonary arterial pressure, with only a minimal increase in the transpulmonary gradient (mean PA pressure – pulmonary capillary wedge pressure), as a reflection of the passive increase in PA pressure necessary to overcome the increased downstream resistance. A preserved right ventricle must generate high systolic pressures to ensure adequate forward blood flow in these patients, and thus moderate degrees of pulmonary hypertension are not only characteristic but also favorable. Other patients will have reactive pulmonary vasoconstriction resulting in marked elevations in pulmonary arterial pressure beyond that which is necessary to maintain cardiac output. These patients are frequently distinguished by a marked elevation in PA diastolic pressure. This has been studied extensively in patients with mitral stenosis but is less well characterized in patients with left ventricular diastolic dysfunction.

TREATMENT. Treatment of HFpEF is difficult (see Chap. 30). The goal is to reduce or remove the elevated pulmonary venous resistance with medications such as nitrates, diuretics, and aggressive treatment of systemic hypertension. When successful, the pulmonary arterial pressure will also fall and the cardiac output will increase. Comorbid diseases such as obesity, diabetes, and obstructive sleep apnea must be addressed. Atrial fibrillation is not well tolerated in these patients and every attempt should be made to maintain sinus rhythm. Pulmonary vasodilators are not indicated, because their major hemodynamic effect is to raise cardiac output, and thus will predictably cause a worsening of pulmonary edema if the pulmonary venous obstruction is not being relieved. There are a number of reports of rapid deterioration and death when pulmonary vasodilators are used in the presence of pulmonary venous hypertension.

Pulmonary hypertension as a result of mitral stenosis has been well characterized, and tends to resolve with time after mitral valve repair or replacement[68] (see Chap. 66). The resolution is highly variable, and can occur immediately or over more than 1 year. Although pulmonary hypertension is associated with an increased operative risk, it should not interfere with appropriate treatment, regardless of severity. Pulmonary hypertension occasionally occurs in the setting of severe aortic stenosis, and portends a worse prognosis. Although severe pulmonary hypertension is an independent predictor of perioperative mortality, aortic valve replacement is associated with a reduction in pulmonary artery pressures and improvement in NYHA functional class. The prognosis of those with pulmonary hypertension and severe aortic stenosis who do not undergo surgery is poor, with a 20% survival after a median of 436 days.

PULMONARY VENOOCCLUSIVE DISEASE

Pulmonary venoocclusive disease (PVOD) is a rare form of PAH. The histopathologic diagnosis is based on the presence of obstructive eccentric fibrous intimal pads in the pulmonary veins and venules. Arterialization of the pulmonary veins is often present and is associated with alveolar capillary congestion.[66] Other changes of chronic pulmonary hypertension, such as medial hypertrophy and muscularization of the arterioles with eccentric intimal fibrosis, may also be seen. The pulmonary venous obstruction explains the increased pulmonary capillary wedge pressure described in patients in the late stages of the disease and the increase in basilar bronchovascular markings noted on the chest radiograph. The chest CT scan may be helpful, revealing smooth interlobular septal thickening, ground-glass opacities, and a mosaic perfusion pattern. A perfusion lung scan showing multiple perfusion defects and a CT scan showing no evidence of pulmonary embolism are highly suggestive of the diagnosis. The treatment of PVOD is unsatisfactory.[69] Warfarin anticoagulation is essential. Anecdotal reports of success with calcium blockers or epoprostenol have been tempered by reports of these treatments producing fulminant pulmonary edema. Any therapy needs particularly close supervision, and early referral of the patient for lung transplantation should be considered.

Pulmonary Arterial Hypertension Associated with Hypoxic Lung Diseases

Diseases of the lung parenchyma associated with hypoxia are a common cause of mild pulmonary hypertension. Hypoxia induces muscularization of distal vessels and medial hypertrophy of more proximal arteries, as well as a loss of vessels, which is compounded by a loss of lung parenchyma in the setting of lung disease. Intimal thickening appears to be an early event that occurs in association with progressive air flow limitation. The development of plexiform lesions is not observed.

CHRONIC OBSTRUCTIVE PULMONARY DISEASE. Chronic obstructive pulmonary disease (COPD) refers to a heterogeneous group of diseases that share a common feature—the airways are narrowed, which results in an inability to exhale completely. Although there are numerous disorders that fall under the heading of COPD, the most common are emphysema and chronic bronchitis. Pulmonary hypertension in COPD has multiple causative factors, including pulmonary vasoconstriction caused by alveolar hypoxia, acidemia, and hypercarbia, compression of pulmonary vessels by the high lung volume, loss of small vessels in the vascular bed in regions of the emphysema and lung destruction, and increased cardiac output and blood viscosity from polycythemia secondary to hypoxia. Of these, hypoxia is the most important factor. Changes in airway resistance may augment pulmonary vascular resistance in patients with COPD by increasing the alveolar pressure. The effect of airway resistance on pulmonary artery pressure may be particularly important when ventilation increases (e.g., in cases of acute exacerbation of COPD). In patients with COPD, even small increases in flow that occur during mild exercise may increase pulmonary artery pressure significantly. Alveolar hypoxia is a potent pulmonary arterial constrictor that reduces perfusion with respect to ventilation in an attempt to restore PaO_2. There is also a positive correlation between the $PaCO_2$ and PA pressure in COPD.

Clinically, patients with COPD present with dyspnea and signs of right heart failure, usually in the setting of marked hypoxemia. At cardiac catheterization, the level of the mean pulmonary arterial pressure is usually less than 30 mm Hg. The mean PA pressure typically seen in these patients is lower than the mean PA pressure in patients with IPAH who respond favorably to pulmonary vasodilator therapy. The fact that these patients are clinically failing may indicate that it is not the severity of the pulmonary hypertension but the degree of hypoxemia that is determining their clinical symptomatology. Because right ventricular failure occurs at this level of pulmonary hypertension, it is probable that the right ventricle in these patients is profoundly affected by the hypoxemia and behaves more like an ischemic right ventricle than a pressure-loaded right ventricle.

Although relatively mild, the level of the pulmonary arterial hypertension is predictive of prognosis in patients with COPD. Nonetheless, there has never been a clinical trial showing a beneficial effect of any pulmonary vasodilator in these patients. Concern over worsening ventilation-perfusion mismatch from vasodilators that has been demonstrated with acute testing is likely why these medications are not used. The only effective treatment for patients with COPD and pulmonary hypertension has been supplemental oxygen, with several studies showing an improvement in morbidity and mortality. Clinicians also need to follow the level of hemoglobin in these patients. Patients with hypoxemia should have reactive polycythemia as a fundamental biologic mechanism to compensate for their cardiopulmonary disease. A hemoglobin in the low-normal range, although well tolerated in patients with normal oxygenation, may not be tolerated in patients with hypoxemia and mild pulmonary hypertension

Patients who present with severe pulmonary hypertension should be evaluated for another disease process responsible for the high pulmonary arterial pressures before it is attributed to the COPD. However, there is a small subset of patients with COPD who do develop severe pulmonary arterial hypertension (mean PA pressure [PAP] > 45 mm Hg).[70] These patients have a distinctive pattern of cardiopulmonary abnormalities with mild to moderate airway obstruction, severe hypoxemia, hypocapnia, and a low DLCO. It is possible that the severe pulmonary hypertension is occurring in the presence of lung disease rather than as a result of the lung disease. Clinically, these patients have a hemodynamic profile more typical of PAH, with a marked increase in PA pressure, normal pulmonary capillary wedge pressures, and markedly elevated pulmonary vascular resistance. Pulmonary vasodilators have been associated with clinical worsening and should not be used.[71]

INTERSTITIAL LUNG DISEASES. Interstitial lung diseases (ILDs) represent various conditions that involve the alveolar walls, perialveolar tissue, and other contiguous supporting structures. Pulmonary hypertension in patients with ILD is often associated with obliteration of the pulmonary vascular bed by lung destruction and fibrosis.[72] The mechanism for pulmonary hypertension may be related to hypoxemia, a loss of effective pulmonary vasculature from lung destruction, and/or by indirectly triggering a pulmonary vasculopathy. Although ILD may be caused by environmental inhalant exposures, drugs, radiation, and recurring aspiration pneumonias, a large number of patients have ILD of unknown origin, the most common being idiopathic pulmonary fibrosis. ILD associated with CTD (e.g., scleroderma), represents an additional diagnostic challenge, because these patients may have only parenchymal disease, only vascular disease, or various stages of both.

The hemodynamic profile of patients with ILD and pulmonary hypertension is distinct from that of patients with IPAH. It is uncommon for the mean PA pressure ever to exceed 40 mm Hg in these patients, whereas it is unusual for the mean PA pressure to be less than 40 mm Hg in patients with IPAH. Consequently, the combination of an abnormality consistent with interstitial lung disease on the chest CT scan and mild pulmonary hypertension should indicate the diagnosis of pulmonary hypertension associated with ILD and not IPAH (**Fig. 78-11**).

Most therapies for ILD have been directed toward halting progression or inducing regression of the interstitial disease process with immunosuppressive and anti-inflammatory agents. Overall, the results

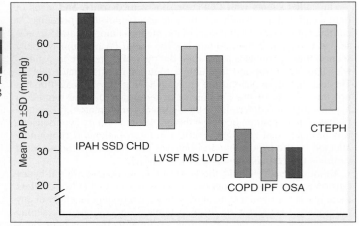

FIGURE 78-11 Mean PAP in patients with different causes of pulmonary hypertension (PH). The mean PAP ± 1 SDs (standard deviations) are shown from published series of patients with pulmonary hypertension from a variety of causes undergoing catheterization. From the graph, it would be difficult to determine the cause of the PH based on the mean PA pressure, with the exception of those with underlying lung disease. CHD = congenital heart disease; IPF = idiopathic pulmonary fibrosis; LVDF = left ventricular diastolic failure; LVSF = left ventricular systolic failure; MS = mitral stenosis; SSD = scleroderma spectrum of diseases.

of these trials have been disappointing, which makes the treatment of any associated pulmonary hypertension an attractive therapeutic target. Although vasodilator therapy has been available for decades, there are no randomized clinical trials showing benefit of these agents in ILD. Given the expense and morbidity associated with these therapies, we would caution against their anecdotal use in any patient until more definitive data support their chronic use. To date, lung transplantation is the only intervention proven to improve survival.

SLEEP-DISORDERED BREATHING. Observational studies have demonstrated a wide variation in the incidence of pulmonary hypertension as a complication of obstructive sleep apnea (OSA), with a wide range of severity (see Chap. 79). OSA is associated with repetitive nocturnal arterial oxygen desaturation and hypercapnia, large intrathoracic negative pressure swings, and acute increases in PA pressure. Mild pulmonary hypertension has been reported to occur in 20% to 40% of patients,[73] although the diagnosis of pulmonary hypertension in OSA is clouded by the frequent coexistence of systemic hypertension, obesity, and diastolic dysfunction. Right heart catheterization is usually necessary to make a clear diagnosis. Acute pulmonary hemodynamic changes during obstructive apneas have been well defined; however, the extent to which these translate into persistent daytime pulmonary hypertension remains less certain. Right ventricular failure from OSA is distinctly uncommon. Treatment with continuous positive airway pressure improves pulmonary hemodynamics in patients with OSA.

ALVEOLAR HYPOVENTILATION DISORDERS. Restrictive lung disease may result from neuromuscular diseases or other factors that affect chest wall expansion, including severe obesity. Chronic alveolar hypoventilation can lead to hypoxemia, hypercapnia, and acidosis and cause pulmonary hypertension. Thoracovertebral deformities that can result in chronic alveolar hypoventilation and pulmonary hypertension include idiopathic kyphoscoliosis, spinal tuberculosis, congenital spinal developmental abnormalities, spinal cord injury, ankylosing spondylitis, or other congenital and acquired muscular skeletal conditions, such as pectus excavatum. Pulmonary hypertension is related to the reduction of the vascular bed caused by hypoventilation and hypoxia. Usually, symptoms are slowly progressive. Hypoxemia can occur from both ventilation-perfusion mismatch and

underlying atelectasis. In patients with advanced disease, intermittent positive pressure breathing and noninvasive ventilation have been used successfully, as well as supplemental oxygen in patients who are hypoxemic. The development of right-sided heart failure is an unusual manifestation of respiratory failure caused solely by respiratory muscle weakness from neuromuscular disease. It usually develops in response to hypoxic and hypercapnic stimuli in patients with chronic forms of these disorders.

Bilateral diaphragmatic paralysis as a result of phrenic nerve injury, which can be traumatic or secondary to an underlying motor neuron disease, is an uncommon and rarely recognized cause of pulmonary hypertension. It may occur after cardiac surgery, as a manifestation of Lyme disease, after radiation therapy, or as a manifestation of other neurologic disorders. When an affected patient is upright, ventilation may be normal or almost normal, but when the patient is supine, gas exchange deteriorates. The diagnosis may be suspected in a patient with supine breathlessness, disturbed sleep pattern, paradoxical motion of the abdomen on inspiration, and low vital capacity in the upright position. Patients with nontraumatic bilateral diaphragmatic paralysis may go unrecognized until they present with respiratory failure or pulmonary hypertension. The diagnosis can be made when the vital capacity is reduced by more than 40% of predicted and paradoxical motion of the hemidiaphragms is noted with fluoroscopy. Patients can also have unilateral paralysis of the diaphragm, which is more common but is associated with fewer symptoms and physiological abnormalities. The treatment should always be directed toward correcting the underlying chronic neuromuscular disease, if present, and addressing nocturnal hypoventilation with noninvasive ventilatory techniques.

Pulmonary Hypertension Caused by Chronic Thromboembolic Disease

Chronic thromboembolic pulmonary hypertension (CTEPH) is an underdiagnosed disorder (see Chap. 77).[74] Pulmonary embolism, either as a single episode or as recurrent events, is thought to be the typical initiating process, followed by progressive vascular remodeling and in situ propagation of the thrombus. However, more than half of patients with CTEPH may not have a history of clinically overt pulmonary embolism. Whereas the incidence was originally believed to be approximately 0.1% to 0.5% of patients who survive an acute pulmonary embolus, more recent data have suggested a higher incidence, as much as 5%. An identifiable hypercoagulable state is found in only a minority of patients. The lupus anticoagulant is present in 10% to 20% of patients with CTEPH whereas inherited deficiencies of protein C, protein S, and antithrombin III as a group can be identified in up to 5% of this population. Other risk factors for the development of chronic thromboembolic pulmonary hypertension have been identified, including chronic inflammatory disorders, myeloproliferative syndromes, presence of a ventriculoatrial shunt, and splenectomy.

Rather than having inherent fibrinolytic resolution of the thromboembolism with restoration of vascular patency, the thromboemboli in these patients fail to resolve adequately. They undergo organization and incomplete recanalization and become incorporated into the vascular wall. Usually, they are in the subsegmental, segmental, and lobar vessels, although it is believed that chronic thromboembolism tends to propagate in a retrograde manner, leading to slowly progressive vascular obstruction. The development of a pulmonary hypertensive arteriopathy, similar to that seen in patients with other forms of pulmonary hypertension, has been documented in nonobstructive lung regions as well as in vessels distal to partially or completely occluded proximal pulmonary arteries. These small-vessel changes therefore appear to be a significant contributor to the hemodynamic progression seen in some patients. The pathology of CTEPH has features that distinguish it from IPAH. The lesions are frequently more variable—that is, there are arterial pathways that appear relatively unaffected by vascular disease and others that typically show recanalized vascular thromboses.

PATIENT EVALUATION. CTEPH involving the proximal pulmonary arteries is a well-characterized entity. The slowly progressive nature of the course of CTEPH allows right ventricular hypertrophy to ensue, which compensates for the increased pulmonary vascular resistance. However, because of progressive thrombosis or vascular changes in the uninvolved vascular bed, the pulmonary hypertension becomes progressive and the patient manifests the clinical symptoms of dyspnea, fatigue, hypoxemia, and right-sided heart failure. Patients may present with progressive dyspnea on exertion and/or signs of right heart failure after a single or recurrent episode of overt pulmonary embolism. Some patients experience a reprieve between the acute event and clinical signs of CTEPH, which may last from a few months to many years. The findings on clinical examination of patients with CTEPH are similar to those of other patients with pulmonary hypertension, with the exception that these patients tend to have lower cardiac outputs than patients with IPAH, which is often reflected in the reduced carotid arterial pulse volume. On occasion, bruits can be heard over areas of the lung that represent vessels with partial occlusions, but they must be carefully listened for. Thrombophilia screening, including testing for antiphospholipid antibodies, lupus anticoagulant, and anticardiolipin antibodies, should be performed.

The perfusion lung scan has a high sensitivity for the detection of CTEPH and is an important reason why lung scans are recommended for all patients who present with pulmonary hypertension (see Fig. 78-8). However, the lung scan typically underestimates the severity of the central pulmonary arterial obstruction. Therefore, patients who present with one or more mismatched segmental or larger defects should undergo contrast-enhanced CT scanning[75] (see Chaps. 19 and 77; **Fig. 78-12**). The contrast-enhanced CT features of CTEPH include evidence of organized thrombus lining the pulmonary vessels in an eccentric or concentric fashion, enlargement of the right ventricle and central pulmonary arteries, variation in size of segmental arteries, bronchial artery collaterals, and parenchymal changes from pulmonary infarcts. Marked variation in the size of the segmental vessels is specific for CTEPH and is believed to represent involvement of the segmental vessels caused by thromboemboli. With nonenhanced CT, areas of increased attenuation that do not obscure the vessels and that have a ground-glass appearance have been characterized as a mosaic pattern corresponding to hypoperfusion of the lung. Although this pattern is consistent with CTEPH, it may also be seen in patients with cystic fibrosis and those with bronchiectasis, but is almost never seen in patients with IPAH.

Pulmonary angiography continues to be the standard for defining the pulmonary vascular anatomy and is performed in patients thought to be amenable to surgical intervention to determine the location and surgical accessibility of the thromboemboli and to rule out other diagnostic possibilities. Maturation and organization of clot results in vessel retraction and partial recanalization, resulting in several angiographic patterns suggestive of chronic thromboembolic disease—pouch defect, pulmonary webs or bands, intimal irregularities, abrupt narrowing of major pulmonary vessels, and obstruction of main, lobar, or segmental pulmonary arteries, frequently at their point of origin. Bronchial artery collaterals may be present. Because CTEPH is usually bilateral, the presence of unilateral central PA obstruction should prompt consideration of other diagnoses, such as pulmonary vascular tumors or extravascular compression from a lung carcinoma, hilar or mediastinal adenopathy, or mediastinal fibrosis.

Hemodynamically, these patients may be indistinguishable from patients with IPAH. However, it can be misleading to rely on the pulmonary capillary wedge pressure, because there is no way for the clinician to know whether the vessel that is used to obtain the wedge pressure tracing has distal thrombus. Thus, these patients need to have a direct measurement of left ventricular end-diastolic pressure when the diagnosis is made. Patients with CTEPH tend to have higher right atrial pressures and lower cardiac outputs than comparable patients with IPAH for the same level of PA pressure. Some patients will have a reactive component to their pulmonary hypertension believed to be attributable to pulmonary vasoconstriction in the vasculature that is uninvolved with pulmonary thromboemboli. One clinical dilemma is the patient with a documented solitary pulmonary embolism who

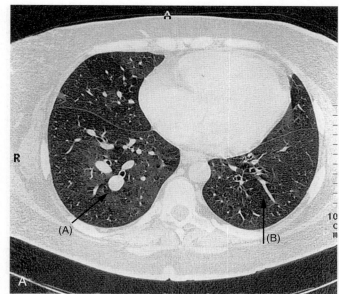

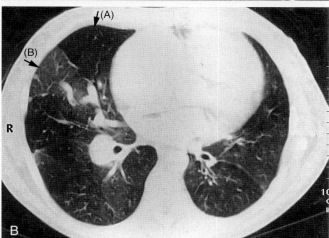

FIGURE 78-12 Chest CT scans in a patient with CTEPH. **A,** Helical scan with contrast medium enhancement of the pulmonary vasculature shows a marked disparity in vessel size between the involved vessels (A), which are enlarged from thrombus, and the uninvolved vessels (B). **B,** Noncontrast-enhanced high-resolution scan illustrates a marked mosaic pattern manifest by differences in density of regions of the lung parenchyma reflecting the perfused areas (B) and the nonperfused areas (A), also consistent with underlying thromboembolic disease.

develops pulmonary hypertension. Whether this represents coincidence, a cause and effect phenomenon, or a subset of genetically susceptible individuals may be impossible to resolve.

TREATMENT. The natural history of CTEPH is poor and is related to the severity of the pulmonary hypertension. It is important to make the diagnostic distinction between patients with CTEPH and those with other forms of pulmonary hypertension because the treatments are so different. For the former group, a potentially curative therapy through pulmonary thromboendarterectomy (PTEA) is available (**Fig. 78-13**). In specialized centers, these patients can have a dramatic improvement in their symptoms, hemodynamics, and survival and is the treatment of choice. Because this disease is generally progressive, the hemodynamic indications for surgical intervention are an elevation of PA pressure and pulmonary vascular resistance for a period of more than 3 months, despite adequate anticoagulation. Operability is determined by the location and extent of proximal thromboemboli and should involve the main, lobar, or proximal segmental arteries. It

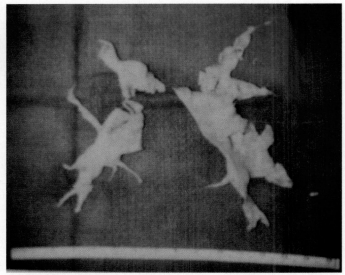

FIGURE 78-13 Specimen removed from a patient undergoing pulmonary thromboendarterectomy. The thrombus is highly organized and fibrous and represents a cast of the pulmonary circulation. Because the procedure is a true endarterectomy, the thrombosis can often be removed as a single unit. The more thrombus removed, the greater clinical improvement expected as a result of the surgery.

is also important to evaluate whether the amount of surgically accessible thrombus is compatible with a degree of hemodynamic impairment. Failure to reduce the pulmonary vascular resistance significantly with PTEA, usually a result of the small-vessel arteriopathy that may accompany this disease, is associated with a higher perioperative mortality rate and worse long-term outcome.

There is a close relationship between preoperative pulmonary vascular resistance and perioperative mortality. Right ventricular dysfunction is not considered a contraindication to surgery because right ventricular function has been noted to improve once the obstruction of the pulmonary blood flow has been removed. The operation is a true endarterectomy, requiring establishment of a dissection plane at the level of the media. The procedure is performed on cardiopulmonary bypass and usually requires periods of complete circulatory arrest to allow for a bloodless field and define an adequate dissection plane.

Postoperative management can be extremely challenging. Patients in whom a large volume of central thrombus is removed (see Fig. 78-13), associated with backbleeding from the distal vascular segments and an immediate fall in the PA pressure, usually have an extremely good postoperative course and long-term follow-up. Patients in whom small amounts of thrombus can be removed, the thrombus becomes fragmented at the time of PTEA, or there is no distal backbleeding from the segment where the thrombus was removed usually have a difficult postoperative course. In addition, lack of a significant fall in PA pressure or increase in cardiac output portends a difficult postoperative recovery. Much of the mortality risk appears to be related to severe right ventricular dysfunction, which actually initially worsens during the surgical procedure. Reperfusion injury, manifest by profound hypoxemia and pulmonary infiltrates corresponding to the segments where thrombus was removed, occurs in approximately 15% to 20% of patients and can be extensive. The only effective management of this complication is sustained assisted ventilation and oxygen supplementation. Survivors who have a good result, with a significant reduction in postoperative pulmonary vascular resistance at 48 hours, can expect to realize an improvement in functional class and exercise tolerance. Lifelong anticoagulation with a goal INR ratio of 2.5 to 3.5 is indicated postoperatively.

Some patients will have extensive disease that is inoperable or only partially amenable to surgical removal. The use of pulmonary vasodilators has been tested in anecdotal short-term studies with some success.[76] Both bosentan and sildenafil have been associated with an improvement in symptoms and exercise tolerance. It is assumed that the drugs affect the uninvolved pulmonary vasculature. Because there have been no prospective randomized trials of vasodilators in CTEPH, it remains unknown whether their use will translate into a clinically meaningful and sustained improvement in these patients. Nonetheless, in patients with inoperable CTEPH a clinical trial of pulmonary vasodilator therapy may be warranted, with the goal of improving the patient's symptomatology and quality of life.

Pulmonary Hypertension from Conditions with Uncertain Mechanisms

SICKLE CELL DISEASE. Cardiopulmonary complications are common in sickle cell disease. The cause of pulmonary hypertension, which has been reported in 20% to 32% of sickle cell disease patients, is multifactorial, with contributing factors that include hemolysis, impaired NO bioavailability, chronic hypoxemia, high cardiac output, thromboembolism, and parenchymal and vascular injury caused by sequestration of sickle erythrocytes, chronic liver disease, and asplenia.[77] In general, the hemodynamic profile of most patients with pulmonary hypertension in the setting of sickle cell disease is distinct from those with IPAH. It is characterized by a more modest elevation in PA pressure, an elevation in left heart filling pressures, and invariably a markedly elevated cardiac output. Left-sided heart disease, or pulmonary venous hypertension, is a contributing factor in most patients. Whether the pulmonary hypertension reduces survival or is simply a marker of more advanced sickle cell disease remains unclear. Intensification of sickle cell disease therapy, such as with hydroxyurea or exchange transfusions, should be the mainstay of treatment. There have been no controlled trials demonstrating benefit from pulmonary vasodilator therapy.

SCHISTOSOMIASIS. Although schistosomiasis is extremely rare in North America, hundreds of millions of people are affected worldwide, particularly in developing countries.[78] The development of pulmonary hypertension almost always occurs in the setting of hepatosplenic disease. Clinical features appear when ova embolize to the lungs, where they induce formation of delayed hypersensitivity granulomas. In addition, deposition of fibrous tissue may cause narrowing, thickening, and occlusion of the pulmonary arterioles. Histologically, focal changes related directly to the presence of schistosome ova may be located in the alveolar tissue or in the pulmonary arteries. However, classic changes typical of IPAH are also found, including plexiform lesions. The clinical symptoms and radiographic findings in these patients who develop pulmonary hypertension are not distinctive. In developing countries, this condition can be confused with IPAH.[79] The diagnosis of schistosomiasis-induced pulmonary hypertension is confirmed by finding the parasite ova in the urine or stool of persons with symptoms. However, the insidious onset of pulmonary vascular disease years after infection makes finding these parasite ova difficult. Active infections are treated with praziquantel, which kills the adult worms and stops further destruction of tissue by ova deposition. However, eradication of the infection does not seem to alter the progression of the pulmonary vascular disease.

SARCOIDOSIS. Sarcoidosis is a multisystemic granulomatous disease of unknown origin characterized by an enhanced cellular immune response at the sites of involvement. Although any organ can be involved, sarcoidosis most commonly affects the lungs and intrathoracic lymph nodes. The clinical manifestation and natural history of sarcoidosis vary greatly, but the lung is involved in more than 90% of patients. The most common presenting symptoms are cough and shortness of breath, which is of a progressive nature. As the disease progresses in the lung parenchyma, extensive interstitial fibrosis is the result. In addition, obstructive airway disease, fibrocystic disease, bronchiectasis, endobronchial granulomas, and lobar atelectasis are common consequences of lung involvement. Cardiac involvement from sarcoidosis appears to be more common than previously thought and may be present in up to one third of cases.[80] Consequently, patients presenting with dyspnea should undergo a thorough cardiac evaluation for the possibility of cardiac involvement. Noncaseating granulomas may infiltrate the myocardium and lead to the development of a restrictive cardiomyopathy (see Chap. 68). Patients with cardiac involvement from sarcoidosis also present with varying degrees of heart block, arrhythmias, and/or clinical features of biventricular diastolic heart failure. The prognosis of patients with cardiac involvement from sarcoidosis is variable but can be poor.

Pulmonary hypertension is usually the result of chronic severe fibrocystic sarcoidosis. Patients have chronic progressive dyspnea with effort, a chest radiograph demonstrating severe diffuse interstitial fibrotic lung disease, and pulmonary function test results that reflect severe restrictive physiology and marked hypoxemia. In these cases, the resulting pulmonary hypertension is usually mild to moderate and typical of patients presenting with restrictive lung disease of any cause. Management is generally focused on reversing any acute exacerbations of the lung disease and giving supplemental oxygen, when indicated. A subset of patients present with severe pulmonary hypertension thought to be caused by pulmonary vascular involvement, often in the setting of quiescent disease. It appears that these patients develop pulmonary vascular disease triggered in some way by the sarcoid disease process. The use of intravenous epoprostenol chronically may reverse the right-sided heart failure and improve hemodynamics, but will not affect the underlying fibrotic lung disease, and most patients will remain symptomatic and dyspneic.[81]

Future Perspectives

It has become apparent that the clinical manifestation of pulmonary hypertension is a final common pathway originating from diverse abnormalities in the pulmonary circulation associated with a number of risk factors. Animal models of pulmonary hypertension have illustrated how changes in specific molecular pathways can produce pulmonary hypertension, and how blocking these pathways can lead to reversal of advanced disease. Whether the reversal of the disease can be achieved in patients with therapy remains unknown, but to date has never been demonstrated. As the molecular pathways involved in pulmonary hypertension are becoming elucidated and understood, drugs that block these pathways will hold promise as future treatment. Although the presence of redundant pathways and multiple abnormalities will make clinical progress more challenging, clinical trials using growth factor inhibitors are being conducted. Many patients with long-standing pulmonary hypertension can function at a reasonable level as long as their right ventricular function remains intact. Novel therapies aimed at improving right ventricular adaptation to pulmonary hypertension with medications, or augmenting right ventricular function with medical devices, is another area that has great potential.

REFERENCES

Normal Pulmonary Circulation

1. Kasper M: Phenotypic characterization of pulmonary arteries in normal and diseased lung. Chest 128:547S, 2005.
2. Bartsch P, Gibbs JS: Effect of altitude on the heart and the lungs. Circulation 116:2191, 2007.
3. Weir EK, Lopez-Barneo J, Buckler KJ, Archer SL: Acute oxygen-sensing mechanisms. N Engl J Med 353:2042, 2005.
4. Ichinose F, Roberts JD Jr, Zapol WM: Inhaled nitric oxide: A selective pulmonary vasodilator: Current uses and therapeutic potential. Circulation 109:3106, 2004.

Pathobiology of Pulmonary Arterial Hypertension

5. Rabinovitch M: Molecular pathogenesis of pulmonary arterial hypertension. J Clin Invest 118:2372, 2008.
6. Morrell NW, Adnot S, Archer SL, et al: Cellular and molecular basis of pulmonary arterial hypertension. J Am Coll Cardiol 54:S20, 2009.
7. Budhiraja R, Tuder RM, Hassoun PM: Endothelial dysfunction in pulmonary hypertension. Circulation 109:159, 2004.
8. McLaughlin VV, Archer SL, Badesch DB, et al: ACCF/AHA 2009 expert consensus document on pulmonary hypertension. Circulation 119:2250, 2009.
9. Pietra GG, Capron F, Stewart S, et al: Pathologic assessment of vasculopathies in pulmonary hypertension. J Am Coll Cardiol 43:25S, 2004.
10. Gorlach A, BelAiba RS, Hess J, Kietzmann T: Thrombin activates the p21-activated kinase in pulmonary artery smooth muscle cells. Role in tissue factor expression. Thromb Haemost 93:1168, 2005.

11. Benisty JI, McLaughlin VV, Landzberg MJ, et al: Elevated basic fibroblast growth factor levels in patients with pulmonary arterial hypertension. Chest 126:1255, 2004.
12. White RJ, Meoli DF, Swarthout RF, et al: Plexiform-like lesions and increased tissue factor expression in a rat model of severe pulmonary arterial hypertension. Am J Physiol Lung Cell Mol Physiol 293:L583, 2007.
13. Barst RJ, McGoon M, Torbicki A, et al: Diagnosis and differential assessment of pulmonary arterial hypertension. J Am Coll Cardiol 43:40S, 2004.
14. Yu Y, Fantozzi I, Remillard CV, et al: Enhanced expression of transient receptor potential channels in idiopathic pulmonary arterial hypertension. Proc Natl Acad Sci USA 101:13861, 2004.
15. Hong Z, Smith AJ, Archer SL, et al: Pergolide is an inhibitor of voltage-gated potassium channels, including Kv1.5, and causes pulmonary vasoconstriction. Circulation 112:1494, 2005.
16. Humbert M, Morrell NW, Archer SL, et al: Cellular and molecular pathobiology of pulmonary arterial hypertension. J Am Coll Cardiol 43:13S, 2004.
17. Bonnet S, Michelakis ED, Porter CJ, et al: An abnormal mitochondrial-hypoxia inducible factor-1alpha-Kv channel pathway disrupts oxygen sensing and triggers pulmonary arterial hypertension in fawn hooded rats: Similarities to human pulmonary arterial hypertension. Circulation 113:2630, 2006.
18. Bonnet S, Rochefort G, Sutendra G, et al: The nuclear factor of activated T cells in pulmonary arterial hypertension can be therapeutically targeted. Proc Natl Acad Sci USA 104:11418, 2007.
19. McMurtry MS, Archer SL, Altieri DC, et al: Gene therapy targeting survivin selectively induces pulmonary vascular apoptosis and reverses pulmonary arterial hypertension. J Clin Invest 115:1479, 2005.
20. Richter A, Yeager ME, Zaiman A, et al: Impaired transforming growth factor-beta signaling in idiopathic pulmonary arterial hypertension. Am J Respir Crit Care Med 170:1340, 2004.
21. Marcos E, Fadel E, Sanchez O, et al: Serotonin-induced smooth muscle hyperplasia in various forms of human pulmonary hypertension. Circ Res 94:1263, 2004.
22. Eddahibi S, Guignabert C, Barlier-Mur AM, et al: Cross talk between endothelial and smooth muscle cells in pulmonary hypertension: Critical role for serotonin-induced smooth muscle hyperplasia. Circulation 113:1857, 2006.
23. de Caestecker M: Serotonin signaling in pulmonary hypertension. Circ Res 98:1229, 2006.
24. Machado RD, Koehler R, Glissmeyer E, et al: Genetic association of the serotonin transporter in pulmonary arterial hypertension. Am J Respir Crit Care Med 173:793, 2006.
25. Hassoun PM, Mouthon L, Barbera JA, et al: Inflammation, growth factors, and pulmonary vascular remodeling. J Am Coll Cardiol 54:S10, 2009.
26. Hamid R, Newman JH: Evidence for inflammatory signaling in idiopathic pulmonary artery hypertension: TRPC6 and nuclear factor-kappaB. Circulation 119:2297, 2009.
27. Csiszar A, Smith KE, Koller A, et al: Regulation of bone morphogenetic protein-2 expression in endothelial cells: Role of nuclear factor-kappaB activation by tumor necrosis factor-alpha, H_2O_2, and high intravascular pressure. Circulation 111:2364, 2005.
28. Marecki JC, Cool CD, Parr JE, et al: HIV-1 Nef is associated with complex pulmonary vascular lesions in SHIV-nef-infected macaques. Am J Respir Crit Care Med 174:437, 2006.
29. Tuder RM, Abman SH, Braun T, et al: Development and pathology of pulmonary hypertension. J Am Coll Cardiol 54:S3, 2009.
30. Newman JH, Trembath RC, Morse JA, et al: Genetic basis of pulmonary arterial hypertension. J Am Coll Cardiol 43:33S, 2004.
31. Cogan JD, Vnencak-Jones CL, Phillips JA 3rd, et al: Gross BMPR2 gene rearrangements constitute a new cause for primary pulmonary hypertension. Genet Med 7:169, 2005.
32. Teichert-Kuliszewska K, Kutryk MJ, Kuliszewski MA, et al: Bone morphogenetic protein receptor-2 signaling promotes pulmonary arterial endothelial cell survival: Implications for loss-of-function mutations in the pathogenesis of pulmonary hypertension. Circ Res 98:209, 2006.
33. Machado RD, James V, Southwood M, et al: Investigation of second genetic hits at the BMPR2 locus as a modulator of disease progression in familial pulmonary arterial hypertension. Circulation 111:607, 2005.
34. Machado RD, Aldred MA, James V, et al: Mutations of the TGF-beta type II receptor BMPR2 in pulmonary arterial hypertension. Hum Mutat 27:121, 2006.
35. Aldred MA, Vijayakrishnan J, James V, et al: BMPR2 gene rearrangements account for a significant proportion of mutations in familial and idiopathic pulmonary arterial hypertension. Hum Mutat 27:212, 2006.
36. Long L, MacLean MR, Jeffery TK, et al: Serotonin increases susceptibility to pulmonary hypertension in BMPR2-deficient mice. Circ Res 98:818, 2006.

Clinical Assessment of the Patient

37. van Wolferen SA, Marcus JT, Westerhof N, et al: Right coronary artery flow impairment in patients with pulmonary hypertension. Eur Heart J 29:120, 2008.
38. Souza R, Bogossian HB, Humbert M, et al: N-terminal-pro-brain natriuretic peptide as a haemodynamic marker in idiopathic pulmonary arterial hypertension. Eur Respir J 25:509, 2005.
39. Li JH, Safford RE, Aduen JF, et al: Pulmonary hypertension and thyroid disease. Chest 132:793, 2007.
40. McGoon M, Gutterman D, Steen V, et al: Screening, early detection, and diagnosis of pulmonary arterial hypertension: ACCP evidence-based clinical practice guidelines. Chest 126:14S, 2004.
41. Fisher MR, Forfia PR, Chamera E, et al: Accuracy of Doppler echocardiography in the hemodynamic assessment of pulmonary hypertension. Am J Respir Crit Care Med 179:615, 2009.
42. Benza R, Biederman R, Murali S, et al: Role of cardiac magnetic resonance imaging in the management of patients with pulmonary arterial hypertension. J Am Coll Cardiol 52:1683, 2008.
43. Salzman SH: The 6-min walk test: clinical and research role, technique, coding, and reimbursement. Chest 135:1345, 2009.
44. Oudiz RJ, Barst RJ, Hansen JE, et al: Cardiopulmonary exercise testing and six-minute walk correlations in pulmonary arterial hypertension. Am J Cardiol 97:123, 2006.
45. Ghofrani HA, Wilkins MW, Rich S: Uncertainties in the diagnosis and treatment of pulmonary arterial hypertension. Circulation 118:1195, 2008.
46. Halpern SD, Taichman DB: Misclassification of pulmonary hypertension due to reliance in pulmonary capillary wedge pressure rather than left ventricular end-diastolic pressure. Chest 136:37, 2009.

47. Simonneau G, Robbins IM, Beghetti M, et al: Updated clinical classification of pulmonary hypertension. J Am Coll Cardiol 54:S43, 2009.

48. Hyduk A, Croft J, Ayala C, et al: Pulmonary hypertension surveillance—United States, 1980-2002. MMRWR Surveill Summ 54:1, 2005.

Pulmonary Arterial Hypertension

49. Mereles D, Ehlken N, Kreuscher S, et al: Exercise and respiratory training improve exercise capacity and quality of life in patients with severe chronic pulmonary hypertension. Circulation 114:1482, 2006.

50. Johnson SR, Mehta S, Granton JT: Anticoagulation in pulmonary arterial hypertension: A qualitative systematic review. Eur Respir J 28:999, 2006.

51. Simonneau G, Rubin LJ, Galie N, et al: Addition of sildenafil to long-term intravenous epoprostenol therapy in patients with pulmonary arterial hypertension: A randomized trial. Ann Intern Med 149:521, 2008.

52. Sitbon O, Humbert M, Jais X, et al: Long-term response to calcium channel blockers in idiopathic pulmonary arterial hypertension. Circulation 111:3105, 2005.

53. Gomberg-Maitland M, Olschewski H: Prostacyclin therapies for the treatment of pulmonary arterial hypertension. Eur Respir J 31:891, 2008.

54. Lang I, Gomez-Sanchez M, Kneussl M, et al: Efficacy of long-term subcutaneous treprostinil sodium therapy in pulmonary hypertension. Chest 129:1636, 2006.

55. Nagendran J, Archer SL, Soliman D, et al: Phosphodiesterase type 5 is highly expressed in the hypertrophied human right ventricle, and acute inhibition of phosphodiesterase type 5 improves contractility. Circulation 116:238, 2007.

56. Galie N, Ghofrani HA, Torbicki A, et al: Sildenafil citrate therapy for pulmonary arterial hypertension. N Engl J Med 353:2148, 2005.

57. Galie N, Brundage BH, Ghofrani HA, et al: Tadalafil therapy for pulmonary arterial hypertension. Circulation 119:2894, 2009.

58. Dupuis J, Hoeper MM: Endothelin receptor antagonists in pulmonary arterial hypertension. Eur Respir J 31:407, 2008.

59. Kurzyna M, Dabrowski M, Bielecki D, et al: Atrial septostomy in treatment of end-stage right heart failure in patients with pulmonary hypertension. Chest 131:977, 2007.

60. Orens JB, Garrity ER Jr: General overview of lung transplantation and review of organ allocation. Proc Am Thorac Soc 6:13, 2009.

61. Dempsie Y, Morecroft I, Welsh DJ, et al: Converging evidence in support of the serotonin hypothesis of dexfenfluramine-induced pulmonary hypertension with novel transgenic mice. Circulation 117:2928, 2008.

62. Berger RMF: Pulmonary hypertension associated with congenital cardiac disease. Cardiol Young 19:311, 2009.

63. Galie N, Beghetti M, Gatzoulis MA, et al: Bosentan therapy in patients with Eisenmenger syndrome: A multicenter, double-blind, placebo-controlled study. Circulation 114:48, 2006.

64. Condliffe R, Kiely DG, Peacock AJ, et al: Connective tissue disease-associated pulmonary arterial hypertension in the modern treatment era. Am J Respir Crit Care Med 179:151, 2009.

65. Krowka MJ: Evolving dilemmas and management of portopulmonary hypertension. Semin Liver Dis 26:265, 2006.

66. Frazier AA, Franks TJ, Mohammed TL, et al: From the Archives of the AFIP: Pulmonary veno-occlusive disease and pulmonary capillary hemangiomatosis. Radiographics 27:867, 2007.

Pulmonary Venous Hypertension

67. Lam CS, Roger VL, Rodeheffer RJ, et al: Pulmonary hypertension in heart failure with preserved ejection fraction: A community-based study. J Am Coll Cardiol 53:1119, 2009.

68. Fawzy ME, Hassan W, Stefadouros M, et al: Prevalence and fate of severe pulmonary hypertension in 559 consecutive patients with severe rheumatic mitral stenosis undergoing mitral balloon valvotomy. J Heart Valve Dis 13:942, 2004.

69. Montani D, Price LC, Dorfmuller P, et al: Pulmonary veno-occlusive disease. Eur Respir J 33:189, 2009.

Pulmonary Arterial Hypertension Associated with Hypoxic Lung Disease

70. Chaouat A, Bugnet AS, Kadaoui N, et al: Severe pulmonary hypertension and chronic obstructive pulmonary disease. Am J Respir Crit Care Med 172:189, 2005.

71. Stolz D, Rasch H, Linka A, et al: A randomised, controlled trial of bosentan in severe COPD. Eur Respir J 32:619, 2008.

72. Behr J, Ryu JH: Pulmonary hypertension in interstitial lung disease. Eur Respir J 31:1357, 2008.

73. Atwood CW, McCrory D, Garcia JGN, et al: Pulmonary artery hypertension and sleep-disordered breathing: ACCP evidence-based clinical practice guidelines. Chest 126:72S, 2004.

Pulmonary Hypertension Caused by Chronic Thromboembolic Disease

74. Auger WR, Fedullo PF: Chronic thromboembolic pulmonary hypertension. Semin Respir Crit Care Med 30:471, 2009.

75. Coulden R: State-of-the-art imaging techniques in chronic thromboembolic pulmonary hypertension. Proc Am Thorac Soc 3:577, 2006.

76. Condliffe R, Kiely DG, Gibbs JS, et al: Improved outcomes in medically and surgically treated chronic thromboembolic pulmonary hypertension. Am J Respir Crit Care Med 177:1122, 2008.

Pulmonary Hypertension with Uncertain or Multifactorial Mechanisms

77. Machado RF, Gladwin MT: Chronic sickle cell lung disease: New insights into the diagnosis, pathogenesis and treatment of pulmonary hypertension. Br J Haematol 129:449, 2005.

78. Butrous G, Ghofrani HA, Grimminger F: Pulmonary vascular disease in the developing world. Circulation 118:1758, 2008.

79. Lapa M, Dias B, Jardim C, et al: Cardiopulmonary manifestations of hepatosplenic schistosomiasis. Circulation 119:1518, 2009.

80. Mehta D, Lubitz SA, Frankel Z, et al: Cardiac involvement in patients with sarcoidosis: Diagnostic and prognostic value of outpatient testing. Chest 133:1426, 2008.

81. Fisher KA, Serlin DM, Wilson KC, et al: Sarcoidosis-associated pulmonary hypertension: Outcome with long-term epoprostenol treatment. Chest 130:1481, 2006.

CHAPTER **79** # Sleep Apnea and Cardiovascular Disease

Virend K. Somers

Normal Sleep Physiology

Sleep, which usually comprises up to one third of our lifetime, is a complex and dynamic physiologic process.[1] Rapid eye movement (REM) sleep makes up about 25% of a night of sleep. It is a tonic state punctuated by periods of phasic activity, during which autonomic and cardiac functions are erratic.[2] Thermoregulation is reduced, and sympathetic neural drive, heart rate, and blood pressure increase. Non–rapid eye movement (NREM) sleep comprises about 75% of sleep. During NREM sleep, in contrast to REM sleep, autonomic and cardiac regulation is stable. Sympathetic neural activity decreases and parasympathetic tone predominates, which decreases the arterial baroreceptor set point, heart rate, blood pressure, cardiac output, and systemic vascular resistance. Because of the predominance of parasympathetic neural tone, it is not unusual for healthy individuals to have sinus bradycardia, marked sinus arrhythmia, sinus pauses, or first-degree and type I second-degree atrioventricular block during sleep. Thus, the majority of sleep is quiescent with respect to cardiac function, with the exception being the dynamic changes of phasic REM sleep.

Sleep Disorders

The two principal sleep disorders with a recognized impact on cardiovascular function and disease are obstructive sleep apnea (OSA) and central sleep apnea (CSA).

Obstructive Sleep Apnea

DEFINITION AND PHYSIOLOGY. OSA is a sleep-related breathing disorder. Its principal feature is upper airway occlusion, which causes partial or complete cessation of air flow. This causes hypoxia and strenuous ventilatory efforts, followed by a transient arousal and restoration of airway patency and air flow. This sequence of events can recur hundreds of times nightly. In symptomatic individuals, the condition is called the obstructive sleep apnea syndrome.

An obstructive apnea is defined as the absence of air flow for at least 10 seconds in the presence of active ventilatory efforts, which are reflected by thoracoabdominal movements. An obstructive hypopnea is defined as a decrease of more than 50% in thoracoabdominal movements for at least 10 seconds associated with a decrease of more than 4% in oxygen saturation. The apnea-hypopnea index (AHI) is the average number of apneic and hypopneic events per hour of sleep, and it is the most common metric to describe the severity of OSA. OSA is present when the AHI is 5 or more and is considered severe when the AHI is 30 or more; however, these are essentially arbitrary thresholds created by expert consensus. In the context of cardiovascular disease and risk assessment,[3,4] low AHI thresholds are reasonable because clinically important cardiovascular outcomes are associated with an AHI as low as (and even lower than) 5 events/hour.[2]

The mechanisms of OSA relate to the structure and function of the pharyngeal musculature and the state of the central nervous system during sleep.[3,5] The patency of the upper airway is determined by pharyngeal dilator and abductor muscle tone competing against negative transmural pharyngeal pressures during inspiration. The supine position makes airway collapse more likely because of the posterior displacement of the tongue, soft palate, and mandible. People with micrognathia, retrognathia, tonsillar hypertrophy, macroglossia, and acromegaly are especially predisposed to OSA. Also, changes in central nervous system activity during sleep, particularly in REM sleep, decrease diaphragmatic activity (i.e., ventilatory drive) and pharyngeal muscle tone, which destabilizes the airway and favors airway collapse. Sedative-hypnotic medications or alcohol may compound these effects and increase the risk of obstructive apneas. Apneas terminate because of transient arousals to a lighter sleep stage, which are demonstrable with electroencephalographic recordings but may not result in subjective awakening or awareness. Chemoreceptors, which are activated by the hypoxemia and hypercapnia of apnea, elicit postapneic hyperventilation, also contributing to arousals.

PATHOPHYSIOLOGIC MECHANISMS LINKING OBSTRUCTIVE SLEEP APNEA TO CARDIOVASCULAR DISEASE. Individuals with OSA demonstrate an increased sensitivity of the peripheral chemoreceptors, which results in an increased ventilatory response to hypoxemia during sleep and wakefulness.[3] Activation of the chemoreceptors also stimulates sympathetic traffic to skeletal muscle vasculature, which results in peripheral vasoconstriction. During apneas, as hypoxemia worsens, peripheral sympathetic activity markedly increases and blood pressure acutely rises.[2] Severe oxygen desaturations may be associated with ventricular ectopy. In some individuals, peripheral sympathetic overactivity may be accompanied by cardiac parasympathetic activation, which results in peripheral vasoconstriction and bradycardia (i.e., the homeostatic "diving reflex" that simultaneously decreases myocardial oxygen demand and increases cerebral and cardiac perfusion).[2,3] Even during daytime wakefulness, individuals with OSA have persistently heightened sympathetic activity, partly because of tonic chemoreflex activation.

These mechanisms may be manifested clinically by a lack of the usual dip in nocturnal blood pressure, drug-resistant hypertension (see Chaps. 45 and 46), automatic tachycardias driven by sympathetic activity, and profound nocturnal bradycardias caused by cardiac vagal activity. Common nocturnal arrhythmias, such as marked sinus arrhythmia and second-degree atrioventricular block (Mobitz type I), are exacerbated, and higher degree conduction abnormalities, such as long sinus pauses and advanced atrioventricular block, may occur transiently (see Chaps. 36 and 39).[2,4] The chronically elevated sympathetic activity results in increased resting heart rates, decreased heart rate variability, and increased blood pressure variability. In conjunction with structural heart disease or heart failure, this may have prognostic implications.

The inspiratory efforts against a collapsed airway during an obstructive apnea generate marked negative intrathoracic pressures, which themselves cause acute cardiac structural and hemodynamic effects.[3,4,6]

Whereas normal inspiratory pressures are about −8 cm H$_2$O, individuals with OSA can generate intrathoracic pressures of −30 cm H$_2$O or lower. This increases venous return to the right side of the heart, produces ventricular interdependence, decreases left ventricular compliance and filling, and results in decreased cardiac output. Coupled with heightened peripheral sympathetic activity, these changes can directly increase cardiac afterload and detrimentally affect left ventricular systolic function. Acute diastolic dysfunction and increases in left atrial transmural pressure also occur, which may cause atrial or pulmonary vein stretch. This is evidenced by increased atrial volume, increases in atrial natriuretic peptide levels, and the common symptom of nocturia in individuals with OSA. The intrathoracic pressure fluctuations may cause chronic diastolic dysfunction and left atrial enlargement,[7] associated with OSA independently of obesity and hypertension. These changes, together with oscillations in sympathetic and parasympathetic tone, may promote the initiation of atrial fibrillation during sleep.[8] OSA also results in the release of important neurohumoral mediators of cardiac and vascular disease.[9] Individuals with OSA have increased production of the potent vasoconstrictor endothelin and impaired endothelial function, which affect vasomotion. OSA has also been associated with systemic inflammation, which may advance atherosclerosis. Perhaps through its effects on sympathetic activity or because of sleep deprivation, OSA may increase insulin resistance, which promotes cardiovascular risk through multiple pathways.[10] Last, OSA is associated with increased levels of leptin, a hormone secreted by fat cells that is also associated with cardiovascular events.[9]

OBSTRUCTIVE SLEEP APNEA AND CARDIOVASCULAR DISEASE ASSOCIATIONS AND OUTCOMES. The true prevalence of OSA in the population is unknown because most people with OSA have not undergone polysomnography and remain undiagnosed. Population-based studies estimate that 1 in 5 middle-aged Western adults with a body mass index (BMI) of 25 to 28 kg/m^2 have OSA, and 1 in 20 are symptomatic with the OSA syndrome. OSA is strongly associated with obesity, and there is a direct relationship between BMI and the AHI.[3] OSA is present in more than 40% of those with a BMI of 30 and is especially common in individuals with a BMI of 40. OSA is also associated with multiple metabolic abnormalities, including abdominal obesity, diabetes, and dyslipidemia, and it is highly prevalent in patients with the metabolic syndrome.[10] Given its putative roles

in predisposing to and exacerbating insulin resistance,[9-11] OSA may conceivably contribute to the underlying pathophysiologic process of the metabolic syndrome.

OSA is highly prevalent in patients with cardiovascular disease (**Table 79-1**). Estimates of prevalence may differ geographically according to the BMI of patient populations. Many of these cardiovascular disease associations may occur because of the comorbidities of OSA, namely, obesity and its metabolic consequences, which together increase the risk of organic heart disease. However, observational studies have suggested that OSA itself may lead to incident cardiovascular disease. In a large population sample, the AHI correlated independently and directly with the development of hypertension during a period of 4 years.[3] OSA may also be a risk factor for new-onset atrial fibrillation. In 3542 people observed for an average of about 5 years after diagnostic polysomnography, non-elderly adults (younger than 65 years) with OSA (AHI = 5) were more likely than those without OSA to have incident atrial fibrillation (**Fig. 79-1**). The severity of nocturnal oxygen desaturation was associated with the magnitude of this risk independently of other atrial fibrillation risk factors, including obesity, hypertension, and heart failure.[12] OSA may be present in up to 50% of patients requiring cardioversion for atrial

TABLE 79-1	Estimated Prevalence of Obstructive Sleep Apnea in Patients with Cardiovascular Diseases	
CARDIOVASCULAR DISEASE		**PREVALENCE (%)**
Hypertension		50
Coronary artery disease		33
Acute coronary syndrome		50
Myocardial infarction		50-60
Heart failure with systolic dysfunction		30-40
Acute stroke		50
Atrial fibrillation requiring cardioversion		50
Lone atrial fibrillation		33

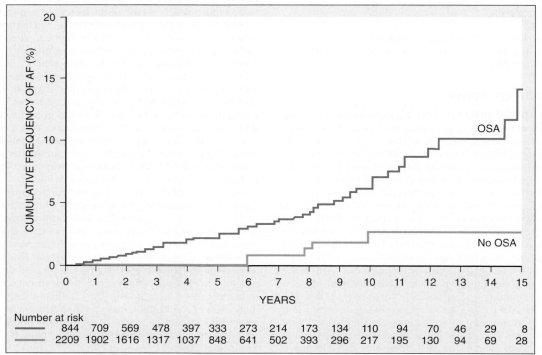

Number at risk															
844	709	569	478	397	333	273	214	173	134	110	94	70	46	29	8
2209	1902	1616	1317	1037	848	641	502	393	296	217	195	130	94	69	28

FIGURE 79-1 The cumulative frequency of new-onset atrial fibrillation (AF) in 3542 adults younger than 65 years, observed for an average of 4.6 years after diagnostic polysomnography. Individuals with OSA are shown with the blue line, and individuals without OSA are shown by the orange line. *(Modified from Gami AS, Hodge DO, Herges RM, et al: Obstructive sleep apnea, obesity, and the risk of incident atrial fibrillation. J Am Coll Cardiol 49:565, 2007.)*

fibrillation,[13] and untreated OSA may increase the likelihood of recurrence of atrial fibrillation after cardioversion.[3] There is emerging evidence implicating obstructive apnea in the pathophysiologic process and complications of hypertrophic cardiomyopathy.[14] Reliable evidence also exists for the direct effects of OSA in heart failure. Interventional studies of continuous positive airway pressure, which can effectively abolish obstructive apneas and hypopneas (see later), have shown increases in left ventricular ejection fraction.[4] OSA also can increase the risk of stroke, myocardial infarction, and death. In 1022 older adults observed for an average of about 3.5 years after diagnostic polysomnography, OSA (AHI = 5) was independently associated with a doubling of the risk of incident stroke or death.[15] In another 1651 men observed for an average of about 10 years, those with untreated severe OSA (AHI = 30) had a nearly three-fold risk of death from stroke or myocardial infarction and a more than threefold risk of coronary revascularization or nonfatal myocardial infarction or stroke, independently of important comorbidities, compared with healthy men (**Fig. 79-2**).[16] Data from the Sleep Heart Health Study of more than 6000 subjects suggest that nocturnal desaturations of 4% or more are independently associated with cardiovascular disease.[17] A prospective cohort of 6441 men and women from the same study demonstrated that sleep disordered breathing was accompanied by an increase in all-cause mortality and coronary artery disease–related mortality in men aged 40 to 70 years (**Fig. 79-3**).[18] Finally, the unique nocturnal pathophysiology of OSA may be associated with an increased risk of nocturnal cardiac events. A retrospective study of 112 individuals who had undergone polysomnography and then had sudden cardiac death found that those with OSA had a peak in sudden cardiac death during the sleeping hours, which contrasted with the nadir of sudden cardiac death during this period in those without OSA and in the general population (**Fig. 79-4**).[19] In a related prospective study of patients admitted for myocardial infarction, patients with nocturnal onset of myocardial infarction had a much greater likelihood of having OSA (**Fig. 79-5**),[20] suggesting that OSA may have triggered the nocturnal myocardial infarction. Of patients with myocardial infarction onset between 12 AM and 6 AM, about 90% had OSA. Currently, however, available evidence does not definitively implicate OSA as an independent cause of cardiovascular events. **Figure 79-6** summarizes the pathophysiology of OSA, its possible intermediate cardiovascular disease mechanisms, and its cardiovascular disease associations and risks.

Central Sleep Apnea (Cheyne-Stokes Respirations)

DEFINITION AND PHYSIOLOGY. CSA refers to multiple forms of periodic breathing in which ventilation waxes and wanes, gradually alternating between hyperpnea and apnea. CSA may occur in infants and in people traveling to high altitudes. CSA, sometimes in the form of Cheyne-Stokes respirations, is also associated with heart failure (see Chaps. 25 to 27).[3,21]

CSA, like OSA, is considered a sleep-related breathing disorder, even though its characteristic ventilatory patterns can also present subtly during wakefulness. Its principal defect is an instability of ventilatory control, which results in oscillations in the arterial partial pressure of carbon dioxide ($PaCO_2$) above and below the apneic threshold, producing periodic hyperpnea and apnea.[5] Ventilation is controlled by feedback loops that integrate information from multiple sources (e.g., central and peripheral chemoreceptors, intrapulmonary receptors, ventilatory muscle afferents) to limit fluctuations in $PaCO_2$ and the arterial partial pressure of oxygen (PaO_2). Control of ventilation becomes unstable when a phase delay exists between the inputs (chemosensors) and responses (ventilatory muscles) in these feedback loops and also when the gain of these feedback loops is increased so that small inputs produce exaggerated responses.[5]

Patients with heart failure (see Chap. 25) have ventilatory instability and CSA because of their heightened chemosensitivity to $PaCO_2$ (high loop gain) and long circulation time (phase delay). Increased chemosensitivity chronically decreases $PaCO_2$ closer to the apneic threshold. Also, stimulation of pulmonary irritant mechanoreceptors by increased left ventricular filling pressures and pulmonary edema causes hyperventilation beyond what is necessary to

normalize the $PaCO_2$.[5] This hyperpnea leads to hypocapnia beyond the apneic threshold, and the central efferents to the ventilatory muscles become suppressed, resulting in apnea. In heart failure, this may be exacerbated by the prolonged lung to periphery circulation time, which is inversely proportional to cardiac output. During apnea, declining PaO_2 and rising $PaCO_2$ ultimately initiate breathing, which may or may not be

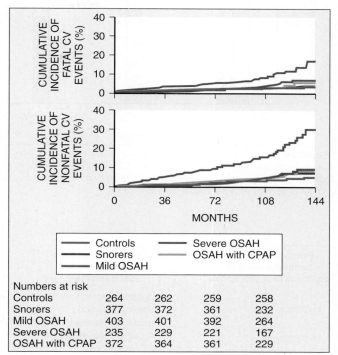

Numbers at risk				
Controls	264	262	259	258
Snorers	377	372	361	232
Mild OSAH	403	401	392	264
Severe OSAH	235	229	221	167
OSAH with CPAP	372	364	361	229

FIGURE 79-2 Cumulative frequency of fatal **(top)** and nonfatal **(bottom)** cardiovascular (CV) events in 1651 men observed for an average of 10.1 years. CPAP = continuous positive airway pressure; OSAH = obstructive sleep apnea–hypopnea syndrome. *(Modified from Marin JM, Carrizo SJ, Vicente E, et al: Long-term cardiovascular outcomes in men with obstructive sleep apnoea–hypopnoea with or without treatment with continuous positive airway pressure: An observational study. Lancet 365:1046, 2005.)*

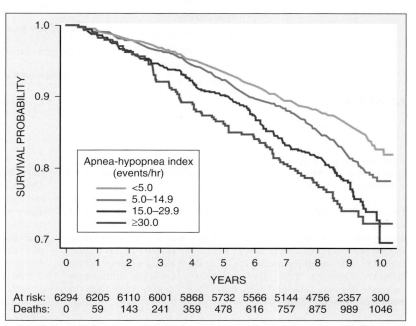

At risk:	6294	6205	6110	6001	5868	5732	5566	5144	4756	2357	300
Deaths:	0	59	143	241	359	478	616	757	875	989	1046

FIGURE 79-3 Kaplan-Meier survival curves across categories of the apnea-hypopnea index. *(Modified from Punjabi NM, Caffo BS, Goodwin JL, et al: Sleep-disordered breathing and mortality: A prospective cohort study. PLoS Med 6:e1000132, 2009.)*

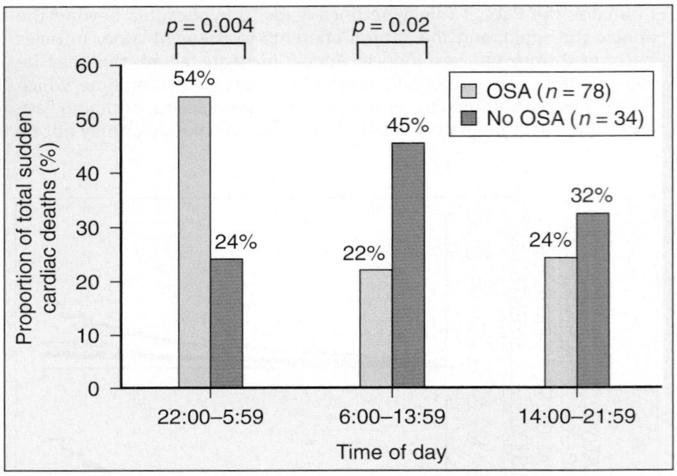

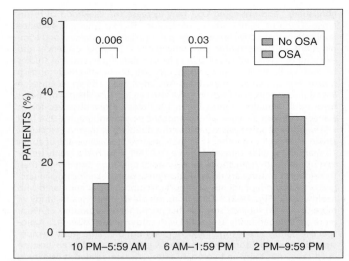

FIGURE 79-4 The day-night pattern of sudden cardiac death in individuals with and without polysomnogram-confirmed OSA. *(Modified from Gami AS, Howard DE, Olson EJ, et al: Day-night pattern of sudden death in obstructive sleep apnea. N Engl J Med 352:1206, 2005.)*

FIGURE 79-5 Day-night pattern of myocardial infarction based on three 8-hour time intervals in OSA (n = 64) and non-OSA (n = 28) patients. *(Reprinted with permission from Kuniyoshi FH, Garcia-Touchard A, Gami AS, et al: Day-night variation of acute myocardial infarction in obstructive sleep apnea. J Am Coll Cardiol 52:343, 2008.)*

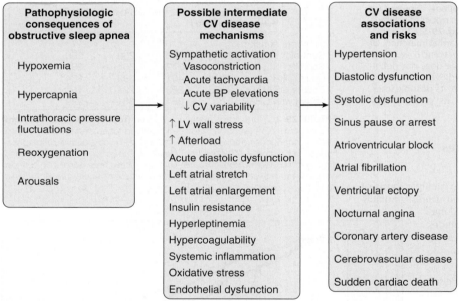

FIGURE 79-6 The pathophysiologic consequences of OSA may acutely and chronically elicit multiple intermediate cardiovascular (CV) disease mechanisms, which may promote the association of OSA with a number of cardiovascular conditions and diseases.

daytime somnolence may be especially problematic sequelae in heart failure patients who already have fatigue and functional limitations. The repetitive episodes of hypoxemia can have detrimental effects on myocardial oxygen supply, ventricular performance, and electrical stability. Individuals with CSA have heightened peripheral muscle sympathetic nerve activity and elevated levels of circulating catecholamines, which may be directly related to the severity of CSA.[3] Heart rate and blood pressure increase gradually with the rate of ventilation and peak with hyperpnea. The mechanisms of the elevated heart rate and blood pressure are not directly related to hypoxemia or sympathetic activity but instead are directly related to the periodic breathing itself and even manifested during periodic breathing in the awake state. Indeed, there is increasing evidence that daytime periodic breathing is itself associated with poor outcomes in heart failure patients.[22] Whereas CSA is associated with sleep fragmentation, cyclical hypoxemia, sympathetic overactivity, and periodicity of increased heart rate and blood pressure, its direct consequences for the cardiovascular system are unclear (see later).

followed by an arousal. Arousals directly lead to hyperpnea and promote the periodic breathing of CSA because the same PCO_2 that was present during sleep is relatively hypercapnic for the awake state.

It is important to note the fundamental physiologic differences between OSA and CSA. In OSA, the principal defect is with pharyngeal muscle structure and function, ventilatory efforts continue during apnea, and arousals lead to airway patency and resumed breathing. In CSA, the principal defect is with central ventilatory control, there are no ventilatory efforts during apnea, and breathing resumes before arousals. Although there are important physiologic differences between the two, OSA and CSA may often coexist, particularly in patients with heart failure.[3,21]

PATHOPHYSIOLOGIC MECHANISMS LINKING CENTRAL SLEEP APNEA TO CARDIOVASCULAR DISEASE. CSA has important clinical implications for heart failure. Sleep deprivation and

CENTRAL SLEEP APNEA AND CARDIOVASCULAR DISEASE ASSOCIATIONS AND OUTCOMES. The prognostic role of CSA, the mechanisms by which it could increase cardiac risk, and the usefulness of targeting these mechanisms for intervention have been debated. CSA is associated with more severe forms of heart failure.[3,21] Individuals with CSA have elevated pulmonary capillary wedge pressure compared with patients with heart failure who do not have CSA. Also, the degree of hypocapnia in patients with CSA and heart failure is directly related to left ventricular filling pressures. However, not all patients with severe heart failure have CSA because the key pathophysiologic elements that cause unstable ventilatory control are not always present. The prevalence of CSA in patients with heart failure has been estimated at 30% to 40%.[23] Some small prospective studies assessing its prognostic value have suggested that the risk of cardiac transplantation and death are directly related to the severity of CSA, represented by the central apnea–hypopnea index.[24] It is possible that this is partly because of the associated increase in sympathetic activity, which is a known prognostic factor in heart failure. Also, patients with heart failure and CSA are more likely to have premature ventricular contractions, which may reflect ventricular electrical instability and a heightened risk of sudden cardiac death. This may not necessarily follow for patients with CSA but without heart failure. In a 10-year follow-up of 130 patients with stroke, OSA but not CSA was associated with an increased risk of early death.[25] However, large prospective systematic analyses of the relationship of CSA with significant heart failure outcomes or sudden cardiac death are lacking.[24]

Screening and Diagnosis of Sleep Disorders

History and Examination

After snoring, which is ubiquitous in people with OSA, the most common symptom of OSA is excessive daytime sleepiness, which is defined as falling asleep during daytime activities such as reading, conversing, eating, and driving. However, for unclear reasons, daytime somnolence may be less common in OSA patients with comorbid cardiovascular disease, such as heart failure. Another related but distinct symptom is tiredness on waking from sleep. An important symptom of OSA is witnessed nocturnal apnea, which is usually reported by the bed partner of the patient. Other symptoms may include nightly gasping or choking episodes, nighttime or morning headaches, morning dry mouth or sore throat, gastroesophageal acid reflux, and nocturia. Cognitive and memory difficulties as well as psychological and behavioral changes may be associated with severe OSA.[1]

The physical examination findings in people with OSA may be normal, but it is usually notable for an overweight or obese body habitus. However, about 40% of obese people do not have OSA (and about 30% of people with OSA are not obese). Increased neck circumference, particularly more than 17 inches, is more specific than the BMI for predicting OSA. Certain cranial features, such as a low soft palate, narrow oropharynx, large uvula, micrognathia, and retrognathia, also predispose to OSA.

Symptoms of CSA are not very specific, particularly in those with symptomatic heart failure. Snoring may not be present in individuals with CSA. Observations of the characteristic crescendo-decrescendo ventilatory pattern by a patient's bed partner may be helpful but may be difficult for them to identify. The physical examination is not specific for CSA beyond the findings of heart failure, although CSA is more common in male or lean heart failure patients.

Screening Tools for Obstructive Sleep Apnea

Even an expert's subjective prediction of OSA based on a patient's history and physical examination alone has a diagnostic accuracy of only about 50%. Multiple prediction models and questionnaires have been developed by researchers to assess the likelihood of OSA. Most agree that age, BMI, neck circumference, hypertension, loud and habitual snoring, and witnessed apneas are the most sensitive and specific characteristics of OSA. However, the predictive accuracy of any model is determined by the prevalence of OSA in the population in which it is applied. In patients with cardiovascular disease, in whom the prevalence of OSA is high, it is especially important to use variables with a high specificity for OSA, such as neck circumference and witnessed apneas. Overnight pulse oximetry has been used to screen for OSA; however, there are several limitations to its use, and more research is necessary to identify its appropriate role.[26]

Polysomnography

Polysomnography is the current gold standard test for the diagnosis of sleep disordered breathing, including OSA and CSA.[1] Traditionally, this is performed during a full night and, if indicated, repeated on another night to apply and to titrate continuous positive airway pressure (CPAP) therapy. Split-night studies, in which the diagnostic study occurs during the first half of the night and CPAP titration occurs during the second half of the night, are increasingly used as a more cost-effective diagnostic-therapeutic strategy. Polysomnography provides comprehensive information about sleep efficiency, sleep architecture, arousals and their causes, disordered breathing events, oscillations in oxygen saturation, and cardiac arrhythmias during specific sleep stages or events. Major limitations to obtaining polysomnography in the large population of patients with cardiovascular disease who probably have OSA or CSA are the cost and access to sleep centers. In fact, it has been estimated that more than 60% of U.S. adults with OSA are undiagnosed. In response to this, the use of portable sleep monitoring[26] for the evaluation of OSA has recently received approval for reimbursement, provided very specific monitoring criteria are met.[3]

Sleep Apnea Therapy

Obstructive Sleep Apnea

POSITIVE AIRWAY PRESSURE THERAPY. Positive airway pressure (PAP) therapy effectively splints open the airway, preventing its collapse and resultant apneas.[1] It is applied by naso-oral masks, nasal masks, or nasal pillows. A memory card records time of use for assessment of adherence. Continuous PAP is the principal therapy used. Autotitrating PAP machines and bilevel PAP machines are sometimes used for patients who do not tolerate standard continuous PAP.

A number of potential drawbacks of PAP therapy create obstacles to widespread acceptance by individual patients. These include claustrophobia, rhinitis or nasal congestion, nose bleeds, abrasions of the bridge of the nose, and air leaks because of poor fit of the device. Usually, these can be managed with conscientious attention to the patient's specific needs and regular follow-up.

Multiple cardiovascular benefits have been demonstrated with effective PAP therapy in individuals with OSA.[27] Nocturnal hypoxemia is relieved and sympathetic activity decreases, not only during sleep but also in daytime normoxic wakefulness. Similarly, PAP can promote decreases in blood pressure during sleep and daytime, particularly in patients with uncontrolled hypertension. PAP therapy is effective in relieving symptoms in some OSA patients with nocturnal myocardial ischemia or angina. In patients with heart failure and OSA, PAP causes direct improvements in left ventricular systolic function and, during several months of therapy, leads to increased left ventricular ejection fraction and improved functional status.[3,4] Long-term observational studies have suggested that OSA patients who use PAP are at decreased risk of major adverse cardiovascular events, such as myocardial infarction, coronary revascularization, stroke, and death.[16] Large randomized controlled trials assessing the effects of PAP on long-term cardiovascular outcomes have not been reported and it is unknown whether PAP will truly reduce cardiovascular events or death.[3,27] Current indications for CPAP therapy in patients with OSA are listed in **Table 79-2**.

OTHER THERAPIES. Treatment of obesity by lifestyle modification is effective in attenuating or curing OSA.[28] Pharmacologic therapy for OSA

TABLE 79-2	Indications for Continuous Positive Airway Pressure (CPAP) for Obstructive Sleep Apnea Treatment

Adults for whom surgery is a likely alternative to CPAP, with either
- An apnea-hypopnea index ≥15

or
- An apnea-hypopnea index ≥5 in a patient with symptoms (e.g., excessive daytime sleepiness, impaired cognition, mood disorders, insomnia), hypertension, ischemic heart disease, or history of stroke

Based on the Centers for Medicare and Medicaid Services, U.S. Department of Health and Human Services: Medicare Coverage Database, National Coverage, Continuous Positive Airway Pressure (CPAP) Therapy for Obstructive Sleep Apnea (OSA) (http://www.cms.hhs.gov/mcd).

is ineffective.[29] Mechanical devices other than PAP include oral appliances that maintain an anterior position of the tongue or the entire mandible.[30] These may be efficacious in patients with OSA that is mild or exclusive to the supine position. For patients with positional (supine) OSA, wearing a well-fitting shirt with a tennis ball sewn tightly to the midback should maintain a nonsupine sleep position, although there are insufficient data to prove its efficacy.

Surgical options exist for the treatment of OSA.[31] Bariatric surgery incidentally cures OSA in most morbidly obese patients; however, OSA returns if weight is regained. A number of surgeries that modify the oropharynx should be considered second-line therapies to weight loss and PAP. These are options for patients with specific craniofacial characteristics amenable to each specific approach. Tonsillectomy is more effective in children or thin adults. Tracheostomy, which was the first treatment ever effectively applied for OSA, is completely successful in abolishing obstructive apneas but should be reserved for patients with the motivation and support to maintain the apparatus.

Central Sleep Apnea

POSITIVE AIRWAY PRESSURE THERAPY. The rationale for use of positive-pressure ventilation in patients with CSA is based not on treatment of CSA per se but rather on treatment of heart failure. The same hemodynamic benefits of continuous PAP therapy shown in OSA patients have been reported in patients with heart failure and CSA, namely, decreased sympathetic activity, decreased ventricular afterload, and increased left ventricular ejection fraction.[32] Concomitant with these changes, the severity of CSA decreases. In the largest controlled trial performed to clarify the potential benefits of continuous PAP in this population, 258 patients with New York Heart Association Class II to IV heart failure and CSA were randomized to effective therapy with continuous PAP or no therapy.[33] The trial was stopped early, in part because of concerns about early divergence of transplantation-free survival favoring the control group, and no survival benefit was observed for the CPAP-treated group. A subsequent post hoc analysis proposed that survival may have been improved in those patients in whom CPAP effectively suppressed CSA, suggesting that alternative effective therapies may improve survival in these patients.[34] Adaptive pressure support servoventilation, another form of PAP, has been shown in short-term controlled trials to improve CSA. However, long-term outcome studies have not been reported.

OTHER THERAPIES. Low-flow oxygen supplementation may abolish CSA in some patients.[24] Two randomized placebo-controlled trials in heart failure patients have shown that nocturnal administration of low-flow oxygen by nasal cannula immediately improved the AHI, oxygen saturation, and sleep architecture and that 1 week of nocturnal oxygen supplementation improved functional capacity. A controlled study of 24 patients with heart failure has shown that implantation of a biventricular permanent pacemaker improves indices of CSA (both the AHI and minimum nocturnal oxygen saturation) and sleep quality after about 4 months.[35]

Small studies have shown improvements in CSA with the administration of theophylline; however, there are no large long-term studies assessing the safety of theophylline, a methylxanthine, in heart failure patients.[24,32] Another experimental intervention successful in directly abolishing CSA is the inhalation of a gas mixture that has a carbon dioxide tension as low as 1 to 3 mm Hg higher than ambient air. This resets the resting hypocapnic state of heart failure further from the apneic threshold.[24] The safety of delivery of carbon dioxide–enriched air to heart failure patients has not been assessed, and this is not applied clinically.

Future Perspectives

Whereas OSA has been implicated in cardiovascular disease generally and hypertension in particular, whether it is an independent risk factor for conditions such as myocardial infarction, stroke, and atrial fibrillation remains to be definitively established. More important, longitudinal controlled intervention trials are needed to ascertain whether treatment of OSA reduces cardiovascular events and mortality. In the meantime, treatment of patients with OSA and coexisting cardiovascular disease will need to be individualized on the basis of the overall clinical context.

Whether CSA is a marker of the severity of the underlying heart disease rather than a mediator of risk and whether it is a worthwhile target for intervention to improve cardiovascular prognosis also remain to be determined. In general, therapies that improve heart failure (e.g., angiotensin-converting enzyme inhibitors, biventricular pacing) also improve CSA. Pending further longitudinal controlled outcome studies, treatment directed specifically at CSA, such as oxygen or PAP, should probably be reserved for patients with severe daytime somnolence or symptoms attributable to nocturnal hypoxemia (angina or significant arrhythmias). Otherwise, optimization of heart failure management should remain the principal goal.

ACKNOWLEDGMENT

The author is grateful to Apoor Gami, MD, for contributions to the earlier edition of this chapter.

REFERENCES

Obstructive Sleep Apnea

1. Kryger MH, Roth T, Dement WC (eds): Principles and Practice of Sleep Medicine. 4th ed. Philadelphia, Elsevier Saunders, 2005.
2. Verrier RL, Josephson ME: Impact of sleep on arrhythmogenesis. Circ Arrhythmia Electrophysiol 2:450, 2009.
3. Somers VK, White DP, Amin R, et al: Sleep apnea and cardiovascular disease: An American Heart Association/American College of Cardiology Foundation Scientific Statement from the American Heart Association Council for High Blood Pressure Research Professional Education Committee, Council on Clinical Cardiology, Stroke Council, and Council on Cardiovascular Nursing. In collaboration with the National Heart, Lung, and Blood Institute National Center on Sleep Disorders Research (National Institutes of Health). Circulation 118:1080, 2008.
4. Bradley TD, Floras JS: Obstructive sleep apnoea and its cardiovascular consequences. Lancet 373:82, 2009.
5. White DP: Pathogenesis of obstructive and central sleep apnea. Am J Respir Crit Care Med 172:1363, 2005.
6. Shivalkar B, Van de Heyning C, Kerremans M, et al: Obstructive sleep apnea syndrome: More insights on structural and functional cardiac alterations, and the effects of treatment with continuous positive airway pressure. J Am Coll Cardiol 47:1433, 2006.
7. Otto ME, Belohlavek M, Romero-Corral A, et al: Comparison of cardiac structural and functional changes in obese otherwise healthy adults with versus without obstructive sleep apnea. Am J Cardiol 99:1298, 2007.
8. Gami AS, Friedman PA, Chung MK, et al: Therapy insight: Interactions between atrial fibrillation and obstructive sleep apnea. Nat Clin Pract Cardiovasc Med 2:145, 2005.
9. Wolk R, Gami AS, Garcia-Touchard A, Somers VK: Sleep and cardiovascular disease. Curr Probl Cardiol 30:625, 2005.
10. Svatikova A, Wolk R, Gami AS, et al: Interactions between obstructive sleep apnea and the metabolic syndrome. Curr Diab Rep 5:53, 2005.
11. McArdle N, Hillman D, Beilin L, Watts G: Metabolic risk factors for vascular disease in obstructive sleep apnea: A matched controlled study. Am J Respir Crit Care Med 175:190, 2007.
12. Gami AS, Hodge DO, Herges RM, et al: Obstructive sleep apnea, obesity, and the risk of incident atrial fibrillation. J Am Coll Cardiol 49:565, 2007.
13. Gami AS, Pressman G, Caples SM, et al: Association of atrial fibrillation and obstructive sleep apnea. Circulation 110:364, 2004.
14. Sengupta PP, Sorajja D, Eleid MF, et al: Hypertrophic obstructive cardiomyopathy and sleep-disordered breathing: An unfavorable combination. Nat Clin Pract Cardiovasc Med 6:14-15, 2009.
15. Yaggi HK, Concato J, Kernan WN, et al: Obstructive sleep apnea as a risk factor for stroke and death. N Engl J Med 353:2034, 2005.
16. Marin JM, Carrizo SJ, Vicente E, Agusti AG: Long-term cardiovascular outcomes in men with obstructive sleep apnoea-hypopnoea with or without treatment with continuous positive airway pressure: An observational study. Lancet 365:1046, 2005.
17. Punjabi NM, Newman AB, Young TB, et al: Sleep-disordered breathing and cardiovascular disease: An outcome-based definition of hypopneas. Am J Respir Crit Care Med 177:1150, 2008.
18. Punjabi NM, Caffo BS, Goodwin JL, et al: Sleep-disordered breathing and mortality: A prospective cohort study. PLoS Med 6:e1000132, 2009.
19. Gami AS, Howard DE, Olson EJ, Somers VK: Day-night pattern of sudden death in obstructive sleep apnea. N Engl J Med 352:1206, 2005.
20. Kuniyoshi FH, Garcia-Touchard A, Gami AS, et al: Day-night variation of acute myocardial infarction in obstructive sleep apnea. J Am Coll Cardiol 52:343, 2008.

Central Sleep Apnea

21. Caples SM, Somers VK: Influence of cardiac function and failure on sleep disordered breathing: Evidence for a causative role. J Appl Physiol 99:2433, 2005.
22. Brack T, Thuer I, Clarenbach CV, et al: Daytime Cheyne-Stokes respiration in ambulatory patients with severe congestive heart failure is associated with increased mortality. Chest 132:1463, 2007.
23. Oldenburg O, Lamp B, Faber L, et al: Sleep-disordered breathing in patients with symptomatic heart failure. A contemporary study of prevalence in and characteristics of 700 patients. Eur J Heart Fail 9:251, 2007.
24. Pepin JL, Chouri-Pontarollo N, Tamisier R, Levy P: Cheyne-Stokes respiration with central sleep apnea in chronic heart failure: Proposals for a diagnostic and therapeutic strategy. Sleep Med Rev 10:33, 2006.
25. Sahlin C, Sandberg O, Gustafson Y, et al: Obstructive sleep apnea is a risk factor for death in patients with stroke: A 10-year follow-up. Arch Intern Med 168:297, 2008.

Screening and Diagnosis of Sleep Disorders

26. Littner MR: Portable monitoring in the diagnosis of the obstructive sleep apnea syndrome. Semin Respir Crit Care Med 26:56, 2005.

Sleep Apnea Therapy

27. Giles TL, Lasserson TJ, Smith BJ, et al: Continuous positive airways pressure for obstructive sleep apnoea in adults. Cochrane Database Syst Rev (1):CD001106, 2006.

28. Veasey SC, Guilleminault C, Strohl KP, et al: Medical therapy for obstructive sleep apnea: A review by the Medical Therapy for Obstructive Sleep Apnea Task Force of the Standards of Practice Committee of the American Academy of Sleep Medicine. Sleep 29:1036, 2006.

29. Smith I, Lasserson TJ, Wright J: Drug therapy for obstructive sleep apnoea in adults. Cochrane Database Syst Rev (2):CD003002, 2006.

30. Ng A, Gotsopoulos H, Darendeliler AM, Cistulli PA: Oral appliance therapy for obstructive sleep apnea. Treat Respir Med 4:409, 2005.

31. Sundaram S, Bridgman SA, Lim J, Lasserson TJ: Surgery for obstructive sleep apnoea. Cochrane Database Syst Rev (2):CD001004, 2005.

32. Javaheri S: Central sleep apnea in congestive heart failure: Prevalence, mechanisms, impact, and therapeutic options. Semin Respir Crit Care Med 26:44, 2005.

33. Bradley TD, Logan AG, Kimoff RJ, et al: Continuous positive airway pressure for central sleep apnea and heart failure. N Engl J Med 353:2025, 2005.

34. Arzt M, Floras JS, Logan AG, et al: Suppression of central sleep apnea by continuous positive airway pressure and transplant-free survival in heart failure: A post hoc analysis of the Canadian Continuous Positive Airway Pressure for Patients with Central Sleep Apnea and Heart Failure Trial (CANPAP). Circulation 115:3173, 2007.

35. Sinha AM, Skobel EC, Breithardt OA, et al: Cardiac resynchronization therapy improves central sleep apnea and Cheyne-Stokes respiration in patients with chronic heart failure. J Am Coll Cardiol 44:68, 2004.

SLEEP APNEA AND CARDIOVASCULAR DISEASE

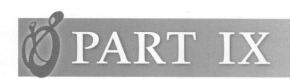

PART IX

CARDIOVASCULAR DISEASE IN SPECIAL POPULATIONS

CHAPTER **80**

Cardiovascular Disease in the Elderly

Janice B. Schwartz and Douglas P. Zipes

Demographics and Epidemiology

The proportion of people aged 65 years and older in the United States is projected to increase from 12.4% (35 million) of the population in 2000 to 19.6% (71 million) in 2030 and to 82 million in 2050 (*www.cdc.gov*). The number of people older than 80 years is projected to double from 9.3 million in 2000 to 19.5 million in 2030 and to more than triple by 2050. Women represented 59% of persons older than 65 years in 2000 and are estimated to compose 56% of the older population in 2030 (**Fig. 80-1**). If current projections hold, there will be increases in the percentage of racial minorities (see Chap. 2). From 2000 to 2030, the proportion of persons aged ≥65 years who are members of racial minority groups (i.e., African American, American Indian–Alaska Native, Asian–Pacific Islander) is expected to increase from 11.3% to 16.5%, and the proportion of Hispanics is expected to increase from 5.6% to 10.9%. Almost half of people older than 65 years in the United States in 2000 had after-tax incomes at the poverty level (41% of 65- to 74-year-olds and 56% of those older than 75 years), and this trend is likely to continue.[1] Global trends are similar, with the worldwide population older than 65 years projected to increase to 973 million or 12% in 2030 and to make up about 20% of the population in 2050 (see Chap. 1). Increases will be greatest in undeveloped nations. Estimates are for twice as many women as men older than 80 years and three times as many women as men older than 90 years.

Cardiovascular disease is both the most frequent diagnosis and the leading cause of death in both men and women older than 65 years. Hypertension occurs in one half to two thirds of people older than 65 years, and heart failure is the most frequent hospital discharge diagnosis among older Americans. The profile of these common cardiovascular diseases in older patients differs from that in younger patients. Systolic but not diastolic blood pressure increases with aging, resulting in increased pulse pressure. Systolic hypertension becomes a stronger predictor of cardiovascular events, especially in women (see Chap. 81). Heart failure with preserved systolic function becomes more common at older ages and is more common in women. Coronary artery disease (CAD) is more likely to involve multiple vessels and the left main artery and is equally likely in women and men older than 65 years. Equal numbers of older men and women present with acute myocardial infarction (MI) until the age of 80 years, after which more women present. Non-ST rather than ST elevation MI accounts for two thirds of MI in older patients. More than 80% of all deaths attributable to cardiovascular disease occur in people older than 65 years, with approximately 60% of deaths in patients older than 75 years.

Importantly, cardiovascular disease in older people is not seen in isolation; 80% of older Americans have at least one chronic medical condition, and 50% have at least two. Arthritis affects about 60% of persons older than 65 years, cancer is present in 34%, and diabetes affects about 20% (**Fig. 80-2**). Also common are ear, nose, and throat problems and vision disorders and orthopedic problems. As U.S. adults live longer, the prevalence and incidence of dementia that impairs memory, decision-making capability, orientation to physical surroundings, and language also increase. The prevalence of dementia is estimated at 13% in community-dwelling white people older than 65 years and is higher in women than in men and African American and Hispanic populations.[2] By the age of 80 years, approximately 40% of people may be affected. Of Medicare beneficiaries with dementias, 60% have hypertension, 26% have CAD, 25% have had a stroke, 23% have diabetes, and 16% have heart failure.[2] Patients with dementia are three times more likely to be hospitalized and to remain in the hospital longer than are Medicare beneficiaries without dementias, such that about one quarter of all hospital patients aged 65 and older have dementia at any one time.[2]

The high morbidity and mortality from cardiovascular disease in the elderly warrant aggressive approaches to prevention and treatment that have been shown to be effective in older patients. Compelling data demonstrate reduced morbidity and mortality rates for the treatment of hypertension, heart failure, atrial fibrillation, acute coronary syndromes, CAD, stroke, diabetes, and lipid abnormalities in older patients 60 to 74 years of age, although data on minorities and women

1727

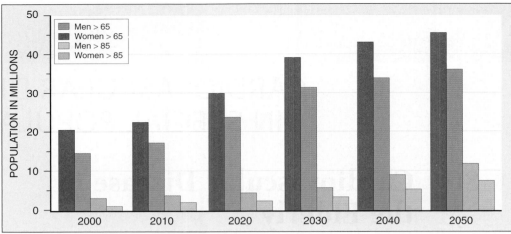

FIGURE 80-1 United States population estimates projected from 2000 until 2050. Dark pink bars represent numbers of women older than 65 years, and dark blue bars represent numbers of men older than 65 years; lighter pink bars represent numbers of women older than 85 years, and lighter blue bars represent numbers of men older than 85 years in millions of people. *(Source: U.S. Census Bureau.)*

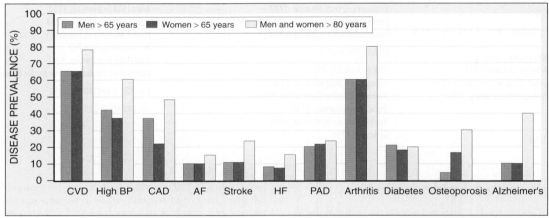

FIGURE 80-2 Prevalence of cardiovascular and other common chronic medical illnesses in older persons in the United States. Data are percentages. AF = atrial fibrillation; CAD = coronary artery disease; CVD = cardiovascular disease; HF = heart failure; high BP = hypertension (all forms); PAD = peripheral artery disease. Blue bars represent data for men older than 65 years, pink bars represent women older than 65 years, and yellow bars represent men and women older than 80 years.

are limited. Fewer trials of cardiovascular therapies have enrolled significant numbers of men or women older than 75 years, elderly patients with multisystem disease, or elderly patients with cognitive impairment, and none has addressed cardiovascular therapies in the nursing home population. When clinical trials enroll older patients, participants differ markedly from the majority of older patients. The projected increase in numbers of older people from previously understudied and undertreated groups presents both medical and economic challenges for cardiovascular disease treatment.

Pathophysiology

No universal definition of "elderly" or an accurate biomarker for aging exists. Whereas physiologic changes associated with aging do not appear at a specific age and do not proceed at the same pace in all individuals, most definitions of elderly are based on chronologic age. The World Health Organization uses 60 years of age to define elderly, whereas most U.S. classifications use the age of 65 years. Gerontologists subclassify older age groups into young old (60 to 74 years), old old (75 to 85 years), and very old (older than 85 years). Cardiovascular society statements have addressed differences in responses of patients younger than 65 years, those 65 to 74 years, and those 75 to 84 years separately from those of patients older than 85 years.[3,4] Clinicians often separate older patients into two subgroups, those 65 to 80 years of age and those older than 80 years, to highlight the frailty, reduced capacity

(physical and mental), and presence of multiple disorders that are more common after 80 years of age.

Hallmarks of cardiovascular aging in humans include progressive increases in systolic blood pressure, pulse pressure, pulse wave velocity, and left ventricular mass and increased incidence of CAD and atrial fibrillation.[5-9] Reproducible age-related decreases are seen in rates of early left ventricular diastolic filling, maximal heart rates, maximal cardiac output, maximum aerobic capacity or maximal oxygen consumption ($\dot{V}O_2$ max), exercise-induced augmentation of ejection fraction, reflex responses of heart rate, heart rate variability, and vasodilation in response to beta-adrenergic stimuli or endothelium-mediated vasodilator compounds.

Cellular, enzymatic, and molecular alterations in the arterial vessel wall include migration of activated vascular smooth muscle cells into the intima, with increased matrix production due to altered activity of matrix metalloproteinases, angiotensin II, transforming growth factor-β, intercellular cell adhesion molecules, and production of collagen and collagen cross-linking. There is also loss of elastic fibers, increases in fibronectin, and calcification. These processes lead to arterial dilation and increased intimal thickness, resulting in increased vascular stiffness. Increased arterial stiffness is manifested by increases in pulse wave velocity away from the heart and increased and earlier pulse wave reflections back toward the heart (often estimated as the aortic augmentation index). Typical arterial and radial waveforms from a young and older individual are shown in **Figure 80-3**. In both animal and human models of aging, endothelial cell production of nitric oxide (NO) decreases with age; there is decreased endothelial cell mass associated with increased cell senescence and apoptosis and increased NO consumption due to an age-dependent increase in vascular superoxide anion production. These changes contribute to reduced endothelial cell NO-mediated vasodilatory responses of the peripheral and coronary vasculature. Vascular responses to beta-adrenergic agonists and alpha-adrenergic blockade are also reduced with aging. In contrast, responses to non–endothelial cell–derived compounds such as nitrates and nitroprusside are preserved with aging but may vary by vascular bed or be altered by diseases such as hypertension and diabetes.

Changes in the extracellular matrix of the myocardium parallel those in the vasculature, with increased collagen, increased fibril diameter and collagen cross-linking, an increase in the ratio of type I to type III collagen, decreased elastin content, and an increase in fibronectin. There may also be a shift in the balance between matrix metalloproteinases and tissue inhibitors of matrix metalloproteinases that favors increased production of extracellular matrix. Fibroblast proliferation is induced by growth factors, in particular angiotensin, transforming growth factors, tumor necrosis factor-α, and platelet-derived growth factor. These changes are accompanied by cell loss and altered cellular function.[5] In the atria, decreased sinus node cells, decreased L-type calcium channels within sinus node cells, and extracellular matrix changes contribute to sinus node dysfunction and atrial fibrillation. Collagen, elastic tissue, and calcification changes in or near the central fibrous body and the atrioventricular (AV) node or proximal bundle branches contribute to conduction abnormalities and annular valvular calcification. In the ventricle, collagen deposition and extracellular matrix changes contribute to loss of cells, hypertrophy of myocytes with changes in myosin subforms, and altered myocardial calcium handling.[9] Changes in myocardial calcium handling include reduced or delayed inactivation of L-type transmembrane calcium current, decreased and delayed intracellular ionized calcium uptake by cardiac myocyte sarcoplasmic reticulum, and reduced and delayed outwardly directed potassium rectifier current activation. The result is prolongation of the membrane action potential and inward calcium current with prolongation of both contraction and relaxation.[5]

Age-related changes are also seen in the intravascular environment. Increases in fibrinogen, coagulation factors (V, VIII and IX, XIIa), and von Willebrand factor are seen without countering increases in anticoagulant factors (see Chap. 87). Platelet phospholipid content is altered and platelet activity is increased with increased binding of platelet-derived growth factor to the arterial wall in older individuals compared with younger individuals. Increased levels of plasminogen activator inhibitor (PAI-1) are seen with aging, especially during stress, resulting in impaired fibrinolysis. Circulating prothrombotic inflammatory cytokines, especially interleukin-6, also increase with age and may play a role in the pathogenesis of acute coronary syndromes. All these changes also potentiate development of atherosclerosis.[9]

Consistent changes in the autonomic nervous system accompany aging and influence cardiovascular function. For the beta-adrenergic system, age-related changes include decreased receptor numbers, altered G protein coupling, and altered G protein–mediated signal transduction. Age-related decreases in alpha-adrenergic platelet receptors and decreased alpha-adrenergic–mediated arterial vasoreactivity of forearm blood vessels occur, whereas alpha-adrenergic–mediated changes in human hand veins appear to be preserved. Dopaminergic receptor content and dopaminergic transporters decrease and cardiac contractile responses to dopaminergic stimulation may be blunted with aging. Decreased sensitivity and responses to parasympathetic stimulation are seen in cardiac and vascular tissues, whereas increased central nervous system effects are frequently seen in aging models. The combined age-related autonomic changes lead to decreased baroreflex function and responses to physiologic stressors with increased sensitivity to parasympathetic stimulation of the central nervous system.

Unifying hypotheses for age-related changes throughout the body include cumulative oxidative damage, inflammatory responses to cellular stress or infection, and programmed cell death. Some age-related cardiovascular changes can be partially if not totally reversed. Exercise improves endothelial function, measures of arterial stiffness, and

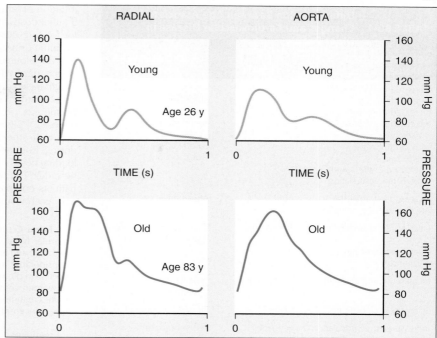

FIGURE 80-3 Directly measured arterial waveforms from a peripheral artery (radial) and calculated aortic pressure waves for a young man aged 26 years in the upper panels and his 83-year-old grandfather in the lower panels. *(Courtesy of Michael O'Rourke, MD, University of Sydney, Australia.)*

baroreceptor function in older people. Calorie restriction slows aging and cardiac changes as well as increasing maximal life span in several small animal models. In humans, calorie restriction decreases weight, blood pressure, and risk factors for atherosclerosis and has improved indices of diastolic function in cross-sectional studies.[10,11] Medications such as angiotensin-converting enzyme (ACE) inhibitors, aldosterone antagonists, and beta blockers may influence the vascular and cardiac remodeling associated with hypertension, atherosclerosis, or heart failure.[9] Pilot studies suggest that combined exercise, stress management, and specialized diets that lower low-density lipoprotein (LDL) also increase telomerase activity and that cellular aging processes can be slowed.[12] Dietary antioxidant intake has been associated with slowing of age-related changes in the vasculature, but pharmacologic approaches with anti-inflammatory and antioxidant vitamin administration or omega-3 free fatty acids for either primary or secondary prevention have not been successful in humans.[13] Similarly, dehydroepiandrosterone has not been shown to have significant beneficial effects in older women or men. The most recent vitamin to be targeted for study is vitamin D. Decreased nutritional intake of vitamin D and sun exposure has resulted in vitamin D deficiency in high proportions of Americans, especially the elderly. A large study of vitamin D supplementation in older men and women to determine effects on cardiovascular events and cancer occurrence is under way. Other potential antiaging agents under investigation include those that directly target advanced glycation end products, inflammation, and collagen cross-links.

Age-related changes create a cardiovascular system faced with increased pulsatile load and one that is less able to increase output in response to stress. Age-related changes also limit maximal capacity and decrease reserve capacity, contributing to lower thresholds for symptoms in the presence of cardiovascular diseases that become more common with increasing age. **Table 80-1** summarizes age-related cardiovascular changes contrasted with cardiovascular disease.

Medication Therapy: Modifications for the Older Patient

Most of the therapeutic interventions for the elderly are pharmacologic, making appropriate drug selection and modification of dosing regimens for the older patient important (see Chap. 5).

TABLE 80-1	Differentiation Between Age-Associated Changes and Cardiovascular Disease in Older People	
AGE-ASSOCIATED CHANGES	ORGAN	CARDIOVASCULAR DISEASE
Increased intimal thickness Arterial stiffening Increased pulse pressure Increased pulse wave velocity Early central wave reflections Decreased endothelium-mediated vasodilation	Vasculature	Systolic hypertension Coronary artery obstruction Peripheral artery disease Carotid artery obstruction
Increased left atrial size Atrial premature complexes	Atria	Atrial fibrillation
Decreased maximal heart rate Decreased heart rate variability	Sinus node	Sinus node dysfunction, sick sinus syndrome
Increased conduction time	Atrioventricular node	Type II block, third-degree block
Sclerosis, calcification	Valves	Stenosis, regurgitation
Increased left ventricular wall tension Prolonged myocardial contraction Prolonged early diastolic filling rate Decreased maximal cardiac output Right bundle branch block Ventricular premature complexes	Ventricle	Left ventricular hypertrophy Heart failure (with or without preserved systolic function) Ventricular tachycardia, fibrillation

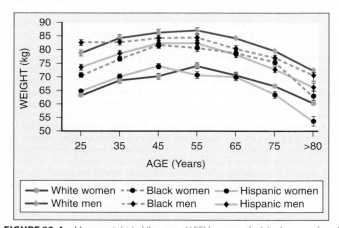

FIGURE 80-4 Mean weight in kilograms (±SE) by age, ethnicity/race, and sex/gender. *(Modified from Schwartz JB: The current state of knowledge on age, sex, and their interactions on clinical pharmacology. Clin Pharmacol Ther 82:87, 2007. Data source: NHANES: www.cdc.gov.)*

Loading Doses of Medications (see Chap. 10)

On average, body size decreases with aging and body composition changes, resulting in decreased total body water, intravascular volume, and muscle mass. Age-related changes are continuous but most pronounced after 75 to 80 years. Women, with the exception of African American women, tend to weigh less and to have smaller body and intravascular volumes and muscle mass than do men at all ages (**Fig. 80-4**). Higher serum concentrations of medications will be

found in older patients, and especially older white and Asian women, if initial doses are the same as in younger patients. Weight adjustment for loading doses of the cardiovascular drugs digoxin, type I antiarrhythmic drugs, and type III antiarrhythmic drugs and for aminoglycoside antibiotics, chemotherapy regimens, and unfractionated heparin are standard. When fibrinolytic drugs have been administered without weight-based dosage adjustments, increased risk of intracranial hemorrhage results in patients with older age, smaller body weight, and female sex (in addition to hypertension and prior cerebrovascular disease).[14] Bleeding with low-molecular-weight heparins in combination with other lytic agents can be reduced by use of weight-based dosing. Routine dosage adjustments for weight should be made in loading doses of medications, especially those with a narrow therapeutic index. The result is usually a loading dose that is lower in older patients compared with younger patients and lowest in older white and Asian women.

Chronic Medication Administration

RENAL CLEARANCE (see Chap. 93). Renal clearance by all routes (glomerular filtration, renal tubular reabsorption and secretion) decreases with age and is lower in women compared with men at all ages. There is considerable intersubject variability, but a general estimate is a 10% decline in glomerular filtration per decade, with 15% to 25% lower rates in women compared with men. The Cockcroft-Gault algorithm to estimate creatinine clearance includes age, sex, weight, and serum creatinine concentration as variables:

$$\text{Creatinine clearance} = (140 - \text{age[yr]} \times \text{weight[kg]})/(\text{creatinine} \times 72)$$
$$\text{multiplied by 0.85 for women}^{15}$$

and highlights that significant decreases in renal elimination can be present in older patients in the presence of normal serum creatinine measurements. With elevations of serum creatinine, severe renal impairment is likely to be present. The Modification of Diet in Renal Disease (MDRD) algorithm incorporates serum creatinine (S_{Cr}), age, race, and sex as variables nonlinearly and may better estimate glomerular filtration rate (eGFR) in community-dwelling elderly and obese people and has been used in risk estimates.[16]

$$\text{eGFR(mL/min/m}^2) = 186.3^* \times S_{Cr}^{-1.154} \times \text{age}^{-0.203} \times \text{sex} (\times 0.742 \text{ if female}) \times$$
$$\text{race} (\times 1.212 \text{ if African American})^\dagger$$

Online creatinine clearance and eGFR calculators are available at *http://www.kidney.org.*

The Cockcroft-Gault formula predicts a linear decrease with age that is steeper than the nonlinear decline predicted by the MDRD eGFR formula (**Fig. 80-5**). The result is underestimates with the Cockcroft-Gault formula and overestimates with the MDRD formula.[17] Most guidelines base dosage adjustments on estimated creatinine clearance (Cockcroft-Gault) to reduce excess dosing. The eGFR (MDRD) algorithm is used to classify renal status, risk of procedures, and renal complications and is reported routinely by most clinical laboratories. Both algorithms predict an "average" white woman older than 65 years to have stage 3 renal function (*http://www.kidney.org*) or moderate renal failure (see Fig. 80-5). Failure to adjust dosages of renally cleared narrow therapeutic index medications, such as thrombolytic agents, low-molecular-weight heparin, and glycoprotein (GP) IIb/IIIa inhibitors, has resulted in increased bleeding and intracerebral hemorrhages.[18-20]

Limitations of current methods to estimate renal clearance include lack of accuracy during hemodynamic instability or acute renal damage and reliance on creatinine measurements. Cystatin is a marker of renal clearance that reflects changes in renal function more rapidly and may reflect age-related changes without sex differences.[21-24] Estimates using cystatin differ from those with creatinine but appear to correlate with outcomes.[25] Incorporation of albuminuria in algorithms may also improve assessment of renal disease.

Even with limitations of current creatinine-based algorithms, routine estimation of creatinine clearance for dosages of renally cleared

---

*Note: use 175 if a standardized serum creatinine assay is used.
†For SI units: eGFR = $(3.1 \times S_{Cr}/88.4)^{-1.154} \times \text{age}^{-0.203} \times \text{sex} \times \text{race}$.

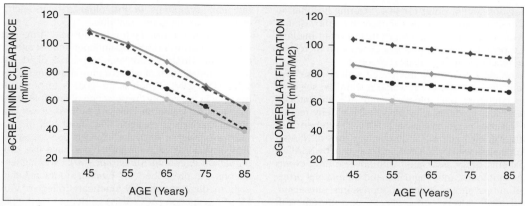

FIGURE 80-5 Estimates of creatinine clearance with the Cockcroft and Gault formula **(left panel)** and estimates of glomerular filtration rate with the MDRD simplified algorithm **(right panel)** for men and women aged 45 to 85 years. For calculations, mean weight and height by decade were obtained from U.S. survey data (NHANES, *http://www.cdc.gov*); serum creatinine is 1.0 mg/dL (average for older than 65 years in NHANES). Pink lines and circles represent estimates for women; blue lines and diamonds are estimates for men; lighter symbols are estimates for whites, and darker symbols represent estimates for African Americans. The shaded areas indicate GFR estimates of 30 to 59 mL/min/m² classified as stage 3 renal disease or moderate GFR decrease. Cockcroft and Gault estimates show a steeper decline with age. Both formulas estimate lower clearance in women compared with men and higher clearances in African Americans compared with whites (based on average height and weights and the same creatinine concentration). *(Modified from Schwartz JB: The current state of knowledge on age, sex, and their interactions on clinical pharmacology. Clin Pharmacol Ther 82:87, 2007.)*

medications and estimates of glomerular filtration for risk assessment before contrast agent administration, procedures, or surgery can guide efforts to reduce adverse effects and provides an opportunity for quality improvement. Consensus guidelines for oral dosing of renally excreted medications used frequently in the elderly may also be helpful.[26]

HEPATIC (AND INTESTINAL) CLEARANCE. No algorithms for estimation of age-related changes in hepatic and extrahepatic drug biotransformation have been validated clinically. In part, this is because hepatic and extrahepatic drug biotransformation processes may be influenced by more complex and heterogeneous factors that include both genetic and environmental influences, and enzymes can be both inhibited and induced (see Chap. 10).

Drugs metabolized by the conjugative reactions of glucuronidation (morphine, diazepam), sulfation (methyldopa), or acetylation (procainamide) do not appear to be affected by aging but show disease-related effects, may show frailty-related decreases, and show consistently lower clearance in women compared with men. Age-related changes are usually in phase I oxidative biotransformations by the membrane-bound cytochrome P-450 oxidative group of enzymes responsible for elimination of more than 50% of metabolized drugs.[27] Cardiovascular drugs showing age-related decreases in cytochrome P (CYP)–mediated clearance in research publications include alpha blockers (doxazosin, prazosin, terazosin), some beta blockers (metoprolol, propranolol, timolol), calcium channel blockers (dihydropyridines, diltiazem, verapamil), several HMG-CoA reductase inhibitors (fluvastatin and, in some studies, atorvastatin), and the benzodiazepine midazolam. Decreases in oxidative drug metabolism or clearance would suggest that lower amounts of drug per unit time (or day) should be given to older patients compared with younger patients, leading to the conventional dosing recommendation to "start low and go slow" for the older patient. Unfortunately, age-related changes have not been found in population studies of patients including women and patients receiving multiple medications.[28] Disease, environment, gender, and co-medications may have greater effects than age alone. Therefore, it is important to titrate to clinical effect if one starts with reduced dosages.

Attention has focused on genetic variation in explaining variability in drug metabolism, and allelic variants for many CYP enzymes have been described (see Chap. 10). Warfarin has polymorphisms of the CYP enzyme responsible for its metabolism (2C9) that are associated with lower warfarin requirements, and variants in the vitamin K epoxide reductase complex (VKORC) can either increase or decrease sensitivity to warfarin (see Fig. 80-e1 on website).[29] Increased age also increases sensitivity to warfarin, and estimates from different series suggest that age explains 40% of the variance in dosing; genetic variation of *VKORC1* can explain 25% of dosing variation, and variants of *CYP2C9* can explain 12% of dosing variation. Lower initial warfarin doses should be used in older patients and women (2 to 5 mg), and most often a loading dose is either not recommended or limited to 5 mg (see Chap. 87 and *www.ags.org*). Algorithms that incorporate age, race, sex, height and weight, and comedications in combination with other factors (including genetics) may help in estimating doses for individual patients. (see *www.warfarindosing.org*). With use of lower initial doses and multiple variable estimation algorithms in older patients, genotyping may not confer additional bleeding risk reduction, and the cost of genotyping for warfarin dosing estimation is not currently reimbursed by the Centers for Medicare and Medicaid Services.

Another drug with important genetic influences is clopidogrel. Clopidogrel is administered as a prodrug that requires metabolism by CYP2C19, and to a lesser extent CYP3A, for antiplatelet effects[29] (see Chap. 87). As with warfarin, age (in combination with body mass index and lipid levels) also contributes to platelet responses, and women tend to respond less well than men.[30]

ELIMINATION HALF-LIVES. In general, elimination half-lives of drugs increase with age, so the time between dosage adjustments needs to be increased in older patients before the full effect of a given dose can be assessed. Conversely, increased time is needed for complete drug elimination from the body and dissipation of drug effects.

Age-related changes in protein binding of drugs are not usually found. Changes in free drug concentrations due to the competition of drugs for binding sites can occur, but changes are predicted to be transitory. Clinically significant examples involve warfarin and changes in anticoagulation when additional drugs are added to warfarin therapy.

Table 80-2 summarizes general guidelines for drug dosing in older patients.

Adverse Drug Events and Drug Interactions

Adverse drug events are estimated to affect millions of people per year and account for up to 5% of total hospital admissions. A recent literature review found adverse drug event admission rates of 10.7% in elderly patients, with cardiovascular drugs accounting for about half of the admissions, nonsteroidal anti-inflammatory drugs (NSAIDs) for

20%, and central nervous system drugs for 14%.[31] During hospitalization, the odds ratio of severe adverse drug events with cardiovascular medications has been reported to be 2.4 times that of other medications. Heart failure, especially in women, is associated with increased risk of adverse drug reactions during hospitalization.[32]

The classes of drugs most commonly associated with adverse drug events in the elderly include diuretics, warfarin, NSAIDs, selective serotonin reuptake inhibitors, beta blockers, and ACE inhibitors.[33] Current pain management guidelines for pain in the elderly recommend NSAID and selective cyclooxygenase 2 (COX-2) inhibitor use only rarely and with extreme caution. Cardiovascular risks of NSAIDs in patients with CAD are less well delineated and may vary by NSAID.[34] In nursing home patients, drugs associated with adverse drug events are more frequently antibiotics, anticoagulants and antiplatelet drugs, atypical and typical antipsychotic drugs, antidepressants, antiseizure medications, or opioids.[35] Adverse drug effects may present with

"atypical" symptoms in the older patient, such as mental status changes and impaired cognition.

The strongest risk factor for adverse drug-related events is the number of drugs prescribed, independent of age. Chronic administration of four drugs is associated with a risk of adverse effects of 50% to 60%; administration of eight or nine drugs increases the risk to almost 100% (**Fig. 80-6**). Whereas the goal is to prescribe as few drugs as possible in the elderly, the presence of multiple diseases and multidrug regimens for common cardiovascular diseases often results in polypharmacy. Surveys estimate that about half of people older than 65 years use three or more medications prescribed on a daily basis, and 20% of patients 75 years and older have five drugs prescribed per outpatient encounter (*www.cdc.gov*). Even higher numbers of medications are prescribed for nursing home patients, averaging six to eight medications per day. American College of Cardiology/American Heart Association (ACC/AHA) guidelines for the pharmacologic treatment of patients after uncomplicated MI and for the management of chronic heart failure recommend use of more than three drugs (available at *ACC.org* or *heart.org*). Current regimens for treatment of the common disorders of diabetes and osteoporosis in the elderly similarly include two to four drugs. Strategies that minimize the chance of drug interactions and adverse drug effects are thus essential.

PHARMACOKINETIC INTERACTIONS. Pharmacokinetic interactions that alter the concentration of concomitantly administered medications are more likely if they are metabolized by or inhibit the same pathway. Tables 10-1 and 10-2 in Chapter 10 list examples of cardiovascular drugs by metabolic pathway with examples of inducers and inhibitors and interactions (also see *www.fda.gov/cder*). The most potent inhibitors of the cytochrome P-450 oxidative enzymes are amiodarone (all CYP isoforms) and dronedarone (CYP3A), the azole antifungal drugs itraconazole and ketoconazole (CYP3A), and protease inhibitors (CYP3A), followed by diltiazem (CYP3A) and erythromycin (CYP3A) (see *http://medicine.iupui.edu/clinpharm/ddis/table.asp*). Oral hypoglycemic agents are commonly prescribed drugs in the elderly, and coadministration of sulfonamide antibiotics with sulfonylureas can lead to hypoglycemia, in part because of CYP2C9 inhibition. Some drugs are administered as prodrugs and metabolized to active agents (cardiovascular examples include many ACE inhibitors and clopidogrel). Inhibition of the antiplatelet effects of clopidogrel has been reported with coadministration of atorvastatin that decreases clopidogrel activation by CYP3A, or proton pump inhibitors that inhibit CYP2C19-mediated clopidogrel activation.

TABLE 80-2	Guidelines for Medication Prescribing in Older Patients

In general, loading doses should be reduced. Weight (or body surface area) can be used to estimate loading dose requirements. Weight differences between the sexes are greatest for white people.

Use estimates of glomerular filtration to guide dosing of renally cleared medications and contrast agent administration. Reduce initial doses of metabolically or hepatically cleared drugs but titrate to effect.

Time between dosage adjustments and evaluation of dosing changes should be longer in older patients than in younger patients.

Routine use of strategies to avoid drug interactions is essential. Incorporation of reference materials, a team approach, and quality improvement efforts are effective strategies.

Knowledge of effects of noncardiac medications is critical.

Assessment of adherence and attention to factors contributing to nonadherence should be part of the prescribing process.

Physicians must be familiar with the patient's source of prescription medication coverage and provide education and assistance with obtaining critical medications.

Multidisciplinary approaches to monitoring of medication therapy may improve outcomes.

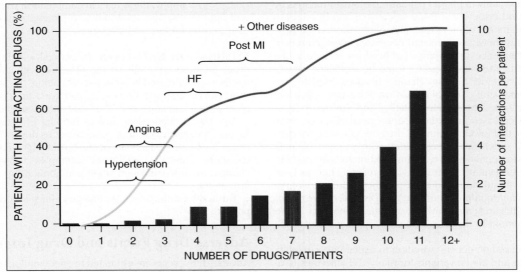

FIGURE 80-6 The relationship between the number of drugs consumed and drug interactions. Current guidelines for the pharmacologic management of patients with heart failure (HF) or myocardial infarction (post MI) place them at high risk for drug interactions. *(From Schwartz JB: Clinical Pharmacology, ACCSAP V, 2003. As modified from Nolan L, O'Malley K: The need for a more rational approach to drug prescribing for elderly people in nursing homes. Age Aging 18:52, 1989; and Denham MJ: Adverse drug reactions. Br Med Bull 46:53, 1990.)*

Inducibility of hepatic enzyme activity can lower concentrations of medications and lead to ineffective therapy. The antituberculous drug rifampin is the most potent inducer of CYP1A and CYP3A. With mandatory screening for tuberculosis, treatment with rifampin may be initiated. Dosages of coadministered drugs cleared by CYP1A and CYP3A may need to be increased during rifampin administration and decreased on discontinuation of rifampin. Markedly decreased cyclosporine levels and reduced clopidogrel inhibition of platelet aggregation during rifampin coadministration have been reported.[36] Other clinically relevant CYP inducers include carbamazepine (all CYPs); dexamethasone and phenytoin (CYP2C); caffeine, cigarette smoke, lansoprazole, omeprazole (CYP1A), and St. John's wort (CYP3A) (see http://medicine.iupui.edu/clinpharm/ddis/table.asp). Diet-drug and herb-drug interactions also occur.[37]

Despite the predictability of some interactions, many hospital admissions of elderly patients for drug toxicity involve administration of drugs known to interact.[38] Because of the multiplicity of potential interactions and release of new medications and discovery of new interactions, use of pharmacy or computerized and online tools that provide comprehensive up-to-date information and guidelines for avoidance of drug interactions is highly recommended. Available tools include the Physicians' Desk Reference (traditional, pocket, or online versions), PDR Guide to Drug Interactions, Side Effects, and Indications (traditional, computer version, or hand-held computer version available free of charge at www.PDR.net), Lexi-comp (software for smartphones, PDAs, and desktops), the Medical Letter and the Medical Letter Drug Interactions Program (computer based), Epocrates for the handheld computer or iPhone (available free of charge at www.epocrates.com), and online pharmacology texts or data bases (the Food and Drug Administration: www.fda.gov/cder, drug reactions section; www.druginteractions.org or http://medicine.iupui.edu/flockhart). Many individual hospitals, health care systems, and pharmacies provide internal reference sources.

Specialized clinics and use of specific algorithms or computer-based dosage programs to monitor oral anticoagulant therapy in outpatients have been shown to reduce bleeding-related complications. Other approaches that have been shown to reduce adverse drug reactions in older patients include involvement of pharmacy-trained individuals to assess the appropriateness of doses and medication counseling by multidisciplinary care team members. Algorithms have been developed for older patients to identify both medications that are potentially inappropriate and should be discontinued (STOPP criteria) and ones that appear indicated and should be initiated (START criteria).[39,40] A major limitation is the frequent lack of complete and readily accessible information on medication consumption and disease states in the older patient with multiple diseases and physicians. Integrated medical record and pharmacy information, interactive data bases, and computerized physician order entry with clinical decision support can reduce adverse drug events and improve medication therapy. Such systems, however, are not yet widely implemented. In contrast, mandated drug use review efforts appear ineffective.[41]

ADVERSE PHARMACODYNAMIC EFFECTS. Age-related changes in cardiovascular physiology and dynamics affect pharmacodynamics (see Table 80-1). Greater age-related nervous system sensitivity to parasympathetic stimulation may explain adverse effects such as urinary retention, constipation and fecal impaction, or worsened cognition in older patients who receive drugs with anticholinergic properties. Gastrointestinal transit time is generally increased in the elderly, and constipation is a frequent complaint of hospitalized elderly, less active elderly, and institutionalized elderly. Drug-induced constipation and bowel obstruction can occur in older patients receiving bile acid sequestrants, anticholinergic medications, opiates, and verapamil.

Pharmacodynamic drug interactions are more likely to occur between drugs acting on the same system. A classic example of additive effects that can produce hypotension and postural hypotension in the elderly is the coadministration of direct vasodilators or nitrates with alpha blockers, beta blockers, calcium channel blockers, ACE inhibitors, angiotensin receptor blockers (ARBs), diuretics, sildenafil,

or tricyclic antidepressants. Other examples are bradycardia with combinations of amiodarone, beta-adrenergic blocking drugs, digoxin, diltiazem, or verapamil; and bleeding due to increased inhibition of platelet and clotting factors with combinations of aspirin, NSAIDs (including some COX-2–selective inhibitors), warfarin, or clopidogrel. Increased potassium concentrations due to combined administration of ACE inhibitors, ARBs, aldosterone and renin antagonists, and potassium-sparing diuretics in older patients are cited as causes of serious adverse drug reactions that are preventable.[35,42] Combinations of NSAIDs, including selective COX-2 inhibitors, with ACE inhibitors can also decrease potassium excretion with resultant hyperkalemia or can cause a decrease in renal function in the older patient. Combinations of drugs that produce QT interval prolongation can result in marked QT interval prolongation and torsades de pointes arrhythmias (see Chap. 39). Importantly, noncardiac drugs such as antibiotics (azithromycin, clarithromycin, erythromycin, gatifloxacin, gemifloxacin, moxifloxacin), antidepressants (amitriptyline, fluoxetine, lithium, venlafaxine), antipsychotics (haloperidol, risperidone), tamoxifen, and vardenafil used in the elderly may have additive effects with cardiovascular drugs such as the class IA, class IC, and class III antiarrhythmic drugs, isradipine, nicardipine, and ranolazine (see Chap. 37; online updated lists of medications that prolong the QT are available at www.Qtdrugs.org).

Examples of pharmacodynamic interactions with antagonistic effects include increased angina when beta agonists and theophylline are given to patients with CAD receiving beta blockers or nondihydropyridine calcium channel antagonists and loss of hypertension control when a drug such as fludrocortisone acetate is given for postural hypotension. Concern has also been raised about the ability of ibuprofen to block aspirin's binding to platelets and to diminish the cardioprotective effects of aspirin. The COX-2–selective NSAIDs rofecoxib and valdecoxib were removed from the market because of increased cardiovascular events, and other selective and nonselective NSAIDs are undergoing scrutiny.[34] Concern has also been raised with the weight gain and edema and possible increased incidence of heart failure with newer thiazolidinedione oral agents for the treatment of diabetes (rosiglitazone and pioglitazone).[43] Nicotinic acid raises high-density lipoprotein (HDL) concentration and reduces triglyceride levels but worsens insulin resistance and can exacerbate hyperglycemia in diabetics, as can beta blockers (with the exception of carvedilol) and thiazides. Selective estrogen receptor modulators and aromatase inhibitors can increase cholesterol and increase the risk of venous thromboembolic events, and serious cardiac events appear increased with some agents.[44] Familiarity with effects of noncardiac medications is necessary during pharmacotherapy of the elderly.

Inappropriate Prescribing in the Elderly

A number of lists of medications considered "inappropriate" for routine use in the elderly because of adverse effects or lack of efficacy have been compiled. The updated 2003 Beers criteria[45] can be accessed online (archinte.ama-assn.org/cgi/reprint/163/22/2716.pdf). Long-acting benzodiazepines, sedative and hypnotic agents, long-acting oral hypoglycemic agents, selected analgesics and NSAIDs, first-generation antihistamines, antiemetics, and gastrointestinal antispasmodics are usually considered inappropriate in the elderly. Amiodarone, clonidine, disopyramide, doxazosin, ethacrynic acid, guanethidine, and guanadrel have been classified as generally inappropriate in the elderly. More recent definitions of "inappropriate drug use" include failure to consider drug-disease interactions and failure to adjust drug dosages for age-related changes (i.e., digoxin at doses above 0.125 mg/day), drug duplication, drug-drug interactions, and duration of use. By use of these criteria, most drug use review studies concluded that inappropriate drug prescribing occurs in a significant fraction of older patients.[35,46] Resources such as the Physicians' Desk Reference may not contain geriatric prescribing information on older medications or present data on minimally effective doses established after drug marketing approval or in guidelines. Disturbingly, analyses suggest that inappropriate prescribing of medications to older patients

TABLE 80-3   Estimation of 4-Year Mortality in Community-Dwelling Elderly by Medical and Function Information

	Points
Age (year)	
60-64	1
65-69	2
70-74	3
75-79	4
80-84	5
>85	7
Male sex	2
Diabetes mellitus	1
Cancer	2
Lung disease	2
Heart failure	2
Body mass index <25	1
Current smoker	2
Assistance needed for	
Bathing	2
Managing finances	2
Difficulty	
Walking several blocks	2
Pushing or pulling heavy objects	1

Score	4-Year Mortality (%)
0	0-1
1	1
2	1.5
3	3.5
4	5
5	5-8
6	9
7	12-15
8	19-20
9	20-24
10	27-28
11	43-45
12	44-48
13	54-59
≥14	64-67

Modified from Lee S, Lindquist K, Segal M, Covinsky K: Development and validation of a prognostic index for 4-year mortality in older adults. JAMA 295:801, 2006.

in both the community and nursing homes has not decreased in recent years.[46-48]

Appropriate prescribing of medications is evolving to include consideration of discontinuing guideline-recommended medications in patients with life expectancy that may be too short to achieve long-term benefits or in whom concomitant diseases such as end-stage dementia result in therapeutic goals related primarily to quality of life. Estimation of life expectancy from both comorbid conditions and functional measures is gaining acceptance in determining appropriateness for screening for diseases, preventive strategies, and therapeutic decision making for older adults.[49-52] Recent models that estimate life expectancy use data likely to be available during routine clinical care or at the time of hospital discharge.[50,53] **Table 80-3** presents one model developed from a large and diverse sample of community-dwelling elderly in the United States. It identifies noncardiac factors that contribute significantly to overall mortality in the elderly. Another overall mortality prediction tool based on common laboratory tests plus age may also be useful in the hospital setting.[53] A logical approach to choosing appropriate medications, as well as other therapies, would incorporate consideration of remaining life expectancy, time until benefit, treatment targets, and goals of care for the individual older patient.

Adherence

Adherence with medications is commonly thought to be lower in older patients compared with younger patients. Contributing factors include the cost of medications; difficulty with understanding directions because of small print of written directions, hearing impairment, or impaired memory; inadequate instructions; complex dosing regimens; difficulties with packaging materials; and insufficient education of the patient, family, or caregiver on medication use. Of these, the most limiting are thought to be the cost of medications, poor education of the patient about medications, and cognitive impairment in elderly patients, especially those living alone. Use of HMG-CoA reductase inhibitors has been directly related to drug payment coverage and copayment requirements in Medicare recipients and in veterans.[54]

Physicians routinely overestimate the patient's adherence with medications. Assessment of adherence should be part of care, and issues related to potential contributors to medication nonadherence

should be addressed by prescribing health care professionals. Unfortunately, there are few trials of interventions to improve medication adherence with resources usually available in clinical settings or that address adherence with multiple medication regimens. Strategies to improve adherence include programs for low-income seniors, visual or memory aids, medication-dispensing tools, use of geriatric-friendly packaging, assessment of cognitive status and the patient's understanding and inclusion of caregivers or family members in discussion about medications, and use of multidisciplinary teams or collaboration with pharmacists. Nonadherence is multifactorial, and it is likely that multiple strategies will need to be used.

Medicare D

January 1, 2006, marked the beginning of prescription drug coverage under the Medicare Prescription Drug and Modernization Act of 2003 in the United States. The Medicare D legislation created a complex plan involving government-contracted private industry coverage requiring individual enrollment. All plans include deductibles of $250 per year and partial payment of annual drug costs up to the estimated average annual drug expenditure for seniors of $2250 per year and then a gap in payment until costs exceed $3600 for all but low-income seniors (i.e., patients "dually eligible" for Medicaid and Medicare and those with incomes of 100% to 150% poverty levels). A multitude of plans are offered in regions that vary in benefits, co-pays, covered formulary medications, and tiers of medications with differing levels of co-pays within formularies. Physicians and pharmacists have had the task of educating a significant number of patients and families. Specific medications excluded from coverage by the law include those inappropriate for use in the elderly (such as barbiturates and benzodiazepines; see earlier) but also over-the-counter medications, vitamins, and products for symptomatic relief of colds or cough and medications not used for "medically accepted" indications. Information for physicians and patients on plans and formularies is available from many sources, including *www.Medicare.gov*, *www.MedicareToday.org*, *www.HLC.org*, *www.cms.hhs.gov*, *www.ama-assn.org*, and *www.accesstobenefits.org* or at 800-Medicare (800-633-4227).

The program created the potential for improving medication access, adherence, and therapy and has achieved some of these goals. Only about 10% of Medicare beneficiaries are currently without prescription coverage compared with 25% to 38% in preceding years, and a small but significant decrease in cost-related medication nonadherence has been documented.[55] Unfortunately, those in the poorest health or with multiple morbidities have not appeared to have improvements in cost-related medication nonadherence.

CURRENT CONTROVERSIES. Current controversies include the following: relative importance of factors influencing drug clearance rates (i.e., age, sex, genetics, environmental factors, disease state, comedications); relative importance of factors influencing drug responses in older patients (age, genetics, disease state, adherence, comedications); most efficacious approaches to decrease adverse medication events; role of electronic prescribing; optimization of medication alert system; and how to achieve universally available medical and medication information.

Vascular Disease

Hypertension (see Chaps. 45 and 46)

PREVALENCE AND INCIDENCE. Either diastolic (>90 mm Hg) or systolic (>140 mm Hg) hypertension occurs in one half to two thirds of people older than 65 years and in 75% of people older than 80 years.[56] The prevalence varies by race (or genetics) and is slightly higher in African Americans and Hispanics compared with non-Hispanic whites (see Chap. 2). The profile of hypertension is altered by aging, with systolic hypertension becoming more prevalent than diastolic hypertension. Systolic blood pressure rises with aging in both men and women but rises more steeply in women (see Chap. 81). After the age of 65 years, average systolic blood pressures are higher in women than in men. In contrast, diastolic blood pressure is relatively constant from 50 to 80 years of age, with average diastolic pressures higher in men than in women from the age of 50 to 80 years. "Isolated" systolic hypertension, without elevation of diastolic blood pressure, is present in about 8% of sexagenarians and more than 25% of the population older than 80 years. A large number of older people are unaware that they have hypertension. Even when it is recognized, hypertension is not controlled in many older patients, and older age is considered one of the strongest risk factors for resistant hypertension.[56,57]

TREATMENT. Relative risks for cardiovascular events associated with increasing blood pressure do not decline with older age, and absolute risk increases markedly in older patients, emphasizing the need for treatment of hypertension in the elderly.[56] Randomized placebo-controlled clinical trials of elderly patients during the past three decades have unequivocally demonstrated that treatment of diastolic or systolic hypertension confers cardiovascular benefits (see Table 80-e1 on website). Most of these studies used thiazide diuretics, beta blockers, or calcium channel blockers as first-line therapy with addition of secondary agents. ARBs were used in one study that showed only stroke benefits, and ACE inhibitors and ARBs have been used in comparative trials of newer drugs to older drugs that show stroke and cardiovascular benefits. Importantly, a recent trial enrolling the very old has demonstrated the safety and efficacy of carefully monitored treatment of systolic hypertension to a target of 150/80 mm Hg using indapamide with or without an ACE inhibitor in patients older than 80 years.[58] The participants were relatively "healthy" elderly (less than 12% had cardiovascular disease, only 7% had prior strokes or diabetes), and beneficial effects of treatment were seen within 1 year. In addition to reduced stroke, heart failure, and deaths from cardiovascular causes, overall mortality was also reduced. These findings counter prior meta-analysis and guideline concerns about risks of treatment of systolic hypertension in people older than 80 years but add to the controversy over the optimal target systolic blood pressure. Whereas other trials and American College of Cardiology clinical performance measures state a target of <140 mm Hg, many participants in the trials showing benefits did not achieve this goal.

There is no clear distinction in relative benefits between one pharmacologic agent or combination of agents and others for the treatment of uncomplicated hypertension in the elderly, although some data support varying benefit of agents on individual cardiovascular outcomes (see Table 80-e1 on website). Morbidity and mortality benefits of treatment of hypertension in the elderly have been seen with the five major antihypertensive classes—diuretics, beta blockers, calcium antagonists, ACE inhibitors, and angiotensin receptor antagonists.[59] Limited data show antihypertensive efficacy for a renin inhibitor, but longer term morbidity and mortality studies have not been completed. It appears that it is the control of both systolic and diastolic blood pressure that confers beneficial outcomes, that more than one

medication has been administered to most trial participants, and that combination regimens are usually required to even approach blood pressure targets in older patients. The emphasis should be on diagnosis and treatment of hypertension rather than on the choice of initial individual therapeutic agents. Most guidelines and societies recommend basing the selection of combinations of pharmacologic agents on individual cardiovascular risk factors, concomitant diseases, side effect profiles, and ease of use.

The impact of common noncardiovascular conditions on both the efficacy and side effects of antihypertensive agents should be considered (**Table 80-4**). Arthritis is second in prevalence to cardiovascular disease in the elderly, and NSAIDs are among the most frequently consumed drugs (prescription and over-the-counter) in older people. In addition to the potential for cardiovascular ischemic events, adverse renal effects or hyperkalemia may occur when NSAIDs are given in combination with ACE inhibitors, ARBs, aldosterone, or renin antagonists. Loss of blood pressure control and heart failure have been precipitated by administration of nonselective NSAIDs as well as COX-2–selective NSAIDs. Age-related bone loss accelerates in older men and women and is the major contributing cause of osteoporosis. Osteoporosis in turn is a major risk factor for fractures in older people; the lifetime risk of osteoporotic fracture in Americans is estimated at 40% for women and 13% for men. Thiazides have been shown to preserve bone mineral density compared with placebo in randomized controlled trials and have been associated with higher bone mineral density and a reduction in risk of hip fractures in epidemiologic studies, providing a noncardiac treatment benefit in older patients.[60,61] Older patients for whom thiazide diuretics may not be a good choice include patients with urinary frequency problems (stress incontinence, urinary frequency with or without incontinence due to prostatic hypertrophy, overactive bladders, and patients needing assistance with toileting) because drugs that do not increase urinary frequency may have higher adherence.

Table 80-4 presents suggested antihypertensive regimens in older patients based on the presence of hypertension *and* concomitant conditions. Further data on frequent geriatric problems and medications to use or to avoid are available at *www.geriatricsatyourfingertips.com.* Education of the patient and caregiver should also be a component of care. A meta-analysis of randomized trials concluded that chronic disease self-management programs for older adults with hypertension produced clinically important benefits but could not identify key features of such programs.[62] A recent large randomized trial to improve blood pressure control in older male hypertensives found the best results with education of the patient on medication adherence, low-sodium diet, exercise, and the frequent need for more than one medication for blood pressure control, in combination with provider education and pharmacy alerts to providers regarding patients' responses to medications.[63]

ADDITIONAL CONSIDERATIONS IN THE OLDER PATIENT WITH HYPERTENSION. Both the Seventh Report of the Joint National Committee on Prevention, Detection, Evaluation, and Treatment of High Blood Pressure (JNC 7)[64] and the European Guidelines for the Management of Arterial Hypertension[65] recommend lower initial drug dosages and slower medication titration in older patients as well as the need to monitor for postural hypotension. A decrease in standing systolic blood pressure is estimated to be present in 15% of 70- to 74-year old community-dwelling men or women and in up to 30% of patients with systolic hypertension. Postural hypotension of >20 mm Hg or 20% of systolic pressure is a risk factor for falls and fractures that carry significant morbidity and mortality. Antihypertensive medications add to the risk of postural hypotension, as do many antiparkinson agents, antipsychotic agents, and tricyclic antidepressant drugs. The frailest and oldest of the elderly may reside in long-term care facilities. It is estimated that 30% to 70% are hypertensive and 30% have postural hypotension. Diuretic therapy appears to be effective in controlling systolic blood pressure in these patients and may also decrease postural hypotension. Postural blood pressure changes should be assessed (after ≥5 minutes supine, immediately after standing, and 2 minutes after standing) in older patients and volume depletion avoided.

TABLE 80-4 Considerations for Pharmacologic Therapy for Older Patients with Hypertension and Other Disorders

HYPERTENSION +	EFFICACY CONSIDERATIONS	TOXICITY OR ADVERSE EFFECT CONSIDERATIONS
Arthritis	—	ACE, ARB, aldosterone, and renin antagonist interactions with NSAIDs
Atrial fibrillation		Interactions with warfarin
Recurrent	ARB, ACE*	
Permanent	Beta blocker, calcium channel blocker (non-DHP)*,†	
Atrioventricular block	—	Beta blockers, non-DHP calcium channel blockers
Carotid disease or stroke	Calcium channel blocker,† ACE*	
Constipation	—	Verapamil
Coronary artery disease	Beta blocker*,† calcium channel blocker*,†	Nitrates and postural hypotension
Dementia	Clonidine‡	
Depression	—	SSRIs and hyponatremia
Diabetes	ACE,*,† ARB,*,† CCB (non-DHP) , beta blocker	Chlorpropamide and hyponatremia ACE or ARB + renin inhibitor and hyperkalemia
Glaucoma	Beta blocker	
Gout		Thiazide diuretics*
Heart failure	ACE,*,† ARB,*,† + loop diuretic,*,† beta blocker,*,† ± aldosterone antagonist*,†,§	Calcium channel blockers (possible)* ACE, ARB, aldosterone antagonist and hyperkalemia
Hyponatremia	—	Diuretic (especially with SSRI)
Incontinence	—	Diuretic
Metabolic syndrome	ACE,* ARB,* calcium channel blocker*	Beta blockers, diuretics
Myocardial infarction	Beta blocker,*,† ± ACE,*,† ± aldosterone antagonist*	ACE, ARB, aldosterone antagonist and hyperkalemia
Osteoporosis	Thiazides (beta blocker, ACE neutral or protect); potassium (K) phosphate (versus KCl)	Furosemide (bone loss)
Peripheral artery disease	Calcium channel blocker (DHP),*,† ACE + diuretics‖	Beta blocker (only if severe)
Postural hypotension	Thiazide¶	Alpha blocker, calcium channel blockers (DHP)
Prostatic hypertrophy	Alpha blocker†	
Pulmonary disease (asthma, COPD)		Beta blocker
Renal failure	ACE,*,† ARB,*,† ACE + ARB; loop diuretic*,†	Aldosterone antagonists (? renin inhibitors) and hyperkalemia
Ventricular arrhythmias	Beta blocker†	Thiazide, loop diuretics and hypokalemia

ACE = angiotensin-converting enzyme inhibitor; ARB = angiotensin receptor blocker; COPD = chronic obstructive pulmonary disease; NSAIDs = nonsteroidal anti-inflammatory drugs; DHP = dihydropyridine; SSRI = selective serotonin reuptake inhibitor.

*Recommendations for second-line agents usually added to thiazide diuretics from Chobanian AV, Bakris GL, Black HR, et al: The Seventh Report of the Joint National Committee on Prevention, Detection, Evaluation, and Treatment of High Blood Pressure. The JNC 7 Report. JAMA 289:2560, 2003.

†Mancia G, De Backer G, Dominiczak A, et al: 2007 Guidelines for the management of arterial hypertension. The Task Force for the management of arterial hypertension of the European Society of Hypertension (ESH) and of the European Society of Cardiology (ESC). Eur Heart J 28:1462, 2007.

‡Only available transdermal formulation for patients unable to swallow or who refuse oral medications.

§Systolic heart failure only.

‖Norgren L, Hiatt W, Dormandy J, et al: Inter-Society consensus for the management of peripheral arterial disease (TASC II). J Vasc Surg 45:S5A, 2007.

¶Nursing home patients.

Postprandial declines in both systolic and diastolic blood pressure occur in hospitalized, institutionalized, and community-dwelling elderly. The greatest decline occurs about 1 hour after eating, with blood pressure returning to fasting levels at 3 to 4 hours after eating. Vasoactive medications with rapid absorption and peaks should not be administered with meals.

New onset or worsening of hypertension occurs in 10% to 40% of cancer patients during administration of inhibitors of the vascular endothelial growth factor (VEGF) signaling pathway (bevacizumab, sunitinib, sorafenib) and has been associated with cardiac events and heart failure. Blood pressure should be controlled before administration of these drugs and monitored during VEGF therapy. If hypertension occurs, it should be promptly treated. Blood pressure has usually been controlled by oral antihypertensive therapy with ACE inhibitors, ARBs, beta blockers, diuretics, and occasionally nitrates. Verapamil and diltiazem are contraindicated in combination with VEGF inhibitors that are metabolized by CYP3A, and nifedipine may induce VEGF

secretion and should be avoided. In cases of severe or persistent hypertension despite the initiation of antihypertensive treatment, temporary or permanent discontinuation of angiogenic inhibitors should be considered.[66]

Table 80-5 summarizes the approach to hypertension in older patients.

CURRENT CONTROVERSIES. Current controversies include the following: target blood pressures for systolic blood pressure in the very old (>80 years); lowest acceptable diastolic blood pressure during antihypertensive therapy; impact of differences in central versus peripheral blood pressure; initial therapy with single agents versus combination regimens; use of lifestyle modifications; impact of blood pressure treatment on development of dementia; safety and efficacy of aldosterone and renin inhibitors in the elderly; and role of aortic stiffness in predicting systolic blood pressure responses or as a target for systolic blood pressure–lowering agents.

Note: Updated JNC 8 recommendations will be published soon and are expected to address some of these controversies.

TABLE 80-5 Approach to Hypertension in Older Patients

Systolic as well as diastolic hypertension should be treated; current recommendations are based on brachial artery measurements:
  Diastolic target is <90 mm Hg.
  Systolic target is <140 mm Hg for most (<150 mm Hg for patients older than 80 years).
The focus should be on achieving blood pressure control, not initial therapy.
Multiple medications are usually required in older patients, and combinations should be based on concomitant diseases.
Drug dosing regimens should be adjusted for age and disease-related changes in drug metabolism and potential drug-drug interactions.
Patients should be monitored for adverse effects and drug interactions, especially
  Postural hypotension and postprandial hypotension
  Hypovolemia with diuretics
  Hyperkalemia with ACE inhibitors, ARBs, aldosterone, renin antagonists

Coronary Artery Disease (see Chaps. 49 and 57)

PREVALENCE AND INCIDENCE. Both the prevalence and severity of atherosclerotic CAD increase with age in men and women. Autopsy studies show that more than half of people older than 60 years have significant CAD, with increasing prevalence of left main or triple-vessel CAD with older age. By use of electrocardiographic evidence of MI, abnormal echocardiogram, carotid intimal thickness, and abnormal ankle-brachial index as measures of subclinical vascular disease in community-dwelling people older than 65 years, abnormalities were detected in 22% of women and 33% of men aged 65 to 70 years and 43% of women and 45% of men older than 85 years (see *http://www.chs-nhlbi.org/*). By 80 years of age, the frequency of symptomatic CAD is about 20% to 30% in both men and women. Because of the increasing proportion of women at older ages, however, there are more older women with angina presenting for care. These women have been less likely to receive evidence-based therapy for stable angina, aggressive therapy for acute coronary syndromes, or diagnostic evaluations.[67-70]

DIAGNOSIS

Estimation of Risk

Risk factors such as hypertension, total cholesterol level, and LDL-cholesterol concentration and tools such as those developed from the Framingham Study in younger populations may be less accurate in the very old or in women.[71,72] The Reynolds Risk Score may improve risk estimates in women up to age 80 years thought to be at intermediate risk (*http://www.reynoldsriskscore.org/*). Data suggest that HDL-cholesterol concentration, increased pulse pressure, and measures of arterial stiffness assume importance in risk assessment in older people. Chronic kidney disease (as defined by eGFR) has also been identified as a risk factor for cardiovascular disease and progression of cardiovascular disease, but it is not yet incorporated into risk models. Predictive models that incorporate both traditional risk factors (such as smoking, blood pressure, selected lipid levels, diabetes) and age-specific markers (such as pulse pressure, arterial stiffness, and possibly albuminuria with further adjustment for sex) may provide the best current estimates of cardiovascular risk in older people without known CAD.[73-75] In estimating risk of all-cause mortality, data from large populations including those undergoing angiography found that sex-specific risk scores combining complete blood count and basic metabolic profile components and age were highly predictive of mortality at 30 days, 1 year, and 5 years.[53] Such risk scores and estimates of life expectancy based on geriatric factors warrant use to assist in therapeutic decision making.

History

Anginal symptoms are more likely to be absent or ischemia silent in older patients compared with young patients. Symptoms are termed atypical because the description differs from the classic description of substernal pressure with exertion. Symptoms may primarily be dyspnea, shoulder or back pain, weakness, fatigue (in women), or epigastric discomfort and may be precipitated by concurrent illnesses. Some older patients describe symptoms with effort, but those with limited physical exertion may not report symptoms, and those with altered manifestations of pain due to concomitant diabetes or age-related changes may have symptoms at rest or during mental stress. Memory impairment may also limit the accuracy of the history. Lack of symptoms during evidence of myocardial ischemia on electrocardiography has been reported in 20% to 50% of patients 65 years or older.

Testing for Ischemia (see Chap. 53)

The prevalence of resting ST-T wave abnormalities on electrocardiography in older people results in a modest age-associated reduction in specificity of exercise electrocardiography (see Chap. 14). Treadmill exercise testing can provide prognostic information in patients able to exercise sufficiently and can also provide information about functional capacity and exercise tolerance. Exercise results can be enhanced by the use of modified protocols beginning with low-intensity exercise. Most series report slightly higher sensitivity (84%) and lower specificity (70%) in patients older than 75 years than in younger patients. Echocardiography and nuclear testing can overcome some of the limitations of electrocardiographic interpretation (see Chaps. 15 and 17). In older patients unable to exercise, pharmacologic agents such as dipyridamole and adenosine can be used with nuclear scintigraphy to assess myocardial perfusion at rest and after vasodilation; or agents such as dobutamine can be combined with echocardiography or other imaging techniques to assess ventricular function at rest and during increased myocardial demand.

The value of screening for asymptomatic CAD in the elderly is not known. The presence of coronary calcifications is high (**Fig. 80-7**), and neither the presence nor degree of coronary calcification has correlated with coronary flow decrease in the older population, and data are especially limited for women.[76-78] The high prevalence of hypertension, diabetes, obesity, and inactivity in the elderly, including those aged 65 to 75 years, would suggest that increased efforts to improve diet and

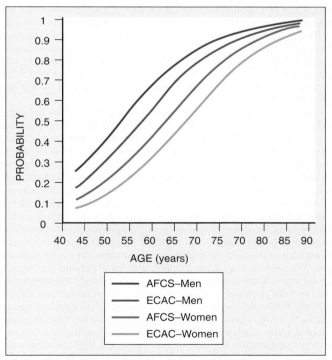

FIGURE 80-7 Predicted probability of presence of detectable coronary artery calcification among Amish Family Calcification Study (AFCS) and Epidemiology of Coronary Artery Calcification (ECAC; Lancaster County, Penn.) study participants. (*From Bielak LF, Yu PF, Ryan KA, et al. Differences in prevalence and severity of coronary artery calcification between two non-Hispanic white populations with diverse lifestyles. Atherosclerosis 196:888, 2008.*)

activity levels, smoking cessation, treatment of hypertension and diabetes, and optimization of renal function would be of greater benefit on overall morbidity and mortality than screening with vascular imaging studies in the asymptomatic elderly.

TREATMENT (see Chaps. 49 and 57)

Medical

Optimization of medical care warrants greater emphasis.[79] Optimal medical therapy for patients with stable coronary disease, including the elderly and diabetics with multivessel CAD, has recently been shown to produce results equivalent to those of percutaneous coronary intervention in reducing the risk of cardiovascular events.[80,81] Therapeutic goals and management goals for chronic stable angina are targeted at (1) symptom relief with nitrates, beta blockers, calcium antagonists, and partial free fatty acid inhibitors and (2) risk reduction and slowing of the progression of disease with control of hypertension and diabetes, weight control, lipid lowering (including triglycerides), exercise, and smoking cessation.[79] Aspirin at 75 to 162 mg/day is recommended, although benefits in women, especially older women, are not as clear as in men.[82] Secondary prevention efforts should be targeted at interventions conferring benefit within the anticipated life span of the patient. Lifestyle changes of smoking cessation, increased activity, and weight control provide improvements in a short time frame, whereas benefits of lipid lowering may take longer. Annual influenza vaccinations reduce cardiovascular events in older populations.

LIPID LOWERING IN THE ELDERLY (see Chaps. 47 and 49). Lipid lowering may not confer benefit until after 3 to 5 years of treatment on the basis of data from secondary prevention trials of HMG-CoA reductase inhibitors that enrolled significant numbers of older patients (summarized in Table 80-e2 on the website). These trials used 40 mg/day pravastatin, 20 to 40 mg/day simvastatin, or 1200 mg/day gemfibrozil (see Table 80-e2 on the website). Whereas increasingly lower LDL-cholesterol targets (<100 mg/dL) are recommended in CAD guidelines with higher doses of statins being used, the major trial on which these recommendations are based explicitly excluded CAD patients older than 75 years (Treating to New Targets [TNT] trial) and enrolled primarily white men.[79,83] Post hoc analyses of patients between the ages of 65 and 75 years showed reduced combined cardiovascular event endpoints (10.3% compared with 12.6%) with 80 mg/day atorvastatin compared with 10 mg/day atorvastatin but no mortality benefit with the higher dose for the elderly subgroup (or the entire group).[83] The optimal lipid target has not been definitively established for patients older than 75 years.

Dose considerations are important because risk factors for statin-induced myopathy include older age (>80 years and in women more than in men), smaller body frame, frailty, and multisystem disease (including chronic renal insufficiency, especially due to diabetes), and myopathy also increases with increasing dosages. Myopathy may be difficult to differentiate from other types of musculoskeletal disorders or pain in the older patient, or it may not be recognized because of cognitive impairment. Complaints may also be nonspecific or described as "flulike," with fatigue nearly as common a complaint as muscle pain. An observational study of 7924 French patients receiving "high"-dose statin therapy (atorvastatin 40 or 80 mg/day, fluvastatin 80 mg/day, pravastatin 40 mg/day, or simvastatin 40 or 80 mg/day), with 30% older than 65 years, found that 10.5% of patients had muscle symptoms, with the incidence of muscle pain related to activity levels. Muscle pain required analgesics in 39%, 38% reported inability to perform moderate exertion, and 4% were either confined to bed or unable to work.[84] Similarly, whereas the incidence of rhabdomyolysis is low with statins in randomized trials, it is higher during clinical use.[85] In older patients, the smallest *effective* dose of a lipid-lowering agent should be used and signs and symptoms monitored. Muscle strength testing may be helpful in evaluation of symptoms in older patients, including simple assessments of ability to rise from a chair or to climb stairs.

STATINS FOR PRIMARY PREVENTION (see Chap. 49). The elderly have not been the target of most primary prevention trials of lipid lowering. Older patients with hypertension and CAD risk factors have not had all-cause mortality benefits when they are studied as part of randomized trials of lipid lowering (see Table 80-e2 on website). Data on reductions in cardiovascular endpoints differ between studies, but in the largest that showed reduction in a composite cardiovascular endpoint (ASCOT-LLA), prespecified subgroups of women, diabetics, patients with metabolic syndrome, nonobese patients, and those with prior vascular diseases did not show coronary heart disease benefit. Aggressive lipid lowering as primary prevention should be reserved for elderly patients with longer life expectancy and should be accompanied by monitoring for adverse effects.

CURRENT CONTROVERSIES: LIPID-LOWERING STRATEGIES IN THE ELDERLY WITH OR AT RISK FOR CAD. Current controversies include the following: primary prevention with statins in the elderly, especially women; optimal targets for lipid lowering, especially in the very old and in nonwhites; frequency and management of statin-induced myalgias or myopathy in older patients; coronary heart disease and mortality and risk related to lipid subfractions (HDL-cholesterol versus LDL-cholesterol or apolipoprotein B).

Additional lipid-lowering agents are discussed in Chapter 47.

Special Considerations with Pharmacologic Treatment of the Elderly CAD Patient

See also Medication Therapy: Modifications for the Older Patient.

Marked vasodilation due to rapid absorption or higher peak effects of isosorbide dinitrates can exacerbate postural hypotension, so agents with smooth concentration versus time profiles such as mononitrates or transdermal formulations may be preferred for daily administration, although cost may be prohibitive. Beta blockers have not been shown to increase the occurrence of depression in randomized trials, but beta blockers that are not lipophilic (e.g., atenolol, nadolol) may produce fewer central nervous system effects. Calcium channel blockers, especially the dihydropyridines, can produce pedal edema more frequently in the older patient. Shorter acting formulations can produce or exacerbate postural hypotension and should be avoided. Verapamil can exacerbate constipation, especially in the inactive elderly. Both beta blockers and nondihydropyridine calcium channel blockers should be avoided in the presence of sick sinus node disease. Hormone replacement therapy is not indicated for either primary prevention of coronary heart disease or treatment of coronary heart disease.[86] Adverse effects of dizziness, constipation, nausea, asthenia, headache, dyspepsia, and abdominal pain with the piperazine derivative ranolazine are more common in elderly patients, and women may have less exercise benefit with ranolazine compared with men.[87] Individual antianginal agents are further discussed in Chapter 57.

Revascularization (see Chaps. 57 and 58)

Revascularization procedures in the elderly are increasing, with greater increases in the numbers of percutaneous coronary intervention (PCI) procedures than in coronary artery bypass grafting (CABG).[88] At least half of PCI procedures and CABG are performed in patients older than 65 years, with one third in patients older than 70 years. In randomized trials, patients aged 65 to 80 years have been reported to have higher early morbidity and mortality after CABG compared with PCI but greater angina relief and fewer repeated procedures after CABG. Stroke is more common after CABG than after PCI (1.7% versus 0.2%), and heart failure and pulmonary edema are more common after PCI (4.0% versus 1.3%). Five-year survival rates are above 80% for both procedures, but there is considerable selection bias in patients undergoing these procedures; women and minorities are underrepresented, and those at lowest and intermediate risk undergo the bulk of procedures.[88]

Information about elderly patients after revascularization as part of "routine" clinical care has emerged from clinical and administrative databases (**Fig. 80-8**). These patients tend to be older and to have more multivessel disease and comorbid conditions than those in randomized studies, and long-term survival rates are lower and complication rates are higher than in randomized trials. Early CABG mortality increases from below 2% in patients younger than 60 years to between

5% and 8% in patients older than 75 years, approaching 10% in patients older than 80 years. Elderly women are at highest risk, in part because of comorbid conditions. For patients older than 90 years, operative mortality has been reported as 11.8% in the Society of Thoracic Surgeons database.[89] An online risk calculator incorporating patient risk factors and risks for specific surgical procedures can be accessed at the Society of Thoracic Surgeons website. The Mayo Clinic Risk Score for PCI also appears to estimate in-hospital mortality risk for CABG.[90]

PCI. Registry data from 2000 found PCI in-hospital mortality risk of less than 1% in patients younger than 60 years that increased to 2% to 5% in patients older than 75 years and to more than 5% in patients older than 80 years. Data on PCI during 2004-2006 found similar in-hospital mortality rates (up to 1% for those up to 70 years of age, about 2% for 70- to 80-year-olds, and 3.2% for those older than 80 years).[90] These represent highly selected older patients, and risk estimates need to be adjusted before application to patients with differing characteristics.[90]

PCI VERSUS CABG. One initial study of nearly 1700 patients older than 80 years (two- or three-vessel disease, excluding left main) found better in-hospital mortality and short-term survival for PCI versus CABG (3% versus 6%),[91] but survival was better after CABG for those surviving 6 months. The larger New York State database of more diverse patients older than 80 years (n = 5550) with multivessel disease (excluding left main) found risk-adjusted mortality and need for revascularization lower in patients treated with CABG (on-pump) compared with those who underwent PCI (bare metal stents).[92] Combined postmarketing registry and trial data compared bare metal stents and paclitaxel drug-eluting stents in patients older than 70 years.[93] Bare metal stents and drug-eluting stents had similar death, MI, and stent thrombosis rates, although repeated revascularization was more common with bare metal stents. A registry-based comparison of drug-eluting stents and CABG for multivessel disease (excluding left main, prior CABG, or recent MI) found that CABG had lower adjusted death rates and MI than drug-eluting stents, with clear advantages of CABG in those older than 80 years.[94] However, death or MI occurred in 16% to 17% of patients older than 80 years at 18-month follow-up.

PCI is associated with a slightly less than 1% risk of permanent stroke or coma, and CABG is associated with a 3% to 6% incidence of permanent stroke or coma in patients older than 75 years.[95] In the immediate postoperative period, longer durations of ventilatory support, greater need for inotropic support and intra-aortic balloon placement, and greater incidence of atrial fibrillation, bleeding, delirium, renal failure, perioperative infarction, and infection are seen in older patients compared with younger patients (see Chap. 84). The highest rate of complications is usually seen in older women and in patients undergoing emergency procedures. The length of disability and rehabilitation after procedures is also usually longer. Postoperative cognitive impairment in older patients detected with neuropsychological testing has been estimated at 25% to 50% after CABG. Randomized trials have reported both improved cognitive outcomes and no difference in cognitive outcomes of off-pump versus on-pump CABG.[96] Pre-revascularization considerations in the older patients should address cognition and the potential need for in-home assistance after the procedure or extended care hospitalization. Postprocedure considerations should also include evaluation for depression (see later).

Comparison of Medical Therapy with Revascularization
(see Chap. 57)

A pivotal randomized study TIME[97] compared invasive (PCI or CABG) versus optimized medical therapy for CAD patients older than 75 years with angina refractory to therapy with at least two antianginal drugs (mean 2.5 ± 0.7) (see Table 80-e3 on website). Initial 6-month analyses

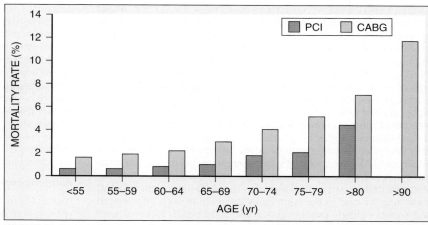

FIGURE 80-8 In-hospital mortality rates reported for revascularization procedures by age group. PCI = percutaneous coronary intervention of all types; CABG = coronary artery bypass graft surgery. *(Data are from the National Cardiovascular Revascularization Network as reported by Alexander K, Anstrom K, Muhlbaier L, et al: Outcomes of cardiac surgery in patients ≥80 years: Results from the National Cardiovascular Network. J Am Coll Cardiol 35:731, 2000; Batchelor W, Anstrom K, Muhlbaier L, et al: Contemporary outcome trends in the elderly undergoing percutaneous coronary interventions: Results in 7,472 octogenarians. National Cardiovascular Network Collaboration. J Am Coll Cardiol 36:723, 2000; and the Society of Thoracic Surgeons data base, Bridges C, Edwards F, Peterson E, et al: Cardiac surgery in nonagenarians and centenarians. J Am Coll Cardiol 197:347, 2003.)* Data were not available for PCI in patients older than 90 years. See text for further discussion of results for drug-eluting stents and newer surgical approaches.

favored revascularization, but the advantage was not present at 1 year. Revascularization presented an early risk of death and complications, and optimized medical therapy carried a chance of later events (hospitalization and revascularization), without a clear advantage of either strategy. Similarly, comparisons of revascularization with medical therapy in diabetics, including women and the elderly[81] (see Table 80-e3 on website), found no significant difference in outcomes between the approaches. Prompt revascularization decreased major cardiovascular events in CABG-treated patients compared with the medically treated but not in prompt PCI patients compared with medical treatment. Evolving data also suggest that PCI may not have fewer neurocognitive consequences.

Clinical Perspective

Age alone should not be the only criterion in considering revascularization procedures. There is a clear role for individualized risk assessment and respect for the patient's preference in the decision-making process. Short-term and long-term benefit should be considered in the context of anticipated life span and quality of life of the patient. Medical therapy has become more aggressive and compares favorably with revascularization in randomized trials of stable CAD patients older than 75 years, especially women. In contrast to the relatively low complication rates of revascularization in randomized trials of highly selected elderly patients, morbidity and mortality with revascularization in routine clinical care in patients older than 75 years are high. PCI is attractive in concept, but even drug-eluting stents may not confer the benefit of CABG in older patients with longer anticipated life spans. The possibility of disability or prolonged hospitalization after interventions and especially surgery must be considered and accurately conveyed to the patient and family. Death, recurrent angina, or MI may not be viewed as carrying the same negative impact as a disabling stroke by many older patients. For the patient unable to make decisions, involvement of family members or agents is key to decisions that reflect the wishes of the patient.

CURRENT ISSUES IN REVASCULARIZATION OF THE ELDERLY. Current issues include the following: appropriate selection criteria for specific therapies for octogenarians and nonagenarians; modifiable risk factors for revascularization mortality and morbidity in older patients; age-adjusted PCI and CABG protocol regimens; role of transradial approaches for PCI; benefits of on-pump versus off-pump CABG surgery (see Chap. 84); prevention of cognitive decline after revascularization procedures; and comparisons between modern medical therapy and revascularization.

ACUTE CORONARY SYNDROMES (see Chaps. 54 and 55). About 60% of hospital admissions for acute myocardial infarction (AMI) are in people older than 65 years, and approximately 85% of deaths due to AMI occur in this group.[98,99] With increasing age, the gender composition of patients presenting with AMI changes: from predominantly men in middle age, to equal numbers of men and women between the ages of 75 and 84 years, to the majority of patients with AMI being women at ages over 80 years (see Chap. 81). Mortality rates are usually higher in older women than in men with AMI, as are adverse outcomes with thrombolytics, fibrinolytics, and GP IIb/IIIa inhibitors. Mortality is at least threefold higher in the patient older than 85 years compared with the patient younger than 65 years. Patients enrolled in trials for treatment of AMI are generally younger, are more often male, and have less renal failure and less heart failure than patients in either the Medicare database or clinical registries. The older old patient with AMI presenting for care in the community differs from both middle-aged and younger elderly patients and is also substantially different from highly selected patients older than 65 years enrolled in randomized clinical trials.[3]

Diagnosis

Chest pain or discomfort is the most common complaint in patients up to the age of 75 years, but after the age of 80 years, complaints of diaphoresis increase and chest discomfort decreases (see Chap. 53). Altered mental status, confusion, and fatigue become common manifestations of MI in the oldest patients. Older patients may also present with sudden pulmonary edema or neurologic symptoms such as syncope or stroke. The electrocardiogram (ECG) is also more likely to be nondiagnostic (see Chap. 13). Nonspecific symptoms and nondiagnostic electrocardiographic findings lead to delays in diagnosis and implementation of therapy and highlight the importance of rapid laboratory testing for circulating markers of myocardial damage.

Treatment

Treatment decisions are often considered separately for ST elevation MI (STEMI) and non–ST elevation MI (NSTEMI) in the older patient analogous to other guidelines.[3,4,98,99] There is general agreement that eligible STEMI patients who receive reperfusion therapy (fibrinolytic therapy or PCI) have a lower risk of death, but few patients older than 75 years were enrolled in trials that serve as the basis for this recommendation. Lack of consensus on the best approach for reperfusion for acute MI in the elderly reflects the lack of data and the comorbidities and delayed presentation of older patients as well as the lack of widespread rapid access to high-volume PCI facilities and the higher incidence of serious adverse effects with pharmacologic reperfusion strategies. For NSTEMI, the debate centers on early versus delayed or selective risk-stratified invasive strategies after antiplatelet and antithrombin therapy and initiation of beta blockade and ACE inhibitors or ARBs in the presence of left ventricular dysfunction. It is unlikely that randomized trials will provide the answers to these questions in the very old patient, and registry data that include significant numbers of women and older patients with comorbidities serve an important role for this group. These data show that results in the community setting do not currently achieve the same results as reported in clinical trials.

REPERFUSION. Non–age-adjusted guidelines recommend reperfusion approaches in STEMI patients without contraindications if they present within 12 hours of symptom onset. PCI and fibrinolytic therapy have similar outcomes when they are delivered within 3 hours from symptom onset. In elderly patients who present in shock or are in a high-risk category or present later, PCI can offer better results.

Thrombolysis or Fibrinolysis (see Chap. 55)

For patients up to the age of 75 years, most trials show that fibrinolytic, antiplatelet, and antithrombin therapy is associated with a survival advantage compared with placebo that may be similar to or less than that seen in younger patients.[3,4,98-100] Bleeding and transfusion rates are higher in older patients, especially with improper dosing of antiplatelet and antithrombin agents.[98,99] Those at high risk for intracerebral hemorrhage include patients older than 75 years, women, African

Americans, smaller patients (<65 kg for women and <80 kg for men), and those with prior stroke or systolic blood pressure >160 mm Hg. Fibrin-specific agents are also associated with increased stroke risk due to intracerebral hemorrhage in those older than 75 to 80 years. Coadministered low-molecular-weight or unfractionated heparin at excess doses contributes to the excess bleeding.[3] Dosage adjustments for weight and estimated renal clearance may decrease but not eliminate risks of bleeding in very old patients and in women. Cardiac rupture risk with thrombolysis is also increased in patients older than 70 years and in women (0.5% to 2%) and does not appear to be related to the intensity of anticoagulation. Risks of reperfusion in patients older than 85 years appear to differ from those in younger patients, supporting individualized clinical decisions.

Antithrombotic Agents

Aspirin (81 to 325 mg/day) reduces mortality in patients older than 70 years and is recommended for older patients with acute coronary syndromes of all types. Clopidogrel is added to aspirin in patients not considered for surgical revascularization, before PCI, or before discharge for medically treated patients. GP IIb/IIIa inhibitors in high-risk non–ST elevation acute coronary syndromes, especially if catheterization and PCI are planned, appear efficacious in patients older than 70 years, although net benefit may decline with increasing age. Bleeding risk including intracerebral hemorrhage is increased about twofold with GP IIb/IIIa inhibitors, rising to 7.2% for eptifibatide in patients older than 80 years.[3]

Antiplatelet and antithrombin agents have narrow therapeutic windows with dosing recommendations based on weight and renal function. More than 65% of patients older than 75 years with acute coronary syndromes receive an excess dose.[18,101] Women are more likely to receive excess GP IIb/IIIa doses than are men in both clinical practice and randomized trials, and about 25% of the bleeding risk in women is attributable to excess dosing.[20,102] These data highlight the need for adjustment of dosing of antithrombotic and antiplatelet agents for estimated renal clearance.

Invasive Strategies

In elderly patients with acute STEMI, primary angioplasty in experienced centers is associated with improved outcomes compared with thrombolytic strategies (see Chap. 55). This potential benefit, however, has not been seen in octogenarians.[103] Acute procedural success rates are somewhat lower in older patients and are associated with increased bleeding and increased risk for contrast-mediated renal dysfunction. Facilitated PCI is not endorsed for elderly patients secondary to increased bleeding risk.[4]

Antiplatelet therapy with clopidogrel (or prasugrel) has a routine role before PCI but should not be used in patients considered for CABG. Prasugrel has increased risk of fatal bleeding events compared with clopidogrel in patients older than 75 years with acute coronary syndromes and should not be used in older patients. Early versus delayed eptifibatide before angiography is not recommended.[104]

In-hospital mortality of patients older than 75 years is estimated to be fourfold to fivefold higher than in younger patients. For those older than 80 years, 2005 registry data for primary PCI for STEMI show in-hospital mortality as 16.6%. Two randomized trials have attempted to compare PCI with fibrinolysis in older patients with STEMI, and both were terminated prematurely because of inability to meet recruitment goals: the Senior PAMI[105] and the recently presented TRIANA trial.[106] It is clear that this question will not be answered in clinical trials. The published data suggest that benefits of invasive strategies relate primarily to later events and need for subsequent revascularization, except in older patients with cardiogenic shock due to left ventricular failure who have improved long-term survival with early invasive strategies.[107] There is growing evidence to support an invasive strategy that can be "delayed" for a period of hours to days to allow stabilization, initiation of pharmacologic therapy, and risk assessment. The Timing of Intervention in Acute Coronary Syndromes (TIMACS) trial[108] included patients older than 75 years and found no difference between early and delayed invasive strategies in low- to intermediate-risk patients (by GRACE score). For higher risk patients, early intervention reduced composite short-term cardiovascular endpoints. A recent randomized comparison of immediate invasive strategy with next working day invasive intervention in patients with NSTEMI using modern antiplatelet regimens found no difference in peak troponin levels between the two strategies in patients older or younger than 75 years.[109] Death rates were the same with both approaches. These data were published after the updated 2007 guidelines,[14] which stated that an initial conservative strategy (selected invasive) could be considered but favored rapid revascularization for older unstable angina/NSTEMI patients. The best strategy currently appears to be to initiate pharmacologic therapy and assess risk at the time of presentation, to consider urgent revascularization for older patients at highest risk and nonurgently for those at intermediate risk, and to be guided by symptoms and evolving clinical status for those at low risk. The patient's preferences should be considered in all scenarios.

For additional information on pharmacologic agents, see Chap. 55.

Current Perspective

Despite increased morbidity and mortality for older patients with CAD and acute coronary syndromes compared with younger patients, risk-adjusted AMI mortality in the United States has decreased from 1995-2006 in the Medicare population.[110] In analyses of community practice outcomes of five recommended therapies (early use of aspirin, beta blockers, heparin, GP IIb/IIIa inhibitors, and cardiac catheterization), in-hospital mortality declined as a function of the number of guideline-recommended therapies given in patients aged 75 years and older, with greater benefit with use of guideline-recommended therapies in older than in younger patients. With special attention to altered dosing for and sensitivity of older patients and close observation for adverse effects of intensive medical and interventional management in elderly subgroups with acute coronary syndromes, short-term morbidity can potentially be further reduced. In contrast to current trends for increased rates of cardiac catheterization and revascularization in lower risk MI patients, use of early invasive strategies should be redirected to high-risk patients, who may have greater benefit.

POST–MYOCARDIAL INFARCTION

Medications

Administration of aspirin, beta blockers, ACE inhibitors, or ARBs in patients with left ventricular dysfunction and lipid-lowering drugs for the post-MI patient is based on clinical trial data showing benefit in populations that have included elderly patients. With the caveat of adjustment of dosing for age and renal status, recommendations are the same as in younger patients (see Chap. 49 and earlier). In contrast, eplerenone did not show either cardiovascular mortality or all-cause mortality benefits for patients older than 65 years with heart failure after MI.[111] The addition of clopidogrel to aspirin after non–ST elevation MI has similar benefits in patients younger and older than 65 years, without significant data on patients older than 75 years.[112] Considerations that may be unique to the elderly patient after MI are the use of antidepressants and hormonal replacement therapy.

Depression affects 10% of community-dwelling older people (see Chap. 91). The prevalence of depression in patients after MI is estimated at 20% to 30% for major depression[113] and up to 50% for potentially significant symptoms of depression.[114] Studies show associations between depression and low perceived social support and increased cardiac morbidity and mortality in post-MI patients and in patients undergoing CABG. Individual trials of counseling interventions in patients with depression have not shown cardiac benefit, but meta-analyses suggest benefit. Trials of selective serotonin reuptake inhibitor (SSRI) antidepressant therapy in patients with depression after acute coronary syndromes or MI suggest benefits of SSRI use on either cardiac events and mortality (perhaps due to antiplatelet properties) or quality of life and overall function, especially in patients with a prior history of depression. Screening for depression can take the form of a simple two-question test followed by additional evaluation for patients with answers suggesting the presence of depression. Alternatively, the nine-item self-report Patient Health Questionnaire screening

instrument can be used in literate patients, or the geriatric depression screen for older patients can be administered.[115] Increasing use of SSRI and mixed-mechanism antidepressants has led to recognition of hyponatremia with SSRIs and that SSRI antiplatelet effects can increase the risk of bleeding in combination with warfarin, low-molecular-weight heparin, or aspirin and in patients with hereditary platelet defects.[116] The first-generation SSRI fluoxetine confers increased risk of syncope in elderly patients.

Randomized trials comparing administration of hormone replacement therapy in the form of combined estrogen and progesterone or estrogen alone have shown overall lack of cardiovascular morbidity or mortality benefit and potential harm for both secondary and primary prevention in postmenopausal women (see Chap. 81).[117] Similar to estrogen, the selective estrogen modulator raloxifene lowered LDL-cholesterol and increased HDL-cholesterol but did not decrease coronary event rates and increased stroke rates and thromboembolism.[118] A comparison of raloxifene to tamoxifen for prevention of breast cancer in women found equivalent efficacy in invasive breast cancer reduction, equivalent risks for ischemic disease and stroke, and lower risk of thromboembolic events with raloxifene.[119] Neither estrogen nor estrogen plus progesterone, raloxifene, or tamoxifen can be recommended for cardiovascular disease prevention or treatment.

Rehabilitation Programs (see Chap. 50)

The feasibility of and improvement with intensive exercise interventions have been shown for the elderly, including the frail elderly, residing in the community as well as in the nursing home. The Cardiac Rehabilitation in Advanced Age (CR-AGE) trial compared hospital-based cardiac rehabilitation with home-based cardiac rehabilitation in cognitively intact patients from the ages of 46 to 86 years with recent MI.[120] Similar improvement in total work capacity and health-related quality of life was seen with home-based rehabilitation and hospital-based rehabilitation in all age groups without improvement in the control group. Improvement was somewhat smaller in the group older than 75 years. Benefits decreased over time after hospital rehabilitation but were maintained with home cardiac rehabilitation, and costs were lower in the home rehabilitation group.

Table 80-6 summarizes the approach to the older patient with CAD.

Carotid Artery Disease and Stroke (see Chap. 62)

PREVALENCE AND INCIDENCE. Stroke is the third leading cause of death and is the most common cause of major adult disability in the United States. The risk of stroke increases with age and doubles for each decade after the age of 55 years. Framingham data estimate the 10-year probability of stroke at 11% for men at the age of 65 years and 7% for women at the age of 65 years. At the age of 80 years, the probability increases to 22% and 24% for men and women, respectively. After the age of 85 years, women are at greater risk than are men. Carotid stenosis is responsible for about 15% to 25% of strokes and atrial fibrillation for about 15%. Whereas a transient ischemic attack (TIA) signals a high short-term risk of stroke, 70% of strokes are first events, stressing the importance of primary prevention and treatment of risk factors.[121] Modifiable risk factors for noncardioembolic ischemic stroke or TIA in the elderly are hypertension, diabetes, smoking and passive smoking, hyperlipidemia, lack of physical activity, inadequate treatment of atrial fibrillation, carotid artery disease, heart failure, estrogen administration to postmenopausal women, and sleep apnea (see Chap. 79). Nonmodifiable risk factors for stroke include age, sex (risk greater in men than in women), race/ethnicity (risk greater in African Americans compared with whites), and family history of stroke.

DIAGNOSIS

Transient Ischemic Attack

The traditional diagnosis of TIA—an episode of neurologic impairment lasting less than 24 hours attributable to focal ischemia in the brain or retina—was usually based on clinical history and was not associated with a new permanent neurologic deficit. Recently, high-resolution computed tomography (CT) and diffusion-weighted magnetic resonance imaging (MRI) studies have demonstrated that 15% to 50% of ischemic episodes with symptoms lasting less than 24 hours

TABLE 80-6	Approach to the Older Patient with Coronary Artery Disease

Optimization of medical care warrants greater emphasis.
  Exercise for all, weight loss for the overweight, and smoking cessation in smokers
  Control of hypertension and diabetes
  For relief of symptoms—beta blockers, nitrates, calcium channel blockers
  For prevention of complications—antiplatelet drugs and lipid lowering
  Pharmacologic treatments must incorporate age-related adjustments in dosing; consider altered reflex responses and drug interactions.
Morbidity and mortality from CAD and CAD treated medically or with revascularization increase with age, especially at ages older than 75 years, and there are no advantages of revascularization over optimal medical care for the older patient with stable or nondisabling CAD or who has a satisfactory quality of life.
  Decisions about medical therapy versus revascularization, or for PCI versus CABG, should be based on the role of CAD in the context of the individual older patient's overall health, lifestyle, projected life span, and preferences.
For acute coronary syndromes
  Older patients presenting with acute coronary syndromes in the community are substantially older, are more often women, and have more comorbidity than patients enrolled in randomized studies that are the basis for care guidelines, and clinical outcomes for the oldest patients are generally worse than trial results.
  ST elevation MI has a high mortality in the oldest patients.
  Immediate invasive strategies show the greatest benefit in higher risk patients.
  For patients at lower or intermediate risk, treatment choices should be based on consideration of patient and family preferences, quality of life issues, end-of-life preferences, sociocultural differences, and the experience and capabilities of the site of care.
  All treatment regimens must be adjusted for renal status and size.
Anticipated procedural complication rates should reflect the age and health status of the patient, not complication rates from randomized studies or younger patients.
  Recovery times will be prolonged from all procedures.
  Depression should be evaluated.
For patients older than 80 years, there are limited data.
  Recommendations are based on extrapolations from younger and less sick populations.
  Incremental benefits between therapies are small.
  Decisions between PCI and fibrinolytics or neither in patients older than 75 years should be individualized.

are associated with new cerebral infarction. These insights have led to tissue-based definitions of TIA and stroke. A recent American Heart Association–endorsed statement defines TIA as "a transient episode of neurological dysfunction caused by focal brain or retinal ischemia without evidence of acute infarction" and has no time limit for symptoms.[122] Ischemic stroke is defined as infarction of central nervous system tissue.

Scoring systems may help estimate short-term risk of stroke after a TIA. The ABCD^2 score (see Table 62-1) is calculated by **A**ge ≥60 years (1 point) and **B**lood pressure ≥140/90 mm Hg (1 point), **C**linical features (1 point for speech impairment without weakness, 2 points for unilateral weakness), **D**uration of TIA (≥60 minutes = 2 points and <60 minutes = 1 point), and **D**iabetes (1 point), with 2-day risk of stroke of 0% for scores of 0 or 1, 1.3% for 2 or 3, 4.1% for 4 or 5, and 8.1% for 6 or 7. High scores also appear to identify patients with moderate or severe carotid stenosis. The presence of a new infarct on brain imaging is also associated with an increased short-term risk of subsequent stroke, but it is unclear whether there is additive predictive value of MRI changes to scoring rules such as the ABCD^2.

Stroke

A lopsided face, weak arm, and garbled speech are the most common warning signs of stroke. The mnemonic FAST (face, arm, speech, time) can help identify patients with a potential stroke. Assessment should include a detailed neurologic examination with a stroke rating scale (see Chap. 62) and rapid triage to neuroimaging. Brain imaging

guides selection of acute interventions. Non–contrast-enhanced CT is most commonly available, but MRI allows greater tissue definition.[123] Specialized or certified stroke centers are not universally available across the United States but provide the best opportunity for optimal care for older patients likely to have multiorgan disease and complex stroke types.[123]

TREATMENT

Acute Stroke Management[123,124]

Intravenous recombinant tissue plasminogen activator (rtPA) is the only medical therapy approved by the Food and Drug Administration proven to reduce effects of an ischemic stroke. Thrombolysis with rtPA is recommended for selected patients with ischemic stroke with a measurable neurologic deficit (see Chap. 62) in whom it can be administered within hours of stroke onset. Recent guidelines extend the time window for administration of rtPA to 3 to 4.5 hours after stroke onset. Because bleeding risk increases with age and with administration of rtPA at increasing times after onset of symptoms, the recommended time window for patients older than 80 years, however, remains within 3 hours of stroke onset.[125] A persistent systolic blood pressure >185 mm Hg or a diastolic blood pressure >110 mm Hg despite treatment is a contraindication to intravenous administration of rtPA. Other contraindications include recent trauma, surgery, MI, active bleeding, anticoagulation, low platelet levels, prior intracranial hemorrhage, and suggestion of subarachnoid hemorrhage. A major neurologic deficit denotes a poor prognosis, and a number of experts consider use of tPA in these patients. Subtypes of ischemic stroke are not thought to influence responses to rtPA. Symptomatic hemorrhagic transformation of the infarction after rtPA administration occurs in 5.2% of patients but can be reduced by proper selection of patients. Orolingual angioedema occurs in about 5% and is more common in patients taking ACE inhibitors and those with ischemia in the frontal cortex and insula. Intra-arterial thrombolysis is an option for selected patients with major stroke of <6 hours in duration who are not candidates for intravenous rtPA if they are at an experienced stroke center with immediate access to cerebral angiography and qualified interventionalists.

Data support administration of aspirin within 24 to 48 hours of stroke for most patients (not within 24 hours of intravenous rtPA) but not early anticoagulation with unfractionated or low-molecular-weight heparin or acute use of clopidogrel or GP IIb/IIIa receptor inhibitors outside the setting of clinical trials. Endovascular techniques and devices to extract thrombus are under evaluation. Current use should be limited to comprehensive stroke centers or clinical trials, as should use of combination pharmacologic regimens for reperfusion.

Blood pressure management in the setting of acute stroke remains controversial. Aggressive reduction in pressure is not generally recommended, but blood pressure control should precede any thrombolytic therapy. Randomized trials of blood pressure control in the acute stroke setting are ongoing and have passed the 1-year follow-up of data safety monitoring without termination, suggesting that judicious lowering of blood pressure does not have excessive risk. When hypertension is treated, intravenous and short-acting agents are recommended in consensus guidelines for initial therapy (labetalol or nicardipine, with nitropaste in ongoing trials). Poststroke management should include the early initiation of rehabilitation therapy, a swallow screening test for dysphagia, an active secondary stroke prevention program, and the proactive prevention of venous thrombi. Evaluation for depression is also strongly recommended.[126]

Prevention

Secondary and primary prevention is targeted at modifiable risk factors.[121] Evidence-based recommendations are for antiplatelet therapy in patients with prior stroke, TIA, or MI and anticoagulation in high-risk patients such as those with atrial fibrillation (see Chap. 39). Carotid artery interventions should be considered for patients with symptomatic disease or severe lesions.[127] Clinical trials with limited numbers of elderly and excluding the very elderly have also demonstrated that LDL-cholesterol reduction reduces the risk of stroke in

TABLE 80-7	**Approach to Anticoagulation in Older Patients**

Obtain complete medication and nutraceutical intake data to anticipate warfarin requirements, interactions, contraindications, and necessary adjustment.

Educate patient, family, and caregivers on diet, alcohol effects, and drug interactions and need for monitoring and communication.

Initiate at low doses—often at 2 mg, not to exceed 5 mg.
   Estimate dosages by multiple variable clinical algorithms (such as *www.warfarindosing.org*).
   Genotyping to guide initial dosing is not currently recommended or reimbursed.

Monitor closely and titrate slowly. Consider use of
   Anticoagulation clinics
   Fingerstick self-testing (patient, family, or caregiver)

Consider warfarin effects of all medications, supplements, and diet changes.

Use preventive measures for osteoporosis.

patients with cardiovascular disease or major cardiovascular disease risk factors and in patients with prior strokes. Smoking cessation and avoidance of second-hand smoke and estrogen therapy, weight control, limited alcohol intake, and increased activity are also part of a preventive strategy.[121]

ANTIPLATELET DRUGS. Aspirin is considered standard therapy after a stroke regardless of the patient's age (see Chap. 62). Combined aspirin and extended-release dipyridamole can prevent slightly more strokes than placebo or aspirin alone but has greater gastrointestinal intolerance, headache, cost, and drug discontinuation.[128] Combined aspirin and clopidogrel has no additive benefit but markedly increases moderate and major bleeding and is not recommended except for limited duration in patients with recent coronary events or prior vascular stenting.[129] Secondary prevention trials with clopidogrel that enrolled stroke patients found reductions in composite endpoints that included stroke but greater reduction in peripheral artery disease events.[130] A direct comparison of low-dose aspirin and extended-release dipyridamole with clopidogrel for recurrent stroke found similar rates of recurrent stroke with either regimen in patients 65 to 75 years old as well as in those older than 75 years.[131] Side effects leading to discontinuation (headache, especially; vomiting, nausea, and dizziness) were more common with aspirin and dipyridamole than with clopidogrel, whereas an unexpectedly lower rate of new or worsening heart failure was found with aspirin plus dipyridamole. A comparison of warfarin with aspirin did not find significant differences in the prevention of recurrent ischemic stroke or death or occurrence of serious adverse events.[132] At this time, aspirin (50 to 325 mg/day), aspirin plus extended-release dipyridamole, and clopidogrel monotherapy are considered options for secondary prevention in patients with noncardioembolic ischemic stroke or TIA. The patient's tolerance, ease of use, cost (highest with clopidogrel), and concomitant diseases or procedures should guide the choice. Bleeding complications are more frequent in older than in younger patients. No dose-response relationship has been observed for the protective effects of aspirin (50 to 1000 mg/day), whereas larger doses increase the risk of gastrointestinal bleeding.[133] The minimally effective dose for aspirin has not been determined, but lower doses of at least 50 mg/day are recommended for the older patient.

ANTICOAGULANT DRUGS. Warfarin is not recommended routinely for ischemic stroke except for patients with thromboembolic stroke (see Chap. 87 for warfarin considerations). For elderly patients with atrial fibrillation and stroke or TIA, the subsequent risk of ischemic stroke is high, and despite a higher risk of hemorrhage, overall benefit is seen with warfarin. See **Table 80-7** for a summary of the approach to anticoagulation in the older patient.

LIPID-LOWERING DRUGS. Recommendations for LDL-cholesterol level reduction are similar to those for post-MI patients (see Chaps. 47 and 49).[129] However, the trial data on

which the recommendations are based did not include significant numbers of older patients and excluded the very old. Benefit with statins for primary and secondary prevention in the elderly is thought to require years of administration. Aggressive lipid lowering can be strongly endorsed only for younger elderly patients with stroke and those with at least 4 or 5 years life expectancy and those with other indications for lipid lowering.

ANTIHYPERTENSIVE DRUGS. Antihypertensive therapy is recommended for prevention of recurrent stroke and prevention of other vascular events in all persons who have had an ischemic stroke or TIA and are beyond the hyperacute period. The optimal blood pressure target and drug regimens for older patients are uncertain, and the choice of agent should be based on the individual patient's characteristics and comorbid conditions (see hypertension, earlier, and Chap. 46).

Surgical and Endovascular Approaches

Several clinical trials have demonstrated that carotid endarterectomy (CEA) in symptomatic patients with 70% to 99% internal carotid artery stenosis with stroke or TIA attributable to the stenosis is safe and effective in reducing the risk of ipsilateral stroke (see Chap. 63).[127] Surgery performed better compared with medical treatment in preventing disabling ipsilateral stroke in a large randomized study, although the medical regimens were not as aggressive as currently recommended and used (**Fig. 80-9**).[134] Benefit is less certain with stenosis of 50% to 69%. Benefit is greatest in those with more severe stenosis, in those older than 75 years, in men, and in those with recent stroke. Revascularization is not recommended for patients with lesions of less than 50%.

Increased risk of perioperative stroke or death is seen with surgery for completed stroke (versus TIA), female sex, age older than 75 years, systolic blood pressure above 180 mm Hg, peripheral vascular disease, intracranial vascular disease, and bilateral carotid disease. These data form the basis for recommendations that CEA should not be considered unless the combined mortality and morbidity rate is less than 3% for asymptomatic patients with at least a 5-year life expectancy and less than 7% for symptomatic patients. Two large trials of highly selected asymptomatic patients showed marginal or modest benefit in stroke prevention (risk reduced from 2% to 1% per year) with CEA and suggested lack of overall benefit in patients older than 75 years because of mortality from other diseases. Selection of surgery for asymptomatic patients should focus on subgroups at increased risk of stroke, such as those with stenosis of higher severity, progressive stenosis, history of

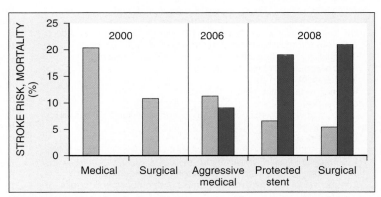

FIGURE 80-9 Risk of stroke (light blue) is compared for medical and surgical therapy for patients with hemispheric transient ischemic attack in the North American Symptomatic Carotid Endarterectomy Trial (*Benevente O, Eliasziw M, Streifler J, et al: Prognosis after transient monocular blindness associated with carotid-artery stenosis. N Engl J Med 345:1084, 2000*) are shown on the left. On the right are more recent data comparing risk of stroke (light blue) and risk of death (dark blue) with surgical carotid endarterectomy with protected stenting (SAPPHIRE long-term follow-up) in high-risk patients (*Gurm HS, Yadav JS, Fayad P, et al: Long-term results of carotid stenting versus endarterectomy in high-risk patients. N Engl J Med 358:1572, 2008*). Earlier medical therapy did not include aggressive lowering of lipids or blood pressure, and the data shown differ for lower risk as well as for older patients (see text for further details).

contralateral symptomatic carotid artery stenosis, or increased serum creatinine concentrations.

CAROTID ENDARTERECTOMY COMPARED WITH CAROTID ARTERY BALLOON ANGIOPLASTY AND STENTING (see Fig. 80-9). Randomized clinical trials and prospective registries have not demonstrated definitive longer term advantages of one approach over the other, except for older patients, who have higher periprocedural rates of stroke and death with angioplasty and stenting (even with distal protection devices) but not with surgical CEA.[135,136] Risk of stroke or death within 30 days of carotid stenting has been reported as between 1% and 2% for patients up to 69 years of age, 5.3% for patients 70 to 79 years of age, and 12.1% for patients older than 80 years.[137] Reocclusion rates are also higher with stents. Large randomized trials comparing surgical and nonsurgical approaches are still ongoing.[138] Currently, carotid angioplasty and stenting with distal protection devices is considered an alternative to CEA in patients who are known to have a higher operative complication rate because of medical or technical contraindications to surgery, in patients with restenosis after endarterectomy, and in patients with intracranial lesions for whom medical therapy has failed and when procedural risks do not exceed acceptable limits defined for CEA.[138] Costs for carotid angioplasty and stenting are currently reimbursed by Centers for Medicare and Medicaid Services only for patients with symptomatic carotid artery stenosis of at least 70% who are at high risk for surgery. Carotid angioplasty and stenting procedures are rapidly increasing worldwide; however, not all centers and registries report major adverse event rates that meet the acceptable major adverse event rate criteria.[138,139] Consensus panels have concluded that the efficacy of carotid revascularization (by any means) in asymptomatic patients ≥75 years has not been established.[138]

Table 80-8 summarizes the general approach to the older patient with stroke.

TABLE 80-8 Approach to the Older Patient with Stroke

Prevention is key.
 Treat hypertension, diabetes, smoking, physical inactivity, elevated lipids, obesity, and sleep apnea and limit alcohol intake and estrogen use.
 Anticoagulate patients with atrial fibrillation (in the absence of contraindications).
Acute stroke treatment
 Evaluate rapidly, in an institution that provides emergency stroke care, if possible.
  Use stroke rating scales and neuroimaging for diagnosis and to guide therapy.
 Administer recombinant tissue plasminogen activator (rtPA) within 3 hours in selected patients with controlled blood pressure.
 Administer aspirin (325 mg) within 24 to 48 hours, but not within 24 hours of rtPA.
 Use low-molecular-weight heparin or heparinoids for prevention of deep venous thrombosis, venous thromboembolism, and pulmonary embolism, with dose adjustment for size and renal clearance.
 Anticoagulation is not recommended.
 Initiate rehabilitation early.
 Routinely evaluate and treat for depression.
Secondary prevention
 Aspirin (at lower doses), or aspirin plus extended-release dipyridamole or clopidogrel
 Lipid lowering
  Usually with a statin in those with at least 3-year anticipated life span
  Consider aggressive lipid lowering.
 The combination of aspirin plus clopidogrel is not recommended.
 Consider warfarin for patients with strokes of thromboembolic origin.
Carotid revascularization
 Role in asymptomatic patients ≥75 years has not been established.
 Symptomatic patients with 70% to 99% internal carotid artery stenosis without other risks for short-term mortality
 Selected patients with high-risk lesions by operators with low mortality rates
 Carotid endarterectomy is the standard for the lower risk older patient. The oldest patients have the worst results with transvascular carotid interventions.
 Carotid artery stenting with protection devices is an alternative for the higher surgical risk symptomatic older patient.

Peripheral Artery Disease (see Chap. 61)

PREVALENCE AND INCIDENCE. Peripheral artery disease (PAD) is the clinical term used to denote stenotic, occlusive, and aneurysmal disease of the aorta and its branch arteries, exclusive of the coronary arteries.[140] Using the ankle-brachial index to identify lower extremity PAD, NHANES found the crude prevalence of PAD in noninstitutionalized U.S. adults aged 60 years and older to be 11.6%. The prevalence was higher in persons aged 80 years and older (23.2%) and 70 to 79 years (12.5%) than in those aged 60 to 69 years. Prevalence also differed with race, with higher rates in non-Hispanic black men (19.2%) and women (19.3%) and Mexican American women (15.6%) compared with white men (12.1%) and women (11.3%). Only 29.6% of those with PAD reported leg pain with walking. Because individuals with PAD have relative risk of death from cardiovascular causes approximately equal to that of patients with coronary or cerebrovascular disease, screening is recommended.

Patients with known atherosclerotic coronary, carotid, or renal artery disease are likely to have concomitant lower extremity PAD. Risk factors are smoking, age, diabetes, dyslipidemia, hypertension, or hyperhomocysteinemia and possibly elevated C-reactive protein. After the age of 70 years, age alone is a risk factor for lower extremity PAD. Whereas a number of community-based studies have demonstrated the prevalence of PAD, risk factor–modifying therapies remain underused.

DIAGNOSIS. Intermittent claudication is the earliest and most frequent presenting symptom in about one third of patients. More than half of patients with abnormal ankle-brachial index measurements have "atypical" leg discomfort. Twenty percent to 30% of patients with PAD are asymptomatic. As disease severity progresses, patients may describe fewer symptoms related to PAD as they avoid activities that precipitate symptoms. Screening for PAD with the ankle-brachial index is recommended in all patients older than 70 years, patients aged 50 to 69 years who smoke or have diabetes, patients with leg symptoms with exertion or abnormal results on vascular examinations of the leg, and patients with coronary, carotid, or renal artery disease.[140] In patients with symptoms of intermittent claudication and normal ankle-brachial index at rest, measurement of the ankle-brachial index after exercise is recommended. In patients with functional impairment, insufficient response to therapies without other diseases that would limit activity, pulse volume recording or duplex ultrasound imaging may assist in evaluating further therapeutic options. Signs of acute limb ischemia include pain, paralysis, paresthesias, pulselessness, and pallor. New appearance of any of these symptoms warrants evaluation.

TREATMENT[140-142]. Initial therapy should be directed at smoking cessation and formal or supervised exercise training programs in all patients and weight loss in overweight patients to improve symptoms and walking impairment. Cilostazol has the best evidence for treatment benefit in patients with claudication, and a 3- to 6-month course is recommended as first-line pharmacotherapy except in the patient with heart failure. Pentoxifylline is a second-line alternative therapy that can be used in patients with heart failure, but it has a lower level of evidence of clinical utility. Naftidrofuryl in oral formulation is available in several European countries, and meta-analyses and international guidelines support its use.[142] To reduce overall mortality risk and to slow progression of disease, diabetes, elevated lipid levels, and other cardiovascular risk factors such as hypertension should be treated.

Antiplatelet therapy with either aspirin or clopidogrel is generally recommended.[142] Aspirin or clopidogrel will not improve claudication but may reduce the risk of cardiovascular events, slow progression of disease, and improve results of revascularization procedures. Whereas the benefit of aspirin for prevention of cardiovascular events in patients with PAD has been questioned, experts appear unlikely to change recommendations until results of a large study of aspirin at low dose (100 mg/day) are available.[143,144] Dual antiplatelet therapy with aspirin and clopidogrel might slightly lower rates of cardiovascular events at the expense of higher rates of minor and moderate bleeding. Warfarin added to antiplatelet therapy provides no additional benefit while increasing life-threatening bleeding.[145] A role for ACE inhibitors even in the absence of hypertension (as defined by older definitions) has been suggested.[140,141] Benefits of L-arginine, carnitine,

TABLE 80-9	Approach to the Older Patient with Peripheral Artery Disease

Treatment of cardiovascular risk factors and supervised walking-based exercise programs are first-line therapy.
   Antiplatelet therapy with aspirin or clopidogrel is usually recommended.
Medications can improve symptoms (cilostazol > pentoxifylline); cilostazol should not be used in patients with heart failure.
Thorough examinations of the feet should be included in examinations.
   Patients with decreased sensation or at risk for lesions should be referred to foot care specialists.
Revascularization options include PCI for iliac disease, but long-term efficacy requires surgical approaches at the femoropopliteal and infrapopliteal level.
Surgical morbidity and mortality increase with age, and postoperative recovery times can be prolonged. All are highest in the setting of surgery for critical ischemia or limb salvage.

and ginkgo biloba are less clear. Supplementation with folate, vitamin E, or omega-3 fatty acids is not recommended, nor is chelation therapy.[142]

Decreased sensation due to age, cognitive impairment, neuropathy or diabetes, increased risk of cutaneous damage from minor trauma with age, and decreased vision increase the chance of missing early signs of critical limb ischemia in older patients. The patient with PAD and the caregiver should be educated on limb hygiene, frequent examination, and early reporting of lesions, and health care professionals must inspect limbs as a routine part of clinical care. It appears that only about a quarter of patients with intermittent claudication will deteriorate significantly, although measured walking time does decrease progressively over time. Multidisciplinary care can help patients with critical limb ischemia avoid limb loss.

Revascularization can be performed by endovascular or surgical techniques for individuals with unacceptable responses to pharmacologic or lifestyle modifications, limiting disability, or critical limb ischemia. For acute limb ischemia, time to diagnosis and initiation of treatment is inversely related to successful outcome (see Chap. 61). Options include percutaneous catheter–directed thrombolytic therapy, percutaneous mechanical thrombus extraction with or without thrombolytic therapy, and surgical thrombectomy or bypass. Initial thrombolytic therapy is recommended for ischemia of ≤14 days' duration or graft occlusions, and initial surgical revascularization is recommended for those with ischemia of >14 days' duration or native arterial occlusions.[146] Interventional procedures have been most successful for disease of the iliac arteries. Guidelines address choices between surgical and catheter-based approaches as well as methods of catheter-based approaches that continue to evolve (see TransAtlantic Inter-Society consensus statements, Chaps. 61 and 63).[140,142,146] Decisions should be based on symptoms, responses to therapies, comorbid conditions, quality of life, and recognition of higher morbidity and longer surgical recovery times of older patients as well as the morbidity and mortality results of the operator.

Table 80-9 presents the general approach to the older patient with lower extremity PAD. Disease of the aorta is discussed in Chapter 60.

CURRENT CONTROVERSIES. Current controversies include the following: optimal pharmacologic therapies for PAD; role of prostaglandins and angiogenesis therapy; optimal endovascular techniques; and role of endovascular procedures versus surgical procedures.

Heart Failure (see Chaps. 25 to 30)

Heart failure has become primarily a disorder of the elderly. Heart failure contributes to at least 20% of hospital admissions of patients older than 65 years, with approximately three quarters of heart failure hospitalizations occurring in patients older than 65 years and more than 85% of heart failure deaths occurring in patients older than 65 years. Heart failure is self-reported by 0.1% of people at ages 18 to 39 years, by about 4% at ages 65 to 74 years, and by about 6% at ages 75 to 105 years. In the Cardiovascular Health Study of independent community-dwelling subjects aged 66 to 103 years, heart failure developed at a rate of 19.3/1000 patient-years. The incidence increased from 10.6/1000 person-years in participants 65 to 69 years of age to 42.5/1000 person-years in those older than 80 years.[147] Similar data have been reported among Medicare beneficiaries (**Fig. 80-10**). Asymptomatic left ventricular systolic dysfunction is estimated to occur in another 3% to 5% of the community, with higher prevalence at older ages. The incidence and prevalence of heart failure are higher in men than in women at all ages, and heart failure is more likely to result from CAD in men than in women. With more women alive at older ages, there are more older women than older men presenting for care for heart failure, and the etiology is less likely to be ischemic (see Chap. 81). Heart failure of any type is associated with a reduction in life span as well as decreased quality of life and recurrent hospitalizations.[148] Average 5-year mortality for heart failure patients with systolic dysfunction is approximately 50% and may be only slightly lower for heart failure patients with preserved systolic function (see Fig. 30-4).[149,150] Prognosis both for systolic heart failure and for heart failure with preserved ejection fraction is worse in patients older than 65 years, and the presence of preserved ejection fraction has less impact on survival than in younger patients. In community-based cohorts, overall survival after onset of heart failure has improved during the past two decades, but there has been less improvement among women and elderly patients with heart failure (**Fig. 80-11**).[151,152]

In contrast to middle-aged patients with heart failure, factors other than left ventricular systolic function contribute to heart failure in the elderly population. Heart failure in the presence of a normal or preserved ejection fraction may be seen in 40% to 80% of older patients with heart failure and is almost twice as frequent in women as in men.[149,153] A history of hypertension is often present, and increased circulating blood volume is present in a subset.[149,154] The pathophysiology is primarily attributed to left ventricular diastolic dysfunction (a leftward- and upward-shifted end-diastolic pressure-volume relationship); left ventricular diastolic chamber size is normal or reduced despite elevated filling pressures,

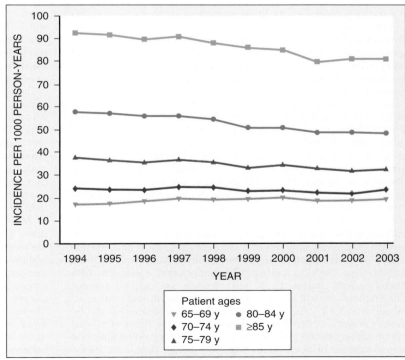

FIGURE 80-10 Incidence rates of heart failure by age in a nationally representative sample of nearly 3 million Medicare beneficiaries. The incidence of heart failure increases with increasing age within the Medicare population. (*From Curtis L, Whellan D, Hammill B, et al: Incidence and prevalence of heart failure in elderly persons, 1994-2003. Arch Intern Med 168:418, 2008.*)

CH 80

CARDIOVASCULAR DISEASE IN THE ELDERLY

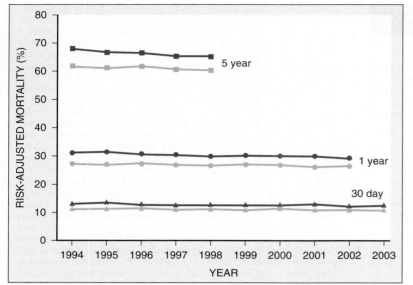

FIGURE 80-11 Risk-adjusted mortality after onset of heart failure by year of incidence and sex in a nationally representative sample of nearly 3 million Medicare beneficiaries. Mortality declined only slightly and was consistently lower for women. *(From Curtis L, Whellan D, Hammill B, et al: Incidence and prevalence of heart failure in elderly persons, 1994-2003. Arch Intern Med 168:418, 2008.)*

resulting in decreased stroke volume and cardiac output (see Fig. 30-10). Thus, some call the disorder diastolic heart failure. Endocardial biopsy specimens from heart failure patients without CAD show structural and functional differences in cardiomyocytes compared with cardiomyocytes from patients with abnormal ejection fraction (systolic heart failure).[155] Myocytes from patients with diastolic heart failure had increased diameter and higher myofibrillar density and developed greater passive force and had greater calcium sensitivity. Myocardial collagen volume fraction was equally elevated.

Exercise intolerance is the primary symptom in chronic heart failure of either systolic (see Chap. 28) or diastolic (see Chap. 30) etiology. Dyspnea and fatigue are prominent symptoms, but fatigue also accompanies many chronic illnesses and is part of the clinical syndrome of frailty in the elderly. Shortness of breath, orthopnea or development of nocturnal cough, and paroxysmal nocturnal dyspnea suggest the presence of heart failure. Less than half of patients with moderate or severe diastolic or systolic dysfunction as measured by Doppler echocardiography had recognized heart failure in a large community-based study.[156] Potential explanations for unrecognized heart failure in the older patient include the nonspecificity of complaints of fatigue, ascribing of symptoms to aging or comorbid conditions, reduction in activities to avoid symptoms, and memory impairment leading to poor historical information. Physical examination may not be as definitive as in younger individuals. Peripheral edema can be due to age-related changes in venous tone, decreased skin turgor, or prolonged sedentary states, and evaluation of volume status based on neck veins may be difficult in the older patient. Rales and a third heart sound may be present only during episodes of acute decompensation, and differentiation of heart failure from pneumonia may be difficult in older patients less likely to present with temperature elevations. With diastolic heart failure, third heart sounds are seldom present. Chest radiography will show pulmonary congestion during acute exacerbations and for some time after an episode; cardiomegaly will be present in systolic heart failure but may or may not be present in heart failure with preserved ejection fraction. Use of echocardiography and serum markers of heart failure takes on greater diagnostic importance.[155,157] Measurement of natriuretic peptides such as B-type natriuretic peptide (BNP) and N-terminal pro-BNP (NT-proBNP) can improve diagnostic accuracy of patients with dyspnea presenting for acute care and may be helpful in evaluating older patients with

dyspnea and nonspecific symptoms or multiple comorbidities. Levels of natriuretic peptides increase with age and with renal decline, and are higher in women than in men, so interpretation requires consideration of these factors. For NT-proBNP, cutoffs for heart failure diagnosis are age specific, with an almost fourfold higher cutoff value for patients older than 75 years compared with those younger than 75 years. For BNP, a twofold higher cutoff value has been suggested for patients with eGFR less than 60 mL/min/1.73 m^2 (the eGFR for most white women older than 65 years; see earlier).

Most data from randomized double-blind studies of therapy for heart failure are from studies of younger middle-aged men with systolic dysfunction resulting from ischemic CAD and few major medical comorbidities. Notably, initial landmark studies of the treatment of systolic heart failure with the ACE inhibitor enalapril as well as hydralazine plus isosorbide excluded patients older than 75 or 80 years. More recent studies have included subsets of elderly (see Chaps. 27 and 28 and **Table 80-10**), and guidelines for the management of patients with chronic heart failure are based on the aggregate data[157-160] and are available at *www.acc.org, www.heart.org* or *www.onlinejcf.com*. Limited trial data are available to guide treatment of the older patient with heart failure and preserved or normal ejection fraction, and recent trials have not demonstrated survival benefits with ACE inhibitors or ARBs in these patients (see Table 80-10). Because the direct applicability of clinical trial findings and heart failure treatment guidelines to the majority of older heart failure patients is unknown and the limited data suggest that outcomes differ from trial results in younger systolic heart failure patients, it is important to consider care in the context of the individual patients and their goals, comorbid conditions, and estimated life expectancy.

HEART FAILURE WITH DECREASED SYSTOLIC FUNCTION (SYSTOLIC HEART FAILURE) (see Chap. 28). Pharmacologic therapy is targeted at control of systolic and diastolic hypertension (see earlier), use of diuretics to control pulmonary congestion and pulmonary edema, and control of ventricular response rate in patients with atrial fibrillation. Most systolic heart failure trials have tested the new therapy or intervention on a background of "usual therapy" that has varied over time. Earlier trials included digitalis and diuretics as usual therapy, but more recent usual therapy is an ACE inhibitor or ARB or beta blocker plus a diuretic, with lower rates of digoxin use.

The DIG trial analyses suggest that a morbidity and hospitalization benefit can accompany digoxin concentrations between 0.5 and 0.9 ng/mL, and the optimal use may be in those with atrial fibrillation.[161,162] Efficacy for ACE inhibitors in post-MI patients with systolic heart failure (SAVE, AIRE, TRACE) and ARBs in systolic heart failure (candesartan in the CHARM programs) has been demonstrated in trials that have included significant numbers of elderly patients.[163-168] In the carefully controlled and monitored setting, dose titration resulted in lower daily doses in older patients, especially those older than 80 years. Caution and close monitoring are necessary with use of ACE inhibitors or ARBs in the elderly, and in general, the "full doses" used in studies of younger patients should not be the target for the oldest patients. Combined use of ACE inhibitors and ARBs has no additive benefit, may have additive adverse effects, and is not recommended. Vasodilating beta blockers are usually considered and should be instituted at low doses during periods of clinical stability. Except for trials with non–U.S.-approved bucindolol, large beta blocker trials excluded patients older than 80 years and have enrolled fewer women than men. Trials with bisoprolol showed benefit at all doses, but doses titrated to tolerance were lower in the oldest enrolled patients with the greater medical comorbidities and in those with the most severe heart failure.[169] At least one trial of a vasodilating beta blocker not available in the United States (nebivolol, see Table 80-10) in exclusively elderly patients with heart failure has reported reduced combined endpoints of all-cause death or hospitalization for heart

Table 80-10 Investigations of Heart Failure Therapies in Elderly Patients

STUDY	PATIENTS	N (% WOMEN)	% >65 YEARS, MEDIAN AGE	DRUG (DOSE)	COMEDICATIONS	MAJOR RESULTS
SENIORS (randomized, placebo controlled) 2005	Heart failure (decreased EF in 64%; preserved EF in 36%)	2128 (37)	100% >70, 76	Nebivolol (10 mg/day)	Diuretic in 86%, ACE or ARB in 88%, aldosterone antagonist in 28%, digoxin in 39%	Overall advantage (low and preserved EF) Subgroups: survival advantage in <75 yr; no advantage in >75 yr
PEP-CHF (randomized, placebo controlled) 2006	Heart failure (preserved EF; hospitalized within 6 months)	850 (56)	100% >70, 76	Perindopril (4 mg/day) (+ diuretic)	Loop diuretics in 44%-47%, thiazide diuretics in 55%, beta blockers in 54%, digoxin in 12%, aldosterone antagonist in 10%	No survival benefit with intention-to-treat analyses but underpowered Reduced heart failure hospitalizations, but 30% not on assigned treatment at 1 yr Equal numbers in both groups taking ACE at end
OPTIMIZE-HF (registry and Medicare data) 2009	Decreased EF	7529 (45)	100%, 78 treated, 80 untreated	Beta blocker compared with no beta blocker	Diuretic in 83%, ACE or ARB in 62%-77%, aldosterone antagonist in 11%-18%, digoxin in 38%	Survival advantage for decreased EF
	Preserved EF	9712 (66)	100%, 80 treated, 81 untreated		Diuretic in 80%, ACE or ARB in 54%-65%, digoxin in 20%-23%, aldosterone antagonist in 7%-9%	No benefit in preserved EF group
I-PRESERVE (randomized, placebo controlled) 2008	Preserved EF	4128 (60)	100% >60, 72 35% >75	Irbesartan (300 mg/day)	Diuretic in 83%, beta blocker in 58%, ACE in 25%, aldosterone antagonist in 15%, digoxin in 13%	No benefit for death from any cause or hospitalization versus placebo

ACE = angiotensin-converting enzyme inhibitor; ARB = angiotensin receptor blocker; EF = ejection fraction.
SENIORS: Flather M, Shibata M, Coats A, et al: Randomized trial to determine the effect of nebivolol on mortality and cardiovascular hospital admission in elderly patients with heart failure (SENIORS). Eur Heart J 26:212, 2005. PEP-CHF: Cleland J, Tendera M, Adamus J, et al: The perindopril in elderly people with chronic heart failure (PEP-CHF) study. Eur Heart J 27:2338, 2006. OPTIMIZE-HF: Hernandez A, Hammill B, O'Connor C, et al: Findings from the OPTIMIZE-HF (Organized Program to Initiate Lifesaving Treatment in Hospitalized Patients with Heart Failure) Registry. Clinical effectiveness of beta-blockers in heart failure. J Am Coll Cardiol 53:184, 2009. I-PRESERVE: Massie B, Carson P, McMurray J, et al: Irbesartan in patients with heart failure and preserved ejection fraction. N Engl J Med 359:359, 2008.

failure, with nonsignificant differences in all-cause death.[170,171] U.S. Registry and Medicare data analyses of exclusively older patients support the conclusion that beta blocker use in clinical populations with heart failure diagnoses is associated with a survival advantage.[150] Ongoing studies are comparing individual beta blockers in elderly heart failure patients.

Studies of aldosterone antagonists have enrolled older patients, primarily white men. Benefit may be seen with these drugs used at lower doses in patients with severe heart failure, but increased use of spironolactone has been accompanied by increased incidence of hyperkalemia in older patients with heart failure, and close monitoring is necessary. Trial data on eplerenone are limited to heart failure in the post-MI setting in younger elderly with the suggestion of no benefit in those older than 65 years.[111] Caution is warranted for its use, especially without data for efficacy and known risks of hyperkalemia in patients with reduced renal clearance common in the elderly. Direct vasodilators such as hydralazine and nitrates have a limited role in older patients because of the increased likelihood of orthostatic hypotension.

Nonpharmacologic Strategies

Dietary sodium restriction is advised, and moderate physical activity should be encouraged if feasible. Supervised exercise training programs based on cardiac rehabilitation algorithms have shown modest benefit on all-cause mortality and hospitalization rates in middle-aged and younger elderly patients with systolic heart failure receiving optimal therapy by heart failure guidelines (age range, 51 to 68 years;

70% were men).[172] Perhaps more relevantly, self-reported health status was improved in the exercise group compared with placebo.[173] Exercise programs similar to those used in cardiac rehabilitation programs should be considered for older patients with systolic heart failure receiving optimal medical therapy to improve heart failure–related quality of life.

Cardiac resynchronization therapy (CRT) can decrease hospitalizations and reduce mortality in selected patients with prolonged cardiac repolarization or QRS intervals on the ECG and symptomatic systolic heart failure despite optimal medical therapy. Most trials excluded patients with atrial fibrillation. CRT trials to determine the efficacy of defibrillator implantation have not included significant numbers of elderly patients. Guidelines as well as clinical judgment dictate that such therapies be considered on an individual basis and when estimated longevity from all causes is long enough to confer benefit (see Chaps. 29 and 38). Revascularization therapies are considered in the setting of ischemia (see Chaps. 31, 32, and 57). The few highly selected patients older than 65 years who have received cardiac transplantation appear to have survival times similar to those of younger patients, with slightly more morbidity and mortality due to the surgical procedure but lower rates of rejection compared with younger patients (see Chap. 31).

HEART FAILURE WITH NORMAL OR PRESERVED LEFT VENTRICULAR EJECTION FRACTION (DIASTOLIC HEART FAILURE). Management is based on control of physiologic factors (blood pressure, heart rate, blood volume, and myocardial ischemia) that are known to exert important effects on ventricular relaxation and the treatment of diseases known to cause diastolic heart failure. Diuretics are effective in the presence of signs and symptoms of volume overload.[157,160] Circulating blood volume is a major determinant of ventricular filling pressure, and the use of diuretics may improve breathlessness in patients with diastolic heart failure (as well as in those with systolic heart failure), but overdiuresis must be avoided. ACE inhibitors and ARBs have been advocated on the basis of the potential for left ventricular regression and reduction of interstitial fibrosis and arterial stiffness. However, larger randomized trials of ACE inhibitors or ARBs for diastolic heart failure in the elderly have not found a survival or hospitalization benefit.[174,175] In these trials, an ACE inhibitor or ARB was added to baseline therapy with diuretics in three quarters of patients, beta blockers in more than half, calcium channel blockers in about one third, spironolactone in 10% to 15%, and digoxin in 15% to 28% (higher in earlier studies). Thus, ACE inhibitors and ARBs may help alleviate symptoms in individual patients, but they have not demonstrated the improved outcomes for diastolic heart failure that they have for systolic heart failure. Their use should be guided by symptomatic responses and the patient's tolerance.

Beta blockers and rate-slowing calcium channel blockers are often advocated on the premise that they decrease blood pressure and afterload and prolong the diastolic filling period. However, a comprehensive study of heart failure registry data linked to Medicare claims data incorporating a broad cohort of patients from all regions of the United States failed to find a survival benefit with the use of a variety of beta blockers in heart failure patients with preserved ejection fraction.[150] Nondihydropyridine calcium channel antagonists can improve measures of diastolic function during short-term use, but definitive data on outcomes with chronic administration for diastolic heart failure are not available. Digoxin was reported to yield symptomatic improvement and decreased hospitalizations (without mortality benefit) in the DIG study of patients with diastolic or systolic heart failure.[176] In analyses of the subset of patients with normal ejection fractions, no benefit of digoxin was detected in patients with mild to moderate heart failure who were in normal sinus rhythm and receiving diuretics and ACE inhibitors.[162] The risk-to-benefit ratio of digoxin in women with heart failure has also been questioned. Data are also lacking on nitrates, but some clinicians find them helpful in reducing orthopnea if they are given at bedtime.

The search for more effective therapies for diastolic heart failure is ongoing with investigations of the aldosterone antagonists spironolactone and eplerenone, the renin inhibitor aliskiren, endothelin receptor antagonists, statins, ion channel inhibitors ivabradine and ranolazine, and use of erythropoietin in patients with anemia. Studies of the collagen cross-link breaker alagebrium were terminated before enrollment was completed, and no other agents of this class are currently under study (*www.clinicaltrials.gov*).

ADDITIONAL CONSIDERATIONS FOR THE OLDER PATIENT WITH HEART FAILURE.

Elderly patients with heart failure have the highest rehospitalization rate of all adult patient groups. Education and involvement of the patient, family members, and caregivers are key to the management of older patients with heart failure. Recognition of warning signs of worsening failure, understanding of medication regimens, diet adjustments, and regular moderate physical activity should be emphasized. Reliance cannot be placed on classic symptoms of heart failure, and weight should be measured daily with a mechanism for rapid communication of information and timely adjustment of diuretic dosages to prevent exacerbations of heart failure. Although diagnosis of heart failure may be improved by measurement of natriuretic peptides, a comparison of symptom-guided therapy with BNP-guided therapy did not improve overall clinical outcomes or quality of life in older patients and cannot be recommended as a routine monitoring strategy.[177] Multidisciplinary team approaches with patient contacts between office visits and more frequent contact during the transitional period after hospital discharge can be highly beneficial and reduce rehospitalization rates.[178,179] Use of primary care preventive strategies such as influenza vaccination can

TABLE 80-11	Approach to the Older Patient with Heart Failure

Symptoms may be nonspecific in the older patient—suspect heart failure.
  Consider heart failure diagnosis in patients with fatigue, dyspnea, exercise intolerance, or low activity.
Diagnosis may be facilitated by use of echocardiography or serum markers of heart failure.
Heart failure may be present in the older patient with preserved systolic function (ejection fraction), especially in older women.
Aggressive treatment of hypertension or diabetes, when present, may improve heart failure outcomes.
Treat symptoms with a goal of improving quality of life and morbidity.
  Control blood pressure—systolic and diastolic.
  Treat ischemia.
  Control atrial fibrillation rate.
  Promote physical activity.
  Adjust medications for age- and disease-related changes in kinetics and dynamics.
Educate and involve patients, family members, or caregivers in management of heart failure.
  Monitor weight.
Consider use of multidisciplinary team approaches.

also reduce hospitalizations for heart failure in older people.[180] For very old patients or those with progressive symptoms of severe heart failure, goals of improving symptoms and quality of life and preventing acute exacerbations and hospitalization rather than prolongation of life become the emphasis. Palliative care programs may have special expertise in the management of symptoms such as dyspnea with opiates and in providing support for family and caregivers as well as for the patient with advanced heart failure.[181] See **Table 80-11** for the approach to the older patient with heart failure.

CURRENT CONTROVERSIES AND ISSUES IN HEART FAILURE IN THE ELDERLY. Current controversies include the following: blood pressure target for older patients with heart failure; efficacious treatment of diastolic heart failure; impact of exercise training on mortality; optimal use of case management teams for heart failure in the elderly; role of nutrition; role of renal dysfunction, anemia, or treatment with erythropoietin on outcomes; role of ultrafiltration; role of devices in patients older than 75 to 80 years or older patients with significant comorbid conditions; role of cross-link breaking agents to reduce ventricular stiffening; and role of testosterone in older men with heart failure.

Arrhythmias

Cell loss and collagen infiltration occur in the area of the sinus node, throughout the atria, the central fibrous body, and the cytoskeleton of the heart with increasing age. Changes are most marked in the area of the sinus node, with destruction of as many as 90% of cells by the age of 75 years. In the center of the sinus node, expression of the L-type calcium channel protein $Ca_v1.2$ responsible for the upstroke of the action potential and depolarization is also decreased with aging.[182] The correlation between pathology and sinus node function, however, is poor, and sinus node function is preserved in most elderly patients, although sinoatrial conduction is decreased. Collagen infiltration and fibrosis are of lesser magnitude in the area of the AV node and more marked in the left and right bundle branches. Conduction times through the AV node increase with aging, with the site of delay above the His bundle. Despite age-related collagen infiltration, His-Purkinje conduction times are not usually increased by aging alone.

Resting heart rate is not altered by age, but maximal heart rate and beat-to-beat variability in heart rate decrease with age because of decreases in sinus node responses to beta-adrenergic and parasympathetic stimulation (see Chap. 94). On the surface ECG, the PR interval increases and the R, S, and T wave amplitudes decrease. The QRS axis shifts leftward. This shift may reflect increased left ventricular mass or interstitial fibrosis of the anterior fascicular radiation. Right bundle branch block is found in 3% of healthy people older than 85 years and in up to 20% of centenarians and in 8% to 10% of older patients with heart disease, but it is not associated with cardiac morbidity or mortality. The presence of left bundle branch block increases with age and is more likely to be associated with cardiovascular disease.

Nonspecific intraventricular conduction delays become more frequent with increasing age and are usually related to underlying myocardial disease. Repolarization times throughout the myocardium increase with age, and surface ECG QT intervals increase.

Atrial ectopy has been found on electrocardiographic recordings in 10% of community-dwelling elderly without known cardiac disease and in up to 80% during 24-hour ambulatory electrocardiographic recordings. Brief episodes of atrial tachyarrhythmias are seen on 24-hour ambulatory ECGs in up to 50% of community-dwelling elderly. Premature ventricular complexes also increase in prevalence and frequency with age. Ventricular ectopic beats are seen on electrocardiography in 6% to 11% of elderly without known cardiovascular disease and in as many as 76% on 24-hour ambulatory electrocardiographic recordings. In the absence of cardiac disease, these age-related changes have not been associated with subsequent cardiovascular events (see Table 80-1).

Sinus Node Dysfunction

Bradycardia due to sinus node dysfunction or AV conduction disease is more common as age increases. The mean age of patients undergoing permanent pacemaker implantation is about 74 years, with 70% of new pacemaker recipients being older than 70 years. In the United States, 85% of pacemaker implantations are in patients older than 65 years, with up to 30% implanted in patients older than 80 years. The most common indication is for sinus node dysfunction.

Atrioventricular Conduction Disease

First-degree AV block is diagnosed in 6% to 10% of healthy elderly. Higher degree AV block is less common. Transient type II AV block occurs on 0.4% to 0.8% of 24-hour ambulatory ECGs of community-dwelling elderly and transient third-degree AV block in less than 0.2%. These arrhythmias usually represent advanced conduction system disease, requiring pacemaker implantation (see Chap. 39). Acquired AV block is the second most important indication for permanent pacemaker implantation.

Studies have compared outcomes with single-chamber versus dual-chamber pacing devices in older patients with sinus node dysfunction or AV node disease (see Chap. 38). The overall conclusion is that dual-chamber pacing does not provide a significant 2- to 6-year survival advantage or benefit with respect to cardiovascular death or stroke. For some patients, quality of life or heart failure symptoms may be improved or atrial fibrillation may be less common with atrial-based pacing, but procedural complication rates and reoperation rates before discharge are higher with dual-chamber pacemaker implantation.[183-185] For further discussion of pacing, see Chap. 38.

CURRENT CONTROVERSIES. Current controversies include the optimal pacing mode for individual patients with sinus and AV node disease and the role of resynchronization therapy in the elderly.

Atrial Arrhythmias

ATRIAL FIBRILLATION (see Chap. 39). Atrial fibrillation is seen on 24-hour ambulatory recordings in 10% of community-dwelling older patients. The incidence doubles with each decade beginning at the age of 60 years, so that by the age of 80 to 89 years, the incidence of atrial fibrillation is currently estimated to be 8% to 10%. Median age of patients with atrial fibrillation in the United States is about 75 years, with approximately 70% of patients with atrial fibrillation between the ages of 65 and 85 years. Atrial fibrillation is projected to increase, with a 2.5-fold increase in the prevalence during the next 50 years. Hospitalizations for atrial fibrillation have already increased.[186] Atrial fibrillation is rarely an isolated condition in the older patient. Hypertension, ischemic heart disease, heart failure, valvular disease, and diabetes are the most common conditions associated with atrial fibrillation, and thyroid disease should also be considered. The risk for stroke associated with atrial fibrillation combined with the high prevalence of other stroke risk factors mandates a focus on antithrombotic therapy (anticoagulation), management of associated conditions, and rate control to improve symptoms.

Currently, warfarin remains the first-line agent in the United States on the basis of long-term experience with its efficacy and adverse effects. Patients should be anticoagulated with warfarin in the absence of contraindications. The target international normalized ratio (INR) is 2 to 2.5 in older patients in whom close monitoring of INRs can be performed. Low fixed warfarin doses of 1 mg are not efficacious. Patients older than 75 years may require less than half the dose of middle-aged patients for equivalent anticoagulation. Warfarin dosing guidelines for the elderly recommend initiation of warfarin at the estimated maintenance dosage of warfarin, usually 2 to 5 mg daily, and it can be better estimated with algorithms that incorporate multiple clinical factors (*www.warfarindosing.org*). As discussed before, genotyping is not currently recommended or reimbursed for warfarin dosing estimation. Drug interaction information should be consulted whenever warfarin is being initiated or a drug is added to or deleted from a patient's medications. Chronic warfarin administration may contribute to osteoporosis. Vitamin K plays a role in bone metabolism, and oral anticoagulation with warfarin antagonizes vitamin K. In analyses of women receiving chronic oral anticoagulation compared with nonanticoagulated cohorts, increased risk of osteoporosis and higher rates of vertebral and rib fractures were associated with oral anticoagulation for more than 12 months.[187] Measures to prevent osteoporosis should accompany long-term anticoagulation with warfarin (calcium and vitamin D in most; bisphosphonates, calcitonin if needed).

In older patients who are unable to tolerate or who are not candidates for warfarin, aspirin combined with clopidogrel (75 mg/day) may reduce the risk of major vascular events, but as with warfarin, the risk of major hemorrhage is increased.[188] A large international trial of elderly patients with atrial fibrillation found the oral direct thrombin inhibitor dabigatran noninferior to warfarin for stroke prevention and to be associated with less bleeding at the lower (110 mg/day) of two doses but with a trend for increased risk of MI; the higher dose (150 mg/day) had lower stroke rates but increased bleeding and increased risk of MI.[189] Hepatotoxicity is stated to be less than that with the previously promising thrombin inhibitor ximelagatran. As experience with and access to dabigatran increase, current antithrombotic strategies may need to be reevaluated.

Randomized studies have found no significant difference in long-term outcome between rate control and rhythm control, even in the presence of heart failure, and it is the unusual older patient who requires rhythm control to provide symptom relief.[190-195] Agents effective in controlling heart rate include beta blockers, non-dihydropyridine calcium channel antagonists, amiodarone, and digoxin (for less active elderly). Dronedarone, an amiodarone-like drug without iodine moieties, has recently become available and is effective for control of heart rate and may improve cardiovascular outcomes with fewer adverse effects than with amiodarone.[196,197] Like amiodarone, it is a strong CYP3A inhibitor and increases digoxin, creatinine, and simvastatin levels. There are limited data on dose response or dose alterations for use in the elderly, and it should not be used in patients with systolic heart failure. Other recent data show that neither ARBs nor statins prevent recurrences of atrial fibrillation and that the beta blocker nebivolol improves atrial fibrillation outcomes in older patients.[171,198]

See **Table 80-12** for a summary of the approach to the older patient with atrial fibrillation.

CURRENT CONTROVERSIES. Current controversies include the following: optimal rate control; optimal use of dronedarone; best strategies to reduce bleeding risk with warfarin; estimating risk of complications of atrial fibrillation; role of self-monitoring of INR to improve warfarin therapy; and role and safety of dabigatran.

Ventricular Arrhythmias

Treatment of premature ventricular contractions with most type I antiarrhythmic agents either has been of no benefit or has decreased survival. If patients have symptoms, administration of a beta blocker may be helpful. Sustained ventricular tachycardia and ventricular fibrillation require treatment in patients of any age[199] (see Chap. 39).

| TABLE 80-12 | Approach to the Older Patient with Atrial Fibrillation |

Atrial fibrillation is frequent in the elderly and confers a risk of stroke.
Routine examinations or electrocardiographic evaluations should be targeted toward detection of atrial fibrillation.
Thyroid disease and medical conditions should be controlled.
Anticoagulation with warfarin is the chief weapon against stroke.
   The potential for both greater benefit and fatal intracranial bleeding is present at ages older than 75 years, especially in women.
   Careful attention to anticoagulation monitoring is needed.
   Aspirin plus clopidogrel (75 mg/day) can reduce stroke risk in patients who are not candidates for warfarin or are warfarin intolerant, with overall bleeding risks similar to those with warfarin.
   Aspirin alone does not increase bleeding risk but increases bleeding risk.
Rate control produces equivalent benefits with lower costs and morbidity than attempts at rhythm control.
   Useful agents in the elderly include digoxin (rest control), beta blockers, nondihydropyridine calcium channel blockers, and amiodarone or dronedarone with dose adjustments for age, weight, and diseases.

Syncope

It is estimated that 40% of people older than 70 years fall at least once a year, and there is significant overlap between falls and syncope in older adults, with an estimated 30% of falls being due to syncope in the elderly. Syncope accounts for 1% to 3% of emergency department visits and as much as 6% of hospital admissions, and it is the sixth most common cause of hospitalization of patients older than 65 years. The cause of syncope often remains undetermined. The San Francisco Syncope Rule (high risk if any of the following are present: history of heart failure or hematocrit lower than 30%, abnormal ECG, shortness of breath, systolic blood pressure <90 mm Hg at presentation) or other more complex algorithms can help identify patients at high and low risk for short-term consequences and guide evaluations.[200] Dedicated syncope units and the rapid access multidisciplinary approach may also increase the diagnostic yield and reduce the need for hospitalization but are not widely available.[201] In a review of diagnostic testing in a series of older patients (mean age, 79 years) with syncope, the lowest likelihood of useful test results was found with electroencephalography, head CT scans, and cardiac enzyme tests.[59] Postural blood pressure recordings had the highest yield but were obtained uncommonly. In addition, carotid ultrasonography and tilt-table testing seldom identify the cause. A careful history and physical examination and use of a risk stratification algorithm can help identify patients likely to benefit from cardiac enzyme and heart rhythm monitoring.

Valvular Disease (see Chap. 66)

Age-related changes in the fibromuscular skeleton of the heart include myxomatous degeneration and collagen infiltration termed sclerosis. Another change is calcification of the aortic valve leaflets, aortic annulus, base of the semilunar cusps, and mitral annulus. The underlying processes involve lipid accumulation, inflammation, remodeling of the extracellular matrix, angiogenesis, and finally calcification.[202] Calcification progresses from the base of the cusps to the leaflets, eventually causing a reduction in leaflet motion and effective valve area without commissural fusion. Increasing calcification with progression to stenosis is now the most common cause of valvular stenoses in older patients, especially at the aortic position. Ischemic or hypertensive disease has become the most common cause of valvular regurgitation, especially at the mitral valve. Similarly, pulmonary regurgitation and tricuspid regurgitation in the elderly are usually secondary to pulmonary hypertension and dilation of the right ventricle resulting from left ventricular ischemia, heart failure, or pulmonary disease. Less common causes of mild to moderate mitral or aortic regurgitation are ruptured chordae, endocarditis, trauma, aortic dissection, and rheumatic heart disease.

Infective endocarditis is seen in about equal frequency in younger and older patients, but it is more likely to be associated with nosocomial infections with the use of intravascular catheters or devices, the presence of prosthetic implants, pacemaker leads, atheromas, or mitral annular calcification in older patients. Polymicrobial infections are uncommon in the elderly, and the most frequent pathogens are group D streptococci and enterococcus, *Staphylococcus epidermidis,* and viridans streptococci (see Chap. 67).

Treatment of symptomatic valvular disease relies on surgical approaches.[203] Surgery in older patients between 70 and 80 years of age is increasingly common, but experience with those older than 90 years is limited and carries a high surgical mortality rate.

Aortic Valve Disease

AORTIC STENOSIS. Sclerosis of the aortic valve is present in as many as 30% of the elderly, and the prevalence increases as age increases from 65 years to more than 85 years. Mild aortic stenosis is present in about 9% of people older than 65 years, moderate stenosis in 5%, and severe aortic stenosis in about 2%. Risk factors for progression from sclerosis to stenosis include a congenitally bicuspid valve, hypertension, hyperlipidemia, smoking, end-stage renal disease, and, in some series, diabetes, shorter stature, or male sex. No correlations have been found between C-reactive protein and calcification or rate of progression of stenosis. Intriguingly, telomere length has been reported to be shorter in older patients with critical calcific aortic valve stenosis compared with age-matched controls.

The pathophysiologic consequences of aortic stenosis are independent of cause and include left ventricular hypertrophy, elevated left ventricular diastolic pressures, and decreased stroke volume in patients of all ages. However, for any given degree of aortic stenosis, left ventricular hypertrophy and decreased left ventricular compliance are greater in patients older than 65 years compared with younger patients. Approximately 50% of patients with severe aortic stenosis will have significant CAD, further influencing left ventricular function, symptoms, and morbidity.

Diagnosis

Symptoms can be exertional angina, syncope, or heart failure and may be precipitated by atrial arrhythmias such as atrial fibrillation. Symptoms may be absent in inactive older patients, may be subtle, or may not be elicited from patients with memory impairment. Physical findings of calcific aortic valve stenosis in older patients differ from those seen with young patients with biscuspid aortic valves or rheumatic aortic stenosis and do not accurately reflect the degree of stenosis. The age-related arterial changes of decreased compliance and increased stiffness mask the carotid artery findings associated with aortic stenosis in younger individuals. The carotid artery upstroke and peak may appear normal, and carotid amplitude may be unaltered or increased even in the presence of severe calcific stenosis. The presence of decreased carotid upstroke and volume (in the absence of carotid disease) usually indicates severe stenosis. Aortic sclerosis and aortic stenosis both produce systolic ejection murmurs, but the murmur of aortic stenosis is late peaking (links to audio examples are found on the website). The volume of the murmur depends on flow as well as the pressure gradient and does not reflect the severity of stenosis. A murmur may be absent in low-output states, reflecting severe aortic valve obstruction. The murmur may also be high pitched and musical as opposed to harsh and low frequency, and the second heart sound may be preserved. Hypertension is common in the elderly, making left ventricular hypertrophy on electrocardiography or ventricular enlargement on chest radiography similarly of little diagnostic help. Thus, Doppler echocardiography has become the clinical standard for diagnosis of aortic stenosis in the elderly. In the patient with low cardiac output (low flow), maneuvers to increase output (exercise or inotropes such as dobutamine) are helpful in quantifying stenosis. Catheterization is less commonly used to make the diagnosis, but coronary angiography is usually performed to evaluate CAD in older patients before valvular interventions.

Management

Management of the older patient with aortic stenosis (**Table 80-13**) is similar to that of younger patients, with recognition of the increased likelihood of concomitant coronary disease and diseases of other organs (see Chap. 66).[203,204] Risk factors should be treated. Neither U.S.

TABLE 80-13	Approach to the Older Patient with Suspected Valvular Disease

Physical examination cannot reliably assess the severity of valvular lesions in most older patients.
Doppler echocardiography is the clinical standard for diagnosis and evaluation of the severity of valve lesions.
  Differentiates sclerosis from stenosis
  Can assist in monitoring progression of stenosis
  Quantitates regurgitation
  Assesses calcification of valves and supporting structures
Age is a predictor of worse outcomes for the natural history of valvular lesions as well as for surgical approaches.
Surgery is definitive therapy for valvular lesions. Age, coronary artery disease, additional diseases, projected life span, and desired lifestyle are factors in evaluation of surgical options.

nor European guidelines recommend routine antibiotic prophylaxis before dental, gastrointestinal (GI), or genitourinary (GU) procedures except in patients at high risk of infection, defined as those with implanted devices or grafts, prior endocarditis, and congenital heart disease.[203,204] The guidelines note the lack of multicenter randomized trial data on the effects of antibiotic prophylaxis and that it may be reasonable to use antibiotic prophylaxis in individual patients. The authors of this chapter might consider this to include older patients with frequent infections with recurrent sepsis, those receiving chemotherapeutic agents with a lowered white blood cell count, or patients within 60 days of implantation of cardiac devices or non-cardiac bioprostheses as examples of patients for whom antibiotic prophylaxis might be considered. In addition to careful clinical monitoring of symptoms, reevaluation with transthoracic echocardiography is currently recommended every 3 to 5 years for patients with mild stenosis, every 1 to 2 years for patients with moderate stenosis, and more frequently in those with severe stenosis.[203] Monitoring for iron deficiency anemia should also be performed because of the acquired coagulopathy and bleeding from intestinal angiodysplasia that is being increasingly recognized in older patients with aortic stenosis. Although valvular calcification processes have similarities to atherosclerotic processes, randomized double-blind placebo-controlled trials have failed to demonstrate slowing of progression of calcific aortic stenosis with lipid-lowering agents.[205-207] Evidence to support the use of ACE inhibitors or ARBs to slow calcification or the use of the selective aldosterone receptor antagonist eplerenone to slow progression of aortic stenosis does not exist. Treatment of symptomatic and severe aortic stenosis requires valve replacement.

Surgical morbidity and mortality relate to the severity and duration of aortic stenosis, degree of left ventricular hypertrophy, presence or absence of heart failure or CAD, comorbidities (especially renal), urgency and complexity of the procedure, and age of the patient. Combined valve replacement and CABG is associated with higher perioperative morbidity and mortality than is isolated valve replacement. Estimates of average operative mortality for older patients who have undergone valve replacement with or without CABG have been reported as 6% for high surgery volume centers and 13% in low surgery volume centers.[208] Operative mortality for aortic valve replacement in patients 80 years and older is estimated at 8% to 15%.[209] Perioperative renal failure, pulmonary insufficiency, stroke, late cognitive impairment, and late death rates are higher than in younger individuals. Postoperative hospitalization and rehabilitation times are also usually longer in older patients (see Chap. 84).

Minimally invasive and percutaneous approaches to the aortic valve are currently under investigation, but this technology is still evolving.[209,209a] Aortic balloon valvotomy is not a substitute for surgery because mortality after aortic valvuloplasty is similar to that in patients with severe symptomatic aortic valvulotenosis who do not undergo surgery. Procedural morbidity and mortality are high (>10%), and initial improvement is followed by rapid restenosis and recurrence of symptoms within months in most series.[203,204] A limited role for valvotomy as a bridge to valve surgery in hemodynamically unstable patients

(cardiogenic shock), in patients undergoing emergent noncardiac surgery, and in patients with severe comorbidities who are too ill to undergo cardiac surgery has been supported by some.[210]

Appropriate selection of patients for aortic valve replacement includes assessment of the burden of disease in addition to the valve disease, anticipated life span independent of valve disease, and symptom status. Surgical risk assessment tools that incorporate comorbidities and clinical status as well as individual and combined procedures in calculations may be helpful[211-213] (online tools are available at *www.sts.org* or *www.euroscore.org*; *http://www.sts.org/sections/stsnationaldatabase/riskcalculator/*, and *http://www.euroscore.org/calc.html*). Although not specifically developed for older patients, they incorporate the major risk factors of New York Heart Association functional class, diabetes, hypertension, renal insufficiency, and low ejection fraction that were identified in a European report on outcomes of valve surgery in octogenarians.[208,214] Combined procedures (CABG or multiple valves) also have almost twofold greater risk than single-valve surgeries in older patients. The more comorbidities and the frailer the patient, and the more complicated the procedure, the more likely that perioperative mortality and postoperative morbidity[214a] will outweigh the benefit (see Chap. 84).

Biologic tissue valves are frequently implanted in elderly patients on the basis of factors including avoidance of chronic anticoagulation, longer bioprosthesis durability with older age, and shorter anticipated life expectancy (see Chap. 66). Estimated structural failure rates of current bioprosthetic valves are about 1% per patient-year in patients older than 65 years.

Asymptomatic older patients with aortic stenosis and their families should be educated on signs and symptoms related to aortic stenosis and observed regularly for development of symptoms and by Doppler echocardiography for changes in aortic valve area. Sudden death in asymptomatic patients with aortic stenosis occurs, but the frequency in prospective studies using echocardiography is estimated at less than 1%, much lower than previous estimates of 3% to 5% in retrospective studies. Operative mortality in older patients exceeds either of these rates. Thus, asymptomatic older patients with severe aortic stenosis are not usually recommended for surgical interventions.[203,204]

CURRENT CONTROVERSIES. Current controversies include the following: role of pharmacotherapy or biologicals in prevention of or slowing of aortic valve calcification; management and frequency of monitoring of asymptomatic older patients with aortic stenosis; potential biomarkers of progression of stenosis; relative risks, benefits, and methods of minimally invasive and percutaneous aortic valve replacement; duration and type of antithrombotic therapy after surgical implantation of a biologic valve; and indications for early valve replacement in asymptomatic elderly patients with very severe aortic stenosis.

Aortic Regurgitation

The prevalence of aortic regurgitation also increases with age. Mild aortic regurgitation was detected by Doppler echocardiography in 13% of patients older than 80 years and moderate or severe regurgitation in 16% in one series.[215] Causes of aortic regurgitation in the older patient include primary valvular disease (myxomatous or infective) or aortic root disease and dilation secondary to hypertension or dissection. Most often, significant aortic regurgitation in older patients is seen in combination with aortic stenosis.

Older age is a predictor of worse outcome for the natural history of aortic regurgitation. The life span of older patients with chronic severe aortic regurgitation who did not undergo valve replacement in the presurgical era was estimated at 2 years after onset of heart failure. When infective aortic regurgitation occurs in the elderly, the clinical manifestations may be insidious and nonspecific and symptoms fewer than in younger patients (see Chap. 67). Central nervous system symptoms are common and may predict a less favorable clinical outcome. Patients who have acute heart failure and pulmonary congestion as the manifestation of aortic valve endocarditis have a mortality rate of 50% to 80%.

Aortic regurgitation can be diagnosed by the classic diastolic murmur on physical examination. The finding of a widened pulse pressure usually associated with aortic regurgitation in younger patients is of limited diagnostic value in the older patient because age-related changes in the vasculature usually produce a widened pulse pressure in older people. Doppler echocardiography is the usual method of quantitation of the regurgitation and assessment of ventricular function. Patients older than 75 years are more likely to develop symptoms or left ventricular dysfunction at earlier stages of left ventricular dilation, have more persistent ventricular dysfunction and heart failure symptoms after surgery, and have worse postoperative survival rates than younger patients.

Mitral Annular Calcification

Mitral annular calcification is a chronic degenerative process that is age related and is seen more commonly in women than in men and in people older than 70 years (see Fig. 16-21). An increased prevalence of mitral annular calcification is seen in patients with systemic hypertension, increased mitral valve stress, mitral valve prolapse, elevated left ventricular systolic pressure, aortic valve stenosis, chronic renal failure, secondary hyperparathyroidism, atrial fibrillation, and aortic atherosclerosis. Like aortic valve calcification, mitral annular calcification is associated with risk factors for the development of atherosclerosis. Mitral annular calcification may produce mitral stenosis, mitral regurgitation, atrial arrhythmias, and AV conduction delay and predispose to infective endocarditis. It is an independent risk factor for systemic embolism and stroke, with the risk of stroke directly related to the degree of mitral annular calcification. It has also been identified as an independent risk factor for cardiovascular death in some series.

Mitral Stenosis

Increasing numbers of older patients now present with symptomatic mitral stenosis. Symptoms are the same as in the younger patient and include exertional dyspnea, orthopnea, paroxysmal nocturnal dyspnea, and pulmonary edema or right-sided heart failure. Atrial fibrillation is more common in older patients. Physical findings of calcific mitral stenosis differ from those of rheumatic mitral stenosis, and neither a loud first heart sound nor opening snap is usually heard. The characteristic diastolic rumbling murmur is usually present. Quantification of stenosis is usually accomplished by Doppler echocardiography. Older patients are more likely to have heavy calcification and fibrosis of the valve leaflets and subvalvular fusion, making them less likely than younger patients to benefit from percutaneous valvotomy. The success rate of valvotomy in older patients is less than 50%; procedural mortality rates approach 3%, and there are higher complication rates including pericardial tamponade in 5% and thromboembolism in 3%. Selected older patients with favorable valve morphology may be candidates for percutaneous approaches, but long-term clinical improvement is considerably less and mortality is higher in older than in younger patients. Mitral valve surgery also carries higher risks in the older patient. In the older patient with concomitant medical problems or pulmonary hypertension at systemic levels, perioperative mortality for surgical mitral valve replacement may be as high as 10% to 20% compared with 6% for the average patient. Decisions must be individualized, but surgical valvular replacement is usually the procedure of choice for the older patient without severe pulmonary hypertension and with a longer projected life span discounting the mitral stenosis.

Mitral Regurgitation

Myxomatous degeneration and functional mitral regurgitation from left ventricular dysfunction after MI as causes of mitral regurgitation in the older patient are increasing (see Chap. 66). Rheumatic mitral disease is declining, and endocarditis etiology is unchanged. Mitral regurgitation may also be seen in the setting of left ventricular dilation due to heart failure.

Acute mitral regurgitation presents with heart failure and pulmonary edema, but this may also be the initial presentation for medical care of the older patient with chronic mitral regurgitation. Chronic mitral regurgitation may be asymptomatic, especially in the sedentary patient. In symptomatic patients, initial complaints are usually easy fatigability and decreasing exercise tolerance because of low forward cardiac output followed by dyspnea on exertion, orthopnea, paroxysmal nocturnal dyspnea, and dyspnea at rest as the left ventricle function fails. Right-sided heart failure may also occur. Findings on examination are not altered by age, and a holosystolic murmur is usually present along with displacement of the left ventricular apical impulse and third heart sound or early diastolic flow rumble. Comprehensive two-dimensional transthoracic echocardiography with Doppler study is recommended to evaluate left ventricular size and function, right ventricular and left atrial size, pulmonary artery pressure, and severity of mitral regurgitation. Transesophageal echocardiography is used when transthoracic echocardiography is suboptimal. Surgical options are based on symptoms, valvular anatomy, left ventricular function, atrial fibrillation, pulmonary hypertension, and extent of comorbid diseases.[203,204] Transesophageal echocardiography is recommended in the evaluation of surgical candidates to assess feasibility and to guide repair. Cardiac catheterization is used when there is a discrepancy between symptoms and noninvasive findings and to evaluate CAD. Medical treatment of chronic mitral regurgitation is age independent and includes therapy for heart failure and management of atrial fibrillation. Older age is a risk factor for hospital mortality with isolated mitral valve surgery. Elderly patients with mitral regurgitation have less successful surgical outcomes than do older patients with aortic stenosis. The average operative mortality for mitral valve replacement in the elderly exceeds 14% in the United States and is above 20% in low-volume centers.[208] Risks are reduced somewhat if mitral repair rather than mitral valve replacement is performed but increased with the need for combined CABG surgery for CAD that is often present in older patients. Mitral valve repair is preferred to mitral valve replacement when possible in the older patient, and repair rates now equal (or exceed) replacement rates. Series reporting mitral valve repair results (alone and with CABG) estimate early death rates in patients older than 70 years of 5%-9%.[216,217] Survival after combined mitral valve replacement and CABG at 5 years may be as low as 50%. When valve repair is not possible, mitral valve replacement is primarily performed with tissue valves in patients older than 65 years.[203,204] Although there is increasing evidence to support early intervention in patients with mitral valve regurgitation, the increased surgical risks related to age, common co-morbid conditions, and the likelihood of concomitant coronary artery disease necessitating a combined procedure with high morbidity and mortality in the older patient are the basis for the current AHA/ACC guideline recommendation that under most circumstances asymptomatic elderly patients or patients with mild symptoms should be treated medically.

Additional Considerations in the Elderly

Drug-induced valve disease is uncommon but was recently associated with chronic therapy with ergot-derived dopamine agonists such as pergolide (and cabergoline) in older patients with Parkinson disease. Fibroproliferative lesions produced valvular insufficiency or regurgitation that necessitated valve replacement in some patients and ultimately resulted in removal of pergolide from the U.S. market. Valvular fibrotic changes have not been seen with non–ergot dopamine agonists used for Parkinson disease. Papillary muscle rupture occurs in 1% to 3% of patients with acute MI and is primarily a disease of the elderly. Surgical treatment is recommended, and in this setting, the outcome of combined CABG plus mitral valve surgery is the same as or better than that of mitral valve repair alone.

Future Directions

Increasing emphasis is being placed on preventive strategies for cardiovascular disease in older patients and improving the quality of care by current therapies that were not designed for the elderly. A major limitation is the lack of understanding of the mechanisms underlying many age-related cardiovascular changes or diseases and the marked differences between older patients enrolled in clinical trials and the much larger population of older patients presenting for care. Increased investigation at both the basic level and the clinical level is needed to identify therapies that will benefit older patients based on both the pathophysiology of age-related cardiovascular disease and the frequent presence of comorbid diseases. Caring for patients near the end of their lives is different from caring for patients with longer life expectancies. Research and training will be needed to achieve coordinated care for the older patient that must consider both medical and social factors to provide optimal care.

REFERENCES

Demographics, Epidemiology, and Pathophysiology

1. U.S. Census Bureau: Income 2001 (http://www.census.gov/hhes/income). Accessed July 15, 2003.
2. 2009 Alzheimer's Disease Facts and Figures (www.alz.org).
3. Alexander K, Newby L, Cannon C, et al: Acute coronary care in the elderly, part I: Non–ST-segment elevation acute coronary syndromes: A scientific statement for healthcare professionals from the American Heart Association Council on Clinical Cardiology: In collaboration with the Society of Geriatric Cardiology. Circulation 115:2549, 2007.
4. Alexander K, Newby L, Armstrong P, et al: Acute coronary care in the elderly, part II: ST-segment-elevation myocardial infarction: A scientific statement for healthcare professionals from the American Heart Association Council on Clinical Cardiology: In collaboration with the Society of Geriatric Cardiology. Circulation 115:2570, 2007.
5. Lakatta E: Arterial and cardiac aging: Major shareholders in cardiovascular disease enterprises: Part III: Cellular and molecular clues to heart and arterial aging. Circulation 107:490, 2003.
6. Lakatta E: Arterial and cardiac aging: Major shareholders in cardiovascular disease enterprises: Part II: The aging heart in health: links to heart disease. Circulation 107:346, 2003.
7. Lakatta E, Levy D: Arterial and cardiac aging: Major shareholders in cardiovascular disease enterprises: Part I: Aging arteries: A "set up" for vascular disease. Circulation 107:139, 2003.
8. O'Rourke M, Hashimoto J: Mechanical factors in arterial aging: A clinical perspective. J Am Coll Cardiol 50:1, 2007.
9. Lakatta E, Wang M, Najjar S: Arterial aging and subclinical arterial disease are fundamentally intertwined at macroscopic and molecular levels. Med Clin North Am 93:583, 2009.
10. Fontana L, Meyer T, Klein S, Holloszy J: Long-term calorie restriction is highly effective in reducing the risk for atherosclerosis in humans. Proc Natl Acad Sci U S A 101:6659, 2004.
11. Meyer TE, Kovacs SJ, Ehsani AA, et al: Long-term caloric restriction ameliorates the decline in diastolic function in humans. J Am Coll Cardiol 47:398, 2006.
12. Ornish D, Lin J, Daubenmier J, et al: Increased telomerase activity and comprehensive lifestyle changes: A pilot study. Lancet Oncol 9:1048, 2008.
13. Honarbakhsh S, Schachter M: Vitamins and cardiovascular disease. Br J Nutr 101:1113, 2009.

Medication Therapy

14. Anderson J, Adams C, Antman E , et al: ACC/AHA 2007 guidelines for the management of patients with unstable angina/non ST-elevation myocardial infarction: Executive Summary: A report of the American College of Cardiology/American Heart Association Task Force on Practice Guidelines (Writing Committee to revise the 2001 guidelines for the management of patients with unstable angina/non ST-elevation myocardial infarction): Developed in collaboration with the American College of Emergency Physicians, the Society for Cardiovascular Angiography and Interventions, the Society of Thoracic Surgeons: Endorsed by the American Association of Cardiovascular and Pulmonary Rehabilitation and the Society for Academic Emergency Medicine. Circulation 116:803, 2007.
15. Cockcroft DW, Gault MH: Prediction of creatinine clearance from serum creatinine. Nephron 16:31, 1976.
16. Stevens L, Coresh J, Greene T, Levey A: Assessing kidney function—measured and estimated glomerular filtration rate. N Engl J Med 354:2473, 2006.
17. Pequignot R, Belmin J, Chauvelier S, et al: Renal function in older hospital patients is more accurately estimated using the Cockcroft-Gault formula than the Modification Diet in Renal Disease formula. J Am Geriatr Soc 57:1638, 2009.
18. Alexander K, Chen A, Roe M, et al: Excess dosing of antiplatelet and antithrombin agents in the treatment of non–ST-segment elevation acute coronary syndromes. JAMA 294:3108, 2005.
19. Lansky A, Pietras C, Costa R, et al: Gender differences in outcomes after primary angioplasty versus primary stenting with and without abciximab for acute myocardial infarction: Results of the Controlled Abciximab and Device Investigation to Lower Late Angioplasty Complications (CADILLAC) trial. Circulation 111:1611, 2005.
20. Kirtane A, Piazza G, Murphy S, et al: Correlates of bleeding events among moderate- to high-risk patients undergoing percutaneous coronary intervention and treated with eptifibatide. Observations from the PROTECT–TIMI-30 Trial. J Am Coll Cardiol 47:2374, 2006.
21. Shlipak M, Wassel Fyr C, Chertow G, et al: Cystatin C and mortality risk in the elderly: The health, aging, and body composition study. J Am Soc Nephrol 17:254, 2006.
22. Ognibene A, Mannucci E, Caldini A, et al: Cystatin C reference values and aging. Clin Biochem 39:658, 2006.
23. Wasen E, Isoaho R, Mattila K, et al: Estimation of glomerular filtration rate in the elderly: A comparison of creatinine-based formulae with serum cystatin C. J Intern Med 256:70, 2004.
24. Grubb A, Bjork J, Lindstrom V, et al: A cystatin-C based formula without anthropometric variables estimates glomerular filtration rate better than creatinine clearance using the Cockcroft-Gault formula. Scand J Clin Lab Invest 65:153, 2005.
25. Shlipak M, Katz R, Kestenbaum B, et al: Rate of kidney function decline in older adults: A comparison using creatinine and cystatin C. Am J Nephrol 30:171, 2009.
26. Hanlon J, Aspinall S, Semla T, et al: Consensus guidelines for oral dosing of primarily renally cleared medications in older adults. J Am Geriatr Soc 57:335, 2009.
27. Schwartz J: The current state of knowledge on age, sex, and their interactions on clinical pharmacology. Clin Pharmacol Ther 82:87, 2007.
28. Schwartz J, Abernethy D: Aging and medications: Past, present, future. Clin Pharmacol Ther 85:3, 2009.
29. Marin F, Gonzalez-Conejero R, Capanzano P, et al: Pharmacogenetics in cardiovascular antithrombotic therapy. J Am Col Cardiol 54:1041, 2009.
30. Shuldiner A, O'Connell J, Bliden K, et al: Association of cytochrome P450 2C19 genotype with the antiplatelet effect and clinical efficacy of clopidogrel therapy. JAMA 302:849, 2009.
31. Kongkaew C, Noyce P, Ashcroft D: Hospital admissions associated with adverse drug reactions: A systematic review of prospective observational studies. Ann Pharmacother 42:1017, 2008.
32. Catananti C, Liperoti R, Settanni S, et al: Heart failure and adverse drug reactions among hospitalized older adults. Clin Pharmacol Ther 86:307, 2009.
33. Cresswell K, Fernando B, McKinstry B, Sheikh A: Adverse drug events in the elderly. Br Med Bull 83:259, 2007.
34. Ray W, Varas-Lorenzo C, Chung C, et al: Cardiovascular risks of nonsteroidal antiinflammatory drugs in patients after hospitalization for serious coronary heart disease. Circ Cardiovasc Qual Outcomes 2:155, 2009.
35. Gurwitz J, Field T, Judge J, et al: The incidence of adverse drug events in two large academic long-term care facilities. Am J Med 118:251, 2005.
36. Lau WC, Waskell LA, Watkins PB, et al: Atorvastatin reduces the ability of clopidogrel to inhibit platelet aggregation: A new drug-drug interaction. Circulation 2002:32, 2003.
37. De Smet P: Herbal remedies. N Engl J Med 347:2046, 2002.
38. Juurlink D, Mamdani M, Kopp A, et al: Drug-drug interactions among elderly patients hospitalized for drug toxicity. JAMA 289:1652, 2003.
39. Barry P, Gallagher P, Ryan C, O'Mahony D: START (screening tool to alert doctors to the right treatment)—an evidence-based screening tool to detect prescribing omissions in elderly patients. Age Ageing 36:632, 2007.
40. Gallagher P, O'Mahony D: STOPP (Screening Tool of Older Persons' potentially inappropriate Prescriptions): Application to acutely ill elderly patients and comparison with Beers' criteria. Age Ageing 37:673, 2008.
41. Briesacher B, Limcangco R, Simoni-Wastila L, et al: Evaluation of nationally mandated drug use reviews to improve patient safety in nursing homes: A natural experiment. J Am Geriatr Soc 53:991, 2005.
42. Juurlink D, Mamdani M, Lee D, et al: Rates of hyperkalemia after publication of the Randomized Aldactone Evaluation Study. N Engl J Med 351:543, 2004.
43. McGuire D, Inzucchi S: New drugs for the treatment of diabetes mellitus. Circulation 117:440, 2008.
44. A comparison of letrozole and tamoxifen in postmenopausal women with early breast cancer. The Breast International Group (BIG) 1-98 Collaborative Group. N Engl J Med 353:2747, 2005.
45. Fick D, Cooper J, Wade W, et al: Updating the Beers criteria for potentially inappropriate medication use in older adults: Results of a US consensus panel of experts. Arch Intern Med 163:2716, 2003.
46. Simon S, Chan K, Soumerai S, et al: Potentially inappropriate medication use by elderly persons in U.S. Health Maintenance Organizations, 2000-2001. J Am Geriatr Soc 53:227, 2005.
47. Rochon P, Lane C, Bronskill S, et al: Potentially inappropriate prescribing in Canada relative to the US. Drugs Aging 21:939, 2004.
48. Curtis L, Ostbye T, Sendersky V, et al: Inappropriate prescribing for elderly Americans in a large outpatient population. Arch Intern Med 164:1621, 2004.
49. Lin O, Kozarek R, Schembre D, et al: Screening colonoscopy in very elderly patients. JAMA 295:2357, 2006.
50. Lee S, Lindquist K, Segal M, Covinsky K: Development and validation of a prognostic index for 4-year mortality in older adults. JAMA 295:801, 2006.
51. Walter L, Lewis C, Barton M: Screening for colorectal, breast, and cervical cancer in the elderly: A review of the evidence. Am J Med 118:1078, 2005.
52. O'Connor P: Adding value to evidence-based clinical guidelines. JAMA 294:741, 2005.
53. Horne B, May H, Muhlestein J, et al: Exceptional mortality prediction by risk scores from common laboratory tests. Am J Med 122:550, 2009.
54. Doshi JA, Zhu J, Lee BY, et al: Impact of a prescription copayment increase on lipid-lowering medication adherence in veterans. Circulation 119:390, 2009.
55. Madden J, Graves A, Zhang F, et al: Cost-related medication nonadherence and spending on basic needs following implementation of Medicare Part D. JAMA 299:1922, 2008.
56. Lloyd-Jones D, Evans J, Levy D: Hypertension in adults across the age spectrum. Current outcomes and control in the community. JAMA 294:466, 2005.

Hypertension

57. Calhoun D, Jones D, Textor S, et al: Resistant hypertension: Diagnosis, evaluation, and treatment. A scientific statement from the American Heart Association Professional Education Committee of the Council for High Blood Pressure Research. Hypertension 51:1403, 2008.
58. Beckett NS, Peters R, Fletcher AE, et al: Treatment of hypertension in patients 80 years of age or older. N Engl J Med 358:1887, 2008.
59. Mendu M, McAvay G, Lampert R, et al: Yield of diagnostic tests in evaluating syncopal episodes in older patients. Arch Intern Med 169:1299, 2009.
60. Lacroix A, Ott S, Ichikawa L, et al: Low-dose hydrochlorothiazide and preservation of bone mineral density in older adults. A randomized double-blind, placebo-controlled trial. Ann Intern Med 133:516, 2000.
61. Bolland M, Ames R, Horne A, et al: The effect of treatment with a thiazide diuretic for 4 years on bone density in normal postmenopausal women. Osteoporos Int 18:479, 2007.
62. Chodosh J, Morton S, Mojica W, et al: Meta-analysis: Chronic disease self-management programs for older adults. Ann Intern Med 143:427, 2005.
63. Roumie C, Elasy T, Greevy R, et al: Improving blood pressure control through provider education, provider alerts, and patient education. A cluster randomized trial. Ann Intern Med 145:165, 2006.
64. Chobanian AV, Bakris GL, Black HR, et al: The Seventh Report of the Joint National Committee on Prevention, Detection, Evaluation, and Treatment of High Blood Pressure. The JNC 7 Report. JAMA 289:2560, 2003.
65. Mancia G, De Backer G, Dominiczak A, et al: 2007 Guidelines for the management of arterial hypertension. The Task Force for the Management of Arterial Hypertension of the European Society of Hypertension (ESH) and of the European Society of Cardiology (ESC). Eur Heart J 28:1462, 2007.

66. Izzedine H, Ederhy S, Goldwasser F, et al: Management of hypertension in angiogenesis inhibitor-treated patients [review]. Ann Oncol 20:807, 2009.

Coronary Artery Disease

67. Daly C, Clemens F, Sendon JLL, et al: Gender differences in the management and clinical outcome of stable angina. Circulation 113:490, 2006.
68. Vaccarino V, Rathore S, Wenger N, et al: Sex and racial differences in the management of acute myocardial infarction, 1994 through 2002. N Engl J Med 353:671, 2005.
69. Anand S, Xie C, Mehta SR, et al: Differences in the management and prognosis of women and men who suffer from acute coronary syndromes. J Am Coll Cardiol 46:1845, 2005.
70. Blomkalns A, Chen A, Hochman J, et al: Gender disparities in the diagnosis and treatment of non–ST-segment elevation acute coronary syndromes: Large-scale observations from the CRUSADE (Can Rapid Risk Stratification of Unstable Angina Patients Suppress Adverse Outcomes With Early Implementation of the American College of Cardiology/American Heart Association Guidelines) National Quality Improvement Inititiative. J Am Coll Cardiol 45:832, 2005.
71. Psaty B, Anderson M, Kronmal R, et al: The association between lipid levels and the risks of incident myocardial infarction, stroke, and total mortality: The Cardiovascular Health Study. J Am Geriatr Soc 52:1639, 2004.
72. Stork S, Feelders R, van den Beld A, et al: Prediction of mortality risk in the elderly. Am J Med 119:519, 2006.
73. Mattace-Raso F, van der Cammen T, Hofman A, et al: Arterial stiffness and risk of coronary heart disease and stroke. The Rotterdam Study. Circulation 113:657, 2006.
74. Hansen T, Staessen J, Torp-Pederson C, et al: Prognostic value of aortic pulse wave velocity as index of arterial stiffness in the general population. Circulation 113:664, 2006.
75. Cao J, Biggs M, Barzilay J, et al: Cardiovascular and mortality risk prediction and stratification using urinary albumin excretion in older adults ages 68-102: The Cardiovascular Health Study. Atherosclerosis 197:806, 2008.
76. Mieres J, Shaw L, Arai A, et al: Role of noninvasive testing in the clinical evaluation of women with suspected coronary artery disease: Consensus statement from the Cardiac Imaging Committee, Council on Clinical Cardiology, and the Cardiovascular Imaging and Intervention Committee, Council on Cardiovascular Radiology and Intervention, American Heart Association. Circulation 111:682, 2005.
77. Redberg R: Coronary artery calcium: Should we rely on this surrogate marker? Circulation 113:336, 2006.
78. Bielak LF, Yu PF, Ryan KA, et al: Differences in prevalence and severity of coronary artery calcification between two non-Hispanic white populations with diverse lifestyles. Atherosclerosis 196:888, 2008.
79. Fraker TD Jr, Fihn SD, Gibbons RJ, et al: 2007 Chronic angina focused update of the ACC/AHA 2002 guidelines for the management of patients with chronic stable angina: A report of the American College of Cardiology/American Heart Association Task Force on Practice Guidelines Writing Group to develop the focused update of the 2002 Guidelines for the management of patients with chronic stable angina. Circulation 116:2762, 2007.
80. Boden W, O'Rourke R, Teo K, et al: Optimal medical therapy with or without PCI for stable coronary artery disease. N Engl J Med 356:1503, 2007.
81. The BARI 2D Study Group: A randomized trial of therapies for type 2 diabetes and coronary artery disease. N Engl J Med 360:2503, 2009.
82. Gasparyan A, Watson T, Lip G: The role of aspirin in cardiovascular prevention. J Am Coll Cardiol 51:1829, 2009.
83. LaRosa J, Grundy S, Waters D, et al: Intensive lipid lowering with atorvastatin in patients with stable coronary disease. N Engl J Med 352:1425, 2005.
84. Bruckert E, Hayem G, Dejager S, et al: Mild to moderate muscular symptoms with high-dosage statin therapy in hyperlipidemic patients—the PRIMO Study. Cardiovasc Drugs Ther 19:403, 2005.
85. Antons K, Williams C, Baker S, Phillips P: Clinical perspectives of statin-induced rhabdomyolysis. Am J Med 119:400, 2006.
86. Ouyang P, Michos E, Karas R: Hormone replacement therapy and the cardiovascular system: Lessons learned and unanswered questions. J Am Coll Cardiol 47:1741, 2006.
87. Chaitman B: Ranolazine for the treatment of chronic angina and potential use in other cardiovascular conditions. Circulation 113:2462, 2006.
88. Dunlay S, Rihal C, Sundt T, et al: Current trends in coronary revascularization. Curr Treat Options Cardiovasc Med 11:61, 2009.
89. Bridges C, Edwards F, Peterson E, et al: Cardiac surgery in nonagenarians and centenarians. J Am Coll Surg 197:347, 2003.
90. Singh M, Peterson E, Milford-Beland S, et al: Validation of the Mayo Clinic Risk Score for in-hospital mortality after percutaneous coronary interventions using the National Cardiovascular Data Registry. Circ Cardiovasc Interv 1:36, 2008.
91. Dacey L, Likosky D, Ryan T, et al: Long-term survival in octogenarians with multivessel coronary disease after surgery versus percutaneous intervention. Ann Thorac Surg 84:1904, 2007.
92. Hannan E, Racz M, Walford G, et al: Long-term outcomes of coronary-artery bypass grafting versus stent implantation. N Engl J Med. 325:2174, 2005.
93. Forman D, Cox D, Ellis S, et al: Long-term paclitaxel-eluting stent outcomes in elderly patients. Circ Cardiovasc Interv 2:178, 2009.
94. Hannan E, Wu C, Walford G, et al: Drug-eluting stents vs coronary artery bypass grafting in multivessel coronary disease. N Engl J Med 358:331, 2008.
95. King S, Smith S, Hirshfeld J, et al: 2007 Focused Update of the ACC/AHA/SCAI 2005 Guideline update for percutaneous coronary intervention: A report of the American College of Cardiology/American Heart Association Task Force on Practice Guidelines: 2007 Writing Group to review new evidence and update the ACC/AHA/SCAI 2005 Guideline Update for Percutaneous Coronary Intervention, Writing on behalf of the 2005 Writing Committee. Circulation 117:261, 2008.
96. Panesar S, Athanasious T, Nair S, et al: Early outcomes in the elderly: A meta-analysis of 4921 patients undergoing coronary artery bypass grafting—a comparison between off-pump and on-pump techniques. Heart 12:1808, 2006.
97. Pfisterer M, Buser P, Osswald S, et al: Outcome of elderly patients with chronic symptomatic coronary artery disease with an invasive vs. optimized medical treatment strategy: One-year results of the randomized TIME trial. JAMA 289:1117, 2003.
98. Antman E, Hand M, Armstrong P, et al: 2007 Focused Update of the ACC/AHA 2004 Guidelines for the Management of Patients With ST-Elevation Myocardial Infarction: A report of the American College of Cardiology/American Heart Association Task Force on Practice Guidelines: Developed in collaboration With the Canadian Cardiovascular Society endorsed by the American Academy of Family Physicians: 2007 Writing Group to Review New Evidence and Update the ACC/AHA 2004 Guidelines for the Management of Patients With ST-Elevation Myocardial Infarction, Writing on Behalf of the 2004 Writing Committee. Circulation 117:296, 2008.
99. Anderson J, Adams C, Antman E, et al: ACC/AHA 2007 guidelines for the management of patients with unstable angina/non–ST-elevation myocardial infarction: A report of the American College of Cardiology/American Heart Association Task Force on Practice Guidelines (Writing Committee to Revise the 2002 Guidelines for the Management of Patients With Unstable Angina/Non–ST-Elevation Myocardial Infarction) developed in collaboration with the American College of Emergency Physicians, the Society for Cardiovascular Angiography and Interventions, and the Society of Thoracic Surgeons endorsed by the American Association of Cardiovascular and Pulmonary Rehabilitation and the Society for Academic Emergency Medicine. J Am Coll Cardiol 50:e1, 2007.
100. Mehta R, Granger C, Alexander K, et al: Reperfusion strategies for acute myocardial infarction in the elderly. State of the art paper. J Am Coll Cardiol 45:471, 2005.
101. Alexander K, Roe M, Kulkarni S, et al: Evolution of cardiovascular care for elderly patients with non–ST-segment elevation acute coronary syndromes. Results from CRUSADE. J Am Coll Cardiol 46:1490, 2005.
102. Alexander K, Chen A, Newby L, et al: Sex differences in major bleeding with glycoprotein IIb/IIIa inhibitors: Results from CRUSADE. Circulation 114:1380, 2006.
103. Sixon S, Grines C, O'Neill W: The year in interventional cardiology. J Am Coll Cardiol 47:1689, 2006.
104. Giugliano RP, White JA, Bode C, et al: Early versus delayed, provisional eptifibatide in acute coronary syndromes. N Engl J Med 360:2176, 2009.
105. Grines C: Senior PAMI Trial. 2002.
106. Bardají A, Bueno H, Fernández-Ortiz A, et al: Type of treatment and short-term outcome in elderly patients with acute myocardial infarction admitted to hospitals with a primary coronary angioplasty facility. The TRIANA (TRatamiento del Infarto Agudo de miocardio eN Ancianos) Registry. Rev Esp Cardiol 58:351, 2005.
107. Hochman J, Sleeper L, Webb J, et al: Early revascularization and long-term survival in cardiogenic shock complicating acute myocardial infarction. JAMA 295:2511, 2006.
108. Mehta S, Granger C, Boden W, et al: Early versus delayed invasive intervention in acute coronary syndromes. N Engl J Med 360:2165, 2009.
109. Montalescot G, Cayla G, Collet JP, et al: Immediate vs. delayed intervention for acute coronary syndromes: A randomized clinical trial. JAMA 302:947, 2009.
110. Krumholz H, Wang Y, Chen J, et al: Reduction in acute myocardial infarction mortality in the United States. Risk-standardized mortality rates from 1995-2006. JAMA 302:767, 2009.
111. Pitt B, Remme W, Zannad F, et al: Eplerenone, a selective aldosterone blocker, in patients with left ventricular dysfunction after myocardial infarction. N Engl J Med 348:1309, 2003.
112. Sabatine M, Cannon C, Gibson C, et al: Addition of clopidogrel to aspirin and fibrinolytic therapy for myocardial infarction with ST-segment elevation. N Engl J Med 352:1179, 2005.
113. Thombs B, Bass E, Ford D, et al: Prevalence of depression in survivors of acute myocardial infarction. J Gen Intern Med 21:30, 2006.
114. Bush D, Ziegelstein R, Patel U, et al: Post–Myocardial Infarction Depression. Evidence Report/Technology Assessment No. 123. (Prepared by the Johns Hopkins University Evidence-based Practice Center under Contract No. 290-02-0018). Rockville, Md, Agency for Healthcare Research and Quality, 2005. AHRQ publication No. 05-E018-2.
115. Whooley M: Depression and cardiovascular disease. JAMA 296:2874, 2006.
116. Serebruany VL: Selective serotonin reuptake inhibitors and increased bleeding risk: Are we missing something? Am J Med 119:113, 2006.
117. Hulley S, Grady D: Postmenopausal hormone treatment. JAMA 301:2493, 2009.
118. Barrett-Connor E, Mosca L, Collins et al: Effects of raloxifene on cardiovascular events and breast cancer in postmenopausal women. N Engl J Med 355:125, 2006.
119. Vogel V, Costantino J, Wickerham D, et al, National Surgical Adjuvant Breast and Bowel Project (NSABP): Effects of tamoxifen vs raloxifene on the risk of developing invasive breast cancer and other disease outcomes: The NSABP Study of Tamoxifen and Raloxifene (STAR) P-2 trial. JAMA 295:2727, 2006.
120. Marchionni N, Fattirolli F, Fumagalli S, et al: Improved exercise tolerance and quality of life with cardiac rehabilitation of older patients after myocardial infarction. Results of a randomized, controlled trial. Circulation 107:2201, 2003.

Carotid Artery Disease and Stroke

121. Goldstein L, Adams R, Alberts M, et al: Primary prevention of ischemic stroke: A guideline from the American Heart Association/American Stroke Association Stroke Council: Cosponsored by the Atherosclerotic Peripheral Vascular Disease Interdisciplinary Working Group; Cardiovascular Nursing Council; Clinical Cardiology Council; Nutrition, Physical Activity, and Metabolism Council; and the Quality of Care and Outcomes Research Interdisciplinary Working Group. Circulation 113:e873, 2006.
122. Easton J, Saver J, Albers G, et al: Definition and evaluation of transient ischemic attack: A Scientific Statement for healthcare professionals from the American Heart Association/American Stroke Association Stroke Council, Council on Cardiovascular Surgery and Anesthesia; Council on Cardiovascular Radiology and Intervention; Council on Cardiovascular Nursing; and the Interdisciplinary Council on Peripheral Vascular Disease. The American Academy of Neurology affirms the value of this statement as an educational tool for neurologists. Stroke 40:2276, 2009.
123. Adams H, Del Zoppo G, Alberts M, et al: Guidelines for the Early Management of Adults With Ischemic Stroke: A guideline from the American Heart Association/American Stroke Association Stroke Council, Clinical Cardiology Council, Cardiovascular Radiology and Intervention Council and the Atherosclerotic Peripheral Vascular Disease and Quality of Care Outcomes in Research Interdisciplinary Working Groups. Stroke 38:1655, 2007.
124. Alberts M, Felberg R, Guterman L, Levine S: Atherosclerotic Peripheral Vascular Disease Symposium II. Stroke intervention: State of the art. Circulation 118:2845, 2008.

125. Del Zoppo G, Saver J, Jauch E, Adams H: Expansion of the time window for treatment of acute ischemic stroke with intravenous tissue plasminogen activator: A science advisory from the American Heart Association Stroke Council. Stroke 40:2945, 2009.
126. Bates B, Choi J, Duncan P, et al: Veterans Affairs/Department of Defense clinical practice guideline for the management of adult stroke rehabilitation care. Executive summary. Circulation 36:2049, 2005.
127. Sacco R, Adams R, Alberts M, et al: Guidelines for prevention of stroke in patients with ischemic stroke or transient ischemic attack. A statement for healthcare professionals from the American Heart Association/American Stroke Association Council on Stroke: Co-sponsored by the Council on Cardiovascular Radiology and Intervention: The American Academy of Nerurology affirms the value of this guideline. Circulation 113:e409, 2006.
128. ESPRIT Study Group: Aspirin plus dipyridamole versus aspirin alone after cerebral ischaemia of arterial origin (ESPRIT): Randomised controlled trial. Lancet 367:1665, 2006.
129. Adams R, Albers G, Alberts M, et al: Update to the AHA/ASA recommendations for the prevention of stroke in patients with stroke and transient ischemic attack. Stroke 39:1647, 2008.
130. CAPRIE Steering Committee: A randomised, blinded, trial of clopidogrel versus aspirin in patients at risk of ischaemic events (CAPRIE). Lancet 348:1329, 1996.
131. Sacco R, Diener H-C, Yusuf S, et al: Aspirin and extended-release dipyridamole versus clopidogrel for recurrent stroke. N Engl J Med 359:1238, 2008.
132. Mohr J, Thompson J, Lazar R, et al: A comparison of warfarin and aspirin for the prevention of recurrent ischemic stroke. N Engl J Med 345:1444, 2001.
133. Antiplatelet Trialists' Collaboration: Collaborative meta-analysis of randomised trials of antiplatelet therapy for prevention of death, myocardial infarction and stroke in high risk patients. BMJ 324:71, 2002.
134. Barnett H, Meldrum H, Eliaszіw M: The appropriate use of carotid endarterectomy. CMAJ 166:1169, 2002.
135. Gurm HS, Yadav JS, Fayad P, et al: Long-term results of carotid stenting versus endarterectomy in high-risk patients. N Engl J Med 358:1572, 2008.
136. Mas J-L, Chatellier G, Beyssen B, et al: Endarterectomy vs. stenting in patients with symptomatic severe carotid stenosis. N Engl J Med 355:1660, 2006.
137. Hobson R, Howard V, Roubin G, et al: Carotid stenting is associated with increased complications in octogenarians: 30 day stroke and death rates in the CREST lead-in phase. J Vasc Surg 40:1106, 2004.
138. White C, Beckman J, Cambria R, et al, American Heart Association Writing Group 5: Atherosclerotic Peripheral Vascular Disease Symposium II. Controversies in carotid artery revascularization. Circulation 118:2852, 2008.
139. Massop D, Dave R, Metzger C, et al, SAPPHIRE Worldwide Investigators: Stenting and angioplasty with protection in patients at high-risk for endarterectomy: SAPPHIRE Worldwide Registry first 2,001 patients. Catheter Cardiovasc Interv 73:129, 2009.

Peripheral Arterial Disease

140. Hirsh A, Haskal Z, Hertzer N, et al: ACC/AHA 2005 Practice Guidelines for the management of patients with peripheral arterial disease (lower extremity, renal, mesenteric, and abdominal aortic): Executive Summary: A collaborative report from the American Association for Vascular Surgery/Society for Vascular Surgery, Society for Cardiovascular Angiography and Interventions, Society for Vascular Medicine and Biology, Society of Interventional Radiology, and the ACC/AHA Task Force on Practice Guidelines (Writing Committee to Develop Guidelines for the Management of Patients with Peripheral Arterial Disease). Circulation 113:1474, 2006.
141. Hankey G, Norman P, Eikelboom J: Medical treatment of peripheral artery disease. JAMA 295:547, 2006.
142. Norgren L, Hiatt W, Dormandy J, et al: Inter-Society Consensus for the Management of Peripheral Arterial Disease (TASC II). J Vasc Surg 45(Suppl 1):S5, 2007.
143. Berger JK, Krantz MJ, Kittelson J, Hiatt W: Aspirin for the prevention of cardiovascular events in patients with peripheral artery disease. A meta-analysis of randomized trials. JAMA 301:1909, 2009.
144. McDermott M, Criqui M: Aspirin and secondary prevention in peripheral artery disease. A perspective for the early 21st century. JAMA 301:1927, 2009.
145. The Warfarin Antiplatelet Vascular Evaluation Trial Investigators: Oral anticoagulant and antiplatelet therapy and peripheral arterial disease. N Engl J Med 357:217, 2007.
146. Gray B, Conte M, Dake M, et al: Atherosclerotic Peripheral Vascular Disease Symposium II. Lower extremity revascularization: State of the art. Circulation 118:2864, 2008.

Heart Failure

147. Gottdiener J, Arnold A, Aurigemma G, et al: Predictors of congestive heart failure in the elderly: The Cardiovascular Health Study. J Am Coll Cardiol 35:1628, 2000.
148. Solomon S, Anavekar N, Skali H, et al: Influence of ejection fraction on cardiovascular outcomes in a broad spectrum of heart failure patients. Circulation 112:3738, 2005.
149. Lee D, Gona P, Vasan R, et al: Relation of disease pathogenesis and risk factors to heart failure with preserved or reduced ejection fraction. Insights from the Framingham Heart Study of the National Heart, Lung, and Blood Institute. Circulation 119:3070, 2009.
150. Hernandez A, Hammill B, O'Connor C, et al: Clinical effectiveness of beta-blockers in heart failure. Findings from the OPTIMIZE-HF (Organized Program to Initiate Lifesaving Treatment in Hospitalized Patients with Heart Failure) Registry. J Am Coll Cardiol 53:184, 2009.
151. Roger VL, Weston S, Redfield M, et al: Trends in heart failure incidence and survival in a community-based population. JAMA 292:344, 2004.
152. Barker W, Mullooly J, Getchell W: Changing incidence and survival for heart failure in a well-defined older population, 1970-1974 and 1990-1994. Circulation 113:799, 2006.
153. Maeder M, Kaye D: Heart failure with normal left ventricular ejection fraction. J Am Coll Cardiol 53:905, 2009.
154. Maurer M, King D, Rumbarger E, et al: Left heart failure with a normal ejection fraction: Identification of different pathophysiologic mechanisms. J Card Fail 11:177, 2005.
155. van Heerebeek L, Borbely A, Niessen H, et al: Myocardial structure and function differ in systolic and diastolic heart failure. Circulation 113:1966, 2006.
156. Redfield M, Jacobsen S, Burnett J, et al: Burden of systolic and diastolic ventricular dysfunction in the community: Appreciating the scope of the heart failure epidemic. JAMA 289:194, 2003.
157. Jessup M, Abraham W, Casey D, et al: 2009 Focused update: ACCF/AHA guidelines for the diagnosis and management of heart failure in adults: A report of the American College of Cardiology Foundation/American Heart Association Task Force on Practice Guidelines. Circulation 119:1977, 2009.
158. Hunt S, Abraham W, Chin M, et al: ACC/AHA 2005 Guideline update for the diagnosis and management of chronic heart failure in the adult. Circulation 112:e154, 2005.
159. Adams K, Lindenfeld J, Arnold J, et al: Executive Summary: HFSA 2006 Comprehensive Heart Failure Practice Guideline. J Card Fail 12:10, 2006.
160. Dickstein K, Cohen-Solal A, Filippatos G, et al: ESC guidelines for the diagnosis and treatment of acute and chronic heart failure 2008: The Task Force for the diagnosis and treatment of acute and chronic heart failure 2008 of the European Society of Cardiology. Developed in collaboration with the Heart Failure Association of the ESC (HFA) and endorsed by the European Society of Intensive Care Medicine (ESICM). Eur J Heart Fail 10:933, 2008.
161. Ahmed A, Waagstein F, Pitt B, et al: Effectiveness of digoxin in reducing one-year mortality in chronic heart failure in the Digitalis Investigation Group trial. Am J Cardiol 103:82, 2009.
162. Ahmed A, Rich M, Fleg J, et al: Effects of digoxin on morbidity and mortality in diastolic heart failure: The ancillary digitalis investigation group trial. Circulation 114:397, 2006.
163. Garg R, Yusuf S: Overview of randomized trials of angiotensin converting enzyme inhibitors on mortality and morbidity in patients with heart failure. JAMA 273:1450, 1995.
164. Flather M, Yusuf S, Kober L, et al: Long-term ACE-inhibitor therapy in patients with heart failure or left-ventricular dysfunction: A systematic overview of data from individual patients. Lancet 355:1575, 2000.
165. Dahlöf B, Devereux RB, Kjeldsen SE, et al: Cardiovascular morbidity and mortality in the Losartan Intervention For Endpoint reduction in hypertension study (LIFE): A randomised trial against atenolol. Lancet 359:995, 2002.
166. Blood Pressure Lowering Treatment Trialists' Collaboration: Effects of different blood-pressure-lowering regimens on major cardiovascular events: Results of prospectively-designed overviews of randomised trials. Lancet 362:1527, 2003.
167. Blood Pressure Lowering Treatment Trialists' Collaboration: Effects of different blood pressure–lowering regimens on major cardiovascular events in individuals with and without diabetes mellitus: Results of prospectively designed overviews of randomized trials. Arch Intern Med 165:1410, 2005.
168. Cohen-Solal A, McMurray J, Swedberg K, et al: Benefits and safety of candesartan treatment in heart failure are independent of age: Insights from the Candesartan in Heart failure–Assessment of Reduction in Mortality and morbidity programme. Eur Heart J 29:3022, 2008.
169. Simon T, Mary-Krause M, Funck-Brentano C, et al: Bisoprolol dose-response relationship in patients with congestive heart failure: A subgroup analysis in the cardiac insufficiency bisoprolol study (CIBIS II). Eur Heart J 24:552, 2003.
170. Flather M, Shibata M, Coats A, et al: Randomized trial to determine the effect of nebivolol on mortality and cardiovascular hospital admission in elderly patients with heart failure (SENIORS). Eur Heart J 26:215, 2005.
171. Ghio S, Magrini G, Serio A, et al, SENIORS Investigators: Effects of nebivolol in elderly heart failure patients with or without systolic left ventricular dysfunction: Results of the SENIORS echocardiographic substudy. Eur Heart J 27:562, 2006.
172. O'Connor C, Whellan D, Lee K, et al: Efficacy and safety of exercise training in patients with chronic heart failure: HF-ACTION Randomized Controlled Trial. JAMA 301:1439, 2009.
173. Flynn K, Pina I, Whellan D, et al: Effects of exercise training on health status in patients with chronic heart failure: HF-ACTION Randomized Controlled Trial. JAMA 301:1451, 2009.
174. Yusuf S, Pfeffer M, Swedberg K, et al: Effects of candesartan in patients with chronic heart failure and preserved left-ventricular ejection fraction: The CHARM-Preserved trial. Lancet 362:777, 2003.
175. Cleland J, Tendera M, Adamus J, et al: The perindopril in elderly people with chronic heart failure (PEP-CHF) study. Eur Heart J 27:2338, 2006.
176. The Digoxin Investigators Group: The effect of digoxin on mortality and morbidity in patients with heart failure. N Engl J Med 336:525, 1997.
177. Pfisterer M, Buser P, Rickli H, et al: BNP-guided vs. symptom-guided heart failure therapy. The Trial of Intensified vs. Standard Medical Therapy in Elderly Patients with Congestive Heart Failure (TIME-CHF) Randomized Trial. JAMA 301:383, 2009.
178. Whellan D, Vic Hasselblad V, Peterson E, et al: Metaanalysis and review of heart failure disease management randomized controlled clinical trials. Am Heart J 149:722, 2005.
179. Sochalski J, Jaarsma T, Krumholz H, et al: What works in chronic care management: The case of heart failure. Health Aff (Millwood) 28:179, 2009.
180. Nichol K, Nordin J, Mullooly J, et al: Influenza vaccination and reduction in hospitalizations for cardiac disease and stroke among the elderly. N Engl J Med 348:1322, 2003.
181. Pantilat S, Steimle A: Palliative care for patients with heart failure. JAMA 291:2476, 2004.

Arrhythmias

182. Jones S, Boyett M, Lancaster M: Declining into failure. The age-dependent loss of the L-type calcium channel within the sinoatrial node. Circulation 115:1183, 2007.
183. Healey J, Toff W, Lamas G, et al: Cardiovascular outcomes with atrial-based pacing compared with ventricular pacing: Meta-analysis of randomized trials, using individual patient data. Circulation 114:11, 2006.
184. Kaszala K, Kalahasty G, Ellenbogen K: Cardiac pacing in the elderly. Am J Geriatr Cardiol 15:77, 2006.
185. Martinez C, Tzur A, Hrachian H, et al: Pacemakers and defibrillators: Recent and ongoing studies that impact the elderly. Am J Geriatr Cardiol 15:82, 2006.
186. Fuster V, Rydén L, Cannom D, et al: ACC/AHA/ESC 2006 Guidelines for the Management of Patients with Atrial Fibrillation: A report of the American College of Cardiology/American Heart Association Task Force on Practice Guidelines and the European Heart Society of Cardiology Committee for Practice Guidelines (Writing Committee to Revise the 2001 Guidelines for the Management of Patients with Atrial Fibrillation). J Am Coll Cardiol 48:e149, 2006.
187. Caraballo P, Heit J, Atkinson E, et al: Long-term use of oral anticoagulants and the risk of fracture. Arch Intern Med 159:1750, 1999.
188. The ACTIVE Investigators: Effect of clopidogrel added to aspirin in patients with atrial fibrillation. N Engl J Med 360:2066, 2009.
189. Connolly S, Ezekowitz M, Yusuf S, et al: Dabigatran versus warfarin in patients with atrial fibrillation. N Engl J Med 361:1139, 2009.

190. Wyse D, Waldo A, DiMarco J, et al: A comparison of rate control and rhythm control in patients with atrial fibrillation. N Engl J Med 347:1825, 2002.

191. Van Gelder I, Hagens V, Bosker H, et al: A comparison of rate control and rhythm control in patients with recurrent persistent atrial fibrillation. N Engl J Med 347:1834, 2002.

192. Carlsson J, Miketic S, Windeler J, et al: Randomized trial of rate-control versus rhythm-control in persistent atrial fibrillation: The strategies of treatment of atrial fibrillation (STAF) study. J Am Coll Cardiol 41:1690, 2003.

193. Opolski G, Torbicki A, Kosior D, et al: Rate control vs rhythm control in patients with nonvalvular persistent atrial fibrillation: The results of the Polish How to Treat Chronic Atrial Fibrillation (HOT CAFE) Study. Chest 126:476, 2004.

194. de Denus S, Sanoski C, Carlsson J, et al: Rate vs. rhythm control in patients with atrial fibrillation: A meta-analysis. Arch Intern Med 165:258, 2005.

195. Roy D, Talajic M, Nattel S, et al: Rhythm control versus rate control for atrial fibrillation and heart failure. N Engl J Med 358:2667, 2008.

196. Hohnloser S, Crijns H, van Eikels M, et al: Effect of dronedarone on cardiovascular events in atrial fibrillation. N Engl J Med 360:668, 2009.

197. Patel C, Yan G-X, Kowey P: Droneradone. Circulation 120:636, 2009.

198. The GISSI-AF Investigators: Valsartan for prevention of recurrent atrial fibrillation. N Engl J Med 360:1606, 2009.

199. Zipes DP, Camm AJ, Borggrefe M, et al: ACC/AHA/ESC 2006 guidelines for management of patients with ventricular arrhythmias and the prevention of sudden cardiac death—executive summary: A report of the American College of Cardiology/American Heart Association Task Force and the European Society of Cardiology Committee for Practice Guidelines (Writing Committee to Develop Guidelines for Management of Patients With Ventricular Arrhythmias and the Prevention of Sudden Cardiac Death). Circulation 114:e385, 2006.

200. Quinn J, McDermott D, Steiell I, et al: Prospective validation of the San Francisco syncope rule to predict patients with serious outcomes. Ann Emerg Med. 47:448, 2006.

201. Chen L, Benditt D, Shen W-K: Management of syncope in adults: An update. Mayo Clin Proc 83:1280, 2008.

202. Akat K, Borggrefe M, Kaden J: Aortic valve calcification: Basic science to clinical practice. Heart 95:616, 2009.

203. Bonow R, Carabello B, Cahatterjee K, et al: 2008 focused update incorporated into the ACC/AHA 2006 Guidelines for the Management of Patients With Valvular Heart Disease. A Report of the American College of Cardiology/American Heart Association Task Force on Practice Guidelines (Writing Committee to Develop Guidelines on Management of Patients With Valvular Heart Disease). J Am Coll Cardiol 52:e1, 2008.

204. Vahanian A, Baumgartner H, Bax J, et al: Guidelines on the management of valvular heart disease: The Task Force on the Management of Valvular Heart Disease of the European Society of Cardiology. Eur Heart J 28:230, 2007.

205. Cowell S, Newby D, Prescott R, et al: A randomized trial of intensive lipid-lowering therapy in calcific aortic stenosis. N Engl J Med 352:2389, 2005.

206. Rossebø A, Pedersen T, Boman K, et al: Intensive lipid lowering with simvastatin and ezetimibe in aortic stenosis. N Engl J Med 359:1343, 2008.

207. Chan KL, Teo K, Dumesnil JG, et al: Effect of lipid lowering with rosuvastatin on progression of aortic stenosis: Results of the Aortic Stenosis Progression Observation: Measuring Effects of Rosuvastatin (ASTRONOMER) Trial. Circulation 121:306, 2010.

208. Goodney P, O'Connor G, Wennberg D, Birkmeyer J: Do hospitals with low mortality rates in coronary artery bypass also perform well in valve replacement? Ann Thorac Surg 76:1131, 2003.

209. Rosengart T, Fedman T, Borger M, et al: Percutaneous and minimally invasive valve procedures. A scientific statement from the American Heart Association Council on Cardiovascular Surgery and Anesthesia, Council on Clinical Cardiology, Functional Genomics and Translational Biology Interdisciplinary Working Group, and Quality of Care and Outcomes Research Interdisciplinary Working Group. Circulation 117:1750, 2008.

209a. Leon MB, Smith CR, Mack M, et al: Transcatheter aortic-valve implantation for aortic stenosis in patients who cannot undergo surgery. N Engl J Med 363:1667, 2010.

210. Kauterman K, Michaels A, Ports T: Is there any indication for aortic valvuloplasty in the elderly? Am J Geriatr Cardiol 12:190, 2003.

211. Nashef S, Roques F, Hammill B, et al: Validation of European System for Cardiac Operative Risk Evaluation (EuroSCORE) in North American cardiac surgery. Eur J Cardiothorac Surg 22:101, 2002.

212. Shroyer A, Coombs L, Peterson E, et al: The Society of Thoracic Surgeons: 30-day operative mortality and morbidity risk models. Ann Thorac Surg 75:1856, 2003.

213. Ambler G, Omar R, Royston P, et al: Generic, simple risk stratification model for heart valve surgery. Circulation 112:224, 2005.

214. Bossone E, Di Bendetto G, Frigiola A, et al: Valve surgery in octogenarians: In-hospital and long-term outcomes. Can J Cardiol 23:223, 2006.

214a. Maillet JM, Sommeb D, Hennel E, et al: Frailty after aortic valve replacement (AVR) in octogenarians. Arch Gerontol Geriatrics 48:391, 2009.

215. Aronow W, Ahn C, Kronzon I: Comparison of echocardiographic abnormalities in African-American, Hispanic, and white men and women aged >60 years. Am J Cardiol 87:1131, 2001.

216. Lee R, Sundt TI, Moon M, et al: Mitral valve repair in the elderly: Operative risk for patients over 70 years of age is acceptable. J Cardiovasc Surg 44:157, 2003.

217. Chikwe J, Goldstone AB, Passage J, et al: A propensity score-adjusted retrospective comparison of early and mid-term results of mitral valve repair versus replacement in octogenarians. Eur Heart J. published ahead of print doi:10.1093/eurheartj/ehq331

CHAPTER **81**   # Cardiovascular Disease in Women

L. Kristin Newby and Pamela S. Douglas

Background

Throughout history, differences between men and women in health and in illness have fascinated researchers and clinicians alike. The Institute of Medicine's Committee on Understanding the Biology of Sex and Gender Differences defined *sex* as "the classification of living things, generally as male or female according to their reproductive organs and functions assigned by the chromosomal complement."[1] *Gender*, on the other hand, was defined as "a person's self-representation as male or female or how that person is responded to by social institutions on the basis of the individual's gender presentation." Women (XX) and men (XY) differ in their genetic complement by a single chromosome of the 46 that define the human species. The influence of this single chromosomal difference affects the mechanisms and expression of disease as well as the psychosocial and behavioral characteristics and environments of individuals, which may protect from or enhance susceptibility to cardiovascular disease. In this discussion of cardiovascular disease in women, both of these definitions help explain differences in the occurrence, presentation, or course of cardiovascular disease—and, in some cases, in treatment and response to therapy.

Scope of the Problem

Cardiovascular disease is the leading cause of death among women, regardless of race or ethnicity, accounting for approximately 455,000 deaths in the United States in 2005 and causing the deaths of 1 in 3 women; this amounts to more deaths from heart disease than from stroke, lung cancer, chronic obstructive lung disease, and breast cancer combined.[2] About half of these deaths (1 in 6) result from coronary heart disease. Estimates of the lifetime costs from coronary heart disease in a woman range from $0.77 million to $1.1 million, depending on the severity of coronary disease.[3] Encouragingly, between 1980 and 2002, age-adjusted mortality from heart disease decreased in both men (52%) and women (49%).[2] For coronary heart disease specifically, mortality rates fell in both men and women by 4.4% from 2000 to 2002.[2] Approximately 47% of this decrease was due to the influence of evidence-based medicine (post–myocardial infarction [MI] secondary prevention, initial treatment of acute coronary syndromes [ACS], heart failure treatment, revascularization for chronic angina, and use of antihypertensive and lipid-lowering therapy) and approximately 44% to a reduction in several risk factors (hypertension, cholesterol, smoking, and physical inactivity) in the general population.[4] However, although overall mortality among women decreased, mortality among young women (between 35 and 44 years of age) increased by 1.3% per year from 1997 to 2002.[5]

Whether there are fundamental differences between women and men in mortality after MI, or whether such observed differences reflect corresponding differences in baseline characteristics, has long been a topic of discussion. In addition to differences in patient-related factors, two studies suggest that mortality may differ among women and men according to the type of ACS at presentation. In an analysis of a population-based cohort (N = 78,254) from the American Heart Association's Get With the Guidelines, after adjustment for baseline confounders, mortality was similar among women and men (adjusted OR, 1.04; 95% CI, 0.99 to 1.10). Among patients with ST-segment elevation MI, however, women had significantly higher mortality even after adjustment for age and other comorbidities (adjusted OR, 1.12; 95% CI, 1.02 to 1.23).[6] Results were similar in a meta-analysis of 136,247 patients randomized in 11 ACS trials from 1993 to 2006. In this analysis, women with ST-segment elevation MI were at a higher 30-day mortality risk than men (adjusted OR, 1.15; 95% CI, 1.06 to 1.24), and women with non–ST-segment elevation MI (adjusted OR, 0.77; 95% CI, 0.63 to 0.95) and unstable angina (adjusted OR, 0.55; 95% CI, 0.43 to 0.70) were at a lower 30-day mortality risk than men.[7] In a subset in which angiographic data were available, these differences may have been explained by the extent of coronary disease. These conclusions warrant caution, given known selection bias in the use of angiography in women, as discussed in later sections. In general, however, these observations suggest that understanding of the differences between men and women in the development or progression of cardiovascular disease, factors associated with outcome, use of proven therapies, and response to therapy is paramount.

Prevention and management of cardiovascular disease in women begin with awareness of the problem. Despite estimates that a 40-year-old woman has a lifetime risk of cardiovascular disease of 32%,[8] only about 55% of women identified cardiovascular disease as their greatest health risk in a 2006 survey conducted by the American Heart Association (AHA).[9] Physician awareness of women's cardiovascular risks is also suboptimal. In one study, only 71.2% of surveyed internists and obstetrics and gynecology specialists responded correctly to all 13 questions assessing knowledge about cardiac risk factors.[10]

Experts in industrialized societies have long recognized that the first presentation with coronary heart disease occurs approximately 10 years later among women than among men, and most commonly after menopause. The worldwide INTERHEART study, a large study of more than 52,000 individuals with MI, first demonstrated that this approximate 8- to 10-year difference in age at onset holds widely around the world, across various socioeconomic, climatic, and cultural environments (see Chap. 1).[11] Although coronary artery disease in general is manifested earlier in less developed countries, the age gap in time of onset between men and women is universal (**Table 81-1**). Despite this delay in onset, mortality from coronary heart disease is increasing more rapidly among women than among men in both the developed and developing world.[12] Risk factors were similar in all regions of the world, although the strength of association of some risk factors with MI varied between women and men, as discussed later.[11] Another important observation that supports the critical role of risk awareness

TABLE 81-1	Comparison of Age at First Myocardial Infarction Among Women and Men Across Geographic Regions	
REGION	MEDIAN AGE, WOMEN	MEDIAN AGE, MEN
Western Europe	68 (59-76)	61 (53-70)
Central and eastern Europe	68 (59-74)	59 (50-68)
North America	64 (52-75)	58 (49-68)
South America and Mexico	65 (56-73)	59 (50-68)
Australia and New Zealand	66 (59-74)	58 (50-67)
Middle East	57 (50-65)	50 (44-57)
Africa	56 (49-65)	52 (46-61)
South Asia	60 (50-66)	52 (45-60)
China and Hong Kong	67 (62-72)	60 (50-68)
Southeast Asia and Japan	63 (56-68)	55 (47-64)

Modified from Yusuf S, Hawken S, Õunpuu S, et al: Effect of potentially modifiable risk factors associated with myocardial infarction in 52 countries (the INTERHEART study): Case-control study. Lancet 364:937, 2004.

is that younger, premenopausal women—not older women—carry a mortality excess compared with similarly aged men presenting with MI in the National Registry of Myocardial Infarction (NRMI).[13]

Experts have widely speculated that this age difference reflects premenopausal protection from the development of atherosclerotic coronary disease afforded by circulating estrogen, which is markedly reduced at menopause. Despite this plausible biologic explanation, replacement of estrogen after menopause does not prevent clinical cardiovascular events.[14-17] An excellent review by Ouyang and colleagues[18] provides a summary of hormonal influence on atherosclerotic vascular disease and the spectrum of observational and clinical trials research on postmenopausal hormone therapy.

Coronary Artery Disease Risk Factors and Risk Factor Modification (see Chaps. 1, 2, 44, and 49)

The classic risk factors for coronary atherosclerosis are commonly divided into those that are potentially modifiable to mitigate risk (diabetes, hypertension, hyperlipidemia, cigarette smoking, obesity, and sedentary lifestyle) and those that are not modifiable (age and family history). With a few exceptions, these factors have similar influence on cardiovascular risk in both sexes.

Unmodifiable Risk Factors

AGE (see Chap. 80). Age is one of the most powerful risk factors for the development of cardiovascular disease and accompanying clinical events. Although the prevalence of cardiovascular disease with increasing age varies modestly by sex (prior to the fifth decade of life, prevalence in men is greater than in women, but prevalence equalizes in the sixth decade and in subsequent decades becomes greater in women), the magnitude of the association of age with clinical cardiovascular events is similar among men and women.[2]

FAMILY HISTORY. Coronary heart disease and death from cardiovascular disease have a hereditary component.[19,20] In a few families, the predilection for coronary disease is monogenic, with transmission occurring in a mendelian pattern (see Chaps. 8 and 44). In contrast, the majority of coronary artery disease is complex, likely reflecting multiple genes, each contributing modestly to a predisposition to atherosclerosis and atherothrombotic clinical events. The current use of genome-wide association studies is shedding considerable light in this regard (see Chaps. 7, 8 and 44).[21]

Whether sex differences exist in the frequency of genetic polymorphisms that influence the occurrence of cardiovascular events remains an open question. The statistical association of gene variants with coronary disease differs in men and women, suggesting that different pathways may operate in the manifestation of cardiovascular disease between the sexes.[22] Two of 112 polymorphisms in 71 candidate genes associated with MI in women: stromelysin 1, a member of the matrix metalloproteinase family of enzymes that are believed to be involved in plaque rupture (RR, 4.7; 99% CI, 2.0 to 12.2), and (much less strongly) plasminogen activator inhibitor 1 (PAI-1). In contrast, in men, two different genes associate with MI: the gap junction protein connexin37 (RR, 1.7; 95% CI, 1.1 to 1.6) and p22 (phox), a component of the NAD(P)H redox system (RR, 0.7; 95% CI, 0.6 to 0.9). This apparent sex-related difference in the association of genetic polymorphisms with clinical disease phenotypes may be less related to the presence or absence of the genetic mutation itself than to the influences of sex on variation in the expression of various genes or the downstream responses to gene products.

Variations in sex hormones and their levels between men and women or other differences related to the presence or absence of Y chromosome genes, including but not limited to those that regulate cellular function, could influence these observed associations. Indeed, ex vivo male macrophages responded to androgens with augmentation of 27 atherosclerosis-associated genes, resulting in increased foam cell formation and enhanced lysosomal low-density lipoprotein (LDL) cholesterol degradation, whereas ex vivo female cells did not show a response in any of the 588 genes tested.[23] Such differences may explain observed differences in the pathophysiology of atherosclerosis, including plaque composition (more cellular and fibrous tissue in women),[24] endothelial function (estrogen-induced coronary vasodilation), and hemostasis (higher fibrinogen and factor VII levels in women).[25-27] Furthermore, the underlying inciting pathophysiologic change of atherothrombotic coronary events varies in women and men and may be influenced by both genetics and sex-based differences, including the effects of estrogen that influence gene expression and protein production or activity. For example, women are twice as likely to have plaque erosion (37% in women versus 18% in men), and men more frequently have plaque rupture as the underlying inciting event (82% in men versus 63% in women).[28] With the continued evolution of ribonucleic acid (RNA) microarray technology, metabolomics, and proteomic capabilities, it will become increasingly feasible to determine expression patterns of tens of thousands of genes and the presence and relative abundance of their protein and metabolite products simultaneously. Although only limited work has explored sex differences in gene expression, proteomics, or metabolomics, further work in these areas may provide important insights into development, diagnosis, and tailored treatment of cardiovascular disease in women and men.

Potentially Modifiable Risk Factors

HYPERTENSION (see Chaps. 45 and 46). Hypertension is an increasingly common risk factor among the U.S. population, with 65 million affected individuals in National Health and Nutrition Examination Surveys (NHANES) from 1999 to 2000.[29] Overall, more than 35 million women had hypertension, a 15% higher prevalence than that in men. The prevalence of hypertension increased with age in both sexes, but from 45 to 54 years of age, the escalation was greater among women than among men, the difference in prevalence reaching statistical significance at 75 years of age and older. In subjects younger than 35 years of age, hypertension was significantly more prevalent among men than among women.

In a meta-analysis of 61 prospective studies of hypertension involving more than 1 million previously healthy adults between 49 and 89 years of age, the association with ischemic heart disease risk was only slightly stronger in women than in men.[30] The slope of the association between ischemic heart disease mortality and blood pressure was fairly constant, arguing against a "threshold" systolic pressure below which disease risk is not further reduced. An analysis of men and women in the Framingham Heart Study supports this position by showing that the gradient of cardiovascular risk extended to high-normal and normal blood pressures in both sexes.[31] .

Unfortunately, women remain one of the populations most likely to be undertreated when they have an established diagnosis of hypertension and, even more concerning, little progress has been made in improving rates of treatment and control during the past decade.

Whereas treatment and control rates in men increased by an absolute 9.8% and 15.3%, respectively, between the NHANE surveys spanning 1988 to 1994 and a follow-up survey from 1999 to 2000, the treatment and control rates in women were essentially unchanged (increases of only 1.9% and 0.5%, respectively).[32]

DIABETES AND THE METABOLIC SYNDROME (see Chaps. 44 and 64). The prevalence of diabetes in the United States is escalating rapidly. Between 2000 and 2001, it rose by 8.2%, and in the 11 years between 1990 and 2001, it rose by 61%; it is expected to double by 2050 across all age and sex groupings.[2] In 2006, women older than 20 years of age represented more than half (9.5 million) of the 17 million patients with known diabetes and accounted for 2.5 million of the estimated 6.4 million with undiagnosed diabetes.[2] Furthermore, of the 57 million people in the United States with prediabetes, defined as impaired glucose tolerance or a fasting blood glucose concentration of 110 to <126 mg/dL, women accounted for 23 million.[2] Cardiovascular disease is twice as common among women with diabetes as among those without, they are four times as likely to be hospitalized, and women have a higher risk for most clinical events and are less likely to be treated to HbA1c goal than men are.[2]

Metabolic syndrome relates closely to insulin resistance and comprises a constellation of at least three of the following risk factors: abdominal obesity, atherogenic lipid profile (excessive triglycerides or inadequate high-density lipoprotein [HDL] cholesterol), blood pressure of 130/85 mm Hg or higher, and fasting glucose concentration of 110 mg/dL or greater. At any given LDL-cholesterol level, metabolic syndrome increases the risk for coronary heart disease. Because of this, the National Cholesterol Education Program (NCEP) Adult Treatment Panel III considers metabolic syndrome a secondary target of risk reduction therapy.[33] After adjustment for age, metabolic syndrome appears to be highly prevalent in both sexes, with little difference in rates between women and men.[34]

HYPERLIPIDEMIA (see Chap. 47). According to summary statistics from the AHA, 47% of women older than 20 years of age have a total serum cholesterol level ≥200 mg/dL, and 31.7% have an LDL-cholesterol level ≥130 mg/dL—incidences similar to those in the general population.[2] More favorably, whereas 15.5% of Americans overall have an HDL level less than 40 mg/dL, only 6.7% of women are in this range.[2] The relative risk for coronary disease events associated with elevation of various lipid variables was determined in a nested case-control study from the Nurses' Health Study. Among 32,826 healthy women who provided blood samples at baseline, the multivariable adjusted relative risks (adjusted for high-sensitivity C-reactive protein [hs-CRP], homocysteine, and other traditional cardiac risk factors) for the highest quintiles of lipid variables were apolipoprotein B (RR, 4.1; 95% CI, 2 to 8.3), low levels of HDL (RR, 2.6; 95% CI, 1.4 to 5), LDL (RR, 3.1; 95% CI, 1.7 to 5.8), and triglycerides (RR, 1.9; 95% CI, 1.0 to 3.9).[35] Adverse changes in lipid profiles accompany menopause.[36] Perimenopausal triglyceride levels are the most erratic but follow roughly the same pattern of increase as total cholesterol and LDL cholesterol, which increase on average by an absolute 10% from levels at 6 months before menopause. Menopause influences HDL cholesterol less dramatically. HDL concentration declines gradually in the two years preceding menopause and then levels off after menopause. The postmenopausal increase in cardiovascular disease risk may result partly from these lipid alterations.

The 1988-1994 NHANES showed that serum cholesterol concentrations in U.S. adults were on a downward trend, but lipid profiles changed little between the 1988-1994 and 1999-2002 NHANES. In the follow-up survey, the prevalence of hypercholesterolemia was similar for men and women, and of all adults with high total cholesterol, only 35% were aware of their diagnosis, and rates were similar among men and women. Only 10.2% of dyslipidemic women were under treatment, compared with 12% overall, and among treated women, only 3.7% achieved a total cholesterol concentration of 5.2 mmol/liter compared with 5.4% overall.[37] As with hypertension, these findings highlight the need for a stronger commitment to prevention, treatment, and control of hypercholesterolemia, with an enhanced focus on women.

Lifestyle Risk Factors

In 2006, 60.5% of American women were overweight or obese, defined as a body mass index (BMI) greater than 25 kg/m².[2] The prevalence of obesity (BMI >30 kg/m²) in women increased gradually but markedly, from 12.2% in 1991 to 20.8% in 2001.[38] The 2005-2006 NHANES identified 35.3% of women as obese.[39] Furthermore, as summarized in the 2009 AHA Heart Disease and Stroke Statistics,[2] in conjunction with the obesity epidemic, the National Center for Health Statistics reported in 2005 that 12% of women engaged in no moderate to vigorous leisure time physical activity, and a 2007 National Health Interview Survey found that 66.3% of women never engaged in vigorous physical activity and only 9.8% of women engaged in vigorous activity 5 days or more per week. Objective NHANES accelerometer data were even more sobering; only 3.2% of women 20 to 59 years of age and only 2.5% older than 60 years of age met recommendations for at least 30 minutes of moderate to vigorous physical activity at least 5 days per week.[40] Perhaps more concerning for the future of heart disease in women, 31.8% of girls in grades 9 through 12 had not engaged in moderate to vigorous physical activity in the preceding 7 days,[41] and in another study, 31% of white girls and 56% of black girls 16 to 17 years of age engaged in no leisure time physical activity at all.[42] In 2006, the estimated prevalence of cigarette smoking among women 18 years of age or older was 18.1%, and 10.7% of girls 12 to 17 years of age and 23.6% 18 years of age or older reported smoking in the past month.[2]

Global Assessment of Risk Factors for Coronary Heart Disease (see Chap. 44)

Primary findings of the large, case-control INTERHEART study provide some of the best data to date on the relation of clinical parameters to the risk of ischemic heart disease worldwide, including patterns of association of MI risk among women compared with men.[11] Overall, after adjustment, nine risk factors accounted for 90.4% of the population attributable risk for MI (94% of the population attributable risk among women and 90% among men). The risk factors were apolipoprotein B/apolipoprotein A-I ratio, cigarette smoking, hypertension, diabetes, abdominal obesity, psychosocial factors (an index based on combining parameter estimates for depression, stress at work or home, financial stress, one or more life events, and locus of control scores), fruit and vegetable intake, exercise, and alcohol intake.

Although the strength of association of most risk factors with MI was similar among women and men, the INTERHEART study confirmed a markedly stronger association of diabetes with MI among women (**Fig. 81-1**).[11] Psychosocial factors also tended to associate more strongly with increased risk among women, although the difference was less in magnitude. In addition, healthy lifestyle choices including regular exercise and modest alcohol consumption provided stronger protection among women than among men, and fruit and vegetable intake tended to more greatly benefit women. Although further work is necessary to define the underpinnings of these observations, they nonetheless have important implications for counseling and management of women to prevent the development of cardiovascular disease.

The Framingham Risk Score remains the most widely used and authoritative tool to estimate global, long-term coronary artery disease risk in women, as in men. However, it may underestimate risk, especially in younger women,[43] and alternative algorithms have been proposed. These include the Reynolds Risk Score, which adds hs-CRP, HbA1c, and family history, increasing the predictive value from a C-statistic of 0.75 to 0.80.[44] Still other data suggest that atherosclerosis imaging may have particular value in women; in the MESA study, 32% of low-risk women had measurable coronary artery calcification, and the likelihood of death was closely related to coronary artery calcification score.[45]

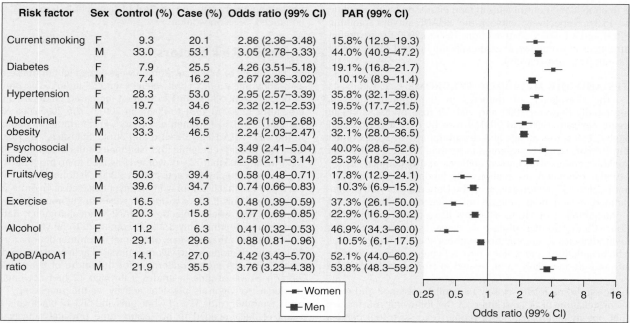

Risk factor	Sex	Control (%)	Case (%)	Odds ratio (99% CI)	PAR (99% CI)
Current smoking	F	9.3	20.1	2.86 (2.36–3.48)	15.8% (12.9–19.3)
	M	33.0	53.1	3.05 (2.78–3.33)	44.0% (40.9–47.2)
Diabetes	F	7.9	25.5	4.26 (3.51–5.18)	19.1% (16.8–21.7)
	M	7.4	16.2	2.67 (2.36–3.02)	10.1% (8.9–11.4)
Hypertension	F	28.3	53.0	2.95 (2.57–3.39)	35.8% (32.1–39.6)
	M	19.7	34.6	2.32 (2.12–2.53)	19.5% (17.7–21.5)
Abdominal obesity	F	33.3	45.6	2.26 (1.90–2.68)	35.9% (28.9–43.6)
	M	33.3	46.5	2.24 (2.03–2.47)	32.1% (28.0–36.5)
Psychosocial index	F	-	-	3.49 (2.41–5.04)	40.0% (28.6–52.6)
	M	-	-	2.58 (2.11–3.14)	25.3% (18.2–34.0)
Fruits/veg	F	50.3	39.4	0.58 (0.48–0.71)	17.8% (12.9–24.1)
	M	39.6	34.7	0.74 (0.66–0.83)	10.3% (6.9–15.2)
Exercise	F	16.5	9.3	0.48 (0.39–0.59)	37.3% (26.1–50.0)
	M	20.3	15.8	0.77 (0.69–0.85)	22.9% (16.9–30.2)
Alcohol	F	11.2	6.3	0.41 (0.32–0.53)	46.9% (34.3–60.0)
	M	29.1	29.6	0.88 (0.81–0.96)	10.5% (6.1–17.5)
ApoB/ApoA1 ratio	F	14.1	27.0	4.42 (3.43–5.70)	52.1% (44.0–60.2)
	M	21.9	35.5	3.76 (3.23–4.38)	53.8% (48.3–59.2)

FIGURE 81-1 Relative risks associated with various cardiac risk factors among men (M) and women (F) in the INTERHEART study. PAR = population attributable risk. *(From Yusuf S, Hawken S, Ôunpuu S, et al: Effect of potentially modifiable risk factors associated with myocardial infarction in 52 countries [the INTERHEART study]: Case-control study. Lancet 364:937, 2004.)*

Presentation with Acute Coronary Disease (see Chap. 53)

Symptoms commonly associated with MI in both sexes include chest pain, pressure, or squeezing; pain radiating to the neck, shoulder, back, arms, or jaw; palpitations; dyspnea; heartburn, nausea, vomiting, or abdominal pain; diaphoresis; and dizziness. Women may experience milder symptoms or describe them somewhat differently and may more frequently experience nonspecific prodromal symptoms, such as fatigue.[46] A study of 127 men and 90 women by Milner and colleagues[47] showed that among patients who presented to the emergency department with symptoms of coronary disease other than chest pain, there were several sex-related differences in symptoms. Dyspnea, nausea and vomiting, indigestion, fatigue, sweating, and arm or shoulder pain as presenting symptoms in the absence of chest pain were all more frequent among women than among men, but the Myocardial Infarction Triage and Intervention (MITI) Project investigators demonstrated that chest pain was present in almost all women (99.6%) and men (99%) who experienced a documented acute MI.[48] In addition to symptom differences, women with MI have more comorbidities, including hypertension, and present later in the course of symptoms and more frequently with high-risk clinical findings of heart failure and tachycardia.[49]

Women (4 million visits/year) are hospitalized more frequently than men (2.4 million visits/year) for the evaluation of chest pain,[2] but women who present with chest pain or even more clearly with ACS are more likely than men to have a noncardiac cause or other nonatherosclerotic causes, such as vasospasm.[50] The National Institutes of Health–sponsored Women's Ischemia Syndrome Evaluation (WISE) study confirmed a marked discordance between observed rates of obstructive coronary artery disease and the predicted probability of coronary disease (**Fig. 81-2**).[51] This discordance was pervasive across age groups, regardless of whether angina was classified as typical or atypical.

Imaging for Diagnosis and Prognosis

Compounding observations of differences in presentation and the discordance between predicted probability of disease and actual disease, there is a paucity of data regarding the best diagnostic strategy for assessment of women with chest pain to establish or to exclude a diagnosis of coronary artery disease. Thus, recommendations for the use of stress testing in women often derive from studies performed predominantly in men. Accuracy in the clinical setting is often confounded by the use of tests among women with low pretest probability, yielding multiple false-positive results. In one small study, however, the results of exercise stress testing according to the Duke Treadmill Score appeared as good for both diagnosis and prognosis in women as in men, with a higher negative predictive value in women.[52]

In general, recommendations for stress testing with imaging in women parallel those in men.[53] In a consensus statement from the AHA on imaging in women, Mieres and colleagues[54] summarized the available data on diagnostic stress testing and derived an algorithm to guide the use of exercise testing with or without cardiac imaging in women with chest pain. **Figure 81-3** demonstrates the algorithm for use in intermediate- or high-risk women with atypical or typical chest pain symptoms. Imaging in symptomatic women generally is recommended for those at intermediate or high risk for coronary artery disease. Both stress echocardiographic and stress gated myocardial single-photon emission computed tomographic nuclear imaging appear to perform similarly in women for diagnosis,[55] and both were given similar recommendations for stress testing in women in the AHA position statement.[54] Evidence suggests that the prognostic utility of either form of imaging with stress testing is similar (**Fig. 81-4**) and describes a gradient of risk that is similar in men and women.[55]

Evidence-Based Therapy in Women

WOMEN IN CLINICAL RESEARCH (see Chaps. 6 and 44). Randomized clinical trials with adequate power to demonstrate clinically meaningful differences between treatments, interventions, or management strategies should guide clinical practice. Assessment of treatment effect within a subgroup is usually underpowered and also fraught with the likelihood of type I error resulting from multiple comparisons. That said, consistency of findings across subgroups provides reassurance that the trial results are generalizable. Use of observational studies to assess treatment benefits and risks is complex and subject to multiple recognized and unrecognized biases, which may lead to erroneous conclusions. The story of hormone replacement therapy for primary and secondary prevention of cardiovascular events is an excellent example of the problems encountered in drawing inferences about treatment effects from nonrandomized cohorts. Multiple observational studies had shown dramatic reductions in coronary heart disease death or MI among users of hormone replacement therapy. However, a series of large randomized clinical trials later demonstrated that not only did hormone replacement therapy fail to reduce coronary heart disease events, but events actually increased in some cases among those randomly assigned to receive hormone therapy compared with those assigned to placebo treatment.[14-17]

Unfortunately, in a systematic review surveying the literature for all randomized controlled trials of MI from 1966 to 2000, Lee and colleagues[56] demonstrated that there was a marked discordance between the representation of women among MI patients and their representation in clinical trials (**Fig. 81-5**). Even in the most recent years of the survey, women sustained 45% of all MIs but represented only 27% of patients enrolled in randomized controlled trials of treatments for acute MI. Women were similarly underrepresented in the randomized controlled trials that formed the evidence base of support for the 2007 update of the AHA cardiovascular prevention guidelines for women.[57] These observations highlight that recruitment of women in proportion to their representation among patients with the cardiovascular disease of interest is paramount to support the application of the results of clinical trials to women. A 2007 "think tank" meeting of representatives from academia, industry, and regulatory agencies led to the suggestion of a number of strategies in four major areas to improve representation of women in the evidence base for the treatment of heart disease: improved clinical trial designs to optimize the study of women; appropriate incentives to conduct research in women; strategies to improve enrollment of women in clinical trials; and mandated reporting of results of clinical trials by sex.[58]

PRACTICE GUIDELINES TO CODIFY TREATMENT RECOMMENDATIONS. In general, American College of Cardiology/American Heart Association (ACC/AHA) guidelines for the management of ST-segment elevation and non–ST-segment elevation MI, as well as for chronic coronary disease, are silent or neutral on treatment by sex.[50,59-61] In addition to these "gender-neutral"

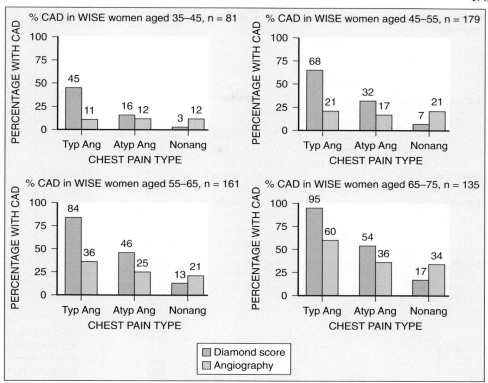

FIGURE 81-2 Observed rates of coronary artery disease (CAD) at angiography (yellow bars) compared with Diamond probability of CAD (purple bars). Atyp Ang = atypical angina; Nonang = nonanginal pain; Typ Ang = typical angina. *(From Shaw LJ, Bairey Merz CN, Pepine CJ, et al: Insights from the NHLBI-sponsored Women's Ischemia Syndrome Evaluation [WISE] Study. Part I: Gender differences in traditional and novel risk factors, symptom evaluation, and gender-optimized diagnostic strategies. J Am Coll Cardiol 47:4S, 2006.)*

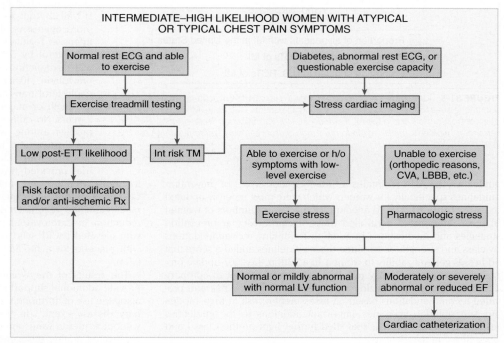

FIGURE 81-3 Algorithm for stress testing in women with moderate to high risk of coronary artery disease presenting with typical or atypical symptoms. CVA = cerebrovascular accident; ECG = electrocardiogram; EF = ejection fraction; ETT = exercise treadmill test; h/o = history of; LBBB = left bundle branch block; LV = left ventricular; TM = treadmill. *(From Mieres JH, Shaw LJ, Arai A, et al: Role of noninvasive testing in the clinical evaluation of women with suspected coronary artery disease: Consensus statement from the Cardiac Imaging Committee, Council of Clinical Cardiology, and the Cardiovascular Imaging and Intervention Committee, Council on Cardiovascular Radiology and Intervention, American Heart Association. Circulation 111:682, 2005.)*

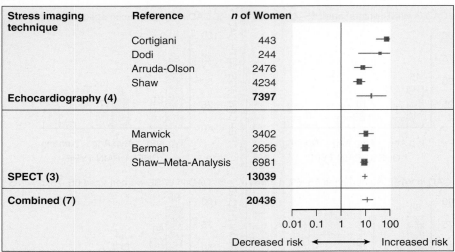

Stress imaging technique	Reference	n of Women	
	Cortigiani	443	
	Dodi	244	
	Arruda-Olson	2476	
	Shaw	4234	
Echocardiography (4)		**7397**	
	Marwick	3402	
	Berman	2656	
	Shaw–Meta-Analysis	6981	
SPECT (3)		**13039**	
Combined (7)		**20436**	

0.01 0.1 1 10 100

Decreased risk ←——→ Increased risk

FIGURE 81-4 Prognostic utility of echocardiographic and nuclear stress imaging among women. SPECT = single-photon emission computed tomography. *(From Shaw LJ, Vasey C, Sawada S, et al: Impact of gender on risk stratification by exercise and dobutamine stress echocardiography: Long-term mortality in 4234 women and 6898 men. Eur Heart J 26:447, 2005.)*

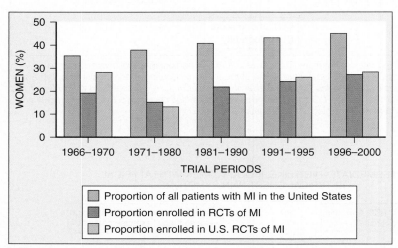

FIGURE 81-5 Underrepresentation of women in clinical trials of acute myocardial infarction (MI) relative to their representation among all patients with acute MI. RCTs = randomized controlled trials. *(From Lee PY, Alexander KP, Hammill BG, et al: Representation of elderly persons and women in published randomized trials of acute coronary syndromes. JAMA 286:708, 2001.)*

guidelines, the AHA maintains a broadly endorsed set of prevention guidelines specifically for women, which were most recently updated in 2007 (**Table 81-2**).[62] To account for the lower numbers of women in most randomized controlled trials of cardiovascular prevention strategies and medications, in addition to ranking recommendations by class and strength of evidence, these guidelines added a score that addresses generalizability to women. In addition, the 2007 update proposed managing the delay relative to men in the onset of coronary heart disease by emphasizing a perspective of lifetime risk and provided recommendations based on assessment of risk in high, moderate, and optimal categories. Important additions to the guidelines resulted from several trials that shed further light on the Class I and Class III recommendations.

The Women's Health Study randomized 39,876 healthy women older than 45 years to low-dose aspirin (100 mg on alternate days) or placebo and observed them for 10 years for first occurrence of death, nonfatal MI, or nonfatal stroke.[63] This trial provided important insights into the use of aspirin for primary prevention in women (see Chap. 44). Although the overall study showed a nonsignificant 9% reduction in the primary composite endpoint (RR, 0.91; 95% CI, 0.80 to 1.03), when the individual endpoints were examined, there was heterogeneity of effect. There was no effect of aspirin on the rate of nonfatal MI (RR, 1.02; 95% CI, 0.84 to 1.25) or cardiovascular death (RR, 0.95; 95% CI, 0.74 to 1.22), but aspirin reduced stroke risk by 17% overall (RR, 0.83; 95% CI, 0.69 to 0.99) and ischemic stroke by 24% (RR, 0.76; 95% CI, 0.63 to 0.93). Hemorrhagic stroke increased nonsignificantly (RR, 1.24; 95% CI, 0.82 to 1.87), but gastrointestinal bleeding requiring transfusion was significantly increased (RR, 1.40; 95% CI, 1.07 to 1.83). This study revealed significant age × treatment interactions for the effect of aspirin on the primary composite endpoint and the individual endpoint of nonfatal MI. Whereas the benefit of aspirin in reducing ischemic stroke was consistent across all age groups, only in those older than 65 years of age did aspirin significantly reduce the risk of nonfatal MI (RR, 0.66; 95% CI, 0.44 to 0.97). Thus, the use of aspirin in primary prevention requires a careful assessment of multiple potential risks and benefits of treatment before prescription in an individual woman. In a subsequent meta-analysis of all randomized trials of aspirin in primary prevention, aspirin reduced the rate of cardiovascular death, MI, or stroke by 12% (OR, 0.88; 95% CI, 0.79 to 0.99), largely because of a reduction in ischemic stroke (OR, 0.76; 95% CI, 0.63 to 0.93). There was no reduction in cardiovascular death or in MI alone, in contrast to men, in whom there was a 14% reduction in the composite of death, MI, or stroke, with a 32% reduction in MI but no reduction in ischemic stroke or cardiovascular death. Rates of bleeding were increased similarly in women and men.[64]

The Pravastatin or Atorvastatin Evaluation and Infection Trial–Thrombolysis In Myocardial Infarction 22 (PROVE IT-TIMI 22) trial demonstrated the safety and effectiveness of more aggressive lipid-lowering therapy with statins.[65] An intensive regimen of 80 mg of atorvastatin reduced LDL cholesterol by 51% to a median of 62 mg/dL, compared with a reduction of 22% to a median of 95 mg/dL in the pravastatin 40-mg arm. This greater reduction of LDL cholesterol translated into a 16% reduction in the hazard for death or major cardiac events at a mean follow-up of 2 years. No differences occurred in the safety or efficacy profiles among women and men. Even more recently, the Rosuvastatin to Prevent Vascular Events in Men and Women with Elevated C-Reactive Protein (JUPITER) trial provided firm evidence in primary prevention that for both women and men, treatment guided by hsCRP was beneficial among individuals whose cholesterol levels would not meet guideline recommendations for treatment. There was a 15% reduction in cardiovascular death, MI, and stroke among patients with elevated hsCRP who were treated with rosuvastatin compared with placebo for a median of 1.9 years (HR, 0.53; 95% CI, 0.40 to 0.69).[66]

The results of the Women's Health Initiative estrogen-only trial provide additional support for the Class III recommendation discouraging the use of hormone replacement therapy to prevent a first coronary disease event.[12] In this trial, 10,739 postmenopausal women without a uterus were randomized to placebo or 0.625 mg of oral conjugated equine estrogens daily. The trial was stopped early by its Data and Safety Monitoring Board in February 2004. At that point, there was no significant benefit of conjugated equine estrogens on the primary composite endpoint of death or nonfatal MI (RR, 0.91; 95% CI, 0.75 to 1.12), but the incidences of stroke (RR, 1.39; 95% CI, 1.10 to 1.77) and pulmonary embolus (RR, 1.34; 95% CI, 0.87 to 2.06) increased in the estrogen arm. Thus, it appears that no cardiovascular

TABLE 81-2 Recommendations from the 2007 American Heart Association Women's Evidence-Based Prevention Guidelines

CLINICAL AREA	RECOMMENDATIONS
Class I Recommendations	
Lifestyle interventions	Smoking cessation; avoid second-hand smoke
	30 minutes of moderate-intensity physical activity on most (preferably all) days of the week
	Cardiac rehabilitation/risk reduction program post-MI, post–coronary intervention, and if chronic angina
	Overall healthy eating pattern; limit saturated fat to <10% of calories, cholesterol to <300 mg/day; limit *trans* fatty acids
	Weight maintenance/reduction to BMI 18.5-24.9 kg/m² and waist circumference ≤35 inches
Major risk factor interventions	Encourage optimal BP <120/80 through lifestyle approaches
	Pharmacotherapy if BP <140/90 or lower if end-organ damage or diabetes
	Use thiazide diuretics unless absolute contraindication
	Optimal lipid targets: LDL <100 mg/dL, HDL <50 mg/dL, triglycerides <150 mg/dL, non–HDL cholesterol <130 mg/dL
	In high-risk women or elevated LDL, reduce intake of saturated fat to <7% of calories and cholesterol to <200 mg/day and reduce *trans* fatty acids
	Drug therapy for lipid abnormalities:
	High risk: initiate if LDL >100 mg/dL; statin therapy if high risk and LDL >100 mg/dL; niacin or fibrate if HDL is low or non–HDL cholesterol is high
	Intermediate risk: initiate if LDL >130 mg/dL; niacin or fibrate if HDL is low or non–HDL cholesterol is high
	Lifestyle approaches and pharmacotherapy to achieve near-normal (<7%) HbA1c in women with diabetes
Preventive drug regimens	Aspirin in high-risk women (75-162 mg daily) or clopidogrel if aspirin allergic or intolerant
	Beta blockers indefinitely post-MI unless contraindicated
	ACE inhibitors in high-risk women (post-MI, EF ≤40, or diabetes) unless contraindicated; ARBs in high-risk women who are intolerant of ACE inhibitors
Aldosterone blockade	Aldosterone blockade after MI if renal function and potassium are normal in women who are receiving therapeutic doses of ACE inhibitors and beta blockers who have EF ≤40 with symptomatic heart failure
Atrial fibrillation/stroke prevention	For chronic or paroxysmal atrial fibrillation, warfarin to INR 2.0-3.0 unless low risk
	Aspirin (325 mg daily) if contraindication to warfarin or at low risk for stroke (<1%/yr)
Class III Recommendations	
Hormone therapy	Do not start or continue estrogen plus progestin for primary or secondary prevention. Do not initiate or continue other forms of hormone therapy for prevention of cardiovascular disease pending results of ongoing trials.
Antioxidants	Do not use antioxidant supplements for cardiovascular disease prevention.
Folic acid	Do not use folic acid, with or without B₆ or B₁₂ supplementation, for cardiovascular disease prevention.
Aspirin	Routine use of aspirin in women <65 years of age is not recommended for MI prevention.

ACE = angiotensin-converting enzyme; ARB = angiotensin receptor blocker; BMI = body mass index; BP = blood pressure; EF = ejection fraction; HbA1c = hemoglobin A1c; HDL = high-density lipoprotein; INR = international normalized ratio; LDL = low-density lipoprotein; MI = myocardial infarction.

Modified from Mosca L, Banka CL, Benjamin EJ, et al: American Heart Association evidence-based guidelines for cardiovascular disease prevention in women: 2007 update. J Am Coll Cardiol 49:1230, 2007.

benefits and potential harm result from postmenopausal administration of conjugated equine estrogens. Because of these and similar results of other studies of hormone replacement therapy, the U.S. Food and Drug Administration has placed a black box warning on the labeling of all estrogen-containing compounds.

Finally, several trials of vitamin supplementation revealed no benefit and potential harm and resulted in Class III recommendations in the 2007 update of the Women's Prevention Guidelines (see Table 81-2).

ACC/AHA STEMI and UA/NSTEMI ACS Guidelines

The ST-segment elevation MI (STEMI) guidelines are silent on sex-specific recommendations, providing completely sex-neutral treatment recommendations.[59] The unstable angina/non–ST-segment elevation MI (UA/NSTEMI) guidelines provide the following Class I summary recommendation regarding the treatment of women: "Women with UA/NSTEMI should be managed in a manner similar to men. Specifically, women, like men with UA/NSTEMI, should receive aspirin and clopidogrel. Indications for noninvasive and invasive testing are similar in women and men. (*Level of Evidence: B*)."[50] However, the literature suggests that subtle differences exist between the sexes and that these have relevance to the care of individual patients (see later discussion).

Invasive Management and Revascularization

A meta-analysis of trials of percutaneous coronary intervention (PCI) confirmed that women suffer vascular complications of their procedures more frequently than men do.[67] In addition, many studies of predominantly elective PCI demonstrated higher in-hospital mortality among women than among men. Late mortality was similar between the sexes. Findings were similar for the use of primary PCI to treat acute MI, showing higher in-hospital mortality but similar late mortality.

Three randomized controlled trials of early invasive strategies for the management of non–ST-segment elevation MI showed conflicting results with regard to treatment benefit in women.[68-70] Although differences in the frequency of use of bypass surgery and the early hazard discussed may have contributed to these observations, Glaser and colleagues[68] demonstrated a critical principle of the relationship of risk-to-treatment benefit that may be even more salient in explaining the results of these trials. For low-risk patients (as evidenced by normal troponin levels), treatment effect becomes neutral, whereas it is modest overall and substantial among high-risk patients with positive troponins. These observations held with use of either the TIMI risk score or the presence or absence of ST-segment shifts to define risk categories. More recently, in a meta-analysis of eight randomized trials enrolling 3075 women and 7075 men (**Fig. 81-6** and Fig. 56-16), O'Donoghue and colleagues[71] confirmed that women benefit significantly from an invasive management strategy if they are biomarker positive (OR for death, MI, or rehospitalization for ACS, 0.67; 95% CI, 0.50 to 0.88) but not when they are biomarker negative (OR, 0.94; 95% CI, 0.61 to 1.44). Men benefited substantially if they were biomarker positive (OR, 0.56, 95% CI, 0.46 to 0.67) and trended toward benefit even when biomarker negative (OR 0.72; 95% CI, 0.51 to 1.01).

For a summary of coronary artery bypass grafting in women, consult the ACC/AHA guidelines for coronary artery bypass graft surgery.[72] In general, women have a higher risk for perioperative morbidity and mortality, but in many studies, much of this difference is explained by presentation of women at older ages and with more severe coronary disease, risk factors, and left ventricular dysfunction. Even at younger ages, and after adjustment for body size and other risk factors, women

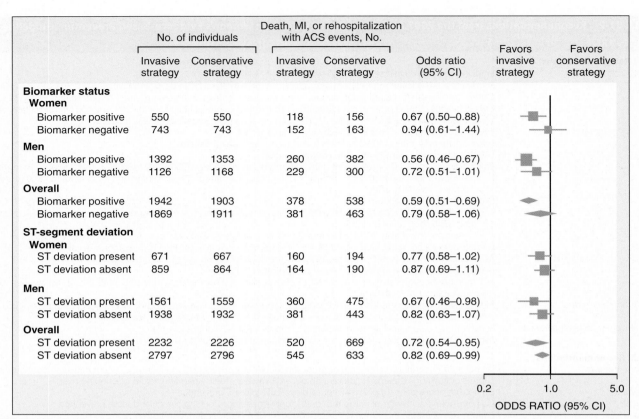

	No. of individuals		Death, MI, or rehospitalization with ACS events, No.		Odds ratio (95% CI)	Favors invasive strategy	Favors conservative strategy
	Invasive strategy	Conservative strategy	Invasive strategy	Conservative strategy			
Biomarker status							
Women							
Biomarker positive	550	550	118	156	0.67 (0.50–0.88)		
Biomarker negative	743	743	152	163	0.94 (0.61–1.44)		
Men							
Biomarker positive	1392	1353	260	382	0.56 (0.46–0.67)		
Biomarker negative	1126	1168	229	300	0.72 (0.51–1.01)		
Overall							
Biomarker positive	1942	1903	378	538	0.59 (0.51–0.69)		
Biomarker negative	1869	1911	381	463	0.79 (0.58–1.06)		
ST-segment deviation							
Women							
ST deviation present	671	667	160	194	0.77 (0.58–1.02)		
ST deviation absent	859	864	164	190	0.87 (0.69–1.11)		
Men							
ST deviation present	1561	1559	360	475	0.67 (0.46–0.98)		
ST deviation absent	1938	1932	381	443	0.82 (0.63–1.07)		
Overall							
ST deviation present	2232	2226	520	669	0.72 (0.54–0.95)		
ST deviation absent	2797	2796	545	633	0.82 (0.69–0.99)		

0.2   1.0   5.0
ODDS RATIO (95% CI)

FIGURE 81-6 Death, MI, or rehospitalization with ACS for biomarker status and ST-segment deviation in trials of an invasive versus conservative treatment strategy in non–ST-segment elevation ACS, from a meta-analysis of several trials. Odds ratios were generated from random-effects models. Size of data markers is weighted on the basis of the inverse variance. The odds ratios and corresponding P values for the interaction terms for the efficacy of an invasive over a conservative strategy in biomarker-positive versus biomarker-negative patients were as follows: for all patients, OR for interaction, 0.79; P for interaction = 0.18; for women, OR for interaction, 0.75; P for interaction = 0.36; and for men, OR for interaction, 0.77; P for interaction = 0.09. The analogous data for patients with versus without ST-segment deviation were as follows: for all patients, OR for interaction, 0.83; P for interaction = 0.07; for women, OR for interaction, 0.87; P for interaction = 0.76; and for men, OR for interaction, 0.79; P for interaction = 0.07. VINO, VANQWISH, and ICTUS trials were excluded from the primary biomarker analysis because they enrolled only patients with elevated biomarkers, thus precluding the comparison of biomarker-positive and biomarker-negative subgroups. The meta-analysis ORs and 95% CIs for the efficacy of an invasive strategy versus conservative strategy if those three trials were also included were as follows: for all patients biomarker positive, OR, 0.72; 95% CI, 0.53-0.98; for all patients biomarker negative, OR, 0.79; 95% CI, 0.60-1.03; for biomarker-positive men, OR, 0.71; 95% CI, 0.49-1.01; for biomarker-negative men, OR, 0.72; 95% CI, 0.54-0.98; for biomarker-positive women, OR, 0.71; 95% CI, 0.56-0.91; and for biomarker-negative women, OR, 0.94; 95% CI, 0.61-1.44. *(From O'Donoghue M, Boden WE, Braunwald E, et al: Early invasive vs conservative treatment strategies in women and men with unstable angina and non–ST-segment elevation myocardial infarction: A meta-analysis. JAMA 300:71, 2008.)*

may be at slightly higher perioperative risk than men are.[73] Women have more postoperative depression than men but ultimately appear to recover similarly, although some reports suggest that quality of life may be rated lower in women than in men as far out as 1 year.[74-76] Long-term survival depends more on concomitant disease and risk factors, and after adjustment, it is similar in women and men. Thus, the guidelines recommend: "Coronary bypass surgery should therefore not be delayed or denied to women who have the appropriate indications for revascularization."[72]

Glycoprotein IIb/IIIa Inhibitors

A similar picture emerges with the small molecule glycoprotein IIb/IIIa inhibitors, with initial studies indicating heterogeneity of treatment effect by sex. Although men appeared to benefit from eptifibatide treatment, women had an increased rate of death or MI at 30 days in the Platelet Glycoprotein IIb/IIIa in Unstable Angina: Receptor Suppression Using Integrilin Therapy (PURSUIT) trial.[77] A subsequent meta-analysis of all small molecule glycoprotein IIb/IIIa inhibitor (eptifibatide or tirofiban) trials revealed similar results in aggregate.[78] However, once patients were stratified by risk with troponin results, it was clear that the treatment benefit extended to both men and women at high risk for adverse outcomes, and that adverse outcomes occurred mostly in low-risk individuals.

The recently completed Early Glycoprotein IIb/IIIa Inhibition in Non–ST-Segment Elevation Acute Coronary Syndrome (EARLY ACS) trial of early versus delayed provisional eptifibatide use among patients with non–ST-segment elevation ACS provides additional assurance of the safety of glycoprotein IIb/IIIa inhibitors among women who are at high risk at presentation.[79] Among patients who had at least two of the following—age ≥60 years, ST-segment shifts on the presenting electrocardiogram, or positive biomarkers of myocardial necrosis (84% of patients were troponin positive)—women and men had similar reductions in the primary endpoint of death, MI, recurrent ischemia requiring urgent revascularization, or thrombotic bailout at 96 hours (8% for men versus 7% for women; P for interaction, 0.949). Surprisingly, there was a trend toward a reduction in death or MI at 30 days among women (OR, 0.80; 95% CI, 0.64 to 1.004; P = 0.052) but not among men (OR, 0.94; 95% CI, 0.81 to 1.09). In aggregate, these results suggest that selected properly, women stand to benefit similarly from glycoprotein IIb/IIIa inhibition, but in situations in which treatment benefit is less certain (e.g., biomarker-negative patients), risks—particularly of bleeding—may predominate.

Bleeding with Antithrombotic Therapy

The differential treatment effects observed among women and men with the small molecule glycoprotein IIb/IIIa inhibitors and the relationship with risk for ischemic complications may be explained partly by the counterbalancing higher risk for complications of therapy, particularly bleeding. In a recent analysis from the Can Rapid Risk Stratification of Unstable Angina Patients Suppress Adverse Outcomes with Early Implementation of the ACC/AHA Guidelines (CRUSADE) registry, of patients receiving antithrombotic therapy with unfractionated heparin, enoxaparin, or a small molecule glycoprotein IIb/IIIa inhibitor, 42% received at least one initial dose outside of recommended dosing ranges.[80] Such overdosing associated with increased likelihood of bleeding that increased with the number of agents that were overdosed. Women were significantly more likely to be overdosed than were men, in part because of advanced age and associated renal impairment as well as lower body weight. Several studies have now shown that bleeding and the use of blood transfusions are associated with increased ischemic outcomes among patients with ACS[81-83]; thus, treatment of women at lower risk for adverse ischemic outcomes exposes them to both inherent bleeding risks of treatment and those associated with inappropriate dosing, to which they are more prone, that may offset or exceed any benefit of therapy. Careful attention, particularly to adjustments in dosing for body weight and estimated creatinine clearance, is critically important to ensure safe use of these therapies.

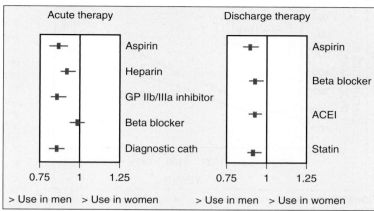

FIGURE 81-7 Use of guidelines-recommended therapies among women compared with men in the CRUSADE registry. ACEI = angiotensin-converting enzyme inhibitor; cath = cardiac catheterization; GP IIb/IIIa = glycoprotein IIb/IIIa. *(From Blomkalns AL, Chen AY, Hochman JS, et al; CRUSADE Investigators: Gender disparities in the diagnosis and treatment of non–ST-segment elevation acute coronary syndromes: Large-scale observations from the CRUSADE [Can Rapid Risk Stratification of Unstable Angina Patients Suppress Adverse Outcomes with Early Implementation of the American College of Cardiology/American Heart Association Guidelines] National Quality Improvement Initiative. J Am Coll Cardiol 45:832, 2005.)*

Sex Differences in Treatment

Despite abundant data in aggregate to support the use of existing evidence-based therapy similarly among women and men and sex-neutral practice guidelines for their use, undertreatment of women relative to men persists. In an analysis from the CRUSADE registry of patients with non–ST-segment elevation ACS, use of all therapies for acute management, including invasive management, and discharge management were suboptimal; but after adjustment for confounders, use of guidelines-recommended therapies and invasive management was lower in women than in men for all agents except beta-adrenergic receptor blockers (beta blockers) in the acute setting (**Fig. 81-7**).[84] These differences do not appear to be influenced by differences in objective measures of risk, such as troponin positivity or level of troponin elevation.[85] Among more than 345,000 patients with ST-segment elevation MI, the NRMI-1 investigators similarly observed lower rates of use of aspirin, beta blockers, and heparin in women compared with men and later administration of fibrinolytic therapy among women.[86] Using data from 78,254 patients in the Guidelines Applied in Practice data base, Jneid and colleagues[87] showed that in addition to lower use of guidelines-recommended medications, women had lower use of reperfusion therapy when eligible and also had longer times to either fibrinolytic therapy or primary PCI for ST-segment elevation MI. Equally important, women appear to have greater risk than men for nonadherence to long-term use of evidence-based medications in secondary prevention, particularly aspirin, statins, and angiotensin-converting enzyme (ACE) inhibitors.[88] Although the cause of these disparities in treatment and adherence is likely multifactorial, concerted efforts to correct them will be necessary for women to achieve the full potential of available therapies.

One important component of the strategy to improve adherence to cardiovascular disease guidelines is women's awareness of disease risk and physicians' awareness of guidelines and ability to correctly assess and assign risk level. Although the number of women who recognize cardiovascular disease as the leading cause of death among women has increased to 55% in a recent survey, in that same survey only 48% of women correctly identified the optimal level for blood pressure, 37% for HDL, 21% for LDL, and 31% for blood glucose concentration.[89] When present, though, individual awareness that one's level was not healthy did prompt initiation of steps to lower risk.

In a related study, 500 randomly selected physicians were surveyed about their awareness of and adherence to cardiovascular prevention guidelines.[90] Surprisingly, fewer than 1 in 5 physicians knew that more women than men die each year from cardiovascular disease. Using

case studies, the investigators evaluated physicians' assessment of a patient's risk. Regardless of specialty, assignment of risk strongly associated with the recommendation for lifestyle or treatment interventions, but more women at calculated intermediate risk were perceived by physicians as being at low risk than occurred for intermediate-risk men. Thus, improved physician assessment of risk may be important in reducing undertreatment relative to guidelines recommendations.

Use of standardized treatment algorithms and participation in quality improvement programs may improve overall adherence to treatment guidelines and lessen sex-related undertreatment. The ACC's Guidelines Applied in Practice discharge tool is one such strategy that appears to be effective in increasing the use of guidelines-recommended therapies at discharge in both men and women.[91] Use of the tool may be associated with lower mortality among women at 1 year.

Cardiac Rehabilitation (see Chap. 50)

In a 2004 systematic review and meta-analysis of randomized controlled trials of exercised-based cardiac rehabilitation after MI that represented 48 trials since 1970, 21 included only men, 26 included both men and women, and 20% of all participants were women.[92] In aggregate, these trials showed a 20% reduction in total mortality and a 26% reduction in cardiac mortality among patients randomized to exercise-based cardiac rehabilitation compared with controls receiving usual care. Improvements in lipid levels and blood pressure and greater rates of smoking cessation were also found. Detailed analyses of men and women were not performed, but conclusions were general regarding the benefits of exercise-based cardiac rehabilitation after MI. In keeping with these findings, the ACC/AHA guidelines for the management of patients with ST-segment elevation MI provide a Class I recommendation for "cardiac rehabilitation/secondary prevention programs, when available … for patients with STEMI, particularly those with multiple modifiable risk factors and/or those moderate- to high-risk patients in whom supervised exercise training is warranted. (*Level of Evidence: C*)."[56] The guidelines for the management of patients with non–ST-segment elevation ACS recommend such programs especially for individuals who smoke.[50] Despite these recommendations, women are less likely than men to participate in cardiac rehabilitation after acute MI.[93]

Heart Failure (see Chaps. 26 to 30)

The prevalence of heart failure is increasing in both sexes. Although both the incidence and prevalence of heart failure are greater among

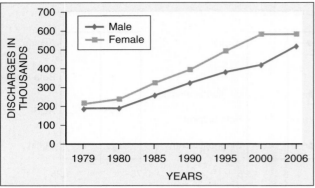

FIGURE 81-8 Trends in hospital discharges for heart failure from 1979 to 2006 by sex. *(From Lloyd-Jones D, Adams R, Carnethon M, et al: Heart disease and stroke statistics—2009 update: A report from the American Heart Association Statistics Committee and Stroke Statistics Subcommittee. Circulation 119:e21, 2009.)*

men than among women, the lifetime risk for development of heart failure among women and men at the age of 40 years is greater among women (1 in 6) than among men (1 in 9).[2] In 2004, women accounted for 57% of heart failure deaths, and heart failure continues to complicate acute MI more frequently in women than in men.[2] Although women accounted for more hospital discharges for heart failure each year than did men through 2000, that gap has narrowed through most recent estimates in 2006 (**Fig. 81-8**).[2]

The underlying pathophysiologic process of heart failure may be different in women and men. In the Medicare population, 80% of patients with heart failure and preserved systolic function are women (see Chap. 30).[94] Alcoholic cardiomyopathy occurs less frequently in women than in men, but this may be because of the lower prevalence of alcoholism among women; alcohol may actually be more toxic to the myocardium in women, with a lower total dose required to produce cardiomyopathy.[95] In a study of 105,388 patients admitted with acute decompensated heart failure, women accounted for 52% of cases but had preserved left ventricular function more frequently than men did (51% versus 28%).[96] Men and women had similar length of stay and adjusted in-hospital mortality; diuretic therapy was used similarly, but women received vasoactive agents less frequently. Although both sexes were undertreated with evidence-based oral therapies for heart failure, women were less likely than men to receive them. Additional data from the Acute Decompensated Heart Failure National Registry (ADHERE) indicate that approximately half of patients admitted for management of heart failure have preserved systolic function, and that these patients are more frequently women.[97] Reports from both the Mayo Clinic and the province of Ontario, Canada, reflect these findings of female prevalence among patients with heart failure with preserved left ventricular function.[98,99] Furthermore, these reports show an increasing prevalence of heart failure with preserved left ventricular function and indicate that its prognosis, which is similar to that of heart failure with systolic dysfunction, has remained essentially unchanged for more than a decade.

Because most evidence for the management of heart failure arises from trials in which left ventricular systolic dysfunction predominated or was a critical inclusion criterion and in which men predominated, assessment of the utility of these therapies in women is challenging—particularly when preserved systolic function is much more prominent among women with heart failure. The Candesartan in Heart Failure: Assessment of Reduction in Mortality and Morbidity (CHARM) clinical trials shed light on the treatment of both women and men with heart failure with preserved systolic function. In an aggregate analysis of CHARM trials, women more frequently had preserved systolic function (50%) than did men (35%). In these trials, despite generally lower use of evidence-based treatments for heart failure, women had lower adjusted mortality and the composite of death or heart failure hospitalization, regardless of cause of heart failure or left ventricular function. Benefit from treatment with candesartan, an angiotensin II receptor blocker, was identical in women and men.[100]

The current ACC/AHA heart failure guidelines recommend the following as a Class I recommendation: "Groups of patients including (a) high-risk ethnic minorities (e.g., blacks), (b) groups underrepresented in clinical trials, and (c) any groups believed to be underserved should, in the absence of specific evidence to direct otherwise, have clinical screening and therapy in a manner identical to that applied to the broader population. (*Level of Evidence: B*)."[101] In women, caution should be used in digoxin dosing, especially among elderly women with diminished renal function, and recognition of different side effect profiles, such as increased frequency of cough with ACE inhibitors, may be important.[101]

Implantable cardioverter-defibrillator (ICD) device implantation and cardiac resynchronization therapy are increasingly important components of the management of patients with heart failure and ischemic heart disease with left ventricular systolic dysfunction. The utility of and indication for ICD implantation and cardiac resynchronization therapy are reviewed in Chaps. 29 and 38. An excellent review on this topic by Goldberger and Lampert[102] is also available. Although multiple studies have provided evidence for use of these therapies, none of the studies, alone or in aggregate, have enrolled sufficient numbers of patients to allow meaningful conclusions about utility in women compared with men. Guidelines are therefore broadly inclusive and recommend use of ICD therapy for secondary prevention in all patients with "otherwise good clinical function and prognosis, for whom prolongation of survival is a goal."[101] As with the application of many therapies discussed previously, however, there is a substantial gap between men and women in the use of ICD therapy. In an analysis from the Guidelines Applied in Practice data base, only 35.4% of eligible patients received ICD therapy after MI. Relative to white men, both white women and black women were substantially less likely to receive an ICD (white women: OR, 0.62; 95% CI, 0.56 to 0.68; black women: OR, 0.56; 95% CI, 0.44 to 0.71).[103] Results were similar in older patients in the 2005 Centers for Medicare and Medicaid Services 5% sample data base. In this analysis of patients older than 65 years of age, men were more than three times as likely as women to receive an ICD when indicated for primary prevention (HR, 3.15; 95% CI, 2.86 to 3.47), but there was no reduction in mortality in the year after implantation among those who received an ICD.[104] For secondary prevention, men also more frequently received ICD therapy than women did (HR, 2.44; 95% CI, 2.30 to 2.59). In this setting, ICD therapy associated with 35% lower mortality among those who received an ICD.

Transplantation for the treatment of heart failure is used less frequently in women than in men. This is in part because of the older age of women with heart failure and differences in women's desires for transplantation.[105] According to AHA statistics, in the United States in 2004, 72.4% of transplant patients were men.[2] Among transplanted patients, 1-year survival rates were only slightly less among women (84.6%) compared with men (86.4%). This gap widened slightly at 3 years (76.1% versus 78.9%, respectively, in women and men) and at 5 years (68.5% versus 72.2%).

For a recent summary of heart failure etiology, diagnosis, and treatment in women, consult the excellent review by Hsich and Piña.[106]

Peripheral Arterial Disease (see Chap. 61)

Approximately 8 million Americans are believed to have lower extremity peripheral arterial disease, and their risk of death from cardiovascular disease is nearly sixfold greater than that of individuals without peripheral arterial disease.[2] As with coronary disease, the prevalence is slightly higher in men than in women.[107] Smoking and diabetes are the most potent risk factors for peripheral arterial disease. According to AHA 2009 summary statistics, only 10% of patients complain of classic intermittent claudication (ranging from 6/10,000 among men 30 to 44 years of age and 3/10,000 among women 30 to 44 years of age to 61/10,000 among men 65 to 74 years of age and 54/10,000 among women 65 to 74 years of age); 40% have no leg symptoms, and 50% have other atypical symptoms.[2] Particularly in elderly women, up to 66% may have no symptoms at all. For an in-depth summary of the epidemiology, diagnosis, and management of peripheral arterial disease, consult the 2005 AHA/ACC practice guidelines.[108] Recommendations for diagnosis and management generally are sex neutral. Interestingly, despite the higher cardiovascular risk among patients with peripheral vascular disease, use of aspirin for primary prevention among patients with ankle-brachial indices below 0.95 did not significantly improve outcomes compared with placebo in the 3350-patient Aspirin for Asymptomatic Atherosclerosis trial (results presented at the 2009 Scientific Sessions of the European Society of Cardiology, August 30, 2009), but the trial may have been underpowered considering the 12% reduction in primary prevention in the recent Antithrombotic Trialists' meta-analysis.[109]

The population prevalence of renal artery stenosis is not well established; but in older adults, it was determined in one study to be 8.4% and was more common in men (9.1%) than in women (5.5%).[110] About 90% of lesions are caused by atherosclerosis, but fibromuscular dysplasia is a particularly prevalent pathophysiologic finding in young women with hypertension and renal artery stenosis.[108] Guidelines for diagnosis and treatment are similar in women and in men.

Mesenteric arterial disease predominates in women; approximately two thirds of acute presentations are in elderly women (median age, 70 years), and 70% of chronic intestinal ischemia occurs in women.[108] Without treatment, acute intestinal ischemia is nearly always fatal. Surgical treatment to remove ischemic bowel and revascularize is given a Class I, B level of evidence recommendation in the guidelines for management of peripheral arterial disease.[108] Despite surgical treatment, mortality remains at approximately 70%. Percutaneous revascularization and surgical revascularization are recommended in the appropriate settings (see Chap. 63).[108] Abdominal aortic aneurysms caused by atherosclerotic disease are more prevalent in men than in women and are more prevalent in both sexes among older individuals and smokers.[108] Although treatment recommendations are sex neutral, screening of asymptomatic individuals is recommended in men but not in women because of the low number of abdominal aortic aneurysm–related deaths in women <75 years and the many competing health risks in older women.[111]

Future Perspectives

Cardiovascular disease is common among women, and as the population ages, the number of women living with coronary disease and its sequelae, such as heart failure, will only increase. In general, although underrepresentation of women in clinical trials persists, most existing treatments appear to be equally effective in women and men. Despite increasing awareness among physicians and women about cardiovascular disease risk, women are more likely to be undertreated and for some therapies are more susceptible to complications. Increased attention to careful selection of therapies according to risk and careful monitoring of dosing will be imperative to modulate the balance of benefit and risk in women. The growth in our understanding of genetic susceptibility to cardiovascular disease and rapid advances in genomic, proteomic, and metabolomic techniques promise to elucidate further the underpinnings of differences in disease pathophysiology in men and women that may ultimately lead to new therapies and perhaps the sex-specific application of new or existing therapies in the coming years.

REFERENCES

General and Risk Factors in Women

1. Wizemann TM, Pardue ML (eds): Institute of Medicine Committee on Understanding the Biology of Sex and Gender Differences. Exploring the Biological Contributions to Human Health. Does Sex Matter? Washington, DC, National Academy Press, 2001.
2. Lloyd-Jones D, Adams R, Carnethon M, et al: Heart disease and stroke statistics—2009 update: A report from the American Heart Association Statistics Committee and Stroke Statistics Subcommittee. Circulation 119:e21, 2009.
3. Shaw LJ, Merz CN, Pepine CJ, et al: The economic burden of angina in women with suspected ischemic heart disease: Results from the National Institutes of Health–National Heart, Lung and Blood Institute–sponsored Women's Ischemia Syndrome Evaluation. Circulation 114:894, 2006.
4. Ford ES, Ajani UA, Croft JB, et al: Explaining the decrease in U.S. deaths from coronary disease, 1980-2000. N Engl J Med 356:2388, 2007.
5. Ford ES, Capewell S: Coronary heart disease mortality among young adults in the U.S. from 1980 through 2002: Concealed leveling of mortality rates. J Am Coll Cardiol 50:2128, 2007.
6. Jneid H, Fonarow GC, Cannon CP, et al: Sex differences in medical care and early death after acute myocardial infarction. Circulation 118:2803, 2008.
7. Berger JS, Elliott L, Gallup D, et al: Sex differences in mortality following acute coronary syndromes. JAMA 302:874, 2009.
8. Lloyd-Jones DM, Larson MG, Beiser A, Levy D: Lifetime risk of developing coronary heart disease. Lancet 353:89, 1999.
9. Mosca L, Mochari H, Christian A, et al: National study of women's awareness, preventive action, and barriers to cardiovascular health. Circulation 113:525, 2006.
10. Barnhart J, Lewis V, Houghton JL, Charney P: Physician knowledge levels and barriers to coronary risk prevention in women: Survey results from the women and heart disease physician education initiative. Women's Health Issues 17:93, 2007.
11. Yusuf S, Hawken S, Ôunpuu S, et al: Effect of potentially modifiable risk factors associated with myocardial infarction in 52 countries (the INTERHEART study): Case-control study. Lancet 364:937, 2004.
12. Yusuf S, Reddy S, Ôunpuu S, Anand S: Global burden of cardiovascular diseases: Part I: General considerations, the epidemiologic transition, risk factors, and impact of urbanization. Circulation 104:2746, 2001.
13. Vaccarino V, Parsons L, Every NR, et al: Sex-based differences in early mortality after myocardial infarction. National Registry of Myocardial Infarction 2 Participants. N Engl J Med 341:217, 1999.

Hormone Therapy

14. Hulley S, Grady D, Bush T, et al: Randomized trial of estrogen plus progestin for secondary prevention of coronary heart disease in postmenopausal women. JAMA 280:605, 1998.
15. Grady D, Herrington D, Bittner V, et al: Cardiovascular disease outcomes during 6.8 years of hormone therapy: Heart and Estrogen/Progestin Replacement Study follow-up (HERS II) [erratum in JAMA 288:1064, 2002]. JAMA 288:49, 2002.
16. Manson JE, Hsia J, Johnson KC, et al: Estrogen plus progestin and the risk of coronary heart disease. N Engl J Med 349:523, 2003.
17. Women's Health Initiative Steering Committee: Effects of conjugated equine estrogen in postmenopausal women with hysterectomy: The Women's Health Initiative randomized controlled trial. JAMA 291:1701, 2004.
18. Ouyang P, Michos ED, Karas RH: Hormone replacement therapy and the cardiovascular system: Lessons learned and unanswered questions. J Am Coll Cardiol 47:1741, 2006.

Genetics

19. Zdravkovic S, Wienke A, Pedersen NL, et al: Heritability of death from coronary heart disease: A 36-year follow-up of 20 966 Swedish twins. J Intern Med 252:247, 2002.
20. Murabito JM, Pencina MJ, Nam BH, et al: Sibling cardiovascular disease as a risk factor for cardiovascular disease in middle-aged adults. JAMA 294:3117, 2005.
21. Paynter NP, Chasman DI, Pare G, et al: Association between a literature-based genetic risk score and cardiovascular events in women. JAMA 303:631, 2010.
22. Yamada Y, Izawa H, Ichihara S, et al: Prediction of the risk of myocardial infarction from polymorphisms in candidate genes. N Engl J Med 347:1916, 2002.

Mechanisms of Coronary Artery Disease in Women

23. Ng MKC, Quinn CM, McCrohon JA, et al: Androgens up-regulate atherosclerosis-related genes in macrophages from males but not females: Molecular insights into gender differences in atherosclerosis. J Am Coll Cardiol 42:1306, 2003.
24. Kramer MC, Rittersma SZ, de Winter RJ, et al: Relationship of thrombus healing to underlying plaque morphology in sudden coronary death. J Am Coll Cardiol 55:122, 2010.
25. English JL, Jacobs LO, Green G, et al: Effect of the menstrual cycle on endothelium dependent vasodilation of the brachial artery in normal young women. Am J Cardiol 82:256, 1998.
26. Sader MA, McCredie RJ, Griffiths KA, et al: Oestradiol improves arterial endothelial function in healthy men receiving testosterone. Clin Endocrinol (Oxf) 54:175, 2001.
27. Weksler B: Hemostasis and thrombosis. In Douglas PS (ed): Cardiovascular Health and Disease in Women. 2nd ed. Philadelphia, WB Saunders, 2002, pp 157-177.
28. Virmani R, Burke AP, Farb A, Kolodgie FD: Pathology of the vulnerable plaque. J Am Coll Cardiol 47(Suppl):C13, 2006.

Specific Risk Factors in Women

29. Fields LE, Burt VL, Cutler JA, et al: The burden of adult hypertension in the United States 1999 to 2000: A rising tide. Hypertension 44:398, 2004.
30. Prospective Studies Collaboration: Age-specific relevance of usual blood pressure to vascular mortality: A meta-analysis of individual data for one million adults in 61 prospective studies. Lancet 360:1903, 2002.
31. Vasan RS, Larson MG, Leip EP, et al: Impact of high-normal blood pressure on the risk of cardiovascular disease. N Engl J Med 345:1291, 2001.
32. Hajjar I, Kotchen TA: Trends in prevalence, awareness, treatment, and control of hypertension in the United States, 1988-2000. JAMA 290:199, 2003.
33. Expert Panel on Detection, Evaluation, and Treatment of High Blood Cholesterol in Adults: Executive Summary of the Third Report of the National Cholesterol Education Program (NCEP) Expert Panel on Detection, Evaluation, and Treatment of High Blood Cholesterol in Adults (Adult Treatment Panel III). JAMA 285:2486, 2001.
34. Ford ES, Giles WH, Dietz WH: Prevalence of the metabolic syndrome among US adults: Findings from the third National Health and Nutrition Examination Survey. JAMA 287:356, 2002.
35. Shai I, Rimm EB, Hankinson SE, et al: Multivariate assessment of lipid parameters as predictors of coronary heart disease among postmenopausal women: Potential implications for clinical guidelines. Circulation 110:2824, 2004.
36. Jensen J, Nilas L, Christiansen C: Influence of menopause on serum lipids and lipoproteins. Maturitas 12:321, 1990.
37. Ford ES, Mokdad AH, Giles WH, Mensah GA: Serum total cholesterol concentrations and awareness, treatment, and control of hypercholesterolemia among US adults: Findings from the National Health and Nutrition Examination Survey, 1999 to 2000. Circulation 107:2185, 2003.

38. Mokdad AH, Ford ES, Bowman BA, et al: Prevalence of obesity, diabetes, and obesity-related health risk factors, 2001. JAMA 289:76, 2003.

39. Ogden CL, Carroll MD, McDowell MA, Flegal KM: Obesity among adults in the United States: No statistically significant change since 2003-2004. NCHS Data Brief No 1. Hyattsville, Md, National Center for Health Statistics, 2007.

40. Troiano RP, Berrigan D, Dodd KW, et al: Physical activity in the United States measured by accelerometer. Med Sci Sports Exerc 40:181, 2008.

41. Eaton DK, Kann L, Kinchen S, et al; Centers for Disease Control and Prevention (CDC): Youth risk behavior surveillance: United States, 2007. MMWR Surveill Summ 57:1, 2008.

42. Kimm SY, Glynn NW, Kriska AM, et al. Decline in physical activity in black girls and white girls during adolescence. N Engl J Med 347:709, 2002.

43. Ford ES, Giles WH, Mokdad AH: The distribution of 10-year risk for coronary heart disease among US adults: Findings from the National Health and Nutrition Examination Survey III. J Am Coll Cardiol 43:1791, 2004.

44. Ridker PM, Buring JE, Rifai N, Cook NR: Development and validation of improved algorithms for the assessment of global cardiovascular risk in women: The Reynolds Risk Score. JAMA 297:611, 2007.

45. Lakoski SG, Greenland G, Wong ND, et al: Coronary artery calcium scores and risk for cardiovascular events in women classified as "low risk" based on Framingham Risk Score: The Multi-Ethnic Study of Atherosclerosis (MESA). Arch Intern Med 167:2437, 2007.

46. Kyker KA, Limacher MC: Gender differences in presentation and symptoms of coronary artery disease. Curr Womens Health Rep 2:115, 2002.

47. Milner KA, Funk M, Richards S, et al: Gender differences in symptom presentation associated with coronary heart disease. Am J Cardiol 84:396, 1999.

48. Kudenchuk PJ, Maynard C, Martin JS, et al: Comparison of presentation, treatment, and outcome of acute myocardial infarction in men versus women (The Myocardial Infarction Triage and Intervention Registry). Am J Cardiol 78:9, 1996.

49. McGuire DK, Newby LK, Biswas MS, Hochman JS: The elderly, women, and patients with diabetes mellitus. In Theroux P (ed): Acute Coronary Syndromes: A Companion to Braunwald's Heart Disease. Philadelphia, Elsevier Science, 2003, pp 553-573.

50. Braunwald E, Antman EM, Beasley JW, et al: ACC/AHA guidelines update for the management of patients with unstable angina and non–ST-segment elevation myocardial infarction. A report of the American College of Cardiology/American Heart Association Task Force on Practice Guidelines (Committee on the Management of Patients with Unstable Angina), 2002. Available at: http://www.acc.org/clinical/guidelines/unstable/unstable.pdf. Accessed June 30, 2006.

51. Shaw LJ, Bairey Merz CN, Pepine CJ, et al: Insights from the NHLBI-sponsored Women's Ischemia Syndrome Evaluation (WISE) Study. Part I: Gender differences in traditional and novel risk factors, symptom evaluation, and gender-optimized diagnostic strategies. J Am Coll Cardiol 47:4S, 2006.

52. Alexander KP, Shaw LJ, DeLong ER, et al: Value of exercise treadmill testing in women. J Am Coll Cardiol 32:1657, 1998.

53. Gibbons RJ, Balady GJ, Bricker JT, et al: ACC/AHA Guidelines update for exercise testing. A report of the American College of Cardiology/American Heart Association Task Force on Practice Guidelines (Committee on Exercise Testing), 2002. Available at: www.acc.org/clinical/guidelines/exercise/dirIndex.htm. Accessed July 16, 2006.

54. Mieres JH, Shaw LJ, Arai A, et al: Role of noninvasive testing in the clinical evaluation of women with suspected coronary artery disease: Consensus statement from the Cardiac Imaging Committee, Council of Clinical Cardiology, and the Cardiovascular Imaging and Intervention Committee, Council on Cardiovascular Radiology and Intervention, American Heart Association. Circulation 111:682, 2005.

55. Shaw LJ, Vasey C, Sawada S, et al: Impact of gender on risk stratification by exercise and dobutamine stress echocardiography: Long-term mortality in 4234 women and 6898 men. Eur Heart J 26:447, 2005.

56. Lee PY, Alexander KP, Hammill BG, et al: Representation of elderly persons and women in published randomized trials of acute coronary syndromes. JAMA 286:708, 2001.

57. Melloni C, Wang TY, Pieper KS, et al: Representation of women in randomized clinical trials of cardiovascular disease prevention [abstract]. J Am Coll Cardiol 51:A249, 2008.

58. Berger JS, Bairey-Merz CN, Redberg RF, Douglas PS: Improving the quality of care for women with cardiovascular disease: Report of a DCRI Think Tank, March 8 to 9, 2007. Am Heart J 156:816; 825.e1, 2008.

Evidence Base for Cardiovascular Therapy in Women

59. Antman EM, Anbe DT, Armstrong PW, et al: ACC/AHA guidelines for the management of patients with ST-elevation myocardial infarction. A report of the American College of Cardiology/American Heart Association Task Force on Practice Guidelines (Committee to Revise the 1999 Guidelines for the Management of Patients with Acute Myocardial Infarction. Circulation 110:e82, 2004.

60. Smith SC Jr, Allen J, Blair SN, et al: AHA/ACC guidelines for secondary prevention for patients with coronary and other atherosclerotic vascular disease: 2006 update. J Am Coll Cardiol 47:2130, 2006.

61. Gibbons RJ, Abrams J, Chatterjee K, et al: ACC/AHA guidelines update for the management of patients with chronic stable angina—summary article. A report of the American College of Cardiology/American Heart Association Task Force on Practice Guidelines (Committee on the Management of Patients with Chronic Stable Angina). Circulation 107:149, 2003.

62. Mosca L, Banka CL, Benjamin EJ, et al: American Heart Association evidence-based guidelines for cardiovascular disease prevention in women: 2007 update. J Am Coll Cardiol 49:1230, 2007.

63. Ridker PM, Cook NR, Lee I-M, et al: A randomized trial of low-dose aspirin in the primary prevention of cardiovascular disease in women. N Engl J Med 352:1293, 2005.

64. Berger JS, Roncaglioni MC, Avanzini F, et al: Aspirin for the primary prevention of cardiovascular events in women and men: A sex-specific meta-analysis of randomized controlled trials. JAMA 295:306, 2006.

65. Cannon CP, Braunwald E, McCabe CH, et al: Intensive versus moderate lipid lowering with statins after acute coronary syndromes [erratum in N Engl J Med 354:778, 2006]. N Engl J Med 350:1495, 2004.

66. Ridker PM, Danielson E, Fonseca FA, et al: Rosuvastatin to prevent vascular events in men and women with elevated C-reactive protein. N Engl J Med 359:2195, 2008.

67. Lansky AJ, Hochman JS, Ward PA, et al: Percutaneous coronary intervention and adjunctive pharmacotherapy in women: A statement for healthcare professionals from the American Heart Association. Circulation 111:940, 2005.

68. Glaser R, Herrmann HC, Murphy SA, et al: Benefit of an early invasive management strategy in women with acute coronary syndromes. JAMA 288:3124, 2002.

69. Lagerqvist B, Safstrom K, Stahle E, et al: Is early invasive treatment of unstable coronary artery disease equally effective for both women and men? FRISC II Study Group Investigators. J Am Coll Cardiol 38:41, 2001.

70. Clayton TC, Pocock SJ, Henderson RA, et al: Do men benefit more than women from an interventional strategy in patients with unstable angina or non–ST-elevation myocardial infarction? The impact of gender in the RITA 3 trial. Eur Heart J 25:1641, 2004.

71. O'Donoghue M, Boden WE, Braunwald E, et al: Early invasive versus conservative treatment strategies in women and men with unstable angina and non–ST-segment elevation myocardial infarction: A metaanalysis. JAMA 300:71, 2008.

72. Eagle KA, Guyton RA, Davidoff R, et al: ACC/AHA guideline update for coronary artery bypass graft surgery. A report of the American College of Cardiology/American Heart Association Task Force on Practice Guidelines (Committee to Update the 1999 Guidelines for Coronary Artery Bypass Graft Surgery), 2004. Available at: http://www.acc.org/clinical/guidelines/cabg/cabg.pdf. Accessed July 12, 2006.

73. Vaccarino V, Abramson JL, Veledar E, Weintraub WS: Sex differences in hospital mortality after coronary artery bypass surgery: Evidence for a higher mortality in younger women. Circulation 105:1176, 2002.

74. Vaccarino V, Lin ZQ, Kasl SV, et al: Sex differences in health status after coronary artery bypass surgery. Circulation 108:2642, 2003.

75. Keresztes PA, Merritt SL, Holm K, et al: The coronary artery bypass experience: Gender differences. Heart Lung 32:308, 2003.

76. Le Grande MR, Elliott PC, Murphy BM, et al: Health related quality of life trajectories and predictors following coronary artery bypass surgery. Health Qual Life Outcomes 4:49, 2006.

77. The PURSUIT Trial Investigators: Inhibition of platelet glycoprotein IIb/IIIa with eptifibatide in patients with acute coronary syndromes. Platelet Glycoprotein IIb/IIIa in Unstable Angina: Receptor Suppression Using Integrilin Therapy. N Engl J Med 339:436, 1998.

78. Boersma E, Harrington RA, Moliterno DJ, et al: Platelet glycoprotein IIb/IIIa inhibitors in acute coronary syndromes: A meta-analysis of all major randomised clinical trials [erratum in Lancet 359:2120, 2002]. Lancet 359:189, 2002.

79. Giugliano RP, White JA, Bode C, et al: Early versus delayed, provisional eptifibatide in acute coronary syndromes. N Engl J Med 360:2176, 2009.

80. Alexander KP, Chen AY, Roe MT, et al: Excess dosing of antiplatelet and antithrombin agents in the treatment of non–ST-segment elevation acute coronary syndromes. JAMA 294:3108, 2005.

81. Rao SV, Jollis JG, Harrington RA, et al: Relationship of blood transfusion and clinical outcomes in patients with acute coronary syndromes. JAMA 292:1555, 2004.

82. Rao SV, O'Grady K, Pieper KS, et al: Impact of bleeding severity on clinical outcomes among patients with acute coronary syndromes. Am J Cardiol 96:1200, 2005.

83. Yusuf S, Mehta SR, Chrolavicius S, et al: Comparison of fondaparinux and enoxaparin in acute coronary syndromes. N Engl J Med 354:1464, 2006.

84. Blomkalns AL, Chen AY, Hochman JS, et al: Gender disparities in the diagnosis and treatment of non–ST-segment elevation acute coronary syndromes: Large-scale observations from the CRUSADE (Can Rapid Risk Stratification of Unstable Angina Patients Suppress Adverse Outcomes with Early Implementation of the American College of Cardiology/American Heart Association Guidelines) National Quality Improvement Initiative. J Am Coll Cardiol 45:832, 2005.

85. Halim SA, Mulgund J, Chen AY, et al: Use of guidelines-recommended management and outcomes among women and men with low-level troponin elevation: Insights from CRUSADE. Circ Cardiovasc Qual Outcomes 2:199, 2009.

86. Vaccarino V, Rathore SS, Wenger NK, et al: Sex and racial differences in the management of acute myocardial infarction, 1994 through 2002. N Engl J Med 353:671, 2005.

87. Jneid H, Fonarow GC, Cannon CP, et al: Sex differences in medical care and early death after acute myocardial infarction. Circulation 118:2803, 2008.

88. Newby LK, Allen LaPointe NM, et al: Long-term adherence to evidence-based secondary prevention therapies in coronary artery disease. Circulation 113:203, 2006.

89. Mosca L, Mochari H, Christian A, et al: National study of women's awareness, preventive action, and barriers to cardiovascular health. Circulation 113:525, 2006.

90. Mosca L, Linfante AH, Benjamin EJ, et al: National study of physician awareness and adherence to cardiovascular disease prevention guidelines. Circulation 111:499, 2005.

91. Jani SM, Montoye C, Mehta R, et al: Sex differences in the application of evidence-based therapies for the treatment of acute myocardial infarction. Arch Intern Med 166:1164, 2006.

92. Taylor RS, Brown A, Ebrahim S, et al: Exercise-based rehabilitation for patients with coronary heart disease: Systematic review and meta-analysis of randomized controlled trials. Am J Med 116:682, 2004.

93. Witt BJ, Jacobsen SJ, Weston SA, et al: Cardiac rehabilitation after myocardial infarction in the community. J Am Coll Cardiol 44:988, 2004.

Heart Failure in Women

94. Masoudi FA, Havranek EP, Smith G, et al: Gender, age, and heart failure with preserved left ventricular systolic function. J Am Coll Cardiol 41:217, 2003.

95. Fernandez-Sola J, Nicolas-Arfelis JM: Gender differences in alcoholic cardiomyopathy. J Gend Specif Med 5:41, 2002.

96. Galvao M, Kalman J, DeMarco T, et al: Gender differences in in-hospital management and outcomes in patients with decompensated heart failure: Analysis from the Acute Decompensated Heart Failure National Registry (ADHERE). J Card Fail 12:100, 2006.

97. Yancy CW, Lopatin M, Stevenson LW, et al: Clinical presentation, management, and in-hospital outcomes of patients admitted with acute decompensated heart failure with preserved systolic function: A report from the Acute Decompensated Heart Failure National Registry (ADHERE) Database [erratum in J Am Coll Cardiol 47:1502, 2006]. J Am Coll Cardiol 47:76, 2006.

98. Owan TE, Hodge DO, Herges RM, et al: Trends in prevalence and outcome of heart failure with preserved ejection fraction. N Engl J Med 355:251, 2006.

99. Bhatia RS, Tu JV, Lee DS, et al: Outcome of heart failure with preserved ejection fraction in a population-based study. N Engl J Med 355:260, 2006.

100. O'Meara E, Clayton T, McEntegart MB, et al: Sex differences in clinical characteristics and prognosis in a broad spectrum of patients with heart failure: Results of the Candesartan in Heart failure: Assessment of Reduction in Mortality and morbidity (CHARM) program. Circulation 115:3111, 2007.

101. Hunt SA, Abraham WT, Chin MH, et al: ACC/AHA Guideline update for the diagnosis and management of chronic heart failure in the adult. A report of the American College of Cardiology/American Heart Association Task Force on Practice Guidelines (Writing Committee to Update the 2001 Guidelines for the Evaluation and Management of Heart Failure), 2005. Available at: http://www.acc.org/clinical/guidelines/failure//index.pdf. Accessed June 25, 2006.

102. Goldberger Z, Lampert R: Implantable cardioverter-defibrillators: Expanding indication and technologies. JAMA 295:809, 2006.

103. Hernandez AF, Fonarow GC, Liang L, et al: Sex and racial differences in the use of implantable cardioverter-defibrillators among patients hospitalized with heart failure. JAMA 298:1525, 2007.

104. Curtis LH, Al-Khatib SM, Shea AM, et al: Sex differences in the use of implantable cardioverter-defibrillators for primary and secondary prevention of sudden cardiac death. JAMA 298:1517, 2007.

105. Aaronson KD, Schwartz JS, Goin JE, et al: Sex differences in patient acceptance of cardiac transplant candidacy. Circulation 91:2753, 1995.

106. Hsich EM, Piña IL: Heart failure in women: A need for prospective data. J Am Coll Cardiol 54:491, 2009.

Peripheral Arterial Disease in Women

107. Criqui MH: Peripheral arterial disease—epidemiological aspects. Vasc Med 6(Suppl):3, 2001.

108. Hirsch AT, Haskal ZJ, Hertzer NR, et al: ACC/AHA 2005 guidelines for the management of patients with peripheral arterial disease (lower extremity, renal, mesenteric, and abdominal aortic): A collaborative report from the American Association for Vascular Surgery/Society for Vascular Surgery, Society for Cardiovascular Angiography and Interventions, Society for Vascular Medicine and Biology, Society of Interventional Radiology, and the ACC/AHA Task Force on Practice Guidelines (Writing Committee to Develop Guidelines for the Management of Patients with Peripheral Arterial Disease), 2005. Available at: http://www.acc.org/clinical/guidelines/pad/index.pdf. Accessed July 16, 2006.

109. Antithrombotic Trialists' Collaboration: Aspirin in the primary and secondary prevention of vascular disease: Collaborative meta-analysis of individual participant data from randomized trials. Lancet 373:1849, 2009.

110. Hansen KJ, Edwards MS, Craven TE, et al: Prevalence of renovascular disease in the elderly: A population-based study. J Vasc Surg 36:443, 2002.

111. U.S. Preventive Services Task Force: Screening for abdominal aortic aneurysm: Recommendation statement. Ann Intern Med 142:198, 2005.

CH
81

CARDIOVASCULAR DISEASE IN WOMEN

CHAPTER 82 **Pregnancy and Heart Disease**

Carole A. Warnes

Approximately 2% of pregnancies involve maternal cardiovascular disease, and as such, this poses an increased risk to both mother and fetus. Most women with cardiovascular disease can have a pregnancy with proper care, but a careful pre-pregnancy evaluation is mandatory. Cardiac disease may sometimes be manifested for the first time in pregnancy because the hemodynamic changes may compromise a limited cardiac reserve.[1] Conversely, the symptoms and signs of a normal pregnancy may mimic the presence of cardiac disease. Lightheadedness, dizziness, shortness of breath, peripheral edema, and even syncope often occur in the course of a normal pregnancy, and for the unwary physician, cardiac disease may be suspected. An understanding of the normal cardiac examination of a pregnant patient is therefore important. For those physicians counseling patients with cardiac disease about the potential risks of a pregnancy, a comprehensive knowledge of the underlying defect as well as of the hemodynamic changes that pregnancy will impose is imperative.

With the declining incidence of rheumatic heart disease in Western countries, most maternal cardiac disease is now congenital in origin. Other cardiovascular problems seen include cardiomyopathies, both dilated and hypertrophic, and valvular disease, such as bicuspid aortic valve and mitral valve prolapse. Less common problems include pulmonary hypertension and, rarely, coronary artery disease. Pre-pregnancy counseling is important to give prospective mothers appropriate information about the advisability of pregnancy and to discuss the risks to her and the fetus. Such patients should be seen in a high-risk pregnancy unit and have a clinical examination, electrocardiogram, and chest radiograph. An echocardiogram facilitates a detailed evaluation of myocardial function, valvular disease, and pulmonary pressures. For patients with congenital heart disease, their perception of normal activity may be skewed, and an exercise test is helpful in delineating their true functional aerobic capacity. In general, patients who cannot achieve more than 70% of their predicted functional aerobic capacity are unlikely to tolerate a pregnancy safely. During this visit, it is important to take a careful family history to assess whether there is any congenital heart disease in the family. Genetic counseling may also be considered, if necessary. A careful discussion of the maternal and fetal risks should be made at the time of pre-pregnancy counseling, and if the mother is going to pursue a pregnancy, a strategy should be outlined regarding the frequency of follow-up by the cardiologist, and a plan should be put in place for labor and delivery.[2]

A multicenter Canadian study has suggested that maternal cardiac risk may be predicted by the use of a risk index.[3] Four predictors of maternal cardiac events are as follows: (1) prior cardiac event (e.g., heart failure, transient ischemic attack, or stroke before pregnancy) or arrhythmia; (2) baseline New York Heart Association (NYHA) class higher than Class II or cyanosis; (3) left-sided heart obstruction (mitral valve area smaller than 2 cm², aortic valve area less than 1.5 cm², or peak left ventricular outflow tract gradient more than 30 mm Hg by echocardiography); and (4) reduced systemic ventricular systolic function (ejection fraction less than 40%). Each of 599 pregnancies was assigned 1 point when each predictor was present. No pregnancy received more than 3 points. The estimated risk of a cardiac event in pregnancies with 0, 1, and more than 1 point was 5%, 27%, and 75%, respectively. It was concluded that those with a low cardiac risk of 0 could safely be delivered in a community hospital, but those at intermediate or high cardiac risk (risk score of 1 or more) should be delivered at a regional center.

During pregnancy, a multidisciplinary team approach is recommended, with close collaboration with the obstetrician so that the mode, timing, and location of delivery can be planned.[4] The management should be tailored to the specific needs of the patient. During pregnancy, fetal growth is monitored by the obstetric team, and for the woman with congenital heart disease, a fetal cardiac echocardiogram is offered at about 22 to 26 weeks of pregnancy to determine whether the baby has a congenital cardiac anomaly.

Hemodynamic Changes

During Pregnancy

The hemodynamic changes are profound and begin early in the first trimester. The plasma volume begins to increase in the sixth week of pregnancy and by the second trimester approaches 50% above baseline (**Fig. 82-1**). The plasma volume then tends to plateau until delivery. This increased plasma volume is followed by a slightly lesser rise in red cell mass, which results in the relative anemia of pregnancy. The heart rate begins to increase to about 20% above baseline to facilitate the increase in cardiac output (**Fig. 82-2**). Uterine blood flow increases with placental growth, and there is a fall in peripheral resistance. This decreased peripheral resistance may result in a slight fall in blood pressure, which also begins in the first trimester. The venous pressure in the lower extremities rises, which is why approximately 80% of healthy pregnant women develop pedal edema. The adaptive changes of a normal pregnancy result in an increase in cardiac output, which also begins in the first trimester and by the end of the second trimester approaches 30% to 50% above baseline.

These hemodynamic changes may cause problems for the mother with cardiac disease. The added volume load may obviously compromise a patient who has impaired ventricular function and limited cardiac reserve. Stenotic valvular lesions (e.g., aortic stenosis) are less well tolerated than regurgitant lesions because the decrease in peripheral resistance exaggerates the gradient across the aortic valve.

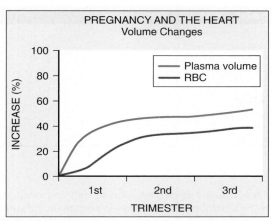

FIGURE 82-1 Plasma volume and red blood cell (RBC) increase during the trimesters of pregnancy. The plasma volume increases to approximately 50% above baseline by the second trimester and then virtually plateaus until delivery.

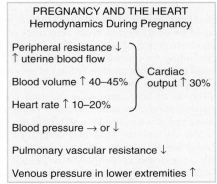

FIGURE 82-2 Hemodynamic changes during pregnancy relate to increased cardiac output and a fall in peripheral resistance. Blood pressure in most patients remains the same or falls slightly. Venous pressure in the legs increases, causing pedal edema in many patients.

Similarly, the tachycardia of pregnancy reduces the time for diastolic filling in a patient with mitral stenosis, with resultant increase in left atrial pressure. In contrast, with a lesion such as mitral regurgitation, the afterload reduction helps offset the volume load on the left ventricle that gestation imposes.

During Labor and Delivery

The hemodynamic changes during labor and delivery are abrupt. With each uterine contraction, up to 500 mL of blood is released into the circulation, prompting a rapid increase in cardiac output and blood pressure. The cardiac output is often 50% above baseline during the second stage of labor and may be even higher at the time of delivery. During a normal vaginal delivery, approximately 400 mL of blood is lost. In contrast, with a cesarean section, about 800 mL of blood is often lost and may pose a more significant hemodynamic burden to the parturient. After delivery of the baby, there is an abrupt increase in venous return, in part because of autotransfusion from the uterus but also because the baby no longer compresses the inferior vena cava. In addition, there continues to be autotransfusion of blood in the 24 to 72 hours after delivery, and this is when pulmonary edema may occur.

All these abrupt changes mandate that for the high-risk patient with cardiac disease, a multidisciplinary approach during labor and delivery is essential. The cardiologist and obstetrician should work with the anesthesiologist to determine the safest mode of delivery.

For most patients with cardiac disease, a vaginal delivery is feasible and preferable; a cesarean section is indicated only for obstetric reasons. Exceptions to this include the patient who is anticoagulated with warfarin because the baby is also anticoagulated, and vaginal

delivery carries an increased risk to the fetus of intracranial hemorrhage. Cesarean section may also be considered in patients who have a dilated unstable aorta (e.g., Marfan syndrome), severe pulmonary hypertension, or a severe obstructive lesion such as aortic stenosis. High-risk patients should be delivered in a center where expertise is available to monitor the hemodynamic changes of labor and delivery and to intervene when necessary. If vaginal delivery is elected, fetal and maternal electrocardiographic monitoring should be performed. Delivery can be accomplished with the mother in the left lateral position so that the fetus does not compress the inferior vena cava, thereby maintaining venous return. The second stage should be assisted, if necessary (e.g., forceps or vacuum extraction), to avoid a long labor. Blood and volume loss should be replaced promptly. For those patients with tenuous hemodynamics, Swan-Ganz catheterization before active labor facilitates optimization of the hemodynamics and should be continued for at least 24 hours after delivery, when pulmonary edema commonly occurs.

Although there is no consensus regarding the administration of antibiotic prophylaxis at the time of delivery for patients with lesions vulnerable to infective endocarditis, many institutions routinely give antibiotics because of the documented bacteremia. This can occur even during an uncomplicated delivery.[5] Patients who are most vulnerable to the deleterious effects of endocarditis are those with cyanotic heart disease and prosthetic valves.[6]

Evaluation

Physical Examination (see Chap. 12)

Because of the altered hemodynamics during pregnancy, the physical examination findings of a healthy pregnant woman change and may mimic cardiac disease. The heart rate increases and the pulse volume is often bounding. By the middle of the second trimester, the jugular venous pressure may be elevated, with brisk descents, because of the volume overload and reduced peripheral resistance. The apical impulse is more prominent, and on auscultation, the first sound may appear loud. Commonly, there is an ejection systolic murmur at the left sternal edge, never more than grade 3/6 in intensity, which relates to increased flow through the left or right ventricular outflow tract. A third sound is very common. There should be no diastolic murmur. The second sound may also appear accentuated, and these combined auscultatory features may suggest an atrial septal defect or pulmonary hypertension. Continuous murmurs may also be heard, from either a cervical venous hum or a mammary souffle. Peripheral edema is common as pregnancy advances. If there is any concern that the physical examination suggests cardiac disease, transthoracic echocardiography should be performed. This facilitates the evaluation of ventricular size and function, valvular heart disease, and any potential shunts (e.g., atrial septal defect, ventricular septal defect) and the noninvasive assessment of pulmonary artery pressure.

Imaging (see Chaps. 15 to 19)

CHEST RADIOGRAPHY. A chest radiograph is not obtained routinely in any pregnant patient because of concern about radiation to the fetus, but it should be considered in any patient when there are concerns about her cardiac status and new onset of dyspnea or failure. The chest radiograph in a normal healthy patient may show slight prominence of the pulmonary artery, and as pregnancy advances, elevation of the diaphragm may suggest an increase in the cardiothoracic ratio.

TRANSTHORACIC ECHOCARDIOGRAPHY. This is the cornerstone of cardiac evaluation in pregnancy and facilitates differentiation of the features of cardiac disease from those of a normal pregnancy. It is used most frequently to determine the ventricular function, to assess the status of native and prosthetic valve disease, and, by use of the tricuspid regurgitant velocity, to assess pulmonary artery pressure. For those patients with congenital heart disease, a detailed assessment of any shunt and complex anatomy may be made.

During pregnancy, because of the increased cardiac output, the velocities across the left and right ventricular outflow tracts increase, which may mimic an increase in outflow tract gradient. Careful examination of the two-dimensional anatomic appearances will help differentiate this from a true valvular abnormality, and calculation of valve area will be helpful. Similarly, because of the increased stroke volume, any valvular regurgitation will appear to be accentuated. Serial echocardiograms may be particularly useful in a patient with a mechanical valve prosthesis who is vulnerable to thrombosis during pregnancy. The valve area calculation, in addition to pressure half-time determination, may be more helpful than a simple measurement of valve gradient; this may appear to be increased as pregnancy advances because the circulation becomes more hyperkinetic and cardiac output increases.

In patients with impaired ventricular function, particularly those with cardiomyopathy, echocardiography plays the most important role in assessing left ventricular function. In a normal pregnancy, the left ventricular end-diastolic measurement is increased, and there may be similar increases in right ventricular size as well as in the volumes of both atria. Measurement of ejection fraction is determined by changes in preload and afterload, and in the supine position, preload may be reduced because the fetus may compress the inferior vena cava.

TRANSESOPHAGEAL ECHOCARDIOGRAPHY. Transesophageal echocardiography is seldom performed during pregnancy but may be necessary to provide more detailed imaging of valvular disease, the presence or absence of a shunt, or intracardiac thrombus. In addition, it may be useful to determine the presence or absence of endocarditis to facilitate the detection of a valvular vegetation or perivalvular abscess. Transesophageal echocardiography can be performed safely, although careful monitoring of maternal oxygen saturation is necessary if midazolam is used for sedation. Antibiotic prophylaxis is unnecessary.

FETAL ECHOCARDIOGRAPHY. Excellent imaging of the fetal heart can usually be obtained by 20 weeks' gestation. The four-chamber view may be obtained in most pregnancies and should demonstrate two atrioventricular valves, the crux of the heart, and whether two ventricles of equal size are present. The patent foramen ovale should also be demonstrated. Typically, the heart should be smaller than one third of the size of the fetal thorax.

Management During Pregnancy

Medical Therapy

Patients who are otherwise healthy may require little or no specific treatment other than the usual obstetric recommendations and monitoring. Patients who are NYHA Class I or II may need to limit strenuous exercise and to have adequate rest, supplementation of iron and vitamins to minimize the anemia of pregnancy, low-salt diet if there is concern about ventricular dysfunction, and regular cardiac and obstetric evaluations, the frequency of which must be individualized. Patients who are NYHA Class III or IV may need hospital admission for bed rest and close monitoring and may require early delivery if there is maternal hemodynamic compromise.

Surgical Management

Cardiac surgery is seldom necessary during pregnancy and should be avoided whenever possible. There is a higher risk of fetal malformation and loss if cardiopulmonary bypass is performed in the first trimester; if it is performed in the last trimester, there is a higher likelihood of precipitating premature labor. The "optimal time" appears to be between 20 and 28 weeks of gestation, and the fetal outcome may be improved by use of normothermic rather than hypothermic extracorporeal circulation, higher pump flows, higher pressures (mean blood pressure of 60 mm Hg), and as short a bypass time as possible. Obstetric monitoring of the fetus during the procedure is recommended so

TABLE 82-1 High-Risk Pregnancies
Pulmonary hypertension
Dilated cardiomyopathy, ejection fraction <40%
Symptomatic obstructive lesions
Aortic stenosis
Mitral stenosis
Pulmonary stenosis
Coarctation of the aorta
Marfan syndrome with aortic root >40 mm
Cyanotic lesions
Mechanical prosthetic valves

that fetal bradycardia may be dealt with promptly and uterine contractions may be controlled. Despite these interventions, the current risk of fetal loss is still at least 10% and is probably higher when the cardiac surgery is emergent. Maternal functional class is an important predictive factor for maternal death. A multidisciplinary approach is preferable to optimize the outcome for both mother and baby.

High-Risk Pregnancies

In some situations, the maternal risk of pregnancy is very high, and the patient should be counseled to avoid pregnancy and sometimes even to consider termination of pregnancy if it occurs (**Table 82-1**). No data exist regarding the precise level of pulmonary hypertension that poses a major threat to the mother, but in my experience, systolic pulmonary artery pressures higher than 60% to 70% of the systemic pressure are likely to be associated with maternal compromise; in these circumstances, pregnancy is best avoided. Women who have a left ventricular ejection fraction less than 40% from any cause are not likely to withstand the volume load that pregnancy imposes and should be advised not to become pregnant. Because pregnancy is associated with a decrease in peripheral resistance, symptomatic patients with significant stenotic cardiac lesions (see Table 82-1) are likely to deteriorate during a pregnancy. Patients with a dilated aortic root more than 40 mm are vulnerable to progressive aortic dilation, dissection, and rupture during pregnancy, particularly those patients with Marfan syndrome. This occurs not only because of the increased stroke volume but probably also because the gestational hormonal changes may be additive to the underlying histologic abnormality in the aortic media. Estrogen inhibits collagen and elastin synthesis in the aorta, and progesterone has been shown to accelerate the deposition of noncollagenous proteins in the aortas of rats.

Cardiovascular Diseases

Congenital Heart Disease (see Chap. 65)

Most maternal cardiac disease in Western societies is now congenital in origin. This relates to the enormous advances in congenital cardiac surgery during the last 50 years, so that most babies born with congenital heart disease, even with complex lesions, now survive to adulthood. Some patients will present for the first time in pregnancy with symptoms and learn that they have congenital heart disease. Other patients with repaired defects may encounter cardiac problems during pregnancy, the most common being heart failure and arrhythmias.[7] All patients, whether or not they have had cardiac repair, should have a detailed evaluation and appropriate counseling before pregnancy is considered.[8]

ATRIAL SEPTAL DEFECT. Secundum atrial septal defect is one of the most common congenital heart defects. Patients with even a large secundum atrial septal defect usually tolerate pregnancy without complication unless there is coexistent pulmonary hypertension or atrial fibrillation. The volume load on the right ventricle is usually well tolerated. Meticulous attention should be paid to the maternal leg veins, particularly during peridelivery, because deep venous thrombosis could precipitate a paradoxical embolus and stroke. Elective closure of an atrial septal defect by device or operative repair is preferable before pregnancy is contemplated.

VENTRICULAR SEPTAL DEFECT. Patients with small defects usually tolerate pregnancy without difficulty. In the setting of a large ventricular septal defect and pulmonary hypertension, patients should be counseled not to proceed with a pregnancy (see later discussion of Eisenmenger syndrome).

PATENT DUCTUS ARTERIO-SUS. Small ducts with normal or near-normal pressures usually cause no hemodynamic perturbations during pregnancy. In the setting of a large shunt, the added volume load of pregnancy might precipitate left ventricular failure. Those with pulmonary hypertension should be counseled not to have a pregnancy.

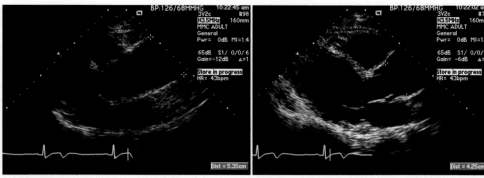

FIGURE 82-3 Long-axis parasternal two-dimensional echocardiographic images of a 30-year-old woman with a normal functioning bicuspid aortic valve. Her ascending aorta measures 4.25 cm at the sinotubular junction (**left**) and 5.35 cm at the mid ascending aorta (**right**). An aortic root replacement (valve sparing) was recommended before pregnancy.

CONGENITAL AORTIC STENOSIS. (see Chap. 66) Aortic stenosis in women of childbearing age usually occurs secondary to a bicuspid aortic valve. A detailed two-dimensional anatomic and Doppler echocardiographic assessment of the valve function should be performed before pregnancy is contemplated. In addition, there should be a careful examination of the entire thoracic aorta because bicuspid aortic valve is associated with an aortopathy, and even with a functionally normal valve, an aortic dilation or ascending aortic aneurysm may be present. Pregnancy is usually considered to be contraindicated if the aortic dimension is larger than 4.5 cm (**Fig. 82-3**).

Mild aortic stenosis is usually well tolerated, provided the patient has a normal exercise capacity and no symptoms.[9] Moderate stenosis is sometimes well tolerated, but the patient needs to be evaluated carefully before pregnancy. In the absence of symptoms, with a normal exercise test without ST-T wave changes, pregnancy with a compliant patient who is carefully managed is likely to be successful. Those with severe aortic stenosis (valve area smaller than 1 cm^2) or a mean gradient greater than 50 mm Hg should be counseled not to have a pregnancy. The decrease in peripheral resistance during pregnancy will exaggerate the aortic gradient and may precipitate symptoms. Patients may respond to bed rest and the administration of beta blockers, but an early delivery may be necessary. The risk to the mother of continuing the pregnancy versus delivery of a baby early by cesarean section needs to be balanced. Labor and delivery can be particularly problematic in such patients because of the abrupt hemodynamic changes, particularly the abrupt fall in afterload when the baby is delivered. Blood loss at the time of parturition can also precipitate maternal collapse. Epidural analgesia needs to be carefully and slowly administered, and spinal block should be avoided because of the potential for hypotension. Delivery may be facilitated by central venous pressure monitoring or the use of a Swan-Ganz catheter to maintain optimum hemodynamics. This should be continued for at least 24 hours after delivery.

Several small reports have reviewed percutaneous aortic balloon valvuloplasty during pregnancy; this can be accomplished, provided the valve anatomy is favorable and the procedure is performed by an experienced interventionalist.[10] Radiation exposure of the fetus can be minimized by lead screening of the mother's abdomen and pelvis. It should be performed in centers with extensive experience and surgical back-up and, if performed after 26 weeks of pregnancy, should have obstetric standby in case of premature labor.

COARCTATION OF THE AORTA. (see Chaps. 60 and 65) Women with coarctation may present for the first time during pregnancy because of systemic hypertension. A significant coarctation causes diminished flow to both the uterus and fetus, which may result in small-for-dates babies or even fetal loss. Therapeutic options include antihypertensive therapies, percutaneous balloon or stenting of the coarctation, or surgical intervention. Because of the associated aortopathy, the entire aorta is vulnerable to dilation, aneurysm, and dissection. When the presence of a coarctation is known, the entire aorta should be imaged at the time of pre-pregnancy counseling. Most women, however, will have a successful pregnancy with proper care.

PULMONARY STENOSIS. Pulmonary stenosis is usually well tolerated during pregnancy, particularly if the right ventricular pressure is less than 70% of systemic pressure and sinus rhythm is maintained. If necessary, balloon pulmonary valvuloplasty can be performed, with shielding of the fetus from radiation.

CYANOTIC HEART DISEASE. Cyanosis poses risks for both mother and fetus.[11] The decrease in peripheral resistance that accompanies pregnancy augments the right-to-left shunt and may exaggerate the maternal cyanosis. Because of the erythrocytosis that accompanies cyanosis and the propensity to thrombosis, women who develop venous thrombosis are at risk of paradoxical embolus and stroke. Maternal hypoxia imposes a pronounced handicap to fetal growth and survival. Presbitero and colleagues[12] have evaluated 44 women with 96 pregnancies (excluding patients with Eisenmenger syndrome) and confirmed earlier study findings that the degree of maternal cyanosis has a profound impact on fetal outcome. When the maternal oxygen saturation is less than 85%, the fetal outcome is poor, with only 2 of 17 pregnancies (12%) resulting in live-born infants (**Table 82-2**). Conversely, when the maternal oxygen saturation is 90% or higher, 92% of the pregnancies result in a live birth. Maternal cardiovascular complications occurred in 14 patients (32%). Eight patients had heart

TABLE 82-2	**Fetal Outcome in Cyanotic Congenital Heart Disease and Its Relationship with Maternal Cyanosis**		
	NO. OF PREGNANCIES	**NO. OF LIVE BIRTHS**	**PERCENTAGE BORN ALIVE**
Hemoglobin, g/dL*			
≤16	28	20	71
17-19	40	18	45
≥20	26	2	8
Arterial oxygen saturation (%)†			
≤85	17	2	12
85-89	22	10	45
≥90	13	12	92

*Hemoglobin concentration unknown in two pregnancies.
†Arterial oxygen saturation unknown in 44 pregnancies.
From Presbitero P, Somerville J, Stone S, et al: Pregnancy in cyanotic congenital heart disease. Outcome of mother and fetus. Circulation 89:2673, 1994.

failure, and bacterial endocarditis occurred in two patients, both with palliated tetralogy of Fallot. Two patients had thrombotic complications, one pulmonary and one cerebral.

In addition to the degree of maternal cyanosis, right ventricular function must be assessed before pregnancy by echocardiography or magnetic resonance imaging. The type of maternal cardiac lesion present will also affect the propensity of the baby to inherit congenital cardiac disease. For those women with conotruncal abnormalities (tetralogy or pulmonary atresia), screening for 22q11 deletion is recommended because this has autosomal dominant transmission, and the offspring have a 50% chance of inheriting the genetic defect.[13]

EBSTEIN ANOMALY. The safety of a pregnancy in these patients depends on right ventricular size and function, degree of tricuspid regurgitation, and presence or absence of an atrial communication. The last is present in approximately 50% of patients, and if the patient is cyanotic at rest, the risk of pregnancy increases considerably. An atrial communication poses the added potential risk of a stroke from a paradoxical embolus, and meticulous attention should be paid to the mother's leg veins for the possibility of deep venous thrombosis. Atrial arrhythmias may not be well tolerated in pregnancy with this anomaly, and both atrial fibrillation and reentry tachycardia are common. Accessory bypass tracts causing preexcitation may precipitate rapid tachycardias, which add to the burden of a poorly functioning right ventricle.

CONGENITALLY CORRECTED TRANSPOSITION (L-TRANSPOSITION). Patients with this anomaly have atrioventricular discordance and ventriculoarterial discordance; thus, the systemic ventricle is the morphologic right ventricle. Patients may have a successful pregnancy as long as the ejection fraction of the systemic ventricle is preserved and there are no significant associated anomalies. The most common of these is systemic atrioventricular valve (tricuspid) regurgitation, which contributes to systemic ventricular dysfunction. Other lesions, such as ventricular septal defect, pulmonary stenosis, and complete heart block, may coexist and may compromise the ability to have a successful pregnancy.

Repaired Congenital Heart Disease (see Chap. 65)

Very few operations for congenital heart disease can be considered curative, and almost all patients have residua and sequelae that must be carefully evaluated at the time of pre-pregnancy counseling.

TETRALOGY OF FALLOT. Most women of childbearing age with tetralogy of Fallot will have had prior surgical repair and should be free of cyanosis. An occasional patient will be seen in adulthood who has not had prior surgery or may have been palliated with a surgically created shunt (e.g., Blalock-Taussig). In these cases, pregnancy may pose a risk, depending on the degree of cyanosis, as noted earlier. The fall in peripheral resistance augments the right-to-left shunt through the ventricular septal defect, causing worsening cyanosis, and this poses a risk for mother and fetus.

For those patients with prior definitive surgical repair, a careful assessment of any hemodynamic residua and sequelae should be undertaken before advice is given about the safety of a pregnancy. The clinical and echocardiographic evaluation should focus on the presence of lesions, such as residual pulmonary regurgitation, which is common after repair, and associated right ventricular dysfunction and tricuspid regurgitation. The volume load of pregnancy may not be well tolerated in these circumstances,[14,15] and superimposed atrial and even ventricular arrhythmias may add to the hemodynamic stresses. Additional volume lesions, such as ventricular septal defects and aortic regurgitation, as well as residual right ventricular outflow tract obstruction should be evaluated. For those women with a good surgical repair, good exercise capacity, and minimal residua, pregnancy may be well tolerated, provided they are properly managed.[15,16] Genetic counseling should be offered during pre-pregnancy counseling to look for 22q11 deletion. If there is no parental chromosomal abnormality and no family history of other congenital cardiac disease,

the risk of the fetus having a congenital cardiac anomaly is approximately 5% to 6%, similar to the risk of inheritance of many congenital cardiac lesions.

TRANSPOSITION OF THE GREAT ARTERIES (D-TRANSPOSITION). All patients will have had surgery in childhood, commonly an atrial baffle procedure (Mustard or Senning operation), which leaves the morphologic right ventricle as the systemic pump. Function of the systemic ventricle should be assessed clinically and echocardiographically before pregnancy, as well as the degree of tricuspid (systemic) atrioventricular valve regurgitation and degree of baffle obstruction, the residual atrial septal defect, and the presence or absence of atrial arrhythmias, which are common complications. Dysfunction of the systemic ventricle may be a contraindication to pregnancy.

COARCTATION. The evaluation of the woman with repaired coarctation should include an assessment of the coarctation repair site to exclude residual or recurrent coarctation or aneurysm formation and an imaging study to assess the entire aorta to rule out dilation or aneurysm formation, which is most common in the ascending aorta. The aortic valve and left ventricular function should also be assessed. The outcome for both mother and baby is usually favorable. For patients with mild dilation of the aorta, vaginal delivery with a short second stage is reasonable, but if there is evidence of aortic instability, a cesarean section is preferable.

UNIVENTRICULAR HEART AND FONTAN OPERATIONS. These women have an increased risk of maternal complications, particularly atrial arrhythmias, which may cause profound hemodynamic deterioration. They are particularly vulnerable to thrombosis in the Fontan circuit because of the sluggish flow and prothrombotic state of pregnancy. Function of the single ventricle may deteriorate because of the volume load of pregnancy, and the risk of miscarriage also appears to be increased.

Pulmonary Hypertension (see Chap. 78)

Pulmonary hypertension, regardless of the cause, carries a high mortality when it is associated with pregnancy.[17] Causes include thromboembolic disease, anorexic drugs, valvular heart disease, and primary pulmonary hypertension. The most common cause in childbearing years, however, is secondary to a shunt in the setting of congenital heart disease (e.g., ventricular septal defect, patent ductus arteriosus, or atrial septal defect). When the pulmonary hypertension exceeds approximately 60% of systemic levels, pregnancy is more likely to be associated with complications. In the setting of severe pulmonary vascular disease (Eisenmenger syndrome, see Chap. 65), maternal mortality may approach 50%. The volume load of pregnancy may compromise the poorly functioning right ventricle and precipitate heart failure. The fall in peripheral resistance augments right-to-left shunting and may precipitate more cyanosis.

The time around labor and delivery is particularly dangerous, and the highest incidence of maternal death is during parturition and the puerperium. There may be an abrupt decrease in afterload as the baby is delivered, and hypovolemia from blood loss can cause hypoxia, syncope, and sudden death. Vagal responses to pain may also be life-threatening. Death may also occur from pulmonary embolism or in situ pulmonary infarction. In the largest retrospective review, Gleicher and associates[18] reported 44 documented cases of Eisenmenger syndrome with 70 pregnancies. Of these patients, 52% died in connection with a pregnancy, and 34% of vaginal deliveries resulted in maternal death. Three of four cesarean sections also resulted in maternal death; however, the numbers were small, and it is likely that those patients represented a higher risk cohort because they were the most hemodynamically unstable. Only 25.6% of pregnancies reached term, and more than half of the deliveries were premature. Perinatal mortality was 28.3% and was significantly associated with prematurity. Current recommendations are still that termination of pregnancy is the safer option, although in patients with pulmonary hypertension, this too may be a more complex procedure, and cardiac anesthesia is probably helpful in this regard. Low-dose subcutaneous heparin may be administered during bed rest, but there is no evidence that it improves maternal survival. The mode of delivery needs to be discussed carefully. If the vaginal route is selected, it should be performed in an intensive care unit. Epidural analgesia must be cautiously administered to minimize peripheral vasodilation. A prolonged second stage should be avoided. Meticulous attention should be paid to the peripheral venous system, and a thromboguard or compression pump may help prevent peripheral venous thrombosis. Cesarean section delivery is probably preferable[19] with cardiac anesthesia. In-hospital monitoring should be continued for at least 2 weeks after delivery.

No studies have suggested a more favorable outcome with the use of pulmonary vasodilators, although case reports have suggested a more successful maternal outcome. Nitric oxide can be administered through nasal cannula or facemask, and successful pregnancy has also been reported with intravenous epoprostenol. Sildenafil has also been used, but with all these agents, maternal death may still occur days or weeks after delivery.[20]

In summary, the mortality for patients with severe pulmonary hypertension and pregnancy is prohibitively high. Appropriate advice about contraception should be given to all patients. Estrogen-containing contraceptives are contraindicated in this setting.

Valvular Heart Disease (see Chap. 66)

Because of the declining incidence of rheumatic heart disease in Western countries, rheumatic heart disease is infrequent in North America but remains prevalent in developing countries. The most common problems encountered are bicuspid aortic stenosis (discussed previously) and mitral stenosis, which tends to worsen during pregnancy because of the increase in cardiac output coupled with the increase in heart rate; this shortens the diastolic filling time and exaggerates the mitral valve gradient. Any decrease in stroke volume causes a further reflex tachycardia, which contributes to an elevated left atrial pressure. The onset of atrial fibrillation may precipitate acute pulmonary edema. Patients should have a careful echocardiographic evaluation of their mitral valve gradient, valve area, and pulmonary pressures before proceeding with a pregnancy. Exercise echocardiography may also be helpful in delineating the hemodynamic response to effort in terms of mitral gradient and the presence or absence of pulmonary hypertension.

The cornerstone of therapy for the symptomatic patient is beta blockade. This slows the heart rate, prolongs the diastolic filling time, and can result in marked improvement in symptoms. Bed rest may also be helpful to slow the heart rate and to minimize cardiac demands. The judicious use of diuretics is appropriate if there is pulmonary edema. Anticoagulants should probably be given if the patient is on bed rest and should certainly be administered in the setting of atrial fibrillation. In unusual circumstances, when the mother is refractory to medical therapy, balloon valvuloplasty may be performed if the valve anatomy is favorable and there is no concomitant mitral regurgitation.[21,22] Rarer still, surgical valvotomy may be performed, with the caveats described earlier.

Mitral and aortic regurgitation are fairly well tolerated in pregnancy, provided the regurgitation is no more than moderate, the mother is symptom free before pregnancy, and ventricular function is well preserved. Closer monitoring during pregnancy is usually warranted, however, particularly for those with mitral regurgitation, because the left ventricle tends to dilate as pregnancy progresses, and this may exacerbate the degree of mitral regurgitation. Early delivery may be necessary if there is maternal hemodynamic compromise.

PROSTHETIC VALVES. Pregnancy for the woman with a prosthetic valve poses risks for mother and baby and has been called a "double jeopardy" situation.[23] The choice of a prosthetic valve for the woman of childbearing age involves a detailed discussion of the relative risks so that she can make an informed decision about whether to select a tissue or mechanical prosthesis. Tissue valves are less thrombogenic

than mechanical valves and therefore are less problematic in pregnancy because they do not routinely involve the use of warfarin. The disadvantage is their tendency to degenerate after an average of 10 years, necessitating a reoperation, with its attendant risks and potential mortality. Mechanical prostheses, in contrast, have a greater longevity but require anticoagulation, and whichever anticoagulant strategy is chosen during pregnancy, there is a higher chance of fetal loss, placental hemorrhage, and prosthetic valve thrombosis. Thus, each type of valve has a risk-to-benefit ratio; the choices are reviewed here.

TISSUE PROSTHESES. The most common types of tissue valves used currently are porcine and pericardial valves. For patients in sinus rhythm, they confer the advantage that warfarin is not required, although many patients take a daily baby aspirin (81 mg). These valves are vulnerable to structural degeneration and calcification, which occurs more rapidly in younger patients. In addition, mitral prostheses tend to degenerate faster than those in the aortic position. There is some evidence that pregnancy may accelerate valve degeneration, and in some retrospective series, a second valve replacement was necessary in approximately one third of patients within 2 years of delivery. This is not universally accepted, however, and other large series have shown no difference in structural valve degeneration in young women who had a pregnancy versus those who did not.[24] Nonetheless, all tissue valves will degenerate, necessitating a second operation with an operative risk that is usually higher than the first. In some series, the mortality of a second valve replacement may be as high as 6%, and it must be recognized that if death occurs after the mother has had a successful pregnancy, the young child is left without a mother. Thus, at the time of counseling women of childbearing age about valve choice, the surgical results from the individual's institution should be reviewed. These may vary considerably on the basis of both surgical volume and expertise.

Homografts pose similar problems of structural deterioration and reoperation. The Ross operation, in which an autograft pulmonary valve is placed in the aortic position and a tissue prosthesis (usually porcine) is implanted in the pulmonary position, is associated with good outcomes during pregnancy when the hemodynamic indices are good. Nonetheless, the Ross procedure essentially exchanges one valvular problem for two, and ultimately the tissue pulmonary prosthesis as well as the aortic prosthesis must be replaced.

MECHANICAL PROSTHESES AND ANTICOAGULANT TREATMENT. The management of pregnancy when the mother has a mechanical valve prosthesis is controversial, and no universal consensus exists. There is no perfect strategy, and each modality is associated with some hazard for the mother or the fetus. Before any approach is adopted, it is crucial to explain the risks to the patient. During pregnancy, maternal blood is highly thrombogenic because there is an increased concentration of clotting factors and increased platelet adhesiveness combined with decreased fibrinolysis. These changes in clotting parameters make the risk of valve thrombosis and thromboembolism significant.

Unfractionated Heparin

Unfractionated heparin is a large molecule that does not cross the placenta and does not cause developmental abnormalities in the fetus. Laboratory control of activated partial thromboplastin time (aPTT) is difficult, however, in part because of the variation in response to standard doses and the wide variation in the reagents used to monitor doses. The aPTT ratio should be maintained at a level of at least 2, which corresponds to an anti–factor Xa (anti-Xa) level of more than 0.55 unit/mL in approximately 90% of patients.[25] Unfractionated heparin has been used subcutaneously and intravenously and is often begun in the first trimester, as soon as pregnancy is diagnosed, to minimize fetal exposure to warfarin at the critical time of fetal embryogenesis. It is usually continued until week 13 or 14 of pregnancy, when fetal embryogenesis is almost complete, and then warfarin is substituted. Some physicians continue heparin throughout pregnancy to avoid any fetal exposure to warfarin, but unfractionated heparin has been shown to be a poor anticoagulant in pregnancy. One large retrospective European study comparing different anticoagulation strategies has shown that most maternal complications (e.g., valve thrombosis, stroke, death) occur while mothers are taking heparin.[26] Most complications occur with mechanical mitral tilting disc prostheses, and this observation has been supported by many other studies, particularly with older generation prostheses.[27] One meta-analysis by Chan and colleagues[28] has shown that use of heparin early in the first trimester virtually eliminates the risk of fetal embryopathy but at the expense of maternal valve thrombosis, which occurred with a frequency of 9%. If unfractionated heparin is the selected treatment strategy, the midinterval aPTT should be at least twice that of the control, or an anti-Xa level of 0.35 to 0.7 unit/mL should be maintained.[25]

Low-Molecular-Weight Heparin

Low-molecular-weight heparin is an attractive alternative to unfractionated heparin because of its ease of use and superior bioavailability. Deaths have been reported with its use, however, usually associated with maternal valve thrombosis. The American College of Chest Physicians has suggested that it may be used and the anticoagulant effect carefully monitored by measuring the anti-Xa level. It is recommended that it be administered subcutaneously every 12 hours and the dose adjusted so that a 4-hour postinjection anti-Xa level is maintained at approximately 1.0 to 1.2 unit/mL, perhaps measured weekly.[25] The addition of low-dose aspirin, 75 to 162 mg/day, has also been recommended. There are no large prospective trials to confirm the usefulness of low-molecular-weight heparin in this setting, however, and reported studies are confined to small groups. Certainly, dosing based on weight alone has been shown to be inadequate to maintain most pregnant women in the therapeutic range as measured by anti-Xa activity,[29] and the pharmacokinetics changes throughout pregnancy. One retrospective study has reviewed published series between 1989 and 2004.[30] There were 74 women with 81 pregnancies, most of whom had mitral prostheses. Thromboemboli occurred in 10 of 81 pregnancies (12%), and all these patients had mitral prostheses. Low-molecular-weight heparin was used throughout in 60 pregnancies; in 21 pregnancies, it was used only in the first trimester and again at term. In 51 pregnancies, anti-Xa levels were monitored, and in 30 pregnancies, a fixed dose was used. All 10 patients with thromboemboli were receiving heparin throughout pregnancy, and 9 of them were on a fixed-dose regimen. This underscores the need for meticulous monitoring of anti-Xa levels, and Oran and associates[30] have recommended that the 4- to 6-hour postinjection level be maintained at 1 IU/mL. Thus, the use of low-molecular-weight heparin remains controversial, with no large prospective series and no evidence-based data to support which levels of anti-Xa should be maintained. It should be discontinued at least 24 hours before delivery if epidural analgesia is to be used because it has a prolonged effect and there is risk of spinal hematoma. Unfractionated heparin can be substituted peridelivery because it can be started and stopped abruptly. With all strategies, anticoagulants should be resumed as soon as possible after delivery.

Warfarin

Fetal exposure to warfarin in the first trimester may be associated with fetal embryopathy. In its mildest form, this may be only bone stippling (chondrodysplasia punctata); but in its most severe form, it may be manifested as nasal hypoplasia, optic atrophy, and mental retardation. The reported fetal risk of embryopathy varies widely but probably averages 6%. This risk is reduced by initiation of heparin before 6 weeks of pregnancy, but the disadvantage is an increased risk of maternal valve thrombosis. Warfarin also appears to increase the risk of fetal loss and spontaneous abortion.

The risk of fetal embryopathy may be dose related, and a study by Vitale and colleagues[31] has suggested that the risk is very low if the maternal warfarin dose is 5 mg or less. Thus, the anticoagulant approach for the woman with a mechanical valve needs to be individualized. For the woman with an older generation or tilting disc mitral prosthesis, particularly if she is in atrial fibrillation, the safer approach may be to treat her with warfarin for the first 34 to 35 weeks

of pregnancy, particularly if her dose is less than 5 mg/day. This must be fully discussed with the patient before she becomes pregnant, not only for the medicolegal implications but so that all the risks and benefits are understood. For those patients at lesser risk, heparin therapy (with the provisos noted earlier) may be selected as soon as pregnancy is diagnosed, warfarin substituted at 13 to 14 weeks, and heparin restarted at approximately 35 weeks in anticipation of delivery.

Connective Tissue Disorders

The most common connective tissue disorder is the Marfan syndrome, a disorder of fibrillin that is inherited in an autosomal dominant pattern (see Chap. 60). Preconception counseling is essential to advise prospective parents about the risks of transmission to the offspring and the risks of cardiovascular complications for the mother. A careful clinical and echocardiographic cardiovascular evaluation should be performed. This would usually include magnetic resonance imaging or computed tomography assessment of the entire aorta to look for aortic dilation or dissection. Pregnancy is usually contraindicated if the ascending aorta is larger than 40 mm in diameter, although the exact dimension is still a matter of debate. It should be underscored to all women with Marfan syndrome that pregnancy is not uniformly safe, and aortic dilation and dissection may be unpredictable although more likely when the aorta is larger than 40 mm. One study has suggested that pregnancy is relatively safe up to a diameter of 45 mm.[32] Associated cardiovascular problems also need to be evaluated, including the presence or absence of aortic regurgitation and mitral valve prolapse with associated regurgitation. Many patients are receiving long-term treatment with beta-adrenergic blockers to slow the progression of aortic regurgitation. These should be continued during pregnancy if there is any aortic dilation. Periodic echocardiographic surveillance every 6 to 8 weeks is recommended to monitor the mother's aortic root size, with the interval dependent on the initial echocardiographic findings. Any chest pain should be promptly evaluated to rule out dissection. During labor and delivery, pushing should be avoided, with an assisted second stage if necessary.

Cardiomyopathies (see Chaps. 68 and 69)

DILATED CARDIOMYOPATHY. Patients with idiopathic dilated cardiomyopathy are usually counseled not to have a pregnancy if the ejection fraction is lower than 40%. Because angiotensin-converting enzyme (ACE) inhibitors are contraindicated in pregnancy, ventricular function must be assessed without this drug. Careful echocardiographic evaluation should be performed before pregnancy. Exercise testing may also be helpful because women with ejection fractions of 40% to 50% may not tolerate pregnancy well if they have a poor functional aerobic capacity. Symptomatic patients who proceed with a pregnancy may need hydralazine for afterload reduction, bed rest, and low-dose diuretics for heart failure. Early delivery may also be necessary.

PERIPARTUM CARDIOMYOPATHY. Peripartum cardiomyopathy (PPCM) is a dilated cardiomyopathy documented with echocardiographic left ventricular dysfunction occurring in the last month of pregnancy or within 5 months of delivery. Patients with a prior history of myocardial disease are excluded from this definition, although this makes the diagnosis challenging in many women who have had neither a chest radiograph nor an echocardiogram to confirm that they had previously normal ventricular function. The actual incidence is unknown, but it is probably approximately 1 in 3000. Risk factors include multiparity, being black, older maternal age, and preeclampsia. In a retrospective study of 123 women with PPCM,[33] a history of hypertension was obtained in 43% of patients, and twin pregnancies were reported in 13%. Consistent with earlier studies, most patients (75%) presented in the first month post partum, perhaps suggesting an autoimmune cause rather than the pregnancy's exacerbating a pre-existing cardiomyopathy. This theory is supported by the documentation of autoantibodies in some cases.

The treatment of PPCM is the same as for other forms of congestive heart failure, except that ACE inhibitors and angiotensin receptor blocking agents are contraindicated in pregnancy. Hydralazine, beta blockers, and digoxin have been used and are safe, and diuretics may decrease preload and improve symptoms.[34] Intracardiac thrombus and embolism are common, and consideration should be given to anticoagulation with unfractionated heparin in those with an ejection fraction lower than 35%.[35] Early fetal delivery may be necessary in women needing hospitalization for heart failure. Myocarditis is a causative factor in some cases, with a reported incidence between 8.8% and 78%. The role of endomyocardial biopsy is controversial, but it probably should be considered and performed by those with considerable experience. Immunosuppressive treatment should be given to those with proven myocarditis.

Normalization of ventricular function occurs in about 50% of patients and appears more likely if the ejection fraction is more than 30% at the time of diagnosis.[33] Most physicians counsel against a second pregnancy, even if the ventricular function does return to normal, because PPCM will recur in approximately 30% of cases. This may result in significant clinical deterioration and even death.[36]

HYPERTROPHIC CARDIOMYOPATHY. A wide spectrum of anatomic and hemodynamic abnormalities exist in hypertrophic cardiomyopathy, including left ventricular outflow tract obstruction, mitral regurgitation, arrhythmias, and diastolic dysfunction. Some patients are asymptomatic with minimal hemodynamic disturbance; others are profoundly limited, with marked hemodynamic perturbations. A careful personal history, review of family history, electrocardiography, exercise test, and transthoracic echocardiography should precede counseling about the advisability of a pregnancy. The prospective parents should be informed about the autosomal dominant inheritance pattern, which has variable penetrance. Currently, more than 200 genetic mutations have been identified, and genetic counseling and family screening are appropriate before pregnancy is contemplated.

Most women with hypertrophic cardiomyopathy tolerate pregnancy well. The decrease in afterload that might exacerbate the outflow gradient is largely offset by the maternal increase in plasma volume. Medications such as beta blockers, which alleviate the outflow tract obstruction, may be continued throughout pregnancy, but the dose may need to be increased. Patients who have significant symptoms before pregnancy (usually related to severe left ventricular outflow tract obstruction) may not do well and become hemodynamically unstable. Common symptoms include palpitation, angina, and breathlessness. In a retrospective study of 127 women with 271 pregnancies, 36 women (28.3%) reported cardiac symptoms but 90% were symptomatic before pregnancy.[37] Heart failure occurred postnatally in two women, but there were no maternal deaths. Arrhythmia-related deaths in pregnancy have been reported, however. Low-dose diuretics may be helpful to treat heart failure in pregnancy, but care must be taken not to volume deplete the patient and exacerbate the left ventricular outflow gradient. Meticulous attention should be paid to hemodynamics at the time of delivery. Epidural anesthesia and spinal block should be avoided in case of hypotension, and blood loss should be promptly replaced. The Valsalva maneuver should be avoided, and the second stage should be facilitated as necessary. Cesarean section is indicated for obstetric reasons only.

Coronary Artery Disease (see Chaps. 54 to 57)

Coronary artery disease is uncommon in women of childbearing age but may occur, particularly in the setting of diabetes and tobacco abuse. Acute myocardial infarction is rare, and when it occurs, pregnancy increases the maternal risk threefold to fourfold. The most common cause is coronary artery dissection,[38] and the most common site is in the left anterior descending coronary artery.[39] The treatment should be urgent coronary angiography, with a consideration of percutaneous coronary intervention and stenting. The vulnerability to coronary artery dissection during pregnancy may relate to the presence of hypertension and also to the changes in elastin and collagen synthesis incurred by the hormonal changes of pregnancy.

A U.S. population-based study[40] has reported 44 deaths related to acute myocardial infarction, for a case fatality rate of 5.1%. The odds of acute myocardial infarction were 30-fold higher for women aged 40 years and older than for women younger than 20 years. The odds were more than fivefold higher for black women aged 35 years and older. Thrombus may also occur without atherosclerotic disease, and atherosclerosis with or without intracoronary thrombus is found in some cases, presumably related to the clotting diathesis that occurs during pregnancy.

Hypertension (see Chaps. 45 and 46)

Hypertension in pregnancy is an important cause of maternal morbidity and mortality. The different types of hypertension seen in pregnancy are defined in **Table 82-3**.[41] Gestational hypertension is distinguished from preeclampsia by the lack of proteinuria. About 50% of patients will develop preeclampsia, however, so close monitoring is warranted. It develops in approximately 25% of patients with chronic hypertension. Preeclampsia is a much more worrisome development and tends to occur more commonly in primiparous women and those with twin pregnancies. They do not usually develop frank hypertension until the second half of gestation. The cause is not entirely clear but may relate to endothelial dysfunction causing abnormal remodeling of the placental spiral arteries. Hypertension is just one feature of the diffuse endothelial dysfunction, which is associated with vasospasm, reduced end-organ perfusion, and activation of the coagulation cascade.

Although antihypertensive medications are effective in treating chronic hypertension that has worsened during pregnancy, they are not effective in preventing preeclampsia. When preeclampsia develops, bed rest is usually initiated, with salt restriction and close monitoring, and magnesium sulfate is often administered in an effort to prevent eclamptic seizures and to prolong the pregnancy, thereby facilitating fetal maturity. Urgent delivery is usually necessary, however, after which the blood pressure usually normalizes rapidly.

The treatment of other types of hypertension in pregnancy involves bed rest, salt restriction, and antihypertensive medications. Beta blockers, particularly labetalol (see Cardiovascular Drug Therapy and **Table 82-4**), have been used with good effect, although there is a

TABLE 82-3	Classification of Hypertension in Pregnancy
Chronic hypertension	Hypertension (blood pressure ≥140 mm Hg systolic or ≥90 mm Hg diastolic) present before pregnancy or that is diagnosed before the 20th week of gestation
Gestational hypertension	New hypertension with a blood pressure of 140/90 mm Hg on two separate occasions, without proteinuria, arising de novo after the 20th week of pregnancy. Blood pressure normalizes by 12 weeks post partum.
Preeclampsia superimposed on chronic hypertension	Increased blood pressure above the patient's baseline, a change in proteinuria, or evidence of end-organ dysfunction
Preeclampsia-eclampsia	Proteinuria (>0.3 g during 24 hours or ++ in two urine samples) in addition to new hypertension. Edema is no longer included in the diagnosis because of poor specificity. When proteinuria is absent, suspect the disease when increased blood pressure is associated with headache, blurred vision, abdominal pain, low platelets, or abnormal liver enzymes.

From Gifford RW, August PA, Cunningham G, et al: Report of the National High Blood Pressure Education Program Working Group on High Blood Pressure in Pregnancy. Am J Obstet Gynecol 183:S1, 2000.

TABLE 82-4	Cardiovascular Drugs in Pregnancy
DRUG	POTENTIAL FETAL SIDE EFFECTS
Amiodarone	Goiter, hypothyroidism and hyperthyroidism, IUGR
Angiotensin-converting enzyme inhibitors	Contraindicated; IUGR, oligohydramnios, renal failure, abnormal bone ossification; FDA class X
Aspirin	Baby aspirin not harmful
Beta blockers	Relatively safe; IUGR, neonatal bradycardia, and hypoglycemia
Calcium channel blockers	Relatively safe; few data; concern regarding uterine tone at the time of delivery
Digoxin	Safe; no adverse effects
Flecainide	Relatively safe; limited data; used to treat fetal arrhythmias
Hydralazine	Safe; no major adverse effects
Lasix	Safe; caution regarding maternal hypovolemia and reduced placental blood flow
Lidocaine	Safe; high doses may cause neonatal central nervous system depression
Methyldopa	Safe; considered by some to be the drug of choice for hypertension in pregnancy
Procainamide	Relatively safe; limited data; has been used to treat fetal arrhythmias, no major fetal side effects
Propafenone	Limited data
Quinidine	Relatively safe; rarely associated with neonatal thrombocytopenia; minimal oxytocic effect
Warfarin	Fetal embryopathy, placental and fetal hemorrhage, central nervous system abnormalities; FDA class X

IUGR = intrauterine growth retardation.

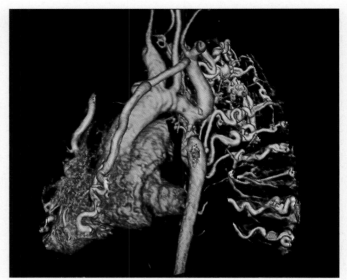

FIGURE 82-4 Magnetic resonance imaging scan of a 34-year-old with severe coarctation of the aorta (near interruption), with multiple and very large collateral vessels. She had had two prior pregnancies with preeclampsia and the coarctation had gone unnoticed.

long safety record with methyldopa, which has no adverse effect on mother or baby.

Coarctation of the aorta needs to be considered (**Fig. 82-4**).

Arrhythmias (see Chaps. 36 to 39)

Because of the physiologic changes of pregnancy, the heart may be more vulnerable to arrhythmias during this time. Potential contributing factors include the increase in preload, causing more myocardial irritability; increased heart rate, which may affect the refractory period; fluid and electrolyte shifts; and changes in catecholamine levels. Worsening of arrhythmias is not a consistent feature, however, and many women with a past history of tachycardia may not notice any change in the frequency of symptoms, and some even improve. The presenting symptom complex may be difficult to separate from the normal symptoms of pregnancy, including a sensation of fast heartbeat and skipped beats, which most commonly are supraventricular ectopics. The general approach should include taking a careful history, looking for any precipitating causes, and ruling out any concomitant medical problems (e.g., thyroid disease) by performing appropriate laboratory tests, such as complete blood count, electrolyte level measurement, and thyroid function determination. The clinical examination may help define whether the arrhythmia occurs in the setting of a normal heart or whether there is any underlying organic heart disease. If there is any doubt after the clinical examination, a transthoracic echocardiogram should be obtained. If the mother has no underlying cardiac disease, pharmacologic treatment should be administered if she is symptomatic or if the arrhythmia poses a risk to the mother or baby. In general, supraventricular and ventricular ectopic beats require no therapy. If there is underlying

organic disease, the precipitating cause should be treated, if possible, and if this does not resolve, the arrhythmia medical therapy should be initiated.

The most common arrhythmia is atrial reentry tachycardia. Treatment of this type of arrhythmia is generally the same as for nonpregnant women, but with added concern about the effects of medications on the fetus (see Table 82-4). In general, the lowest dose necessary to treat the arrhythmia should be administered, and there should be a periodic evaluation of whether it is necessary to continue treatment. Atrial fibrillation is usually an indication that there is underlying structural heart disease. If the arrhythmia is unresponsive to medical therapy, electrical cardioversion may be performed and is not usually harmful to the fetus. Some have recommended that during elective cardioversion, fetal monitoring should be performed in case transient fetal bradycardia is present.

Premature ventricular complexes are common during pregnancy and usually require no treatment. Ventricular tachycardia is rare but may be a consequence of ischemic heart disease or cardiomyopathy. The treatment depends on the rate of tachycardia and the hemodynamic status of the mother. The choices of medications are listed in Table 82-4; electrical cardioversion should be performed if there is hemodynamic compromise.

Cardiovascular Drug Therapy (see Chap. 10)

When administration of cardiovascular drugs is being contemplated during pregnancy, the U.S. Food and Drug Administration (FDA) classification of these drugs must be considered. The reader is referred to more detailed information in this regard. Category X drugs are those for which fetal abnormalities have been demonstrated in animal or human studies, and the drug is contraindicated (e.g., warfarin). Almost all cardiovascular drugs are classified as category C, which means that animal studies have revealed adverse fetal effects, but there are no controlled data in women. A medication should be given only if the benefits outweigh the potential risk to the fetus. Important principles to be considered in using cardiovascular medications for pregnant women include the use of drugs with the longest safety record, the use of the lowest dose and shortest duration necessary, and in general the avoidance of a multidrug regimen, if possible. All these issues need to be reviewed carefully with the prospective mother at the time of pre-pregnancy counseling. A list of cardiovascular medications that might be considered in pregnancy is given in Table 82-4.

ASPIRIN. Aspirin crosses the placenta, and concern exists about its effect on fetal prostaglandins, which might cause closure of the fetal ductus arteriosus. Baby aspirin (81 mg), however, has been used safely in pregnancy without premature closure of the fetal duct. It may be useful adjunctive therapy when the mother has a mechanical valve prosthesis, and it can help prevent valve thrombosis.

AMIODARONE. Amiodarone and its iodine component cross the placenta and may cause neonatal goiter. The risks and benefits of its use, however, need to be balanced. If it has proved effective in controlling serious maternal arrhythmias, it may be safer for the mother to continue its use during pregnancy.

ANGIOTENSIN-CONVERTING ENZYME INHIBITORS. These are contraindicated in pregnancy because they are associated with abnormal renal development in the fetus as well as oligohydramnios and intrauterine growth retardation.

BETA-ADRENERGIC RECEPTOR BLOCKERS. These have been used extensively during pregnancy for treatment of arrhythmias, hypertrophic cardiomyopathy, and hypertension. They cross the placenta but are not teratogenic. Concern exists, however, particularly regarding fetal growth, because they have been demonstrated to cause fetal growth retardation. They may also be associated with neonatal bradycardia and hypoglycemia. More concern exists with regard to atenolol than some of the other beta-blocking agents. From a practical perspective, however, although the risk-to-benefit ratio needs to be considered, beta blockers have been used safely during pregnancy, although it is recommended that fetal growth be monitored more carefully.

CALCIUM CHANNEL BLOCKERS. These have been used to treat both arrhythmias and hypertension. There are limited data regarding their use. Most experience probably exists with verapamil, and no major adverse fetal effects have been recorded. Diltiazem and nifedipine have also been used, but studies are limited.

DIGOXIN. Digoxin has been used during pregnancy for many decades, and although it does cross the placenta, no adverse effects with its use have been reported.

DIURETICS. These agents, most commonly furosemide, may be used to treat congestive heart failure during pregnancy and sometimes are used for the treatment of hypertension. Aggressive use of diuretics, however, may cause reduction in placental blood flow and have a detrimental effect on fetal growth.

WARFARIN. Warfarin is usually contraindicated in the first trimester of pregnancy because it crosses the placenta and may cause fetal embryopathy. As noted earlier (see Mechanical Prostheses and Anticoagulant Treatment), however, there may be some high-risk situations in which the mother and physician determine that the safer approach is to continue warfarin therapy, particularly when the maternal dose is 5 mg or lower. Concern exists in the third trimester about labor and delivery because the immature fetal liver does not metabolize warfarin as rapidly as the mother's liver. After discontinuation of warfarin, reversal of anticoagulation occurs more rapidly in the mother, whereas reversal of anticoagulation in the fetus may take up to 1 week because of the immature fetal liver. Vaginal delivery when the fetus is anticoagulated is contraindicated because of the risk of fetal hemorrhage. Therefore, switching to an alternative anticoagulant such as heparin must be done well before labor is anticipated.

Contraception

For women with cardiac disease, appropriate contraceptive advice should be given before they become sexually active. This is particularly true for those with congenital heart disease, who, like other adolescents without heart disease, often become sexually active in their early teens. For some, pregnancy may pose a high risk of morbidity and even mortality. Patients need to be given detailed advice about various contraceptive methods and their effectiveness, and each patient should understand the relative risks and benefits of each modality.[42] The approach should be individualized, also bearing in mind the patient's likely compliance.[43]

BARRIER CONTRACEPTION. Male and female condoms help protect against sexually transmitted disease but must be used correctly and require some dexterity. Even when used appropriately, they have a recognized failure rate of approximately 15 pregnancies/100 woman-years of use. The decision to use a barrier method therefore depends on how critical it is for the woman to avoid pregnancy and on compliance and the ability to use a condom correctly.

INTRAUTERINE DEVICES. Intrauterine devices (IUDs) may be used in parous women, with failure rates of approximately 3 pregnancies/100 woman-years. Complications include infection and arrhythmia at the time of insertion. A vasovagal response occurring in a patient with idiopathic pulmonary arterial hypertension or secondary pulmonary hypertension, such as Eisenmenger syndrome, could be life-threatening, and many physicians therefore avoid use of an IUD in such patients. More recently developed IUDs are more effective than earlier devices in preventing pregnancy, particularly those that are loaded with progesterone, which suppresses endometrial activity and thickens cervical mucus.

Oral Contraceptives

Combination estrogen-progesterone oral preparations are very effective, with an extremely low failure rate, and for this reason, coupled with ease of use, are widely taken. For the woman with heart disease, however, concern exists because of increased risk of venous thromboembolism, atherosclerosis, hyperlipidemia, hypertension, and ischemic heart disease, particularly for those who are older than 40 years and for those who smoke. In addition, patients with congenital heart disease who have cyanosis, atrial fibrillation or flutter, mechanical prosthetic heart valves, or a Fontan circulation probably should avoid estrogen-containing preparations. Those with impaired ventricular function from any cause (probably an ejection fraction less than 40%) or with a history of any prior thromboembolic event should avoid estrogen.

Progesterone-only contraceptives are less reliable than combined preparations, with failure rates of 2 to 5 pregnancies/100 woman-years. The woman must take the pill at the same time every day for optimum efficacy, and this requires considerable motivation on the part of the patient. There is a paucity of data about adverse effects of progesterone agents on the cardiovascular system, but these are probably safe for most women with heart disease.

ALTERNATIVE COMBINED HORMONAL PREPARATIONS. Newer modalities include a vaginal ring, which is a once-monthly device that is removed after three weeks. A contraceptive patch containing estrogen and progesterone is also available as well as an injectable preparation, both of which have similar efficacy rates.

DEPOT PROGESTERONE. Injectable progesterone, given once every 3 months, is effective and is an attractive alternative for patients who may have problems with compliance with oral medications. Some patients find fluid retention and irregular menstruation to be problems, but cardiovascular contraindications are otherwise the same as those for progesterone.

ALTERNATIVE PROGESTERONE MODALITIES. Subdermal implants, which are inserted into the arm, are also available.

Tubal Sterilization

Tubal sterilization may be performed laparoscopically or through a laparotomy. For patients who have tenuous cardiac hemodynamics, there may be some risk of cardiac instability, and cardiac anesthesia may be preferable. This is particularly important, for example, in patients with primary or secondary pulmonary hypertension when general anesthesia may be hazardous and insufflation of the abdomen may elevate the diaphragm and contribute to unstable cardiorespiratory function. More recently, tubal sterilization has been accomplished with the use of an intrafallopian plug, which is inserted endoscopically.[44]

Future Perspectives

Appropriate pregnancy counseling for women with cardiac disease is problematic. Few physicians have expertise or training to manage such patients, particularly those women with congenital heart disease. Few evidence-based guidelines are available, and most published data involve isolated case reports or small cohort studies. Many questions remain unanswered. Although successful pregnancy is possible in many women with heart disease, does the volume load cause subtle long-term deterioration in ventricular function in those with limited cardiac reserve?[45] What is the ideal management strategy for women with mechanical valve prostheses? These continued uncertainties emphasize the need for multicenter research initiatives to answer prospectively the many questions that remain.

REFERENCES

General

1. Roos-Hesselink JW, Duvekot JJ, Thorne SA: Pregnancy in high risk cardiac conditions. Heart 95:680, 2009.
2. Connolly H, Warnes C: Pregnancy and contraception. In Gatzoulis MA, Webb GD, Daubeney PE (eds): Diagnosis and Management of Adult Congenital Heart Disease. Edinburgh, Churchill Livingstone, 2003, pp 135-177.
3. Siu SC, Sermer M, Colman JM, et al: Prospective multicenter study of pregnancy outcomes in women with heart disease. Circulation 104:515, 2001.
4. Thorne SA: Pregnancy in heart disease. Heart 90:450, 2004.
5. Elkayam U, Bitar F: Valvular heart disease and pregnancy part I: Native valves. J Am Coll Cardiol 46:223, 2005.

Congenital Heart Disease

6. Warnes CA, Williams RG, Bashore TM, et al: ACC/AHA 2008 Guidelines for the Management of Adults with Congenital Heart Disease: A report of the American College of Cardiology/American Heart Association Task Force on Practice Guidelines (writing committee to develop guidelines on the management of adults with congenital heart disease). Circulation 118:e714, 2008.
7. Drenthen W, Pieper PG, Roos-Hesselink JW, et al: Outcome of pregnancy in women with congenital heart disease: A literature review. J Am Coll Cardiol 49:2303, 2007.
8. Stout K: Pregnancy in women with congenital heart disease: The importance of evaluation and counselling [comment]. Heart 91:713, 2005.
9. Silversides CK, Colman JM, Sermer M, et al: Early and intermediate-term outcomes of pregnancy with congenital aortic stenosis. Am J Cardiol 91:1386, 2003.
10. Myerson SG, Mitchell AR, Ormerod OJ, Banning AP: What is the role of balloon dilatation for severe aortic stenosis during pregnancy? [see comment]. J Heart Valve Dis 14:147, 2005.
11. Warnes CA: Cyanotic congenital heart disease. In Oakley C, Warnes CA (eds): Heart Disease in Pregnancy. Malden, Mass, Blackwell, 2007, pp 43-58.
12. Presbitero P, Somerville J, Stone S, et al: Pregnancy in cyanotic congenital heart disease. Outcome of mother and fetus. Circulation 89:2673, 1994.
13. Beauchesne LM, Warnes CA, Connolly HM, et al: Prevalence and clinical manifestations of 22q11.2 microdeletion in adults with selected conotruncal anomalies [see comment]. J Am Coll Cardiol 45:595, 2005.
14. Khairy P, Ouyang DW, Fernandes SM, et al: Pregnancy outcomes in women with congenital heart disease. Circulation 113:517, 2006.
15. Meijer JM, Pieper PG, Drenthen W, et al: Pregnancy, fertility, and recurrence risk in corrected tetralogy of Fallot [see comment]. Heart 91:801, 2005.
16. Veldtman GR, Connolly HM, Grogan M, et al: Outcomes of pregnancy in women with tetralogy of Fallot [see comment]. J Am Coll Cardiol 44:174, 2004.
17. Warnes CA: Pregnancy and pulmonary hypertension. Int J Cardiol 97(Suppl 1):11, 2004.
18. Gleicher N, Midwall J, Hochberger D, Jaffin H: Eisenmenger's syndrome and pregnancy. Obstet Gynecol Surv 34:721, 1979.
19. Bonnin M, Mercier FJ, Sitbon O, et al: Severe pulmonary hypertension during pregnancy: Mode of delivery and anesthetic management of 15 consecutive cases [see comment]. Anesthesiology 102:1133; discussion 5A, 2005.
20. Lacassie HJ, Germain AM, Valdes G, et al: Management of Eisenmenger syndrome in pregnancy with sildenafil and L-arginine. Obstet Gynecol 103:1118, 2004.

Rheumatic and Acquired Valvular Heart Disease

21. Routray SN, Mishra TK, Swain S, et al: Balloon mitral valvuloplasty during pregnancy. Int J Gynaecol Obstet 85:18, 2004.
22. Aggarwal N, Suri V, Goyal A, et al: Closed mitral valvotomy in pregnancy and labor. Int J Gynaecol Obstet 88:118, 2005.
23. Elkayam U, Singh H, Irani A, Akhter MW: Anticoagulation in pregnant women with prosthetic heart valves. J Cardiovasc Pharmacol Ther 9:107, 2004.
24. Jamieson WR, Miller DC, Akins CW, et al: Pregnancy and bioprostheses: Influence on structural valve deterioration. Ann Thorac Surg 60:S282; discussion S287, 1995.
25. Bates SM, Greer IA, Hirsh J, Ginsberg JS: Use of antithrombotic agents during pregnancy: The Seventh ACCP Conference on Antithrombotic and Thrombolytic Therapy. Chest 126:627S, 2004.
26. Sbarouni E, Oakley CM: Outcome of pregnancy in women with valve prostheses. Br Heart J 71:196, 1994.
27. Elkayam U, Bitar F: Valvular heart disease and pregnancy: Part II: Prosthetic valves. J Am Coll Cardiol 46:403, 2005.
28. Chan WS, Anand S, Ginsberg JS: Anticoagulation of pregnant women with mechanical heart valves: A systematic review of the literature. Arch Intern Med 160:191, 2000.
29. Barbour LA, Oja JL, Schultz LK: A prospective trial that demonstrates that dalteparin requirements increase in pregnancy to maintain therapeutic levels of anticoagulation. Am J Obstet Gynecol 191:1024, 2004.
30. Oran B, Lee-Parritz A, Ansell J: Low molecular weight heparin for the prophylaxis of thromboembolism in women with prosthetic mechanical heart valves during pregnancy. Thromb Haemost 92:747, 2004.
31. Vitale N, De Feo M, De Santo LS, et al: Dose-dependent fetal complications of warfarin in pregnant women with mechanical heart valves [see comment]. J Am Coll Cardiol 33:1637, 1999.

Connective Tissue Disorders

32. Meijboom LJ, Vos FE, Timmermans J, et al: Pregnancy and aortic root growth in the Marfan syndrome: A prospective study [see comment]. Eur Heart J 26:914, 2005.

Cardiomyopathies

33. Elkayam U, Akhter MW, Singh H, et al: Pregnancy-associated cardiomyopathy: Clinical characteristics and a comparison between early and late presentation. Circulation 111:2050, 2005.
34. Sliwa K, Fett J, Elkayam U: Peripartum cardiomyopathy. Lancet 368:687, 2006.
35. Phillips SD, Warnes CA: Peripartum cardiomyopathy: Current therapeutic perspectives. Curr Treat Options Cardiovasc Med 6:481, 2004.
36. Sliwa K, Forster O, Zhanje F, et al: Outcome of subsequent pregnancy in patients with documented peripartum cardiomyopathy. Am J Cardiol 93:1441, 2004.
37. Thaman R, Varnava A, Hamid MS, et al: Pregnancy related complications in women with hypertrophic cardiomyopathy. Heart 89:752, 2003.

Coronary Artery Disease

38. Roth A, Elkayam U: Acute myocardial infarction associated with pregnancy. J Am Coll Cardiol 52:171, 2008.
39. Maeder M, Ammann P, Angehrn W, Rickli H: Idiopathic spontaneous coronary artery dissection: Incidence, diagnosis and treatment. Int J Cardiol 101:363, 2005.
40. James AH, Jamison MG, Biswas MS, et al: Acute myocardial infarction in pregnancy: A United States population-based study. Circulation 113:1564, 2006.

Hypertension

41. Gifford RW, August PA, Cunningham G, et al: Report of the National High Blood Pressure Education Program Working Group on High Blood Pressure in Pregnancy. Am J Obstet Gynecol 183:S1, 2000.

Contraception

42. Wald R, Colman J: Pregnancy and contraception. In Warnes C (ed): The AHA Clinical Series: Adult Congenital Heart Disease. Hoboken, NJ, Wiley-Blackwell, 2009, pp 237-259.
43. Thorne S, MacGregor A, Nelson-Piercy C: Risks of contraception and pregnancy in heart disease. Heart 92:1520, 2006.
44. Famuyide AO, Hopkins MR, El-Nashar SA, et al: Hysteroscopic sterilization in women with severe cardiac disease: Experience at a tertiary center. Mayo Clin Proc 83:431, 2008.
45. Guedes A, Mercier LA, Leduc L, et al: Impact of pregnancy on the systemic right ventricle after a Mustard operation for transposition of the great arteries. J Am Coll Cardiol 44:433, 2004.

 GUIDELINES CAROLE A. WARNES AND THOMAS H. LEE

Pregnancy and Heart Disease

Recommendations for the management of heart disease in pregnancy appear in various American College of Cardiology/American Heart Association (ACC/AHA) guidelines. These include guidelines on valvular heart disease,[1] atrial fibrillation,[2] and stroke.[3] The European Society of Cardiology also published guidelines on the management of valvular heart disease[4] as well as a position paper on use of anticoagulants in heart disease.[5]

ATRIAL FIBRILLATION

Atrial fibrillation is rare during pregnancy and is usually associated with another underlying cause, such as mitral stenosis, congenital heart disease, or hyperthyroidism. Diagnosis and treatment of the underlying condition causing the dysrhythmia are of utmost importance. Antithrombotic therapy is recommended for all pregnant women with atrial fibrillation.

The type of therapy should be chosen with regard to the stage of pregnancy (**Table 82G-1**).[2] The ventricular rate should be controlled with digoxin, calcium channel antagonist, or beta blocker. Direct-current cardioversion can be performed without fetal damage in women who become hemodynamically unstable because of atrial fibrillation. Administration of quinidine or procainamide is a reasonable approach for cardioversion in pregnant women with atrial fibrillation who are hemodynamically stable.

VALVULAR DISEASE

Many women with valvular heart disease can be successfully managed throughout pregnancy, labor, and delivery with conservative medical measures. Symptomatic or severe valvular lesions should be addressed and rectified before conception and pregnancy whenever possible. Drugs should be avoided when possible.[1]

Mitral Stenosis

Pregnant women with mild to moderate mitral stenosis can almost always be managed with judicious use of diuretics and beta blockade. A cardioselective beta blocker may prevent deleterious effects of epinephrine blockade on myometrial tissue. Women with severe mitral stenosis should be considered for percutaneous balloon mitral valvotomy before conception, if possible. Percutaneous balloon valvotomy is a reasonable option for women who develop severe symptoms during pregnancy.

Mitral Regurgitation

Mitral regurgitation can usually be managed medically with diuretics and vasodilator therapy. If surgery is required, repair is always preferred.

Aortic Stenosis

Pregnant women with mild obstruction and normal left ventricular systolic function can be managed conservatively throughout pregnancy. Those with moderate to severe obstruction or symptoms should be advised to delay conception until aortic stenosis can be corrected. Women with severe aortic stenosis who develop symptoms may require either early delivery of the baby or percutaneous aortic balloon valvotomy or surgery before delivery.

Aortic Regurgitation

Isolated aortic regurgitation can usually be managed with diuretics and vasodilator therapy when needed. Surgery during pregnancy should be contemplated only for control of refractory symptoms.

Endocarditis Prophylaxis

The guidelines do not recommend routine antibiotic prophylaxis in patients with valvular heart disease undergoing uncomplicated vaginal delivery or cesarean section unless infection is suspected. For high-risk patients, such as those with cyanotic heart disease, prosthetic heart valves, or a prior history of endocarditis, antibiotics are considered optional.[6]

SUPRAVENTRICULAR TACHYCARDIAS

Premature atrial beats, which are commonly observed during pregnancy, are generally benign and well tolerated. In patients with mild symptoms and structurally normal hearts, no treatment other than reassurance should be provided. Given that all commonly used antiarrhythmic drugs cross the placental barrier to some extent, antiarrhythmic drug therapy should be used only if symptoms are intolerable or if the tachycardia causes hemodynamic compromise (**Table 82G-2**).[7]

Catheter ablation should be recommended for women with symptomatic tachyarrhythmias before they contemplate pregnancy. Because of the potential problem of recurring tachyarrhythmias during pregnancy, the policy of withdrawing antiarrhythmic drugs and resuming them later can be recommended only as an alternative in selected cases. Catheter ablation is the procedure of choice for drug-refractory, poorly tolerated supraventricular tachycardia. If needed, it should be performed in the second trimester.

TABLE 82G-1 ACC/AHA Recommendations for Management of Atrial Fibrillation (AF) During Pregnancy

CLASS	INDICATION	LEVEL OF EVIDENCE
Class I (indicated)	Control the rate of ventricular response with digoxin, a beta blocker, or a calcium channel antagonist.	C
	Perform electrical cardioversion in patients who become hemodynamically unstable because of the dysrhythmia.	C
	Administer antithrombotic therapy (anticoagulant or aspirin) throughout pregnancy to all patients with AF (except those with lone AF).	C
Class IIb (weak supportive evidence)	Attempt pharmacologic cardioversion by administration of quinidine, procainamide, or sotalol in hemodynamically stable patients who develop AF during pregnancy.	C
	Administer heparin to patients with risk factors for thromboembolism during the first trimester and last month of pregnancy. Unfractionated heparin may be administered either by continuous intravenous infusion in a dose sufficient to prolong the activated partial thromboplastin time to 1.5 to 2 times the control (reference) value or by intermittent subcutaneous injection in a dose of 10,000 to 20,000 units every 12 hours, adjusted to prolong the midinterval (6 hours after injection) activated partial thromboplastin time to 1.5 times control. Limited data are available to support the subcutaneous administration of low-molecular-weight heparin for this indication.	C
	Administer an oral anticoagulant during the second trimester to patients at high thromboembolic risk.	C

TABLE 82G-2 ACC/AHA Recommendations for Treatment Strategies for Supraventricular Tachycardias During Pregnancy

INDICATION	CLASS I (INDICATED) [LEVEL OF EVIDENCE]	CLASS IIa (STRONG SUPPORTIVE EVIDENCE) [LEVEL OF EVIDENCE]	CLASS IIb (WEAK SUPPORTIVE EVIDENCE) [LEVEL OF EVIDENCE]	CLASS III (NOT INDICATED) [LEVEL OF EVIDENCE]
Acute conversion of PSVT	Vagal maneuver [C] Adenosine [C] Direct-current cardioversion [C]	Metoprolol,* propranolol* [C]	Verapamil [C]	
Prophylactic therapy	Digoxin [C] Metoprolol*	Propranolol* [B] Sotalol,* flecainide† [C]	Quinidine, propafenone,† verapamil [C] Procainamide [B] Catheter ablation [C]	Atenolol‡ [B] Amiodarone [C]

*Beta-blocking agents should not be taken in the first trimester, if possible.
†Consider atrioventricular node–blocking agents in conjunction with flecainide and propafenone for certain tachycardias.
‡Atenolol is categorized in class C (drug classification for use during pregnancy) by legal authorities in some European countries.
PSVT = paroxysmal supraventricular tachycardia.

STROKE

Pregnancy increases the risk for stroke and complicates the selection of acute and preventive treatments. Guidelines for acute treatment have not yet been established. Recommendations for stroke prevention in pregnant women made by the American Heart Association and American Stroke Association (AHA/ASA)[4] focus on anticoagulation and antiplatelet strategies (**Table 82G-3**), which are similar to those for management of valvular heart disease during pregnancy.

HYPERTENSION

The European Society of Hypertension and the European Society of Cardiology (ESH/ESC) issued guidelines in 2007 that address the management of hypertension in pregnancy (**Table 82G-4**).[8]

ANTICOAGULATION

The 2006 ACC/AHA guidelines on valvular heart disease emphasize the importance of pre-pregnancy counseling about anticoagulation strategies

before pregnancy and the need for meticulous and frequent monitoring of anticoagulation once pregnancy occurs. The guidelines reflect the high complication rates in pregnant women with mechanical prosthetic heart valves managed with subcutaneous heparin and support the use of intravenous heparin during the first trimester. After the 36th week of pregnancy, transition from warfarin to heparin is recommended in anticipation of labor. There is no consensus on the ideal management strategy for women with mechanical prosthetic heart valves given the paucity of data regarding their comparative efficacy. A menu of options is proposed for anticoagulation strategies (**Table 82G-5**).

These strategies are complicated by the fact that low-molecular-weight heparin is not approved by the U.S. Food and Drug Administration (FDA) for use in any patient with a mechanical prosthetic heart valve, and the FDA has issued an advisory warning against the use of enoxaparin (Lovenox) in pregnant women with mechanical prosthetic heart valves. The guidelines note that some data indicate that low-molecular-weight heparin appears to be safe in nonpregnant patients with mechanical heart valves, but the expert panel could not recommend its use directly, given the status of FDA-approved indications. The ACC/AHA Guidelines for Adult Congenital Heart Disease emphasize that whichever anticoagulant

TABLE 82G-3	AHA/ASA Recommendations for Stroke Prevention During Pregnancy	
CLASS	**INDICATION**	**LEVEL OF EVIDENCE**
Class IIb (weak supportive evidence)	For pregnant women with ischemic stroke or TIA and high-risk thromboembolic conditions, such as known coagulopathy or mechanical heart valves, the following options may be considered: adjusted-dose UFH throughout pregnancy, e.g., a subcutaneous dose every 12 hours with activated partial thromboplastin time monitoring; adjusted-dose LMWH with factor Xa monitoring throughout pregnancy; or UFH or LMWH until week 13, followed by warfarin until the middle of the third trimester, when UFH or LMWH is then reinstituted until delivery.	C
	Pregnant women with lower risk conditions may be considered for treatment with UFH or LMWH in the first trimester, followed by low-dose aspirin for the remainder of the pregnancy.	C

LMWH = low-molecular-weight heparin; TIA = transient ischemic attack; UFH = unfractionated heparin.

TABLE 82G-4	ESH/ESC Guidelines for the Management of Hypertension During Pregnancy

Nonpharmacologic treatment (including close supervision and restriction of activities) should be considered with SBP 140-149 mm Hg or DBP 90-95 mm Hg. In the presence of gestational hypertension (with or without proteinuria), drug treatment is indicated at blood pressure ≥140/90 mm Hg. SBP levels ≥170 or DBP >110 mm Hg should be considered an emergency requiring hospitalization.

In nonsevere hypertension, oral methyldopa, labetalol, calcium antagonists, and (less frequently) beta blockers are drugs of choice.

In preeclampsia with pulmonary edema, nitroglycerin is the drug of choice. Diuretic therapy is inappropriate because plasma volume is reduced.

As emergency, IV labetalol, oral methyldopa, and oral nifedipine are indicated; IV hydralazine is no longer the drug of choice because of excess perinatal adverse effects. IV infusion of sodium nitroprusside is useful in hypertensive crises, but prolonged administration should be avoided.

Calcium supplementation, fish oil, and low-dose aspirin are not recommended. However, low-dose aspirin may be used prophylactically in women with a history of early-onset preeclampsia.

DBP = diastolic blood pressure; IV = intravenous; SBP = systolic blood pressure.

TABLE 82G-5	ACC/AHA Recommendations for Anticoagulation Regimens in Pregnant Patients with Mechanical Prosthetic Valves	
CLASS	**INDICATION**	**LEVEL OF EVIDENCE**
Class I (indicated)	Continuous therapeutic anticoagulation with frequent monitoring	B
	If warfarin is discontinued between weeks 6 and 12 of gestation, replace with continuous intravenous UFH, dose-adjusted UFH, or dose-adjusted subcutaneous LMWH.	C
	Up to 36 weeks of gestation, the therapeutic choice of continuous intravenous or dose-adjusted subcutaneous UFH, dose-adjusted LMWH, or warfarin should be discussed fully.	C
	If dose-adjusted LMWH is used, the LMWH should be administered twice daily subcutaneously to maintain the anti-Xa level between 0.7 and 1.2 unit/mL 4 hours after administration.	C
	If dose-adjusted UFH is used, the aPTT should be at least twice control.	C
	If warfarin is used, the INR goal should be 3.0 (range, 2.5 to 3.5).	C
	Warfarin should be discontinued starting 2 to 3 weeks before planned delivery and continuous intravenous UFH given instead.	C
Class IIa (strong supportive evidence)	It is reasonable to avoid warfarin between weeks 6 and 12 of gestation because of the high risk of fetal defects.	C
	It is reasonable to resume UFH 4 to 6 hours after delivery and begin oral warfarin in the absence of significant bleeding.	C
	It is reasonable to give low-dose aspirin (75 to 100 mg/day) in the second and third trimesters of pregnancy in addition to anticoagulation with warfarin or heparin.	C
Class III (not indicated)	LMWH should not be administered unless anti-Xa levels are monitored 4 to 6 hours after administration.	C
	Dipyridamole should not be used instead of aspirin as an alternative antiplatelet agent because of its harmful effects on the fetus.	B

aPTT = activated partial thromboplastin time; INR = international normalized ratio; LMWH = low-molecular-weight heparin; UFH = unfractionated heparin.

strategy is chosen, women with mechanical prosthetic heart valves should be cared for at tertiary care centers where a multidisciplinary team with expertise and training in the management of such patients is responsible for their care.[6]

REFERENCES

1. Bonow RO, Carabello BA, Chatterjee K, et al: ACC/AHA 2006 guidelines for the management of patients with valvular heart disease: A report of the American College of Cardiology/American Heart Association Task Force on Practice Guidelines (writing committee to revise the 1998 Guidelines for the Management of Patients With Valvular Heart Disease): Developed in collaboration with the Society of Cardiovascular Anesthesiologists: Endorsed by the Society for Cardiovascular Angiography and Interventions and the Society of Thoracic Surgeons [erratum appears in Circulation 115:e409, 2007]. Circulation 114:e84, 2006.

2. Fuster V, Ryden LE, Cannom DS, et al: ACC/AHA/ESC 2006 Guidelines for the Management of Patients with Atrial Fibrillation: A report of the American College of Cardiology/American Heart Association Task Force on Practice Guidelines and the European Society of Cardiology Committee for Practice Guidelines (Writing Committee to Revise the 2001 Guidelines for the Management of Patients With Atrial Fibrillation): Developed in collaboration with the European Heart Rhythm Association and the Heart Rhythm Society [erratum appears in Circulation 116:e138, 2007]. Circulation 114:e257, 2006.

3. Adams H, Adams R, Del Zoppo G, Goldstein LB: Guidelines for the early management of patients with ischemic stroke: 2005 guidelines update. A scientific statement from the Stroke Council of the American Heart Association/American Stroke Association [erratum appears in Stroke 36:1626, 2005]. Stroke 36:916, 2005.

4. Vahanian A, Baumgartner H, Bax J, et al: Guidelines on the management of valvular heart disease: The Task Force on the Management of Valvular Heart Disease of the European Society of Cardiology [see comment]. Eur Heart J 28:230, 2007.

5. De Caterina R, Husted S, Wallentin L, et al: Anticoagulants in heart disease: Current status and perspectives [see comment]. Eur Heart J 28:880, 2007.

6. Warnes CA, Williams RG, Bashore TM, et al: ACC/AHA 2008 Guidelines for the Management of Adults with Congenital Heart Disease: A report of the American College of Cardiology/American Heart Association Task Force on Practice Guidelines (writing committee to develop guidelines on the management of adults with congenital heart disease). Circulation 118:e714, 2008.

7. Blomstrom-Lundqvist C, Scheinman MM, Aliot EM, et al: ACC/AHA/ESC guidelines for the management of patients with supraventricular arrhythmias—executive summary. A report of the American College of Cardiology/American Heart Association Task Force on Practice Guidelines and the European Society of Cardiology Committee for Practice Guidelines (writing committee to develop guidelines for the management of patients with supraventricular arrhythmias) developed in collaboration with NASPE—Heart Rhythm Society. J Am Coll Cardiol 42:1493, 2003.

8. Mancia G, De Backer G, Dominiczak A, et al: 2007 Guidelines for the management of arterial hypertension: The Task Force for the Management of Arterial Hypertension of the European Society of Hypertension (ESH) and of the European Society of Cardiology (ESC). Eur Heart J 28:1462, 2007.

CHAPTER 83 **Exercise and Sports Cardiology**

Gary J. Balady and Philip A. Ades

The importance of exercise and sports were recognized by the ancient Greeks thousands of years ago, but an interesting paradox now exists. A large volume of evidence from epidemiologic observational studies, cohort studies, randomized controlled trials, and basic research, primarily conducted during the past four decades, demonstrates unequivocal evidence that exercise and physical activity confer health. The publication of the seminal 1996 Surgeon General's Report on Physical Activity and Health[1] moved the promotion of physical activity to the top of America's national public health agenda. Physical inactivity is now recognized as an independent risk factor for the development of cardiovascular disease (CVD)[2] (see Chap. 49). In the face of these events, however, only a small proportion of Americans engage in adequate physical activity. The Centers for Disease Control and Prevention has indicated that approximately 31% of adult Americans participate in recommended levels of physical activity, and almost 40% report no regular leisure time physical activity whatsoever.[3] Although the world benefits from advancements in technology that lead to increased productivity and improved quality of life, the price is paid in part by the generation of a sedentary society that spends much of its time in cars, at computer stations, and in front of televisions and video screens.

Medical professionals and public health and community leaders continue their unprecedented efforts to promote increased physical activity through venues that range from casual walks to participation in organized sports, and health care providers need to support these efforts for their patients in regard to optimizing the benefits of participation while minimizing the small but potential associated risks. This chapter presents these issues with an overview of the classifications of exercise and sports, data regarding the benefits of exercise and mechanisms by which these benefits occur, risks of exercise, exercise prescription, and screening and recommendations for participation in exercise and athletic competition with a particular emphasis on those with specific cardiovascular conditions.

Physical Activity, Exercise, and Sports

To understand the many issues regarding exercise and sports, and subsequently make important activity-related clinical decisions, a review of standard definitions[1] is essential. Physical activity refers to any activity in which skeletal muscle contraction and relaxation result in bodily movement and require energy. The intensity of physical activity can be described in terms of the energy required per unit of time for the performance of the activity. This variable can be quantified in absolute terms by measuring the oxygen uptake during the activity using respiratory gas analysis. It can also be estimated using standard regression equations as a multiple of resting energy expenditure (MET), where one MET is defined as the oxygen requirement in the resting awake individual (3.5 mL/kg of body weight/min). The intensity of a physical activity can also be defined in relative terms by expressing it as a proportion of the individual's maximal capacity (e.g., the percentage of maximal oxygen uptake or the percentage of maximum heart rate). Alternatively, activity intensity can be expressed as a measure of the force of muscle contraction required (in pounds or kilograms). When defining the amount of physical activity or exercise, an important interrelationship exists between the total dose of activity and the intensity at which the activity is performed. Dose refers to the total amount of energy expended in physical activity expressed in terms of kilocalories or MET-hours, whereas intensity reflects the rate of energy expenditure during such activity.

Exercise or exercise training is planned physical activity performed with the goal of improving or preserving physical fitness. Physical fitness is a set of attributes that enables an individual to perform physical activity. Physical fitness is best assessed by directly measuring peak or maximum oxygen uptake during a graded exercise test. Although this is not always practical, it is more commonly estimated from the peak MET level attained or reporting the peak work rate (e.g., speed and grade of a treadmill, watts on a stationary cycle) during graded exercise tests.[1]

Most types of exercise involve both endurance and resistance training, but one training type usually predominates (**Table 83-1**). The physiologic responses to exercise depend on the type of exercise performed. Endurance exercise, also referred to as aerobic, dynamic, or isotonic exercise, consists of activity involving high-repetition movements against low resistance. Regular endurance exercise is also referred to as endurance training, because it usually leads to an improved exercise capacity, thereby enabling the individual to exercise for a longer duration or at a higher work rate. Resistance exercise involves low-repetition movements against high resistance, in which muscle tension develops predominantly without much muscle shortening. Regular resistance training leads to increased strength and is also referred to as power or strength training. **Figure 83-1** demonstrates the classification of several types of sports as related to the peak static and dynamic components achieved during competition.[4] The classification does not take into account differences in environment (e.g., altitude, temperature, air quality) in which the sport is performed. Each of these variables can influence the physiologic responses during sports activity as well.

Finally, a distinction must be made between competitive and recreational sports, because the physiologic and emotional demands during training and performance may differ markedly.[5] Competitive athletes participate in an organized sport that places a high premium on athletic excellence and achievement, and requires systematic training and regular competition. These athletes characteristically extend themselves to high levels of effort for long periods of time,

TABLE 83-1	Exercise Prescription for Endurance and Resistance Training

Endurance Training

Frequency	3-5 days/wk	**Modality***
		Aerobics
		Arm ergometry
		Cross country ski machines
		Combined arm-leg cycle
Intensity	55%-90% maximum HR *or*	Elliptical machines
	40%-85% maximum Vo_2 or HRR	Jogging, running
		Rowing
		Stair climber
		Swimming
Duration:	20-60 min	Walking

Resistance Training

Frequency	2-3 days/wk	**All Major Muscle Groups**
		Arms and shoulders
		Biceps curl
Intensity	One to three sets of 8-15 RM	Tricep extension
	for each muscle group	Overhead press
		Lateral raises
		Chest and back
		Bench press
		Lateral pull-downs, pull-ups
		Bent over, seated row
		Legs
		Leg extensions, curls, press
		Adductor, abductor

*Modalities listed are not all-inclusive.
HR = heart rate; maximum HR= 220 − age, or peak HR on exercise test; HRR = heart rate reserve = [(peak HR minus resting HR) × %] plus (resting HR); RM = maximum number of times a load can be lifted before fatigue; Vo_2 = measured oxygen uptake.
Modified from American College of Sports Medicine: ASCM's Guidelines for Exercise Testing and Prescription: 8th ed. Philadelphia, Lippincott Williams & Wilkins, 2009; and Fletcher GF, Balady GJ, Amsterdam EA, et al: Exercise standards for testing and training: A statement for health professionals from the American Heart Association. Circulation 104:1694, 2001.

often doing so regardless of other considerations. Recreational athletes engage in activities, on a regular or inconsistent basis, which do not require regular systematic training or the pursuit of excellence. Hence, they do not have the same pressure to excel as do competitive athletes.

Benefits of Exercise

Physical activity is associated with lower all-cause mortality rates in healthy individuals,[2,4,6,7] individuals with chronic diseases,[8] diabetic persons,[9] and older adults (see Chaps. 49 and 50).[10] Although studies of men and women have demonstrated that physical activity performed decades earlier without subsequent maintenance appears to have no long-term benefit, the risk for all-cause mortality decreases in inactive men and women who subsequently become more physically active.[2] Physical fitness can be more readily measured than physical activity. A consistent and graded relationship exists between peak exercise capacity attained during exercise testing and subsequent mortality in both men and women.[4,6] Regular exercise training in patients with coronary artery disease has demonstrated a reduction in mortality and cardiovascular events in meta-analyses[11] and in a recent large cross -sectional study,[12] but this benefit has not yet been conclusively demonstrated in any single, prospective, randomized trial. In the recently reported HF-ACTION trial, such training in patients with heart failure yielded modest significant reductions in the combined endpoint of all-cause mortality and hospitalizations after prespecified adjusted analysis.[13]

The specific mechanisms whereby physical activity reduces mortality and cardiovascular events are likely multifactorial, and extend beyond a reduction in cardiovascular risk factors, because beneficial effects have been shown on thrombosis, endothelial function, inflammation, and autonomic tone. The magnitude of blood pressure reduction attained with exercise is modest and, in mildly hypertensive persons, yields an effect that resembles that of pharmacologic monotherapy.[14] Physical activity and exercise induce several important and beneficial effects on glucose metabolism, including increased insulin sensitivity, decreased hepatic glucose production, preferential use of glucose over fatty acids by exercising muscle, and reduced obesity.[15] In addition, regular exercise may prevent the onset of diabetes mellitus.[16] Overweight and obesity are associated with significant increases in cardiovascular morbidity and mortality.[17] Exercise training appears to be an important component of weight loss programs, although most randomized controlled trials have shown only modest reductions in weight. Studies have suggested that physical activity and exercise help prevent obesity, maintain weight loss, and prevent weight regain after diet-induced weight loss.[18] The effects of exercise on lipid profiles demonstrate the greatest benefit on triglyceride levels, modest changes in high-density lipoprotein (HDL) levels, and little to no change in low-density lipoprotein (LDL) levels.[2] However, some data have suggested that exercise training reduces the concentration of atherogenic, small, dense LDL particles.[19] A unique study of monozygotic twins has shown that there is a strong genetic component to HDL levels that can be slightly but favorably modified by vigorous activity.[20]

Further evidence suggests that exercise training has beneficial effects on the fibrinolytic system, and many studies have reported an inverse relationship between physical activity or fitness and inflammatory markers.[21] Chronic exercise training appears to have an important and favorable influence on endothelial function in the peripheral arteries[22] as well as the coronary circulation.[23] This effect may depend in part on increased nitric oxide production, and yield a net reduction in oxidative stress[24] and an increase in endothelial progenitor cells.[25] Such improvements have been linked to a reduction in adverse cardiovascular events.[26] Finally, exercise training appears to modulate the balance between sympathetic and parasympathetic tone favorably, an effect associated with improvements in survival.[27]

Changes in the muscular, cardiovascular, and neurohumoral systems that result from exercise training lead to improvement in functional capacity and strength. These changes are referred to as the training effect, and they enable an individual to exercise to higher peak work rates with lower heart rates at each submaximal level of exercise. Aging is associated with a decline in maximal exercise capacity, and a longitudinal study has demonstrated that this decline accelerates with each successive decade of life.[28] Although regular exercise may attenuate this loss of exercise capacity at any age, it does not appear to prevent the progressively greater decline with advancing age.[28]

Risks of Exercise

Although there are many benefits to exercise, the risks during exercise and sports activities are low.[29] Most hazards involve the cardiovascular and musculoskeletal systems. These differ relative to the participant's age, sex, physical fitness, underlying cardiovascular and medical conditions, and the particular activity or sport. Accordingly, the cardiovascular risk-benefit ratio should be assessed for each individual for any given activity.

Age exerts a major influence on cardiovascular risk during exercise. Exercise-related death in persons older than 35 years of age usually results from atherosclerotic coronary artery disease, whereas genetic or congenital cardiac malformations are the predominant causes in younger individuals.[29] Although no centralized program requires mandatory reporting of sudden death in young athletes in the United States, the best available data come from the U.S. National Registry of Sudden Death in Athletes.[30] A recent comprehensive report from this registry has demonstrated that among 1866 sudden deaths in athletes younger than 40 years (mean, 19 years), 56% were deemed to be caused by a cardiovascular cause, at a rate of less than 100 cases/year and an incidence of 0.61/100,000 person-years. A prospective series of somewhat older Italian athletes (mean age, 26 years) who had undergone a national preparticipation screening program has reported the rate of sudden death to be 2.3/100,000 athletes/year, with a rate in men that is more than twice that in women.[31] The cardiovascular causes of sudden death in young athletes younger than 40 years of age are shown in **Table 83-2**, and a detailed report of sudden deaths per specific sport is provided in **Table 83-3**.

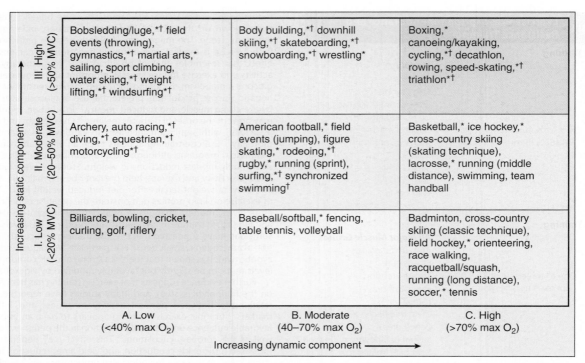

FIGURE 83-1 Classification of sports. This classification is based on peak static and dynamic components achieved during competition. The increasing dynamic component is related to the estimated percentage of maximal oxygen uptake (max O_2) achieved and results in an increasing cardiac output. The increasing static component is related to the estimated percentage of maximal voluntary contraction (MVC) attained and results in an increasing blood pressure. The lowest total cardiovascular demands are shown in green and the highest in red. Blue, yellow, and lavender depict low moderate, moderate, and high moderate total cardiovascular demands. *Danger of bodily collision. †Increased risk if syncope occurs. *(From Mitchell JH, Haskell W, Snell P, Van Camp SP: Task Force 8: Classification of sports. J Am Coll Cardiol 45:1364, 2005.)*

TABLE 83-2	Cardiovascular Causes of Sudden Death in Young Athletes (N = 690)
CAUSE	**PROPORTION OF ALL CAUSES (%)**
Hypertrophic cardiomyopathy	36
Coronary artery anomalies	17
Possible hypertrophic cardiomyopathy*	8
Myocarditis	6
Arrhythmogenic right ventricular cardiomyopathy	4
Ion channel disease	4
Mitral valve prolapse	3
Bridged left anterior descending coronary artery	3
Atherosclerotic coronary artery disease	3
Aortic rupture	3
Aortic stenosis	2
Dilated cardiomyopathy	2
Wolff-Parkinson-White syndrome	2
Other	5

*Findings suggestive but not diagnostic of hypertrophic cardiomyopathy.
Data from Maron BJ, Doerer JJ, Haas TS, et : Sudden death in young competitive athletes: Analysis of 1866 deaths in the United States, 1980-2006. Circulation 119:1085, 2009 (see Chap. 69).

The reported rates of exertionally related sudden death among middle-aged persons vary in part because of the method of data collection and reporting the type of activity involved, and the population studied. Prospectively collected data on men[32] and women[33] have demonstrated that the risk of sudden death during moderate to vigorous exertion is low. Among middle-aged men without known CVD in the Physicians' Health Study, the absolute risk during any episode of vigorous exertion was 1/1.51 million episodes of exertion,[32] whereas that reported in middle-aged women of the Nurses' Health Study during moderate to vigorous exertion was 1/36.5 million hours of exertion.[33] There is also evidence that heavy exertion may trigger an acute myocardial infarction; however, even less precise estimates are available for this occurrence in the general population. Importantly, these studies[32,33] and others clearly demonstrate that the risk of an adverse event increases transiently during the period of exertion, particularly in sedentary persons with occult or known coronary artery disease when performing an unaccustomed, vigorous physical activity. Conversely, the overall risk is significantly lower among those who engage in habitual moderate to vigorous physical activity and exercise.

Traumatic and musculoskeletal injuries during exercise and sports activities constitute an important and sometimes disabling risk of participation, but exceed the scope of this chapter. However, blunt, nonpenetrating chest blows may trigger ventricular fibrillation and sudden cardiac death. This condition is known as commotio cordis and causes approximately 3% of sudden deaths in young athletes in the United States.[30] It most commonly occurs in baseball, ice hockey, lacrosse, football, and martial arts, and is often the result of direct bodily contact from the ball or puck, or between players. Methods for preventing this devastating and often fatal event are discussed in detail elsewhere[34] (see Chap. 41).

Although the risks of each sport vary, long-distance marathon racing deserves special mention. Marathoning in the United States is becoming widely popular, particularly among middle-aged individuals. Of the 340 marathons that took place in 2007, there were 403,000 finishing times recorded. Approximately 69% of male marathoners and 55% of female marathoners are 35 years of age or older, and 6% of men and 3% of female are 60 years of age or older.[35] Studies have demonstrated that the risk of sudden cardiac death during marathon road racing is

TABLE 83-3 Demographics of Sudden Death in Young Athletes

SPORT	NO. (%)	AGE, yr	MALE, N (%)	FEMALE, N (%)	WHITE	BLACK	OTHER*	SURVIVORS, N (%)	TRAUMA INJURY	COMMOTIO CORDIS	CV DISEASES[†]
Football	565 (30)	17 ± 4	564 (99.8)	1 (0.2)	280	205	80	13 (2)	140 (25)	12 (2)	281 (50)
Basketball	405 (22)	17 ± 4	364 (90)	41 (10)	142	243	20	30 (7)	4 (1.0)	0	349 (86)
Soccer	115 (6)	16 ± 4	93 (81)	22 (19)	81	14	20	7 (6)	11 (10)	4 (4)	80 (70)
Baseball	111 (6)	16 ± 4	111 (100)	0	95	5	11	14 (13)	16 (14)	30 (27)	54 (49)
Motor vehicle racing[‡]	104 (6)	28 ± 8	103 (99)	1 (1)	102	0	2	0	97 (93)	0	5 (5)
Track and field	96 (5)	17 ± 4	74 (77)	22 (23)	62	22	12	3 (3)	25 (26)	0	61 (64)
Wrestling	69 (4)	22 ± 8	69 (100)	0	56	4	9	2 (3)	7 (10)	1 (1.4)	37 (54)
Boxing	56 (3)	25 ± 6	55 (98)	1 (2)	21	19	16	0	42 (75)	0	11 (1.8)
Swimming[§]	46 (2)	17 ± 4	30 (65)	16 (35)	43	1	2	1 (2)	0	0	35 (76)
Cross country	38 (2)	17 ± 4	29 (76)	9 (24)	30	6	2	2 (5)	0	0	29 (76)
Hockey	29 (1.5)	18 ± 5	29 (100)	0	28	1	0	3 (10)	4 (14)	7 (24)	11 (38)
Horse riding[∥]	27 (1.4)	27 ± 8	17 (63)	10 (37)	21	1	5	0	24 (89)	0	2 (7)
Softball	22 (1.2)	19 ± 6	6 (27)	16 (73)	19	0	3	2 (9)	3 (14)	1 (5)	12 (55)
Marathon	20 (1.1)	28 ± 7	15 (75)	5 (25)	16	0	4	3 (15)	0	0	13 (65)
Lacrosse	19 (1.0)	18 ± 2	19 (100)	0	18	1	0	2 (11)	1 (5)	8 (42)	9 (47)
Skiing[¶]	19 (1.0)	25 ± 8	14 (74)	5 (26)	19	0	0	0	15 (79)	0	1 (5)
Triathlon	17 (0.9)	32 ± 5	15 (88)	2 (12)	16	0	1	0	3 (18)	0	8 (47)
Rugby	16 (0.9)	21 ± 3	16 (100)	0	13	2	1	0	3 (19)	0	7 (44)
Martial arts	15 (0.8)	23 ± 7	14 (93)	1 (7)	12	3	0	0	5 (33)	2 (13)	2 (13)
Others**	14 (0.8)	26 ± 9	12 (86)	2 (14)	14	0	0	2 (14)	3 (21)	0	5 (36)
Rowing	11 (0.6)	22 ± 6	8 (73)	3 (27)	10	0	1	0	0	0	9 (82)
Cycling	10 (0.5)	29 ± 8	8 (80)	2 (20)	7	2	1	0	7 (70)	0	3 (30)
Tennis	10 (0.5)	19 ± 4	8 (80)	2 (20)	8	0	2	0	0	0	8 (80)
Volleyball	10 (0.5)	18 ± 5	1 (10)	9 (90)	5	3	2	1 (10)	0	0	10 (100)
Gymnastics	9 (0.5)	15 ± 3	5 (56)	4 (44)	6	0	3	0	4 (44)	0	3 (33)
Surfing	9 (0.5)	23 ± 8	9 (100)	0	7	0	2	0	2 (22)	0	1 (11)
Figure skating	2 (0.1)	24 ± 6	2 (100)	0	2	0	0	0	0	0	1 (50)
Golf	2 (0.1)	18 ± 0.7	2 (100)	0	2	0	0	0	0	0	2 (100)
Totals	1866	19 ± 6	1692	174	1135	532	199	85	416	65	1049

*Hispanic (n = 103); Asian (n = 20); Native American (n = 5); Pacific Islander (n = 5); Middle Eastern (n = 3); Indian (n = 1); Japanese (n = 1); mixed (n = 6); unknown (n = 55).
[†]Documented by autopsy and/or clinical findings.
[‡]Includes automobile (n = 63) and motorcycle (n = 41) racing.
[§]Swimming (n = 40); water polo (n = 6).
[∥]Jockey (n = 16); equestrian (n = 11).
[¶]Skiing (n = 12); snowboarding (n = 5); ski-jumping (n = 2).
** Skateboarding (n = 5); jai-alai (n = 4); field hockey (n = 2); bobsledding (n = 1); bowling (n = 1); riflery (n = 1).
From Maron BJ, Doerer JJ, Haas TS, et al: Sudden death in young competitive athletes: Analysis of 1866 deaths in the United States, 1980-2006. Circulation 119:1085, 2009.

approximately 0.8 to 1.1/100,000 race participants,[36,37] and that this risk appears to be decreasing relative to prior estimates, while the likelihood of survival is increasing. Improved survival may result from the greater availability of automated cardiac defibrillators at these events.[36] The risk of marathon racing among persons with recognized or occult CVD is not known, but it would be expected to be greater. Although marathon racing can lead to metabolic derangements, hyponatremia caused by overhydration recently has been recognized as an important and preventable risk.[38] Several studies have demonstrated structural and biochemical evidence of transient myocardial injury and systolic and diastolic dysfunction in the right and left ventricles. Some of these abnormalities may persist up to 1 month after a race,[39,39a] but the clinical significance of these findings is uncertain.

Exercise Prescription for Health and Fitness

Consensus papers and guidelines from the American Heart Association and the American College of Sports Medicine,[2,40,41] Institute of Medicine,[42] and U.S. Surgeon General[1] all recommend that adults exercise for 30 to 60 minutes at moderate-intensity levels (e.g., brisk walking) on most, if not all, days of the week, with the goal of achieving a weekly energy expenditure of at least 1000 kcal. This is considered the most basic exercise prescription. It is simple, effective, and based on scientific evidence. This recommendation has been further modified to specify that alternatively, vigorous-intensity aerobic physical activity should be performed for a minimum of 20 minutes on 3 days/

week, and that every adult should perform activities that maintain or increase muscular strength and endurance a minimum of 2 days/week.[40] The recommended daily physical activity can be accomplished in a single session or during multiple shorter intervals throughout the day. If exercise is of low intensity (e.g., slow walking), it should be performed more frequently and for longer duration.

Numerous exercise training studies have evaluated the frequency, intensity, and duration of the training sessions required to achieve physical fitness and muscular strength (see Table 83-1). Improvements in peak oxygen uptake of 15% to 30% are usually achieved for sedentary individuals using the regimen as outlined for endurance training. Intermittent activity at comparable exercise intensity and total duration can confer fitness benefits similar to those of continuous activity.[2] Details regarding the exercise prescription are provided elsewhere.[41]

The prescription for exercise training in persons with known CVD is presented in detail in Chap. 50. Issues regarding exercise and sports participation in those with specific cardiovascular conditions are discussed later in this chapter. Exercise tests should be performed on all cardiac patients who are about to begin an exercise training program, and should be repeated periodically or whenever the patient's condition warrants. Exercise intensity can be ascertained by an exercise test using the heart rate reserve method and peak heart rate (see Table 83-1). If angina or ischemic ST-segment depression occurs during the exercise test, the training heart rate should be a minimum of 10 beats/min below the heart rate at which the abnormality occurs. Modalities for training can be categorized by the specific muscle groups that are exercised, such as arms, legs, or both. In addition, different modalities emphasize predominantly endurance or resistance exercises (see Table 4.1.3 on website).

Screening

Concerted efforts to promote physical activity and exercise aim to increase levels of regular physical activity throughout the U.S. population, including the almost 25% of adult Americans who have some form of CVD. Although the benefits of exercise generally outweigh the risks, adequate screening and evaluation are important to identify and counsel persons with underlying CVD to minimize those risks before they begin exercising at vigorous levels ($\geq$60% heart rate reserve or $\geq$77% peak heart rate; see Table 83-1). However, screening should not constitute an impediment to the widespread implementation of physical activity.

Screening can take place in many different settings and venues, such as the following: during office visits to the health care provider[40,41,43]; at health and fitness centers on enrollment or periodic guest use[44]; using self-screening tools from the American Heart Association and other organizations; and during preseason physical examinations for young athletes about to engage in a particular sport.[45,46] If underlying CVD is suspected or detected by any of these evaluations, then appropriate medical referral for further assessment is needed.

Medical Office Setting

Details regarding medical screening are provided elsewhere.[41,43,45,46] Abnormalities in any of the key elements of the history and physical examination, as shown in **Table 83-4**, should prompt further evaluation and testing. Using the American Heart Association risk classification scheme (**Table 83-5**), health care providers can assess whether vigorous exercise training can be permitted and what level of supervision and monitoring, if any, are needed.[47] Exercise testing is important in the risk stratification process for those deemed to be at greater risk of having underlying heart disease, particularly coronary artery disease, or those with diabetes. It also allows the establishment of appropriate and specific safety precautions, target exercise training heart rate, and initial levels of exercise training work rates.

Health and Fitness Facilities

The American Heart Association recommends that all facilities offering exercise equipment or services should conduct cardiovascular

TABLE 83-4	American Heart Association Consensus Panel Recommendations for Preparticipation Athletic Screening

Family History
1. Premature sudden cardiac death
2. Heart disease in surviving relatives < 50 yr

Personal History
3. Heart murmur
4. Systemic hypertension
5. Fatigue
6. Syncope, near-syncope
7. Excessive, unexplained exertional dyspnea
8. Exertional chest pain

Physical Examination
9. Heart murmur (supine/standing)
10. Femoral arterial pulses (to exclude coarctation of aorta)
11. Stigmata of Marfan syndrome
12. Brachial blood pressure measurement (sitting)

From Maron BJ, Douglas PS, Graham TP, et : Task Force 1: Preparticipation screening and diagnosis of cardiovascular disease in athletes. J Am Coll Cardiol 45:1322, 2005.

screening of all new members and/or prospective users.[44] The use of simple screening tools, such as the Physical Activity Readiness Questionnaire (PAR-Q), are recommended, with appropriate medical evaluation and follow-up as indicated.

Athletes

Screening of competitive athletes prior to participation in organized sports is a particularly challenging issue, and is discussed in detail elsewhere.[43,45,46,48,49] There are approximately 10 to 15 million athletes in the United States. Although sudden cardiac death among these athletes is uncommon, it is nonetheless a tragic and potentially avoidable event. The risk for sudden death during exercise in young persons is much lower than in middle-aged adults because few young persons have advanced coronary artery disease, and because congenital and genetic cardiovascular problems that cause sudden cardiac death (e.g., hypertrophic cardiomyopathy, anomalous coronary arteries, congenital long-QT syndrome) are so rare (see Table 83-2). The estimated prevalence of these conditions in the young athletic population is 0.2%.[48] Mass screening of athletes can be particularly difficult, because individuals with these life-threatening conditions are often asymptomatic and their physical examination is generally unrevealing. In addition, the evaluation can be confounded by the normal physiologic changes in autonomic tone and in cardiac size and structure that occur with prolonged and intense training, known as the athlete's heart.[45] These changes are reflected in the electrocardiogram (ECG), which can appear abnormal in about 40% of elite athletes, and in the echocardiogram, which may demonstrate increased cardiac mass, chamber dimensions, and wall thickness. Chap. 69 discusses criteria for distinguishing hypertrophic cardiomyopathy from the athlete's heart.

Because no screening test or procedure will yield 100% sensitivity and specificity for the detection of a life-threatening cardiovascular abnormality or guarantee a zero-risk outcome, what more can be done to promote their detection and reduce the occurrence of adverse events? Although the specifics of screening remain controversial,[50] the American Heart Association does not recommend routine electrocardiography or echocardiography in the initial mass screening evaluation of young athletes because of their diagnostic and cost limitations when applied to this population.[46] However, these tests may be an important part of subsequent evaluations in the medical office setting, as clinically indicated. Those responsible for screening evaluations and supervision of athletes should be informed about the most common causes of sudden death in athletes (see Table 83-2). This will heighten their awareness of the signs and symptoms of associated cardiac conditions during the initial assessment and at any time during athletic participation. The initial medical history and physical should include

TABLE 83-5 American Heart Association Risk Classification for Exercise Training

Class A: Apparently healthy individuals.

This classification includes the following:

A1. Children, adolescents, men < 45 yr, and women < 55 yr who have no symptoms or known presence of heart disease or major coronary risk factors.

A2. Men ≥ 45 yr and women ≥55 yr who have no symptoms or known presence of heart disease and with less than two major cardiovascular risk factors.

A3. Men ≥ 45 yr and women ≥ 55 yr who have no symptoms or known presence of heart disease and with two or more major cardiovascular risk factors.

Activity guidelines: No restrictions other than basic guidelines

Supervision required: None

ECG and blood pressure monitoring: Not required

NOTE: It is suggested that persons classified as Class A2, and particularly Class A3, undergo a medical examination and possibly a medically supervised exercise test before engaging in vigorous exercise.

Class B: Presence of known, stable cardiovascular disease with low risk for complications with vigorous exercise, but slightly greater than for apparently healthy individuals.

This classification includes individuals with any of the following diagnoses:

1. Coronary artery disease (angina, myocardial infarction, coronary revascularization, abnormal exercise test, and abnormal coronary angiograms), whose condition is stable and who have the clinical characteristics outlined below
2. Valvular heart disease, excluding severe valvular stenosis or regurgitation with the clinical characteristics as outlined below
3. Congenital heart disease—risk stratification for patients with congenital heart disease should be guided by 36th Bethesda Conference recommendations[60]
4. Cardiomyopathy—ejection fraction ≤ 30%; includes stable patients with heart failure with clinical characteristics as outlined below; not hypertrophic cardiomyopathy or recent myocarditis
5. Exercise test abnormalities that do not meet any of the high-risk criteria outlined in class C, below

Clinical characteristics (must include all of the following):

1. NYHA Class I or II
2. Exercise capacity ≥ 6 METs
3. No evidence of "congestive" heart failure
4. No evidence of myocardial ischemia or angina at rest nor on the exercise test ≤ 6 METs
5. Appropriate rise in systolic blood pressure during exercise
6. Absence of sustained or nonsustained ventricular tachycardia at rest or with exercise
7. Ability to self-monitor intensity of activity satisfactorily

Activity guidelines: Activity should be individualized with exercise prescription provided by qualified individuals and approved by primary health care provider.

Supervision required: Medical supervision during initial prescription session is beneficial. Supervision by appropriate trained nonmedical personnel for other exercise sessions is recommended until the individual understands how to monitor his or her activity. Medical personnel should be trained and certified in Advanced Cardiac Life Support (ACLS). Nonmedical personnel should be trained and certified in basic life support, which includes cardiopulmonary resuscitation.

ECG and blood pressure monitoring: Useful during the early prescription phase of training, usually 6 to 12 sessions.

Class C: Those at moderate to high risk for cardiac complications during exercise and/or unable to self-regulate activity or to understand recommended activity level.

This classification includes individuals with any of the following diagnoses:

1. CAD with the clinical characteristics outlined below
2. Valvular heart disease—excluding severe valvular stenosis or regurgitation with the clinical characteristics as outlined below
3. Congenital heart disease—risk stratification for patients with congenital heart disease should be guided by 36th Bethesda Conference recommendations[60]
4. Cardiomyopathy—ejection fraction < 30%; includes stable patients with heart failure with clinical characteristics as outlined below; not hypertrophic cardiomyopathy or recent myocarditis
5. Complex ventricular arrhythmias not well controlled

Clinical characteristics (any of the following):

1. NYHA Class III or IV
2. Exercise test results:
   • Exercise capacity < 6 METs
   • Angina or ischemic ST depression at a workload < 6 METs
   • Fall in systolic blood pressure below resting levels during exercise
   • Nonsustained ventricular tachycardia with exercise
3. Previous episode of primary cardiac arrest (i.e., cardiac arrest that did not occur in the presence of an acute myocardial infarction or during a cardiac procedure)
4. A medical problem that the physician believes may be life-threatening

Activity guidelines: Activity should be individualized with exercise prescription provided by qualified individuals and approved by primary health care provider.

Supervision: Medical supervision during all exercise sessions until safety is established.

ECG and blood pressure monitoring: Continuous during exercise sessions until safety is established, usually 12 sessions or more.

NOTE: Class C patients who have successfully completed a series of supervised exercise sessions may be reclassified to Class B, providing that the safety of exercise at the prescribed intensity is satisfactorily established by appropriate medical personnel, and that the patient has demonstrated the ability to self-monitor.

Class D: Unstable disease with activity restriction. Exercise for conditioning purposes is not recommended.

This classification includes individuals with any of the following:

1. Unstable ischemia
2. Severe and symptomatic valvular stenosis or regurgitation
3. Congenital heart disease—criteria for risk that would prohibit exercise conditioning in patients with congenital heart disease should be guided by 36th Bethesda Conference recommendations[60]
4. Heart failure that is not compensated
5. Uncontrolled arrhythmias
6. Other medical conditions that could be aggravated by exercise

Activity guidelines: No activity is recommended for conditioning purposes. Attention should be directed to treating and restoring patient to Class C or better. Daily activities must be prescribed based on individual assessment by the patient's personal physician.

Modified from Fletcher GF, Balady GJ, Amsterdam EA, et : Exercise standards for testing and training: A statement for health professionals from the American Heart Association. Circulation 104:1694, 2001.

all the key elements as defined by the American Heart Association (see Table 83-4). Abnormal findings should prompt appropriate medical referral and further cardiovascular testing, as indicated. Finally, athletes and coaches should be advised that if the athlete develops chest discomfort, syncope or near-syncope, excessive dyspnea, palpitations, or other unusual symptoms during training or competition, they should report to medical personnel for an appropriate evaluation.

Exercise and Sports in Persons with Cardiovascular Disease

The presence of structural heart disease once signified the imposition of a sedentary lifestyle and an almost total avoidance of physical activity and competitive sports. There is now compelling evidence that regular exercise can reduce cardiovascular events and cardiovascular mortality in individuals with known coronary heart disease (CHD).[11,12] Furthermore, in the setting of other cardiovascular conditions, such as arterial hypertension, valvular heart disease, and chronic heart failure, regular exercise results in an increased functional capacity, improved quality of life, and improved cardiovascular risk factors.[13,51,52] Thus, after careful evaluation, most individuals with structural heart disease can safely participate in prescribed physical activity. Participation in competitive sports for individuals with structural heart disease depends on its type and severity, the type and intensity of the sport being pursued, and the level of risk or harm that could occur pursuant to participation.[5] Details regarding recommendations for participation have been presented in the 36th Bethesda Conference report.[53] Participation in competitive sports should be precluded only after a full cardiovascular examination and a knowledgeable assessment of potential harm from participation. In the heat of competition, however, individuals participating in competitive sports may not properly judge the significance of cardiac-related symptoms or if is prudent to terminate physical exertion.

Coronary Artery Disease

A large body of scientific evidence developed since the 1970s, primarily in cardiac rehabilitation programs, has shown that regular exercise reduces total and cardiovascular mortality in individuals with recently diagnosed CHD[11,12] (see Chap. 50). However, a relative paucity of data exists for competitive athletes with established CHD regarding the risk of athletic participation. The risk of competitive athletics likely increases to some degree in all patients with established CHD, and the risk of exercise-related events parallels the extent of disease, presence of left ventricular (LV) dysfunction, inducible ischemia, and electrical instability, along with the intensity of the competitive sport and intensity of effort.[54] Athletes with CHD diagnosed by any method should have their LV function assessed and undergo maximal exercise testing to assess exercise capacity, the presence of angina or inducible ischemia, and the presence of exercise-induced arrhythmias. In general, two levels of risk can be defined on the basis of testing.[54] First, mildly increased risk is predicted by the presence of preserved LV function at rest, normal exercise tolerance for age, absence of exercise-induced ischemia or complex ventricular arrhythmias, absence of hemodynamically significant coronary stenosis, and/or having undergone successful coronary revascularization. Second, substantially increased risk is identified by the presence of any of the following: impaired LV systolic function at rest (ejection fraction < 50%); evidence of exercise-induced myocardial ischemia or complex ventricular arrhythmias; and hemodynamically significant stenosis of a major coronary artery to 50% or more luminal narrowing if coronary angiography was performed. The 36th Bethesda Conference recommendations for participation in competitive sports have suggested that athletes in the mildly increased risk group can participate in low dynamic and low to moderate static competitive sports such as golf, bowling, diving, or motorcycling, but not in more strenuous competitive sports such as cycling, running, or basketball[54] (see Fig. 83-1). Athletes in the substantially increased risk category should generally be restricted to only the lowest intensity competitive sports. They

should be reminded of the nature of prodromal symptoms and instructed to cease sports activity promptly should such symptoms appear.

Hypertension

Arterial hypertension is the most common cardiovascular condition observed in competitive athletes. Regular physical activity benefits individuals with systemic hypertension because it reduces blood pressure,[14] protects against stroke,[51] and protects against obesity-induced hypertension.[55] The presence of stage I hypertension in the absence of target organ damage, including left ventricular hypertrophy (LVH) on echocardiography, should not limit eligibility for any competitive sport, assuming that blood pressure has been adequately controlled with medication or lifestyle therapies. Athletes with more severe hypertension (stage 2), even without target organ damage such as LVH, should be restricted particularly from high static sports until blood pressure is controlled by lifestyle modification or drug therapy.[56] Hypertension per se has not been incriminated as a cause of sudden cardiac death in young competitive athletes; thus, the goal of treatment is to prevent target organ damage and long-term sequelae such as stroke or myocardial infarction.

Valvular Heart Disease

In general, patients with mild left-sided valvular regurgitation or stenosis who are asymptomatic with exercise testing, without other contraindications, can participate in regular physical activity and in essentially all competitive sports (see Chap. 66). In mitral stenosis, most patients with significant stenosis are sufficiently symptomatic, so that participation in competitive sports is not an issue. If atrial fibrillation and anticoagulation are present, the patient should not participate in sports with a risk for bodily contact. Individuals with mild to moderate mitral regurgitation who are in sinus rhythm, with normal LV size and function and normal pulmonary artery pressures, can participate in all competitive sports.[57] Patients with significant mitral regurgitation should be followed longitudinally with serial echocardiograms for changes in LV ejection fraction and end-systolic volume.[57] Individuals with severe mitral regurgitation and definite LV enlargement, pulmonary hypertension, or LV systolic dysfunction should not participate in any competitive sports.

Aortic stenosis can cause sudden death in young competitive athletes.[30] The severity of aortic stenosis is assessed by echocardiography or Doppler. It is important to note that most, but not all, episodes of exertional sudden death have occurred in individuals in whom aortic stenosis is severe. Because aortic stenosis is often progressive, follow-up should be longitudinal with serial echocardiography. Although athletes with mild aortic stenosis (valve area > 1.5 cm^2) can participate in exercise and competitive sports, those with asymptomatic, moderate aortic stenosis should engage only in lower-intensity sports and/or competition limited to sports with a moderate or low component of static or dynamic effort (see Fig. 83-1). Individuals with severe aortic stenosis or moderate stenosis with symptoms should not engage in any competitive sports and should also limit the intensity of regular exercise. Finally, the risk of exercise and competitive sports in patients with aortic insufficiency depends on its severity and clinical setting. For example, in the setting of a dilated proximal aorta, even with only mild regurgitation, only low-intensity exercise or sports can be recommended.[57] On the other hand, in the setting of mild or moderate aortic insufficiency, with normal or only mildly increased end-diastolic volume and a normal aorta, athletes can participate in all competitive sports. Finally, patients with severe aortic insufficiency and LV diastolic diameters larger than 67 mm, or mild to moderate insufficiency with symptoms, should not participate in any competitive sports.

Cardiomyopathy

Hypertrophic cardiomyopathy (see Chap. 69), myocarditis, and arrhythmogenic right ventricular dysplasia are known antecedents to sudden cardiac death in young athletes,[30] and thus are a contraindication to intense exercise and most competitive sports, with the possible exception of those of low intensity.[58] On the other hand, patients with stable New York Heart Association (NYHA) Class II or III chronic heart failure caused by ischemic cardiomyopathy or idiopathic dilated cardiomyopathy appear to be able to participate in supervised cardiac rehabilitation training programs safely, with transition to home programs without a substantially increased risk of cardiac death (see Chap. 50).[13] These programs have demonstrated clinical benefits, including an increased exercise capacity, improved quality of life, and possible survival benefit.[13] Individuals with NYHA Class II or III chronic heart failure and systolic LV dysfunction are generally too symptomatic to participate in high-intensity competitive sports.

Arrhythmias

A complaint of syncope or of palpitations occurring during physical exertion or sports participation mandates full evaluation. In particular, structural heart disease needs to be ruled out and the cause of these symptoms needs to be determined, if possible. These evaluations should include, but not be limited to, echocardiography, electrocardiography, exercise stress testing, and ambulatory monitoring. In the presence of structural heart disease, individuals with ventricular or supraventricular tachyarrhythmias should generally be excluded from intensive exercise or sports competition until definitive therapy can be accomplished.[59] In some cases, depending on the severity of the structural heart disease, if arrhythmias are controlled with medications or ablation, exercise and competition can be reconsidered. However, the presence of an intracardiac defibrillator to prevent sudden cardiac death has not been deemed to be an adequately tested therapy in a setting in which sudden cardiac death might otherwise be brought on by exercise.[59] Sinus bradycardia, sinus pause, and sinus arrest of less than 3 seconds are common in endurance-trained athletes and generally require no further evaluation or preclusion of exercise. When vasovagal syncope is diagnosed, despite its favorable prognosis, athletes with this condition should not participate in sports in which even a momentary loss of consciousness could be hazardous, such as automobile racing or downhill ski racing. For more details relating to the risk of specific arrhythmias, see the 36th Bethesda Conference report.[59]

Congenital Heart Disease

The most common congenital heart diseases that have been associated with untoward events during sports competition are hypertrophic cardiomyopathy (see Chap. 69), coronary artery anomalies, Marfan syndrome, and congenital aortic valve stenosis.[60] Other congenital lesions that are frequently associated with elevated pulmonary resistance also need to be considered (see Chap. 65). Hypertrophic cardiomyopathy is the most common underlying cause of sudden cardiac death during sports participation in young athletes and therefore is considered a disqualifying diagnosis for sports competition and intensive exercise.[30] Congenital coronary anomalies of wrong sinus origin, in which a coronary artery passes between great arteries, are the second most common cause of sudden death in young athletes.[30] As such, this diagnosis should result in exclusion from all participation in sports. Participation can be reconsidered after successful surgical correction in an athlete without ischemia or arrhythmias during maximal exercise testing. Coronary anomalies should be considered in athletes with exertional syncope, chest pain, or symptomatic ventricular arrhythmias and can be diagnosed by echocardiography, computed tomography, magnetic resonance imaging, or coronary arteriography.

Marfan syndrome is an autosomal dominant disorder of connective tissue, with an estimated prevalence of 1/5,000 to 10,000 (see Chaps. 8 and 60). Cardiac manifestations include progressive dilation of the aortic root or descending aorta, which predisposes to dissection and rupture, and mitral valve prolapse with associated mitral regurgitation. The risk for aortic rupture is usually linked to dilation of the proximal aorta to more than 50 mm, although even lesser levels of dilation increase risk. Athletes with aortic root dilations of more than

40 mm, moderate or worse mitral regurgitation, or a family history of dissection or sudden death in a relative with Marfan syndrome can only participate in low-intensity competitive sports (see Fig. 83-1). Weightlifting has been specifically linked with aortic dissection in athletes with cystic medial necrosis, and it should be considered relatively contraindicated in Marfan syndrome.[61]

Finally, a variety of congenital heart lesions linked to pulmonary hypertension present a risk during exercise and competitive sports.[60] In general, in the absence of other contraindications, if the pulmonary artery systolic pressure is less than 30 mm Hg, athletes can participate in all sports. If, however, the pulmonary systolic pressure is more than 30 mm Hg in the presence of an uncorrected intracardiac shunt, a full evaluation and individual exercise prescription are required for athletic participation. Patients with cyanotic congenital heart disease are generally too symptomatic to participate in intense exercise or competitive sports, although from a medical point of view, they should be precluded from participation. Variants of tetralogy of Fallot, atrial septal defects, ventricular septal defects, and Ebstein anomaly all require full evaluation on an individual basis before a decision can be made regarding athletic participation. The final decision should be based on the severity of the lesion, pulmonary pressure at rest and during exercise, and intensity of the sport being considered. In cases of mild or fully corrected lesions with normal pulmonary pressures, full participation can be considered. Details of these and other congenital conditions can be reviewed in the proceedings of the 36th Bethesda Conference report.[60]

Future Perspectives

As our society becomes more sedentary, and adverse health consequences such as obesity and diabetes increase, major and sustained efforts at physical activity promotion are needed. Whereas a broad approach requires concerted and multifaceted efforts that involve health policy makers, schools, worksites, insurers, the media, and others, health care providers have a primary responsibility to the individual. Medical education of physicians, nurses, and other health care providers needs to incorporate training in physical activity and exercise counseling, as well as screening for exercise- and sports-related risks. Health care providers need to evaluate the activity status of their patients routinely and promote the adoption of a physically active lifestyle. Accordingly, health care providers must be familiar with the physiologic demands of exercise and specific sports so that they may evaluate and mitigate risk appropriately, while not unduly proscribing participation.

Many of the recommendations made regarding screening and counseling individuals about their participation in exercise and sports are based on expert consensus. Because of the wide range and varied nature of the physiologic demands of sports and associated training, and the great variation in the presence and severity of underlying CVD and comorbidities of prospective participants, it is unlikely that there will ever be adequate scientific data to define individual risk precisely. However, the continued generation of carefully collected outcome data regarding adverse event rates during specific sports-related activities, and the underlying cause of those events, can fill many gaps in the available information and help further refine risk assessment. In the meantime, available guidelines need to be implemented by the medical community and those involved with athletic screening and training. Standardization of medical screening forms to contain key elements of the history and physical examination (see Table 83-4), and algorithms that outline steps for further evaluation, should be established for athletic screening at all levels of competition, from school to professional athletics. Finally, all those involved with directly supervising exercise and sports-related activities in any venue need to be facile with the prompt recognition of an adverse event, alerting of emergency medical systems, provision of cardiopulmonary resuscitation, and use of the automated external defibrillator (AED), where available. The American Heart Association and 36th Bethesda Conference Report[62] have outlined recommendations regarding the availability of AEDs at health and fitness facilities, sports arenas, and other venues of competitive athletic programs.

REFERENCES

Physical Activity, Benefits, and Risks of Exercise

1. U.S. Department of Health and Human Services: Physical Activity and Health: A Report of the Surgeon General. Atlanta, Centers for Disease Control and Prevention, 1996.
2. Thompson PD, Buchner D, Pina IL, et al: Exercise and physical activity in the prevention and treatment of atherosclerotic cardiovascular disease: A statement from the Council on Clinical Cardiology (Subcommittee on Exercise, Rehabilitation, and Prevention) and the Council on Nutrition, Physical Activity, and Metabolism (Subcommittee on Physical Activity). Circulation 107:3109, 2003.
3. Centers for Disease Control and Prevention: Exercise or Physical Activity, 2009 (http://www.cdc.gov/nchs/fastats/exercise.htm).
4. Kodama S, Saito K, Tanaka S, et al: Cardiorespiratory fitness as a quantitative predictor of all-cause mortality and cardiovascular events in healthy men and women: A meta-analysis. JAMA 301:2024, 2009.
5. Mitchell JH, Haskell W, Snell P, Van Camp SP: Task Force 8: Classification of sports. J Am Coll Cardiol 45:1364, 2005.
6. Gulati M, Pandey DK, Arnsdorf MF, et al: Exercise capacity and the risk of death in women: The St. James Women Take Heart Project. Circulation 108:1554, 2003.
7. Paffenbarger RS, Hyde RT, Wing A, et al: Physical activity, all-cause mortality, and longevity of college alumni. N Eng J Med 314:605-613, 1986.
8. Martinson BC, O'Connor PJ, Pronk NP: Physical inactivity and short-term all-cause mortality in adults with chronic disease. Arch Intern Med 161:1173, 2001.
9. Tanasescu M, Leitzmann MF, Rimm EB, et al: Physical activity in relation to cardiovascular disease and total mortality among men with type 2 diabetes. Circulation 107:2435, 2003.
10. Landi F, Cesari M, Lattanzio F, et al: Physical activity and mortality in frail, community-living, elderly patients. J Gerontol A Biol Sci Med Sci 59:833, 2004,
11. Taylor RS, Brown A, Ebrahim S, et al: Exercise-based rehabilitation for patients with coronary heart disease: Systematic review and meta-analysis of randomized controlled trials. Am J Med 116:682, 2004.
12. Suaya JA, Stason WB, Ades PA, et al: Cardiac rehabilitation and survival in older coronary patients. J Am Coll Cardiol 54:25, 2009.
13. O'Connor CM, Whellan DJ, Lee KL, et al: Efficacy and safety of exercise training in patients with chronic heart failure: HF-ACTION randomized controlled trial. JAMA 301:1439, 2009.
14. Whelton SP, Chin A, Xin X, et al: Effect of aerobic exercise on blood pressure: A meta-analysis of randomized, controlled trials. Ann IntERN Med 136:493, 2002.
15. Sigal RJ, Kenney GP, Wasserman DH, et al: Physical activity/exercise and type 2 diabetes: A consensus statement from the American Diabetes Association. Diabetes Care 29:1433, 2006.
16. Knowler WC, Barrett-Connor E, Fowler SE, et al: Reduction in the incidence of type 2 diabetes with lifestyle intervention or metformin. N Eng J Med 346:393, 2002.
17. Klein S, Burke LE, Bray GA, et al: Clinical implications of obesity with specific focus on cardiovascular disease. A statement for professionals from the American Heart Association Council on Nutrition, Physical Activity, and Metabolism. Circulation 110:2952, 2004.
18. Kumayika SK, Obarzanek E, Stettler J, et al: Population-based prevention of obesity: The need for comprehensive promotion of healthful eating, physical activity, and energy balance: A scientific statement from the American Heart Association. Circulation 118:428, 2008.
19. Slentz CA, Houmard JA, Johnson JL, et al: Inactivity, exercise training and detraining, and plasma lipoproteins. STRIDE: A randomized, controlled study of exercise intensity and amount. J Appl Physio 103:432, 2007.
20. Williams PT, Blanche PJ, Krauss RM: Behavioral versus genetic correlates of lipoproteins and adiposity in identical twins discordant for exercise. Circulation 112:350, 2005.
21. Kasapis C, Thompson PD: The effects of physical activity on C-reactive protein and inflammatory markers: A systematic review. J Am Coll Cardiol 45:1563, 2005.
22. Vona M, Codeluppi GM, Iannino T, et al: Effects of different types of exercise training followed by detraining on endothelium-dependent dilation in patients with recent myocardial infarction. Circulation 119:1601, 2009.
23. Hambrecht R, Wolf A, Geilen S, et al: Effect of exercise on coronary endothelial function in patients with coronary artery disease. N Eng J Med 342:454, 2000.
24. Adams V, Linke A, Krankel N, et al: Impact of regular physical activity on the NAD(P)H kinase and angiotensin receptor system in patients with coronary artery disease. Circulation 111:555, 2005.
25. Steiner S, Neissner A, Ziegler S, et al: Endurance training increases the number of endothelial progenitor cells in patients with cardiovascular risk and coronary disease. Atherosclerosis 181:305, 2005.
26. Halcox JP, Schenki WH, Zalos G, et al: Prognostic value of coronary vascular endothelial dysfunction. Circulation 106:653, 2002.
27. Adamson PB, Smith AL, Abraham WT, et al: Continuous autonomic assessment in patients with symptomatic heart failure: prognostic value of heart rate variability measured by implanted cardiac resynchronization device. Circulation 110:2389, 2004.
28. Fleg JL, Morrell CH, Bos AG, et al: Accelerated longitudinal decline of aerobic capacity in healthy older adults. Circulation 112:674, 2005.
29. Thompson PS, Franklin BA, Balady GJ, et al: Exercise and acute cardiovascular events: Placing the risks into perspective. A scientific statement from the American Heart Association. Circulation 115:2358, 2007.
30. Maron BJ, Doerer JJ, Haas TS, et al: Sudden death in young competitive athletes: Analysis of 1866 deaths in the United States, 1980-2006. Circulation 119:1085, 2009.
31. Corrado D, Hasso C, Rizzoli G, et al: Does sports activity enhance the risk of sudden death in adolescents and young adults? J Am Coll Cardiol 42:1959, 2003.
32. Albert CM, Mittleman MA, Chae CU, et al: Triggering of sudden death from cardiac causes by vigorous exertion. N Engl J Med 343:1355, 2000.
33. Whang W, Manson JE, Hu FB, et al: Physical exertion, exercise, and sudden cardiac death in women. JAMA 295:1399, 2006.
34. Maron BJ, Estes NAM, Link MA: Task Force 11: Commotio cordis Task Force 8: Classification of sports. J Am Coll Cardiol 45:1371, 2005.
35. MarathonGuide.com Staff: USA Marathoning: 2007 Overview (http://www.marathonguide.com/features/Articles/2007RecapOverview.cfm).
36. Roberts WO, Maron BJ: Evidence for decreasing occurrence of sudden cardiac death associated with the marathon. J Am Coll Cardiol 46:1373, 2005.
37. Redelmeier DA, Greenwald JA: Competing risks of mortality with marathons: Retrospective analysis. BMJ 335:1275, 2007.
38. Almond CSD, Shin AY, Fortescue EB, et al: Hyponatremia among runners in the Boston Marathon. N Engl J Med 352:1550, 2005.
39. Neilan TG, Yoerer DM, Douglas PS, et al: Persistent and reversible cardiac dysfunction among amateur marathon runners. Eur Heart J 27:1079, 2006.
39a. Saravia SG, Knebel F, Schroeckh S, et al: Cardiac troponin T release and inflammation demonstrated in marathon runners. Clin Lab 56:51, 2010.

Exercise Prescription and Screening

40. Haskell WL, Lee IM, Pate RR, et al: Physical activity and public health. Updated recommendation for adults from the American College of Sports Medicine and the American Heart Association. Circulation 116:1081, 2007.
41. American College of Sports Medicine: ASCM's Guidelines for Exercise Testing and Prescription. 8th ed. Philadelphia, Lippincott Williams & Wilkins, 2009.
42. Brooks GA, Butte NF, Rand WM, et al: Chronical of the Institute of Medicine physical activity recommendation: How a physical activity recommendation came to be among dietary recommendations. Am J Clin Nutr 79(Suppl):921S, 2004.
43. Maron B, Arujo C, Thompson P, et al: Recommendations for preparticipation screening and the assessment of cardiovascular disease in master athletes. Circulation 103:327, 2001.
44. Balady GJ, Chaitman B, Driscoll D, et al: American Heart Association/American College of Sports Medicine joint scientific statement: Recommendations for cardiovascular screening, staffing, and emergency policies at health/fitness facilities. Circulation 97:2283, 1998.
45. Maron BJ, Douglas PS, Graham TP, et al: Task Force 1: Preparticipation screening and diagnosis of cardiovascular disease in athletes. J Am Coll Cardiol 45:1322, 2005.
46. Maron BJ, Thompson PD, Ackerman MJ, et al: Recommendations and considerations related to preparticipation screening for cardiovascular abnormalities in competitive athletes: 2007 update: A scientific statement from the AHA. Circulation 115:1643, 2007.
47. Fletcher GF, Balady GJ, Amsterdam EA, et al: Exercise standards for testing and training: A statement for health professionals from the AHA. Circulation 104:1694, 2001.
48. Maron BJ, Zipes DP: Introduction: Eligibility recommendations for competitive athletes with cardiovascular abnormalities—general considerations. J Am Coll Cardiol 45:1318, 2005.
49. Maron BJ, Chaitman BR, Ackerman MJ, et al: Recommendations for physical activity and recreational sports participation for young patients with genetic cardiovascular diseases. Circulation 109:2807, 2004.
50. Thompson PD: Preparticipation screening of competitive athletes: Seeking simple solutions to a complex problem. Circulation 119:1072, 2009.

Exercise and Cardiovascular Disease

51. Ades PA: Cardiac rehabilitation and the secondary prevention of coronary heart disease. N Engl J Med 345:892, 2001.
52. Flynn KE, Piña IL, Whellan DJ, et al: Effects of exercise training on health status in patients with chronic heart failure: HF-ACTION randomized controlled trial. JAMA 301:1451, 2009.
53. Mitten MJ, Zipes DP: 36th Bethesda Conference: Eligibility recommendations for competitive athletes with cardiovascular abnormalities. J Am Coll Cardiol 45:1318, 2005.
54. Thompson PD, Balady GJ, Chaitman BR, et al: Task Force 6: Coronary artery disease. J Am Coll Cardiol 45:1348, 2005.
55. Lee CD, Folsom AR, Blair SN: Physical activity and stroke risk: A meta-analysis. Stroke 34:2475, 2003.
56. Kaplan NM, Gidding SS, Pickering TG, Wright JT Jr: Task Force 5: Systemic hypertension. J Am Coll Cardiol 45:1346, 2005.
57. Bonow RO, Cheitlin MD, Crawford MH, Douglas PS: Task Force 3: Valvular heart disease. J Am Coll Cardiol 45:1334, 2005.
58. Maron BJ, Ackerman MJ, Nishimura RA, et al: Task Force 4: HCM and other cardiomyopathies, mitral valve prolapse, myocarditis, and Marfan syndrome. J Am Coll Cardiol 45:1340, 2005.
59. Zipes DP, Ackerman MJ, Estes NA 3rd, et al: Task Force 7: Arrhythmias. J Am Coll Cardiol 45:1354, 2005.
60. Graham TP Jr, Driscoll DJ, Gersony WM, et al: Task Force 2: Congenital heart disease. J Am Coll Cardiol 45:1326, 2005.
61. Elefteriades JA, Hatzaras I, Tranquilli MA, et al: Weight lifting and rupture of silent aortic aneurysms [letter]. JAMA 290:2803, 2003.
62. Myerberg RJ, Estes NAM, Fontaine JM, et al: Task Force 10: Automated external defibrillators. J Am Coll Cardiol 45:1369, 2005.

CHAPTER **84** # Medical Management of the Patient Undergoing Cardiac Surgery

Richard J. Gray and Dhun H. Sethna

Organization of the Program

Organization of the most successful programs, defined by low surgical mortality and morbidity, is generally characterized by larger surgical volume (and large per-surgeon volume), often with a single or small number of separate surgical practice groups under an enlightened surgical leadership. Application of goal-directed, multidisciplinary protocols and a quality improvement program have been shown to be associated with lower mortality after cardiac surgery. This decline may be less prominent in patients with diabetes, and focused quality improvement protocols are often required for this subset of patients.[1,2] The process of cardiac surgery has been shown to benefit from interventions to improve teamwork and communication, such as preoperative briefings, revised approach to structuring of operative teams to favor members who have gained familiarity with the operating surgeon, standardized communication practices, multidisciplinary grand rounds, and postoperative debriefings. Such forums may also be the venue to discuss ethical issues in cardiac surgery, such as refusal to operate on a noncompliant intravenous drug–abusing patient with recurrent prosthetic valve infections. Quality assurance is a must in any program; given the scope of the usual team, inclusion of nursing, anesthesia, cardiology, critical care, and others is important, with time spent reviewing data on surgical outcomes.

In a retrospective study using the Medicare Provider Analysis and Review file of 114,233 Medicare beneficiaries who survived coronary artery bypass graft (CABG) surgery without concomitant valve repair during a hospitalization for fiscal year 2005,[3] the mean cost of a hospitalization was $32,201 ± $23,059, and the mean length of stay was 9.9 ± 7.8 days. After adjustment for patient demographics and comorbid conditions, 13.6% of Medicare beneficiaries who were experiencing complications consumed significantly more hospital resources (incremental cost, $15,468) and had a longer length of stay (incremental stay, 5.3 days). In the Commonwealth of Virginia, the baseline cost of isolated CABG cases with no complications between 2004 and 2007 was $26,056.[4] Isolated atrial fibrillation (AF) was the most frequently cited complication and had the lowest additive cost ($2,574). Additive costs were greatest for prolonged ventilation ($40,704), renal failure ($49,128), mediastinitis ($62,773), and operative mortality ($49,242). The average hospital costs related to excessive postoperative hemorrhage in cardiac surgery are substantial. These observations suggest that the significant cost currently spent on treatment of complications of cardiac surgery can be better contained by redirecting resources to patient safety initiatives, such as evidence-based preoperative risk

stratification, and perioperative best practices guidelines that have been shown to reduce selected complications.

Preoperative Risk Analysis

Advanced Age and Gender

Long-term survival of octogenarians submitted to a wide variety of cardiac operations is satisfactory despite substantial rates of early complications and deaths (see Chap. 80).[5] Most survivors are free from cardiac symptoms. Postoperative complications are stronger risk factors for hospital deaths and long-term survival than are preoperative comorbidities and procedural variables. Time spent on cardiopulmonary bypass (CPB) is associated with long-term survival.[6] Notwithstanding, with optimal perioperative patient management and patient selection, octogenarians can expect a long-term survival and quality of life similar to that of their younger colleagues after primary and redo cardiac surgery. Surviving octogenarians remain at home, function independently, and engage in regular leisure activities years after cardiac surgery.[7] Octogenarians undergoing aortic valve replacement (AVR) can experience a life expectancy similar to that of the general population based on actuarial curves, with more than half the patients surviving more than 6 years after their surgery.[8] More perioperative complications occur in patients older than 75 years who have low body mass index (BMI <23).[9] Off-pump CABG (OPCAB) using only arterial conduits confers an operative survival benefit leading to an enhanced long-term quality of life.[10] High operative mortality (13%) and postoperative complication (43%) rates are to be expected in nonagenarians.[11] However, select nonagenarians can also undergo elective CABG with a 95% 30-day survival; the main risk factor for death is emergency surgery. Physiologic indicators, social factors, and patient preferences should be integrated in the patient selection process, with more proactive intervention in symptomatic nonagenarian patients as it relates to earlier consideration of elective rather than emergency cardiac operations. Notwithstanding, complications result in prolonged average intensive care unit (ICU) stay (12 days; median, 5 days) and longer average hospital stay (17.5 days; median, 11 days).

In retrospective cohort studies of large data bases involving 15,000 to 54,425 patients undergoing CABG, early mortality was found to be significantly higher in women (see Chap. 81) after adjustment for confounding factors, including low body surface area.[12,13] This gender differential increases from top- to bottom-tier hospitals, suggesting that female patients could benefit from having CABG performed at tertiary care medical centers rather than at small community hospitals. On the other hand, a survey conducted between 1992 and 2002 of 3760 consecutive patients who underwent isolated CABG showed no differences in in-hospital mortality or 5-year survival between men and women.[14] Malignant ventricular arrhythmias, calcified aorta, and preoperative renal failure are poor prognostic signs in women. The benefit of open heart surgery at 2-year follow-up is equivalent in both genders in terms of quality of life as assessed by the 36-item short-form health survey questionnaire (SF-36), although women show lower baseline scores. Although women have more late strokes after valve replacement, they undergo fewer reoperations and have better overall long-term survival compared with men.[15]

Ethnicity and Race

In a survey conducted between 1997 and 2007 involving 12,874 consecutive CABG patients including 2033 (15.8%) blacks and 10,841 (84.2%) whites, survival at 3, 5, and 10 years for blacks was significantly lower than for whites (see Chap. 2).[16] Off-pump surgery did not narrow the disparity in outcomes between blacks and whites. In the Bypass Angioplasty Revascularization Investigation trial, clinical outcomes of black patients after coronary revascularization were worse than those of white patients in a clinical trial setting with similar treatment and access to care.[17] The differences in outcome between black and white patients were not completely attributable to the greater levels of comorbidity among black patients at study entry. Black patients were also less likely to be admitted at cardiac hospitals for coronary revascularization compared with general hospitals in the same area.[18]

SOCIOECONOMIC AND IQ STATUS. Lower socioeconomic status is associated with a poorer early outcome after CABG and is independent of other recognized risk factors. Lower scores on measures of IQ at two time points have been shown to be associated with general cardiovascular morbidity and, particularly, total mortality, at a level of magnitude greater than several other established risk factors.[19]

BODY WEIGHT. Underweight is an independent predictor for early mortality, and morbid obesity is an independent predictor for late mortality after CABG.[20]

CASE VOLUME. As a discriminator of quality of care and mortality, the use of hospital volumes of cardiac surgery, which may combine the experience of a wide range of individual surgeons, has been said to be "only slightly better than a coin flip."[21] There is considerable outcomes variability not explained by hospital volume, and low volume does not preclude excellent performance. Except for internal thoracic artery (ITA) use, care processes and morbidity rates are not associated with volume.[22] A retrospective cohort of 948,093 Medicare patients undergoing CABG with CPB in 870 U.S. hospitals from 1996 to 2001 showed considerable variation in adjusted mortality within the low-volume group (1% to 17%) as well as within the high-volume group (2% to 11%) so that the volume criterion alone was a poor discriminator of mortality (C-statistic = 0.51). Of the 660 low-volume hospitals, 253 (38%) had risk-adjusted mortality rates that were similar to or lower than the overall risk-adjusted mortality of some of the high-volume hospitals. Volume statistics of individual surgeons seem to be a better quality criterion of early mortality and postoperative complications. In a study of first-time isolated CABG operations, patients treated by low-volume surgeons (1 to 50 cases annually) had significantly higher mortality rates than those treated by medium-volume surgeons (51 to 100 cases annually; 7.0% versus 3.8%), high-volume surgeons (101 to 150 cases annually; 7.0% versus 2.7%), or very-high-volume surgeons (>151 cases annually; 7.0% versus 3.2%).[23] The adjusted odds ratio of hospital in-patient deaths declined with increasing surgeon volume. Hospital volume and surgeon volume effects on CABG outcomes are probably interdependent. High-volume hospitals invariably have some processes, infrastructure and personnel factors, or both that seem to produce not only better short-term outcomes but also better long-term outcomes.[24] Despite significant reduction in the volume of patients referred for surgical revascularization, risk profiles of patients undergoing isolated CABG in Washington State changed only modestly, and CABG mortality was not adversely affected and morbidity was reduced.[25] Thus, although minimal volume standards might be effective to improve quality to some extent, volume has limitations as a marker of quality because of its wide range of variance. In terms of case volume, for hospitals in the highest percentage OPCAB quartile, adjusted mortality and complication rates for patients having OPCAB were significantly

lower than for the on-pump group; by contrast, for hospitals in the lowest percentage OPCAB quartile, mortality and complications were similar in off-pump and on-pump groups.[26] A surgeon performance index has been described that, with appropriate feedback, has been shown to improve performance of an individual surgeon with improvements in the range and mean of the overall performance of the surgical team.[27]

SURGICAL TECHNIQUE. Conventional sternotomy with CPB is still the standard in most institutions (see Chap. 57). Alternative approaches should be used as tools within a decision-making algorithm driven by patient-related factors of coronary anatomy and comorbidity and the surgeon's experience, wherein thinking "better bypass" must override thinking "off pump." Beating-heart OPCAB has the potential to eliminate intraoperative global myocardial ischemia and to be an acceptable surgical option for patients after acute myocardial infarction (MI). It is associated with lower postoperative mortality and morbidity—the cytokine and chemokine production profile of the inflammatory response associated with CABG is largely similar with the off-pump and on-pump techniques in low-risk patients, but slightly higher concentrations of eotaxin, macrophage inflammatory protein 1ß, and interleukin (IL)–12 were found in the on-pump group.[28] Minimally invasive direct CABG (MIDCAB), conducted through a left thoracotomy, is limited to patients with amenable coronary anatomy.[29] Port-access CABG requires CPB with cardiac arrest but avoids sternotomy. OPCAB may be considered with a median sternotomy or with MIDCAB procedures.

Meta-analysis indicates that OPCAB appears to be as good as or superior to on-pump CABG in terms of reduced length of hospital stay and operative morbidity and mortality, including decreased need for intra-aortic balloon pump placement, rate of postoperative renal failure, hemorrhage-related reexploration, and stroke, especially in high-risk patients (see Chap. 57).[30] A very short preoperative course of erythropoietin administration is a safe and easy method to reduce the need for blood transfusions at OPCAB.[31] Although both OPCAB and on-pump CABG can be performed in high-risk patients with low short-term complications at 30-day follow-up,[32] a randomized trial by the Veterans Affairs study group showed the 1-year composite outcome to be higher for OPCAB than for on-pump CABG. The proportion of patients with fewer grafts completed than originally planned was higher with OPCAB than with on-pump CABG. Follow-up angiograms in 1371 patients who underwent 4093 grafts revealed that the overall rate of graft patency was lower in the OPCAB group than in the on-pump group. There were no treatment-based differences in neuropsychological outcomes or short-term use of major resources.[33] Risk factors for wound infection after OPCAB are comparable to those previously reported for conventional bypass grafting. In one study, diabetic patients had a comparative operative mortality and perioperative MI rate to that of nondiabetic patients.[34] However, they had an increased prevalence of postoperative acute renal insufficiency and infections. In patients with diabetes, the use of bilateral ITA conduits, even when they are harvested in a skeletonized fashion, is a risk factor. OPCAB is associated with favorable early outcomes in the elderly population, but these early benefits may not be maintained in the long term, and OPCAB shows trends toward worse long-term results. High-risk patients undergoing beating-heart myocardial revascularization with left ventricular (LV) assisted technique show reduced inflammatory response compared with patients treated with minimal extracorporeal circulation. Although the benefit of OPCAB increases as the relative use of the procedure at a hospital increases, OPCAB today can be safely implemented across numerous hospitals.

After risk adjustment, patients with critical left main stem stenosis or those with diffuse coronary artery disease (CAD) requiring endarterectomy can undergo OPCAB safely, with results comparable to those of on-pump CABG. Anatomic factors against OPCAB include target vessel size less than 1.25 mm, calcification, intramyocardial location of target vessels, and multiple stenoses. The risk of reduced graft patency also needs to be considered in choosing OPCAB as a tailored strategy in selected patients. Given that OPCAB can be performed safely, patients in the moderate- or high-risk range (i.e., elderly with multiple comorbidities or emergency patients operated on within the first 48 hours of acute MI) could preferentially be treated by use of OPCAB. Compared with men, women are a high-risk group and benefit from off-pump operation in terms of early mortality after CABG. Conversely, during follow-up, women have high adjusted risks of major cardiac and cerebral events after OPCAB.[35] Experienced OPCAB surgeons have a low risk of acute conversion to CPB. Acutely converted patients have a moderately increased risk of in-hospital death and serious complications that are difficult to quantify because conversion is infrequent and unpredictable.

REOPERATION. Although hospital mortality for reoperative CABG is approaching that of primary CABG in many centers, it still remains a significant risk factor for operative mortality in contemporary practice. Aggressive risk-factor reduction (see Chap. 49) and complete arterial coronary revascularization at primary CABG should result in fewer coronary reoperations. In a study of elective redo CABG patients, minimal tissue dissection and target vessel revascularization without CPB did not add significant benefit with regard to perioperative morbidity and mortality. Routine use of preoperative multidetector computed tomography (CT) angiography to detect high-risk findings (see Chap. 19) has a strong association with adoption of preventive surgical strategies in high-risk patients undergoing redo cardiac surgery.[36]

SEASONAL VARIATION. Hospital mortality and ICU stay after CABG have been shown to be increased during the winter season compared with the rest of the year.[37]

Baseline Laboratory Values

A lower preoperative hemoglobin level (13 g/dL for men and 12 g/dL for women) is an independent predictor of late mortality in patients undergoing CABG, whereas anemia is a risk factor for early and late mortality. In another analysis, preoperative hemoglobin level less than 10 g/dL was not a strong independent predictor of 30-day operative mortality or perioperative morbidity in multivariate models for on-pump CABG-only patients.[38] Preoperative anemia is also independently associated with acute kidney injury (AKI) after CABG. Moderate or severe anemia may be intertwined with other risk factors, such as serum creatinine concentration or heart failure, making risk assessment in complex patients difficult. Elevated preprocedural systemic markers of inflammation have been associated with adverse clinical outcomes after CABG. Higher preoperative white blood cell count has been independently associated with higher perioperative myocardial necrosis (creatine kinase MB isoenzyme [CK-MB] release) and 1-year mortality,[39] and it can have a significant impact on the risk for perioperative cerebrovascular accident and neuropsychological outcomes. However, reducing the perioperative inflammatory response with leukocyte filtration does not seem to be efficacious in improving short-term outcomes. High residual platelet reactivity as estimated by the PFA-100 point-of-care test independently correlates with a worse clinical outcome in patients undergoing CABG.[40] Poor preoperative glycemic control, as measured by an elevated hemoglobin A1c level, is associated with reduced in-hospital and lower long-term survival after CABG. For each unit increase in hemoglobin A1c, there is a significantly increased risk of perioperative MI and deep sternal wound infection.[41] Preoperative C-reactive protein (CRP) concentration greater than 1.0 mg/dL carries a higher risk of overall postoperative death, cardiac death, low cardiac output syndrome, and any cerebrovascular complication, with reduced overall long-term survival.[42] A CRP level greater than 10 mg/liter is a risk factor for early mortality, whereas a level greater than 5 mg/liter is a risk factor for late mortality.[43] Patients with high baseline CRP levels are also at higher risk of having postoperative AF after on-pump and off-pump surgery. Low basal free triiodothyronine (T_3) concentration has been shown to reliably predict the occurrence of postoperative AF in CABG patients (see Chap. 86).[44] Preoperative plasma B-type natriuretic peptide independently predicted in-hospital ventricular dysfunction, hospital stay, and up to 5-year all-cause mortality after primary CABG, but it does not predict the occurrence of postoperative AF.[45,46] The serum level of cardiac troponin I (cTnI) measured within 24 hours before elective CABG further identifies a subgroup of patients with higher risk for perioperative MI, low cardiac output syndrome, and high in-hospital mortality. Meta-analysis also shows an association between postoperative troponin release with mid- and short-term all-cause mortality after adult cardiac surgery.[47] Preoperative cTnI measurement before emergency CABG is a powerful and independent determinant of in-hospital mortality and major adverse cardiac events in acute coronary syndromes (see Chap. 56).[48]

Preoperative Drug Therapy

Preoperative aspirin taken within 5 days preceding CABG is associated with significantly lower in-hospital mortality without increased risk of reoperation for bleeding or need for blood transfusion. In patients who have had OPCAB, it does not increase bleeding-related complications, mortality rate, or other morbidities.

The risk versus benefit of preoperative administration of clopidogrel remains unresolved. On the basis of multivariable models, preoperative clopidogrel is an independent risk factor for increased transfusion requirements and prolonged ICU and hospital length of stay. Among in-hospital referral patients, preoperative clopidogrel administered within 5 days before CABG has been shown to increase early mortality and morbidity, and the risk of death is greatest when the drug is given within 48 hours of surgery.[49] Preoperative use of aspirin plus clopidogrel may be associated with an increased risk of infection after CABG. On the other hand, preoperative use of clopidogrel has also been shown not to be associated with increased major or life-threatening bleeding or need for surgical reexploration or higher risk of blood and blood product transfusion after CABG.[50] The ACUITY trial concluded that clopidogrel therapy in acute coronary syndrome in patients who underwent early CABG led to less ischemic events after surgery with no increased risk of bleeding.[51] A post hoc analysis of the CURE trial reported that patients who underwent early CABG after non–ST elevation acute coronary syndrome showed significant improvement in cardiovascular outcomes with preoperative clopidogrel therapy, with no significant increase in life-threatening postoperative bleeding.[52] It is recommended that surgery in patients receiving clopidogrel be performed with standard heparinization and antifibrinolytic strategies; platelets transfused before chest closure have a beneficial effect on hemostasis. Aprotinin may reduce bleeding and transfusion requirements of packed red blood cells, platelets, and total blood units in patients receiving clopidogrel who need urgent or elective CABG.[53] Recent use of clopidogrel before OPCAB is associated with greater risk for bleeding with similar mortality rate.[54] However, discontinuation of clopidogrel 3 days (72 hours) before the operation demonstrated a similar blood loss pattern compared with a control group.[55]

Preoperative enoxaparin given less than 12 hours before CABG is associated with lower postoperative hemoglobin values and higher rates of transfusion compared with preoperative continuous unfractionated heparin administration. Intraoperative heparin resistance may also be increased, requiring more heparin to maintain the desired activated clotting time, leading to higher heparin concentrations and lower antithrombin values compared with control patients. Patients with heparin-induced antibodies (heparin/PF4 antibodies) are more likely to develop thrombosis after cardiac surgery. Patients in whom antibodies are present before surgery show longer persistence of antibodies and increased incidence of thrombotic events over time and may be at risk for development of thrombosis, and therefore further exposure to heparin should be limited.

The multiple benefits of perioperative use of statins in cardiac surgery have been reviewed.[56] Preoperative statin therapy confers a protective benefit on postoperative outcomes in patients undergoing CABG regardless of inflammatory markers, with additional protection observed in patients with positive troponin T levels (see Chaps. 47 and 49). Myocardial damage is reduced, and both short- and long-term results can be improved.[57] Statin therapy in patients undergoing cardiac valve procedures has been associated with decreased postoperative morbidity and death,[58] even in the absence of CAD.[59] One large series (10,061 patients) failed to detect a protective effect of preoperative statin therapy on perioperative outcomes or long-term survival in patients undergoing isolated valve surgery. Valve patients undergoing concomitant CABG, however, appeared to receive a long-term survival benefit from statins.[60] The influence of preoperative statin therapy on postoperative AF has been reviewed,[61] with studies showing a higher or a lower incidence after elective CABG. Higher dose statins may offer the best preventive effect for AF as low-dose statins do not influence postoperative AF.

Preoperative angiotensin-converting enzyme inhibitors are associated with a reduced rate of AKI after on-pump CABG surgery.[62] Meta-analysis of 3323 patients from 50 randomized controlled trials shows that low-dose (1000 mg) corticosteroid prophylaxis given before CPB is as effective as higher doses in reducing the risk of AF and the duration of mechanical ventilation in adults undergoing cardiac surgery but with a higher incidence of postoperative hyperglycemia requiring insulin infusion.[63] The risk of all-cause infection is not increased. High-dose insulin therapy, titrated to maintain blood glucose concentrations below 180 mg/dL, has also been shown to blunt the early postoperative surge in inflammatory response to CPB as reflected by decreased levels of IL-6, IL-8, and tumor necrosis factor.[64]

Preoperative Medical Conditions

Pregnancy

Cardiac surgery during pregnancy is associated with increased maternal (8.6%) and fetal (18.6%) mortality rates. Poor functional class has been associated with a higher risk of maternal death, as is the use of vasoactive drugs, age, type of surgery, and reoperation. Maternal age older than 35 years, functional class, reoperation, emergency surgery, type of myocardial protection, and anoxic time can have adverse effects on fetal survival.

Cardiovascular Risk Factors (see Chap. 44)

CIGARETTE SMOKING. Smoking is a strong risk factor for the development of postoperative respiratory complications, which are twice as common in smokers (29.5%) as in nonsmokers (13.6%) and ex-smokers (14.7%). Patients who have stopped smoking for more than 6 months have complication rates similar to those who have never smoked. Even smoking cessation for more than 2 months can significantly reduce the rate of respiratory complications (57.1% versus 14.5%).

OBESITY. Despite the perception that obesity increases the risk of in-hospital and early (1 year) mortality and morbidity in CABG operations, the clinical outcomes of these patients are not so different from those of other patients when proper attention is given to detail. However, long-term survival may be reduced, and higher rates of AF, bleeding, reoperation, renal dysfunction, and gastrointestinal complications may occur. In addition, the relationship of BMI with post-CABG mortality and morbidity is U shaped, with the minimum risk located around a BMI of 30 kg/m², indicating that patients classified as overweight have the lowest risk, and those in the lower end of the obese range may not have seriously elevated risk.[65] BMI greater than 40 leads to significantly more complications, including a higher incidence of postoperative sternal wound infections, prolonged ventilation, and longer hospital stay.

DIABETES. The outcome in patients after cardiac surgery using CPB is negatively influenced by the presence of diabetes (see Chap. 64), with insulin-dependent type 2 diabetics showing a significantly higher rate of major postoperative complications including AKI, deep sternal wound infection, and prolonged postoperative stay compared with nondiabetics and those not taking insulin.[66] Patients with undiagnosed and insulin-treated diabetes have a higher risk of pulmonary complications in the perioperative course of CABG than do nondiabetic patients. These results may be explained if one considers the lung as another target organ of the diabetic disease. Although there may not be a higher risk of in-hospital mortality, longevity has been shown to be significantly reduced during a 5-year follow-up period. In-hospital resource use may be expected to be higher in diabetics; each 50 mg/dL blood glucose increase has been shown to be associated with longer postoperative days, higher hospitalization charges by $2824, and increased hospitalization cost by $1769. OPCAB in diabetic patients can significantly reduce postoperative morbidity and length of stay compared with coronary operation on CPB. The absence of diabetes-related target organ damage, specifically renal failure or peripheral vascular disease, is associated with long-term survival after CABG that is similar to or only slightly less than that of patients without diabetes. Diabetes does not affect the early postoperative and midterm results, including 1-year graft patency, in patients with multivessel disease undergoing total arterial revascularization and OPCAB.

METABOLIC SYNDROME. Postoperative stroke occurs in 4.7% of patients with metabolic syndrome and 2.1% of patients without metabolic syndrome, and postoperative AKI occurs in 3.8% of patients with metabolic syndrome and 1.1% of patients without metabolic syndrome, both of which are significantly high.[67]

PERIPHERAL VASCULAR DISEASE. Patients with peripheral vascular disease (see Chap. 61) undergoing CABG have better intermediate survival out to 3 years than do similar patients undergoing percutaneous coronary intervention. It is an independent risk factor for late mortality but not for early mortality.[68] OPCAB is safe in such patients with acceptable results and a reduced incidence of postoperative stroke. However, they are at higher risk for limb ischemia, impaired leg wound healing, and infection, especially after intra-aortic balloon counterpulsation therapy. About 10% of patients scheduled for CABG have associated unsuspected abdominal aortic aneurysm (see Chap. 60); whether this justifies routine preoperative echocardiographic screening remains undetermined. When calcification of the ascending aorta is detected on chest radiography, multidetector CT evaluation should be considered to map out the locations of calcium. Alternatively, intraoperative epiaortic ultrasound may be useful to avoid vascular disruption or stroke during cannulation or proximal anastomoses of bypass grafts. The most severe aortic calcification, known as porcelain aorta, may require OPCAB or an alternative approach to cannulation or proximal grafting.

Renal Dysfunction (see Chap. 93)

The RIFLE (R, renal risk; I, injury; F, failure; L, loss of kidney function; E, end-stage renal disease) classification or its recent modification, the Acute Kidney Injury Network definition and classification system, is becoming the standard for determination of postoperative AKI after cardiac surgery and is an independent risk factor for 90-day mortality.[69] In a small study of elderly cardiac surgery patients, serum cystatin C, a protease inhibitor, and plasma creatinine correlated equally in the detection of mild postoperative AKI as defined by the RIFLE criteria.[70] The Thakar scoring system for predicting the incidence of postoperative AKI requiring dialysis (AKI-D) allows the discrimination between patients with higher or lower risks of AKI-D.[71] Preoperative serum creatinine concentration between 1.47 and 2.25 mg/dL is an important predictor of worse in-hospital mortality, morbidity, and midterm survival after CABG, isolated valve surgery, and combined valve and CABG procedures. Mild elevation of preoperative creatinine level (1.3 to 2.0 mg/dL) can significantly increase the probability of perioperative mortality, low cardiac output, hemodialysis, and prolonged hospital stay. Total mortality in patients with lower calculated glomerular filtration rate (<71.1 mL $\cdot$ min^{-1} $\cdot$ 1.73 m^{-2}) is significantly increased, and its impact on these patients is evident at up to 15 years of follow-up. Mini-CPB is associated with a lower incidence of AKI compared with conventional CPB among patients undergoing CABG. Bilateral ITA grafting provides better long-term survival than single ITA grafting in patients with chronic kidney disease.[72]

Atrial Fibrillation

Preoperative AF is associated with an increased risk for perioperative mortality and morbidity, late mortality, and recurrent cardiovascular events in patients undergoing cardiac surgery.[73] The negative effect of AF might be more significant in patients with an ejection fraction greater than 40%. Both the EuroSCORE and, until recently, the Society of Thoracic Surgeons (STS) risk calculator do not include AF as a potential risk modifier; however, it should be identified as a variable to be investigated and incorporated into future risk calculators (see Chap. 40). Spontaneous cardioversion to sinus rhythm during surgery is transient in the majority of patients and is not associated with midterm survival benefit. Notwithstanding, if patients in AF require surgical revascularization, it is appropriate to consider performing a concomitant surgical ablation procedure. Preoperative values of atrial natriuretic peptide, angiotensin II, the sialylated carbohydrate antigen KL-6, hyaluronic acid, and pyridinoline cross-linked telopeptide of type I collagen in the blood have been proposed as new indices to predict the occurrence of AF after CABG.[74] Subclinical hypothyroidism appears to influence the development of transient postoperative AF after CABG. However, it is still unproven whether preoperative thyroxine replacement therapy might prevent this event.

Pulmonary Disease

Preoperative assessment of chronic obstructive pulmonary disease (COPD), currently reported to the STS data base by either clinical interview including medication and oxygen use or spirometric testing, may result in underestimation of risk.[75] COPD is associated with a higher mortality (7%) and higher incidence (50%) of postoperative respiratory complications, especially pneumonia, requiring prolonged ICU and hospital stay. Although not an independent predictor of increased early mortality and morbidity, it is a continuing detrimental risk factor for long-term survival. The subgroup of elderly patients (>75 years) with COPD who are receiving steroids have prohibitive postoperative mortality. A logistic risk model to predict the development of respiratory failure after valve surgery has been described,[76] as has also a simple score to identify patients with a strong likelihood of success in rapid weaning from mechanical ventilation.[77]

Neurologic Disease

The National Institutes of Health Stroke Scale and Mini-Mental State Examination scores can be used to predict both serious adverse neurologic outcome and deterioration of intellectual function in type I (clinically diagnosed stroke, transient ischemic attack, encephalopathy, or coma) or type II (deterioration of intellectual function) neurologic outcomes after CABG.[78] Preoperative stroke carries a higher risk for development of postoperative neurologic complications. An accepted rule of thumb is to wait 2 or 3 months after a stroke before placing a patient on CPB. Patients with remote cerebrovascular accident, even though they may have completely recovered, often exhibit signs of reactivation whereby some or all of the previous symptoms reappear, albeit in a milder form. Although the prognosis for recovery is good, several weeks are sometimes needed.

Carotid artery occlusive disease occurs in 1.5% to 6% of patients with CAD and may be associated with postoperative stroke. Although mandatory preoperative screening with bilateral duplex ultrasound of all patients is still done in some institutions, limiting this process to patients older than 65 years, those with a carotid bruit, or those with suspected or established cerebrovascular disease can reduce the screening load by nearly 40% with negligible impact on surgical management or neurologic outcomes. In those patients in whom critical, symptomatic carotid artery stenosis coexists at the time of scheduled CABG, a combined or staged CABG and carotid endarterectomy procedure can be done with excellent results. It still remains unclear whether a combined or staged technique shows superior outcomes over the other.

Patients with advanced parkinsonism require considerable nursing care after cardiac surgery, and their inability to generate a good cough effort requires aggressive respiratory care. ICU and hospital stay may be prolonged, and discharge to an extended care facility is often necessary. Abnormal peripheral vascular tone secondary to autonomic dysfunction, manifested in its extreme form as the Shy-Drager syndrome, can cause hemodynamic problems in the perioperative period. Although there is no absolute score from the Mini-Mental State Examination that provides a cutoff for declaring a patient inoperable, the indications for surgery in patients with Alzheimer disease who are severely disoriented, confused, and incapable of independent living should be strongly considered on an individual basis with a view against operation. Preoperative depression is an independent risk factor for postoperative mortality.

Hepatic Cirrhosis

Liver disease may be associated with complex multifactorial coagulopathies. Cardiac operation can be performed safely in patients with mild or moderately advanced hepatic cirrhosis with a 6% early mortality. Complication rates can be high at 39% for Pugh class A patients and 80% for Pugh class B and C on the basis of one study,[79] but rates may be lower for OPCAB in such patients.[80] Careful consideration of operative indications and methods is necessary in cirrhotic patients with low platelet counts or high MELD (the Model for End-Stage Liver Disease) scores. A high incidence of hospital morbidity is predicted in patients with platelet counts of less than $9.6 \times 10^4/\mu L$ or MELD scores exceeding 13.[81]

Connective Tissue Disease

CABG appears to be safe in patients with connective tissue diseases (see Chap. 89; rheumatoid arthritis and systemic lupus) with acceptable early results. Wound complications may be a problem, and the use of steroids or other immunomodulating agents is associated with increased postoperative complications. Chronic steroid therapy in general does not increase mortality or overall morbidity, but it may be associated with a greater chance for development of atrial arrhythmias or of requiring prolonged ventilation.

Human Immunodeficiency Virus Type 1

Although the incidence of active infectious endocarditis in patients with human immunodeficiency virus type 1 (HIV-1) has been reduced, noninfectious valvular disease and CAD are on the rise in such patients (see Chap. 72). Those patients requiring cardiac surgery show a high (22%) overall mortality with 58% actuarial 15-year survival and no blunting of the CD4 response induced by antiretrovirals.[82] The late causes of death are usually not AIDS related.

Hematology and Oncology

Whether cardiac surgery is justifiable in patients with malignant tumors is determined by the long-term outcome of the treated malignant neoplasm. Fatal progression of the tumor can occur if the time interval between the occurrence of the malignant neoplasm and cardiac surgery is short. Cardiac operations can be performed with acceptable mortality (4.1%) in patients with hematologic malignant neoplasms but with significant morbidity rates (50%), most often bleeding and infection.[83]

Antiphospholipid syndrome (APS) is a rare coagulation disorder associated with recurrent arterial and venous thrombotic events (see Chap. 87). The effects of surgery in APS have been reviewed.[84] Patients with APS undergoing cardiac surgery belong to a high-risk subgroup, and some patients with unexplained perioperative thromboembolic complications, such as graft occlusion, may turn out to have undiagnosed APS. Patients with glucose-6-phosphate dehydrogenase deficiency who are undergoing cardiac surgery may have a more complicated course with a longer ventilation time, more hypoxia, increased hemolysis, and a need for more blood transfusion. Because this difference may be caused by subnormal free radical deactivation, strategies that minimize bypass in general and free radicals specifically may be beneficial. Patients with glycoprotein IIIa allele $PI^{A1/A2}$ genetic polymorphism (PI^{A1} homozygotes) who undergo CABG show increased postoperative bleeding that is further accentuated by preoperative aspirin therapy.[85] Heart valve surgery and surgery for congenital heart diseases can be performed safely in patients with sickle cell disease or sickle cell trait with acceptable outcome and survival rates. Perioperative anemia from excessive hemodilution during CPB is a risk factor for major morbidity even in the absence of blood transfusions.

Preoperative Risk Calculation

On a background of increasingly complex preoperative profiles, outcomes after first CABG seem to have improved in routine clinical practice since the 1990s and compare well to those seen in clinical trials. Three mortality measures have traditionally been used to estimate perioperative outcomes: in-hospital, 30-day, and procedural (either in-hospital or 30-day) mortality. In the same population of patients, the in-hospital mortality is generally the lowest rate, whereas the procedural mortality rate is usually the highest. In addition, because complications occur more frequently than death, risk-adjusted major morbidity may differentially affect quality of care and enhance a surgical team's ability to assess their quality. A limitation of standard risk models is that risk associated with some preoperative variables can change significantly over time after surgery, and assessments that assume constant risk during the postoperative follow-up period may substantially overestimate or underestimate risk. Diabetes adds little incremental risk immediately after surgery, but the risk increases steadily and doubles at 9.5 years after surgery (see Chap. 64). Age, COPD, and urgent or emergent status also show risk, changing by 50% to 60% during a decade. Avoidance of CPB does not confer significant clinical advantages in all high-risk coronary patients; instead, there are particular subsets of patients for whom beating-heart surgery can be particularly indicated and others for whom on-pump revascularization seems a better solution (see Chap. 57). Off-pump surgery improves in-hospital outcome only in the subset of patients at highest risk. Off-pump patients have more early and late cardiac complications, whereas patients operated on-pump exhibit a higher incidence of postoperative systemic organ dysfunction. Adaptation of the operation to the individual patient is probably the best way to improve outcomes.

Two successful and widely used risk models are the EuroSCORE additive model, which also comes in a full logistic version, and the STS model. Notwithstanding, preoperative risk calculation remains an imperfect art. With use of the STS data base, models have been developed for postoperative mortality and composite endpoint and for postoperative morbidity, including stroke, renal failure, reoperation, prolonged ventilation, and sternal infection.[86] Severe diastolic dysfunction is a strong predictor of adverse outcome and mortality after on-pump CABG, and this high risk is not adequately predicted by EuroSCORE and the STS model. Measures of diastolic function should be included in routine preoperative risk assessment.[87] A preoperative echocardiographic wall motion score index is a surrogate measure of residual remote myocardial function and is a promising tool for better selection of patients to improve results after surgical ventricular restoration procedures for advanced ischemic heart failure.[88]

EuroSCORE. The EuroSCORE (**Table 84-1**) is the most rigorously evaluated scoring system in modern cardiac surgery. It has a significantly better discriminatory power to predict 30-day mortality than the STS risk algorithm for patients undergoing CABG. It has been used not only to estimate perioperative mortality risk but also to assess 3-month mortality, length of stay, and specific postoperative complications such as renal failure, sepsis or endocarditis, and respiratory failure in the whole context of cardiac surgery and to predict ICU cost and ICU stay of more than 2 days after open heart surgery. The additive EuroSCORE gives excellent discrimination that is as good as the logistic version of the model, but it greatly underestimates risk in high-risk patients compared with the logistic version. Recalibration of the logistic EuroSCORE in high-risk patients is needed because of its tendency to overestimate the mortality risk.[89] Internationally, the evidence is highly suggestive that the additive version generally overestimates mortality at lower scores (EuroSCORE 6) and underestimates mortality at higher values (EuroSCORE >13). The additive model is also less precise and exhibits a predictive distortion, which should be accounted for, particularly when it is employed at the individual patient level. The logistic EuroSCORE is more accurate at predicting mortality in simultaneous CABG and valve surgery as the additive EuroSCORE significantly underpredicts in this high-risk group. The logistic version should be used to predict mortality when possible. If this is not feasible, a modified additive score could be employed at the bedside. It may be necessary to validate the EuroSCORE when it is applied to new international populations. In addition, certain independent risk factors obtained in the standard logistic EuroSCORE may not be as important in a newly calibrated EuroSCORE based on current information. An example given is that of age. Whereas previous data would have suggested a significantly increased risk for an octogenarian undergoing isolated CABG, improvements in surgical technique and perioperative care have improved the outcomes associated with CABG in this elderly group. All of this has important implications when an individual surgeon's performance is analyzed in the current era, in which risk stratification may actually be different when a risk stratification model derived from obsolete data is used. A modified EuroSCORE with only five variables has been suggested.[90]

For valvular heart disease, the EuroSCORE has been used to predict not only in-hospital mortality, for which it was originally designed, but also long-term mortality in the whole context of heart valve surgery (see Chap. 66). Meta-analysis shows that the EuroSCORE has low discrimination ability for valve surgery, and it overpredicts risk.[91] Moreover, EuroSCORE risk stratification may be inferior to the STS model in patients undergoing AVR,[92] and it has been shown to be imprecise for prediction of perioperative mortality among octogenarian AVR patients, but it may be useful for predicting mortality during medium-term follow-up. The Northern New England Cardiovascular Disease Study Group risk model and the Providence Health System Cardiovascular Study Group risk model are additional commonly applied algorithms for valvular heart disease. Both allow similar assessment of prevalence and mortality, and a new unified model has been proposed.[93] A scoring system using blood tests and clinical risk factors to determine thromboembolic risk after heart valve replacement has been described and may be used to guide prosthesis choice and antithrombotic management.[94]

The "Normal" Postoperative Convalescence

The usual postoperative course is influenced by physiologic changes as a result of anesthesia, surgical trauma, and CPB, which make these

---

TABLE 84-1 The Additive EuroSCORE

RISK FACTOR	DEFINITION	SCORE
Patient-Related Factors		
Age	Per 5 years or part thereof (>60 yr)	1
Sex	Female	1
Chronic pulmonary disease	Long-term use of bronchodilators or steroids for lung disease	1
Extracardiac arteriopathy	Any one or more of the following: claudication; carotid occlusion or >50% stenosis; previous or planned intervention on the abdominal aorta, limb arteries, or carotid arteries	2
Neurologic dysfunction	Disease severely affecting ambulation or day-to-day functioning	2
Previous cardiac surgery	Requiring opening of the pericardium	3
Serum creatinine	>200 mmol/liter preoperatively	2
Active endocarditis	Patient still receiving antibiotic treatment for endocarditis at the time of surgery	3
Critical preoperative state	Any one or more of the following: ventricular tachycardia or fibrillation or aborted sudden death, preoperative cardiac massage, preoperative ventilation before arrival in the operating room, preoperative inotropic support, intra-aortic balloon counterpulsation, or preoperative acute renal failure (anuria or oliguria <10 mL/hr)	3
Cardiac-Related Factors		
Unstable angina	Rest angina requiring IV nitrates until arrival in the operating room	2
LV dysfunction	Moderate or LVEF 0.30-0.50	1
	Poor or LVEF <0.30	3
Recent myocardial infarct	<90 days	2
Pulmonary hypertension	Systolic PA pressure >60 mm Hg	2
Operation-Related Factors		
Emergency	Carried out on referral before the beginning of the next working day	2
Other than isolated CABG	Major cardiac procedure other than or in addition to CABG	2
Surgery on thoracic aorta	For disorder of ascending, arch, or descending aorta	3
Postinfarct septal rupture		4

EUROSCORE	PATIENTS	DIED (%)	OBSERVED	EXPECTED
0-2 (low risk)	4,529	36 (0.8)	(0.56-1.10)	(1.27-1.29)
3-5 (medium risk)	5,977	182 (3.0)	(2.62-3.51)	(2.90-2.94)
6 or greater (high risk)	4,293	480 (11.2)	(10.25-12.16)	(10.93-11.54)
Total	14,799	698 (4.7)	(4.37-5.06)	(4.72-4.95)

CABG = coronary artery bypass grafting; IV = intravenous; LV = left ventricular; LVEF = left ventricular ejection fraction; PA = pulmonary artery.
Modified from Nashef SA, Rogues F, Michel P, et al: European system for cardiac operative risk evaluation (EuroSCORE). Eur J Cardiothorac Surg 16:9, 1999.

patients unique from other hospitalized medical and surgical patients. The use of CPB and ischemia-reperfusion injury can be associated with a systemic inflammatory response syndrome. Significant activation of complement, platelets, neutrophils, monocytes and macrophages, coagulation, fibrinolysis, and kallikrein cascades results in elevated concentrations of tumor necrosis factor, CRP, IL-6, and IL-8 within the first few days after operation. This "whole-body inflammation" can lead to a "post-pump syndrome" that is clinically expressed as fever, leukocytosis, abnormal coagulation, hypoxemia (from neutrophil aggregation and lysis in pulmonary vasculature), increased pulmonary capillary permeability, renal dysfunction, and cognitive dysfunction. Preoperative treatment with statins is associated with lower biochemical parameters of systemic inflammatory response and myocardial damage after cardiac surgery with CPB.

Cardiovascular Convalescence

Sinus tachycardia of 100 to 120 beats/min may occur a few hours after surgery without apparent cause and should lead to assessment of adequacy of blood volume, low cardiac output syndrome, pericardial effusion or tamponade, infection (even without fever), and occult hyperthyroidism. Orthostatic hypotension can be a problem in some patients, persisting for up to 2 weeks or so after surgery. It may be associated with persistent sinus tachycardia with the heart rate relatively fixed at 100 to 120 beats/min. Investigation of intravascular volume status, liberalization of salt intake, and reevaluation of antihypertensive medications or diuretics that may have been ordered are indicated. Tightly fitting veno-occlusive stockings as well as instructions to the patient about slowly arising from lying or sitting positions are occasionally helpful.

Pulmonary Convalescence

Current practice is to extubate patients ideally within 4 to 6 hours after operation. Such rapid weaning or "fast tracking" should be encouraged in elective, hemodynamically stable patients with adequate gas exchange who have no evidence of heart failure, excessive bleeding, or neurologic complications. In one study, the 30-day mortality rate for fast tracked patients was 0.34%, mean intensive care time was 5 hours 52 minutes, mean time to extubation was 3 hours 10 minutes, mean readmission rate to intensive care was 0.34%, and mean hospital stay from day of operation (inclusive) was 5.7 days. This process increased throughput by 14.6% (compared with standard practices), allowing intensive care beds to be used by more than one patient each day, leading to significant cost savings by reducing the nursing ratio per patient. Immediate extubation after OPCAB appears to reduce the incidence of postoperative AF independent of comorbidities. Periextubation tachycardia should be controlled with intravenous esmolol.

Atelectasis is common. The usual suspects include general anesthesia; manual compression of the lung during operation; one-lung ventilation during minimally invasive surgery; apnea during CPB; and postoperative poor coughing or deep inspirations, gastric distention, interstitial lung water, and pleural effusions. Systematic literature reviews and a randomized study have failed to show that routine, prophylactic use of incentive spirometry, continuous positive airway pressure, or physical therapy lowers pulmonary morbidity in the usual patient, reflecting the low morbidity of most cases of postoperative atelectasis. However, preoperative inspiratory muscle training in high-risk patients may reduce the incidence of postoperative pulmonary complications. Pleural effusions occurring 2 to 3 weeks after surgery may represent a postpericardiotomy syndrome that occurs in 10% to 40% of patients; they, too, resolve spontaneously during a few months.

The incidence of pneumothorax after pleural and mediastinal drain removal is very low. The decision to obtain routine chest radiographs could be based on clinical judgment. Although the presence of an air leak is currently a contraindication to chest tube removal, a retrospective study of 6038 patients demonstrated that patients with air leaks can be safely discharged home with their chest tubes, which can then be safely removed even in the presence of a small pneumothorax if the patients are asymptomatic and have no subcutaneous emphysema after 14 days on a portable device at home and the pleural space deficit has not increased in size.[95]

Neurologic Convalescence

Ulnar and median nerve injury has been described after CABG in 1.9% to 18% of patients as a result of a fractured first rib after sternotomy, stretch or compression injury of the brachial plexus from sternal retraction, awkward arm positioning, or needle trauma at internal jugular puncture. In one small study, fracture of the first rib or of the costotransverse articulation as diagnosed by radionuclide bone scan was described in 15% of patients. Ulnar involvement follows the typical pattern of sensory distribution, generally numbness of the small finger and the medial portion of the ring finger in the affected limb. Median neuropathy results in motor weakness of the muscles of the hand and forearm, typically noted when the patient is unable to grasp a cup or eating cutlery. Resolution occurs in even the most serious cases, usually by 2 to 3 months. Numbness or tingling related to the leg incision wound has been reported in 61% of patients, of whom 37% improve within 3 months. However, up to 41% may have persistent numbness beyond 2 years. Incisional leg pain has been reported by 46% of patients, of whom 77% show improvement by 3 months and only 10% experience pain persisting beyond 2 years.

Neurologic dysfunction may occur in 32% of patients because of surgical trauma or ischemic neuropathy after the radial artery is removed as a conduit for CABG. There are no major neurologic hand complications in the presence of adequate collateral arterial blood supply. All reported neurologic complaints were associated with sensory conduction deceleration of no clinical significance in electromyographic investigations of median nerve sensory-motor and ulnar nerve motor conduction. Preoperative and postoperative radial nerve motor and sensory conduction records were statistically similar. The technique of radial artery harvesting does not seem to influence outcomes.

Visual symptoms are common and often consist of poor visual acuity, blurring, or scotoma. Many patients will describe prominent "floaters" that they had not experienced previously; others report seeing various spots and stripes. Because spontaneous recovery may take up to 6 months, it is ill-advised to change eyeglasses during this time in all but the most severely affected patients.

Postoperative Laboratory Values

Perioperative hematocrit levels are usually in the low 30s; even though the root cause of the usual postoperative anemia is related to hemodilution and blood loss, there may be features of anemia of "chronic disease." Platelet count <100,000 is common, but thrombocytopenia much below 50,000 should be investigated. Postoperative thrombotic thrombocytopenic purpura should be recognized as a possible pathophysiologic mechanism for unexplained postoperative thrombocytopenia, and treatment should be initiated once the diagnosis is established. Mild metabolic acidosis with serum bicarbonate levels of 18 to 26 mEq/liter and pH of 7.3 or above may occur and usually resolve with rewarming and improvement in cardiac output. Potassium levels can change rapidly and need regular and frequent surveillance and a replacement protocol. Calcium levels may often be depressed to 7.0 mg/dL or less because of hemodilution; this rarely requires treatment, but more profound lowering, especially in the presence of hypotension, should be treated. Phosphate levels should be routinely measured immediately after surgery and appropriate therapy instituted because significant hypophosphatemia is common (34.3%) and may be associated with considerable morbidity, including prolonged ventilation, increased cardioactive drug requirements, and prolonged hospital stay.[96] CPB is associated with increases in insulin consumption, and high catecholamine and cortisol levels exacerbate hyperglycemia; these changes are induced to a lesser degree by OPCAB. High serum glucose levels during and after CPB are independent risk factors for early death and morbidity in both diabetic and nondiabetic patients, but especially in diabetic women. An insulin nomogram or protocol is needed at least briefly to avoid diabetic ketoacidosis in diabetic patients and to improve leukocyte chemotaxis. Cardiac troponin T (cTnT) elevation is observed in nearly all subjects, with a median cTnT concentration of 1.08 ng/mL overall.[97] Direct predictors of postoperative cTnT values include preoperative MI; preoperative, intraoperative, or postoperative intra-aortic balloon pump; number of distal anastomoses; bypass time; and number of intraoperative defibrillations. Glomerular filtration rate, OPCAB, and use of warm cardioplegia are inversely associated with cTnT values. A linear association is seen between cTnT levels and length of stay and ventilator hours, and in an analysis adjusted for the STS risk model, cTnT remained independently prognostic for death, death or heart failure, death or need for vasopressors, and the composite of all three. In contrast to consensus-endorsed cTnT cut points for postoperative evaluation, a cTnT <1.60 ng/mL has a negative predictive value of 93% to 99% for exclusion of various post-CABG complications. Serum cTnI levels measured 24 hours after cardiac surgery predict short-, medium-, and long-term mortality and remain independently predictive when adjusted for all other potentially confounding variables. CABG is associated with a marked reduction in serum homocysteine and folate levels in the early postoperative period. This reduction is, at least in part, independent of hemodilution and may be caused by an altered homocysteine turnover because of an increased consumption of gluta-thione during and soon after CABG.

Perioperative Electrocardiographic Changes

Hemiblocks are the most common postoperative anomaly and are generally transient; many are gone within 48 hours and the majority by hospital discharge. There is dispute about the long-term significance, with some believing that they do not worsen prognosis. Conversely, left bundle branch block and nonspecific interventricular conduction delay, both seen less often, are associated with a worse long-term prognosis and may be associated with a significant risk of cardiac death in the first year after surgery. The appearance of new Q waves should raise the concern of an MI, but unmasking of previously evident Q waves of a remote inferior wall MI has been reported, as has disappearance of anterior Q waves. Atrioventricular (AV) block is a common complication of AVR. There is also a 23% incidence of postoperative complete AV block after mitral valve surgery, which may be the outcome of damage of the AV node artery.

Postoperative Drug Therapy

The use of antiplatelet therapy after CABG has been reviewed.[98] Clopidogrel (75 mg/day for 5 days) may not inhibit platelet aggregation in the first 5 postoperative days and therefore should not be used as a sole antiplatelet agent early after CABG.[99] However, there is also evidence that either clopidogrel plus aspirin or clopidogrel alone can maintain high graft patency in the early postoperative phase after CABG.[100] OPCAB patients can safely receive clopidogrel in the early postoperative period without increased risk for mediastinal hemorrhage when it is started 4 hours postoperatively, if the chest tube output is <100 mL/hr for 4 hours, and then daily. Clopidogrel therapy was independently associated with decreased symptom recurrence and reduced adverse cardiac events after OPCAB. Extending clopidogrel use beyond 30 days does not have a significant effect on defined endpoints. Early postoperative use of enoxaparin or unfractionated heparin is associated with a significant increase in reexploration for postoperative bleeding, often at a significantly delayed time after the initial surgery. Statin treatment initiated early after grafting improves long-term survival in patients with a single ITA graft but not in those with bilateral ITA grafts. Survival of statin-treated patients with single ITA grafts was similar to that of patients with bilateral ITA grafts. Calcium channel blockers may be associated with significantly reduced mortality after cardiac surgery, including CABG.

Hospital Course

Fast-track anesthesia routinely allows early (<24 hours) transfer out of the ICU. Virtually all patients are suitable for fast-track recovery. Patients with advanced age, high APACHE score, and reexploration are likely to have prolonged ICU stays (>3 days) with higher ICU mortality when renal, respiratory, or heart failure is present. Readmission to the ICU after fast-track anesthesia, although uncommon at 3.3%, is associated with a longer second ICU stay and significant mortality.[101] Forty-three percent of ICU readmissions occur within 24 hours of discharge and are commonly the result of pulmonary problems (47%), usually difficulty in clearing secretions, or arrhythmias (20%).

Although length of hospital stay will vary with the surgical procedure and many other factors, hospital discharge on the third to fifth postoperative day should be the goal for the patient having a

straightforward CABG or valve procedure with CPB. Earlier discharge is possible in OPCAB patients; in one study, 55.8% of patients were discharged on the day after OPCAB with no deaths, but they had a high readmission rate of 12.7%. Early discharge is unusual in patients with diabetes, renal failure, or recent MI. Previous bypass, obesity, acute MI, and hypertension are associated with readmission. Prolonged ICU stay (>10 days) leads to high early mortality (33%), especially in patients who require dialysis, and quality of life is worse compared with the general population in both physical and mental aspects, but the difference is moderate. Discharge medications should include aspirin (81 to 325 mg), other antithrombotic drugs as dictated by a valve procedure or prior drug-eluting coronary stent, statins for those with CAD, oral analgesic such as acetaminophen with codeine, stool softener, beta blocker, and short-term use of any special agents used for arrhythmia management.

A nationwide inpatient sample of 8,398,554 discharges after CABG conducted between 1988 and 2005 showed that whereas median length of stay decreased from 11 to 8 days between 1988 and 2005 ($P < 0.0001$), there was a simultaneous increase in nonroutine discharges (patients discharged with continued health care needs) from 12% in 1988 to 45% in 2005 ($P < 0.0001$), primarily comprising home health care and long-term facility use. Multivariable regression models showed age, female gender, comorbidities, concurrent valve surgery, and surgery in lower volume hospitals to be associated with nonroutine discharge.[102] Thus, the significant shortening of length of stay during CABG may be counterbalanced by the increased requirement for additional expensive postoperative health care resources and services. Frailty is a newly recognized risk for postoperative complications and an independent predictor of in-hospital mortality, institutional discharge, and reduced midterm survival.[103]

Postoperative Morbidity

Cardiovascular Morbidity

HYPOTENSION AND LOW CARDIAC OUTPUT. Preoperative LV dysfunction is the most important determinant of postoperative low output. Additional determinants of low cardiac output include poor myocardial preservation with a long CPB pump run resulting in myocardial edema, loss of high-energy phosphates, and accumulation of oxygen free radicals; surgical technical mishap; and perioperative MI. Distinction between intrinsic cardiac dysfunction and pericardial tamponade is essential and can present challenges not seen in nonsurgical patients. Although equalized right atrial and pulmonary capillary wedge pressures may be the presenting situation in the surgical patient when both are low (8 to 10 mm Hg), clots can form in the pericardium, resulting in nonuniform cavity compression. A common area for such clots is around the right atrium at the site of venous cannulation. This can result, for instance, in compression of the right atrium with cervical vein distention with low cardiac filling pressures. Selective restriction of left atrial filling has also been observed in association with high right-sided filling pressures and low left atrial pressures. With intravenous fluid administration, pulmonary capillary wedge pressure should increase out of proportion to right atrial pressure (eventually exceeding the right atrial pressure by 5 mm Hg) in the absence of tamponade. The exception will be the patient with single-chamber (right atrial) compression by pericardial clot or even a lower pulmonary capillary wedge pressure caused by clot in the region of the left atrium. Transthoracic or transesophageal bedside echocardiography is useful to confirm normal LV contraction and the presence of pericardial blood. Technetium-tagged red blood cell nuclear studies with delayed imaging have proved useful in difficult cases. Many surgeons simply prefer taking the patient back for exploration if tamponade is suspected but cannot be confirmed. The diagnosis of postoperative diastolic dysfunction has been reviewed.[104]

Hemodynamic monitoring is essential in the management of postoperative low output syndromes; however, there are pitfalls, some unique to the cardiac surgical patient. The correlation of pulmonary capillary wedge pressure or pulmonary artery diastolic pressure with LV end-diastolic pressure has been questioned in the early hours after surgery because of altered ventricular compliance from hypothermia and myocardial edema and elevated pulmonary vascular resistance. Pulmonary ventilation using positive end-expiratory pressure in excess of the left atrial pressure will also invalidate this relationship. Directly measured diastolic systemic or pulmonary pressures can be falsely low because of underdamping of monitoring systems. Pulmonary capillary wedge pressures can appear spuriously low because of over-wedging of the balloon device. Thermodilution output calculations can be inaccurate in the setting of severe tricuspid regurgitation. For these reasons, overall clinical assessment of the patient and the trend of hemodynamic performance are more important than any single measurement.

Management of hypotension or low output syndrome starts with ensuring adequate oxygenation and hematocrit and a check for acidosis. Filling pressures should then be optimized with intravenous volume to raise pulmonary capillary wedge pressure to 18 to 20 mm Hg, but this may need to be higher if there is LV hypertrophy or other cause of LV diastolic stiffness. There may be a blunted elevation of filling pressures with fluid administration in the vasodilated patient caused by sedation, fever, rewarming, or other factors. The heart rate may need to be adjusted with atrial or AV sequential pacing to a maximum of 90 to 100 beats/min. AV synchrony is vital to maintenance of cardiac function at this time.

VASOACTIVE DRUGS. There is marked hospital variation in the use of vasoactive therapies in high-risk CABG patients in clinical practice. Hospital-level risk-adjusted rates of any inotrope use can vary from 35% to 100%, and vasodilator rates vary from 10% to 100%. If low output or hypotension persists, vasoactive drugs are needed and should be chosen on the basis of the framework shown in **Table 84-2**. Dobutamine is a good choice; because it does not release norepinephrine from endogenous stores (unlike dopamine), it may be useful when endogenous stores of norepinephrine are depleted, as in chronic heart failure. Epinephrine is generally reserved for unresponsiveness to dopamine or dobutamine; there is significant renal vascular constriction with epinephrine. Norepinephrine raises blood pressure with little effect on heart rate or tachyarrhythmias. It can also be used in conjunction with other agents, such as phentolamine (a weak alpha blocker and direct vascular smooth muscle relaxant) or dopamine, to blunt the intense alpha constricting effects, resulting in increases in blood pressure and vascular resistance with no change in heart rate, cardiac output, or filling pressures and with less renal vascular constriction. The "inodilators" amrinone and milrinone improve cardiac output by a reduction in vascular resistance and some increase in inotropy with little increase in heart rate. Unlike virtually all other vasoactive drugs, their relatively long duration of action must be kept in mind (<3 hours for amrinone; <2 hours for milrinone) during weaning to fully appreciate intrinsic cardiac performance. Levosimendan (12 μg/kg bolus, followed by an infusion of 0.2 μg/kg/min) started immediately after induction can significantly enhance primary weaning from CPB compared with placebo in patients undergoing three-vessel on-pump CABG. The need for additional inotropic or mechanical therapy is decreased.

RIGHT VENTRICULAR FAILURE. Acute right ventricular decompensation can lead to LV failure with catastrophic results. As with LV dysfunction, checking for oxygen saturation, optimizing heart rate and maintaining AV synchrony, correcting acidosis, and optimizing preload, afterload, and intrinsic ventricular performance are all important. Maintaining ventilator settings to avoid high peak inspiratory pressures will help reduce pulmonary vascular resistance. However, there are certain caveats. In the surgical patient, unlike the medical patient with right ventricular infarction, fluid administration can be useful to improve right ventricular function, but the limits of right atrial pressure elevation are less forgiving and can lead to rapid deterioration of LV function. Because the right-sided cardiac chambers are capacious, significant volume increase may occur

with only modest increases in right atrial pressure, resulting in leftward shift of the intraventricular septum, thereby encroaching on LV filling. Inotropic agents that improve ventricular function but reduce pulmonary artery pressures are important, so dobutamine would be preferred to dopamine and epinephrine would be preferred to norepinephrine.

Phosphodiesterase inhibitors such as vardenafil may play a useful role, depending on systemic pressure (see Chap. 78).[105] They generally improve ventricular contractility and reduce pulmonary artery pressures and also may have positive lusitropic effects on diastolic relaxation. However, they may also lower blood pressure, which as a rule is the limiting factor in managing severe right-sided failure. This usually requires a combination of agents with careful titration of each. Prostaglandin E_1 given in smaller doses will have a selective effect on pulmonary vascular resistance with little systemic effects. The selective infusion of different drugs into the right side (intravenous vasodilator/inotrope) and left side (inotrope/constrictor into the left atrium), although attractive, has not been successful in the authors' experience because of the dominantly systemic effect of these agents, especially in the presence of poor cardiac function. Exceptions would be various inhaled agents such as nitric oxide, which because of its unique route of administration and short half-life results in a decrease in pulmonary resistance with little effect on systemic vascular resistance (SVR) and systemic blood pressure. Epoprostenol (prostacyclin, prostaglandin I_2) is a short-acting, selective pulmonary vasodilator that, when inhaled, will lower pulmonary afterload with little effect on systemic pressure. Iloprost, another prostacyclin analogue, lowers pulmonary vascular resistance for up to 2 hours with little effect on systemic pressures when it is given by aerosol.

CARDIAC ARREST. MI is the predominant precipitating cause of cardiac arrest after CABG or AVR, and ventricular fibrillation or tachycardia is the most common mechanism. Despite aggressive resuscitation, outcome is poor (69% survival after respiratory arrest and 50% after cardiac arrest). Young patients with good LV function have a better probability of survival if they do not suffer a postoperative MI. Guidelines for resuscitation in cardiac arrest after cardiac surgery have been released by the EACTS Clinical Guidelines Committee.[106] Resternotomy at the bedside may be lifesaving. In an international survey from 53 countries, the incidence of cardiac arrest reported was 1.8%; emergency resternotomy after arrest, 0.5%; and emergency reinstitution of bypass, 0.2%.[107] Respondents indicated that they would perform three attempts at defibrillation for ventricular fibrillation without intervening external cardiac massage and for all arrests perform emergency resternotomy within 5 minutes if within 24 hours of the operation. Fifty percent of respondents would give epinephrine immediately, 58% would permit a nonsurgeon to perform an emergency resternotomy, and 76% would allow a surgeon's assistant and 30% an anesthesiologist to do this.

MECHANICAL CIRCULATORY SUPPORT. The preoperative use of intra-aortic balloon pumping appears to shift high-risk patients undergoing CABG on pump and off pump into a lower risk category and is associated with comparable perioperative troponin leakage and short-term and long-term outcomes similar to those of low-risk patients not receiving intra-aortic balloon pumping. It can be placed preoperatively to stabilize the patient with high-risk ischemic heart disease, including those with recurring ischemia with precarious coronary anatomy, severe LV dysfunction, or mechanical complications of MI, such as ventricular septal rupture or acute mitral regurgitation. The postoperative indication is persistent low output or hypotension, despite safely tolerated dosages of inotropic drugs. As cardiac function improves in anticipation of balloon removal, drug support should be reduced and maintained at low levels.

Other devices can be used short term when maximal medical therapy and intra-aortic balloon counterpulsation are not sufficient, including extracorporeal membrane oxygenation and ventricular assist devices (see Chap. 32).

POSTOPERATIVE HYPERTENSION. Defined by a mean arterial pressure of 105 mm Hg, an increase of 20 mm Hg over baseline, or a systolic pressure above 140 mm Hg, postoperative hypertension is especially common and severe after valve surgery, particularly after relief of aortic stenosis. Patients who were hypertensive preoperatively and those receiving beta blockers preoperatively are also more prone to exhibit postoperative hypertension. Because it usually is manifested early (within 1 to 2 hours), the risk is that of arterial anastomosis disruption and mediastinal bleeding, myocardial ischemia caused by excessive afterload, and, if severe, the risk of stroke. Integrity of saphenous vein or ITA grafts may also be compromised.

Elevated serum catecholamines have been implicated as an etiologic factor, along with elevation of renin, angiotensin, vasopressin, and

TABLE 84-2	Hemodynamic Manipulation			
BP	**PCWP**	**CO**	**SVR**	**TREATMENT**
↓	N or ↑	↓	↑	Inotrope
↓	N	N or ↑	↓	Alpha agent
↑	↑	↓	↑	Vasodilator

BP = blood pressure; CO = cardiac output; N = normal; PCWP = pulmonary capillary wedge pressure; SVR = systemic vascular resistance.

sympathetic activity. Although it is epinephrine levels that are most profoundly elevated in the first several hours after surgery, the norepinephrine levels remain elevated for several days. Further evidence of the central role played by norepinephrine is the observation that patients with postoperative hypertension have norepinephrine levels that are consistently elevated at twofold to sevenfold the upper limits of normal, whereas epinephrine levels are normal in some and only modestly elevated in others.

The hemodynamic picture is often that of normal or slightly reduced cardiac output and significant elevation of SVR. Consequently, a vasodilator, most commonly nitroglycerin, is used in this situation. Postoperative hypertension can also be seen in the setting of hyperdynamic cardiovascular function with sinus tachycardia, normal or elevated cardiac output, and normal or slightly elevated SVR. Esmolol or labetalol given as a continuous infusion is a common choice in this setting.

PERIOPERATIVE MYOCARDIAL INFARCTION. Common genetic variants in the 9p21 locus, previously known to be associated with MI in nonsurgical populations, are also associated with perioperative myocardial injury after CABG.[108] Acute ischemic injury of the myocardium is caused primarily by the limitations of myocardial protection during the procedure. Because coronary blood flow is absent during aortic cross-clamping for surgery with CABG, success depends directly on the ability to reduce myocardial oxygen requirements to a negligible level. The STS data base reports the national incidence of perioperative MI for 2005 to be 1.1%, based on the diagnostic criteria of CK-MB (or CK) at least five times the upper limits of normal at <24 hours postoperatively and one of the following if >24 hours: evolutionary ST-segment elevation, new Q waves in two or more contiguous leads or new left bundle branch block, or CK-MB (or CK) at least three times the upper limits of normal. The clinical risk factors appear to be older age and longer pump time as well as elevated LV end-diastolic pressure, unstable angina, and left main CAD.

The patient with perioperative MI usually emerges from the surgery with new Q waves that persist. "Pseudo" Q waves mimicking inferior wall MI may occur as a result of a marked left axis shift. The occurrence of perioperative MI seems to have an adverse impact on survival acutely, but there is disagreement about any impact on long-term survival, with some reporting reduced survival and others showing impact related only to enzyme level.

The mechanism of MI occurring days or weeks after the procedure is often bypass graft closure. The pattern of enzyme release, climbing to a peak a few hours after surgery rather than the more common immediate tapering, suggests a mechanism other than the expected enzyme release from inadequate myocardial preservation and other operative events. In one report, cTnI cutoff levels of 13 ng/mL identified patients at higher risk of hospital death (9.5% versus 0.7%) and were the only independent predictor but had no influence on mortality at 2 years' follow-up. In the case of CK-MB, a cutoff of >40 ng/mL was associated with higher perioperative mortality, but this association no longer persisted at 1 year. OPCAB appears to be associated with less release of cardiac enzymes but with no influence on survival at 1 year.

PERICARDIAL EFFUSION AND POSTCARDIOTOMY SYNDROME. Pericardial effusion occurs in 1.5% of patients, and symptoms are nonspecific. Several factors, mainly related to preoperative characteristics and type of operation, predispose patients to effusion. Echocardiography-guided pericardiocentesis is effective and safe in these patients.

Controversy still exists about the etiology of the postcardiotomy syndrome. Anti–heart antibodies, present in high titers in virtually all cases, have implicated an autoimmune response. Antibody to adenovirus or coxsackievirus B1 to B6 is present in 70% of affected patients, leading to the speculation that this is an immunologic reaction triggered by acute or latent virus infection. Signs and symptoms (**Table 84-3**) range from a low-grade fever, with or without white blood cell count elevation, to a profound illness with pericardial and pleuritic pain, myalgias, and lassitude with fever up to 104°F. A pericardial friction rub and often a pleural rub along with effusions are common. Elevated white cell count with a leftward shift and elevated sedimentation rate are also seen commonly. The electrocardiogram may show diffuse ST-segment elevation or can be entirely normal. The echocardiographic finding of a small pericardial effusion is also not specific.

TABLE 84-3	Typical Signs and Symptoms in Postpericardiotomy Syndrome Patients	
SIGN OR SYMPTOM	**NO. OF PATIENTS**	**INCIDENCE, %**
Fever	45	100
Increased incisional pain	43	95
Pericardial or pleural rub	43	95
Malaise and weakness	31	69
Increased white blood cell count	38	84
Increased erythrocyte sedimentation rate	36	80
Pericardial or pleural fluid	30	67
Asymptomatic	2	4

Modified from Urschel HC, Razzuk MA, Gardner M: Coronary artery bypass occlusion secondary to postcardiotomy syndrome. Ann Thorac Surg 22:528, 1976.

The time of appearance can be as early as 1 week after surgery, but most cases appear 2 to 3 weeks after surgery and can appear for up to 2 months. The most serious consequences are pericardial constriction, bypass graft closure, and tamponade. Tamponade itself is uncommon. Therapy with oral prednisone 70 to 80 mg/day with tapering during 10 to 14 days is indicated. In the early phase of the presentation, inpatient treatment is appropriate unless the symptoms and involvement are very mild. Specifically, the systolic pressure should be above 100 mm Hg, the pulse pressure above 30 mm Hg, and the heart rate no higher than 110 beats/min. The patient should be examined frequently for evidence of increasing pulsus paradoxus or decreased urine output. Pericardial drainage is indicated when these parameters suggest tamponade (see Chap. 75), although, as noted, tamponade is uncommon. Pericardiocentesis poses special risks in patients with anteriorly placed coronary grafts. The fluid can be loculated, and catheter drainage should not be attempted unless there is echocardiographic evidence of fluid anteriorly or around the cardiac apex. For these reasons, pericardiocentesis should be done in the operating room or in an ICU setting, with use of echocardiographic guidance and only by experienced individuals. Special care is needed in skin preparation to avoid bacterial contamination. Fluid accumulation recurs with a reported incidence of 13% in a pediatric population to as high as 50% in adults in one report. A significant rate of early bypass graft occlusion as a consequence of postpericardiotomy syndrome has been reported with and without constriction and, along with the goal of symptomatic relief, is a reason for aggressive medical therapy.

CONSTRICTIVE PERICARDITIS. The diagnosis and management of postoperative constrictive pericarditis have been reviewed.[109] Constrictive pericarditis after open heart surgery may appear as early as 2 weeks or as late as several years after the procedure, the majority appearing between 3 and 12 months postoperatively. The presentation is similar to that of other causes of constriction (see Chap. 75), in which the hallmarks are distended neck veins, peripheral edema, ascites, and hepatosplenomegaly. Echocardiography is valuable in making the diagnosis (see Chap. 15), and definitive diagnosis by cardiac CT has also been reported (see Chap. 19). When constriction is suspected but cannot be confirmed by equalized diastolic pressures, rapid intravenous volume infusion may illustrate the true hemodynamic features. Most patients will require surgery, consisting of either localized or radical pericardiectomy, and the surgical results are generally favorable. Patients presenting within 2 months of surgery warrant a trial of medical therapy consisting of diuretics and steroids because of the high likelihood of a more inflammatory component with less fibrosis. The mechanisms proposed for constriction include the postpericardiotomy syndrome, the use of povidone-iodine pericardial irrigation, and the late effects of hemopericardium.

PERIOPERATIVE ARRHYTHMIAS

Atrial Fibrillation

The prevalence, risks, and management of perioperative AF have been reviewed.[110] The incidence of atrial tachyarrhythmias is 33% after CABG and 35% to 50% after valve-related procedures. AF is the most common arrhythmia, with an incidence of 20% to 40%, usually occurring between postoperative days 3 and 5. Age-related myocardial fibrosis is believed to be closely related to the occurrence of AF after

CABG. Independent predictors of AF include age older than 75 years, history of AF, diabetes, duration of CPB and crossclamp time, bicaval cannulation, inadequate protection of the atria during crossclamping, postoperative serum elevation of both epinephrine and norepinephrine, and postoperative high doses of nonsteroidal anti-inflammatory drugs. Meta-analysis of 14 studies (16,505 patients) has shown a slightly lower incidence of AF (19%) with OPCAB than with CABG with CPB (24%), including the elderly. Similar arrhythmias also occur in patients having noncardiac thoracic surgical procedures, but at reduced frequency. New-onset post-CABG AF is associated with increased long-term risk of mortality independent of the patient's preoperative severity. After control for a comprehensive array of risk factors associated with post-CABG adverse outcomes, risk of long-term mortality in patients who developed new-onset post-CABG AF after isolated CABG is 29% higher than in patients without it.[111]

No preventive strategies have been successful in eliminating the problem of postoperative AF, and the most successful approaches reduce the incidence by about half. Sotalol has been shown to be more effective than beta blockers in prevention but is a negative inotropic agent and can cause QT prolongation with polymorphic ventricular tachycardia including torsades de pointes. In a meta-analysis, beta blockers decreased the incidence of AF by approximately 40%. Amiodarone is effective when it is started preoperatively, intraoperatively, or postoperatively. Routine use of postoperative prophylactic intravenous bolus and subsequent 5 days of oral amiodarone therapy after CABG decrease the total cost of care.[112] Biatrial pacing has also shown efficacy when it is applied for the first 3 days postoperatively. Continuous monitoring of oxygen saturation and subsequent oxygen therapy for hypoxia have been shown to reduce the incidence of AF.

The management of AF after cardiac surgery has been reviewed.[113] Treatment of AF or atrial flutter begins with control of the heart rate (see Chap. 40) by use of intravenous metoprolol or esmolol, which has the advantage of rapid onset of action and 50% likelihood of conversion to sinus rhythm. Diltiazem affects rate control and cardioversion to a lesser extent and may be associated with hypotension or worsening heart failure. There is the possibility of complete AV block when intravenous beta blockers and calcium antagonists are combined, so that pacing wires should be in place and connected to a pacing device. Digoxin is not a first-line agent for prophylaxis, but it may be given intravenously in low daily doses (0.125 mg) to supplement beta blocker effects. Other approaches to acute pharmacologic conversion include procainamide, propafenone, ibutilide, and dofetilide. The last two agents are useful when negative inotropism is not tolerated or if bronchospasm is an issue with beta-blocking agents. Both prolong the QT interval and exhibit proarrhythmic properties and should be stopped as soon as cardioversion takes place.

Low-energy cardioversion with use of biatrial epicardial wires implanted during surgery is effective and safe in conscious patients. Overdrive atrial pacing is effective with use of temporary epicardial atrial pacing wires placed at surgery if the underlying rhythm is atrial flutter or paroxysmal atrial tachycardia. When the type of rhythm is not clear, an atrial electrogram can be helpful. Bipolar electrograms can be recorded by attaching one epicardial lead to each of the two arm leads of the electrocardiographic patient cable by an alligator clip. By recording standard lead I on the lead selector, a bipolar atrial electrogram is recorded. A unipolar recording can be performed by attaching the atrial lead to the precordial patient monitoring lead. If there is any sign of organized regular depolarization of the left atrium, a trial of overdrive pacing is indicated. Starting at a pacing rate of just under the atrial flutter rate with maximal stimulus output, the pacing rate is slowly increased by 10-beat increments until atrial entrainment occurs. Failure to correct the rhythm can be caused by a number of factors, including a broken pacemaker wire or loss of contact with the epicardial surface. If only one such wire is broken or available, unipolar pacing is possible with use of the functioning wire as a negative pole and an electrode patch close to the wire as the other electrode. The threshold for capture may rise above the level of output of commercially available pacing units (which is usually 20 mA), in which case repeated attempts after dosing with an antiarrhythmic agent may be successful. On occasion, atrial pacing will convert atrial flutter to AF. Because the ventricular response rate is often slower and more responsive to negative chronotropic agents, this is usually a preferred rhythm.

Rapid atrial pacing that is unable to be converted to sinus rhythm may induce a level of higher grade AV blockade, resulting in a more controlled ventricular response rate despite persistent flutter. Heparin anticoagulation should be considered for the patient who has not converted in 24 hours and earlier if there is a history of atrial tachyarrhythmias before surgery. Cardioversion is reserved for patients exhibiting acute hemodynamic instability. It is desirable to have an anesthesiologist performing the sedation if possible. For elective cardioversion, anterior-posterior paddles are preferred, with the posterior paddle placed at the lower tip of the scapula. In one study of 640 consecutive CABG patients, amiodarone and early electrical cardioversion were more effective than non-amiodarone therapies for restoration of sinus rhythm. Hemodynamic compromise, systemic embolism, and anticoagulation-related complications, including pericardial tamponade, may complicate the management of AF.

VENTRICULAR ARRHYTHMIAS. Ventricular ectopy including nonsustained ventricular tachycardia requiring at least a short course of therapy has been reported in up to 50% of patients, with high occurrence between postoperative days 3 and 5. Possible mechanisms include the previously mentioned elevation of circulating catecholamines, clinical or subclinical myocardial necrosis, and electrolyte abnormalities. Until more definitive data are available, it is prudent to individualize therapy on the basis of known or suspected risk factors, such as LV function and the patient's medical history. An initial approach is to use atrial pacing, which will often reduce the ectopy without resorting to drugs. For nonsustained ventricular tachycardia, magnesium and amiodarone are commonly used. For sustained ventricular tachycardia, overdrive pacing, cardioversion, or intravenous amiodarone is used.

CONDUCTION DEFECTS. Complete AV block, like lesser degrees of AV block, can be caused by incomplete washout of cardioplegia solution and antiarrhythmic drugs or their toxicity and is generally transient. Surgical transection of the node during AVR is a well-known complication and leads to permanent AV blockade. Improvement in preoperative complete heart block may occur in up to 29% of patients after successful AVR and can occur for up to 18 months after surgery. Factors weighing against recovery with the potential need for a permanent pacemaker include a heavily calcified AV node or aortic valve ring with extension into the septum, appearance of AV block hours or days after surgery, and, to a lesser extent, a significant preoperative conduction defect. In the absence of excessive calcification, optimism is warranted, and it may be realistic to wait for up to 10 days for recovery before implantation of a permanent pacemaker. Surgically placed epicardial pacemaker wires are commonly used and can be lifesaving. Paired placement on the right atrium and right ventricle enhances diagnostic capability and allows pacing of all modes of bradycardia and for overdrive pacing.

Postoperative Pulmonary Morbidity

Pulmonary complications after cardiac surgery have been reviewed in detail.[114] In a large, multicenter administrative data base of 51,351 patients who underwent CABG, the incidence of adult respiratory distress syndrome/pulmonary edema was 4.9%; pneumonia, 0.8%; and other respiratory complications, 3.0%. Clinical observations suggest a 7.5% incidence of pulmonary morbidity, with an associated 21% mortality, in cardiac surgery patients with use of CPB. Heart failure is a major cause of postoperative pulmonary morbidity, and preoperative LV systolic dysfunction has a greater correlation than reduced preoperative pulmonary function with postoperative respiratory failure. Observational and randomized studies, and one propensity analysis study from the STS data base, suggest that the incidence of pulmonary complications is lower in patients receiving OPCAB. Small studies of patients undergoing mini-sternotomy or anterior thoracotomy have not convincingly shown reductions in respiratory complications.

Data from the STS data base indicate that 6.0% of patients undergoing CABG by median sternotomy require mechanical ventilation for more than 48 hours, with higher incidence of 2-week hospital stay (6%) and higher mortality (11.3%) than in patients undergoing OPCAB, including patients with COPD. Factors that predispose to prolonged ventilation include low albumin, low cardiac output state, persistent postoperative bleeding, neurologic complications, acute renal failure, bloodstream infections, and intra-abdominal complications. Postoperative AF may lead to hemodynamic instability requiring reintubation.

PNEUMONIA. Pneumonia has been reported in 2% to 22% of cardiac surgery patients and may be associated with up to 27% mortality. Clinical presentation occurs, on average, 4 days after surgery and ranges from fever with productive cough to acute respiratory failure requiring prolonged ventilation. Silent aspiration leading to pneumonia occurs commonly in the elderly, especially those with neurologic or cognitive impairment. Other reported predisposing factors include use of H2 receptor blockers (which increase colonization of gastric fluid with gram-negative organisms, which are then microaspirated) or broad-spectrum antibiotics, presence of nasogastric tube (which facilitates microaspiration), reintubation, prolonged mechanical ventilation, and transfusion of four or more units of blood products. Diagnosis is difficult because of frequent concomitant atelectasis and pleural effusions, and hence a high index of suspicion is warranted. Gram-negative organisms are the most common, but gram-positive bacteria appearing in the sputum before surgery are often the culprits in pneumonia occurring within 3 days of CABG. Resistant strains are emerging. Ventilator-associated pneumonia occurs in 8% of patients after cardiac surgery, rising to 9% to 21% in those with respiratory failure and 44% when intubation is longer than 7 days. It has been suggested that the risk of pneumonia increases by 1% with each day of mechanical ventilation. Mortality of ventilator-associated pneumonia can be as high as 75% because of associated multiorgan failure.

ACUTE RESPIRATORY DISTRESS SYNDROME. Acute respiratory distress syndrome (ARDS) is characterized by the presence of bilateral interstitial infiltrates on the chest radiograph, a pulmonary capillary wedge pressure of less than 18 mm Hg, and the presence of arterial hypoxemia leading to PaO_2/FiO_2 ratio less than 200. It occurs in less than 2% of patients undergoing CPB but is associated with mortality up to 80% because of associated multiorgan failure. It remains unclear whether off-pump or minimally invasive procedures reduce the occurrence of ARDS. The etiology of ARDS is multifactorial and includes pulmonary endothelial trauma caused by the whole-body inflammation on CPB, cessation of ventilation during CPB, translocation of enteric endotoxins secondary to intestinal hypoperfusion, and ischemia-reperfusion injury and hypothermia, with contributions from untoward reactions to protamine and transfusion products. Management is aimed at general multiorgan supportive care. Prevention of ventilator-associated pulmonary mechanotrauma through the use of small tidal volumes (6 mL/kg) has been shown to reduce mortality by 25%; the associated permissive hypercapnia is not detrimental. The use of heparin-coated circuits, hollow-fiber membrane oxygenators, or high-dose steroids to modulate the systemic inflammatory response has not been shown consistently to improve outcomes.

Postoperative Bleeding

Coagulopathy is common after CPB and is related to reductions in coagulation factors, fibrinolysis, inadequate reversal of heparinization, excessive protamine administration, other perioperative drugs, and defective platelet formation. It has been suggested that CPB-induced platelet aggregation may not be caused by factors released from the tubing or its coating but may be initiated by short bouts of high shear stress, and its continuation is critically dependent on adenosine diphosphate. Patients undergoing OPCAB show protection against activation of coagulation and fibrinolysis and against endothelial injury only during the intraoperative period; this is followed by the development of a prothrombotic pattern comparable to that of patients undergoing on-pump surgery lasting at least as late as 30 days after surgery. In addition, in patients undergoing OPCAB, the intraoperative administration of hetastarch increases the postoperative transfusion requirement and the volume of blood drained postoperatively. Hemodilution with low intraoperative hematocrit levels (<19%) has been shown not to contribute to postoperative bleeding. In contrast to standard coagulation testing (prothrombin time, fibrinogen level, D-dimer, and platelet count), platelet function as assessed by thromboelastography and whole-blood aggregometry may predict both bleeding and thrombosis after OPCAB.

Pharmacologic approaches and perioperative use of antithrombotic drugs (see Chap. 87) to reduce blood loss and transfusions in the perioperative period have been reviewed.[115] Meta-analysis has shown no significant difference in efficacy between the inexpensive lysine analogues, such as epsilon–aminocaproic acid or tranexamic acid, and more expensive serine protease inhibitors, such as high-dose aprotinin.

The specific use of aprotinin during cardiac surgery and its safety remain unresolved; cumulative evidence suggests that the risk associated with aprotinin may not be worth the hemostatic benefit. In a retrospective study of 1524 cardiac surgery patients at high risk for postoperative stroke, the administration of full-dose aprotinin but not half-dose aprotinin was associated with a lower incidence of stroke.[116] It has been proposed that the higher level of kallikrein inhibition obtained with full dosing may be required for end-organ protection. Another study concluded that its use is not associated with a change in mortality, MI, or renal failure risk but is associated with a reduced risk of stroke and a trend toward reduced incidence of AF.[117] The drug reduces perioperative bleeding during OPCAB. However, there is evidence showing an increased risk of death associated with aprotinin. A multicenter, blinded, randomized trial in high-risk cardiac surgery patients demonstrated a significantly higher occurrence of all-cause 30-day mortality with aprotinin compared with aminocaproic acid or tranexamic acid.[118] Analysis of electronic administrative records showed a 64% higher mortality on the day of CABG in patients who received aprotinin alone (n = 33,517) than in those who received aminocaproic acid alone (n = 44,682).[119] In another retrospective analysis of patients who underwent isolated CABG or combined CABG with valve operations, those who received aprotinin had a higher mortality rate and larger increases in serum creatinine levels than did patients who received aminocaproic acid or no antifibrinolytic agent.[120] On the other hand, there are studies indicating that full-dose aprotinin use is not associated with MI, neurologic dysfunction, renal insufficiency, or death after CABG or valve operations but does result in less postoperative bleeding and blood product transfusion and early extubation.[121] In another single-institution observational study involving 7836 consecutive patients (1998-2006), aprotinin was effective in reducing bleeding after cardiac surgery, was safe, and did not affect short- or medium-term survival.[122] The risk of hypersensitivity reactions is low (0.09%) after primary exposure to aprotinin. This risk after reexposure reaches a maximum between the 4th day and the 30th day after previous exposure and declines considerably after 6 months.

Desmopressin acetate (DDAVP) causes a 2- to 20-fold increase in plasma levels of factor VIII and von Willebrand factor and releases tissue plasminogen activator and prostacyclin from vascular endothelium. The drug may be useful in mild to moderate forms of hemophilia or von Willebrand disease, in uremic patients with platelet dysfunction, and in certain forms of postoperative platelet dysfunction based on specific testing.

Recombinant activated factor VII (rFVIIa) as rescue therapy in severe, uncontrollable hemorrhage after cardiac surgery is efficacious and safe and is not associated with adverse neurologic or cardiovascular effects. The median dose is 93 µg/kg, and 85% of patients need a single dose. In a registry cohort of 304 patients, the documented response rate to a single dose of rFVIIa was 84%, of which 23% experienced cessation of bleeding and 61% showed a reduction in bleeding. The percentage of patients alive at 28 days was 95% if bleeding ceased after rFVIIa, 86% if bleeding was reduced, and 60% if there was no response.[123]

Risk factors for surgical reexploration include advanced age, smaller BMI, nonelective cases, and five or more distal anastomoses. Preoperative aspirin and heparin are risk factors for the on-pump CABG group. Patients needing reexploration are at higher risk of complications if the time to reexploration is prolonged. Chest reexploration in the ICU for bleeding or tamponade after heart surgery can be a safe alternative to return to the operating room.

The main determinant of morbidity and mortality for patients requiring a surgical reexploration after cardiac operations is the amount of packed red blood cells transfused. Packed red blood cells must be used judiciously as perioperative packed red blood cell transfusion carries the potential for exposure to a variety of cellular and humoral antigens, disease transmission, and immunomodulation. A multidisciplinary approach to blood conservation has been proposed and can result in lower transfusion rates and equivalent patient outcomes. Transfusion is associated with reduced risk-adjusted 1-year survival after CABG, with the largest proportion of deaths occurring within 30 days. In a group of cardiac surgery patients, the risk of pneumonia increased by 5% per unit of red blood cells or platelets received, with higher risk for each day that the blood was stored. However, the administration of blood per se may not lead to increased postoperative infection. Point-of-care coagulation monitoring using thromboelastography has been shown to reduce postoperative transfusion requirements. Preoperative erythropoietin administered during weeks is associated with higher postoperative hemoglobin concentrations with modest reductions in transfusion requirements. Alternatively, intraoperative autologous heparinized blood removal before CPB in hemodynamically stable patients and retransfusion after CPB, intraoperative cell salvage, and autotransfusion of washed salvaged red blood cells also reduce need for transfusion. The mechanical cell salvage procedure reduces the red blood cell deformability and the cell 2,3-diphosphoglycerate content. Retransfusion of the processed blood by a cell-saving device does not further compromise the red blood cell function in patients undergoing cardiac surgery with CPB. Based on IL-6 and free hemoglobin washout, the quality of the processed blood remains constant even with multiple runs of the cell-saving device.

The volume remaining in the oxygenator and tubing set should be returned without cell processing or hemofiltration. Using the hard shell cardiotomy reservoir from the heart-lung machine, autotransfusion of the shed mediastinal blood can be continued hourly up to 18 hours after operation. By these methods, homologous red blood cell transfusion may be avoided in up to 98.6% of patients. However, cardiotomy suction and autotransfusion of mediastinal shed blood may contribute to the perioperative inflammatory response. Lipid particles in the size range of 10 to 60 μm in shed mediastinal blood with more than 300,000 particles per milliliter of blood can certainly contribute to microembolic complications.[124] Triglyceride profiles in these lipid particles and in adipose tissue are similar, suggesting that their origin is the mediastinum. Closed circuit extracorporeal circulation (CCECC) for CABG is associated with a significant reduction of red blood cell damage and activation of coagulation cascades similar to off-pump surgery compared with conventional CPB; in contrast, fibrinolysis markers and IL-6 were markedly increased in CCECC postoperatively. A substantially lower need for postoperative blood transfusions and a comparable hemorrhage-related reexploration rate suggest that OPCAB may avoid the morbidity and mortality associated with excessive postoperative blood loss. There is a tendency toward less activation of coagulation and fibrinolysis in low-risk patients during elective OPCAB compared with on-pump surgery.

Postoperative Renal Dysfunction

The development of AKI after cardiac surgery (see Chap. 93) is a devastating complication with high morbidity and up to 42% 30-day mortality.[125] Risk factors for the development of AKI include advanced age, diabetes, COPD, peripheral vascular disease, emergency operation, previous cardiac surgery, low preoperative hemoglobin level, high preoperative CRP level, perioperative MI, reexploration, and number of blood transfusions.[126] In the immediately postoperative period, neutrophil gelatinase–associated lipocalin and cystatin C correlate with and are independent predictors of duration and severity of AKI and duration of intensive care stay after adult cardiac surgery; however, the combination of both renal biomarkers does not add predictive value. The risk of adverse clinical events is not associated with ITA and saphenous vein graft failure, suggesting that factors other than graft failure account for the worse clinical outcomes, at least during the first year. In one study, three thresholds of AKI (>25%, >50%, and >75% decrease in estimated glomerular filtration rate within 1 week of surgery or need for postoperative dialysis) occurred in 24%, 7%, and 3% of the cohort, respectively. All three thresholds were independently associated with a more than fourfold increase in the odds of dying.[127] Early recovery of renal function is associated with improved long-term survival. Significant risk factors for death are complex procedures, gastrointestinal complications, long crossclamp time (>88 minutes), reexploration, advanced age (>75 years), elevated preoperative creatinine, postoperative pulmonary edema, sepsis, multiple organ failure, and hypotension. Although CPB is considered to be an important contributor to AKI, OPCAB improves only early mortality; long-term survival has been shown to be better in those revascularized on-pump, possibly because of more complete revascularization with CPB.

The use of various forms of renal replacement therapy after cardiac surgery (hemodialysis, hemofiltration, or combination) has been reviewed.[128] Patients with normal preoperative renal function can develop unexpected postoperative AKI requiring dialysis when they undergo urgent or emergent surgery or experience intraoperative technical complications requiring longer CPB and crossclamp times. Patients with even mild preoperative renal dysfunction commonly experience worsening of renal function even when the perioperative course is uncomplicated and often require dialysis in the hospital or after discharge. The decision to initiate dialysis in renal failure patients not on dialysis who develop further postoperative AKI can be difficult. Dialysis in such patients has been shown to reduce neurologic and gastrointestinal complications, to reduce major adverse events with lower length of stay, and probably to lower the rate of multiorgan failure. However, although in-hospital mortality may be relatively low, midterm mortality is increased compared with those who do not undergo dialysis. Preoperative renal failure patients on dialysis show a significant increase in hospital mortality, postoperative sepsis, and respiratory failure after cardiac surgery. The risk of dialysis dependence may be reduced with OPCAB. Patients who have undergone kidney transplantation show better survival than those on dialysis. Patients with serum creatinine concentration >2.0 mg/dL or dialysis dependence who have had an acute or recent MI and undergo CABG show an 8% to 10% hospital mortality and a higher risk of pulmonary complications and AF.

In patients with elevated preoperative serum creatinine, mannitol (25 g) or dopamine infusion at 3.0 to 4.5 μg/kg/min is often given intraoperatively; furosemide (20 to 100 mg) or hemofiltration should be considered during CPB. Sustained mild hypothermia does not improve renal outcomes. However, rewarming on CPB is associated with increased renal injury and should be avoided. N-Acetylcysteine is not beneficial in the prevention of renal dysfunction after cardiac surgery, and its routine use should be avoided. Likewise, there is no benefit of high-dose furosemide (Lasix) given postoperatively. Fenoldopam mesylate (0.08 μg/kg/min) infusion starting at the induction of anesthesia and continued for at least the next 24 hours may reduce the risk of acute renal failure in high-risk patients.[129] Maintaining high mean perfusion pressure (around 80 mm Hg), reducing pump time, and optimizing hemodynamics with pharmacologic or mechanical support are also beneficial. Infection control and renal protection must be stressed. Early and aggressive use of continuous venovenous hemofiltration postoperatively in patients with volume overload and high serum creatinine concentration is associated with better than expected survival. Off-pump surgery offers better early and late outcomes in patients with normal preoperative creatinine concentration. When the preoperative creatinine concentration is abnormal, the surgical strategy does not seem to have any influence.[130]

Postoperative Neurologic Morbidity

COGNITIVE DYSFUNCTION. Cognitive dysfunction after cardiac surgery has been reviewed.[131] It is a common short-term (33% to 83%) and long-term (20% to 60%) occurrence and may resolve after days to weeks or may remain as a permanent disorder, especially in terms of memory impairment. Often, longitudinal cognitive performance of patients with CABG shows a two-stage course with early improvement followed by later decline. Long-term cognitive deficit is predicted by early cognitive decline but not by ischemic brain lesions on magnetic resonance imaging (MRI). However, small studies indicate that prospective longitudinal neuropsychological performance of patients with CABG may be no different from that of comparable nonsurgical control subjects with CAD at 3 months or 1 year after baseline examination. This suggests that the generally reported cognitive decline during the early postoperative period after CABG may be transient and reversible. Subjective memory assessments have been correlated with objective performance on several memory tests.[132] Although subjective memory complaints are more common in patients with depression, they cannot be explained by depression alone. Baseline impairment before surgery in patients with CAD may also be higher than generally suspected. Pathologic findings point to a complex etiology involving the interplay of anesthesia effects, systemic inflammation, cerebral microemboli, and cerebral hypoperfusion with cerebral oxygen desaturation. Intraoperative hemodynamic instability, hypoxia, elevated preoperative creatinine, poor preoperative LV function, medications, postoperative infections, and intraoperative hyperglycemia in nondiabetic patients have been described as additional risk factors. Reduced preoperative endotoxin immunity has been proposed as a predictor of postoperative cognitive dysfunction in the elderly; a significant positive association between serum concentrations of S100B protein and neuropsychological function has been reported. Preoperative cerebral MRI may be used to predict the risk for cognitive dysfunction after CABG. Long-term cognitive function and MRI evidence of brain injury are similar after off-pump and on-pump CABG. OPCAB does not appear to consistently offer immunity from adverse neurocognitive outcomes, suggesting that the clinical decline may not be specific to the use of CPB but may also occur in patients with similar risk factors for cardiovascular and cerebrovascular disease.[133]

Cognitive dysfunction is clinically expressed as impairment of memory, concentration, language comprehension, and social integration and is usually evaluated with a battery of neuropsychological tests assessing the cognitive domains of attention, language, verbal and visual memory, visual construction, executive function, and psychomotor and motor speed. The clinical syndrome occurs more commonly in the elderly and those with low educational status, limited social support, diabetes, and severe noncoronary atherosclerotic disease. Women appear more likely to suffer injury to brain areas subserving visuospatial processing. The success of neuroprotective therapeutic interventions, including high-dose steroids, has been limited.

STROKE. Stroke and encephalopathy after cardiac surgery have been reviewed in detail.[134] Early stroke after CPB is independently associated with higher stroke-related death and is associated with increased need for skilled rehabilitation at discharge. Neuroprotective strategies aimed at reducing early postoperative stroke may have a positive impact on death and neurologic disability after CPB. Stroke after cardiac surgery is defined as any new permanent (manifest stroke) or temporary neurologic deficit or deterioration (transient ischemic attack or prolonged reversible ischemic neurologic deficit) and is confirmed by CT or MRI whenever possible. Brain MRI with diffusion-weighted imaging is the most sensitive and accurate neurologic imaging technique and is preferred to conventional MRI (T2 and FLAIR) because it can reveal significantly more lesions, especially in a "watershed" distribution. Stroke patients with hypoperfused brain tissue may be identified by comparing the mismatch between diffusion-weighted imaging and perfusion-weighted imaging. If diffusion-weighted imaging is not feasible, then head CT should be obtained.

The development of major stroke after CABG has been reported to be 1.5% to 5% in prospective studies and about 0.8% to 3.2% in retrospective analysis. When neurologic or psychometric analyses are performed before and after the operation, the occurrence of cerebral damage has varied from 15% to 40%. When more sensitive biochemical markers of brain cell damage are used, there is evidence of neurologic abnormality in more than 60% of patients. Clinically silent infarction may be far more frequent and could contribute to long-term cognitive dysfunction in patients after cardiac procedures. Serial measurement of serum S100B protein in the initial 12 hours after CPB has been used to predict early postoperative brain injury. Preoperative assessment of white matter disease by cerebral MRI may also help predict the patient's risk for development of cerebral injury. Use of a risk prediction model for stroke indicates that most strokes occur among patients at low or medium preoperative risk, suggesting that many of these strokes may be preventable.

Most strokes develop within the first 2 days after surgery and are up to two times more common in combined cardiac procedures or technically challenging operations. Multivariable analysis has identified 10 variables that were independent predictors of stroke: history of cerebrovascular disease, peripheral vascular disease, diabetes, hypertension, previous cardiac surgery, preoperative infection, urgent operation, CPB time more than 2 hours, need for intraoperative hemofiltration, and high transfusion requirement. The temperature at which CPB is performed is not a significant factor. Undergoing OPCAB reduces the incidence of perioperative stroke mainly by minimizing early strokes; however, the risk of delayed strokes is not different between patients undergoing on-pump and off-pump CABG.[135] Perioperative stroke confers significant mortality and morbidity. The 30-day mortality for stroke patients can be 10 times greater than that for those who do not suffer stroke. The greatest risk of death is noted within the first year after surgery. Five-year survival is lower among patients who had major functional limitations before discharge, among those who had hypoperfusion strokes, and among patients who were discharged to locations other than home or rehabilitation facilities. Patients with ascending aortic atherosclerosis, older age (>70 years), preoperative unstable angina, COPD, and carotid artery disease are at risk for late postoperative stroke (new strokes during 5-year follow-up) after CABG. Approximately 20% of patients with valve prostheses have a late embolic stroke within 15 years after valve replacement. Some risk factors, such as smoking, mitral mechanical prostheses, aortic tilting disc valves, and mitral valve surgery in the setting of LV dysfunction, are potentially modifiable.

ENCEPHALOPATHY. Encephalopathy, defined as diffuse brain injury, occurs in 8% to 32% of patients, depending on its manifestation, which can range from coma to confusion, agitation, and combativeness. Like stroke, it is associated with high mortality and prolonged length of hospital stay, with additional convalescence often required in a nursing home or assisted living facility. Psychotic symptoms are independently associated with prolonged ICU length of stay, multiorgan failure or shock, cardiac arrest, and higher in-hospital death after surgery. Important risk factors are advanced age, carotid bruits, hypertension, diabetes, and previous history of stroke. Perioperative hypothermia (<33°C), hypoxemia, low hematocrit, renal failure, increased serum sodium levels, infection, and stroke can be independent precipitating factors. Postoperative delirium is frequent after cardiac operations, especially in the elderly, and is associated with a higher mortality and readmissions, memory and concentration problems, and sleep disturbances. The Delirium Observation Screening (DOS) scale is a checklist developed for use before and after surgery to assess whether delirium has developed in patients.[136] The increased use of beating-heart surgery without CPB may lead to a lower occurrence of this complication.

REDUCING RISK OF POSTOPERATIVE STROKE AND ENCEPHALOPATHY. Evidence is accumulating that patients with perioperative encephalopathy and stroke have more pre-existing cerebrovascular disease than was recognized earlier, as evidenced by routine preoperative MRI scans. The main perioperative causes of neurologic dysfunction are microemboli caused by air, blood cell aggregates, calcium, or aortic atheroma associated with the pump oxygenator; the potential risk of air embolization during aortic cannulation; atheroembolism from the ascending aorta; and clots from the left ventricle. There is an independent, direct association between degree of hemodilution during CPB and risk of perioperative stroke, with each percentage decrease in hematocrit being associated with a 10% increase in the odds of suffering perioperative stroke. CT studies of the head suggest that a main mechanism of brain injury is cerebral embolization rather than cerebral hypoperfusion. Studies have also demonstrated a higher incidence of perioperative stroke (5%) in patients with abnormal preoperative regional cerebral perfusion, which is associated with older age, current tobacco use, and diabetes mellitus. The role of atheroembolism as a recognized complication of cardiac surgery has been reviewed by Djaiani.[137] Prophylactic cerebrovascular interventions and the selective use of aorta no-touch OPCAB can significantly reduce the incidence of perioperative stroke. Carbon dioxide field flooding can efficiently reduce air emboli released from incompletely deaired cardiac chambers and should be advocated for patients undergoing open heart surgery. AF after CABG has also been shown to be associated with the development of embolic postoperative stroke, usually occurring late (>7 days) after operation.

Although macroembolization is less common during modern cardiac surgery, microembolization remains a problem despite attention to routine precautions such as arterial filtration, reservoir filtration, filtration within the pump oxygenator, venting of the aorta, and (in the case of a diseased aorta) use of femoral cannulation, retrograde cardioplegia through the coronary sinus, bilateral ITA conduits, and insertion of proximal anastomoses on the carotid or innominate arteries. Transesophageal echocardiography, epiaortic scanning, and transcranial Doppler studies have documented embolic showers to the head during aortic crossclamping and unclamping. Superior neurologic outcomes are achieved by use of intra-aortic filters to capture particulate debris and avoidance of partial aortic clamping during OPCAB (no-touch technique). In one study of 700 consecutive patients, the incidence of stroke was significantly lower in the no-touch group.[138] Logistic regression has identified partial aortic clamping as the only independent predictor of stroke, influencing this risk 28-fold. Pulsatile flow, despite modest improvements in cerebral perfusion, does not seem to offer benefits in the incidence of stroke. Maintenance of high mean arterial pressure (80 to 100 mm Hg) on CPB does lead to fewer strokes than with lower mean pressure (50 to 60 mm Hg). The role of perioperative lidocaine for cerebral protection remains uncertain. Magnesium administration is safe and improves short-term postoperative neurologic function after cardiac surgery, particularly in preserving short-term memory and cortical control over brainstem functions.

NEUROPATHY. Phrenic nerve injury is a function of pericardial slush use and surgical dissection of the ITA. When no topical ice slush is used, an elevated left hemidiaphragm, manifested as the diaphragm's being two or more intercostal spaces higher than the opposite side, occurs in 2.5% of cases. This incidence is increased to 26% when topical ice slush is used and is further raised to 39% when the left ITA is dissected. The right phrenic nerve is at risk of injury in 4% of patients during high mobilization of the right ITA. Phrenic nerve injury can be prevented if the pericardiophrenic branch of the ITA is preserved. The hemidiaphragm remains elevated in 80% of patients at the end of 1 month and in 22% at the end of 1 year. Spontaneous recovery may be anticipated in two thirds of patients in whom the injury is identified postoperatively. High right ITA harvesting should be used with caution in patients with preoperative pulmonary dysfunction, in whom phrenic nerve injury would be poorly tolerated. Bilateral diaphragmatic paralysis has a prolonged time course of recovery.

Vocal cord palsy after adult cardiac surgery has been comprehensively reviewed.[139] The cumulative incidence is 1.1% (33 of 2980 patients). It may also be caused by injury of the recurrent laryngeal nerves by surgical dissection or nonsurgical mechanisms such as tracheal intubation and central venous catheterization. Other reported surgical mechanisms of injury are harvesting of ITA and topical cold cardioprotection. Bilateral nerve palsy has been lethal on at least one occasion.

The risk of perioperative optic neuropathy associated with cardiac surgery in which CPB is used is low (roughly 0.1%), but the outcomes can be devastating. Factors that lead to the condition remain unknown, although the presence of systemic vascular disease and both an absolute and relative drop in hemoglobin during the perioperative period seem to be important. Because this condition often causes profound permanent visual loss, it has been recommended that patients, particularly those with systemic vascular disease, be made aware of this potential complication when cardiac surgery with CPB is planned. In one study of neurologic complications after CABG, 17% had evidence of retinal infarction. Half were asymptomatic; others complained of visual disturbances such as reading difficulty or haziness in the peripheral vision. Despite the presence of definite pathologic changes, recovery of visual acuity can be expected. Cortical blindness can occur and may be missed during brief daily hospital visits with patients. One should be alerted when the patient appears to stare through rather than to focus on the objects of intended vision. When asked, the patient is unable to read or comprehend the content, often turning the reading material in various directions to help clarify confusion. Despite profound dysfunction, patients may not spontaneously mention such symptoms and occasionally may flatly deny their presence (Anton syndrome). CT or diffusion-weighted MRI may be useful in differentiating retinal from cortical causes of visual disturbances. The prognosis for symptomatic improvement is good, but detectable visual abnormalities often remain.

NEUROPSYCHIATRIC CHANGES. Depression is common after surgery, especially in patients with the tendency preoperatively. It can start in the first week, worsens for 2 to 3 weeks, and usually resolves by 6 weeks. Clinically significant depression such as that which interferes with daily activity and postoperative recovery, not showing signs of improvement by 4 to 6 weeks, should be formally evaluated and treated, especially if it is present before surgery. Severe psychotic symptoms are seen in 2.1% of postoperative patients. Higher age, renal failure, dyspnea, heart failure, and LV hypertrophy are independent preoperative predisposing factors. Perioperative hypothermia (<33°C), hypoxemia, low hematocrit, renal failure, hypernatremia, infection, and stroke are independent

precipitating factors. Psychotic symptoms have been shown to be independently associated with a prolonged length of stay in the ICU, multiorgan failure or shock, cardiopulmonary resuscitation, and in-hospital death after surgery.

Postoperative Gastrointestinal Morbidity

Abdominal organ morbidity after cardiac surgery has been thoughtfully reviewed by Hessel.[140] In his analysis of 37 reports between 1976 and 2004 covering more than 172,000 operations, the incidence of gastrointestinal complications averaged about 1.2% (range, 0.2% to 5.5%) and was associated with a high 33% average mortality (range, 13% to 87%), accounting for nearly 15% of all cardiac surgery deaths. In the STS data base for 1997 (www.sts.org/doc/2986), the incidence was 2.8% in 206,143 reported cases, which was about the same frequency as reoperation for bleeding, renal failure, and stroke and nearly two to three times more frequent than sternal infection, perioperative MI, acute respiratory failure, dialysis, and multiorgan failure. Gastrointestinal bleeding was the most common; mesenteric ischemia, pancreatitis, and cholecystitis were next in frequency; paralytic ileus, perforated peptic ulcer, hepatic failure, diverticular disease, pseudo-obstruction of the colon, small bowel obstruction, and multiorgan failure were less common. Intestinal infarction was invariably fatal, and high mortalities, averaging 70%, were associated with intestinal ischemia (which is usually of the nonocclusive type) and hepatic failure.

Damage to gastrointestinal organs can occur from hypoperfusion caused by vasoconstriction on CPB, atheroembolism, or perioperative hemodynamic instability leading to reduced mucosal blood flow with mucosal ischemia characterized by low mucosal pH. The systemic inflammatory response syndrome from endotoxemia, which can be initiated by splanchnic ischemia, has also been proposed as a mechanism. Complement activation on CPB, release of leukotriene B_4 and tumor necrosis factor, and plasmin formation result in damage to endothelial and mucosal cells and extracellular matrix as well as capillary leakage and microthrombi.

Identification of patients at higher risk for gastrointestinal morbidity and optimization of their perioperative hemodynamic management are the cornerstones for lowering of this complication. Prolonged postoperative mechanical ventilation longer than 24 hours is a risk factor; others include advanced age, low ejection fraction, perioperative inotropic or mechanical support, transfusions, arrhythmias, history of renal dysfunction, reoperation, emergency surgery, and poor New York Heart Association functional classification. Splanchnic blood flow may be improved with preoperative volume loading (1.5 mL/kg/hr of crystalloid or up to 600 mL of 6% hetastarch), phosphodiesterase inhibitors (milrinone), and selective gut decontamination (oral polymyxin, tobramycin, and amphotericin preoperatively for 3 days). Vasopressors should be avoided; the benefits of dopamine and dobutamine remain uncertain. The conduct of CPB may be of value; high flows, minimized circuits with low prime volumes, pulsatile flow, maintenance of hematocrit >25%, minimization of atheroembolization, and perioperative administration of aspirin have been shown to contribute to reduced gastrointestinal morbidity. Early diagnosis of bowel ischemia is difficult, although very high lactate levels, persistent metabolic acidosis, leukocytosis, and ileus may be clues. An aggressive approach including early use of colonoscopy, peritoneal lavage, and early interventional angiography with dilation or papaverine infusion and, occasionally, surgical intervention may be lifesaving.

Postoperative Wound Infection

The incidence of deep sternal wound infection appears to be decreasing, partly from the use of perioperative intravenous insulin.[141] Obesity is still the single most important risk factor for postoperative sternal dehiscence, with or without infection, after any type of cardiac operation. In a multivariate analysis, preoperative AF and an elevated CRP level were found to be significant predictors of mediastinitis in patients undergoing CABG.[142] Postoperative sternal wound complications after cardiac surgical procedures are classified as uninfected dehiscence (El Oakley class 1), superficial infections (El Oakley class 2A), and deep sternal wound infections (El Oakley class 2B). Recurrence rates of sternal infections remain high at nearly 20%. An algorithm for the management of poststernotomy complications has been proposed.[143] Prophylactic sternal reinforcement seems to prevent this complication by preventing nonunion or malunion, which can subsequently lead to deep sternal wound infections and mediastinitis. The current standard for sternotomy closure remains the method of wire cerclage. Bilateral ITA harvesting has carried a higher risk of sternal infection; skeletonization of both ITAs, in contrast to harvesting in a pedicled fashion, significantly reduces this risk.[144] There is no difference in the incidence of sternal dehiscence or superficial or deep sternal infection among diabetic patients receiving a single ITA or double skeletonized ITAs. Moreover, a study did not find tracheostomy to confer additional risk, suggesting that early tracheostomy may be considered in postoperative patients in respiratory failure.[145] Prophylactic antibiotics, usually cefazolin, are traditionally given at induction and a second dose before wound closure, with *Staphylococcus aureus* as the indicator microorganism. It has been shown that conventional doses do not provide targeted antimicrobial cefazolin plasma levels during the entire surgical procedure when CPB time exceeds 120 minutes. Patients with shorter bypass times and those undergoing profound hypothermic circulatory arrest are better protected, but the generally used protocol of prophylaxis is not optimal for all patients.

Leg wound complications are common, with an incidence of about 32% after traditional saphenous vein harvesting, with 65% of the patients requiring antibiotics. Single-dose cefazolin used as antibiotic prophylaxis in cardiac surgery is associated with a higher surgical site infection rate than a 24-hour, multiple-dose cefazolin regimen. Endoscopic saphenous vein harvesting of a short vein segment from the thigh results in less wound morbidity and better cosmetic results compared with open venous harvesting of a short vein segment from the calf. Prophylactic application of low-energy shock wave therapy may improve wound healing after vein harvesting for CABG. A retrospective analysis concluded that application of platelet-rich and platelet-poor plasma significantly reduced occurrences of chest wound infection, chest drainage, and leg wound drainage.[146] Radial artery infections secondary to catheterization for blood pressure monitoring are rare (0.2%) but potentially serious complications. Strict, systematic changing of arterial lines on a timely basis is warranted. A high suspicion index, aggressive surgical treatment of bacterial arteritis, and appropriate intravenous antibiotics are critical. Early surgical intervention is necessary in cases of infected radial artery pseudoaneurysms.

Postoperative Endocrine Abnormalities

Tight glucose control, defined as glucose concentration below 130 mg/dL for more than 50% of measurements, is mandatory after cardiac surgery and requires a standard protocol and metrics to track protocol performance. Reduced postoperative infections, especially mediastinitis, are experienced in diabetic patients and even in nondiabetic patients when intensive insulin therapy is used to keep blood glucose concentration below 110 mg/dL.

Diabetes insipidus after CABG has been ascribed to altered left atrial non-osmoreceptor function that provokes altered antidiuretic hormone activity during the period of asystole on CPB.[147] The euthyroid sick syndrome (non–thyroid illness syndrome) in CABG patients is considered to be a nonspecific response to stress. Reduction in serum total T_3 and free T_3 levels is associated with substantially elevated reversed T_3 levels, with values of thyroid-stimulating hormone, thyroxine, and free thyroxine remaining within normal limits. Off-pump surgery is associated with thyroid hormone changes similar to conventional surgical revascularization. It has been proposed that intravenous T_3 may have a potential role in the management of postoperative low cardiac output states (see Chap. 86).

REFERENCES

1. Stamou SC, Camp SL, Stiegel RM, et al: Quality improvement program decreases mortality after cardiac surgery. J Thorac Cardiovasc Surg 136:494, 2008.
2. Auerbach AD, Hilton JF, Maselli J, et al: Shop for quality or volume? Volume, quality, and outcomes of coronary artery bypass surgery. Ann Intern Med 150:696, 2009.
3. Brown PP, Kugelmass AD, Cohen DJ, et al: The frequency and cost of complications associated with coronary artery bypass grafting surgery: Results from the United States Medicare program. Ann Thorac Surg 85:1980, 2008.
4. Speir AM, Kasirajan V, Barnet SD, et al: Additive costs of postoperative complications for isolated coronary artery bypass grafting patients in Virginia. Ann Thorac Surg 88:40, 2009.

Preoperative Risk Analysis

5. Nissinen J, Wistbacka J-O, Loponen P, et al: Coronary artery bypass surgery in octogenarians: Long-term outcome can be better than expected. Ann Thorac Surg 89:1119, 2010.
6. Rohde SL, Baker RA, Tully PJ, et al: Preoperative and intraoperative factors associated with long-term survival in octogenarian cardiac surgery patients. Ann Thorac Surg 89:105, 2010.
7. Chaturvedi RK, Blaise M, Verdon J, et al: Cardiac surgery in octogenarians: Long-term survival, functional status, living arrangements, and leisure activities. Ann Thorac Surg 89:805, 2010.
8. Likosky DS, Sorensen MJ, Dacey LJ, et al: Long-term survival of the very elderly undergoing aortic valve surgery for valvular heart disease. Circulation 120(Suppl 1):S127, 2009.
9. Maurer MS, Luchsinger JA, Wellner R, et al: The effect of body mass index on complications of cardiac surgery in the oldest old. J Am Geriatr Soc 50:988, 2002.
10. Matsuura K, Kobayashi J, Tagusari O, et al: Off-pump coronary artery bypass grafting using only arterial grafts in elderly patients. Ann Thorac Surg 80:144, 2005.
11. Speziale G, Nasso G, Barattoni MC, et al: Operative and middle-term results of cardiac surgery in nonagenarians: A bridge toward routine practice. Circulation 121:208, 2010.
12. Guru V, Fremes SE, Tu JV, et al: Time-related mortality for women after coronary artery bypass graft surgery: A population-based study. J Thorac Cardiovasc Surg 127:1158, 2004.
13. Blankstein R, Ward RP, Arnsdorf M, et al: Female gender is an independent predictor of operative mortality after coronary artery bypass graft surgery. Circulation 112(Suppl I):I-323, 2005.
14. Ioannis K, Toumpoulis CE, Anagnostopoulos SK, et al: Assessment of independent predictors for long-term mortality between women and men after coronary artery bypass grafting: Are women different from men? J Thorac Cardiovasc Surg 131:343, 2006.
15. Kulik A, Lam B-K, Rubens FD, et al: Gender differences in the long-term outcomes after valve replacement surgery. Heart 95:318, 2009.
16. Cooper WA, Thourani VH, Guyton RA, et al: Racial disparity persists after on-pump and off-pump coronary artery bypass grafting surgery for coronary artery disease. Circulation 120(Suppl 1):S59, 2009.
17. Melsop K, Brooks MM, Boothroyd DB, et al: Effect of race on the clinical outcomes in the Bypass Angioplasty Revascularization Investigation trial. Circ Cardiovasc Qual Outcomes 12:186, 2009.
18. Nallamothu BK, Lu X, Vaughan-Sarrazin MS, et al: Coronary revascularization at specialty cardiac hospitals and peer general hospitals in black Medicare beneficiaries. Circ Cardiovasc Qual Outcomes 1:116, 2009.
19. Batty GD, Shipley MJ, Gale CR, et al: Does IQ predict total and cardiovascular disease mortality as strongly as other risk factors? Comparison of effect estimates using the Vietnam Experience Study. Heart 94:1541, 2008.
20. van Straten AHM, Bramer S, Soliman Hamad MA, et al: Effect of body mass index on early and late mortality after coronary artery bypass grafting. Ann Thorac Surg 89:30, 2010.
21. Karl F, Welke MJ, Barnett MS, et al: Limitations of hospital volume as a measure of quality of care for coronary artery bypass graft surgery. Ann Thorac Surg 80:2114, 2005.
22. Shahian DM, O'Brien SM, Normand SL, et al: Association of hospital coronary artery bypass volume with processes of care, mortality, morbidity, and the Society of Thoracic Surgeons composite quality score. Thorac Cardiovasc Surg 139:273, 2010.
23. Wen HC, Tang CH, Lin HC, et al: Association between surgeon and hospital volume in coronary artery bypass graft surgery outcomes: A population-based study. Ann Thorac Surg 81:835, 2006.
24. Lin HC, Xirasagar S, Tsao NW, et al: Volume-outcome relationships in coronary artery bypass graft surgery patients: 5-year major cardiovascular event outcomes. J Thorac Cardiovasc Surg 135:923, 2008.
25. Aldea GS, Mokadam NA, Melford R Jr, et al: Changing volumes, risk profiles, and outcomes of coronary artery bypass grafting and percutaneous coronary interventions. Ann Thorac Surg 87:1828, 2009.
26. Konety SH, Rosenthal GE, Vaughan-Sarrazin MS: Surgical volume and outcomes of off-pump coronary artery bypass graft surgery: Does it matter? J Thorac Cardiovasc Surg 137:1116, 2009.
27. Hartrumpf M, Claus T, Erb M, et al: Surgeon performance index: Tool for assessment of individual surgical quality in total quality management. Eur J Cardiothorac Surg 35:751, 2009.
28. Castellheim A, Hoel TN, Videm V, et al: Biomarker profile in off-pump and on-pump coronary artery bypass grafting surgery in low-risk patients. Ann Thorac Surg 85:1994, 2008.
29. Biancari F, Rimpiläinen R: Meta-analysis of randomised trials comparing the effectiveness of miniaturised versus conventional cardiopulmonary bypass in adult cardiac surgery. Heart 95:964, 2009.
30. Abu-Omar Y, Taggart DP: The present status of off-pump coronary artery bypass grafting. Eur J Cardiothorac Surg 36:312, 2009.
31. Weltert L, D'Alessandro S, Nardella S, et al: Preoperative very short-term, high-dose erythropoietin administration diminishes blood transfusion rate in off-pump coronary artery bypass: A randomized blind controlled study. J Thorac Cardiovasc Surg 139:621, 2010.
32. Molle CH, Perko MJ, Lund JT, et al: No major differences in 30-day outcomes in high-risk patients randomized to off-pump versus on-pump coronary bypass surgery: The Best Bypass Surgery Trial. Circulation 121:498, 2010.
33. Shroyer AL, Grover FL, Hattler B, et al: On-pump versus off-pump coronary artery bypass surgery. N Engl J Med 361:1827, 2009.
34. Marcheix B, Vanden Eynden F, Demers P, et al: Influence of diabetes mellitus on long-term survival in systematic off-pump coronary artery surgery. Ann Thorac Surg 86:1181, 2008.
35. Fu SP, Zheng Z, Yuan X, et al: Impact of off-pump techniques on sex differences in early and late outcomes after isolated coronary artery bypass grafts. Ann Thorac Surg 87:1090, 2009.
36. Kamdar AR, Meadows TA, Roselli EE, et al: Multidetector computed tomographic angiography in planning of reoperative cardiothoracic surgery. Ann Thorac Surg 85:1239, 2008.
37. Shuhaiber JH, Goldsmith K, Nashef SA: The influence of seasonal variation on cardiac surgery: A time-related clinical outcome predictor. J Thorac Cardiovasc Surg 136:894, 2008.
38. Bell ML, Grunwald GK, Baltz JH, et al: Does preoperative hemoglobin independently predict short-term outcomes after coronary artery bypass graft surgery? Ann Thorac Surg 86:1415, 2008.
39. Newall N, Grayson AD, Oo AY, et al: Preoperative white blood cell count is independently associated with higher perioperative cardiac enzyme release and increased 1-year mortality after coronary artery bypass grafting. Ann Thorac Surg 81:583, 2006.

40. Bevilacqua S, Alkodami A, Volpi E, et al: Risk stratification after coronary artery bypass surgery by a point-of-care test of platelet function. Ann Thorac Surg 87:496, 2009.
41. Halkos ME, Puskas JD, Lattouf OM, et al: Elevated preoperative hemoglobin A1c level is predictive of adverse events after coronary artery bypass surgery. J Thorac Cardiovasc Surg 136:631, 2008.
42. Kangasniemi OP, Biancari F, Luukkonen F, et al: Preoperative C-reactive protein is predictive of long-term outcome after coronary artery bypass surgery. Eur J Cardiothorac Surg 29:983, 2006.
43. van Straten AHM, Soliman Hamad MA, van Zundert AJ, et al: Preoperative C-reactive protein levels to predict early and late mortalities after coronary artery bypass surgery: Eight years of follow-up. J Thorac Cardiovasc Surg 138:954, 2009.
44. Cerillo AG, Bevilacqua S, Storti S, et al: Free triiodothyronine: A novel predictor of postoperative atrial fibrillation. Eur J Cardiothorac Surg 24:487, 2003.
45. Fox AA, Shernan SS, Collard CD, et al: Preoperative B-type natriuretic peptide is an independent predictor of ventricular dysfunction and mortality after primary coronary artery bypass grafting. J Thorac Cardiovasc Surg 136:452, 2008.
46. Tavakol M, Hassan KZ, Abdula RK, et al: Utility of brain natriuretic peptide as a predictor of atrial fibrillation after cardiac operations. Ann Thorac Surg 88:802, 2009.
47. Lurati Buse GA, Koller MT, Grapow M, et al: The prognostic value of troponin release after adult cardiac surgery: A meta-analysis. Eur J Cardiothorac Surg 37:399, 2010.

Preoperative Laboratory Values and Drug Treatment

48. Thielmann M, Massoudy P, Neuhauser M, et al: Prognostic value of preoperative cardiac troponin I in patients undergoing emergency coronary artery bypass surgery with non ST-elevation or ST-elevation acute coronary syndromes. Circulation 114(Suppl I):I-448, 2006.
49. Herman CR, Buth KJ, Kent BA, et al: Clopidogrel increases blood transfusion and hemorrhagic complications in patients undergoing cardiac surgery. Ann Thorac Surg 89:397, 2010.
50. Karabulut H, Toraman F, Evrenkaya S, et al: Clopidogrel does not increase bleeding and allogenic blood transfusion in coronary artery surgery. Eur J Cardiothorac Surg 25:419, 2004.
51. Ebrahimi R, Dyke C, Mehran R, et al: Outcomes following pre-operative clopidogrel administration in patients with acute coronary syndromes undergoing coronary artery bypass surgery: The ACUITY (Acute Catheterization and Urgent Intervention Triage strategy) Trial. J Am Coll Cardiol 53:1965, 2009.
52. Fox KA, Mehta SR, Peters R, et al: Benefits and risks of the combination of clopidogrel and aspirin in patients undergoing surgical revascularization for non–ST-elevation acute coronary syndrome: The Clopidogrel in Unstable angina to prevent Recurrent ischemic Events (CURE) Trial. Circulation 110:1202, 2004.
53. Lindvall G, Sartipy I, van der Linden J: Aprotinin reduces bleeding and blood product use in patients treated with clopidogrel before coronary artery bypass grafting. Ann Thorac Surg 80:922, 2005.
54. Vaccarino GN, Thierer J, Albertal M, et al: Impact of preoperative clopidogrel in off pump coronary artery bypass surgery: A propensity score analysis. J Thorac Cardiovasc Surg 137:309, 2009.
55. Maltais S, Perrault LP, Do QB: Effect of clopidogrel on bleeding and transfusions after off-pump coronary artery bypass graft surgery: Impact of discontinuation prior to surgery. Eur J Cardiothorac Surg 34:127, 2008.
56. Paraskevas KI: Applications of statins in cardiothoracic surgery: More than just lipid-lowering. Eur J Cardiothorac Surg 33:377, 2008.
57. Mannacio VA, Iorio D, de Amicis V, et al: Effect of rosuvastatin pretreatment on myocardial damage after coronary surgery: A randomized trial. J Thorac Cardiovasc Surg 136:1541, 2009.
58. Fedoruk LM, Wang H, Conaway MR, et al: Statin therapy improves outcomes after valvular heart surgery. Ann Thorac Surg 85:1521, 2008.
59. Tabata M, Khalpey Z, Cohn LH, et al: Effect of preoperative statins in patients without coronary artery disease who undergo cardiac surgery. J Thorac Cardiovasc Surg 136:1510, 2009.
60. Borger MA, Seeburger J, Walther T, et al: Effect of preoperative statin therapy on patients undergoing isolated and combined valvular heart surgery. Ann Thorac Surg 89:773, 2010.
61. Liakopoulos OJ, Choi Y-H, Kuhn EW, et al: Statins for prevention of atrial fibrillation after cardiac surgery: A systematic literature review. J Thorac Cardiovasc Surg 138:678, 2009.
62. Benedetto U, Sciarretta S, Roscitano A, et al: Preoperative angiotensin-converting enzyme inhibitors and acute kidney injury after coronary artery bypass grafting. Ann Thorac Surg 86:1160, 2008.
63. Ho KM, Tan JA: Benefits and risks of corticosteroid prophylaxis in adult cardiac surgery: A dose-response meta-analysis. Circulation 119:1853, 2009.
64. Albacker T, Carvalho G, Schricker T, et al: High-dose insulin therapy attenuates systemic inflammatory response in coronary artery bypass grafting patients. Ann Thorac Surg 86:20, 2008.

Preoperative Medical Conditions

65. Wagner BD, Grunwald GK, Rumsfeld J, et al: Relationship of body mass index with outcomes after coronary artery bypass graft surgery. Ann Thorac Surg 84:10, 2007.
66. Alserius T, Hammar N, Nordqvist T, et al: Improved survival after coronary artery bypass grafting has not influenced the mortality disadvantage in patients with diabetes mellitus. J Thorac Cardiovasc Surg 138:1115, 2009.
67. Kajimoto K, Miyauchi K, Kasai T, et al: Metabolic syndrome is an independent risk factor for stroke and acute renal failure after coronary artery bypass grafting. J Thorac Cardiovasc Surg 137:658, 2009.
68. van Straten AHM, Firanescu C, Soliman Hamad MA, et al: Peripheral vascular disease as a predictor of survival after coronary artery bypass grafting: Comparison with a matched general population. Ann Thorac Surg 89:414, 2010.
69. Haase M, Bellomo R, Matalanis G, et al: A comparison of the RIFLE and Acute Kidney Injury Network classifications for cardiac surgery–associated acute kidney injury: A prospective cohort study. Thorac Cardiovasc Surg 138:1370, 2009.
70. Ristikankare A, Pöyhiä R, Kuitunen A, et al: Serum cystatin C in elderly cardiac surgery patients. Ann Thorac Surg 89:689, 2010.
71. Heise D, Sundermann D, Braeuer A, et al: Validation of a clinical score to determine the risk of acute renal failure after cardiac surgery. Eur J Cardiothorac Surg 37:710, 2010.
72. Kinoshita T, Asai T, Murakami Y, et al: Efficacy of bilateral internal thoracic artery grafting in patients with chronic kidney disease. Ann Thorac Surg 89:1106, 2010.
73. Ad N, Barnett SD, Haan CK, et al: Does preoperative atrial fibrillation increase the risk for mortality and morbidity after coronary artery bypass grafting? J Thorac Cardiovasc Surg 137:901, 2009.
74. Sezai A, Hata M, Niino T, et al: Study of the factors related to atrial fibrillation after coronary artery bypass grafting: A search for a marker to predict the occurrence of atrial fibrillation before surgical intervention. J Thorac Cardiovasc Surg 137:895, 2009.
75. Ad N, Henry L, Halpin L, et al: The use of spirometry testing prior to cardiac surgery may impact the Society of Thoracic Surgeons risk prediction score: A prospective study in a cohort of patients at high risk for chronic lung disease. J Thorac Cardiovasc Surg 139:686, 2010.
76. Filsoufi F, Rahmanian PB, Castillo JG, et al: Logistic risk model predicting postoperative respiratory failure in patients undergoing valve surgery. Eur J Cardiothorac Surg 34:953, 2008.
77. Trouillet J-L, Combes A, Vaissier E, et al: Prolonged mechanical ventilation after cardiac surgery: Outcome and predictors. J Thorac Cardiovasc Surg 138:948, 2009.
78. Nussmeier NA, Miao Y, Roach GW, et al: Predictive value of the National Institutes of Health Stroke Scale and the Mini-Mental State Examination for neurologic outcome after coronary artery bypass graft surgery. J Thorac Cardiovasc Surg 139:901, 2010.
79. Lin CH, Lin FY, Wang SS, et al: Cardiac surgery in patients with liver cirrhosis. Ann Thorac Surg 79:1551, 2005.
80. Hayashida N, Shoujima T, Teshima H, et al: Clinical outcome after cardiac operations in patients with cirrhosis. Ann Thorac Surg 77:500, 2004.
81. Morisaki A, Hosono M, Sasaki Y, et al: Risk factor analysis in patients with liver cirrhosis undergoing cardiovascular operations. Ann Thorac Surg 89:811, 2010.
82. Mestres CA, Chuquiure JE, Claramonte X, et al: Long-term results after cardiac surgery in patients infected with the human immunodeficiency virus type-1 (HIV-1). Eur J Cardiothorac Surg 23:1007, 2003.
83. Fecher AM, Birdas TJ, Haybron D, et al: Cardiac operations in patients with hematologic malignancies. Eur J Cardiothorac Surg 25:537, 2004.
84. Gorki H, Malinovski V, Stanbridge RDL: The antiphospholipid syndrome and heart valve surgery. Eur J Cardiothorac Surg 33:168, 2008.
85. Morawski W, Sanak M, Cisowski M, et al: Prediction of the excessive perioperative bleeding in patients undergoing coronary artery bypass grafting: Role of aspirin and platelet glycoprotein IIIa polymorphism. J Thorac Cardiovasc Surg 130:791, 2005.

Preoperative Risk Calculation

86. Laurie A, Shroyer W, Coombs LP, et al: The society of thoracic surgeons: 30-day operative mortality and morbidity risk models. Ann Thorac Surg 75:1856, 2003.
87. Merello L, Riesle E, Alburquerque J, et al: Risk scores do not predict high mortality after coronary artery bypass surgery in the presence of diastolic dysfunction. Ann Thorac Surg 85:1247, 2008.
88. Klein P, Holman ER, Versteegh MIM, et al: Wall motion score index predicts mortality and functional result after surgical ventricular restoration for advanced ischemic heart failure. Eur J Cardiothorac Surg 35:847, 2009.
89. Ranucci M, Castelvecchio S, Menicanti L, et al: An adjusted EuroSCORE model for high-risk cardiac patients. Eur J Cardiothorac Surg 36:791, 2009.
90. Ranucci M, Castelvecchio S, Menicanti L, et al: Accuracy, calibration and clinical performance of the EuroSCORE: Can we reduce the number of variables? Eur J Cardiothorac Surg 37:724, 2010.
91. Parolari A, Pesce LL, Trezzi M, et al: EuroSCORE performance in valve surgery: A meta-analysis. Ann Thorac Surg 89:787, 2010.
92. Wendt D, Osswald BR, Kayser K, et al: Society of Thoracic Surgeons Score is superior to the EuroSCORE determining mortality in high risk patients undergoing isolated aortic valve replacement. Ann Thorac Surg 88:468, 2009.
93. Jin R, Grunkemeier GL, Starr AS, et al: Validation and refinement of mortality risk models for heart valve surgery. Ann Thorac Surg 80:471, 2005.
94. Butchart EG, Ionescu A, Payne N, et al: A new scoring system to determine thromboembolic risk after heart valve replacement. Circulation 108(Suppl II):II-68, 2003.

The "Normal" Postoperative Convalescence

95. Cerfolio RJ, Minnich DJ, Bryant AS: The removal of chest tubes despite an air leak or a pneumothorax. Ann Thorac Surg 87:1690, 2009.
96. Cohen J, Kogan A, Sahar G, et al: Hypophosphatemia following open heart surgery: Incidence and consequences. Eur J Cardiothorac Surg 26:306, 2004.
97. Mohammed AA, Agnihotri AK, van Kimmenade RRJ, et al: Prospective, comprehensive assessment of cardiac troponin T testing after coronary artery bypass graft surgery. Circulation 120:843, 2009.
98. Zimmermann N, Gams E, Hohlfeld T: Aspirin in coronary artery bypass surgery: New aspects of and alternatives for an old antithrombotic agent. Eur J Cardiothorac Surg 34:93, 2008.
99. Lim E, Cornelissen J, Routledge T, et al: Clopidogrel did not inhibit platelet function early after coronary bypass surgery: A prospective randomized trial. J Thorac Cardiovasc Surg 128:432, 2004.
100. Gao C, Ren C, Li D, et al: Clopidogrel and aspirin versus clopidogrel alone on graft patency after coronary artery bypass grafting. Ann Thorac Surg 88:59, 2009.
101. Kogan A, Cohen J, Raanani E, et al: Readmission to the intensive care unit after "fast-track" cardiac surgery: Risk factors and outcomes. Ann Thorac Surg 76:503, 2003.
102. Swaminathan M, Phillips-Bute BG, Patel UD, et al: Increasing healthcare resource utilization after coronary artery bypass graft surgery in the United States. Circ Cardiovasc Qual Outcomes 2:305, 2009.
103. Lee DH, Buth KJ, Martin B-J, et al: Frail patients are at increased risk for mortality and prolonged institutional care after cardiac surgery. Circulation 121:973, 2010.

Postoperative Morbidity

104. Alsaddique AA: Recognition of diastolic heart failure in the postoperative heart. Eur J Cardiothorac Surg 34:1141, 2008.
105. Jing Z-C, Jiang X, Wu BX, et al: Vardenafil treatment for patients with pulmonary arterial hypertension: A multicentre, open-label study. Heart 95:1531, 2009.
106. Dunning J, Fabbri A, Kolh PH, et al: Guideline for resuscitation in cardiac arrest after cardiac surgery. Eur J Cardiothorac Surg 36:3, 2009.

107. Adam Z, Adam S, Everngam RL, et al: Resuscitation after cardiac surgery: Results of an international survey. Eur J Cardiothorac Surg 36:29, 2009.

108. Liu K-Y, Muehlschlegel JD, Perry TE, et al: Common genetic variants on chromosome 9p21 predict perioperative myocardial injury after coronary artery bypass graft surgery. J Thorac Cardiovasc Surg 139:483, 2010.

109. Schwefer M, Aschenbach R, Heidemann J, et al: Constrictive pericarditis, still a diagnostic challenge: Comprehensive review of clinical management. Eur J Cardiothorac Surg 36:502, 2009.

110. Kaireviciute D, Aidietis A, Lip GY: Atrial fibrillation following cardiac surgery: Clinical features and preventative strategies. Eur Heart J 30:410, 2009.

111. Filardo G, Hamilton C, Hebeler RF Jr, et al: New-onset postoperative atrial fibrillation after isolated coronary artery bypass graft surgery and long-term survival. Circ Cardiovasc Qual Outcomes 2:164, 2009.

112. Zebis LR, Christensen TD, Kristiansen IR, et al: Amiodarone cost effectiveness in preventing atrial fibrillation after coronary artery bypass graft surgery. Ann Thorac Surg 85:28, 2008.

113. Rho RW: The management of atrial fibrillation after cardiac surgery. Heart 95:422, 2009.

114. Weissman C: Pulmonary complications after cardiac surgery. Semin Cardiothorac Vasc Anesth 8:185, 2004.

115. Dunning J, Versteegh M, Fabbri A, et al: Guideline on antiplatelet and anticoagulation management in cardiac surgery. Eur J Cardiothorac Surg 34:73, 2008.

116. Frumento RJ, O'Malley CM, Bennett-Guerrero E, et al: Stroke after cardiac surgery: A retrospective analysis of the effect of aprotinin dosing regimens. Ann Thorac Surg 75:479, 2003.

117. Sedrakyan A, Treasure T, Elefteriades JA: Effect of aprotinin on clinical outcomes in coronary artery bypass graft surgery: A systematic review and meta-analysis of randomized clinical trials. J Thorac Cardiovasc Surg 128:442, 2004.

118. Fergusson DA, Hébert PC, Mazer CD, et al: A Comparison of aprotinin and lysine analogues in high-risk cardiac surgery. N Engl J Med 358:2319, 2008.

119. Schneeweiss S, Seeger JD, Landon J, et al: Aprotinin during coronary-artery bypass grafting and risk of death. N Engl J Med 358:771, 2008.

120. Shaw AD, Stafford-Smith M, White WD, et al: The effect of aprotinin on outcome after coronary-artery bypass grafting. N Engl J Med 358:784, 2008.

121. Later AFL, Maas JJ, Engbers FHM, et al: Tranexamic acid and aprotinin in low- and intermediate-risk cardiac surgery: A non-sponsored, double-blind, randomised, placebo-controlled trial. Eur J Cardiothorac Surg 36:322, 2009.

122. Pagano D, Howell NJ, Freemantle N, et al: Bleeding in cardiac surgery: The use of aprotinin does not affect survival. J Thorac Cardiovasc Surg 135:495, 2008.

123. Dunkley C, Phillips L, McCall P, et al: Recombinant activated factor VII in cardiac surgery: Experience from the Australian and New Zealand Haemostasis Registry. Ann Thorac Surg 85:836, 2008.

124. Eyjolfsson A, Scicluna S, Johnsson P, et al: Characterization of lipid particles in shed mediastinal blood. Ann Thorac Surg 85:978, 2008.

125. Mehta R, Hafley GE, Gibson CM, et al: Influence of preoperative renal dysfunction on one-year bypass graft patency and two-year outcomes in patients undergoing coronary artery bypass surgery. J Thorac Cardiovasc Surg 136:1149, 2009.

126. van Straten AHM, Soliman Hamad MA, van Zundert AAAJ, et al: Risk factors for deterioration of renal function after coronary artery bypass grafting. Eur J Cardiothorac Surg 37:106, 2010.

127. Karkouti K, Wijeysundera DN, Yau TM, et al: Acute kidney injury after cardiac surgery: Focus on modifiable risk factors. Circulation 119:495, 2009.

128. Elahi M, Asopa A, Pflueger A, et al: Acute kidney injury following cardiac surgery: Impact of early versus late haemofiltration on morbidity and mortality. Eur J Cardiothorac Surg 35:854, 2009.

129. Ranucci M, Soro G, Barzaghi N, et al: Fenoldopam prophylaxis of postoperative acute renal failure in high-risk cardiac surgery patients. Ann Thorac Surg 78:1332, 2004.

130. Di Mauro M, Gagliardi M, Iacò AL, et al: Does off-pump coronary surgery reduce postoperative acute renal failure? The importance of preoperative renal function. Ann Thorac Surg 84:1496, 2007.

131. Gao L, Taha R, Gauvin D, et al: Postoperative cognitive dysfunction after cardiac surgery. Chest 128:3664, 2005.

132. McKhann GM, Selnes OA, Grega MA, et al: Subjective memory symptoms in surgical and nonsurgical coronary artery patients: 6-year follow-up. Ann Thorac Surg 87:27, 2009.

133. Selnes OA, Grega MA, Bailey MM, et al: Do management strategies for coronary artery disease influence 6-year cognitive outcomes? Ann Thorac Surg 88:445, 2009.

134. McKhann GM, Grega MA, Borowicz LM Jr, et al: Stroke and encephalopathy after cardiac surgery: An update. Stroke 37:562, 2006.

135. Nishiyama K, Horiguchi M, Shizuta S, et al: Temporal pattern of strokes after on-pump and off-pump coronary artery bypass graft surgery. Ann Thorac Surg 87:1839, 2009.

136. Koster S, Oosterveld FCJ, Hensens AG, et al: Delirium after cardiac surgery and predictive validity of a risk checklist. Ann Thorac Surg 86:1883, 2008.

137. Djaiani GN: Aortic arch atheroma: Stroke reduction in cardiac surgical patients. Semin Cardiothorac Vasc Anesth 10:143, 2006.

138. Lev-Ran O, Braunstein R, Sharony R, et al: No-touch aorta off-pump coronary surgery: The effect on stroke. J Thorac Cardiovasc Surg 129:307, 2005.

139. Dimarakis I, Protopapas AD: Vocal cord palsy as a complication of adult cardiac surgery: Surgical correlations and analysis. Eur J Cardiothorac Surg 26:773, 2004.

140. Hessel EA II: Abdominal organ injury after cardiac surgery. Semin Cardiothorac Vasc Anesth 8:243, 2004.

141. Matros E, Aranki SF, Bayer LR, et al: Reduction in incidence of deep sternal wound infections: Random or real? J Thorac Cardiovasc Surg 139:680, 2010.

142. Elenbaas TW, Soliman Hamad MA, Schönberger JP, et al: Preoperative atrial fibrillation and elevated C-reactive protein levels as predictors of mediastinitis after coronary artery bypass grafting. Ann Thorac Surg 89:704, 2010.

143. Doyle AJ, Large SR, Murphy F: Sternal wound dehiscence after internal mammary artery harvesting. Logical management. Part 2. Interact Cardiovasc Thorac Surg 4:511, 2005.

144. De Paulis R, de Notaris S, Scaffa R, et al: The effect of bilateral internal thoracic artery harvesting on superficial and deep sternal infection: The role of skeletonization. J Thorac Cardiovasc Surg 129:536, 2005.

145. Parwis B, Rahmanian DH, Adams JG, et al: Tracheostomy is not a risk factor for deep sternal wound infection after cardiac surgery. Ann Thorac Surg 84:1984, 2007.

146. Khalafi RS, Bradford DW, Wilson MG: Topical application of autologous blood products during surgical closure following a coronary artery bypass graft. Eur J Cardiothorac Surg 34:360, 2008.

147. Kuan P, Messenger JC, Ellestad MH: Transient central diabetes insipidus after aortocoronary bypass operations. Am J Cardiol 52:1181, 1983.

CHAPTER **85** # Anesthesia and Noncardiac Surgery in Patients with Heart Disease

Lee A. Fleisher and Joshua Beckman

Cardiovascular morbidity and mortality represent a special concern in the patient with known (or risk factors for) cardiovascular disease who undergoes noncardiac surgery. The costs of perioperative myocardial injury add substantially to total health care expenditures, with an average increased length of stay of 6.8 days for patients with perioperative myocardial ischemic injury. Perioperative cardiovascular complications not only affect the immediate period, but also may influence outcome over subsequent years. The evidence base for managing patients with cardiovascular disease peri–noncardiac surgery has grown in recent decades, beginning with identification of those at greatest risk and progressing to recent randomized trials to identify strategies to reduce perioperative cardiovascular complications. Guidelines provide information for the management of high-risk patients and disseminate best practices. This chapter attempts to distill this information, incorporating the available guidelines from the American College of Cardiology (ACC)/American Heart Association (AHA) and from the European Society of Cardiology (ESC) while acknowledging that these guidelines undergo constant evolution.[1,2]

Assessment of Risk

The identification of perioperative cardiac risk has been studied for three decades, and much of the work has focused on the development of clinical risk indices. The most recent index was developed in a study of 4315 patients 50 years of age or older undergoing elective major noncardiac procedures in a tertiary-care teaching hospital. Six independent predictors of complications were identified and included in a revised cardiac risk index (RCRI): high-risk type of surgery, history of ischemic heart disease, history of congestive heart failure, history of cerebrovascular disease, preoperative treatment with insulin, and preoperative serum creatinine higher than 2 mg/dL, with increasing cardiac complication rates noted with an increasing number of risk factors. Patients can be stratified into low, intermediate, and high cardiovascular risk on the basis of having zero, one or two, or three or more RCRI risk factors, respectively. The RCRI has become the standard tool for assessing the probability of perioperative cardiac risk in a given individual, and directs the decision to perform cardiovascular testing and implement perioperative management protocols. The RCRI has been validated in vascular surgery populations and predicts long-term outcome and quality of life, although one group has advocated inclusion of age as a risk factor. The RCRI is discussed throughout the rest of this chapter.

Ischemic Heart Disease

A patient may be evaluated by those in a number of health care systems before undergoing noncardiac surgery; he or she may be seen by a primary caregiver or a cardiologist. However, many patients are only evaluated immediately before surgery by the surgeon or anesthesiologist. The stress of noncardiac surgery may raise heart rate (HR) preoperatively, which associates with a high incidence of symptomatic and asymptomatic myocardial ischemia. Therefore, the preoperative clinical evaluation of the patient may identify stable or unstable coronary artery disease (CAD). Patients with acute coronary syndromes, such as unstable angina or decompensated heart failure of ischemic origin, have a high risk of developing further decompensation or myocardial necrosis and of death during the perioperative period. Such patients clearly warrant further evaluation and medical stabilization. If the noncardiac surgery is truly emergent, there are several older case series using intra-aortic balloon bump counterpulsation to provide short-term myocardial protection beyond maximal medical therapy, although this measure is rarely used today.

If the patient does not have unstable symptoms, the identification of known or symptomatic stable CAD or risk factors for CAD can guide further diagnostic evaluation or changes in perioperative management. In determining the extent of the preoperative evaluation, it is important not to perform testing unless the results will affect perioperative management. These management changes include cancellation of surgery for prohibitive risk compared with benefit, delay of surgery for further medical management, coronary interventions before surgery, use of an intensive care unit, and changes in monitoring. As discussed later, the potential benefit of preoperative coronary revascularization has been questioned, often limiting the need for extensive testing.

The patient with stable angina represents a continuum from mild angina with extreme exertion to dyspnea with angina after walking up a few stairs. The patient who only manifests angina after strenuous exercise often does not demonstrate signs of left ventricular dysfunction and generally can be stabilized with adequate medical therapy, particularly treatment with aspirin, beta-adrenergic blocking agents (beta blockers), and statins (see Chaps. 49 and 57). In contrast, a patient with dyspnea on mild exertion would be at high risk for developing perioperative ventricular dysfunction, myocardial ischemia, and possible myocardial infarction (MI). Such patients have a high probability of having extensive CAD, and additional monitoring or cardiovascular testing should be considered (see Chap. 17), depending on the surgical procedure, institutional factors, and prior evaluation.

Traditionally, coronary risk assessment for noncardiac surgery in patients with a prior MI was based on the time interval between the MI and surgery. Multiple studies have demonstrated an increased incidence of reinfarction after noncardiac surgery if the prior MI was within 6 months of the operation. Improvements in perioperative care have shortened this time interval, but its relative importance is less relevant in the current era of thrombolytics, angioplasty, and routine coronary risk stratification after an acute MI. Although some patients with a recent MI may continue to have myocardium at risk for subsequent ischemia and infarction, most patients in the United States will have had their critical coronary stenosis evaluated and revascularized or will be on maximal medical therapy. The AHA/ACC Task Force on Perioperative Evaluation of the Cardiac Patient Undergoing Noncardiac Surgery has suggested that the highest risk cohort is made up of patients within 30 days of MI, during which plaque and myocardial healing occur. After that period, risk stratification is based on the presentation of disease (i.e., those with active ischemia are at highest risk).

Hypertension

In the 1970s, a series of case studies changed the prevailing concept that antihypertensive agents should be discontinued before surgery. The reports suggested that poorly controlled hypertension was associated with untoward hemodynamic responses, and that antihypertensive agents should be continued perioperatively. However, several large prospective studies did not establish mild to moderate hypertension as an independent predictor of postoperative cardiac complications such as cardiac death, postoperative MI, heart failure, or arrhythmias. The approach to the patient with hypertension therefore mostly relies on management strategies from the nonsurgical literature.

A hypertensive crisis in the postoperative period, defined as a diastolic blood pressure (BP) higher than 120 mm Hg and clinical evidence of impending or actual end organ damage, poses a definite risk of MI and cerebrovascular accident (see Chap. 45). Diagnostic criteria include papilledema or other evidence of increased intracranial pressure, myocardial ischemia, or acute renal failure. Several precipitants of hypertensive crises have been identified, including preeclampsia or eclampsia, pheochromocytomas, abrupt clonidine withdrawal before surgery, use of chronic monoamine oxidase inhibitors with or without sympathomimetic drugs in combination, and inadvertent discontinuation of antihypertensive therapy.

Chronic hypertension may predispose patients to perioperative myocardial ischemia because CAD is more prevalent in these patients. Recent clinical trials have yielded mixed conclusions regarding the relevance of hypertension to perioperative outcomes. A retrospective evaluation of 2462 patients undergoing vascular surgery has shown that adding hypertension to a risk prediction model improved its prognostic ability.[3] In contrast, in the Perioperative Ischemic Evaluation (POISE) trial of beta-adrenergic blockade, chronic hypertension was present in 62% of the 8351 subjects, yet was not a predictor of postoperative stroke or death.[4] Thus, hypertensive patients with known peripheral and coronary vascular disease should have preoperative BP levels monitored and controlled.

Whether patients with mild to moderate hypertension should be considered at greater risk for perioperative myocardial ischemia remains uncertain. Surgery generally need not be postponed or canceled in the otherwise uncomplicated patient with mild to moderate hypertension. Antihypertensive medications should be continued perioperatively, and BP should be maintained near preoperative levels to reduce the risk of myocardial ischemia. In patients with more severe hypertension, such as diastolic BP higher than 110 mm Hg, the potential benefits of delaying surgery to optimize antihypertensive medications should be weighed against the risk of delaying the surgical procedure. With rapid-acting intravenous agents, BP can usually be controlled within several hours. Weksler and colleagues studied 989

chronically treated hypertensive patients who presented for noncardiac surgery with diastolic BP between 110 and 130 mm Hg and with no previous MI, unstable or severe angina pectoris, renal failure, pregnancy-induced hypertension, left ventricular hypertrophy, previous coronary revascularization, aortic stenosis, preoperative dysrhythmias, conduction defects, or stroke. The control group had their surgery postponed and remained in the hospital for BP control, and the study patients received 10 mg of nifedipine, delivered intranasally.[1] No statistically significant differences in postoperative complications were observed, suggesting that this subset of patients without significant cardiovascular comorbidities can proceed with surgery despite elevated BP on the day of surgery.

Heart Failure

Heart failure associates with perioperative cardiac morbidity after noncardiac surgery in almost all studies. Goldman and colleagues have identified a third heart sound or signs of heart failure as portending the highest perioperative risks. For patients who present for noncardiac surgery with signs or symptoms of heart failure, its underpinnings require characterization.[1] The preoperative evaluation should aim to identify the underlying coronary, myocardial, and/or valvular heart disease and assess the severity of systolic and diastolic dysfunction. Hammill and associates[5] have evaluated short-term outcomes in patients with heart failure, CAD, or neither who underwent major noncardiac surgery, using Medicare Claims data. Older patients with heart failure who undergo major surgical procedures have substantially higher risks of operative mortality and hospital readmission than other patients, including those with coronary disease, admitted for the same procedures. Treatment of decompensated hypertrophic cardiomyopathy is different than treatment for dilated cardiomyopathy (see Chap. 69), and thus the preoperative evaluation can influence perioperative management; in particular, this assessment may influence perioperative fluid and vasopressor management. Ischemic cardiomyopathy is of greatest concern because the patient has a substantial risk for developing further ischemia, leading to myocardial necrosis and potentially a downward spiral. A pulmonary artery catheter or transesophageal echocardiography may be helpful for such patients.

Obstructed hypertrophic cardiomyopathy was formerly regarded as a high-risk condition associated with high perioperative morbidity. A retrospective review of perioperative care in 35 patients, however, has suggested that the risk of general anesthesia and major noncardiac surgery is low in such patients. This study did suggest relative contraindication of spinal anesthesia in view of the sensitivity of cardiac output to preload in this condition. Haering and coworkers have studied 77 patients with asymmetrical septal hypertrophy who were retrospectively identified from a large database.[1] Of these patients, 40% had one or more adverse perioperative cardiac events, including one patient who had an MI and ventricular tachycardia that required emergent cardioversion. Most of the events were perioperative congestive heart failure, and no perioperative deaths occurred. Unlike in the original cohort of patients, the type of anesthesia was not an independent risk factor. Important independent risk factors for adverse outcomes (as seen generally) included major surgery and increasing duration of surgery.

Valvular Heart Disease

Aortic stenosis places a patient at increased risk, with those with critical stenosis associated with the highest risk of cardiac decompensation in patients undergoing elective noncardiac surgery (see Chap. 66). Kertai has reported a substantially higher rate of perioperative complications in patients with severe aortic stenosis, compared with patients with moderate aortic stenosis—31% (5/16) versus 11% (10/92).[1,6] The presence of any of the classic triad of angina, syncope, and heart failure in a patient with aortic stenosis should prompt further evaluation and potential interventions, usually valve replacement. Many patients with severe or critical aortic stenosis are asymptomatic.

Preoperative patients with aortic systolic murmurs warrant a careful history and physical examination, and often further evaluation. Several recent case series of patients with critical aortic stenosis have demonstrated that when necessary, noncardiac surgery can be performed with acceptable risk. For the most part, these series have included patients with few or no symptoms but a valve area smaller than $0.5 \, cm^2$. Aortic valvuloplasty is an alternative option for some patients. Although the long-term outcome of patients who undergo aortic balloon valvuloplasty is generally poor, primarily because of restenosis, this procedure can provide temporary benefit surrounding noncardiac surgery in patients who cannot undergo valve replacement in the short term. The considerable procedure-related morbidity and mortality risk must be carefully considered before recommending this strategy to lower the risk of noncardiac surgery.

Mitral valve disease tends to cause less risk of perioperative complications than aortic stenosis, although occult mitral stenosis from rheumatic heart disease is still encountered on occasion and can lead to severe left heart failure in the presence of tachycardia (e.g., uncontrolled atrial fibrillation) and/or volume loading. In contrast to aortic valvuloplasty, mitral valve balloon valvuloplasty often yields short-term and long-term benefit, especially in younger patients with predominant mitral stenosis but without severe mitral valve leaflet thickening or significant subvalvular fibrosis and calcification.

In the perioperative patient with a functioning prosthetic heart valve, antibiotic prophylaxis and anticoagulation are major issues. All patients with prosthetic valves who undergo procedures that can cause transient bacteremia should receive prophylaxis (see Chap. 67). In patients with prosthetic valves, the risk of increased bleeding during a procedure while receiving antithrombotic therapy must be weighed against the increased risk of a thromboembolism caused by stopping the therapy. The common practice for patients undergoing noncardiac surgery with a mechanical prosthetic valve in place is cessation of oral anticoagulants 3 days before surgery (see Chap. 66). This allows the international normalized ratio (INR) to fall to less than 1.5 times normal; oral anticoagulants can then be resumed on postoperative day 1. An alternative approach in patients at high risk for thromboembolism is conversion to heparin during the perioperative period, which can then be discontinued 4 to 6 hours before surgery and resumed shortly thereafter. The use of low-molecular-weight heparins (LMWHs) in preoperative warfarin anticoagulation bridging was investigated in a multicenter, single-arm cohort study[7] of 224 high-risk patients (prosthetic valves, atrial fibrillation, and a major risk factor). Warfarin was held for 5 days; LMWHs were given 3 days preoperatively and at least 4 days postoperatively. The overall rate of thromboembolism was 3.6%, and the overall rate of cardioembolism was 0.9%. Major bleeding was seen in 6.7% of subjects, although only 8 of 15 episodes occurred during LMWH administration. LMWHs are cost-effective because of reduction in hospital admission duration, but two studies have shown a residual anticoagulation effect in as many as two thirds of patients.[8,9]

Many current prosthetic valves have a lower risk of valve thrombosis than the older ball-in-cage valves, so the risk of heparin may outweigh the benefit in the perioperative setting. According to the AHA/ACC guidelines, heparin can usually be reserved for high-risk patients. High risk is defined by the presence of a mechanical mitral or tricuspid valve or mechanical aortic valve and of risk factors (e.g., atrial fibrillation, previous thromboembolism, hypercoagulable condition, older generation mechanical valves, ejection fraction less than 30%, or more than one mechanical valve).[10] Subcutaneous LMWHs or unfractionated heparin offers an alternative outpatient approach but receives a tentative recommendation. Discussion between the surgeon and cardiologist regarding the optimal perioperative management is critical.

Congenital Heart Disease in Adults

Congenital heart disease afflicts 500,000 to 1 million U.S. adults (see Chap. 65). The nature of the underlying anatomy and any anatomic correction affect the perioperative plan and incidence of complications, which include infection, bleeding, hypoxemia, hypotension, and paradoxical embolization. A major concern in the patient with congenital heart disease is the presence of pulmonary hypertension and Eisenmenger syndrome. Regional anesthesia traditionally has been avoided in these patients because of the potential for sympathetic blockade and worsening of the right to left shunt. However, a review of the published literature incorporating 103 cases has found that overall perioperative mortality is 14%; patients receiving regional anesthesia had a mortality of 5%, whereas those receiving general anesthesia had a mortality of 18%.[6] The authors concluded that most deaths probably occurred as a result of the surgical procedure and disease, and not from anesthesia. Although perioperative and peripartum mortalities were high, many anesthetic agents and techniques had been used with success. Patients with congenital heart disease are at risk for infective endocarditis and should receive antibiotic prophylaxis. This recent review discusses the anesthetic management of these patients in detail.

Arrhythmias

Cardiac arrhythmias are common in the perioperative period, particularly in older patients or in patients undergoing thoracic surgery (see Chaps. 36 to 41). Predisposing factors include prior arrhythmias, underlying heart disease, hypertension, perioperative pain (e.g., hip fracture), severe anxiety, and other situations that heighten adrenergic tone. A prospective study of 4181 patients aged 50 years or older found supraventricular arrhythmia in 2% of patients during surgery and in 6.1% of patients after surgery. Perioperative atrial fibrillation raises several concerns, including an incidence of stroke (see Chap. 40). Winkel and colleagues[11] evaluated 317 patients undergoing major vascular surgery without atrial fibrillation to determine the incidence of new-onset atrial fibrillation and its association with adverse cardiovascular outcomes. They reported an incidence of 4.7% and a more than sixfold increase in cardiovascular death, MI, unstable angina, and stroke in the first 30 days, and a fourfold increase over the next 12 months. Early treatment to restore sinus rhythm or to control the ventricular response and initiate anticoagulation is therefore indicated. Prophylactic intravenous diltiazem in randomized, placebo-controlled trials in high-risk thoracic surgery has reduced the incidence of clinically significant atrial arrhythmias.[1] Balser and associates have studied 64 cases of postoperative supraventricular tachyarrhythmia. After adenosine administration, patients who remained in supraventricular tachyarrhythmia were prospectively randomized to receive intravenous diltiazem or intravenous esmolol for ventricular rate control; it was reported that intravenous esmolol produces a more rapid (2-hour) conversion to sinus rhythm than does intravenous diltiazem.[1] **Figure 85-1** presents an algorithm for atrial fibrillation management.

Although ventricular arrhythmias were originally identified as a risk factor for perioperative morbidity, recent studies have not confirmed this finding. O'Kelly studied a consecutive sample of 230 male patients with known CAD or at high risk of CAD who were undergoing major noncardiac surgical procedures.[1] Preoperative arrhythmias associated with intraoperative and postoperative arrhythmias, but nonfatal MI and cardiac death were not substantially more frequent in those with prior perioperative arrhythmias. Amar and coworkers[12] studied 412 patients undergoing major thoracic surgery and determined that the incidence of nonsustained ventricular tachycardia is 15% but is not associated with poor outcome. Despite this finding, the presence of an arrhythmia in the preoperative setting should provoke a search for underlying cardiopulmonary disease, ongoing myocardial ischemia or infarction, drug toxicity, or metabolic derangements.

Conduction abnormalities can increase perioperative risk and may require the placement of a temporary or permanent pacemaker. On the other hand, patients with intraventricular conduction delays, even in the presence of a left or right bundle branch block, and with no history of advanced heart block or symptoms, rarely progress to complete heart block perioperatively. The availability of transthoracic pacing units has decreased the need for temporary transvenous pacemakers.

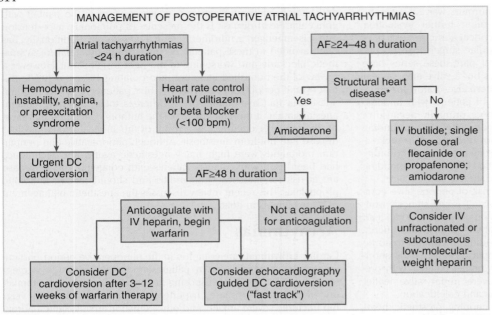

FIGURE 85-1 Proposed algorithm for the treatment of postoperative atrial tachyarrhythmias. AF = atrial fibrillation or flutter; bpm = beats/min; DC = direct current. *Structural heart disease is defined as the presence of one of the following: left ventricular hypertrophy with wall thickness > 1.4 cm, mitral valve disease, coronary artery disease, or heart failure. *(From Amar D: Perioperative atrial tachyarrhythmias. Anesthesiology 97:1618, 2002.)*

Diagnostic and Nondiagnostic Testing

Decision to Undergo Diagnostic Testing

The ACC/AHA[1] and ESC[2] guidelines have both proposed algorithms based on the available evidence and incorporating class of recommendations and level of evidence in each step (**Fig. 85-2**). The current algorithms use a stepwise bayesian strategy that relies on assessment of clinical markers, prior coronary evaluation and treatment, functional capacity, and surgery-specific risk (see later). Successful use of the algorithms requires an appreciation for different levels of risk attributable to certain clinical circumstances, levels of functional capacity, and types of surgery, and for how the information from any diagnostic testing will influence perioperative management.

A number of studies have attempted to identify clinical risk markers for perioperative cardiovascular morbidity and mortality. As noted, patients with unstable coronary syndromes and severe valvular disease have active cardiac conditions. Patients with known stable CAD have intermediate risk. Other clinical risk factors in the RCRI make up the remainder of the intermediate risk predictors (e.g., history of congestive heart failure, history of cerebrovascular disease, preoperative treatment with insulin, preoperative serum creatinine level > 2 mg/dL). Cardiovascular disease has clinical risk markers, each associated with variable levels of perioperative risk, which have been classified as low-risk factors. The classification of perioperative clinical risk markers for assessing the need for further testing is shown in **Table 85-1**.

As described with regard to anginal pattern, exercise tolerance is one of the strongest determinants of perioperative risk and the need for invasive monitoring (see Chap. 14). In one study of outpatients referred for evaluation before major noncardiac procedures,[1] patients were asked to estimate the number of blocks they could walk and how many flights of stairs they could climb without experiencing cardiac symptoms (**Table 85-2**). Patients who could not walk four blocks and could not climb two flights of stairs were considered to have poor exercise tolerance, and had twice as many perioperative cardiovascular complications as those with better functional status. The likelihood of a serious complication occurring was inversely related to the number of blocks that could be walked or flights of stairs that could be climbed. Several scales based on activities of daily living have been proposed to assess exercise tolerance. Current guidelines advocate one such scale (the Duke Activity Scale Index; see Chaps. 50 and 83).

The type of surgical procedure itself has a significant impact on perioperative risks and the amount of preparation required to perform anesthesia safely. For surgical procedures not associated with significant stress or a high incidence of perioperative myocardial ischemia or morbidity, the costs of the evaluation often exceed any benefits from the information gained by preoperative assessment. For example, outpatient procedures cause little morbidity and mortality; in such patients, perioperative management is rarely changed by cardiovascular status unless the patient demonstrates unstable angina or overt congestive heart failure. In fact, 30-day mortality after outpatient surgery may actually be lower than expected if the patients did not have surgery. In contrast, open surgery for vascular disease entails a high risk of morbidity and ischemic potential (see Chap. 61). Intra-abdominal, thoracic, and orthopedic procedures entail intermediate risk (**Table 85-3**). Endovascular procedures fall into this intermediate-risk category on the basis of their perioperative morbidity and mortality, although long-term survival appears similar to that in patients who undergo open procedures.

In addition to the risk of the surgical procedure itself, risk also correlates with the surgical volume in a given center. Several studies have demonstrated differential mortality rates in cancer and vascular surgeries, with higher mortality seen in low-volume centers, although recent studies have demonstrated that low-volume centers may also have low mortality rates if proper care systems are in place. Therefore, surgical mortality rates may be institution specific, which may influence the decision to perform further perioperative evaluations and interventions.

The AHA/ACC guidelines[1] presented their recommendations in algorithmic form as a framework for determining which patients are candidates for cardiac testing (see Fig. 85-2). Given the availability of the evidence, the Writing Committee chose to include the level of the recommendations and strength of evidence for each of the pathways:

- Step 1: The consultant should determine the urgency of noncardiac surgery. In many cases, patient-specific or surgery-specific factors dictate an obvious strategy (e.g., emergent surgery) that may not allow for further cardiac assessment or treatment.
- Step 2: Does the patient have an active cardiac condition? In patients being considered for elective noncardiac surgery, the presence of unstable coronary disease, decompensated heart failure, or severe arrhythmia or valvular heart disease usually leads to cancellation or delay of surgery until the cardiac problem has been clarified and treated appropriately. Examples of unstable coronary syndromes include previous MI with evidence of important ischemic risk by clinical symptoms or noninvasive study, unstable or severe angina, and new or poorly controlled ischemia-mediated heart failure. Depending on the results of tests or interventions and the risk of delaying surgery, it may be appropriate to proceed to the planned surgery with maximal medical therapy.
- Step 3: Is the patient undergoing low-risk surgery? Interventions based on cardiovascular testing in stable patients would rarely result in a change in management, and it would be appropriate to proceed with the planned surgical procedure.

■ Step 4: Does the patient have moderate functional capacity without symptoms? In highly functional asymptomatic patients, management will rarely change on the basis of results of any further cardiovascular testing, and it is therefore appropriate to proceed with the planned surgery. If the patient has poor functional capacity, is symptomatic, or has unknown functional capacity, the presence of clinical risk factors will determine the need for further evaluation. If the patient has no clinical risk factors, it is appropriate to proceed with the planned surgery, and no further change in management is indicated.

If the patient has one or two clinical risk factors, it is reasonable to proceed with the planned surgery (with heart rate control) or to consider testing if it will change management. In patients with three or more clinical risk factors, if the patient is undergoing vascular surgery, it has been suggested that testing should only be considered if it will change management. In nonvascular surgery in which the perioperative morbidity related to the procedure ranges from 1% to 5% (intermediate-risk surgery), there are insufficient data to determine the best strategy—proceeding with the planned surgery with tight heart rate control with beta blockade, or further cardiovascular testing if it will change management.

Falcone and coworkers performed a small randomized trial of 99 patients undergoing elective vascular surgery.[1] Patients at low or intermediate clinical risk were randomized to testing or no testing, with no difference in perioperative or long-term outcome. The vast majority of these patients were highly functional and placed on perioperative beta blocker therapy, suggesting that exercise capacity can help determine the need for further diagnostic testing preoperatively.

Poldermans and colleagues[13] randomized 770 intermediate-risk patients to cardiac stress testing ($N = 386$) or no testing. Those with extensive stress-induced ischemia were considered for revascularization, with the choice of procedure at the discretion of the primary physician. HR was tightly controlled with beta blockers in all patients. Patients assigned to no testing had similar incidences of cardiac death or MI at 30 days after surgery, as did those assigned to testing (1.8% versus 2.3%; odds ratio [OR], 0.78; 95% confidence interval [CI], 0.28 to 2.1; $P = 0.62$). Regardless of allocated strategy, patients with a HR less than 65 beats/min had lower risk than the remaining patients (1.3% versus 5.2%; OR, 0.24; 95% CI, 0.09 to 0.66; $P < 0.003$). The authors suggested that testing is not required in patients at intermediate risk if HR is controlled; however, we believe that testing may still be indicated if the results will change management.

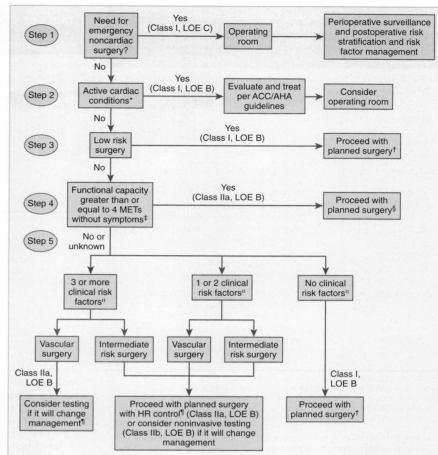

FIGURE 85-2 American College of Cardiology/American Heart Association (ACC/AHA) Task Force on Perioperative Evaluation of Cardiac Patients Undergoing Noncardiac Surgery proposed algorithm for decisions regarding the need for further evaluation. This represents one of a number of such algorithms in the literature. This incorporates the class of recommendation for each step and level of evidence (LOE). *See Table 85-1 for active cardiac conditions. †See Class III recommendations in Section 5.2.3. Noninvasive Stress Testing in the guidelines. ‡See Table 85-2 for estimated MET level equivalent. §Noninvasive testing may be considered before surgery in specific patients with risk factors if it will change management. ‖Clinical risk factors include ischemic heart disease, compensated or prior heart failure, diabetes mellitus, renal insufficiency, and cerebrovascular disease. ¶Consider perioperative beta blockade (see Table 11 in the source article listed below for populations in which this has been shown to reduce cardiac morbidity/mortality. MET = metabolic equivalent. *(From Fleisher LA, Beckman JA, Brown KA, et al: 2009 ACCF/AHA focused update on perioperative beta blockade incorporated into the ACC/AHA 2007 guidelines on perioperative cardiovascular evaluation and care for noncardiac surgery: A report of the American College of Cardiology Foundation/American Heart Association Task Force on Practice Guidelines. Circulation 120:e169, 2009.)*

Tests to Improve Identification and Definition of Cardiovascular Disease

Several noninvasive diagnostic methods can evaluate the extent of CAD before noncardiac surgery. The exercise electrocardiogram has traditionally evaluated individuals for the presence of CAD, but as noted, patients with excellent exercise tolerance in daily life will rarely benefit from further testing. Patients with poor exercise capacity, in contrast, may not achieve adequate HR and BP for diagnostic purposes on electrocardiographic stress tests. Such patients often require concomitant imaging.

A substantial number of high-risk patients either cannot exercise or have contraindications to exercise (e.g., patients with claudication or an abdominal aortic aneurysm undergoing vascular surgery, both of which have a high rate of perioperative cardiac morbidity). Pharmacologic stress testing therefore has become popular, particularly as a preoperative test in vascular surgery patients. Several studies have shown that the presence of a redistribution defect on dipyridamole or adenosine thallium or sestamibi imaging in patients undergoing peripheral vascular surgery predicts postoperative cardiac events (see Chap. 17). Pharmacologic stress imaging is best used in patients at moderate clinical risk. Several strategies may increase the predictive value of such tests. The redistribution defect can be quantitated, with larger areas of defect associating with increased risk. Additionally, both increased lung uptake and left ventricular cavity dilation indicate ventricular dysfunction with ischemia. It has been shown that the delineation of low-risk and high-risk thallium scans (larger area of defect, increased lung uptake, and left ventricular cavity dilation) markedly improve the test's predictive value; patients with high-risk thallium scans have particularly increased risk for perioperative morbidity and long-term mortality.

TABLE 85-1	Active Cardiac Conditions Requiring Evaluation and Treatment Before Noncardiac Surgery (Class I, level of evidence: B)
CONDITION	**EXAMPLES**
Unstable coronary syndromes	Unstable or severe angina* (CCS class III or IV)† Recent MI‡
Decompensated HF (NYHA functional class IV; worsening or new-onset HF)	
Significant arrhythmias	High-grade atrioventricular block Mobitz II atrioventricular block Third-degree atrioventricular heart block Symptomatic ventricular arrhythmias Supraventricular arrhythmias (including atrial fibrillation) with uncontrolled ventricular rate (HR higher than 100 beats per minute at rest) Symptomatic bradycardia Newly recognized ventricular tachycardia
Severe valvular disease	Severe aortic stenosis (mean pressure gradient higher than 40 mm Hg, aortic valve area less than 1 cm², or symptomatic) Symptomatic mitral stenosis (progressive dyspnea on exertion, exertional presyncope, or HF)

*According to Campeau L: Letter: grading of angina pectoris. Circulation 54:522, 1976.
†May include "stable" angina in patients who are unusually sedentary.
‡The American College of Cardiology National Cardiovascular Data Registry defines recent MI as >7 days but ≤1 month (within 30 days).
CCS = Canadian Cardiovascular Society; HF = heart failure; NYHA = New York Heart Association.
From Fleisher LA, Beckman JA, Brown KA, et al: 2009 ACCF/AHA focused update on perioperative beta blockade incorporated into the ACC/AHA 2007 guidelines on perioperative cardiovascular evaluation and care for noncardiac surgery: A report of the American College of Cardiology Foundation/American Heart Association Task Force on Practice Guidelines. Circulation 120:e169, 2009.

TABLE 85-2	Estimated Energy Requirements for Various Activities
NO. OF METS	**QUESTION: CAN YOU ...**
1	Take care of yourself? Eat, dress, or use the toilet? Walk indoors around the house? Walk a block or two on level ground at 2 to 3 mph (3.2-4.8 kph)?
4	Do light work around the house like dusting or washing dishes? Climb a flight of stairs or walk up a hill? Walk on level ground at 4 mph (6.4 kph)? Run a short distance? Do heavy work around the house, like scrubbing floors or lifting or moving heavy furniture? Participate in moderate recreational activities like golf, bowling, dancing, doubles tennis, or throwing a baseball or football?
>10	Participate in strenuous sports like swimming, singles tennis, football, basketball, or skiing?

kph = km/hr; MET = metabolic equivalent; mph = miles/hr.
Modified from Fleisher LA, Beckman JA, Brown KA, et al: 2009 ACCF/AHA focused update on perioperative beta blockade incorporated into the ACC/AHA 2007 guidelines on perioperative cardiovascular evaluation and care for noncardiac surgery: A report of the American College of Cardiology Foundation/American Heart Association Task Force on Practice Guidelines. Circulation 120:e169, 2009.

TABLE 85-3	Cardiac Risk Stratification for Noncardiac Surgical Procedures*
RISK STRATIFICATION	**EXAMPLES OF PROCEDURES**
Vascular (reported cardiac risk often >5%)	Aortic and other major vascular surgery Peripheral vascular surgery
Intermediate (reported cardiac risk generally = 1%-5%)	Intraperitoneal and intrathoracic surgery Carotid endarterectomy Head and neck surgery Orthopedic surgery Prostate surgery
Low (reported cardiac risk generally <1%)†	Endoscopic procedures Superficial procedure Cataract surgery Breast surgery Ambulatory surgery

*Combined incidence of cardiac death and nonfatal MI.
†These procedures generally do not require further preoperative cardiac testing.
From Fleisher LA, Beckman JA, Brown KA, et al: 2009 ACCF/AHA focused update on perioperative beta blockade incorporated into the ACC/AHA 2007 guidelines on perioperative cardiovascular evaluation and care for noncardiac surgery: A report of the American College of Cardiology Foundation/American Heart Association Task Force on Practice Guidelines. Circulation 120:e169, 2009.

Stress echocardiography has also been widely used as a preoperative test (see Chap. 15). One advantage of this test is that it assesses myocardial ischemia dynamically in response to increased inotropy and HR, such as may occur during the perioperative period. The presence of new wall motion abnormalities that occur at low HR is the best predictor of increased perioperative risk, with large areas of defect being of secondary importance. Boersma and colleagues have assessed the value of dobutamine stress echocardiography with respect to the extent of wall motion abnormalities and the ability of preoperative beta blocker treatment to attenuate risk in patients undergoing major aortic surgery.[1] They assigned one point for each of the following characteristics: age older than 70 years, current angina, MI, congestive heart failure, prior cerebrovascular disease, diabetes mellitus, and renal failure. As the total number of clinical risk factors increases, perioperative cardiac event rates also increase.

So, which diagnostic test should be used for preoperative risk assessment? Several groups have published meta-analyses examining the various preoperative diagnostic tests. Good predictive values for ambulatory electrocardiogram monitoring, radionuclide angiography, dipyridamole thallium imaging, and dobutamine stress echocardiography have been demonstrated. Shaw and associates have also demonstrated excellent predictive values for dipyridamole thallium imaging and dobutamine stress echocardiography.[1] Beattie and coworkers have performed a meta-analysis of 25 stress echocardiography studies and 50 thallium imaging studies.[1] The likelihood ratio for stress echocardiography was more indicative of a postoperative cardiac event than that for thallium imaging (likelihood ratio, 4.09; 95% CI, 3.21 to 6.56, versus likelihood ratio, 1.83; 95% CI, 1.59 to 2.10; $P < 0.001$). The difference was attributable to fewer false-negative stress echocardiograms. A moderate to large perfusion defect by either test predicted postoperative MI and death. An important determinant with respect to the choice of preoperative testing is the expertise at the local institution. Another factor is whether assessment of valve function or myocardial thickness is of interest, where echocardiography may be preferred. Stress nuclear imaging may have slightly higher sensitivity, but stress echocardiography may be less likely to yield false–positive results. The role in preoperative risk assessment of newer imaging modalities for preoperative assessment using magnetic resonance imaging, multislice computed tomography, coronary calcium scores, and positron emission tomography is rapidly evolving.

Anesthesia Used in Cardiac Patients Undergoing Noncardiac Surgery

There are three classes of anesthetics: general, regional, and monitored anesthesia care (MAC). General anesthesia can best be defined as a state including unconsciousness, amnesia, analgesia, immobility, and attenuation of autonomic responses to noxious stimulation. General anesthesia can be achieved with inhalational agents, intravenous agents, or a combination (frequently known as a balanced technique). Additionally, general anesthesia can be achieved with or without an endotracheal tube. Laryngoscopy and intubation were traditionally thought to be the greatest stress and risk for myocardial ischemia, but extubation may involve greater risk. Alternative methods for delivering general anesthesia are via a mask or a laryngeal mask airway, a device that fits above the epiglottis and does not require laryngoscopy or intubation.

Five inhalational anesthetic agents (in addition to nitrous oxide) are currently approved in the United States, although enflurane and halothane are rarely used today. All inhalational agents have reversible myocardial depressant effects and lead to decreases in myocardial oxygen demand. The degree to which they depress cardiac output depends on their concentration, effects on systemic vascular resistance, and effects on baroreceptor responsiveness; agents therefore differ in their specific effects on HR and BP. Isoflurane causes negative inotropic effects and potent vascular smooth muscle relaxation, and has minimal effects on baroreceptor function. Desflurane has the fastest onset and is commonly used in the outpatient setting. Sevoflurane's onset and offset of action is intermediate to that of isoflurane and desflurane. Its major advantage is its extremely pleasant smell, making it the agent of choice for children.

Issues have been raised regarding the safety of inhalational agents in patients with CAD. Several large-scale randomized and nonrandomized studies of inhalational agents in patients undergoing coronary artery bypass grafting (CABG) have not demonstrated any increased incidence of myocardial ischemia or infarction in patients receiving inhalation agents versus narcotic-based techniques.

The safety of desflurane has also raised some concerns. Desflurane can cause airway irritability and has led to tachycardia in volunteer studies. In a large-scale study comparing a narcotic-based anesthetic to a desflurane-based anesthetic, the desflurane group had a significantly higher incidence of myocardial ischemia, although there was no difference in the incidence of MI.[1] Including a narcotic with desflurane can avoid this tachycardia. Sevoflurane has been studied in one randomized trial compared with isoflurane in patients at high risk for cardiovascular disease.[1] No differences in the incidence of myocardial ischemia were observed, but the study was underpowered to detect any difference in the incidence of MI. Overall, at this time, there appears to be no one best inhalation anesthetic for the patient with CAD.

The use of inhalational anesthetics in patients with CAD has theoretical advantages. Several investigative groups have demonstrated in vitro and in animals that these agents have protective effects on the myocardium similar to those of ischemic preconditioning.[1] This favorable effect on myocardial oxygen demand would serve to offset the theoretical effects of coronary steal in patients with chronic coronary occlusion.

High-dose narcotic techniques offer far advantages of hemodynamic stability and lack of myocardial depression. Narcotic-based anesthetics were frequently considered for cardiac anesthesia and were advocated for use in all high-risk patients, including those undergoing noncardiac surgery. The disadvantage of these traditional high-dose narcotic techniques is the requirement for postoperative ventilation. An ultrashort-acting narcotic (remifentanil) was introduced into clinical practice, obviating the need for prolonged ventilation. This agent can assist early extubation in patients undergoing cardiac surgery, and may aid in the management of short periods of intense intraoperative stress in high-risk patients.

Despite the theoretical advantages of a high-dose narcotic technique, several large-scale trials in patients undergoing CABG have shown no difference in survival or major morbidity compared with the inhalation-based technique.[1] This observation has in part led to the abandonment of high-dose narcotics in much of cardiac surgery and to an emphasis on early extubation. Most anesthesiologists use a balanced technique involving the administration of lower doses of narcotics with an inhalational agent. This approach allows the anesthesiologist to derive the benefits of each of these agents while minimizing the side effects.

An alternative mode of delivering general anesthesia is with the intravenous agent propofol. Propofol is an alkyl phenol that can be used for induction and maintenance of general anesthesia. It can result in profound hypotension caused by reduced arterial tone, with no change in HR. The major advantage of propofol is its rapid clearance with few residual effects on awakening, but because it is expensive, its current use tends to be limited to operations of brief duration. Despite its hemodynamic effects, it has been used extensively to assist early extubation after coronary artery bypass surgery. Current evidence indicates that there is no one best general anesthetic technique for patients with CAD undergoing noncardiac surgery, and has led to the abandonment of the concept of a cardiac anesthetic.

Spinal and Epidural Anesthesia

Regional anesthesia includes the techniques of spinal, epidural, and peripheral nerve blocks. Each technique has its advantages and risks. Peripheral techniques, such as a brachial plexus or Bier block, offer the advantage of causing minimal or no hemodynamic effects. In contrast, spinal or epidural techniques can produce sympathetic blockade, which can reduce BP and slow HR. Spinal anesthesia and lumbar or low thoracic epidural anesthesia can also evoke reflex sympathetic activation mediated above the level of blockade, which might lead to myocardial ischemia.

The primary clinical difference between epidural and spinal anesthesia is the ability to provide continuous anesthesia or analgesia via placement of an epidural catheter, as opposed to a single dose in spinal anesthesia, although some clinicians will place a catheter in the intrathecal space. Although the speed of onset depends on the local anesthetic agent used, spinal anesthesia and its associated autonomic effects occur sooner than the same agent administered epidurally. A catheter, usually left in place for epidural anesthesia, permits titration of the agent. Epidural catheters can also be used postoperatively to provide analgesia.

A great deal of research has compared regional with general anesthesia for patients with CAD, particularly in patients undergoing infrainguinal bypass surgery. In one meta-analysis, overall mortality was reduced by about one third in patients allocated to neuraxial blockade, although the findings were controversial because most of the benefit was observed in older studies.[14] Reductions in MI and renal failure also occurred. A recent large-scale study of regional versus general anesthesia in noncardiac surgery patients was unable to demonstrate a difference in outcome.[1]

Monitored Anesthesia Care

MAC encompasses local anesthesia administered by the surgeon, with or without sedation. In a large-scale cohort study, MAC was associated with increased 30-day mortality in a univariate analysis compared with general anesthesia, although it did not remain significant in multivariate analysis once patient comorbidity was taken into account. The major issue with MAC is the ability to block the stress response adequately, because inadequate analgesia associated with tachycardia may be worse than the potential hemodynamic effects of general or regional anesthesia. Since the introduction of newer, short-acting intravenous agents, general anesthesia can now be administered essentially without an endotracheal tube. This allows the anesthesiologist to provide intense anesthesia for short or peripheral procedures without the potential effects of endotracheal intubation and extubation, and therefore blurs the distinction between general anesthesia and MAC. Using an analysis of closed insurance claims, Bhananker and colleagues[15] have demonstrated a high incidence of respiratory complications with MAC.

Intraoperative Hemodynamics and Myocardial Ischemia

Over the last two decades, numerous studies have explored the relationship between hemodynamics and perioperative ischemia and MI. Tachycardia is the strongest predictor of perioperative ischemia.

Although traditionally an HR higher than 100 beats/min defines tachycardia, slower HRs may result in myocardial ischemia. As described later, control of HR using beta blockers decreases the incidence of myocardial ischemia and infarction. Feringa and associates[16] have demonstrated that control of HR lowers the incidence of perioperative MI, with the greatest benefit if HR is controlled to less than 70 beats/min. Although concern about beta blockers causing intraoperative hypotension in patients with CAD has been raised, no evidence supports such a contention. During CABG, the vast majority of episodes of intraoperative ischemia do not correlate with hemodynamic changes. In the absence of tachycardia, hypotension has not been shown to be associated with myocardial ischemia.

Postoperative Management

Response to Surgery

To determine the best approach to preoperative testing, it is important to understand the pathophysiology of perioperative cardiac events. A full discussion of the pathophysiology of perioperative MI has been published.[17] All surgical procedures cause a stress response, although the extent of the response depends on the extent of the surgery and the use of anesthetics and analgesics to reduce the response. The stress response can increase HR and BP, which can precipitate episodes of myocardial ischemia in areas distal to coronary artery stenoses. Prolonged myocardial ischemia (either prolonged individual episodes or cumulative duration of shorter episodes) can cause myocardial necrosis and perioperative MI and death. Identification of patients with a high risk of coronary artery stenoses, through either history or cardiovascular testing, can lead to the implementation of strategies to reduce morbidity from supply-demand mismatches. As noted, beta blockers can reduce the increased demand, whereas coronary revascularization may improve supply-related issues in patients with critical stenoses.

A major mechanism of MI in the nonoperative setting is plaque rupture of a noncritical coronary stenosis, with subsequent coronary thrombosis (see Chaps. 43 and 54). Because the perioperative period is marked by tachycardia and a hypercoagulable state, plaque disruption and thrombosis may commonly occur. Because the nidus for the thrombosis is a noncritical stenosis, preoperative cardiac evaluation may fail to identify such a patient before surgery, although control of HR may decrease the propensity of the plaque to rupture. The areas distal to the noncritical stenosis would not be expected to have collateral coronary flow, and therefore any acute thrombosis may have a greater detrimental effect than it would in a previously severely narrowed vessel. In the absence of fixed coronary narrowing elsewhere, preoperative cardiovascular testing will clearly not identify these patients. On the other hand, if the postoperative MI is caused by prolonged increase in myocardial oxygen demand in patients with one or more critical fixed stenosis, preoperative testing likely would identify such patients.

Evidence from several autopsy and postinfarction angiography studies after surgery supports both mechanisms. Ellis and coworkers have demonstrated that one third of all patients sustained events in areas distal to noncritical stenoses.[1] Dawood and colleagues have demonstrated that fatal perioperative MI occurs predominantly in patients with multivessel coronary disease, especially left main and three-vessel disease, but the severity of preexisting underlying stenosis does not predict the resulting infarct territory.[1] This analysis suggested that fatal events occur primarily in patients with advanced fixed stenoses, but that the infarct may result from plaque rupture in a mild or only moderately stenotic segment of diseased vessel.

Intensive Care

Over the last several years, provision of intensive care by intensivists has become a patient safety goal. Pronovost and associates have performed a systematic review of the literature on physician staffing patterns and clinical outcomes in critically ill patients.[18] They grouped intensive care unit (ICU) physician staffing into low-intensity (no

intensivist or elective intensivist consultation) or high-intensity (mandatory intensivist consultation or closed ICU; all care directed by intensivist) groups. High-intensity staffing was associated with lower hospital mortality in 16 of 17 studies (94%) and with a pooled estimate of the relative risk for hospital mortality of 0.71 (95% CI, 0.62 to 0.82). High-intensity staffing was associated with a lower ICU mortality in 14 of 15 studies (93%) and with a pooled estimate of the relative risk for ICU mortality of 0.61 (95% CI, 0.50 to 0.75). High-intensity staffing reduced hospital length of stay (LOS) in 10 of 13 studies and reduced ICU LOS in 14 of 18 studies without case-mix adjustment. High-intensity staffing was associated with reduced hospital LOS in two of four studies and reduced ICU LOS in both studies that adjusted for case mix. No study found increased LOS with high-intensity staffing after case mix adjustment. High-intensity versus low-intensity ICU physician staffing is associated with reduced hospital and ICU mortality and reduced hospital and ICU LOS.

Pain Management

Postoperative analgesia may reduce perioperative cardiac morbidity. Because postoperative tachycardia and catecholamine surges probably promote myocardial ischemia and/or coronary plaque rupture, and because postoperative pain can produce tachycardia and increased catecholamines, effective postoperative analgesia may reduce cardiac complications. Postoperative analgesia also may reduce the hypercoagulable state. Epidural anesthesia may reduce platelet aggregability, as compared with general anesthesia. Whether this reduction is related to intraoperative or postoperative management is unclear. In an analysis of Medicare claims data, the use of epidural analgesia (as determined by billing codes for postoperative epidural pain management) was associated with decreased risk of death at 7 days. Future research will focus on how best to deliver postoperative analgesia to maximize the potential benefits in reducing complications.

Surveillance and Implications of Perioperative Cardiac Complications

The optimal and most cost-effective strategy for monitoring high-risk patients for major morbidity after noncardiac surgery is unknown. Myocardial ischemia and infarctions that occur postoperatively are usually silent, most likely because of the confounding effects of analgesics and postoperative surgical pain. Creatine kinase (CK)-MB is also less specific for myocardial necrosis postoperatively, because this marker can rise during aortic surgery and after mesenteric ischemia. Further confounding the issue, most perioperative MIs do not cause ST-segment elevation, and nonspecific ST-T wave changes are common after surgery with or without MI. The diagnosis of a perioperative MI is therefore particularly difficult using these traditional tests.

A marked elevation in mortality associated with postoperative myocardial infarction provides continuing impetus for improving methods of detection. Similar to the detection of MI on presentation for chest pain, biomarkers been used to identify myocardial necrosis. Lee and coworkers measured CK-MB and troponin T levels in 1175 patients undergoing noncardiac surgery and created receiver-operating characteristic curves.[1] They found that troponin T had a similar performance for diagnosing perioperative MI, but significantly better correlation for major cardiac complications developing after an acute MI. Metzler and colleagues examined the sensitivity of troponin assay at variable cutoff levels; a value higher than 0.6 ng/mL demonstrated a positive predictive value of 87.5% and a negative predictive value of 98%. Le Manach and associates studied 1152 consecutive patients who underwent abdominal infrarenal aortic surgery and identified four patterns of cardiac troponin I (cTn-I) release after surgery.[1] One group did not have any abnormal levels, whereas a second group had only mild elevations of cTn-I levels. Interestingly, two groups demonstrated elevations of cTn-I consistent with a perioperative MI (PMI). One demonstrated acute (<24-hour) and early elevations of cTn-I above threshold, and the other demonstrated prolonged low levels of cTn-I release, followed by a delayed

(>24-hour) elevation of cTnI. The authors suggested that these two patterns represent two distinct pathophysiologies—acute coronary occlusion for early morbidity and prolonged myocardial ischemia for late events. Mohler and coworkers[19] evaluated cTn-I and CK-MB in 784 high-risk vascular surgery patients on the day of surgery and at 24, 72, and 120 hours postoperatively. They reported a sensitivity of 51% and a specificity of 91% for the defined cardiovascular event, using a receiver operating characteristic (ROC)–defined cut point for CK-MB of 3.1 ng/mL.

Recently, brain natriuretic peptide (BNP) has been studied in the perioperative period. Mahla and colleagues[20] measured preoperative and postoperative N-terminal pro-BNP (NT-proBNP) in 218 vascular surgery patients. Using ROC analysis-defined cut points, patients with elevated NT-proBNP had an almost 20-fold in-hospital and fivefold long-term risk of cardiac events. Goei and associates[21] have evaluated the predictive capacity of preoperative levels of NT-proBNP in 356 vascular surgery patients; they found that BNP elevations are associated with adverse 30-day cardiovascular events in subjects with normal renal function but not in those with severe renal impairment. In a meta-analysis of seven prospective observational studies, BNP or NT-proBNP above the ROC-determined optimal threshold was associated with marked increases in 30-day and intermediate-term cardiac death, nonfatal MI, and major adverse cardiac events.[22] A subsequent meta-analysis demonstrated that preoperative BNP measurement independently predicts perioperative cardiovascular events in studies that only considered the outcomes of death, cardiovascular death, or MI (OR, 44.2; 95% CI, 7.6 to 257.0; I(2) = 51.6%) and studies that included other outcomes (OR, 14.7; 95% CI, 5.7 to 38.2; I(2) = 62.2%); the *P* value for interaction was 0.28.[23]

Traditionally, PMIs were associated with a 30% to 50% short-term mortality, but recent series have reported a fatality rate of perioperative MIs of less than 20%. Whether these shifts in timing relate to reductions or better detection of hypotension-related subendocardial ischemia, or a change in the timing of true plaque rupture events, remains unclear. Studies from the 1980s suggested a peak incidence of the second and third postoperative days. Badner and coworkers, using troponin I as a marker for MI, have suggested that the immediate and first postoperative days show the highest incidence, as confirmed in other studies.[1] The finding that postanesthetic care unit hypotension best predicted troponin release suggests a hemodynamic rather than plaque rupture event. Thus, the change likely relates to more robust surveillance methods, not a fundamental shift in how or when myocardial ischemia or infarct occur.

Increasing evidence associates a perioperative MI or biomarker elevation with worse long-term outcome. Lopez-Jimenez and colleagues found that abnormal troponin T levels were associated with an increased incidence of cardiovascular complications within 6 months of surgery.[1] Kim and associates studied perioperative troponin I levels in 229 patients having aortic or infrainguinal vascular surgery or lower extremity amputation.[1] Twenty-eight patients (12%) had postoperative troponin I levels higher than 1.5 ng/mL, which was associated with a sixfold increased risk of 6-month mortality and a 27-fold increased risk of MI. Furthermore, they observed a relationship between troponin I concentration and mortality. Landesberg and coworkers demonstrated that postoperative CK-MB and troponin, even at low cutoff levels, are independent and complementary predictors of long-term mortality after major vascular surgery.[1] Mahla and colleagues[20] also demonstrated that elevations in BNP levels are associated with a fivefold long-term risk of cardiac events. The appropriate use of screening biomarkers in current preoperative risk assessment algorithms remains unstudied.

Reducing Cardiac Risk of Noncardiac Surgery

Surgical Revascularization

Coronary revascularization has been suggested as a means of reducing perioperative risk surrounding noncardiac surgery. Retrospective

evidence indicates that prior successful preoperative revascularization may decrease postoperative cardiac risk two- to four-fold in patients undergoing elective vascular surgery. The strongest evidence comes from the Coronary Artery Surgery Study (CASS) Registry, which enrolled patients from 1978 to 1981.[1] The operative mortality for patients with CABG before noncardiac surgery was 0.9% but was significantly higher (2.4%) in patients without prior CABG. However, a 1.4% mortality rate was associated with the CABG procedure itself. Eagle and associates have reported a long-term analysis of patients entered into CASS and assigned to medical or surgical therapy for CAD for more than 10 years who subsequently underwent 3368 noncardiac operations in the years following assignment of coronary treatment.[1] Intermediate-risk surgery such as abdominal, thoracic, or carotid endarterectomy associated with a combined morbidity and mortality of 1% to 5%, with a small but substantial improvement in outcome in patients who had undergone prior revascularization. The most improvement in outcome occurred in patients undergoing major vascular surgery, such as abdominal or lower extremity revascularization. This observational study did not randomize patients, however, and was undertaken in the 1970s and 1980s, before significant advances in medical, surgical, and percutaneous coronary strategies.

Several cohort studies have examined the benefit of percutaneous coronary intervention (PCI) before noncardiac surgery. Posner and colleagues used an administrative data set of patients who underwent PCI and noncardiac surgery in Washington State.[1] They matched patients with coronary disease undergoing noncardiac surgery with and without prior PCI and looked at cardiac complications. In this nonrandomized design, they noted a significantly lower rate of 30-day cardiac complications in patients who underwent PCI at least 90 days before the noncardiac surgery. PCI within 90 days of noncardiac surgery did not improve outcome. The advent of drug-eluting stents requiring prolonged antiplatelet therapy may promote operative bleeding complications or increase subacute stent thrombosis if antiplatelet treatment stops perioperatively (see Chap. 58).

Several randomized trials have addressed the value of both CABG and PCI in a subset of patients. McFalls and colleagues[24] reported the results of a multicenter randomized trial in the Veterans Affairs Health System in which patients with documented CAD on coronary angiography, excluding those with left main disease or severely depressed ejection fraction (<20%), were randomized before elective major vascular surgery to CABG (59%) or PCI (41%) versus routine medical therapy. At 2.7 years after randomization, mortality in the revascularization group was not significantly different (22%) compared with the no-revascularization group (23%). Within 30 days after the vascular operation, a postoperative MI, defined by elevated troponin levels, occurred in 12% of the revascularization group and 14% of the no-revascularization group (*P* = 0.37). The authors suggested that coronary revascularization is not indicated in patients with stable CAD, and further support the lack of efficacy of PCI or CABG for single- or double-vessel disease before noncardiac surgery. In a reanalysis of the data, the completeness of the revascularization affects the rate of perioperative MI, with CABG being more effective than PCI.

Poldermans and associates[25] have evaluated the role of coronary artery revascularization in 101 vascular surgery patients with three or more Lee index risk factors and extensive stress-induced ischemia, on a background of beta blocker therapy. Coronary angiography showed two-vessel disease in 12 patients (24%), three-vessel disease in 33 patients (67%), and left main disease in 4 patients (8%). Revascularization improved neither 30-day nor 1-year outcome (*P* > 0.2 for both). Long-term benefit was only shown in those with corrected left main disease.[26] Most recently, Garcia and coworkers[27] analyzed randomized and nonrandomized patients who had preoperative coronary angiography, and unprotected left main CAD was present in 4.6% of patients who underwent coronary angiography before vascular surgery; this was the only subset of patients showing a benefit with preoperative coronary artery revascularization.

As described earlier, Poldermans and colleagues[13] randomized vascular patients at intermediate risk to testing and interventions or no testing, and found no difference in 30-day cardiac events with beta blocker therapy provided to all subjects. Monaco and associates[28] studied 208 patients at moderate clinical risk who were undergoing major vascular surgery and were randomly allocated to a selective strategy group, in whom coronary angiography was performed based on the results of noninvasive tests, or to a systematic strategy group, who systematically underwent preoperative coronary angiography. The strategy of routine coronary angiography had no effect on short-term outcome, but positively affected long-term outcome of peripheral arterial disease surgical patients at medium to high risk.

One issue in interpreting the results is that the length of time between coronary revascularization and noncardiac surgery most likely affects its protective effect and potential risks. Back and coworkers[29] have studied 425 consecutive patients undergoing 481 elective major vascular operations at an academic Veterans Affairs Medical Center. Coronary revascularization was classified as recent (CABG, <1 year; percutaneous transluminal coronary angioplasty [PTCA], <6 months) in 35 cases, as prior (CABG, 1 to 5 years; PTCA, 6 months to 2 years) in 45 cases, and as remote (CABG, >5 years; PTCA, >2 years) in 48 cases. Outcomes in patients with previous PTCAs were similar to those after CABG. Significant differences in adverse cardiac events and mortality were found between patients with CABG done within 5 years or PTCA within 2 years (6.3% and 1.3%, respectively), individuals with remote revascularization (10.4% and 6.3%, respectively), and non-revascularized patients stratified at high risk (13.3% and 3.3%, respectively) or intermediate or low risk (2.8% and 0.9%, respectively). The authors concluded that previous coronary revascularization (CABG, >5 years; PTCA, >2 years) provides only modest protection against adverse cardiac events and mortality following major arterial reconstruction.

Coronary Stenting and Noncardiac Surgery

PCI using coronary stenting poses several special issues. Kaluza and colleagues reported the outcome in 40 patients who underwent prophylactic coronary stent placement less than six weeks before major noncardiac surgery requiring general anesthesia.[1] They reported 7 MIs, 11 major bleeding episodes, and 8 deaths. All of the deaths and MIs, as well as 8 of the 11 bleeding episodes, occurred in patients who underwent surgery fewer than 14 days after stenting. Four patients died after undergoing surgery 1 day after stenting. Wilson and associates reported on 207 patients who underwent noncardiac surgery within 2 months of stent placement.[1] Eight patients died or suffered an MI, and all of those were among the 168 patients undergoing surgery 6 weeks after stent placement. Vincenzi and coworkers studied 103 patients and reported that the risk of a perioperative cardiac event was 2.11-fold greater in patients with recent stents (<35 days before surgery) as compared with PCI more than 90 days before surgery.[1] The importance of delaying surgery was reported, even though the investigators either continued antiplatelet drug therapy or only briefly interrupted it; heparin was administered to all patients. Leibowitz and colleagues studied 216 consecutive patients who had PCI within 3 months of noncardiac surgery (112 had PTCA and 94 had stenting).[1] A total of 26 patients (12%) died, 13 in the stent group (14%) and 13 in the PTCA group (11%)—a nonsignificant difference. The incidence of acute MI and death within 6 months did not differ significantly (7% and 14% in the stent group and 6% and 11% in the PTCA group, respectively). Many more events occurred in the two groups when noncardiac surgery was performed within 2 weeks of PCI. On the basis of the accumulating data, elective noncardiac surgery after PCI, with or without stent placement, should be delayed for 4 to 6 weeks.

Drug-eluting stents may represent an even greater problem during the perioperative period. Emerging data from a series of recent analyses in the nonoperative setting and several perioperative case reports suggest that the risk of thrombosis continues for at least one year after insertion (see Chap. 58).[1] Several reports have suggested that drug-eluting stents may represent an additional risk over a prolonged period (up to 12 months), particularly if antiplatelet agents are discontinued. Schouten and colleagues[30] retrospectively evaluated 192 patients who underwent noncardiac surgery and had a successful PCI because of unstable CAD within 2 years of the procedure. Drug-eluting stents accounted for 52% of the stents placed. Of the 192 patients, 30

underwent surgery prior to the recommended discontinuation of dual antiplatelet therapy for the particular stent (30 days for bare metal stents and up to 6 months for sirolimus-eluting stents). In patients in whom antiplatelet therapy was stopped before the required time for clopidogrel use (early surgery group), the incidence of death or non-fatal MI was 30.7%, compared with 0% in patients who continued antiplatelet therapy. The elevated risk of stent thrombosis and cardiovascular events, however, seems to abate over time. Godet and associates[31] investigated the risk of postoperative adverse cardiovascular events at a mean of 14 months after drug-eluting stent placement in 96 consecutive patients, noting a 2% in-stent thrombosis rate. More recently, Anwaruddin and coworkers[32] determined the risk of postoperative complications in 481 patients with drug-eluting stent placement an average of 1.1 years prior to the operation. They reported a 9% risk of death, nonfatal MI, or stent thrombosis by 30 days. A 2007 science advisory from the AHA, ACC, Society for Cardiovascular Angiography and Interventions, American College of Surgeons, and American Dental Association stressed the importance of 12 months of dual antiplatelet therapy after placement of a drug-eluting stent.[1] This advisory also recommended postponing elective surgery for 1 year and, if surgery cannot be deferred, considering the continuation of aspirin during the perioperative period in high-risk patients with drug-eluting stents. In patients with illness requiring more timely surgery, strategies for bridging the cessation of antiplatelet therapy until the procedure include the use of intravenous eptifibatide and tirofiban, but these have not been tested in adequate numbers to permit recommendation.

Pharmacologic Interventions

BETA-ADRENERGIC BLOCKING AGENTS. Beta blockers (Table 85-4) are the best-studied medical treatment, and guidelines for their use in the perioperative period have been published recently. Mangano and colleagues administered atenolol or placebo, beginning on the morning of surgery and continuing for 7 days postoperatively, in a cohort of 200 patients with known coronary disease or risk factors for CAD who were undergoing high-risk noncardiac surgery.[1] They demonstrated a marked reduction in the incidence of perioperative myocardial ischemia, although no differences in the rates of perioperative MI. Survival improved markedly at 6 months in the atenolol group and continued for at least 2 years. The authors speculated that the lower incidence of myocardial ischemia resulted from less plaque destabilization, with a resultant reduction in subsequent MI or death in the 6 months after noncardiac surgery. Issues of randomization and uneven distribution of risk factors and treatment at baseline and on discharge with beta blockers may account for the findings, at least in part. However, Poldermans and associates have studied the perioperative use of bisoprolol versus routine care in elective major vascular surgery in the Dutch Echocardiographic Cardiac Risk Evaluation Applying Stress Echo (DECREASE) trial.[1] This medication was started at least 7 days preoperatively, titrated to achieve a resting HR less than 60 beats/min, and continued postoperatively for 30 days. The study was confined to patients with at least one clinical marker of cardiac risk (prior MI, diabetes, angina pectoris, heart failure, age older than 70 years, or poor functional status), and evidence of inducible myocardial ischemia on a preoperative dobutamine stress echocardiogram. Patients with extensive regional wall abnormalities (large zones of myocardial ischemia) were excluded. Bisoprolol reduced perioperative MI or cardiac death by almost 80% in this high-risk population. Because of the selection criteria, the efficacy of bisoprolol in the highest risk group—those who would be considered for coronary revascularization or modification or cancellation of the surgical procedure—cannot be determined from this trial. The event rate in the placebo group (almost 40%) suggests, however, that all but the highest risk patients were enrolled in the trial.

Boersma and coworkers have reevaluated the value of dobutamine stress echocardiography with respect to the extent of wall motion abnormalities and the use of beta blockers during surgery for the entire cohort of patients screened for the DECREASE trial.[1] They assigned one point for each of the following characteristics: age older

TABLE 85-4 Beta-Adrenergic Blocking Agents

STUDY	NO. OF PATIENTS IN STUDY	BETA BLOCKER REGIMEN	PATIENT RISK GROUP	SURGICAL PROCEDURE	DURATION OF BETA BLOCKADE	WERE BETA BLOCKERS FULLY TITRATED?	WERE BETA BLOCKERS OF BENEFIT?
MSCPI	200	Atenolol, 50-100 mg	Known CAD or at risk for CAD with ≥ two risk factors	Vascular, abdominal, orthopedic, neurosurgery	Duration of hospitalization	No	Yes, at 6-8 mo
DECREASE I	112	Bisoprolol, varying doses	≥ One or more RCRI risk factor and positive DBA stress echo	Major vascular surgery	1 wk before until 30 days after surgery	Yes, to heart rate of 60 beats/min	Yes, 90% reduction in MI and death
MaVS	496	Metoprolol, single dose	ASA class 1-3	Major vascular surgery	2 hr before until 5 days after surgery	No. Metoprolol dosed by patient weight.	No; more intraoperative treatment requiring bradycardia in metoprolol arm
DIPOM	921	Metoprolol succinate, two doses	Diabetic patients; <10% had history of CAD	Intermediate risk surgery	1 day before until a maximum of 8 days after surgery (mean 4.6 days)	Two doses; 100 mg/day or 50 mg/day if heart rate = 55-65 beats/min	No benefit or harm
POISE	8351	Metoprolol succinate	History of CAD, PVD, stroke, CHF, undergoing vascular surgery, or ≥ three or more RCRI risk factors	Noncardiac surgery (major vascular surgery 36%, intraperitoneal 21%, orthopedic 21%)	2-4 hr before surgery to 30 days after surgery	No, dose limitation for low heart rate	Yes and no; reduction in CV death, NFMI, NF cardiac arrest; increase in mortality and stroke
DECREASE IV	1066	Bisoprolol	Intermediate risk (risk estimate, 1%-6% MI or death)	General, urologic, orthopedic, ENT surgery	Within 30 days of surgery until 30 days after	Yes, to target heart rate 50-70 beats/min	Yes, 66% reduction in NFMI and cardiac death

DBA = dobutamine; ENT = ear, nose, and throat; NFMI = nonfatal MI.
Modified from Chopra V, Eagle KA: Perioperative beta-blockers for cardiac risk reduction: Time for clarity. JAMA 303:551, 2010.

than 70 years, current angina, MI, congestive heart failure, prior cerebrovascular event, diabetes mellitus, and renal failure. As the total number of clinical risk factors increased, perioperative cardiac event rates also increased. When the risk of death or MI was stratified by perioperative beta blocker usage, there was no significant improvement in those without any of the prior risk factors. In those with a risk factor score between 1 and 3, which represented more than half of all patients, the rate of cardiac events fell from 3% to 0.9% by effective beta blockade. Most importantly, in those with fewer than three risk factors, comprising 70% of the population, beta blocker therapy was effective in reducing cardiac events in those with new wall motion abnormalities in one to four segments (33% versus 2.8%), having a smaller effect in those without new wall motion abnormalities (5.8% versus 2%). Beta blockers were not protective in those patients with new wall motion abnormalities in more than five segments. This group with risk factors and extensive wall motion abnormalities on preoperative stress echo may be the group to consider for prophylactic coronary revascularization. Dunkelgrun and colleagues[33] investigated the role of beta blockade in intermediate-risk noncardiac surgery patients (defined as a predicted risk of cardiac event of 1% to 6%) in an open-label randomized trial. Bisoprolol, titrated to a heart rate of 50 to 70 beats/min preoperatively and maintained during the hospitalization, reduced the rate of perioperative cardiac death and nonfatal MI from 66% to 2.1%.

The trial data supporting the use of beta blockers are not uniformly positive. Brady and associates randomized 103 patients without previous MI who had infrarenal vascular surgery to oral metoprolol or placebo from admission until 7 days after surgery.[1] Perioperative beta blockade with metoprolol did not seem to reduce 30-day cardiovascular events, but it was underpowered to do so. The study did show that metoprolol reduced the time from surgery to discharge. Lindenauer and colleagues[34] retrospectively reviewed the records of 782,969 patients and determined who received beta blocker treatment during the first 2 hospital days. The relationship between perioperative beta blocker treatment and the risk of death varied directly with cardiac risk; among the 580,665 patients with an RCRI score of 0 or 1, treatment was associated with no benefit and possible harm, whereas among the patients with an RCRI score of 2, 3, or 4 or higher, the adjusted odds ratios for death in the hospital were 0.88 (95% CI, 0.80 to 0.98), 0.71 (95% CI, 0.63 to 0.80), and 0.58 (95% CI, 0.50 to 0.67), respectively.

A study of 497 vascular surgery patients randomized to a fixed dose of metoprolol versus placebo demonstrated no difference in perioperative outcome. A trial of metoprolol in diabetic patients without known coronary disease undergoing a diverse group of surgical procedures was unable to demonstrate any difference in perioperative outcomes.[1] In the POISE trial, Devereaux and colleagues randomized 8351 high-risk patients undergoing noncardiac surgery to metoprolol succinate 200 mg daily, or matching placebo.[4] The long-acting metoprolol was first administered at 100 mg 2 to 4 hours before surgery, within 6 hours after surgery, and then at 200 mg daily thereafter. Active treatment with a beta blocker reduced the composite of cardiovascular death, nonfatal MI, and nonfatal cardiac arrest at 30 days after randomization by 1.1%, but increased mortality by 0.8% and stroke by 0.5%. Why was this variance seen? One prominent difference among these trials is the use of titration. In the clinical trials showing reductions in events, beta blockers were titrated to ensure appropriate effect, whereas in the trials in which beta blockers did not improve outcomes or instead worsened them, titration was limited or absent. The timing of medication administration is another possible cause; preoperative titration associated with better outcomes than administration at or just after surgery.

In 2009, an update to the ACC/AHA guidelines on perioperative beta blockade modified previous recommendations based on recent evidence.[1] The continuation of beta blockers in patients undergoing surgery who are receiving beta blockers remains a Class I recommendation. No other Class I recommendations are stated. The use of beta

ANESTHESIA AND NONCARDIAC SURGERY IN PATIENTS WITH HEART DISEASE

TABLE 85-5	Recommendations for Perioperative Beta Blocker Therapy

Class I

1. Beta blockers should be continued in patients undergoing surgery who are receiving beta blockers for treatment of conditions with ACCF/AHA Class I guideline indications for the drugs (level of evidence: C).

Class IIa

1. Beta blockers titrated to heart rate and blood pressure are probably recommended for patients undergoing vascular surgery who are at high cardiac risk because of coronary artery disease or the finding of cardiac ischemia on preoperative testing (level of evidence: B).
2. Beta blockers titrated to heart rate and blood pressure are reasonable for patients in whom preoperative assessment for vascular surgery identifies high cardiac risk, as defined by the presence of more than one clinical risk factor* (level of evidence: C).
3. Beta blockers titrated to heart rate and blood pressure are reasonable for patients in whom preoperative assessment identifies coronary artery disease or high cardiac risk, as defined by the presence of more than one clinical risk factor,* who are undergoing intermediate-risk surgery (level of evidence: B).

Class IIb

1. The usefulness of beta blockers is uncertain for patients who are undergoing intermediate-risk procedures or vascular surgery in whom preoperative assessment identifies a single clinical risk factor in the absence of coronary artery disease* (level of evidence: C).
2. The usefulness of beta blockers is uncertain in patients undergoing vascular surgery with no clinical risk factors who are not currently taking beta blockers (level of evidence: B).

Class III

1. Beta blockers should not be given to patients undergoing surgery who have absolute contraindications to beta blockade (level of evidence: C).
2. Routine administration of high-dose beta blockers in the absence of dose titration is not useful and may be harmful to patients not currently taking beta blockers who are undergoing noncardiac surgery (level of evidence: B).

*Clinical risk factors include history of ischemic heart disease, history of compensated or prior heart failure, history of cerebrovascular disease, diabetes mellitus, and renal insufficiency (defined in the Revised Cardiac Risk Index as a preoperative serum creatinine of 2 mg/dL).
From Fleischmann KE: Perioperative focused update. J Am Coll Cardiol 54:2102, 2009.

blockers titrated to heart rate and blood pressure are all Class IIa recommendations for the following: (1) patients undergoing vascular surgery who are at high cardiac risk because of CAD; (2) the finding of cardiac ischemia on preoperative testing in patients for whom preoperative assessment for vascular surgery identified high cardiac risk, as defined by the presence of more than one RCRI clinical risk factor; and (3) for patients in whom preoperative assessment identified CAD or high cardiac risk, as defined by the presence of more than one clinical risk factor, who are undergoing intermediate-risk surgery. A new Class III recommendation is that the routine administration of high-dose beta blockers in the absence of dose titration is not useful, and may be harmful to patients not currently taking beta blockers who are undergoing noncardiac surgery (**Table 85-5**).

Several pragmatic considerations pertain to the use of perioperative beta blockers in those not currently taking these agents. Several authors have recently demonstrated that most patients presenting for noncardiac surgery, and even for vascular surgery, have not been started on beta blockers.[1] One concern of anesthesiologists is related to the acute administration of beta-blocking agents on the morning of surgery. The combined effect of acute HR decrease and the induction of anesthesia in a patient who had previously been beta blocker–naïve has anecdotally been associated with marked bradycardia and hypotension. Treatment of these events may lead to wide swings in HR and BP and less HR control than desired. Thus, the approach to the use of beta blockers depends on the preoperative status, type of surgery, cardiac risk factors, and any results of cardiac stress testing. Ideally, beta blocker therapy should be initiated more than seven days in advance,[35]

and longer-acting agents such as atenolol or bisoprolol should be used. Analyzing a large data base, Redelmeier and associates have demonstrated improved perioperative survival in patients given atenolol as compared with metoprolol.[1] If the patient is undergoing nonvascular surgery or vascular surgery and has indications for beta blocker therapy independent of surgery, but is not currently taking beta blockers, then initiation of beta blockers several days preoperatively by the internist, cardiologist, or other primary care provider is appropriate to ensure a stable beta blocker level on the day of surgery. If several days of beta blocker therapy cannot be achieved, the potential risks of new-onset beta blocker therapy during induction of general, epidural, or spinal anesthesia may outweigh the benefits of beginning drug therapy the morning of surgery. Because the study by Mangano and coworkers did not demonstrate any difference in in-hospital outcome, and the approach of Raby and colleagues demonstrated similar efficacy with respect to perioperative ischemia,[1] we suggest inducing general anesthesia or providing regional anesthesia before starting beta blocker therapy. If the induction is associated with tachycardia, then administration of esmolol is appropriate. After adequate anesthesia and analgesia are achieved, HR should be controlled and maintained below 70 beats/min. Feringa and coworkers[16] have demonstrated that higher doses of beta blockers and tight HR control are associated with reduced perioperative myocardial ischemia and troponin T release and with improved long-term outcome in vascular surgery patients.

STATIN THERAPY. In addition to their cholesterol-lowering properties, statins have anti-inflammatory and plaque-stabilizing properties (see Chap. 47). Given the potential mechanisms of perioperative MIs, statins could have theoretical benefits. Poldermans and colleagues performed a case-control study of 2816 patients who underwent major vascular surgery from 1991 to 2000. Statin therapy was significantly less common in patients experiencing a postoperative MI compared with controls (8% versus 25%; $P < 0.001$).[1] The adjusted odds ratio for perioperative mortality among statin users as compared with nonusers was 0.22 (95% CI, 0.10 to 0.47). Lindenauer and associates used administrative data to study a cohort of 780,591 patients; 77,082 patients (9.9%) received lipid-lowering therapy perioperatively, and 23,100 (2.96%) died during hospitalization.[1] Using multivariate modeling and propensity matching, the number needed to treat to prevent a postoperative death was 85 (95% CI, 77 to 98) and varied from 186 among patients at lowest risk to 30 among those with an RCRI score of 4 or more. Durazzo and colleagues randomized 100 patients to receive 20 mg atorvastatin or placebo once a day for 45 days.[1] The incidence of cardiac events was more than three times higher with placebo (26%) compared with atorvastatin (8%; $P < 0.031$). Patients given atorvastatin exhibited a significant decrease in the rate of cardiac events, compared with the placebo group, within 6 months after vascular surgery ($P < 0.018$). In DECREASE IV, Dunkelgrun and coworkers[33] used a 2 × 2 factorial design to evaluate high-dose fluvastatin and beta blockade in intermediate-risk patients. Nonsignificant reductions in cardiovascular death and MI were noted. Accumulating evidence suggests that statin therapy should continue during the perioperative period, and consideration should be given for starting statin therapy in high-risk patients, particularly those who meet the National Cholesterol Education Program's Adult Treatment Panel III's recommendations, because it could be argued that the patient should have been on a statin already.

NITROGLYCERIN. Only two randomized trials have evaluated the potential protective effect of prophylactic nitroglycerin for reducing perioperative cardiac complications after noncardiac surgery. In a small study by Coriat and colleagues in patients undergoing carotid endarterectomy, high-dose (1 µg/kg/min) nitroglycerin was more effective than low-dose (0.5 µg/kg/min) nitroglycerin in reducing the incidence of myocardial ischemia, but MI did not occur in either group.[1] The anesthetic used in this study was an oxygen-pancuronium-fentanyl method, and therefore inhalational agents were not administered. Dodds and associates have studied nitroglycerin versus placebo using a balanced anesthetic technique and reported no difference in the rates of myocardial ischemia or infarction.[1] Taken together, the evidence suggests that prophylactic nitroglycerin does not reduce the incidence of perioperative cardiac morbidity, although neither trial was powered to detect a modest benefit of nitroglycerin. Because prophylactic nitroglycerin has considerable hemodynamic effects and is not known to prevent MI or cardiac death, it would seem prudent to avoid the prophylactic use of nitroglycerin, although there are clear indications for its use once myocardial ischemia develops.

Nonpharmacologic Interventions

TEMPERATURE. Frank and coworkers completed a randomized trial of regional versus general anesthesia for lower extremity vascular bypass procedures and noted an association between hypothermia (temperature < 35°C) and myocardial ischemia.[1] They subsequently performed a trial in 300 high-risk patients undergoing a diverse group of intermediate-risk and high-risk procedures, randomizing patients to maintenance of normothermia or routine care. They observed a significantly reduced incidence of perioperative cardiac morbidity and mortality within 24 hours of surgery in the group that was kept normothermic.

ELECTROCARDIOGRAPHIC, HEMODYNAMIC, AND ECHO-CARDIOGRAPHIC MONITORING. A number of studies have demonstrated the predictive value of correlating perioperative ST-segment changes and major cardiac events (see earlier). Furthermore, the duration of cumulative or continuous perioperative ST changes strongly predicts poor outcomes. ST-segment monitoring therefore has become a standard during the intraoperative and ICU periods for high-risk patients. Patients at low to moderate risk may also develop ST-segment changes, but these changes may not reflect true myocardial ischemia, as suggested in a recent series.[1]

The time of greatest risk of a postoperative cardiac event may be when the patient is on the ward and unmonitored. ST-segment telemetry monitors have not been tested to any large degree in the perioperative period. The issue of whether early treatment of prolonged ST-segment changes leads to improved outcomes remains unresolved. Until such studies are completed, the efficacy of such monitors remains debatable.

Much controversy surrounds the value of pulmonary artery catheterization for noncardiac surgery. Several small randomized trials did not demonstrate a significant reduction in major cardiac morbidity and mortality in patients undergoing aortic surgery. A large-scale cohort study by Polanczyk and colleagues, in which patients who had pulmonary catheters placed were matched to those who did not, that used a propensity score also failed to demonstrate any significant benefit.[1] An increased incidence of congestive heart failure and untoward noncardiac outcomes in the pulmonary artery catheter group were observed. A total of 1994 patients were randomized to goal-directed therapy guided by a pulmonary catheter, with standard care without the use of a pulmonary catheter for patients undergoing urgent or elective major surgery. No difference in survival occurred, but there was a higher rate of pulmonary embolism in the catheter group compared with the standard-care group. Therefore, current evidence does not support the routine use of pulmonary artery catheterization for high-risk patients undergoing major noncardiac surgery. Further work will be required to understand whether these results can be generalized to the high-risk vascular surgical population and to determine the benefits of pulmonary artery catheters in specific clinical situations.

Transesophageal echocardiography (TEE) represents another means of assessing intraoperative cardiac function (see Chap. 15). It is an extremely sensitive, noninvasive tool to monitor intraoperative wall motion abnormalities and fluid status. In patients undergoing aortic cross clamping, TEE proved to have a significantly better sensitivity for detecting intraoperative ischemia than electrocardiographic monitoring. For noncardiac surgery, a study of TEE, two-lead electrocardiography, and 12-lead electrocardiography demonstrated minimal additive value of TEE over two-lead electrocardiography. Although TEE for the routine monitoring of intraoperative ischemia in noncardiac surgery may have minimal additive value over ST-segment recording for predicting patients who will sustain perioperative morbidity, TEE

monitoring may be valuable to guide treatment in patients with unstable hemodynamics for whom filling status and/or myocardial function are uncertain.

TRANSFUSION THRESHOLD. Much controversy surrounds the optimal hemoglobin level at which to transfuse high-risk noncardiac surgical patients. No randomized trials have evaluated the optimal transfusion threshold, although there is a great deal of anecdotal evidence. Several small cohort studies have shown that hematocrits in the 27% to 29% range represent the point below which the incidence of myocardial ischemia and potentially MI increases. A large-scale trial of transfusion triggers in the ICU did not document increased morbidity and mortality with a transfusion threshold of hemoglobin less than 7 g/dL, but there were trends toward increased morbidity in the subset of patients with ischemic heart disease.[1] The evidence suggests that patients with known ischemic heart disease that has not been revascularized should be maintained perioperatively with a hemoglobin level higher than 9 g/dL.

REFERENCES

Assessment of Risk

1. Fleisher LA, Beckman JA, Brown KA, et al: 2009 ACCF/AHA focused update on perioperative beta blockade incorporated into the ACC/AHA 2007 guidelines on perioperative cardiovascular evaluation and care for noncardiac surgery: A report of the American College of Cardiology Foundation/American Heart Association Task Force on Practice Guidelines. Circulation 120:e169, 2009.
2. Poldermans D, Bax JJ, Boersma E, et al: Guidelines for pre-operative cardiac risk assessment and perioperative cardiac management in non-cardiac surgery: The Task Force for Preoperative Cardiac Risk Assessment and Perioperative Cardiac Management in Non-cardiac Surgery of the European Society of Cardiology (ESC) and endorsed by the European Society of Anaesthesiology (ESA). Eur Heart J 30:2769, 2009.
3. Welten GM, Schouten O, van Domburg RT, et al: The influence of aging on the prognostic value of the revised cardiac risk index for postoperative cardiac complications in vascular surgery patients. Eur J Vasc Endovasc Surg 34:632, 2007.
4. Devereaux PJ, Yang H, Yusuf S, et al: Effects of extended-release metoprolol succinate in patients undergoing non-cardiac surgery (POISE trial): A randomised controlled trial. Lancet 371:1839, 2008.

Congenital and Valvular Heart Disease

5. Hammill BG, Curtis LH, Bennett-Guerrero E, et al: Impact of heart failure on patients undergoing major noncardiac surgery. Anesthesiology 108:559, 2008.
6. Cannesson M, Earing MG, Collange V, Kersten JR: Anesthesia for noncardiac surgery in adults with congenital heart disease. Anesthesiology 111:432, 2009.
7. Kovacs MJ, Kearon C, Rodger M, et al: Single-arm study of bridging therapy with low-molecular-weight heparin for patients at risk of arterial embolism who require temporary interruption of warfarin. Circulation 110:1658, 2004.
8. O'Donnell MJ, Kearon C, Johnson J, et al: Brief communication: Preoperative anticoagulant activity after bridging low-molecular-weight heparin for temporary interruption of warfarin. Ann Intern Med 146:184, 2007.
9. Douketis JD, Woods K, Foster GA, Crowther MA: Bridging anticoagulation with low-molecular-weight heparin after interruption of warfarin therapy is associated with a residual anticoagulant effect prior to surgery. Thromb Haemost 94:528, 2005.
10. Bonow RO, Carabello BA, Chatterjee K, et al: 2008 Focused update incorporated into the ACC/AHA 2006 guidelines for the management of patients with valvular heart disease: A report of the American College of Cardiology/American Heart Association Task Force on Practice Guidelines (Writing Committee to Revise the 1998 Guidelines for the Management of Patients With Valvular Heart Disease): Endorsed by the Society of Cardiovascular Anesthesiologists, Society for Cardiovascular Angiography and Interventions, and Society of Thoracic Surgeons. Circulation 118:e523, 2008.

Arrhythmias

11. Winkel TA, Schouten O, Hoeks SE, et al: Prognosis of transient new-onset atrial fibrillation during vascular surgery. Eur J Vasc Endovasc Surg 38:683, 2009.
12. Amar D, Zhang H, Roistacher N: The incidence and outcome of ventricular arrhythmias after noncardiac thoracic surgery. Anesth Analg 95:537, 2002.

Diagnostic Testing

13. Poldermans D, Bax JJ, Schouten O, et al: Should major vascular surgery be delayed because of preoperative cardiac testing in intermediate-risk patients receiving beta-blocker therapy with tight heart rate control? J Am Coll Cardiol 48:964, 2006.

Anesthesia and Postoperative Management

14. Rodgers A, Walker N, Schug S, et al: Reduction of postoperative mortality and morbidity with epidural or spinal anaesthesia: Results from overview of randomised trials. BMJ 321:1493, 2000.
15. Bhananker SM, Posner KL, Cheney FW, et al: Injury and liability associated with monitored anesthesia care: A closed claims analysis. Anesthesiology 104:228, 2006.
16. Feringa HH, Bax JJ, Boersma E, et al: High-dose beta-blockers and tight heart rate control reduce myocardial ischemia and troponin T release in vascular surgery patients. Circulation 114:I344, 2006.
17. Landesberg G, Beattie WS, Mosseri M, et al: Perioperative myocardial infarction. Circulation 119:2936, 2009.

18. Pronovost PJ, Angus DC, Dorman T, et al: Physician staffing patterns and clinical outcomes in critically ill patients: a systematic review. JAMA 288:2151, 2002.

19. Mohler ER 3rd, Mantha S, Miller AB, et al: Should troponin and creatinine kinase be routinely measured after vascular surgery? Vasc Med 12:175, 2007.

Reducing Cardiac Risks

20. Mahla E, Baumann A, Rehak P, et al: N-terminal pro-brain natriuretic peptide identifies patients at high risk for adverse cardiac outcome after vascular surgery. Anesthesiology 106:1088, 2007.

21. Goei D, Schouten O, Boersma E, et al: Influence of renal function on the usefulness of N-terminal pro-B-type natriuretic peptide as a prognostic cardiac risk marker in patients undergoing noncardiac vascular surgery. Am J Cardiol 101:122, 2008.

22. Rodseth RN, Padayachee L, Biccard BM: A meta-analysis of the utility of pre-operative brain natriuretic peptide in predicting early and intermediate-term mortality and major adverse cardiac events in vascular surgical patients. Anaesthesia 63:1226, 2008.

23. Karthikeyan G, Moncur RA, Levine O, et al: Is a pre-operative brain natriuretic peptide or N-terminal pro-B-type natriuretic peptide measurement an independent predictor of adverse cardiovascular outcomes within 30 days of noncardiac surgery? A systematic review and meta-analysis of observational studies. J Am Coll Cardiol 54:1599, 2009.

24. McFalls EO, Ward HB, Moritz TE, et al: Coronary-artery revascularization before elective major vascular surgery. N Engl J Med 351:2795, 2004.

25. Poldermans D, Schouten O, Vidakovic R, et al: A clinical randomized trial to evaluate the safety of a noninvasive approach in high-risk patients undergoing major vascular surgery: The DECREASE-V Pilot Study. J Am Coll Cardiol 49:1763, 2007.

26. Schouten O, van Kuijk JP, Flu WJ, et al: Long-term outcome of prophylactic coronary revascularization in cardiac high-risk patients undergoing major vascular surgery (from the randomized DECREASE-V Pilot Study). Am J Cardiol 103:897, 2009.

27. Garcia S, Moritz TE, Ward HB, et al: Usefulness of revascularization of patients with multivessel coronary artery disease before elective vascular surgery for abdominal aortic and peripheral occlusive disease. Am J Cardiol 102:809, 2008.

28. Monaco M, Stassano P, Di Tommaso L, et al: Systematic strategy of prophylactic coronary angiography improves long-term outcome after major vascular surgery in medium- to high-risk patients: A prospective, randomized study. J Am Coll Cardiol 54:989, 2009.

29. Back MR, Leo F, Cuthbertson D, et al: Long-term survival after vascular surgery: specific influence of cardiac factors and implications for preoperative evaluation. J Vasc Surg 40:752, 2004.

30. Feringa HH, Elhendy A, Karagiannis SE, et al: Improving risk assessment with cardiac testing in peripheral arterial disease. Am J Med 120:531, 2007.

31. Godet G, Le Manach Y, Lesache F, et al: Drug-eluting stent thrombosis in patients undergoing non-cardiac surgery: is it always a problem? Br J Anaesth 100:472, 2008.

32. Anwaruddin S, Askari AT, Saudye H, et al: Characterization of post-operative risk associated with prior drug-eluting stent use. JACC Cardiovasc Interv 2:542, 2009.

33. Dunkelgrun M, Boersma E, Schouten O, et al: Bisoprolol and fluvastatin for the reduction of perioperative cardiac mortality and myocardial infarction in intermediate-risk patients undergoing noncardiovascular surgery: A randomized controlled trial (DECREASE-IV). Ann Surg 249:921, 2009.

34. Lindenauer PK, Pekow P, Wang K, et al: Perioperative beta-blocker therapy and mortality after major noncardiac surgery. N Engl J Med 353:349, 2005.

35. Chopra V, Eagle KA: Perioperative beta-blockers for cardiac risk reduction: Time for clarity. JAMA 303:551, 2010.

GUIDELINES LEE A. FLEISHER AND JOSHUA BECKMAN

Reducing Cardiac Risk with Noncardiac Surgery

Currently, specialty societies have published two sets of guidelines on perioperative cardiovascular evaluation and management for noncardiac surgery. An American College of Cardiology/American Heart Association (ACC/AHA) task force published guidelines in 1996, and updated them in 2009.[1] The Task Force for Preoperative Cardiac Risk Assessment and Perioperative Cardiac Management in Non-cardiac Surgery of the European Society of Cardiology (ESC), and endorsed by the European Society of Anaesthesiology (ESA), published guidelines in 2009.[2] The two sets of guidelines are similar and use a sequential algorithmic approach to testing, but differ in how they rate the evidence on beta-adrenergic receptor blocking agents (beta blockers). For details of the European guidelines, see additional content on the website.

The ACC/AHA guidelines emphasize the importance of a directed history and physical examination, including assessment of functional capacity and the revised cardiac risk index (RCRI) or Lee index risk factors. Risk factors include age older than 70 years, prior myocardial infarction, angina, congestive heart failure, prior cerebrovascular event, diabetes mellitus, and renal insufficiency. Clinicians should give attention to noncardiac comorbid conditions as well as cardiac issues. The ACC/AHA guidelines do not endorse any single risk prediction decision aid, but instead recommend a stepwise algorithm to identify patients most appropriate for noninvasive testing for further risk stratification (see Fig. 85-2). Each step includes the class of recommendation and the level of evidence.

ANCILLARY TESTING

ACC/AHA recommendations for the use of tests in patients undergoing noncardiac surgery are summarized in **Table 85G-1**. In the ACC/AHA guidelines, the routine 12-lead electrocardiogram (ECG) is recommended for patients undergoing vascular surgery or with at least one RCRI clinical risk factor. They recommend restraint in the use of ECGs for asymptomatic patients undergoing low-risk procedures. Routine use of echocardiography to assess left ventricular (LV) function is discouraged unless patients have worsening heart failure or dyspnea of unknown cause. Similarly, routine use of exercise or pharmacologic stress testing in asymptomatic patients without evidence of coronary artery disease is considered a Class III indication (not supported by evidence).

The ACC/AHA recommendations for the use of coronary revascularization (**Table 85G-2**) aim to improve the patient's long-term cardiovascular prognosis and minimize the risk of an acute complication during the procedure. In general, the same indications determine whether a nonsurgical patient warrants coronary angiography in the preoperative setting. For patients who require percutaneous revascularization, a strategy using balloon angioplasty alone or in conjunction with a bare metal stent is recommended because of the mandate for 12 months of dual antiplatelet therapy after drug-eluting stent deployment.[3] The ESC guidelines recommended that percutaneous coronary intervention (PCI) or coronary artery bypass grafting (CABG) be performed according to the applicable guidelines for management in stable angina pectoris. **Table 85G-3** lists the recommendations regarding timing of noncardiac surgery after coronary revascularization, particularly PCI. Both the ACC/AHA and ESC guidelines propose algorithms regarding the optimal management of surgery based on previous PCI (**Fig. 85G-1**; see website).[2]

RISK REDUCTION INTERVENTIONS

The ACC/AHA guidelines emphasize that "It is almost never appropriate to recommend coronary bypass surgery or other invasive interventions such as coronary angioplasty in an effort to reduce the risk of noncardiac surgery when they would not otherwise be indicated." Thus, they give more attention to medical therapies and monitoring interventions for higher-risk patients.

In 2009, ACC/AHA published a focused update on the perioperative use of beta blockers that responded to new data from clinical trials.[4] The updated guidelines support the use of beta blockers in various patient subgroups (**Fig. 85G-2**), especially patients with coronary heart disease or at high cardiac risk who are undergoing vascular surgery; those who are taking a beta blocker to treat angina, hypertension, or symptomatic arrhythmias; and those with other ACC/AHA Class I guideline recommendations. The guidelines are somewhat less supportive of beta blocker use in other populations, for whom the ideal target populations, doses, and routes of administration have yet to be delineated. The answers to practical questions, such as how, when, and how long to continue perioperative beta blocker therapy, also remain uncertain. The guidelines are uniform in the recommendation of dose titration to heart rate and blood pressure. A large clinical trial has shown that administration of oral, long-acting beta blockers initiated at the time of surgery in the absence of dose titration results in increased total mortality and stroke.[5] This strategy received a Class III (not supported by the evidence and may be harmful) recommendation. The ESC guidelines are more supportive of perioperative beta blockers; they are recommended for patients who have known ischemic heart disease (IHD) or myocardial ischemia according to preoperative stress testing, and for patients scheduled for high-risk surgery.

TABLE 85G-1 Recommendations for Noninvasive Stress Testing Before Noncardiac Surgery

Class I

1. Patients with active cardiac conditions in whom noncardiac surgery is planned should be evaluated and treated per ACC/AHA guidelines* before noncardiac surgery (level of evidence: B).

Class IIa

1. Noninvasive stress testing of patients with three or more clinical risk factors and poor functional capacity (less than 4 METs) who require vascular surgery[†] is reasonable if it will change management (level of evidence: B).

Class IIb

1. Noninvasive stress testing may be considered for patients with at least one or two clinical risk factors and poor functional capacity (less than 4 metabolic equivalents [METs]) who require intermediate risk or vascular surgery if it will change management (level of evidence: B).

Class III

1. Noninvasive testing is not useful for patients with no clinical risk factors undergoing intermediate-risk noncardiac surgery (level of evidence: C).
2. Noninvasive testing is not useful for patients undergoing low-risk noncardiac surgery (level of evidence: C).

*See Fleisher and colleagues[1] for the following references: ACC/AHA/ESC Guidelines for the Management of Patients With Atrial Fibrillation,[108] ACC/AHA/ACP Guidelines for the Management of Patients with Chronic Stable Angina,[188] ACC/AHA 2005 Guideline Update for the Diagnosis and Management of Chronic Heart Failure in the Adult,[189] ACC/AHA Guidelines for the Management of Patients With ST-Elevation Myocardial Infarction,[49] ACC/AHA/ESC Guidelines for the Management of Patients With Supraventricular Arrythmias,[190] ACC/AHA 2002 Guideline Update for the Management of Patients With Unstable Angina and Non-ST-Segment Elevation Myocardial Infarction[187] ACC/AHA 2006 Guidelines for the Management of Patients With Valvular Heart Disease,[102] and ACC/AHA/ESC Guidelines for the Management of Patients With Ventricular Arrhythmias and the Prevention of Sudden Cardiac Death.[191]
[†]Vascular surgery is defined by emergency aortic and other major vascular surgery and peripheral vascular surgery.

From Fleisher LA, Beckman JA, Brown KA, et al: 2009 ACCF/AHA focused update on perioperative beta blockade incorporated into the ACC/AHA 2007 guidelines on perioperative cardiovascular evaluation and care for noncardiac surgery. J Am Coll Cardiol 54:e13, 2009.

TABLE 85G-2 Preoperative Coronary Revascularization with CABG or Percutaneous Coronary Intervention

Class I*

1. Coronary revascularization before noncardiac surgery is useful in patients with stable angina who have significant left main coronary artery stenosis (level of evidence: A).
2. Coronary revascularization before noncardiac surgery is useful in patients with stable angina who have three-vessel disease (survival benefit is greater when LV ejection fraction [EF] is less than 0.50; level of evidence: A).
3. Coronary revascularization before noncardiac surgery is useful in patients with stable angina who have two-vessel disease with significant proximal left anterior descending artery stenosis and either EF less than 0.50 or demonstrable ischemia on noninvasive testing (level of evidence: A).
4. Coronary revascularization before noncardiac surgery is recommended for patients with high-risk unstable angina or non–ST-segment elevation myocardial infarction (MI; level of evidence: A).
5. Coronary revascularization before noncardiac surgery is recommended for patients with acute ST-elevation MI (level of evidence: A).

Class IIa

1. In patients in whom coronary revascularization with PCI is appropriate for mitigation of cardiac symptoms and who need elective noncardiac surgery in the subsequent 12 months, a strategy of balloon angioplasty or bare metal stent placement followed by 4 to 6 weeks of dual antiplatelet therapy is probably indicated (level of evidence: B).
2. In patients who have received drug-eluting coronary stents and who must undergo urgent surgical procedures that mandate the discontinuation of thienopyridine therapy, it is reasonable to continue aspirin if at all possible and restart the thienopyridine as soon as possible (level of evidence: C).

Class IIb

1. The usefulness of preoperative coronary revascularization is not well established in high-risk ischemic patients (e.g., abnormal dobutamine stress echocardiogram, with at least five segments of wall motion abnormalities; level of evidence: C).
2. The usefulness of preoperative coronary revascularization is not well established for low-risk ischemic patients with an abnormal dobutamine stress echocardiogram (segments 1 to 4; level of evidence: B).

Class III

1. It is not recommended that routine prophylactic coronary revascularization be performed in patients with stable coronary artery disease (CAD) before noncardiac surgery (level of evidence: B).
2. Elective noncardiac surgery is not recommended within 4 to 6 weeks of bare metal coronary stent implantation or within 12 months of drug-eluting coronary stent implantation in patients for whom thienopyridine therapy, or aspirin and thienopyridine therapy, will need to be discontinued perioperatively (level of evidence: B).
3. Elective noncardiac surgery is not recommended within 4 weeks of coronary revascularization with balloon angioplasty (level of evidence: B).

*All Class I indications are consistent with the ACC/AHA 2004 Guideline Update for Coronary Artery Bypass Graft Surgery. (Eagle KA, Guyton RA, Davidoff R, et al: ACC/AHA 2004 guideline update for coronary artery bypass graft surgery: A report of the American College of Cardiology/American Heart Association Task Force on Practice Guidelines [Committee to Update the 1999 Guidelines for Coronary Artery Bypass Graft Surgery]. Circulation 110:e340-437, 2004).

From Fleisher LA, Beckman JA, Brown KA, et al: 2009 ACCF/AHA focused update on perioperative beta blockade incorporated into the ACC/AHA 2007 guidelines on perioperative cardiovascular evaluation and care for noncardiac surgery. J Am Coll Cardiol 54:e13, 2009.

TABLE 85G-3	Recommendations on Timing of Noncardiac Surgery in Cardiac-Stable or Asymptomatic Patients with Prior Revascularization		
RECOMMENDATIONS		**CLASS OF RECOMMENDATION**	**LEVEL OF EVIDENCE**
It is recommended that patients with previous CABG in the last 5 years be sent for noncardiac surgery without further delay.		I	C
It is recommended that noncardiac surgery be performed in patients with recent bare metal stent implantation after a minimum of 6 weeks and optimally 3 months following the intervention.		I	B
It is recommended that noncardiac surgery be performed in patients with recent drug-eluting stent implantation no sooner than 12 months following the intervention.		I	B
Consideration should be given to postponing noncardiac surgery in patients with recent balloon angioplasty until at least 2 weeks following the intervention.		IIa	B

From Poldermans D, Bax JJ, Boersma E, et al: Guidelines for pre-operative cardiac risk assessment and perioperative cardiac management in non-cardiac surgery: The Task Force for Preoperative Cardiac Risk Assessment and Perioperative Cardiac Management in Non-cardiac Surgery of the European Society of Cardiology (ESC) and endorsed by the European Society of Anaesthesiology (ESA). Eur Heart J 30:2769-812, 2009.

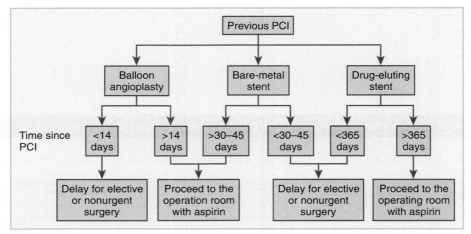

FIGURE 85G-1 Proposed approach to the management of patients with previous PCI requiring noncardiac surgery. (*From Fleisher LA, Beckman JA, Brown KA, et al: 2009 ACCF/AHA focused update on perioperative beta blockade incorporated into the ACC/AHA 2007 guidelines on perioperative cardiovascular evaluation and care for noncardiac surgery. J Am Coll Cardiol 54:e13, 2009.*)

Similar to the ACC/AHA guidelines, continuation of beta blockers is recommended for patients previously treated with beta blockers because of IHD, arrhythmias, or hypertension (see website).

Intraoperative nitroglycerin is supported for patients with acute ischemic syndromes who must undergo urgent noncardiac procedures. The ACC/AHA guidelines warn that prophylactic use of nitroglycerin must take into account the anesthetic plan and patient's hemodynamics, and must recognize the risk of vasodilation and hypovolemia during anesthesia and surgery. The ACC/AHA task force did not find sufficient evidence to balance risks and benefits of intra-aortic balloon counterpulsation for patients with myocardial ischemic syndromes or routine use of transesophageal echocardiography.

The ACC/AHA guidelines acknowledge that the use of a pulmonary artery catheter (PAC) may be reasonable for patients at risk for major hemodynamic disturbances easily detected by a PAC. However, because incorrect interpretation of data from a PAC may cause harm, the decision must be based on three parameters—patient disease, surgical procedure (i.e., intraoperative and postoperative fluid shifts), and practice setting (experience in PAC use and interpretation of results). ST-segment monitoring to detect perioperative ischemia in patients with coronary heart disease can be useful, but the guidelines acknowledge that no studies have shown that this intervention directs therapy that improves outcome.

According to the ACC/AHA guidelines, perioperative surveillance for acute coronary syndromes using routine electrocardiography and cardiac serum biomarkers is unnecessary for clinically low-risk patients undergoing low-risk procedures. In patients with high or intermediate clinical risk with known or suspected coronary artery disease who are undergoing high- or intermediate-risk procedures, the guidelines recommend performance of electrocardiography at baseline, immediately after the surgical procedure, and daily on the first 2 days after surgery. The guidelines support cardiac troponin measurements for detection of myocardial injury in patients with evidence of myocardial ischemia, but not their routine measurement.

2007 Perioperative guideline recommendations	2009 Perioperative focused update recommendations	Comments
Class I		
1. Beta blockers should be continued in patients undergoing surgery who are receiving beta blockers to treat angina, symptomatic arrhythmias, hypertension, or other ACC/AHA Class I guideline indications. (Level of Evidence: C)	1. Beta blockers should be continued in patients undergoing surgery who are receiving beta blockers for treatment of conditions with ACCF/AHA Class I guideline indications for the drugs. (Level of Evidence: C)	2007 recommendation remains current in 2009 update with revised wording.
2. Beta blockers should be given to patients undergoing vascular surgery who are at high cardiac risk owing to the finding of ischemia on preoperative testing. (Level of Evidence: B)		Deleted/combined recommendation (class of recommendation changed from I to IIa for patients with cardiac ischemia on preoperative testing).
Class IIa		
1. Beta blockers are probably recommended for patients undergoing vascular surgery in whom preoperative assessment indentifies coronary heart disease. (Level of Evidence: B)	1. Beta blockers titrated to heart rate and blood pressure are probably recommended for patients undergoing vascular surgery who are at high cardiac risk owing to coronary artery disease or the finding of cardiac ischemia on preoperative testing. (Level of Evidence: B)	Modified/combined recommendation (wording revised and class of recommendation changed from I to IIa for patients with cardiac ischemia on preoperative testing).
2. Beta blockers are probably recommended for patients in whom preoperative assessment for vascular surgery identifies high cardiac risk, as defined by the presence of more than 1 clinical risk factor.* (Level of Evidence: B)	2. Beta blockers titrated to heart rate and blood pressure are reasonable for patients in whom preoperative assessment for vascular surgery identifies high cardiac risk, as defined by the presence of more than 1 clinical risk factor.* (Level of Evidence: C)	Modified recommendation (level of evidence changed from B to C).
3. Beta blockers are probably recommended for patients in whom preoperative assessment identifies coronary heart disease or high cardiac risk, as defined by the presence of more than 1 clinical risk factor,* who are undergoing intermediate-risk or vascular surgery. (Level of Evidence: B)	3. Beta blockers titrated to heart rate and blood pressure are reasonable for patients in whom preoperative assessment identifies coronary artery disease or high cardiac risk, as defined by the presence of more than 1 clinical risk factor,* who are undergoing intermediate-risk surgery. (Level of Evidence: B)	2007 recommendation remains current in 2009 update with revised wording.
Class IIb		
1. The usefulness of beta blockers is uncertain for patients who are undergoing either intermediate-risk procedures or vascular surgery, in whom preoperative assessment identifies a single clinical risk factor.* (Level of Evidence: C)	1. The usefulness of beta blockers is uncertain for patients who are undergoing either intermediate-risk procedures or vascular surgery in whom preoperative assessment identifies a single clinical risk factor in the absence of coronary artery disease.* (Level of Evidence: C)	2007 recommendation remains current in 2009 update with revised wording.
2. The usefulness of beta blockers is uncertain in patients undergoing vascular surgery with no clinical risk factors who are not currently taking beta blockers. (Level of Evidence: B)	2. The usefulness of beta blockers is uncertain for patients undergoing vascular surgery with no clinical risk factors* who are not currently taking beta blockers. (Level of Evidence: B)	2007 recommendation remains current in 2009 update.
Class III		
1. Beta blockers should not be given to patients undergoing surgery who have absolute contraindications to beta blockade. (Level of Evidence: B)	1. Beta blockers should not be given to patients undergoing surgery who have absolute contraindications to beta blockade. (Level of Evidence: C)	2007 recommendation remains current in 2009 update.
	2. Routine administration of high-dose beta blockers in the absence of dose titration is not useful and may be harmful to patients not currently taking beta blockers who are undergoing noncardiac surgery. (Level of Evidence: B)	New recommendation

* Clinical risk factors include history of ischemic heart disease, history of compensated or prior heart failure, history of cerebrovascular disease, diabetes mellitus, and renal insufficiency (defined in the Revised Cardiac Risk Index as a preoperative serum creatinine of >2 mg/dL). ACC indicates American College of Cardiology; and AHA, American Heart Association.

FIGURE 85G-2 ACC/AHA recommendations for use of perioperative beta blockers. (From Fleischmann KE, Beckman JA, Buller CE, et al: 2009 ACCF/AHA focused update on perioperative beta blockade. J Am Coll Cardiol 54:2102, 2009.)

REFERENCES

1. Fleisher LA, Beckman JA, Brown KA, et al: 2009 ACCF/AHA focused update on perioperative beta blockade incorporated into the ACC/AHA 2007 guidelines on perioperative cardiovascular evaluation and care for noncardiac surgery. J Am Coll Cardiol 54:e13, 2009.
2. Poldermans D, Bax JJ, Boersma E, et al: Guidelines for pre-operative cardiac risk assessment and perioperative cardiac management in non-cardiac surgery: The Task Force for Preoperative Cardiac Risk Assessment and Perioperative Cardiac Management in Non-cardiac Surgery of the European Society of Cardiology (ESC) and endorsed by the European Society of Anaesthesiology (ESA). Eur Heart J 30:2769, 2009.
3. Grines CL, Bonow RO, Casey DE Jr, et al: Prevention of premature discontinuation of dual antiplatelet therapy in patients with coronary artery stents: A science advisory from the American Heart Association, American College of Cardiology, Society for Cardiovascular Angiography and Interventions, American College of Surgeons, and American Dental Association, with representation from the American College of Physicians. J Am Coll Cardiol 49:734, 2007.
4. Fleischmann KE, Beckman JA, Buller CE, et al: 2009 ACCF/AHA focused update on perioperative beta blockade. J Am Coll Cardiol 54:2102, 2009.
5. Devereaux PJ, Yang H, Yusuf S, et al: Effects of extended-release metoprolol succinate in patients undergoing non-cardiac surgery (POISE trial): A randomised controlled trial. Lancet 371:1839, 2008.

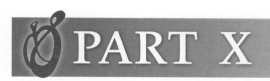

PART X

CARDIOVASCULAR DISEASE AND DISORDERS OF OTHER ORGANS

CHAPTER 86

Endocrine Disorders and Cardiovascular Disease

Irwin Klein

Medical science has few areas in which basic science investigation is linked more closely to clinical observations and therapy than in cardiovascular endocrinology. As our understanding of the cellular and molecular effects of various hormones has evolved, we can better understand the clinical manifestations that arise from excess hormone secretion and glandular failure, leading to hormone deficiency states. More than 200 years ago, English physician Caleb Hillier Parry described a woman with goiter and palpitations whose "each systole shook the whole thorax." He was the first to suggest a connection between diseases of the heart and enlargement of the thyroid gland. The cardiovascular abnormalities associated with pathologic changes of endocrine glands were recognized before the identification of the specific hormones produced by these glands. This chapter reviews the spectrum of cardiac disease states that arise from changes in specific endocrine function. This approach allows us to explore the cellular mechanisms whereby various hormones can alter the cardiovascular system through actions on cardiac myocytes, vascular smooth muscle cells, and other target cells and tissues.

Pituitary Gland

The pituitary gland consists of two distinct anatomic portions. The anterior pituitary, or adenohypophysis, contains six different cell types; five of these produce polypeptide or glycoprotein hormones, and the sixth is classically referred to as being composed of nonsecretory chromophobic cells. Of these cell types, the somatotropic cells, which secrete human growth hormone (hGH), and the corticotropic cells, which produce adrenocorticotropic hormone (ACTH), can contribute to cardiac disease. The posterior pituitary, or neurohypophysis, is the anatomic location for the nerve terminals that secrete vasopressin (antidiuretic hormone) or oxytocin.

Growth Hormone

In adults, excessive growth hormone secretion before the fusion of bony epiphysis leads to gigantism, whereas increased secretion of hGH after maturation of the long bones leads to acromegaly. Growth hormone exerts its cellular effects through two major pathways. The first is by

hormone binding to specific growth hormone receptors on target cells. These receptors have been identified in the heart, skeletal muscle, fat, liver, and kidneys, as well as in many additional cell types throughout fetal development.[1] The second growth-promoting effect of hGH results from stimulation of synthesis of insulin-like growth factor type 1 (IGF-1). This protein is produced primarily in the liver, but other cell types can produce IGF-1 under the influence of hGH.

Shortly after the identification of the IGF family, it was proposed that most actions of growth hormone are mediated through this second messenger. Clinical disease activity of patients with growth hormone excess (acromegaly) correlates better with serum levels of IGF-1 than with hGH levels. The ability to promote glucose uptake and cellular protein synthesis gave rise to the term *insulin-like*. IGF-1 binds to its cognate IGF-1 receptor, localized on almost all cell types. Transgenic experiments have demonstrated that the presence of IGF-1 receptors on cell types is closely linked to the ability of those cells to divide. Studies in which the IGF-1 receptor was overexpressed in cardiac myocytes reportedly produced an increased myocyte number and mitotic rate, and enhanced the replication of postdifferentiated myocytes. The harnessing of this action potentially could benefit genetic manipulation and repair of the diseased myocardium.

Infusion of hGH or IGF-1 acutely changes hemodynamics. The acute increases in cardiac contractility and cardiac output may be caused, at least in part, by a decrease in systemic vascular resistance and cardiac afterload.[2] Short-term administration of hGH and IGF-1 does not increase blood pressure, implying that the increase in cardiac output results from changes in systemic vascular resistance.[3,4]

Cardiovascular Manifestations of Acromegaly

Acromegaly is a relatively uncommon condition (approximately 900 new cases each year in the United States). Acromegaly and pituitary-dependent human gigantism are associated with markedly increased morbidity and mortality, primarily from cardiovascular disease. Untreated acromegaly, identified by its characteristic clinical signs and symptoms and by increased hGH secretion, markedly shortens life expectancy, with less than 20% of patients surviving beyond 60 years. Multiple studies have implicated increased neoplasia arising from the gastrointestinal tract, colon polyps, colon cancer, and pulmonary disease in this increased mortality.[5] However, cardiovascular and cerebrovascular changes, including hypertension, cardiomegaly, congestive heart failure, and cerebral vascular accidents, are the major events that limit survival.[6]

The cardiovascular and hemodynamic effects of acromegaly vary considerably depending on age, severity of disease, and disease duration.[7] Patients diagnosed with less than 5 years of disease activity had no significant change in systolic or diastolic blood pressure, but echocardiographic determination of left ventricular mass index increased almost 35% and cardiac index increased 24%.[8] Measures of systolic function, including stroke index, increased significantly, and systemic vascular resistance rose by 20%. Left ventricular diastolic function was normal.[6] These studies contrast with reports that longer duration of acromegaly produces left ventricular dysfunction and cardiomyopathy. In untreated acromegaly, global left ventricular diastolic dysfunction accompanies cardiac hypertrophy. Regional myocardial systolic strain abnormalities, identified by Doppler imaging, reversed with treatment.[9]

Known cardiac disease risk factors—including hypertension, insulin resistance, diabetes mellitus, and hyperlipidemia—frequently occur in patients with acromegaly. Although initial reports suggested that accelerated atherosclerosis caused impairment of cardiac function in long-standing acromegaly, a postmortem study revealed significant coronary artery disease in only 11% of patients dying from disease-related causes. Angiography shows normal or dilated coronary arteries in most cases. Nuclear stress testing is positive in less than 25% of patients, indicating that atherosclerosis and ischemic heart disease are unlikely to account for the marked degrees of biventricular cardiac hypertrophy, cardiac failure, and cardiovascular mortality. A rather specific functional and histologic myocyte change appears to arise from prolonged excess serum levels of hGH and IGF-1.[8] As many as two thirds of acromegaly patients have echocardiographic criteria for left ventricular hypertrophy (LVH).[6,7] Right ventricular mass also increases in acromegaly, indicating a more generalized process beyond systemic hypertension.[9] Asymmetrical septal hypertrophy, initially thought to be common in patients with acromegaly, is an unusual finding. Acromegaly increases the prevalence of aortic and mitral valve disease, which persists despite disease cure.[10] Progressive mitral valve regurgitation and left ventricular strain occur in patients with uncontrolled acromegaly.[11] Acromegaly patients may present with dilation of the aortic root and/or defects of the cardiac conduction system.[7,12]

Histologic evaluation of acromegaly cardiac tissue reveals an increase in myocyte size (hypertrophy) without an increase in cell number. Acromegaly produces interstitial fibrosis and infiltration of a variety of inflammatory cells, including mononuclear cells consistent with myocarditis.[6] The absence of cell necrosis in the presence of an inflammatory reaction has raised the question of whether some of these histologic findings can be accounted for by IGF-1–promoted programmed cell death (apoptosis).

Functional changes accompany pathologic involvement of the heart in acromegaly.[8,9] Although approximately 10% of newly diagnosed patients have signs and symptoms of cardiac compromise, this percentage increases markedly with disease duration.[11-13] Some studies have reported a low incidence of overt left ventricular failure, suggesting that supervening factors, including hypertension, type 2 diabetes, and hyperlipidemia, are necessary to impair function. In acromegaly, LVH and congestive heart failure can occur in long-standing disease without hypertension, indicating that high levels of growth hormone and/or IGF-1 can produce cardiac myopathic changes per se. Successful therapy reverses many, if not all, of these findings.[14,15]

Abnormalities on the electrocardiogram (ECG), including left axis deviation, septal Q waves, ST-T wave depression, abnormal QT dispersion, and conduction system defects, occur in up to 50% of acromegaly patients. A variety of dysrhythmias can occur, including atrial and ventricular ectopic beats, sick sinus syndrome, and supraventricular and ventricular tachycardias.[6] Fourfold increases in complex ventricular arrhythmias and late potentials observed in a signal-averaged ECG, thought to be predictors of ventricular irritability, were also more common in active acromegaly when compared with treated patients.[12]

In contrast, exercise stress testing with electrocardiographic monitoring did not show inducible rhythm disturbances or evidence of ischemia, suggesting that left ventricular rhythm disturbances are not related to any underlying ischemia.

Secondary hypertension associated with acromegaly occurs in 20% to 40% of patients.[5-7] Given the overall high prevalence rate of hypertension in the adult population and the insidious onset of acromegaly, determining whether hypertension is secondary or merely coincidental is difficult. Improvement with therapy, however, suggests that they are related.[15] Although observational studies of survival in acromegaly initially suggested that hypertension was not an independent risk factor for mortality, a survey of patients dying of the disease found that mean blood pressures were higher than in those who survived.[5] The mechanism underlying hypertension in acromegaly is not clearly understood. Newly diagnosed patients with short-duration disease had systolic and diastolic blood pressures no different from those in age- and sex-matched controls, whereas the cardiac index was significantly increased. In long-standing acromegaly patients, the arterial intimal thickness is increased, and these changes respond to hGH lowering.[2]

Growth hormone administration promotes sodium retention and volume expansion, and appears to have a potent antinatriuretic effect independent of any effect on aldosterone.[3,16] Studies of the renin-angiotensin-aldosterone system have shown a failure to inhibit renin release optimally by volume expansion. Angiotensin II inhibitors cause a paradoxical increase in blood pressure in patients with acromegaly. The role of hyperinsulinemia in the hypertension of acromegaly has been questioned. Increased serum insulin can contribute to urinary sodium retention, impairment of endothelial-dependent vasodilation, and increased sympathetic activity.

DIAGNOSIS. In 99% of cases, acromegaly arises from benign adenomas of the anterior pituitary gland.[5,15] At diagnosis, most of these neoplasms are classified as macroadenomas (>10 mm), and patients have clinical evidence of disease for longer than 10 years. The diagnosis can be confirmed by demonstrating a serum growth hormone level higher than 5 ng/dL and a serum IGF-1 level higher than 300 mIU/mL, measured 1 hour after a 100-g glucose load. In most patients, fasting growth hormone levels are higher than 10 ng/mL. Tumor localization can be established by magnetic resonance imaging (MRI) dedicated to the pituitary gland. Rarely, growth hormone–releasing hormone (GH-RH) can be secreted, causing diffuse hyperplasia of the pituitary. Such changes must prompt consideration of a neoplastic lesion residing in other parts (ectopic) of the endocrine system.

THERAPY. Transsphenoidal surgery with resection of the adenoma is the procedure of choice for initial management. If hGH and/or IGF-1 levels remain elevated, radiotherapy in older patients or dopamine or somatostatin receptor agonists in younger patients can restore normal serum growth hormone and IGF-1 levels. Octreotide acetate is a pharmacologic analogue to somatostatin and is effective in the vast majority of patients to lower hGH to less than 5 ng/mL. Primary therapy might involve lowering IGF-1 levels and shrinking tumor size in selected cases.[15,17] The cardiovascular complications of acromegaly, including hypertension, LVH, and left ventricular dysfunction, improve with treatment, and survival is significantly better in patients achieving disease remission.[7,11] Pegvisomant, a growth hormone receptor antagonist, can normalize IGF-1 levels in long-term therapy and may play a role in somatostatin-resistant patients.[14]

Adrenal Gland

Adrenocorticotropic Hormone and Cortisol

The adrenocorticotropic cells in the anterior pituitary synthesize a large protein (pro-opiomelanocortin), which is then processed within the corticotroph cell into a family of smaller proteins that include alpha-melanocyte–stimulating hormone, beta-endorphin, and ACTH. ACTH, in turn, binds to specific cells within the adrenal gland. The adrenal gland anatomically consists of two major segments, the cortex and medulla.

The cortex zona glomerulosa produces aldosterone and the zona fasciculata produces primarily cortisol and some androgenic steroids. The zona reticularis also produces cortisol and androgens. ACTH regulates the synthesis of cortisol in the zona fasciculata and reticularis. The zona glomerulosa shows much less ACTH responsiveness and responds primarily to angiotensin II by increased aldosterone secretion.

Cushing Disease

Excess cortisol secretion and its attendant clinical disease states can arise from excess pituitary release of ACTH (Cushing disease) or through the adenomatous or rarely malignant neoplastic process arising in the adrenal gland itself (Cushing syndrome). Well-characterized conditions of adrenal glucocorticoid and mineralocorticoid excess appear to result from the excessively high levels of (ectopic) ACTH produced by small cell carcinoma of the lung, carcinoid tumors, pancreatic islet cell tumors, medullary thyroid cancer, and other adenocarcinomas and hematologic malignancies.

Cortisol, a member of the glucocorticoid family of steroid hormones, binds to monomeric receptors located within the cytoplasm of many cell types (**Fig. 86-1**). The unliganded glucocorticoid receptors are bound to heat shock protein complexes. After binding cortisol, the receptors dissociate from these complexes, homodimerize or occasionally heterodimerize, translocate to the

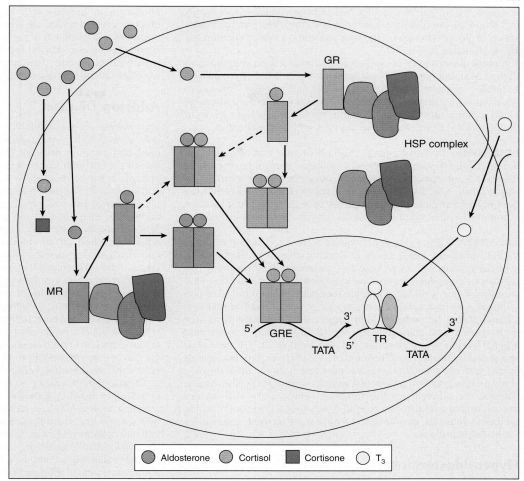

FIGURE 86-1 Schematic representation of a generalized nuclear hormone receptor mechanism of action. The mineralocorticoid receptor (MR) has similar affinities for aldosterone and cortisol. Circulating levels of cortisol are 100 to 1000 times greater than that of aldosterone. In MR-responsive cells, the enzyme 11-beta-hydroxysteroid dehydrogenase metabolizes cortisol to cortisone, thereby allowing aldosterone to bind to MR. MR and the glucocorticoid receptor (GR) are cytoplasmic receptors that after binding ligand, translocate to the nucleus and bind to glucocorticoid response elements (GREs) in the promoter regions of responsive genes. T_3 is transported into the cell via specific membrane proteins and binds to thyroid hormone receptors (TRs), which are bound to TREs in the promoter regions of T_3-responsive genes. HSP = heat shock protein; TATA = TATA box promoter region. *(Courtesy of Dr. S. Danzi.)*

nucleus, and function as transcription factors. Several cardiac genes contain glucocorticoid response elements in their promoter regions that confer glucocorticoid responsiveness.[18] These genes include those that encode the voltage-gated potassium channel, as well as protein kinases, which serve to phosphorylate and regulate voltage-gated sodium channels. This expression may be chamber-specific and play a role in the developing fetal heart.[19]

The cardiac effects of glucocorticoid excess in Cushing disease rise from the effects of glucocorticoids on the heart, liver, skeletal muscle, and fat tissue.[18-20] Accelerated atherosclerosis can result from abnormal glucose metabolism with hyperglycemia and hyperinsulinemia, hypertension, and altered clotting and platelet function. The mechanism for cortisol-mediated hypertension is multifactorial. In contrast to aldosterone-induced hypertension, the central administration of glucocorticoids lowers blood pressure.[21] Thus, cortisol-mediated hypertension appears not to result from activation of the mineralocorticoid receptor. In addition, antagonism of glucocorticoid effects via its cytosolic receptor can block cortisol-induced elevations of glucose and insulin levels, but not those related to blood pressure.[22,23] Interestingly, one study has suggested that inhibition of sodium retention is also insufficient to block the cortisol-mediated rise in blood pressure, pointing to the changes in vascular reactivity, systemic vascular resistance, and nitric oxide–mediated vasodilation as candidates for the hypertensive effect.[18]

The rise in serum glucose levels and the development of insulin resistance may activate proinflammatory cytokines such as tumor necrosis factor-α and interleukin-6 (IL-6), which may underlie the accelerated

atherosclerosis of insulin resistance found in other endocrine disease states.[22] Thus, although typically acting as an anti-inflammatory hormone, cortisol excess can promote inflammation and accelerate atherosclerosis by producing insulin resistance, changes in corticosteroid binding protein, and regulation of proinflammatory cytokines.[24] The centripetal obesity characteristic of glucocorticoid excess resembles that seen in the insulin resistance syndromes. Excess androgen production resulting from increased ACTH stimulation of the adrenal cortex may also accelerate atherosclerosis in men and women.

The increased cardiovascular morbidity and mortality of Cushing syndrome can in large part be explained by cerebrovascular disease, peripheral vascular disease, coronary artery disease with myocardial infarction, and chronic congestive heart failure.[20,23] All expected changes in the setting of accelerated atherosclerosis result from hypertension and hyperlipidemia. Studies of left ventricular structure and function have shown hypertrophy and impaired contractility in 40% of patients.[25] Cushing syndrome can present as dilated cardiomyopathy.[26] In addition, the marked muscle weakness resulting from corticosteroid-induced skeletal myopathy contributes to impaired exercise tolerance.

Patients with Cushing disease can exhibit a variety of electrocardiographic changes. The duration of the P-R interval appears to correlate inversely with adrenal cortisol production rates. The mechanism underlying this may relate to the expression or regulation of the voltage-gated sodium channel (SCN5A). Changes in ECGs, specifically in P-R and QT intervals, may also arise from the direct (nongenomic) effects of glucocorticoids on the voltage-gated potassium channel (Kv 1.5) in excitable tissues.[18,20]

A particular complex of cardiac and adrenal lesions, referred to as Carney complex, combines Cushing syndrome, cardiac myxoma, and a variety of pigmented dermal lesions (not café-au-lait).[27] This monogenic autosomal dominant trait maps to the Q2 region of chromosome 17. Myxomas most commonly occur in the left atrium but can occur throughout the heart, occur at young ages, and be multicentric.

DIAGNOSIS. The diagnosis of Cushing disease and Cushing syndrome require the demonstration of increased cortisol production as reflected by an elevated 24-hour, urinary-free cortisol or nocturnal salivary cortisol level.[24] ACTH measurements to determine whether the disease is pituitary, adrenal, or ectopically based, and anatomic localization with MRI of the suspected lesions, confirm the laboratory findings.

TREATMENT. The treatment of excess cortisol production depends on the underlying mechanisms. In Cushing disease, transsphenoidal hypophysectomy with or without postoperative radiation therapy can partially or completely reverse the increased ACTH production of the anterior pituitary. Cushing syndrome requires surgical removal of one (adrenal adenoma, adrenal carcinoma) or both (multiple nodular) adrenal glands. Immediately after surgery, it is necessary to replace both cortisol and mineralocorticoid (fludrocortisone) to prevent adrenal insufficiency. Treatment of the ectopic ACTH syndrome requires identification and treatment of the neoplastic process. Patients treated with exogenous steroids for more than 1 month often develop clinical signs and symptoms of Cushing syndrome. In nonsurgical patients, the adrenal enzyme inhibitor ketoconazole can reverse excess cortisol production. Even mild or subclinical degrees of Cushing syndrome (adrenal incidentaloma) appear to increase the risk for cardiovascular disease.

Hyperaldosteronism

Aldosterone production by the zona glomerulosa is under the control of the renin-angiotensin system. Renin secretion responds primarily to changes in intravascular volume. Aldosterone synthesis and secretion is primarily regulated by angiotensin II, which binds to the angiotensin II type I receptor on the cells of the zona glomerulosa.[28]

The mechanism of action of aldosterone on target tissues resembles that reported for glucocorticoids (see Fig. 86-1). Aldosterone enters cells and binds to the mineralocorticoid receptor, which then translocates to the nucleus and promotes the expression of aldosterone-responsive genes. In addition to kidney cells, in which mineralocorticoid receptors control sodium transport, in vitro studies have demonstrated these receptors in rat cardiac myocytes; they respond to mineralocorticoid stimulation with an increase in protein synthesis. Whether these changes correspond to any relevant in vivo cardiac effects is unclear, but aldosterone may augment the development of cardiac hypertrophy in hypertension.[29]

The aldosterone antagonists spironolactone and eplerenone compete for receptor binding in the cytosol (see Fig. 86-1). They are the most recent class of compounds approved for the treatment of heart failure.[30] Recent studies have defined a role for these agents after acute myocardial infarction and for the treatment of left ventricular dysfunction, heart failure, and hypertension.[31,32]

Although the major cause of increased serum aldosterone levels is in the physiologic response to the activation of the renin-angiotensin system, there are well-recognized aldosterone-producing benign adrenal adenomas (Conn syndrome). Primary hyperaldosteronism augments sodium retention, causes hypertension, increases renal loss of magnesium and potassium, decreases arterial compliance with a rise in systemic vascular resistance and resulting vascular damage, and alters the sympathetic and parasympathetic neural regulation. Many of the changes in the heart and cardiovascular system in hyperaldosteronism result from the associated hypertension.[32] A recent report has linked primary aldosteronism to the development of atrial

fibrillation in patients with hypertension but no structural heart disease. A recent review has discussed the approach to the detection, diagnosis, and treatment of patients with primary aldosteronism.[33] The hyperaldosterone-mediated hypokalemia and much of the associated hypertension respond to the surgical removal of a unilateral (or occasionally bilateral) benign adrenal adenoma(s).[34]

Addison Disease

Long before recognition that the glands situated just above the upper pole of each kidney (suprarenal) synthesize and secrete glucocorticoids and mineralocorticoids, Thomas Addison described the association of atrophy with loss of function of these structures, with marked changes in the cardiovascular system. The hypovolemia, hypotension, and acute cardiovascular collapse resulting from renal sodium wasting, hyperkalemia, and loss of vascular tone are the hallmarks of acute addisonian crisis, one of the most severe endocrine emergencies. Adrenal insufficiency most commonly arises from bilateral loss of adrenal function on an autoimmune basis, as a result of infection, hemorrhage, or metastatic malignancy—or in selected cases, of inborn errors of steroid hormone metabolism.[35] In contrast, secondary adrenal insufficiency, which results from pituitary-dependent loss of ACTH secretion, leads to a fall in glucocorticoid production while mineralocorticoid production, including aldosterone, remains at relatively normal levels. Studies have addressed the issue of relative hypothalamic-pituitary-adrenal insufficiency in acutely ill patients.[36] Although the actual existence of such an entity and diagnostic criteria for establishing this occurrence remain to be validated, it has reopened the question of the need for stress-dose cortisol treatment of critical illness.

Addison disease can occur at any age. The noncardiac symptoms, including increased pigmentation, abdominal pain with nausea and vomiting, and weight loss, can be chronic, whereas the tachycardia, hypotension, and electrolyte abnormalities herald impending cardiovascular collapse and crisis.[35] Blood pressure measurements uniformly show low diastolic pressure (<60 mm Hg), with significant orthostatic changes reflecting volume loss. Laboratory findings of hyponatremia and hyperkalemia indicate loss of aldosterone production (renin levels are high). Hyperkalemia can alter the ECG, producing low-amplitude P waves and peaked T waves.[36] Newly diagnosed untreated patients with Addison disease have reduced left ventricular, end-systolic, and end-diastolic dimensions compared with controls. Cardiac atrophy is an unusual condition; it is seen in malnutrition caused by anorexia, in astronauts after prolonged space flight, in populations with sodium-deficient diets, and characteristically with Addison disease (teardrop heart; **Fig. 86-2**). This atrophy reflects a response to decreases in cardiac workload, because restoration of normal plasma volume with mineralocorticoid and glucocorticoid replacement increases ventricular mass.

DIAGNOSIS. Acute adrenal insufficiency characteristically occurs in the setting of acute stress, infection, or trauma in a patient with chronic autoimmune adrenal insufficiency, or in children with congenital abnormalities of cortisol metabolism. It can also occur from bilateral adrenal hemorrhage in patients with severe systemic infection or diffuse intravascular coagulation.[35] Secondary adrenal insufficiency can occur in the setting of hypopituitarism, which is usually chronic, but acute changes caused by pituitary hemorrhage (apoplexy) or pituitary inflammation (lymphocytic hypophysitis) can occur. Patients treated with long-term suppressive doses of corticosteroids (>10 mg of prednisone for more than 1 month) can develop acute adrenal insufficiency if treatment is precipitously stopped.

The diagnosis is established when, in the morning or during severe stress, cortisol levels are low (<8 mg/dL) and fail to rise above 20 µg/dL 30 minutes after an intravenous (IV) injection of 0.25 mg of cosyntropin. Diagnosis in the setting of acute illness may be more difficult, and a low (<10 µg/dL) morning serum level of cortisol may suffice to suggest impaired control of secretion.[36]

TREATMENT. Management of acute addisonian crisis needs to address three major issues. The first is adequate hydrocortisone

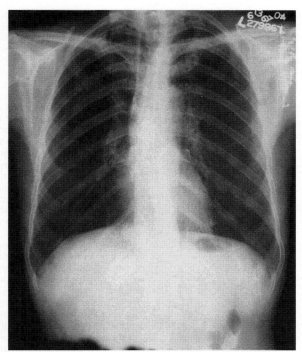

FIGURE 86-2 Routine chest radiograph of a patient with Addison disease related to tuberculosis. In addition to the small cardiac silhouette, there are calcified lymph nodes in the hilum of the right lung. *(Courtesy of Dr. J. B. Naidich.)*

replacement—100 mg given as an initial IV bolus, then 100 mg every 8 hours for the first 24 hours, tapering the dose for the next 72 to 96 hours. The second is the restoration of intravascular fluid deficit using large volumes of normal saline with 5% dextrose. The third is identifying and treating any underlying precipitating cause, including infection, acute cardiac or cerebral ischemia, or intra-abdominal emergency. Chronic treatment is oral corticosteroid and mineralocorticoid (fludrocortisone, 0.1 mg/day) replacement, but these patients are at increased risk for all-cause and cardiovascular mortality.[37]

Parathyroid Disease

Diseases of the parathyroid glands can produce cardiovascular disease and alter cardiac function by two mechanisms. The first is changes in the secretion of parathyroid hormone (PTH), a protein hormone, which affects the heart, vascular smooth muscle cells, and endothelial cells. The second mechanism is changes in serum calcium levels. Serum ionized calcium regulates the synthesis and secretion of PTH by an exquisitely sensitive negative feedback mechanism.[38]

PTH can bind to its receptor and alter the spontaneous beating rate of neonatal cardiac myocytes through an increase in intracellular cyclic adenosine monophosphate (cAMP). PTH can also alter calcium influx and cardiac contractility in adult cardiac myocytes and relaxation of vascular smooth muscle cells. In addition to PTH, a structurally related parathyroid hormone–related peptide (PTHrP) is synthesized and secreted in a variety of tissues, including cardiac myocytes. PTHrP can bind to the PTH receptor on cardiac cells and stimulate cAMP accumulation and contractile activity, as well as regulate L-type calcium currents. Thus, the direct effects of increased serum levels of PTHrP on the heart and systemic vasculature can accompany paraneoplastic syndromes characterized by hypercalcemia.[38]

Hyperparathyroidism

Classic primary hyperparathyroidism producing hypercalcemia most often results from the adenomatous enlargement of one of the four parathyroid glands. The cardiovascular actions of hypercalcemia include the following: an increase in cardiac contractility; shortening of the ventricular action potential duration, primarily through changes in phase 2; and blunting of the T wave and changes in the ST segment, occasionally suggesting cardiac ischemia.[39] The Q-T interval is shortened and occasionally accompanied by decreases in the P-R interval. Treatment with digitalis glycosides appears to increase sensitivity of the heart to hypercalcemia.

Hypercalcemia has been linked to pathologic changes in the heart, including the myocardial interstitium, conducting system, and calcific deposits in the valve cusps and annuli. Although initially observed in fairly long-standing and severe hypercalcemia, so-called metastatic calcifications can also occur in secondary parathyroid disease arising from chronic renal failure, in which the serum calcium–phosphorus product constant is exceeded. Whereas left ventricular systolic function is generally maintained in primary hyperparathyroidism, severe or chronic disease may impair diastolic function. Changes in left ventricular structure and function do not appear to improve by 1 year after successful parathyroid surgery.[39]

A simultaneous increase in serum immunoreactive PTH (best represented by the intact PTH assay), with an elevation of the serum calcium level, establishes the diagnosis of primary hyperparathyroidism. Other causes include hypercalcemia of malignancy with an increased level of PTHrP or arising from direct bony metastasis, or neoplastic (lymphoma) or non-neoplastic (sarcoidosis) disease leading to an increase in synthesis and release of 1,25-dihydroxyvitamin D_3. Treatment for hyperparathyroidism is the surgical removal of the parathyroid adenoma.

Hypocalcemia

Low serum levels of total and ionized calcium directly alter myocyte function. Hypocalcemia prolongs phase 2 of the action potential duration and the Q-T interval. Severe hypocalcemia can impair cardiac contractility and gives rise to a diffuse musculoskeletal syndrome, including tetany and rhabdomyolysis. Primary hypoparathyroidism is rare and can be seen after surgical removal of the parathyroid glands, in the setting of polyglandular dysfunction syndromes, as the result of glandular agenesis (DiGeorge) syndrome, and in the rare heritable disorder pseudohypoparathyroidism.

The most common cause of low serum calcium levels is chronic renal failure and high PTH levels. In such patients, the effects of chronically high levels of PTH (secondary hyperparathyroidism) on the heart and cardiovascular system predominate.[38] The ability of PTH to stimulate G protein–coupled receptors may impair myocyte contractility and contribute to the LVH commonly observed in patients with chronic renal failure. Cinacalcet, a recently approved calcimimetic agent, can treat the secondary hyperparathyroidism associated with chronic renal failure. A trial to assess its effectiveness on cardiovascular events is ongoing.[40]

Vitamin D

Recent evidence has suggested that lower levels of vitamin D (<30 ng/mL of 25-hydroxyvitamin D) are associated with increased all-cause and cardiovascular morbidity.[41] In postmenopausal women, increased vitamin D intake reduces the relative risk of developing cancer. Although low levels of vitamin D occur in chronic renal disease and heart failure, it is too soon to draw conclusions regarding vitamin D supplementation to prevent cardiac disease.[42]

Thyroid Gland

The thyroid gland and heart share a close relationship, arising in embryology. In ontogeny, the thyroid and heart anlage migrate together. The close physiologic relationship is affirmed by predictable changes in cardiovascular function across the entire range of thyroid disease states; cardiovascular manifestations are some of the most common and characteristic findings of hyperthyroidism. The diagnosis and management of thyroid hormone–mediated cardiac disease states require understanding of the cellular mechanisms of thyroid hormone on the heart and vascular smooth muscle cells.[43]

Cellular Mechanisms of Thyroid Hormone Action on the Heart

Under the regulation of thyroid-stimulating hormone (thyrotropin, TSH), the thyroid gland has the unique property of concentrating iodide and, through a series of enzymatic steps, synthesizes predominantly tetraiodothyronine (T_4, 85%) and a smaller percentage of triiodothyronine (T_3, 15%; **Fig. 86-3**). The major source of T_3 synthesis is by conversion by 5′-monodeiodination, primarily in the liver and skeletal muscle and in the kidneys. Studies have confirmed T_3 as the active form of thyroid hormone that accounts for the vast majority of biologic effects, including stimulation of tissue thermogenesis, alterations in the expression of various cellular proteins, and actions on the heart and vascular smooth muscle cells.[44,45] Serum-free T_3, in turn, is taken up by transport proteins (**Fig. 86-4**). Most data indicate that the cardiac myocyte cannot metabolize T_4 to T_3. Therefore, despite the presence of the relevant enzymes, all the observed nuclear actions and changes in gene expression result from changes in blood levels of T_3. As reported for the steroid and retinoic acid families of receptor proteins, the thyroid hormone receptors (TRs) bind as homodimers or heterodimers to the thyroid hormone response elements (TREs) in a promoter region of specific genes. Binding to the promoter regions can activate or repress gene expression.[46]

Thyroid hormone transcriptionally regulates many cardiac proteins (**Table 86-1**). These include structural and regulatory proteins, cardiac membrane ion channels, and cell surface receptors, thus providing a molecular mechanism to explain many of the diverse effects of thyroid hormone on the heart. The first reported and best studied to date have been the myosin heavy chain isoforms (alpha and beta). The human ventricle expresses primarily beta myosin, and there are limited alterations in isoform expression accompanying thyroid disease states. Changes in myosin heavy chain isoform expression occur in the human atria in various

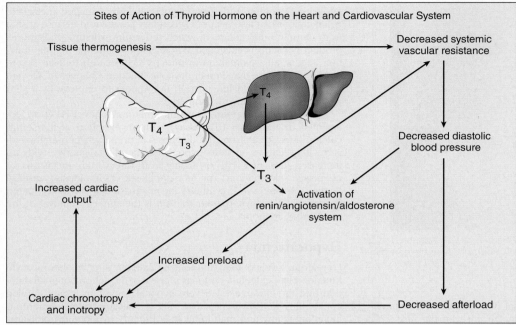

FIGURE 86-3 Schematic representation of thyroid hormone metabolism and the effects of T_3 on the heart and systemic vasculature.

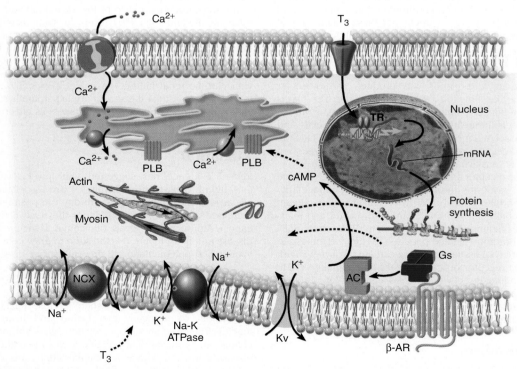

FIGURE 86-4 T_3 enters the cell via specific membrane transporters and binds to nuclear T_3 receptors. The complex binds to thyroid hormone response elements and regulates transcription of specific genes. Non-nuclear T_3 actions on channels for Na^+, K^+, and Ca^{2+} ions are indicated. AC = adenylyl cyclase; ATPase = adenosine triphosphatase; β-AR = beta-adrenergic receptor; Gs = guanine nucleotide binding protein subunit; Kv = voltage-gated potassium channel; mRNA = messenger RNA; NCX = sodium calcium exchanger; PLB = phospholamban; TR = T_3 receptor protein.

TABLE 86-1	Thyroid Hormone Regulation of Cardiac Gene Expression

Positively Regulated

Alpha-myosin heavy chain
Sarcoplasmic reticulum Ca^{2+}-ATPase
Na^+, K^+-ATPase
Voltage-gated potassium channels (Kv 1.5, Kv 4.2, Kv 4.3)
Atrial and brain natriuretic peptide
Malic enzyme
Beta-adrenergic receptor
Guanine nucleotide-binding protein G_s
Adenine nucleotide transporter 1

Negatively Regulated

Beta-myosin heavy chain
Phospholamban
Na^+, Ca^{2+} exchanger
Thyroid hormone receptor alpha$_1$
Adenylyl cyclase (AC) types V, VI
Guanine nucleotide-binding protein G_i
Monocarboxylate transporters 8 and 10

ATPase = adenosine triphosphatase.

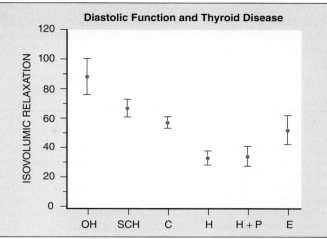

FIGURE 86-5 Diastolic function, as measured by the isovolumic relaxation time, varies over the entire range of thyroid disease, including overt hypothyroidism (OH), subclinical hypothyroidism (SCH), control (C), hyperthyroidism (H), hyperthyroidism after beta-adrenergic blockade (H + P), and hyperthyroidism after treatment to restore normal thyroid function (E).

diseases, including congestive heart failure, and whether these changes are thyroid hormone–mediated remains to be determined.[47]

Sarcoendoplasmic reticulum Ca^{2+}-ATPase (SERCA) is an important ion pump that determines the magnitude of myocyte calcium cycling (see Chap. 24). The reuptake of calcium into the sarcoendoplasmic reticulum early in diastole in part determines the rate at which the left ventricle relaxes (isovolumetric relaxation time [IVRT]).[43] The activity of SERCA2 in turn is regulated by the polymeric protein phospholamban, with its ability to inhibit SERCA activity further modified by the level of phosphorylation of the individual phospholamban monomers.[48] Inotropic agents that enhance cardiac contractility through increases in myocyte cAMP do so by stimulating the phosphorylation of phospholamban. Thyroid hormone inhibits the expression of phospholamban and increases phospholamban phosphorylation.[49] Genetically engineered animals deficient in phospholamban do not increase cardiac contractility further after exposure to excess thyroid hormone.[48] These data indicate that thyroid hormone exerts most of its direct effects on cardiac contractility by regulating calcium cycling through the SERCA-phospholamban system transcriptionally and post-transcriptionally. This molecular mechanism can explain why diastolic function varies inversely across the entire spectrum of thyroid disease states, including even mild subclinical hypothyroidism (**Fig. 86-5**).[50,51] In addition, beta-adrenergic blockade of the heart in hyperthyroidism does not decrease the rapid diastolic relaxation, further dissociating the thyroid hormone from the adrenergic effects of thyrotoxicosis.

Changes in other myocyte genes, including Na^+,K^+-ATPase, account for the increase in basal oxygen consumption of the experimental hyperthyroid heart and explain the decrease in digitalis sensitivity of hyperthyroid patients. Studies have shown that thyroid hormone can regulate the genetic expression of its own nuclear receptors and plasma membrane transport proteins (MCT8 and 10) within the cardiac myocyte (see Table 86-1).

In addition to the well-characterized nuclear effects of thyroid hormone, some cardiac responses to thyroid hormone appear to be mediated through nongenomic mechanisms,[52] as suggested by their relatively rapid onset of action—faster than can be accounted for by changes in gene expression and protein synthesis—and failure to be affected by inhibitors of gene transcription. The significance of these diverse actions remains to be established, but may explain the ability of acute T_3 treatment to alter cardiovascular hemodynamics. They may alter the functional properties of membrane ion channels and pumps, including the sodium channel and inward rectifying potassium current (I_K).

Thyroid Function Testing

A number of sensitive and specific laboratory tests can establish a diagnosis of thyroid disease with a high degree of precision. The serum TSH level is the most widely used and sensitive measure for the diagnosis of hypothyroidism and hyperthyroidism.[53] Serum TSH levels uniformly increase (>5 mIU/mL) in patients with primary hypothyroidism and, conversely, because of the normal feedback of excess levels of T_4 (and T_3) on the pituitary synthesis and secretion of TSH, the levels are low in hyperthyroidism (<0.1 mIU/mL). Measures of free T_4 can be useful when coexistent hepatic, nutritional, or genetic disease may alter thyroxine-binding globulin content. Autoimmune thyroid disease (Hashimoto and Graves) can be further diagnosed by the use of serologic measures of antithyroid antibodies, most specifically antithyroid peroxidase (anti-TPO) or antithyroglobulin antibodies.

Thyroid Hormone–Catecholamine Interaction

Early observations of the heart in hyperthyroidism emphasized the similarity to that of hyperadrenergic states, and moreover proposed enhanced sensitivity to catecholamines in this setting. This postulate formed the basis for the test described by Emil Goetsch in 1918, in which hyperthyroidism could be diagnosed by demonstrating a marked cardioacceleration and blood pressure response to small subcutaneous doses of epinephrine. Hyperthyroid subjects have decreased circulating catecholamine concentrations, despite the appearance of increased adrenergic signs and symptoms. Increased beta$_1$-adrenergic receptors on cardiac myocytes observed in experimental hyperthyroidism provide a mechanism for enhanced catecholamine sensitivity. A carefully controlled study of nonhuman primates, however, found no increase in sensitivity of the heart or cardiovascular system to catecholamines in experimental hyperthyroidism.[54] Accompanying the increased levels of beta$_1$-adrenergic receptors and guanosine triphosphate–binding proteins, thyroid hormone decreases the expression of cardiac-specific adenylyl cyclase catalytic subunit isoforms (V, VI), and thereby maintains the cellular response to beta-adrenergic agonists within normal limits.[55]

Hemodynamic Alterations in Thyroid Disease

Changes in myocardial contractility and hemodynamics occur across the entire spectrum of thyroid disease (**Table 86-2**; see Fig. 86-5). Multiple studies, including those in experimental animals, as well as invasive and noninvasive measurements in patients, have indicated that T_3 regulates cardiac inotropy and chronotropy through both direct and indirect mechanisms.[56-59] T_3 acts on tissues throughout the body to increase tissue thermogenesis (see Fig. 86-3). Direct effects on vascular smooth muscle cells decrease systemic vascular resistance of the arterioles of the peripheral circulation. A decrease in mean

TABLE 86-2 Cardiovascular Changes with Thyroid Disease

PARAMETER	NORMAL	HYPERTHYROID	HYPOTHYROID
Systemic vascular resistance (dyne-cm · sec^{-5})	1500-1700	700-1200	2100-2700
Heart rate (beats/min)	72-84	88-130	60-80
Cardiac output (liter/min)	5.8	>7.0	<4.5
Blood volume (% of normal)	100	105.5	84.5

arterial pressure and activation of the renin-angiotensin-aldosterone system occurs, as does an increase in renal sodium reabsorption. The increase in plasma volume, coupled with an increase in erythropoietin, leads to an increase in blood volume and a rise in cardiac preload. Thus, a combination of lower systemic vascular resistance (by as much as 50%), coupled with increases in venous return and preload, increases cardiac output. Cardiac output may more than double in hyperthyroidism and, conversely, may decrease by as much as 30% to 40% in hypothyroidism. Studies using positron emission tomography (PET) measurements of acetate metabolism have demonstrated that the marked increase in cardiac output in hyperthyroidism causes no change in energy efficiency.[60]

T$_3$ appears to reduce systemic vascular resistance by direct effects on vascular smooth muscle cells and through changes in the vascular endothelium potentially involving the synthesis and secretion of nitric oxide.[56] T$_3$ can produce vasodilation within hours after administration to patients undergoing coronary artery bypass grafting (CABG) and to patients with chronic congestive heart failure.[47,59] Arterial compliance also falls in hyperthyroidism, and may explain why mean arterial and diastolic pressures are low and peak systolic pressures increase.[57] Thus, the combination of increased cardiac output and decreased arterial compliance, which may be more pronounced in older patients with some degree of arterial vascular disease, leads to systolic hypertension in up to 30% of patients. In hypothyroidism, systemic vascular resistance may increase as much as 30%. Mean arterial pressure rises, with up to 20% of patients having diastolic hypertension. Even mild hypothyroidism may decrease endothelial-derived relaxing factors.[61] The diastolic hypertension of hypothyroidism is frequently associated with a low renin level and a decrease in hepatic synthesis of renin substrate. This leads to a characteristically low level of salt sensitivity, again reinforcing the importance of an increase in systemic vascular resistance underlying the mechanism for diastolic hypertension.

Hyperthyroidism

Cardiovascular symptoms are an integral and often the predominant clinical presentation of patients with hyperthyroidism. Most patients experience palpitations resulting from increases in the rate and force of cardiac contractility. The increase in heart rate results from a decrease in parasympathetic stimulation and an increase in sympathetic tone. Heart rates higher than 90 beats/min at rest and during sleep commonly occur, the normal diurnal variation in heart rate is blunted, and the increase during exercise is exaggerated. Many hyperthyroid patients experience exercise intolerance and exertional dyspnea, caused in part by skeletal and respiratory muscle weakness.[62,63] In the setting of a low vascular resistance and increased preload, cardiac functional reserve is compromised and cannot rise further to accommodate the demands of submaximal or maximal exercise.

A subset of thyrotoxic patients can experience angina-like chest pain. In older patients with known or suspected coronary artery disease, the increase in cardiac work associated with the increase in cardiac output and cardiac contractility of hyperthyroidism can produce myocardial ischemia, which can respond to beta-adrenergic blocking agents (beta blockers) or the restoration of a euthyroid state. Rare patients, usually younger women, experience a syndrome of chest pain at rest associated with ischemic electrocardiographic changes. Cardiac catheterization has demonstrated that most of these patients have angiographically normal coronary arteries, but coronary vasospasm similar to that found in variant angina can occur. Myocardial

infarction rarely develops, and these patients appear to respond to calcium channel blockers or nitroglycerin.[43] Recent reports have documented cerebrovascular ischemic symptoms in young, primarily Asian women with Graves disease. This syndrome, Moyamoya disease, is characterized by anatomic occlusion of the terminal portions of internal carotid arteries. Treatment of hyperthyroidism can prevent further cerebral ischemic symptoms and reinforces the importance of routine thyroid function tests, including TSH, in patients who present with cardiac or cerebral vascular ischemic symptoms.

Hyperthyroidism is associated with a substantial degree of pulmonary hypertension (pulmonary artery systolic pressure > 75 mm Hg), which is reversible after treatment of Graves disease.[64] This observation implies that although systemic vascular resistance is decreased with thyrotoxicosis, pulmonary vascular resistance is not. Evaluation for thyroid disease with measurement of the serum TSH level may benefit all patients with unexplained pulmonary hypertension.[57]

ATRIAL FIBRILLATION. The most common rhythm disturbance in patients with hyperthyroidism is sinus tachycardia,[43] but its clinical impact is overshadowed by patients with atrial fibrillation resulting from thyrotoxicosis (see Chap. 40). The prevalence of atrial fibrillation and the less common forms of supraventricular tachycardia in this disease ranges from 2% to 20%.[65,66] When compared with a control population with normal thyroid function and a 2.3% prevalence of atrial fibrillation, the prevalence of atrial fibrillation in overt hyperthyroidism was 13.8%. In a study of more than 13,000 hyperthyroid patients, the prevalence for atrial fibrillation was less than 2%, perhaps because of earlier recognition and disease treatment.[65] When that same group of patients was analyzed for age distribution, prevalence increased stepwise in each decade, peaking at approximately 15% in patients older than 70 years. This study confirms that atrial fibrillation caused by hyperthyroidism is more common with advancing age. In a study of unselected patients presenting with atrial fibrillation, less than 1% of cases was caused by overt hyperthyroidism. Thus, the yield of abnormal thyroid function testing, including a low serum TSH level, appears to be low in patients with new-onset atrial fibrillation. However, the ability to restore thyrotoxic patients to a euthyroid state and sinus rhythm justifies TSH testing in most patients with recent onset of otherwise unexplained atrial fibrillation or other supraventricular arrhythmias.

Treatment of atrial fibrillation in the setting of hyperthyroidism includes beta-adrenergic blockade using a beta$_1$ selective or nonselective agent to control the ventricular response (**Table 86-3**). This symptomatic measure can be accomplished rapidly, whereas treatments leading to restoration of the euthyroid state require more time. Digitalis has been used to control the ventricular response in hyperthyroidism-associated atrial fibrillation, but because of the increased rate of digitalis clearance, decreased sensitivity of the drug action resulting from high cellular levels of Na$^+$,K$^+$-ATPase, and decreased parasympathetic tone, patients usually require higher doses of this medication. Anticoagulation in patients with hyperthyroidism and atrial fibrillation is controversial.[43,67] The potential for systemic or cerebral embolization must be weighed against the risk of bleeding and complications. Whether hyperthyroid patients are at increased risk for systemic embolization per se is not totally resolved.[68] In a retrospective study of patients with hyperthyroidism, age rather than atrial fibrillation was the main risk factor for embolization. Retrospective analysis of large series of patients has not demonstrated a prevalence of thromboembolic

TABLE 86-3 Beta-Adrenergic Receptor Blockade in the Treatment of Hyperthyroidism*

DRUG	DOSAGE	FREQUENCY	CONSIDERATIONS
Propranolol	10-40 mg	tid or qid	Nonselective β-AR blockade; longest experience
Atenolol	25-100 mg	bid	Relative beta₁ selectivity; increased patient compliance
Metoprolol	25-50 mg	qid	Relative beta₁ selectivity
Nadolol	40-160 mg	qd	Nonselective β-AR blockade; once daily; least experience to date
Esmolol	IV pump, 50-100 μg/kg/min		In ICU setting of severe hyperthyroidism or storm

*Each of these drugs has been approved for the treatment of cardiovascular diseases, but to date none has been approved for the treatment of hyperthyroidism.
β-AR = beta-adrenergic receptor; ICU = intensive care unit.

events greater than the reported risk of major bleeding from warfarin treatment. Thus, in younger patients with hyperthyroidism and atrial fibrillation in the absence of other heart disease, hypertension, or other independent risk factors for embolization, the benefits of anticoagulation have not been proven and might be outweighed by the risk. Aspirin provides an alternative for lowering the risk for embolic events in younger individuals and can be used safely.

Successful treatment of hyperthyroidism with radioiodine or antithyroid drugs and restoration of normal serum levels of T_4 and T_3 are associated with reversion to sinus rhythm in two thirds of patients within 2 to 3 months.[65] In older patients or in the setting of atrial fibrillation of longer duration, the rate of reversion to sinus rhythm is lower and electrical or pharmacologic cardioversion therefore should be attempted, but only after the patient has been rendered euthyroid. Most patients (90%) can be restored to sinus rhythm by electrical cardioversion or pharmacologic measures, and many will remain in sinus rhythm for up to 5 years or more. In a regimen that added disopyramide, 300 mg/day, for 3 months after successful cardioversion, patients were more likely to remain in sinus rhythm than those not treated.[67]

HEART FAILURE IN THYROID DISEASE. The cardiovascular alterations in hyperthyroidism include increased resting cardiac output and enhanced cardiac contractility (**Fig. 86-6**; see Table 86-2). Nevertheless, a minority of patients presents with symptoms, including dyspnea on exertion, orthopnea, and paroxysmal nocturnal dyspnea, as well as signs demonstrating peripheral edema, elevated jugular venous pressure, or an S_3 indicative of heart failure. This complex of findings, coupled with a failure to increase the LV ejection fraction with exercise, has suggested a hyperthyroid cardiomyopathy. The term often used in this setting, *high-output failure*, is not appropriate, because although resting cardiac output is as much as two to three times normal, the exercise intolerance does not appear to be a result of cardiac failure, but rather of skeletal muscle weakness[43,63] and perhaps associated pulmonary hypertension.[64] High-output states, however, can increase renal sodium reabsorption, expand plasma volume, and cause development of peripheral edema, pleural effusions, and venous hypertension. Whereas systemic vascular resistance falls with hyperthyroidism, the pulmonary vascular bed is not similarly affected and, as a result of the increase in output to the pulmonary circulation, there is an increase in pulmonary artery pressures.[57] This results in a rise in mean venous pressure, jugular venous hypertension, hepatic congestion, and peripheral edema of the type associated with primary pulmonary hypertension or right heart failure.

Patients with long-standing hyperthyroidism and marked sinus tachycardia or atrial fibrillation can develop low cardiac output, impaired cardiac contractility with a low ejection fraction, an S_3, and pulmonary congestion, all consistent with congestive heart failure.[43] Review of such cases suggests that impairment in left ventricular function results from prolonged high heart rate and the development of rate-related heart failure. When the left ventricle becomes dilated, mitral regurgitation may also develop (see Chap. 66). Recognition of this entity is important because treatment aimed at slowing heart rate or controlling the ventricular response in atrial fibrillation appears to improve left ventricular function, even before initiation of antithyroid therapy. Because these patients are critically ill, they should be managed in an intensive care unit setting. Some patients

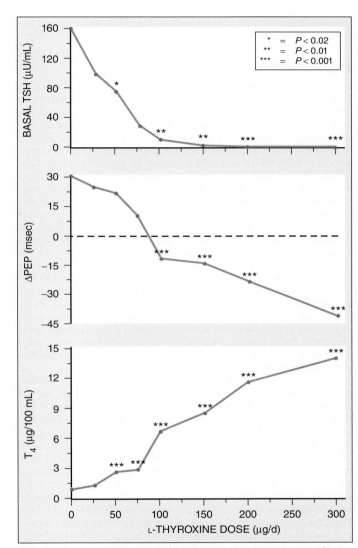

FIGURE 86-6 Response to stepwise L-thyroxine sodium treatment of hypothyroid patients as assessed by serum TSH and T_4 levels and by improvement in left ventricular contractility as measured noninvasively by the change in the pre-ejection period (PEP). *(From Crowley WF Jr, Ridgway EC, Bough EW, et al: Noninvasive evaluation of cardiac function in hypothyroidism. Response to gradual thyroxine replacement. N Engl J Med 296:1, 1977.)*

with hyperthyroidism, similar to the overall congestive heart failure population, do not tolerate initiation of beta blockers in full doses. Treatment can be started with lower doses of short-acting beta blockers in conjunction with classic forms of treatment of acute congestive heart failure, including diuresis.

The increase in rate-pressure product and oxygen consumption that results from hyperthyroidism can impair cardiac function in older patients with known or suspected ischemic, hypertensive, or valvular heart disease. It is important to recognize hyperthyroidism in older patients promptly, because they are at higher risk of cardiovascular and cerebral vascular events before[69] and subsequent to treatment.[70]

TREATMENT. Treatment of patients with thyrotoxic cardiac disease should include a beta-adrenergic antagonist to lower the heart rate to 10% or 15% above normal. This causes the tachycardia-mediated component of ventricular dysfunction to improve, whereas the direct inotropic effects of thyroid hormone will persist (see Table 86-3 and Fig. 86-4).[43] The rapid onset of action and improvement in many of the signs and symptoms of hyperthyroidism indicate that most patients with overt symptoms should receive beta blockers. Definitive therapy can then be accomplished safely with iodine-131 alone or in combination with an antithyroid drug.

Hypothyroidism

In contrast to the dramatic clinical signs and symptoms of hyperthyroidism, the cardiovascular findings of hypothyroidism are more subtle.[71] Mild degrees of bradycardia, diastolic hypertension, narrow pulse pressure and relatively quiet precordium, and decreased intensity of the apical impulse are all characteristic. Hemodynamic changes of hypothyroidism are diametrically opposite to those of hyperthyroidism (see Table 86-2) and explain many of the physical findings. Despite the decrease in cardiac output and contractility of the hypothyroid myocardium, studies of myocardial metabolism by PET scan have shown energy inefficiency of the hypothyroid myocardium. The oxygen cost of work increases primarily as a result of the increase in afterload.[72] Treatment of hypothyroid patients with the restoration of a euthyroid state resolves these changes in parallel with a return of systemic vascular resistance to lower levels.

Hypothyroidism also produces increases in total and low-density lipoprotein (LDL) cholesterol in proportion to the rise in serum TSH levels.[73] Although thyroid hormone can alter cholesterol metabolism through multiple mechanisms, including a decrease in biliary excretion, it appears that changes in LDL metabolism caused by decreases in LDL receptor number are a primary mechanism.[74] A recent study has noted that a liver-selective thyroid hormone agonist, eprotirome, can further lower cholesterol levels in statin-treated patients, which supports this concept.[75]

The serum creatine kinase (CK) level is elevated by 50% to 10-fold in up to 30% of patients with hypothyroidism. Analysis of isoform specificity indicates that more than 96% is CK-MM, consistent with a skeletal muscle origin of increased enzyme release.[74] The serum level of creatine kinase in hypothyroidism after initiation of standard oral thyroid hormone replacement declines slowly over weeks. Pericardial effusions can occur consistent with the observation that patients with hypothyroidism have an increase in the volume of distribution of albumin and a decrease in lymphatic clearance function. Occasionally, the pericardial effusions are large, causing the appearance of cardiomegaly on chest radiograph. Although rare, tamponade with hemodynamic compromise can occur. Echocardiography demonstrates small to moderate effusions in up to 30% of overtly hypothyroid patients, which resolve over a period of weeks to months after initiation of thyroid hormone replacement.[71]

As a result of changes in ion channel expression, the ECG in hypothyroidism is characterized by sinus bradycardia, low voltage, and prolongation of the action potential duration and QT interval. The latter predisposes patients to ventricular arrhythmias, and some patients with acquired torsade de pointes have improved or completely resolved with thyroid hormone replacement.[43]

Increases in risk factors for atherosclerosis, including hypercholesterolemia, hypertension, and elevated levels of homocysteine, may elevate the risk for atherosclerosis and coronary and systemic vascular disease in patients with hypothyroidism (see Chaps. 44 and 47).[73,74] One study has reported increases in abdominal aortic atherosclerosis in older female patients with even mild hypothyroidism.[76] Whether patients with hypothyroidism have an increase in coronary artery

disease is an important clinical issue. One report has suggested increased cardiovascular morbidity and mortality with untreated subclinical hypothyroidism,[77] and that increases in carotid intimal medial thickness resolve with thyroid hormone replacement.[78] Noninvasive studies, including nuclear scans, have demonstrated abnormalities in perfusion suggestive of myocardial ischemia, but these defects appear to resolve with thyroid hormone treatment.

In patients younger than 50 years of age with no history of heart disease, it is possible to initiate full replacement doses of L-thyroxine (100 to 150 µg/day) without concern for untoward cardiac effects. In patients older than 50 years of age with known or suspected coronary artery disease, the issue is more complicated.

In patients with known coronary artery disease and coexistent hypothyroidism, three major issues need to be addressed. The first is whether coronary artery revascularization is required before initiating thyroid hormone replacement. If patients are not candidates for percutaneous intervention, CABG can be accomplished in patients with unstable angina, left main coronary artery disease, or three-vessel disease with impaired left ventricular function, even in the setting of overt hypothyroidism. Rarely, a patient has sufficiently profound hypothyroidism to prolong bleeding times and partial thromboplastin times, requiring preoperative supplementation of clotting factors. Thyroid hormone replacement can be delayed until the postoperative period, when it can be administered in full doses parenterally or orally.[43]

The second issue is in patients with known stable cardiac disease, in whom cardiac revascularization is not clinically indicated. Treatment of such patients should begin with low doses (12.5 µg) of L-thyroxine and increased stepwise (12.5 to 25 µg) every 6 to 8 weeks until the serum TSH level is normal. Thyroid hormone replacement in this setting and its ability to lower systemic vascular resistance and decrease afterload, as well as improve myocardial efficiency, can actually decrease clinical signs of myocardial ischemia. Beta blockers are an ideal concomitant therapy to control heart rate.

The third important issue involves patients who, although potentially at risk for coronary artery disease, exhibit no clinical signs or symptoms. In this group, thyroid hormone replacement can be started at low doses, generally in the range of 25 to 50 µg/day, and increased by 25 µg every 6 to 8 weeks until the serum TSH level is normal. If signs or symptoms of ischemic heart disease develop, the same recommendations apply as to patients with known underlying heart disease.

In all patients, thyroid hormone replacement should be sufficient to restore the serum TSH level to normal and the patients are clinically euthyroid. The concept that these patients benefit from maintenance of mild hypothyroidism is not supported by the known effects of thyroid hormone on the heart and cardiovascular system.[43,71,72] Thyroid hormone replacement should be accomplished by purified preparations of levothyroxine sodium. Preparations containing T_4 with T_3 (thyroid extract) or the existing purified preparations of T_3 do not offer benefit. The short half-life of T_3 and the inability to maintain serum levels within the normal range in patients so treated can add to cardiac risk.[78] An interesting issue is whether some patients with statin-induced myopathy have underlying thyroid disease as a contributing factor. The myopathy or myalgia symptoms of both conditions are similar (**Table 86-4**), and thyroid function testing with TSH should be part of the evaluation of these patients.[74]

DIAGNOSIS. Hashimoto disease, post–radioiodine therapy for Graves disease, and iodine deficiency (in parts of the world where that remains a public health problem) are the leading causes of hypothyroidism and produce diagnostic elevation in serum TSH levels.[53] Thus, the finding of an elevated TSH level is sufficient to establish the diagnosis and form the basis for treatment. In routine practice, additional testing with a serum T_4 and T_3 resin uptake is confirmatory. The prevalence of hypothyroidism is estimated at 3% to 4% for overt disease and 7% to 10% for the milder forms of disease, and increases with advancing age. TSH screening can therefore be advised for all adults, particularly patients with hypertension, hypercholesterolemia, hypertriglyceridemia, coronary or peripheral vascular disease, and unexplained pericardial or pleural effusions and for various musculoskeletal syndromes or statin-associated myopathy.[43,74]

TABLE 86-4	Clinical Characterization of Muscle Disease Syndromes
STATIN-INDUCED	**HYPOTHYROID-RELATED**
Myopathy—any associated disease	Myalgia—nonspecific muscle symptoms, cramping, especially nocturnal, variable CK level
Myalgia—muscle aches, weakness without CK level elevation	Myopathy—impaired endurance usually with CK level elevation; pseudomyotonia
Myositis—symptoms plus elevated CK level	Hoffmann syndrome—impaired function; pseudohypertrophy; often marked CK level elevations
Rhabdomyolysis—symptoms plus markedly elevated CK levels	

CK = creatine kinase.

TREATMENT. The response to treatment of hypothyroidism is predictable, especially from a cardiovascular perspective. Stepwise thyroid hormone replacement using levothyroxine sodium (Levoxyl, Synthroid) incrementally decreases serum TSH, serum cholesterol, and serum creatine kinase levels and improves left ventricular performance. Full replacement is accomplished when the serum TSH level is normal.[53] In the rare condition of myxedema coma, characterized by the development of hypothermia, altered mental status, hypotension, bradycardia, and hypoventilation in patients with severe and long-standing hypothyroidism, the need for thyroid hormone replacement is more emergent, and treatment can be accomplished with 100 μg of T_4 or 25 to 50 μg of T_3 daily, administered intravenously. These patients often require intensive care unit monitoring with volume repletion, gentle warming, and ventilatory support in the face of CO_2 retention. Administration of hydrocortisone (100 mg three times daily) should be undertaken until results of serum cortisol testing are obtained. When treated in this manner, hemodynamics including systemic vascular resistance, cardiac output, and heart rate improve within 24 to 48 hours.

Subclinical Disease

In contrast to overt symptomatic thyroid disease, subclinical thyroid disease implies the absence of classic hyperthyroid- or hypothyroid-related symptoms in patients with thyroid dysfunction. The definition has been further refined to include the demonstration of an abnormal TSH level in the face of normal serum levels of total T_4, free T_4, total T_3, and free T_3.[53,80,81] With the advent of widespread TSH screening, the magnitude of subclinical thyroid disease may exceed that of overt disease by threefold to fourfold.

SUBCLINICAL HYPOTHYROIDISM. Subclinical hypothyroidism, defined as a TSH level above the upper range of the reference population (usually >5 mIU/mL), is seen in up to 9% of unselected populations, and prevalence increases with advancing age. In contrast to younger patients, in whom there is a strong female predilection, this difference is lost in older populations. Subclinical hypothyroidism alters lipid metabolism, atherosclerosis, cardiac contractility, and systemic vascular resistance. Cholesterol levels rise in parallel with increments in TSH level elevations, starting at 5 mIU/liter. A large study of women in Rotterdam has shown that atherosclerosis and myocardial infarction increase with odds ratios of 1.7 and 2.3, respectively, in subclinical hypothyroid women. Of note, the presence of antithyroid antibodies as a measure of autoimmune thyroid disease indicated heightened risk.[76] Restoration of serum TSH levels to normal after thyroid hormone replacement improves lipid levels, lowers systemic vascular resistance, and improves cardiac contractility. Patients with subclinical hypothyroidism have prolonged isovolumic relaxation times, whereas systolic contractile function does not change (see Fig. 86-6). Replacement with L-thyroxine sodium at a mean dose of 68 μg/

day (range, 50 to 100 μg/day) restored isovolumic relaxation times to normal, and when compared with the same patients before therapy, systemic vascular resistance declined and systolic function significantly improved.[81] A variety of studies have indicated that the changes in systemic vascular resistance result from alterations in endothelium-dependent vasodilation.[50,61] Taken together, it seems appropriate from a cardiovascular perspective to recommend thyroid hormone replacement for all patients with subclinical hypothyroidism.[82] A decrease in carotid intimal medial thickness in these patients also supports replacement strategies.[78] The lack of untoward cardiac effects observed when serum TSH levels normalize indicates that the potential benefits far outweigh the risks of treatment.[43,73,80]

SUBCLINICAL HYPERTHYROIDISM. Subclinical hyperthyroidism is diagnosed when the serum TSH level is low (<0.1 mIU/mL) and T_4 and T_3 levels are normal.[53] The significance of subclinical hyperthyroidism was conclusively established from a study of atrial fibrillation in patients 60 years of age or older in the Framingham cohort.[83] Prevalence of atrial fibrillation after 10 years was 28% in the subclinical hyperthyroid patient population, compared with 11% in patients with normal thyroid function, with a relative risk of 3.1. A large U.S. study of patients 65 years of age or older confirmed and extended this result. This population-based study of more than 1000 individuals with subclinical hyperthyroidism not receiving L-thyroxine therapy or antithyroid medication demonstrated that a TSH level lower than 0.5 mIU/mL associated with twofold increased mortality, with a relative risk of 2.3 to 3.3 from all causes, which in turn was largely accounted for by increases in cardiovascular mortality.[84,85]

Although the cardiovascular changes are well established, the management of patients with subclinical hyperthyroidism is controversial. Therapy can be individualized with regard to three specific groups. The first group includes patients receiving thyroid hormone replacement for hypothyroidism, in which the low TSH level is believed to be the result of excess medication, and reduction of the dose is indicated. The second group includes patients with a prior diagnosis of thyroid cancer currently receiving L-thyroxine for the express purpose of TSH suppression. In younger patients, beta blockers can reverse many (if not all) cardiovascular manifestations, including heart rate control, LVH, and atrial ectopy. In older patients, the degree of TSH suppression can be relaxed by lowering the T_4 dosage. The third group includes patients in whom subclinical hyperthyroidism results from endogenous thyroid gland overactivity, including Graves disease or nodular goiter. Younger patients in this category appear to have little or no untoward effects, whereas older patients are potentially at risk from atrial fibrillation. In patients older than 60 years of age, antithyroid therapy (methimazole, 5 to 10 mg/day) can produce improvement and, in patients who respond or require long-term treatment, consideration should be given to the use of radioiodine for definitive therapy.[43,86]

Amiodarone and Thyroid Function (see Chap. 37)

Amiodarone is an iodine-rich antiarrhythmic agent effective for the treatment of ventricular and atrial tachyarrhythmias. Its 30% by weight iodine content and its structural similarity to levothyroxine cause abnormalities in thyroid function test results in as many as 60% of patients treated for short or long periods of time.[87] The finding that dronedarone, a recently approved noniodinated benzofuran antiarrhythmic, does not alter thyroid function reinforces this concept.[88] Similar to other iodinated drugs, amiodarone inhibits the 5′-monodeiodination of T_4 in the liver and pituitary.[44] Inhibition of T_4 metabolism in the liver decreases serum T_3 and increases serum T_4 levels, whereas serum TSH levels initially remain normal. With more chronic treatment and as the total iodide content of the body rises, T_4 synthesis and release from the thyroid gland can be inhibited, producing a rise in TSH levels. In patients with underlying goiter, autoimmune thyroid disease, or enzymatic defects in thyroid hormone biosynthesis, and in some patients without any risk factors, there is a progression to overt chemical and clinical hypothyroidism with a marked rise in serum TSH

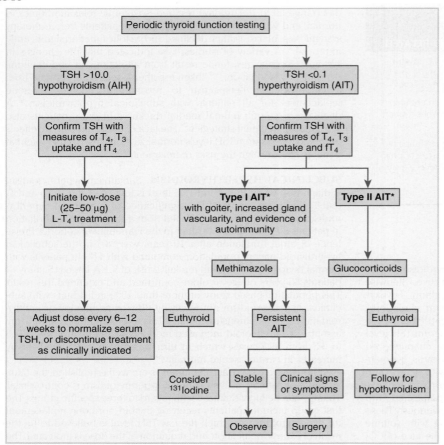

FIGURE 86-7 Amiodarone-induced thyroid disease (AIT) can be diagnosed based on classic signs and symptoms of hypothyroidism or hyperthyroidism, or more commonly by routine (every 3 to 6 months) thyroid function testing. Any single abnormal TSH level should be confirmed. Clinical hypothyroidism with a TSH level > 10 mIU/mL should be treated. AIT management is described and depends on the severity and duration of clinical findings. *Mixed types I and II forms of AIT may require combination therapy with thionamides and corticosteroids. fT_4 = free T_4.

by a variety of proinflammatory cytokines, including IL-6. This is primarily a destructive process causing release of preformed thyroid hormone, which may continue for weeks or months and most often is associated with low to absent radioiodine uptake. Further experience has shown that these two types have substantial overlap for many of the distinguishing parameters. Amiodarone-induced thyrotoxicosis is associated with a threefold increased risk for major adverse cardiovascular events, underscoring its clinical importance.[90] Prompt and effective treatment is indicated.[87]

Because of the increased thyroidal and total body iodine content, use of iodine-131 is almost always ineffective.[43] Similarly, treatment with antithyroid drugs has marginal effectiveness.[89] Corticosteroids (prednisone, 20 to 40 mg/day) provide benefit, perhaps with increased usefulness for patients with type II disease who have high serum levels of IL-6.[87] But corticosteroids can be instituted in all patients because, when effective, the response usually occurs within 2 to 4 weeks of initiating treatment. In patients unresponsive to glucocorticoids with evidence of hyperthyroidism, including weight loss, tachycardia, palpitations, worsening angina, ventricular tachycardia, or other untoward cardiac effects, treatment with antithyroid therapy (methimazole [Tapazole], 10 to 30 mg/day) and potassium perchlorate (if available) is variably effective and can cause significant side effects. One study[91] and growing clinical experience have confirmed that total thyroidectomy can be performed safely and is an effective means of reversing the hyperthyroidism rapidly. Preoperative treatment with beta blockers is indicated, and there have been no reported cases of resulting thyroid storm.

Whether amiodarone-mediated thyroid dysfunction should mandate discontinuation of the drug is an important issue. There is no evidence that stopping amiodarone hastens the resolution of chemical hyperthyroidism. Because certain patients require amiodarone therapy to manage arrhythmias, and because the duration of drug retention in the body in lipid-soluble stores is in excess of 6 months, it seems prudent to continue amiodarone therapy while making separate management plans to treat thyroid dysfunction. Substitution of dronedarone for amiodarone may prevent these untoward effects in situations in which dronedarone has shown antiarrhythmic efficacy.[88]

Changes in Thyroid Hormone Metabolism That Accompany Cardiac Disease

In addition to the changes in thyroid function that can result from classic thyroid disease, there are primary alterations in serum total and free T_3 and occasionally serum T_4 levels that accompany a variety of acute and chronic illnesses, including sepsis, starvation, and cardiac disease. In the absence of thyroid gland abnormality, changes in serum T_3 levels result from alterations in thyroid hormone metabolism. These cases have been referred to as nonthyroidal illness. The mechanism for this decrease in serum T_3 levels is multifactorial and in part related to a decrease in 5′-monodeiodination in the liver.[44]

A population-based study of patients with cardiac disease has shown that a low serum T_3 level strongly predicts all-cause and cardiovascular mortality.[92] Following uncomplicated acute myocardial infarction, serum T_3 levels fall by about 20% and reach a nadir after approximately 96 hours. Experimental myocardial infarction in animals produces a similar decrease in serum T_3 levels, and replacement of T_3 levels to normal has been reported to increase left ventricular

levels.[89] The overall prevalence of hypothyroidism in amiodarone-treated patients is between 15% and 30%. The symptoms of hypothyroidism in this setting can be subtle, and significant hypothyroidism can occur even in their absence.[71]

Thyroid function should be measured every 3 months in all patients receiving amiodarone (**Fig. 86-7**). The effect on thyroid function does not depend on dose and can occur at any time after initiating treatment—and because of the high lipid solubility and long half-life of the drug, still can occur up to 1 year after discontinuing therapy.[87,89]

Less common, but perhaps more challenging, is the development of amiodarone-induced thyrotoxicosis. Although initially not observed in the iodine-replete American population, the experience from Italy suggested that it occurred with a prevalence as high as 10%.[89] The onset was often sudden and could occur shortly after drug initiation, during chronic treatment, or up to 1 year after stopping therapy. Clinical clues to the development of this condition include the new onset or recurrence of ventricular irritability (increased firing of an implantable cardioverter-defibrillator [ICD]), decreased coumadin dose requirements, or the return or worsening of the obstructive physiology of hypertrophic cardiomyopathy (see Chap. 69). Although the pathogenesis is multifactorial, early studies distinguished two forms of amiodarone-induced thyrotoxicosis. Type I occurs primarily in patients with preexisting thyroid disease and most commonly in iodine-deficient areas. These patients may rarely have an increase in 24-hour radioiodine uptake measures and frequently some measures of thyroid autoimmunity, including antithyroid antibodies. In contrast, type II disease was identified as a form of thyroiditis presumably mediated

contractile function.[43] A recent study of T_3 treatment of humans with NYHA Class III or IV heart failure has shown similar results.[93]

Children and adults undergoing cardiac surgery with cardiopulmonary bypass demonstrate a predictable fall in serum T_3 levels in the perioperative period.[94] Although treatment strategies using acute administration of intravenous T_3 to adults after CABG have shown an improvement in cardiac output and a fall in systemic vascular resistance, there was no alteration in overall mortality. In this group of patients, atrial fibrillation decreased by as much as 50% when compared with age-matched controls.[95] Pediatric cardiac patients, especially those undergoing surgery in the neonatal period, demonstrate an even greater decline in serum T_3 levels that can last longer. The low postoperative T_3 level identifies patients at increased risk for morbidity and mortality.[96] A prospective randomized study has shown that especially in neonates, the degree of therapeutic intervention and the need for postoperative inotropic agents is decreased by the administration of T_3 in doses sufficient to restore serum T_3 levels to normal.[97]

In patients with chronic congestive heart failure, the fall in serum T_3 levels correlates with the severity of heart failure as assessed by NYHA classification.[47,93] Up to 30% of patients with heart failure have a low serum T_3 level, which occurs in patients treated with amiodarone and in those who are not. In view of the deleterious effects of hypothyroidism on the myocardium, T_3 replacement may provide benefit. Human studies using a novel form of T_3 that can restore serum T_3 levels to normal and avoid the peaks and valleys of drug levels currently associated with existing drug preparations are needed to answer this question.

Pheochromocytoma

Pheochromocytomas (see Chaps. 45 and 94) are primarily benign tumors arising from neuroectodermal chromaffin cells usually within the adrenal medulla and abdomen, but they may arise anywhere within the plexus of sympathetic adrenergic nerves. Although the prevalence is probably less than 1/2000 cases of diastolic hypertension, the importance of pheochromocytoma derives from the dramatic mode in which symptoms can present. Autopsy studies have shown that in 75% of patients, the diagnosis was not clinically suspected and, in more than 50% of patients, it contributed to mortality.[98]

Most pheochromocytomas are 1 cm or larger, the vast majority arise as a unilateral adrenal lesion, and extra-adrenal tumors are more common in children.[99] Although most tumors are sporadic, approximately 10% are familial, and the latter are more often bilateral or occur in an extra-adrenal location. When pheochromocytoma coexists with medullary thyroid carcinoma or occasionally with hyperparathyroidism, it is designated as multiple endocrine neoplasia (MEN) syndrome type 2. These patients have a mutation in the RET proto-oncogene. In patients with MEN 2B, pheochromocytomas coexist with medullary thyroid cancer and mucosal neuromas frequently seen on the lips and tongue. In patients with neurofibromatosis, pheochromocytoma may be present in up to 1% of patients; in von Hippel–Lindau disease, pheochromocytoma develops in association with cerebellar or retinal angiomas and may have specific gene expression indicating a propensity for malignancy.[100]

Pheochromocytoma presents clinically with headache, palpitations, excessive sweating, tremulousness, chest pain, weight loss, and a variety of other constitutional complaints. Hypertension may be episodic but is usually constant, and is paradoxically associated with orthostatic hypotension on arising in the morning. The paroxysmal attacks and classic symptoms result from episodic excess catecholamine secretion.[98]

The first onset of hypertension caused by pheochromocytoma can be at the time of elective surgical intervention for an unrelated condition. As a result of norepinephrine release, with an increase in systemic vascular resistance, cardiac output is minimally (if at all) increased, despite increases in heart rate. The ECG can show LVH as well as the presence of inverted T waves, suggesting left ventricular strain. Although ventricular and atrial ectopy and episodes of supraventricular tachycardia can occur, there is little to distinguish the LVH from that of essential hypertension.[98]

Impaired left ventricular function and cardiomyopathy have occurred in patients with pheochromocytoma. The mechanism underlying this is complex and includes the following: increased left ventricular work and LVH from associated hypertension; potential adverse effects of excess catecholamines on myocyte structure and contractility; and changes in coronary arteries, including thickening of the media, presumably potentially impairing blood flow to the myocardium. Histologic evidence of myocarditis is present postmortem in patients with previously diagnosed or undiagnosed disease.[98] The possibility of catecholamine-stimulated tachycardia in turn mediating left ventricular dysfunction should be addressed, because treatments designed to slow heart rate may improve left ventricular function.

The release of catecholamines from pheochromocytomas involves diffusion out of chromaffin cells, as well as release of storage vessels, accounting for the demonstration of chromogranin A in the circulation. The primary catecholamine released is norepinephrine, but epinephrine can also increase. Demonstration of elevated serum dopamine levels implies malignant transformation, which in turn suggests that the tumor may arise in an extra-adrenal site and have certain gene expression profiles.[100] Rarely, pheochromocytoma can arise within the heart, presumably from chromaffin cells, which are part of the adrenergic autonomic paraganglia.[101]

DIAGNOSIS. Diagnosis is established by demonstrating an increase in norepinephrine or epinephrine or its metabolites in serum or blood. Quantitative 24-hour urinary metanephrine levels are the most reliable screening procedures, and plasma catecholamine levels, when determined under proper conditions, are also fairly sensitive.[101,102] Provocative tests aim to increase plasma catecholamine levels in patients with episodic disease; in contrast, the clonidine suppression test is safe and suppresses plasma norepinephrine levels by more than 50% in essential hypertensive patients, but not in those with pheochromocytoma.[99] Imaging modalities include MRI, which has a high degree of specificity, and computed tomography (CT), which has a high degree of sensitivity because adrenal lesions are large enough to be detected. Further studies with isotopic precursors of catecholamine biosynthesis, including ^{131}I-metaiodobenzylguanidine (MIBG), can confirm that anatomic lesions are producing catecholamines.

TREATMENT. Definitive treatment of pheochromocytoma requires removal of the lesion. Accurate preoperative localization reduces operative mortality and eliminates the need for exploratory laparotomy. Endoscopic procedures are now standard.[103] Preoperative pharmacologic management includes 7 to 14 days of alpha-adrenergic blockade, usually with prazosin or phenoxybenzamine. Beta blocker therapy is contraindicated before establishing sufficient alpha blockade. If supraventricular arrhythmias or unremitting tachycardia is present, beta$_1$-selective agents such as atenolol are preferred.[102] Operative intervention requires constant blood pressure monitoring and intravenous phentolamine or sodium nitroprusside may be required to treat episodic hypertension.[98] Postoperative management includes the use of large volumes of crystalloid-containing fluids to maintain blood volume and prevent hypotension. Glucose may be necessary to replace depleted liver glycogen stores. Success of surgery can be determined by effective blood pressure and symptomatic improvement, but also with measurement of urinary catecholamines 4 weeks after the procedure. In patients who are not candidates for surgical treatment, metyrosine can decrease catecholamine synthesis and improve most cardiovascular signs and symptoms.

Future Perspectives

The recognition that a variety of naturally occurring hormones have such profound effects on the heart and cardiovascular system suggests that these actions can be captured to treat a variety of cardiovascular diseases. The ability of thyroid hormone to lower cholesterol levels,[75] enhance cardiac contractility (especially diastolic function) via novel transcription-based mechanisms,[104] and at the same time lower systemic vascular resistance provides a platform for developing novel therapies. Similarly, the ability of vasoactive intestinal peptide to lower pulmonary artery pressure opens the possibility of treating patients with pulmonary hypertension from many different causes.

REFERENCES

(For references to the older literature, please consult the 8th edition of *Braunwald's Heart Disease*, Chap. 81.)

Acromegaly

1. Lu C, Schwartzbauer G, Sperling MA, et al: Demonstration of direct effects of growth hormone on neonatal cardiomyocytes. J Biol Chem 276:22892, 2001.
2. Napoli R, Guardasole V, Angelini V, et al: Acute effects of growth hormone on vascular function in human subjects. J Clin Endocrinol Metab 88:2817, 2003.
3. Colao A, Vitale G, Pivonello R, et al: The heart: An end-organ of GH action. Eur J Endocrinol 151(Suppl):S93, 2004.
4. Brevetti G, Marzullo P, Silvestro A, et al: Early vascular alterations in acromegaly. J Clin Endocrinol Metab 87:3174, 2002.
5. Mestron A, Webb SM, Astorga R, et al: Epidemiology, clinical characteristics, outcome, morbidity and mortality in acromegaly based on the Spanish Acromegaly Registry (Registro Espanol de Acromegalia, REA). Eur J Endocrinol 151:439, 2004.
6. Clayton RN: Cardiovascular function in acromegaly. Endocr Rev 24:272, 2003.
7. Bruch C, Herrmann B, Schmermund A, et al: Impact of disease activity on left ventricular performance in patients with acromegaly. Am Heart J 144:538, 2002.
8. Colao A, Spinelli L, Cuocolo A, et al: Cardiovascular consequences of early-onset growth hormone excess. J Clin Endocrinol Metab 87:3097, 2002.
9. Di Bello V, Bogazzi F, Di Cori A, et al: Myocardial systolic strain abnormalities in patients with acromegaly: A prospective color Doppler imaging study. J Endocrinol Invest 29:544, 2006.
10. Colao A, Spinelli L, Marzullo P, et al: High prevalence of cardiac valve disease in acromegaly: An observational, analytical, case-control study. J Clin Endocrinol Metab 88:3196, 2003.
11. van der Klaauw AA, Bax JJ, Roelfsema F, et al: Uncontrolled acromegaly is associated with progressive mitral valvular regurgitation. Growth Horm IGF Res 16:101, 2006.
12. Herrmann BL, Bruch C, Saller B, et al: Acromegaly: Evidence for a direct relation between disease activity and cardiac dysfunction in patients without ventricular hypertrophy. Clin Endocrinol (Oxf) 56:595, 2002.
13. Damjanovics SS, Neskovic AN, Petakov MS, et al: High output heart failure in patients with newly diagnosed acromegaly. Am J Med 112:610, 2002.
14. Trainer PJ, Drake WM, Katznelson L, et al: Treatment of acromegaly with the growth hormone-receptor antagonist pegvisomant. N Engl J Med 342:1171, 2000.
15. Clemmons DR, Chihara K, Freda PU, et al: Optimizing control of acromegaly: Integrating a growth hormone receptor antagonist into the treatment algorithm. J Clin Endocrinol Metab 88:4759, 2003.
16. Fazio S, Cittadini A, Biondi B, et al: Cardiovascular effects of short-term growth hormone hypersecretion. J Clin Endocrinol Metab 85:179, 2000.
17. Colao A, Pivonello R, Auriemma RS, et al: Predictors of tumor shrinkage after primary therapy with somatostatin analogues in acromegaly: A prospective study in 99 patients. J Clin Endocrinol Metab 91:2112, 2006.

Adrenal Cortex

18. Whitworth JA, Mangos GJ, Kelly JJ: Cushing, cortisol, and cardiovascular disease. Hypertension 36:912, 2000.
19. Wintour EM: Cortisol as a growth hormone for the fetal heart. Endocrinology 147:3641, 2006.
20. Colao A, Pivonello R, Spiezia S, et al: Persistence of increased cardiovascular risk in patients with Cushing disease after five years of successful cure. J Clin Endocrinol Metab 84:2664, 1999.
21. Maron BA, Leopold JA: Mineralocorticoid receptor antagonists and endothelial function. Curr Opin Investig Drugs 9:963, 2008.
22. Fernandez-Real J, Ricard W: Insulin resistance and chronic cardiovascular inflammatory syndrome. Endocr Rev 24:278, 2003.
23. Suzuki T, Shibata H, Ando T, et al: Risk factors associated with persistent postoperative hypertension in Cushing syndrome. Endocr Res 26:791, 2000.
24. Dekker MJ, Koper JW, van Aken MO, et al: Salivary cortisol is related to atherosclerosis of carotid arteries. J Clin Endocrinol Metab 93:3741, 2008.
25. Muiesan ML, Lupia M, Salvetti M, et al: Left ventricular structural and functional characteristics in Cushing syndrome. J Am Coll Cardiol 41:2275, 2003.
26. Marazuela M, Aguilar-Torres R, Benedicto A, et al: Dilated cardiomyopathy as a presenting feature of Cushing syndrome. Int J Cardiol 88:331, 2003.
27. Bertherat J: Carney complex (CNC). Orphanet J Rare Dis 6:21, 2006.
28. Carey RM, Siragy HM: Newly recognized components of the renin-angiotensin system: Potential roles in cardiovascular and renal regulation. Endocr Rev 24:261, 2003.
29. Young MJ, Funder JW: Mineralocorticoid receptors and pathophysiological roles for aldosterone in the cardiovascular system. J Hypertens 20:1465, 2002.
30. Szucs TD, Holm MV, Schwenkglenks M, et al: Cost-effectiveness of eplerenone in patients with left ventricular dysfunction after myocardial infarction—an analysis of the Ephesus Study from a Swiss perspective. Cardiovasc Drugs Ther 20:193, 2006.
31. Verma A, Solomon SD: Optimizing care of heart failure after acute MI with an aldosterone receptor antagonist. Curr Heart Fail Rep 4:183, 2007.
32. Matsumura K, Fujii K, Oniki H, et al: Role of aldosterone in left ventricular hypertrophy in hypertension. Am J Hypertens 19:13, 2006.
33. Watson T, Karthikeyan VJ, Lip GYH, Beevers DG: Atrial fibrillation in primary aldosteronism. J Renin Angiotensin Aldosterone Syst 10:190, 2009.
34. Funder JW, Carey RM, Fardella C: Case detection, diagnosis, and treatment of patients with primary aldosteronism: An endocrine society clinical practice guideline. J Clin Endocrinol Metab 93:3266, 2008.
35. Espinosa G, Santos E, Cervera R, et al: Adrenal involvement in the antiphospholipid syndrome: Clinical and immunologic characteristics of 86 patients. Medicine (Baltimore) 82:106, 2003.
36. Cooper MS, Stewart PM: Corticosteroid insufficiency in acutely ill patients. N Engl J Med 348:727, 2003.
37. Bergthorsdottir R, Leonsson-Zachrisson M, Oden A, Johannsson G: Premature mortality in patients with Addison's disease: A population-based study. J Clin Endocrinol Metab 91:4849, 2006.

Parathyroid Disease

38. Stefenelli T, Abela C, Frank H, et al: Cardiac abnormalities in patients with primary hyperparathyroidism: Implications for follow-up. J Clin Endocrinol Metab 82:106, 1997.
39. Birgander M, Bondeson A-G, Bondeson L, et al: Cardiac structure and function before and after parathyroidectomy in patients with asymptomatic primary hyperparathyroidism. Endocrinologist 19:154, 2009.
40. Floege J, Raggi P, Block GA, et al: Study design and subject baseline characteristics in the ADVANCE Study: Effects of cinacalcet on vascular calcification in haemodialysis patients. Nephrol Dial Transplant 25:1916, 2010.

Vitamin D

41. Holick MF: Vitamin D deficiency. New Engl J Med 357:266, 2007.
42. Vanga SR, Good M, Howard PA, Vacek JL: Role of vitamin D in cardiovascular health. Am J Cardiol 106:798, 2010.

Thyroid Disease

43. Klein I, Danzi S: Thyroid disease and the heart. Circulation 116:1725, 2007.
44. Gereben B, Zavacki AM, Ribich S, et al: Cellular and molecular basis of deiodinase-regulated thyroid hormone signaling. Endocr Rev 29:898, 2008.
45. Bassett JH, Harvey CB, Williams GR: Mechanisms of thyroid hormone receptor–specific nuclear and extra nuclear actions. Mol Cell Endocrinol 213:1, 2003.
46. Danzi S, Dubon P, Klein I: Effect of serum triiodothyronine on regulation of cardiac gene expression: Role of histone acetylation. Am J Physiol Heart Circ Physiol 289:H1506, 2005.
47. Danzi S, Klein I: Changes in thyroid hormone metabolism and gene expression in the failing heart: Therapeutic implications. *In* Iervasi G, Pingitore A (eds): Thyroid and Heart Failure: From Pathophysiology to Clinics. Milan, Italy, Springer-Verlag, 2009, pp 97-108.
48. Carr AN, Kranias EG: Thyroid hormone regulation of calcium cycling proteins. Thyroid 12:453, 2002.
49. Ojamaa K, Kenessey A, Klein I: Thyroid hormone regulation of phospholamban phosphorylation in the rat heart. Endocrinology 141:2139, 2000.
50. Biondi B, Klein I: Hypothyroidism as a risk factor for hypothyroidism. Endocrine 24:1, 2004.
51. Virtanen VK, Saha HH, Groundstroem KW, et al: Thyroid hormone substitution therapy rapidly enhances left-ventricular diastolic function in hypothyroid patients. Cardiology 96:59, 2001.
52. Davis PJ, Davis FB, Lin HY, et al: Translational implications of nongenomic actions of thyroid hormone initiated at its integrin receptor. Am J Physiol Endocrinol Metab 297:E1238, 2009.
53. Demers LM, Spencer CA: Laboratory medicine practice guidelines, laboratory support for the diagnosis and monitoring of thyroid disease. Thyroid 13:3, 2003.
54. Hoit BD, Khoury SF, Shao Y, et al: Effects of thyroid hormone on cardiac beta-adrenergic responsiveness in conscious baboons. Circulation 96:592, 1997.
55. Ojamaa K, Klein I, Sabet A, et al: Changes in adenylyl cyclase isoforms as a mechanism for thyroid hormone modulation of cardiac beta-adrenergic receptor responsiveness. Metabolism 49:275, 2000.
56. Park KW, Kai HB, Ojamaa K, et al: The direct vasomotor effect of thyroid hormones on rat skeletal muscle resistance arteries. Anesth Analg 85:734, 1997.
57. Danzi S, Klein I: Thyroid hormone and blood pressure regulation. Curr Hypertens Rep 5:513, 2003.
58. Biondi B, Palmieri EA, Lombardi G, et al: Effects of thyroid hormone on cardiac function: The relative importance of heart rate, loading conditions, and myocardial contractility in the regulation of cardiac performance in human hyperthyroidism. J Clin Endocrinol Metab 87:968, 2002.
59. Schmidt B, Martin N, Georgens AC, et al: Nongenomic cardiovascular effects of triiodothyronine in euthyroid male volunteers. J Clin Endocrinol Metab 87:1681, 2002.
60. Bengel FM, Lehnert J, Ibrahim T, et al: Cardiac oxidative metabolism, function, and metabolic performance in mild hyperthyroidism: A noninvasive study using positron emission tomography and magnetic resonance imaging. Thyroid 13:471, 2003.
61. Taddei S, Caraccio N, Virdis A, et al: Impaired endothelium-dependent vasodilatation in subclinical hypothyroidism: Beneficial effect of levothyroxine therapy. J Clin Endocrinol Metab 88:3731, 2003.
62. Kahaly GJ, Kampmann C, Mohr-Kahaly S: Cardiovascular hemodynamics and exercise tolerance in thyroid disease. Thyroid 12:473, 2002.
63. Im SH, Oh CW, Kwon OK, et al: Moyamoya disease associated with Graves' disease: Special considerations regarding clinical significance and management. J Neurosurg 102:1013, 2005.
64. Marvisi M, Zambrelli P, Brianti M: Pulmonary hypertension is frequent in hyperthyroidism and normalizes after therapy. Eur J Intern Med 17:267, 2006.
65. Shimizu T, Koide S, Noh JY, et al: Hyperthyroidism and the management of atrial fibrillation. Thyroid 12:489, 2002.
66. Auer J, Scheibner P, Mische T, et al: Subclinical hyperthyroidism as a risk factor for atrial fibrillation. Am Heart J 142:838, 2001.
67. Nakazawa H, Lythall DA, Noh J, et al: Is there a place for the late cardioversion of atrial fibrillation? A long-term follow-up study of patients with post-thyrotoxic atrial fibrillation. Eur Heart J 21:327, 2000.
68. Fuster V, Ryden LE, Asinger RW, et al: ACC/AHA/ESC guidelines for the management of patients with atrial fibrillation. J Am Coll Cardiol 38:1266, 2001.
69. Franklyn JA, Maisonneuve P, Sheppard MC, et al: Mortality after the treatment of hyperthyroidism with radioactive iodine. N Engl J Med 338:712, 1998.
70. Flynn RW, MacDonald TM, Jung RT, et al: Some cardiovascular diseases occur with increased frequency in patients treated for hyperthyroidism or hypothyroidism. J Clin Endocrinol Metab 91:2159, 2006.
71. Klein I: The cardiovascular system in hypothyroidism. *In* Braverman LE, Utiger RD (eds): Werner & Ingbar's The Thyroid: A Fundamental and Clinical Text. 9th ed. Philadelphia, Lippincott Williams & Wilkins, 2005, pp 774-780.

72. Bengel FM, Nekolla SC, Ibrahim T, et al: Effect of thyroid hormones on cardiac function, geometry, and oxidative metabolism assessed noninvasively by positron emission tomography and magnetic resonance imaging. J Clin Endocrinol Metab 85:1822, 2000.

73. Cappola AR, Ladenson PW: Hypothyroidism and atherosclerosis. J Clin Endocrinol Metab 88:2438, 2003.

74. Rush J, Danzi S, Klein I: Role of thyroid disease in the development of statin-induced myopathy. Endocrinologist 16:279, 2006.

75. Ladenson PW, Kristensen JD, Ridgway EC, et al: Use of the thyroid hormone analogue eprotirome in statin-treated dyslipidemia. N Engl J Med 362:906, 2010.

76. Hak AE, Pols HAP, Visser TJ, et al: Subclinical hypothyroidism is an independent risk factor for atherosclerosis and myocardial infarction in elderly women: The Rotterdam Study. Ann Intern Med 132:270, 2000.

77. Walsh JP, Bremmer AP, Bulsara MK, et al: Subclinical thyroid dysfunction as a risk factor for cardiovascular disease. Arch Intern Med 165:2467, 2005.

78. Kim SD, Kim SH, Park KS, et al: Regression of the increased common carotid artery-intima media thickness in subclinical hypothyroidism after thyroid hormone replacement. Endocr J 56:753, 2009.

79. Rodondi N, Bauer DC, Cappola AR: Subclinical thyroid dysfunction, cardiac function, and the risk of heart failure. The Cardiovascular Health study. J Am Coll Cardiol 52:1152, 2008.

80. Rodondi N, den Elzen WPJ, Bauer DC, et al: Subclinical hypothyroidism and the risk of coronary heart disease and mortality. JAMA 304:1365, 2010.

81. Biondi B, Cooper DS: The clinical significance of subclinical thyroid dysfunction. Endocr Rev 29:76, 2008.

82. Razvi SS, Pearce SH: Treatment of subclinical hypothyroidism and cardiovascular morbidity and mortality—analysis of the United Kingdom General Practitioner Research Database. Abstract, International Thyroid Congress, 2010.

83. Sawin CT: Subclinical hyperthyroidism and atrial fibrillation. Thyroid 12:501, 2002.

84. Cappola AR, Fried LP, Arnold AM, et al: Thyroid status, cardiovascular risk, and mortality in older adults. JAMA 295:1033, 2006.

85. Parle JV, Maisonneuve P, Sheppard MC, et al: Prediction of all-cause and cardiovascular mortality in elderly people from one low serum thyrotropin result: A 10-year cohort study. Lancet 358:861, 2001.

86. Mitchell AL, Pearce SH: How should we treat patients with low serum thyrotropin concentrations? Clin Endocrinol (Oxf) Epub Sept 10, 2009.

Amiodarone

87. Cohen-Lehman J, Dahl P, Danzi S, Klein I: Effects of amiodarone on thyroid function. Nat Rev Endocrinol 6:34, 2010.

88. Multaq (Dronedarone): Briefing Document: Advisory Committee Meeting of the Cardiovascular and Renal Drugs Division of the US Food and Drug Administration, March 18, 2009 (http://www.fda.gov/downloads/AdvisoryCommittees/CommitteesMeetingMaterials/Drugs/CardiovascularandRenalDrugsAdvisoryCommittee/UCM134981.pdf).

89. Bogazzi F, Bartalena L, Cosci C, et al: Treatment of type II amiodarone-induced thyrotoxicosis by either iopanoic acid or glucocorticoids: A prospective, randomized study. J Clin Endocrinol Metab 88:1999, 2003.

90. Yiu KH, Jim MH, Siu CW, et al: Amiodarone-induced thyrotoxicosis is associated with a nearly threefold increased risk for major adverse cardiovascular events that must be identified and treated. J Clin Endocrinol Metab 94:109, 2009.

91. Williams M, Lo Gerfo P: Thyroidectomy using local anesthesia in critically ill patients with amiodarone-induced thyrotoxicosis: A review and description of the technique. Thyroid 12:523, 2002.

Changes in Thyroid Hormone Metabolism in Cardiac Disease

92. Iervasi G, Pingitore A, Landi P, et al: Low-T_3 syndrome: A strong prognostic predictor of death in patients with heart disease. Circulation 107:708, 2003.

93. Pingitore A, Galli E, Barison A, et al: Acute effects of triiodothyronine (T_3) replacement therapy in patients with chronic heart failure and low-T3 syndrome: A randomized, placebo-controlled study. J Clin Endocrinol Metab 93:1351, 2008.

94. Portman MA, Fearneyhough C, Ning W, et al: Triiodothyronine repletion in infants during cardiopulmonary bypass for congenital heart disease. J Thorac Cardiovasc Surg 120:604, 2000.

95. Klemperer JD, Klein I, Ojamaa K, et al: Triiodothyronine therapy lowers the incidence of atrial fibrillation after cardiac operations. Ann Thorac Surg 61:1323, 1996.

96. Portman MA, Slee A, Olson AK, et al: Triiodothyronine supplementation in infants and children undergoing cardiopulmonary bypass (TRICC): A multicenter placebo-controlled randomized trial: Age analysis. Circulation 122(suppl 1):S224, 2010.

97. Chowdhury D, Parnell V, Ojamaa, K, et al: Usefulness of triiodothyronine (T_3) treatment after surgery for complex congenital heart disease in infants and children. Am J Cardiol 84:1107, 1999.

Pheochromocytoma

98. Bravo EL: Pheochromocytoma. Cardiol Rev 10:44, 2002.

99. Manger WM, Gifford RW: Pheochromocytoma. J Clin Hypertens (Greenwich) 4:62, 2002.

100. Brouwers FM, Elkahloun AG, Munson PJ, et al: Gene expression profiling of benign and malignant pheochromocytoma. Ann N Y Acad Sci 1073:541, 2006.

101. Lenders JW, Pacak K, Eisenhofer G: New advances in the biochemical diagnosis of pheochromocytoma: Moving beyond catecholamines. Ann N Y Acad Sci 970:29, 2002.

102. Schiff RL, Welsh GA: Perioperative evaluation and management of the patient with endocrine dysfunction. Med Clin North Am 87:175, 2003.

103. Eigelberger MS, Duh QY: Pheochromocytoma. Curr Treat Options Oncol 2:321, 2001.

104. Danzi S, Klein I: Thyroid hormone treatment to mend a broken heart. J Clin Endocrinol Metab 93:1172, 2008.

CHAPTER **87**

Hemostasis, Thrombosis, Fibrinolysis, and Cardiovascular Disease

Jeffrey I. Weitz

Hemostasis preserves vascular integrity by balancing the physiologic processes that maintain blood fluidity under normal circumstances and prevent excessive bleeding after vascular injury. Preservation of blood fluidity depends on an intact vascular endothelium and a complex series of regulatory pathways that maintain platelets in a quiescent state and keep the coagulation system in check. In contrast, arrest of bleeding requires rapid formation of hemostatic plugs at sites of vascular injury to prevent exsanguination. Perturbation of hemostasis can lead to thrombosis, which can occur in arteries or veins and is a major cause of morbidity and mortality. Arterial thrombosis is the most common cause of acute coronary syndromes, ischemic stroke, and limb gangrene, whereas thrombosis in the deep veins of the leg leads to the postphlebitic syndrome and to pulmonary embolism, which can be fatal.

Most arterial thrombi form on top of disrupted atherosclerotic plaques, because plaque rupture exposes thrombogenic material in the plaque core to the blood. This material then triggers platelet aggregation and fibrin formation, which results in the generation of a platelet-rich thrombus that temporarily or permanently occludes blood flow.[1,2] Temporary occlusion of blood flow in coronary arteries may trigger unstable angina, whereas persistent obstruction causes myocardial infarction. The same processes can occur in the cerebral circulation, where temporary arterial occlusion may manifest as a transient ischemic attack and permanent occlusion can lead to a stroke.

In contrast to arterial thrombi, venous thrombi rarely form at sites of obvious vascular disruption.[2] Although they can develop after surgical trauma to veins, or secondary to indwelling venous catheters, they usually originate in the valve cusps of the deep veins of the calf or in the muscular sinuses, where there is stasis. Sluggish blood flow in these veins reduces the oxygen supply to the avascular valve cusps. Hypoxemia induces endothelial cells lining the valve cusps to express adhesion molecules, which tether tissue factor–bearing leukocytes and microparticles onto their surface. Tissue factor–bearing leukocytes and microparticles adhere to these activated cells and induce coagulation. Impaired blood flow exacerbates local thrombus formation by reducing clearance of activated clotting factors. Calf vein thrombi that extend into the proximal veins of the leg can dislodge and travel to the lungs to produce pulmonary embolism.

Arterial and venous thrombi contain platelets and fibrin, but the proportions differ. Arterial thrombi are rich in platelets because of the high shear in the injured arteries. In contrast, venous thrombi, which form under low shear conditions, contain relatively few platelets and consist mostly of fibrin and trapped red cells.[2] Because of the predominance of platelets, arterial thrombi appear white, whereas venous thrombi appear red, reflecting the trapped red cells.

The antithrombotic drugs used for prevention and treatment of thrombosis target components of thrombi, and include antiplatelet drugs, which inhibit platelets; anticoagulants, which attenuate coagulation; and fibrinolytic agents, which induce fibrin degradation (**Fig. 87-1**). With the predominance of platelets in arterial thrombi, strategies to inhibit or treat arterial thrombosis focus mainly on antiplatelet agents,[2] although in the acute setting, strategies often include anticoagulants and fibrinolytic agents. When arterial thrombi are occlusive and rapid restoration of blood flow is required, mechanical and pharmacologic methods enable thrombus extraction, compression, or degradation. Although rarely used for this indication, anticoagulants can also prevent recurrent ischemic events after acute myocardial infarction. Anticoagulants are the mainstay for prevention and treatment of venous thromboembolism because fibrin is the predominant component of venous thrombi. Antiplatelet drugs are less effective than anticoagulants because of the limited platelet content of venous thrombi. Selected patients with venous thromboembolism benefit from fibrinolytic therapy[3]—for example, patients with massive or submassive pulmonary embolism—achieve more rapid restoration of pulmonary blood flow with systemic or catheter-directed fibrinolytic therapy than with anticoagulant therapy alone (see Chap. 77). Selected patients with extensive deep vein thrombosis in the iliac and/or femoral veins also may have a better outcome with catheter-directed fibrinolytic therapy and/or mechanical thrombus extraction in addition to anticoagulants.

Building on a review of hemostasis and thrombosis that highlights the processes involved in platelet activation and aggregation, blood coagulation, and fibrinolysis, this chapter focuses on antiplatelet, anticoagulant, and fibrinolytic drugs in common use. It also provides a brief overview of new antithrombotic drugs in advanced stages of development.

Hemostatic System

The major components of the hemostatic system are the vascular endothelium, platelets, and the coagulation and fibrinolytic systems.

Vascular Endothelium

A monolayer of endothelial cells lines the intimal surface of the circulatory tree and separates the blood from the prothrombotic subendothelial components of the vessel wall. As such, the vascular endothelium (see Chap. 43) encompasses about 10^{13} cells and covers a vast surface area. Rather than serving as a static barrier, the healthy vascular endothelium is a dynamic organ that actively regulates hemostasis by inhibiting platelets, suppressing coagulation, and promoting fibrinolysis.[1,2]

PLATELET INHIBITION. Endothelial cells synthesize prostacyclin and nitric oxide and release them into the blood. These agents not

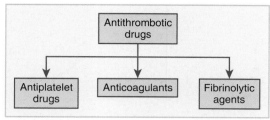

FIGURE 87-1 Classification of antithrombotic drugs.

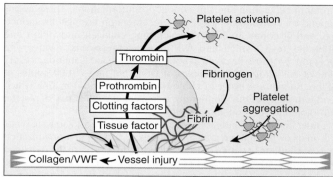

FIGURE 87-3 Central role of thrombin in thrombogenesis. Vascular injury simultaneously triggers platelet adhesion and activation, as well as activation of the coagulation system. Platelet activation is initiated by exposure of subendothelial collagen and vWF, onto which platelets adhere. Adherent platelets become activated and release ADP and thromboxane A₂, platelet agonists that activate ambient platelets and recruit them to the site of injury. Coagulation, which is triggered by tissue factor exposed at the site of injury, results in thrombin generation. Thrombin not only converts fibrinogen to fibrin, but also serves as a potent platelet agonist. When platelets are activated, glycoprotein IIb/IIIa on their surface undergoes a conformational change that endows it with the capacity to ligate fibrinogen and mediate platelet aggregation. Fibrin strands then weave the platelet aggregates together to form a platelet-fibrin thrombus (see Fig. 56-3).

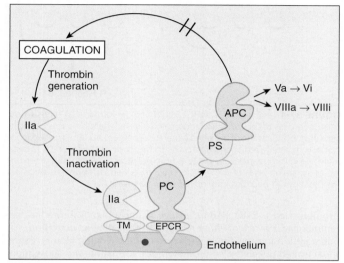

FIGURE 87-2 Protein C pathway. Activation of coagulation triggers thrombin (IIa) generation. Excess thrombin binds to thrombomodulin (TM) on the endothelial cell surface. Once bound, the substrate specificity of thrombin alters such that it no longer acts as a procoagulant, but becomes a potent activator of protein C (PC). EPCR binds protein C and presents it to thrombomodulin-bound thrombin for activation. Activated protein C (APC), together with its cofactor, protein S (PS), binds to the activated platelet surface and proteolytically degrades factors Va and VIIIa into inactive fragments (Vi and VIIIi). Degradation of these activated cofactors inhibits thrombin generation (double bar).

only serve as potent vasodilators, but also inhibit platelet activation and subsequent aggregation by stimulating adenylate cyclase and increasing intracellular levels of cyclic adenosine monophosphate (cAMP). In addition, endothelial cells express CD39 on their surface, a membrane-associated ecto adenosine diphosphatase (ADPase). By degrading ADP, a platelet agonist, CD39 attenuates platelet activation.[4]

ANTICOAGULANT ACTIVITY. Intact endothelial cells play an essential part in the regulation of thrombin generation through various mechanisms. Endothelial cells produce heparan sulfate proteoglycans, which bind circulating antithrombin and accelerate the rate at which it inhibits thrombin and other coagulation enzymes.[5] Tissue factor pathway inhibitor (TFPI), a naturally occurring inhibitor of coagulation, binds heparan sulfate on the endothelial cell surface.[6] Administration of heparin or low-molecular-weight heparin (LMWH) displaces glycosaminoglycan-bound TFPI from the vascular endothelium, and released TFPI may contribute to the antithrombotic activity of these drugs.[7] Endothelial cells express thrombomodulin and endothelial cell protein C receptor (EPCR) on their surface.[8]

Thrombomodulin binds thrombin and alters this enzyme's substrate specificity so that it no longer acts as a procoagulant, but becomes a potent activator of protein C (**Fig. 87-2**). Activated protein C serves as an anticoagulant by degrading and inactivating activated factors V and VIII (factor Va and VIIIa, respectively), key cofactors involved in thrombin generation. EPCR on the endothelial cell surface enhances this

pathway by binding protein C and presenting it to the thrombin–thrombomodulin complex for activation.[9]

FIBRINOLYTIC ACTIVITY. The vascular endothelium promotes fibrinolysis by synthesizing and releasing tissue and urokinase plasminogen activator (t-PA and u-PA, respectively), which initiate fibrinolysis by converting plasminogen to plasmin.[10] Endothelial cells in most vascular beds synthesize t-PA constitutively. In contrast, perturbed endothelial cells produce u-PA in the settings of inflammation and wound repair.

Endothelial cells also produce type 1 plasminogen activator inhibitor (PAI-1), the major regulator of t-PA and u-PA. Therefore, net fibrinolytic activity depends on the dynamic balance between the release of plasminogen activators and PAI-1. Fibrinolysis localizes to the endothelial cell surface because these cells express annexin II, a coreceptor for plasminogen and t-PA that promotes their interaction. Therefore, healthy vessels actively resist thrombosis and help maintain platelets in a quiescent state.[10]

Platelets

Platelets are anucleate particles released into the circulation after fragmentation of bone marrow megakaryocytes. Because they are anucleate, platelets have limited capacity to synthesize proteins. Thrombopoietin, a glycoprotein synthesized in the liver and kidneys, regulates megakaryocytic proliferation and maturation as well as platelet production.[11] Once they enter the circulation, platelets have a life span of 7 to 10 days.

Damage to the intimal lining of the vessel exposes the underlying subendothelial matrix. Platelets home to sites of vascular disruption and adhere to the exposed matrix proteins. Adherent platelets undergo activation and not only release substances that recruit additional platelets to the site of injury, but also promote thrombin generation and subsequent fibrin formation (**Fig. 87-3**). A potent platelet agonist, thrombin amplifies platelet recruitment and activation. Activated platelets then aggregate to form a plug that seals the leak in the vasculature. Understanding the steps in these highly integrated processes helps pinpoint the sites of action of the antiplatelet drugs and rationalizes the usefulness of anticoagulants for the treatment of arterial thrombosis and venous thrombosis.

ADHESION. Platelets adhere to exposed collagen and von Willebrand factor (vWF) and form a monolayer that supports and promotes thrombin generation and subsequent fibrin formation.[12] These events depend on constitutively expressed receptors on the platelet surface, $\alpha_2\beta_1$ and glycoprotein (GP) VI, which bind collagen, and GPIbα and GPIIb/IIIa ($\alpha_{IIb}\beta_3$), which bind vWF. The platelet surface is crowded with receptors, but those involved in adhesion are the most abundant: every platelet has about 80,000 copies of GPIIb/IIIa and 25,000 copies of GPIbα. Receptors cluster in cholesterol-enriched subdomains, which render them more mobile, thereby increasing the efficiency of platelet adhesion and subsequent activation.[13]

Under low shear conditions, collagen can capture and activate platelets on its own. Captured platelets undergo cytoskeletal reorganization that causes them to flatten out and adhere more closely to the damaged vessel wall. Under high shear conditions, however, collagen and vWF must act in concert to support optimal platelet adhesion and activation. vWF synthesized by endothelial cells and megakaryocytes assembles into multimers that range from 550 to over 10,000 kDa.[14] When released from storage in the Weibel-Palade bodies of endothelial cells or the alpha granules of platelets, most of the vWF enters the circulation, but the vWF released from the abluminal surface of endothelial cells accumulates in the subendothelial matrix, where it binds collagen via its A3 domain. This surface-immobilized vWF can simultaneously bind platelets via its A1 domain. In contrast, circulating vWF does not react with unstimulated platelets. This difference in reactivity likely reflects vWF conformation; circulating vWF is in a coiled conformation that prevents access of its platelet-binding domain to vWF receptors on the platelet surface, whereas immobilized vWF assumes an elongated shape that exposes the A1 domain. In their extended conformation, large vWF multimers act as the molecular glue that tethers platelets to the damaged vessel wall with sufficient strength to withstand higher shear forces. Large vWF multimers provide additional binding sites for collagen, and heighten platelet adhesion because platelets have more vWF receptors than collagen receptors.[15] Adhesion to collagen or vWF results in platelet activation, the next step in platelet plug formation.

ACTIVATION. Adhesion to collagen and vWF initiates signaling pathways that result in platelet activation. These pathways induce cyclooxygenase-1 (COX-1)–dependent synthesis and release of thromboxane A$_2$, and trigger the release of ADP from storage granules. Thromboxane A$_2$ is a potent vasoconstrictor and, like ADP, locally activates ambient platelets and recruits them to the site of injury. This process results in expansion of the platelet plug. To activate platelets, thromboxane A$_2$ and ADP must bind to their respective receptors on the platelet membrane. The thromboxane receptor (TP) is a G protein–coupled receptor that is found on platelets and on the endothelium, which explains why thromboxane A$_2$ induces vasoconstriction as well as platelet activation.[16] ADP interacts with a family of G protein–coupled receptors on the platelet membrane.[17,18] Most important of these is P2Y$_{12}$, which is the target of the thienopyridines, but P2Y$_1$ also contributes to ADP-induced platelet activation, and maximal ADP-induced platelet activation requires activation of both receptors. A third ADP receptor, P2X$_1$, is an ATP-gated calcium channel. Platelet storage granules contain ATP and ADP; ATP released during the platelet activation process may contribute to the platelet recruitment process in a P2X$_1$-dependent fashion.

Although TP and the various ADP receptors signal through different pathways, they all increase the intracellular calcium concentration in platelets. This in turn induces shape change via cytoskeletal rearrangement, granule mobilization and release, and subsequent platelet aggregation. Activated platelets promote coagulation by expressing phosphatidyl serine on their surface, an anionic phospholipid that supports assembly of coagulation factor complexes. Once assembled, these clotting factor complexes trigger a burst of thrombin generation and subsequent fibrin formation. In addition to converting fibrinogen to fibrin, thrombin amplifies platelet recruitment and activation and promotes expansion of the platelet plug. Thrombin binds to protease-activated receptors types 1 and 4 (PAR1 and PAR4, respectively) on the platelet surface and cleaves their extended amino termini (**Fig. 87-4**), thereby generating new amino termini that serve as tethered ligands that bind and activate the receptors.[17,19] Whereas low concentrations of

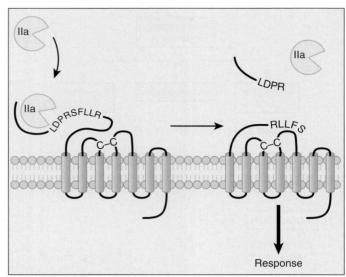

FIGURE 87-4 Activation of PAR1 by thrombin. Thrombin (IIa) binds to the amino terminus of the extracellular domain of PAR1, where it cleaves a specific peptide bond. Cleavage of this bond generates a new amino-terminus sequence that acts as a tethered ligand and binds to the body of the receptor, thereby activating it. Thrombin then dissociates from the receptor. Analogues of the first five or six amino acids of the tethered ligand sequences, known as thrombin receptor agonist peptides, can independently activate PAR1.

thrombin cleave PAR1, PAR4 cleavage requires higher thrombin concentrations. Cleavage of either receptor triggers platelet activation.

In addition to providing a surface on which clotting factors assemble, activated platelets also promote fibrin formation and subsequent stabilization by releasing factor V, factor XI, fibrinogen, and factor XIII. Thus, there is coordinated activation of platelets and coagulation, and the fibrin network that results from thrombin action helps anchor the platelet aggregates at the site of injury. Activated platelets also release adhesive proteins, such as vWF, thrombospondin, and fibronectin, which may augment platelet adhesion at sites of injury, as well as growth factors, such as platelet-derived growth factor (PDGF) and transforming growth factor-β (TGF-β), which promote wound healing. Platelet aggregation is the final step in the formation of the platelet plug.

AGGREGATION. Platelet aggregation links platelets to each other to form clumps. GPIIb/IIIa mediates these platelet-to-platelet linkages. On nonactivated platelets, GPIIb/IIIa exhibits minimal affinity for its ligands. On platelet activation, GPIIb/IIIa undergoes a conformational transformation, which reflects transmission of inside-out signals from its cytoplasmic domain to its extracellular domain.[15] This transformation enhances the affinity of GPIIb/IIIa for its ligands, fibrinogen, and under high shear conditions, vWF. Arg-Gly-Asp (RGD) sequences located on fibrinogen and vWF, as well as a platelet-binding Lys-Gly-Asp (KGD) sequence on fibrinogen, mediate their interaction with GPIIb/IIIa. When subjected to high shear, circulating vWF elongates and exposes its platelet-binding domain, which enables its interaction with the conformationally activated GPIIb/IIIa.[14] Divalent fibrinogen and multivalent vWF molecules serve as bridges and bind adjacent platelets together. Once bound to GPIIb/IIIa, fibrinogen and vWF induce outside-inside signals that augment platelet activation and result in the activation of additional GPIIb/IIIa receptors, creating a positive feedback loop. Because GPIIb/IIIa acts as the final effector in platelet aggregation, it is a logical target for potent antiplatelet drugs. Fibrin, the ultimate product of the coagulation system, tethers the platelet aggregates together and anchors them to the site of injury.

Coagulation

Coagulation results in the generation of thrombin, which converts soluble fibrinogen to fibrin. Coagulation occurs through the action of discrete enzyme complexes, which are composed of a vitamin K–dependent enzyme and a nonenzyme cofactor, and assemble on anionic phospholipid membranes in a calcium-dependent fashion. Each enzyme complex activates a vitamin K–dependent substrate that becomes the enzyme component of the subsequent complex (**Fig. 87-5**). Together, these complexes generate a small amount of thrombin that amplifies its own generation by activating the nonenzyme cofactors and platelets, which then provide an anionic surface on which the complexes assemble. The three enzyme complexes involved in thrombin generation are extrinsic tenase, intrinsic tenase, and prothrombinase. Although extrinsic tenase initiates the system under most circumstances, the contact system also plays a role in some situations.

EXTRINSIC TENASE. This complex forms on exposure of tissue factor–expressing cells to the blood. Tissue factor exposure occurs after atherosclerotic plaque rupture because the core of the plaque is rich in cells that express tissue factor. Denuding injury to the vessel wall also exposes tissue factor constitutively expressed by subendothelial fibroblasts and smooth muscle cells. In addition to cells in the vessel wall, circulating monocytes and monocyte-derived microparticles (small membrane fragments) also provide a source of tissue factor.[20] When tissue factor–bearing monocytes or microparticles bind to platelets or other leukocytes and their plasma membranes fuse, tissue factor transfer occurs. By binding to adhesion molecules expressed on activated endothelial cells or to P-selectin on activated platelets, these tissue factor–bearing cells or microparticles can initiate or augment coagulation.[21] This phenomenon likely explains how venous thrombi develop in the absence of obvious vessel wall injury.[2]

Tissue factor is an integral membrane protein that serves as a receptor for factor VIIa. The blood contains trace amounts of factor VIIa, which has negligible activity in the absence of tissue factor.[22] With tissue factor exposure on anionic cell surfaces, factor VIIa binds in a calcium-dependent fashion to form the extrinsic tenase complex, which is a potent activator of factors IX and X. Once activated, factors IXa and Xa serve as the enzyme components of intrinsic tenase and prothrombinase, respectively.

INTRINSIC TENASE. Factor IXa binds to factor VIIIa on anionic cell surfaces to form the intrinsic tenase complex. Factor VIII circulates in blood in complex with vWF. Thrombin cleaves factor VIII and releases it from vWF, converting it to its activated form. Activated platelets express binding sites for factor VIIIa. Once bound, factor VIIIa binds factor IXa in a calcium-dependent fashion to form the intrinsic tenase complex, which then activates factor X. The reduction in catalytic efficiency of factor IXa–mediated activation of factor X that occurs with deletion of individual components of the intrinsic tenase complex highlights their importance. Absence of the membrane or factor VIIIa almost completely abolishes enzymatic activity, and the catalytic efficiency of the complete complex is 10^9-fold greater than that of factor IXa alone. Because intrinsic tenase activates factor X at a rate 50- to 100-fold faster than extrinsic tenase, it plays a critical role in the amplification of factor Xa and subsequent thrombin generation.

PROTHROMBINASE. Factor Xa binds to factor Va, its activated cofactor, on anionic phospholipid membrane surfaces to form the prothrombinase complex. Activated platelets release factor V from their alpha granules, and this platelet-derived factor V may be more important in hemostasis than its plasma counterpart. Whereas plasma factor V requires thrombin activation to exert its cofactor

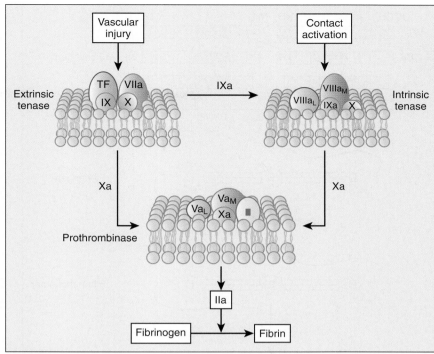

FIGURE 87-5 Coagulation system. Coagulation occurs through the action of discrete enzyme complexes, which are composed of a vitamin K–dependent enzyme and a nonenzyme cofactor. These complexes assemble on anionic phospholipid membranes in a calcium-dependent fashion. Vascular injury exposes tissue factor (TF), which binds factor VIIa to form extrinsic tenase. Extrinsic tenase activates factors IX and X. Factor IXa binds to factor VIIIa to form intrinsic tenase, which activates factor X. Factor Xa binds to factor Va to form prothrombinase, which converts prothrombin (II) to thrombin (IIa). Thrombin then converts soluble fibrinogen into insoluble fibrin.

activity, the partially activated factor V released from platelets already exhibits substantial cofactor activity. Activated platelets express specific factor Va binding sites on their surface, and bound factor Va serves as a receptor for factor Xa. The catalytic efficiency of factor Xa activation of prothrombin increases by 10^9-fold when factor Xa is incorporated into the prothrombinase complex. Prothrombin binds to the prothrombinase complex, where it undergoes conversion to thrombin in a reaction that releases prothrombin fragment 1.2 (F1.2). Plasma levels of F1.2, therefore, provide a marker of prothrombin activation.

FIBRIN FORMATION. The final effector in coagulation is thrombin. Thrombin converts soluble fibrinogen into insoluble fibrin. Fibrinogen is a dimeric molecule, each half of which is composed of three polypeptide chains—the Aα, Bβ, and γ chains. Numerous disulfide bonds covalently link the chains together and join the two halves of the fibrinogen molecule (**Fig. 87-6**). Electron micrographic studies of fibrinogen reveal a trinodular structure, with a central E domain flanked by two D domains. Crystal structures show symmetry of design with the central E domain, which contains the amino termini of the fibrinogen chains joined to the lateral D domains by coiled coil regions.

Fibrinogen, the most abundant plasma protein involved in coagulation, circulates in an inactive form. Thrombin binds to the amino termini of the Aα and Bβ chains of fibrinogen, where it cleaves specific peptide bonds to release fibrinopeptide A and fibrinopeptide B and generates fibrin monomer (see Fig. 87-6). Because they are products of thrombin action on fibrinogen, plasma levels of these fibrinopeptides provide an index of thrombin activity. Fibrinopeptide release creates new amino termini that extend as knobs from the E domain of one fibrin monomer and insert into preformed holes in the D domains of other fibrin monomers. This creates long strands known as protofibrils, consisting of fibrin monomers noncovalently linked together in a half-staggered overlapping fashion.

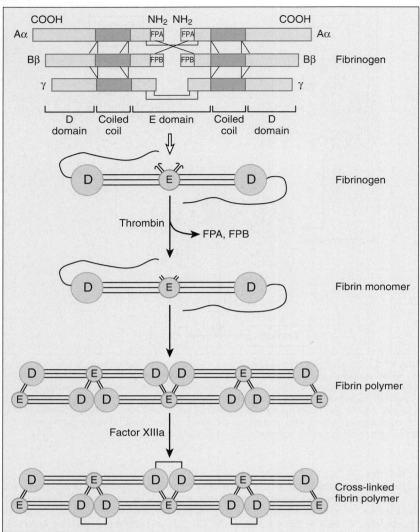

FIGURE 87-6 Fibrinogen structure and conversion of fibrinogen to fibrin. A chimeric molecule, each half of fibrinogen is composed of three polypeptide chains—the Aα, Bβ, and γ chains. Numerous disulfide bonds (lines) covalently link the chains together and join the two halves of the fibrinogen molecule to yield a trinodular structure with a central E domain linked via the coiled coil regions to two lateral D domains. To convert fibrinogen to fibrin, thrombin cleaves specific peptide bonds at the amino (NH₂) termini of the Aα and Bβ chains of fibrinogen to release fibrinopeptide A (FPA) and fibrinopeptide B (FPB), thereby generating fibrin monomer. Fibrin monomers polymerize to generate protofibrils arranged in a half-staggered overlapping fashion. By covalently cross-linking α and γ chains of adjacent fibrin monomers, factor XIIIa stabilizes the fibrin network and renders it resistant to degradation.

Noncovalently linked fibrin protofibrils are unstable. By covalently cross-linking alpha and gamma chains of adjacent fibrin monomers, factor XIIIa stabilizes the fibrin in a calcium-dependent fashion and renders it relatively resistant to degradation. Factor XIII circulates in blood as a heterodimer consisting of two A and two B subunits. The active site and calcium binding site of factor XIII are localized to the A subunit. Platelets contain large amounts of factor XIII in their cytoplasm, but platelet-derived factor XIII consists only of A subunits. Both plasma and platelet factor XIII are activated by thrombin.

CONTACT PATHWAY. Current thinking is that tissue factor exposure represents the sole pathway for activation of coagulation and that the contact system, which includes factor XII, prekallikrein, and high-molecular-weight kininogen, is unimportant for hemostasis because patients deficient in these factors do not have bleeding problems. The physiologic role of factor XI is more difficult to assess because the plasma level of factor XI does not predict the propensity for bleeding.

Although the capacity of thrombin to feed back and activate platelet-bound factor XI may explain this phenomenon, platelet-derived factor XI may be more important for hemostasis than circulating factor XI.

The contact pathway cannot be ignored, however, because coronary catheters and other blood-contacting medical devices, such as stents or mechanical valves, likely trigger clotting through this mechanism.[23] Factor XII bound to the surface of catheters or devices undergoes a conformational change that results in its activation. Factor XIIa converts prekallikrein to kallikrein in a reaction accelerated by high-molecular-weight kininogen, and factor XIIa and kallikrein then feed back to activate additional factor XII. Factor XIIa propagates coagulation by activating factor XI (**Fig. 87-7**).

In addition to its role in device-related thrombosis, the contact pathway may also contribute to arterial thrombosis. RNA released from damaged cells in atherosclerotic plaques activates factor XII, and mice given RNA-degrading enzymes exhibit attenuated thrombosis at sites of arterial injury. Polyphosphates released from activated platelets also activate factor XII, and may provide another stimulus for contact pathway activation. Mice deficient in factor XI or XII form small unstable thrombi at sites of arterial damage, suggesting that factors XI and XII contribute to thrombogenesis.[24] It is unknown whether the same is true in humans. Patients with unstable angina have increased plasma levels of factor XIa,[25] but it is unclear whether this reflects activation by factor XIIa or thrombin. Although the contribution of the contact pathway to thrombin generation remains uncertain, the final product of coagulation is fibrin. Hemostasis depends on the dynamic balance between the formation of fibrin and its degradation. The fibrinolytic system mediates fibrin breakdown.

Fibrinolytic System

Fibrinolysis is initiated when plasminogen activators convert plasminogen to plasmin, which then degrades fibrin into soluble fragments (**Fig. 87-8**). Blood contains two immunologically and functionally distinct plasminogen activators, t-PA and u-PA. t-PA mediates intravascular fibrin degradation, whereas u-PA binds to a specific u-PA receptor (u-PAR) on the surface of cells, where it activates cell-bound plasminogen.[10] Consequently, pericellular proteolysis during cell migration and tissue remodeling and repair are the major functions of u-PA.

Regulation of fibrinolysis occurs at two levels. PAI-1 and, to a lesser extent, PAI-2, inhibit the plasminogen activators, whereas alpha₂-antiplasmin inhibits plasmin. Endothelial cells synthesize PAI-1, which inhibits both t-PA and u-PA, whereas monocytes and the placenta synthesize PAI-2, which specifically inhibits u-PA.[10] Thrombin-activated fibrinolysis inhibitor (TAFI) also modulates fibrinolysis and provides a link between fibrinolysis and coagulation.[26] Thrombosis can occur if there is impaired activation of the fibrinolytic system, whereas excessive activation leads to bleeding. Therefore, a review of the mechanisms of action of t-PA, u-PA, and TAFI is worthwhile.

MECHANISM OF ACTION OF TISSUE PLASMINOGEN ACTIVATOR. t-PA, a serine protease, contains five discrete domains—a fibronectin-like finger domain, an epidermal growth factor (EGF) domain, two kringle domains, and a protease domain. Synthesized as a single-chain polypeptide, plasmin readily converts t-PA into a two-chain form. Single- and two-chain forms of t-PA convert plasminogen to plasmin. Native Glu-plasminogen is a single-chain polypeptide with

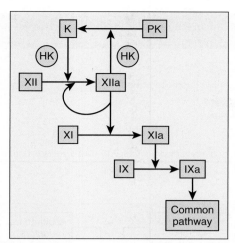

FIGURE 87-7 Contact system. Factor XII (fXII) is activated by contact with negatively charged surfaces. XIIa converts prekallikrein (PK) to kallikrein (K) and can feed back to activate more XII. Similarly, XIIa also can feed back to amplify its own generation. About 75% of circulating PK is bound to high-molecular-weight kininogen (HK), which localizes it to anionic surfaces and promotes PK activation. XIIa propagates clotting by activating XI, which then activates IX. The resultant IXa assembles into the intrinsic tenase complex, which activates X to initiate the common pathway of coagulation.

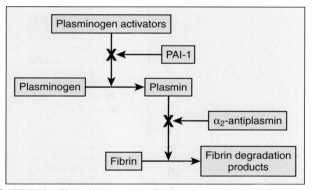

FIGURE 87-8 Fibrinolytic system and its regulation. Plasminogen activators convert plasminogen to plasmin. Plasmin then degrades fibrin into soluble fibrin degradation products. The system is regulated at two levels. Type 1 plasminogen activator inhibitor (PAI-1) regulates the plasminogen activators, whereas alpha₂-antiplasmin serves as the major inhibitor of plasmin.

a Glu residue at its amino-terminus. Plasmin cleavage at the amino terminus generates Lys-plasminogen, a truncated form with a Lys residue at its new amino terminus. t-PA cleaves a single peptide bond to convert single-chain Glu- or Lys-plasminogen into two-chain plasmin, composed of a heavy chain containing five kringle domains and a light chain containing the catalytic domain. Because its open conformation exposes the t-PA cleavage site, Lys-plasminogen is a better substrate than Glu-plasminogen, which assumes a circular conformation that renders this bond less accessible.

t-PA has little enzymatic activity in the absence of fibrin, but its activity increases by at least three orders of magnitude when fibrin is present.[10] This increase in activity reflects the capacity of fibrin to serve as a template that binds t-PA and plasminogen and promotes their interaction. t-PA binds to fibrin via its finger and second kringle domains, whereas plasminogen binds fibrin via its kringle domains. Kringle domains are looplike structures that bind Lys residues on fibrin. As fibrin undergoes degradation, more Lys residues are exposed, which provide additional binding sites for t-PA and plasminogen. Consequently, degraded fibrin stimulates t-PA activation of plasminogen more than intact fibrin.

Alpha₂-antiplasmin rapidly inhibits circulating plasmin by docking to its first kringle domain and then inhibiting the active site.[10] Because

plasmin binds to fibrin via its kringle domains, plasmin generated on the fibrin surface resists inhibition by alpha₂-antiplasmin. This phenomenon endows fibrin-bound plasmin with the capacity to degrade fibrin. Factor XIIIa cross-links small amounts of alpha₂-antiplasmin onto fibrin, which prevents premature fibrinolysis.

Like fibrin, annexin II on endothelial cells binds t-PA and plasminogen and promotes their interaction. Cell-surface gangliosides and alpha-enolase also may bind plasminogen and promote its activation by altering its conformation into the more readily activated open form. Plasminogen binds to endothelial cells via its kringle domains. Lipoprotein(a), which also possesses kringle domains, impairs cell-based fibrinolysis by competing with plasminogen for cell-surface binding. This phenomenon may explain the association between elevated levels of lipoprotein(a) and atherothrombosis.[27]

MECHANISM OF ACTION OF UROKINASE PLASMINOGEN ACTIVATOR. Synthesized as a single-chain polypeptide, single-chain u-PA (scu-PA) has minimal enzymatic activity. Plasmin readily converts scu-PA into a two-chain form that is enzymatically active and capable of binding u-PAR on cell surfaces. Further cleavage at the amino terminus of two-chain u-PA yields a truncated, lower molecular weight form that lacks the u-PAR binding domain.[10]

Two-chain forms of u-PA readily convert plasminogen to plasmin in the absence or presence of fibrin. In contrast, scu-PA does not activate plasminogen in the absence of fibrin, but it can activate fibrin-bound plasminogen, because plasminogen adopts a more open and readily activatable conformation when immobilized on fibrin. Like the higher molecular weight form of two-chain u-PA, scu-PA binds to cell surface u-PAR, where plasmin can activate it. Many tumor cells elaborate u-PA and express u-PAR on their surface. Plasmin generated on these cells endows them with the capacity for metastasis.[28]

MECHANISM OF ACTION OF THROMBIN-ACTIVATED FIBRINOLYSIS INHIBITOR. TAFI, a procarboxypeptidase B–like molecule synthesized in the liver, circulates in blood in a latent form where thrombin bound to thrombomodulin can activate it. Unless bound to thrombomodulin, thrombin activates TAFI inefficiently.[26] TAFI attenuates fibrinolysis by cleaving Lys residues from the carboxy termini of chains of degrading fibrin, thereby removing binding sites for plasminogen, plasmin, and t-PA. TAFI links fibrinolysis to coagulation because the thrombin-thrombomodulin complex not only activates TAFI, which attenuates fibrinolysis, but also activates protein C, which mutes thrombin generation.

TAFI has a short half-life in plasma because the enzyme is unstable.[26] Genetic polymorphisms can result in synthesis of more stable forms of TAFI. Persistent attenuation of fibrinolysis by these variant forms of TAFI may render patients susceptible to thrombosis.

Thrombosis

A physiologic host defense mechanism, hemostasis focuses on arrest of bleeding by forming hemostatic plugs composed of platelets and fibrin at sites of vessel injury. In contrast, thrombosis reflects a pathologic process associated with intravascular thrombi that fill the lumens of arteries or veins.

Arterial Thrombosis

Most arterial thrombi occur on top of disrupted atherosclerotic plaques (see Chap. 43). Coronary plaques with a thin fibrous cap and a lipid-rich core are most prone to disruption.[1,2] Rupture of the fibrous cap exposes thrombogenic material in the lipid-rich core to the blood and triggers platelet activation and thrombin generation. The extent of plaque disruption and the content of thrombogenic material in the plaque determine the consequences of the event, but host factors also contribute. Breakdown of regulatory mechanisms that limit platelet activation and inhibit coagulation can augment thrombosis at sites of plaque disruption.

Decreased production of nitric oxide and prostacyclin by diseased endothelial cells can trigger vasoconstriction and platelet activation.[29]

TABLE 87-1	Classification of Hypercoagulable States		
HEREDITARY		**MIXED**	**ACQUIRED**
Loss of Function			
Antithrombin deficiency		Hyperhomocysteinemia	Advanced age
Protein C deficiency			Previous venous thromboembolism
Protein S Deficiency			Surgery
Gain of Function			Immobilization
Factor V Leiden			Obesity
Prothrombin gene mutation			Cancer
Elevated factor VIII, IX, or XI levels			Pregnancy, puerperium; drug-induced—L-asparaginase, hormone therapy

Proinflammatory cytokines lower thrombomodulin expression by endothelial cells, which promotes thrombin generation, and stimulate PAI-1 expression, which inhibits fibrinolysis.[30]

Products of blood coagulation contribute to atherogenesis, as well as to its complications. Microscopic erosions in the vessel wall trigger the formation of tiny platelet-rich thrombi. Activated platelets release PDGF and TGF-β, which promote a fibrotic response.[31] Thrombin generated at the site of injury not only activates platelets and converts fibrinogen to fibrin, but also activates PAR-1 on smooth muscle cells and induces their proliferation, migration, and elaboration of extracellular matrix. Microthrombi incorporation into plaques promotes their growth, and decreased endothelial cell production of heparan sulfate, which normally limits smooth muscle proliferation, contributes to plaque expansion. The multiple links between atherosclerosis and thrombosis have prompted the term *atherothrombosis*.

Venous Thrombosis

The causes of venous thrombosis (see Chap. 77) include those associated with hypercoagulability, which can be genetic or acquired, and the mainly acquired risk factors, such as advanced age, obesity, or cancer, which are associated with immobility (**Table 87-1**). Inherited hypercoagulable states and these acquired risk factors combine to establish the intrinsic risk of thrombosis for each individual. Superimposed triggering factors, such as surgery, pregnancy, or hormonal therapy, modify this risk, and thrombosis occurs when the combination of genetic, acquired, and triggering forces exceed a critical threshold (**Fig. 87-9**).

Some acquired or triggering factors entail a higher risk than others. For example, major orthopedic surgery, neurosurgery, multiple trauma, and metastatic cancer (particularly adenocarcinoma) associate with the highest risk, whereas prolonged bed rest, antiphospholipid antibodies, and the puerperium are associated with an intermediate risk, and pregnancy, obesity, long-distance travel, or the use of oral contraceptives or hormonal replacement therapy are mild risk factors. Up to 50% of patients who present with venous thromboembolism before 45 years of age have inherited hypercoagulable disorders—so-called thrombophilia—particularly those whose events occurred in the absence of risk factors or with minimal provocation, such as after minor trauma or a long-haul flight or with estrogen use. The following sections describe the inherited and acquired hypercoagulable states.

Hypercoagulable States

INHERITED HYPERCOAGULABLE STATES. Inherited hypercoagulable states fall into two categories. Some are associated with gain of function in procoagulant pathways (e.g., factor V Leiden, the prothrombin gene mutation, and increased levels of procoagulant proteins); others are associated with loss of function of endogenous anticoagulant proteins (e.g., deficiencies of antithrombin, protein C, and protein S). Although all these inherited hypercoagulable disorders increase the risk of venous thromboembolism, only increased levels of procoagulant proteins are clearly associated with an increased risk of arterial thrombosis.

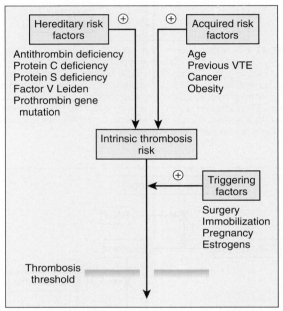

FIGURE 87-9 Thrombosis threshold. Hereditary and acquired risk factors combine to create an intrinsic risk of thrombosis for each individual. This risk is increased by extrinsic triggering factors. If the intrinsic and extrinsic forces exceed a critical threshold where thrombin generation overwhelms protective mechanisms, thrombosis occurs. VTE = venous thromboembolism.

Factor V Leiden

Factor V Leiden mutation, present in about 5% of whites, is the most common inherited thrombophilia. Because of a founder effect, the mutation is less common in Hispanics and blacks and rare in Asians. Caused by a point mutation in the factor V gene, the defect results in the synthesis of a factor V molecule with a Gln residue in place of an Arg residue at position 506, one of three sites at which activated protein C cleaves factor Va to inactivate it. Consequently, activated factor V Leiden resists rapid proteolysis and persists 10-fold longer in the presence of activated protein C than its wild-type counterpart. Inherited in an autosomal dominant fashion, individuals heterozygous for the factor V Leiden mutation have a fivefold increase in the risk of venous thromboembolism; those homozygous for the mutation have a higher risk. However, the absolute risk of venous thrombosis is low with factor V Leiden, and with an annual risk of 0.1% to 0.3%, subjects with this disorder have a lifetime risk of thrombosis of only 5% to 10%.

An activated protein C resistance assay establishes the diagnosis of factor V Leiden in most cases. This assay involves calculation of the ratio of the activated partial thromboplastin time (aPTT) measured after activated protein C addition, divided by that determined prior to its addition. Use of factor V–deficient plasma increases the specificity of the test. If the clotting assay result is equivocal, genetic testing using a polymerase chain reaction (PCR)–based assay confirms the diagnosis.

Prothrombin Gene Mutation

The second most common thrombophilic disorder, the prothrombin gene mutation, reflects a G to A nucleotide transition at position 20210 in the 3'-untranslated region of the prothrombin gene. This mutation causes elevated levels of prothrombin, which enhance thrombin generation and may limit factor Va inactivation by activated protein C. The exact mechanism whereby the G20210A mutation increases prothrombin levels remains controversial. Enhanced protein synthesis may result from more efficient 3'-end formation, increased messenger RNA stability, increased translation efficiency, or some combination of these mechanisms.

The prevalence of the prothrombin gene mutation is about 3% in whites and lower in Asians and blacks. The mutation increases the risk of venous thrombosis to a similar extent as factor V Leiden. Laboratory diagnosis depends on genetic screening after PCR amplification of the 3'-untranslated region of the prothrombin gene. Although heterozygotes have 30% higher levels of prothrombin than noncarriers, the wide range of prothrombin levels in healthy individuals precludes the use of this phenotype for carrier identification.

Elevated Levels of Procoagulant Proteins

Elevated levels of factor VIII and other coagulation factors, including fibrinogen and factors IX and XI, appear to be independent risk factors for venous thrombosis. Increased levels of factor VIII also have been associated with up to a threefold increase in the risk of myocardial infarction.[32] Although the molecular bases for the high levels of these coagulation factors have yet to be identified, genetic mechanisms likely contribute because these quantitative abnormalities have high hereditability.

Antithrombin Deficiency

Synthesized in the liver, antithrombin regulates coagulation by forming a 1:1 covalent complex with thrombin, factor Xa, or other activated clotting factors. Heparan sulfate or heparin accelerates the rate of antithrombin interaction with its target proteases. Inherited antithrombin deficiency is rare, occurring in about 1/2000 people, and can be caused by decreased synthesis of a normal protein or synthesis of a dysfunctional protein. A parallel reduction in the levels of antithrombin antigen and activity identifies deficiencies caused by decreased synthesis, whereas decreased antithrombin activity in the face of normal antigen levels identifies dysfunctional forms of antithrombin. A measurement of antithrombin activity, with or without added heparin, identifies variants with impaired heparin-binding capacity.

Acquired antithrombin deficiency results from decreased synthesis, increased consumption, or enhanced clearance. Decreased synthesis can occur in patients with severe hepatic disease, particularly cirrhosis, or in those given L-asparaginase. Increased activation of coagulation can result in antithrombin consumption in disorders such as extensive thrombosis, disseminated intravascular coagulation, severe sepsis, disseminated malignancy, or prolonged extracorporeal circulation. Heparin treatment also can reduce antithrombin levels up to 20% by enhancing its clearance. Severe antithrombin deficiency can occur in some patients with nephrotic syndrome caused by loss of protein in the urine.

Protein C Deficiency

Thrombin initiates the protein C pathway when it binds thrombomodulin on the endothelial cell surface (see Fig. 87-2). Thrombin bound to thrombomodulin activates protein C about 1000-fold more efficiently than free thrombin.[8] EPCR augments this process 20-fold by binding protein C and presenting it to the thrombin-thrombomodulin complex for activation.[9] Activated protein C then dissociates from the activation complex and decreases thrombin generation by inactivating factors Va and VIIIa on the activated platelet surface. For efficient inactivation of these factors, activated protein C must bind to protein S, its cofactor.

There are inherited and acquired forms of protein C deficiency. About 1 in 200 adults has heterozygous protein C deficiency inherited in an autosomal dominant fashion, but most have no history of thrombosis.[8] The variable phenotypic expression of hereditary protein C deficiency suggests the existence of other, yet unrecognized, modifying factors. In contrast to antithrombin deficiency, in which the homozygous state is embryonic lethal, homozygous or doubly heterozygous protein C deficiency can occur. Newborns with these disorders often present with purpura fulminans characterized by widespread thrombosis.

Inherited protein C deficiency can result from decreased synthesis of normal protein or synthesis of dysfunctional forms of protein C. Identification of the type of deficiency requires simultaneous measurement of protein C antigen and activity; reduced synthesis of a normal protein results in a parallel reduction in protein C antigen and activity, whereas synthesis of a dysfunctional protein results in normal antigen and reduced activity.

Acquired protein C deficiency can be caused by decreased synthesis or increased consumption. Decreased synthesis can occur in patients with liver disease or in those given warfarin. Protein C consumption can occur with severe sepsis, with disseminated intravascular coagulation, and after surgery. Whereas antithrombin levels can be low in patients with nephrotic syndrome, protein C levels are normal or elevated in such patients.

Protein S Deficiency

Protein S serves as a cofactor for activated protein C (see Fig. 87-3). In addition, protein S may directly inhibit prothrombin activation because of its capacity to bind factor Va or Xa, components of the prothrombinase complex. The importance of the direct anticoagulant activity of protein S is uncertain.

In the circulation, about 60% of total protein S is bound to C4b-binding protein, a complement component; only the remaining free 40% is functionally active. Diagnosis of protein S deficiency requires measurement of the free and bound forms of protein S. Inherited protein S deficiency can result from reduced synthesis of the protein or synthesis of a dysfunctional protein. Acquired protein S deficiency can be caused by decreased synthesis, increased consumption, loss, or shift of free protein S to the bound form. Decreased synthesis can occur in patients with severe liver disease or in those given warfarin or L-asparaginase. Increased consumption of protein S occurs in patients with acute thrombosis or disseminated intravascular coagulation. Patients with nephrotic syndrome can excrete free protein S in their urine, causing decreased protein S activity. Total protein S levels in these patients are often normal because the levels of C4b-binding protein increase, shifting more protein S to the bound form. C4b-binding protein levels also increase in pregnancy and with the use of oral contraceptives. This shifts more protein S to the bound form and lowers the levels of free protein S and protein S activity. The consequences of this phenomenon are uncertain.

Other Hereditary Disorders

A polymorphism in the gene that encodes EPCR is associated with venous thrombosis. Linked to EPCR shedding and high levels of soluble EPCR, this polymorphism reduces endothelial EPCR, and soluble EPCR competes with its endothelial cell counterpart for protein C binding.[33]

A polymorphism in factor XIII that results in more rapid activation by thrombin is associated with a reduced risk of thrombosis.[34] Unexpectedly, in some case-control studies, this polymorphism was associated with a small reduction in the risk of myocardial infarction. The mechanism responsible for this protection is unclear.

ACQUIRED HYPERCOAGULABLE STATES. These states include surgery and immobilization, advanced age, obesity, cancer, pregnancy and estrogen therapy (oral contraception or hormone replacement therapy), prior history of venous thromboembolism, antiphospholipid antibody syndrome, and hyperhomocysteinemia (see Table 87-1). These conditions can occur in isolation or in conjunction with hereditary hypercoagulable states.

Surgery and Immobilization

Surgery can directly damage veins, and immobilization after surgery leads to stasis in the deep veins of the leg. The risk of venous

CH
87

HEMOSTASIS, THROMBOSIS, FIBRINOLYSIS, AND CARDIOVASCULAR DISEASE thromboembolism in surgical patients depends on patient age, type of surgery, and presence of active cancer. Patients older than 65 years of age are at greater risk; high-risk types of surgery include major orthopedic procedures, neurosurgery, or extensive abdominal or pelvic surgery, especially for cancer. Because the risk of venous thromboembolism increases up to 20-fold in these patients, they require vigorous thromboprophylaxis until they are fully mobile.

Hospitalization and nursing home confinement account for about 60% of cases of venous thromboembolism, again reflecting the impact of immobilization. Hospitalization for medical illness accounts for a similar proportion of cases as hospitalization for surgery, highlighting the need for thromboprophylaxis in medical patients and in surgical patients.

Advanced Age

Predominantly a disease of older age, venous thromboembolism in those younger than 50 years of age has an incidence of 1/10,000 and increases about 10-fold/decade thereafter. Men have an overall age-adjusted incidence rate about 1.2-fold higher than that in women. Although incidence rates are higher in women during their reproductive years, men have higher incidence rates after 45 years of age. There are many potential reasons for the increase in the incidence of venous thromboembolism with advanced age, including decreased mobility, intercurrent diseases, and a vascular endothelium that is less resistant to thrombosis. Levels of procoagulant proteins also increase with age.

Obesity

The risk of venous thromboembolism increases about 1.2-fold for every 10-kg/m^2 increase in body mass index, but the basis for the association between obesity and venous thromboembolism is unclear. Obesity leads to immobility; in addition, adipose tissue, particularly visceral fat, expresses proinflammatory cytokines and adipokines, which may promote coagulation by increasing levels of procoagulant proteins or may impair fibrinolysis by elevating PAI-1 levels. With the growing epidemic of obesity, the incidence of venous thromboembolism may increase.

Cancer

About 20% of patients with venous thromboembolism have cancer (see Chap. 90).[35] Cancer patients who develop venous thromboembolism have reduced survival compared with those without venous thromboembolism. Patients with brain tumors and advanced ovarian or prostate cancer have particularly high rates of venous thromboembolism. Treatment with chemotherapy, hormonal therapy, and biologic agents (e.g., erythropoietin and antiangiogenic drugs) further increases the risk, as do central venous catheters and surgery for cancer.

The pathogenesis of thrombosis in cancer patients is multifactorial in origin and represents a complex interplay between the tumor, patient characteristics, and hemostatic system.[35] Many types of tumor cells express tissue factor or other procoagulants that can initiate coagulation. In addition to its role in coagulation, tissue factor also acts as a signaling molecule that promotes tumor proliferation and spread.[36]

Patient characteristics that contribute to venous thromboembolism include immobility and venous stasis secondary to extrinsic compression of major veins by tumor. Surgical procedures, central venous catheters, and chemotherapy can injure vessel walls. In addition, tamoxifen and selective estrogen receptor modulators (SERMs) induce an acquired hypercoagulable state by reducing the levels of natural anticoagulant proteins.

A proportion of patients who present with unprovoked venous thromboembolism have occult cancer. This observation has prompted some experts to recommend extensive screening for cancer in such patients, but potential harm—including procedure-related morbidity, the psychological impact of false-positive tests, and the cost of screening—offsets any benefits of this approach. Small studies comparing extensive cancer screening with no screening in patients with unprovoked venous thromboembolism have not demonstrated a reduction in cancer-related mortality with screening. Therefore, unless there are symptoms suggestive of underlying cancer, only age-appropriate screening for

breast, cervical, colon, and possibly prostate cancer is indicated, because screening for these cancers may reduce mortality.

Pregnancy

Pregnant women have a five- to sixfold higher risk of venous thromboembolism than age-matched nonpregnant women (see Chap. 82). Venous thromboembolism occurs in about 1 in 1000 pregnancies, and about 1 in 1000 women develop venous thromboembolism in the postpartum period. Venous thromboembolism is the leading cause of maternal morbidity and mortality. Patient-related factors influence the risk of venous thromboembolism in pregnancy and the puerperium. These include age older than 35 years, body mass index higher than 29, cesarean delivery, thrombophilia, and personal or family history of venous thromboembolism. Ovarian hyperstimulation and multiparity also are risk factors.

More than 90% of deep vein thrombi in pregnancy occur in the left leg, because the enlarged uterus compresses the left iliac vein by exerting pressure on the overlying right iliac and ovarian arteries. Hypercoagulability occurs in pregnancy because of the combination of venous stasis and changes in the blood. Uterine enlargement reduces venous blood flow from the lower extremities. This is not the only mechanism responsible for venous stasis, however, because blood flow from the lower extremities begins to decrease by the end of the first trimester, likely reflecting hormonally induced venous dilation. Systemic factors also contribute to hypercoagulability. Thus, the levels of procoagulant proteins, such as factor VIII, fibrinogen, and vWF, increase in the third trimester of pregnancy. Coincidentally, there is suppression of natural anticoagulant pathways. The net effect of these changes is enhanced thrombin generation, as evidenced by elevated levels of F1.2 and thrombin-antithrombin complexes.

About half of the episodes of venous thromboembolism in pregnancy occur in women with thrombophilia. The risk of venous thromboembolism in women with thrombophilic defects depends on the type of abnormality and the presence of other risk factors. The risk appears to be highest in women with antithrombin, protein C, or protein S deficiency, and lower in those with factor V Leiden or the prothrombin gene mutation. In general, the daily risk of venous thromboembolism in these women is higher in the postpartum period than during pregnancy. The risk during pregnancy is similar in all three trimesters. Therefore, women needing thromboprophylaxis require treatment throughout pregnancy and for at least 6 weeks postpartum.

Sex Hormone Therapy

Oral contraceptives, estrogen replacement therapy, and SERMs all associate with an increased risk of venous thrombosis (see Chap. 81). The relatively high risk of venous thromboembolism associated with first-generation oral contraceptives prompted the development of low-dose formulations. Currently available low-estrogen combination oral contraceptives contain 20 to 50 µg of ethinylestradiol and one of several different progestins. Even these low-dose combination contraceptives are associated with a three- to fourfold increased risk of venous thromboembolism compared with nonusers. In absolute terms, this translates to an incidence of 3 to 4/10,000 compared with 5 to 10/100,000 in nonusers of reproductive age.

Whereas smoking increases the risk of myocardial infarction and stroke in women taking oral contraceptives, it is unclear whether smoking affects the risk of venous thromboembolism. Obesity, however, affects the risk of arterial and venous thrombosis. The risk of venous thromboembolism is highest during the first year of oral contraceptive use and persists only for the duration of use.

Case-control studies have suggested a 20- to 30-fold higher risk of venous thromboembolism in women with inherited thrombophilia who use oral contraceptives compared with nonusers with thrombophilia or users without these defects. Despite the increased risk, there is no need for routine screening for thrombophilia in young women considering oral contraceptive use. Based on the incidence and case fatality rate of thrombotic events, estimates have suggested that screening 400,000 women would detect 20,000 factor V Leiden carriers and that prevention of a single death would necessitate withholding oral contraceptives in all these women. Even larger numbers of women with less prevalent thrombophilic defects would require screening. Based on these considerations, routine screening is not recommended.

Evidence has mounted that hormonal replacement therapy with conjugated equine estrogen, with or without a progestin, increases the risk of myocardial infarction, ischemic stroke, and venous thromboembolism. Consequently, the use of hormone replacement therapy has markedly decreased. SERMs, such as tamoxifen, are estrogen-like compounds that serve as an estrogen antagonist in the breast but as estrogen agonists in other tissues, such as bone and the uterus. Like estrogens, tamoxifen increases the risk of venous thromboembolism three- to fourfold. The risk is higher in postmenopausal women, particularly those receiving systemic combination chemotherapy. Aromatase inhibitors are replacing tamoxifen for the treatment of estrogen receptor–positive breast cancer. These newer agents are associated with a lower risk of venous thromboembolism than tamoxifen. Raloxifene, a SERM used to prevent osteoporosis, increases the risk of venous thromboembolism threefold compared with placebo, which contraindicates raloxifene for the prevention of osteoporosis in women with a history of venous thromboembolism.

History of Prior Venous Thromboembolism

A history of previous venous thromboembolism places patients at risk for recurrence. When anticoagulation treatment stops, patients with unprovoked venous thromboembolism have a risk of recurrence of about 10% at 1 year and 30% at 5 years. This risk appears to be independent of whether or not there is an underlying thrombophilic defect, such as factor V Leiden or the prothrombin gene mutation.

The risk of recurrent venous thromboembolism is lower in patients whose incident event occurred in association with a transient risk factor, such as major surgery or prolonged immobilization. These patients have a risk of recurrence of about 4% at 1 year and 10% at 5 years. Patients whose venous thromboembolism occurred on the background of minor risk factors, such as oral contraceptive use or a long-haul flight, likely have an intermediate risk of recurrence. Patients at the highest risk for recurrence are those with inherited deficiencies of antithrombin, protein C, or protein S, antiphospholipid antibody syndrome, or advanced malignancy, or those homozygous for factor V Leiden or the prothrombin gene mutation. Their risk of recurrence is likely to be 15% at 1 year and up to 50% at 5 years.

Antiphospholipid Antibody Syndrome (see Chap. 89)

A heterogeneous group of autoantibodies directed against proteins that bind phospholipid, antiphospholipid antibodies can be categorized into those that prolong phospholipid-dependent coagulation assays, so-called lupus anticoagulants (LAs) or anticardiolipin antibodies (ACLs), which target cardiolipin. A subset of ACLs recognizes other phospholipid-bound proteins, particularly beta$_2$-glycoprotein I.

Patients with thrombosis in association with a persistent LA and/or ACL antibody have antiphospholipid syndrome. Primary antiphospholipid syndrome occurs in isolation, whereas secondary forms are associated with autoimmune disorders, such as systemic lupus erythematosus or other connective tissue diseases. Thrombosis in these patients can be arterial, venous, or placental. Arterial thrombosis can manifest as a transient ischemic attack, stroke, or myocardial infarction. In addition to deep vein thrombosis and pulmonary embolism, saggital sinus thrombosis also can occur. Placental thrombosis is likely the root cause of the pregnancy-related complications that characterize antiphospholipid syndrome. These complications include fetal loss before 10 weeks' gestation and unexplained fetal death after 10 weeks' gestation. Intrauterine growth retardation, pre-eclampsia, and eclampsia also can occur. Treatment with aspirin and/or LMWH during pregnancy may reduce the risk of these complications in women with documented thrombophilic defects.

Laboratory diagnosis of antiphospholipid syndrome requires the presence of an LA or ACL antibody on tests done at least 6 weeks apart. Diagnosis of a LA requires a battery of phospholipid-dependent clotting tests, whereas immunoassays detect ACL antibodies. Only antibodies of medium to high titer and of the IgG or IgM subclass are associated

with thrombosis. About 3% to 10% of healthy individuals have ACL antibodies. Such antibodies also occur with certain infections, such as mycobacterial pneumonia, malaria, or parasitic disorders, and after exposure to some medications. Often, these antibodies are of low titer and are transient. About 30% to 50% of patients with systemic lupus erythematosus or other connective tissue disorders have ACL antibodies, and 10% to 20% have an LA.

The mechanism whereby antiphospholipid antibodies trigger thrombosis is unclear. These antibodies directly activate endothelial cells in culture and induce the expression of adhesion molecules that can tether tissue factor-bearing leukocytes or microparticles onto their surface. ACL antibodies also interfere with the protein C pathway, inhibit antithrombin catalysis by endothelial heparan sulfate, and impair fibrinolysis. The importance of these mechanisms in humans remains unclear.

Hyperhomocysteinemia

Homocysteine is an intermediate sulfur-containing amino acid that serves as a methyl group donor during the metabolism of methionine, an essential amino acid derived from the diet. The interconversion of methionine and homocysteine depends on the availability of 5-methyltetrahydrofolate, a methyl group donor; vitamin B$_{12}$ and folate, cofactors in the interconversion; and the enzyme methionine synthase. Increased levels of homocysteine can result from increased production or reduced metabolism. Severe hyperhomocysteinemia and cystinuria, which are rare, usually result from deficiency of cystathionine in beta-synthetase. Mild to moderate hyperhomocysteinemia is more common, and can be caused by genetic mutations in methylenetetrahydrofolate reductase (MTHFR) when they are accompanied by nutritional deficiency of folate, vitamin B$_{12}$, or vitamin B$_6$. Common polymorphisms in MTHFR, C677T and A1298C, are associated with reduced enzymatic activity and increased thermolability, which increase the requirement for nutritional cofactors. Hyperhomocysteinemia also can be associated with certain drugs, such as methotrexate, theophylline, cyclosporine, and most anticonvulsants, as well as some chronic diseases, such as end-stage renal disease, severe hepatic dysfunction, and hypothyroidism.

A fasting serum homocysteine level higher than 15 mmol/liter is considered elevated. Although elevated levels once were a common finding, routine fortification of flour in North America with folic acid has resulted in lower homocysteine levels in the general population. Elevated serum levels of homocysteine may be associated with an increased risk of myocardial infarction, stroke, and peripheral arterial disease, as well as venous thromboembolism.

Although administration of folate, along with vitamin B$_{12}$ and vitamin B$_6$, reduces levels of homocysteine, randomized trials have shown that such therapy does not lower the risk of recurrent cardiovascular events in patients with coronary artery disease or stroke, nor does it lower the risk of recurrent venous thromboembolism (see Chap. 49). Based on these negative trials and the declining incidence of hyperhomocysteinemia, enthusiasm for screening for hyperhomocysteinemia has declined.

Treatment of Thrombosis

Antiplatelet Drugs

The commonly used antiplatelet drugs include aspirin, thienopyridines (e.g., ticlopidine, clopidogrel, prasugrel), dipyridamole, and GPIIb/IIIa antagonists, with distinct sites of action (see Fig. 87-9).

ASPIRIN. The most widely used antiplatelet agent worldwide is aspirin. As an inexpensive and effective drug, aspirin serves as the foundation of most antiplatelet strategies.

Mechanism of Action

Aspirin produces its antithrombotic effect by irreversibly acetylating and inhibiting platelet COX-1 (**Fig. 87-10**), a critical enzyme in the biosynthesis of thromboxane A$_2$. At high doses (about 1 g/day), aspirin also inhibits COX-2, an inducible COX isoform found in

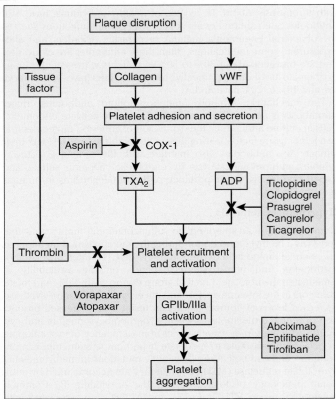

FIGURE 87-10 Sites of action of antiplatelet drugs. Aspirin inhibits thromboxane A_2 (TXA_2) synthesis by irreversibly acetylating COX-1. Reduced TXA_2 release attenuates platelet activation and recruitment to the site of vascular injury. Ticlopidine, clopidogrel, and prasugrel irreversibly block $P2Y_{12}$, a key ADP receptor on the platelet surface; cangrelor and ticagrelor are reversible inhibitors of $P2Y_{12}$. Abciximab, eptifibatide, and tirofiban inhibit the final common pathway of platelet aggregation by blocking fibrinogen and vWF binding to activated GPIIb/IIIa. Vorapaxar and atopaxar inhibit thrombin-mediated platelet activation by targeting PAR1, the major thrombin receptor on platelets.

endothelial cells and inflammatory cells.[37] In endothelial cells, COX-2 initiates the synthesis of prostacyclin, a potent vasodilator and inhibitor of platelet activation, which antagonizes the effects of thromboxane A_2.

Indications

Aspirin is widely used for the secondary prevention of cardiovascular events in patients with coronary artery disease, cerebrovascular disease, or peripheral vascular disease (see Chaps. 55-57 and 61). Compared with placebo, aspirin produces a 25% reduction in the risk of cardiovascular death, myocardial infarction, or stroke in these patients.[37] Aspirin also is used for primary prevention in patients whose estimated annual risk of myocardial infarction is in excess of 1%, a point at which benefits are likely to outweigh harms.[38] This includes patients older than 40 years, with two or more major risk factors for cardiovascular disease, or those older than 50 years, with one or more such risk factors. Aspirin is equally effective in men and women. In men, aspirin mainly reduces the risk of myocardial infarction, whereas in women, aspirin lowers the risk of stroke.

Dosage

Usually administered at doses of 75 to 325 mg once daily, there is no evidence that higher dose aspirin is more effective than lower doses, and some meta-analyses have suggested reduced efficacy with higher doses.[37] Because the side effects of aspirin depend on dose, daily aspirin doses of 75 to 150 mg are recommended for most indications. When rapid platelet inhibition is required, the initial dose of aspirin should be at least 160 mg.

Side Effects

Most common side effects are gastrointestinal and range from dyspepsia to erosive gastritis or peptic ulcers with bleeding and perforation.[37] Use of enteric-coated or buffered aspirin in place of plain aspirin does not eliminate the risk of gastrointestinal side effects. The risk of major bleeding with aspirin is 1% to 3% per year.[37] With concomitant use of aspirin and anticoagulants such as warfarin, the risk of bleeding increases. When combined with warfarin, use of low-dose aspirin (75 to 100 mg daily) is best. Eradication of *Helicobacter pylori* infection and administration of proton pump inhibitors may reduce the risk of aspirin-induced gastrointestinal bleeding in patients with peptic ulcer disease.

Patients with a history of aspirin allergy characterized by bronchospasm should not be given aspirin. This problem occurs in about 0.3% of the general population but is more common in patients with chronic urticaria or asthma, particularly those with coexisting nasal polyps or chronic rhinitis.[39] Aspirin overdose is associated with hepatic and renal toxicity.

Aspirin Resistance

The term *aspirin resistance* is used to describe clinical and laboratory phenomena.[40] A diagnosis of clinical aspirin resistance, defined as the failure of aspirin to protect patients from ischemic vascular events, can only be made after such an event occurs. This retrospective diagnosis provides no opportunity to modify therapy. Furthermore, it is unrealistic to expect aspirin, which selectively blocks thromboxane A_2–induced platelet activation, to prevent all vascular events.

Aspirin resistance also has been described biochemically as failure of the drug to produce its expected inhibitory effects on tests of platelet function, such as thromboxane A_2 synthesis or arachidonic acid–induced platelet aggregation.[37] However, the tests of platelet function used for the diagnosis of biochemical aspirin resistance have not been standardized.[37,40] Furthermore, no definitive evidence shows that these tests identify patients at risk of recurrent vascular events, or that resistance can be reversed either by giving higher doses of aspirin or by adding other antiplatelet drugs. Until such information is available, testing for aspirin resistance remains a research tool.

THIENOPYRIDINES. The thienopyridines include ticlopidine, clopidogrel, and prasugrel—drugs that target $P2Y_{12}$, a key ADP receptor on platelets. Prasugrel is the newest addition to the thienopyridine class.

Mechanism of action

The thienopyridines selectively inhibit ADP-induced platelet aggregation by irreversibly blocking P2Y12 (see Fig. 87-10). Ticlopidine and clopidogrel, are prodrugs that require metabolism by the hepatic cytochrome P-450 (CYP450) enzyme system to be activated. Consequently, when given in usual doses, ticlopidine and clopidogrel have a delayed onset of action. Although prasugrel also is a prodrug that requires metabolic activation, its onset of action is more rapid than ticlopidine or clopidogrel, and it produces greater and more predictable inhibition of ADP-induced platelet aggregation.[41] These characteristics reflect the rapid and complete absorption of prasugrel from the gut and its more efficient activation pathways. Whereas all the absorbed prasugrel undergoes activation, only 15% of absorbed clopidogrel undergoes metabolic activation, with the remainder inactivated by esterases.

The active metabolites of all of the thienopyridines bind irreversibly to the receptor $P2Y_{12}$. Consequently, these drugs have prolonged action—a problem if patients require urgent surgery. Such patients have increased risk for bleeding, which necessitates stopping the thienopyridine at least 5 days prior to the procedure.

Indications

Like aspirin, ticlopidine is more effective than placebo at reducing the risk of cardiovascular death, myocardial infarction, and stroke in patients with atherosclerotic disease.[42] Because of its delayed onset of action, ticlopidine is not recommended for patients with acute myocardial infarction. Ticlopidine is used little because of the risk of myelosuppression and because of the greater potency and better safety profile of newer drugs.[42]

When compared with aspirin in patients with recent ischemic stroke, myocardial infarction, or peripheral arterial disease, clopidogrel reduced the risk of cardiovascular death, myocardial infarction, and stroke by 8.7%. Therefore, clopidogrel is more effective than aspirin, but at greater cost. The combination of clopidogrel and aspirin capitalizes on their capability to block complementary pathways of platelet activation. For example, this combination is recommended for at least 4 weeks after implantation of a bare-metal stent in a coronary artery and for at least 1 year in those with a drug-eluting stent.[42] Recent concerns about late in-stent thrombosis with drug-eluting stents have led some experts to recommend long-term use of clopidogrel plus aspirin for this indication (see Chap. 58).[43,44]

The combination of clopidogrel and aspirin also is effective in patients with unstable angina (see Chap. 56). In 12,562 such patients, the risk of cardiovascular death, myocardial infarction, or stroke was 9.3% in those randomized to the combination of clopidogrel and aspirin, and 11.4% in those given aspirin alone. This 20% relative risk reduction with combination therapy was highly statistically significant, but combining clopidogrel with aspirin increases the risk of major bleeding to about 2% per year—a risk that persists even with a daily aspirin dose of 100 mg or less.[45] Therefore, clopidogrel plus aspirin use should be restricted to situations in which there is clear evidence of benefit. For example, this combination has not proven to be superior to clopidogrel alone in patients with acute ischemic stroke[46] or to aspirin alone for primary prevention in those at risk for cardiovascular events.[47]

Prasugrel was compared with clopidogrel in 13,608 patients with acute coronary syndromes who were scheduled to undergo a percutaneous coronary intervention (PCI).[48] The incidence of the primary efficacy endpoint, a composite of cardiovascular death, myocardial infarction, and stroke, was significantly lower with prasugrel than with clopidogrel (9.9% and 12.1%, respectively), mainly reflecting a reduction in the incidence of nonfatal myocardial infarction. The incidence of stent thrombosis also was significantly lower with prasugrel than with clopidogrel (1.1% and 2.4%, respectively). These advantages, however, were at the expense of significantly higher rates of fatal bleeding (0.4% and 0.1%, respectively) and life-threatening bleeding (1.4% and 0.9%, respectively) with prasugrel. Because patients older than 75 years of age and those with a history of prior stroke or transient ischemic attack have a particularly high risk of bleeding, prasugrel should generally be avoided in older patients, and the drug is contraindicated in those with a history of cerebrovascular disease. Caution is required if prasugrel is used for patients weighing less than 60 kg or those with renal impairment.

DOSAGE. Ticlopidine is given twice daily at a dose of 250 mg. The more potent clopidogrel is given once daily at a dose of 75 mg.[42] Because its onset of action is delayed for several days, loading doses of clopidogrel are given when rapid ADP receptor blockade is desired (see Chap. 58). After a loading dose of 60 mg, prasugrel is given once daily at a dose of 10 mg. Patients older than 75 years of age or weighing less than 60 kg may do better with a daily prasugrel dose of 5 mg.[49]

SIDE EFFECTS. The most common side effects of ticlopidine are gastrointestinal. More serious are the hematologic side effects, which include neutropenia, thrombocytopenia, and thrombotic thrombocytopenic purpura. These side effects usually occur within the first few months of starting treatment. Therefore, blood counts must be carefully monitored when initiating therapy with ticlopidine. Gastrointestinal and hematologic side effects are rare with clopidogrel[42] and prasugrel.[49]

THIENOPYRIDINE RESISTANCE. The capacity of clopidogrel to inhibit ADP-induced platelet aggregation varies among subjects.[50] This variability reflects, at least in part, genetic polymorphisms in the CYP isoenzymes involved in the metabolic activation of clopidogrel. The most important of these is *CYP2C19*.[51,52] Clopidogrel-treated patients with the loss-of-function *CYP2C19*2* allele exhibit reduced platelet inhibition compared with those with the wild-type *CYP2C19*1* allele, and experience a higher rate of cardiovascular events.[53,54] This is important because estimates suggest that up to 25% of whites, 30% of blacks, and 50% of Asians carry the loss-of-function allele, which would render them resistant to clopidogrel. Even patients with reduced-function CYP2C19*3, *4, or *5 alleles may derive less benefit from clopidogrel than those with the full-function *CYP2C19*1* allele. Concomitant administration of clopidogrel and proton pump inhibitors, which are inhibitors of *CYP2C19*, produces a small reduction in the inhibitory effects of clopidogrel on ADP-induced platelet aggregation. This interaction does not appear to increase the risk of cardiovascular events.[55]

In contrast to their effect on the metabolic activation of clopidogrel, *CYP2C19* polymorphisms appear to be less important determinants of the activation of prasugrel. There was no association between the loss-of-function allele and decreased platelet inhibition or increased rate of cardiovascular events with prasugrel.[56,57]

Although *CYP3A4* also contributes to the metabolic activation of clopidogrel, polymorphisms in this enzyme do not appear to influence clopidogrel responsiveness. However, a small study in patients undergoing PCI has revealed that atorvastatin, a competitive inhibitor of *CYP3A4*, reduces the inhibitory effect of clopidogrel on ADP-induced platelet aggregation. This finding was not confirmed in a subsequent study.[58] The impact of this interaction on clinical outcomes is unknown. Clopidogrel-treated patients with polymorphisms in *ABCB1* may exhibit reduced drug absorption, which may render them at higher risk for cardiovascular events.

The observation that genetic polymorphisms affecting clopidogrel absorption or metabolism influence clinical outcomes raises the possibilities that pharmacogenetic profiling may help identify clopidogrel resistant patients, and that point-of-care assessment of the extent of clopidogrel-induced platelet inhibition may help detect patients at higher risk for subsequent cardiovascular events.[59] It is unknown whether administration of higher doses of clopidogrel to such patients will overcome this resistance. Instead, prasugrel or newer P2Y$_{12}$ inhibitors may be better choices for these patients. For an update on recent experience with newer P2Y12 antagonists, including ticagrelor, see below and Chaps. 55 and 56.

DIPYRIDAMOLE. A relatively weak antiplatelet agent on its own,[37] an extended-release formulation of dipyridamole combined with low-dose aspirin, a preparation marketed as Aggrenox, is used for the prevention of stroke in patients with transient ischemic attacks.

Mechanism of Action

By inhibiting phosphodiesterase, dipyridamole blocks the breakdown of cAMP. Increased levels of cAMP reduce intracellular calcium and inhibit platelet activation. Dipyridamole also blocks the uptake of adenosine by platelets and other cells. With more extracellular adenosine, there is a further increase in local cAMP levels because the platelet adenosine A$_2$ receptor and adenylate cyclase are coupled (**Fig. 87-11**).

DOSAGE. Aggrenox is given twice daily. Each capsule contains 200 mg of extended-release dipyridamole and 25 mg of aspirin.[37]

SIDE EFFECTS. Because dipyridamole has vasodilatory effects, caution is necessary in patients with coronary artery disease. Gastrointestinal

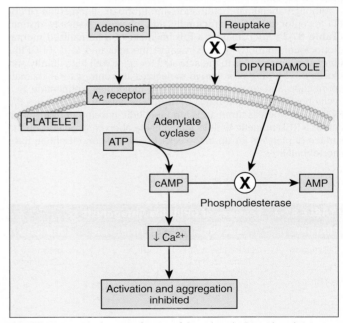

FIGURE 87-11 Mechanism of action of dipyridamole. Dipyridamole increases levels of cAMP in platelets by blocking the reuptake of adenosine, thereby increasing the concentration of adenosine available to bind to the A2 receptor, and by inhibiting phosphodiesterase-mediated cAMP degradation. By promoting calcium uptake, cAMP reduces intracellular levels of calcium. This, in turn, inhibits platelet activation and aggregation.

complaints, headache, facial flushing, dizziness, and hypotension also can occur. These symptoms often subside with continued use of the drug.

INDICATIONS. Dipyridamole plus aspirin was compared with aspirin or dipyridamole alone, or with placebo, in patients with an ischemic stroke or transient ischemic attack (see Chap. 62). The combination reduced the risk of stroke by 22.1% compared with aspirin and by 24.4% compared with dipyridamole. A second trial compared dipyridamole plus aspirin with aspirin alone for secondary prevention in patients with ischemic stroke. Vascular death, stroke, or myocardial infarction occurred in 13% of patients given combination therapy and in 16% of those treated with aspirin alone.[60] Although the combination of dipyridamole plus aspirin compares favorably with aspirin, the combination is not superior to clopidogrel. In a large randomized trial that compared dipyridamole plus aspirin with clopidogrel for secondary prevention in patients with ischemic stroke,[61] recurrent stroke event rates were similar (9.0% and 8.8%, respectively), as were the rates of vascular death, stroke, and myocardial infarction (13.1% in both treatment arms). However, there was a trend for more hemorrhagic strokes with dipyridamole plus aspirin than with clopidogrel (0.8% and 0.4%, respectively) and more major bleeding (4.1% and 3.8%, respectively).

Although Aggrenox can replace aspirin for stroke prevention, because of the vasodilatory effects of dipyridamole and the paucity of data supporting the usefulness of this drug in patients with symptomatic coronary artery disease, Aggrenox should be avoided in such patients. Clopidogrel is a better choice for patients with coronary artery disease.

GPIIb/IIIa RECEPTOR ANTAGONISTS. As a class, parenteral GPIIb/IIIa receptor antagonists have an established niche in patients with acute coronary syndromes. The three agents in this class are abciximab, eptifibatide, and tirofiban.

Mechanism of Action

A member of the integrin family of adhesion receptors, GPIIb/IIIa is expressed on the surface of platelets and megakaryocytes. With about 80,000 copies per platelet, GPIIb/IIIa is the most abundant receptor.[15] Consisting of a noncovalently linked heterodimer, GPIIb/IIIa is inactive on resting platelets. With platelet activation, inside-outside signal transduction pathways trigger conformational activation of the receptor. Once activated, GPIIb/IIIa binds fibrinogen and, under high shear conditions, vWF. Once bound, fibrinogen and vWF bridge adjacent platelets together to induce platelet aggregation.

Although abciximab, eptifibatide, and tirofiban all target the GPIIb/IIIa receptor, they are structurally and pharmacologically distinct (**Table 87-2**). Abciximab is a Fab fragment of a humanized murine monoclonal antibody directed against the activated form of GPIIb/IIIa.[62] Abciximab binds to the activated receptor with high affinity and blocks the binding of adhesive molecules. In contrast to abciximab, eptifibatide and tirofiban are synthetic molecules. Eptifibatide is a cyclic heptapeptide that binds GPIIb/IIIa because it incorporates the KGD motif, whereas tirofiban is a nonpeptidic tyrosine derivative that acts as a RGD mimetic. With its long half-life, abciximab persists on the surface of platelets for up to 2 weeks. Eptifibatide and tirofiban have shorter half-lives.

TABLE 87-2	Features of GPIIb/IIIa Antagonists		
FEATURE	**ABCIXIMAB**	**EPTIFIBATIDE**	**TIROFIBAN**
Description	Fab fragment of humanized mouse monoclonal antibody	Cyclical KGD-containing heptapeptide	Nonpeptidic RGD mimetic
Specific for GPIIb/IIIa	No	Yes	Yes
Plasma half-life	Short (min)	Long (2.5 hr)	Long (2.0 hr)
Platelet-bound half-life	Long (days)	Short (sec)	Short (sec)
Renal clearance	No	Yes	Yes

In addition to targeting the GPIIb/IIIa receptor, abciximab (but not eptifibatide or tirofiban) also inhibits the closely related $\alpha_v\beta_3$ receptor, which binds vitronectin, and $\alpha_M\beta_2$, a leukocyte integrin. Inhibition of $\alpha_v\beta_3$ and $\alpha_M\beta_2$ may endow abciximab with anti-inflammatory and/or antiproliferative properties that extend beyond platelet inhibition.[62]

DOSAGE. All the GPIIb/IIIa antagonists are given as an intravenous bolus followed by an infusion. Because of their renal clearance, eptifibatide and tirofiban doses require reduction in patients with renal insufficiency.[62]

SIDE EFFECTS. In addition to bleeding, thrombocytopenia is the most serious complication. Antibodies directed against neoantigens on GPIIb/IIIa that are exposed on antagonist binding[63] cause thrombocytopenia, which is immune-mediated. With abciximab, thrombocytopenia occurs in up to 5% of patients and is severe in about 1% of these individuals. Thrombocytopenia is less common with the other two agents, occurring in about 1% of patients.

INDICATIONS. Abciximab and eptifibatide are used in patients undergoing PCI, particularly those with acute myocardial infarction, whereas tirofiban and eptifibatide are used for high-risk patients with unstable angina (see Chaps. 55, 56, and 58).[64,65]

NEWER ANTIPLATELET AGENTS. New agents in advanced stages of development include cangrelor and ticagrelor, direct-acting reversible P2Y$_{12}$ antagonists, and vorapaxar and atopaxar, orally active inhibitors of PAR-1, the major thrombin receptor on platelets (see Fig. 87-10). Cangrelor is an adenosine analogue that binds reversibly to P2Y$_{12}$ and inhibits its activity. The drug has a half-life of 3 to 6 minutes and is given intravenously as a bolus followed by an infusion. When stopped, platelet function recovers within 60 minutes. Recent trials comparing cangrelor with placebo during PCI or comparing cangrelor with clopidogrel after such procedures revealed little or no advantage of cangrelor.[66,67] Consequently, identification of a role for cangrelor requires additional studies.

Ticagrelor is an orally active, reversible inhibitor of P2Y$_{12}$. The drug is given twice daily and not only has a more rapid onset and offset of action than clopidogrel, but also produces greater and more predictable inhibition of ADP-induced platelet aggregation. When compared with clopidogrel in patients with acute coronary syndromes,[68] ticagrelor produced a greater reduction in the primary efficacy endpoint, a composite of cardiovascular death, myocardial infarction, and stroke at 1 year, than clopidogrel (9.8% and 11.7%, respectively; $P = 0.001$). This difference reflected a significant reduction in cardiovascular death (4.0% and 5.1%, respectively; $P = 0.001$) and myocardial infarction (5.8% and 6.9%, respectively; $P = 0.005$) with ticagrelor relative to clopidogrel. Rates of stroke were similar with ticagrelor and clopidogrel (1.5% and 1.3%, respectively) and there was no difference in rates of major bleeding. When minor bleeding was added to the major bleeding results, however, ticagrelor showed an increase relative to clopidogrel (16.1% and 14.6%, respectively; $P = 0.008$). Ticagrelor also was superior to clopidogrel in patients with acute coronary syndrome who underwent PCI or cardiac surgery. Although not yet licensed, in one study, ticagrelor demonstrated a reduction in cardiovascular death compared with clopidogrel in patients with acute coronary syndromes (see Chaps. 55 and 56).

Vorapaxar, an orally active inhibitor of the thrombin receptor PAR-1,[69] is under investigation as an adjunct to aspirin or aspirin plus clopidogrel. Two large phase III trials are underway. Atopaxar, a second oral PAR-1 antagonist, also is in development.[70]

Anticoagulants

There are parenteral and oral anticoagulants. Currently available parenteral anticoagulants include heparin, LMWH and fondaparinux, a synthetic pentasaccharide. The only available oral anticoagulants in the United States are vitamin K antagonists; of these, warfarin is the agent most often used in North America.

Dabigatran etexilate, an oral thrombin inhibitor, and rivaroxaban, an oral factor Xa inhibitor, are available in Europe and Canada for short-term thromboprophylaxis after elective hip or knee replacement surgery.[71]

TABLE 87-3	Comparison of the Features of Heparin, Low-Molecular-Weight Heparin, and Fondaparinux		
FEATURE	HEPARIN	LMWH	FONDAPARINUX
Source	Biologic	Biologic	Synthetic
Molecular weight	15,000	5000	1728
Target	Xa and IIa	Xa and IIa	Xa
Bioavailability (%)	30	90	100
Half-life (hr)	1	4	17
Renal excretion	No	Yes	Yes
Antidote	Complete	Partial	No
HIT	<5%	<1%	Never

PARENTERAL ANTICOAGULANTS

HEPARIN. A sulfated polysaccharide, heparin is isolated from mammalian tissues rich in mast cells (**Table 87-3**). Most commercial heparin is derived from porcine intestinal mucosa and is a polymer of alternating D-glucuronic acid and N-acetyl-D-glucosamine residues.[72]

Mechanism of Action

Heparin acts as an anticoagulant by activating antithrombin (previously known as antithrombin III) and accelerating the rate at which it inhibits clotting enzymes, particularly thrombin and factor Xa.[72] Antithrombin, the obligatory plasma cofactor for heparin, is a member of the serine protease inhibitor (serpin) superfamily. Synthesized in the liver and circulating in plasma at a concentration of $2.6 \pm 0.4 \,\mu M$, antithrombin acts as a suicide substrate for its target enzymes.

To activate antithrombin, heparin binds to the serpin via a unique pentasaccharide sequence found on one third of the chains of commercial heparin (**Fig. 87-12**). Heparin chains lacking this pentasaccharide sequence have little or no anticoagulant activity.[72] Once bound to antithrombin, heparin induces a conformational change in the reactive center loop of antithrombin that renders it more readily accessible to its target proteases. This conformational change enhances the rate at which antithrombin inhibits factor Xa by at least two orders of magnitude, but has little effect on the rate of thrombin inhibition by antithrombin. To catalyze thrombin inhibition, heparin serves as a template that binds antithrombin and thrombin simultaneously. Formation of this ternary complex brings the enzyme in close apposition to the inhibitor, thereby promoting the formation of a stable covalent thrombin-antithrombin complex.

Only pentasaccharide-containing heparin chains composed of at least 18 saccharide units, which correspond to a molecular weight of 5400, are long enough to bridge thrombin and antithrombin together.[72] With a mean molecular weight of 15,000 (range, 5000 to 30,000), almost all the chains of unfractionated heparin are long enough to provide this bridging function. Consequently, by definition, heparin has equal capacity to promote the inhibition of thrombin and factor Xa by antithrombin, and has an anti-factor Xa–to–anti–factor IIa (thrombin) ratio of 1:1. Heparin causes the release of TFPI from the endothelium. A factor Xa–dependent inhibitor of tissue factor–bound factor VIIa,[6] TFPI may contribute to the antithrombotic activity of heparin. Longer heparin chains induce the release of more TFPI than shorter chains.

Pharmacology of Heparin

Heparin requires parenteral administration; it usually is administered subcutaneously or by continuous intravenous infusion. The intravenous route is most often used for therapeutic purposes. If given subcutaneously for the treatment of thrombosis, the dose must be high enough to overcome the limited bioavailability associated with this method of delivery.[72]

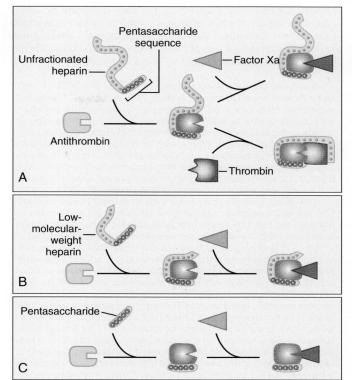

FIGURE 87-12 Mechanism of action of heparin, LMWH, and fondaparinux, a synthetic pentasaccharide. **A,** Heparin binds to antithrombin via its pentasaccharide sequence. This induces a conformational change in the reactive center loop of antithrombin that accelerates its interaction with factor Xa. To potentiate thrombin inhibition, heparin must simultaneously bind to antithrombin and thrombin. Only heparin chains composed of at least 18 saccharide units, which corresponds to a molecular weight of 5400, are of sufficient length to perform this bridging function. With a mean molecular weight of 15,000, all the heparin chains are long enough to do this. **B,** LMWH has greater capacity to potentiate factor Xa inhibition by antithrombin than thrombin because, with a mean molecular weight of 4500 to 5000, at least half of the LMWH chains are too short to bridge antithrombin to thrombin. **C,** The pentasaccharide only accelerates factor Xa inhibition by antithrombin because the pentasaccharide is too short to bridge antithrombin to thrombin.

In the circulation, heparin binds to the endothelium and to plasma proteins other than antithrombin. Heparin binding to endothelial cells explains its dose-dependent clearance. At low doses, the half-life of heparin is short because it rapidly binds to the endothelium. With higher doses of heparin, the half-life is longer, because heparin clearance is slower once the endothelium is saturated. Clearance is mainly extrarenal; heparin binds to macrophages, which internalize and depolymerize the long heparin chains and secrete shorter chains back into the circulation. Because of its dose-dependent clearance mechanism, the plasma half-life of heparin ranges from 30 to 60 minutes with bolus intravenous doses of 25 and 100 U/kg, respectively.[72]

Once heparin enters the circulation, it binds to plasma proteins other than antithrombin—a phenomenon that reduces the anticoagulant activity of heparin. Some of the heparin-binding proteins found in plasma are acute-phase reactants whose levels are elevated in ill patients. Activated platelets or endothelial cells release other proteins that can bind heparin, such as large multimers of vWF. Activated platelets also release platelet factor 4 (PF4), a highly cationic protein that binds heparin with high affinity. The large amounts of PF4 associated with platelet-rich arterial thrombi can neutralize the anticoagulant activity of heparin. This phenomenon may attenuate heparin's capacity to suppress thrombus growth.

Because the levels of heparin-binding proteins in plasma vary from person to person, the anticoagulant response to fixed or weight-adjusted doses of heparin is unpredictable. Consequently, coagulation monitoring is essential to ensure the response is therapeutic. This is particularly important when heparin is administered for the treatment of established thrombosis because a subtherapeutic anticoagulant response may render patients at risk for recurrent thrombosis, whereas excessive anticoagulation increases the risk of bleeding.[72]

MONITORING THE ANTICOAGULANT EFFECT OF HEPARIN. The aPTT or anti–factor Xa level is used to monitor heparin. Although the aPTT is the test most often used for this purpose, there are problems with the assay; aPTT reagents vary in their sensitivity to heparin, and the type of coagulometer used for testing can influence the results.[72] Consequently, laboratories must establish a therapeutic aPTT range with each reagent-coagulometer combination by measuring the aPTT and anti–factor Xa level in plasma samples collected from heparin-treated patients. With most aPTT reagents and coagulometers in current use, heparin levels are therapeutic, with a two- to threefold prolongation of the aPTT.

Anti–factor Xa levels also can be used to monitor heparin therapy. With this test, therapeutic heparin levels range from 0.3 to 0.7 units/mL. Although this test is gaining in popularity, anti–factor Xa assays have yet to be standardized, and results can vary widely between laboratories.

Up to 25% of patients with venous thromboembolism are heparin-resistant; they require more than 35,000 units/day to achieve a therapeutic aPTT. It is useful to measure anti–factor Xa levels in heparin-resistant patients because many will have a therapeutic anti–factor Xa level despite a subtherapeutic aPTT. This dissociation in test results occurs because elevated plasma levels of fibrinogen and factor VIII, both acute-phase proteins, shorten the aPTT but have no effect on anti–factor Xa levels.[72] Anti–factor Xa levels are better than the aPTT for heparin monitoring in patients who exhibit this phenomenon. Patients with congenital or acquired antithrombin deficiency and those with elevated levels of heparin-binding proteins also may need high doses of heparin to achieve a therapeutic aPTT or anti–factor Xa level. If there is good correlation between the aPTT and the anti–factor Xa level, either test can be used for monitoring heparin therapy.

DOSAGE. For prophylaxis, heparin is usually given in fixed doses of 5000 units subcutaneously two or three times daily. With these low doses, coagulation monitoring is unnecessary.[73] In contrast, monitoring is essential when the drug is given in therapeutic doses. Fixed-dose or weight-based heparin nomograms are used to standardize heparin dosing and to shorten the time required to achieve a therapeutic anticoagulant response. At least two heparin nomograms have been validated in patients with venous thromboembolism, and both reduce the time required to achieve a therapeutic aPTT. Weight-adjusted heparin nomograms also have been evaluated in patients with acute coronary syndromes. After an intravenous heparin bolus of 5000 units, or 70 units/kg, a heparin infusion rate of 12 to 15 units/kg/hour is usually administered.[72] In contrast, weight-adjusted heparin nomograms for patients with venous thromboembolism use an initial bolus of 5000 units, or 80 units/kg, followed by an infusion of 18 units/kg/hour. Thus, achievement of a therapeutic aPTT requires higher doses of heparin in patients with venous thromboembolism than in those with acute coronary syndromes. This may reflect differences in the thrombus burden. Heparin binds to fibrin, and the fibrin content of extensive deep vein thrombi is more than that of small coronary thrombi.

Heparin manufacturers in North America measure heparin potency in USP units, with a unit defined as the concentration of heparin that prevents 1 mL of citrated sheep plasma from clotting for 1 hour after calcium addition. In contrast, manufacturers in Europe measure heparin potency with anti–factor Xa assays using an international heparin standard for comparison. Because of problems with heparin contamination with oversulfated chondroitin sulfate,[74] which the USP assay system does not detect, North American heparin manufacturers now use the anti–factor Xa assay to measure heparin potency. Use of international units in place of USP units results in a 10% to 15% reduction in heparin dose. This change is unlikely to affect patient care because heparin has been dosed this way in Europe for many years. Furthermore, heparin monitoring ensures a therapeutic anticoagulant response in high-risk situations, such as cardiopulmonary bypass surgery or PCI.

Limitations of Heparin

Heparin has pharmacokinetic and biophysical limitations (**Table 87-4**). The pharmacokinetic limitations reflect heparin's propensity to bind in a pentasaccharide-independent fashion to cells and plasma proteins. Heparin binding to endothelial cells explains its dose-dependent clearance, whereas binding to plasma proteins results in a variable anticoagulant response and can lead to heparin resistance.

TABLE 87-4	Pharmacokinetic and Biophysical Limitations of Heparin
LIMITATION	**MECHANISM**
Poor bioavailability	Limited absorption of long heparin chains
Dose-dependent clearance	Binds to endothelial cells
Variable anticoagulant response	Binds to plasma proteins; levels vary from patient to patient
Reduced activity in the vicinity of platelet-rich thrombi	Neutralized by platelet factor 4 released from activated platelets
Limited activity against factor Xa incorporated into the prothrombinase complex and thrombin bound to fibrin	Reduced capacity of heparin-antithrombin complex to inhibit factor Xa bound to activated platelets and thrombin bound to fibrin

The biophysical limitations of heparin reflect the inability of the heparin-antithrombin complex to inhibit factor Xa when it is incorporated into the prothrombinase complex that converts prothrombin to thrombin, and to inhibit thrombin bound to fibrin.[72] Consequently, factor Xa bound to activated platelets within platelet-rich thrombi can generate thrombin, even in the face of heparin. Thrombin bound to fibrin is protected from inhibition by the heparin-antithrombin complex. Clot-associated thrombin can then trigger thrombus growth by locally activating platelets and amplifying its own generation through feedback activation of factors V, VIII, and XI. Heparin neutralization by the high concentrations of PF4 released from activated platelets within the platelet-rich thrombus further compounds this problem.

Side Effects

The most common side effect of heparin is bleeding. Other complications include thrombocytopenia, osteoporosis, and elevated levels of transaminases.

BLEEDING. The risk of heparin-induced bleeding increases with higher heparin doses. Concomitant administration of drugs that affect hemostasis, such as antiplatelet or fibrinolytic agents, increases the risk of bleeding, as does recent surgery or trauma.[75] Protamine sulfate will neutralize heparin in patients with serious bleeding. A mixture of basic polypeptides isolated from salmon sperm, protamine sulfate binds heparin with high affinity to form protamine-heparin complexes that undergo renal clearance. Typically, 1 mg of intravenous protamine sulfate neutralizes 100 units of heparin. Anaphylactoid reactions to protamine sulfate can occur, but administration by slow intravenous infusion reduces the risk of these problems.[72]

THROMBOCYTOPENIA. Heparin-induced thrombocytopenia (HIT) is an antibody-mediated process triggered by antibodies against neoantigens on PF4 that are exposed when heparin binds to this protein.[76] These antibodies, which usually are of the IgG subtype, bind simultaneously to the heparin-PF4 complex and to platelet Fc receptors. Such binding activates the platelets and generates platelet microparticles. Circulating microparticles are procoagulant because they express anionic phospholipids on their surface and can bind clotting factors, thereby promoting thrombin generation.

Typically, HIT occurs 5 to 14 days after initiation of heparin therapy, but can manifest earlier if the patient has received heparin within the past 3 months (**Table 87-5**). It is rare for the platelet count to fall below 100,000/μL in patients with HIT, and even a 50% decrease in the platelet count from the pretreatment value should raise the suspicion of HIT in those receiving heparin. HIT is more common in surgical patients than in medical patients and, like many autoimmune disorders, occurs more frequently in women than in men.[77]

HIT can be associated with arterial or venous thrombosis. Venous thrombosis, which manifests as deep vein thrombosis and/or pulmonary embolism, is more common than arterial thrombosis. Arterial thrombosis can manifest as ischemic stroke or acute myocardial

TABLE 87-5	Features of Heparin-Induced Thrombocytopenia
FEATURE	**DETAILS**
Thrombocytopenia	Platelet count of 100,000/μL or less or decrease in platelet count of 50% or more from baseline
Timing	Platelet count falls 5-10 days after starting heparin
Type of heparin	More common with unfractionated heparin than with LMWH
Type of patient	More common in surgical patients than medical patients; more common in women than in men
Thrombosis	Venous thrombosis more common than arterial thrombosis

TABLE 87-6	Management of Heparin-Induced Thrombocytopenia

- Stop all heparin.
- Give an alternative anticoagulant, such as lepirudin, argatroban, bivalirudin, or fondaparinux.
- Do not give platelet transfusions.
- Do not give warfarin until the platelet count returns to baseline levels; if warfarin was administered, give vitamin K to restore INR to normal.
- Evaluate for thrombosis, particularly deep vein thrombosis.

TABLE 87-7	Advantages of Low-Molecular-Weight Heparin and Fondaparinux over Heparin	
ADVANTAGE	**CONSEQUENCE**	
Better bioavailability and longer half-life after subcutaneous injection	Can be given subcutaneously once or twice daily for both prophylaxis and treatment	
Dose-independent clearance	Simplified dosing	
Predictable anticoagulant response	Coagulation monitoring unnecessary for most patients	
Lower risk of heparin-induced thrombocytopenia	Safer than heparin for short- or long-term administration	
Lower risk of osteoporosis	Safer than heparin for long-term administration	

infarction. Rarely, platelet-rich thrombi in the distal aorta or iliac arteries can cause critical limb ischemia.[76,77]

The diagnosis of HIT is established with enzyme-linked assays to detect antibodies against heparin-PF4 complexes or with platelet activation assays. Enzyme-linked assays are sensitive, but can be positive in the absence of any clinical evidence of HIT.[78] The most specific diagnostic test is the serotonin release assay. This test involves quantification of serotonin release after exposure of washed platelets loaded with labeled serotonin to patient serum in the absence or presence of varying concentrations of heparin. If the patient serum contains HIT antibody, heparin addition induces platelet activation and subsequent serotonin release.

To manage HIT, heparin should be stopped in patients with suspected or documented HIT, and an alternative anticoagulant should be administered to prevent or treat thrombosis (**Table 87-6**).[79] The agents most often used for this indication are parenteral direct thrombin inhibitors, such as lepirudin, argatroban, or bivalirudin, or factor Xa inhibitors, such as fondaparinux.

Patients with HIT, particularly those with associated thrombosis, often have evidence of increased thrombin generation that can lead to consumption of protein C. If these patients receive warfarin without a concomitant parenteral anticoagulant, the further decrease in protein C levels induced by the vitamin K antagonist can trigger skin necrosis.[80] To avoid this problem, patients with HIT require treatment with a direct thrombin inhibitor or fondaparinux until the platelet count returns to normal levels. At this point, low-dose warfarin therapy can be introduced and the thrombin inhibitor can be discontinued when the anticoagulant response to warfarin has been therapeutic for at least 2 days.[76-79]

OSTEOPOROSIS. Treatment with therapeutic doses of heparin for longer than 1 month can cause a reduction in bone density. This occurs in up to 30% of patients given long-term heparin therapy,[72] and symptomatic vertebral fractures occur in 2% to 3% of these individuals.

Studies in vitro and in laboratory animals have provided insights into the pathogenesis of heparin-induced osteoporosis. These investigations suggest that heparin causes bone resorption by decreasing bone formation and enhancing bone resorption. Thus, heparin affects the activity of osteoclasts and osteoblasts.[72]

ELEVATED LEVELS OF TRANSAMINASES. Therapeutic doses of heparin frequently cause modest elevations in the serum levels of hepatic transaminases, without a concomitant increase in the level of bilirubin. The levels of transaminases rapidly return to normal when the drug is stopped. The mechanism responsible for this phenomenon is unknown.

LOW-MOLECULAR-WEIGHT HEPARIN. Consisting of smaller fragments of heparin, LMWH is prepared from unfractionated heparin by controlled enzymatic or chemical depolymerization. The mean molecular weight of LMWH is about 5000, one third the mean molecular weight of unfractionated heparin.[72] Because of its advantages over heparin (**Table 87-7**), LMWH has replaced heparin for many indications.

Mechanism of Action

Like heparin, LMWH exerts its anticoagulant activity by activating antithrombin. With a mean molecular weight of about 5000, which corresponds to about 17 saccharide units, at least half of the pentasaccharide-containing chains of LMWH are too short to bridge thrombin to antithrombin (see Fig. 87-12). These chains retain the capacity to accelerate factor Xa inhibition by antithrombin, because this activity largely results from the conformational changes in antithrombin evoked by pentasaccharide binding. Consequently, LMWH catalyzes factor Xa inhibition by antithrombin more than thrombin inhibition.[72] Depending on their unique molecular weight distributions, LMWH preparations have anti–factor Xa–to–anti–factor IIa ratios ranging from 2:1 to 4:1 (see Table 87-3).

Pharmacology of Low-Molecular-Weight Heparin

Although usually given subcutaneously, LMWH can be administered intravenously if a rapid anticoagulant response is needed. LMWH has pharmacokinetic advantages over heparin. These advantages arise because the shorter heparin chains bind less avidly to endothelial cells, macrophages, and heparin-binding plasma proteins.[72] Reduced binding to endothelial cells and macrophages eliminates the rapid, dose-dependent, and saturable mechanism of clearance that is a characteristic of unfractionated heparin. Instead, the clearance of LMWH is dose-independent and its plasma half-life is longer. Based on the measurement of anti–factor Xa levels, LMWH has a plasma half-life of about 4 hours. Because of its renal clearance, LMWH can accumulate in patients with renal insufficiency.

LMWH exhibits about 90% bioavailability after subcutaneous injection.[72] Because LMWH binds less avidly than heparin to heparin-binding proteins in plasma, LMWH produces a more predictable dose response, and resistance to LMWH is rare. With a longer half-life and more predictable anticoagulant response, LMWH can be given subcutaneously once or twice daily without coagulation monitoring, even when the drug is given in treatment doses. These properties render LMWH more convenient than unfractionated heparin. Capitalizing on this feature, studies in patients with venous thromboembolism have shown that home treatment with LMWH is as effective and safe as in-hospital treatment with continuous intravenous infusions of heparin. Outpatient treatment with LMWH streamlines care, reduces health care costs, and increases patient satisfaction.

LOW-MOLECULAR-WEIGHT HEPARIN MONITORING. In most patients, LMWH does not require coagulation monitoring. If monitoring is necessary, the anti–factor Xa level is measured, because most LMWH preparations have little effect on the aPTT. Therapeutic anti–factor Xa levels with LMWH range from 0.5 to 1.2 units/mL when measured 3 to 4 hours after drug administration. With prophylactic doses of LMWH, peak anti–factor Xa levels of 0.2 to 0.5 units/mL are desirable.[72]

Situations that may require LMWH monitoring include renal insufficiency and obesity. LMWH monitoring in patients with a creatinine clearance of 50 mL/min or less is advisable to ensure that there is no drug accumulation. Although weight-adjusted LMWH dosing appears to produce therapeutic anti–factor Xa levels in overweight patients, this approach has not been well studied in those with morbid obesity. It may also be advisable to monitor the anticoagulant activity of LMWH during pregnancy because dose requirements can change, particularly in the third trimester. Monitoring also should be considered in high-risk settings, such as in patients with mechanical heart valves who are given LMWH for the prevention of valve thrombosis.

DOSAGE. The doses of LMWH recommended for prophylaxis or treatment vary depending on the preparation. For prophylaxis, once-daily subcutaneous doses of 4000 to 5000 units are often used, whereas doses of 2500 to 3000 units are given when the drug is administered twice daily. For treatment of venous thromboembolism, a dose of 150 to 200 units/kg is given if the drug is administered once daily. If a twice-daily regimen is used, a dose of 100 units/kg is given. In patients with unstable angina, LMWH is given subcutaneously on a twice-daily basis at a dose of 100 to 120 units/kg. The dose is reduced in patients with renal impairment.

SIDE EFFECTS. The major complication of LMWH is bleeding. Meta-analyses have suggested that the risk of major bleeding may be lower with LMWH than with unfractionated heparin.[81] HIT and osteoporosis are less common with LMWH than with unfractionated heparin.[76-78]

BLEEDING. The risk of bleeding with LMWH increases when antiplatelet or fibrinolytic drugs are given concomitantly. Recent surgery, trauma, or underlying hemostatic defects also increase the risk of bleeding with LMWH.[75]

Although protamine sulfate serves as an antidote for LMWH, it incompletely neutralizes the anticoagulant activity of LMWH because it only binds the longer chains.[72] Because longer chains are responsible for the catalysis of thrombin inhibition by antithrombin, protamine sulfate completely reverses the anti–factor IIa activity of LMWH. In contrast, protamine sulfate only partially reverses the anti–factor Xa activity of LMWH because the shorter pentasaccharide-containing chains of LMWH do not bind protamine sulfate. Consequently, continuous intravenous unfractionated heparin may be safer than subcutaneous LMWH for patients at high risk for bleeding.

THROMBOCYTOPENIA. The risk of HIT is about fivefold lower with LMWH than with heparin.[76-78] LMWH binds less avidly to platelets and causes less PF4 release. Furthermore, with lower affinity for PF4 than heparin, LMWH is less likely to induce the conformational changes in PF4 that trigger the formation of HIT antibodies. LMWH should not be used to treat HIT patients because most HIT antibodies exhibit cross-reactivity with LMWH. This in vitro cross-reactivity is not simply a laboratory phenomenon; there are case reports of thrombosis in HIT patients treated with LMWH.

OSTEOPOROSIS. The risk of osteoporosis is lower with long-term LMWH than with heparin.[72] For extended treatment, therefore, LMWH is a better choice than heparin because of the lower risk of osteoporosis and HIT.

FONDAPARINUX. A synthetic analogue of the antithrombin-binding pentasaccharide sequence, fondaparinux differs from LMWH in several ways (see Table 87-3). Fondaparinux is licensed for thromboprophylaxis in medical, general surgical, or high-risk orthopedic patients and as an alternative to heparin or LMWH for the initial treatment of patients with established venous thromboembolism. The drug is not yet licensed in the United States as an alternative to heparin or LMWH in patients with acute coronary syndromes.

Mechanism of action

As a synthetic analogue of the antithrombin-binding pentasaccharide sequence found in heparin and LMWH, fondaparinux has a molecular weight of 1728. Fondaparinux binds only to antithrombin (see Fig. 87-12) and is too short to bridge thrombin to antithrombin. Consequently, fondaparinux catalyzes factor Xa inhibition by antithrombin and does not enhance the rate of thrombin inhibition.[72]

PHARMACOLOGY OF FONDAPARINUX. Fondaparinux exhibits complete bioavailability after subcutaneous injection. With no binding to endothelial cells or plasma proteins, the clearance of fondaparinux is dose-independent and its plasma half-life is 17 hours. The drug is given subcutaneously once daily. Because of its renal clearance, fondaparinux is contraindicated in patients with a creatinine clearance less than 30 mL/min, and it should be used with caution in those with a creatinine clearance less than 50 mL/min.[72]

Fondaparinux produces a predictable anticoagulant response after administration in fixed doses because it does not bind to plasma proteins. It is given at a dose of 2.5 mg once daily for prevention of venous thromboembolism. For initial treatment of established venous thromboembolism, fondaparinux is given at a dose of 7.5 mg once daily. The dose can be reduced to 5 mg once daily for those weighing less than 50 kg and increased to 10 mg for those weighing more than 100 kg. When given in these doses, fondaparinux is as effective as heparin or LMWH for the initial treatment of patients with deep vein thrombosis or pulmonary embolism, and produces similar rates of bleeding.[82]

Fondaparinux is used at a dose of 2.5 mg once daily in patients with acute coronary syndromes. When this prophylactic dose of fondaparinux was compared with treatment doses of enoxaparin in patients with non–ST-segment elevation acute coronary syndromes, there was no difference in the rate of cardiovascular death, myocardial infarction, or stroke at 9 days.[83] In one study, however, the rate of major bleeding, was 50% lower with fondaparinux than with enoxaparin, a difference that likely reflects that the dose of fondaparinux was lower than that of enoxaparin. In acute coronary syndrome patients who require PCI, there is a risk of catheter thrombosis with fondaparinux unless adjunctive heparin is given.[84]

SIDE EFFECTS. Although fondaparinux can induce the formation of HIT antibodies, HIT does not occur.[85] This apparent paradox reflects the fact that induction of HIT requires heparin chains of sufficient length to bind multiple PF4 molecules. Fondaparinux is too short to do this. In contrast to LMWH, there is no cross-reactivity of fondaparinux with HIT antibodies. Consequently, fondaparinux appears to be effective for the treatment of HIT,[86,87] although large clinical trials supporting its use are lacking.

The major side effect of fondaparinux is bleeding, and it has no antidote. Protamine sulfate has no effect on the anticoagulant activity of fondaparinux because it fails to bind to the drug. Recombinant activated factor VII reverses the anticoagulant effects of fondaparinux in volunteers,[72] but it is unknown whether this agent controls fondaparinux-induced bleeding.

PARENTERAL DIRECT THROMBIN INHIBITORS

Heparin and LMWH indirectly inhibit thrombin because they require antithrombin to exert their anticoagulant activity. In contrast, direct thrombin inhibitors do not require a plasma cofactor; instead, they bind directly to thrombin and block its interaction with its substrates. Approved parenteral direct thrombin inhibitors include lepirudin, argatroban, and bivalirudin (**Table 87-8**). Lepirudin and argatroban are licensed for the treatment of patients with HIT, whereas bivalirudin is approved as an alternative to heparin in patients undergoing PCI, including those with HIT.

LEPIRUDIN. A recombinant form of hirudin, lepirudin is a bivalent direct thrombin inhibitor that interacts with the active site of thrombin and exosite 1, the substrate binding site.[72] For rapid anticoagulation, lepirudin is given by continuous intravenous infusion, but the drug can

TABLE 87-8	Comparison of the Properties of Hirudin, Bivalirudin, and Argatroban		
PARAMETER	**HIRUDIN**	**BIVALIRUDIN**	**ARGATROBAN**
Molecular mass	7000	1980	527
Site(s) of interaction with thrombin	Active site and exosite 1	Active site and exosite 1	Active site
Renal clearance	Yes	No	No
Hepatic metabolism	No	No	Yes
Plasma half-life (min)	60	25	45

be given subcutaneously for thromboprophylaxis. Lepirudin has a plasma half-life of 60 minutes after intravenous infusion and is cleared by the kidneys. Consequently, lepirudin accumulates in patients with renal insufficiency. A high proportion of lepirudin-treated patients develop antibodies against the drug. Although these antibodies rarely cause problems, in a small subset of patients they can delay lepirudin clearance and enhance its anticoagulant activity; some of these patients experience serious bleeding.

Lepirudin is usually monitored using the aPTT, and the dose is adjusted to maintain an aPTT that is 1.5 to 2.5 times the control. The aPTT is not an ideal test for monitoring lepirudin therapy because the clotting time plateaus with higher drug concentrations. Although the ecarin clotting time provides a better index of lepirudin dose than the aPTT, the ecarin clotting time has yet to be standardized and the test is not available in all coagulation laboratories.

ARGATROBAN. Argatroban, a univalent inhibitor that targets the active site of thrombin, is metabolized in the liver.[72] Consequently, it must be used with caution in patients with hepatic insufficiency. Because it is not cleared by the kidneys, argatroban is safer than lepirudin for HIT patients with renal impairment.

Argatroban is administered by continuous intravenous infusion and has a plasma half-life of about 45 minutes. The aPTT is used to monitor its anticoagulant effect, and the dose is adjusted to achieve an aPTT 1.5 to 3 times the baseline value, but not to exceed 100 seconds. Argatroban also prolongs the international normalized ratio (INR), a feature that can complicate the transitioning of patients to warfarin. This problem can be circumvented by using the levels of factor X to monitor warfarin in place of the INR. Alternatively, argatroban can be stopped for 2 to 3 hours before INR determination.

BIVALIRUDIN. A synthetic 20–amino acid analogue of hirudin, bivalirudin is a divalent thrombin inhibitor.[72] Thus, the N-terminal portion of bivalirudin interacts with the active site of thrombin, whereas its C-terminal tail binds to exosite 1, the substrate-binding domain on thrombin. Bivalirudin has a plasma half-life of 25 minutes, the shortest half-life of all the parenteral direct thrombin inhibitors. Bivalirudin is degraded by peptidases and is partially excreted via the kidneys. When given in high doses in the cardiac catheterization laboratory, the anticoagulant activity of bivalirudin is monitored using the activated clotting time. With lower doses, its activity can be assessed using the aPTT.

Studies comparing bivalirudin with heparin have suggested that bivalirudin produces less bleeding. This feature, plus its short half-life, renders bivalirudin an attractive alternative to heparin in patients undergoing PCI. Bivalirudin also has been used successfully in HIT patients who require PCI.[72]

ORAL ANTICOAGULANTS

Vitamin K antagonists were identified more than 60 years ago during investigations into the cause of hemorrhagic disease in cattle. Characterized by decreased prothrombin levels, this disorder occurs after ingestion of hay containing spoiled sweet clover. Hydroxycoumarin, which was isolated from bacterial contaminants in the hay, interferes with vitamin K metabolism, thereby causing a syndrome similar to vitamin K deficiency. This compound spawned the development of other vitamin K antagonists, including warfarin.

WARFARIN. A water-soluble vitamin K antagonist initially developed as a rodenticide, warfarin is the coumarin derivative most often prescribed in North America. Like other vitamin K antagonists, warfarin interferes with the synthesis of the vitamin K–dependent clotting proteins, which include prothrombin (factor II) and factors VII, IX, and X. Warfarin also impairs synthesis of the vitamin K–dependent anticoagulant proteins C and S.[88]

Mechanism of Action

All the vitamin K–dependent clotting factors possess glutamic acid residues at their N termini. A post-translational modification adds a

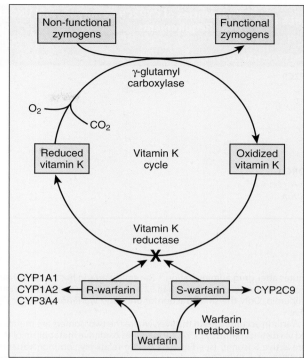

FIGURE 87-13 Mechanism of action of warfarin. A racemic mixture of S and R enantiomers, S-warfarin is most active. By blocking vitamin K epoxide reductase, warfarin inhibits the conversion of oxidized vitamin K into its reduced form. This inhibits vitamin K–dependent γ-carboxylation of factors II, VII, IX, and X, because reduced vitamin K serves as a cofactor for a γ-glutamyl carboxylase that catalyzes the γ-carboxylation process, thereby converting prozymogens to zymogens capable of binding calcium and interacting with anionic phospholipid surfaces. S-warfarin is metabolized by *CYP2C9*. Common genetic polymorphisms in this enzyme can influence warfarin metabolism. Polymorphisms in the C1 subunit of vitamin K reductase (VKORC1) also can affect the susceptibility of the enzyme to warfarin-induced inhibition, thereby influencing warfarin dosage requirements.

carboxyl group to the γ carbon of these residues to generate γ-carboxyglutamic acid. This modification is essential for expression of the activity of these clotting factors because it permits their calcium-dependent binding to anionic phospholipid surfaces.[88] The γ-carboxylation process is catalyzed by a vitamin K–dependent carboxylase. Thus, vitamin K from the diet is reduced to vitamin K hydroquinone by vitamin K reductase (**Fig. 87-13**). Vitamin K hydroquinone serves as a cofactor for the carboxylase enzyme, which in the presence of carbon dioxide, replaces the hydrogen on the γ carbon of glutamic acid residues with a carboxyl group. During this process, vitamin K hydroquinone is oxidized to vitamin K epoxide, which is then reduced to vitamin K by vitamin K epoxide reductase (VKOR).

Warfarin inhibits VKOR, thereby blocking the γ-carboxylation process. This results in the synthesis of vitamin K–dependent clotting proteins that are only partially γ-carboxylated.[88] Warfarin acts as an anticoagulant because these partially γ-carboxylated proteins have reduced or absent biologic activity. The onset of action of warfarin is delayed until the newly synthesized clotting factors with reduced activity gradually replace their fully active counterparts.

The antithrombotic effect of warfarin depends on a reduction in the functional levels of factor X and prothrombin, clotting factors that have half-lives of 24 and 72 hours, respectively.[88] Because of the delay in achieving an antithrombotic effect, initial treatment with warfarin is supported by concomitant administration of a rapidly acting parenteral anticoagulant, such as heparin, LMWH, or fondaparinux, in patients with established thrombosis or at high risk for thrombosis.

PHARMACOLOGY OF WARFARIN. Warfarin is a racemic mixture of R and S isomers. Warfarin is rapidly and almost completely absorbed from the gastrointestinal tract. Levels of warfarin in the blood peak about 90

TABLE 87-9 Frequencies of CYP2C9 Genotypes and VKORC1 Haplotypes in Different Populations and Their Effect on Warfarin Dose Requirements

GENOTYPE/HAPLOTYPE	WHITES	Frequency % BLACKS	ASIANS	DOSE REDUCTION COMPARED WITH WILD TYPE
CYP2C9				
*1/*1	70	90	95	—
*1/*2	17	2	0	22
*1/*3	9	3	4	34
*2/*2	2	0	0	43
*2/*3	1	0	0	53
*3/*3	0	0	1	76
VKORC 1				
Non-A, non-A	37	82	7	—
Non-A/A	45	12	30	26
A/A	18	6	63	50

minutes after drug administration.[88] Racemic warfarin has a plasma half-life of 36 to 42 hours, and more than 97% of circulating warfarin is bound to albumin. Only the small fraction of unbound warfarin is biologically active.

Warfarin accumulates in the liver, where the two isomers are metabolized via distinct pathways. CYP2C9 mediates oxidative metabolism of the more active S isomer (see Fig. 87-12). Two relatively common variants, CYP2C9*2 and CYP2C9*3, encode an enzyme with reduced activity. Patients with these variants require lower maintenance doses of warfarin. Approximately 25% of whites have at least one variant allele of CYP2C9*2 or CYP2C9*3, whereas these variant alleles are less common in blacks and Asians (**Table 87-9**). Heterozygosity for CYP2C9*2 or CYP2C9*3 decreases the warfarin dose requirement by 20% to 30% relative to that required in subjects with the wild-type CYP2C9*1/*1 alleles, whereas homozygosity for the CYP2C9*2 or CYP2C9*3 allele reduces the warfarin dose requirement by 50% to 70%. Consistent with their decreased warfarin dose requirement, subjects with at least one CYP2C9 variant allele are at increased risk for bleeding. Compared with individuals with no variant alleles, the relative risks for warfarin-associated bleeding in CYP2C9*2 or CYP2C9*3 carriers are 1.91 and 1.77, respectively.[89,90]

Polymorphisms in VKORC1 also can influence the anticoagulant response to warfarin.[90-94] Several genetic variations of VKORC1 are in strong linkage disequilibrium and have been designated as non-A haplotypes. VKORC1 variants are more prevalent than variants of CYP2C9. Asians have the highest prevalence of VKORC1 variants, followed by whites and blacks (see Table 87-9). Polymorphisms in VKORC1 likely explain 30% of the variability in warfarin dose requirements. Compared with VKORC1 non-A, non-A homozygotes, the warfarin dose requirement decreases by 25% and 50% in A/A heterozygotes and homozygotes, respectively. These findings prompted the U.S. Food and Drug Administration (FDA) to amend the prescribing information for warfarin to indicate that lower initiation doses should be considered for patients with CYP2C9 and VKORC1 genetic variants. In addition to genotype data, other pertinent patient information has been incorporated into warfarin dosing algorithms. Although such algorithms help predict suitable warfarin doses, it remains unclear whether better dose identification improves patient outcome in terms of reducing hemorrhagic complications or recurrent thrombotic events.

In addition to genetic factors, diet, drugs, and various disease states influence the anticoagulant effect of warfarin. Fluctuations in dietary vitamin K intake affect the activity of warfarin. A wide variety of drugs can alter absorption, clearance, or metabolism of warfarin.[88] Because of the variability in the anticoagulant response to warfarin, coagulation monitoring is essential to ensure a therapeutic response.

Monitoring

Warfarin therapy is most often monitored using the prothrombin time, a test sensitive to reductions in the levels of prothrombin, factor VII, and factor X. The test involves the addition of thromboplastin, a reagent that contains tissue factor, phospholipid, and calcium, to citrated plasma and determining the time to clot formation. Thromboplastins vary in their sensitivity to reductions in the levels of the vitamin

K–dependent clotting factors. Consequently, less sensitive thromboplastins will trigger the administration of higher doses of warfarin to achieve a target prothrombin time. This is problematic, because higher doses of warfarin increase the risk of bleeding.

The INR was developed to circumvent many of the problems associated with the prothrombin time. To calculate the INR, the patient's prothrombin time is divided by the mean normal prothrombin time, and this ratio is then multiplied by the international sensitivity index (ISI), an index of the sensitivity of the thromboplastin used for prothrombin time determination to reductions in the levels of the vitamin K–dependent clotting factors. Highly sensitive thromboplastins have an ISI of 1.0. Most current thromboplastins have ISI values that range from 1.0 to 1.4.[88]

Although the INR has helped standardize anticoagulant practice, problems persist. The precision of INR determination varies depending on reagent-coagulometer combinations, leading to variability in the INR results. Also complicating INR determination is unreliable reporting of the ISI by thromboplastin manufacturers. Furthermore, every laboratory must establish the mean normal prothrombin time with each new batch of thromboplastin reagent. To accomplish this, the prothrombin time must be measured in fresh plasma samples from at least 20 healthy volunteers using the same coagulometer used for patient samples.

For most indications, warfarin is administered in doses that produce a target INR of 2.0 to 3.0. An exception is patients with high-risk mechanical heart valves, for whom a target INR of 2.5 to 3.5 is recommended.[88] Studies in atrial fibrillation have demonstrated an increased risk of cardioembolic stroke when the INR falls below 1.7, and an increase in bleeding with INR values above 4.5.[95] These findings highlight the narrow therapeutic window of vitamin K antagonists. In support of this concept, a study in patients receiving long-term warfarin therapy for unprovoked venous thromboembolism has demonstrated a higher rate of recurrent venous thromboembolism with a target INR of 1.5 to 1.9 compared with a target INR of 2.0 to 3.0.[88]

Dosing

Warfarin is usually started at a dose of 5 to 10 mg. Lower doses are used for patients with CYP2C9 or VKORC1 polymorphisms that affect the pharmacodynamics or pharmacokinetics of warfarin and render patients more sensitive to the drug. The dose is then titrated to achieve the desired target INR.[88] Because of its delayed onset of action, patients with established thrombosis or those at high risk for thrombosis are given concomitant treatment with a rapidly acting parenteral anticoagulant, such as heparin, LMWH, or fondaparinux. Initial prolongation of the INR reflects a reduction in the functional levels of factor VII. Consequently, concomitant treatment with the parenteral anticoagulant should be continued until the INR has been therapeutic for at least 2 consecutive days. A minimum 5-day course of parenteral anticoagulation is recommended to ensure that the levels of prothrombin have fallen into the therapeutic range with warfarin.[72]

Because warfarin has a narrow therapeutic window, frequent coagulation monitoring is essential to ensure that the anticoagulant response is therapeutic. Even patients with stable warfarin dose requirements should have their INR determined every 3 to 4 weeks. More frequent monitoring is necessary with the introduction of new medications, because many drugs enhance or reduce the anticoagulant effects of warfarin.

Side Effects

Like all anticoagulants, the major side effect of warfarin is bleeding; a rare complication is skin necrosis. Warfarin crosses the placenta and can cause fetal abnormalities, so it should not be used during pregnancy.[88]

BLEEDING. At least half of bleeding complications with warfarin occur when the INR exceeds the therapeutic range. Bleeding complications may be mild, such as epistaxis or hematuria, or more severe, such as retroperitoneal or gastrointestinal bleeding. Life-threatening intracranial bleeding also can occur.[75]

To minimize the risk of bleeding, the INR should be maintained in the therapeutic range. In asymptomatic patients whose INR is between 3.5 and 4.5, warfarin should be withheld until the INR returns to the therapeutic range. If the INR is over 4.5, a therapeutic INR can be achieved more rapidly by administration of low doses of sublingual vitamin K.[96] A vitamin K dose of 1 mg usually is adequate for patients with an INR between 4.9 and 9, whereas 2 to 3 mg can be used for those with an INR higher than 9. Higher doses of vitamin K can be administered if more rapid reversal of the INR is required, or if the INR is excessively high. Although vitamin K administration results in a more rapid reduction in the INR, there is no evidence that it reduces the risk of hemorrhage.[96]

Patients with serious bleeding need additional treatment. These patients should be given 10 mg of vitamin K by slow intravenous infusion. Additional vitamin K should be given until the INR is in the normal range. Treatment with vitamin K should be supplemented with fresh-frozen plasma as a source of vitamin K–dependent clotting proteins. For life-threatening bleeds, or if patients cannot tolerate the volume load, prothrombin complex concentrates can be used.[88]

Warfarin-treated patients who experience bleeding when their INR is in the therapeutic range require investigation into the cause of the bleeding. Those with gastrointestinal bleeding often have underlying peptic ulcer disease or a tumor. Similarly, investigation of hematuria or uterine bleeding in patients with a therapeutic INR may unmask a tumor of the genitourinary tract.

SKIN NECROSIS. A rare complication of warfarin, skin necrosis usually occurs 2 to 5 days after initiation of therapy. Well-demarcated erythematous lesions form on the thighs, buttocks, breasts, or toes. Typically, the center of the lesion becomes progressively necrotic. Examination of skin biopsies taken from the borders of these lesions reveals thrombi in the microvasculature.

Warfarin-induced skin necrosis occurs in patients with congenital or acquired deficiencies of protein C or protein S.[88] Initiation of warfarin therapy in these patients produces a precipitous fall in plasma levels of proteins C or S, thereby eliminating this important anticoagulant pathway before warfarin exerts an antithrombotic effect through lowering of the functional levels of factor X and prothrombin. The resultant procoagulant state triggers thrombosis, but the reason that the thrombosis localizes to the microvasculature of fatty tissues is unclear.

Treatment involves discontinuation of warfarin and reversal with vitamin K, if needed. An alternative anticoagulant, such as heparin or LMWH, should be given to patients with thrombosis. Protein C concentrates or recombinant activated protein C may accelerate healing of the skin lesions in protein C deficient patients; fresh-frozen plasma may be of value for those with protein S deficiency. Occasionally, skin grafting is necessary when there is extensive skin loss.

Because of the potential for skin necrosis, patients with known protein C or protein S deficiency require overlapping treatment with a parenteral anticoagulant when initiating warfarin therapy. Warfarin should be started in low doses in these patients, and the parenteral anticoagulant should be continued until the INR is therapeutic for at least 2 to 3 consecutive days.

Pregnancy

Warfarin crosses the placenta and can cause fetal abnormalities or bleeding. The fetal abnormalities include a characteristic embryopathy, which consists of nasal hypoplasia and stippled epiphyses. The risk of embryopathy is highest with warfarin administration in the first trimester of pregnancy.[97] Central nervous system abnormalities also can occur with warfarin exposure at any time during pregnancy. Finally, maternal administration of warfarin produces an anticoagulant effect in the fetus that can cause bleeding. This is of particular concern at delivery, when trauma to the head during passage through the birth canal can lead to intracranial bleeding. Because of these potential problems, warfarin is contraindicated in pregnancy, particularly in the first and third trimesters (see Chaps. 66 and 82). Instead, heparin, LMWH, or fondaparinux can be given during pregnancy for prevention or treatment of thrombosis. Warfarin does not pass into breast milk, and thus is safe for nursing mothers.

Special Problems

Patients with an LA or those who need urgent or elective surgery present special challenges. Although observational studies have suggested that patients with thrombosis complicating APL require higher-intensity warfarin regimens to prevent recurrent thromboembolic events, two randomized trials have demonstrated that targeting an INR of 2.0 to 3.0 is as effective as higher-intensity treatment and produces less bleeding.[98] Monitoring warfarin therapy can prove difficult in patients with APL if the LA prolongs the baseline INR. Warfarin can be dosed based on measurements of factor X levels in such patients.

If patients receiving long-term warfarin treatment require an elective invasive procedure, warfarin can be stopped 5 days prior to the procedure to allow the INR to return to normal levels. Those at high risk for recurrent thrombosis can be bridged with once- or twice-daily subcutaneous injections of LMWH when the INR falls below 2.0. The last dose of LMWH should be given 12 to 24 hours prior to the procedure, depending on whether LMWH is administered twice or once daily, respectively. After the procedure, warfarin can be restarted.

NEW ORAL ANTICOAGULANTS

New oral anticoagulants that target thrombin or factor Xa are under development.[99-102] These drugs have a rapid onset of action and have half-lives that permit once- or twice-daily administration. Designed to produce a predictable level of anticoagulation, these new oral agents are given in fixed doses without routine coagulation monitoring. Therefore, these drugs are more convenient to administer than warfarin.

Dabigatran etexilate, an oral thrombin inhibitor, and rivaroxaban, an oral factor Xa inhibitor, are licensed in Europe and Canada for short-term thromboprophylaxis after elective hip or knee replacement surgery, and in the United States for atrial fibrillation. Phase III trials with apixaban, another oral factor Xa inhibitor, also have been completed in patients undergoing major orthopedic surgery (**Table 87-10**).

The recently reported RE-LY trial[101] shows the promise of these new agents for long-term indications. This trial compared two different dose regimens of dabigatran etexilate (110 or 150 mg twice daily) with warfarin (dose-adjusted to achieve an INR between 2.0 and 3.0) for stroke prevention in 18,113 patients with nonvalvular atrial fibrillation. The annual rates of the primary efficacy outcome, stroke or systemic embolism, were 1.7% with warfarin, 1.5% with the lower dose dabigatran regimen, and 1.1% with the higher-dose regimen. Thus, the lower-dose dabigatran regimen was noninferior to warfarin, whereas the higher-dose regimen was superior. Annual rates of major bleeding were 3.4% with warfarin, compared with 2.7% and 3.1% with the lower-dose and higher-dose dabigatran regimens, respectively. Thus, the lower-dose dabigatran regimen was associated with less major bleeding than warfarin, whereas the rate of major bleeding with the higher-dose regimen was not significantly different from that with warfarin. Rates of intracerebral bleeding were significantly lower with both doses of dabigatran than with warfarin, as were rates of life-threatening bleeding. There was no evidence of hepatotoxicity with dabigatran.

TABLE 87-10	Comparison of Features of New Oral Anticoagulants in Advanced Stages of Development		
FEATURE	**RIVAROXABAN**	**APIXABAN**	**DABIGATRAN ETEXILATE**
Target	Xa	Xa	IIa
Molecular weight	436	460	628
Prodrug	No	No	Yes
Bioavailability (%)	80	50	6
Time to peak (hr)	3	3	2
Half-life (hr)	9	9-14	12-17
Renal excretion (%)	65	25	80
Antidote	None	None	None

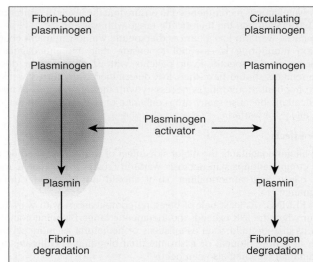

FIGURE 87-14 Consequences of activation of fibrin-bound or circulating plasminogen. The fibrin specificity of plasminogen activators reflects their capacity to distinguish between fibrin-bound and circulating plasminogen, which depends on their affinity for fibrin. Plasminogen activators with high affinity for fibrin preferentially activate fibrin-bound plasminogen. This results in the generation of plasmin on the fibrin surface. Fibrin-bound plasmin, which is protected from inactivation by alpha$_2$-antiplasmin, degrades fibrin to yield soluble fibrin degradation products. In contrast, plasminogen activators with little or no affinity for fibrin do not distinguish between fibrin-bound and circulating plasminogen. Activation of circulating plasminogen results in systemic plasminemia and subsequent degradation of fibrinogen and other clotting factors.

Unmonitored dabigatran etexilate (150 mg twice daily) was compared with warfarin for treatment of venous thromboembolism in the RE-COVER trial.[102] The primary efficacy outcome, recurrent venous thromboembolism and related deaths, occurred in 2.4% of patients randomized to dabigatran and in 2.1% of those given warfarin. Major bleeding episodes occurred in 1.5% of patients randomized to dabigatran and in 1.9% of those assigned to warfarin. Therefore, dabigatran appears to be as effective and safe as warfarin for the treatment of venous thromboembolism. The promising results of these trials indicate that replacements for warfarin will soon be available.

Fibrinolytic Drugs

Used to degrade thrombi, fibrinolytic drugs (see Chap. 55) can be administered systemically or delivered via catheters directly into the substance of the thrombus. Currently approved fibrinolytic agents include streptokinase, acylated plasminogen streptokinase activator complex (anistreplase), urokinase, recombinant tissue plasminogen activator (rt-PA; also known as alteplase or activase), and two recombinant derivatives of rt-PA, tenecteplase and reteplase. All these agents act by converting the proenzyme, plasminogen, to plasmin, the active enzyme.[10] There are two pools of plasminogen: circulating plasminogen and fibrin-bound plasminogen (**Fig. 87-14**). Plasminogen activators that preferentially activate fibrin-bound plasminogen are fibrin-specific. In contrast, nonspecific plasminogen activators do not discriminate between fibrin-bound and circulating plasminogen.[103] Activation of circulating plasminogen results in the generation of unopposed plasmin that can trigger the systemic lytic state. Alteplase and its derivatives are fibrin-specific plasminogen activators, whereas streptokinase, anistreplase, and urokinase are nonspecific agents.

STREPTOKINASE. Unlike other plasminogen activators, streptokinase is not an enzyme and does not directly convert plasminogen to plasmin. Instead, it forms a 1:1 stoichiometric complex with plasminogen, thus inducing a conformational change in plasminogen that exposes its active site (**Fig. 87-15**). This conformationally altered plasminogen then converts additional plasminogen molecules to plasmin.[10] Streptokinase has no affinity for fibrin, and the streptokinase-plasminogen complex activates free and fibrin-bound plasminogen. Activation of circulating plasminogen generates sufficient amounts of plasmin to overwhelm alpha$_2$-antiplasmin. Unopposed plasmin not only degrades fibrin in the occlusive thrombus, but also induces a systemic lytic state.[103]

When given systemically to patients with acute myocardial infarction, streptokinase reduces mortality. For this indication, the drug is usually given as an intravenous infusion of 1.5 million units over 30 to 60 minutes. Patients who receive streptokinase can develop antibodies against it, as can patients with prior streptococcal injection. These antibodies can reduce the effectiveness of streptokinase.

Allergic reactions occur in about 5% of patients treated with streptokinase. These may manifest as a rash, fever, chills, and rigors; rarely, anaphylactic reactions can occur. Transient hypotension is common with streptokinase and likely reflects plasmin-mediated release of bradykinin.

The hypotension usually responds to leg elevation and administration of intravenous fluids and low doses of vasopressors, such as dopamine or norepinephrine.

ANISTREPLASE. To generate this drug, streptokinase is mixed with equimolar amounts of Lys-plasminogen, a plasmin-cleaved form of plasminogen with a Lys residue at its N terminal. The active site of Lys-plasminogen exposed on combination with streptokinase is blocked with an anisoyl group. After intravenous infusion, the anisoyl group is slowly removed by deacylation, giving the complex a half-life of about 100 minutes. This allows drug administration via a single bolus infusion. Although it is more convenient to administer, anistreplase offers few mechanistic advantages over streptokinase. Like streptokinase, anistreplase does not distinguish between fibrin-bound and circulating plasminogen. Consequently, anistreplase produces a systemic lytic state. Similarly, allergic reactions and hypotension are just as frequent with anistreplase as they are with streptokinase.[104]

When anistreplase was compared with alteplase in patients with acute myocardial infarction, reperfusion was obtained more rapidly with alteplase than with anistreplase.[104] Improved reperfusion was associated with a trend toward better clinical outcomes and reduced mortality with alteplase. These results and the high cost of anistreplase have dampened enthusiasm for its use.

UROKINASE. Derived from cultured fetal kidney cells, urokinase is a two-chain serine protease with a molecular weight of 34,000.[105] Urokinase directly converts plasminogen to plasmin. Unlike streptokinase, urokinase is not immunogenic, and allergic reactions are rare. Urokinase produces a systemic lytic state because it does not discriminate between fibrin-bound and circulating plasminogen.[103] Despite many years of use, systemic urokinase has never been evaluated for coronary fibrinolysis; instead, it is used for catheter-directed lysis of thrombi in the deep veins or in coronary or peripheral arteries.

ALTEPLASE. A recombinant form of single-chain t-PA, alteplase has a molecular weight of 68,000. Plasmin rapidly converts alteplase into its two-chain form. The interaction of alteplase with fibrin is mediated by the finger domain and, to a lesser extent, by the second kringle domain (**Fig. 87-16**).[10] The affinity of alteplase for fibrin is considerably higher than that for fibrinogen. Consequently, the catalytic efficiency of plasminogen activation by alteplase is two to three orders of magnitude higher in the presence of fibrin than in the presence of fibrinogen.[103]

Although alteplase preferentially activates plasminogen in the presence of fibrin, alteplase is not as fibrin-selective as was first predicted. Its

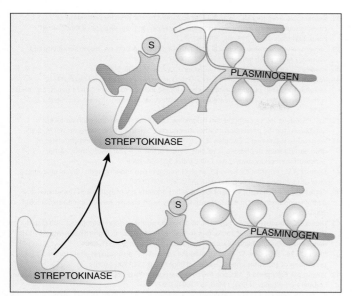

FIGURE 87-15 Mechanism of action of streptokinase. Streptokinase binds to plasminogen and induces a conformational change in plasminogen that exposes its active site. The streptokinase-plasmin(ogen) complex then serves as the activator of additional plasminogen molecules.

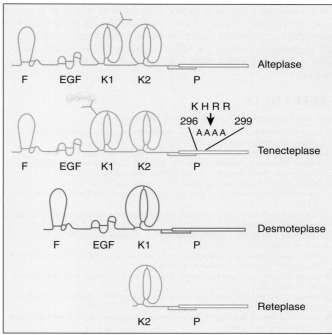

FIGURE 87-16 Domain structures of alteplase, tenecteplase, desmoteplase, and reteplase (see Fig. 55-14). The finger (F), epidermal growth factor (EGF), first and second kringles (K1 and K2, respectively), and protease (P) domains are illustrated. The glycosylation site (Y) on K1 has been repositioned in tenecteplase to endow it with a longer half-life. In addition, a tetra-alanine substitution in the protease domain renders tenecteplase resistant to PAI-1 inhibition. Desmoteplase differs from alteplase and tenecteplase in that it lacks a K2 domain. Reteplase is a truncated variant that lacks the F, EGF, and K1 domains.

fibrin specificity is limited because like fibrin, (DD)E, the major soluble degradation product of cross-linked fibrin, binds alteplase and plasminogen with high affinity. Consequently, (DD)E is as potent as fibrin as a stimulator of plasminogen activation by alteplase. Whereas plasmin generated on the fibrin surface results in thrombolysis, plasmin generated on the surface of circulating (DD)E degrades fibrinogen. Fibrinogenolysis results in the accumulation of fragment X, a high-molecular-weight clottable fibrinogen degradation product. Incorporation of fragment X into hemostatic plugs formed at sites of vascular injury renders them susceptible to lysis.[106] This phenomenon may contribute to alteplase-induced bleeding.

A trial comparing alteplase with streptokinase for the treatment of patients with acute myocardial infarction demonstrated significantly lower mortality with alteplase than with streptokinase, although the absolute difference was small.[106a] Patients younger than 75 years of age with anterior myocardial infarction who presented less than 6 hours after symptom onset derived the greatest benefit from alteplase. For treatment of acute myocardial infarction or acute ischemic stroke, alteplase is given as an intravenous infusion over 60 to 90 minutes. The total dose of alteplase usually ranges from 90 to 100 mg. Allergic reactions and hypotension are rare, and alteplase is not immunogenic.

TENECTEPLASE. A genetically engineered variant of t-PA, tenecteplase was designed to have a longer half-life than t-PA and to be resistant to inactivation by PAI-1.[107] To prolong its half-life, a new glycosylation site was added to the first kringle domain (see Fig. 87-16). Because addition of this extra carbohydrate side chain reduced fibrin affinity, the existing glycosylation site on the first kringle domain was removed. To render the molecule resistant to inhibition by PAI-1, a tetra-alanine substitution was introduced at residues 296-299 in the protease domain, the region responsible for the interaction of t-PA with PAI-1.

Tenecteplase is more fibrin-specific than t-PA. Although both agents bind to fibrin with similar affinity, the affinity of tenecteplase for (DD)E is significantly lower than that of t-PA.[107] Consequently, (DD)E does not stimulate systemic plasminogen activation by tenecteplase to the same extent as t-PA. As a result, tenecteplase produces less fibrinogenolysis than t-PA.

For coronary fibrinolysis, tenecteplase is given as a single intravenous bolus. In a large phase III trial that enrolled more than 16,000 patients, the 30-day mortality rate with single-bolus tenecteplase was similar to that with accelerated dose t-PA. Although rates of intracranial hemorrhage also were similar with both treatments, patients given tenecteplase had fewer noncerebral bleeds and a reduced need for blood transfusions compared with those treated with t-PA.[107] The improved safety profile of tenecteplase likely reflects its enhanced fibrin specificity.

RETEPLASE. A recombinant t-PA derivative, reteplase is a single-chain variant that lacks the finger, epidermal growth factor, and first kringle domains (see Fig. 87-16). This truncated derivative has a molecular weight of 39,000. Reteplase binds fibrin more weakly than t-PA because it lacks the finger domain. Because it is produced in *Escherichia coli*, reteplase is not glycosylated; this endows it with a plasma half-life longer than that of t-PA. Consequently, reteplase is given as two intravenous boluses separated by 30 minutes. Clinical trials have demonstrated that reteplase is at least as effective as streptokinase for treatment of acute myocardial infarction,[108] but is not superior to t-PA.

NEWER FIBRINOLYTIC AGENTS. Newer fibrinolytic agents include desmoteplase (see Fig. 87-16), a recombinant form of the full-length plasminogen activator isolated from the saliva of the vampire bat,[109] and alfimeprase, a truncated form of fibrolase, an enzyme isolated from the venom of the southern copperhead snake.[110] Clinical studies with these agents have proven disappointing. Desmoteplase, which is more fibrinspecific than t-PA, was investigated for the treatment of acute ischemic stroke.[111] Patients presenting 3 to 9 hours after symptom onset were randomized to one of two doses of desmoteplase or to placebo. Overall response rates were low, and were no different with desmoteplase than with placebo. Mortality was higher in the desmoteplase arms.

Alfimeprase is a metalloproteinase that degrades fibrin and fibrinogen in a plasmin-independent fashion.[110] In the circulation, alfimeprase is inhibited by alpha$_2$-macroglobulin, so it must be delivered via a catheter directly into the thrombus. Despite promising phase III results,[112] studies of alfimeprase for the treatment of peripheral arterial occlusion or for restoration of flow in blocked central venous catheters were stopped because of lack of efficacy. The disappointing results with desmoteplase and alfimeprase highlight the challenges of introducing new fibrinolytic drugs.

Conclusions and Future Directions

Thrombosis in the arteries or veins reflects a complex interplay among the vessel wall, platelets, coagulation system, and fibrinolytic pathways. Activation of coagulation also triggers inflammatory pathways that may contribute to thrombogenesis. A better understanding of the biochemistry of platelet aggregation and blood coagulation and advances in structure-based drug design have identified new targets and resulted in the development of novel antithrombotic drugs. Well-designed clinical trials have provided detailed information on which drugs are most efficacious. Despite these advances, however, arterial and venous thromboembolic disorders remain a major cause of morbidity and mortality. The search for better targets and more potent, safer, or more convenient antiplatelet, anticoagulant, and fibrinolytic drugs continues.

REFERENCES

Basic Mechanisms of Thrombosis and Hemostasis

1. Libby P: The molecular mechanisms of the thrombotic complications of atherosclerosis. J Intern Med 263:517, 2008.
2. Mackman N: Triggers, targets and treatments of thrombosis. Nature 451:914, 2008.
3. Emmerich J, Meyer G, Decousus H, et al: Role of fibrinolysis and interventional therapy for acute venous thromboembolism. Thromb Haemost 96:251, 2006.
4. Marcus AJ, Broekman MJ, Drosopoulos JH, et al: Role of CD39 (NTPDase-1) in thromboregulation, cerebroprotection, and cardioprotection. Semin Thromb Hemost 31:234, 2005.
5. Li JP, Vlodavsky I: Heparin, heparan sulfate and heparanase in inflammatory reactions. Thromb Haemost 102:823, 2009.
6. Lwaleed BA, Bass PS: Tissue factor pathway inhibitor: Structure, biology and involvement in disease. J Pathol 208:327, 2006.
7. Tobu M, Ma Q, Iqbal O, et al: Comparative tissue factor pathway inhibitor release potential of heparins. Clin Appl Thromb Hemost 11:37, 2005.
8. Esmon CT: Inflammation and the activated protein C anticoagulant pathway. Semin Thromb Hemost 32:49, 2006.
9. Esmon CT: Structure and functions of the endothelial cell protein C receptor. Crit Care Med 32:S298, 2004.
10. Rijken DC, Lijnen HR: New insights into the molecular mechanisms of the fibrinolytic system. J Thromb Haemost 7:4, 2009.
11. Kaushansky K: The molecular mechanisms that control thrombopoiesis. J Clin Invest 115:3339, 2005.
12. Watson SP: Platelet activation by extracellular matrix proteins in haemostasis and thrombosis. Curr Pharm Des 15:1358, 2009.
13. López JA, del Conde I, Shrimpton CN: Receptors, rafts, and microvesicles in thrombosis and inflammation. J Thromb Haemost 3:1737, 2005.
14. Turner NA, Nolasco L, Ruggeri ZM, Moake JL: Endothelial cell ADAMTS-13 and VWF: Production, release, and VWF string cleavage. Blood 114:5102, 2009.
15. Sadler JE: von Willebrand factor assembly and secretion. J Thromb Haemost 7(Suppl 1):24, 2009.
16. Nakahata N: Thromboxane A2: Physiology/pathophysiology, cellular signal transduction and pharmacology. Pharmacol Ther 118:18, 2008.
17. Smyth SS, Woulfe DS, Weitz JI, et al: G-protein-coupled receptors as signaling targets for antiplatelet therapy. Arterioscler Thromb Vasc Biol 29:449, 2009.
18. Cattaneo M: Platelet P2 receptors: Old and new targets for antithrombotic drugs. Expert Rev Cardiovasc Ther 5:45, 2007.
19. McEachron TA, Pawlinski R, Richards KL, et al: Protease-activated receptors mediate cross-talk between coagulation and fibrinolysis. Blood Aug. 24, 2010 [Epub ahead of print].
20. Butenas S, Orfeo T, Mann KG: Tissue factor in coagulation: Which? Where? When? Arterioscler Thromb Vasc Biol 29:1989, 2009.
21. Blann A, Shantsila E, Shantsila A: Microparticles and arterial disease. Semin Thromb Hemost 35:488, 2009.
22. Morrissey J, Mackman N: Tissue factor and factor VIIa: Understanding the molecular mechanism. Thromb Res 122(Suppl 1):S1, 2008.
23. Vogler EA, Siedecki CA: Contact activation of blood-plasma coagulation. Biomaterials 30:1857, 2009.
24. Müller F, Renné T: Novel roles for factor XII-driven plasma contact activation system. Curr Opin Hematol 15:516, 2008.
25. Butenas S, Undas A, Gissel MT, et al: Factor XIa and tissue factor activity in patients with coronary artery disease. Thromb Haemost 99:142, 2008.
26. Marx PF, Verkleij CJ, Seron MV, Meijers JC: Recent developments in thrombin-activatable fibrinolysis inhibitor research. Mini Rev Med Chem 9:1165, 2009.
27. Tziomalos K, Athyros VG, Wierzbicki AS, Mikhallidis DP: Lipoprotein a: Where are we now? Curr Opin Cardiol 24:351, 2009.
28. McMahon B, Kwaan HC: The plasminogen activator system and cancer. Pathophysiol Haemost Thromb 36:184, 2008.
29. Tang EH, Vanhoutte PM: Prostanoids and reactive oxygen species: Team players in endothelium-dependent contractions. Pharmacol Ther 122:140, 2009.
30. Zhang C: The role of inflammatory cytokines in endothelial dysfunction. Basic Res Cardiol 103:398, 2008.
31. Jennings LK: Role of platelets in atherothrombosis. Am J Cardiol 103:4A, 2009.
32. Bank I, Libourel EJ, Middeldorp S, et al: Elevated levels of FVIII:C within families are associated with an increased risk for venous and arterial thrombosis. J Thromb Haemost 1:79, 2005.
33. Saposnik B, Reny JL, Gaussem P, et al: A haplotype of the EPCR gene is associated with increased plasma levels of sEPCR and is a candidate risk factor for thrombosis. Blood 103:1311, 2004.
34. Kobbervig C, Williams E: FXIII polymorphisms, fibrin clot structure and thrombotic risk. Biophys Chem 112:223, 2004.
35. Falanga A, Marchetti M: Venous thromboembolism in the hematologic malignancies. J Clin Oncol 27:4848, 2009.
36. Kasthuri RS, Taubman MB, Mackman N: Role of tissue factor in cancer. J Clin Oncol 27:4834, 2009.

Antiplatelet Agents

37. Patrono C, Baigent C, Hirsh J, et al: Antiplatelet drugs: American College of Chest Physicians Evidence-Based Clinical Practice Guidelines (8th Edition). Chest 133:199S, 2008.

38. Berger JS, Roncaglioni MC, Avanzini F, et al: Aspirin for the primary prevention of cardiovascular events in women and men: A sex-specific meta-analysis of randomized controlled trials. JAMA 295:306, 2006.
39. Stevenson DD, Szczeklik A: Clinical and pathologic perspectives on aspirin sensitivity and asthma. J Allergy Clin Immunol 118:773, 2006.
40. Hankey GJ, Eikelboom JW: Aspirin resistance. Lancet 367:606, 2006.
41. Wallentin L, Varenhorst C, James S, et al: Prasugrel achieves greater and faster P2Y12 receptor-mediated platelet inhibition than clopidogrel due to more efficient generation of its active metabolite in aspirin-treated patients with coronary artery disease. Eur Heart J 29:21, 2008.
42. Savi P, Herbert JM: Clopidogrel and ticlopidine: P2Y12 adenosine diphosphate-receptor antagonists for the prevention of atherothrombosis. Semin Thromb Haemost 31:174, 2005.
43. Wenaweser P, Daemen J, Zwahlen M, van Domburg R, et al: Incidence and correlates of drug-eluting stent thrombosis in routine clinical practice: 4-year results from a large 2-institutional cohort study. J Am Coll Cardiol 52:1134, 2008.
44. Eisenstein EL, Anstrom KJ, Kong DF, et al: Clopidogrel use and long-term clinical outcomes after drug-eluting stent implantation. JAMA 297:159, 2007.
45. Cooke GE, Goldschmidt-Clermont PJ: The safety and efficacy of aspirin and clopidogrel as a combination treatment in patients with coronary heart disease. Expert Opin Drug Saf 5:815, 2006.
46. Diener HC, Bogousslavsky J, Brass LM, et al: Aspirin and clopidogrel compared with clopidogrel alone after recent ischemic stroke or transient ischemic attack in high-risk patients (MATCH): Randomised, double-blind, placebo-controlled trial. Lancet 364:331, 2004.
47. Bhatt DL, Fox KA, Hacke W, et al: Clopidogrel and aspirin versus aspirin alone for the prevention of atherothrombotic events. N Engl J Med 354:1706, 2006.
48. Wiviott SD, Braunwald E, McCabe CH, et al: Prasugrel versus clopidogrel in patients with acute coronary syndromes. N Engl J Med 357:2001, 2007.
49. Tantry US, Bliden KP, Gurbel PA: Prasugrel. Expert Opin Invest Drugs 15:1627, 2006.
50. Nguyen TA, Diodati JG, Pharand C: Resistance to clopidogrel: A review of the evidence. J Am Coll Cardiol 45:1157, 2005.
51. Hulot JS, Bura A, Villard E, et al: Cytochrome P450 2C19 loss-of-function polymorphism is a major determinant of clopidogrel responsiveness in healthy subjects. Blood 108:2244, 2006.
52. Angiolillo DJ, Fernandez-Ortiz A, Bernardo E, et al: Contribution of gene sequence variations of the hepatic cytochrome P450 3A4 enzyme to variability in individual responsiveness to clopidogrel. Arterioscler. Thromb. Vasc. Biol 26:1895, 2006.
53. Simon T, Verstuyft C, Mary-Krause M, et al: Genetic determinants of response to clopidogrel and cardiovascular events. N Engl J Med 360:363, 2009.
54. Mega JL, Close SL, Wiviott SD, et al: Cytochrome P-450 polymorphisms and response to clopidogrel. N Engl J Med 360:354, 2009.
55. O'Donoghue ML, Braunwald E, Antman EM, et al: Pharmacodynamic effect and clinical efficacy of clopidogrel and prasugrel with or without a proton-pump inhibitor: An analysis of two randomized trials. Lancet 374:989, 2009.
56. Varenhorst C, James S, Erlinge D, et al: Genetic variation of CYP2C19 affects both pharmacokinetic and pharmacodymamic responses to clopidogrel but not prasugrel in aspirin-treated patients with coronary artery disease. Eur Heart J 30:1744, 2009.
57. Mega JL, Close SL, Wiviott SD, et al: Cytochrome P450 genetic polymorphisms and the response to prasugrel: Relationship to pharmacokinetic, pharmacodynamic, and clinical outcomes. Circulation 119:2553, 2009.
58. Malmstrom RE, Ostergren J, Jorgensen L, Hjemdahl P, et al: Influence of statin treatment on platelet inhibition by clopidogrel—a randomized comparison of rosuvastatin, atorvastatin and simvastatin co-treatment. J Intern Med 266:457, 2009.
59. Michelson AD: Platelet function testing in cardiovascular diseases. Circulation 119:e489, 2004.
60. ESPRIT Study Group; Halkes PH, van Gijn J, Kappelle LJ, et al: Aspirin plus dipyridamole versus aspirin alone after cerebral ischaemia of arterial origin (ESPRIT): Randomised controlled trial. Lancet 367:1665, 2006.
61. Diener HC, Sacco RL, Yusuf S, Cotton D, et al: Effects of aspirin plus extended-release dipyridamole versus clopidogrel and telmisartan on disability and cognitive function after recurrent stroke in patients with ischemic stroke in the Prevention Regimen for Effectively Avoiding Second Strokes (PRoFESS) trial: A double-blind, active and placebo-controlled study. Lancet Neurol 7:875, 2008.
62. Rossi ML, Zavalloni D: Inhibitors of platelets glycoprotein IIb/IIIa (GPIIb/IIIa) receptor: Rationale for their use in clinical cardiology. Mini Rev Med Chem 4:703, 2004.
63. Aster RH: Immune thrombocytopenia caused by glycoprotein IIb/IIIa inhibitors. Chest 127:53S, 2005.
64. Harrington RA, Becker RC, Cannon CP, Gutterman D, et al: Antithrombotic therapy for non-ST-segment elevation acute coronary syndromes: American College of Chest Physicians Evidence-Based Clinical Practice Guidelines (8th Edition). Chest 133:670S, 2008.
65. Goodman SG, Menon V, Cannon CP, Steg G, et al: Acute ST-segment elevation myocardial infarction: American College of Chest Physicians Evidence-Based Clinical Practice Guidelines (8th Edition). Chest 133:708S, 2008.
66. Bhatt DL, Lincoff MA, Gibson CM, et al: Intravenous platelet blockade with cangrelor during PCI. N Engl J Med 361:2330, 2009.
67. Harrington RA, Stone GW, McNulty S, et al: Platelet inhibition with cangrelor in patients undergoing PCI. N Engl J Med 361:2318, 2009.
68. Wallentin L, Becker RC, Budaj A, Cannon CP, et al: Ticagrelor versus clopidogrel in patients with acute coronary syndromes. N Engl J Med 361:1045, 2009.
69. Oestreich J: SCH-530348, a thrombin receptor (PAR-1) antagonist for the prevention and treatment of atherothrombosis. Curr Opin Invest Drugs 10:988, 2009.
70. Serebruany VL, Kogushi M, Dastros-Pitei D, Flather M, et al: The in-vitro effects of E5555, a protease-activated receptor (PAR)-1 antagonist, on platelet biomarkers in healthy volunteers and patients with coronary artery disease. Thromb Haemost 102:111, 2009.

Anticoagulants

71. Gross PL, Weitz JI: New antithrombotic drugs. Clin Pharmacol Ther 86:139, 2009.
72. Hirsh J, Bauer KA, Donati MB, Gould M, et al: Parenteral anticoagulants: American College of Chest Physicians Evidence-Based Clinical Practice Guidelines (8th Edition). Chest 133:141S, 2008.

73. Geerts WH, Bergqvist D, Pineo, GF, et al: Prevention of venous thromboembolism: American College of Chest Physicians Evidence-Based Clinical Practice Guidelines (8th Edition). Chest 133:381S, 2008.
74. Blossom DB, Kallen AJ, Patel PR, et al: Outbreak of adverse reactions assocated with contaminated heparin. N Engl J Med 359:2674, 2008.
75. Schulman S, Beyth RJ, Kearon C, Levine MN: Hemorrhagic complications of anticoagulant and thrombolytic treatment: American College of Chest Physicians Evidence-based Clinical Practice Guidelines (8th Edition). Chest 133:257S, 2008.
76. Shantsila E, Lip GY, Chong BH: Heparin-induced thrombocytopenia. A contemporary clinical approach to diagnosis and management. Chest 135:1651, 2009.
77. Greinacher A: Heparin-induced thrombocytopenia. J Thromb Haemost 7(Suppl 1):9, 2009.
78. Warkentin TE, Linkins LA: Immunoassays are not created equal. J Thromb Haemost 7:1256, 2009.
79. Hirsh J, Heddle N, Kelton JG: Treatment of heparin-induced thrombocytopenia: A critical review. Arch Intern Med 164:361, 2004.
80. Srinivasan AF, Rice L, Bartholomew JR, et al: Warfarin-induced skin necrosis and venous limb gangrene in the setting of heparin-induced thrombocytopenia. Arch Intern Med 164:66, 2004.
81. Quinlan DJ, McQuillan A, Eikelboom JW: Low-molecular-weight heparin compared with intravenous unfractionated heparin for treatment of pulmonary embolism: A meta-analysis of randomized, controlled trials. Ann Intern Med 140:175, 2004.
82. Buller HR, Davidson BL, Decousus H, et al: Fondaparinux or enoxaparin for the initial treatment of symptomatic deep venous thrombosis: A randomized trial. Ann Intern Med 140:867, 2004.
83. Fifth Organization to Assess Strategies in Acute Ischemic Syndromes Investigators: Comparison of fondaparinux and enoxaparin in acute coronary syndromes. N Engl J Med 354:1464, 2006.
84. Yusuf S, Mehta SR, Chrolavicius S, et al: Effects of fondaparinux on mortality and reinfarction in patients with acute ST-segment elevation myocardial infarction: The OASIS-6 randomized trial. JAMA 295:1519, 2006.
85. Warkentin TE, Cook RJ, Marder VJ, et al: Anti-platelet factor 4/heparin antibodies in orthopedic surgery patients receiving antithrombotic prophylaxis with fondaparinux or enoxaparin. Blood 106:3791, 2005.
86. Kuo KH, Kovacs MJ: Fondaparinux: A potential new therapy for HIT. Hematology 10:271, 2005.
87. Grouzi E, Kyriakou E, Panagou I, Spilliotopoulou I: Fondaparinux for the treatment of acute heparin-induced thrombocytopenia: A single-center experience. Clin Appl Thromb Hemost 16:663, 2010.
88. Ansell J, Hirsh J, Hylek E, Jacobson A, et al: Pharmacology and management of the vitamin K antagonists: American College of Chest Physicians Evidence-Based Clinical Practice Guidelines (8th Edition). Chest 133:160S, 2008.
89. Sanderson S, Emery J, Higgins J: CYP2C9 gene variants; drug dose and bleeding risk in warfarin-treated patients: A HUGEnet™ systematic review and meta-analysis. Genet Med 7:97, 2005.
90. Sconce EA, Khan TI, Wynne HA, et al: The impact of CYP2C9 and VKORC1 genetic polymorphism and patient characteristics on warfarin dose requirements: Proposal for a new dosing regimen. Blood 106:2329, 2005.
91. Wadelius M, Chen LY, Eriksson N, et al: Association of warfarin dose with genes involved in its action and metabolism. Hum Genet 121:23, 2007.
92. McClain M, Palomaki GE, Piper M, et al: A rapid-ACCE review of CYP2C9 and VKORC1 alleles testing to inform warfarin dosing in adults at elevated risk for thrombotic events and to avoid serious bleeding. Genet Med 10:89, 2008.
93. Rieder MJ, Reiner AP, Gage BF: Effects of VKORC1 haplotypes on the transcriptional regulation and warfarin dose. N Engl J Med 352:2285, 2005.
94. International Warfarin Pharmacogenetics Consortium: Estimation of the warfarin dose with clinical and pharmacogenetic data. N Engl J Med 360:753, 2009.
95. Singer DE, Albers GW, Dalen JE, Fang MC, et al: Antithrombotic therapy in atrial fibrillation: American College of Chest Physicians Evidence-Based Clinical Practice Guidelines (8th Edition). Chest 133:546S, 2008.
96. Crowther MA, Ageno W, Garcia D, et al: Oral vitamin K versus placebo to correct excessive anticoagulation in patients receiving warfarin: A randomized trial. Ann Intern Med 150:293, 2009.
97. Bates SM, Greer IA, Pabinger I, Sofaer S, et al: Venous thromboembolism, thrombophilia, antithrombotic therapy, and pregnancy: American College of Chest Physicians Evidence-Based Clinical Practice Guidelines (8th Edition). Chest 133:844S, 2008.
98. Finazzi G, Marchioli R, Brancaccio V, et al: A randomized clinical trial of high-intensity warfarin vs. conventional antithrombotic therapy for the prevention of recurrent thrombosis in patients with the antiphospholipid syndrome (WAPS). J Thromb Haemost 3:848, 2005.
99. Bates SM, Weitz JI: The status of new anticoagulants. Br J Haematol 134:3, 2006.
100. Gross PL, Weitz JI: New antithrombotic drugs. Clin Pharmacol Ther 86:139, 2009.
101. Connolly SJ, Ezekowitz MD, Yusuf S, et al: Dabigatran versus warfarin in patients with atrial fibrillation. N Engl J Med 361:1139, 2009.
102. Schulman S, Kearon C, Kakkar AK, Mismetti P, et al: Dabigatran versus warfarin in the treatment of acute venous thromboembolism. N Engl J Med 361:2342, 2009.

Fibrinolytic Drugs

103. Longstaff C, William S, Thelwell C: Fibrin binding and the regulation of plasminogen activators during thrombolytic therapy. Cardiovasc Hematol Agents Med Chem 6:212, 2008.
104. Bell WR Jr: Evaluation of thrombolytic agents. Drugs 54:11, 1997.
105. Vincenza Carriero M, Franco P, Vocca I, Alfano D, et al: Structure, function and antagonists of urokinase-type plasminogen activators. Front Biosci 14:3782, 2009.
106. Schaefer AV, Leslie BA, Rischke JA, et al: Incorporation of fragment X into fibrin clots renders them more susceptible to lysis by plasmin. Biochemistry 45:4257, 2006.
106a. The Gusto Investigators: An international randomized trial comparing four thrombolytic strategies for acute myocardial infarction. N Engl J Med 329:673, 1993.
107. Melandri G, Vagnarelli F, Calabrese D, Semprini F, et al: Review of tenecteplase (TNKase) in the treatment of acute myocardial infarction. Vasc Health Risk Manag 5:249, 2009.
108. Simpson D, Siddiqui MA, Scott LJ, Hilleman DE: Spotlight on reteplase in thrombotic occlusive disorders. BioDrugs 21:65, 2007.
109. Paciaroni M, Medeiros E, Bogousslavsky J: Desmoteplase: Expert Opin Biol Ther 9:773, 2009.
110. Deitcher SR, Funk WD, Buchanan J, et al: Alfimeprase: A novel recombinant direct-acting fibrinolytic. Expert Opin Biol Ther 6:1361, 2006.
111. Hacke W, Furlan AJ, Al-Rawi Y, Davalos A, et al: Intravenous desmoteplase in patients with acute ischaemic stroke selected by MRI perfusion-diffusion weighted imaging or perfusion CT (DIAS-2): A prospective, randomized, double-blind, placebo-controlled study. Lancet Neurol 8:141, 2009.
112. Moll S, Kenyon P, Bertolli L, De Maio J, et al: Phase II trial of alfimeprase, a novel-acting fibrin degradation agent, for occluded central venous access devices. J Clin Oncol 24:3056, 2006.

CH
87

HEMOSTASIS, THROMBOSIS, FIBRINOLYSIS, AND CARDIOVASCULAR DISEASE

CHAPTER **88** # Rheumatic Fever

B. Soma Raju and Zoltan G. Turi

Rheumatic fever (RF) is an autoimmune disorder that remains incompletely characterized with regard to its basic elements—cause, pathophysiology, diagnosis, and treatment—despite evidence of its existence dating to at least the 1600s. The classic understanding that the disease is a post–suppurative streptococcal pharyngitis cascade, leading variably to arthritis, chorea, dermal manifestations, and, most important, carditis, has largely withstood challenge. Immunologic studies have confirmed the presence of epitopes on the bacterial surface that mimic cardiac myosin as well as antigens found in valve, skin, joint, and brain tissue that account for the immunologic cross-reactive attack characteristic of RF. No single diagnostic tool or laboratory test exists for RF. Hence, the diagnosis depends on a composite of clinical criteria.

The sequelae of only one manifestation, carditis, account for most of the morbidity and essentially all of the mortality associated with RF. As a cause of heart disease in adults, RF has declined dramatically in industrialized nations but remains a major source of morbidity and mortality in developing countries and in some selected aboriginal populations in wealthy nations. The primary consequences of RF, rheumatic mitral and aortic valve disease in adults, are also declining worldwide but remain a major burden on the limited health care resources of the countries where the disease is most prevalent (see Chap. 1). The diagnostic and treatment algorithms for RF are still largely based on descriptive series and expert opinion panels. Because failure to diagnose RF and to institute secondary prophylaxis results in rheumatic heart disease (RHD), increasing attention is being focused on improving sensitivity of diagnosis in areas where the disease is endemic.

Epidemiology

Streptococcus pyogenes is responsible for diseases ranging from pharyngitis to glomerulonephritis, necrotizing fasciitis, and toxic shock syndrome. Suppurative pharyngitis is the only clearly established prequel to RF. In 2005, 15.6 million people were estimated to have RF or RHD on the basis of traditional clinical measures that may represent substantial underestimation.[1] The majority of these cases are from sub-Saharan Africa and south central Asia, which along with indigenous populations in Australia and New Zealand represent the world's highest prevalence.

Given a causal association between group A beta-hemolytic streptococci (GABHS) and RF, their epidemiology is also linked. Whereas most pharyngitis (80%) is viral in etiology, GABHS is isolated in up to 75% of cases from children with symptoms of severe bacterial pharyngitis.[2] Antistreptolysin O titers more than 200 Todd units are found in up to 50% of asymptomatic children 6 to 15 years old, the prime age group for RF. This reflects the frequent occurrence of pharyngitis in this age group (estimated to be once yearly), approximately 15% to 20% of which is caused by GABHS.[3] Recurrence is most common in adolescents and young adults and is uncommon beyond the age of 34 years. Data from the early antibiotic era suggest that 0.3% to 3% of those with untreated GABHS pharyngitis develop RF. Although there is no clear gender predisposition, postpubertal chorea and the

development of mitral stenosis are more common in females. GABHS is present in 10% to 30% of asymptomatic individuals in the prime RF age groups in the United States, but it is higher in many countries. A history of pharyngitis has been reported in approximately two thirds of RF cases. Carriers (patients with positive throat cultures without clinical history or rise in antibody titers) do not appear predisposed to RF. The possibility that RF may follow nonpharyngeal streptococcal infection, in particular pyoderma, continues to be explored.

DECLINE IN RHEUMATIC FEVER. The decline in RF began before the antibiotic era. Explanations include improvement in environmental factors, decrease in rheumatogenicity of streptococcal strains, and improved specificity in diagnosis. The last was largely due to the introduction of the Jones criteria, before which children with minor manifestations such as isolated arthralgias were frequently assigned a diagnosis of RF. The decrease in mortality from acute carditis in the preantibiotic era suggests that the virulence of rheumatogenic strains decreased as well. **Figure 88-1** demonstrates the dramatic decline in mortality associated with RF in the United States in the past century along with milestones in diagnosis and management. Whereas the incidence of RF in industrialized states is now estimated to be less than 1/100,000 people, it is 100-fold higher in endemic areas.[4] RHD occurs in up to 3% of children in some developing nations.[1] Socioeconomic, epidemiologic, cultural, and other factors influence applicability of some of the standard RF algorithms in these countries. As a cause of valvular disease seen at autopsy or surgery, RHD has declined exponentially since the 1920s, when 39.5% of New England cardiac admissions were related to RHD; it now accounts for less than 0.5% of primary discharge diagnoses in the United States. In contrast, rates remain comparable to those of the 1950s in the poorest nations as well as in isolated subpopulations such as the aboriginal people of Australia. Crowding, inadequate medical facilities, lack of antibiotics for primary therapy and secondary prevention, and lack of medical personnel have sustained the prevalence of RF and RHD. There is a trend in some developing nations toward declining frequency, in part because of better availability of basic care, sometimes associated with over-the-counter dispensing of antibiotics.

The outbreaks of RF in the United States in the 1980s prompted extensive investigation of the disease in an industrialized nation. RF occurred in areas without the risk factors attributed to susceptible populations, and some evidence suggests an association with the reappearance of rheumatogenic strains of *S. pyogenes*.[5] The diagnosis remains rare in industrialized countries, accounting for approximately 0.1% of pediatric hospitalizations in the United States, with geographic clusters and some evidence of ethnic susceptibility, in particular Asians and Pacific Islanders.

Pathobiology

The classic triad of agent, host, and environment plays a major role in the pathogenesis of RF. GABHS has more than 130 subtypes defined by M-protein surface molecules.[3] Some of these appear to be rheumatogenic, typically mucoid strains that adhere well to pharyngeal tissue and have antiphagocytic properties that allow persistence of bacteria in tissues for up to 2 weeks, until specific antibodies are created. M protein, *N*-acetylglucosamine, and several other epitopes mimic myocardium (myosin and tropomyosin), heart valves (laminin),

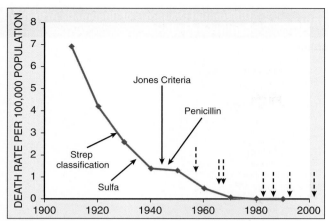

FIGURE 88-1 Decline in mortality from rheumatic fever in the United States during the 20th century. Note that the decline began well before the availability of penicillin. Dashed arrows mark the multiple modifications or revisions of the Jones criteria or World Health Organization expert opinion reviews and recommendations. *(Modified from Gordis L: The virtual disappearance of rheumatic fever in the United States: Lessons in the rise and fall of disease. T. Duckett Jones memorial lecture. Circulation 72:1155, 1985.)*

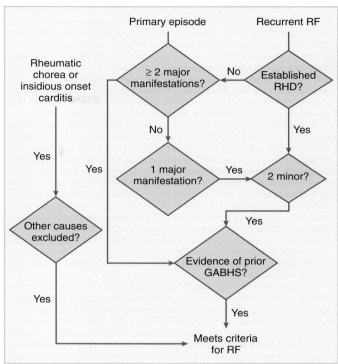

FIGURE 88-2 Algorithm for diagnosis of acute rheumatic fever, incorporating the 1992 revision of the Jones criteria and the World Health Organization (WHO) expert consultation report (2002-2003). The WHO modifications incorporated in the flow chart are more sensitive and less specific than those incorporated in the American Heart Association criteria. GABHS = group A beta-hemolytic streptococci; RF = rheumatic fever; RHD = rheumatic heart disease.

synovia (vimentin), skin (keratin), and subthalamic and caudate nuclei in the brain (lysogangliosides).[6] Superantigenic activity triggered by M-protein fragments as well as streptococcal toxins have also been implicated in autoimmune reactivity mediated by B cells and T cells. T cells activated against myosin and bacterial epitopes react to valve tissue with as yet incompletely defined host factors that may enhance the inflammatory response in heart valves. Considerable heterogeneity exists in the epitopes associated with RF in different geographic areas as well as in the genes that encode M proteins, in particular the chromosomal *emm* sequence types that have been associated with GABHS pharyngitis and RF. Other properties of GABHS, such as production of serum opacity factor, differentiate strains associated with RF from those associated with glomerulonephritis. Patients who develop RF appear to manifest a hyperimmune response to GABHS, the level of which appears to correlate with the severity of RF manifestations. The decline in incidence of RF has paralleled the decrease in rheumatogenic M-protein strains isolated from the throats of children with pharyngitis, whereas conversely, the reappearance of RF in the United States has been associated with an increase in strains known to be rheumatogenic.[5] Unfortunately, strains that vary from those classically associated with rheumatogenicity continue to be isolated, confounding development of a widely applicable vaccine; there is evidence that GABHS may have evolved to prevent clearance by the immune system.

The risk for development of RF after GABHS pharyngitis is associated with genetic susceptibility and is also much higher in those with prior RF, in whom risk is as high as 50%. This provides a strong mandate for long-term secondary antibiotic prophylaxis. The evidence that hosts are genetically predisposed to RF is significant, with varying human leukocyte antigen (HLA) class II alleles and tumor necrosis factor-α as well as other genetic markers identified in populations known to be susceptible.[7] The issue of susceptibility is confounded by markers that either may reflect genetic susceptibility or may be expressed as a consequence of repeated exposure to group A streptococci.[8] In particular, a B-cell alloantigen, D8/17, appears to be both sensitive and specific in some endemic areas for screening of patients with RF as well as patients with prior RF in first-degree relatives.

Finally, environmental elements correlate strongly with development of RF. Where epidemic pharyngitis has been documented, such as in military barracks before antibiotic availability, approximately 3% developed RF. With the element of overcrowding removed, during the same period, the RF rate was approximately one tenth as common. It has been hypothesized that there is increased virulence associated with rapid transmission across multiple hosts.

Pathology

In patients dying of rheumatic carditis, autopsy examination has demonstrated verrucous vegetations on the valve leaflets, along with extensive inflammation and edema.[9] In the exudative phase, during the first few weeks after the onset of RF, fibrinoid degeneration of collagen is noted. Inflammation is seen in left ventricular (LV) endocardium, with lymphocytic, macrophage, and, in a minority of cases, plasma cell, polymorphonuclear leukocyte, eosinophil, and mast cell infiltration. In the proliferative phase, 1 to 6 months after the onset of RF, Aschoff bodies, granulomatous lesions pathognomonic for rheumatic carditis, are seen and can be found in valve tissue as well as in endocardium, myocardium, and pericardium. Although Aschoff bodies can be demonstrated as early as the second week of onset of RF, they may be present chronically without evidence of carditis. Rheumatic arthritis is manifested by edema, lymphocytic and polymorphonuclear infiltration, and fibrinoid lesions that resolve. In patients with chorea, inflammatory changes have been noted in the cerebral cortex, cerebellum, and basal ganglia.

Diagnosis

Jones Criteria (Fig. 88-2)

Before the initial 1944 Jones criteria, RF diagnosis was based on a wide, inconsistent range of nonspecific symptoms, including minor arthralgias, fevers, and abdominal pain. Because RF was a major cause of mortality, the criteria were designed to address the need for accurate diagnosis to allow assessment of disease incidence and treatment outcomes. Thus, specificity was emphasized over sensitivity, which remained the prevailing focus of multiple revisions. The major criteria—carditis, polyarthritis, chorea, erythema marginatum, and subcutaneous nodules—have been unchanged since the first revision in 1956. Minor criteria include the clinical findings of arthralgia and fever and elevated acute-phase reactants. Evidence of a prior group A streptococcal infection was incorporated in 1965 as an *essential* criterion. Although it is not specific for an acute attack of GABHS pharyngitis, the requirement adds to the overall specificity of the Jones criteria. The subsequent modifications continued to favor increased specificity by emphasizing arthritis over arthralgia and eliminated nonspecific elements from the minor criteria, such as epistaxis, abdominal and precordial pain, pulmonary findings, prolonged PR interval, anemia, and elevated white blood cell counts. The original revisions also emphasized evidence of prior RF, based on the much greater susceptibility for recurrence. With the 1992 revision, the guidelines placed emphasis on diagnosis of an *initial* attack of RF.

In the past decade, the focus has shifted to concerns that the criteria now lack sufficient sensitivity. The 2004 World Health Organization (WHO) report addressed the issue of recurrent RF, in particular for patients with established RHD, and suggested algorithms for increasing the overall sensitivity.[3] Whereas two major or one major and two minor manifestations plus evidence of preceding GABHS infection are required for a primary episode of RF or recurrent RF without established RHD, two minor criteria are deemed to be sufficient to make the diagnosis with reasonable specificity in the setting of RHD if there is evidence of recent streptococcal infection. There are two exceptions to the requirement that evidence for antecedent GABHS infection be established because laboratory evidence may be absent: chorea, in which there is a long latency period before symptoms occur; and the chronic low-grade carditis that follows many cases of RF.

The prior emphasis on specificity warned against the use of a single finding, such as fever, monarthritis, arthralgia, or elevation of the erythrocyte sedimentation rate or C-reactive protein level, to make the diagnosis of RF.[10] However, in countries where the disease is prevalent, laboratory data may not be available, the patient's presentation may be too late for some elements of the Jones criteria to be observed, and over-the-counter treatment with anti-inflammatory or antibiotic agents may obscure elements of the criteria. In this setting, clinical findings such as monarthritis or polyarthralgias are used by practitioners to make a diagnosis of "probable rheumatic fever" in vulnerable age groups when a number of minor manifestations are present, in particular if there is evidence of antecedent GABHS infection. The importance of such a controversial "probable" category is the suspicion raised for possible subsequent development of carditis, with the benefits of serial follow-up examinations and, in particular, the administration of chronic secondary antibiotic prophylaxis.

A number of clinical conditions mimic RF, including some associated with GABHS infections (**Table 88-1**).[11] Special considerations apply if a first attack of RF occurs in adulthood. In this setting, arthritis dominates, with a lower incidence of carditis; the other major manifestations are rare. Although the Jones criteria may be met, they become less specific, and other causes need to be excluded.

Carditis

Approximately 40% to 60% of RF episodes result in RHD,[4,11] with progression dependent on the severity of carditis, recurrences of RF, and availability of and compliance with secondary prophylaxis. Carditis typically is manifested as valvulitis, classically detected by the presence of mitral regurgitation (MR) or, less commonly, aortic regurgitation (AR). It can be responsible for acute and chronic myocardial dysfunction and acute, although not chronic, pericardial disease. Neither myocarditis nor pericarditis appears to occur in the absence of valvulitis, and if evidence of valvular involvement is not present, nonrheumatic causes must be considered. Whereas carditis typically is manifested in children as MR, with AR seen in approximately 20% to 40%, mitral stenosis is the most frequent clinically important valvular lesion in adults. Rheumatic tricuspid stenosis is less common and isolated rheumatic aortic stenosis is rare.

The severity of LV dysfunction appears to correlate with the extent of valvulitis rather than myocardial injury. A clinical syndrome suggesting rheumatic myocarditis is not associated with the troponin level elevation seen in viral myocarditides. When severe heart failure does occur in RF, both echocardiographic data and postmortem pathology findings point to altered myocardial mechanics caused by valvular regurgitation rather than by myocarditis. Traditionally, the diagnosis has been made on the basis of auscultation of MR or, less commonly, AR in the setting of heart failure, with cardiomegaly in the most severe cases. Severe MR is most commonly associated with the worst prognosis, acute and sometimes refractory and fatal heart failure.[12] This

TABLE 88-1	Differential Diagnosis of Rheumatic Arthritis, Carditis, and Chorea

Arthritis
Infectious
   Staphylococcal, gonococcal
   Endocarditis
   Lyme disease
   Mycobacterial, fungal
   Viral
Reactive
   Poststreptococcal
   Enteric infection
   Reiter syndrome
   Inflammatory bowel
Connective tissue disease
   Rheumatoid arthritis
   Systemic lupus
   Systemic vasculitis
Miscellaneous
   Gout
   Leukemia, lymphoma
   Sarcoidosis
   Cancer
   Familial Mediterranean fever
   Henoch-Schönlein purpura
   Mucocutaneous disorders
   "Growth pains" in children
   Serum sickness

Carditis
Murmur
   Physiologic murmur
   Mitral valve prolapse
   Bicuspid aortic valve
   Anemia
   Straight back syndrome
Congenital heart disease
   Ventricular septal defect
   Subvalvular aortic stenosis
   Primum atrial septal defect
Viral myocarditis
Endocarditis
Pericarditis

Chorea
Familial chorea—Huntington
Hormone induced
   Oral contraceptives
   Pregnancy
Drug induced
   Anticonvulsants
   Antidepressants
   Metoclopramide
   Phenothiazines
Connective tissue
   Systemic lupus
   Periarteritis
Lyme disease
Wilson disease
Atypical seizures
Hyperthyroidism
Hypoparathyroidism
Tourette syndrome
PANDAS

PANDAS = *p*ediatric *a*utoimmune *n*europsychiatric *d*isorders *a*ssociated with *s*treptococcal infection.
Modified from Pinals RS: Polyarthritis and fever. N Engl J Med 330:769, 1994; Kothari SS: Active rheumatic carditis. *In* Narula J, Virman R, Srinath Reddy K, Tandon R (eds): Rheumatic Fever. Washington, DC, American Registry of Pathology, Armed Forces Institute of Pathology, 1999, p 265; and Swedo SE: Sydenham's chorea: A model for childhood autoimmune neuropsychiatric disorders. JAMA 272:1788, 1994.

subgroup is most likely to develop significant chronic RHD, with an incidence as high as 90%. There is a linear relationship between the severity of MR during the first episode of RF and subsequent RHD.

Because valvulitis can be transient, serial evaluation is appropriate. In a significant percentage of patients, the carditis is subclinical, setting the stage for scarring of the mitral or aortic valve apparatus with manifestations occurring years or decades later. Although valvulitis does account for the majority of myocardial dysfunction, there is a characteristic regional wall motion abnormality in the inferobasal segment adjacent to the mitral valve. The inflammatory process typically involves the leaflets and often extends into the submitral apparatus. Because pericarditis alone is not diagnostic of rheumatic carditis, detection of an associated valvular lesion is important. Pericardial involvement may result in effusion, but large effusions, chronic constriction, and tamponade are rare. Tachycardia and various arrhythmias are nonspecific. The use of endomyocardial biopsy or radionuclide tracers for detection of inflammation has not been of additional diagnostic benefit.

Recurrent episodes of RF result in a very high incidence of carditis. The diagnosis of recurrent or "mimetic" carditis has traditionally been based on new cardiac murmurs, pericarditis, and an increase in cardiac silhouette size. The greater environmental exposure to infections in a population already susceptible to RF makes exclusion of endocarditis in patients with fever and heart murmurs especially important, particularly when other major Jones criteria are absent.

PHYSICAL EXAMINATION. There are a number of hallmarks of acute carditis on physical examination during an initial episode of RF. There may be a prominent LV impulse secondary to cardiac enlargement but not as localized as with chronic MR. Because of recent onset, there is usually at most only mild LV dilation. Sinus tachycardia is common, but atrial fibrillation is rare. The first heart sound may vary in intensity from normal to diminished because of MR, prolonged PR interval, or both. The second heart sound is normally or widely or variably split, depending on degree of the MR. The pulmonary component of the second sound is accentuated with the presence of pulmonary hypertension in severe MR. Whereas the aortic second sound is classically diminished in chronic AR, it is usually normal in RF because mobility of the aortic valve is not affected early. A third heart sound is common, but not specific for severity of MR, because children frequently have an S_3 without associated disease.

The soft, blowing, high-pitched pansystolic murmur of MR is a hallmark of carditis in RF, best heard at the apex and selectively transmitted to the axilla and back; the latter suggests severe MR. A non-pansystolic murmur may occur when MR is mild, although it retains its high-frequency, soft, blowing character, distinguishing it from physiologic murmurs. The apical diastolic murmur of Carey Coombs is often related to the severity of MR but is also associated with flow disturbances caused by mitral valve deformity secondary to valvulitis, in addition to the increased flow in diastole. Unlike the late diastolic accentuation seen with mitral stenosis, this murmur is typically mid-diastolic. When the aortic valve is involved, there is an early decrescendo diastolic murmur best heard along the base and left sternal border. AR in the absence of MR is uncommon. A murmur of functional tricuspid regurgitation may occur in the setting of severe heart failure, pulmonary hypertension, and right ventricular dilation, with associated neck vein distention and other hallmarks of tricuspid insufficiency. It has been suggested that echocardiography may be helpful in settings such as concomitant pericarditis, in which auscultation may be difficult. However, MR is usually moderate or severe when pericarditis is secondary to RF and the murmur is often detectable, despite a friction rub, which may be intermittent.

ECHOCARDIOGRAPHY. Increasing attention has been paid to echocardiography as a more sensitive tool than auscultation to detect carditis and RHD. Studies in developing countries have suggested that the increased sensitivity provided by ultrasound may be as high as 10-fold.[1] Defining echocardiographic Doppler findings that are specific for rheumatic valvulitis in the absence of auscultatable murmurs is a subject of controversy, as is the use of echocardiography alone to justify a diagnosis of carditis for this major Jones criterion.[10] MR is the most common echocardiographic finding. Mitral valve thickening or concomitant AR is seen with moderate frequency in the period after RF.[13] Several sets of echocardiographic criteria have been developed to differentiate pathologic from functional MR, including posterior direction, length and velocity of the mitral jet, holosystolic flow, significant turbulence, and MR seen in orthogonal planes. Consensus recommendations for diagnosis of MR secondary to RHD include a regurgitant jet >1 cm in length seen in at least two planes and a mosaic pattern with peak velocity >2.5 m/sec persistent throughout systole.[3] Specificity can be increased by the addition of morphologic valve features consistent with rheumatic deformities, such as valvular or subvalvular thickening or restricted leaflet

mobility. Nodular lesions are seen in roughly 25%. Use of morphologic abnormalities consistent with RHD combined with concomitant regurgitation (without the Doppler features described before) results in up to a fourfold increase in sensitivity compared with use of Doppler criteria alone.[14]

Echocardiography is useful to confirm findings on auscultation, to exclude nonrheumatic causes, and to sequentially follow up valvular insufficiency, cardiac chamber size, pulmonary hypertension, valve thickening, and LV systolic function (see Chaps. 15 and 66). Importantly, in patients without clinical findings for carditis, an important minority of those with arthritis and, in particular, chorea manifest echocardiographic abnormalities. An additional argument for the routine use of echocardiography is a reduction in the false-positive rate. The latter is substantial when only auscultation and other clinical criteria are used for diagnosis of valvulitis.[1]

It has been argued that diagnosis of carditis on the basis of echocardiography without physical examination findings ("echocarditis") results in overdiagnosis. In particular, MR may be detected by echocardiography in other febrile illnesses. Longitudinal studies of such patients will shed light on the long-term implications of "silent carditis." There is modest evidence that these patients may have a milder course, but study design issues make this uncertain.[15] Whereas WHO consensus criteria do not accept echocardiographic findings alone for the major Jones criterion of carditis, the controversy has led some workers in endemic areas to establish independent criteria that do. The potential benefits of long-term antibiotic prophylaxis and serial cardiac evaluation in these patients need to be weighed against cost and logistics; relatively less expensive echocardiographic equipment may tip the balance.

Arthritis

Polyarthritis is the earliest and most frequent manifestation of RF, occurring in up to 75% of those with acute symptoms. It is typically migratory, very painful, and limited to the major joints of the arms and legs. Arthritis occurs within 2 to 3 weeks after onset of RF and is the only clinically apparent manifestation in one third to one half of patients. The arthritis is self-limited, with symptoms and findings varying from minor arthralgias to severe arthritis with erythema, warmth, and swelling. Joint aspiration may reveal moderate leukocytosis. Commonly, tenderness is out of proportion to other findings. During the migratory phase, multiple joints can be involved in different phases of inception and resolution. Inflammation in individual joints lasts 1 to 2 weeks, and the polyarthritis as a whole resolves in 1 month or less. Chronic sequelae and disability do not appear to occur, with the rare exception of Jaccoud arthropathy, an unusual periarticular fibrosis that is not specific for RF. The arthritis phase frequently overlaps the onset of carditis, and the two manifestations appear to be inversely related in severity—patients with severe arthritis appear to have less severe manifestations of carditis, and vice versa. Considerable debate has taken place over the differing patterns of joint manifestations in industrialized and developing countries and whether arthralgias or single-joint arthritis should be made a major criterion in areas where the diagnosis may otherwise be missed, largely because of late presentation. In general, because it resolves completely, the long-term importance of the arthritis of RF is that it draws attention to the presence of carditis, which may otherwise be missed in asymptomatic individuals.

A number of conditions resemble the migratory polyarthritis of RF (see Table 88-1). In general, failure to respond to salicylates suggests nonrheumatic etiology. If salicylates (or nonsteroidals) are given early, they may blunt the full appearance of the syndrome, resulting in monoarthritis. Other forms of infectious arthritis including Lyme disease, other autoimmune disorders, and acute leukemia can present with polyarthritis, ironically including a serum sickness syndrome induced by penicillin. Bacterial endocarditis with joint involvement is especially important to consider. Because the peak antistreptolysin O titer typically occurs at the same time as the onset of rheumatic arthritis, joint inflammation in the absence of an elevated antistreptolysin O titer is unlikely to be related to RF.

A major consideration in the differential diagnosis is poststreptococcal reactive arthritis (PSRA). It occurs early after streptococcal pharyngitis without other manifestations of RF, may affect the small joints of the upper extremities, is much less responsive to salicylates, and has longer duration. There is substantial commonality between RF and PSRA, including evidence of similar genetic susceptibility. A formula based on laboratory data, clinical course, and response to anti-inflammatory agents helps differentiate this entity from RF.[16] The consensus has been that these patients should be monitored for the development of RHD, and secondary prophylaxis is recommended for children. However, serial echocardiography in adults with PSRA has not demonstrated increased development of RHD compared with matched controls.[17]

Chorea

Sydenham chorea is manifested as involuntary irregular movements, fibrillation of the tongue, characteristic spooning with external rotation of the hands, and abolition of the movements with sleep. It occurs as the sole manifestation of RF in 20% of patients and in conjunction with arthritis in 30%. Concomitant subclinical carditis detected by echocardiography appears to be as high as 70%.[18] Chorea is a uniquely delayed manifestation of RF, with a wide range in reported incidence between 5% and 35%, latency of 1 to 7 months, and choreiform manifestations that may last for months and occasionally years. Importantly, there is a substantial risk of subsequent RHD in these patients, found in one study to be more than 50%.[19] Attention has focused on psychological manifestations of the disease, including short- and long-term emotional lability, obsessive-compulsive behavior, attention deficit/hyperactivity disorder, and other central nervous system manifestations such as seizures and chronic migraine. These too appear to be immunologically mediated, with evidence of antibodies to brain tissue. Although neurologic deficits typically resolve within 2 years, residual psychiatric disturbances occur in a small but significant number of patients in the subsequent decades. Recurrences are common. Because of the late manifestation of chorea, laboratory evidence of prior streptococcal infection is far less common than with carditis or arthritis. Thus, consideration of the differential diagnosis is particularly relevant; this includes epilepsy, connective tissue diseases, other choreas, primary psychiatric disorders, Lyme disease, and toxic reactions to various drugs including oral contraceptives. The diagnosis is made on clinical grounds, as neuroimaging has not been diagnostic. A syndrome of pediatric autoimmune neuropsychiatric disorders associated with streptococcal infections (PANDAS), in a fashion similar to poststreptococcal reactive arthritis, has a temporal relationship to GABHS infection but is not associated with other features of RF. Immunologic cross-reactivity between basal ganglia and GABHS epitopes has been hypothesized, but the evidence base is incomplete and the diagnostic and therapeutic management algorithms used for patients with Sydenham chorea, including secondary antibiotic prophylaxis, are not recommended.[2]

Cutaneous Manifestations

Both major cutaneous criteria of RF occur in less than 10% of cases, and neither is specific for RF. Subcutaneous nodules are usually seen concomitant with moderate to severe rheumatic carditis, occur several weeks after onset of cardiac findings, consist of firm nodules found over major joints and bone prominences, are asymptomatic and sometimes evanescent, and typically resolve within a few weeks to 2 months. They can be seen with other autoimmune disorders. Erythema marginatum typically also occurs in conjunction with carditis, with a milder course, but it may last for months or years. It tends to occur early in the course of RF and localizes over the trunk or proximal extremities. It resembles the cutaneous findings associated with juvenile rheumatoid arthritis and Lyme disease and is seen in settings that include sepsis and drug reactions.

Laboratory Findings

There is no specific laboratory test for RF. Erythrocyte sedimentation rate and C-reactive protein are reliable markers for the severity of the autoimmune response and inflammatory activity, and the time course generally correlates with activity of the disease, although masking may be induced by anti-inflammatory agents. Because of the late onset of chorea, the acute-phase reactants, like the anti-GABHS titers, are frequently no longer elevated at presentation. The electrocardiographic findings of RF include sinus arrhythmias, with tachycardia related to fever, pericarditis, or myocarditis; bradycardia occurs in a minority. First-degree but occasionally second- or third-degree AV block occurs in 30% or more of patients but is not specific for valvular involvement or carditis. Heart block is secondary to inflammation of peri–atrioventricular nodal tissues and possibly increased vagal tone; lesions in or around the His bundle have been demonstrated. There is no correlation with prognosis or subsequent valvular manifestations. The QT interval is frequently prolonged, and QT dispersion has been reported to correlate with acute rheumatic carditis. There have been rare episodes of torsades de pointes and sudden death.

In general, the most important test in the diagnostic algorithm relates to detection of GABHS.[2] A positive throat culture is of limited value because many individuals are carriers; conversely, a negative culture may be secondary to elimination of GABHS from the pharynx because of immune response or antibiotics. The rapid streptococcal antigen detection test (RADT) is highly specific but less sensitive. Immunoassays that are both sensitive and specific have not been widely adopted.

Because only a minority of pharyngitis is secondary to GABHS, and because GABHS is present in a significant number of patients in a carrier state, the decision to treat with antibiotics is ultimately based on the clinical manifestations of pharyngitis and perceived risk, including the age of the patient and prevalence of RF in the community. A clinical spectrum that suggests bacterial infection, including lymphadenopathy, fever, headache, severe throat symptoms, and tonsillar-pharyngeal swelling or exudate in the absence of viral upper respiratory symptoms, makes the clinical diagnosis relatively specific. The highest sensitivity and specificity and the least antibiotic overuse appear to be associated with treatment of patients with acute pharyngitis who have a positive RADT result or negative RADT result but positive subsequent throat culture. In adults, in regions where RF risk is low, empiric treatment without positive throat culture or RADT is generally unnecessary and associated with substantial overtreatment. In general, use of the formal criteria for diagnosis and treatment of GABHS pharyngitis has led to undertreatment in developing countries; the opposite is true in industrialized nations, where thousands need to be treated with antibiotics to prevent one case of RF.

Baseline antibody levels exhibit substantial age and geographic variability, with high levels during the peak ages of vulnerability to RF. In contrast, *rising* streptococcal antibody titers, including antistreptolysin O, anti-deoxyribonuclease B, antihyaluronidase, and streptozyme, are more specific although variably affected by non-GABHS infections. Up to 20% of patients developing RF may have negative antistreptolysin O titers. The time course of antibody level increase is within 1 month of onset of streptococcal pharyngitis and plateaus for 3 to 6 months, after which a decline is seen, with levels elevated from the patient's baseline that typically last 1 year or less. A variety of increasingly sophisticated laboratory tests, many not available in areas where RF is endemic, are specific for a host of other rheumatic disorders that can be differentiated from RF and its sequelae.

Treatment

The sine qua non of treatment is acute antimicrobial therapy to eliminate GABHS from the pharynx and subsequent continuous antibiotics for secondary prevention (**Table 88-2**). Primary prevention, with effective antibiotic treatment starting less than 10 days after the onset of pharyngitis, largely eliminates risk of RF and is the most cost-effective approach. Once the RF is manifested, the treatment algorithm varies, depending on manifestations of major criteria (**Fig. 88-3**). The course of RF covers a spectrum from mild, resolving without treatment, to severe and recurrent with consequent end-stage RHD. Long-term monitoring is warranted, even if symptoms resolve early, because approximately half of carditis patients develop RHD.[4,11] The first line of symptomatic therapy has traditionally been anti-inflammatory agents, ranging from salicylates to steroids, although the course of the disease is not influenced by anti-inflammatory therapy.[20] Evidence for bed rest is from the preantibiotic era, and many practitioners now treat RF patients on an outpatient basis, except for those presenting with carditis, for whom bed rest, at a minimum during the symptomatic stage, is empirically applied.

TABLE 88-2 Antibiotic Therapy for Acute Rheumatic Fever and Long-Term Prophylaxis

Initial Treatment of Group A Beta-Hemolytic Streptococcal Pharyngitis (Adult Dosages)

ANTIBIOTIC	DOSE	FREQUENCY	DURATION	COMMENTS	CLASS
Benzathine penicillin G	1.2 million units IM	One time	Acutely only	↓ Compliance issues ↑ Pain	I
Penicillin V	500 mg PO	Twice daily	10 days		I
Amoxicillin	1000 mg PO	Daily	10 days		I
Penicillin Allergic					
Narrow-spectrum cephalosporins*	Varies by drug	Varies by drug	10 days	Avoid if history of anaphylaxis secondary to penicillin	I
Clindamycin*,†	300 mg PO	Twice daily	10 days		IIa
Azithromycin*,‡	500 mg PO day 1 250 mg PO days 2-5	Daily	5 days		IIa
Clarithromycin*,‡	250 mg PO	Twice daily	10 days		IIa

Secondary Prophylaxis Regimen for Patients with Documented RF (Adult Dosages)§

ANTIBIOTIC	DOSE	FREQUENCY	COMMENTS	CLASS
Benzathine penicillin G	1.2 million units IM	Every 3 to 4 weeks¶	↓ Compliance issues ↑ Pain	I
Penicillin V	250 mg PO	Twice daily		I
Erythromycin*,‡	250 mg PO	Twice daily		I
Sulfadiazine*	1 g PO	Daily		I
Sulfisoxazole*	1 g PO	Daily		IIa

*Alternative for penicillin-allergic patients. Erythromycin for secondary prophylaxis is an alternative for patients allergic to both penicillin and sulfa.

†Dosage is empiric. For severe pharyngitis, doses up to 1.2 g daily in two to four divided doses.

‡Some areas have a high rate of macrolide-resistant group A streptococci. In addition, erythromycin toxicity, including gastrointestinal intolerance and long-QT syndrome, limits its use.

§Duration of therapy ranges from 5 years to life-long (see text). For patients with poststreptococcal reactive arthritis, recommended duration is 1 year in nonendemic areas, 5 years where RF is prevalent if no evidence of carditis appears.

¶In endemic areas, benzathine penicillin every 3 weeks should be considered to maintain optimal drug levels (Class I indication). In nonendemic areas, benzathine penicillin is given every 3 weeks if RF recurs on the regimen of every 4 weeks (Class I).

Modified from Gerber MA, Baltimore RS, Eaton CB, et al: Prevention of rheumatic fever and diagnosis and treatment of acute streptococcal pharyngitis. A scientific statement from the American Heart Association Rheumatic Fever, Endocarditis, and Kawasaki Disease Committee. Circulation 119:1541, 2009; and Rheumatic fever and rheumatic heart disease. World Health Organ Tech Rep Ser 923:1, 2004.

Prevention Strategies

PRIMARY PREVENTION. Effective eradication of GABHS from the pharynx defines the role of primary prevention. Patients with apparent bacterial pharyngitis and positive test results for GABHS should be treated as early as possible in the suppurative phase. The differential diagnosis, in addition to viral infection, includes non-GABHS and gonococcal pharyngitis. Penicillin is uniformly effective for GABHS if it is taken orally for a full 10-day course or if intramuscular benzathine penicillin is administered because penicillin-resistant GABHS has not been demonstrated. The particular advantage of intramuscular benzathine penicillin G is that it avoids compliance issues. Oral cephalosporins, indicated for penicillin-allergic patients, have been used in shorter than 10-day courses with high compliance, with bacterial elimination and clinical response that may be superior to penicillin treatment, but the evidence base is insufficient to recommend this regimen for treatment in endemic areas. Aggressive antibiotic therapy for primary prevention is essential in areas where RF is prevalent and may represent the best hope for decreasing the overall health care burden of RHD.[21] In contrast, in populations where RF is rare, antibiotic use results in modest therapeutic benefit, and the risk-to-benefit ratio has been called into question.

SECONDARY PREVENTION. The method of choice for prevention of RF recurrence is continuous administration of benzathine penicillin G every 4 weeks. Because of low penicillin levels during the fourth week, 3-week intervals should be considered in endemic areas or for patients at high risk. Those with documented RF should have continuous secondary prevention as soon as the primary GABHS treatment regimen has been completed. An oral regimen should be reserved primarily for patients deemed to be at low risk for recurrent RF or those allergic to penicillin or otherwise intolerant of intramuscular therapy. The duration of therapy depends on the patient's age, known RHD, time since last episode of RF, number of episodes, family history, occupational exposure, and environmental factors, such as living in endemic areas.[3] The Class I recommendations are 5 years or until the age of 21 years (whichever is longer) in the absence of carditis, 10 years or until the age of 21 years for patients with mild or apparently healed carditis, and 10 years or until the age of 40 years for patients who develop RHD.[2] Patients at high risk for repeated episodes of RF, such as those at significant risk of recurrent exposure to GABHS infection, should be considered for life-long antibiotic prophylaxis. Confounding factors have been reluctance of rural practitioners to administer parenteral antibiotics for fear of allergic reactions and, for similar reasons, regulations prohibiting parenteral administration in hospitals in some developing countries. The actual risk of anaphylaxis, estimated to be 0.2%, is less in children younger than 12 years.

Therapeutic Modalities

CARDITIS. Salicylates and nonsteroidals have no specific role in rheumatic carditis, with the exception of treatment of concomitant pericarditis. Acute carditis has generally been treated with steroids even though a meta-analysis of eight randomized controlled trials failed to demonstrate superiority of steroids, immunoglobulins, or salicylates over placebo in the progression of RHD.[20] Nevertheless, in the setting of severe, potentially life-threatening heart failure, steroid administration is widespread. Withdrawal of steroids or salicylates can result in rebound or relapse. Treatment of cardiac manifestations otherwise follows established guidelines, including management of congestive heart failure and severe valvular regurgitation, although special attention should be paid to use of digitalis because these patients are sensitive to development of heart block.

Unless valvular regurgitation and severe congestive heart failure are refractory to drug therapy, valve surgery is avoided whenever possible during RF. Surgical morbidity and mortality have been significant, and failed repair leading to valve replacement has been frequent. However, when surgery is necessary, LV function generally improves significantly, consistent with valve regurgitation rather than myocardial dysfunction being the primary mechanism leading to heart failure.

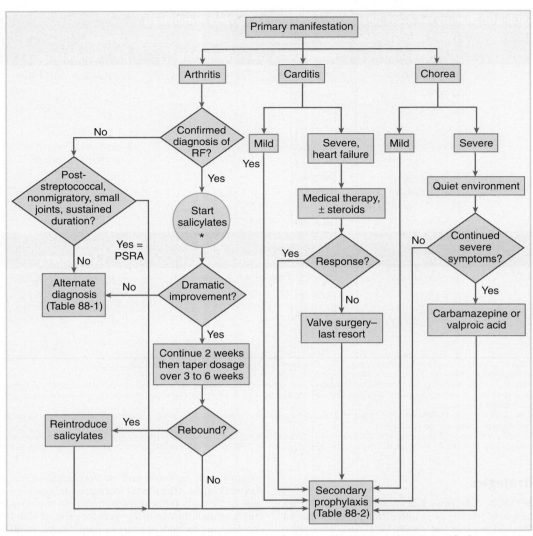

FIGURE 88-3 Algorithm for management of rheumatic fever and its primary manifestations. *Salicylates are also indicated for fever and arthralgia, but there is no evidence of effectiveness for carditis or chorea. PSRA = poststreptococcal reactive arthritis; RF = rheumatic fever. *(Modified from Thatai D, Turi ZG: Current guidelines for the treatment of patients with rheumatic fever. Drugs 57:545, 1999.)*

ARTHRITIS. Salicylates are the first line of therapy for migratory poly-arthritis because of their highly effective analgesic, anti-inflammatory, and antipyretic properties. Nonsteroidals are effective alternatives. Aspirin (up to 100 mg/kg/day in four or more divided doses) is both therapeutic and diagnostic; failure of the pain to resolve within 24 hours suggests alternative causes of arthritis. Although salicylate levels can be followed (15 to 30 mg/dL is the therapeutic range), these data are usually not available in endemic areas; instead, patients are monitored for tinnitus and gastrointestinal toxicity. Early administration does have the potential to mask the evolving clinical picture (e.g., arthritis when medication is given for arthralgias). Steroids are typically not used because they offer no therapeutic advantage and may mask the presence of other illnesses causing arthritis, such as lupus, or exacerbate other causes, such as infectious arthritis.

CHOREA. Traditional treatment has included sedation and empiric use of antiseizure or antipsychotic medications. Small series have studied corticosteroids, along with plasmapheresis and intravenous immuno-globulins, to assess their influence on the severity and time course of symptoms. The duration of symptoms does appear to be shortened with treatment. However, the evidence base is not conclusive, some of the interventions are potentially toxic, and, pending larger studies, a conservative approach to a largely self-limited disorder has been deemed appropriate. For patients with refractory symptoms, there is modest evidence favoring use of carbamazepine or valproic acid. Because of the high incidence of carditis,[18] whether clinical or subclinical, and potential progression to RHD, these patients require long-term antibiotic therapy.

Future Directions

A universal streptococcal vaccine has been elusive, partly because of the number and variability of antigenic stimulants, making the use of a vaccine that identifies specific epitopes ineffective. A simple and inexpensive screening test for identification of patients and populations genetically susceptible to RF has not been developed, nor is there a readily available, universally applicable, and inexpensive screening test for GABHS antibodies. Given the relatively modest cost of secondary prophylaxis and the prohibitive expense associated with RHD in developing countries where RF remains endemic, systematic longitudinal studies of more sensitive diagnostic tools, in particular portable echocardiography, have been an important research focus in the past decade.[1] RF still receives <0.4% of research funds aimed at the so-called neglected diseases. Competition for limited health care resources, with a growing prevalence of ischemic heart disease in developing countries (see Chap. 1), has limited the financing of potentially highly cost-effective preventive health care programs.

REFERENCES

Epidemiology

1. Marijon E, Ou P, Celermajer DS, et al: Prevalence of rheumatic heart disease detected by echocardiographic screening. N Engl J Med 357:470, 2007.

2. Gerber MA, Baltimore RS, Eaton CB, et al: Prevention of rheumatic fever and diagnosis and treatment of acute Streptococcal pharyngitis: A scientific statement from the American Heart Association Rheumatic Fever, Endocarditis, and Kawasaki Disease Committee. Circulation 119:1541, 2009.
3. Rheumatic fever and rheumatic heart disease. World Health Organ Tech Rep Ser 923:1, 2004.
4. Carapetis JR, Steer AC, Mulholland EK, et al: The global burden of group A streptococcal diseases. Lancet Infect Dis 5:685, 2005.
5. Shulman ST, Stollerman G, Beall B, et al: Temporal changes in streptococcal M protein types and the near-disappearance of acute rheumatic fever in the United States. Clin Infect Dis 42:441, 2006.

Pathobiology and Pathology

6. Martins TB, Veasy LG, Hill HR: Antibody responses to group A streptococcal infections in acute rheumatic fever. Pediatr Infect Dis J 25:832, 2006.
7. Guilherme L, Kalil J: Rheumatic fever: From innate to acquired immune response. Ann N Y Acad Sci 1107:426, 2007.
8. Bryant PA, Robins-Browne R, Carapetis JR, et al: Some of the people, some of the time: Susceptibility to acute rheumatic fever. Circulation 119:742, 2009.
9. Virmani R, Farb A, Burke AP, Narula J: Pathology of acute rheumatic carditis. In Narula J, Virmani R, Reddy KS, Tandon R (eds): Rheumatic Fever. Washington, DC, American Registry of Pathology, 1999, pp 217-234.

Diagnosis

10. Ferrieri P: Proceedings of the Jones Criteria workshop. Circulation 106:2521, 2002.
11. Lee JL, Naguwa SM, Cheema GS, et al: Acute rheumatic fever and its consequences: A persistent threat to developing nations in the 21st century. Autoimmun Rev 9:117, 2009.

12. Kamblock J, N'Guyen L, Pagis B, et al: Acute severe mitral regurgitation during first attacks of rheumatic fever: Clinical spectrum, mechanisms and prognostic factors. J Heart Valve Dis 14:440, 2005.
13. Caldas AM, Terreri MT, Moises VA, et al: The case for utilizing more strict quantitative Doppler echocardiographic criterions for diagnosis of subclinical rheumatic carditis. Cardiol Young 17:42, 2007.
14. Marijon E, Celermajer DS, Tafflet M, et al: Rheumatic heart disease screening by echocardiography: The inadequacy of World Health Organization criteria for optimizing the diagnosis of subclinical disease. Circulation 120:663, 2009.
15. Tubridy-Clark M, Carapetis JR: Subclinical carditis in rheumatic fever: A systematic review. Int J Cardiol 119:54, 2007.
16. Barash J, Mashiach E, Navon-Elkan P, et al: Differentiation of post-streptococcal reactive arthritis from acute rheumatic fever. J Pediatr 153:696, 2008.
17. van Bemmel JM, Delgado V, Holman ER, et al: No increased risk of valvular heart disease in adult poststreptococcal reactive arthritis. Arthritis Rheum 60:987, 2009.
18. Demiroren K, Yavuz H, Cam L, et al: Sydenham's chorea: A clinical follow-up of 65 patients. J Child Neurol 22:550, 2007.
19. Carapetis JR, McDonald M, Wilson NJ: Acute rheumatic fever. Lancet 366:155, 2005.

Treatment

20. Cilliers AM, Manyemba J, Saloojee H: Anti-inflammatory treatment for carditis in acute rheumatic fever. Cochrane Database Syst Rev (2):CD003176, 2003.
21. Karthikeyan G, Mayosi BM: Is primary prevention of rheumatic fever the missing link in the control of rheumatic heart disease in Africa? Circulation 120:709, 2009.

CHAPTER 89

Rheumatic Diseases and the Cardiovascular System

Alexandra Villa-Forte and Brian F. Mandell

Systemic rheumatologic disorders may involve the cardiovascular system directly or indirectly. Patients often seek medical attention because of constitutional symptoms, musculoskeletal pain, fever, peripheral or visceral ischemia, or organ failure without apparent involvement of the cardiovascular system. Involvement of the heart and vessels can range from clinically silent to catastrophic. Alternatively, the cardiovascular specialist may first recognize that cardiovascular symptoms may have a primary immunologic basis. Examples include patients who present with claudication, ischemic heart disease, or aortic aneurysms caused by arteritis, and patients with systemic lupus erythematosus (SLE) who develop acute myocarditis, pericarditis, or valvular dysfunction. Patients with several systemic inflammatory diseases have a documented elevated risk for coronary and cerebrovascular events in the absence of excessive traditional cardiovascular risk factors.

Vasculitis

Discrimination among the various forms of vasculitis begins with the concept of primary (immune dysregulation, without a known trigger) versus secondary. Secondary vasculitis is associated with another condition (e.g., drug allergy, viral hepatitis, bacterial endocarditis) or with rheumatic disease. Secondary vasculitis requires treatment of the underlying disease or removal of the causative agent. Misclassification could lead to inappropriate use of immunosuppressive therapy, with adverse or lethal consequences. Examples include vasculitis secondary to sepsis, particularly endocarditis, drug toxicity, and poisonings, malignancies, cardiac myxomas, and multifocal emboli from large-vessel aneurysms (**Table 89-1**). These conditions can mimic vasculitis or cause multifocal ischemia or infarction, with accompanying vasculitis.

The greatest certainty in the diagnosis of primary vasculitis is in the setting of classic clinical and laboratory patterns with supportive histopathology—for example, a 70-year-old woman with new-onset severe headache, temporal region pain, hip and shoulder girdle stiffness, visual aberration (amaurosis or blindness), and a high erythrocyte sedimentation rate (ESR). This picture would be so compatible with giant cell arteritis that empiric therapy could be started without biopsy evidence of the diagnosis, but a positive biopsy would remove any doubt and would be useful if the response to steroids is delayed. Unfortunately, many patients with vasculitis do not present with such recognizable features. Instead, one may have to depend on combinations of less typical clues. A patient with ischemic digits, active urinary sediment, and peripheral neuropathy is likely to have vasculitis, especially if mimics have already been ruled out. The presence of a purpuric rash, particularly if it is palpable (**Fig. 89-1**), furthers the probability of a small-vessel vasculitis but will not exclude a secondary cause, such as a malignancy or hepatitis C–associated vasculitis.

Approach to Proving the Diagnosis of Vasculitis

Definitive diagnosis depends on documenting lesions in affected tissue. The greatest success in achieving a tissue diagnosis comes from a biopsy of abnormal or symptomatic sites. In patients with proven vasculitis, the yield from biopsies of clinically normal sites (i.e., blind biopsy) is considerably less than 20%. Therefore, a biopsy of apparently normal tissue is not recommended. Biopsies of abnormal organs provide diagnostically useful information in about 65% of cases. Needle biopsies are small and often do not contain affected tissue; uniform involvement of vessels in affected viscera is uncommon.

A biopsy may not be practical in certain circumstances, such as systemic illness with symptoms of intestinal ischemia, carotidynia, or findings of unequal pulses or blood pressures. Because biopsy of large vessels is usually impractical, angiography may be helpful. In this setting, vascular stenoses and/or aneurysms that cannot be explained by atherosclerosis or infection may provide sufficient circumstantial evidence to proceed with treatment for primary vasculitis.

Forms of Vasculitis Relevant to Cardiologists and Cardiovascular Surgeons

TAKAYASU ARTERITIS

Takayasu arteritis (TA) is an idiopathic large-vessel vasculitis of young adults that affects the aorta and its major branches.

EPIDEMIOLOGY. Women are affected about 10 times more often than men. The median age at onset is 25 years. Best known in Asia, TA can occur worldwide and can affect individuals of all races and ethnicities. The prevalence of TA is estimated as 2.6/1,000,000 persons in the United States and 1.26/1,000,000 in northern Europe.[1] An autopsy series from Japan noted features of TA in 1 in every 3000 autopsies.[2]

PATHOGENESIS. The cause of TA is unknown. Acute lesions contain mononuclear cell infiltrates that appear to have entered the vessel wall through the vasa vasorum and subsequently migrate to the arterial intima. These cells are predominantly macrophages and T cells (gamma-delta, cytotoxic, and natural killer). The presence of various cytokines, including interleukin-6 (IL-6) and tumor necrosis factor (TNF) in these granulomatous lesions has prompted various therapeutic approaches using cytokine-targeted biologic agents.[3]

TABLE 89-1	Diseases That Can Mimic Primary Systemic Vasculitis

Sepsis, especially endocarditis
Drug toxicity, poisoning
  Cocaine
  Amphetamines
  Ephedra
  Phenylpropanolamine
Coagulopathy
  Anticardiolipin antibody syndrome
  Disseminated intravascular coagulation
Malignancy (solid organ or liquid tumors)
Cardiac myxoma
Multifocal emboli from large-vessel aneurysms (cholesterol, mycotic)
Ehlers-Danlos syndrome (vascular ectatic type)
Fibromuscular dysplasia

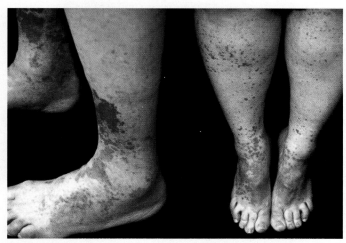

FIGURE 89-1 Palpable purpura. Vascular inflammation at the level of capillaries and venules leads to exudation of formed elements and the color and texture of lesions noted in these patients. The person on the right is a young woman with Henoch-Schönlein vasculitis or purpura (HSP). The older man on the left has a similar lesion, but in this case, it was associated with hepatitis C, acquired in the course of transfusions for heart surgery. HCV infection led to cryoglobulinemia and secondary vasculitis. The treatment for each patient is different. The patient with HSP, who does not have extracutaneous disease, only requires reassurance and monitoring for her usually self-limiting problem, whereas the patient with HCV and vasculitis requires antiviral therapy.

CLINICAL FEATURES. In TA, arterial stenoses occur three to four times more often than aneurysms. Claudication (>60% upper versus 30% lower extremities) is the most common complaint and bruits (approximately 80%), blood pressure, or pulse asymmetries (60 to 80%) are the most common findings. Aneurysms are most common and clinically most significant in the aortic root, where they can lead to valvular regurgitation (**Fig. 89-2A**, left; see Fig. 89-2B). Hypertension results most often from renal artery stenosis, but can also be associated with suprarenal aortic stenosis or a chronically damaged, rigid aorta. Cardiac, renal, and central nervous system (CNS) vascular complications cause most severe morbidity and mortality. Estimates of mortality range from a low of approximately 3% to approximately 35% at 5-year follow-up.[1,4]

Symptoms of claudication, Raynaud phenomenon, ischemia, or the finding of hypertension, especially in young patients, necessitate examination for asymmetry of extremity pulses, blood pressure, and bruits. Increasing extremity or visceral ischemia, malaise, myalgias, arthralgias, night sweats, and fever may indicate active disease. Occurrence of such symptoms in the setting of an elevated ESR indicates active disease. Many patients still experience progressive disease[1,4] but do not have any constitutional or new vascular symptoms, and as

many as 50% may have normal ESRs. Active disease in these patients is suggested by the following:

1. New vascular abnormalities on sequential angiographic studies despite suspected remission.
2. Presence of inflammatory changes in bypass biopsy specimens from patients in whom surgery was performed because of critical flow abnormalities in the setting of clinically quiescent disease.[1,4]

Determining disease activity in TA is a major challenge because of poor correlation among clinical, laboratory, radiologic, and histologic data. Studies using refinements in magnetic resonance imaging (MRI)[5] may enable the clinician to detect qualitative abnormalities in the vessel wall that imply inflammatory change. ^{18}F-fluorodeoxyglucose–positron emission tomography (FDG-PET) has been evaluated in the assessment of disease activity; preliminary results were encouraging, showing high sensitivity and specificity for the presence of inflammation.[6] However, the clinical usefulness of this test remains uncertain, and its correlation with disease activity has been questioned.[7] The value of FDG-PET may be limited by the presence of atherosclerotic disease and other conditions that could lead to false-positive results. Prospective studies with large numbers of patients to define the operating characteristics of PET clearly are necessary.

Cardiac sequelae of TA result more often from aortic regurgitation and inadequately treated hypertension than from arteritis affecting the coronary vessels.[1,4] Indirect evidence from echocardiography suggests that left ventricular systolic dysfunction caused by myocarditis may affect approximately 18% of patients.[8] When coronary artery vasculitis is detected (less than 5%), it is most frequent in the ostial regions. More distal involvement may also occur, and both types of lesions may affect the same patient. These observations underscore the importance of considering vasculitis in the differential diagnosis of young patients with ischemic symptoms.

DIFFERENTIAL DIAGNOSIS. Certain congenital diseases cause abnormalities of arterial extracellular matrix and aortic regurgitation (e.g., Marfan syndrome, Ehlers-Danlos syndrome). However, these conditions do not cause stenotic lesions in large vessels, the most common feature of TA. Inborn genetic errors that affect arterial matrix do not cause systemic symptoms, abnormal acute-phase reactants, anemia, or thrombocytosis, which may accompany large-vessel vasculitis. The young female predominance of TA distinguishes it from patients with typical atherosclerosis, a disease much more likely to affect the lower extremity large vessels than the arms, and the abdominal aorta more than the aortic root. Infectious causes of large-vessel aneurysms (e.g., bacterial, syphilitic, mycobacterial, fungal) must be considered in both sexes and all age groups, but are not usually associated with vascular stenoses affecting the arch vessels. Other autoimmune diseases may be complicated by large-vessel vasculitis, but they are discerned by their associated characteristics (e.g., SLE, Cogan syndrome, Behçet disease, spondyloarthropathies) and age predilections (e.g., Kawasaki disease in younger individuals or giant-cell arteritis in older adults). Sarcoidosis can closely mimic TA. Making the correct diagnosis depends on finding other characteristic features of sarcoidosis (e.g., proliferative synovitis, skin lesions, Bell's palsy, adenopathy). There are no specific diagnostic tests for TA. The diagnosis depends on clinical features in conjunction with vascular imaging abnormalities. In patients who undergo vascular surgery, histopathologic abnormalities may support the diagnosis, but the surgeon must recognize the need to send tissue for this purpose.

TREATMENT. Almost all patients with TA improve when treated with high doses of a corticosteroid (e.g., prednisone, 1 mg/kg/day); relapses are common with tapering of corticosteroid therapy. Corticosteroid-resistant or relapsing patients may respond to the addition to daily therapy of cyclophosphamide (approximately 2 mg/kg) or weekly therapy with methotrexate (approximately 20 mg).[1,4,9] Approximately 40% of patients who receive a cytotoxic agent and corticosteroids will achieve remission but, over time, about half these patients will also relapse, leading to the need for chronic immunosuppressive therapy

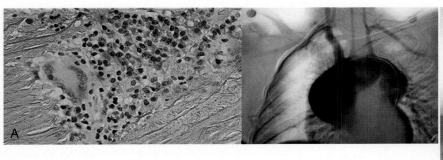
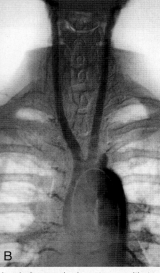

FIGURE 89-2 Takayasu disease. **A,** Takayasu arteritis. Granulomatous inflammation and medial destruction (left) has led to marked aortic root dilation (right) in a 17-year-old female high school student who developed symptoms of congestive heart failure and exertional angina. She also had diffuse narrowing of the left common carotid artery and irregular dilation of the innominate artery. (Hematoxylin-eosin stain; magnification ×40.) **B,** Occlusion of both subclavian arteries led to leg pressures being the only reliable measure of central aortic pressure.

in many patients. Such unsatisfactory results have led to ongoing studies that seek to take advantage of new insights into pathogenesis. Preliminary studies have shown that treatment designed to block TNF may dramatically improve most patients (14 of 15) with TA who have relapsed during tapering of steroid therapy.[10,11]

A discussion of pharmacologic therapy for TA only addresses one important aspect of care. Other important issues include treatment of the anatomic effects of vascular lesions; fibrotic stenosis and thrombosed vessels will not respond to corticosteroids. Patients with TA may have signs of clinical deterioration caused by fixed critical stenoses or aneurysms. Hypertension affects approximately 40% to 90% of patients.[1,4] In Asia, India, and Mexico, TA is one of the most common causes of hypertension in adolescents and young adults. One of the most common traps in clinical management relates to not knowing whether blood pressure recordings in an extremity represent aortic root pressure. Because more than 90% of patients have stenotic lesions, and the most common site of stenosis is the subclavian and innominate arteries, blood pressure in one or both arms may underestimate pressure in the aorta. Elevated aortic root pressure, when unrecognized and untreated, enhances the risks of hypertensive complications. Intravascular pressure recordings during angiographic procedures can address this issue. The importance of knowing the distribution and severity of all vascular lesions cannot be overemphasized. In the setting of renal insufficiency, the potential of contrast agents to cause further renal impairment may limit exploring the extent of all potential vascular lesions. However, in the absence of contraindications, patients should have the entire aorta and its primary branches included in vascular imaging studies. MR angiography does not affect the opportunity to measure intravascular pressures, but may suffice to delineate vascular lesions without resorting to catheter-guided angiography.

Whenever feasible, anatomic correction of clinically significant lesions should be considered, especially in the setting of renal artery stenosis and hypertension. In about 20% of patients, aortic root involvement may lead to valvular insufficiency, angina, and congestive heart failure (see Fig. 89-2).[1,4] Severe or progressive changes may require aortic surgery, with or without valve replacement. Because of the high prevalence of subclavian and carotid stenoses in TA, severe symptomatic stenoses of these vessels should be treated by grafts that originate from the aortic root and not from an arch vessel to another arch vessel. The latter may be followed by loss of the graft because of new stenosis in an initially spared subclavian or carotid artery. Conversely, a graft from the ascending aorta is a safer long-term conduit

because the ascending aorta in TA essentially never becomes stenotic. Mesenteric and celiac artery stenoses are usually asymptomatic and only rarely require surgery. Angioplasty and intravascular stents have met with restenosis far more often than bypass, which is preferred whenever feasible. It is always best to operate on patients who are in remission; however, judgment of disease activity in TA may be difficult. Consequently, all bypass surgeries should include vascular biopsy specimens for histopathologic evaluation. Findings from surgical specimens may help guide the need for postoperative immunosuppressive treatment. Even high-flow grafts can occlude spontaneously soon after surgery, often for unclear reasons.

The care of patients with TA requires a team approach that includes clinicians familiar with the proper use of immunosuppressive therapies, vascular imaging and intervention specialists and, in the setting of critical stenoses or aneurysms, cardiovascular surgeons. For most patients, medical and surgical therapies provide important palliation.

GIANT CELL ARTERITIS OF OLDER ADULTS

Giant cell arteritis (GCA) and Takayasu arteritis are the principal diseases associated with sterile granulomatous inflammation of large and medium-sized vessels.

EPIDEMIOLOGY. In the United States, GCA affects approximately 18/100,000 population older than 50 years of age (mean, 74 years of age). GCA is more common in northern latitudes. In Iceland and Denmark, the prevalence is 27 and 21/100,000, respectively, in the group older than 50 years of age. Although females predominate (2 to 3:1), this sex difference is less striking than in TA (6 to 10:1). The demographic characteristics of GCA are the same as for patients with polymyalgia rheumatica (PMR), and 30% to 50% of patients with GCA concurrently have features of PMR.[12]

PATHOGENESIS. The cause of GCA remains unknown; the inflammatory lesion begins in the adventitia. The vasa vasorum furnish the conduit for the mononuclear cells (dendritic cells, macrophages, and Th1-type lymphocytes) that mediate vascular injury. Dendritic cells participate in the process by presenting to lymphocytes the putative antigen that is believed to promote the development of GCA. The finding of clonality of approximately 4% of T lymphocytes without clonality of peripheral blood lymphocytes in the vessel wall supports this conjecture. Vascular lesions initially overexpress proinflammatory cytokines such as IL-1, IL-6, TNF, and interferon-γ (IFN-γ). Intermediate

TABLE 89-2 Clinical Profile of Giant Cell Arteritis

ABNORMALITY	FREQUENCY (%)
Atypical headache	60-90
Tender temporal artery	40-70
Systemic symptoms not attributable to other diseases	20-50
Fever	20-50
Polymyalgia rheumatica	30-50
Acute visual abnormalities	12-40
Transient ischemic attack or stroke	5-10
Claudication	
Jaw	30-70
Extremity	5-15
Aortic aneurysm	15-20
Dramatic response to corticosteroid therapy	~100
Positive temporal artery biopsy	~50-80

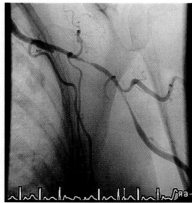

FIGURE 89-3 Giant cell arteritis. Here, Takayasu-like lesions involving the subclavian and axillary arteries are shown.

lesions harbor mediators of matrix destruction (e.g., metalloproteinases, reactive oxygen and nitrogen species). In later stages, growth factors such as platelet-derived growth factor (PDGF) and fibroblast growth factor (FGF) participate in stimulating myointimal proliferation, leading to vessel stenosis.

CLINICAL FEATURES. The most characteristic features of GCA are new onset of atypical and often severe headaches, scalp and temporal artery tenderness, acute visual loss, polymyalgia rheumatica, and pain in the muscles of mastication (**Table 89-2**). Concurrence of such abnormalities with an increase in the ESR supports a clinical diagnosis of GCA and mandates treatment, even without proof of diagnosis from a temporal artery biopsy. The diagnosis is doubtful if dramatic improvement does not occur within 24 to 72 hours. The yield of positive temporal artery biopsies in patients clinically diagnosed with GCA is about 50% to 80%, depending on the clinical pattern of disease. Patients with a high ESR who have presented to an ophthalmologist with symptoms of new-onset atypical headache and visual loss are more likely to have a positive biopsy than patients who present with symptoms of vague limb girdle pain, chronic headache, and malaise, or patients with predominant aortitis.

GCA may produce clinically apparent aortitis in at least 15% of cases and involve the primary branches of the aorta, especially the subclavian arteries, in a similar number of individuals.[12,13] Postmortem studies have suggested that large-vessel involvement is far more common than clinically appreciated. Consequently, some patients with GCA may present with features that resemble those of TA. Among older adults with inflammatory large-vessel disease, the same considerations and precautions must be applied in GCA as in patients with TA—the need to identify an extremity that provides a reliable blood pressure equivalent to aortic root pressure and follow-up to include careful observation for new bruits, pulse, and blood pressure asymmetry. Patients with GCA are more than 17 times more likely than age-matched controls to have thoracic aortic aneurysms, and about 2.5 times more likely than age-matched controls to have abdominal aortic aneurysms. Half of patients with thoracic aortic aneurysms die as a result of those lesions. Because aneurysms were found in the course of routine care or at postmortem, these may be conservative estimates. The finding of large-vessel disease, including aortic aneurysms, in older adults with GCA should not be assumed to be caused by atherosclerosis. It is not surprising that about half of patients with GCA have objective features of cardiac disease. Myocardial infarction (MI) caused by GCA is rare or rarely appreciated; histopathologic findings in coronary arteries are infrequently sought in the group of patients whose mean age is 74 years.

DIFFERENTIAL DIAGNOSIS. Mimics of GCA include other vasculitides that may cause musculoskeletal pain, headache, visual aberrations, fever, and malaise. Although these include Wegener granulomatosis, microscopic polyangiitis, and others, it is relatively simple to exclude these based on the presence of more characteristic features of those illnesses (e.g., upper and/or lower airway disease and features of small-vessel vasculitis). Rarely, the GCA phenotype may be part of a paraneoplastic process. If polymyalgia rheumatica is the most compelling symptom of GCA, the differential then also includes polymyositis and proximal-onset rheumatoid arthritis. No precise serologic test exists for GCA. Diagnosis is based on a clinically compatible presentation, concurrent elevated acute-phase reactants (more than 80% of cases), a positive temporal artery biopsy (50% to 80% of cases) or angiographic abnormalities of large vessels (**Fig. 89-3**) compatible with GCA.

TREATMENT. Corticosteroid treatment continues to be the most effective therapy for GCA. Prednisone (≈0.7 to 1 mg/kg/day) will reduce symptoms within 1 to 2 days and often eliminate symptoms within 1 week. Approximately 2 to 4 weeks after clinical and laboratory measurement, particularly of the ESR, normalized tapering of corticosteroids can begin. Unfortunately, the ESR does not always normalize, even with disease control, so it should not be relied on as the only measure of disease activity. Occasional patients may either not achieve complete remission or not tolerate weaning of corticosteroid therapy. Cytotoxic and other immunosuppressive agents, including anti-TNF agents, have not proved efficacious in controlled comparative trials.[14,15] Two retrospective studies have demonstrated that the use of low-dose aspirin reduces cranial ischemic events (blindness and stroke) three- to fourfold compared with patients who had not received such therapy; in the absence of contraindications, all patients with GCA should receive low-dose aspirin.[16,17]

IDIOPATHIC AORTITIS

Aortitis can occur in TA and GCA, Behçet disease, and Cogan syndrome, and in children as a complication of Kawasaki disease. Occasionally, it is an unanticipated finding in patients undergoing surgery for aortic valve regurgitation, aneurysm resection, or coarctation.[18] Little is known about the frequency and clinical characteristics of idiopathic aortitis. Aortitis in the context of retroperitoneal fibrosis is a separate topic that will not be discussed in this chapter.

EPIDEMIOLOGY. A 20-year review of pathologic specimens from consecutive aortic surgeries at the Cleveland Clinic Foundation has revealed that 52 of 1204 specimens (4.3%) showed findings of idiopathic aortitis. Of patients with idiopathic aortitis, 67% were women.[18]

PATHOGENESIS. Unless the patient with idiopathic aortitis had a past history of GCA or TA, the mechanisms of disease remain unexplored.

CLINICAL FEATURES. In our series, 96% of patients with idiopathic aortitis had findings limited to the thoracic aorta. These data resemble those from large postmortem series in which aortas were examined in spite of the absence of overt aortic disease during life. In 69% of cases, idiopathic aortitis was not related to a current or past history of systemic disease. However, in 31% (16 of 52), aortitis was associated with a past history of GCA, TA, SLE, Wegener granulomatosis, or various other disorders.

DIFFERENTIAL DIAGNOSIS. Patients with idiopathic aortitis vary in age from childhood to the very elderly. Consequently, differential diagnosis should consider Kawasaki disease, TA, GCA, SLE, sarcoidosis, Cogan syndrome, Behçet disease, spondyloarthropathies, rheumatoid arthritis, rheumatic fever, and aortitis caused by infectious agents (e.g., tuberculosis, syphilis, mycoses, bacteria). Symptoms or findings of these diseases may immediately allow prioritization of diagnostic choices. However, some processes may be clinically silent, and ancillary laboratory studies (e.g., rapid plasma reagin [RPR], antinuclear antibody [ANA], skin tests such as purified protein derivative [PPD]), cultures, and special stains of surgical specimens may aid diagnosis. The diagnosis of idiopathic aortitis requires ruling out all causes of aortitis that may have specific therapies.

TREATMENT. In our experience with 36 patients, followed for a mean period of 42 months and analyzed retrospectively, new aneurysms were identified in 6 of 25 patients not treated with corticosteroids and in 0 of 11 patients treated postoperatively with corticosteroids. Although this observation could suggest that such therapy is warranted, there were marked variations of dose and duration of therapy that led to uncertainty about corticosteroid efficacy. Because only 17% of all patients subsequently developed new aneurysms over 3.5 years, we do not believe that all such patients require medical treatment.[18] These observations suggest isolated inflammatory disease of the aortic root in most patients. Treatment should depend on documentation of ongoing inflammatory disease. We approach this by history and physical examination, laboratory evaluation (complete blood count [CBC], ESR, C-reactive protein [CRP]), and imaging studies (MRI or MR angiography of the entire aorta and its primary branches). These tests should not be done in the immediate postoperative period. Because new lesions may occur over time, patients with idiopathic aortitis identified at the time of surgery should be periodically evaluated for recurrence. If disease definitely recurs, treatment should be pursued as recommended for TA and GCA. Although proof of the effectiveness of this approach is lacking, it can be defended based on the similarities of these conditions and demonstrated efficacy in GCA and TA.

KAWASAKI DISEASE

Kawasaki disease (KD) is an acute febrile systemic illness of childhood. It is the principal cause of acquired heart disease in children in Japan and the United States.

EPIDEMIOLOGY. KD occurs primarily in children younger than 4 or 5 years of age. Peak incidence is in children younger than 2 years of age. Boys are affected 1.5 times more often than girls. KD almost never occurs beyond 8 years of age (mean age in Japan is 12 months and, in the United States, 2.8 years of age). Although all racial groups can be affected, Asian children have the highest incidence of KD (50 to 200/100,000 children younger than 5 years of age versus 6 to 15/100,000 in the United States). Asian Americans have a higher incidence of KD than black Americans, in whom the incidence exceeds that of white Americans.[19] Although siblings of patients with KD are infrequently affected, KD does affect siblings more often than the general age-matched population (2.1% versus 0.19%). When siblings are affected, symptoms often occur shortly after their family member becomes ill. This raises questions about an infectious cause in the setting of an immunologic predisposition.[19-22]

PATHOGENESIS. Fever, rash, conjunctivitis, adenopathy, and geographic clustering suggest an infectious cause, but no agent has yet

---

TABLE 89-3 Definition of Kawasaki Disease

Fever ≥ 5 days, without other explanation, plus at least four of the following:[21]
1. Bilateral conjunctival injection
2. Mucous membrane changes—injected or fissured lips; injected pharynx or strawberry tongue
3. Extremity abnormality—erythema of palms, soles, edema of hands, feet, or generalized or peripheral desquamation (hands, feet)
4. Rash (polymorphous)
5. Cervical lymphadenopathy (usually a single node > 1.5 cm)

Associated manifestations
  Irritability
  Sterile pyuria, meatitis
  Perineal erythema and desquamation
  Arthralgias, arthritis
  Abdominal pain, diarrhea
  Aseptic meningitis
  Hepatitis
  Obstructive jaundice
  Hydrops of gallbladder
  Uveitis
  Sensorineural hearing loss
  Cardiovascular changes

80% cases < 4 years; rare, >8 years.
CDC = Centers for Disease Control and Prevention.
Modified from Barron K: Kawasaki disease: Etiology, pathogenesis and treatment. Cleve Clin J Med 69(Suppl 2):69, 2002.

---

been identified. The essential absence of disease in neonates invites speculation about protection from maternal antibodies, and the rarity of KD in adults suggests protection through acquired immunity.[21,22]

The acute phase of illness is characterized by immunoinflammatory activation. This includes high levels of acute-phase reactants, leukocytosis with a left shift, lymphocytosis with a predominance of polyclonal B cells, and thrombocytosis that frequently reaches 1,000,000/mm^3. Blood T lymphocytes, including CD4$^+$ and CD8$^+$ cells, increase in number and show signs of activation. In spite of these observations, children with acute KD are often transiently anergic. Increased blood levels of a broad range of cytokines and soluble forms of endothelial cell adhesion molecules indicate immune activation. Cytokine-mediated endothelial cell activation and cytotoxic factors to endothelial cells may play an important early role in pathogenesis. Tissue specimens reveal vasculitis with endothelial cell edema, necrosis, desquamation, and a changing profile of leukocytes in the vessel wall—first, neutrophils and later, macrophages and T lymphocytes. After months, the inflammatory infiltrate diminishes and, as it fades, myointimal proliferation may produce stenoses or wall weakening resulting in coronary aneurysm formation. Either situation sets the stage for subsequent thrombosis.[21,22]

CLINICAL FEATURES. The most prominent features of KD are included in the case definition guidelines of the Centers for Disease Control and Prevention (**Table 89-3**). These guidelines lack any specific serologic diagnostic test. The illness is usually self-limiting, within 4 to 8 weeks, and mortality is 2%.

Cardiac abnormalities include pericardial effusions (approximately 30%), myocarditis, mitral regurgitation (approximately 30%), aortitis and aortic regurgitation (infrequent), congestive heart failure, and atrial and ventricular arrhythmias.[21,22] Electrocardiographic findings include decreased R wave voltage, ST-segment depression, and low-amplitude or inverted T waves. Slowed atrioventricular conduction can occur. In untreated patients or patients treated with aspirin alone, coronary artery aneurysms occur in 20% to 25% of cases within 2 weeks and are associated with a mortality rate of approximately 2%. Early diagnosis and treatment with aspirin and intravenous immune globulin (IVIG) have reduced the death rate to well below 1% and the prevalence of coronary artery aneurysms to approximately 5%. Deaths usually result from acute coronary artery thrombosis in aneurysms that form following vasculitis. Noninvasive techniques disclose coronary artery aneurysms in approximately 20% of patients, compared with

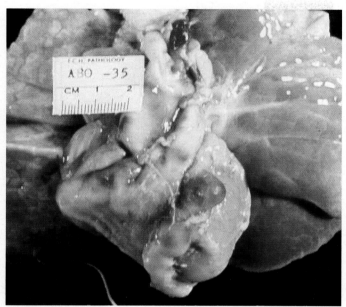

FIGURE 89-4 Giant coronary artery aneurysms caused by Kawasaki disease. Note the bulbous protrusion from the left anterior descending coronary artery. *(Courtesy of Dr. Karyl Barron.)*

60% shown by angiography. Aneurysms usually appear 1 to 4 weeks after onset of fever. New aneurysms seldom form after 6 weeks. Aneurysms are more common in the proximal than distal coronary arteries. Giant aneurysms (larger than 8 mm; **Fig. 89-4**) are the most likely to thrombose later and occlude, leading to infarction and even sudden death; endothelial abnormalities and intimal proliferation in smaller lesions (<4 mm) may lead to cardiac ischemia as well. About half of all small aneurysms will undergo angiographic regression within 1 to 2 years. Giant aneurysms rarely regress. MI may result from thrombus formation in aneurysms or severe stenoses and occurs most commonly in the first year after illness, but may occur years later.[19]

Postmortem studies have also demonstrated vasculitis of the aorta and of the celiac, carotid, subclavian, and pulmonary arteries. Rare case reports of gut vasculitis in KD exist. Gastrointestinal (GI) morbidity may depend more on small-vessel than large-vessel disease.

DIFFERENTIAL DIAGNOSIS. Given the resemblance of KD to infectious diseases, competing diagnoses include bacterial, spirochetal (e.g., leptospirosis), rickettsial (e.g., Rocky Mountain spotted fever), and viral illnesses. Drug reactions, poisonings, juvenile rheumatoid arthritis, SLE, other vasculitides, and malignancies, especially lymphomas and leukemias, may also share aspects of KD.

TREATMENT. Before the use of high dosages of aspirin and IVIG, coronary artery aneurysms were relatively common. The current standard of care consists of 2 g/kg of IVIG as a single infusion. Treatment provided within the first 10 days of illness shows efficacy most convincingly. Aspirin (80 to 100 mg/kg/day until the patient is afebrile) has both anti-inflammatory and antithrombotic effects. After fever subsides, the dose of aspirin is reduced (3 to 5 mg/kg/day) to achieve primarily antiplatelet effects. This treatment should continue until the platelet count and other inflammatory markers return to normal (about 8 weeks). Long-term, low-dose aspirin is recommended for children with echocardiographically demonstrated aneurysms, although controlled studies have not proved the efficacy of such therapy. A small subset of KD patients resists conventional therapy and is prone to aneurysm formation and long-term disease sequelae. The use of corticosteroids in this group and other patients remains controversial. The increased frequency of coronary artery aneurysms in an early report of corticosteroid-treated patients has not been seen by others.[21]

Recommendations for long-term follow-up by the American Heart Association include consideration of anticoagulation therapy in children with multiple giant aneurysms and known obstructive lesions, and evaluation by stress testing during adolescence. Severe coronary artery lesions have been treated by bypass, but if disease is widespread and bypass not possible, transplantation should be considered.[19] Coronary artery bypass procedures have been reserved for patients with severe obstructive lesions, such as those involving the main left coronary artery (LCA) or at least two of three major coronary arteries. Internal thoracic artery grafts appear to fare better than saphenous vein grafts. Data on percutaneous interventions, including those using drug-eluting stents, are limited.

Vasculitis of Small or Medium-Sized Vessels That May Affect the Cardiovascular System

Churg-Strauss Syndrome

Churg-Strauss syndrome (CSS; allergic angiitis and granulomatosis) is a very rare syndrome that typically includes a history of asthma; eosinophilia; pulmonary infiltrates; upper airway inflammation; and variable renal, neurologic, cutaneous, and cardiac involvement. Histopathologic observations from involved lesions reveal eosinophilic granulomatous infiltrates and vasculitis.

EPIDEMIOLOGY. The most generous estimates of incidence of CSS are 2.4 cases/1,000,000 persons annually. Those affected may be children or adults, with the peak group being 35 to 50 years of age and with no sex bias.[23]

PATHOGENESIS. The cause of CSS remains unknown. Nonetheless, authorities have recommended withdrawal of any newly introduced drugs or treatments (e.g., desensitization), and avoidance of new environmental stimuli (e.g., farm, workplace, if relevant to the medical history). A role for leukotriene antagonists, as used in the treatment of asthma, in precipitating CSS is the subject of controversy. Most would agree that if such an agent were introduced just before the emergence of CSS, it should be discontinued.

The granulomatous nature of CSS lesions suggests an involvement of Th1 lymphocytes and macrophages, although antineutrophil cytoplasmic antibody (ANCA), if relevant, and eosinophils argue for a role of Th2-biased lymphocytes. The latter produce IL-5, a cytokine that increases eosinophil production and release from the bone marrow.

CLINICAL FEATURES. By definition, the diagnosis of CSS requires a past or present history of atopy, usually asthma. Systemic symptoms are present in 70% to 100% of cases from different series. Chest imaging reveals infiltrates, usually multifocal, in 30% to 75%. Much less often, pulmonary nodules may be seen, as in Wegener granulomatosis (WG). In CSS, nodules seldom cavitate, a finding that is common in WG. Cardiac disease in CSS is the most common cause of death. It is reported in 15% to 55% of cases and may include pericarditis, myocarditis, and coronary arteritis. Congestive heart failure occurs in 15% to 30% of cases. Mesenteric ischemia (≈5%) contributes significantly to morbidity and mortality, and may cause frank blood per rectum, melena, or bowel perforation. Many more patients have abdominal pain (30% to 60%) for which the ultimate cause is suspected to be CSS. The small intestine and colon are the sites more often affected. Peripheral neurologic abnormalities (sensory and/or motor) affect more than two thirds of patients. Approximately 50% of patients have musculoskeletal symptoms and rashes, and renal disease (glomerulonephritis) affects at least one third.

DIFFERENTIAL DIAGNOSIS. CSS may be confused with WG. Patients who suffer from WG do not have an unusually high frequency of allergies, asthma, and striking eosinophilia, but some patients with WG have a more modest peripheral eosinophilia (≈10%).

Other considerations in the differential diagnosis include parasitic infections, especially helminths (e.g., larvae and adults of hookworm, ascaris, trichinella, strongyloides, filaria, flukes) that may produce chronic eosinophilia by stimulating IL-5 in affected organs. Because helminths may migrate through the lungs, infiltrates and bronchospasm may result, producing a picture of eosinophilic pneumonia and asthma. Idiopathic hypereosinophilic syndrome (HES) is a diagnosis to be considered only after exclusion of all other causes of eosinophilia. In some cases, HES is part of a leukoproliferative syndrome and may be associated with splenomegaly, cytogenetic abnormalities, myelofibrosis, myelodysplasia, anemia, and abnormal red blood cell forms. The absence of vasculitis and asthma distinguishes HES from CSS. HES has particular interest for cardiologists because of the risks of cardiac fibrosis, ventricular apical necrosis, valvular dysfunction, and intraventricular thrombus formation. Myocarditis and cardiac fibrosis may lead to a restrictive cardiomyopathy.

TREATMENT. Corticosteroids (usually prednisone, 1 mg/kg/day orally) usually produce dramatic improvement. In patients with critical organ system involvement (heart, brain, kidneys, gut), it may be prudent to provide pulse IV therapy (methylprednisolone, 1 g/day) for 1 to 3 days. Although recommended, this regimen has never been the subject of controlled clinical trials. Patients who are critically ill should also receive a second agent (usually cyclophosphamide). Cyclophosphamide is used daily in a dose of 2 mg/kg, assuming normal renal function. In the presence of renal impairment, the dose must be proportionately reduced to avoid severe bone marrow suppression. Long-term cyclophosphamide therapy carries many risks, and cyclophosphamide is now used to induce remission. Then, after 3 to 6 months, if remission continues, cyclophosphamide is switched to maintenance therapy with daily azathioprine or weekly methotrexate.

Polyarteritis Nodosa

Polyarteritis nodosa (PAN) is a nongranulomatous disease of only medium-sized arteries. The older PAN literature has been a source of confusion. Those series included patients with both PAN and microscopic polyangiitis (MPA), a disease that can have features of PAN but is defined by the presence of small-vessel vasculitis (capillaries, venules, and arterioles). Today, cases of nongranulomatous vasculitis with glomerulonephritis (renal capillaritis) and pulmonary infiltrates (alveolitis or capillaritis) would be considered MPA and not PAN, according to the Chapel Hill Consensus Conference (CHCC) on Nomenclature. The guidelines also stress that PAN and MPA are not mediated by immune complex and are not secondary forms of vasculitis, although hepatitis B and C can produce similar syndromes.

EPIDEMIOLOGY. Because not all researchers strictly adhere to the CHCC guidelines, it is difficult to know the incidence of PAN. Even liberal application of these guidelines indicates that PAN is a rare disease, with an annual incidence of less than 1/100,000. Some include vasculitis caused by hepatitis, mediated by immune complexes and cryoglobulins, in this figure. Men and women are equally affected. PAN may affect people of any age, but the incidence peaks between 40 and 60 years of age.

PATHOGENESIS. When one properly excludes cases associated with hepatitis, the cause of medium-sized vessel vasculitis compatible with PAN is unknown. The histopathology of lesions varies and often evolves over time, at first having a predominance of neutrophils and later, of mononuclear cells. Granulomas and increased numbers of eosinophils are not present. Necrotizing changes may follow, with weakening of the vessel wall and aneurysm formation (**Fig. 89-5**) or myointimal proliferation, causing stenosis and occlusion.

CLINICAL FEATURES. Systemic symptoms occur in at least half of patients in different series. Any organ system can be involved. However, if one adheres to CHCC guidelines, several features should not be included because they reflect microvascular (capillary or venule) disease—palpable purpura, pulmonary infiltrates, or

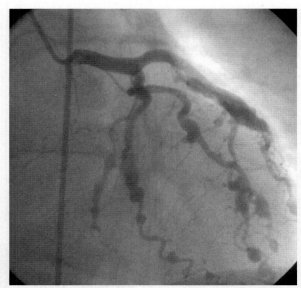

FIGURE 89-5 Coronary artery aneurysms caused by PAN.

hemorrhage and glomerulonephritis. In contrast, these findings occur in MPA.

PAN would more typically include deep skin inflammatory changes that may produce painful nodules (similar to erythema nodosum) or progress to infarction and gangrene (30% to 50%), neuropathy (especially mononeuritis multiplex, 20% to 50%), renal infarction and insufficiency (≈10% to 30%), hypertension (approximately 30%), segmental pulmonary infarctions (<40%), and cardiac disease (10% to 30%—congestive failure, angina, infarction, pericarditis). Although musculoskeletal symptoms occur in over 50% of all PAN patients, they are not a helpful differential diagnostic feature. As noted for CSS, markers of poor prognosis include ischemia or infarction of critical organs (brain, gut, kidneys, and heart). Although clinically apparent heart disease may only affect less than one third of cases, postmortem examination may reveal medium-sized vessel vasculitis or consequences of hypertension (left ventricular hypertrophy, congestive heart failure) in up to 75%.

DIFFERENTIAL DIAGNOSIS. It is important to reemphasize that certain infections may cause inflammation of medium-sized vessels. All patients with clinical findings that resemble those of PAN should be tested for hepatitis B and C. A PAN-like presentation is usually associated with hepatitis B virus (HBV) and cryoglobulinemia, whereas an MPA-like presentation occurs more frequently in association with hepatitis C virus (HCV) infection and cryoglobulinemia. Rarely, infection with human immunodeficiency virus (HIV) may present in this fashion. In immunocompromised hosts, cytomegalovirus (CMV) should also be sought as a possible cause of small and medium-sized vessel disease. The PAN-MPA–like spectrum obligates a search for bacterial and fungal infections as causes of endocarditis or endovascular vegetations. Use and abuse of vasoactive drugs (e.g., cocaine, amphetamines, ephedrine) should also be considered (see Chap. 73). PAN is not associated with ANCA. No serologic diagnostic tests exist for PAN; the diagnosis depends on biopsy or angiographic proof of medium-sized vessel inflammation (**Fig. 89-6**), but the angiograms are not specific for PAN.

TREATMENT. The guidelines for treatment are the same as those for CSS. Not all patients with PAN require the addition of a cytotoxic agent (cyclophosphamide, methotrexate, or azathioprine) to the corticosteroid. In the setting of critical organ disease, however, one should not hesitate to use these agents.

Other primary vasculitides such as hypersensitivity vasculitis, Henoch-Schönlein purpura, and WG may all have cardiac consequences. However, because vasculitis-mediated heart disease is infrequent in these disorders, they will not be addressed further here. The principles of treatment resemble those noted for CSS and PAN, except that WG therapy always requires the addition of a cytotoxic agent. Although primary cardiac involvement from vasculitis is not common in WG, accelerated atherosclerosis may occur in these patients, compared with controls that are matched for age, sex, and conventional risk factors.[24,25]

Systemic Rheumatologic Disorders

Rheumatoid Arthritis

Rheumatoid arthritis (RA) is the most common form of chronic inflammatory polyarthritis. Approximately 70% of patients have rheumatoid factor (RF). The presence of RF does not confirm the diagnosis of RA, because some healthy persons and those with other diseases, including chronic viral hepatitis and bacterial endocarditis, may also have RF. Use of the anticyclic citrullinated peptide (anti-CCP) test, adds some specificity to the serologic diagnosis; it is not detected in RF-positive patients with hepatitis C. Similar to RF, anti-CCP in a patient with RA marks more aggressive disease. Systemic complications of RA include pericarditis, pleuritis, vasculitis, interstitial lung disease, atherosclerotic cardiovascular disease, and Sjögren and Felty

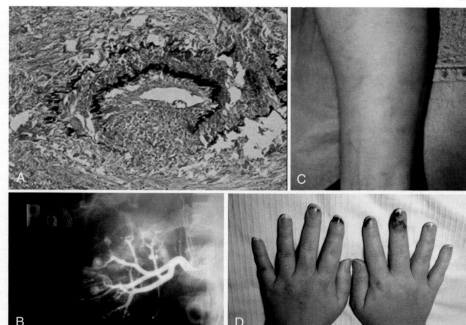

FIGURE 89-6 In PAN, the likelihood of having adequate collateral circulation to maintain tissue viability following vasoocclusion is less than that seen in other vasculitides. **A,** Section of a muscular artery showing destruction of the internal elastic lamina (from 5 to 8 o'clock), as well as intimal thickening and stenosis. **B,** Although aneurysms may be visually more striking on angiography, renovascular occlusive lesions may contribute to high-renin hypertension and renal failure. **C,** Palpable subcutaneous nodules on the patient's forearms that were painful. **D,** Infarcts on the fingers caused by severe digital artery involvement. **A,** Hematoxylin-eosin stain; magnification ×20.

syndromes. Patients with RA also have a slightly increased prevalence of lymphoma, an important consideration when estimating the risk of drug-induced lymphoproliferative disease in patients with RA.

EPIDEMIOLOGY. RA affects approximately 1% to 3% of the population. The disease affects those of all ages, but is most frequently diagnosed in women (>2:1) during their third to fifth decades of life.

PATHOGENESIS. The cause of RA is unknown. There is a genetic predisposition, but this is seemingly polygenic. There may be an infectious trigger, but no agent has been identified. An abnormal and persistent T-cell response triggers macrophage activation. TNF, IL-1, and other cytokines sustain the chronic inflammatory response, which includes angiogenesis, proliferation of synovial tissue, and bone remodeling. The dramatic efficacy of specific anti-TNF and anti–B-cell therapies suggest a dominant role for these targets in the pathogenesis of the disease.

CLINICAL FEATURES. RA is a chronic symmetrical polyarthritis that affects small and large joints, especially the metacarpophalangeal joints and wrists, sparing the lumbar and thoracic spine and distal interphalangeal joints. It affects the pericardium in approximately 40% of patients, as indicated by echocardiographic and necropsy studies (see Chap. 75). Chronic, asymptomatic effusive pericardial disease is far more common than acute pericarditis.[26] Asymptomatic pericardial abnormalities were commonly observed by echocardiography in the era before current aggressive approaches to treatment of the disease. The electrocardiogram (ECG) is usually normal in patients with chronic pericardial disease, but may show characteristic changes in acute pericarditis. Coexistent small pleural effusions are common and may reflect rheumatoid serositis or hemodynamic effects of the pericarditis. Pericardial calcification can occur, mimicking tuberculous pericarditis, but this is rare.

Limited data describe the nature of pericardial fluid in RA. Fluid is frequently blood-tinged, with leukocyte counts ranging from scant to more than 30,000/mm³, generally with a neutrophil predominance. The

glucose level in the pericardial fluid may be low when compared with serum glucose levels, similar to markedly depressed glucose levels reported in rheumatoid pleural effusions. The presence of rheumatoid factor in the fluid does not confirm the diagnosis of RA pericarditis. Constrictive pericarditis can occur and must be distinguished from restrictive cardiomyopathy, a rare complication of secondary amyloidosis in patients with longstanding RA.

Treatment of clinical pericarditis includes the use of nonsteroidal anti-inflammatory drugs (NSAIDs), intensified systemic immunosuppressive therapy, pericardial steroid injections, or pericardiocentesis if hemodynamic compromise occurs. If systemic therapy is ineffective or already at an intense level, patients with recurrent pericardial effusions may require a pericardial window. There are no data on colchicine therapy in RA pericarditis. The current use of aggressive medical therapy early in the course of rheumatoid disease may decrease the frequency of extra-articular complications of RA, including pericardial involvement.

RA does not usually cause clinically apparent myocarditis, but congestive heart failure probably occurs with increased prevalence. Secondary amyloidosis is rare in rheumatoid disease, but can cause cardiomyopathy and atrioventricular block. Focal cardiac involvement with rheumatoid nodules can occur and may be associated with conduction block. All levels of block have been described and, once established, may not respond to anti-inflammatory or immunosuppressive therapies.

Autopsy studies have indicated frequent involvement of the cardiac valves and aorta, but valve abnormalities in RA rarely cause clinical problems. Slowly progressive granulomatous valvulitis may be difficult, if not impossible, to distinguish from disease unrelated to RA. A rapidly progressive aortic valvulitis, advancing to the need for valve replacement caused by regurgitation for less than 5 years, has been described. Rheumatoid aortitis, with involvement of the aortic valve, has been reported, but aortitis is not frequently recognized antemortem. Pulmonary hypertension (PHtn) may result from rheumatoid lung disease.

Patients with RA have an increased incidence of coronary artery disease (CAD), which may be masked by limited physical activity because of joint disease. Hence, special consideration should be given to the patient with RA about to undergo major noncardiac surgery. Although currently unsupported by adequate evidence, it is reasonable to consider longstanding RA as an intermediate risk factor in assessing preoperative risk, similar to patients with renal insufficiency in the American Heart Association (AHA) guidelines. Coronary arteritis is a rarely reported complication of RA.

DIFFERENTIAL DIAGNOSIS. Rheumatoid arthritis, in the absence of characteristic radiographic erosive changes, remains a diagnosis of exclusion. Other conditions that can cause a symmetrical small and large joint polyarthritis include chronic hepatitis B and C, SLE, several vasculitides, and crystal-induced arthropathies. Early or acute RA can also be confused with bacterial endocarditis and other infections, such as parvovirus or rubella. Lyme disease (*Borrelia* sp. infection), which can cause cardiac conduction disease, produces an oligoarticular large joint arthritis that does not mimic RA.

TREATMENT. Current treatment regimens for the treatment of RA emphasize aggressive disease-modifying therapy as soon as the diagnosis is made. Combination therapy with agents such as methotrexate, sulfasalazine, leflunomide, hydroxychloroquine, and low-dose prednisone is frequently used. NSAIDs are not a mainstay of therapy because of the following: (1) they have not been shown to alter the course of RA; (2) they can increase risk of GI bleeding; and (3) chronic use of cyclooxygenase 1 (COX-1) or COX-2 inhibitors can cause renal dysfunction and hypertension.

Antagonists of TNF are extremely effective agents, although cost and the unknown long-term effects of therapy are of concern in their use. The increased use of effective therapy may be associated with a decreased incidence of extra-articular complications of RA. The use of high-dose infliximab in patients with severe CHF and RA has raised a concern over increased cardiac morbidity and mortality.[27] The data available do not clearly preclude the use of anti-TNF agents in patients with mild and controlled CHF, but warrant increased vigilance.

HLA-B27—Associated Spondyloarthropathies

The RF-negative spondyloarthropathies include ankylosing spondylitis, psoriatic arthritis, inflammatory bowel disease–associated arthritis, and postinfectious reactive arthritis.

EPIDEMIOLOGY. The vast majority of white patients with ankylosing spondylitis and many patients with other spondyloarthropathies have the HLA-B27 gene; however, most who carry this gene do not have spondyloarthritis, and gene typing should not be a routine diagnostic test. Patients with spondyloarthropathy share several features that distinguish them from rheumatoid arthritis. Although females do suffer from these disorders, ankylosing spondylitis and reactive arthritis are male-dominant diseases. The spondyloarthropathies are less common than RA.

PATHOGENESIS. The spondyloarthropathies have been historically grouped together because of some shared clinical characteristics and the disproportionate presence of the B27 antigen. Studies with transgenic rats expressing the human B27 antigen have shown that these animals, when raised in a non–germ-free environment, exhibit inflammation of skin, spine, and other tissues similar to that seen in human patients. These observations support a role for B27 in the pathogenesis of the inflammation. The B27 gene may permit an abnormal immune response to gut or mucosal bacterial antigens, which cross-react with tissue antigens present in joints, skin, and other tissues. The abnormal response includes the breakdown of tolerance to unknown self-antigens and the perpetuation of localized inflammation, a conjecture that lacks confirmation. Not all patients with spondyloarthropathies have the B27 antigen; either there are alternative pathogenic mechanisms, or the current ability to define the HLA-B locus at a molecular rather than serological level limits our full understanding of its pathogenetic role.

CLINICAL FEATURES. Unlike rheumatoid arthritis, the entire spine, not just the cervical region, may be involved. Sacroiliac joint involvement is frequent, and may be the only musculoskeletal manifestation. Large peripheral joints are commonly involved, but unlike in RA, involvement tends to be asymmetrical. There frequently is inflammation of the tendons, ligaments, or joint capsules at the point of attachment to bone (enthesis; thus, the term *enthesitis*). Diffuse tendon sheath involvement may produce sausage digits (not seen in RA). In the United States, 90% of white patients with ankylosing spondylitis and approximately 60% of patients with inflammatory bowel disease–related spondylitis have the HLA-B27 gene. The carriage rate of HLA-B27 in healthy U.S. whites is approximately 10%. It is much lower in blacks and Asians. Presence of the gene predisposes to anterior uveitis and perhaps cardiac conduction disease and proximal aortitis. Thus, patients with psoriatic arthritis, enteropathic arthritis, and reactive arthritis, as well as ankylosing spondylitis, are predisposed to these complications. Patients may express extraskeletal B27-associated complications without overt rheumatic disease.

Pericarditis, although reported, is not characteristic of the spondyloarthropathies. CAD occurs at an increased rate in psoriasis and psoriatic arthritis, but it has not been well studied in other disorders. Diastolic dysfunction may occur in patients who have HLA-B27 but rarely has clinical significance. Cardiac conduction disease can complicate ankylosing spondylitis and other B27-associated disorders. Up to one third of patients with ankylosing spondylitis develop conduction disease. Atrioventricular (AV) conduction block may initially be intermittent, but tends to progress. Conduction disease is more common in male patients, and as many as 20% of men with permanent pacemakers carry the HLA-B27 gene. Conduction disease may be the only abnormality associated with the HLA-B27 gene. Electrophysiologic studies have indicated that the level of block is usually at the AV node and is not fascicular.[28] Atrial fibrillation may occur more commonly than expected in patients with the HLA-B27 gene.

Aortic root disease has been reported in up to 100% of ankylosing spondylitis patients who also had aortic valve involvement in an autopsy series.[29] Characteristic findings include thickening of the aortic root, with subsequent dilation. Aortic cusp nodularity with proximal thickening comprises the subaortic hump, which was found in 74% of 44 selected patients with ankylosing spondylitis[30] using transesophageal echocardiography. In this study, aortic regurgitation developed in 50% of patients, and 20% of patients developed congestive heart failure, underwent valve replacement, had a stroke, or died, as compared with only 3% of age- and sex-matched volunteers. The aortic lesions progressed in 24% of patients and resolved in an additional 20% over an approximately 2-year follow-up. The severity of aortic root disease was associated with the patient's age and duration of spondylitis. Dilation and stiffening of the aortic root may contribute to the aortic regurgitation. Hence, the regurgitant murmur, as in syphilitic aortitis, may be best heard along the right sternal border. However, an electrocardiographic and transthoracic echocardiographic study of 100 Swiss men with ankylosing spondylitis of more than 15 years' duration has shown no significant increase in valvular or conduction disease.[30]

DIFFERENTIAL DIAGNOSIS. The B27-associated spondyloarthropathies are characterized by inflammation of the spine, with morning stiffness of the involved areas. Unlike RA, the peripheral arthritis is usually asymmetrical, with frequent involvement of large joints. The specific spondyloarthropathies are clinically distinguished by their associated extra-articular features (e.g., psoriasis, balanitis, urethritis, oral and/or genital ulcers). Psoriatic arthritis may be present, and severe, in the absence of significant cutaneous psoriasis. Cardiac involvement seems linked more to the presence of the HLA-B27 gene than to any specific rheumatic disorder.

TREATMENT. For years, the spondyloarthropathies have been treated symptomatically, with marginal success, with NSAIDs and physical therapy. Modification of the disease course has not been well documented with such therapy. The disease-modifying drugs used successfully in patients with RA (methotrexate, sulfasalazine) have minimal efficacy in relieving the symptoms and findings of spinal inflammation, although they often successfully relieve peripheral arthritis. The B27 extra-articular manifestations are treated, as needed, with corticosteroids (uveitis) or surgery (aortic regurgitation, aortitis). Anti-TNF agents (etanercept, infliximab, adalimumab) have demonstrated impressive clinical efficacy in treating the symptoms of spondylitis; whether they will be beneficial for treating or preventing cardiovascular manifestations is currently unknown. As noted, the use of these agents in patients with heart failure warrants vigilance.

Systemic Lupus Erythematosus

SLE is a systemic autoimmune disease characterized by the presence of immune complexes, autoantibodies, and ANAs in the setting of a constellation of clinical features, which may include serositis, arthritis, glomerulonephritis, CNS dysfunction, hemolytic anemia, thrombocytopenia, and leukopenia. More than 20% of patients with SLE have antiphospholipid antibodies (APLAs) that predispose to arterial and venous thrombosis, pulmonary hypertension, valvular dysfunction, or miscarriage (see Chap. 87).

EPIDEMIOLOGY. SLE is more common in women and can occur at any age. Both idiopathic and drug-induced SLE have cardiac manifestations. Reversible drug-induced SLE is well recognized following treatment with various cardiac medications, including procainamide, hydralazine, and quinidine.

PATHOGENESIS. Over 95% of patients with SLE have a positive ANA; however, even high titers of ANA are not diagnostic of SLE. Anti–double-stranded DNA is more specific for SLE but is present in only 50% to 70% of patients with idiopathic SLE, often in those with glomerulonephritis. SLE is an autoantibody and immune complex disorder, with immunoglobulin and complement deposition in involved organs, including the heart. The serologic findings may be detectable years before clinical disease manifests. However, the view of SLE as only an immune complex disorder is an oversimplification. Some animal models of SLE have been associated with retroviral infections, but there are no consistently demonstrable viral agents in humans with SLE. Studies of twins have suggested a role for genetic factors, and recent data support the involvement of IFN-α in SLE pathogenesis.

CLINICAL FEATURES. Pericarditis is the most commonly recognized cardiac problem in SLE (see Chap. 75).[31] Imaging and autopsy series have demonstrated pericardial involvement in more than 60% of patients, although clinically significant pericarditis occurs in less than 30%. Unexplained chest pain is common in patients with SLE, but is more likely caused by manifestations other than pericarditis. Pericarditis may occur as the initial manifestation of SLE, appear at any point during the disease course, or occur as a complication of chronic renal disease. Pericardial fluid has generally demonstrated a neutrophil predominance, elevated protein level, and low or normal glucose concentration. Complement levels in pericardial fluid tend to be low, but this is not a characteristic unique to SLE. The fluid is indistinguishable from that obtained from patients with bacterial pericarditis, and infection must therefore be excluded. Pericardial tamponade may (rarely) occur at any point in the course of SLE, including the initial presentation. When effusions occur in the setting of chronic renal failure, it is difficult to distinguish uremic from SLE pericarditis. Pericarditis, as well as tamponade, can occur with drug-induced lupus. Constrictive pericarditis, presumably as a sequela of SLE pericarditis, can occur.

Coronary arteritis, resulting in ischemic syndromes, occurs rarely in patients with SLE. The distinction between atherosclerotic CAD, which is far more common, and coronary arteritis has been inferred from sequential angiographic studies that show more rapid changes in luminal images with arteritis than those characteristic of CAD.

Additional causes of acute coronary syndromes in SLE include thrombosis, often related to the presence of APLAs and, very rarely, embolism from nonbacterial vegetative endocarditis (Libman-Sacks).

APLAs are associated in some echocardiographic studies with valve thickening and nonbacterial endocarditis. Antiendothelial cell antibodies may accelerate atherogenesis (see Fig. 15-62). The presence of APLAs independently predicted CAD in a subset analysis of the Helsinki heart study. The rare patient with coronary arteritis should be treated with high-dose corticosteroids, and patients with thrombotic disease related to APLAs should receive long-term anticoagulation. Aspirin is probably not sufficient as an anticoagulant, although therapeutic trial evidence is lacking in patients with APLAs. Thrombocytopenia is common in patients with APLAs, and may complicate therapeutic decisions.

Myocardial dysfunction in SLE is usually multifactorial and may result from immunologic injury, ischemia, valvular disease, or coexistent problems such as hypertension. Acute myocarditis is infrequent, but can be the initial presentation of SLE. Patients with peripheral skeletal myositis are reportedly at increased risk for myocarditis. Measurement of troponin I may help in the assessment of cardiac involvement, but the MB fraction of creatine kinase (CK) may be significantly elevated in the presence of skeletal myositis, even in the absence of myocarditis. Noninvasive studies have demonstrated abnormal systolic and diastolic function in patients with active SLE. These changes often reverse with control of disease activity. Acute or chronic congestive heart failure caused by SLE, in the absence of other contributing factors, is not common. Endomyocardial biopsy of the patient with cardiomyopathy and suspected SLE will not likely provide a specific diagnosis of SLE. The biopsy generally reveals patches of myocardial fibrosis, sparse interstitial mononuclear cell infiltrates, and occasional myocyte necrosis with immune complex deposition, even in areas devoid of inflammatory changes. Unexplained acute left ventricular (LV) failure in a patient with active SLE warrants a trial of corticosteroid therapy. Hydroxychloroquine-induced cardiomyopathy should be considered in patients on this drug.

Tachyarrhythmias can occur in patients with SLE with pericarditis. Sinus tachycardia may be the earliest manifestation of myocarditis. Abnormal heart rate variability may be caused by autonomic dysfunction or occult myocarditis. Unexplained sinus tachycardia, which resolves with treatment of SLE, can occur in the presence of active SLE, even when evidence of cardiac dysfunction is absent. Occult pulmonary embolism should be considered as a cause of tachycardia in patients with SLE, especially in the presence of APLAs. Abnormal myocardial single-photon emission computed tomography (SPECT) scans have been noted, even in some patients with a normal resting echocardiogram.[32]

Conduction disease is not expected in adults with SLE, but infants born to mothers with SLE, and some other systemic autoimmune diseases, have an increased incidence of congenital complete AV block. The pathogenic mechanism is the transmission of maternal anti-Ro and anti-La antibodies in utero, causing myocardial inflammation and fibrosis of the conduction system.[33] The risk for developing complete AV block in infants born to mothers carrying this antibody is low. However, women with systemic autoimmune diseases known to be associated with this antibody should be screened for its presence prior to pregnancy. If present, the fetus should be followed throughout pregnancy with ultrasound studies to detect fetal conduction abnormality or hydrops. AV block usually appears early in pregnancy and is almost always irreversible. If recognized early, dexamethasone may reverse fetal myocarditis in utero. Data to support this intervention are limited.

Valvular pathology in SLE is common. Recognized 50 years ago as noninfectious vegetations (Libman-Sacks endocarditis), transesophageal studies have shown valvular abnormalities in over 50% of patients with SLE.[34] Valvular thickening is the most common echocardiographic finding, followed by vegetations and valvular insufficiency. The vegetations generally localize on the atrial side of the mitral valve and the arterial side of the aortic valve and are usually nonmobile. Over time, the lesions may resolve or worsen; fibrosis may cause retraction of the valve, causing regurgitation. Less commonly, the vegetations on the valve may occlude the orifice, causing stenosis. Valvulitis (**Fig. 89-7**), with valve fenestrations and rapidly progressing dysfunction, can occur. The nonbacterial vegetations rarely embolize

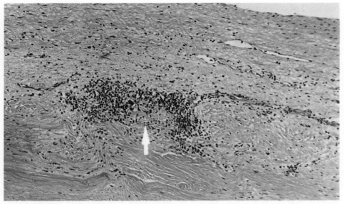

FIGURE 89-7 Valvulitis in SLE. Patients with SLE can develop valve dysfunction caused by bland vegetations (Libman-Sacks endocarditis), valve-associated thrombosis, and rarely true valvulitis. This photomicrograph illustrates aortic valve valvulitis that was discovered at the time of surgery for aortitis and aortic insufficiency (×400). The white arrow indicates a cluster of infiltrating leukocytes.

and cause stroke syndromes. Several studies have demonstrated an increased prevalence of cardiac valve dysfunction in the presence of APLA, with or without SLE. Because vegetations may occur in APLA-negative patients with SLE, multiple mechanisms may affect heart valve damage in SLE patients. Because of the high prevalence of valvular abnormalities in patients with SLE, it has been suggested that antibiotic prophylaxis for endocarditis be considered for all patients with SLE before high-risk procedures are carried out. Adequate studies do not exist to provide evidence for this proposal. There are reports of mitral and aortic valve replacement in patients with SLE.[35] Valve repair has also been described.[36] Recurrence of valve disease, particularly thrombosis, may affect prosthetic valves.

Pulmonary artery hypertension is common in SLE.[37] Clinically significant pulmonary hypertension is less common. Causes of the development of pulmonary hypertension include thromboembolic disease associated with APLAs, intimal proliferation of the pulmonary artery and, very rarely, arteritis of the pulmonary vessels. Successful heart-lung transplantation has been reported in a patient with SLE and progressive pulmonary hypertension. Aortitis with associated valvular insufficiency can occur rarely in SLE.[38]

DIFFERENTIAL DIAGNOSIS. Among the most common features of SLE are ANAs (>95%), arthralgias and arthritis (60% to 90%), constitutional symptoms (50% to 75%), rash (50% to 80%), Raynaud vasospasm (30% to 60%), and glomerulonephritis (30% to 75%). Characteristic features that enhance diagnostic likelihood include butterfly rash, sun-sensitive skin eruptions, discoid skin lesions, cytopenias (especially thrombocytopenia and leukopenia), antibodies to double-stranded DNA and Sm (anti-Smith), hypocomplementemia, and characteristic findings on biopsies of involved sites. Diseases that can be confused with SLE include dermatomyositis, infections, particularly endocarditis, lymphomas, thrombotic thrombocytopenic purpura, immune thrombocytopenic purpura, Still disease, and sarcoidosis. The pattern of cardiac involvement in SLE is not diagnostic.

TREATMENT. There is no single treatment for SLE. The specific manifestations are managed on an individual basis. Life-threatening organ involvement is controlled by high-dose corticosteroids, often with the addition of cyclophosphamide, azathioprine, or mycophenolate. Patients with mild pericarditis without threat of hemodynamic compromise are generally treated with a short course of NSAID therapy, unless there is a contraindication, such as renal insufficiency. Corticosteroids are used for more severe disease. There are no data on colchicine for the treatment of lupoid pericarditis. If prompt response to steroid therapy does not occur, large sterile pericardial effusions, particularly those accompanied by fever and/or hemodynamic compromise, are best treated with drainage and, if recurrent,

consideration of a pericardial window. Arteritis and myocarditis are treated with high-dose corticosteroids, with or without adjunctive cyclophosphamide or azathioprine. Corticosteroid therapy may be tried for acute valvulitis; the indications for surgery are the same as for other causes of valvular dysfunction.

Antiphospholipid Antibody Syndrome

APLA syndrome (APLAS; see Chap. 87) is defined as the presence of either APLA or a lupus anticoagulant and a history of otherwise unexplained recurrent venous or arterial thrombosis, or frequent second- or third-trimester miscarriages. Thrombocytopenia, hemolytic anemia, and livedo reticularis are commonly present. APLAs are common (10% to 30%) in SLE, although not all these patients will exhibit the clinical syndrome. Low to moderate levels of APLA can also accompany a number of infectious and other autoimmune diseases, usually without clinical consequence. In the absence of an underlying systemic disease, APLAS is termed *primary*. The presence of APLA or a lupus anticoagulant, in the absence of sequelae, does not routinely warrant therapy.

EPIDEMIOLOGY. The true prevalence of the antiphospholipid antibody syndrome is unknown. The demonstration of a lupus anticoagulant or APLAs alone does not define the clinical syndrome, which requires a coincident clinical thrombotic or embolic event(s).

PATHOGENESIS. (see Chap. 87)

CLINICAL FEATURES. Venous thromboembolic disease is the most common manifestation and usually occurs in the legs and lungs (see Chap. 77). Arterial thrombosis often causes stroke, but can occur in a wide range of locations. Primary APLAS is not associated with pericarditis, myocarditis, or conduction disease. Cardiac manifestations include thrombotic CAD, intracardiac thrombi, and nonbacterial endocarditis.[39] Heart valve abnormalities occur in approximately 30% of patients with primary APLAS and include leaflet thickening, thrombotic masses extending from the valve ring or leaflets, or vegetations. The mitral valve is affected more frequently than the aortic valve and regurgitation is far more common than stenosis (**Fig. 89-8**). Most valvular involvement is clinically silent. The first manifestation of valvular involvement with APLAS may be a thromboembolic event, such as stroke. The incidence of superimposed bacterial endocarditis is not known. Treatment of clinically significant valvular or intracardiac thrombotic masses is high-dose anticoagulation with heparin and then chronic warfarin,[40] with or without the addition of aspirin. Management of heparin dosing, in the setting of a lupus anticoagulant, which prolongs the baseline partial thromboplastin time (PTT), may require consultation with the coagulation laboratory[41] and use of special assays. Vegetations may resolve with anticoagulation therapy over several months,[42] but may also resolve spontaneously. Patients with APLAS have elevated risk for MI and reocclusion following coronary intervention or bypass grafting. Aggressive prophylactic anticoagulation should be used perioperatively in patients with APLAS and previous thrombosis. Pulmonary hypertension can occur in patients with APLAS secondary to chronic thromboembolic disease, or pulmonary arteriolar intimal proliferation.

DIFFERENTIAL DIAGNOSIS. The differential diagnosis of APLAS includes SLE, thrombocytopenic purpura (TTP), idiopathic thrombocytopenic purpura (ITP), and occult neoplasia. SLE can involve the heart, as discussed earlier. TTP can cause myocardial ischemia, but not valvular disease; occult neoplasia is associated with nonbacterial thrombotic endocarditis.

TREATMENT. The primary therapy of APLAS is anticoagulation, generally to a level similar to that for patients with prosthetic valves. Preliminary studies have supported aspirin treatment for arterial disease, although many clinicians prefer to use warfarin, and prospective trials have indicated that an international normalized ratio (INR) of approximately 2.0 to 2.5 is sufficient (older, retrospective studies

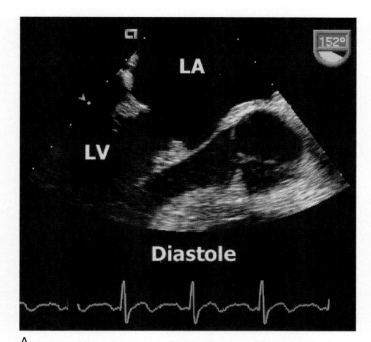

FIGURE 89-8   A, B, Transesophageal echocardiogram demonstrating large masses representing sterile vegetations in a 41-year-old male with a previous history of deep venous thrombosis, symptoms of dyspnea on exertion, and a holosystolic apical murmur. A transthoracic echocardiogram demonstrated severe mitral regurgitation. The presence of opposing lesions on both the anterior (right) and posterior (left) leaflets of the mitral valve, also known as kissing vegetations, is characteristic of the anticardiolipin antibody syndrome. *(Courtesy of Dr. Mario Garcia, Cleveland Clinic, Cleveland.)*

had suggested a target INR of 3.0) for venous thrombosis. Monitoring the anticoagulation level can be difficult in the presence of a prolonged PTT, but use of weight-based algorithms or low-molecular-weight heparin while waiting for a full warfarin effect makes this easier. There are no long-term controlled studies on the effect of chronic anticoagulation and valve disease. Valve replacement can be successful in these patients; the indications for surgery are the same as for other patients. The need for lifelong anticoagulation in these

patients may influence the choice of valve. Patients with baseline prolonged PT or INR because of the presence of lupus anticoagulant may require that warfarin therapy be monitored by the activity levels of factors II and X.

Scleroderma

Scleroderma (progressive systemic sclerosis [PSS]; CREST syndrome) and its variants are characterized by microvascular occlusive disease with vasospasm and intimal proliferation in conjunction with various patterns of cutaneous and parenchymal fibrosis. Although early lesions are inflammatory, the most obvious clinical manifestations result from enhanced fibrosis.

EPIDEMIOLOGY. Scleroderma is a rare disease. An increased prevalence occurs in certain populations, such as the Choctaw Native Americans. The average onset occurs between 45 and 65 years of age. Children are infrequently affected. Among younger individuals, there is a female bias (approximately 7:1 versus 3:1 for entire scleroderma cohorts).

PATHOGENESIS. The cause of scleroderma is unknown. An increased frequency of autoimmune disorders and autoantibodies in relatives of patients suggests the importance of genetic factors. Nonetheless, scleroderma affects both members of twin pairs extremely rarely, indicating that if inheritance plays a role, it is complex, almost certainly polygenic, and perhaps influenced by environmental factors. The latter view is supported by the association of scleroderma-like conditions with exposure to tainted oils (e.g., rapeseed oil) and drugs (e.g., certain preparations of L-tryptophan).

The earliest lesions are mononuclear infiltrates, primarily T lymphocytes, surrounding small arteries. Endothelial injury and vascular leak probably accounts for the edema seen in the early stages of scleroderma in some patients. Immunocyte and endothelial cell activation yields release of cytokines (e.g., transforming growth factor-β, PDGF, IL-4), stimulating an increase in fibroblast production of extracellular matrix macromolecules, especially types I and III collagen and glycosaminoglycans. Over 90% of patients are ANA-positive in both PSS and the more limited CREST (**c**alcinosis, **R**aynaud phenomenon, **e**sophageal dysmotility, **s**clerodactyly, **t**elangiectasia) variant.

CLINICAL FEATURES. Raynaud phenomenon usually precedes skin hardening and ultimately occurs in more than 90% of patients, supporting the initial and critical role of vascular dysfunction. Common features among patients with limited CREST or generalized PSS are arthralgias (more than 90%), esophageal dysmotility (more than 80%), telangiectasias (90% with CREST, approximately 60% with generalized disease) and pulmonary fibrosis (35% of CREST, 70% generalized). Renal crisis[43] is 20-fold more common in generalized disease than in CREST (20% versus 1%). Calcinosis may occur in both subtypes, but is twice as common in the CREST variant (40% versus 20%). Generalized PSS is distinguished by proximal cutaneous fibrosis. Thus, the term *limited* is not meant to indicate the absence of risk of visceral disease, but only refers to the distribution of skin involvement. The pattern of visceral involvement differs somewhat between CREST and PSS.

Pericardial involvement is common in PSS, and includes fibrinous pericarditis in up to 70% of patients at autopsy (see Chap. 75).[44] Echocardiography demonstrates small pericardial effusions in less than 40% of patients. Acute pericarditis syndromes, including large effusions, occasionally occur. Pericarditis with effusions may require corticosteroid therapy, but there is concern over the risk of inducing scleroderma renal crisis with the use of corticosteroids.

Necropsy and endomyocardial biopsies have demonstrated the presence of patchy fibrosis, occasionally with contraction band necrosis. These findings may result from intermittent intense ischemia produced by microvascular occlusion, perhaps caused by vasospasm. The epicardial coronary arteries are generally angiographically normal. However, approximately 80% of PSS and 65% of CREST patients have fixed perfusion defects on scintigraphic imaging. MIs can occur in PSS patients who have angiographically normal coronary arteries. Ventricular conduction abnormalities are common and, along with a septal pseudoinfarct pattern, correlate with reduced myocardial function with exercise. Abnormalities can be found throughout the conduction system, and more than 60% of patients have ventricular ectopy. Patients with scleroderma, especially those with a history of palpitations or syncope, are prone to sudden death.[45] The risk of sudden death is further increased in patients with coexistent skeletal myositis. Primary valvular disease is not common. Renal crisis[43] may be associated with minimal or extreme hypertension, rapidly rising creatinine level, microangiopathy, thrombocytopenia, and left ventricular failure. Treatment is with angiotensin-converting enzyme (ACE) inhibitors, and other antihypertensive medications, if needed—not with corticosteroids. The goal is rapid control of the blood pressure in the low-normal range.

Pulmonary hypertension occurs in limited scleroderma and PSS and is a major clinical problem (see Chap. 78). This complication may result from intrinsic pulmonary artery disease or from interstitial fibrosis.[46] Patients with CREST, as well as PSS, should undergo periodic echocardiography to screen for asymptomatic pulmonary hypertension.

DIFFERENTIAL DIAGNOSIS. Initially, before skin hardening occurs, SLE, RA, or severe primary Raynaud disease can be confused with scleroderma. Buerger disease does not lead to thick tight skin and is more often seen in male smokers, but can cause Raynaud phenomenon and digital necrosis (see Chap. 61). Cryoglobulinemia and its primary causes (hepatitis, malignancy, other systemic autoimmune diseases) should be excluded in patients who present with principally vascular symptoms and ischemic lesions. Eosinophilic fasciitis, carcinoid syndrome, nephrogenic sclerosis associated with gadolinium exposure, and several paraneoplastic syndromes can, rarely, also cause some diagnostic confusion. In time, the emergence of features typical of scleroderma usually enables clarification of diagnosis.

TREATMENT. At present, there is no proven effective treatment to limit the progression of PSS. A controlled trial has suggested that cyclophosphamide may slightly slow the progression of pulmonary involvement in some patients. Treatment of Raynaud vasospasm is symptomatic. Gastric reflux is often severe and can be improved by avoiding food and liquid intake before reclining, not assuming a fully horizontal position (wedged pillows for beds or raising the head of the bed), and by aggressive antacid regimens with proton pump inhibitors. Renal crisis usually responds to aggressive control of blood pressure; ACE inhibitors are the initial agents of choice, and the need for renal replacement therapy may be temporary. A few complications (e.g., myositis, alveolitis, pericarditis) may respond to corticosteroids, but steroid use increases the risk for renal crisis. Conduction disease and arrhythmias are treated as they would be in the absence of PSS. Pulmonary hypertension may respond to vasodilator therapy with endothelin antagonists or prostanoids.

Polymyositis and Dermatomyositis

Weakness of proximal more than distal skeletal muscles characterizes polymyositis (PM) and dermatomyositis. The CK level is usually elevated. Respiratory muscles can be clinically involved. Both conditions can be associated with fever, interstitial lung disease, and sometimes myalgias. Other visceral organ involvement is uncommon in adults. Dermatomyositis has characteristic skin lesions, which include extensor surface and extensor tendon erythema; Gottron papules overlying the knuckles, elbows, and knees; edema of the eyelids; and a photosensitive diffuse papular eruption with scaling. Dermatomyositis may be a paraneoplastic syndrome in patients older than 40 years of age.

EPIDEMIOLOGY. The incidence of inflammatory myositis is about 2 to 10 new cases/1,000,000 population annually. People of all races and ethnicities may develop PM or dermatomyositis. There is a female dominance of 2.5:1. In children, there is less sex bias (1:1), but

when myositis coexists with other autoimmune diseases (e.g., SLE, scleroderma—overlap syndromes), the bias is enhanced (10:1 females). When myositis coexists with malignancy in the adult population (mean age, 60 years), it is not sex-biased. Inflammatory myositis can affect patients of all ages. Juvenile dermatomyositis has no association with malignancy, but may be associated with arteritis, which can cause bowel ischemia.

PATHOGENESIS. The cause of these disorders is unknown. Involved muscles are infiltrated with lymphocytes, and the lymphocyte subsets and histopathologic pattern of inflammation differ between the two disorders. PM is characterized by endomysial mononuclear cell infiltration, although in dermatomyositis there is a greater amount of perivascular inflammation and perifascicular atrophy is seen. Autoantibodies are demonstrable, and certain antibody profiles may be associated with specific clinical patterns of presentation of PM and response to therapy; currently, however, these autoantibodies cannot be used to dictate therapeutic decisions.

CLINICAL FEATURES. Both diseases affect skeletal muscle, but can also affect the heart. Pericarditis is not common but can occur when polymyositis occurs as part of an overlap syndrome with other autoimmune diseases, such as SLE or PSS. Localized or generalized myocardial dysfunction is common by echocardiographic assessment, but infrequently causes clinical heart failure. The cardiomyopathy may be steroid-responsive. Corticosteroid myopathy, a complication of treatment that can mimic PM, although with a normal CK level, generally affects skeletal but not respiratory or cardiac muscle. PM and dermatomyositis frequently affect the conduction system. In an electrocardiographic study of 77 patients, 23% had conduction block,[47] which can occur in the absence of cardiomyopathy. Pulmonary hypertension can occur, but is usually related to interstitial lung disease. Acute alveolitis can at times mimic acute heart failure. Acute dysphagia caused by muscle dysfunction can predispose to aspiration.

DIFFERENTIAL DIAGNOSIS. PM causes a chronically elevated CK level and/or proximal weakness. Statin therapy can cause myopathy, and occasionally an elevated CK level, and thus can mimic PM. Myalgias are more common than in PM, and weakness less common in statin-associated myopathy. Other drugs (e.g., colchicine, hydroxychloroquine, azidothymidine [AZT]) can also induce elevations in the CK level, and drug-induced myopathy should always be considered before proceeding with diagnostic tests for PM (e.g., electromyography, biopsy). Hypothyroidism can mimic PM. Inclusion body myositis causes an elevated CK level, but usually is more indolent than PM and frequently also involves the distal muscles. The distinction is important, because it is less responsive to therapy. Polymyalgia rheumatica is not associated with an increase in muscle enzyme levels or weakness, but causes proximal muscle stiffness and pain. Dermatomyositis is recognized by one of several characteristic rashes, although SLE can mimic the rash in some patients.

TREATMENT. There are no controlled trials to guide treatment decisions. Nonetheless, initial therapy of inflammatory myositis when an underlying malignancy is not identified includes high doses of daily oral corticosteroids. In severe disease—that is, in the setting of dysphagia or myocarditis—a pulse regimen of several grams of methylprednisolone is often prescribed. Many clinicians frequently use a second agent (e.g., methotrexate, azathioprine, cyclosporine, tacrolimus) along with corticosteroids from the outset or if the patient demonstrates a chronic requirement for high-dose corticosteroid therapy. Long-term immunosuppressive therapy is frequently required. Refractory cases may respond to the addition of monthly high-dose IVIG therapy (~2 g/kg).

Sarcoidosis

Sarcoidosis is a granulomatous inflammatory disease of unknown cause that primarily affects the lung parenchyma, but can cause

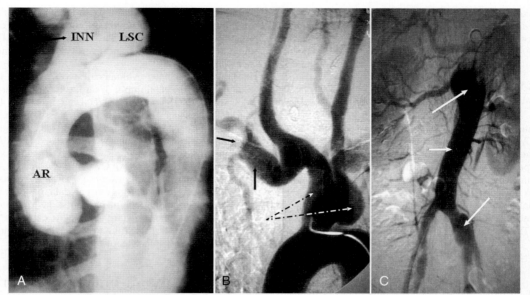

FIGURE 89-9 Sarcoid vasculitis shown in this aortogram from a 20-year-old black man who presented with chronic polyarthritis, uveitis, Bell's palsy, and upper extremity claudication. The angiogram shows aneurysmal dilation of the innominate and proximal subclavian arteries (dashed arrows), the entire aortic root (AR; **A**), occlusion of both subclavian vessels (arrows) associated with arm claudication **(B)**, and stenosis of the iliac vessels **(C)**. Note how sarcoid vasculitis can mimic TA. However, TA is associated with stenoses three to four times more often than aneurysms. Therefore, this angiographic picture should raise the differential diagnosis of TA. INN = innominate artery; LSC = left subclavian artery.

adenopathy, arthropathy, myositis, fever, renal, CNS, liver, skin, eye, aortitis, and cardiac disease.

EPIDEMIOLOGY. Sarcoidosis can affect men and women of all ages; peak incidence is in the second to fourth decade. The prevalence varies with the degree of vigilance applied to screening and susceptibility of populations. Consequently, in Sweden, the prevalence is 64/100,000, although in the United States it has variably been reported as 10 to 40/100,000. The manifestations of the disease are seemingly different in different populations. Scandinavians seem more predisposed to acute sarcoid (Löfgren syndrome). There is a preponderance of cases with cardiac involvement reported from Japan. Blacks and Hispanics seem more prone to severe multisystem disease.

PATHOGENESIS. The cause of sarcoidosis is unknown. A multicenter U.S. study has found limited evidence to support an environmental or occupational exposure cause. In contrast, studies have linked infectious agents, including mycobacterial and propionibacterial organisms, with sarcoidosis. Evidence of polyclonal B-cell activation in the blood and several reports of transmission of sarcoidosis to recipients of organs donated by patients with sarcoidosis have also supported the presence of a transmissible agent, despite the generally successful use of immunosuppressive therapy. There is evidence for a genetic predisposition to sarcoidosis, including familial clustering and shared HLA haplotypes in different populations. Some data link TNF to the pathogenesis of sarcoidosis—hence, the use of anti-TNF therapies for severe manifestations. Scarring from granulomatous inflammation may result in a focus for arrhythmia.

CLINICAL FEATURES. Pericarditis has been described and necropsy studies have documented cardiac involvement in 27% of patients. Clinically significant pericarditis is uncommon. The granulomatous infiltrative disease of the myocardium is often asymptomatic, but can cause arrhythmias, conduction disease and, rarely, otherwise unexplained congestive heart failure (see Chap. 70). Granulomatous infiltration may be patchy, with a predilection toward involvement of the left ventricle, particularly the upper septal area. This distribution influences the likelihood of obtaining a diagnostic right-sided endomyocardial biopsy. MRI with gadolinium may be helpful in

determining and the need for and duration of immunosuppressive therapy, but this approach has not been proven in any formal trial (see Chap. 18 and Fig. 18-13). Sarcoid-dilated cardiomyopathy may be difficult to distinguish from idiopathic cardiomyopathy or occasionally from giant cell myocarditis. Conduction disease is more common than pump dysfunction in patients with sarcoidosis.[48] Biopsy may help distinguish sarcoidosis from idiopathic or giant cell myocarditis, but the diagnostic yield of endomyocardial biopsy is low.[49] Active sarcoidosis is generally believed to be steroid-responsive. However, myocardial involvement with sarcoid can result in large patches of fibrotic scar that may be arrhythmogenic and not responsive to steroids.

Pulmonary artery hypertension and cor pulmonale can occur in sarcoidosis, generally as a result of pulmonary fibrosis. Systemic vasculitis is an uncommon complication of sarcoidosis. Its prevalence remains unknown. Sarcoid vasculitis can affect small- to large-caliber vessels, including the aorta. The latter presentation can be easily confused with Takayasu arteritis (**Fig. 89-9**). Black patients appear predisposed to developing large-vessel involvement.

DIFFERENTIAL DIAGNOSIS. Clinically, there are many mimics of systemic sarcoidosis, including chronic viral hepatitis, granulomatous hepatitis, SLE, Still disease, lymphoma, HIV infection, fungal infections, and Sjögren syndrome. When tissue specimens are available, special stain and culture assays should be performed to seek fungal and mycobacterial infection. The ACE level should not be relied on as a diagnostic test. Cardiac sarcoidosis is usually diagnosed by the presence of otherwise unexplained cardiomyopathy or conduction disease in the presence of documented pulmonary or hepatic sarcoidosis. Patients thought to have arrhythmogenic right ventricular dysplasia have a high (15%) prevalence of probable sarcoidosis on biopsy.

TREATMENT. Although corticosteroid therapy may be palliative for all forms of sarcoidosis, including vasculitis, relapses of the disease are common and may preclude total withdrawal of treatment. Myocardial involvement is generally treated with long-term therapy, and frequently steroid-sparing therapies such as methotrexate are added empirically. Morbidity from disease and treatment is common. There are no controlled trials of therapeutic interventions in cardiac sarcoidosis, and specifically there is no evidence to guide the duration of therapy. The serum ACE level is an imperfect guide to therapy.

Because ventricular arrhythmias may result from scarring, they may not respond to anti-inflammatory therapies and may require an implantable device.

Cardiovascular Risk in Rheumatic Diseases

Systemic rheumatic diseases have been associated with increased cardiovascular (CV) morbidity and mortality and a high prevalence of subclinical atherosclerosis. These chronic inflammatory diseases may share some pathogenic pathways with atherosclerosis, a disease that shares inflammatory mechanisms.

Patients with RA have an increased mortality rate as compared with the general population,[50] mostly attributable to cardiovascular disease (CVD), with a relative risk of at least 2 compared with age-matched normal controls. The risk remains similar after adjusting for known and potential CV risk factors.[51,52] Coronary artery atherosclerosis, as detected by the presence of calcification on cardiac computed tomography (CT) of the coronary arteries (see Chap. 19), appears more severe and prevalent in patients with RA present for more than 10 years than in those with early RA (<5 years) and control subjects.[53] Subclinical atherosclerosis detected as an increase in the intima-media thickness of the carotid artery was also higher in patients with RA than in controls.[54] Excess CV morbidity, with increased prevalence of MI and congestive heart failure, and a higher event fatality, also occurs in RA. The cause of increased atherosclerosis in patients with RA is not known and cannot be explained solely by traditional CV risk factors. Epidemiologic studies have not shown a strikingly higher prevalence of traditional CV risk factors in patients with RA, and corticosteroid use does not explain the increased risk, although dyslipidemia may precede the development of clinical RA. RA may be associated with proatherogenic lipid profiles such as low total and high-density lipoprotein (HDL) cholesterol and high triglyceride levels, a pattern that is associated with a more atherogenic low-density lipoprotein particle.[55] HDL in patients with RA may not exert antioxidant activity and thus may not be protective.[56] Inflammation may contribute to the increased CVD in RA. Elevated systemic levels of proinflammatory cytokines as seen in RA may promote the development of atherosclerosis. Patients with more severe and active RA, advanced joint damage, extra-articular disease, and rheumatoid factor positivity appear to have a higher risk of CV mortality.[57-59] Other confounding risk factors in patients with RA include use of selective or nonselective NSAIDs, underusage of aspirin, and use of corticosteroids, which may accelerate atherosclerosis. The observation that psoriasis and psoriatic arthritis also increase CVD and the possibility that anti-inflammatory therapies may reduce CVD risk strengthen the argument that systemic inflammation (or its mediators) exacerbates atherosclerotic CVD.

The use of disease-modifying agents may reduce risk for heart failure hospitalization in RA patients.[60] Despite the known proatherogenic effects of corticosteroids, they may actually decrease the risk for CV complications in RA by decreasing inflammation. Given the limited interventional data, aggressive prevention and treatment of traditional risk factors and suppression of systemic inflammation in RA are reasonable goals.

Premature MI in patients with SLE, observed in 1976 by Urowitz and colleagues, still occurs.[61] Patients with SLE have significantly increased morbidity and mortality from CVD. The incidence of CAD in SLE patients has been estimated to be 50-fold higher than in age- and sex-matched controls without SLE. In several studies, CVD led the causes of death in patients with SLE.[62-64]

MI may be the initial manifestation of CAD in young patients with SLE. The prevalence of subclinical CAD is high, as determined by scintigraphy, cardiac CT, and autopsy studies. Evidence is increasing that traditional CV risk factors do not fully account for the increased rate of atherosclerosis in these patients, and the disease appears to be an independent risk factor. Atherosclerosis in SLE has been associated with longer duration of disease and less aggressive immunosuppressive therapy.[65] Dyslipidemia with raised triglyceride and lipoprotein(a) levels and nonprotective forms of HDL have been described in patients with SLE.[66] Treatment of SLE patients should include close monitoring and aggressive management of traditional risk factors for CVD.

Many studies have evaluated the risk of CVD in hyperuricemic patients, and a small number of studies have suggested an association between clinical gout and CVD. Data from two large prospective studies have suggested an independent association of gout with CVD and mortality.[67,68] Individuals with gout have a higher risk of death from all causes. Among men without preexisting CAD, the increased mortality risk is primarily caused by an elevated risk of CV death. The mechanism for excess risk of CV death is not clear. Although a cause-and-effect relationship between gout and cardiovascular disease cannot be determined from current data, patients with gout should have aggressive management of CV risk factors. The components of the metabolic syndrome are extremely common in patients with gout.[69] Animal and a few human studies have demonstrated a direct role for hyperuricemia in causing hypertension.

Nonsteroidal Anti-Inflammatory Drugs and the Risk of Cardiovascular Disease

There has been great interest in the CV effect of nonselective NSAIDs and selective COX-2 inhibitors. Published data have supported either a detrimental or salubrious effect on CV events. Initially, attention was given to the selective COX-2 inhibitors after rofecoxib was shown to increase the risk of major coronary events.[70] Epidemiologic studies have raised concern over the use of NSAIDs and have suggested that these drugs may increase CVD by increasing systolic blood pressure, exacerbating congestive heart failure, antagonizing the beneficial effect of aspirin, or promoting thrombosis.[71] Despite anti-inflammatory and (generally reversible) antiplatelet effects, the nonselective NSAIDs do not seem to protect against MI. Instead, one large-population, case-control study has shown an increased risk of MI with the use of rofecoxib, diclofenac, and ibuprofen, even when adjusted for many potential confounders.[72] Another large population-based, matched, case-control study has found that traditional NSAIDs and COX-2 inhibitors are associated with an increased risk of first MI of approximately 40%.[73] A major potential confounder in nonrandomized studies is related to the study populations. Many patients may have an increased baseline risk of CVD and, without appropriate control data, even randomized trials are difficult to interpret. In addition, the timing of exposure of patients to the drugs, in relation to the cardiac event, is often unclear.

In contrast, the use of naproxen is associated with reduced rates of CVD events in patients with RA, and a meta-analysis of observational studies has suggested a modest CVD protective association with naproxen.[74] In a relatively small cohort of patients with early inflammatory polyarthritis, NSAID use was not associated with increased risk of all-cause mortality or CV mortality. Patients who were exposed to NSAIDs tended to have a lower risk of dying than patients who did not receive NSAIDs. This relationship was particularly strong for CV mortality, and ever being exposed to NSAIDs was associated with a 2.5-fold reduction in the risk of CV death. Control of inflammation may result in a beneficial effect on the CV system, although the anti-inflammatory efficacy of these drugs in the doses used is arguable. The study did not show any further CVD benefit from increasing duration of NSAID exposure. Despite the lack of evidence of a true cardioprotective effect of NSAIDs, this study suggested that NSAID use alone does not explain the increased risk of CVD in patients with arthritis.[75]

Despite the concerns from observational and a few prospective trials, the absolute risk of an NSAID inducing a cardiovascular event in a given patient seems to be low, and the benefits of pain reduction must be taken into consideration. Nonetheless, when using NSAIDS, their tendency to increase blood pressure and water retention, cause renal insufficiency, and induce gastropathy and enteritis must always be taken into consideration.

ACKNOWLEDGMENT

We gratefully acknowledge the contributions of Dr. Gary S. Hoffman to an earlier version of this chapter, and to our understanding of the vasculitic disorders.

REFERENCES

Takayasu Arteritis

1. Kerr GS, Hallahan CW, Giordano J, et al: Takayasu's arteritis. Ann Intern Med 120:919, 1994.
2. Hashimoto Y, Tanaka M, Hata A, et al: Four years follow-up study in patients with Takayasu arteritis and severe aortic regurgitation; assessment by echocardiography. Int J Cardiol 54(Suppl):173, 1997.
3. Seko Y, Sato O, Takagi A, et al: Restricted usage of T-cell receptor V alpha-V beta genes in infiltrating cells in aortic tissue of patients with Takayasu's arteritis. Circulation 93:1788, 1996.
4. Maksimowicz-McKinnon K, Clark TM, Hoffman GS: Takayasu's arteritis: Limitations of therapy and guarded prognosis in an American cohort. Arthritis Rheum 56:1000, 2007.
5. Tso E, Flamm SD, White RD, et al: Takayasu's arteritis: Utility of magnetic resonance imaging in diagnosis and treatment. Arthritis Rheum 46:1634, 2002.
6. Webb M, Chambers A, Al-Nahhas A, et al: The role of F-FDG PET in characterizing disease activity in Takayasu arteritis. Eur J Nucl Med Mol Imaging 31:627, 2004.
7. Arnaud L, Haroche J, Malek Z, et al: Is ^{18}F-Fluorodeoxyglucose positron emission tomography scanning a reliable way to assess disease activity in Takayasu arteritis? Arthritis Rheum 60:1193, 2009.
8. Pfizenmaier DH, Al Atawi FO, Castillo K, et al: Predictor of left ventricular dysfunction in patients with Takayasu's arteritis or giant cell aortitis. Clin Exp Rheumatol 22(Suppl 36):S41, 2004.
9. Hoffman GS, Leavitt RY, Kerr GS, et al: Treatment of Takayasu's with methotrexate. Arthritis Rheum 37:578, 1994.
10. Hoffman GS, Merkel PA, Brasington RD, et al: Anti-tumor necrosis factor therapy in patients with difficult to treat Takayasu arteritis. Arthritis Rheum 50:2296, 2004.
11. Molloy ES, Langford CA, Clark TM, et al: Anti-tumour necrosis factor therapy in patients with refractory Takayasu arteritis: long-term follow-up. Ann Rheum Dis 67:1567, 2008.

Giant Cell Arteritis

12. Weyand CM, Goronzy JJ: Medium and large vessel vasculitis. N Engl J Med 349:160, 2003.
13. Evans JM, O'Fallon WM, Hunder GG: Increased incidence of aortic aneurysm and dissection in giant cell (temporal) arteritis. Ann Intern Med 122:502, 1995.
14. Hoffman GS, Cid MC, Rendt-Zagar KE, et al: Infliximab-GCA Study Group: Infliximab for maintenance of glucocorticosteroid-induced remission of giant cell arteritis: a randomized trial. Ann Intern Med 146:621, 2007.
15. Hoffman GS, Cid MC, Hellmann DB, et al: A multicenter, randomized, double-blind, placebo-controlled trial of adjuvant methotrexate treatment for giant cell arteritis. Arthritis Rheum 46:1309, 2002.
16. Nesher GN, Berkun Y, Mates M, et al: Low-dose aspirin and prevention of cranial ischemic complications in GCA. Arthritis Rheum 50:1332, 2004.
17. Lee MS, Smith SD, Galor A, Hoffman GS: Antiplatelet and anticoagulant therapy in patients with giant cell arteritis. Arthritis Rheum 54:3306, 2006.

Idiopathic Aortitis

18. Rojo-Leyva F, Ratliff N, Cosgrove DM, Hoffman GS: Study of 52 patients with idiopathic aortitis from a cohort of 1,204 surgical cases. Arthritis Rheum 43:901, 2000.

Kawasaki Disease

19. Newburger JW, Takahashi M, Gerber MA, et al: Diagnosis, treatment, and long-term management of Kawasaki disease: A statement for health professionals from the Committee on Rheumatic Fever, Endocarditis and Kawasaki Disease, Council on Cardiovascular Disease in the Young, American Heart Association. Circulation 110:2747, 2004.
20. Davis RL, Waller PL, Mueller BA, et al: Kawasaki syndrome in Washington state: Race-specific incidence rates and residential proximity to water. Arch Pediatr Adolesc Med 149:66, 1995.
21. Barron K: Kawasaki disease: Etiology, pathogenesis and treatment. Cleve Clin J Med 69(Suppl 2):69, 2002.
22. Barron KS: Kawasaki disease. *In* Hoffman GS, Weyand CM (eds): Inflammatory Disease of Blood Vessels. New York, Marcel Dekker, 2002, pp 305-319.

Churg-Strauss Syndrome and Polyarteritis Nodosa

23. Watts RA, Scott DG, Lane SE: Epidemiology of Wegener's granulomatosis, microscopic polyangiitis, and Churg-Strauss syndrome. Cleve Clin J Med 69 (Suppl 2):SII84, 2002
24. deLeeuw K, Sanders J-S, Stegeman C, et al: Accelerated atherosclerosis in patients with Wegener's granulomatosis. Ann Rheum Dis 64:753, 2005.
25. Faurschou M, Mellemkjaer L, Sorensen IJ, et al: Increased morbidity from ischemic heart disease in patients with Wegener's granulomatosis. Arthritis Rheum 60:1187, 2009.

Rheumatoid Arthritis

26. Kitas G, Banks MJ, Bacon PB: Cardiac involvement in rheumatoid disease. Clin Med 1:18, 2001.
27. Sarzi-Puttini P, Atzeni F, Shoenfeld Y, Ferraccioli G: TNF-alpha, rheumatoid arthritis, and heart failure: A rheumatological dilemma. Autoimmun Rev 4:153, 2005.

HLA-B27—Associated Spondyloarthropathies

28. Bergfeldt L: HLA-B27–associated cardiac disease. Ann Intern Med 127:621, 1997.
29. Roldan CA, Chavez J, Wiest PW, et al: Aortic root disease associated with ankylosing spondylitis. J Am Coll Cardiol 32:1397, 1998.
30. Brunner F, Kunz A, Weber U, Kissling R: Ankylosing spondylitis and heart abnormalities: Do cardiac conduction disorders, valve regurgitation and diastolic dysfunction occur more often in male patients with diagnosed ankylosing spondylitis for over 15 years than in the normal population? Clin Rheumatol 25:24, 2005.

Systemic Lupus Erythematosus

31. Moder KG, Miller TD, Tazelaar HD: Cardiac involvement in systemic lupus erythematosus. Mayo Clin Proc 74:275, 1999.
32. Laganà B, Schillaci O, Tubani L, et al: Lupus carditis: Evaluation with technetium-99m MIBI myocardial SPECT and heart rate variability. Angiology 50:143, 1999.
33. Finkelstein Y, Adler Y, Harel L, et al: Anti-Ro (SSA) and anti-La (SSB) antibodies and complete congenital heart block. Ann Intern Med 148:204, 1997.
34. Roldan CA, Shively BK, Crawford MH: An echocardiographic study of valvular heart disease associated with systemic lupus erythematosus. N Engl J Med 335:1424, 1996.
35. Fluture A, Chaudhari S, Frishman WH: Valvular heart disease and systemic lupus erythematosus: Therapeutic implications. Heart Dis 5:349, 2003.
36. Perez-Villa F, Font J, Azqueta M, et al: Severe valvular regurgitation and antiphospholipid antibodies in systemic lupus erythematosus: A prospective, long-term follow-up study. Arthritis Rheum 53:460, 2005.
37. Johnson SR, Gladman DD, Urowitz MB, et al: Pulmonary hypertension in systemic lupus. Lupus 13:506, 2004.
38. Ohara N, Myiata T, Kurata A, et al: Ten years' experience of aortic aneurysm associated with systemic lupus erythematosus. Eur J Vasc Endovasc Surg 19:288, 2000.

Antiphospholipid Antibody Syndrome

39. Hojnik M, George J, Ziporen L, Shoenfeld Y: Heart valve involvement (Libman- Sacks endocarditis) in the antiphospholipid syndrome. Circulation 92:1579, 1996.
40. Lim W, Crowther MA, Eikelboom JW: Management of antiphospholipid antibody syndrome: A systematic review. JAMA 295:1050, 2006.
41. Bartholomew J: Dosing of heparin in the presence of a lupus anticoagulant. J Clin Rheumatol 4:307, 1998.
42. Agirbasli MA, Hansen DE, Byrde BF: Resolution of vegetations with anticoagulation after myocardial infarction in primary antiphospholipid syndrome. Echocardiography 10:877, 1997.

Scleroderma

43. Rhew EY, Barr WG: Scleroderma renal crisis: New insights and developments. Curr Rheumatol Rep 6:129, 2004.
44. Byers RJ, Marshall DAS, Freemont AJ: Pericardial involvement in systemic sclerosis. Ann Rheum Dis 45:393, 1997.
45. Kahan A, Coghlan G, McLaughlin V: Cardiac complications of systemic sclerosis. Rheumatology 48(Suppl 3):iii45, 2009.
46. Chang B, Schachna L, White B, et al: Natural history of mild-moderate pulmonary hypertension and the risk factors for severe pulmonary hypertension in scleroderma. J Rheumatol 33:269, 2006.

Polymyositis and Dermatomyositis

47. Stern R, Godblold J, Chess Q, Kagen L: ECG abnormalities in polymyositis. Arch Intern Med 144:2185, 1984.

Sarcoidosis

48. Kim Jessica SD, Hudson MA, Donnino R, et al: Cardiac sarcoidosis. Am Heart J 157:9, 2009.
49. Uemura A, Morimoto SI, Hiramissu S, et al: Histological diagnostic rate of cardiac sarcoidosis: Evaluation of endomyocardial biopsies. Am Heart J 138:299, 1999.
50. Avina-Zubieta JA, Choi HK, Sadatsafavi M, et al: Risk of cardiovascular mortality in patients with rheumatoid arthritis: A meta-analysis of observational studies. Arthritis Rheum 59:1690, 2008.
51. del Rincon ID, Williams K, Stern MP, et al: High incidence of cardiovascular events in a rheumatoid arthritis cohort not explained by traditional cardiac risk factors. Arthritis Rheum 44:2737, 2001.
52. Solomon DH, Karlson EW, Rimm EB, et al: Cardiovascular morbidity and mortality in women diagnosed with rheumatoid arthritis. Circulation 11:1307, 2003.
53. Chung CP, Oeser A, Raggi P, et al: Increased coronary-artery atherosclerosis in rheumatoid arthritis. Arthritis Rheum 52:3045, 2005.
54. Salmon JE, Roman MJ: Subclinical atherosclerosis in rheumatoid arthritis and systemic lupus erythematosus. Am J Med 121:S3, 2008.
55. Nurmohamed MT: Atherogenic lipid profiles and its management in patients with rheumatoid arthritis. Vasc Health Risk Manag 3:845, 2007.
56. Nurmohamed MT, Dijkmans BAC: Dyslipidemia, statins and rheumatoid arthritis. Ann Rheum Dis 68:453, 2009.
57. Gabriel SE, Crowson CS, Maradit-Kremers H, et al: Survival in rheumatoid arthritis: A population-based analysis of trends over 40 years. Arthritis Rheum 48:54, 2003.
58. Navarro-Cano G, del Rincon I, Pogosian S, et al: Association of mortality with disease severity in rheumatoid arthritis, independent of comorbodity. Arthritis Rheum 48:2425, 2003.
59. Gonzalez A, Icen M, Maradit-Kramers H, et al: Mortality trends in rheumatoid arthritis: The role of rheumatoid factor. J Rheumatol 35:1009, 2008.
60. Bernatsky S, Hudson M, Suissa S: Anti-rheumatic drug use and risk of hospitalization for congestive heart failure in rheumatoid arthritis. Rheumatology 44:677, 2005.
61. Urowitz, MB, Bookman AA, Koehler BE, et al: The bimodal mortality pattern of systemic lupus erythematosus. Am J Med 60:221, 1976.
62. Manzi S, Meilahn EN, Rairie JE, et al: Age-specific incidence rates of myocardial infarction and angina in women with systemic lupus erythematosus: Comparison with the Framingham study. Am J Epidemiol 145:408, 1997.
63. Asanuma Y, Oeser A, Shintani AK, et al: Premature coronary artery atherosclerosis in systemic lupus erythematosus. N Engl J Med 349:2407, 2003.
64. Roman MJ, Shanker BA, Davis A, et al: Prevalence and correlates of accelerated atherosclerosis in systemic lupus erythematosus. N Engl J Med 349:2399, 2003.
65. Roman MJ, Crow MK, Lockshin MD, et al: Rate and determinants of progression of atherosclerosis in systemic lupus erythematosus. Arthritis Rheum 56:3412, 2007.
66. Magadmi ME, Ahmad X, Tuskie W et al: Hyperinsulinemia, Insulin resistance and circulating oxidized low density lipoprotein in women with systemic lupus erythematosus. J Rheumol 33:50, 2006.
67. Krishnan E, Baker JF, Furst DE, et al: Gout and the risk of acute myocardial infarction. Arthritis Rheum 54:2688, 2006.

68. Choi HK, Curhan G: Independent impact of gout on mortality and risk for coronary artery disease. Circulation 116:894, 2007.

69. Feig DI, Kang DH, Johnson RJ: Uric acid and cardiovascular risk. N Engl J Med 359:1811, 2008.

70. Bresalier RS, Sandler RS, Quan H, et al: Cardiovascular events associated with rofecoxib in a colorectal adenoma chemoprevention trial. N Engl J Med 352:1092, 2005.

71. Scott PA, Kingsley GH, Scott DL: Non-steroidal anti-inflammatory drugs and cardiac failure: Meta-analyses of observational studies and randomised controlled trials. Eur J Heart Fail 10:1102, 2008.

72. Hippisley-Cox J, Coupland C: Risk of myocardial infarction in patients taking cyclo-oxygenase-2 inhibitors or conventional non-steroidal anti-inflammatory drugs: Population based nested case-control analysis. BMJ 330:1366, 2005.

73. Helin-Salmivaara A, Virtanen A, Vesalainen R, et al: NSAID use and the risk of hospitalization for first myocardial infarction in the general population: A nationwide case-control study from Finland. Eur Heart J 27:1657, 2006.

74. Watson DJ, Rhodes T, Cai B, Guess HA. Lower risk of thromboembolic cardiovascular events with naproxen among patients with rheumatoid arthritis. Arch Intern Med 162:1105, 2002.

75. Goodson NJ, Brookhart AM, Symmons DPM, et al: Non-steroidal anti-inflammatory drug use does not appear to be associated with increased cardiovascular mortality in patients with inflammatory polyarthritis: results from a primary care based inception cohort of patients. Ann Rheum Dis 68:367, 2009.

CHAPTER **90** # The Cancer Patient and Cardiovascular Disease

Thomas Force and Ming Hui Chen

Patients with cancer frequently develop complications in the cardiovascular system. These complications can occur as a result of locally invasive disease or distant spread. Pericardial effusions with tamponade and superior vena cava syndrome are relatively common manifestations of advanced cancers. The cardiovascular system can also be affected by indirect complications, most notably hyperviscosity syndromes, resulting from myeloproliferative disorders or leukemias. Finally, several of the therapies used to treat cancer, including radiation, traditional chemotherapeutics, and so-called targeted therapeutics aimed at factors that are causal or that promote cancer growth and metastasis, can also be toxic to the heart and cardiovascular system. Because cardiovascular disease and cancer are common diseases and share common risk factors, they often coexist in patients. It has become increasingly clear that optimal care of oncology patients by cardiologists and oncologists requires an understanding of both disciplines.

Direct Complications of Neoplasia

Cardiac Tumors

Primary tumors of the heart are uncommon and are usually benign (see Chap. 74). Briefly, the classes of primary tumors that involve the heart include myxomas (which account for 25% to 50% of all primary cardiac tumors), papillary fibroelastomas (10%), rhabdomyomas (of which approximately 50% occur in association with tuberous sclerosis), and lipomas and hemangiomas (5% to 10%).[1] Malignant tumors are usually sarcomas (angiosarcoma being most common) or lymphomas, although primary lymphomas of the heart occur much less frequently than secondary involvement.

In contrast, direct extension of tumors, hematogenous spread, and retrograde lymphatic extension to the heart are common.[2] Based on autopsy studies, involvement of the heart or pericardium occurs in 10% to 12% of all patients with malignant neoplasms. Tumors most likely to involve the heart are primary lung tumors (36% of all patients with cardiac involvement). The grouping of lymphoma, leukemia, and Kaposi sarcoma accounts for 20%, breast cancer for 7%, and esophageal cancer for 6%. Most of these involve the heart by direct extension or regional lymphatic invasion. Metastases to the myocardium are much less common and are often caused by hematogenous spread of melanomas or lymphomas (see Figs. 18-18 and 72-4). From 46% to 71% of patients with melanoma have metastases to the myocardium or pericardium. Although a relatively rare cancer, mesotheliomas commonly invade the pericardium (74% of patients) or myocardium (25% of patients). Patients with myocardial metastases of any origin often present with sudden onset of arrhythmia or, more rarely, conduction abnormalities.

Pericardial Involvement (see Chap. 75)

PERICARDIAL EFFUSION. The differential diagnosis of a pericardial effusion in a patient with a known malignant neoplasm includes malignant effusion, radiation-induced or drug-induced pericarditis, idiopathic pericarditis, infectious (including tuberculosis, fungal, or bacterial), and iatrogenic secondary to procedures. In one series, approximately 40% of patients with cancer and a pericardial effusion were found to have either radiation-induced (10%) or idiopathic (32%) effusions,[2] although other series have reported even higher rates.[3] Drug-induced pericarditis is typically seen after high-dose anthracycline or cyclophosphamide therapy (see later, Cardiovascular Complications of Cancer Therapeutic Agents).

CARDIAC TAMPONADE. Approximately one third of patients with pericardial involvement will present with impaired cardiac function, and cardiac compression can progress to tamponade, demanding immediate drainage. Patients' symptoms include chest pain, fever, dyspnea, cough, and peripheral edema. Tamponade without two or more signs of an inflammatory process (typical pain, friction rub, fever, diffuse ST-segment elevation) is more likely to be malignant (2.9-fold increase in risk).[3] Findings on physical examination, electrocardiography, and chest radiography are typically similar to those of pericardial effusions due to any cause. Echocardiography demonstrates the effusion, which is usually large, although it does not have to be if the fluid has accumulated quickly. However, tamponade can occur with loculated effusions, and in these cases, typical echocardiographic signs may be absent.

The acute treatment of tamponade includes careful fluid replacement as a temporizing measure if the patient is believed to be volume depleted and hemodynamic status is compromised.[3] Echocardiography-guided pericardiocentesis is required. Fluid should be sent for a full battery of diagnostic tests because, as noted, the cause is commonly noncancerous, even in patients with known cancer. If the effusion is malignant, cytologic examination of the pericardial fluid is positive in approximately 85% of patients.

Although no randomized clinical trials of various strategies have been done, the risk of recurrence of the effusion appears to be reduced by extended catheter drainage (3 ± 2 days; 11.5% recurrence) as opposed to simple pericardiocentesis (36% recurrence).[4] Recurrence of pericardial effusion can often be treated with repeated pericardiocentesis with extended catheter drainage. Some have used intrapericardial instillation of chemotherapeutic agents or sclerosing agents, but it is not clear that this approach is more effective than extended catheter drainage. On occasion, percutaneous balloon pericardiotomy or pericardiectomy may be required, but patients with malignant effusions have such a poor prognosis (median survival of

135 days in one series of 275 patients) that invasive procedures should be avoided, if possible. Therapy is directed at the underlying tumor.

CONSTRICTIVE PERICARDITIS. Constrictive or effusive-constrictive pericarditis is a late complication of chest irradiation that may be becoming more common because of the longer survival of patients with breast cancer and Hodgkin disease who typically receive chest irradiation. In a retrospective study of 635 patients with Hodgkin disease, 44 patients developed delayed pericarditis, and pericardiectomy was required in 12.[5] This study included patients who had received mantle irradiation with and without subcarinal block, and rates are lower when blocking is used (see later). The median range for time between radiation therapy and pericardiectomy is 7 to 13 years.[6] In a series of 163 patients undergoing pericardiectomy for constrictive pericarditis of various causes, prior irradiation significantly adversely affected both perioperative mortality (21.4% versus 2.7% for postradiation versus idiopathic constrictive pericarditis) and long-term survival.[3,6] Reasons for this include mediastinal fibrosis from the radiation, which limits the amount of pericardium that can be removed, increasing the risk of residual constriction. In addition, a restrictive myopathy that can follow chest irradiation and can accompany constrictive pericarditis adds significant morbidity and mortality. Patients may have underlying myocardial fibrosis and should be evaluated for this before consideration of pericardiectomy because exclusion of these patients reduces perioperative mortality.[3]

Superior Vena Cava Obstruction

Superior vena cava syndrome (SVCS) occurs when obstruction of the thin-walled superior vena cava (SVC) interrupts venous return of blood to the right atrium from the head, upper extremities, and thorax. The SVC is encircled by lymph nodes that drain from the right thoracic cavity and the lower left thorax (**Fig. 90-1**; see Fig. 16-7). SVCS often is manifested with slowly progressive symptoms worsening during weeks and recruitment of collateral circulation through several venous systems, including the azygos and internal mammary. When symptoms occur abruptly, SVCS can constitute a medical emergency.[7]

SYMPTOMS. Obstruction of the SVC can be caused by malignant or benign disease. Clinically, patients report the progressive development of shortness of breath (60%), facial swelling (50%), cough (24%), arm swelling (18%), chest pain (15%), and dysphagia (9%) as well as distorted vision, hoarseness, nausea, headache, and syncope. Physical findings include venous distention over the neck (66%) and chest wall (54%), facial edema (46%), plethora (19%), and cyanosis (19%). Symptoms may be exacerbated by lying in a supine position or bending forward. Patients with this syndrome may develop life-threatening complications, such as laryngeal or cerebral edema.

CAUSATIVE FACTORS. Seventy-five percent to 85% of cases of SVCS result from neoplasia (**Table 90-1**), with lung cancer

TABLE 90-1	Malignant Neoplasms Associated with Superior Vena Cava Syndrome in Adults*	
NEOPLASTIC DIAGNOSIS	**PERCENTAGE OF SVCS**	**DISEASE-ASSOCIATED SVCS (%)**
Lung cancer, stage 3B or 4	48-81	
Small cell lung cancer		15-45
Squamous cell cancer		20-25
Adenocarcinoma		5-25
Large cell carcinoma		4-30
Lymphoma	2-21	
Diffuse large cell lymphoma		64
Lymphoblastic lymphoma		33
Breast cancer	11	

*Includes lung cancer, lymphomas, and metastases from other solid tumors; 75% to 85% of patients with SVCS have neoplastic disease.

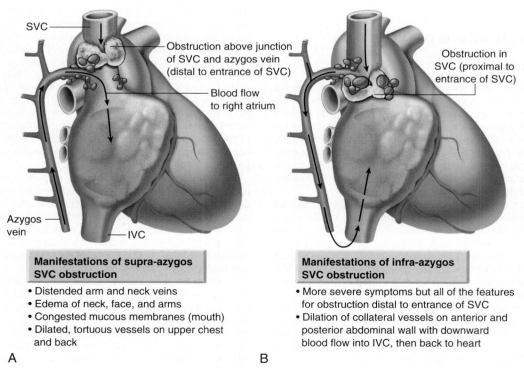

A

B

FIGURE 90-1 Anatomy of superior vena cava (SVC) syndrome. Lymph nodes may obstruct blood return above the entrance of the azygos vein (**A**), resulting in edema of the face, neck, and arms and distended veins in the neck and arms and over the upper chest. Obstruction below the return of the azygos vein (**B**) results in retrograde flow through the azygos through collateral veins to the inferior vena cava (IVC), with all the symptoms and signs in **A** plus dilation of the veins over the abdomen as well. (*Modified from Skatin AT [ed]: Atlas of Diagnostic Oncology. 3rd ed. Philadelphia, Elsevier Science, 2003.*)

accounting for most cases.[7] Of patients with lung cancer, 2% to 5% develop SVCS. However, 10% to 20% of patients with small cell lung cancer (SCLC), which constitutes only 20% of lung cancers, develop SVCS, accounting for almost 40% of patients with SVCS and lung cancer. Of patients with lung cancer–associated SVCS, 80% have right-sided primary lesions.

Lymphoma is the second most common cause of neoplasia-associated SVCS, occurring in 2% to 21% of SVCS patients. Similar to patients with lung cancer, only 1% to 5% of patients with lymphoma develop SVCS (21% of lymphoblastic lymphomas and 7% of diffuse large cell lymphomas). Of patients with primary mediastinal B-cell lymphoma with sclerosis, 57% developed SVCS. Although Hodgkin lymphoma often involves the mediastinum, SVCS rarely develops. Thymoma and germ cell tumors are other primary mediastinal malignant neoplasms that occasionally cause SVCS. The most common metastatic disease that causes SVCS is breast cancer, accounting for 11% of SVCS cases.

DIFFERENTIAL DIAGNOSIS. Benign causes of SVC obstruction not associated with neoplasia result from mediastinal fibrosis caused by radiotherapy or histoplasmosis, tuberculosis, collagen-vascular disease, arteriovenous shunts, or SVC thrombosis as a complication of central venous catheters, pacemaker leads, peritoneovenous shunts, Swan-Ganz catheters, or hyperalimentation catheters. Pacemakers and implantable cardioverter-defibrillators result in up to 30% of local venous thrombosis, in some cases associated with infection; however, SVC obstruction is uncommon and relates to acute or previous lead infection or retention of a severed lead.[8] Other benign causes include granulomas, congenital anomalies, and mediastinal fibrosis from histoplasmosis.

DIAGNOSTIC PROCEDURES. In a patient with characteristic symptoms of SVC obstruction, physical evaluation is usually informative and raises a high level of suspicion. In patients with SVCS caused by neoplasia, 60% lack a prior history of cancer. A mass is generally present on the chest radiograph, with superior mediastinal widening and often pleural effusions. Computed tomography (CT) provides critical additional information. Contrast-enhanced CT can document the presence of obstruction and establish the level, extent, and therapeutic options by mapping collateral and patent vasculature to aid interventional access and to document any pulmonary emboli. Increased use of imaging in patients with cancer has identified many asymptomatic patients with impending SVC obstruction, allowing early radiation therapy to prevent or to delay obstruction. The CT scan can illustrate the strategic relationship of growing tumor masses or the development of nonocclusive, early intraluminal thrombus. Cardiac magnetic resonance imaging (CMR) can also perform this role effectively.

The causes of SVCS include intraluminal, mural, and extraluminal obstruction. Intraluminal causes include bland and neoplastic thrombus as well as direct tumor extension. Bland thrombus is usually associated with intravenous lines or infected pacemaker leads, although it is an uncommon cause of complete occlusion. A paraneoplastic bland thrombus can also occur, and tumor vascularization can be used to differentiate a bland from a neoplastic thrombus. Mural causes include strictures resulting from radiation therapy. Extraluminal causes are usually direct compression by bronchogenic tumors or malignant lymphadenopathy and represent the most common causes detected by imaging.

Because the underlying cause will guide any therapeutic recommendations, obtaining tissue samples to define the cause is essential. Sputum cytology can establish the diagnosis in almost half of patients. Biopsy of enlarged lymph nodes, when present, is frequently a relatively noninvasive method to obtain reliable tissue diagnosis. Thoracentesis can establish the diagnosis of malignancy in 70% of patients with pleural effusions. A diagnosis is made in most of the remaining cases with bronchoscopy, including brushing, washing, and biopsy samples. A marrow biopsy may be diagnostic of lymphoma or SCLC. If the diagnosis remains obscure, percutaneous transthoracic CT-guided fine-needle biopsy is a safe and effective method of diagnosis. When other methods have been unsuccessful, mediastinoscopy has

a high diagnostic yield but a somewhat higher risk of complications (5%).

MANAGEMENT. During medical evaluation and before institution of specific therapy, oxygen is administered to reduce the cardiac output and venous pressure; head elevation, diuretics, and a low-salt diet are used to reduce edema. Dehydration increases the risk of further thrombosis, however. In patients with SVCS caused by malignant tumors, radiotherapy and chemotherapy are the most common first-line treatment options. Steroids can, in some cases, decrease inflammation or tumor-associated obstruction but may obscure the diagnosis of lymphoma.

Increasingly, endovascular stenting is proving to provide more rapid and longer lasting relief of the obstruction (see Chap. 63).[9] Stent insertion has a high percentage of technical success, with rapid relief of symptoms. Adjuvant radiation therapy and chemotherapy can be used. Anticoagulation has not been proven to provide benefit in patients with neoplasia-associated SVCS and may interfere with diagnostic biopsies and interventions. Surgical treatment involves the insertion of a bypass graft between the left innominate or jugular vein and the right atrial appendage, with use of an autologous or Dacron graft. However, this operation is very invasive and difficult. In the chronic situation devoid of vascular interventions, patients may develop a network of chest wall and azygos-hemiazygos collateral vessels that effectively restore venous return to the right side of the heart.

Oncologic treatment of SVCS focuses on determining as rapidly as possible the histologic type of the primary lesion so that curative therapy for lymphomas, germ cell tumors, and even SCLC can be instituted or so that palliation for advanced non-SCLCs and other metastatic solid tumors can be provided. The prognosis of patients who present with SVCS depends greatly on the prognosis of the underlying neoplasm. Combination chemotherapy with or without radiation therapy relieves SVCS symptoms within 1 to 2 weeks in patients with newly diagnosed SCLC and lymphoma.

Valvular Heart Disease

Cardiac valves can be involved directly by primary or metastatic tumor, by bacterial or candidal infections, with nonbacterial thrombotic endocarditis, by trauma from semipermanent catheters inserted to facilitate treatment, and as a late effect of radiation therapy (see later, Complications of Radiation Therapy).

Nonbacterial thrombotic endocarditis can be seen in autoimmune disorders and can also complicate the course of various malignant neoplasms, most commonly adenocarcinomas from the gastrointestinal tract and lung.[10] Morbidity and mortality mainly result from systemic embolism. In one study of 200 nonselected ambulatory patients with solid tumors evaluated for evidence of thromboembolic events and for plasma D-dimer levels, 38 patients had cardiac valvular vegetations. The valves affected were mitral (19), aortic (18), and tricuspid (1). Primary lesions were lymphoma (10), lung (9), and pancreatic (3). Thromboembolism to extremities was diagnosed in 4 patients, cerebrovascular accidents were diagnosed in 2, and 4 patients had silent segmental left ventricular (LV) wall motion abnormalities on echocardiography. Nine of 38 patients (24%) with vegetations developed thromboembolism. D-Dimer levels were increased in 19 of 21 patients (90%) with thromboembolism.[10] Treatment of cancer-related nonbacterial thrombotic endocarditis remains difficult.

Ischemic Heart Disease

Given the similar risk factors for certain cancers and coronary artery disease (CAD), especially smoking, particulate matter air pollution, and age, patients will commonly have both diseases. Furthermore, as discussed in detail later, several cancer therapies can be toxic to the cardiovascular system, producing unstable angina, myocardial infarction (MI), and heart failure (HF). Depending on the type and level of aggressiveness of the chosen cancer therapeutic approach and the risk factor profile of the patient, it is reasonable to consider a baseline evaluation for the presence and severity of CAD or LV dysfunction before initiation of the therapy, even in the absence of symptoms or objective signs of disease. Although there are no firm guidelines that address this issue, patients who will receive agents known to induce unstable angina or MI (see later) should probably undergo stress and imaging studies to screen for CAD before treatment.

Arrhythmias

Arrhythmias in cancer patients are caused most commonly by coexisting abnormalities rather than by the cancer itself. Thus, although arrhythmia-inducing metastases to the myocardium or pericardium certainly occur, more commonly arrhythmias will be caused by hypoxemia (as a result of extensive carcinomas of the lung, metastases to the lung, or pulmonary infection), electrolyte imbalances, cardiotoxic radiation and cancer therapeutics, or comorbidities such as chronic obstructive pulmonary disease. Resuscitation of patients with end-stage cancer is often attempted, but the chance of survival is low. In one series, 0 of 171 patients in whom cardiac arrest was anticipated because of worsening metabolic status survived to discharge. In contrast, 22% survived in whom the arrest was not anticipated.[11] These findings highlight the need for careful attention to end-of-life decisions with end-stage patients, thereby avoiding painful and costly interventions that are usually futile.

Indirect Cardiovascular Complications of Neoplasia

Hyperviscosity

Hyperviscosity can result from a number of causes, including erythrocytosis (from polycythemia vera); thrombocytosis, which can be reactive or secondary to a myeloproliferative disorder (essential thrombocytosis); leukocytosis, occasionally seen in acute leukemias; and an increase in plasma protein levels (seen with multiple myeloma and Waldenström macroglobulinemia). For further information on the cardiovascular complications of hyperviscosity and its treatment, see Chap. 90 Online Supplement on the website.

Cardiovascular Complications of Cancer Therapeutic Agents

Drug development in cancer therapeutics has changed more dramatically in the last decade than in any other era. In this section, the cardiovascular toxicity of traditional chemotherapeutic agents and of the newer targeted therapeutic agents are discussed (see Chap. 73).

Traditional Chemotherapeutic Agents

ANTHRACYCLINES. The anthracyclines currently approved in the United States, doxorubicin (Adriamycin), daunorubicin (Cerubidine), epirubicin (Ellence), and idarubicin (Idamycin PFS), are key components of many chemotherapeutic regimens, having demonstrated efficacy in lymphomas and many solid tumors, including breast and SCLC.[12] This class of agents is clearly the most cardiotoxic to date (**Table 90-2**; see Table 73-7), acutely producing arrhythmias, LV dysfunction, and pericarditis and chronically producing LV dysfunction and HF. The toxicity is strongly dose related. Initial retrospective analyses have suggested that the incidence of HF is 2.2% overall and 7.5% in patients receiving a cumulative dose of 550 mg/m². However, more recent studies have suggested that the incidence is higher than this.[13] The incidence rises significantly for cumulative doses above 400 to 450 mg/m² for doxorubicin. Consequently, for most tumors, oncologists typically limit the dose to 450 to 500 mg/m².[12] If patients develop anthracycline cardiomyopathy, it is often within the first year of completing therapy, with a median of 5 to 9 months. However, the cardiomyopathy may be progressive during years.

Risk factors for cardiotoxicity, in addition to doses above 450 mg/m², include advanced age, history of cardiac disease, and prior mediastinal irradiation (**Fig. 90-2**). Predictors of cardiotoxicity based on assessment of LV function include a baseline LV ejection fraction (LVEF) less than 50% or a decline in LVEF of more than 10% on treatment to a level less than 50%. Diastolic dysfunction may be the first abnormality noted. Children may be particularly susceptible to anthracycline cardiotoxicity; in one series, 5% developed HF at 15 years of follow-up, and the incidence increased to 10% for cumulative doses of 550 mg/m².[14] In addition to dose and mediastinal irradiation, age at diagnosis and female gender are predictors for adverse outcomes in children. Unlike in adults, HF may appear years after treatment has been stopped and may be progressive.[15]

Endomyocardial biopsy is the most sensitive method to detect anthracycline cardiotoxicity, with typical findings being cytosolic vacuolization, lysis of myofibrils, and cellular swelling, findings more typical of a necrotic form of cell death. However, abnormalities on electron microscopy have not been shown to correlate highly with risk for development of HF and are often present in patients at cumulative doses well below those associated with an increased risk of HF. Given the technical nature of the procedure and inherent risks, this is not a practical way to detect or to observe patients with anthracycline cardiotoxicity, and serial determination of LV function, although insensitive, is the currently accepted method.

The cellular mechanisms leading to anthracycline cardiotoxicity remain unclear but are believed, in part, to involve oxidant stress leading to iron oxidation and generation of free radicals that damage cell and organelle membranes through peroxidation of lipids.[16] The oxidized iron hypothesis has led to the use of dexrazoxane (Zinecard), a chelator of intracellular iron. Although the compound does reduce the incidence of cardiotoxicity, concerns were raised in one trial that it might also reduce efficacy of the anthracycline.[17] This was not seen in a later meta-analysis, however, and the drug is approved in the United States. American Society of Clinical Oncology recommendations have suggested that the use of dexrazoxane be limited to patients who have received more than 300 mg/m² of doxorubicin or the equivalent.

Other strategies have been used to limit anthracycline cardiotoxicity, including the use of epirubicin, a stereoisomer of doxorubicin. This agent has less cardiotoxicity than doxorubicin at comparable doses, and 900 to 1000 mg/m² of epirubicin produces cardiotoxicity comparable to 450 to 500 mg/m² of doxorubicin. However, efficacy of the two agents appears to be comparable at equivalent doses. Patients should have a baseline determination of LV function before initiation of anthracycline therapy and should be monitored periodically after that, especially when the cumulative dose rises above 300 to 350 mg/m² for doxorubicin or above the comparable doses for the other anthracyclines. The criteria noted earlier concerning risk factors, baseline LV function, and deterioration of LV function, in combination with dosage consideration, can be used to risk stratify patients for the development of HF. Routine use of troponin measurements is not highly predictive except in patients receiving high-dose chemotherapy (for treatment of aggressive malignant neoplasms). In those patients, an elevated troponin I level predicted those going on to develop LV dysfunction with high sensitivity albeit low predictive accuracy. A negative troponin I strongly predicted patients whose LV function would not deteriorate.[18] A recent report has suggested that prophylactic angiotensin-converting enzyme inhibitor therapy in patients with elevated troponin I levels can prevent progression to HF. Earlier studies of anthracycline cardiotoxicity have suggested a high mortality rate, but with more modern approaches to the management of patients with HF, the prognosis is better (see Fig. 90-2).

TAXANES. The taxanes paclitaxel (Taxol) and docetaxel (Taxotere) disrupt microtubular networks as their mechanism of antitumor activity and are effective in breast cancer. Used alone, they have relatively little cardiotoxicity (see Table 90-2). In one large study, cardiac toxicity occurred in 14% of patients, but 76% of these events were asymptomatic bradycardia. Heart block can also occur. However, when paclitaxel is combined with doxorubicin, cardiotoxicity is increased, and 18% of patients developed HF in one trial. This was found to be secondary to retardation of metabolism of the doxorubicin. When paclitaxel was administered 30 minutes after doxorubicin and the

TABLE 90-2   Clinical Syndromes of Cardiotoxicity

PARAMETER	FREQUENCY	COMMENTS
Left Ventricular Dysfunction–Heart Failure		
Chemotherapeutics		
Anthracyclines		
Doxorubicin	+++	Highly dose dependent
Epirubicin	+	Risk factors include age (old and young), prior mediastinal XRT, history of heart disease, decreased EF, drop
Idarubicin	++	in EF on drug therapy, female gender (for children), and other agents (especially trastuzumab)
		Risk decreased by liposomal encapsulation or dexrazoxane
Alkylating agents		
Cyclophosphamide	+++	Primarily seen with high-dose "conditioning" regimens
Ifosfamide	+++	Risk factors are prior mediastinal XRT or anthracycline drug therapy
		Also can have myocarditis, pericarditis, myocardial necrosis
Taxanes		
Paclitaxel	+	Also employed in paclitaxel-eluting stent
Docetaxel	+/++	
Proteasome inhibitor		
Bortezomib	+/++	Moderately high rates of HF seen in trials (5%), but rates only minimally higher than in patients receiving dexamethasone
Targeted Therapeutics		
Monoclonal antibodies		
Trastuzumab	++	Not common as single agent
		Increased risk with anthracyclines, paclitaxel, cyclophosphamide
Pertuzumab	+/++	Targets HER2
		Rates of LV dysfunction as high as ~25% in one series
Bevacizumab	+/++	Targets VEGF-A (ligand for VEGFRs) and serves as a trap, not allowing VEGF-A to interact with receptor
		HF can be seen in setting of severe hypertension, which occurs in 10%-25% of patients, depending on dose; anthracyclines may increase HF risk
Tyrosine kinase inhibitors		
Imatinib, nilotinib	+	Can cause severe fluid retention with peripheral edema, pleural and pericardial effusion not secondary to LV dysfunction
Dasatinib	++	Same as above re fluid retention
Sunitinib	+++	LV dysfunction common; hypertension likely plays role
Ischemic Syndromes		
Fluorouracil, capecitabine	++	ACS; patients with CAD at increased risk
		Recurs with rechallenge; multiple mechanisms proposed; etiology remains unknown
Cisplatin, carboplatin	+	ACS caused by vasospasm or vascular injury
		Hypertension common; thromboembolism more common (see below)
Interferon-α	+	Risk of ischemia increased in patients with CAD; hypertension common
Paclitaxel	+	Myocardial ischemia in 1%-5%; serious ischemic cardiac events not common
Docetaxel	+	Limited data but rate probably ~1%
Bevacizumab	++	Arterial thrombotic events not common but occurred in 8.5% of patients >65 yr
Vinca alkaloids	+	~1% risk of cardiac events; ischemia possibly caused by coronary spasm
Sorafenib	+ – ++	~2.5% risk of ACS
Erlotinib	+ – ++	Limited data but rate ~2%
Hypertension		
Cisplatin	++++	
Bevacizumab	++++	Extremely common with all anti-VEGF therapeutics to date
Sunitinib	++++	Intrinsic in mechanism of action of these agents
Sorafenib	++++	
Venous Thrombosis		
Cisplatin	+++	DVT or PE in 8.5%; most occur early in treatment; additional risk factors for DVT are often present
Thalidomide	++++	Uncommon with monotherapy but risk rises with concurrent chemotherapy
Lenalidomide	+++	See comments re thalidomide
Erlotinib	++	Rate with erlotinib plus gemcitabine ~2% over that seen with gemcitabine alone

Relative frequency of the cardiotoxicity is scored as follows: + = ≤1%; ++ = 1% to 5%; +++ = 6% to 10%; ++++ = >10%.
ACS = acute coronary syndromes; CAD = coronary artery disease; DVT = deep venous thrombosis; EF = ejection fraction; HF = heart failure; LV = left ventricular; PE = pulmonary embolism; VEGF = vascular endothelial cell growth factor; VEGFR = vascular endothelial cell growth factor receptor; XRT = radiation therapy.
Modified from Yeh ET, Bickford CL: Cardiovascular complications of cancer therapy: Incidence, pathogenesis, diagnosis, and management. J Am Coll Cardiol 53:2231, 2009.

doxorubicin dose was kept to 360 mg/m², the decline in LVEF was greater than that with the combination of doxorubicin plus cyclophosphamide, although the rates of HF were low and not statistically different between the groups.[19] Docetaxel does not retard metabolism of doxorubicin and appears to lead to only a minimal increase in HF.

ALKYLATING AGENTS AND ANTIMETABOLITES. These classes of agents generally have low incidences of cardiotoxicity (see Table 90-2). Cyclophosphamide (Cytoxan) is relatively well tolerated when it is used at conventional doses, but in patients receiving conditioning regimens before autologous stem cell transplantation, which use high-dose cyclophosphamide, acute cardiotoxicity can occur.[20] As opposed to the total cumulative dosage for anthracyclines, dosage of an individual course of treatment is more predictive for cyclophosphamide. Risk factors include prior anthracycline therapy or mediastinal irradiation and possibly prior imatinib therapy.[21] Clinically, patients may present with HF, myocarditis, or pericarditis. In one series of 17 consecutive patients receiving induction therapy, none of whom devel-

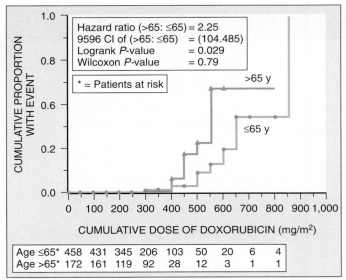

FIGURE 90-2 Risk of doxorubicin-associated congestive heart failure by patient age. This graphically depicts the cumulative doxorubicin dose at the onset of doxorubicin-associated congestive heart failure in 630 patients according to patient age older or younger than 65 years. *(Redrawn from Swain SM, Whaley FS, Ewer MS: Congestive heart failure in patients treated with doxorubicin: A retrospective analysis of three trials. Cancer 97:2869, 2003.)*

oped HF, LV dilation by CMR was evident from the onset.[20] Mechanisms underlying the toxicity are believed to be injury of both endothelial cells and myocytes, and a picture of hemorrhagic myocardial necrosis can emerge. Those who survive the acute phase typically do not have residual LV dysfunction. High-dose ifosfamide (Ifex) induced HF in 17% of patients.[22]

Cisplatin (Platinol)–based regimens are the cornerstone of therapy for testicular germ cell cancer, the most common malignant neoplasm in men aged 20 to 40 years; 80% of those with disseminated nonseminoma achieve long-term survival. Thus, in addition to short-term toxicity, long-term toxicity is a concern in this group. Cisplatin is notable for causing hypertension, which is sometimes severe. Acute chest pain syndromes, including MI, have also been reported, possibly related to coronary spasm. Because cisplatin is often used in combination with bleomycin, an agent that can induce Raynaud phenomenon in approximately one third of patients, long-term vascular toxicity is particularly a concern. Indeed, after a median 10-year follow-up of patients treated with platinum-based regimens (cisplatin or carboplatin [Paraplatin]) versus radiation therapy, 6.7% of patients after chemotherapy and 10% of patients after irradiation suffered a cardiac event, for a relative risk of 2.4- to 2.8-fold compared with patients treated with surgery only. Changes in the ratio of carotid intima-media thickness were detected as early as 10 weeks after a course of cisplatin-based chemotherapy. The morbidity data have led to calls for more conservative approaches to patients at low risk for cancer recurrence.

Fluorouracil (Adrucil) is used in the treatment of many solid tumors, and regimens based on this agent are the mainstay for treatment of colorectal cancer. Fluorouracil can cause acute ischemic syndromes ranging from angina to MI, and this can occur in patients without CAD (approximately 1% of patients), although it is more common in patients with pre-existing disease (4% to 5%). Overall, rates range from 0.55% to 8%, although more sensitive methods of detecting possible subclinical ischemia (ambulatory electrocardiographic monitoring) find much higher rates. Discontinuation of treatment and standard antianginal therapies usually lead to resolution of symptoms, but ischemia often recurs if therapy is reinitiated. An alternative agent, capecitabine (Xeloda), is metabolized to fluorouracil, preferentially in tumor cells, suggesting that it may have less cardiotoxicity. However, one retrospective review (that excluded patients with "significant"

cardiac disease) has found an incidence of 6.5% major cardiac events for the combination, including angina (4.6%), MI, ventricular tachycardia, and sudden death.[21] Vasospasm is believed to be the mechanism triggering ischemia, although thromboembolic events are also increased. It is not clear at this point whether prophylactic nitrates prevent ischemic events. Capecitabine monotherapy appears to have a lower incidence of cardiac toxicity compared with fluorouracil monotherapy.

OTHER CHEMOTHERAPEUTIC AGENTS

Tamoxifen

Tamoxifen (Nolvadex) is widely used in the treatment of breast cancer. On the basis of largely experimental data, it had been proposed to have cardioprotective effects. However, in a large trial of 13,388 patients, in women both with and without CAD, tamoxifen therapy did not reduce or increase the incidence of fatal MI, nonfatal MI, unstable angina, or severe angina.[23] Concerns have been raised, however, that stroke risk might be increased somewhat.

Proteasome Inhibitors

Bortezomib (Velcade) is an inhibitor of the proteasome system responsible for degrading improperly folded proteins and proteins that are no longer needed in the cell. The drug is approved for use in patients with multiple myeloma. The concept behind its use is that malignant cells have altered proteins regulating the cell cycle, leading to more rapid cell division and increased accumulation of damaged proteins as a result. Therefore, the continued health of the malignant cell, as opposed to normal cells, may be more dependent on degradation of the damaged proteins. In support of this concept, proteasome inhibitors are more toxic to proliferating malignant cells in culture than to normal cells. Targets include activation of endoplasmic reticulum stress pathways leading to activation of proapoptotic factors and inactivation of survival factors. Cardiomyocytes have an active proteasome system, raising concerns that inhibitors may be cardiotoxic. However, in the phase III trials of bortezomib, HF was reported in 5% of patients but was also reported in 4% of patients in the dexamethasone arm of the trial.[24]

Additional Agents

A discussion of the cardiotoxicity of additional agents, including cytokines (interleukin-2, aldesleukin [Proleukin], and denileukin diftitox) and interferons, histone deacetylase inhibitors (trichostatin A and suberoylanilide hydroxamic acid), topoisomerase inhibitors (etoposide and teniposide), purine analogues (pentostatin and cladribine), all-*trans*-retinoic acid, arsenic trioxide, and thalidomide and lenalidomide, can be found in the Chap. 90 Online Supplement on the website.

Targeted Therapeutics

The treatment of a number of malignant neoplasms has changed radically during the past few years with the advent of so-called targeted therapies. As opposed to traditional chemotherapeutics, which target basic cellular processes present in most cells, these therapies target factors that are specifically dysregulated in cancerous cells. It was hoped that this approach would reduce toxicities typical of standard chemotherapeutics (e.g., alopecia, gastrointestinal toxicity, myelotoxicity) and at the same time be more effective at treating the cancer. In some situations, this has been the case, but concerns about cardiotoxicity have surfaced for some agents.[25,26]

Most of the targeted cancer therapeutics inhibit the activity of tyrosine kinases (**Table 90-3**).[27] Tyrosine kinases (TKs) attach phosphate groups to tyrosine residues of other proteins, thereby changing the activity, subcellular localization, or rate of degradation of the protein. In the normal cell, these wild-type (i.e., normal) tyrosine kinases play many roles in regulating basic cellular functions. However, in leukemias and cancers, the gene encoding the causal (or contributory) TK is amplified (leading to overexpression) or mutated, leading to a constitutively activated state that drives proliferation of the cancerous

TABLE 90-3 Kinase Inhibitors in Cancer, Their Targets, and Representative Malignant Neoplasms

| AGENT (TRADE NAME) | Targets | | REPRESENTATIVE MALIGNANT NEOPLASMS |
	PRIMARY	OTHER	
Tyrosine Kinase Inhibitors			
FDA Approved			
Imatinib (Gleevec)	Bcr-Abl	Abl, c-Kit, PDGFRs, DDR1, Cdc2	CML, Ph⁺ ALL, CMML, HES, GIST
Nilotinib (Tasigna)	Bcr-Abl and most IRMs	Abl, c-Kit, PDGFRs	Imatinib-resistant CML, ALL, GIST
Dasatinib (Sprycel)	Bcr-Abl and most IRMs	Abl, c-Kit, PDGFRs, DDR1, SFKs, EphB4	Imatinib-resistant CML, ALL, GIST
Sunitinib (Sutent)	VEGFRs	*PDGFRs, c-Kit, CSF-1R, FLT3, RET	RCC, GIST
Sorafenib (Nexavar)	VEGFRs	†PDGFRs, c-Kit, FLT3, Raf-1/B-Raf	RCC, hepatocellular carcinoma
Lapatinib (Tykerb)	EGFR (ERBB1), HER2 (ERBB2)	NI	HER2⁺ breast cancer, ovarian cancer, gliomas, NSCLC
Gefitinib (Iressa)	EGFR	NI	NSCLC, gliomas
Erlotinib (Tarceva)	EGFR	NI	NSCLC, pancreatic cancer, gliomas
Temsirolimus (Torisel)	mTOR	NI	RCC
Everolimus (Afinitor)	mTOR	NI	RCC
Sirolimus (Rapamune)	mTOR	NI	RCC
Projected			
Bosutinib	Bcr-Abl and several IRMs	Abl, SFKs, DDR1, EphB4	Imatinib-resistant CML
Lestaurtinib	JAK2, FLT3	TrkA/B/C	MPD (PCV, ET, IMF), AML
Pazopanib	VEGFR, PDGFR, c-Kit	NK	RCC
Vandetanib	VEGFR, EGFR	NK	NSCLC
Cediranib	VEGFR	NK	Colorectal cancer
Alvocidib	CDK	NK	CLL
Enzastaurin	PKCβ	NK	Diffuse large B-cell lymphoma
Deforolimus	mTOR	NK	RCC, metastatic sarcomas
Monoclonal Antibodies			
Trastuzumab (Herceptin)	HER2/ErbB2	NI	Breast
Pertuzumab (Omnitarg)	HER2/ErbB2	NI	Breast
Bevacizumab (Avastin)	VEGF-A	NI	Colon, renal cell, NSCLC, other

*≥50 targets.
†≥15 targets.
ALL = acute lymphoblastic leukemia; AML = acute myeloid leukemia; CDK = cyclin-dependent kinase; CLL = chronic lymphocytic leukemia; CML = chronic myeloid leukemia; CMML = chronic myelomonocytic leukemia; EGFR = epidermal growth factor receptor; EphB4 = ephrin receptor tyrosine kinase B4; ET = essential thrombocytosis; FDA = Food and Drug Administration; FLT3 = FMS-like tyrosine kinase 3; GIST = gastrointestinal stromal tumors; HES = hypereosinophilic syndrome; IMF = idiopathic myelofibrosis; IRMs = imatinib-resistant Abl mutants; JAK2 = Janus kinase 2; MPDs = myeloproliferative disorders; mTOR = mammalian target of rapamycin; NI = none identified; NK = not known; NSCLC = non–small cell lung cancer; PCV = polycythemia vera; PDGFR = platelet-derived growth factor receptor; Ph⁺ ALL = Philadelphia chromosome–positive acute lymphocytic leukemia; PKCβ = protein kinase C β; RCC = renal cell carcinoma; RET = rearranged during transfection; SFKs = SRC family kinases; VEGF = vascular endothelial cell growth factor; VEGFR = vascular endothelial cell growth factor receptor.
From Cheng H, Force T: Molecular mechanisms of cardiovascular toxicity of targeted cancer therapeutics. Circ Res 106:21, 2010.

clonal cells or blocks their normal death (see Table 90-3).[27] Inhibition of these kinases could then retard cell proliferation or induce cell death. Cardiotoxicity arises when the normal kinase, which is often present in cardiomyocytes and is also inhibited by the agent, plays a central role in maintenance of cardiomyocyte homeostasis. In some cases, cardiotoxicity of these drugs may be predictable, but usually it is not. This is because the targeted kinase is typically not known to provide an important function in the heart or because of off-target effects (i.e., inhibition of TKs other than those the drug was designed to target). Most tyrosine kinase inhibitors (TKIs) compete with ATP for binding to a pocket in the kinase that is moderately well conserved across many TKs. There are approximately 500 protein kinases in the human genome, of which approximately 90 are TKs. Although these drugs are typically designed to target two to five kinases, in truth it is unusual for this class of drugs to inhibit fewer than 10 kinases, and some in use inhibit 30 or more kinases. Furthermore, there may be several additional TKs that are inhibited and many additional serine or threonine kinases (the other major family) that are inhibited, and these will generally not be known to the oncologist or cardiologist caring for the patient. Therefore, if patients present with HF after initiation of therapy, the possibilities of off-target effects accounting for toxicity versus HF from other causes must be considered.

DRUGS AND THEIR TARGETS. Table 90-3 lists approved TKIs, several others that are well along in development, and the monoclonal antibodies most relevant to the heart. The first molecularly targeted therapies, trastuzumab (Herceptin) and imatinib (Gleevec), illustrate the two general classes of these agents—humanized monoclonal antibodies targeting growth factor receptors on the surface of the cancer cell (trastuzumab) and small molecule inhibitors of

receptors or of intracellular pathways regulating growth of the cancer cells (imatinib) (**Fig. 90-3**). All generic names for monoclonal antibodies end in -mab, and all small molecule inhibitors end in -nib.

HER2 Receptor and Its Antagonists: Trastuzumab, Lapatinib, and Pertuzumab

The growth factor receptor HER2 (human epidermal growth factor receptor 2) is amplified in 15% to 30% of breast cancers, and HER2-positive cancers carry a worse prognosis. This amplification, and the resulting overexpression (up to 100-fold) and activation of HER2, both enhances cell cycle progression (and thus proliferation) and inhibits apoptosis of the cancer cells. Trastuzumab is a humanized monoclonal antibody that binds to and inhibits the activity of the HER2 receptor.[25] Treatment with trastuzumab improves survival in patients with metastatic disease and, when used in the adjuvant setting after surgery, reduces recurrences of the cancer.

Trastuzumab is well tolerated as far as its side effect profile. However, it can induce HF in a percentage of patients. The original trials with trastuzumab indicated that 3% to 7% of patients developed LV dysfunction, and this incidence was increased to 27% by concomitant use of doxorubicin (with 16% being New York Heart Association [NYHA] Class III or IV).[25] This is in comparison to rates of 8% total and 3% NYHA Class III or IV HF with anthracyclines plus cyclophosphamide. When trastuzumab was used with paclitaxel, 13% of patients developed cardiotoxicity versus only 1% with paclitaxel alone.

More recently, trastuzumab cardiotoxicity has been analyzed in three key trials in breast cancer patients that assessed efficacy of the agent in the adjuvant setting. In one trial, patients who underwent surgery plus adjuvant or neoadjuvant chemotherapy or radiotherapy were randomized to receive trastuzumab or simply observation. At 1 year of follow-up, 7.1%

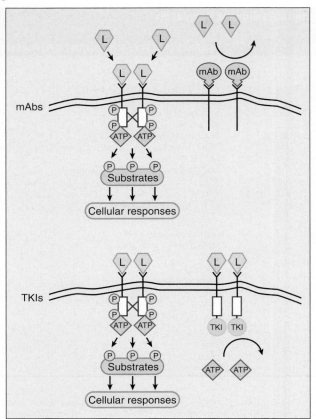

FIGURE 90-3 Mechanisms of action of monoclonal antibodies (mAbs) versus small molecule tyrosine kinase inhibitors (TKIs). Ligand (L) binding to receptor tyrosine kinases leads to receptor dimerization, cross-phosphorylation (purple lines and P), and activation of the intracellular tyrosine kinase domain. Substrates are then phosphorylated, leading to cellular responses. Monoclonal antibodies **(top)** interfere with ligand binding to receptor or receptor dimerization and cross-phosphorylation, blocking activation of the receptor tyrosine kinases.[17] TKIs **(bottom)** do not prevent ligand binding or dimerization. By preventing adenosine triphosphate (ATP) from binding to the kinase domain, they block cross-phosphorylation of receptors and phosphorylation of substrates. *(From Chen MH, Kerkelä R, Force T: Mechanisms of cardiac dysfunction associated with tyrosine kinase inhibitor cancer therapeutics. Circulation 118:86, 2008.)*

of patients in the trastuzumab arm versus 2.2% in the observation arm had significant declines in LVEF, and only 1.7% in the trastuzumab arm versus 0% in the observation arm developed symptomatic HF. These figures represent short-term risks for trastuzumab in otherwise healthy patients with no cardiac morbidities and normal LV function who had received moderate doses of adjuvant chemotherapy and no mediastinal irradiation.

The other two studies, which also excluded patients with a cardiac history and low ejection fraction or a decline in ejection fraction on doxorubicin-cyclophosphamide therapy, examined patients treated with more aggressive regimens. Follow-up was for a mean of 27 months. In this trial, 8.7% of patients in the trastuzumab arm versus 1.6% in the no-trastuzumab arm developed symptomatic HF. Furthermore, 2.2% to 4.1% developed severe HF on trastuzumab versus 0.2% to 0.8% on placebo. The lower rates in these later three trials, compared with earlier studies, reflect not only enrollment of more highly selected patients but also administration of doxorubicin and trastuzumab sequentially rather than concurrently. Even given the lower rates, overall approximately 20% of patients were withdrawn from this trial for cardiac reasons.[28] The more recent trials largely enrolled node-positive patients. However, it is possible that clinical practice will move toward treatment of node-negative patients, for whom the prognostic significance of HER2 positivity is only modest. It will be important to analyze risk-benefit in node-negative patients, in whom even the relatively low rates of HF may outweigh benefits.

MECHANISMS OF TRASTUZUMAB CARDIOTOXICITY. That trastuzumab was cardiotoxic is not altogether surprising because mice

in which the HER2 gene (designated ErbB2 in mice) was knocked out developed a dilated cardiomyopathy.[29] Thus, the ErbB2 receptor, at least in mice, appears to serve a "maintenance" function in cardiomyocytes. Furthermore, cardiomyocytes isolated from the knockout hearts were more susceptible to anthracycline toxicity, consistent with the concept that inhibition of HER2 in patients may have amplified the severity of doxorubicin toxicity by preventing repair. Consistent with this, neuregulin, the endogenous ligand for HER2, can decrease anthracycline cardiotoxicity.[16] Cellular mechanisms of the toxicity of ErbB2 inhibition remain a matter of debate.[30] That the story is more complex is underscored by the reported very low rates of LV dysfunction (1.4%) and HF (0.2%) in a review of trials with lapatinib, the TKI that targets HER2.[30] In contrast, the monoclonal antibody pertuzumab, which interferes with dimerization of HER2 with the HER3 receptor, has induced LV dysfunction (defined as a decline in ejection fraction of ≥10%) in as many as 27% of patients.[31] This highlights the point that not all HER2 antagonists appear to be equivalent in inducing LV dysfunction, with lapatinib being the apparent outlier. This apparent difference could be due to the different mechanisms of action of the TKIs versus monoclonal antibodies or to distinct differences in trial design.[30]

NATURAL HISTORY OF TRASTUZUMAB TOXICITY. Debate continues about the degree to which trastuzumab cardiotoxicity is reversible. Clearly, ultrastructural abnormalities on biopsy appear to be minimal, and patients respond well to standard HF regimens.[32] Some can continue on treatment without recurrence of HF. In follow-up in one of the adjuvant trials, of 27 patients with trastuzumab-induced HF (trastuzumab given after anthracycline plus cyclophosphamide, with or without paclitaxel), only one patient was persistently symptomatic.[28] Furthermore, overall LV function at more than 6 months of follow-up improved for the group versus on-treatment values. However, LV function remained depressed compared with baseline in 17 of 24 patients. Longer term follow-up is required to evaluate this issue fully.

Bcr-Abl and Imatinib

The first targeted small molecule kinase inhibitor to be used successfully in malignant neoplasms was imatinib. This agent inhibits the activity of the fusion protein Bcr-Abl, which arises from the chromosomal translocation that creates the Philadelphia chromosome and is the causal factor in approximately 90% of cases of chronic myeloid leukemia and some cases of B-cell acute lymphoblastic leukemia.[27] This translocation creates a constitutively active protein kinase that drives proliferation and inhibits apoptosis in bone marrow stem cells, leading to the leukemias. Imatinib has revolutionized the treatment of chronic myeloid leukemia, and now 90% of patients are alive 5 years after diagnosis with a disease that was uniformly fatal before the development of imatinib. Imatinib was the first TKI to be associated with HF, although the overall incidence is low.[21,25]

Dasatinib and nilotinib are more potent Bcr-Abl inhibitors, with dasatinib being decidedly less selective than the others. HF is uncommon with imatinib and nilotinib, but HF or LV dysfunction can occur in as many as 4% of patients receiving dasatinib.[21] Furthermore, the median duration of treatment in this trial was only 6 months. However, patients need to be on treatment for life because chronic myeloid leukemia recurs when the drug is stopped. Patients were excluded from the trial if they had abnormal cardiac function, again highlighting the fact that patients in clinical trials may not reflect the population of patients as a whole that will be receiving the drug. Nilotinib also prolongs the QT interval by 15 to 30 milliseconds.

Epidermal Growth Factor Receptor Antagonists

Epidermal growth factor receptor (EGFR) antagonists are in fairly widespread use for a number of solid tumors, although their efficacy has been generally modest. These agents are either monoclonal antibodies (e.g., cetuximab [Erbitux], panitumumab) or small molecule inhibitors (gefitinib [Iressa] or erlotinib [Tarceva]). In contrast to inhibition of HER2, cardiotoxicity with EGFR inhibitors seems to be quite rare. Thus, other causes of HF should be aggressively sought in patients receiving these agents presenting with HF. However, acute MI has been reported with erlotinib (2.3% risk versus 1.2% in patients receiving gemcitabine). Erlotinib is also associated with venous thromboembolism, with rates varying from ~4% to 10%.[21]

Vascular Endothelial Growth Factor and Vascular Endothelial Growth Factor Receptor Antagonists

There is great interest in drug development for agents targeting the vascular supply of tumors. Because vascular endothelial cell growth factor (VEGF) and two of its receptors, VEGFR1 and VEGFR2, are key regulators of angiogenesis and are overexpressed in many solid tumors, they represent prime candidates.[33] The monoclonal antibody bevacizumab (Avastin) targets VEGF-A and, combined with chemotherapy, enhanced survival in metastatic colorectal cancer and metastatic, nonsquamous, non-SCLC,[33] leading many to suggest that "antivascular" therapies may soon be incorporated into many regimens for solid tumors. Sunitinib and sorafenib are TKIs that also target VEGFRs, and many others are in development. Sunitinib and sorafenib are part of a recent trend toward targeting of multiple kinases involved in cancer progression. Although this makes sense for treatment of cancers, multitargeted TKIs raise additional concerns about cardiotoxicity. Hypertension is very common with all three of these VEGF/VEGFR antagonists and can be severe in 8% to 20% of patients. Thus, hypertension appears to be a class effect related to VEGFR inhibition.

All three agents are associated with HF; bevacizumab and sorafenib appear to be less problematic than sunitinib. Rates of HF with bevacizumab monotherapy are low but rise when patients have received prior anthracyclines or irradiation. In one case series of sunitinib-treated patients, 8% developed NYHA Class III or IV HF and an additional 10% suffered asymptomatic but significant declines in ejection fraction.[34]

On the basis of a meta-analysis of five trials, concerns have also been raised about the approximately twofold increase in arterial (but not venous) thromboembolic events with bevacizumab.[35] Age and prior thromboembolic events were risk factors. In patients older than 65 years, 8.5% developed arterial thromboembolic events versus 2.9% for the chemotherapy-alone arm. Stroke risk was increased approximately fourfold (1.9% versus 0.5%).

Sorafenib is also associated with acute coronary syndromes; in one study, the rate was 2.9% for patients receiving sorafenib compared with 0.4% in the placebo arm (*www.univgraph.com/bayer/inserts/nexavar.pdf*; Bayer Pharmaceuticals, Inc., 2006).

There are no guidelines at present concerning screening evaluations and follow-up of patients who will receive VEGF/VEGFR-targeted therapeutics. Until more data are available, a baseline evaluation of LV function should be considered for patients who will receive sunitinib if there are significant risk factors. Patients receiving therapy, especially those with cardiac disease, should be observed closely, and obviously, strict attention should be paid to hypertension management for all of the VEGF/VEGFR therapeutics.

Vascular Disrupting Agents

Another class of agents, the so-called vascular disrupting agents, target endothelial cells. A phase I trial of one such agent, ZD6126, which targets the tubulin network of the endothelial cell, was complicated by pulmonary thromboembolism, asymptomatic creatine kinase MB release, and declines in LVEF. An additional clinical trial of this agent, which appears to target normal as well as tumor vasculature, found an 11% incidence of cardiac events.

Histone Deacetylase Inhibitors

This relatively new class of agents negatively regulates cell proliferation by preventing the removal of acetyl moieties by histone deacetylases. Vorinostat has been approved for use in cutaneous T-cell lymphoma, but several additional trials are ongoing for this and other histone deacetylase inhibitors. In one trial, pulmonary embolism was noted in 5.4% of patients (*http://www.cancer.gov/cancertopics/druginfo/fda-vorinostat*). It is not clear if this is an on-target or off-target effect of the drug, nor is the mechanism known.

CONCERNS ABOUT DRUGS IN DEVELOPMENT. There are literally hundreds of agents in development, but one area of significant concern is inhibition of multiple factors along the phosphoinositide 3-kinase (PI3K)/Akt pathway. Indeed, the most active drug development in cancer is probably directed at the many components that make up this pathway. This pathway is very notable in that all of the major factors in it have been found to be mutated or amplified in a wide range of cancers, making this pathway an ideal target in cancer therapy.[36] Furthermore, it is believed that effective cancer therapy will require targeting of multiple components of the pathway.[36] Whereas this is undoubtedly true from a cancer perspective, with the central role played by the PI3K/Akt pathway in cardiomyocyte survival in the setting of stress, concerns about aggressive targeting of this pathway are obvious. In spite of that, several agents are currently in clinical trials.[36] This PI3K/Akt pathway, more than any other, epitomizes the similarity between cancer signaling and survival signaling in cardiomyocytes.

Complications of Radiation Therapy

Cardiovascular disease is one of the leading causes of mortality in long-term cancer survivors treated with mediastinal irradiation. Patients with lymphomas and breast, lung, and esophageal cancers frequently receive high doses of radiation to the heart and vasculature. Late cardiovascular effects range from valvular heart disease to premature CAD, stroke, cardiomyopathy, HF, constrictive pericarditis, and complete heart block.[37] Similar to anthracycline cardiomyopathy, radiation-induced cardiovascular dysfunction is progressive with time after radiation therapy, with cardiac events typically occurring 10 to 20 years after radiation therapy.[38] In approaching cardiac complications in patients exposed to chest radiation, however, it is important to recognize that the distribution of disease is defined by the geometry of the radiation portal. In other words, it predominantly involves cardiac structures that happen to fall within the portal while leaving nonirradiated adjacent structures relatively intact, hence occasionally producing atypical clinical presentations.[38]

PATHOPHYSIOLOGY. Radiation is believed to cause endothelial dysfunction of the microvasculature leading to thrombosis and small-vessel disease. Furthermore, irradiation of larger vessels included in the field, such as the proximal coronary arteries, results in intimal hyperplasia, eventually leading to premature atherosclerosis and coronary stenosis.[39] Irradiation of the myocardium leads to progressive fibrosis resulting in diastolic dysfunction and finally restrictive cardiomyopathy in long-term survivors.[40]

Much of our understanding of late cardiac effects of radiation therapy comes from the study of Hodgkin lymphoma, in which therapy entails a relatively stereotyped radiation portal and generally good longer term survival. Furthermore, many long-term Hodgkin lymphoma survivors receive radiation therapy alone, separating the contribution of radiation therapy from the additive effects of chemotherapy on the heart.[5,41]

STROKE AND TRANSIENT ISCHEMIC ATTACKS. Long-term cancer survivors who have received head and neck irradiation have a twofold to threefold increased risk of stroke and transient ischemic attacks.[42,43] At 25 years after treatment, the cumulative risk for ischemic cerebral events (cerebrovascular accident, transient ischemic attack) approaches 6% to 7%.[42,43] Importantly, peripheral vascular complications of radiation therapy may also include arterial stenoses and occlusions of any vessels in the radiation fields. Depending on the type of cancer, the subclavian, internal mammary, and coronary arteries also may have been irradiated.

CORONARY ARTERY DISEASE. Premature cardiovascular disease accounts for 25% of non–primary cancer–related deaths in long-term survivors of mantle irradiation.[44] Risk of cardiovascular disease increases with time elapsed since exposure to radiation. Radiation-associated relative risk of ischemia, sudden death, or HF is 2.9% at 10 years and increases with time since exposure to 24.7% at 25 years.[45] Nineteen years after exposure to radiation therapy, standardized incidence ratios for CAD in Hodgkin lymphoma survivors are 3.6 times greater than those in an age- and gender-matched population.[46] Importantly, radiation-associated coronary disease may be difficult to diagnose because many patients do not experience anginal "warning" symptoms after mediastinal irradiation, apparently reflecting irradiation of sensory nerves in the chest.[38] Therefore, a high index of suspicion along with an understanding of cardiovascular risk for CAD is important in the care of this population. The combination of radiation therapy with anthracycline exposure and the presence of traditional cardiac risk factors further increase the risk of cardiovascular disease in long-term survivors.[46,47]

VALVULAR HEART DISEASE. As previously discussed, chest irradiation also increases risk for clinically significant valvular disease, especially involving the aortic valve. Sixty percent of Hodgkin lymphoma survivors treated with high-dose radiation therapy have moderate to severe valvular dysfunction 20 years after treatment.[44] Patients who have received <30 Gy of radiation are less likely to have significant valve disease.[40] Anthracycline chemotherapy also further increases the risk of valve disease and HF after mediastinal radiation therapy.[37,46] Therefore, routine periodic screening for valve disease in patients treated with radiation has been recommended because many patients who are asymptomatic have been found to have subclinical valvular disease.[48]

CARDIOMYOPATHY. Patients who have received radiation therapy are at risk for development of diastolic dysfunction, restrictive cardiomyopathy, and subsequent HF. Systolic dysfunction is relatively infrequent with radiation therapy alone, occurring in >10% of patients.[40,44] Childhood survivors of radiation therapy demonstrate a complex of decreased LV mass, decreased chamber size, and decreased wall thickness.[49] Diastolic dysfunction was also common in adult long-term survivors and associated with worsened event-free survival.[37] Furthermore, significant decrease in peak oxygen uptake to <20 mL/kg/m^2, values that are graded as severely reduced in typical HF populations, may be seen in 30% of childhood survivors of Hodgkin lymphoma.[40]

CONDUCTION BLOCK. Bundle branch block and even complete heart block requiring pacemaker placement may occur, presumably reflecting radiation-induced fibrosis of the conduction system.

Breast cancer survivors may also be at risk for radiation-associated cardiovascular disease, including MI[21,50]; however, late cardiac effects in this population may vary according to the dose, the laterality of the radiation field (left versus right breast), and the era in which the patient was treated.[51] With improved radiation technique, cardiovascular disease deaths declined from 13% to 5.5% in patients treated before 1980 versus those treated after 1985.[52] Survivors treated with older radiation techniques have a higher risk for fatal cardiovascular disease than do patients treated more recently. In contrast, survivors treated with modern techniques of radiation therapy have not shown an increase in cardiovascular disease after 10 to 15 years compared with those who received no breast irradiation.[52] However, longer follow-up is necessary to confirm the lack of increased cardiovascular risk in those treated with modern radiation therapy protocols.

MONITORING. Subclinical cardiovascular disease is common in long-term cancer survivors.[44] Noninvasive cardiac imaging is important in the long-term follow-up of cancer survivors.[38] Echocardiography with tissue Doppler imaging is important for detection of systolic and diastolic dysfunction and for assessment of valvular and pericardial disease. Stress testing, with or without imaging, should be considered in long-term survivors of mediastinal irradiation. Recommendations for cardiac assessment of children and adults are available.[21,48,53]

PREVENTION. Alterations in radiation treatment technique, such as reductions in dose-volume, field size, and cardiac shielding, have decreased cardiac irradiation.[53] Additional approaches to reduce cardiac irradiation at time of therapy include deep inspiratory breath-holding that decreases the amount of myocardium in the field without altering irradiation of the breast.[54-56] These techniques have been validated in clinical trials and are beginning to be implemented in radiation treatment protocols (*www.ClinicalTrials.gov*). Beyond improvements in radiation delivery, however, treatment of modifiable cardiac risk factors in long-term survivors remains central to the reduction of overall cardiovascular risk.[46,48]

Management of Heart Failure Induced by Cancer Therapeutic Agents

At present, the guidelines of the Heart Failure Society of America and the American Heart Association/American College of Cardiology (AHA/ACC) do not contain specific recommendations for treatment of patients with what is presumed to be cancer therapeutic–induced HF. However, it is probably most reasonable at this time to approach the patient as one would any patient with newly diagnosed HF, as discussed in Chap. 28. In this regard, it is critical to exclude other potential causes of HF before assuming that chemotherapy has caused the HF. Several of the agents discussed earlier, including trastuzumab and sunitinib, appear to have some degree of reversibility of LV dysfunction with aggressive treatment with angiotensin-converting enzyme inhibitors and beta blockers. In many cases, patients need to continue the cancer treatment, and a number of anecdotal case reports have suggested that patients whose LV dysfunction largely resolves after withdrawal of the agent and institution of an HF regimen may be safely rechallenged with the agent, although continuing the HF regimen. Clearly, however, at this point there is insufficient evidence to conclude whether this approach is generally safe, so no clear recommendations can be made, and any rechallenge should be undertaken with great caution.

Future Perspectives

Many more targets exist for drug development for leukemias and solid tumors. Given the intense interest in this area by the pharmaceutical industry, inhibitors will likely become available at some point. Clinicians will be faced with a host of novel therapeutics and the prospect of trying to predict which will have adverse effects on the cardiovascular system. The key for the future will be to develop better strategies to identify targets to be avoided, thereby limiting cardiotoxicity. When the target cannot be avoided (i.e., when it is causal), the goal will be to develop prophylactic therapies to prevent or to minimize cardiotoxicity in high-risk patients. When that fails, we need to develop effective approaches to the management of patients with cardiotoxicity so that progression of HF can be prevented and patients can continue on what is often lifesaving treatment. In this endeavor, oncologists and cardiologists must collaborate.

REFERENCES

Direct and Indirect Complications of Neoplasia

1. Luna A, Ribes R, Caro P, et al: Evaluation of cardiac tumors with magnetic resonance imaging. Eur Radiol 15:1446, 2005.
2. Chiles C, Woodard PK, Gutierrez FR, Link KM: Metastatic involvement of the heart and pericardium: CT and MRI imaging. Radiographics 21:439, 2001.
3. Maisch B, Seferovic PM, Ristic AD, et al: Guidelines on the diagnosis and management of pericardial diseases. Eur Heart J 25:587, 2004.
4. Tsang TS, Barnes ME, Gersh BJ: Outcomes of clinically significant idiopathic pericardial effusion requiring intervention. Am J Cardiol 91:704, 2002.
5. Lee PJ, Mallik R: Cardiovascular effects of radiation therapy. Cardiol Rev 13:80, 2005.
6. Bertog SC, Thambidorai SK, Prarakh K, et al: Constrictive pericarditis: Etiology and cause-specific survival after pericardiectomy. J Am Coll Cardiol 43:1445, 2004.
7. Wudel LJ, Nesbitt JC: Superior vena cava syndrome. Curr Treat Options Oncol 2:77, 2001.
8. Teo N, Sabharwal T, Rowland E, et al: Treatment of superior vena cava obstruction secondary to pacemaker wires with balloon venoplasty and insertion of metallic stents. Eur Heart J 23:1465, 2002.
9. Rowell NP, Gleeson FV: Steroids, radiotherapy, chemotherapy and stents for superior vena cava obstruction in carcinoma of the bronchus: A systematic review. Clin Oncol 14:338, 2002.
10. Edoute Y, Haim N, Rinkevich D, et al: Cardiac valvular vegetations in cancer patients: A prospective echocardiographic study of 200 patients. Am J Med 102:252, 1997.
11. Ewer MS, Kish SK, Martin CG, et al: Characteristics of cardiac arrest in cancer patients as a predictor of survival after cardiopulmonary resuscitation. Cancer 92:1905, 2001.

Cardiovascular Complications of Cancer Therapeutic Agents

12. Ng R, Better N, Green MD: Anticancer agents and cardiotoxicity. Semin Oncol 33:2, 2006.
13. Swain SM, Whaley FS, Ewer MS: Congestive heart failure in patients treated with doxorubicin: A retrospective analysis of three trials. Cancer 97:2869, 2003.
14. Kremer LC, van Dalen EC, Offringa M, et al: Anthracycline-induced clinical heart failure in a cohort of 607 children: Long-term follow-up study. J Clin Oncol 19:191, 2001.
15. Lipshultz SE, Lipsitz SR, Sallan SE, et al: Chronic progressive cardiac dysfunction years after doxorubicin therapy for childhood acute lymphoblastic leukemia. J Clin Oncol 23:2629, 2005.
16. Peng X, Chen B, Lim CC, Sawyer DB: The cardiotoxicity of anthracycline chemotherapeutics. Mol Interv 5:163, 2005.
17. Swain SM, Whaley FS, Gerber MC, et al: Cardioprotection with dexrazoxane for doxorubicin-containing therapy in advanced breast cancer. J Clin Oncol 15:1318, 1997.
18. Cardinale D, Sandri MT, Colombo A, et al: Prognostic value of troponin I in cardiac risk stratification of cancer patients undergoing high-dose chemotherapy. Circulation 109:2749, 2004.

19. Biganzoli L, Cufer T, Bruning P, et al: Doxorubicin-paclitaxel: A safe regimen in terms of cardiac toxicity in metastatic breast carcinoma patients. Results from a European Organization for Research and Treatment of Cancer multicenter trial. Cancer 97:40, 2003.

20. Kuittinen T, Husso-Saastamoinen M, Sipola P, et al: Very acute cardiac toxicity during BEAC chemotherapy in non-Hodgkin's lymphoma patients undergoing autologous stem cell transplantation. Bone Marrow Transplant 36:1077, 2005.

21. Yeh ET, Bickford CL: Cardiovascular complications of cancer therapy: Incidence, pathogenesis, diagnosis, and management. J Am Coll Cardiol 53:2231, 2009.

22. Pai VB, Nahata MC: Cardiotoxicity of chemotherapeutic agents: Incidence, treatment and prevention. Drug Safety 22:263, 2000.

23. Reis SE, Costantino JP, Wickerham DL, et al: Cardiovascular effects of tamoxifen in women with and without heart disease: Breast cancer prevention trial. National Surgical Adjuvant Breast and Bowel Project Breast Cancer Prevention Trial Investigators. J Natl Cancer Inst 93:16, 2001.

24. Richardson PG, Sonneveld P, Schuster MW, et al: Bortezomib or high-dose dexamethasone for relapsed multiple myeloma. N Engl J Med 352:2487, 2005.

25. Chen MH, Kerkela R, Force T: Mechanisms of cardiac dysfunction associated with tyrosine kinase inhibitor cancer therapeutics. Circulation 118:84, 2008.

26. Force T, Krause DS, Van Etten RA: Molecular mechanisms of cardiotoxicity of tyrosine kinase inhibition. Nat Rev Cancer 7:332, 2007.

27. Krause DS, Van Etten RA: Tyrosine kinases as targets for cancer therapy. N Engl J Med 353:172, 2005.

28. Tan-Chiu E, Yothers G, Romond E, et al: Assessment of cardiac dysfunction in a randomized trial comparing doxorubicin and cyclophosphamide followed by paclitaxel, with or without trastuzumab as adjuvant therapy in node-positive, human epidermal growth factor receptor 2–overexpressing breast cancer: NSABP B-31. J Clin Oncol 23:7811, 2005.

29. Crone SA, Zhao YY, Fan L, et al: ErbB2 is essential in the prevention of dilated cardiomyopathy. Nat Med 8:459, 2002.

30. De Keulenaer GW, Doggen K, Lemmens K: The vulnerability of the heart as a pluricellular paracrine organ: Lessons from unexpected triggers of heart failure in targeted ErbB2 anticancer therapy. Circ Res 106:35, 2010.

31. Agus DB, Sweeney CJ, Morris MJ, et al: Efficacy and safety of single-agent pertuzumab (rhuMAb 2C4), a human epidermal growth factor receptor dimerization inhibitor, in castration-resistant prostate cancer after progression from taxane-based therapy. J Clin Oncol 25:675, 2007.

32. Ewer MS, Vooletich MT, Durand JB, et al: Reversibility of trastuzumab-related cardiotoxicity: New insights based on clinical course and response to medical treatment. J Clin Oncol 23:7820, 2005.

33. Morabito A, De Maio E, Di Maio M, et al: Tyrosine kinase inhibitors of vascular endothelial growth factor receptors in clinical trials: Current status and future directions. Oncologist 11:753, 2006.

34. Chu T, Rupnick MA, Kerkela R, et al: Cardiotoxicity associated with the tyrosine kinase inhibitor sunitinib. Lancet 270:2011, 2007.

35. Scappaticci FA, Skillings JR, Holden SN, et al: Arterial thromboembolic events in patients with metastatic carcinoma treated with chemotherapy and bevacizumab. J Natl Cancer Inst 99:1232, 2007.

36. Yuan TL, Cantley LC: PI3K pathway alterations in cancer: Variations on a theme. Oncogene 27:5497, 2008.

Cardiovascular Complications of Radiation Therapy

37. Heidenreich PA, Kapoor JR: Radiation induced heart disease: Systemic disorders in heart disease. Heart 95:252, 2009.

38. Chen MH, Diller L: Cardiovascular disease in cancer survivors: From bench to bedside. Circ Res 2010; in press.

39. Fajardo LF: The pathology of ionizing radiation as defined by morphologic patterns. Acta Oncol 44:13, 2005.

40. Adams MJ, Lipsitz SR, Colan SD, et al: Cardiovascular status in long-term survivors of Hodgkin's disease treated with chest radiotherapy. J Clin Oncol 22:3139, 2004.

41. Hull MC, Morris CG, Pepine CJ, Mendenhall NP: Valvular dysfunction and carotid, subclavian, and coronary artery disease in survivors of Hodgkin lymphoma treated with radiation therapy. JAMA 290:2831, 2003.

42. De Bruin ML, Dorresteijn LD, van't Veer MB, et al: Increased risk of stroke and transient ischemic attack in 5-year survivors of Hodgkin lymphoma. J Natl Cancer Inst 101:928, 2009.

43. Bowers DC, Liu Y, Leisenring W, et al: Late-occurring stroke among long-term survivors of childhood leukemia and brain tumors: A report from the Childhood Cancer Survivor Study. J Clin Oncol 24:5277, 2006.

44. Heidenreich PA, Hancock SL, Lee BK, et al: Asymptomatic cardiac disease following mediastinal irradiation. J Am Coll Cardiol 42:743, 2003.

45. Glanzmann C, Kaufmann P, Jenni R, et al: Cardiac risk after mediastinal irradiation for Hodgkin's disease. Radiother Oncol 46:51, 1998.

46. Aleman BM, van den Belt-Dusebout AW, De Bruin ML, et al: Late cardiotoxicity after treatment for Hodgkin lymphoma. Blood 109:1878, 2007.

47. Swerdlow AJ, Higgins CD, Smith P, et al: Myocardial infarction mortality risk after treatment for Hodgkin disease: A collaborative British cohort study. J Natl Cancer Inst 99:206, 2007.

48. Shankar SM, Marina N, Hudson MM, et al: Monitoring for cardiovascular disease in survivors of childhood cancer: Report from the Cardiovascular Disease Task Force of the Children's Oncology Group. Pediatrics 121:e387, 2008.

49. Adams MJ, Lipshultz SE: Pathophysiology of anthracycline- and radiation-associated cardiomyopathies: Implications for screening and prevention. Pediatr Blood Cancer 44:600, 2005.

50. Carver JR, Shapiro CL, Ng A, et al: American Society of Clinical Oncology clinical evidence review on the ongoing care of adult cancer survivors: Cardiac and pulmonary late effects. J Clin Oncol 25:3991, 2007.

51. Early Breast Cancer Trialists' Collaborative Group: Favourable and unfavourable effects on long-term survival of radiotherapy for early breast cancer: An overview of the randomised trials. Lancet 355:1757, 2000.

52. Giordano SH, Kuo YF, Freeman JL, et al: Risk of cardiac death after adjuvant radiotherapy for breast cancer. J Natl Cancer Inst 97:419, 2005.

53. Ng D, Constine LS, Deming RL, et al: American College of Radiology ACR Appropriateness Criteria. Follow-up of Hodgkin's Lymphoma. Available at: http:www/acr.org/ SecondaryMainMenuCategories/quality_safety/app_criteria/pdf/Expert PanelonRadiationOncologyHodgkinsWorkGroup/FollowUpofHodgkinsDiseaseDoc2.aspx.

54. Chen MH, Chuang ML, Bornstein BA, et al: Impact of respiratory maneuvers on cardiac volume within left-breast radiation portals. Circulation 96:3269, 1997.

55. Lu HM, Cash E, Chen MH, et al: Reduction of cardiac volume in left-breast treatment fields by respiratory maneuvers: A CT study. Int J Radiat Oncol Biol Phys 47:895, 2000.

56. Korreman SS, Pedersen AN, Aarup LR, et al: Reduction of cardiac and pulmonary complication probabilities after breathing adapted radiotherapy for breast cancer. Int J Radiat Oncol Biol Phys 65:1375, 2006.

CHAPTER 91 # Psychiatric and Behavioral Aspects of Cardiovascular Disease

Viola Vaccarino and J. Douglas Bremner

Stress, Emotions, and Cardiovascular Disease: General Considerations

The cardiovascular system has long been considered vulnerable to the effects of psychological factors, and popular wisdom holds stress and emotions as important risk factors for cardiovascular disease (CVD). There are ample physiologic and experimental data to substantiate this belief and to support a link between a number of psychosocial factors and cardiovascular risk.

The stress response, an adaptive physiologic mechanism that allows the organism to counteract potentially damaging stimuli, results in stimulation of the sympathoadrenal system and the hypothalamus-pituitary-adrenal axis with release of cortisol and norepinephrine. Activation of the stress system is physiologically useful to counteract the stressor. However, repeated or excessive activation due to psychological stress is believed to be damaging because of adverse effects of neuroendocrine activation on hemodynamics, metabolism, and immune function.[1] For the cardiovascular system, psychological factors have been implicated both as triggers of acute coronary events and as promoters of the atherosclerotic process. Potential underlying biologic mechanisms are numerous and include repeated or sustained increase in blood pressure and heart rate, effects on insulin resistance and other metabolic abnormalities, enhanced platelet activity, endothelial dysfunction, increased systemic vascular resistance, autonomic dysfunction, ventricular arrhythmias, plaque instability, and disruption of coronary flow dynamics.[2] Furthermore, inflammation and immune function are emerging as key intermediary factors of the stress response in many biologic systems.[3]

From Animal Models to Human Populations

Research in nonhuman primates has provided some of the strongest experimental evidence of the adverse cardiovascular effects of chronic stress. Spanning many decades, these studies have demonstrated that chronic psychosocial stress causes endothelial damage and accelerated atherosclerosis; they have also indicated that males and females may be affected differently. Cynomolgus monkeys under social stress develop endothelial injury, and this effect is blocked by propranolol, the beta-adrenergic receptor antagonist, indicating that it is mediated by norepinephrine. Among males, dominant individuals develop more extensive atherosclerosis than subordinates do when housed in recurrently reorganized (unstable) social groups. By contrast, it is the subordinate females who develop more atherosclerosis, rather than the dominants.[4] Subordinate females are more likely than dominant ones to have visceral obesity and to have behavioral and physiologic characteristics consistent with a stressed state.

In humans, the adverse effects of experimentally induced stress on the cardiovascular system are well documented (described later; see Mental Stress); yet, the effects of naturally occurring stressors on cardiovascular function and CVD risk have been more difficult to demonstrate. One problem is the definition of exposure. Under the general term of psychosocial stress, investigators have included interrelated but different elements, encompassing a variety of environmental exposures (from traumatic events to job or family difficulties to minor everyday hassles) as well as individuals' responses or emotional states, such as depression and anxiety. Another problem is the lack of standardized measures to consistently define and to quantify type and severity of psychological stress. As discussed in this chapter, the most robust evidence to date implicates low socioeconomic status, work stress, caregiving stress, social isolation, and depression as risk factors for CVD. In addition to manifest disease, many of these factors have been associated with subclinical markers of atherosclerosis. Findings related to other psychosocial and psychiatric factors, such as other forms of chronic stress, anxiety, and anger or hostility, have been less consistent.

Psychological and Psychiatric Conditions in the Cardiac Patient

Recognition of psychological and psychiatric factors is important in the management of the cardiac patient not only because many of these conditions are prevalent and have been linked to adverse cardiovascular outcomes but also because they are related to health behaviors and lifestyle risk factors that have prognostic significance. These include factors such as lower adherence to treatment recommendations, lower physical activity, unhealthy diet, and tobacco smoking. However, psychological and psychiatric conditions are less likely than traditional CVD risk factors to be recognized and managed in current cardiology practice. This is because of complexities in definition and assessment, as mentioned before, but also because many symptoms of psychological distress are easily confused with physical disease, for example, fatigue, weight loss, poor appetite, or trouble sleeping.

Current recommendations call for cardiologists to be more proactive in addressing this important domain of patient care.[5,6] The goals of this chapter, therefore, are to review key epidemiologic and pathophysiologic evidence linking psychological factors to CVD and to discuss their management in the current practice of cardiology. For clarity, we classify psychological and psychiatric conditions into general categories of acute stressful events, chronic stressors, emotional factors (including affective disorders), and personality traits.

Acute Stress

Stressful and Emotional Triggers of Acute Ischemia (see Chaps. 54 and 56)

A key pathophysiologic event underlying acute cardiac ischemia is the disruption of a vulnerable atherosclerotic plaque because of plaque rupture or plaque erosion with superimposed thrombus formation. However, plaque disruption does not always result in an acute coronary syndrome. It is hypothesized that stressful, emotional episodes act as triggers of acute coronary events by causing pathophysiologic derangements that are necessary for an ischemic event to occur in susceptible individuals. These pathophysiologic effects, discussed later, include hemodynamic responses to cardiovascular activation, coronary vasoconstriction, inflammation, and prothrombotic effects (**Fig. 91-1**).[2]

Many studies, albeit not all, have demonstrated an increase in hospital admissions for acute coronary syndromes after emotionally stressful events, such as natural and industrial disasters, terrorist attacks, and sporting events.[2] During the 1994 Northridge earthquake in the Los Angeles area, there was a 35% increase in hospital admissions for acute myocardial infarction in the week after the earthquake compared with the week before. On the basis of coroners' records, sudden cardiac death increased from an average of 4.6 events per day in the week before the earthquake to 24 events on the day of the earthquake and then fell to 2.7 per day in the next 6 days. Only three of these cases were associated with unusual physical exertion. An analysis of all deaths in Los Angeles County confirmed these data and showed that coronary deaths tended to be clustered around the epicenter of the earthquake; by contrast, there was no increase in noncoronary deaths.[7] Studies of the 1995 Hanshin-Awaji earthquake in Japan showed similar results. However, the 1989 Loma Prieta earthquake in the San Francisco Bay Area was not associated with an increase in coronary events. One explanation may be the timing of the earthquakes. Both the Northridge and Hanshin-Awaji quakes occurred in winter and early in the morning, when there is a greater susceptibility to acute coronary syndromes, whereas the Loma Prieta earthquake struck on an October afternoon.

War and terrorist attacks have also been associated with an increase in acute coronary events, but again, results are mixed. During the initial phases of the Gulf War in the Tel Aviv area in 1991, there was an increase in the incidence of acute myocardial infarction and sudden death. By contrast, the World Trade Center terrorist attack in New York City on September 11, 2001, was not linked to an increase in cardiac death or admissions to acute coronary care in New York City immediately after the attack. It is possible that this event, which was observed by most New Yorkers through news reports on television, did not cause acute stress to the same extent as an incident that poses a direct threat to personal safety. However, the incidence of cardiovascular ailments diagnosed by physicians increased by more than 50% in the next 3 years, therefore suggesting a more chronic impact of the attack rather than an acute triggering effect. In addition, after the attack, ventricular arrhythmias increased by more than twofold among patients with implantable cardioverter-defibrillators (ICDs), but this increase did not occur until 3 days after the event and persisted in the next 30 days.[8] These data again suggest that subacute stress may have played a role.

A limitation of these studies is the lack of information on the circumstances surrounding cardiac events, making it difficult to rule out alternative explanations. Apart from emotional stress, cardiac events could be triggered by concomitant factors, for example, vigorous physical exertion (such as running away) or heavy eating and drinking. In this respect, studies of individual emotional triggers, in which patients are asked about their experiences before symptom onset, provide more information. On the other hand, self-reports of patients may be affected by recall bias.

Among individual emotional triggers, acute anger has been studied most extensively.[2] In the Determinants of Myocardial Infarction Onset study, 2.4% of patients reported being very angry or furious in the 2 hours before acute myocardial infarction. In comparison with a matched control period 24 hours earlier, the odds of acute myocardial infarction after acute anger were increased fourfold, and the risk of anger triggering was particularly high in subjects of lower socioeconomic status. The Stockholm Heart Epidemiology Program (SHEEP) study and other studies found similar results, but the incidence of an acute anger episode before symptom onset varies substantially in all these reports, from 1% to 17%, depending on the definition of the anger episode.

In addition to anger, episodes of acute stress or emotions have been reported as triggers of CVD events. Acute work-related stress has been linked to myocardial infarction. In the SHEEP study, patients reporting a sudden, short-term increase in workload, such as a high-pressure deadline, exhibited a sixfold increase in the odds of myocardial infarction during the next 24 hours in comparison with the period between 24 and 48 hours before the infarction.[9] Exposure to heavy traffic has also been associated with increased risk of myocardial infarction.[10] The time the subjects spend in cars or public transportation is directly related to the risk; in addition to stress, however, pollution and noise may contribute to this effect. Stressful life events have been linked to acute myocardial stunning in susceptible individuals with severe, reversible left ventricular dysfunction.[11] These patients, almost all women, also show exaggerated sympathetic nervous system stimulation as indicated by markedly elevated plasma catecholamine levels. Finally, episodes of depression and sadness have also been linked to the triggering of acute myocardial ischemia. Such episodes appear to be common (18%) in the 2 hours before onset of cardiac symptoms[12] and are associated with substantially increased odds of acute coronary syndromes, between 2.5 and 5 (depending on the severity of depression), compared with a control period for each patient.

Mental Stress

A useful method of assessing the effects of stress and emotion on cardiac function is to measure transient ischemic responses to a

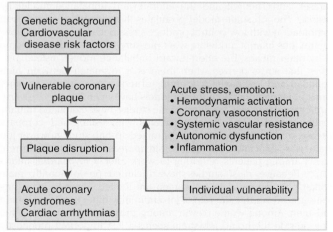

FIGURE 91-1 Potential mechanisms underlying the acute triggering of adverse cardiac events by psychological factors.

standardized psychological stress challenge in the laboratory, or "mental stress test," using mental arithmetic, color naming, public speeches, and similar tasks. Mental stress–induced myocardial ischemia is analogous to exercise stress ischemia, except that the stimulus is psychological rather than physical.[13]

Mental stress ischemia has been studied with a variety of imaging techniques and a range of stressful stimuli.[14] This literature indicates that mental stress ischemia can be induced in one third to two thirds of coronary heart disease patients. It is typically painless and occurs at lower levels of oxygen demand than ischemia due to physical exertion. In addition, mental stress ischemia is generally not related to the severity of coronary artery disease, suggesting that it is not simply a reflection of coronary disease severity. Patients may develop ischemia with mental stress but not with exercise or pharmacologic stress,[15] although results vary. Ischemic responses are induced not only by severe emotional stress but also by milder challenges similar to those that might be encountered in everyday life. In fact, mental stress–induced (but not exercise-induced) myocardial ischemia correlates with ischemia measured in daily life ambulatory monitoring. Thus, mental stress testing could potentially provide a means for the identification of patients vulnerable to myocardial ischemia in everyday life.

In addition to ischemia, mental stress may affect the electrical properties of the heart; a mental stress task in coronary heart disease patients with defibrillators was associated with an increase in T wave alternans and with lower heart rates than with exercise.[16] Mental stress was also associated with a decrease in heart rate variability.[17]

All the results published to date have indicated that mental stress–induced ischemia is a predictor of poor prognosis. Several patient series followed from 1 to 5 years have found substantial increases, between 70% and threefold, in cardiovascular events, revascularization procedures, and death comparing coronary patients with mental stress ischemia with those without, independent of coronary disease severity and CVD risk factors.[13,14] Although the samples of patients followed up longitudinally to date are relatively small, current evidence indicates that myocardial ischemic responses to standardized mental stress are prognostically important at least as much as exercise-induced ischemia.

Potential Mechanisms of Acute Stress

The mechanisms behind emotional triggering of cardiac events are likely to be multiple and may include hemodynamic changes, such as increases in blood pressure, heart rate, systemic vascular resistance, and coronary artery vasoconstriction.[2,13,14] It is clear, however, that different hemodynamic responses underlie ischemia triggered by psychological stress compared with exercise stress. Myocardial ischemic responses to mental stress occur at a lower rate-pressure product than does exercise-induced ischemia in the same patients, although the hemodynamic response tends to be larger than in patients who do not become ischemic. Both people with and without pre-existing coronary heart disease who develop mental stress ischemia show an increase in systemic vascular resistance, suggesting that a rise in afterload caused by peripheral vasoconstriction may play a role in ischemia induced by psychological stress. By contrast, systemic vascular resistance is decreased by exercise. These effects may be secondary to a centrally mediated neurogenic peripheral vasoconstriction; in fact, plasma catecholamines increase rapidly with mental stress and correlate with hemodynamic changes.[18]

Abnormal coronary artery vasomotor response is also observed during mental stress. Patients with atherosclerosis may undergo a paradoxical constriction during mental stress, particularly at points of stenosis, which may reduce myocardial blood flow and thus result in ischemia. This vasomotor response correlates with the endothelium-dependent response to an infusion of acetylcholine, suggesting coronary endothelial dysfunction as a mechanism. The degree of constriction may not, however, be sufficient to explain the decrease in coronary flow during mental stress, which can be reversed by alpha-adrenergic blockade through intracoronary administration of phentolamine; in the absence of epicardial

coronary artery constriction, this suggests sympathetically mediated coronary microvascular dysfunction.[13,14,18] Thus, both coronary endothelial dysfunction and vasomotor abnormalities in the coronary microvasculature appear to play a role in myocardial ischemia triggered by psychological stress.

Autonomic dysfunction is another likely process underlying the acute effects of stress on the heart. Both sympathetic activation and parasympathetic withdrawal can stimulate arrhythmias and lower the threshold for ventricular fibrillation. Heart rate variability, a measure of the beat-to-beat changes in heart rate as the heart responds to internal and external stimuli, is an accepted noninvasive measure of overall cardiac autonomic function. Reduced heart rate variability predicts coronary heart disease incidence in population studies as well as mortality, particularly sudden death, in patients after acute myocardial infarction.[19] Heart rate variability is reduced by acute mental stress in the laboratory and was found to be reduced during major disasters, such as earthquakes and terrorist attacks, in studies of patients who were undergoing ambulatory electrocardiographic monitoring at the time of the event.[2]

Inflammation and immunity are increasingly recognized as key factors in mediation of cellular responses to acute psychological stress. Norepinephrine-dependent adrenergic stimulation due to stress activates the transcription factor nuclear factor κB in circulating monocytes, resulting in initiation of the inflammation cascade.[3] Thus, psychosocial stress stimulates mononuclear cell activation and subsequent immune and inflammatory response, which may result in myocardial ischemia.

On the basis of current evidence, therefore, psychological stress induces physiologic responses that could trigger cardiac ischemia or sudden death. However, it is likely that this risk affects only a subset of vulnerable individuals. In one study, patients who reported emotional triggers of their acute coronary syndrome had more prolonged systolic blood pressure responses and enhanced platelet activation in response to a laboratory stressful challenge compared with the non-trigger group.[20] Therefore, some patients may be particularly susceptible to physiologic responses to emotional stimuli and therefore be at higher risk of unfavorable cardiovascular consequences due to stress. If such patients could be identified in advance, specific procedures could be put in place to minimize their exposure to emotional triggers as well as to reduce their risks associated with such exposure.

Chronic Stress

Work Stress

The belief that work-related stress may be harmful to the heart is highly rooted in popular wisdom; thus, work stress has been extensively studied for its potential adverse cardiovascular effects. Two dominant models of work stress include the job strain model developed by Karasek and Theorell and the effort-reward imbalance model by Siegrist.[5] The job strain model postulates that high work demands in combination with low control produce stress because workers in low-control jobs cannot moderate work pressure by organizing their time or by other means. The effort-reward imbalance model, instead, proposes that stress derives when there is a mismatch between high workload and low payback in terms of money, job security, or other forms of recognition. Both these models have been linked to adverse cardiovascular events, but most of the studies have examined initially healthy populations.[21] Among patients with established coronary disease, studies are few and results mixed. In one study, however, job strain was associated with a twofold increase in risk of recurrent events among patients returning to work after a myocardial infarction.[22] Because most studies have included predominantly male worker populations, data on women are limited. There is some suggestion, however, that the role of job strain may differ between women and men. Among women, even among those who are working full time outside the home, job strain seems a less important prognostic factor than for men, whereas stress in other life domains, such as family and social relations, may be more important.[23]

Low Socioeconomic Status

Socioeconomic status is generally defined by interrelated factors such as occupational status, economic resources, education, and social class. The existence of a social gradient in health and disease has long been recognized.[24] Beginning many decades ago, the Whitehall study of British civil servants reported that even among people who are not poor, there is a social gradient in mortality and morbidity, including CVD, from the bottom to the top of society. Such results have been confirmed in many other contexts including the United States. Low socioeconomic status is accompanied by poorer health habits and higher frequencies of standard CVD risk factors, such as hypertension, obesity, smoking, and unhealthy diet, which, however, only partially account for the CVD gradient due to social class. Many adverse psychosocial characteristics are also related to socioeconomic status. These include financial hardship, poorer housing, neighborhood status, social discrimination and isolation, depression, and adverse working conditions. Thus, low socioeconomic status can be viewed as a composite of chronic stressors that may result in adverse behavioral and physiologic consequences.

Hypothalamic-pituitary-adrenal axis and autonomic dysfunction is observed as socioeconomic status levels decline and may increase the risk for central obesity and metabolic risk factors. The Whitehall II study, for example, described a close relationship between lower social position and increased prevalence of metabolic syndrome, an association that was minimally affected by differences in health behaviors.[25,26] Disturbances in neuroendocrine and cardiac autonomic activity, compatible with activation of the neuroendocrine stress axes, were also noted in subjects with metabolic syndrome and subjects of lower socioeconomic status. Notably, psychosocial factors (socioeconomic status and job-related stress) explained a large portion of the association between adrenal or autonomic disturbances and metabolic syndrome.

Marital and Caregiving Stress

Whereas work stress has been primarily studied among men, marital stress and caregiving stress have been primarily studied among women. In the Stockholm Female Coronary Risk Study, women who underwent a myocardial infarction and reported marital stress had an almost threefold higher risk of recurrent cardiac events than did women with less marital stress after adjustment for other risk factors.[23] Marital stress has also been linked to atherosclerosis progression in women[27]; thus, it appears to be an important risk factor for women. Overall, however, few studies are available on this dimension of chronic stress, and data on sex differences in the response to this stressor are also needed.

Caregiving for an ill family member is common, particularly among women, can be quite stressful, and has been associated with CVD risk and mortality.[5,28] In the Nurses' Health Study, caregiving for an ill or disabled spouse was associated with nearly double increased risk of coronary events after adjustment for other risk factors. Similarly, in the Caregiver Health Effects Study, caregiving was associated with a 63% higher adjusted mortality risk. The adverse effects of caregiving, however, apply only to caregivers who report strain; caregivers not experiencing strain do not have elevated mortality rates. Looking at potential mechanisms, the San Diego Caregiver Study showed that distressed caregivers had an increased likelihood of developing hypertension during the follow-up than controls; they also had higher levels of D-dimer (a circulating procoagulant factor), more sleep disruption, and higher levels of plasma inflammatory cytokines.[28]

Early Life Stress

Psychological trauma, particularly if it occurs early in life, such as childhood maltreatment, is an emerging risk factor for CVD. Its effects may be in part mediated by symptoms of depression, which is associated with trauma exposure. Anda and colleagues, in a series of studies, showed that early adverse life experiences are associated with dramatic increases in anxiety, substance abuse, obesity, and smoking and predict incident coronary heart disease in adulthood independent of these factors.[29] Having 7 or more (of 10) adverse childhood events was associated with an adjusted 3.6-fold increased risk of coronary heart disease. A large proportion of early adverse experiences include childhood sexual or physical abuse, which is common particularly among girls; such history is found in about 20% of women.

A recent meta-analysis confirmed a link between childhood maltreatment and a number of medical outcomes in adulthood, including CVD.[30] Despite heterogeneity of effects across studies, the association is seen both when abuse is measured by self-report and when it is measured objectively. Many potential behavioral, emotional, and biologic explanations may underlie this relationship. Recently, a prospective study linked childhood maltreatment to adult inflammation.[31] Maltreated children showed a significant and graded increase in the risk of having elevated C-reactive protein and other markers of inflammation 20 years later, which persisted after accounting for co-occurring early life risks and health behaviors. This study provides evidence for a long-term effect of early life stress on physical health.

Social Isolation and Lack of Support

Both the size and the quality of a person's social contacts have been related to CVD and total mortality. Social relationships may improve health in a variety of ways, including provision of instrumental and emotional support and encouragement toward a healthy lifestyle and health care seeking. Emotional support may also buffer the adverse effects of psychological stressors. Reverse causation is also possible, however, because individuals who are diseased or otherwise at risk may be less socially engaged.

Despite scientific interest in this construct, there is little theoretical integration on its meaning and little consensus on measurement and mechanisms. Although a number of population studies have shown elevated risk of CVD associated with social isolation or lack of support, results are not consistent, perhaps reflecting variations in measurements and definitions.[21] The effects appear more robust in prognostic studies of patients with coronary heart disease. Factors such as living alone, lacking a confidant, being socially isolated, and perceiving low support have been linked to increased mortality in cardiac populations; in general, the association persisted after adjustment for lifestyle behaviors and disease severity.[21] Thus, instrumental and emotional aspects of social contacts may be particularly beneficial for high-risk individuals such as cardiac patients.

General Stress

Relatively few studies have examined the relationship between nonspecific perceived daily life stress and the onset or exacerbation of CVD. In general, these studies are limited in their measurement of stress and have yielded conflicting results in terms of effect size, sex differences, and other subgroup analyses. For example, the Copenhagen City Heart Study found a relative risk of 2.6 for incident ischemic heart disease comparing high stress versus low stress in men younger than 55 years but no association in women and older men.[32] The largest study addressing this question was the INTERHEART, a large international case-control study of risk factors for myocardial infarction.[33] This study included brief assessments of depression, locus of control, perceived stress at home or work, financial stress, and adverse life events. High general stress at home or work was significantly associated with myocardial infarction, with an odds ratio of 1.55, adjusted for geographic region, age, sex, and smoking. This estimate was similar across regions, ethnic groups, and sex. Permanent general stress, representing the highest severity level of the general stress classification, had an odds ratio of 2.17 for myocardial infarction. The study also evaluated a composite score of psychosocial risk factors and found that in terms of both odds ratio and population attributable risk, the risk associated with psychosocial factors was comparable to that of standard CVD risk factors.[34]

Emotional Factors and Psychiatric Diagnoses

Depression and anxiety differ from other psychological factors considered in this chapter because they are psychiatric disorders and as such amenable to drug treatment or other types of clinical management. Most of the evidence linking these factors to CVD risk, however, has involved the measurement of symptom scales rather than psychiatric diagnoses. In this group, depression has received particular attention and has shown the most robust results for a relationship with CVD.

Depression

Depression is a highly prevalent condition and growing global problem. By 2030, depression is projected to be the second leading cause of disability worldwide (after HIV infection and AIDS) and the number one cause of disability in high-income countries.[35] Depression is three times more common among cardiac patients than among controls, and 15% to 30% of cardiac patients have significant depression. This prevalence is higher in women than in men; among myocardial infarction patients, the prevalence of depression is particularly high, about 40%, among younger women (<60 years old).[36]

Depression as a risk factor varies from mild (subclinical) depressive symptoms to a clinical diagnosis of major depression. As defined by the *Diagnostic and Statistical Manual of Mental Disorders*, fourth edition, major depression is characterized by depressed mood or anhedonia (inability to experience pleasure from normally pleasurable life activities) for at least 2 weeks accompanied by significant functional impairment and additional somatic or cognitive symptoms.

Many meta-analyses of observational studies have provided evidence for an association between clinical depression (or depressive symptoms) and CVD risk, both among individuals initially free of heart disease[37] and in a variety of populations of heart disease patients, including patients with acute coronary syndromes,[37,38] congestive heart failure,[39] stable coronary heart disease,[40] and post–coronary bypass surgery.[37] However, individual studies have produced significantly heterogeneous risk estimates and have varied in their ability to adjust for potential confounding factors such as smoking, physical inactivity, and severity of coronary heart disease. Among individuals initially free of heart disease, a recent meta-analysis reported a pooled unadjusted relative risk for future coronary events of 1.81 (95% confidence interval, 1.53-2.15) comparing depressed with nondepressed persons.[37] Among coronary heart disease patients, the pooled relative risk for recurrent events or mortality was similar, 1.80 (95% confidence interval, 1.50-2.15). However, adjustment for disease severity attenuated the association in coronary heart disease patients by almost 50%, suggesting possible reverse causation (severe coronary heart disease leading to depression).

Most epidemiologic studies of depression as a risk factor for CVD have examined depressive symptoms rather than major depression. Those that did consider major depression tended to find larger risk estimates than those assessing symptom scales, although many were limited in their adjustment for potential confounding factors.[37,40] There is evidence for a gradient of risk linking level of depressive symptoms to likelihood of adverse cardiac events, beginning at relatively low levels of depressive symptoms.

Many potential mechanisms have been postulated for the relationship between depression and CVD.[41] Depression is associated with other cardiovascular risk factors including smoking, sedentary lifestyle, obesity, diabetes, and hypertension, but many studies have shown an independent effect of depression on cardiac outcomes after adjustment for these factors. In heart disease patients, depression is also associated with severity of functional impairment. If functional limitations translate into a decrement in physical activity or self-care, this could accelerate progression of coronary heart disease. In addition, depressed patients show lower adherence to medication regimens, lifestyle risk factor modification, and cardiac rehabilitation. Thus, depression may affect cardiac outcomes through behavioral mechanisms involving healthy lifestyle, delay in seeking treatment, and nonadherence to secondary prevention.[42]

Depression is characterized by an overactivity of the hypothalamic-pituitary-adrenal axis and the sympathoadrenal system that resembles the neuroendocrine response to stress, with increased, or prolonged, release of cortisol and norepinephrine and disruption of normal circadian patterns. These abnormalities may lead to repeated or sustained elevations in blood pressure, heart rate, and plasma glucose concentration and insulin resistance and dyslipidemia.[43]

Depressed individuals also show reduced parasympathetic flow, which contributes to autonomic nervous system dysregulation in depression.[43] Heart rate variability, a noninvasive measure of cardiac autonomic function, is lower in depressed patients. Other indications of autonomic dysfunction in depressed cardiac patients include increased heart rate response to orthostatic challenge, abnormal heart rate response to premature ventricular contractions, and abnormal ventricular repolarization. All these factors are predictors of mortality in cardiac patients.

Enhanced platelet activity in depression has also been proposed as a potential link between depression and cardiac events, but data are limited and results mixed.[44] Other postulated mechanisms involve endothelial dysfunction and inflammation. Psychological stress has been related to impaired endothelial function both in primates and in humans; these findings have been extended to depression.[45] Many studies have shown an association between depression and elevated levels of acute-phase proteins, such as C-reactive protein, and inflammatory cytokines, such as interleukin-6, in subjects with and without CVD. However, results in CVD patients are somewhat inconsistent, and to date there is no evidence that inflammation is a mechanism in the link between depression and cardiovascular outcomes.[46]

Finally, growing evidence suggests that depression and CVD may be different phenotypic expressions of the same genetic substrates.[47] Genetic pleiotropy, however, does not eliminate other causal possibilities, for example, the fact that certain genes cause depression and depression, in turn, causes or complicates CVD.

Despite the important comorbidity between depression and physical illness, less than half of depressed medical patients are recognized by their physicians.[48] During an admission for acute myocardial infarction, less than 15% of patients with depression are identified.[49] One reason for this may be uncertainty about whether depression treatment will improve outcomes and thus whether systematic depression screening is warranted in cardiac patients.[50] Indeed, studies to date have not proved that treatment of depression can improve cardiovascular outcomes. Investigation in this area has been limited, however. Furthermore, depression remains an important illness in and of itself that deserves proper evaluation and treatment. In addition to prognosis, depression substantially affects the quality of life of cardiac patients and is one of the strongest predictors of nonadherence with medical treatment regimens.[51] By recognizing and treating depression, we can improve patients' overall well-being and their adherence to medical treatments and healthy lifestyle behaviors.

Anxiety

Anxiety, like depression, includes a large spectrum of conditions, from psychiatric diagnoses amenable to clinical treatment to subthreshold symptoms that are common in the general population. As for depression, most studies examining the relationship between anxiety and coronary heart disease have considered anxiety symptom scales rather than a clinical diagnosis of anxiety disorder. A systematic review of both etiologic and prognostic studies found highly inconsistent results.[21] About half of the studies failed to find an association between anxiety and CVD risk, both in initially healthy populations and among patients with established coronary heart disease. As with other psychosocial factors, these inconsistencies may be due to differences in the measurement of anxiety and the fact that symptom scales may not discriminate among anxiety disorders that may differ in their biologic substrate and therefore their relationship with CVD. For example, phobic anxiety, rather than other forms of anxiety, has shown more consistent associations with CVD risk, particularly sudden death, in population studies. There is emerging evidence that another anxiety disorder, post-traumatic stress disorder, may increase CVD risk, but studies to date are few and methodologically limited.[52]

Other Psychosocial Characteristics and Personality Traits

Anger and Hostility

Anger and hostility have been intensively studied for their relation with CVD. Despite being different constructs, anger and hostility are often used interchangeably, and their interconnection is poorly defined. Hostility is one of the dimensions of type A personality that was believed, in early research, to be a risk factor for CVD, a relationship not supported by later investigation. Hostility is a personality/cognitive trait characterized by a negative attitude toward others. Anger is an emotional state characterized by feelings ranging from mild irritation to intense fury or rage toward others. A recent meta-analysis found substantial heterogeneity of results, with half to two thirds of the studies failing to find a significant association between anger or hostility and CVD risk.[53] The summary combined estimate for anger and hostility indicated a modest but significant 19% increase in coronary heart disease incidence in initially healthy populations and a 24% increase in recurrent coronary heart disease events in patients with preexisting coronary heart disease. However, studies of higher quality tended to show smaller and nonsignificant effects. The risk associated with anger or hostility appears to be more marked in men and is in large part explained by behavioral factors such as smoking and physical activity.[53]

Type D Personality

Type D (or "distressed") personality, first introduced in 1995 by Denollet and colleagues, is a personality type that combines negative affectivity and social inhibition.[54] It describes individuals who tend to experience negative emotions (dysphoria, tension, worry) and at the same time are inhibited in their expression of emotions, thoughts, and behaviors in a social context. These investigators were able to link this construct to adverse cardiovascular outcomes and total death in a number of studies of CVD patients. Because type D personality is related to other psychosocial characteristics (hostility, anger, depression, and social isolation), its interconnection with and independence from these other factors need more evaluation. However, this personality type seems to be a predictor even after depression and other psychosocial stressors are accounted for. These authors propose that it is the combination of these two traits (negative affect and social inhibition) that is damaging, rather than either one alone.

Psychiatric Care of the Cardiac Patient

Psychotherapy for Depression

In many cases, life events contribute to the development of symptoms of depression and anxiety. Early life stress plays an important role in the development of depression for many people. Relationships and stress in the workplace are also important contributors, and often these factors combine. Dysfunctional relationships or jobs can also contribute to depression. In many cases, medication alone may not suffice for the treatment of depression; psychotherapy plus medication is often better than taking medication alone.

Psychotherapy helps people with depression understand the behaviors, emotions, and ideas that contribute to depression, regain a sense of control and pleasure in life, and learn coping skills. Psychodynamic therapy is based on the assumption that a person is depressed because of unresolved, generally unconscious conflicts, often stemming from childhood. Interpersonal therapy focuses on the behaviors and interactions a depressed patient has with family and friends. The primary goal of this therapy is to improve communication skills and increase self-esteem during a short time. Cognitive-behavioral therapy involves

examination of thought patterns that can be negative and self-defeating and going over the basis of such thoughts and how they contribute to emotions. Psychotherapy has been shown to be as effective for depression as medications, and some people, especially with early life stress issues, may not respond to medication without psychotherapy.

Because of the increased risk of mortality in cardiac patients with depression, it was assumed that successful treatment of depression would reduce this risk. The ENRICHD (Enhancing Recover in Coronary Heart Disease Patients) trial, however, did not find such a beneficial effect of cognitive-behavioral therapy for cardiac outcomes[55]; however, the improvement in depression in comparison to placebo was modest.

Other types of therapy have been shown to be useful for depression and anxiety. These include interpersonal therapy, stress management, and stress reduction. In addition, yoga, meditation, and mindfulness-based stress reduction training can be useful.

Antidepressant Medications

Antidepressant medications are another proven method for the treatment of depression. Antidepressants act on the serotonin and norepinephrine systems as well as other neurotransmitter systems in the brain. Drugs that increase brain levels of serotonin and norepinephrine have been shown to be effective treatment of depression and anxiety. Antidepressants typically bind to proteins called transporters that are responsible for taking the neurotransmitter back up into the neuron after it has been released into the synapse, the space between neurons. Drugs that block uptake of the transmitter by the transporter result in an increase in neurotransmitter in the synapse, which accounts for at least part of the reason that these drugs work. Many of the antidepressant drugs block the serotonin transporter, the norepinephrine transporter, or a combination of the two. The original drugs, the tricyclics, had a more general effect on blockage of neurotransmitter uptake.

TRICYCLIC ANTIDEPRESSANTS. The first medication found to work for the treatment of depression was discovered by accident. The tricyclic drug imipramine (Tofranil) was developed in the 1940s for the treatment of tuberculosis. It was noticed that a number of the depressed patients on the tuberculosis wards were getting better in terms of their depression (if not tuberculosis). This led psychiatrists in France, and later the United States, to try this drug for patients hospitalized for depression, demonstrating its usefulness. This was the birth of the tricyclic medications.

Tricyclics, in addition to imipramine, include doxepin (Sinequan), amoxapine (Asendin), and amitriptyline (Elavil). Tricyclics increase norepinephrine and serotonin levels in the synapse. The most common side effects of the tricyclics are the anticholinergic side effects, which include dry mouth, constipation, memory problems, confusion, blurred vision, sexual dysfunction, and decreased urination. Specific cardiac effects include heart arrhythmias and hypotension. Tricyclics have properties like quinidine, leading to an increase in the PR interval, a prolongation of QRS duration and QT interval, and a flattening of the T wave on the electrocardiogram (see Chap. 36). These effects are usually not of clinical significance. However, tricyclics should be avoided in patients with preexisting cardiac conduction defects, congestive heart failure, or recent myocardial infarction. Prolongation of the QT interval beyond 0.44 second is associated with an increased risk of malignant ventricular arrhythmias (torsades de pointes; see Chap. 39).

The anticholinergic side effects of the tricyclics are especially troublesome for the elderly because they are more susceptible to the memory impairment and orthostatic hypotension that can be associated with these medications. For this reason, it is recommended that the tricyclics amitriptyline and doxepin not be prescribed to the elderly.

Tricyclic medications have been associated with an increased risk of malignant ventricular arrhythmias and sudden cardiac death[56] (see Chap. 41). For patients who suffer a cardiac event while being treated with a tricyclic, abrupt withdrawal from the tricyclic medication can be associated with an increased risk of arrhythmias. Therefore, these medications should be tapered slowly. If prolongation of the QT interval or development of hypotension in patients treated with a tricyclic becomes a problem, tricyclics should be slowly tapered and patients treated with a selective serotonin reuptake inhibitor, venlafaxine, or bupropion (see later). These medications are preferred in patients with new onset of depression after an acute myocardial infarction.

NOREPINEPHRINE REUPTAKE INHIBITORS. Antidepressant medications designed specifically to block reuptake of norepinephrine into the synapse are called norepinephrine reuptake inhibitors (NRIs). Medications in this group include desipramine (Norpramin) and nortriptyline (Aventyl, Pamelor). They have a more favorable profile in terms of anticholinergic side effects and effects on the heart and blood pressure than the tricyclics.

MONOAMINE OXIDASE INHIBITORS. Drugs that block the monoamine oxidase inhibitor enzyme (MAOI drugs) and therefore boost the monoamines (serotonin, norepinephrine) include phenelzine (Nardil) and tranylcypromine (Parnate). They have a more favorable cardiovascular profile than the tricyclics, with little or no effect on cardiac conduction, although they can be associated with orthostatic hypotension and weight gain. They can cause a "wine and cheese reaction" of potentially life-threatening elevations of blood pressure if taken with foods that are high in tyramine content, including wine, cheese, chocolate, and beer. Medications that can precipitate hypertensive reactions if a patient is also taking an MAOI include those with sympathomimetic effects (e.g., amphetamines, ephedrine, cocaine). MAOIs should also not be taken together with meperidine (Demerol). Because of the risk of hypertensive crises, the MAOIs are not recommended for use in cardiac patients and indeed they are no longer commonly prescribed in general.

ANTIDEPRESSANTS WITH NOVEL MECHANISMS OF ACTION. Some drugs act on various neurotransmitter systems or in general are poorly understood in terms of mechanism of action. These include bupropion (Wellbutrin), which primarily acts on dopamine systems and is used for both depression and smoking cessation under the brand name Zyban. Side effects include weight loss and restlessness as well as possible increases in blood pressure. High doses of bupropion can rarely cause seizures. A randomized controlled trial of bupropion versus placebo for the treatment of depression in patients hospitalized after cardiovascular events did not find an increase in mortality or cardiovascular events with bupropion.[57]

Drugs with mixed actions are trazodone (Desyrel) and maprotiline (Ludiomil). These medications have lesser degrees of anticholinergic side effects and effects on the heart and blood pressure than other antidepressant medications do. Trazodone can rarely cause priapism (extended painful erection that requires emergency treatment), however.

Nefazodone (Serzone) has both serotonin reuptake inhibition and postsynaptic serotonin receptor blockade properties. It blocks the reuptake of serotonin into the neuron and also blocks a receptor for serotonin on the neuron on the receiving end. It therefore has a chemically unique mode of action. Nefazodone has been associated with several cases of fatal liver failure. It also has been shown to have teratogenic effects in animal studies and is therefore contraindicated for use in pregnancy. Other side effects include dry mouth, nausea, headache, and upset stomach. Nefazodone has mild effects on the alpha-adrenergic receptor, which means that it can cause mild orthostatic hypotension. Given that alternative antidepressants that do not cause liver failure are just as effective, nefazodone should not be used except as a last resort in the cardiac patient.

Mirtazapine (Remeron) is a tetracyclic antidepressant that has actions on a number of different receptor systems. It blocks presynaptic noradrenergic alpha$_2$ receptors with associated enhancement of norepinephrine release. Mirtazapine also increases serotonin release. Side effects include sweating and shivering, tiredness, strange dreams, dyslipidemia, weight gain, upset stomach, anxiety, and agitation. It can be associated with mild orthostatic hypotension and anticholinergic side effects. It has not been shown to have effects on the heart's electrical properties. In the Myocardial Infarction and Depression-Intervention Trial (MIND-IT), 91 post–myocardial infarction patients with depression were randomly assigned to 8 weeks of mirtazapine or placebo. There was no difference in cardiovascular events between the two groups. Mirtazapine was associated with an increase in fatigue and appetite changes.

SELECTIVE SEROTONIN REUPTAKE INHIBITORS. As the tricyclics went off patent, a new generation of drugs, the selective serotonin reuptake inhibitors (SSRIs), were developed. These medications more specifically act on the serotonin transporter and therefore have a side effect profile different from that of the older tricyclic medications, specifically fewer anticholinergic and cardiac effects, which makes them the antidepressant medications of choice in the population of cardiac patients.

SSRI medications include fluoxetine (Prozac, Sarafem), paroxetine (Paxil), fluvoxamine (Luvox), citalopram (Celexa), escitalopram (Lexapro), and sertraline (Zoloft). They act by blocking the transporter that brings the serotonin back from the synapse into the neuron, effectively increasing the levels of serotonin in the synapse. Fluoxetine, paroxetine, sertraline, and other SSRIs are free of anticholinergic side effects and have no known effects on blood pressure and the heart.

The SSRI medications have not been shown to have greater efficacy than the older tricyclics in the treatment of depression, although a larger number of patients drop out of treatment while receiving tricyclics because of side effects. For example, the Danish Study Group found that the older tricyclic medication clomipramine worked better for severe depression than did paroxetine, although it had more side effects. In general, SSRIs, like the older tricyclics, have only modest efficacy over placebo. A review from 15 years ago showed that more than 80% of the improvement with fluoxetine was accounted for by a placebo effect. A more recent meta-analysis from data submitted to the Food and Drug Administration (FDA) also showed that 80% of the improvement with antidepressants comes from the placebo response.[58] Patients with mild or moderate depression do not have clinically meaningful responses to antidepressants, whereas those with severe depression do.[59]

The primary advantage of SSRIs in the cardiac patient is lesser risk of cardiovascular and anticholinergic side effects. Side effects of SSRIs include nausea, diarrhea, headache, insomnia, and agitation. One of the most troubling side effects of the SSRIs is sexual dysfunction, which includes loss of libido, delayed ejaculation, and erectile dysfunction. Antidepressants without sexual dysfunction side effects can be given instead of an SSRI in these cases, including bupropion, mirtazapine, and trazodone, drugs not in the SSRI class.

SSRI treatment, especially fluoxetine, is also associated with an increase in risk of bleeding.[60] For the cardiac patient taking an aspirin or other antiplatelet or anticoagulation treatment, this can be an important issue; therefore, potential bleeding risks should be carefully evaluated.

SSRIs stopped suddenly can result in a potent withdrawal syndrome, including agitation, nervousness, and sometimes suicidal thoughts. SSRIs can cause akathisia and other extrapyramidal side effects, like the antipsychotics. Akathisia includes feelings of restlessness, pacing, and internal stiffness, which subjectively are very uncomfortable. However, these symptoms are not common and are treatable with benzodiazepines or low doses of propranolol.

A more troubling problem is the potential for suicidality associated with SSRIs. Several recent meta-analyses have shown an increase in suicidal attempts in adults taking SSRIs, and the FDA recently added a warning that SSRI antidepressants may increase the risk of suicidal thoughts or suicide. Studies, however, have shown no difference between SSRIs and the older tricyclic antidepressants in suicide risk, suggesting that *all* antidepressant medications may carry an increased risk of suicide.

Short-term trials of SSRIs have found them to be safe and effective for cardiac patients.[55,61] For instance, in the Sertraline Antidepressant Heart Attack Randomized Trial (SADHART), 369 patients hospitalized for a myocardial infarction or unstable angina with the diagnosis of depression were randomly assigned to receive sertraline at a flexible dose or placebo for 24 weeks. There was no difference in cardiovascular parameters (ejection fraction, QT interval, premature ventricular contractions), cardiovascular events, or death between the two groups. Treatment responders, however, appeared to have better cardiac outcomes than nonresponders. The Canadian Cardiac Randomized Evaluation of Antidepressant and Psychotherapy Efficacy (CREATE) trial found 12 weeks of treatment with the SSRI citalopram to be more efficacious than placebo for the treatment of depression and not to be associated with an increased risk for cardiovascular events.[62] Other studies have not shown differences in cardiovascular outcomes after short-term treatment with fluoxetine in comparison to placebo.[55]

Several cohort studies, however, have shown increased cardiac risk with longer term use of SSRIs. For example, the Nurses' Health Study, which looked at more than 60,000 women without a history of heart disease, found that women taking antidepressants were three times as likely as women not taking antidepressants to have a sudden cardiac death, even after adjustment for severity of depression and risk factors for heart disease.[63] Furthermore, there was an equal risk for SSRIs and other antidepressants outside of the SSRI class. However, sudden cardiac death in healthy women is fairly rare, and in this study, only 46 of 100,000 women taking an SSRI had a sudden cardiac death. The Women's Ischemia Syndrome Evaluation (WISE) study compared women with and without antidepressant and anxiolytic therapy.[64] Antidepressant use was associated with a doubling of risk for cardiovascular events and death. Although anxiolytic use alone was not associated with an increased risk, women who were taking both antidepressants and anxiolytics had a fourfold or greater risk of cardiovascular events and mortality.

SEROTONIN AND NOREPINEPHRINE DUAL REUPTAKE INHIBITORS. The latest group of antidepressants has dual reuptake inhibition for serotonin and norepinephrine (SNRIs) and includes venlafaxine (Effexor) and duloxetine (Cymbalta). In general, these drugs have shown better treatment response for depression than SSRIs and tricyclics. When multiple studies were combined, with treatment response defined as a 50% reduction in symptoms of depression, venlafaxine had a success rate of 74% that was significantly better than that of SSRIs (a 61% success rate) and tricyclics (a 58% success rate).

Both venlafaxine and duloxetine can cause dizziness, constipation, dry mouth, headache, and changes in sleep or more rarely a serotonin syndrome, with restlessness, shivering, and sweating. Venlafaxine has been associated with a dose-dependent increase in blood pressure, which is of particular concern for cardiac patients, especially those with pre-existing hypertension. Although not well studied, there is a good possibility that duloxetine has similar effects. Venlafaxine seems to carry the greatest risk of suicidality among all of the antidepressants, with a threefold increased risk of attempted or completed suicides.

Mood-Stabilizing Agents

Mood-stabilizing agents are used conventionally in the treatment of epilepsy, but they may have efficacy in the stabilization of mood in patients with psychiatric disorders, especially patients with bipolar disorder. Bipolar disorder (formerly known as manic-depressive disorder) is a condition that affects more than 2 million Americans. People who have this illness tend to experience extreme mood swings along with other specific symptoms and behaviors.

It is not known how mood-stabilizing drugs work for bipolar disorder, but many of them modulate function of the excitatory amino acid glutamate, a brain neurotransmitter that plays a critical role in memory and has been implicated in both epilepsy and mood and anxiety disorders. Mood-stabilizing agents include valproic acid (Valproate), carbamazepine (Tegretol), topiramate (Topamax), lamotrigine (Lamictal), phenytoin (Dilantin), and neurontin (Gabapentin). These are commonly used in clinical practice, often in combination with SSRI medications. Valproate can cause a potentially fatal liver failure,

although this is very rare. Side effects of carbamazepine include ataxia, diplopia, and sedation, which are dose related. It can also cause neutropenia and hyponatremia, and in rare cases it is associated with aplastic anemia or life-threatening hepatic toxicity. Carbamazepine has quinidine-like effects on cardiac conduction, similar to the tricyclics, and should be used with caution in cardiac patients. It has interactions with numerous other medications and can affect blood levels of other medications. Lamotrigine in rare cases can cause Stevens-Johnson syndrome, a potentially lethal disease. Lithium (Eskalith, Lithobid, Lithonate) is a primary mineral that has been shown to stabilize the mood of patients with bipolar disorder. Dose-dependent side effects include diarrhea, increased thirst, nausea, trembling, rash, and fatigue. Dose adjustments can eliminate these symptoms. In rare cases, lithium can unmask or exacerbate a sinus node arrhythmia.

Electroconvulsive Therapy

Electroconvulsive therapy (ECT) is used as a last resort for the treatment of depression in patients who have had multiple failed trials of psychotherapy and medication. ECT has an 80% response rate, which is a better response rate than for medications, and contrary to popular belief, it is a safe procedure. ECT causes profound hemodynamic changes, including bradycardia (up to frank asystole, which may last for a few seconds), followed by tachycardia and hypertension. These effects, however, are transient and typically resolve within 20 minutes. Possible complications include persistent hypertension, arrhythmias, asystole lasting more than 5 seconds, chest pain, ischemia, and heart failure. Older age and pre-existing CVD, including hypertension, coronary artery disease, congestive heart failure, aortic stenosis, implanted cardiac devices, and atrial fibrillation, have been associated with increased complication rates. However, most complications remain minor and transient, and most patients can safely complete treatment.[65]

There are no absolute contraindications to ECT. However, the procedure should be delayed in patients who are hemodynamically unstable or have new-onset or uncontrolled hypertension. In patients with stable coronary heart disease and controlled hypertension, medications can be continued through the morning of the procedure. In patients with an implanted pacemaker, the pacemaker should be tested before and after ECT; the magnet should be placed at the patient's bedside in the event that electrical interference leads to pacemaker inhibition and bradycardia. ECT appears safe in patients with an ICD. Detection mode of the ICD should be turned off during ECT, and continuous electrocardiographic monitoring should be performed, with resuscitative equipment by the patient's bedside in the event that external defibrillation is necessary.[65]

Antipsychotics

The typical antipsychotic medications block the dopamine D_2 receptor in the brain, which is thought to be involved in the symptoms of psychosis. Probably more important, antipsychotics (previously known as major tranquilizers) are very sedating, which leads to their use in patients who have agitated behavior.

The antipsychotic drugs developed for schizophrenia are also used as an adjunct to antidepressants for treatment-resistant depression. Some studies, however, have shown an increased risk of death when antipsychotics are used in the elderly. Therefore, they should be used with caution in this population.

The first generation of antipsychotic medications included chlorpromazine (Thorazine), haloperidol (Haldol), thioridazine (Mellaril), and perphenazine (Trilafon). These medications can be associated with troubling extrapyramidal side effects, including twitching, jerking movements, and lip smacking. They also can cause orthostatic hypotension and have anticholinergic side effects and therefore may interfere with memory in the elderly, especially the low-potency antipsychotics thioridazine and chlorpromazine. Typical antipsychotics have mild effects on cardiac conduction, to a lesser degree than tricyclics and greater in the low-potency antipsychotics. High doses of haloperidol have been associated with rare cases of ventricular arrhythmia (torsades de pointes) when given to the agitated, delirious patient.

The second generation of antipsychotic medications, atypical antipsychotics, act by blocking a wide range of different dopamine receptors in addition to other receptors like the serotonin receptors. It is thought that this is the reason they are not associated with risks of extrapyramidal side effects similar to those with the older antipsychotic medications. The first atypical to be produced, clozapine (Clozaril), is associated in rare cases with agranulocytosis, which can be fatal. For this reason, patients taking clozapine have to have their blood counts tested on a regular basis. Clozapine is also associated with anticholinergic side effects and orthostatic hypotension and is not ideal for the cardiac patient. Other atypicals include olanzapine (Zyprexa), risperidone (Risperdal), and quetiapine (Seroquel). These medications have fewer neurologic side effects, although they are not without their own problems. They can interfere with glucose metabolism, increasing the tendency to development of type 2 diabetes.[66] They can also increase lipids and cause weight gain. All of these side effects are particularly adverse for patients with coronary heart disease. Increased diabetes has been seen with olanzapine and clozapine, with less risk with risperidone. There are conflicting results for quetiapine.

Anxiolytic Medications

BENZODIAZEPINE MEDICATIONS. In the 1960s, benzodiazepines displaced barbiturates as the most commonly used treatment of insomnia and became commonly used in patients with anxiety and depression. They were originally marketed as having less potential for dependence and abuse, although this did not bear out over time. Benzodiazepines act on a receptor in the brain called the gamma-aminobutyric acid (GABA)–benzodiazepine receptor complex. This is the same complex to which alcohol and the inhibitory transmitter GABA bind, although benzodiazepines have their own binding site. Like alcohol, they act by increasing a general inhibition on neurons in the brain that results in a calming effect.

Benzodiazepines most commonly prescribed today include alprazolam (Xanax), which is mainly used for anxiety attacks and panic disorder; clonazepam (Klonopin), which is used for epilepsy; and temazepam (Restoril). Triazolam (Halcion) is a very short acting benzodiazepine that was formerly widely prescribed, but it can cause patients to wake up in the night. It also has been associated with a number of negative psychiatric side effects, including violence and aggression thought to be related to disinhibition, especially in the elderly, for which it dropped out of favor.

Other benzodiazepine medications that are longer acting and that are still sometimes used in the treatment of insomnia include oxazepam (Serax), lorazepam (Ativan), chlordiazepoxide (Librium), clorazepate (Tranxene), halazepam (Paxipam), prazepam (Centrax), quazepam (Doral), estazolam (Prosom), diazepam (Valium), and flurazepam (Dalmane). Differences in the individual benzodiazepines are related to the time of onset of action and duration of effect.

Benzodiazepines have not been shown to be better in terms of inducing sleep than other drugs such as diphenhydramine and promethazine. They decrease the average time it takes to fall asleep by just 4 minutes. However, individuals taking benzodiazepines report that they *feel* like they fall asleep faster than they actually do. On average, benzodiazepines increase the user's sleep time by about 1 hour per night.

The side effects from benzodiazepines during the day can cause serious problems. Compared with placebo, individuals taking benzodiazepines had 80% more daytime drowsiness, dizziness, and lightheadedness. Other side effects are problems the next day with memory and increased motor vehicle accidents. Use of benzodiazepine medications is associated with a 60% increase in road traffic accidents. This increased risk is not seen with other psychotropics, including antidepressants. Risk is increased further with concurrent alcohol use and in older age.

The long-acting benzodiazepines can cause significant mental impairment the next day in older patients and are associated with a 50% increase in hip fracture because older people who take them do not have full motor skills back the following day, and this increases the risk of falls. Oxazepam has the least effect on memory and as a result is recommended as the best benzodiazepine for use as a sleeping pill, although it should be used for less than 4 weeks. Long-term use is not recommended for all medications for insomnia.

The primary concern in the cardiac patient using benzodiazepines is a potential risk of respiratory suppression. For this reason, benzodiazepines with shorter half-lives should be preferred to those with longer half-lives in cardiac patients. In patients with cardiac disease and associated pulmonary impairment, these medications should be used with caution.

NONBENZODIAZEPINE "Z-DRUG" MEDICATIONS. The newer generation of insomnia medications, zaleplon (Sonata), zolpidem (Ambien), eszopiclone (Lunesta), and zopiclone (Imovane), or Z drugs, act on specific subsets of the GABA receptor. They are commonly called nonbenzodiazepine medications, but the name is misleading because they bind to the same GABA-benzodiazepine receptor complex in the brain as benzodiazepines and alcohol do. The difference is that they bind to a different part of the same receptor complex. They have been marketed as having less dependency and fewer side effects than the older generation of benzodiazepine medications, and some argue that these drugs have less potential for abuse than the benzodiazepines do. However, studies have not shown them to be more effective or safe than the benzodiazepines, and no difference between the different Z drugs for safety or efficacy has been established. As for benzodiazepines, general side effects for all of these medications include memory impairment, drowsiness, headache, dizziness, nausea, and nervousness. An increased risk of road traffic accidents was also seen with zopiclone. Zaleplon has a much shorter half-life (1 hour) than zolpidem (2.5 hours) and eszopiclone (6 hours) and is therefore promoted as being associated with less drowsiness the next day.

A side effect that has been seen in some patients taking zolpidem is sleepwalking. Zolpidem increases slow-wave sleep, which has been associated with sleepwalking. Cases have been reported of people getting out of bed after taking zolpidem, driving, and getting into car accidents, with no memory of what happened. Patients taking zolpidem should not drink any alcohol, as that can increase the risk of having a dangerous sleepwalking accident.

ANTIHISTAMINES. Drugs developed for the treatment of allergies were found to have sedative properties that are useful for insomnia, and versions for this purpose are available both by prescription and over-the-counter. The most commonly prescribed antihistamine for insomnia is hydroxyzine (Atarax, Vistaril). Over-the-counter diphenhydramine (Benadryl, Simply Sleep, Tylenol PM, Excedrin PM, and their "store brand" counterparts) is often used as a sleep aid and is effective for many people. These medications are relatively free of potential for addiction or abuse. Side effects are less common than for benzodiazepines or Z drugs and include dry mouth, urinary retention, and more rarely confusion, nightmares, nervousness, and irritability.

MEDICATIONS WITH OTHER ACTIONS. Ramelteon (Rozerem) is a melatonin receptor agonist that is used for insomnia. Melatonin is a hormone involved in the sleep-wake cycle. Side effects include headache, drowsiness, fatigue, nausea, dizziness, and more rarely diarrhea and depression. Advantages of this medication are the absence of abuse potential and the lack of withdrawal symptoms.

Buspirone (BuSpar), an agonist of the serotonin 1A receptor, is relatively free of next-day drowsiness and memory impairment or the potential for dependence or abuse. Buspirone is efficacious in the treatment of anxiety and is preferable to the benzodiazepines for the treatment of the cardiac patient as it lacks respiratory suppressive effects. Side effects are minimal and include nausea, headache, and lightheadedness. There are no known adverse cardiac effects.

Anxiolytic medications, when used alone, have not been shown to be associated with increased mortality or cardiovascular events in cardiac patients. However, as mentioned before, when used in combination with antidepressants, they have been associated with a fourfold or greater increase in cardiovascular events and mortality in an observational study.[64] Although treatment of anxiety has not been shown to decrease cardiovascular mortality, it does lead to an improvement in wellness and quality of life, which is an important consideration in cardiac patients with anxiety.[67]

Alternative Medicines, Herbs, and Supplements

There are some natural remedies that have been recommended for depression and anxiety (see Chap. 51).

ST. JOHN'S WORT. St. John's wort (*Hypericum perforatum*) is a popular medication for the over-the-counter treatment of mild depression; 12% of Americans report using it at least once a year. St. John's wort has action similar to that of antidepressants, including monoamine oxidase inhibition, serotonin reuptake inhibition, and actions on sigma receptors. St. John's wort has been shown to be better than placebo in some earlier controlled studies and as effective as tricyclic antidepressants in the treatment of depression. However, most of these earlier studies were poorly controlled and did not use standard definitions of depression, making it difficult to draw conclusions about the efficacy of St. John's wort.

A large placebo-controlled randomized trial using appropriate methodology in patients with severe cases of major depression showed no difference between St. John's wort and placebo. However, a direct head-to-head comparison of St. John's wort with the SSRI paroxetine showed that it was better in reducing symptoms of depression in patients with severe major depression; 71% of St. John's wort–treated patients had a 50% reduction in symptoms compared with 60% of those taking paroxetine. In this study, headache was the only side effect with St. John's wort that was more common than with placebo.

A second study funded by the National Institutes of Health and performed by the Hypericum Depression Trial Study Group (HDTSG) showed that St. John's wort was not more effective than placebo but not worse than an antidepressant comparison. In fact, the placebo effect did best; it was effective in 32% of patients compared with 25% for sertraline and 24% for St. John's wort. However, patients taking St. John's wort experienced fewer side effects than did those who took the antidepressant. St. John's wort caused an increase in swelling, frequent urination, and sexual dysfunction; sertraline caused diarrhea, nausea, sexual dysfunction, forgetfulness, frequent urination, and sweating.

Critics of these studies said that selection of only patients with severe depression obscured the potential benefits for patients with mild depression. One recent meta-analysis of patients with severe depression did not show consistent effects for St. John's wort. There was about a 15% increase in efficacy over placebo for severe depression. Another meta-analysis of St. John's wort for both major and minor depression was consistent with greater efficacy, about a 60% increase over placebo. Finally, a recent Cochrane review noted substantial heterogeneity of results across trials but nonetheless concluded that on the basis of the available evidence, the *Hypericum* extracts are 28% superior to placebo in patients with major depression, are similarly effective as standard antidepressants, and have fewer side effects than standard antidepressants.[68]

St. John's wort can interact with a number of medications, including digoxin, theophylline, protease inhibitors, and cyclosporine.

SAMe. *S*-Adenosylmethionine (SAMe), a molecule found in all human cells, is also promoted as a supplement for the treatment of depression. It plays a role in methylation reactions, including gene expression, maintenance of cell membranes, and neurotransmitter synthesis. Administration of SAMe has been shown to increase levels of serotonin in the brain. A meta-analysis from Italy that pooled data from several small studies concluded that SAMe was better than placebo and equivalent to tricyclic antidepressants in efficacy with fewer side effects. However, there was considerable variability in the studies conducted. Studies have also not had adequate long-term

follow-up to determine long-term benefits of SAMe for depression, although it does not appear that SAMe has potential long-term toxicity.

KAVA. Kava (or kava-kava) is an extract of the roots of the Polynesian plant *Piper methysticum* used in the South Pacific for its sedative, aphrodisiac, and stimulatory effects. Active compounds include the kava pyrones, which may have effects on the brain. Some controlled trials have shown that kava reduces anxiety in patients with anxiety disorders. Side effects of kava, however, are not insignificant and include dizziness, dry mouth, gastric disturbance, diarrhea, drowsiness, depression, and more rarely liver failure, which has caused it to be banned in some countries. Because of the real risk of liver failure, kava is not recommended for the treatment of mood disorders.

OMEGA-3 FATTY ACIDS. Low dietary intake and low serum or red blood cell levels of omega-3 fatty acids are associated with depression in patients with and without coronary heart disease and with an increased risk for cardiac mortality. Two omega-3 fatty acids, eicosapentaenoic acid and docosahexaenoic acid, are found in high concentrations at neuronal synapses in the human brain and are essential for neuronal functioning. In depressed psychiatric patients who were otherwise medically healthy, some studies have indicated that supplementation with omega-3 fatty acids dramatically improves the efficacy of antidepressants; however, few controlled studies have been conducted. A study in patients with stable coronary heart disease and depression, however, showed no improvement in depression after 10 weeks of treatment with omega-3 fatty acids plus sertraline versus a placebo plus sertraline.[69]

VITAMINS. Vitamin E, because of its antioxidant properties, was initially thought to have beneficial effects on the inflammatory processes related to plaque formation in the brains of patients with Alzheimer disease. Trials, however, have not found that vitamin E is beneficial for cognition. Both vitamin E and vitamin A have been associated with increased risk of CVD in several large placebo-controlled trials, contrary to initial theories that they would have the opposite effect.

The use of B vitamins has also been advocated as a way to improve cognition and depression because high plasma levels of the amino acid homocysteine have been associated with Alzheimer disease and depression. Because homocysteine is involved in vitamin B pathways, it was thought that lowering homocysteine with vitamin B therapy would lead to an improvement in cognition and depression. In one study, 276 healthy persons older than 65 years with elevated homocysteine concentrations were given folate and vitamins B_{12} and B_6 or a placebo. Neither folate nor vitamin B supplementation resulted in an improvement in scores of cognition after 2 years.[70]

VALERIAN. Valerian is an extract of the valerian root (*Valeriana officinalis*) and is widely prescribed in Europe for the treatment of insomnia. Valerian is available as a supplement in the United States. In an early study, 166 volunteers were given a valerian-containing commercial product or placebo. After three doses, valerian was associated with a significant decrease in the time it takes to fall asleep and improvement in sleep quality. This study did not measure, however, how well the blinding worked, which is important because valerian has a strong and distinctive smell.

An uncontrolled study of 54 subjects showed a reduction in heart rate, blood pressure, and subjective distress to a stressful task after receiving valerian. This study suggests that valerian may have sedative properties. Valerian does not have major side effects and is probably safe in cardiac patients. However, few data are available to prove its efficacy.

Exercise

A number of studies, dating from the mid-1990s to more recently, show that cardiovascular and resistance or weight training improves depression. These effects may be related in part to an increased growth in brain cells. Regular exercise has favorable effects on the immune system as well, which may promote health, especially in stressed or depressed individuals.

A study of 12,028 randomly selected individuals aged 20 to 79 years showed that increasing physical activity was associated with a 70% reduction in self-reported stress as well as a decrease in life dissatisfaction. Even 2 to 4 hours of walking per week was associated with significant gains. Another study of a group of employees showed reductions in stress levels and depression and improvements in feelings of health and vitality after a 24-week program of aerobic exercise compared with a control group. A 1985 study looked at 43 patients with depression; about half were treated for the condition with antidepressants. Patients were randomized to receive 9 weeks of exercise training (aerobic for 1 hour, three times a week, at 50% to 70% maximum aerobic capacity) or occupational therapy. Exercise was associated with a statistically significant greater decrease in depressive symptoms. In another study, 86 patients with depression who were treated with antidepressants but did not have a therapeutic response were randomized to exercise or health education classes. Exercise involved weight bearing for 45 minutes twice a week for 10 weeks. More patients treated with exercise had an improvement in depression, as defined by a 30% lower Hamilton Depression Scale score; 55% got better with exercise versus 33% without, a difference that was statistically significant. In another study, 156 patients with major depression older than 50 years were randomly assigned to aerobic exercise, antidepressants (sertraline), or a combination of the two for 16 weeks. All patients showed an improvement in symptoms of depression with an essentially identical response between the groups, suggesting that the effect of exercise is at least as large as that of antidepressant medications.

A study found that a half-hour a day of exercise 6 days a week is an effective exercise "dose" to improve the mood of people who have mild to moderate depression, whereas a lower dose is comparable to placebo effect. The study compared two exercise regimens in depressed patients and found that whereas the group that performed 80 minutes of exercise a week received little or no mental health benefit (30% reduction in depressive symptoms versus 29% reduction in the control group), the 3-hour-a-week group had a substantial (47%) reduction in depressive symptoms.[71] Therefore, aerobic exercise at a dose consistent with public health recommendations for CVD prevention is also an effective treatment of mild to moderate depression. Exercise may also complement the effects of antidepressant medication in depressed patients who do not have a complete response to medication.

Treatment Approaches to the Cardiac Patient with Depression and Anxiety

Even though treatment of depression or anxiety has not been shown to improve cardiovascular outcomes in the cardiac patient, it is still necessary to evaluate and to manage these problems to promote the patient's wellness and quality of life as well as to improve patients' ability to adhere to treatments and lifestyle recommendations.

In many cases in which the cardiac patient reports symptoms of depression or anxiety, the cardiologist can address the problem without the need for an immediate referral to a psychiatrist. Many patients complaining of "anxiety" may actually have worry about their cardiac condition. In this situation, education about the cardiac condition, listening to the patient's concerns, and allowing patients to ventilate their worries may go a long way to relieving distress. The next step is to determine if the patient is having thoughts of taking his or her own life or is having severe impairment in functioning that would necessitate referral to a psychiatrist.

A referral to a psychologist or social worker for psychotherapy or counseling may be useful for cardiac patients with symptoms of depression or anxiety. In addition, these patients may benefit from training in stress reduction and stress management techniques, such as yoga, meditation, or mindfulness-based stress reduction classes. The cardiologist may also start a trial of medication. Benzodiazepines

can be used short term but should be limited to less than 2 weeks to reduce the risk for development of dependence. They can be useful, however, in the period before antidepressants start working. An alternative for the treatment of anxiety that does not have the risk of dependence or respiratory suppression is buspirone. Antidepressants useful in the cardiac patient include SSRIs (paroxetine, fluoxetine, sertraline, and others), mirtazapine, and bupropion. Patients who fail to respond to these medications may respond to venlafaxine or duloxetine, with careful monitoring of blood pressure. Healthy lifestyle, especially physical activity, should always be recommended, tailored to patients' functional capabilities, to decrease depression and to improve well-being.

REFERENCES

Stress, Emotions, and Cardiovascular Disease: General Considerations

1. McEwen BS: Central effects of stress hormones in health and disease: Understanding the protective and damaging effects of stress and stress mediators. Eur J Pharmacol 583:174, 2008.
2. Steptoe A, Brydon L: Emotional triggering of cardiac events. Neurosci Biobehav Rev 33:63, 2009.
3. Bierhaus A, Wolf J, Andrassy M, et al: A mechanism converting psychosocial stress into mononuclear cell activation. Proc Natl Acad Sci U S A 100:1920, 2003.
4. Kaplan JR, Chen H, Manuck SB: The relationship between social status and atherosclerosis in male and female monkeys as revealed by meta-analysis. Am J Primatol 71:732, 2009.
5. Rozanski A, Blumenthal JA, Davidson KW, et al: The epidemiology, pathophysiology, and management of psychosocial risk factors in cardiac practice: The emerging field of behavioral cardiology. J Am Coll Cardiol 45:637, 2005.
6. Lichtman JH, Bigger JT Jr, Blumenthal JA, et al: Depression and coronary heart disease: Recommendations for screening, referral, and treatment: A science advisory from the American Heart Association Prevention Committee of the Council on Cardiovascular Nursing, Council on Clinical Cardiology, Council on Epidemiology and Prevention, and Interdisciplinary Council on Quality of Care and Outcomes Research: Endorsed by the American Psychiatric Association. Circulation 118:1768, 2008.

Acute Stress

7. Kloner RA: Natural and unnatural triggers of myocardial infarction. Prog Cardiovasc Dis 48:285, 2006.
8. Steinberg JS, Arshad A, Kowalski M, et al: Increased incidence of life-threatening ventricular arrhythmias in implantable defibrillator patients after the World Trade Center attack. J Am Coll Cardiol 44:1261, 2004.
9. Moller J, Theorell T, de Faire U, et al: Work related stressful life events and the risk of myocardial infarction. Case-control and case-crossover analyses within the Stockholm heart epidemiology programme (SHEEP). J Epidemiol Community Health 59:23, 2005.
10. Peters A, von Klot S, Heier M, et al: Exposure to traffic and the onset of myocardial infarction. N Engl J Med 351:1721, 2004.
11. Wittstein IS, Thiemann DR, Lima JAC, et al: Neurohumoral features of myocardial stunning due to sudden emotional stress. N Engl J Med 352:539, 2005.
12. Steptoe A, Strike PC, Perkins-Porras L, et al: Acute depressed mood as a trigger of acute coronary syndromes. Biol Psychiatry 60:837, 2006.
13. Holmes SD, Krantz DS, Rogers H, et al: Mental stress and coronary artery disease: A multidisciplinary guide. Prog Cardiovasc Dis 49:106, 2006.
14. Strike PC, Steptoe A: Systematic review of mental stress-induced myocardial ischaemia. Eur Heart J 24:690, 2003.
15. Ramachandruni S, Fillingim RB, McGorray SP, et al: Mental stress provokes ischemia in coronary artery disease subjects without exercise- or adenosine-induced ischemia. J Am Coll Cardiol 47:987, 2006.
16. Kop WJ, Krantz DS, Nearing BD, et al: Effects of acute mental stress and exercise on T-wave alternans in patients with implantable cardioverter defibrillators and controls. Circulation 109:1864, 2004.
17. Hamer M, Steptoe A: Association between physical fitness, parasympathetic control, and proinflammatory responses to mental stress. Psychosom Med 69:660, 2007.
18. Soufer R, Jain H, Yoon AJ: Heart-brain interactions in mental stress–induced myocardial ischemia. Curr Cardiol Rep 11:133, 2009.
19. Thayer JF, Lane RD: The role of vagal function in the risk for cardiovascular disease and mortality. Biol Psychol 74:224, 2007.
20. Strike PC, Magid K, Whitehead DL, et al: Pathophysiological processes underlying emotional triggering of acute cardiac events. Proc Natl Acad Sci U S A 103:4322, 2006.
21. Kuper H, Marmot M, Hemingway H: Systematic review of prospective cohort studies of psychosocial factors in the etiology and prognosis of coronary heart disease. Semin Vasc Med 2:267, 2002.

Chronic Stress

22. Aboa-Eboule C, Brisson C, Maunsell E, et al: Job strain and risk of acute recurrent coronary heart disease events. JAMA 298:1652, 2007.
23. Orth-Gomer K: Psychosocial and behavioral aspects of cardiovascular disease prevention in men and women. Curr Opin Psychiatry 20:147, 2007.
24. Siegrist J, Marmot M: Health inequalities and the psychosocial environment—two scientific challenges. Soc Sci Med 58:1463, 2004.
25. Brunner EJ, Hemingway H, Walker BR, et al: Adrenocortical, autonomic, and inflammatory causes of the metabolic syndrome: Nested case-control study. Circulation 106:2659, 2002.
26. Hemingway H, Shipley M, Brunner E, et al: Does autonomic function link social position to coronary risk? The Whitehall II study. Circulation 111:3071, 2005.
27. Wang HX, Leineweber C, Kirkeeide R, et al: Psychosocial stress and atherosclerosis: Family and work stress accelerate progression of coronary disease in women. The Stockholm Female Coronary Angiography Study. J Intern Med 261:245, 2007.

28. Dimsdale JE: Psychological stress and cardiovascular disease. J Am Coll Cardiol 51:1237, 2008.

29. Dong M, Giles WH, Felitti VJ, et al: Insights into causal pathways for ischemic heart disease: Adverse childhood experiences study. Circulation 110:1761, 2004.

30. Wegman HL, Stetler C: A meta-analytic review of the effects of childhood abuse on medical outcomes in adulthood. Psychosom Med 71:805, 2009.

31. Danese A, Pariante CM, Caspi A, et al: Childhood maltreatment predicts adult inflammation in a life-course study. Proc Natl Acad Sci U S A 104:1319, 2007.

32. Nielsen NR, Kristensen TS, Schnohr P, Gronbaek M: Perceived stress and cause-specific mortality among men and women: Results from a prospective cohort study. Am J Epidemiol 168:481; discussion 492, 2008.

33. Rosengren A, Hawken S, Ounpuu S, et al: Association of psychosocial risk factors with risk of acute myocardial infarction in 11 119 cases and 13 648 controls from 52 countries (the INTERHEART study): Case-control study. Lancet 364:953, 2004.

34. Yusuf S, Hawken S, Ounpuu S, et al: Effect of potentially modifiable risk factors associated with myocardial infarction in 52 countries (the INTERHEART study): Case-control study. Lancet 364:937, 2004.

Emotional Factors and Psychiatric Diagnoses

35. Mathers CD, Loncar D: Projections of global mortality and burden of disease from 2002 to 2030. PLoS Med 3:e442, 2006.

36. Mallik S, Spertus JA, Reid KJ, et al: Depressive symptoms after acute myocardial infarction: Evidence for highest rates in younger women. Arch Intern Med 166:876, 2006.

37. Nicholson A, Kuper H, Hemingway H: Depression as an aetiologic and prognostic factor in coronary heart disease: A meta-analysis of 6362 events among 146 538 participants in 54 observational studies. Eur Heart J 27:2763, 2006.

38. van Melle JP, de Jonge P, Spijkerman TA, et al: Prognostic association of depression following myocardial infarction with mortality and cardiovascular events: A meta-analysis. Psychosom Med 66:814, 2004.

39. Rutledge T, Reis VA, Linke SE, et al: Depression in heart failure: A meta-analytic review of prevalence, intervention effects, and associations with clinical outcomes. J Am Coll Cardiol 48:1527, 2006.

40. Barth J, Schumacher M, Herrmann-Lingen C: Depression as a risk factor for mortality in patients with coronary heart disease: A meta-analysis. Psychosom Med 66:802, 2004.

41. Skala JA, Freedland KE, Carney RM: Coronary heart disease and depression: A review of recent mechanistic research. Can J Psychiatry 51:738, 2006.

42. Whooley MA, de Jonge P, Vittinghoff E, et al: Depressive symptoms, health behaviors, and risk of cardiovascular events in patients with coronary heart disease. JAMA 300:2379, 2008.

43. Carney RM, Freedland KE, Veith RC: Depression, the autonomic nervous system, and coronary heart disease. Psychosom Med 67:S29, 2005.

44. von Kanel R: Platelet hyperactivity in clinical depression and the beneficial effect of antidepressant drug treatment: How strong is the evidence? Acta Psychiatr Scand 110:163, 2004.

45. Sherwood A, Hinderliter AL, Watkins LL, et al: Impaired endothelial function in coronary heart disease patients with depressive symptomatology. J Am Coll Cardiol 46:656, 2005.

46. Vaccarino V, Johnson BD, Sheps DS, et al: Depression, inflammation, and incident cardiovascular disease in women with suspected coronary ischemia: The National Heart, Lung, and Blood Institute–sponsored WISE study. J Am Coll Cardiol 50:2044, 2007.

47. de Geus EJ: Genetic pleiotropy in depression and coronary artery disease. Psychosom Med 68:185, 2006.

48. Cepoiu M, McCusker J, Cole MG, et al: Recognition of depression by non-psychiatric physicians: A systematic literature review and meta-analysis. J Gen Intern Med 23:25, 2008.

49. Huffman JC, Smith FA, Blais MA, et al: Recognition and treatment of depression and anxiety in patients with acute myocardial infarction. Am J Cardiol 98:319, 2006.

50. Thombs BD, de Jonge P, Coyne JC, et al: Depression screening and patient outcomes in cardiovascular care: A systematic review. JAMA 300:2161, 2008.

51. Rieckmann N, Gerin W, Kronish IM, et al: Course of depressive symptoms and medication adherence after acute coronary syndromes: An electronic medication monitoring study. J Am Coll Cardiol 48:2218, 2006.

52. Qureshi S, Pyne J, Magruder K, et al: The link between post-traumatic stress disorder and physical comorbidities: A systematic review. Psychiatr Q 80:87, 2009.

Other Psychosocial Characteristics and Personality Traits

53. Chida Y, Steptoe A: The association of anger and hostility with future coronary heart disease: A meta-analytic review of prospective evidence. J Am Coll Cardiol 53:936, 2009.

54. Kupper N, Denollet J: Type D personality as a prognostic factor in heart disease: Assessment and mediating mechanisms. J Pers Assess 89:265, 2007.

Psychiatric Care of the Cardiac Patient

55. Shimbo D, Davidson KW, Haas DC, et al: Negative impact of depression on outcomes in patients with coronary artery disease: Mechanisms, treatment considerations, and future directions. J Thromb Haemost 3:897, 2005.

56. Sala M, Coppa F, Cappucciati C, et al: Antidepressants: Their effects on cardiac channels, QT prolongation and torsades de pointes. Curr Opin Investig Drugs 7:256, 2006.

57. Rigotti NA, Thorndike AN, Regan S, et al: Bupropion for smokers hospitalized with acute cardiovascular disease. Am J Med 119:1080, 2006.

58. Kirsch I, Deacon BJ, Huedo-Medina TB, et al: Initial severity and antidepressant benefits: A meta-analysis of data submitted to the Food and Drug Administration. PLoS Med 5:e45, 2008.

59. Fournier JC, DeRubeis RJ, Hollon SD, et al: Antidepressant drug effects and depression severity: A patient-level meta-analysis. JAMA 303:47, 2010.

60. Ziegelstein RC, Parakh K, Sakhuja A, Bhat U: Platelet function in patients with major depression. Intern Med J 39:38, 2009.

61. Carney RM, Freedland KE: Depression in patients with coronary heart disease. Am J Med 121:S20, 2008.

62. Lesperance F, Frasure-Smith N, Koszycki D, et al: Effects of citalopram and interpersonal psychotherapy on depression in patients with coronary artery disease. JAMA 297:367, 2007.

63. Whang W, Kubzansky LD, Kawachi I, et al: Depression and risk of sudden cardiac death and coronary heart disease in women: Results from the Nurses' Health Study. J Am Coll Cardiol 53:950, 2009.

64. Krantz DS, Whittaker KS, Francis JL, et al: Psychotropic medication use and risk of adverse cardiovascular events in women with suspected coronary artery disease: Outcomes from the Women's Ischemia Syndrome Evaluation (WISE) study. Heart 95:1901, 2009.

65. Tess AV, Smetana GW: Medical evaluation of patients undergoing electroconvulsive therapy. N Engl J Med 360:1437, 2009.

66. Newcomer JW: Abnormalities of glucose metabolism associated with atypical antipsychotic drugs. J Clin Psychiatry 18:36, 2004.

67. Janeway DDO: An integrated approach to the diagnosis and treatment of anxiety within the practice of cardiology. Cardiol Rev 17:36, 2009.

Alternative Medicines, Herbs, and Supplements

68. Linde K, Berner MM, Kriston L: St John's wort for major depression. Cochrane Database Syst Rev (4):CD000448, 2008.

69. Carney RM, Freedland KE, Rubin EH, et al: Omega-3 augmentation of sertraline in treatment of depression in patients with coronary heart disease: A randomized controlled trial. JAMA 302:1651, 2009.

70. McMahon JA, Green TJ, Skeaff CM, et al: A controlled trial of homocysteine lowering and cognitive performance. N Engl J Med 354:2764, 2006.

71. Dunn AL, Trivedi MH, Kampert JB, et al: Exercise treatment for depression: Efficacy and dose response. Am J Prev Med 28:1, 2005.

CHAPTER 92

Neurologic Disorders and Cardiovascular Disease

William J. Groh and Douglas P. Zipes

Cardiac disease occurring secondary to an underlying neurologic disorder is related either to a direct involvement of the heart or is caused by induced neurohormonal abnormalities that act on the heart. In several neurologic disorders, the cardiovascular manifestations are responsible for a greater risk of morbidity and mortality than the neurologic manifestations. This chapter will review those neurologic disorders associated with important cardiovascular sequelae.

Muscular Dystrophies

The muscular dystrophies are a diffuse group of heritable disorders in which direct involvement of cardiac muscle is present to a variable degree. The muscular dystrophies that manifest cardiovascular involvement can be classified into the following:
1. Duchenne and Becker muscular dystrophies
2. Myotonic dystrophies
3. Emery-Dreifuss muscular dystrophies and associated disorders
4. Limb-girdle muscular dystrophies
5. Facioscapulohumeral muscular dystrophy

Duchenne and Becker Muscular Dystrophies

GENETICS. Both Duchenne and Becker muscular dystrophy are X-linked recessive disorders in which the genetic locus has been identified as an abnormality in the dystrophin gene. The dystrophin protein and dystrophin-associated glycoproteins provide a structural link between the myocyte cytoskeleton and extracellular matrix functioning to link contractile proteins to the cell membrane. Dystrophin messenger RNA is expressed predominantly in skeletal, cardiac, and smooth muscle with lower levels in the brain. Absence of dystrophin can lead to membrane fragility, resulting in myofibril necrosis and eventual loss of muscle fibers, with fibrotic replacement. Abnormalities in dystrophin and in dystrophin-associated glycoproteins underlie the degeneration of cardiac and skeletal muscle in several inherited myopathies, including X-linked dilated cardiomyopathy. Beyond the inherited disorders, the loss of dystrophin plays a role in myocyte failure in other cardiomyopathies, including sporadic idiopathic, viral myocarditis, and those associated with coronary artery disease. In Duchenne muscular dystrophy, dystrophin is almost absent whereas in Becker muscular dystrophy, dystrophin is present but reduced in size or amount. This leads to the characteristic rapidly progressive skeletal muscle disease in Duchenne and the more benign course in Becker muscular dystrophy. The heart as a muscle is involved in both disorders. Specific dystrophin gene mutations are associated with a higher prevalence of cardiomyopathy.[1]

CLINICAL PRESENTATION. Duchenne muscular dystrophy is the most common inherited neuromuscular disorder, with an incidence of 1/3,500 live male births. Patients typically become symptomatic before the age of 5 years, presenting with skeletal muscle weakness that progresses if untreated so that the boy becomes wheelchair-bound before the age of 13 years (**Fig. 92-1**). Historically, death occurs commonly by age 25 years, primarily from respiratory dysfunction and, less commonly, from heart failure. A multidisciplinary treatment approach including steroids, cardiac therapy, and ventilatory support has lengthened survival. Becker muscular dystrophy is less common, with an incidence of 1/33,000 live male births, has a more variable presentation of skeletal muscle weakness (see Fig. 92-1), and has a better prognosis, with most patients surviving to age 40 to 50 years.

In both Duchenne and Becker muscular dystrophies, elevated serum creatine kinase activity is observed, over 10- and fivefold normal values, respectively.

CARDIOVASCULAR MANIFESTATIONS. Most patients with Duchenne muscular dystrophy develop a cardiomyopathy, but symptoms can be masked by severe skeletal muscle weakness. Preclinical cardiac involvement is present in 25% by age 6, with the onset of clinically apparent cardiomyopathy after age 10 years common. Up to 90% of Duchenne muscular dystrophy patients 18 years of age or older have a dilated cardiomyopathy by echocardiography. Predilection for involvement in the inferobasal and lateral left ventricle has been observed (**Fig. 92-2**). As with the skeletal muscle weakness, cardiac involvement in Becker muscular dystrophy is more variable than in Duchenne muscular dystrophy, ranging from none or subclinical to severe cardiomyopathy requiring transplantation. Cardiac involvement in Becker muscular dystrophy is independent of the severity of skeletal muscle involvement, with some but not all investigators observing increased likelihood of cardiovascular disease in older patients. More than 50% of patients with subclinical or benign skeletal muscle disease were noted to have cardiac involvement if carefully evaluated. Progression in the severity of cardiac involvement is common. Cardiomyopathy can initially involve only the right ventricle.

Thoracic deformities and a high diaphragm can alter the cardiovascular examination in Duchenne muscular dystrophy. A reduction in the anterior-posterior chest dimension is commonly responsible for a systolic impulse displaced to the left sternal border, a grade 1-3/6 short midsystolic murmur in the second left interspace, and a loud pulmonary component of the second heart sound. In Duchenne and Becker muscular dystrophies, mitral regurgitation is commonly observed. The presence of mitral regurgitation is related to posterior papillary muscle dysfunction in Duchenne muscular dystrophy and to mitral annular dilation in Becker muscular dystrophy.

Female carriers of Duchenne and Becker muscular dystrophies are at increased risk of dilated cardiomyopathy.

Electrocardiography

In most patients with Duchenne muscular dystrophy, the electrocardiogram (ECG) is abnormal (see Chap. 13). The classically described electrocardiographic pattern shows distinctive tall R waves and increased R/S amplitude in V_1 and deep narrow Q waves in the left precordial leads, possibly related to the posterolateral left ventricular involvement (**Fig. 92-3**). Other common findings include a short PR interval and right ventricular hypertrophy. There does not appear to be an association between the presence of a dilated cardiomyopathy and electrocardiographic abnormalities.[2] In patients with Becker muscular dystrophy, electrocardiographic abnormalities are present in up to 75%. These include tall R waves and increased R/S amplitude in V_1, akin to that seen in Duchenne muscular dystrophy, but can also show frequent incomplete right bundle branch block. This may be related to early involvement of the right ventricle. In patients with congestive heart failure, left bundle branch block is common.

Echocardiography

Diastolic dysfunction and regional wall motion abnormalities as observed by echocardiography (see Chap. 15) can precede the global systolic dysfunction in Duchenne and Becker muscular dystrophies. Regional abnormalities in the posterobasal and lateral wall typically occur earlier than in other areas (see Fig. 92-2). A process akin to left ventricular noncompaction can be observed, possibly resulting from compensatory mechanisms in response to the failing dystrophic myocardium. Mitral regurgitation can result from dystrophic changes in the posterior leaflet papillary muscles.

Arrhythmias

In Duchenne muscular dystrophy, persistent or labile sinus tachycardia is the most common arrhythmia recognized (see Chap. 39). Atrial arrhythmias, including atrial fibrillation and atrial flutter, occur primarily as a preterminal rhythm. Abnormalities in atrioventricular conduction have been observed, with both short and prolonged PR intervals recognized. Ventricular arrhythmias occur on monitoring in 30%, primarily ventricular premature beats. Complex ventricular arrhythmias have been reported, more commonly in patients with severe skeletal muscle disease. Sudden

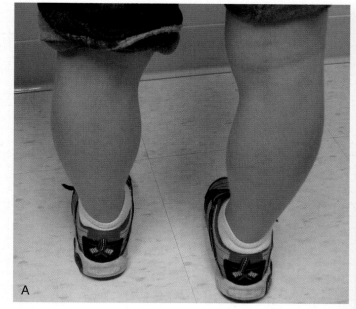
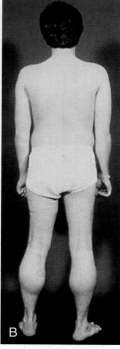

FIGURE 92-1 A, Calf pseudohypertrophy in an 8-year-old boy with Duchenne muscular dystrophy. **B,** Becker muscular dystrophy in a 24-year-old man. There is dystrophy of the shoulder girdle and calf pseudohypertrophy. (**A** courtesy of Dr. Laurence E. Walsh; **B** courtesy of Dr. Robert M. Pascuzzi.)

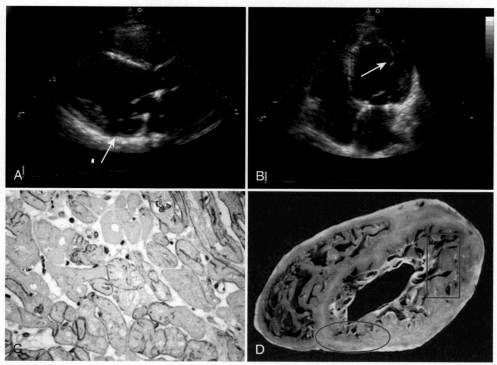

FIGURE 92-2 Cardiac involvement in a 32-year-old man with Becker muscular dystrophy. **A, B,** Transthoracic echocardiogram showing localized thinning and noncompaction in the inferobasal (A, arrow) and apicolateral left ventricle (B, arrow). **C,** Myocardial biopsy showing discontinuous and absent staining consistent with Becker muscular dystrophy. **D,** Explanted heart obtained at transplantation correlating with the echocardiogram with involvement in the inferobasal (oval) and apicolateral left ventricle (rectangle). (**C** stained for dystrophin antibody.) (From Rapezzi C, Leone O, Biagini E, et al: Echocardiographic clues to diagnosis of dystrophin-related dilated cardiomyopathy. Heart 93:10, 2007.)

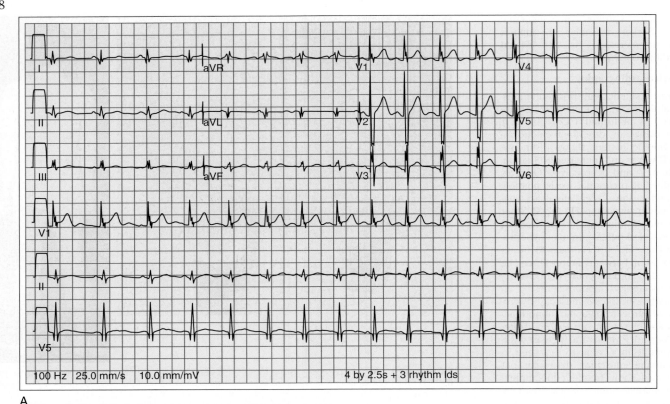

A

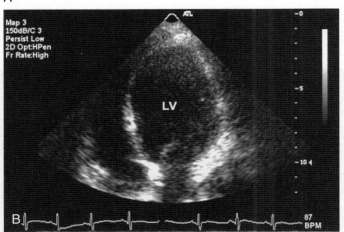

FIGURE 92-3 Dilated cardiomyopathy in a 19-year-old man with Duchenne muscular dystrophy. **A,** ECG showing a QRS complex that is typical of Duchenne dystrophy, with tall R waves in V_1 and deep narrow Q waves in leads I and aVL. **B,** Two-dimensional echocardiogram (parasternal four chamber) showing a dilated, thinned left ventricle (LV).

death occurs in Duchenne muscular dystrophy, typically in patients with end stage muscular disease. Whether the sudden death is caused by arrhythmias is unclear. Several follow-up studies have shown a correlation between sudden death and the presence of complex ventricular arrhythmias. The presence of ventricular arrhythmias was not a predictor for all-cause mortality.

Arrhythmia manifestations in Becker muscular dystrophy typically relates to the severity of the associated structural cardiomyopathy. Distal conduction system disease with complete heart block and bundle branch reentry ventricular tachycardia has been observed.

TREATMENT AND PROGNOSIS. Duchenne muscular dystrophy is a progressive disorder, with death from a respiratory or cardiac cause. Steroids and steroid derivatives are effective in delaying skeletal muscle disease progression and appear also to decrease the progression of the dilated cardiomyopathy.[3] Gene replacement therapy holds

future promise. A primary cardiac cause of death occurs in 25% of patients but appears to be playing an increasingly significant role because of delayed mortality with improved respiratory support. There is an equal distribution of cardiac death from heart failure and sudden death. Annual imaging for assessment of left ventricular function should be initiated in patients at approximately 10 years of age. Angiotensin-converting enzyme (ACE) inhibitors and beta blockers can improve left ventricular function in patients treated early.[1,4] Whether these heart failure therapies improve long-term outcomes is unclear.

In patients with Becker muscular dystrophy, an improvement in left ventricular function is also observed after treatment with ACE inhibitors and beta blockers.[1] Screening left ventricular imaging should occur as in Duchenne muscular dystrophy. Female carriers of Duchenne and Becker muscular dystrophies do not develop a cardiomyopathy during childhood and screening can be delayed until later in

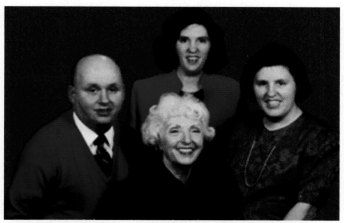

FIGURE 92-4 Myotonic muscular dystrophy in three siblings. The mother (front) is unaffected. Premature balding (left) and characteristic thin facies (rear) are demonstrated.

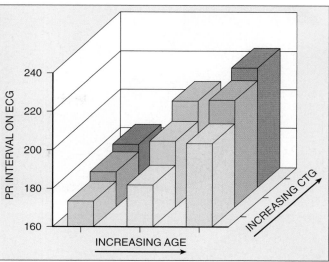

FIGURE 92-5 Relationship between the PR interval on the ECG and age and CTG repeat sequence expansion in 342 patients with myotonic dystrophy type 1. There is a direct relationship between age and CTG repeat sequence expansion and the severity of cardiac conduction disease as quantified by the PR interval. The relationship suggests that cardiac involvement in myotonic dystrophy type 1 is a time-dependent degenerative process, with the rate of progression modulated by the extent of CTG repeat expansion. *(From Groh WJ, Lowe MR, Zipes DP: Severity of cardiac conduction involvement and arrhythmias in myotonic dystrophy type 1 correlates with age and CTG repeat length. J Cardiovasc Electrophysiol 13:444, 2002.)*

adolescence. Whether carriers benefit from afterload reduction therapy is unknown but would seem reasonable based on shared mechanisms. Once heart failure is established, conventional therapy is indicated. Cardiac transplantation has been reported.

Myotonic Dystrophies

GENETICS. The myotonic dystrophies are autosomal dominant inherited disorders characterized by reflex and percussion myotonia, weakness and atrophy of distal skeletal muscles, and systemic manifestations including endocrine abnormalities, cataracts, cognitive impairment, and cardiac involvement (**Fig. 92-4**). Two distinct genetic mutations are known to be responsible for the myotonic dystrophies and are reflected in an updated disease classification. In myotonic dystrophy type 1, the gene mutation is an amplified and unstable trinucleotide, cytosine-thymine-guanine (CTG) repeat found on chromosome 19q13.3. Whereas unaffected patients have 5 to 37 copies of the repeat, patients with myotonic dystrophy have 50 to several thousand repeats. A direct correlation exists between an increasing number of CTG repeats and earlier age of onset and increasing severity of neuromuscular involvement. Cardiac involvement, including conduction disease and arrhythmias, also correlates with the length of repeat expansion (**Fig. 92-5**). It is typical for the CTG repeat to expand as it is passed from parents to their offspring, giving the characteristic worsening clinical manifestations in subsequent generations that is termed *anticipation*.

Myotonic dystrophy type 2, also called proximal myotonic myopathy, has generally less severe skeletal muscle and cardiac involvement than type 1.[5] There is no congenital presentation or cognitive impairment in myotonic dystrophy type 2, typically the most severely involved subsets of the type 1 patients. The genetic mutation responsible for myotonic dystrophy type 2 is a large and unstable tetranucleotide repeat expansion, cytosine-CTG, found on chromosome 3q21. Intergenerational contraction of the repeat expansion has been reported and there is no apparent relationship between the degree of expansion and clinical severity.

The molecular mechanism whereby both myotonic dystrophies exert their similar phenotypic presentations is by the toxic effects of the large mutant RNA expansion on nuclear RNA binding proteins.[6]

CLINICAL PRESENTATION. The myotonic dystrophies are the most common inherited neuromuscular disorders in patients presenting as adults. Until recently, studies have not genetically differentiated myotonic dystrophy types 1 and 2, and therefore the clinical characteristics described are likely for a mixed group. Type 1 is significantly more common than type 2, except possibly in certain areas of northern Europe. The global incidence of myotonic dystrophy type 1 has been estimated to be 1/8000, although it is higher in certain populations, such as French Canadians, and lower to nonexistent in other populations, such as African blacks. The age at onset of symptoms and diagnosis averages 20 to 25 years. Common early manifestations are weakness in the muscles of the face, neck, and distal extremities. On examination, myotonia (delayed muscle relaxation) can be demonstrated in the grip, thenar muscle group, and tongue (**Fig. 92-6**). Diagnosis when the patient is asymptomatic is possible using electromyography and genetic testing. In general, cardiac symptoms occur after the onset of skeletal muscle weakness but can be the initial manifestation of the disease.

Myotonic dystrophy type 2 also manifests with myotonia, muscle weakness, cataracts, and endocrine abnormalities, as in type 1. Age at symptom onset is typically older in myotonic dystrophy type 2.

CARDIOVASCULAR MANIFESTATIONS. Cardiac pathology in the myotonic dystrophies primarily involves degeneration, fibrosis, and fatty infiltration of the specialized conduction tissue, including the sinus node, atrioventricular node, and His-Purkinje system. Degenerative changes are observed in working atrial and ventricular tissue but only rarely progress to a symptomatic dilated cardiomyopathy (**Fig. 92-7**). It is not clear whether there are differences in the cardiac pathology observed between myotonic dystrophy types 1 and 2. The primary cardiac manifestations of the myotonic dystrophies are arrhythmias.

ELECTROCARDIOGRAPHY. Most adult patients with myotonic dystrophy type 1 have electrocardiographic abnormalities. In a large, unselected middle-aged myotonic population followed in a U.S. neuromuscular clinic setting, 65% of patients had an abnormal ECG.[7] Abnormalities included first-degree atrioventricular block in 42%, right bundle branch block in 3%, left bundle branch block in 4%, and nonspecific intraventricular conduction delay in 12%. Q waves not associated with a known myocardial infarction are common. Electrocardiographic abnormalities progress as the patient ages (**Fig. 92-8**).

Electrocardiographic abnormalities are less common in myotonic dystrophy type 2, occurring in approximately 20% of middle-aged patients.

ECHOCARDIOGRAPHY. Left ventricular systolic and diastolic dysfunction, left ventricular hypertrophy, mitral valve prolapse, regional

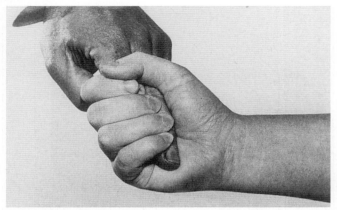

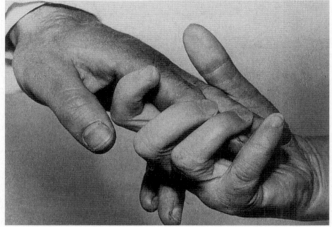

FIGURE 92-6 Grip myotonia in myotonic muscular dystrophy. This patient had an inability to release (bottom) after exerting grip (top). *(From Engel AG, Franzini-Armstrong C [eds]: Myology: Basic and Clinical. 2nd ed. vol. II. New York, McGraw Hill, 1994.)*

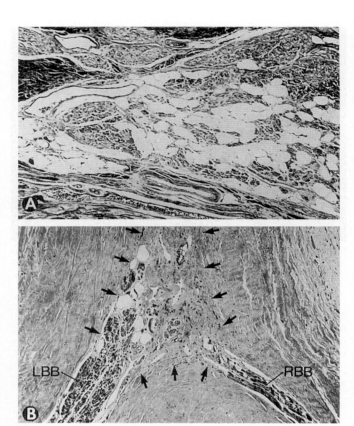

FIGURE 92-7 Histopathology of the atrioventricular bundle in myotonic dystrophy. **A,** Fatty infiltration in a 57-year-old man. **B,** Focal replacement fibrosis and atrophy in a 48-year-old woman. Arrows demarcate expected size and shape of the branching atrioventricular bundle. (**A,** Masson trichrome stain, ×90; **B,** hematoxylin-eosin stain, ×90). LBB = left bundle branch; RBB = right bundle branch. *(From Nguyen HH, Wolfe JT III, Holmes DR Jr, Edwards WD: Pathology of the cardiac conduction system in myotonic dystrophy: A study of 12 cases. J Am Coll Cardiol 11:662, 1988.)*

wall motion abnormalities, and left atrial dilation have been reported in myotonic dystrophy type 1 patients with moderate prevalence rates, as observed by echocardiography (see Chap. 15).[8] However, the prevalence of clinical heart failure is significantly lower, estimated at 2%. Left ventricular hypertrophy and ventricular dilation have been reported in myotonic dystrophy type 2.

Arrhythmias

Patients with myotonic dystrophy type 1 demonstrate a wide range of arrhythmias. With a cardiac electrophysiologic study, the most commonly found abnormality is a prolonged His-ventricular (H-V) interval. Conduction system disease can progress to symptomatic atrioventricular block and necessitate pacemaker implantation. The prevalence of permanent cardiac pacing in patients with myotonic dystrophy type 1 varies widely among studies based on referral patterns and the indications used for implantation. Updated practice guidelines have recognized that asymptomatic conduction abnormalities in neuromuscular diseases such as myotonic dystrophy may warrant special consideration for pacing.

Atrial arrhythmias, primarily atrial fibrillation and atrial flutter, are the most common arrhythmias observed.[7] Ventricular tachycardia can occur. Myotonic dystrophy type 1 patients are at risk of ventricular tachycardia because of reentry in the diseased distal conduction system, as characterized by bundle branch reentry and interfascicular reentry tachycardia (**Fig. 92-9**). Therapy with right bundle branch or fascicular radiofrequency ablation can be curative.

The incidence of sudden death in patients with myotonic dystrophy type 1 is substantial and thought to be caused by primarily arrhythmias. In a prospective registry of 406 myotonic dystrophy type 1

patients from the United States, one third of deaths were sudden, presumably caused by arrhythmias.[7] Sudden death was secondary only to respiratory failure as a cause of death. The mechanisms leading to sudden death in myotonic dystrophy type 1 are not clear. Distal conduction disease producing atrioventricular block can result in the lack of an appropriate escape rhythm and asystole or bradycardia-mediated ventricular fibrillation. Sudden death can occur in myotonic dystrophy type 1, despite previous permanent cardiac pacing, implicating the role of ventricular arrhythmias. Whether a nonarrhythmic cause of sudden death plays a role remains uncertain.

Arrhythmias and sudden death have been reported in myotonic dystrophy type 2 but seem to be rarer than in type 1.[9]

TREATMENT AND PROGNOSIS. Because cardiac manifestations can occur in myotonic dystrophy types 1 and 2, diagnostic evaluation and appropriate therapy should be done for both. However, cardiac management in patients with the myotonic dystrophies is not well established. An echocardiogram can determine whether structural abnormalities are present. In the unusual patient with a dilated cardiomyopathy, standard therapy, including ACE inhibitors and beta blockers, has improved symptoms. Patients presenting with symptoms indicative of arrhythmias, such as syncope and palpitations, should undergo an evaluation, often including a cardiac electrophysiologic study, to determine a cause. Annual ECGs and 24-hour ambulatory monitoring have been recommended for asymptomatic patients. Significant or progressive electrocardiographic abnormalities, despite a lack of symptoms, can be an indication for prophylactic pacing or further diagnostic testing. The presence of significant electrocardiographic conduction

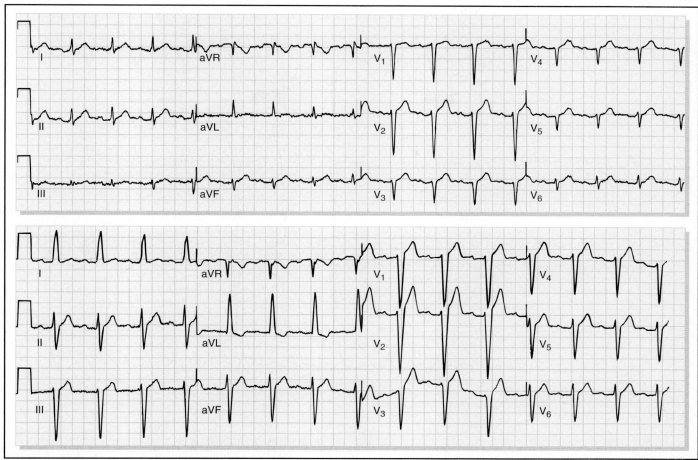

FIGURE 92-8 ECGs obtained 1 year apart in a 36-year-old man with myotonic dystrophy (the top set is older). Note the abnormal Q waves in the precordial leads. An increasing PR interval and QRS duration are observed, consistent with increasing severity of conduction disease.

abnormalities and clinical atrial arrhythmias have been determined to be independent risk factors for sudden death.[7] Whether permanent pacemakers protect against sudden death is unclear, and whether implantable cardioverter-defibrillators (ICDs) would be a more appropriate prophylactic therapy in the myotonic dystrophy patient is untested. Certain families may be more prone to arrhythmia manifestations of myotonic dystrophy. Anesthesia in patients with myotonic dystrophy can increase the risk of atrioventricular block and other arrhythmias. Careful monitoring during the perioperative period, with a low threshold for prophylactic temporary pacing, is recommended.

In patients presenting with wide complex tachycardia, a cardiac electrophysiologic study with particular evaluation for bundle branch reentry tachycardia should be carried out. ICDs are being increasingly used in myotonic dystrophy patients.

The course of neuromuscular abnormalities in the myotonic dystrophies is variable. Death from respiratory dysfunction can occur in advanced skeletal muscle disease. Other patients may be only minimally limited by weakness, up to 60 to70 years of age. Sudden death can reduce survival in patients with the myotonic dystrophies, including those minimally symptomatic from a neuromuscular status. Which evaluation and interventions are appropriate and the degree of effectiveness needed to decrease the risk of sudden death are unclear.

Emery-Dreifuss Muscular Dystrophy and Associated Disorders

GENETICS AND CARDIAC PATHOLOGY. Emery-Dreifuss muscular dystrophy is a rare familial disorder in which skeletal muscle symptoms are often mild, but with cardiac involvement that is common and life-threatening. The disease is typically inherited in an X-linked recessive fashion but there is heterogeneity, in that families have been reported that fit an X-linked dominant, autosomal dominant, and autosomal recessive inheritance pattern. The gene responsible for the X-linked Emery-Dreifuss muscular dystrophy, *STA*, encodes a nuclear membrane protein termed *emerin*. The lack of emerin in skeletal and cardiac muscle is responsible for the disease phenotype. Mutations in genes found on chromosome 1 encoding two other nuclear membrane proteins, lamins A and C, have been identified as being responsible for a variety of other disorders, with a phenotypic expression related to X-linked Emery-Dreifuss muscular dystrophy. These disorders include autosomal dominant and recessive Emery-Dreifuss muscular dystrophy, autosomal dominant dilated cardiomyopathy with conduction disease, autosomal dominant limb-girdle muscular dystrophy with conduction disease, and lipodystrophy with associated cardiac abnormalities.[10]

Nuclear membrane proteins, such as emerin and lamins A and C, provide structural support for the nucleus and interact with the cell's cytoskeletal proteins. Mutations in the tail regions of lamins A and C are responsible for most cases of autosomal dominant Emery-Dreifuss muscular dystrophy, with a phenotype of cardiac and skeletal muscle involvement. Mutations in the rod domain of the lamin A/C gene primarily cause isolated cardiac disease, including dilated cardiomyopathy, conduction system degeneration, and atrial and ventricular arrhythmias.

CLINICAL PRESENTATION. Emery-Dreifuss muscular dystrophy is characterized by a triad of the following: (1) early contractures of the elbow, Achilles tendon, and posterior cervical muscles; (2) slowly progressing muscle weakness and atrophy, primarily in humeroperoneal muscles; and (3) cardiac involvement (**Fig. 92-10**). The disorder has been labeled benign X-linked muscular dystrophy to differentiate the slowly progressive muscular weakness from that of Duchenne muscular dystrophy. A definitive diagnosis can be made in

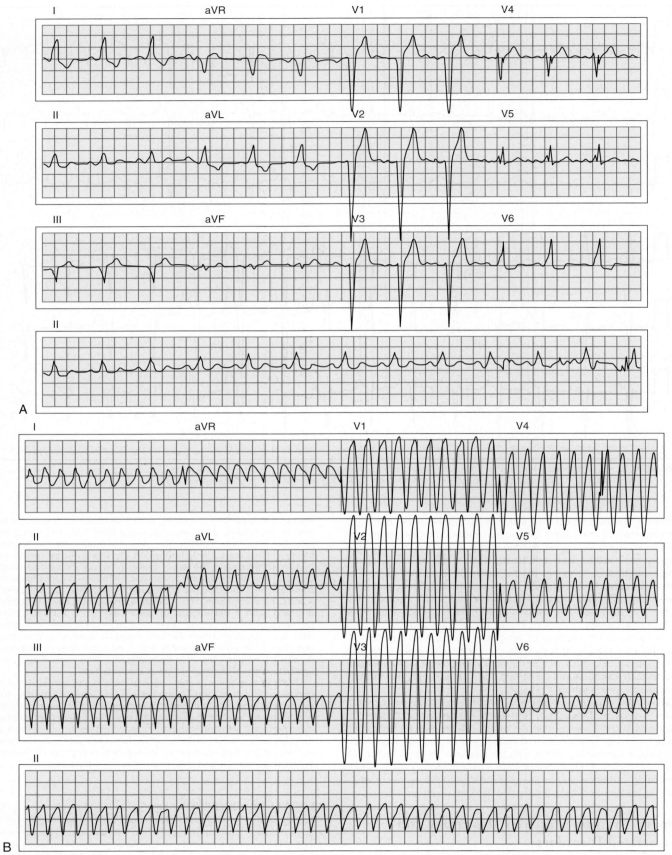

FIGURE 92-9 Bundle branch reentry tachycardia in a 34-year-old woman with myotonic dystrophy type 1 presenting with a symptomatic (recurrent syncope) wide-complex tachycardia. **A,** ECG showing sinus rhythm and a QRS complex with left bundle branch block. **B,** ECG showing a rapid monomorphic tachycardia easily inducible at electrophysiologic study, with left bundle morphology.

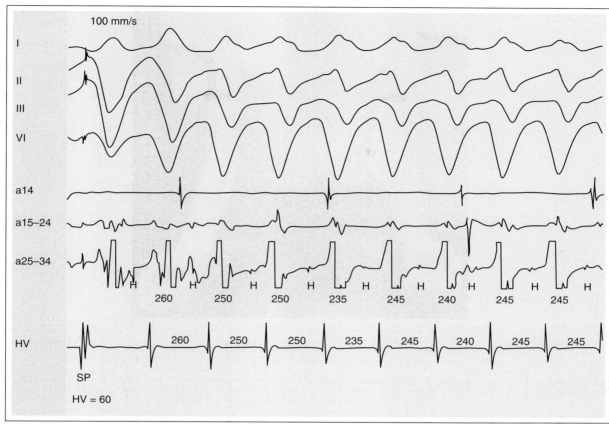

FIGURE 92-9, cont'd **C,** Recordings during electrophysiologic study, including the surface ECG (leads I, II, III, V1) and intracardiac ECGs. A monomorphic ventricular tachycardia is induced with atrial-ventricular (A-V) dissociation and His association consistent with bundle branch reentry tachycardia. H = His recording; HRA = high right atrium; HV = RV; RV = right ventricle; a14 = HRA; a15-24 = His proximal; a25-34 = His distal.

Emery-Dreifuss muscular dystrophy with genetic testing and anti–emerin antibody staining in skeletal muscle biopsy.

In the autosomal dominant and recessive inheritance of Emery-Dreifuss muscular dystrophy, a more variable phenotypic expression and penetrance are typically observed.

A mutation in the lamin A/C gene is also responsible for an autosomal dominant inherited familial partial lipodystrophy, characterized by marked loss of subcutaneous fat, diabetes, hypertriglyceridemia, and cardiac abnormalities.

CARDIOVASCULAR MANIFESTATIONS. Arrhythmias and dilated cardiomyopathy are the major manifestations of cardiac disease in Emery-Dreifuss muscular dystrophy and associated disorders. In X-linked recessive Emery-Dreifuss muscular dystrophy, abnormalities in impulse generation and conduction are exceedingly frequent. ECGs are generally abnormal by age 20 to 30 years, commonly showing first-degree atrioventricular block. The atria appear to be involved earlier than the ventricles, with atrial fibrillation and atrial flutter or, more typically, permanent atrial standstill and junctional bradycardia observed. Abnormalities in impulse generation or conduction are present in the ECG of virtually all patients by age 35 to 40 years and pacing is often required. Ventricular arrhythmias, including sustained ventricular tachycardia and ventricular fibrillation, have been reported in this rare condition. Invasive cardiac electrophysiologic study data are limited in this rare condition. Mild prolongation of the H-V interval and atrial, atrioventricular nodal, and ventricular refractory periods have been observed. Sudden, presumably cardiac, death before age 50 years is common. The incidence of sudden death may decrease with prophylactic pacing.

A nonrandomized study has shown frequent appropriate therapies for ventricular arrhythmias in patients with conduction disease who received prophylactic ICDs.[11] Female carriers of X-linked recessive Emery-Dreifuss muscular dystrophy do not develop skeletal muscle disease but late cardiac disease, including conduction abnormalities and sudden death, can occur. Although arrhythmia disease is the most common presentation of cardiac involvement in X-linked recessive Emery-Dreifuss muscular dystrophy, a dilated cardiomyopathy can rarely develop. The dilated cardiomyopathy is more common in patients in whom survival has been improved with pacemaker implantation. Both autopsy and endomyocardial biopsies have shown abnormal cardiac fibrosis.

An X-linked dominant Emery-Dreifuss muscular dystrophy with incomplete and age-dependent penetrance has been reported.[12] In the families observed, skeletal muscle involvement was absent or mild and the primary cardiac manifestations were atrial fibrillation, heart block, and sudden death. Women were affected later in life than men.

Patients with disorders caused by lamin A and C mutations typically present at age 20 to 40 years with cardiac conduction disease, atrial fibrillation, and dilated cardiomyopathy. Skeletal muscle disease is typically subclinical or absent. Progression of a cardiomyopathy to an extent that heart transplantation is required has been observed. Sudden death in patients with a dilated cardiomyopathy is common. Pacing is often required for symptomatic heart block.

TREATMENT AND PROGNOSIS. Affected patients should be monitored for the development of electrocardiographic conduction abnormalities and other arrhythmias. Atrioventricular block can occur with anesthesia. In X-linked recessive Emery-Dreifuss muscular dystrophy, permanent pacing is recommended once conduction disease is evident, and can be lifesaving. Sudden death, even in patients with pacemakers, can occur. Prophylactic placement of an ICD has been advocated for patients with disorders caused by lamin A and C

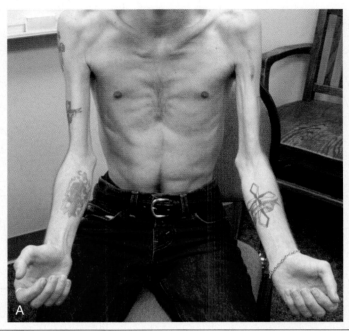

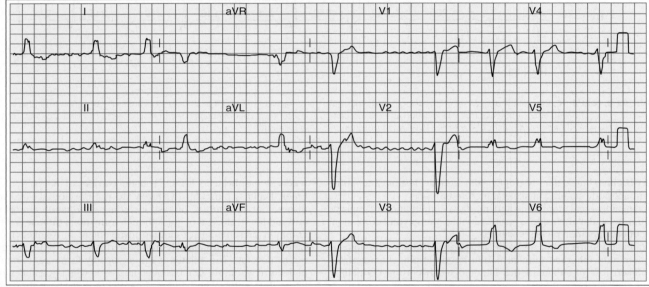

FIGURE 92-10 Emery-Dreifuss muscular dystrophy in a 28-year-old man presenting with syncope. **A,** Contractures of the elbow and atrophy in the humeroperoneal muscles. **B,** ECG at patient presentation showing atrial fibrillation with slow ventricular rate and a QRS complex with left bundle branch block. *(Courtesy of Dr. Robert M. Pascuzzi.)*

mutations if significant electrocardiographic conduction disease is present and pacing is being considered.[11] Whether prophylactic ICDs should be considered only for a certain subgroups of patients or in all patients with Emery-Dreifuss muscular dystrophy and associated disorders, with significant conduction disease or cardiomyopathy, is not clear. History, examination, and cardiac imaging for evaluation of left ventricular function are appropriate for all patients with Emery-Dreifuss muscular dystrophy and associated disorders. Patients with left ventricular dysfunction should benefit from appropriate pharmacologic therapy. Patients appear to benefit from heart transplantation. Female carriers of X-linked recessive Emery-Dreifuss muscular dystrophy develop conduction disease and electrocardiographic monitoring on a routine basis is appropriate.

Limb-Girdle Muscular Dystrophies

GENETICS. The limb-girdle muscular dystrophies constitutes a group of disorders with a limb–pelvic girdle distribution of weakness, but with otherwise heterogeneous inheritance and genetic cause.[13] Inheritance is

most commonly autosomal recessive (limb-girdle muscular dystrophy type 2) but sporadic and autosomal dominant (limb-girdle muscular dystrophy type 1) inheritance is also observed. A genetically based nomenclature (e.g., 1A, 1B, 2A) was introduced to categorize an increasing number of recognized disorders. The genes involved encode dystrophin-associated glycoproteins, sarcomeric proteins, nuclear membrane proteins, and cellular enzymes.

CLINICAL PRESENTATION. The onset of muscle weakness is variable but usually occurs before 30 years of age. The recessive disorders tend to cause earlier and more severe weakness than the dominant disorders. Creatine kinase levels are typically moderately elevated. Patients commonly present with complaints of difficulty with walking or running secondary to pelvic girdle involvement. As the disease progresses, involvement of the shoulder muscles and then more distal muscles occurs, with sparing of facial involvement. Slow progression to severe disability and death can occur.

CARDIOVASCULAR MANIFESTA-TIONS. As with many of the features of the limb-girdle muscular dystrophies, there is heterogeneity observed in the presence and degree of cardiac involvement.

Limb-girdle muscular dystrophies types 2C to F are autosomal recessive disorders caused by mutations in a subunit of the sarcoglycan complex. Patients with sarcoglycanopathies commonly manifest a dilated cardiomyopathy. ECGs show similar abnormalities as in Duchenne and Becker muscular dystrophies, including an increased R wave in V_1 and lateral Q waves. Using electrocardiographic or echocardiographic evaluations, cardiac abnormalities are detected in up to 80% of patients with a smaller proportion symptomatic. A severe cardiomyopathy, including presentation with heart failure in childhood, can occur. Sudden death associated with the cardiomyopathy has been reported. Mechanisms whereby sarcoglycan abnormalities lead to a dilated cardiomyopathy may include a direct myopathic effect exacerbated by vascular spasm and ischemia, increasing cellular dysfunction, and death.[14]

Limb-girdle muscular dystrophy type 2I is an autosomal recessive disorder caused by a mutation in the fukutin-related protein gene located on chromosome 19. The mutation is also responsible for a form of congenital muscular dystrophy. The gene abnormality affects glycosylation of a dystrophin-associated glycoprotein. The age at disease onset and severity of skeletal muscle involvement in limb-girdle muscular dystrophy type 2I is variable, with some patients symptomatic in childhood but, more typically, symptoms developing between age 20 and 40 years. Similar to the sarcoglycanopathies, a high proportion of patients with limb-girdle muscular dystrophy type 2I develop a dilated cardiomyopathy (**Fig. 92-11**).[15] In one series, almost all patients had evidence of cardiac involvement by age 60 years. About 50% of all patients had heart failure symptoms and some were being considered for cardiac transplantation. In limb-girdle muscular dystrophy type 2I, conduction disease did not occur separately from the structural cardiac involvement.

Autosomal dominant limb-girdle muscular dystrophy type 1B is caused by mutations in the gene encoding lamins A and C, similar to that observed in Emery-Dreifuss muscular dystrophy. It is not surprising that the clinical phenotype is also similar to that of Emery-Dreifuss muscular dystrophy, with mild skeletal muscle symptoms and more severe cardiac involvement, primarily arrhythmias. Affected patients develop atrioventricular block by early middle age, often necessitating pacing. Sudden death, thought to be cardiac, is common, including in those in whom pacing was previously instituted. A dilated cardiomyopathy can occur.

TREATMENT AND PROGNOSIS. Because of the heterogeneous nature of limb-girdle muscular dystrophy, specific recommendations for routine cardiac evaluation and therapy are based on the genetic classification. Genetic testing can determine those with limb-girdle types 2C to F, 2I, or 1B, who are at the highest risk for cardiac involvement. In these patients (and their families), cardiac evaluation for arrhythmias and ventricular dysfunction should be done. Patients with dilated cardiomyopathies respond to standard heart failure therapy.[15] Prophylactic placement of an ICD instead of a pacemaker has been recommended in those with lamin A and C mutations after conduction disease is observed.[11]

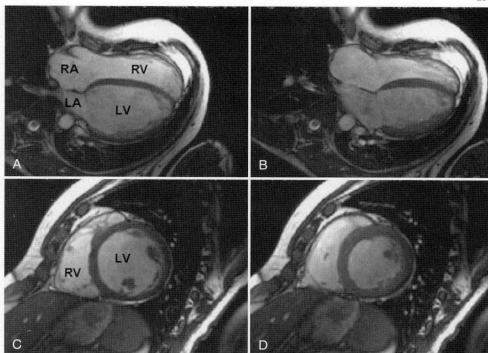

FIGURE 92-11 Cardiac involvement in a 33-year-old man with limb-girdle muscular dystrophy type 2I demonstrated by magnetic resonance imaging. Four-chamber view in diastole **(A)** and systole **(B)**; midventricular short axis in diastole **(C)** and systole **(D)**. The images demonstrate enlarged left and right ventricles, with moderately impaired left ventricular function (calculated ejection fraction = 39%). RA = right atrium; RV = right ventricle; LA = left atrium; LV = left ventricle. (*From Gaul C, Deschauer M, Tempelmann C, et al: Cardiac involvement in limb-girdle muscular dystrophy 2I: Conventional cardiac diagnostic and cardiovascular magnetic resonance. J Neurol 253:1317, 2006.*)

Facioscapulohumeral Muscular Dystrophy

GENETICS. Facioscapulohumeral muscular dystrophy is the third most common muscular dystrophy after Duchenne and myotonic dystrophy, with a prevalence of 1/20,000 persons. It is an autosomal dominant disorder in which the genetic locus has been mapped to chromosome 4q35. Genetic heterogeneity has been reported. The diagnosis can be confirmed by a 4q35 EcoRI allele size of 38 kb or smaller. This repeat region, known as D4Z4, is responsible for binding to a regulatory protein complex that suppresses transcription of adjacent genes. The lack of an appropriate number of D4Z4 repeats results in an overexpression of 4q35 genes and is proposed as the mechanism leading to the facioscapulohumeral muscular dystrophy phenotype. The exact genes that are overexpressed and their protein products are not clear.

CLINICAL PRESENTATION. Muscle weakness tends to follow a slowly progressive but variable course, presenting with facial and/or shoulder girdle muscle weakness and progressing to involve the pelvic musculature. Major disability affecting walking eventually occurs in 20% of patients.

CARDIOVASCULAR MANIFESTATIONS. Cardiac involvement in facioscapulohumeral muscular dystrophy is reported but does not constitute as much of a problem in prevalence or severity as in other muscular dystrophies. In some series, no evidence of cardiac abnormalities were found. Other series have reported a propensity toward arrhythmias, primarily atrial in origin, with atrioventricular conduction abnormalities less common.[16]

TREATMENT AND PROGNOSIS. Because significant clinical cardiac involvement is rare in facioscapulohumeral muscular dystrophy, specific monitoring or treatment recommendations are not well defined. Annual ECGs have been recommended.

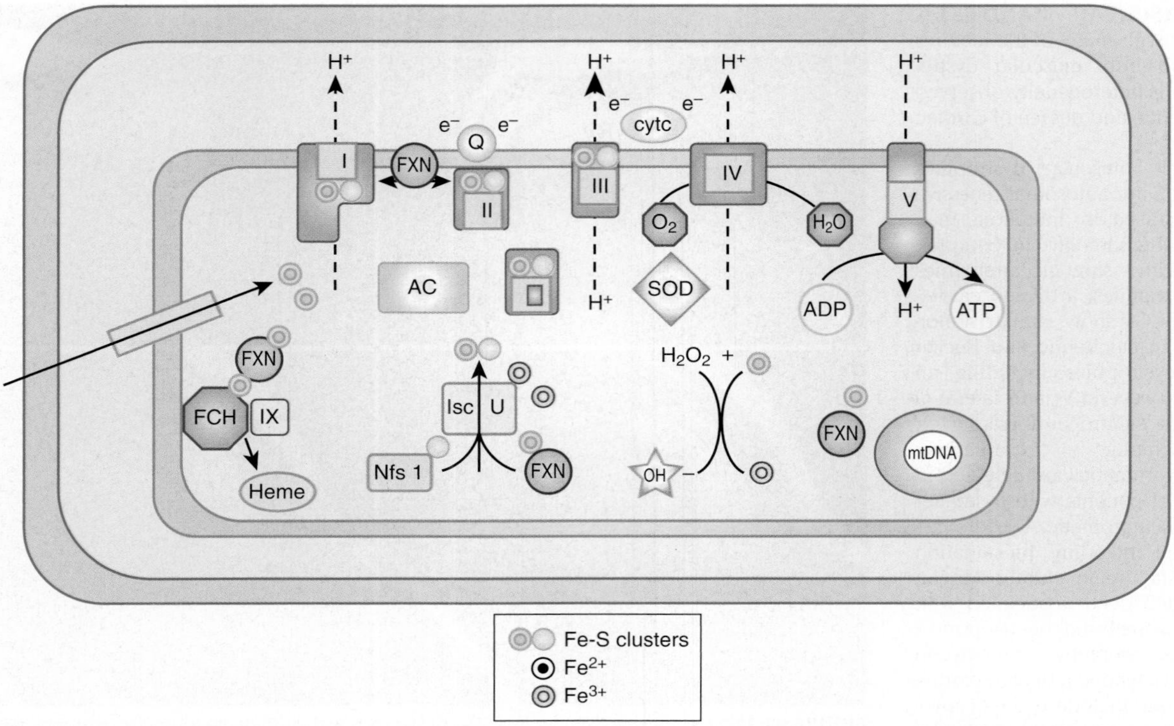

FIGURE 92-12 Postulated functions of frataxin (FXN). 1. Frataxin is a general iron chaperone, providing Fe^{2+} to ferrochelatase (FCH) for heme biosynthesis, mitochondrial iron-sulfur (Fe-S) clusters biogenesis, and maintenance of the mitochondrial aconitase (AC) Fe-S cluster. 2. Frataxin may have a direct interaction with respiratory chain complexes (I-V). 3. Frataxin prevents oxidative stress and protects mitochondrial proteins and mitochondrial DNA (mtDNA) from free Fe^{2+}. It prevents the Fenton reaction by converting Fe^{2+} to Fe^{3+} and thus prevents hydroxyl radical formation. ADP = adenosine diphosphate; ATP = adenosine triphosphate; cytc = cytochrome C; e^- = electron; Q = coenzyme Q (ubiquinone); SOD = superoxide dismutase. *(From Pandolfo M: Friedreich ataxia. Arch Neurol 65:1296, 2008.)*

Friedreich Ataxia

GENETICS. Friedreich ataxia is an autosomal recessive, spinocerebellar, degenerative disease characterized clinically by ataxia of the limbs and trunk, dysarthria, loss of deep tendon reflexes, sensory abnormalities, skeletal deformities, diabetes mellitus, and cardiac involvement.[17] The disease is linked to chromosome 9, with the gene mutation affecting the encoding of a 210–amino acid protein, frataxin. Frataxin is a mitochondrial protein important in iron homeostasis and respiratory function (**Fig. 92-12**). Messenger RNA for frataxin is highly expressed in the heart. The mutation responsible for Friedreich ataxia is an amplified trinucleotide (guanine-adenine-adenine [GAA]) repeat found in the first intron of the gene encoding frataxin. Whereas normal patients have fewer than 33 repeats, patients with Friedreich ataxia have 66 to 1500 GAA repeats. In 95% of patients, both alleles of the gene have the expanded repeat. In 5% of patients, a point mutation occurs on one allele in association with an expanded repeat on the other. The GAA repeat disrupts transcription, severely decreasing frataxin synthesis. The decrease in frataxin leads to mitochondrial dysfunction, poor cellular response to oxidative stress, and apoptosis. Endomyocardial biopsies in patients with Friedreich ataxia have shown deficient function in mitochondrial respiratory complex subunits and in aconitase, an iron-sulfur enzyme involved in iron homeostasis. Abnormal cardiac bioenergetics appear to result from the abnormalities in respiratory function and iron handling. As the GAA triplet size increases, an earlier age of symptom onset, increasing severity of neurologic symptoms, and worsening left ventricular hypertrophy by echocardiography are observed.

CLINICAL PRESENTATION. Friedreich ataxia is the most common inherited spinocerebellar degenerative disease, with a prevalence of 1/50,000. Neurologic symptoms usually manifest around puberty and almost always before the age of 25 years. Progressive loss of neuromuscular function, with the patient wheelchair-bound 10 to 20 years after symptom onset, is the norm. Neurologic symptoms precede cardiac symptoms in most but not all cases.

CARDIOVASCULAR MANIFESTATIONS. Friedreich ataxia is generally associated with a concentric hypertrophic cardiomyopathy (**Fig. 92-13**). Less commonly, asymmetric septal hypertrophy is observed (see Chap. 69). The presence of a left ventricular outflow gradient associated with the septal hypertrophy has been reported. Presentation with a dilated cardiomyopathy is rarer but can occur (**Fig. 92-14**). The dilated cardiomyopathy appears to occur as a progressive transition from a hypertrophic cardiomyopathy. The prevalence of hypertrophy varies among studies but increases in prevalence with a younger age at diagnosis and with increasing GAA trinucleotide repeat length. Up to 95% of neurologically symptomatic patients have abnormalities on electrocardiographic and echocardiographic evaluation. Findings are primarily consistent with ventricular hypertrophy. Left ventricular hypertrophy is not always present on ECGs despite echocardiographic evidence. Widespread T wave inversions are common (**Fig. 92-15**). Patients with left ventricular hypertrophy without systolic dysfunction typically have no cardiac symptoms.

Arrhythmias occur in Friedreich ataxia but are less common than what might be expected considering the high incidence of cardiac hypertrophy. Atrial arrhythmias, including atrial fibrillation and flutter, are associated with the progression to a dilated cardiomyopathy. Ventricular tachycardia, again in the setting of a dilated cardiomyopathy, has been observed. The hypertrophic cardiomyopathy of Friedreich ataxia is not associated with serious ventricular arrhythmias as observed in the other types of heritable hypertrophic cardiomyopathies. Myocardial fiber disarray is not commonly seen in the hypertrophic cardiomyopathy of Friedreich ataxia. Sudden death has been reported but a mechanism has not been well characterized.

Endomyocardial biopsies in Friedreich ataxia have demonstrated myocyte hypertrophy and interstitial fibrosis. Histopathologic examination has revealed myocyte hypertrophy and degeneration, interstitial fibrosis, active muscle necrosis, bizarre pleomorphic nuclei, and periodic acid-Schiff–positive deposition in large and small coronary arteries. Degeneration and fibrosis in cardiac nerves and ganglia and in the conduction system have also been observed. Deposition of calcium salts and iron has been reported.

TREATMENT AND PROGNOSIS. Idebenone, a free radical scavenger, modestly decreases left ventricular hypertrophy and mass in Friedreich ataxia patients.[18] Patients with a greater degree of hypertrophy respond best. It is not clear if idebenone improves left ventricular systolic function. Whether the modest improvement in cardiac imaging parameters with idebenone also leads to any alteration in the clinical cardiovascular course has not been tested. Idebenone does not appear to improve neurologic outcomes.

In most patients with Friedreich ataxia, progressive neurologic dysfunction is the norm, with death from respiratory failure or infection in the fourth or fifth decade. Cardiac death occurs primarily in those developing a dilated cardiomyopathy. These patients tend to do poorly with rapid progression to end-stage congestive heart failure. It is unclear whether pharmacologic or ICD therapy improves outcomes in Friedreich ataxia and dilated cardiomyopathy.

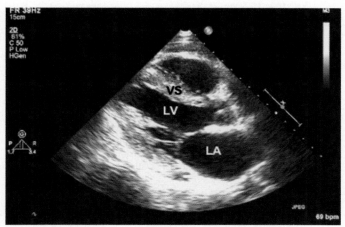

FIGURE 92-13 Hypertrophic cardiomyopathy in a 28-year-old man with Friedreich ataxia. This two-dimensional echocardiogram (parasternal two chamber) shows a thickened ventricular septum (VS) and a dilated left atrium (LA). LV = left ventricle.

Less Common Neuromuscular Diseases Associated with Cardiac Manifestations

Periodic Paralyses

GENETICS. The primary periodic paralyses are rare, nondystrophic, autosomal dominant disorders that result from abnormalities in ion channel genes.[19] They can be classified into hypokalemic, hyperkalemic, and normokalemic periodic paralyses, with several subclassifications in each. In addition, acquired hypokalemic periodic paralysis may complicate thyrotoxicosis, especially in men of Asian descent.

Hypokalemic periodic paralysis is characterized by episodic attacks of weakness in association with decreased serum potassium levels. Penetrance is almost complete in males and approximately 50% in females. Most hypokalemic periodic paralysis have mapped to chromosome 1q31-32, with mutations occurring in the alpha$_1$ subunit of the dihydropyridine-sensitive calcium channel. The disease is genetically heterogeneous, with a mutation at chromosome 17q23 causing abnormalities in the alpha subunit of the skeletal muscle sodium channel (SCN4A).

Hyperkalemic periodic paralysis also manifests with episodic weakness but with symptoms worsening with potassium supplementation. Complete penetrance is observed. Potassium levels are usually high but may be normal during an attack. Hyperkalemic periodic paralysis is caused primarily by mutations in the alpha subunit of SCN4A found at chromosome 17q23. Multiple different mutations in this gene have been reported that result in a potassium-sensitive failure of inactivation (gain of function) in the sodium channel. Hyperkalemic periodic paralysis is genetically heterogeneous, with most affected individuals having an SCN4A mutation but with other loci also identified.

Andersen-Tawil syndrome is a distinct periodic paralysis associated with characteristic dysmorphic physical features, an abnormal QT-U wave pattern, and ventricular arrhythmias (**Fig. 92-16**).[20] The periodic paralysis can be hypo-, hyper-, or normokalemic. Phenotypic variability and incomplete penetrance is observed, making the diagnosis in a family difficult. Approximately two thirds of Andersen-Tawil syndrome patients link to chromosome 17q23, with the mutations responsible occurring in the KCNJ2 gene encoding the inward rectifier potassium protein, Kir2.1. The result of the mutation is a loss of function in the inward rectifier potassium channel, I$_{Kir}$, affecting terminal repolarization of the cardiac action potential. The genetic cause of Andersen-Tawil syndrome in the other third of patients remains unknown. Andersen-Tawil syndrome has been given a long-QT syndrome 7 nomenclature.

CLINICAL PRESENTATION. The primary manifestation of all the periodic paralyses is episodic weakness. Attacks of weakness tend to be more severe and of longer duration with hypokalemic periodic

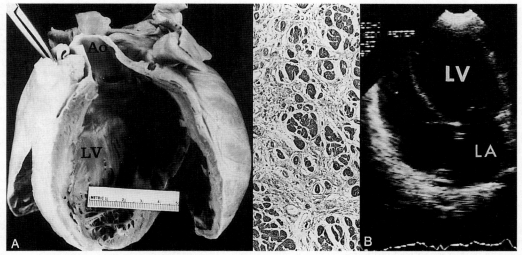

FIGURE 92-14 **A,** Gross and histologic specimens from a 17-year-old boy with Friedreich ataxia whose echocardiogram progressed from normal at age 13 years to a minimally dilated, hypocontractile left ventricle (LV) 3 to 4 years later. The gross specimen shows a mildly dilated LV with normal wall thickness; the walls were flabby. The microscopic section from the left ventricular free wall **(middle panel)** shows marked connective tissue replacement. Although specifically sought, small-vessel coronary artery disease was not identified. **B,** Two-dimensional echocardiogram (apical window) showing the mildly dilated, thin-walled LV. LA = left atrium. (**A, B,** From Child JS, Perloff JK, Bach PM, et al: Cardiac involvement in Friedreich ataxia. J Am Coll Cardiol 7:1370, 1986.)

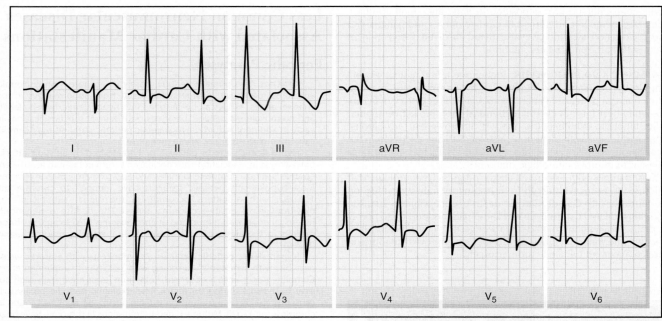

FIGURE 92-15 ECG from a 34-year-old man with Friedreich ataxia. Widespread ST and T changes are observed. *(Courtesy of Dr. Charles Fisch, Indiana University School of Medicine, Indianapolis.)*

paralysis than with hyperkalemic periodic paralysis. In all the periodic paralyses, cold, exercise, and rest after exercise can trigger an attack. Ingestion of carbohydrates can trigger an attack in hypokalemic periodic paralysis but may ameliorate an attack in hyperkalemic periodic paralysis.

CARDIOVASCULAR MANIFESTATIONS. The periodic paralyses are associated with ventricular arrhythmias. Arrhythmias occur primarily in hyperkalemic periodic paralysis and Andersen-Tawil syndrome. Bidirectional ventricular tachycardia has been observed independently of digitalis intoxication. The episodes of bidirectional ventricular tachycardia are independent of attacks of muscle weakness, do not correlate with serum potassium levels, and can convert to sinus rhythm with exercise. Ventricular ectopy is common.

A prolonged QT interval can be observed. In some reports, the prolonged QT interval is episodic and associated with weakness, hypokalemia, or antiarrhythmia therapy. In other cases, a prolonged QT interval can be constant. Andersen-Tawil syndrome is associated with a modest prolongation in the QT interval but more specifically a prolonged and prominent U wave. Ventricular arrhythmias, including premature ventricular contractions, ventricular bigeminy, and nonsustained polymorphic ventricular tachycardia, primarily bidirectional tachycardia, is commonly observed in Andersen-Tawil syndrome. Cardiac conduction abnormalities, atypical of long-QT syndromes, have been observed in Andersen-Tawil syndrome. Torsades de pointes is observed in Andersen-Tawil syndrome but is less common than in the other long-QT syndromes. A family with Andersen-Tawil syndrome and a dilated cardiomyopathy, with an unknown interrelationship, has been reported.

Syncope, cardiac arrest, and sudden death have been reported in the periodic paralyses, most prominently in the Andersen-Tawil syndrome. The factors that portend an increased risk of life-threatening arrhythmias are not clear.

TREATMENT AND PROGNOSIS. The episodes of weakness typically respond to measures that normalize potassium levels. Weakness in hyperkalemic periodic paralysis can respond to mexiletine. Weakness in hypokalemic periodic paralysis can respond to acetazolamide. Treatment of electrolytes usually does not improve arrhythmias or, if it does, only transiently. Improvement in symptomatic nonsustained ventricular tachycardia associated with a prolonged QT interval has

been reported with beta blocker therapy. Class 1A antiarrhythmic agents can worsen muscle weakness and exacerbate arrhythmias associated with a prolonged QT interval. Bidirectional ventricular tachycardia, not associated with a prolonged QT interval, may not respond to beta blocker therapy. Amiodarone has been observed to decrease episodes of polymorphic ventricular tachycardia in Andersen-Tawil syndrome. ICDs have been used for patients with Andersen-Tawil syndrome.

Mitochondrial Disorders

GENETICS. The mitochondrial disorders are a heterogeneous group of diseases resulting from abnormalities in mitochondrial DNA and respiratory chain function.[21] The number of distinct disorders is extensive. Mitochondrial DNA is inherited maternally and most of these disorders are thus transmitted from mother to children of both genders. Some of the disorders occur sporadically or are inherited in an autosomal fashion. Disease severity can vary between patients and family members because both mutant and normal mitochondrial DNA can be present in tissue in a variable proportion. It is not surprising, based on the important metabolic function of mitochondria, that these disorders manifest with systemic pathology. Tissue with a high respiratory workload such as the brain, skeletal muscle, and cardiac muscle are especially affected.

Mitochondrial disorders that have cardiac manifestations present as several clinical phenotypes, including the following: chronic progressive external ophthalmoplegia, which includes the Kearns-Sayre syndrome; *m*yoclonus *e*pilepsy with *r*ed *r*agged *f*ibers (MERRF); *m*itochondrial *m*yopathy, *e*ncephalopathy, *l*actic *a*cidosis, and *s*trokelike episodes, abbreviated MELAS; and Leber hereditary optic neuropathy. Other, rarer mitochondrial point mutation disorders present primarily with cardiac manifestations, typically a hypertrophic or dilated cardiomyopathy. Chronic progressive external ophthalmoplegia is primarily a sporadic disease, whereas the others are maternally inherited.

CLINICAL PRESENTATION. Kearns-Sayre syndrome is characterized by the clinical triad of progressive external ophthalmoplegia, pigmentary retinopathy, and atrioventricular block. Diabetes, deafness, and ataxia can also be associated. Clinical features of MERRF include myoclonus, seizures, ataxia, dementia, and skeletal muscle weakness. MELAS is the most common of the maternally inherited mitochondrial disorders and is characterized by encephalopathy, subacute strokelike events, migraine-like headaches, recurrent emesis, extremity weakness, and short stature. Leber hereditary optic neuropathy manifests as a severe, subacute, painless loss of central vision, predominantly affecting young men.

CARDIOVASCULAR MANIFESTATIONS. In chronic progressive external ophthalmoplegia, most commonly in the Kearns-Sayre syndrome, cardiac involvement manifests primarily as conduction abnormalities. A

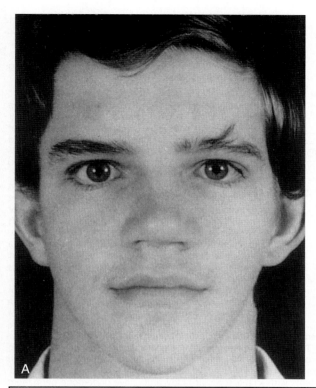

A

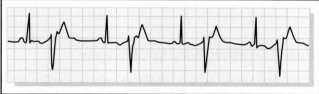

B

FIGURE 92-16 Andersen-Tawil syndrome in a 22-year-old man. **A,** Characteristic low-set ears and hypoplastic mandible. **B,** Electrocardiographic recording revealing ventricular bigeminy. *(From Tawil R, Ptacek LJ, Pavlakis SG, et al: Andersen's syndrome: Potassium-sensitive periodic paralysis, ventricular ectopy, and dysmorphic features. Ann Neurol 35:326, 1994.)*

dilated cardiomyopathy has been reported. In the Kearns-Sayre syndrome, atrioventricular block is observed, usually presenting after eye involvement. The H-V interval is prolonged, consistent with distal conduction disease. Permanent pacing is often required by age 20. An increased prevalence of electrocardiographic preexcitation has also been reported.

Leber hereditary optic neuropathy can be associated with a short PR interval on the ECG and preexcitation. Supraventricular tachycardia has been reported.

In MERRF and MELAS, cardiac involvement manifesting as hypertrophic (symmetrical or asymmetrical) or dilated cardiomyopathy is observed. Other disorders caused by mitochondrial point mutations can present with a similar cardiac phenotype. Patients can present with chest pain with electrocardiographic abnormalities and myocardial perfusion defects. Whether the dilated cardiomyopathy represents a progression from the hypertrophic cardiomyopathy or a separate syndrome is not clear. The dilated cardiomyopathy can result in heart failure and death. MELAS is also associated with an increased risk of preexcitation and Wolff-Parkinson-White syndrome.[22]

TREATMENT AND PROGNOSIS. In Kearns-Sayre syndrome, the implantation of a pacemaker has been advocated when significant or progressive conduction disease is evident, including in asymptomatic patients. The degree of conduction disease that warrants prophylactic pacing is not clear. In Leber hereditary optic neuropathy, a baseline ECG is prudent. In the other mitochondrial disorders, an understanding of the potential for cardiac involvement is necessary. Screening echocardiography has been recommended. Whether other specific screening evaluations are warranted in these disorders is uncertain. Therapy directed at improvement

in the respiratory chain defects—for example, with coenzyme Q10—have not been uniformly demonstrated to be of benefit.

Spinal Muscular Atrophy

GENETICS AND CLINICAL PRESENTATION. Spinal muscular atrophy is a lower motor neuron disorder presenting as progressive, symmetrical proximal muscular weakness.[23] Spinal muscular atrophy is the leading hereditary cause of infant death. The disorder is inherited in an autosomal recessive fashion or is sporadic. Spinal muscular atrophy is classified clinically by the age at symptom onset and disease severity into type I (Werdnig-Hoffman disease), type II (intermediate form), type III (Kugelberg-Welander disease), and type IV (adult onset).

Spinal muscular atrophy links to chromosome 5q13. Mutations or deletions in the telomeric *SMN* (survival of motor neuron) gene occur in more than 98% of patients. The loss of functional SMN protein results in premature neuronal cell death.

CARDIOVASCULAR MANIFESTATIONS. Cardiac involvement in spinal muscular atrophy includes coexisting complex congenital heart disease, cardiomyopathy, and arrhythmias. Congenital heart disease has been associated with types I and III spinal muscular atrophy. The most common abnormality is atrial septal defect, with other abnormalities reported. In spinal muscular atrophy type III, a dilated cardiomyopathy can occur, with endomyocardial biopsies demonstrating fibrosis. Progression leading to a fatal outcome has been reported. Arrhythmia abnormalities, including atrial standstill, atrial fibrillation, atrial flutter, and atrioventricular block, appear to be the most common cardiac manifestation in these diseases. Permanent pacing for atrial standstill and atrioventricular block has been reported.

TREATMENT AND PROGNOSIS. In spinal muscular atrophy type I, severe skeletal muscle involvement with respiratory failure can limit the life span to a significant degree, so that treatment of associated cardiac abnormalities is often not indicated. In spinal muscular atrophy type III, awareness of the potential for associated cardiac abnormalities is necessary. Permanent pacing may be required. Directed therapy to improve functional SMN protein holds future promise.

Desmin-Related Myopathy

GENETICS AND CLINICAL PRESENTATION. Desmin-related myofibrillar myopathy is a rare inherited skeletal muscle dystrophic disorder associated with a cardiomyopathy in more than 50% of affected patients. The disorder is inherited in an autosomal dominant fashion or is sporadic. Desmin mutations are the cause of 1% to 2% of cases of familial dilated cardiomyopathy.[24] Desmin is a cytoskeletal protein that functions as the chief intermediate filament providing support to contracting skeletal and cardiac muscle. Mutations in the desmin gene lead to the inability for the protein to form functioning intermediate filaments. Some mutations cause a cardiomyopathy without an apparent skeletal myopathy.

Patients typically present in their late 20s, with distal weakness that progresses proximally. Difficulty with ambulation and, in severe cases, with respiration, can occur. Creatine kinase levels are mildly elevated in some patients. Muscle biopsy is diagnostic, showing desmin and other myofibrillar protein deposition with immunostaining. Genetic testing is available.

CARDIOVASCULAR MANIFESTATIONS. The cardiomyopathy associated with the desmin-related myopathies can occur before or after the diagnosis of a skeletal myopathy. The cardiac involvement observed typically consists of conduction system dysfunction prior to the onset of a dilated or restrictive cardiomyopathy. Syncope, with the need for pacemaker implantation, has been described. Both sudden and heart failure–related deaths can occur. Sudden death can occur despite pacemaker implantation.

TREATMENT AND PROGNOSIS. The desmin-related myopathies should be considered in the differential diagnosis of individuals or families presenting with skeletal and cardiac myopathies. Monitoring for the development of cardiac conduction and structural disease is indicated in affected families. Prophylactic pacemakers or ICDs should be considered for those patients with significant conduction disease, as in other neuromuscular disorders. Heart failure therapy for appropriate patients is indicated.

Guillain-Barré Syndrome

CLINICAL PRESENTATION. Guillain-Barré syndrome is an acute inflammatory demyelinating neuropathy characterized by peripheral, cranial, and autonomic nerve dysfunction.[25] It is the most common acquired demyelinating neuropathy, with an annual incidence of 1 to 2/100,000 population. Men are more commonly affected than women. In two thirds of affected patients, an acute viral or bacterial illness, typically respiratory or gastrointestinal, precedes the onset of neurologic symptoms by up to 6 weeks. The disorder typically presents with pain, paresthesias, and

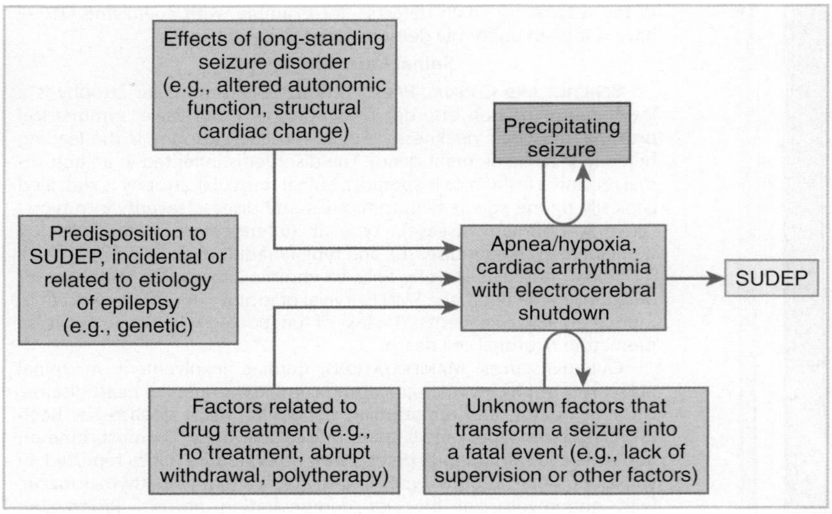

FIGURE 92-17 Interaction between proposed risk factors and triggers for sudden unexpected death in epilepsy. (*From Tomson T, Nashef L, Ryvlin P: Sudden unexpected death in epilepsy: Current knowledge and future directions. Lancet Neurol 7:1021, 2008.*)

symmetrical limb weakness that progresses proximally and can involve cranial and respiratory muscles. Approximately 25% of patients require assisted ventilation.

CARDIOVASCULAR MANIFESTATIONS. Nonambulatory patients are at increased risk for deep venous thrombosis and pulmonary emboli. Cardiac involvement in Guillain-Barré syndrome is related to accompanying autonomic nervous system dysfunction that manifests as hypertension, orthostatic hypotension, resting sinus tachycardia, loss of heart rate variability, electrocardiographic ST-segment abnormalities and both bradycardia and tachycardias. Significant autonomic nervous system dysfunction occurs in about 20% of patients with Guillain-Barré syndrome, primarily in severe cases.[25] Microneurographic recordings have shown increased sympathetic outflow during the acute illness, which normalizes with recovery.

Life-threatening arrhythmias are common in severe cases of Guillain-Barré syndrome, primarily those requiring assisted ventilation. Arrhythmias observed include asystole, symptomatic bradycardia, rapid atrial fibrillation, and ventricular tachycardia or fibrillation. Deaths caused by arrhythmias can occur. Asystole has been commonly associated with tracheal suctioning.

TREATMENT AND PROGNOSIS. Supportive care should include deep venous thrombosis prophylaxis in nonambulatory patients. Early plasmapheresis or intravenous immunoglobulin can improve recovery. In severely affected patients, especially those requiring assisted ventilation, cardiac rhythm monitoring is mandatory. If serious bradycardia or asystole is observed, temporary or permanent pacing can improve survival. Atropine or isoproterenol during tracheal suctioning can be of benefit. The mortality rate in patients hospitalized with Guillain-Barré syndrome is as high as 15%. In patients who recover from Guillain-Barré syndrome, autonomic function also recovers and long-term arrhythmia risk has not been observed.

Myasthenia Gravis

CLINICAL PRESENTATION. Myasthenia gravis is a disorder of neuromuscular transmission resulting from the production of antibody targeted against the nicotinic acetylcholine receptor. The primary symptom, fluctuating weakness, usually begins with the eye and facial muscles and later can involve the large muscles of the limbs. Patients can present at any age, typically at a younger age in women and an older age in men. Myasthenia gravis is usually associated with hyperplasia or a benign or malignant tumor (thymoma) of the thymus gland. The prevalence of myasthenia gravis is 50 to 125 cases/1,000,000.

CARDIOVASCULAR MANIFESTATIONS. A myocarditis can occur in patients with myasthenia gravis, especially in those with thymoma.[26] Up to 16% of patients with myasthenia gravis have cardiac manifestations not explained by another cause. Presentation with arrhythmia symptoms, including atrial fibrillation, atrioventricular block, asystole, ventricular tachycardia, sudden death, or heart failure is typical. Autopsy findings are consistent with myocarditis.

TREATMENT AND PROGNOSIS. Myasthenia gravis is treated with anticholinesterase and immunosuppressive agents. Thymectomy is often indicated. Anticholinesterase agents may slow heart rate and cause

hypotension. Whether immunosuppressive agents or thymectomy improve associated cardiac disease is unknown. Case reports have described patients developing rapidly progressive and fatal heart failure within weeks after thymoma resection, with histology showing giant cell myocarditis.

EPILEPSY

CARDIOVASCULAR MANIFESTATIONS. Epilepsy is a complex brain disorder characterized by chronic seizures. Patients with epilepsy are at an increased risk of sudden death of unknown cause. Sudden unexpected death in epilepsy (SUDEP) is responsible for 2% to 17% of deaths, with an incidence ranging from 0.1 to 9.3/1,000 patient-years, depending on the population studied.[27] The underlying mechanisms leading to sudden death in epilepsy are not clear but may involve apnea, excessive respiratory secretions, acute pulmonary edema, or arrhythmias (**Fig. 92-17**). Most witnessed sudden deaths occur at or in proximity to the time of a seizure. Severe bradycardia with sinus arrest has been documented in a small number of monitored patients during seizures. Whether bradycardia has a role in epileptic patients undergoing sudden death is not clear.

Observational studies have assessed risk factors for sudden unexpected death in epilepsy. These include a high seizure frequency, long duration of epilepsy, poor compliance with antiepileptic drug therapy, and the need for polytherapy to control seizures.

TREATMENT AND PROGNOSIS. A primary arrhythmia disorder needs to be considered in the differential diagnosis of epilepsy. Patients with poorly controlled epilepsy should be aggressively evaluated and treated. Patients with ictal-associated bradycardia have undergone permanent pacemaker implantation. Nighttime supervision of the epileptic patient may decrease the risk of sudden unexpected death.

Acute Cerebrovascular Disease

CARDIOVASCULAR MANIFESTATIONS. Acute cerebrovascular diseases, including subarachnoid hemorrhage, other stroke syndromes, and head injury, can be associated with severe cardiac manifestations.[28] The mechanism whereby cardiac abnormalities occur with brain injury is related to autonomic nervous system dysfunction, with increased sympathetic and parasympathetic output. Excessive myocardial catecholamine release is primarily responsible for the observed cardiac pathology. Hypothalamic stimulation can reproduce the electrocardiographic changes observed in acute cerebrovascular disease. Electrocardiographic changes associated with hypothalamic stimulation or blood in the subarachnoid space can be diminished with spinal cord transection, stellate ganglion blockade, vagolytics, and adrenergic blockers.

Electrocardiographic abnormalities are observed in approximately 70% of patients with subarachnoid hemorrhage. Abnormalities, including ST-segment elevation and depression, T wave inversion, and pathologic Q waves are observed. Peaked inverted T waves and a prolonged QT interval can occur in a significant proportion of patients with abnormal ECGs (**Fig. 92-18**). Hypokalemia can be seen in patients with subarachnoid hemorrhage and can increase the likelihood of QT interval prolongation. Other stroke syndromes are often associated with abnormal ECGs but whether these are related to the stroke syndrome or to underlying intrinsic cardiac disease is often difficult to discern. A prolonged QT interval is more common in subarachnoid hemorrhage than other stroke syndromes. Closed head trauma can cause electrocardiographic abnormalities similar to those of subarachnoid hemorrhage, including a prolonged QT interval.

Myocardial damage, with liberation of enzymes and subendocardial hemorrhage or fibrosis at autopsy, can occur in the setting of acute cerebral disease.[28,29] The term *neurogenic stunned myocardium* is used to describe the reversible syndrome. The process can present with selective apical involvement, a takotsubo cardiomyopathy (see Chap. 68). Cardiac troponin I level elevation and echocardiographic evidence of left ventricular dysfunction is present in a significant proportion of patients with subarachnoid hemorrhage. Patients with poorer

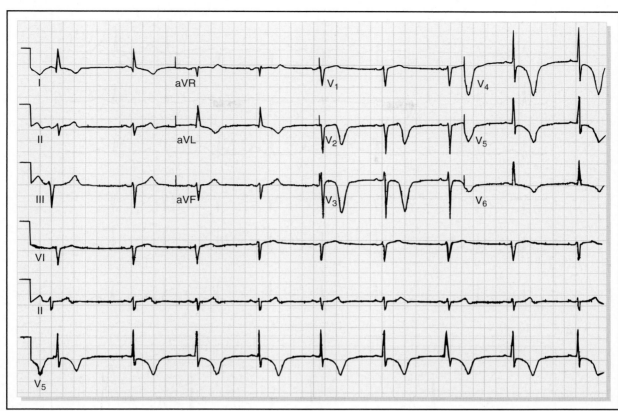

FIGURE 92-18 ECG from a patient with cerebral hemorrhage. Deep and symmetrical T wave inversions are observed. *(Courtesy of Dr. Charles Fisch, Indiana University School of Medicine, Indianapolis.)*

neurologic status at admission are more likely to have an increased peak troponin level. Women are at higher risk of myocardial necrosis.

Pulmonary edema may accompany the acute neurologic insult. The edema can have both a cardiogenic component, related to systemic hypertension and left ventricular dysfunction, and a neurogenic (pulmonary capillary leak) component.

Life-threatening arrhythmias can occur in the setting of acute cerebrovascular disease. Ventricular tachycardia or fibrillation has been observed in patients with subarachnoid hemorrhage and head trauma. A torsades de pointes–type ventricular tachycardia can occur (**Fig. 92-19**). This is often observed in the setting of a prolonged QT interval and hypokalemia. Stroke syndromes, other than subarachnoid hemorrhage, appear to be only rarely associated with serious ventricular tachycardias. Atrial arrhythmias, including atrial fibrillation and regular supraventricular tachycardia, have been observed. Atrial fibrillation is most common in patients presenting with an acute thromboembolic stroke. Separating an effect from the cause can be difficult. Bradycardias, including sinoatrial block, sinus arrest, and atrioventricular block, occur in up to 10% of patients with subarachnoid hemorrhage.

TREATMENT AND PROGNOSIS. Beta-adrenergic blockers appear to be effective for decreasing myocardial damage and controlling supraventricular and ventricular arrhythmias associated with subarachnoid hemorrhage and head trauma. Beta-adrenergic blockers increase the likelihood of bradycardia and cannot be used in patients with hypotension requiring vasopressors. Life-threatening arrhythmias occur primarily in the first day following a neurologic event. Continuous electrocardiographic monitoring during this period is indicated. Careful monitoring of potassium levels, especially in patients with subarachnoid hemorrhage, is warranted. Refractory ventricular arrhythmias have been controlled effectively with stellate ganglion blockade. Electrocardiographic abnormalities reflect unfavorable intracranial factors but do not appear to portend a poor cardiovascular outcome. The magnitude of peak troponin level elevation is predictive for adverse patient outcomes, including severe disability at hospital discharge and death.[28] Other than the mortality occurring secondary to acute arrhythmias, the myocardial necrosis does not appear to play a major factor affecting outcome.

Head injury (e.g., blunt trauma, gunshot wound) and cerebrovascular accidents are the leading causes of brain death in patients being considered as heart donors. These donors can manifest electrocardiographic abnormalities, hemodynamic instability, and myocardial dysfunction related primarily to adrenergic storm and not to intrinsic cardiac disease. Experimental studies on whether contractile performance recovers with transplantation are still controversial. Optimization of volume status and inotropic support, with careful echocardiographic evaluation and possibly left heart catheterization, can allow the use of some donor hearts that would otherwise have been rejected.

Future Perspectives

The molecular mechanisms responsible for cardiac involvement in the neurologic diseases are increasingly better understood. Patients with dystrophic muscular diseases will continue to have their quality and quantity of life improved by supportive clinical care. A prolonged life span will result in a greater proportion of patients manifesting symptoms related to cardiac involvement. Cardiologists and electrophysiologists will be increasingly consulted about the management of these patients. Controversies regarding the appropriate use of pharmacotherapy and device therapy to manage cardiac manifestations in the neurologic diseases will be addressed further with patient series and nonrandomized trials. Gene therapy continues to hold future promise.

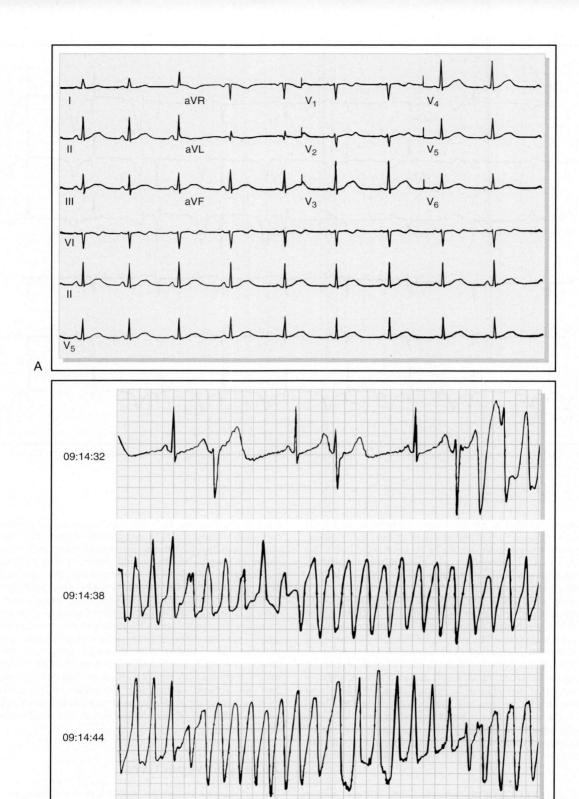

FIGURE 92-19 49-year-old patient with cerebral hemorrhage. **A,** ECG recorded within 3 hours of admission and 4 hours after onset of symptoms. QT interval prolongation is observed. **B,** Electrocardiographic monitoring 6 hours after admission. Ventricular bigeminy precedes the onset of polymorphic ventricular tachycardia. Cardioversion was required. The patient was subsequently treated with a beta-adrenergic blocker without further ventricular tachycardia.

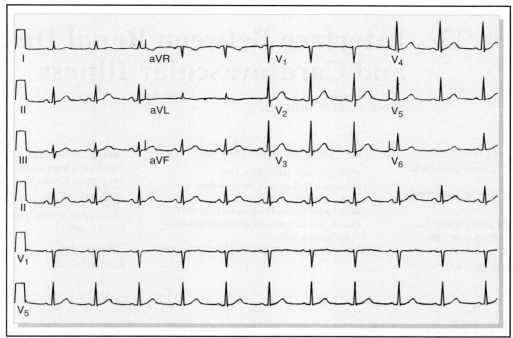

FIGURE 92-19, cont'd **C,** ECG obtained 2 weeks after admission. The QT interval has normalized.

REFERENCES

Duchenne and Becker Muscular Dystrophies

1. Jefferies JL, Eidem BW, Belmont JW, et al: Genetic predictors and remodeling of dilated cardiomyopathy in muscular dystrophy. Circulation 112:2799, 2005.
2. Thrush PT, Allen HD, Viollet L, et al: Re-examination of the electrocardiogram in boys with Duchenne muscular dystrophy and correlation with its dilated cardiomyopathy. Am J Cardiol 103:262, 2009.
3. Manzur AY, Kuntzer T, Pike M, et al: Glucocorticoid corticosteroids for Duchenne muscular dystrophy. Cochrane Database System Rev (1):CD003725, 2008.
4. Duboc D, Meune C, Lerebours G, et al: Effect of perindopril on the onset and progression of left ventricular dysfunction in Duchenne muscular dystrophy. J Am Coll Cardiol 45:855, 2005.

Myotonic Dystrophies

5. Meola G, Moxley RT: Myotonic dystrophy type 2 and related myotonic disorders. J Neurol 251:1173, 2004.
6. Day JW, Ranum LP: RNA pathogenesis of the myotonic dystrophies. Neuromusc Disord 15:5, 2005.
7. Groh WJ, Lowe MR, Chandan S, et al: Electrocardiographic abnormalities and risk of sudden death in myotonic dystrophy type 1. N Engl J Med 358:2688, 2008.
8. Bhakta D, Lowe MR, Groh WJ: Prevalence of structural cardiac abnormalities in patients with myotonic dystrophy type I. Am Heart J 147:224, 2004.
9. Schoser BG, Ricker K, Schneider-Gold C, et al: Sudden cardiac death in myotonic dystrophy type 2. Neurology 63:2402, 2004.

Emery-Dreifuss Muscular Dystrophy and Associated Disorders

10. Worman HJ, Bonne G: "Laminopathies": A wide spectrum of human diseases. Exper Cell Res 313:2121, 2007.
11. Meune C, Van Berlo JH, Anselme F, et al: Primary prevention of sudden death in patients with lamin A/C gene mutations. N Engl J Med 354:209, 2006.
12. Sakata K, Shimizu M, Ino H, et al: High incidence of sudden cardiac death with conduction disturbances and atrial cardiomyopathy caused by a nonsense mutation in the STA gene. Circulation 111:3352, 2005.

Limb-girdle Muscular Dystrophies

13. Guglieri M, Straub V, Bushby K, et al: Limb-girdle muscular dystrophies. Curr Opin Neurol 21:576, 2008.

14. Wheeler MT, Allikian MJ, Heydemann A, et al: Smooth muscle cell-extrinsic vascular spasm arises from cardiomyocyte degeneration in sarcoglycan-deficient cardiomyopathy. J Clin Invest 113:668, 2004.
15. Poppe M, Bourke J, Eagle M, et al: Cardiac and respiratory failure in limb-girdle muscular dystrophy 2I. Ann Neurol 56:738, 2004.

Facioscapulohumeral Muscular Dystrophy

16. Trevisan CP, Pastorello E, Armani M, et al: Facioscapulohumeral muscular dystrophy and occurrence of heart arrhythmia. Eur Neurol 56:1, 2006.

Friedreich Ataxia

17. Pandolfo M: Friedreich ataxia. Arch Neurol 65:1296, 2008.
18. Ribai P, Pousset F, Tanguy ML, et al: Neurological, cardiological, and oculomotor progression in 104 patients with Friedreich ataxia during long-term follow-up. Arch Neurol 64:558, 2007.

Less Common Neuromuscular Diseases Associated with Cardiac Manifestations

19. Finsterer J: Primary periodic paralyses. Acta Neurol Scand 117:145, 2008.
20. Yoon G, Oberoi S, Tristani-Firouzi M, et al: Andersen-Tawil syndrome: Prospective cohort analysis and expansion of the phenotype. Am J Med Genet 140:312, 2006.
21. DiMauro S: Mitochondrial myopathies. Curr Opin Rheum 18:636, 2006.
22. Sproule DM, Kaufmann P, Engelstad K, et al: Wolff-Parkinson-White syndrome in patients with MELAS. Arch Neurol 64:1625, 2007.
23. Lunn MR, Wang CH: Spinal muscular atrophy. Lancet 371:2120, 2008.
24. Taylor MR, Slavov D, Ku L, et al: Prevalence of desmin mutations in dilated cardiomyopathy. Circulation 115:1244, 2007.
25. Hughes RA, Cornblath DR: Guillain-Barré syndrome. Lancet 366:1653, 2005.
26. Joudinaud TM, Fadel E, Thomas-de-Montpreville V, et al: Fatal giant cell myocarditis after thymoma resection in myasthenia gravis. J Thor Cardiovasc Surg 131:494, 2006.
27. Tomson T, Nashef L, Ryvlin P: Sudden unexpected death in epilepsy: Current knowledge and future directions. Lancet Neurol 7:1021, 2008.

Acute Cerebrovascular Disease

28. Naidech AM, Kreiter KT, Janjua N, et al: Cardiac troponin elevation, cardiovascular morbidity, and outcome after subarachnoid hemorrhage. Circulation 112:2851, 2005.
29. Tung P, Kopelnik A, Banki N, et al: Predictors of neurocardiogenic injury after subarachnoid hemorrhage. Stroke 35:548, 2004.

CHAPTER 93 Interface Between Renal Disease and Cardiovascular Illness

Peter A. McCullough

Cardiorenal Intersection

Hemodynamic and regulatory functions inextricably link the heart and kidneys. In a normal 70-kg man, each kidney weighs about 130 to 170 g and receives blood flow of 400 mL/min/100 g, which is approximately 20% to 25% of the cardiac output, allowing the needed flow to maintain glomerular filtration by approximately 1 million nephrons (**Fig. 93-1**). This flow exceeds by severalfold the blood flow through most other organs on a weight basis. Although the oxygen extraction is low, the kidneys account for about 8% of the total oxygen consumption of the body. The kidney has a central role in electrolyte balance, volume, and blood pressure regulation. Communication between these two organs occurs at multiple levels, including the sympathetic nervous system, the renin-angiotensin-aldosterone system (RAAS), antidiuretic hormone, endothelin, and the natriuretic peptides (**Fig. 93-2**). In addition, the kidneys produce active hormones, including 1,25-dihydroxyvitamin D and erythropoietin (EPO), which have cardiovascular sites of action. With the understanding of these systems has come the development of key diagnostic and therapeutic targets in cardiovascular medicine.

The obesity pandemic in developed countries is a central driver of secondary epidemics of type 2 diabetes (DM) and hypertension (HTN), often leading to combined chronic kidney disease (CKD) and cardiovascular disease (CVD).[1] Among those who have DM for 25 years or longer, the prevalence of diabetic nephropathy in types 1 and 2 DM is 57% and 48%, respectively.[2] Approximately 50% of all cases of end-stage renal disease (ESRD) are caused by diabetic nephropathy. With the aging of the general population and cardiovascular care shifting toward the older population, an understanding of why decreasing levels of renal function act as a major adverse prognostic factor after a variety of cardiac events is imperative. Considerable evidence has shown that CKD accelerates atherosclerosis, myocardial disease, and valvular disease and promotes an array of cardiac arrhythmias that can lead to sudden death.[3]

Chronic Kidney Disease as a Cardiovascular Risk State

Chronic kidney disease is defined through a range of estimated glomerular filtration rate (eGFR) values by the National Kidney Foundation Kidney Disease Outcomes Quality Initiative (KDOQI).[4] A common definition for CKD stipulates an eGFR of less than 60 mL/min/1.73 m^2 or the presence of kidney damage (**Fig. 93-3**). Although with normative aging (age 20 to 80 years), the eGFR declines from about 130 to

60 mL/min/1.73 m^2, a variety of pathobiologic processes appear to begin when the eGFR drops below 60 mL/min/1.73 m^2. Most studies of cardiovascular outcomes have found that a critical cut point for the development of contrast-induced acute kidney injury (CI-AKI), restenosis after percutaneous coronary intervention (PCI), recurrent myocardial infarction (MI), diastolic or systolic heart failure (HF), arrhythmias, and cardiovascular death is an eGFR of 60 mL/min/1.73 m^2—which roughly corresponds to a serum creatinine (Cr) level higher than 1.5 mg/dL in the general population (**Fig. 93-4**).[4,8] Because Cr is a crude indicator of renal function and often underestimates renal dysfunction in women and older adults, calculated measures of eGFR or creatinine clearance (CrCl) using the Cockcroft-Gault equation or the modification of diet in renal disease equation are superior methods for the assessment of renal function. The four-variable modification of diet in renal disease equation for eGFR is the preferred method because it does not rely on body weight. The equation is given by the following:

$$eGFR = 186.3 \times \left(serum\ Cr^{-1.154}\right) \times \left(age^{-0.203}\right)$$

Calculated values are multiplied by 0.742 for women and by 1.21 for blacks. Another blood test reflecting renal filtration function is cystatin C.[9] Cystatin C is a nonglycosylated protein with low molecular mass (13-kDa) produced by all nucleated cells. Its low molecular mass and high isoelectric point allow it to be filtered freely by the glomerular membrane and 100% reabsorbed by the proximal tubule. The serum concentration of cystatin C correlates with renal filtration, and because of a stable production rate, it provides a more accurate marker of renal filtration function than the serum Cr level. Serum levels of cystatin C do not depend on weight and height, muscle mass, age, or sex making it less variable than the Cr level. Furthermore, measurements can be made and interpreted from a single random sample, with reference values of 0.54 to 1.21 mg/liter (median, 0.85 mg/liter; range, 0.42 to 1.39 mg/liter).

In addition, microalbuminuria at any level of eGFR indicates CKD and may reflect endothelial dysfunction in glomerular capillaries caused by the metabolic syndrome, DM, or HTN (see Chaps. 45 and 64). Microalbuminuria can be defined as a random urine albumin-to-Cr ratio (ACR) of 30 to 300 mg/g. An ACR higher than 300 mg/g is considered gross proteinuria. The random, spot urine ACR is the office test for microalbuminuria recommended as part of the cardiovascular risk assessment done by cardiologists and other specialists. Microalbuminuria as an independent CVD risk factor for diabetics and those without DM is discussed in Chap. 64. The Seventh Report of the Joint National Committee on Prevention, Detection, Evaluation, and Treatment of High Blood Pressure (JNC 7) has recognized CKD as an

Implications of Anemia Caused by Chronic Kidney Disease

There is increasing recognition of the associations between the blood hemoglobin (Hb) level, CKD, and CVD. The most common cut point for the definition of anemia by the World Health Organization is a Hb level lower than 13 g/dL in men and lower than 12 g/dL in women. Approximately 9% of the general adult population meets the definition of anemia at these levels. In general, anemia caused by CKD is present in 20% of patients with stable coronary disease and 30% to 60% of patients with HF. Hence, anemia is a common and easily identifiable potential diagnostic and therapeutic target.[12,13]

Anemia contributes to multiple adverse outcomes, in part because of decreased tissue oxygen delivery and uptake.[13] The cause of anemia in patients with CKD can be multifactorial, with a central component being a relative deficiency of EPO as well as an increase in hepcidin produced by the liver, resulting in attenuated maturation of hemangioblasts combined with an iron reuptake defect. In response to oxygen tension, the kidneys produce 90% of plasma EPO levels and maintain a range between 10 and 30 IU/mL; however, during anemic periods, these levels may exceed 100 IU/mL. Patients with CKD and HF appear to have a relative EPO deficiency, with an inappropriately low EPO level for the measured blood Hb level. In the setting of CKD and HF, there are increased levels of tumor necrosis factor-α, interleukin-1 (IL-1) and interleukin-6 (IL-6), endothelin, matrix metalloproteinases, and other inflammation-related proteins produced by many organs. These factors can reduce directly red cell production at the level of the bone marrow and aggravate the anemia. Of 29 large prospective studies of HF, 28 found anemia to predict mortality independently.[14] On average, in those patients with HF, for each 1-g/dL decrement in Hb, there is a 13% increase in risk for all-cause mortality. In addition, patients with anemia and CKD will more likely progress to ESRD irrespective of their baseline level of renal function. As Hb drops over time, there is a graded increase in HF hospitalizations and death. Conversely, those patients who have had a rise in Hb—whether as a result of improved nutrition, reduced neurohormonal factors, or other unknown factors—enjoy a significant reduction in endpoints over the next several years. This improvement has been associated with a significant reduction in left ventricular mass index, suggesting a favorable change in left ventricular remodeling.[15] The observational data suggest that changes in Hb, either up or down, are associated with clinical consequences. Hence, there is a rationale for therapeutic intervention on the Hb level to change the natural history of cardiorenal disease.

In addition to the effect on Hb levels, the pleiotropic effects of erythrocyte-stimulating proteins (ESPs) include positive effects on coronary endothelium, resulting in an increase in coronary flow

independent cardiovascular risk state,[10] which has many vascular and metabolic abnormalities (see later; **Fig. 93-5**).[11]

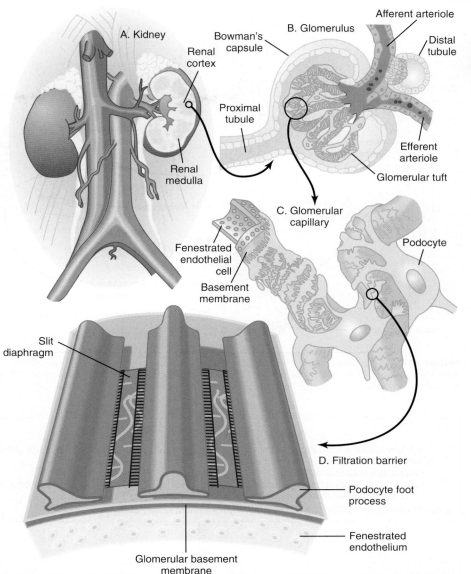

FIGURE 93-1 Normal structure of the glomerular vasculature. **A,** Each kidney contains about 1 million glomeruli in the renal cortex. **B,** Afferent arteriole entering Bowman's capsule and branching into several capillaries that form the glomerular tuft. The walls of the capillaries constitute the actual filter. The plasma filtrate (primary urine) is directed to the proximal tubule, whereas the unfiltered blood returns to the circulation through the efferent arteriole. **C,** The filtration barrier of the capillary wall contains an innermost fenestrated endothelium, the glomerular basement membrane, and a layer of interdigitating podocyte foot processes. **D,** Cross section through the glomerular capillary depicts the fenestrated endothelial layer and the glomerular basement membrane, with overlying podocyte foot processes. An ultrathin slit diaphragm spans the filtration slit between the foot processes, slightly above the basement membrane. To show the slit diaphragm, the foot processes are drawn smaller than actual scale. (*Modified from Tryggvason K, Patrakka J, Wartiovaara J: Hereditary proteinuria syndromes and mechanisms of proteinuria. N Engl J Med 354:1387, 2006.*)

reserve. This effect may be mediated through the activation of endothelial nitric oxide synthase via protein kinase B phosphorylation and by preventing endothelial cell apoptosis. These proteins may also enhance myocardial repair in patients with myocardial injury. This could minimize the progression of left ventricular dysfunction by recruiting vascular progenitor cells, which can become functional myocardial cells, thereby increasing the contractile function of the injured ventricle. The molecular targets for ESPs include receptors expressed on cardiac myocytes, endothelial cells, and endothelial progenitor cells, in addition to hematopoietic stem cells.

Treatment of anemia with exogenous ESPs (EPO and darbepoetin alfa) in CKD has been disappointing in reducing morbidity, particularly that of cardiovascular origin, and in improving survival and quality of

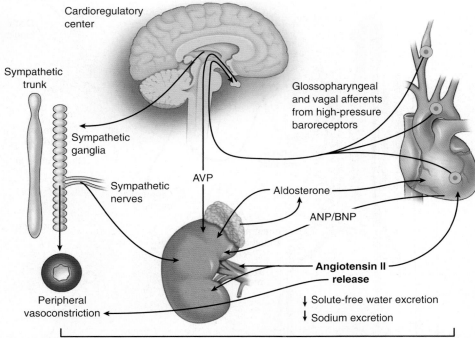

FIGURE 93-2 Major neurohumoral communication systems between the heart and kidney. ANP = A-type natriuretic peptide; AVP = arginine vasopressin; BNP = B-type natriuretic peptide. *(Modified from Schrier RW, Abraham WT: Hormones and hemodynamics in heart failure. N Engl J Med 341:577, 1999.) (see Fig. 45-10)*

Criteria
1. Kidney damage for ≥ 3 months, as defined by structural or functional abnormalities of the kidney, with or without decreased GFR, manifest by *either:* • Pathological abnormalities; or • Markers of kidney damage, including abnormalities in the composition of the blood or urine, or abnormalities in imaging tests 2. eGFR <60 mL/min/1.73m² for ≥ 3 months, with or without kidney damage

Markers of kidney damage	Findings indicating kidney damage
Proteinuria	Albumin-to-creatinine ratio >30 mg/g
Urine sediment abnormalities	Cellular casts, coarse granular casts, fat
Imaging tests	Abnormalities in kidney size Asymmetry in kidney size or function Irregularities in shape (cysts, scars, mass lesions) Stones Hydronephrosis and other abnormalities of the urinary tract Arterial stenosis and other vascular lesions
Abnormalities in blood or urine composition	Nephrotic syndrome Tubular syndromes (renal tubular acidosis, potassium secretory defects, renal glycosuria, renal phosphaturia, Fanconi's syndrome)

FIGURE 93-3 Diagnostic criteria for chronic kidney disease and kidney damage.

consumption with exercise testing. These biomarkers may not reflect clinical outcomes, because treatment with EPO and supplemental iron, which is needed in approximately 70% of patients, can cause three problems: (1) increased platelet activity, thrombin generation, and resultant increased risk of thrombosis; (2) increased endothelin levels and increased asymmetrical dimethylarginine, which theoretically reduces nitric oxide availability, and results in HTN; and (3) worsened measures of oxidative stress. Three randomized trials in CKD have indicated that treatment with ESPs to a higher hemoglobin results in higher CVD events. The Cardiovascular Risk Reduction by Early Anemic Treatment with Epoetin beta in Chronic Kidney Disease Patients (CREATE) trial randomized 603 patients to treatment with EPO to a target of 13.0 to 15.0 g/dL versus 10.5 to 11.5 g/dL for 2.5 years, and found higher rates of CVD and progression to ESRD in the 13.0 to 15.0 g/dL group.[16] The Correction of Hemoglobin and Outcomes in Renal Insufficiency (CHOIR) trial randomized 1432 patients with CKD and treated with EPO to a target of 13.5 versus 11.3 g/dL.[17] The composite endpoint, a combination of mortality and cardiovascular outcomes (stroke, MI, hospitalization because of HF), occurred in 125 events in the 13.5-g/dL arm and 97 events in the 11.3-g/dL arm (*P* = 0.03). A placebo-controlled trial on this issue is critical because it appears that treatment to higher hemoglobin targets results in worsened CVD outcomes. The Trial to Reduce Cardiovascular Events with Aranesp Therapy (TREAT), a multicenter, double-blind, placebo-controlled randomized trial, was specifically designed to determine whether patients with CKD (eGFR = 20 to 60 mL/min/1.73 m²), type 2 DM, and anemia (Hb < 11 g/dL) would experience a reduction in the risk of the composite endpoint of death or cardiovascular morbidity (nonfatal MI, hospitalization for myocardial ischemia, HF, or stroke) when treated with darbepoetin alfa to raise the Hb level to

life. Darbepoetin alfa (Aranesp) is a genetically engineered form of EPO designed to have a longer half-life, making once-monthly injections an attractive treatment option.[13] Increasing the Hb level from below 10 to 12 g/dL has been linked to favorable changes in biomarkers, such as left ventricular remodeling, improved ejection fraction, improved functional classification, and higher levels of peak oxygen

13 g/dL. This study did not show a reduction in the risk of cardiovascular or renal events or death, but showed an excess of stroke in the darbepoetin alfa group.[18] Until there is clear evidence that the partial correction of anemia has favorable outcomes in CVD, this form of treatment is not recommended for the primary purpose of improving the natural history of CVD.

Contrast-Induced Acute Kidney Injury

Contrast-induced acute kidney injury has been defined as a composite rise in the serum Cr level of more than 25% or 0.5 mg/dL, or an increase of 50% (or 0.3 mg/dL) or more from baseline, with a reduction in urine output to less than 0.5 mL/kg/hour for 6 hours after intravascular administration of iodinated contrast (see Chap. 20).[19] The frequency of CI-AKI is approximately 13% in nondiabetics and 20% in diabetics undergoing PCI (see Chap. 58). It is critical to understand that the risk of CI-AKI is related in a curvilinear fashion to the eGFR (**Fig. 93-6**).[20] Fortunately, in patients undergoing PCI, cases of CI-AKI leading to dialysis are rare (0.5% to 2.0%). When this does occur, it portends a catastrophic outcome, including a 36% in-hospital mortality rate and a 2-year survival of only 19%.[21] Although not always attributed to CI-AKI, transient rises in the Cr level relate directly to longer intensive care unit and hospital ward stays (3 and 4 more days, respectively) after bypass surgery. Even transient rises in the Cr level translate to differences in mortality after PCI (**Fig. 93-7**).[22]

Three core elements contribute to the pathophysiology of CI-AKI: (1) direct toxicity of iodinated contrast material to nephrons; (2) microshowers of atheroemboli to the kidneys; and (3) contrast material- and atheroemboli-induced intrarenal vasoconstric-

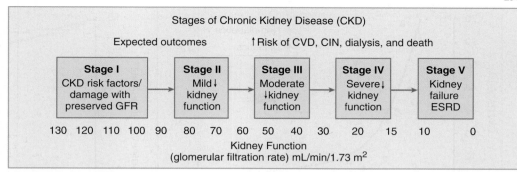

FIGURE 93-4 Classification of CKD according to the KDOQI. Increased rates of adverse events are generally seen below an eGFR of 60 mL/min/1.73 m². CIN = contrast-induced nephropathy. *(From McCullough PA, Sandberg KR: Epidemiology of contrast-induced nephropathy. Rev Cardiovasc Med 4[Suppl 5]: S3, 2003.)*

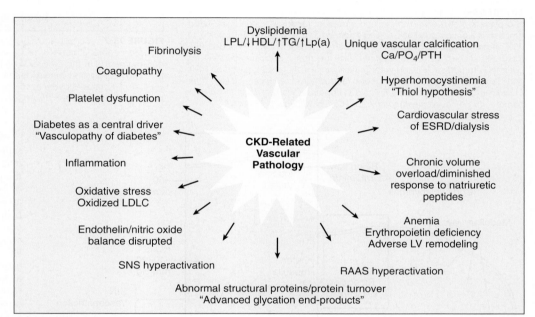

FIGURE 93-5 Pathobiology of the CKD state and its effects on the cardiovascular system. Lp(a) = lipoprotein(a); LPL = lipoprotein lipase; LV = left ventricle; NO = nitric oxide; SNS = sympathetic nervous system. *(Modified from McCullough PA: Why is chronic kidney disease the "spoiler" for cardiovascular outcomes? J Am Coll Cardiol 41:725, 2003.)*

tion. Furthermore, as renal function declines, a host of chronic perturbations occur in hemostasis, lipids, endothelial function, protein metabolism, calcium-phosphorus balance, and oxidative stress.[23] Direct toxicity to nephrons with iodinated contrast media appears to be related to the ionic strength and osmolality of the contrast media.[24] Microshowers of cholesterol emboli occur in about 50% of PCIs when a guiding catheter is passed through the aorta.[25] Most of these showers are clinically silent. In approximately 1% of high-risk cases, however, an acute cholesterol emboli syndrome can develop, manifested by acute renal failure, mesenteric ischemia, decreased microcirculation to the extremities and, in some cases, embolic stroke. Because acute renal failure occurs after coronary artery bypass surgery with almost the same risk predictors as in procedures involving contrast media, atheroembolism represents a common pathogenic feature of both causes of renal failure.[26] Intrarenal vasoconstriction as a pathologic vascular response to contrast medium and perhaps as an organ response to cholesterol emboli is a final hypoxic-ischemic injury to the kidney in PCI. Hypoxia triggers activation of neurohumoral systems and results in further reduction in renal blood flow. When contrast agents are given to animals, there is transient vasodilation caused by nitric oxide release from endothelial cells followed by sustained vascular smooth muscle cell constriction.[27-29] But when there is vascular disease, endothelial dysfunction, and a reduction in the overall number of nephron units,

contrast agents evoke longer periods of renal vasoconstriction and have a prolonged transit time in the kidney in the vascular and urinary spaces. Thus, there is extravasation of iodinated contrast molecules from the renal tubules into the vascular peritubular space, causing additional vasoconstriction and cellular injury (**Fig. 93-8**). The most important predictor of CI-AKI is underlying renal dysfunction. The remnant nephron theory postulates that after sufficient chronic kidney damage has occurred and the eGFR is reduced to less than 60 mL/min/1.73 m², the remaining nephrons are vulnerable. Residual nephrons have increased oxygen demands and are more susceptible to ischemic and oxidative injury. Emerging blood and urine biomarkers become elevated before the rise in the serum Cr level, including neutrophil–gelatinase-associated lipocalin (siderocalin), kidney injury molecule-1, interleukin-18 (IL-18), liver fatty acid binding protein, a variety of tubular enzymes, and cystatin C (see earlier). The clinical use of such markers for CI-AKI is expected in the future.[30]

Prevention of Contrast-Induced Acute Kidney Injury (see Chap. 20)

A prevention strategy for CI-AKI should be used for patients with pre-existing CKD (baseline eGFR < 60 mL/min/1.73 m²), and in particular,

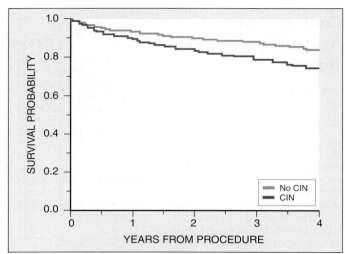

FIGURE 93-6 Rates of contrast-induced acute kidney injury (CI-AKI) by eGFR and diabetic status from the placebo groups of randomized trials. The fitted function is a drawn quadratic. CIN was defined as a serum Cr level increase of 25% and/or 0.5 mg/dL. Trials including less than 25 patients were excluded. Risk for CI-AKI according to the baseline renal function is shown separately for patients with (red circles) and without (yellow circles) diabetes, based on trials and registries that presented these populations separately. *(Data from McCullough PA, Adam A, Becker CR, et al; CIN Consensus Working Panel: Risk prediction of contrast-induced nephropathy. Am J Cardiol 98[Suppl 1]:27, 2006.)*

FIGURE 93-7 Mortality in 7230 patients with and without CKD and contrast-induced nephropathy (CIN), or CI-AKI, after PCI. CIN is defined as ≥25% or ≥0.5-mg/dL rise in the Cr level at 48 hours after PCI. Patients with STEMI and those on hemodialysis were excluded. *(Modified from Dangas G, Iakovou I, Nikolsky E, et al: Contrast-induced nephropathy after percutaneous coronary interventions in relation to chronic kidney disease and hemodynamic variables. Am J Cardiol 95:13, 2005.)*

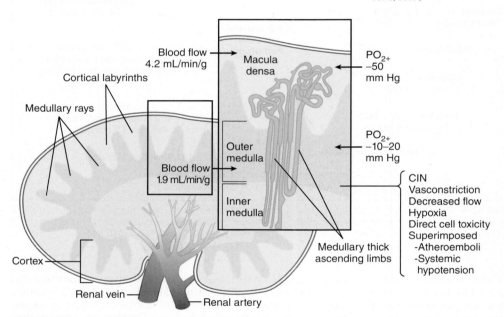

FIGURE 93-8 Pathophysiology of CI-AKI demonstrating, in the presence of a reduced nephron mass, that the remaining nephrons are vulnerable to injury. Iodinated contrast, after causing a brief (minutes) period of vasodilation, causes sustained (hours to days) intrarenal vasoconstriction and ischemic injury. The ischemic injury sets off a cascade of events, largely driven by oxidative injury, causing death of renal tubular cells. If a sufficient mass of nephron units is affected, a recognizable rise in the serum Cr level will occur. *(Modified from McCullough PA: Contrast-induced acute kidney injury. J Am Coll Cardiol 51:1419, 2008.)*

those with CKD and DM. The presence of CKD, DM, and other risk factors including hemodynamic instability, use of intra-aortic balloon counterpulsation, HF, older age, hyperglycemia, and anemia in the same patient can produce a predicted probability of CI-AKI more than 50% (**Fig. 93-9**).[31] Thus, CI-AKI must be discussed in detail during the informed consent process of high-risk patients before the use of intravascular iodinated contrast. Four basic concepts apply to CI-AKI prevention: (1) hydration and volume expansion; (2) choice and quantity of contrast material; (3) pre-, intra-, and postprocedural end-organ protection with pharmacotherapy; and (4) postprocedural monitoring and expectant care.

Hydration with intravenous normal saline or isotonic sodium bicarbonate is reasonable, starting 3 to 12 hours before the procedure at a rate of 1.5 mL/kg/hr or more.[32,33] Those at risk should receive at least 300 to 500 mL of intravenous hydration before administration of the contrast material. If there are particular concerns regarding volume overload or HF in individuals in whom clinical assessment of volume status is difficult, a right-heart catheterization may aid management during and after the procedure. The postprocedure hydration target is a urine output of 150 mL/hr. If patients have a diuresis of more than 150 mL/hr, their extra losses should be replaced with more intravenous fluid. In general, this strategy calls for hydration orders of normal saline or sodium bicarbonate at 150 mL/hr for at least 6 hours after the procedure. Achieving adequate urine flow rates may reduce the rate of CI-AKI by 50%.

Head-to-head randomized trials of iodinated contrast agents have demonstrated the lowest rates of CI-AKI with nonionic, iso-osmolar iodixanol, particularly in those with CKD and DM. A meta-analysis included 16 prospective, double-blind, randomized controlled trials that compared iodixanol with low-osmolar contrast media (LOCM) in adult patients undergoing angiographic examinations and reported Cr values at baseline and following CM administration.[34] The pooled data demonstrated a reduced risk of CI-AKI (≥0.5 mg/dL rise at 72 hours) with iodixanol (overall odds ratio [OR] = 0.39; 95% confidence interval [CI], 0.23 to 0.66; *P* = 0.0004). A 2009 tabular meta-analysis restricted to trials of iodixanol and nonionic LOCM found an overall nonsignificant trend in favor of iodixanol; however, the impact on the subset with CKD and DM could not be evaluated (**Fig. 93-10**).[35] These data support the hypothesis that iodixanol (290 mOsm/kg) is less nephrotoxic than LOCM agents with osmolality ranging from 600 to 800 mOsm/kg; however, this finding applies only to those who have both CKD and DM.

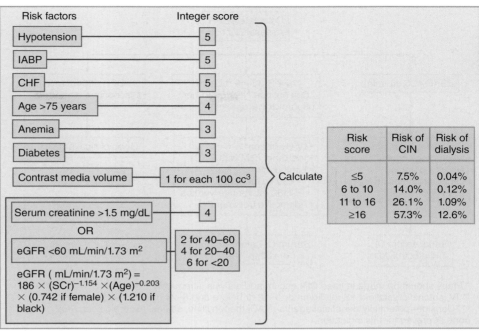

FIGURE 93-9 Risk prediction scheme for the development of contrast-induced nephropathy (CIN), also referred to as CI-AKI, and for renal failure requiring dialysis after coronary angiography or PCI. Anemia is defined as a baseline hematocrit value < 39% for men and < 36% for women; CHF is functional Class III or IV and/or history of pulmonary edema; hypotension = SBP < 80 mm Hg for at least 1 hour, requiring inotropic support with medications or intra-aortic balloon pump (IABP) within 24 hours periprocedurally. *(From Mehran R, Aymong ED, Nikolsky E, et al: A simple risk score for prediction of contrast-induced nephropathy after percutaneous coronary intervention: Development and initial validation. J Am Coll Cardiol 44:1393, 2004.)*

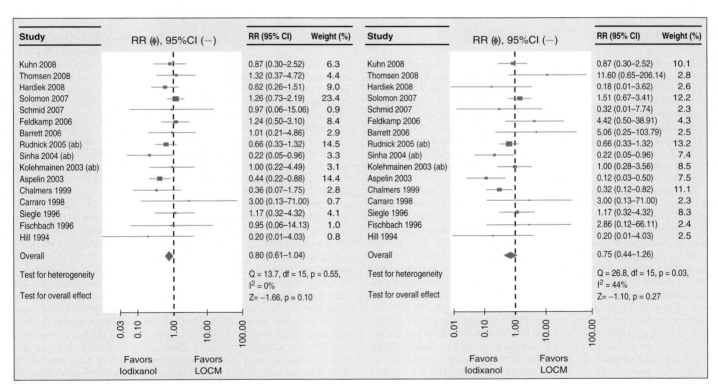

FIGURE 93-10 Incidence of CI-AKI from a 2009 meta-analysis of trials comparing iso-osmolar iodixanol with all nonionic low-osmolar agents, demonstrating an overall trend in favor of a treatment effect with iodixanol (not statistically significant). **Left and right panels,** Results for ≥25% and ≥0.5-mg/dL rise in serum Cr level, respectively. *(From Heinrich MC, Häberle L, Müller V, et al: Nephrotoxicity of iso-osmolar iodixanol compared with nonionic low-osmolar contrast media: Meta-analysis of randomized controlled trials. Radiology 250:68, 2009.)*

The American College of Cardiology/American Heart Association (ACC/AHA) guidelines for the management of acute coronary syndrome (ACS) recommends iodixanol for patients with CKD at risk for CI-AKI undergoing urgent angiography.[36] Although it is desirable to limit contrast to the smallest volume possible in any setting, there is disagreement about a safe contrast limit. The lower the eGFR, the smaller the amount of contrast material needed to cause CI-AKI. In general, contrast medium should be limited to less than 30 mL for a

diagnostic and less than 100 mL for an interventional procedure. If staged procedures are planned, it is advantageous to have more than 10 days between the first and second contrast exposures if contrast nephropathy has occurred with the first procedure.

More than 40 randomized trials have tested various adjunctive strategies for the prevention of CI-AKI.[37] Most of these trials were small, underpowered, and did not find the preventive strategy under investigation superior to placebo. These trials permit several conclusions: (1)

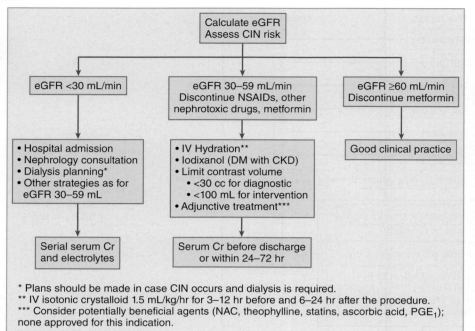

FIGURE 93-11 Algorithm for the management of patients receiving iodinated contrast media. PGE_1 = prostaglandin E_1. *(Modified from McCullough PA: Contrast-induced acute kidney injury. J Am Coll Cardiol 51:1419, 2008.)*

Postprocedural monitoring is critical in the current era of short hospital stays and outpatient procedures. In general, high-risk patients in the hospital should have hydration started 12 hours before the procedure and continued for at least 6 hours afterward. A serum Cr level should be measured 24 hours after the procedure. For outpatients, particularly those with eGFR less than 60 mL/min/1.73 m^2, either an overnight stay or discharge to home with 48-hour follow-up and Cr level measurement is advised. Individuals in whom severe CI-AKI develops have an increased Cr level greater than 0.5 mg/dL in the first 24 hours after the procedure.[39] Thus, for those who do not have this degree of Cr level elevation and an otherwise uneventful course, discharge to home may be considered. For those with eGFR lower than 30 mL/min/1.73 m^2, the possibility of dialysis should be discussed with the patient; preprocedure nephrology consultation is advised for possible pre- and postprocedure hemofiltration and dialysis management.

Acceleration of Vascular Calcification

Atherosclerotic calcification begins as early as the second decade of life, just after fatty streak formation.[40] Coronary artery lesions of young adults have revealed small aggregates of crystalline calcium within the necrotic lipid core of a plaque.[40] Calcium phosphate—the mineral form is hydroxyapatite, $Ca_5(PO_4)_3(OH)$—which contains 40% calcium by weight, is deposited by modulated vascular smooth muscle cells by a mechanism similar to that found in osteogenesis and remodeling.[41] Hydroxyapatite, the predominant crystalline form in calcium deposits, forms primarily in vesicles that pinch off from arterial wall cells, analogous to how matrix vesicles pinch off from chondrocytes in developing bone.[41] Coronary artery calcification (CAC) occurs in atherosclerotic arteries but not in the normal vessel wall (see Chaps. 19 and 43).

When the eGFR falls below 60 mL/min/1.73 m^2, the filtration and elimination of phosphorus are reduced. Subtle degrees of hyperphosphatemia can trigger the increased release of fibroblast growth factor 23, liberating calcium stores from bone and potentially accelerating vascular calcification. Patients with ESRD have the greatest absolute values and rates of accumulation of CAC of any patient population.[42] A variety of stimuli can induce vascular smooth muscle cells to assume osteoblast-like functions in vitro, including phosphorus, which stimulates the Pit-1 receptor on vascular smooth muscle cells, oxidized low-density lipoprotein (LDL), and a number of other factors. Neither calcium intake nor blood levels of calcium are related to vascular calcification. Clinical studies in ESRD have suggested that vascular calcification is driven much more by age, length of time on dialysis, dyslipidemia, and phosphate retention. A systematic review of the literature in CKD and ESRD ($N = 2919$) found 31 studies that were split on finding or not finding the significance of serum Ca, serum phosphate (PO_4), calcium-phosphate product, parathyroid hormone (PTH), or treatments for Ca-PO_4 balance, including phosphate binders, calcium, and vitamin D analogues, in relation to CAC.[43] When taken into consideration, the lipid profiles (primarily reduced high-density lipoprotein cholesterol [HDL-C], elevated triglyceride [TG], elevated LDL-C, and elevated total cholesterol levels) were the most predictive factors of CAC in ESRD.

There have been 10 randomized trials (N = 2612) of therapies aimed to attenuate CAC measured by electron beam, helical, and multislice computed tomography (CT) (see Chap. 19).[44] Therapies included the following: statins, $n = 1113$; placebo, $n = 829$; and antihypertensives, $n = 201$. In patients with CKD ($N = 477$), treatments included

diuretics in the form of loop diuretics or mannitol can worsen CI-AKI if there is inadequate volume replacement for the diuresis that follows; (2) low-dose or renal dose dopamine does not provide protection, despite its popularity in practice, given the counterbalancing forces of intrarenal vasodilation through the dopamine-1 receptor and the vasoconstricting forces of the dopamine-2, alpha, and beta receptors; and (3) renal toxic agents including nonsteroidal antiinflammatory drugs (NSAIDs), metformin, aminoglycosides, and cyclosporine should not be administered in the periprocedural period. There are currently no approved agents for the prevention of CI-AKI.

A suggested algorithm for risk stratification and prevention of CI-AKI is shown in **Figure 93-11**. When the eGFR is less than 60 mL/min/1.73 m^2, then optimal hydration, iodixanol as the contrast agent of choice, and prophylactic agents—including N-acetylcysteine (NAC), statins, aminophylline, ascorbic acid, and prostaglandin E_1—can be considered. Based on many small randomized trials, oral or intravenous NAC, a cytoprotective agent against oxidative injury, may be effective for the prevention of CI-AKI.[37] A trial of NAC in patients with acute MI undergoing primary angioplasty assigned 354 patients (eGFR, ~78 mL/min; ~15% diabetics) to one of three groups: (1) 116 patients were assigned to a standard dose of NAC (600-mg intravenous bolus before primary angioplasty and 600 mg orally twice daily for the 48 hours after angioplasty); (2) 119 patients to a double dose of NAC (1200-mg intravenous bolus and 1200 mg orally twice daily for the 48 hours after intervention); and (3) 119 patients to placebo.[38] The rates of CI-AKI (>25% rise in the Cr level from baseline) were 39 (33%) in controls, 17 (15%) for standard-dose NAC, and 10 (8%) for double-dose NAC ($P < 0.001$). Overall in-hospital mortality was as follows: 13 (11%) in the control group died, 5 (4%) in the standard-dose NAC group, and 3 (3%) in the high-dose NAC group ($P = 0.02$). The rate for the composite endpoint of death, acute renal failure requiring temporary renal replacement therapy, or the need for mechanical ventilation was 21 (18%), 8 (7%), and 6 (5%) in the three groups, respectively ($P = 0.002$). Most operators believe—given the seriousness of CI-AKI, the relative safety of the strategies used, and the evolution of clinical trials shaping our practice—that the combination of hydration, use of iodixanol, and use of prophylactic NAC is a reasonable three-pronged approach to minimize CI-AKI and the risk of acute renal failure requiring dialysis.

low-phosphorus diet (n = 29), sevelamer phosphate binder (n = 229), and calcium-based phosphate binders (n = 219). The overall mean weighted annualized CAC progression was 17.2% ± 6.7%. Patients with CVD and CKD had rates of 16.9% ± 5.2% and 18.4% ± 11.1%, respectively (P < 0.0001). Progression rates ranged among classes of therapy from 13.5% to 19.3% and 14.2% to 24.1%. In contrast, the rate of CAC progression in patients assigned to placebo was 13.5%. Thus, despite earlier enthusiasm about statins, calcium restriction in ESRD, and sevelamer, it appears that no management approach influences the steady progression of arterial calcification.

Sevelamer was also tested in the Dialysis Clinical Outcomes Revisited (DCOR) trial.[45] This 3-year trial involving more than 2100 patients found no difference in mortality and morbidity for those receiving sevelamer hydrochloride versus those using calcium-based phosphate binders (9% relative risk reduction with sevelamer; P = 0.30). There have been two large outcomes trials testing statins in ESRD. The 4D Trial (Deutsche Diabetes Dialyse Studie) randomized 1255 type 2 DM patients with new ESRD to atorvastatin 20 mg daily or placebo for a median of 4 years.[46] The statin was effective in reducing the median serum LDL-C by 42% throughout the study period. The primary endpoint, however, defined as the composite of cardiac death, nonfatal MI, and fatal or nonfatal stroke, was only reduced by 8% with atorvastatin (P = 0.37). The AURORA Trial (A Study to Evaluate the Use of Rosuvastatin in Subjects on Regular Hemodialysis: An Assessment of Survival and Cardiovascular Events) randomized 2776 hemodialysis patients 50 to 80 years of age to rosuvastatin 10 mg daily or placebo over 4 years.[47] The mean reduction in LDL-C was 43% in patients receiving rosuvastatin, from a baseline level of 100 mg/dL. The combined primary endpoints of death from cardiovascular causes, nonfatal MI, or nonfatal stroke were similar (9.2 and 9.5 events/100 patient-years, respectively; hazard ratio, 0.96; P = 0.59). Rosuvastatin had no effect on individual components of the primary endpoint. There was also no significant effect on all-cause mortality (13.5 versus 14.0 events/100 patient-years; hazard ratio, 0.96; P = 0.51). It appears from DCOR, 4D, and AURORA that avoidance of calcium-based phosphate binders or LDL-C reduction in ESRD does not affect cardiovascular events or mortality. Explanations for this lack of effect include the following: advanced calcific atherosclerosis that is not influenced by reductions in LDL-C; nonischemic cardiovascular mechanisms unaffected by lipid status in terminal events in ESRD (e.g., pump failure, non-ischemic arrhythmias); and competing non-cardiovascular causes of mortality (e.g., sepsis, venous thromboembolism). Thus, as of this writing, using statins or any particular phosphate binder in patients with ESRD cannot be expected to influence CAC or clinical outcomes. There have been no trials testing the degree of phosphate lowering or control of PTH on CAC progression and CVD events.

Renal Disease and Hypertension

The kidney is a central regulator of blood pressure and controls intraglomerular pressure through autoregulation. Glomerular injury activates a variety of pathways that increase systemic blood pressure. This effect sets up a vicious circle of more glomerular and tubulointerstitial injury and worsened HTN (see Chap. 45). A cornerstone of management of combined CKD and CVD is strict blood pressure control (**Fig. 93-12**). An optimal blood pressure can be defined as less than 120/80 mm Hg (with systolic blood pressure [SBP] being the more important target), and most patients with CKD and HTN require three or more antihypertensive agents to achieve a goal blood pressure lower than 130/80 mm Hg.[11] The key lifestyle issues with CKD and HTN include dietary changes with sodium restriction, weight reduction to a target body mass index lower than 25 kg/m[2], and exercise for 60 minutes/day most days of the week. Pharmacologic therapy aims for strict blood pressure control with an agent that antagonizes the RAAS,

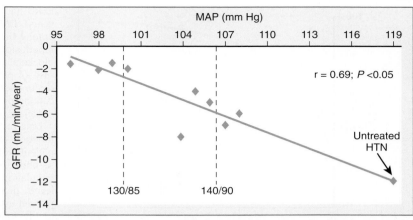

FIGURE 93-12 Influence of SBP on the rate of decline in renal function. MAP = mean arterial pressure. *(Modified from Bakris GL, Williams M, Dworkin L, et al: Preserving renal function in adults with hypertension and diabetes: A consensus approach. National Kidney Foundation Hypertension and Diabetes Executive Committees Working Group. Am J Kidney Dis 36:646, 2003.)*

often in combination with a thiazide-type diuretic. ONTARGET (ONgoing Telmisartan Alone and in combination with Ramipril Global Endpoint Trial) randomized 25,620 participants with DM or known vascular disease to ramipril 10 mg orally every day (n = 8,576), telmisartan 80 mg every day (n = 8,542), or a combination of the two (n = 8,502) over 4.7 years.[48] The secondary renal outcome, dialysis or doubling of the serum Cr level, was similar with telmisartan (2.21%) and ramipril (2.03%) and more frequent with combination therapy (2.49%; P = 0.038). The eGFR decreased least with ramipril compared with telmisartan (-2.82 ± 17.2 versus -4.12 ± 17.4 mL/min/1.73 m[2]; P < 0.0001) or combination therapy (-6.11 ± 17.9 mL/min/1.73 m[2]; P < 0.0001). Thus, unless a patient has systolic HF and meets the criteria for prior angiotensin-converting enzyme inhibitor (ACEI) + angiotensin receptor blocker (ARB) trials, patients with DM and CVD should be treated with an ACEI or an ARB, but not both. Dihydropyridine calcium channel blockers alone should also be avoided because of the relative afferent arteriolar dilation, which increases intraglomerular pressure and worsens glomerular injury. Special diagnostic consideration should be given to the possibility of underlying bilateral renal artery stenosis from the clinical clues of poorly controlled blood pressure on more than three agents, abdominal bruits, smoking history, peripheral arterial disease, and a marked change in the serum Cr level with the administration of an ACEI or ARB.[49] Although renal artery stenosis accounts for less than 3% of ESRD cases, it represents a potentially treatable condition[50] (see Chaps. 45 and 63).

Acute Coronary Syndromes

Diagnosis in Patients with Chronic Kidney Disease

Patients with CKD have shown a higher burden of silent ischemia, which clusters with serious arrhythmias, HF, and other cardiac events. Hemodialysis patients bear considerable hemodynamic stress three times weekly during dialysis sessions. Several studies have demonstrated a relationship between ST-segment depression and release of cardiac biomarkers (primarily troponin) before or during dialysis and poor long-term survival.[51] From a practical perspective, it is important to realize that patients with CKD presenting to the hospital with chest discomfort represent a high-risk group, having a 40% cardiac event rate at 30 days.[52] In making the diagnosis of acute MI (AMI) in patients with CKD or ESRD, troponin I is the preferred biomarker on the basis of its kinetic profile in patients with renal impairment.[53] The skeletal myopathy of CKD can elevate creatine kinase, myoglobin, and some troponin T assay results, making these tests less desirable. In addition to an elevated biomarker of cardiac injury, supporting evidence of the

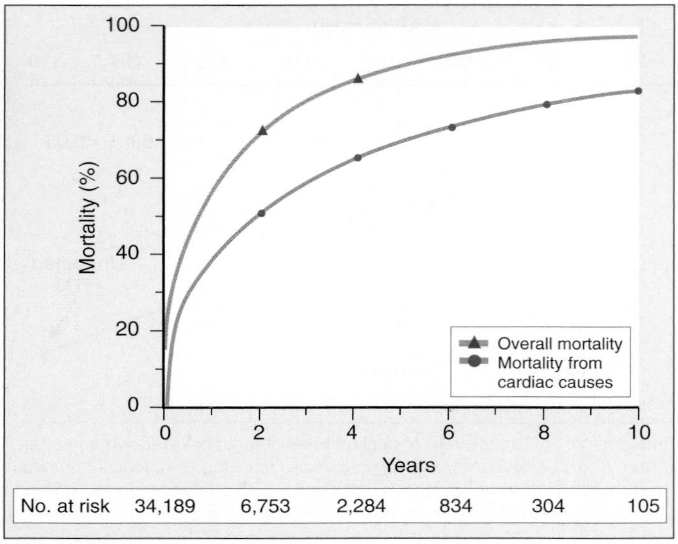

FIGURE 93-13 Cumulative mortality after myocardial infarction in patients with end-stage renal disease from the U.S. Renal Data System. *(Modified from Herzog CA, Ma JZ, Collins AJ: Poor long-term survival after acute myocardial infarction among patients on long-term dialysis. N Engl J Med 339:799, 1998.)*

diagnosis of AMI could be characteristic chest pain, electrocardiographic changes (ST-segment elevation or depression, new Q waves), or the identification of a culprit lesion on angiography. Because of the high event rate and prevalence of CVD in patients with CKD, it is advisable to consider admission to the hospital when the presenting symptom is chest discomfort and the eGFR is lower than 60 mL/min/1.73 m^2 or the patient has ESRD and is receiving dialysis.[54]

Renal Dysfunction as a Prognostic Factor

In the last several decades, considerable advances have been made in the diagnosis and treatment of ACS in the general population (see Chaps. 55 and 56). These advances include early paramedic response and defibrillation, coronary care units, and pharmacotherapy, including antiplatelet agents, antithrombotics, beta-adrenergic receptor blocking agents (beta blockers), ACEIs, and intravenous thrombolytic agents. Primary angioplasty for ST-segment elevation MI (STEMI) has become a well-accepted mode of treatment. These advances, however, have not been tested in patients with CKD or ESRD, primarily because these patients have generally been excluded from randomized treatment trials. Retrospective studies of patients in coronary care units have identified renal dysfunction as the most significant prognostic factor for long-term mortality when adjusting for other clinical factors, including age, sex, and comorbidities.[55] In addition, retrospective studies of patients with AMI consistently identify renal dysfunction as an independent predictor of death, with a greater impact on mortality than baseline demographics or therapies received.[55] Patients with ESRD have the highest mortality after AMI of any large chronic disease population (**Fig. 93-13**).[56]

Reasons for Poor Outcomes in Patients with Renal Dysfunction

Four reasons may underlie poor cardiovascular outcomes in patients with renal dysfunction after an ACS: (1) excess comorbidities associated with CKD and ESRD, in particular DM and HF; (2) therapeutic nihilism; (3) toxicity of therapies; and (4) special biologic and pathophysiologic factors in renal dysfunction that worsen outcomes.[55] In one study by Beattie and coworkers, the comorbidities of patients with STEMI and CKD (mean Cr = 2.7 mg/dL) included older age (mean, 70.2 years), DM (38.1%), and prior HF (23.2%).[6] Those with

ESRD had similar rates of comorbidities, including age (mean, 64.9 years), DM (40.4%), and prior HF (31.7%). This study found that among the CKD and ESRD groups, there are lower rates of use of reperfusion therapy (thrombolysis or primary angioplasty) and beta blockers, suggesting some contribution to poor outcomes from underuse of proven therapies (therapeutic nihilism). Patients with renal dysfunction may present later in their course, have more contraindications, or have other aspects about their presentations that prompt clinicians to use fewer therapies or take a more conservative approach.

Data on the toxicity of treatments for an ACS related to renal dysfunction are often unavailable, primarily because of exclusion of patients with CKD from these trials. The primary defects in thrombosis attributable to uremia are excess thrombin generation, increased circulating thrombin-antithrombin complexes, lower antithrombin III levels, increased plasminogen activation inhibitor, and decreased platelet aggregation. Decreased platelet aggregation is further related to the following: (1) reductions in the dense granule content of adenosine triphosphate, serotonin, and von Willebrand factor; (2) diminished thromboxane A2 generation in response to thrombin; and (3) diminished availability and function of glycoprotein IIb/IIIa. In the balance, patients with CKD and ESRD, when untreated, are more susceptible to atherothrombosis; however, after receiving any form of antiplatelet or antithrombotic therapy, these patients are more prone to bleeding complications.[57] In patients with renal dysfunction, the best measure of bleeding risk is the bleeding time. Unfortunately, the bleeding time is not a practical test for the ACS patient; consequently, clinicians cannot readily assess the a priori bleeding risk for any given CKD or ESRD patient. It is unlikely that bleeding complications alone account for the large differences seen in mortality between CKD and ESRD and those with preserved renal function with AMI.

The final and most important reason why patients with CKD and ESRD have poor outcomes after an ACS is the enhanced vascular pathobiology induced by the chronic renal failure state.[55] The processes that contribute to accelerated atherosclerosis include a dyslipidemia characterized by decreased function of lipoprotein lipase and decreased HDL-C and elevated TG and LDL levels. Levels of homocysteine and other thiols rise when the eGFR drops below 60 mL/min/1.73 m^2, enhancing the oxidation of LDL-C and progression of atherosclerotic lesions.[23] Renal dysfunction is a systemic inflammatory state, associated with higher rates of plaque rupture and incident CVD events. Finally, chronic hyperactivation of the sympathetic nervous system and an imbalance between endothelin, a powerful vasoconstrictor, and nitric oxide, a local paracrine vasodilator, may worsen HTN and may augment intravascular wall stress, which could further contribute to incident CVD events.

Treatment in Patients with Renal Dysfunction

Clinicians must confront ACS in high-risk populations with CKD and ESRD with little evidence on which to base treatment decisions (see Chaps. 55 and 56). Therapies that benefit the general population often yield enhanced benefit in patients with CKD and ESRD. A favorable risk-benefit ratio has now been demonstrated for aspirin, beta blockers, ACEIs, ARBs, aldosterone receptor antagonists, and statins.[58] Therapies that require dose adjustment on the basis of CrCl include low-molecular-weight heparins, bivalirudin, and glycoprotein IIb/IIIa antagonists (**Table 93-1**). Given that the major inputs for bleeding risks include older age, low body weight, and renal dysfunction, Table 93-1 also lists agents that are approved in a weight-adjusted dose form and gives the currently recommended dose adjustments for commonly used antiplatelet and antithrombotic agents.[57] Greater use of such therapies, despite the heightened risk for complications, may attenuate the excess mortality reported in the CKD and ESRD populations. There have been no randomized trials of PCI or bypass surgery in patients with CKD or ESRD. In the Bypass Angioplasty Revascularization Investigation (BARI) trial, however, whether PCI or surgery was used in the management of multivessel coronary disease, CKD and DM associated with worsened long-term survival (**Fig. 93-14**).[8] Further research is needed into the particular pathogenic mechanisms in the renal failure

TABLE 93-1 **Recommended Dose Adjustment of Conventional Antithrombotics Used for Acute Coronary Syndromes***

ANTITHROMBOTIC AGENT	eGFR (mL/min/1.73 m²) (CrCl in mL/min)			
	60-90	30-60	<30	DIALYSIS-DEPENDENT
Aspirin	No adjustment needed	No adjustment needed	No adjustment needed	No adjustment needed
Clopidogrel	No adjustment needed	No adjustment needed	No adjustment needed	No adjustment needed
Ticlopidine	No adjustment needed	No adjustment needed	No adjustment needed	No adjustment needed
Heparin	No guidelines	No guidelines	No guidelines	No guidelines
LMWH	No guidelines	No guidelines	Reduce dose by 30%; factor Xa monitoring advocated	No guidelines
Lepirudin	No guidelines	CrCl = 45-60 mL/min or SrCr = 1.6-2 mg/dL—reduce bolus to 0.2 mg/kg IV + decrease infusion rate by 50% (0.075 mg/kg/hr IV) CrCl = 30-44 mL/min or SrCr = 2.1-3 mg/dL—reduce bolus to 0.2 mg/kg IV + decrease standard initial infusion rate by 70% (0.045 mg/kg/hr IV)	CrCl = 15-29 mL/min or SrCr = 3.1-6 mg/dL—reduce bolus to 0.2 mg/kg IV + decrease infusion rate by 85% (0.0225 mg/kg/hr IV) CrCl < 15 mL/min or SrCr > 6 mg/dL—reduce bolus to 0.2 mg/kg IV; no infusion	Reduce bolus dose to 0.2 mg/kg IV; no infusion
Bivalirudin	No guidelines	Reduce infusion dose by 20%	Reduce infusion dose by 60%	Reduce infusion dose by 90%
Argatroban	No dose adjustment	No dose adjustment	No dose adjustment	
Abciximab	No guidelines Monitoring advocated	No guidelines Monitoring advocated	No guidelines Monitoring advocated	No guidelines; monitoring advocated
Eptifibatide	No guidelines	SrCr = 2-4 mg/dL—135 mg/kg IV bolus + 0.5 mg/kg/min IV infusion	SrCr > 4.0 mg/dL; contraindicated	No clinical data; in vitro data demonstrate clearance
Tirofiban	No dose adjustment	No dose adjustment	0.2 mg/kg/min IV for 30 min, followed by 0.05 mg/kg/min IV	No clinical data; in vitro data demonstrate clearance

*In patients with CKD and ESRD.
LMWH = low-molecular-weight heparin; SrCr = serum creatinine.
Modified from Sica D: The implications of renal impairment among patients undergoing percutaneous coronary intervention. J Invasive Cardiol 14(Suppl B):30B, 2002.

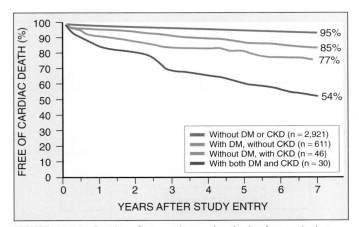

FIGURE 93-14 Freedom from cardiovascular death after angioplasty or bypass surgery in the BARI trial and registry (N = 3608). (*Modified from Szczech LA, Best PJ, Crowley E, et al: Outcomes of patients with chronic renal insufficiency in the Bypass Angioplasty Revascularization Investigation. Circulation 105:2253, 2002.*)

state that promote plaque rupture, accelerate atherosclerosis, lead to ACS complications, and promote the development of HF and arrhythmias.

Chronic Kidney Disease

Complicating Heart Failure

The diagnosis of HF with concomitant renal failure presents a particular challenge. Patients with CKD, and in particular ESRD, frequently have three key mechanical contributors to HF—pressure overload (related to HTN), volume overload, and cardiomyopathy. Approximately 20% of patients approaching hemodialysis have a diagnosis of HF.[59] It is unclear how much of this diagnosis results from chronic volume overload from renal failure or from impaired systolic or diastolic function. Notably, CKD influences the levels of BNP, a diagnostic blood test for HF. In general, when the eGFR is lower than 60 mL/min/1.73 m², a higher BNP cut point of 200 pg/mL should be used in the diagnosis of HF.[60] CKD (eGFR < 60 mL/min/1.73 m²), when present in patients with HF, independently predicts poor outcomes.[61] Estimated and actual GFRs clearly can be reduced by decreased renal blood flow related to low cardiac output. However, multiple studies of patients with classes II and III HF who do not have a low cardiac output state have shown decreased survival in a graded fashion related to renal impairment.

The combination of HF and CKD presents a challenge to cardiologists with respect to proven treatment options. ACEIs, if tolerated (or ARBs if ACEIs are not tolerated) beta blockers, aldosterone antagonists, and loop diuretics are all acceptable combination therapies (see Chap. 28).[62] Caveats in the use of ACEIs and ARBs are the marked elevation in the serum Cr level and acute renal failure, which are more likely to occur when the patient is volume-depleted or in the presence of occult bilateral renal artery stenosis or its equivalent (e.g., unilateral renal artery stenosis present in a renal transplant recipient).[63] When initiating therapy to block the RAAS, it is advisable to have the SBP stable and greater than 90 mm Hg, euvolemia, and a drug regimen without concurrent renal toxic agents. Clinicians should realize that CKD patients enjoy an improved survival and reduced rates of ESRD on ACEIs or ARBs, even though the serum Cr level is chronically elevated on these agents because of reduced intraglomerular pressure. Discontinuation of ACEIs or ARBs because of moderate asymptomatic rises in the Cr level is a common management error. In general, an attempt should be made to use ACEIs or ARBs in patients down to an eGFR of 15 mL/min/1.73 m². Below this level, case reports suggest a high rate

TABLE 93-2 Recommended Dose Adjustment of Selected Medical Therapy for Hypertension, Dyslipidemia, Heart Failure, and Arrhythmias*

AGENT USED	ELIMINATION ROUTE	eGFR (mL/min/1.73 m²) (CrCl in mL/min)			
		90-60	60-30	<30	DIALYSIS-DEPENDENT
Central Adrenergic Blockers					
Clonidine	Renal				↓ Dose 50%
Methyldopa	Renal	qid	qid	↓ tid	↓ bid or qd
Angiotensin-Converting Enzyme Inhibitors					
Captopril	Renal				↓ Dose 50%
Enalapril	Hepatic			↓ Dose 25%	↓ Dose 50%
Lisinopril	Renal			↓ Dose 25%	↓ Dose 50%
Ramipril	Renal, GI			↓ Dose 75%	↓ Dose 75%
Benazepril	Renal			↓ Dose 25%	↓ Dose 75%
Inotropic Agents					
Digoxin	Renal, nonrenal		↓ Dose 50%	↓ Dose 50%	↓ Dose 75%; change to qod
Milrinone	Renal		↓ Dose 25%	↓ Dose 50%	↓ Dose 75%
Antiarrhythmics					
Disopyramide	Renal, hepatic	bid	bid	↓ qd	↓ qod
Flecainide	Renal, hepatic				↓ Dose 25%-50%
Mexiletine	Renal, hepatic				↓ Dose 50%-75%
Procainamide	Renal, hepatic	qid	↓ tid	↓ bid	↓ bid or qd
Dofetilide	Renal, nonrenal		↓ Dose 50%	↓ Dose 75%	Contraindicated
Beta Blockers					
Atenolol	Renal			↓ Dose 50%	↓ Dose 75%; ↓ qod
Sotalol	Renal			↓ Dose 50%	↓ Dose 75%
Others					
Verapamil	Hepatic				↓ Dose 50%-75%
Hydralazine	Hepatic	qid	↓ tid	↓ tid	↓ bid
Gemfibrozil	Renal			↓ Dose 50%	↓ Dose 75%
Fenofibrate	Renal				Contraindicated
Nicotinic acid	Renal, hepatic			↓ Dose 25%	↓ Dose 25%

*In patients with CKD and ESRD.
GI = gastrointestinal.

of hyperkalemia and the concern of accelerating the course to ESRD and dialysis.

The management of the patient who is already receiving dialysis and has HF requires particular care. In general, proven HF therapies, provided they are tolerated, should be used along with regular and ad hoc dialysis as needed to control volume overload. In a randomized trial, carvedilol did provide additional benefit in this scenario.[64] In addition, a retrospective analysis has supported the use of ACEIs in patients with ESRD admitted with HF.[65] Finally, the acute management of decompensated HF in patients with impaired eGFR poses a particularly difficult challenge.[66] In fact, an elevated Cr level is the single most common reason for using positive inotropes or inodilators in hospitalized patients with HF.[67] There are no published reports of dobutamine leading to long-term favorable outcomes and, in the short term, it increases arrhythmias and mortality. Similarly, milrinone has not been shown to reduce mortality, causes arrhythmias, and must be dose-adjusted when the eGFR drops below 45 mL/min/1.73 m² (**Table 93-2**). Another option is the use of intravenous BNP (nesiritide), which causes primarily venodilation and natriuresis.[68] Completed studies with nesiritide have evaluated the CKD subgroups and found benefit in CKD equal to that in those with preserved renal function, although the overall effect is modestly better than that with intravenous nitroglycerin.[69] Patients with advanced HF have reduced renal blood flow, decreased glomerular filtration rate, enhanced proximal reabsorption of water, and an overall reduced capacity of the nephron to excrete water (**Fig. 93-15**). Furthermore, reduced effective arterial blood volume is a stimulus for antidiuretic hormone release, which plays a dominant role in worsening water retention. The clinical signs of this cardiorenal syndrome are an elevation in the serum Cr and blood urea nitrogen levels, hyponatremia, volume retention, and excessive thirst.

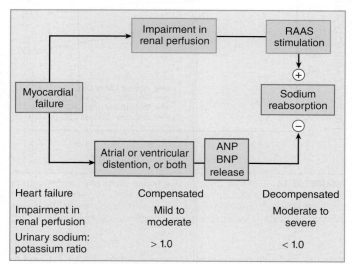

Heart failure	Compensated	Decompensated
Impairment in renal perfusion	Mild to moderate	Moderate to severe
Urinary sodium: potassium ratio	> 1.0	< 1.0

FIGURE 93-15 Pathophysiologic processes in combined heart and kidney failure. ANP = A-type natriuretic peptide; BNP = B-type natriuretic peptide. (From Weber KT: Aldosterone in congestive heart failure. N Engl J Med 345:1689, 2001.)

Treatment efforts should be aimed at improving left ventricular systolic function, often in the hospital setting, with the intravenous therapies mentioned earlier (see Chap. 28). Small trials using continuous venovenous ultrafiltration have demonstrated short-term reductions in symptoms, shorter hospital stays, and reductions in rehospitalizations.[70] Until larger trials confirm longer-term benefits in hospitalization and mortality, ultrafiltration can be considered a last-line approach for the patient with refractory cardiorenal failure.

In summary, CKD and HF present a particularly challenging scenario for clinicians and patients. Frequent monitoring and the combined use of renal and cardioprotective strategies are critical. Future research is needed to confirm anemia correction and ultrafiltration as additional strategies in patients who have cardiorenal syndrome. Dialysis patients, despite having volume reduction with mechanical fluid removal, should have medical therapy with ACEIs or ARBs, beta blockers, and additional agents for blood pressure control if needed.

Complicating Valvular Heart Disease

Impaired renal function has been linked to mitral annular calcification and aortic sclerosis (see Chap. 66). Advanced thickening of the cardiac valves and calcification can accompany ESRD.[71] Approximately 80% of patients with ESRD have the murmur of aortic sclerosis. Neither of these lesions usually progresses to the point where studies beyond echocardiography are needed. Bacterial endocarditis may develop in patients with ESRD who have temporary dialysis access catheters.[72] Endocarditis with common pathogens, including *Staphylococcus*, *Streptococcus*, and *Enterococcus* spp., in the aortic or mitral position, is associated with a mortality rate higher than 50% in this setting (see Chap. 67). It becomes difficult to treat given the continued need for dialysis access and the delay in surgical placement of permanent arteriovenous shunts or fistulas. Unfortunately, surgical mortality associated with valve replacement in ESRD related to endocarditis is high. In the setting of ESRD, when valve surgery is carried out for endocarditis or other causes of valve failure, there has been no difference in survival among those who received tissue or mechanical valve prostheses. Thus, tissue valves are a reasonable choice given the complicating issue of chronic anticoagulation and bleeding with dialysis vascular access.

Renal Function and Arrhythmias

Uremia, hyperkalemia, acidosis, and disorders of calcium-phosphate balance have all been linked to higher rates of atrial and ventricular arrhythmias.[73] Given a concurrent substrate of left ventricular hypertrophy, left ventricular dilation, HF, and valvular disease, it is not surprising that higher rates of almost all arrhythmias have been reported in CKD, including bradyarrhythmias and heart block. Caveats for practical management include dose adjustment for many antiarrhythmic medications, including digoxin, sotalol, and procainamide (see Table 93-2). Of concern, CKD, and ESRD in particular, may cause elevated defibrillation thresholds and failure of implantable cardioverter-defibrillators (ICDs).[74] Until this association is better understood, patients receiving ICDs should have frequent surveillance and consideration for noninvasive programmed stimulation for appropriate antitachycardia and defibrillation therapy. Considering the high rates of sudden death in patients with ESRD, clinical trials of prophylactic ICDs in this population are under consideration.

Consultative Approach to the Hemodialysis Patient

The prevalence of angiographically significant coronary artery disease (CAD) ranges from 25% in young, nondiabetic hemodialysis patients to 85% in older ESRD patients with long-standing DM.[75,76] Cardiac death in dialysis patients younger than age 45 years is approximately 100-fold greater than that in the general population. The prevalence and severity of CAD among patients with ESRD is daunting in terms of occurrence and extent of poor outcomes. Medicare beneficiaries with CKD prior to the initiation of dialysis are 60% more likely to have a billing claim submitted for the diagnosis of CVD and 70% more likely to have a claim submitted for atherosclerotic heart disease.[77] Of those receiving dialysis, a substantial proportion, perhaps the most of them, have established CAD. In diabetic renal transplant candidates, 30%

will have one or more coronary artery lesions with more than 75% stenosis. When comparing the patients who undergo evaluation for CAD, those with ESRD have substantially more numerous and severe coronary artery lesions, as well as more severe left ventricular dysfunction.[76]

The patient with incipient ESRD who has been placed on dialysis can be considered to be the highest cardiovascular risk patient in medicine, with expected rates of CVD death that are many times higher than that expected for a non-ESRD patient, even those with a burden of several cardiovascular risk factors. ESRD is more than a cardiovascular risk equivalent, warranting meticulous efforts to achieve goals mandated by guidelines (**Table 93-3**).

Despite the use of multiple medications, most published series of ESRD patients from clinical trials or registries have indicated that the mean systolic blood pressure is approximately 155 mm Hg. Indeed, 80% of ESRD patients have HTN, but only 30% achieve adequate control.[78] Long-term cardiorenal protection involves two important concepts—blood pressure control to a much lower target (SBP < 130 mm Hg), and use of an agent that blocks the RAAS, such as an

TABLE 93-3	Therapeutic Opportunities to Improve Cardiovascular Care in Patients with Chronic Kidney Disease	
THERAPEUTIC OPPORTUNITY	**RATIONALE**
Weight loss, weight maintenance at BMI < 25 kg/m²	Improve dysmetabolic syndrome and diabetes
Low sodium intake	Reduce blood pressure Make blood pressure more responsive to medications Reduce volume retention between dialysis sessions
Aspirin 81 mg qd or clopidogrel 75 mg orally qd if aspirin-intolerant	Primary prevention of AMI and stroke
Lipid control (e.g., diet, statin, fibrates, niacin) ■ LDLC < 70 mg/dL ■ Non–HDL-C < 100 mg/dL ■ Apo B < 80 mg/dL	Possible prevention of AMI, stroke, and CVD death in CKD Possible reduction in progression of CKD No proven impact on outcomes in ESRD
Blood pressure control to target SBP < 130 mm Hg (optimal, ~120 mm Hg) ■ RAAS blocking agents (ACE or ARB) ■ Beta-blocking agents ■ Diuretics ■ Calcium channel blockers ■ Other add-on agents	Primary prevention of AMI, stroke, heart failure, and CVD death Preserve residual urine volume in peritoneal dialysis patients Reduce LVH Treat subclinical cardiac ischemia
Blood glucose control in diabetes (target HbA1C, 7.0%)	Reduction in risk of AMI, stroke, and CVD death Reduction in worsened nephropathy, retinopathy
Treatment of anemia (target < 12 g/dL and/or lowest ESP or iron doses) ■ ESPs ■ Iron	Improve symptoms of anemia Improve quality of life Possible reduction in LVH Unproven impact on AMI, stroke, HF, and CVD death
Treatment of CKD mineral and bone disorder (targets for ESRD: PO₄ = 3.5-5.5 mg/dL; iPTH = 150-300 pg/mL; Ca × PO₄ product < 55) ■ Phosphate binders ■ Calcitriol, vitamin D analogues	Reduce the risk of soft tissue calcification Reduce risk of symptomatic hyper- or hypocalcemia Possible reduction in all-cause mortality Unproven impact on skeletal fractures, bone pain, AMI, stroke, HF, and CVD death

BMI = body mass index; ESP = erythrocyte-stimulating protein; HbA1C = hemoglobin A1C; non-HDL-C = non-HDL cholesterol.

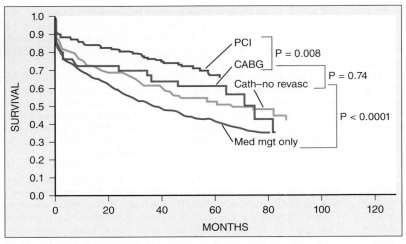

FIGURE 93-16 Long-term survival according to CAD management strategy in patients with CrCl < 60 mL/min or ESRD on dialysis. *(From Keeley EC, Kadakia R, Soman S, et al: Analysis of long-term survival after revascularization in patients with chronic kidney disease presenting with acute coronary syndromes. Am J Cardiol 92:509, 2003.)*

ACEI or ARB as the base of therapy. How can an ACEI or ARB be effective in a patient with ESRD, particularly one who is anephric? The RAAS appears to have considerable redundancy and is able to maintain its function, if not increase its overall level of activity, without participation by the kidneys.[79] Hence, this hyperactivation of the RAAS is a target for therapy in ESRD because ACEIs and ARBs have been demonstrated to reduce left ventricular hypertrophy (LVH) and possibly improve survival in ESRD.[80] A small trial has demonstrated that ramipril is related to preservation of residual urine output in those receiving peritoneal dialysis, which is a consistently favorable management issue in ESRD.[81] A retrospective study has found that although only approximately 20% of patients with ESRD and CAD receive ACEI, those who are given these agents after CAD events have improved all-cause mortality over the next 5 years.[82] The common difficulty with ACEIs or ARBs is worsened hyperkalemia in patients with ESRD. As tolerated, the clinician should consider adjusting the dialytic regimen to improve potassium removal. From all sources of evidence to date, patients with ESRD appear to benefit from ACEI or ARB therapy, provided the serum potassium level and blood pressure can be adequately controlled.

With an ACEI or ARB as a base of therapy, the antihypertensive regimen can be further modified according to blood pressure–lowering efficacy and CAD event reduction. Beta blockers can be used as antihypertensive and anti-ischemic agents.[83] In those with HF, beta blockers improve left ventricular ejection fraction and reduce rates of hospitalization, sudden death, and all-cause mortality.[84,85] Large relative risk reductions in all-cause mortality have been reported for patients who receive beta blockers with ESRD after CAD events.

After inclusion of an ACEI or ARB and beta blockers in the ESRD blood pressure regimen, the remaining choices should be based on ease of management, compliance, and lack of adverse effects. The goal is to create a blood pressure environment for the cardiovascular system in which the mean SBP—on 24-hour monitoring, for example—is at least lower than 130 mm Hg. Guidelines for non-ESRD patients state that the optimal systolic blood pressure should be approximately 120 mm Hg.[11] The difficult task in the ESRD patient is to achieve these goals without having hypotension during dialysis sessions. Given the high rates of severe CAD in ESRD, hypotension during dialysis can worsen clinical and subclinical ischemia recognized as chest discomfort, shortness of breath, ST-segment depression on electrocardiography, and elevations of cardiac troponin on blood testing.[86]

The National Kidney Foundation guidelines support LDL-C reduction, in most cases with a statin, in patients with CKD despite the lack of risk reductions in CVD events observed to date in clinical trials such as 4-D and AURORA.[87,88] In addition, agents that reduce non–HDL-C, including nicotinic acid and fibrates, can be used according to the National Cholesterol Education Project Adult Treatment Panel III (NCEP-ATP-III) guidelines.[89]

In ESRD with DM, blood glucose control to a target glycohemoglobin level lower than 7 mg/dL can be expected to reduce rates of microvascular (retinopathy) and, to a lesser extent, clinically important atherosclerotic disease elsewhere (AMI, stroke, CVD death).[90] Similarly, smoking cessation is recommended for patients with ESRD.[91] The effect of aspirin on renal endpoints is unknown; however, given its CVD protective effect, it is recommended for adult patients with ESRD.[92] For those who are aspirin-intolerant, general cardiology guidelines recommend the use of clopidogrel, although there are no published studies of clopidogrel on cardiovascular outcomes in ESRD.

Several analyses have suggested that ESRD patients with CAD who receive conservative medical management fare the worst of all groups (**Fig. 93-16**).[92-95] Thus, the first step after stress imaging in an ESRD patient with symptomatic CAD is to make an attempt at angiography and revascularization. Usually, multivessel CAD is found, so the next question is, what is the optimal approach—multivessel PCI or coronary artery bypass grafting (CABG)? It is widely accepted that patients with ESRD undergoing mechanical coronary revascularization procedures are at increased risk for adverse events, including death. Dialysis-dependent patients undergoing CABG face a 4.4 times greater risk of in-hospital death, a 3.1 times greater risk of mediastinitis, and a 2.6 times greater risk of stroke compared with those patients undergoing CABG who were not on dialysis.[96] Although newer surgical techniques have been successful in high-risk patients with renal failure, the long-term results, compared with traditional surgical and percutaneous techniques, are not yet known. In general, despite this significant up-front risk of surgery, the literature suggests the superiority of CABG compared with PCI in patients with ESRD. In single-vessel CAD and multivessel CAD without good bypass targets, recent trends have suggested that PCI with stenting is a favorable approach for patients with ESRD. Drug-eluting stents have reduced restenosis rates in this population and may tip the risk-benefit scale in favor of PCI.[97]

In summary, patients with ESRD have more than coronary artery disease risk-equivalent status in their baseline CAD risk assessment. An aggressive approach to medical management for CAD is warranted, even in the case of subclinical CAD. A low threshold for diagnostic testing should apply to ESRD patients (**Fig. 93-17**). When significant CAD is found, ESRD patients appear to benefit from revascularization compared with conservative medical management and, if clinically reasonable, should be given that opportunity for improved survival and reduction in future cardiac events.

Summary

Recognition that patients with CKD have an elevated CVD risk has increased over the last decade. Frequent clinical scenarios in which renal function influences care include CI-AKI, ACS, HF, valvular disease, and arrhythmias. Results from retrospective studies and clinical trial

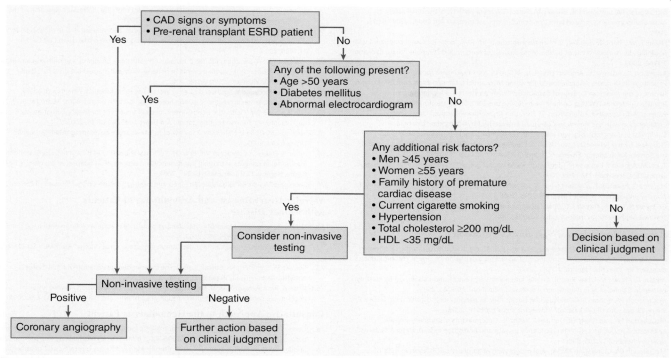

FIGURE 93-17 Approach to the ESRD patient with CAD or being considered for renal transplantation. HDL = high-density lipoprotein cholesterol. *(Modified from McCullough PA: Evaluation and treatment of coronary artery disease in patients with end-stage renal disease. Kidney Int Suppl [95]:S51, 2005.)*

subgroups form the basis of current recommendations, given the lack of prospective randomized trials of CKD and ESRD. Further study of the adverse metabolic milieu of CKD is likely to lead to generalizable diagnostic and therapeutic targets for the future management of renal patients with cardiovascular illness.

REFERENCES

Epidemiology and Outcomes

1. Lewis CE, Jacobs DR Jr, McCreath H, et al: Weight gain continues in the 1990s: 10-year trends in weight and overweight from the CARDIA study. Am J Epidemiol 151:1172, 2000.
2. Bakris GL, Williams M, Dworkin L, et al: Preserving renal function in adults with hypertension and diabetes: A consensus approach. National Kidney Foundation Hypertension and Diabetes Executive Committees Working Group. Am J Kidney Dis 36:646, 2000.
3. McCullough PA: Cardiorenal risk: An important clinical intersection. Rev Cardiovasc Med 3:71, 2002.
4. National Kidney Foundation: Clinical practice guidelines for chronic kidney disease: Evaluation, classification, and stratification. Am J Kidney Dis 2(Suppl 1):S46, 2002.
5. McCullough PA, Soman SS, Shah SS, et al: Risks associated with renal dysfunction in patients in the coronary care unit. J Am Coll Cardiol 36:679, 2000.
6. Beattie JN, Soman SS, Sandberg KR, et al: Determinants of mortality after myocardial infarction in patients with advanced renal dysfunction. Am J Kidney Dis 37:1191, 2001.
7. Chertow GM, Lazarus JM, Christiansen CL, et al: Preoperative renal risk stratification. Circulation 95:878, 1997.
8. Szczech LA, Best PJ, Crowley E, et al: Outcomes of patients with chronic renal insufficiency in the Bypass Angioplasty Revascularization Investigation. Circulation 105:2253, 2002.
9. Filler G, Bokenkamp A, Hofmann W, et al: Cystatin C as a marker of GFR–history, indications, and future research. Clin Biochem 38:1, 2005.
10. Sarnak MJ, Levey AS, Schoolwerth AC, et al: Kidney disease as a risk factor for development of cardiovascular disease: A statement from the American Heart Association Councils on Kidney in Cardiovascular Disease, High Blood Pressure Research, Clinical Cardiology, and Epidemiology and Prevention. Circulation 108:2154, 2003.
11. Chobanian AV, Bakris GL, Black HR, et al: The Seventh Report of the Joint National Committee on Prevention, Detection, Evaluation, and Treatment of High Blood Pressure: The JNC 7 report. JAMA 289:2560, 2003.

Anemia and Chronic Kidney Disease

12. NKF-DOQI clinical practice guidelines for the treatment of anemia of chronic renal failure. National Kidney Foundation-Dialysis Outcomes Quality Initiative. Am J Kidney Dis 30(Suppl 3):S192, 1997.
13. McCullough PA, Lepor NE: The deadly triangle of anemia, renal insufficiency, and cardiovascular disease: Implications for prognosis and treatment. Rev Cardiovasc Med 6:1, 2005.
14. Silverberg DS, Wexler D, Iaina A: The role of anemia in the progression of congestive heart failure. Is there a place for erythropoietin and intravenous iron? J Nephrol 17:749, 2004.

15. Anand I, McMurray JJ, Whitmore J, et al: Anemia and its relationship to clinical outcome in heart failure. Circulation 110:149, 2004.
16. Drüeke TB, Locatelli F, Clyne N, et al: Normalization of hemoglobin level in patients with chronic kidney disease and anemia. N Engl J Med 355:2071, 2006.
17. Singh A, Reddan D: Correction of Hemoglobin and Outcomes in Renal Insufficiency (CHOIR) trial. Presented at the National Kidney Foundation 2006 Spring Clinical Meeting, Chicago, April 19-23, 2006.
18. Pfeffer MA, Burdmann EA, Chen CY, et al: A trial of darbepoetin alfa in type 2 diabetes and chronic kidney disease. N Engl J Med 361:2019, 2009.

Percutaneous Coronary Interventions and Contrast-Induced Acute Kidney Injury

19. McCullough P: Outcomes of contrast-induced nephropathy: Experience in patients undergoing cardiovascular intervention. Catheter Cardiovasc Interv 67:335, 2006.
20. McCullough PA, Manley HJ: Prediction and prevention of contrast nephropathy. J Interv Cardiol 14:547, 2001.
21. Pannu N, Wiebe N, Tonelli M, Alberta Kidney Disease Network: Prophylaxis strategies for contrast-induced nephropathy. JAMA 295:2765, 2006.
22. Rihal CS, Textor SC, Grill DE, et al: Incidence and prognostic importance of acute renal failure after percutaneous coronary intervention. Circulation 105:2259, 2002.
23. Yerkey MW, Kernis SJ, Franklin BA, et al: Renal dysfunction and acceleration of coronary disease. Heart 90:961, 2004.
24. Andersen KJ, Christensen EI, Vik H: Effects of iodinated x-ray contrast media on renal epithelial cells in culture. Invest Radiol 29:955, 1994.
25. Keeley EC, Grines CL: Scraping of aortic debris by coronary guiding catheters: A prospective evaluation of 1,000 cases. J Am Coll Cardiol 32:1861, 1998.
26. Wijeysundera DN, Karkouti K, Beattie WS, et al: Improving the identification of patients at risk of postoperative renal failure after cardiac surgery. Anesthesiology 104:65, 2006.
27. Denton KM, Shweta A, Anderson WP: Preglomerular and postglomerular resistance responses to different levels of sympathetic activation by hypoxia. J Am Soc Nephrol 13:27, 2002.
28. Uder M, Humke U, Pahl M, et al: Nonionic contrast media iohexol and iomeprol decrease renal arterial tone: Comparative studies on human and porcine isolated vascular segments. Invest Radiol 37:440, 2002.
29. Rauch D, Drescher P, Pereira FJ, et al: Comparison of iodinated contrast media-induced renal vasoconstriction in human, rabbit, dog, and pig arteries. Invest Radiol 32:315, 1997.
30. Endre ZH: Acute kidney injury: Definitions and new paradigms. Adv Chronic Kidney Dis 15:213, 2008.
31. Mehran R, Aymong ED, Nikolsky E, et al: A simple risk score for prediction of contrast-induced nephropathy after percutaneous coronary intervention: Development and initial validation. J Am Coll Cardiol 44:1393, 2004.
32. McCullough PA: Contrast-induced acute kidney injury. J Am Coll Cardiol 51:1419, 2008.
33. Stevens MA, McCullough PA, Tobin KJ, et al: A prospective randomized trial of prevention measures in patients at high risk for contrast nephropathy: Results of the P.R.I.N.C.E. Study. Prevention of Radiocontrast-Induced Nephropathy Clinical Evaluation. J Am Coll Cardiol 33:403, 1999.

34. McCullough PA, Bertrand ME, Brinker JA, Stacul F: A meta-analysis of the renal safety of isosmolar iodixanol compared with low-osmolar contrast media. J Am Coll Cardiol 48:692, 2006.

35. Heinrich MC, Häberle L, Müller V, et al: Nephrotoxicity of iso-osmolar iodixanol compared with nonionic low-osmolar contrast media: Meta-analysis of randomized controlled trials. Radiology 250:68, 2009.

36. Anderson JL, Adams CD, Antman EM, et al: ACC/AHA 2007 Guidelines for the Management of Patients With Unstable Angina/Non-ST-Elevation Myocardial Infarction-Executive Summary: A Report of the American College of Cardiology/American Heart Association Task Force on Practice Guidelines (Writing Committee to Revise the 2002 Guidelines for the Management of Patients With Unstable Angina/Non-ST-Elevation Myocardial Infarction) Developed in Collaboration with the American College of Emergency Physicians, the Society for Cardiovascular Angiography and Interventions, and the Society of Thoracic Surgeons: Endorsed by the American Association of Cardiovascular and Pulmonary Rehabilitation and the Society for Academic Emergency Medicine. J Am Coll Cardiol 50:652, 2007.

37. Tepel M, Aspelin P, Lameire N: Contrast-induced nephropathy: A clinical and evidence-based approach. Circulation 113:1799, 2006.

38. Marenzi G, Assanelli E, Marana I, et al: N-acetylcysteine and contrast-induced nephropathy in primary angioplasty. N Engl J Med 354:2773, 2006.

39. Guitterez N, Diaz A, Timmis GC, et al: Determinants of serum creatinine trajectory in acute contrast nephropathy. J Interv Cardiol 15:349, 2002.

Accelerated Atherosclerotic Vascular Calcification

40. McCullough PA, Agrawal V, Danielewicz E, Abela GS: Accelerated atherosclerotic calcification and Monckeberg's sclerosis: A continuum of advanced vascular pathology in chronic kidney disease. Clin J Am Soc Nephrol 3:1585, 2008.

41. Aikawa E, Aikawa M, Libby P, et al: Arterial and aortic valve calcification abolished by elastolytic cathepsin S deficiency in chronic renal disease. Circulation 119:1785, 2009.

42. McCullough PA, Soman S: Cardiovascular calcification in patients with chronic renal failure: Are we on target with this risk factor? Kidney Int Suppl (90):S18, 2004.

43. McCullough PA, Sandberg KR, DumLer F, Yanez JE: Determinants of coronary vascular calcification in patients with chronic kidney disease and end-stage renal disease: A systematic review. J Nephrol 17:205, 2004.

44. McCullough PA, Chinnaiyan KM: Annual progression of coronary calcification in trials of preventive therapies. Arch Int Med 169:2064, 2009.

45. Suki WN, Zabaneh R, Cangiano JL, et al: Effects of sevelamer and calcium-based phosphate binders on mortality in hemodialysis patients. Kidney Int 72:1130, 2007.

46. Wanner C, Krane V, Marz W, et al: Atorvastatin in patients with type 2 diabetes mellitus undergoing hemodialysis. N Engl J Med 353:238, 2005.

47. Fellström BC, Jardine AG, Schmieder RE, et al: Rosuvastatin and cardiovascular events in patients undergoing hemodialysis. N Engl J Med 360:1395, 2009.

Renal Disease and Hypertension

48. Mann JF, Schmieder RE, McQueen M, et al: Renal outcomes with telmisartan, ramipril, or both, in people at high vascular risk (the ONTARGET study): A multicentre, randomised, double-blind, controlled trial. Lancet 372:547, 2008.

49. Cohen MG, Pascua JA, Garcia-Ben M, et al: A simple prediction rule for significant renal artery stenosis in patients undergoing cardiac catheterization. Am Heart J 150:1204, 2005.

50. Fatica RA, Port FK, Young EW: Incidence trends and mortality in end-stage renal disease attributed to renovascular disease in the United States. Am J Kidney Dis 37:1184, 2001.

Ischemic Heart Diseases in Patients with Impaired Renal Function

51. Freda BJ, Tang WH, Van Lente F, et al: Cardiac troponins in renal insufficiency: Review and clinical implications. J Am Coll Cardiol 40:2065, 2002.

52. McCullough PA, Nowak RM, Foreback C, et al: Emergency evaluation of chest pain in patients with advanced kidney disease. Arch Intern Med 162:2464, 2002.

53. McCullough PA, Nowak RM, Foreback C, et al: Performance of multiple cardiac biomarkers measured in the emergency department in patients with chronic kidney disease and chest pain. Acad Emerg Med 9:1389, 2002.

54. McCullough PA: Acute coronary syndromes in patients with renal failure. Curr Cardiol Rep 5:266, 2003.

55. McCullough PA: Why is chronic kidney disease the "spoiler" for cardiovascular outcomes? J Am Coll Cardiol 41:725, 2003.

56. Herzog CA, Ma JZ, Collins AJ: Poor long-term survival after acute myocardial infarction among patients on long-term dialysis. N Engl J Med 339:799, 1998.

57. Sica D: The implications of renal impairment among patients undergoing percutaneous coronary intervention. J Invasive Cardiol 14(Suppl B):30B, 2002.

58. McCullough PA: Evaluation and treatment of coronary artery disease in patients with end-stage renal disease. Kidney Int Suppl (95):S51, 2005.

Heart Failure in Patients with Kidney Disease

59. Schreiber BD: Congestive heart failure in patients with chronic kidney disease and on dialysis. Am J Med Sci 325:179, 2003.

60. McCullough PA, Duc P, OmLand T, et al: B-type natriuretic peptide and renal function in the diagnosis of heart failure: An analysis from the Breathing Not Properly Multinational Study. Am J Kidney Dis 41:571, 2003.

61. Al-Ahmad A, Rand WM, Manjunath G, et al: Reduced kidney function and anemia as risk factors for mortality in patients with left ventricular dysfunction. J Am Coll Cardiol 38:955, 2001.

62. Shlipak MG: Pharmacotherapy for heart failure in patients with renal insufficiency. Ann Intern Med 138:917, 2003.

63. Schoolwerth AC, Sica DA, Ballermann BJ, et al: Renal considerations in angiotensin converting enzyme inhibitor therapy: A statement for healthcare professionals from the Council on the Kidney in Cardiovascular Disease and the Council for High Blood Pressure Research of the American Heart Association. Circulation 104:1985, 2001.

64. Cice G, Ferrara L, D'Andrea A, et al: Carvedilol increases two-year survival in dialysis patients with dilated cardiomyopathy: A prospective, placebo-controlled trial. J Am Coll Cardiol 41:1438, 2003.

65. McCullough PA, Sandberg KR, Yee J, Hudson MP: Mortality benefit of angiotensin-converting enzyme inhibitors after cardiac events in patients with end-stage renal disease. J Renin Angiotensin Aldosterone Syst 3:188, 2002.

66. Smith GL, Vaccarino V, Kosiborod M, et al: Worsening renal function: What is a clinically meaningful change in creatinine during hospitalization with heart failure? J Card Fail 9:13, 2003.

67. Jain P, Massie BM, Gattis WA, et al: Current medical treatment for the exacerbation of chronic heart failure resulting in hospitalization. Am Heart J 145(Suppl):S3, 2003.

68. Keating GM, Goa KL: Nesiritide: A review of its use in acute decompensated heart failure. Drugs 63:47, 2003.

69. Butler J, Emerson C, Peacock WF, et al: The efficacy and safety of B-type natriuretic peptide (nesiritide) in patients with renal insufficiency and acutely decompensated congestive heart failure. Nephrol Dial Transplant 19:391, 2004.

70. Thorsgard M, Bart BA: Ultrafiltration for congestive heart failure. Congest Heart Fail 15:136, 2009.

Valvular Heart Disease and Arrhythmias in Patients with Kidney Disease

71. Umana E, Ahmed W, Alpert MA: Valvular and perivalvular abnormalities in end-stage renal disease. Am J Med Sci 325:237, 2003.

72. Manian FA: Vascular and cardiac infections in end-stage renal disease. Am J Med Sci 325:243, 2003.

73. Soman SS, Sandberg KR, Borzak S, et al: The independent association of renal dysfunction and arrhythmias in critically ill patients. Chest 122:669, 2002.

74. Wase A, Basit A, Nazir R, et al: Impact of chronic kidney disease upon survival among implantable cardioverter-defibrillator recipients. J Interv Card Electrophysiol 11:199, 2004.

Consultative Approach to the Hemodialysis Patient

75. Centers for Disease Control and Prevention (CDC): Incidence of end-stage renal disease among persons with diabetes–United States, 1990-2002. MMWR Morb Mortal Wkly Rep 54:1097, 2005.

76. Reddan DN, Szczech LA, Tuttle RH, et al: Chronic kidney disease, mortality, and treatment strategies among patients with clinically significant coronary artery disease. J Am Soc Nephrol 14:2373, 2003.

77. Szczech LA, Reddan DN, Owen WF, et al: Differential survival following coronary revascularization procedures among patients with renal insufficiency. Kidney Int 60:292, 2001.

78. Agarwal R, Nissenson AR, Batlle D, et al: Prevalence, treatment, and control of hypertension in chronic hemodialysis patients in the United States. Am J 115:291, 2003.

79. Vlahakos DV, Hahalis G, Vassilakos P, et al: Relationship between left ventricular hypertrophy and plasma renin activity in chronic hemodialysis patients. J Am Soc Nephrol 8:1764, 1997.

80. Hampl H, Sternberg C, Berweck S, et al: Regression of left ventricular hypertrophy in hemodialysis patients is possible. Clin Nephrol 58(Suppl 1):S73, 2002.

81. Li PK, Chow KM, Wong TY, et al: Effects of an angiotensin-converting enzyme inhibitor on residual renal function in patients receiving peritoneal dialysis. A randomized, controlled study. Ann Intern Med 139:105, 2003.

82. McCullough PA: Opportunities for improvement in the cardiovascular care of patients with end-stage renal disease. Adv Chronic Kidney Dis 11:294, 2004.

83. Bakris GL: Role for beta-blockers in the management of diabetic kidney disease. Am J Hypertens 16(Pt 2):7S, 2003.

84. Cice G, Ferrara L, D'Andrea A, et al: Carvedilol increases two-year survival in dialysis patients with dilated cardiomyopathy: A prospective, placebo-controlled trial. J Am Coll Cardiol 41:1438, 2003.

85. McCullough PA, Sandberg KR, Borzak S, et al: Benefits of aspirin and beta-blockade after myocardial infarction in patients with chronic kidney disease. Am Heart J 144:226, 2002.

86. Porter GA, Norton TL, Lindsley J, et al: Relationship between elevated serum troponin values in end-stage renal disease patients and abnormal isotopic cardiac scans following stress. Ren Fail 25:55, 2003.

87. Buemi M, Senatore M, Corica F, et al: Statins and progressive renal disease. Med Res Rev 22:76, 2002.

88. National Kidney Foundation: K/DOQI Clinical Practice Guidelines For Managing Dyslipidemias in Chronic Kidney Disease. Executive Summary. New York, National Kidney Foundation, 2003.

89. Grundy SM, Cleeman JI, Merz CN, et al: Implications of recent clinical trials for the National Cholesterol Education Program Adult Treatment Panel III guidelines. Circulation 110:227, 2004.

90. American Diabetes Association: Standards of medical care for patients with diabetes mellitus. Diabetes Care 26(Suppl 1):S33, 2003.

91. Biesenbach G, Zazgornik J: Influence of smoking on the survival rate of diabetic patients requiring hemodialysis. Diabetes Care 19:625, 1996.

92. Winchester JF: Therapeutic uses of aspirin in renal diseases. Am J Kidney Dis 28(Suppl 1):S20, 1996.

93. Keeley EC, McCullough PA: Coronary revascularization in patients with coronary artery disease and chronic kidney disease. Adv Chronic Kidney Dis 11:254, 2004.

94. Reddan DN, Szczech LA, Tuttle RH, et al: Chronic kidney disease, mortality, and treatment strategies among patients with clinically significant coronary artery disease. J Am Soc Nephrol 14:2373, 2003.

95. Keeley EC, Kadakia R, Soman S, et al: Analysis of long-term survival after revascularization in patients with chronic kidney disease presenting with acute coronary syndromes. Am J Cardiol 92:509, 2003.

96. Opsahl JA, Husebye DG, Helseth HK, et al: Coronary artery bypass surgery in patients on maintenance dialysis: Long-term survival. Am J Kidney Dis 12:271, 1988.

97. Mishkel GJ, Varghese JJ, Moore AL, et al: Short- and long-term clinical outcomes of coronary drug-eluting stent recipients presenting with chronic renal disease. J Invasive Cardiol 19:331, 2007.

CHAPTER 94 Cardiovascular Manifestations of Autonomic Disorders

Virend K. Somers*

Cardiovascular function is closely linked and responsive to numerous endogenous and exogenous factors. This interplay is mediated through rapid and often subtle neurohormonal changes. One of the most important mechanisms whereby rapid circulatory control is achieved is the autonomic nervous system, which modulates cardiac function through direct effects on the heart and vascular tone.

Overview of Neural Circulatory Control

The autonomic nervous system can be subdivided into sympathetic, parasympathetic, and enteric components. The principal cardiovascular influences are mediated through the sympathetic and parasympathetic systems. The interplay between these two systems and their relative balance help determine cardiovascular responses under a variety of conditions. These responses usually take the form of changes in blood pressure or heart rate. The physiology whereby blood pressure and heart rate react to autonomic modulation is important to understanding how disorders of the autonomic nervous system can affect cardiovascular function.[1]

Baroreceptors
Autonomic responses, capillary shift mechanisms, hormonal responses, and kidney and fluid balance mechanisms all interact to maintain blood pressure control. Of these, the autonomic nervous system offers the most rapid response system. Neural circulatory regulation occurs via increased contractility of the heart or vasoconstriction of the arterial or venous circulations in response to information received from baroreceptors. This afferent information is synthesized and integrated, and appropriate responses are generated, in the vasomotor center of the brain.

The reflexes by which blood pressure is maintained are collectively known as the baroreflex, which includes arterial baroreceptors (also known as the high pressure receptors) and cardiopulmonary receptors (the low pressure receptors). Under normal physiologic circumstances, sympathetic activity is inhibited and parasympathetic activity predominates.

ARTERIAL BARORECEPTORS. Arterial baroreceptors, which are the most sensitive, are located in the carotid sinuses, aortic arch, and at the origin of the right subclavian artery. The carotid sinus baroreceptors are innervated by the glossopharyngeal nerve (CN IX), and the aortic arch baroreceptors are innervated by the vagus nerve (CN X). Baroreceptors are stretch-dependent mechanoreceptors that sense changes in pressure, transmitting via afferents to the nucleus tractus solitarius (NTS) in the brainstem. When distended, the baroreceptors are activated and generate action potentials increasing in frequency in correlation to the amount of stretch. Thus, spike frequency is used as a surrogate measure of blood pressure at the level of the NTS, with higher frequency correlating with higher blood pressure.

The arterial baroreceptors are tonically active under normal circumstances at a mean arterial pressure (MAP) above 70 mm Hg, which is termed the *baroreceptor set point*. With MAPs below the set point, baroreceptors become essentially silent. However, the set point may vary with persistent blood pressure changes, such as in chronic hypertension, in which the set point is increased, or in chronic hypotension, in which it is decreased (see Chap. 45). The set point may vary, depending on other endogenous factors and disease states.

Integration of baroreceptor afferent signals is achieved at the level of the NTS. The NTS sends inhibitory fibers to the vasomotor center, which regulates the sympathetic nervous system, and excitatory fibers to vagal nuclei that regulate the parasympathetic system. Activation of the NTS (associated with increased action potential frequency from arterial baroreceptors) stimulates parasympathetic outflow while an inactive nucleus induces sympathetic activation and parasympathetic inhibition. Sympathetic activation leads to increased cardiac contractility, increased heart rate, venoconstriction, and arterial vasoconstriction, ultimately leading to increased blood pressure via elevation of total peripheral resistance and cardiac output. Parasympathetic activation leads to a decrease in heart rate and a minor decrease in contractility, resulting in a decrease in blood pressure.

Coupling of sympathetic inhibition with parasympathetic activation allows the baroreflex to maximize blood pressure reduction. Conversely, sympathetic activation with parasympathetic inhibition allows for an increase in blood pressure.

Cardiopulmonary Baroreceptors
Although the arterial baroreceptors are the most sensitive receptors, low-pressure receptors in the heart and venae cavae termed *cardiopulmonary receptors* also play a role in blood pressure modulation. They primarily respond to changes in volume but also to chemical stimuli. They project via vagal afferents to the NTS and via spinal sympathetic afferents to the spinal cord. Stimulation results in vasodilation and inhibition of vasopressin release. Furthermore, a stretch stimulus depresses renal sympathetic nerve activity[2] and has been shown to play a role in modulating renin release, resulting in diuresis and natriuresis,[3] thus regulating whole-body fluid volume to maintain blood pressure homeostasis.[1]

*The author is grateful to Drs. Rose Marie Robertson, David Robertson, and Suraj Kapa for contributions to the prior editions of this chapter.

Heart Rate Modulation

Modulation of heart rate is another means whereby the autonomic nervous system maintains normal blood pressure and exerts control over the cardiovascular system. Increases in heart rate are achieved through increases in contractile frequency via sympathetic activation. This is in part mediated through the arterial baroreflex. The cardiopulmonary receptors have only limited direct influence on heart rate control.

Under normal circumstances, at rest, the intrinsic sinus nodal rate is 95 to 110 beats/min, but efferent parasympathetic input via the vagus nerve suppresses the sinus nodal rate to 60 to 70 beats/min. During rest, there is little sympathetic efferent input and a low concentration of catecholamines. This changes with any movement away from the resting state, as with physical exertion, when sympathetic activity increases and parasympathetic activity decreases. On termination of exertion, the recovery of resting heart rate is again largely governed by parasympathetic dominance.

Although cardiac automaticity is intrinsic to pacemaker activity (see Chap. 35), the autonomic nervous system plays a primary role under normal conditions in defining heart rate and rhythm. The parasympathetic influence is achieved via acetylcholine release from the vagus nerve, which increases conductance of potassium across the cell membrane. In addition, acetylcholine inhibits the hyperpolarization-activated pacemaker current. This effect is quickly dispersed because of the high acetylcholinesterase concentration around the sinus node. The sympathetic influence is achieved by release of epinephrine and norepinephrine, which causes cAMP-mediated phosphorylation of membrane proteins and a resultant increase in the inward calcium current, resulting in accelerated slow diastolic depolarization. Also, other endogenous factors, such as nitric oxide, influence channel function and further modulate autonomic control of heart rate.

Breathing and Chemoreflexes

The chemoreflexes are modulators of sympathetic activation and play an important role in cardiovascular autonomic tone. The chemoreceptors are most simply divided into their central and peripheral components. The peripheral chemoreceptors are located in the carotid bodies and respond to hypoxemia, whereas the central chemoreceptors are in the brainstem and respond mostly to hypercapnia. Hypoxemia or hypercapnia results in hyperventilation and vascular sympathetic activation. Inhibitory influences on the chemoreflex drive are seen with stretch of the pulmonary afferents and with activation of the baroreflex, both of which have a greater influence on peripheral rather than central chemoreflexes.[4,5]

In numerous clinical conditions there is a substantial role of the chemoreflexes in the modulation of neural circulatory control. One is sleep apnea (see Chap. 79), in which the sympathetic vasoconstrictor response to hypoxia is potentiated because of elimination of the inhibitory influence on the chemoreflexes by stretch of the pulmonary afferents.[5] Another is hypertension, in which the ventilatory response to hypoxemia is increased and there is also an increase in sympathetic tone. This may be caused in part by impaired baroreflex sensitivity in hypertensive patients, but also by an increased chemoreflex drive. The tornic chemoreflex drive in obstructive sleep apnea patients can be reversed by the use of 100% oxygen, with which reductions in heart rate, blood pressure, and sympathetic outflow are seen. Administering 100% oxygen to patients with borderline hypertension and to spontaneously hypertensive rats also reduces not only ventilation but vasoconstrictor tone.

DIVING REFLEX. Under circumstances of prolonged apnea, a unique state of simultaneous increased parasympathetic drive to the heart and increased sympathetic drive to the vasculature occurs (**Fig. 94-1**). This is seen in diving mammals and sometimes in humans during prolonged submersion in water. In response to hypoxia, the body usually seeks to increase ventilation and blood flow to end-organs to maintain tissue oxygenation. However, in response to prolonged hypoxia in the absence of breathing, the body no longer experiences replenishment of oxygen stores and the normal homeostatic mechanisms alter so as to maintain oxygen delivery to organs vital to life—the brain and heart. This is achieved by decreasing oxygen delivery to much of the rest of the body via increased sympathetic vasoconstriction. This increased sympathetic outflow, however, does not constrict the cerebral vasculature because cerebral vascular tone is under autoregulatory control. Furthermore, myocardial oxygen demand is decreased because of bradycardia caused by an increase in parasympathetic tone. Thus, it is possible for individuals under exceptional circumstances to survive for prolonged periods of up to 5 minutes or more under anoxic conditions.

Autonomic Testing

Testing of autonomic function may occur at the bedside or via sophisticated instrumentation and long-term studies. Experimental evidence for an association between lethal arrhythmias and increased sympathetic or reduced vagal activity has spurred development of several quantitative markers of autonomic activity. Generally, the two easiest and most economical means of studying the interplay between autonomic and cardiac function are via orthostatics and the Valsalva maneuver, although both are nonspecific. When a patient presents with syncope, a cost-effective means of exploring a neurocardiogenic cause is with a tilt-table test (see Chaps. 36 and 42). Furthermore, studies of baroreflex sensitivity, heart rate variability, heart rate recovery, and chemoreflexes have been shown to help in direct assessment of autonomic dysfunction. Finally, blood levels of norepinephrine and its metabolites may assist in discriminating between different types of dysautonomias.

Orthostatics

Orthostatic hypotension is defined as a decrease of more than 20 mm Hg in systolic pressure or a decrease of more than 10 mm Hg in diastolic pressure

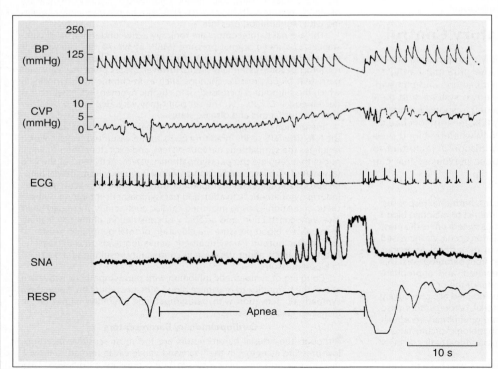

FIGURE 94-1 Components of the diving reflex. Shown are recordings of intra-arterial BP, central venous pressure (CVP), electrocardiogram (ECG), sympathetic nerve activity (SNA), and respiration (RESP) during apnea lasting 30 seconds. SNA is reflected by frequency and amplitude of bursts. Toward the end of the apneic period increases in BP, CVP, and SNA are noted, in addition to progressive bradycardia with eventual complete heart block. Furthermore, O_2 saturation fell to 92%. With release of apnea, electrocardiographic and SNA changes resolve, with some temporarily continued elevation in BP. (*From Somers VK, Dyken ME, Mark AL, Abboud FM: Parasympathetic hyperresponsiveness and bradyarrhythmias during apnoea in hypertension. Clin Auton Res 2:171, 1992.*)

after rising to a standing position from a supine position. Blood pressure and heart rate measurement should be done once symptoms develop or after 3 minutes have passed after rising to the standing position. If the patient is unable to stand, then orthostatics may be done after the patient has risen to a sitting position, with the feet dangling over the edge of the bed. Orthostatic hypotension is an inability of the cardiopulmonary system to maintain sufficient blood pressure and adequate cerebral perfusion against gravity. Generally, on rising from a supine position, an average person may lose about 700 mL of blood from the thorax. This results in decreased stroke volume, as well as a decreased systolic pressure and increased diastolic pressure. Compensation occurs via an increase in heart rate and slight peripheral vasoconstriction. Individuals intolerant of orthostasis may get venous pooling secondary to decreased muscle and vascular tone and develop a decreased circulating blood volume in response to standing. When testing orthostatics, it is important to note that a significant decrease in blood pressure without a corresponding rise in heart rate suggests abnormal autonomic innervation to the heart and may represent an underlying neuropathy, chronotropic incompetence or drug therapy, such as beta blockade, that blunts the heart rate response.

Valsalva Maneuver

The Valsalva maneuver becomes useful for testing patients at the bedside when done in conjunction with continuous electrocardiographic monitoring. During monitoring, the patient will blow continuously into a closed system for 12 seconds at 40 mm Hg and the fastest heart rate during the maneuver is divided by the slowest heart rate immediately afterward. A quotient of less than 1.4 is suggestive of autonomic impairment. However, this is nonspecific. For example, patients with congestive heart failure are less able to restrict blood return to the right atrium and do not exhibit the typical hemodynamic response.[1] Recovery of BP after the Valsalva may provide a useful measure of adrenergic vasoconstrictor reserve (see later).

Other Tests of Autonomic Function

BAROREFLEX SENSITIVITY. Baroreflex sensitivity is a measure of parasympathetic input to the sinus node. Testing baroreflex control of heart rate involves measuring the reflex increase in R-R interval in response to an increase in blood pressure. The increase in blood pressure has historically been achieved by the use of an alpha-adrenergic agonist, most often phenylephrine. Intravenous injection of a bolus of phenylephrine induces a 20- to 30-mm Hg increase in systolic pressure. Generally, a linear relationship exists between the increase in the R-R interval and increase in systolic pressure. The slope is used to quantify the sensitivity of the arterial baroreflex; it is typically steep in healthy individuals but decreases with advancing age and flattens even more with severe cardiovascular disease, such as hypertension or heart failure.

As a measure of autonomic function, baroreflex sensitivity decreases (i.e., shows a flatter slope) with sympathetic dominance and increases (i.e., shows a steeper slope) with parasympathetic dominance. In the search for noninvasive ways to measure baroreflex sensitivity, various devices and maneuvers have been used. The FINAPRES (from finger arterial pressure) device is one such example and has been used in the Autonomic Tone and Reflexes After Myocardial Infarction (ATRAMI) study. Spontaneous increases and decreases in blood pressure, as well as associated RR changes, have been used to determine the spontaneous baroreflex. Furthermore, spectral techniques used to analyze the relationship between beat to beat oscillations of blood pressure (BP) and R-R intervals are being studied as possible alternatives to the more invasive method of phenylephrine infusion.

Generally, autonomic testing evaluates the baroreflex by measuring heart rate changes in response to increases and decreases in BP. However, the baroreflex regulates BP by changing not only heart rate (vagal component) but also peripheral resistance (adrenergic component). A potentially useful nuance in baroreflex testing has been the differentiation between adrenergic and vagal baroreflex sensitivity.[6] Adrenergic baroreflex sensitivity relates the BP recovery time to the preceding BP decrease induced by the Valsalva maneuver, in a sense measuring the sympathetic

vasoconstrictor response to hypotension. This may provide a helpful index for evaluating and following patients with adrenergic failure.

CHEMOREFLEXES. Studies of chemoreflex function are one way of determining the dominant respiratory response, as well as the breathing–heart rate–blood pressure interactions, in certain diseases. As noted, the hypercapnic response is mediated mainly by central chemoreceptors, whereas the hypoxemic response is mediated by peripheral chemoreceptors.

HEART RATE VARIABILITY. Heart rate variability has become a commonly used but difficult to interpret means of studying the interplay between the autonomic nervous system and cardiovascular function. The phenomenon being measured in heart rate variability is that of the oscillation in the interval between consecutive heartbeats, as well as the variance of heart rates. Thus, heart rate variability studies the oscillation of heart rate and R-R intervals.

The actual measurement of heart rate variability has been achieved via multiple different modalities, most notably using time domain and frequency domain methods. It is usually calculated by analyzing the time series of beat to beat intervals from electrocardiographic or arterial pressure tracings. A simple example of time domain measurement of heart rate variability is calculation of the standard deviation of beat to beat intervals. The time domain graph of a value shows how the signal varies over time. The frequency domain graph, however, shows how much of a signal lies within given frequency bands over a range of frequencies. It involves the use of mathematical transforms, such as the Fourier transform, to decompose a function into an infinite or finite number of frequencies. Spectral density analysis is the most common frequency domain method used and involves measurement of how the power of a signal or time series is distributed at any particular frequency.

A common frequency domain method involves application of the discrete Fourier transform to the beat to beat interval time series. The frequency bands of most interest in humans are the high-frequency (HF) band, low-frequency (LF) band, very low frequency (VLF) band, and the ultralow-frequency (ULF) band, each of which has its own physiologic correlate. The HF band lies between 0.15 and 0.4 Hz and is driven by respiration, appearing to derive mainly from vagal activity. The LF band, which lies between 0.04 and 0.15 Hz, appears to derive from vagal and sympathetic activity and is believed to reflect delay in the baroreceptor loop. The VLF band lies between 0.0033 and 0.04 Hz and has been attributed to physical activity. Finally, the ULF band lies between 0 and 0.0033 Hz and is associated with day-night variation.

Other means of calculating heart rate variability include phase domain measurement and other nonlinear dynamic methods. The information provided by each measuring method, however, is complementary and ought to be taken together to define and understand the characteristics of heart rate variability in a given disorder.

The usefulness of heart rate variability as a measure of autonomic function and as a predictor of mortality has been suggested by a number of studies. In the 1970s, Wolf and colleagues showed a higher risk of postinfarction mortality with reduced heart rate variability, and Ewing and associates developed simple bedside tests to use short-term R-R differences as a means of detecting autonomic neuropathy in diabetics. In the late 1980s, heart rate variability was shown to be an independent predictor of post–myocardial infarction mortality. More recently, altered heart rate variability has been associated with other pathologic conditions such as hypertension, hemorrhagic shock,[7] and septic shock.[8] Heart rate variability has been accepted via international consensus as an independent predictor of mortality after myocardial infarction and as an early warning sign for diabetic neuropathy.

Heart rate turbulence, thought to be a reflection of baroreflex sensitivity, may also provide prognostically useful information. Abnormal heart rate turbulence has been linked to total mortality and sudden death in patients after myocardial infarction and patients with heart failure.[9]

HEART RATE RECOVERY. During exercise, heart rate rises, initially secondary to a reduction in vagal tone and then because of increased sympathetic activity. After exercise, parasympathetic reactivation and reduced sympathetic activity contribute to the recovery of resting heart rate. The rate at which the heart rate returns to baseline, measured over the first minute after exercise, is termed the *heart rate recovery*. A delayed heart rate recovery is a marker of decreased vagal activity, which has been shown to be an independent risk factor for sudden cardiac death.[10]

TILT-TABLE TESTING. Tilt-table testing is often conducted in patients presenting with a history of syncope to diagnose possible dysautonomic causes of syncope (see Chap. 42). The test is considered positive if the patient experiences symptoms associated with a blood pressure drop or an arrhythmia. These abnormalities are suggestive of dysfunction of the autonomic system. Normally, blood pressure will compensate via an increase in heart rate and constriction of blood vessels in the legs. In some patients, fainting or syncope could be associated with a precipitous drop in blood pressure (vasodepressor syncope) or pulse rate (cardioinhibitory syncope), or a mixed response, thus requiring continuous monitoring of both.

ORTHOSTATIC HYPOTENSION. Orthostatic hypotension (not the same as orthostatic intolerance; see later) is secondary to neurogenic and non-neurogenic conditions.[11] Neurogenic causes are addressed later (see Autonomic Dysregulation). Non-neurogenic causes include hypovolemia, cardiac dysfunction, and medications (including those used to treat hypertension, myocardial ischemia, depression, psychosis, and Alzheimer and Parkinson disease). It is especially prevalent in older adults, in whom the consequences of the predisposing factors noted can be magnified. Orthostatic hypotension and tachycardia may also occur after prolonged bed rest or after exposure to microgravity, such as in space flight. In some patients, orthostatic hypotension may be accompanied by fatigue, cognitive dysfunction, and emotional difficulties, as well as by gait abnormalities and falls.[12,13] Symptoms can be debilitating and confine patients to bed; the consequent physical deconditioning may worsen the overall problem. Longitudinal studies have suggested that orthostatic hypotension can increase the risk of stroke, myocardial ischemia, and mortality. The therapeutic goal is to attenuate or eliminate symptoms, rather than restore normotension. Pharmacologic therapy is often suboptimal and should be combined with interventions such as compression of venous capacitance beds, use of physical countermaneuvers, and intermittent water bolus treatment. Treatment can be difficult and development of supine hypertension should be minimized, especially in patients with diabetes, heart failure, or cardiac ischemia.

Autonomic Dysregulation

Dysautonomias refer to any dysfunction of the autonomic nervous system, whether central, peripheral, or secondary to other disease processes. In general, the most common dysautonomias are those affecting the sympathetic system. However, the parasympathetic system and conditions of increased parasympathetic tone, such as during sleep or with endurance training, are also important to understand because they can have significant implications for cardiovascular health.

The sympathetic dysautonomias are the most common and may be characterized by disorders of release, function, or reuptake of the main sympathetic chemical messenger, norepinephrine. Furthermore, local blood flow and clearance of norepinephrine from the circulation can manifest as a dysautonomia. The sympathetic dysautonomias can be generally divided into two groups—those associated with decreased function, in which orthostasis often occurs, and those associated with increased outflow, in which hypertension and/or tachycardia may be present.

Primary Chronic Autonomic Failure

Orthostatic intolerance is a key manifestation of neurocirculatory failure. It often serves as the presenting symptom. However, not all orthostatic hypotension is symptomatic of neurocirculatory failure. Most cases of orthostatic hypotension result from blood loss, volume depletion, or a prolonged bedridden state. Only rarely does it result from true autonomic failure.

Chronic autonomic failure is distinguishable from acute-onset autonomic dysfunction syndromes by its progressive nature and prognosis. Generally, chronic autonomic failure can be subdivided into secondary and primary failure, with secondary failure being far more common. In cases of secondary failure, the cause is usually clear and treatment involves therapy for the underlying disorder. However, when autonomic failure dominates the clinical presentation and a clear cause is not apparent, this is termed *primary chronic autonomic failure.*[1]

Primary autonomic failure may be subdivided into three major syndromes—pure autonomic failure, multisystem atrophy, and Parkinson disease. Major overlap among these three syndromes exists, and treatment differs between them.

PURE AUTONOMIC FAILURE. Pure autonomic failure involves orthostatic hypotension in the absence of symptoms or signs of central neurodegeneration. Thus, the dysfunction occurs at the level of peripheral neurons and not in the central nervous system. The functional error lies in available levels of norepinephrine, which are low when supine and rise minimally with standing.[1] Orthostatic hypotension and an inadequate chronotropic response to standing and the Valsalva maneuver are therefore evident. No direct effect on longevity occurs in these patients.

MULTISYSTEM ATROPHY. Multisystem atrophy includes autonomic failure with signs and symptoms of progressive central neurodegeneration. It is generally divided into Parkinsonian, cerebellar, and mixed forms. Patients develop symptoms in the sixth or seventh decade of life, exhibiting sympathetic and parasympathetic dysfunction.[1] In addition to orthostatic hypotension, findings may include impotence, loss of sweating, abnormal pupillary responses, reduced intraocular pressure, sleep apnea, and urinary incontinence. In some patients, orthostatic angina, which is actually exacerbated by the use of nitroglycerin, may occur. The angina appears to be caused by severe orthostatic hypotension and resultant inadequate coronary perfusion. Furthermore, urine production is greater in these patients during the night, leaving patients more hypovolemic in the morning and exaggerating symptoms further.

Orthostatic changes in this disease may be striking, with as much as a 100-mm Hg fall in systolic pressure on standing and a minimal rise in heart rate. Because of the progressive nature and the chronicity, patients may tolerate this precipitous drop in blood pressure relatively well. Patients often exhibit hypertension when supine, suggesting an inappropriate level of circulating catecholamines. In fact, plasma levels of catecholamines and their metabolites are preserved but not appropriately elevated on standing.

Lifespan in multisystem atrophy is diminished, and patients live on average 9 years from diagnosis. Movement abnormalities are centrally mediated and do not often respond to pharmacologic intervention. Furthermore, respiratory compromise can occur progressively, with development of nocturnal stridor that may require continuous positive airway pressure.[1]

PARKINSON DISEASE WITH AUTONOMIC FAILURE. This entity is similar in clinical appearance to multisystem atrophy with parkinsonian features. The most common cause is diffuse disease of autonomic centers in the brain, resulting in autonomic dysfunction similar to that described earlier, affecting organs diffusely.

DIAGNOSIS AND THERAPY. Distinguishing pure autonomic failure from multisystem atrophy and from Parkinson disease with autonomic failure tends to be easier than distinguishing between the latter two. Magnetic resonance imaging (MRI) of the brain in pure autonomic failure will not reveal any central nervous system abnormalities, whereas in the other two it will demonstrate central lesions. Differentiating between multisystem atrophy and Parkinson disease is important, because the prognosis in multisystem atrophy is much worse. It has been suggested that levodopa-carbidopa can be used to distinguish patients with Parkinson disease, but this drug can worsen orthostatic hypotension and there have been reports of patients diagnosed with multisystem atrophy showing some improvement with therapy.

Neuroimaging techniques have been used to distinguish the three types of autonomic failure. Cardiac sympathetic nerves take up ^{123}I-metaiodobenzylguanidine (^{123}I-MIBG) and 6-(^{18}F) fluorodopamine, postganglionic adrenergic markers that radiolabel vesicles in the sympathetic nerve terminals, thus allowing for visualization of cardiac innervation. In patients with multisystem atrophy, normal uptake and hence intact cardiac sympathetic innervation are noted. However, patients with Parkinson disease or pure autonomic failure show no detectable activity in the myocardium on emission scans, consistent with loss of sympathetic innervation of the heart. Thus, even though Parkinson disease with autonomic failure may demonstrate central lesions, there is a suggestion of an additional postganglionic lesion in these patients, which is distinct from the isolated preganglionic lesion of multisystem atrophy (MSA).

The recently updated consensus statement for the diagnosis of MSA reflects the advances and challenges in this field.[14] Preliminary results of an ongoing prospective study comparing patients with MSA to those with Parkinson disease have shown that autonomic defects are more strikingly abnormal in MSA versus those in Parkinson disease.[15] These differences were sustained and greater at 1-year follow-up, suggesting a more rapid progression of dysautonomia in multisystem atrophy than in Parkinson disease. These findings further support the concept that the primary lesion in multisystem atrophy is preganglionic and in Parkinson disease is ganglionic and postganglionic.

Therapy depends on changes in lifestyle in addition to pharmacologic therapy. Ingestion of carbohydrates can lower blood pressure, and a meal before bedtime may be helpful in reducing nighttime supine hypertension. This depressor effect can be difficult for patients after meals during the day, so caffeine ingestion or use of somatostatin in the case of severe blood pressure decreases can be used to attenuate the hemodynamic response to food. Furthermore, water intake can help increase blood pressure. Physical maneuvers that cause compression of the lower extremities have also been noted to help patients symptomatically.[1]

Pharmacologically, the two main areas of intervention include volume expansion and pressor administration. Use of fludrocortisone and adding sodium to the diet can help with volume expansion. The use of pressor agents should be considered in the context of the postganglionic or preganglionic nature of the different diseases. In patients with sympathetic cardiac denervation (i.e., pure autonomic failure or Parkinson disease with autonomic failure), midorine (an alpha-adrenoreceptor agonist) or L-threo-3,4-dihydroxyphenylserine (a norepinephrine precursor converted by parenchymal cells) may be useful. However, patients with MSA in whom sympathetic innervation is intact may benefit from use of a sympathomimetic amine or alpha$_2$-adrenoreceptor blocker. Also, ma-huang or yohimbine may be useful because it induces release of norepinephrine from the sympathetic nerve terminal, but could cause acute hypertension if used improperly.[1]

Secondary Autonomic Failure

More commonly, autonomic failure occurs in the context of some other disease process and treatment of the underlying process may or may not relieve the autonomic dysfunction. The most common cause of secondary autonomic failure is diabetes (see Chap. 64). Diabetic neuropathy is a well-known, long-term complication and all nerves may be affected, both somatic and autonomic. Cardiovascular complications secondary to dysfunction of autonomic control have been described in patients with and without orthostatic hypotension. Heart rate variability and baroreflex testing[16] may help in the detection of diabetic autonomic neuropathy. Nerve conduction abnormalities may not be the only component of autonomic dysfunction in diabetes. Relationships between vascular stiffness and dysfunction of the baroreflex have also been noted. Furthermore, some studies have suggested that the primary dysfunction may be in defective activation of central parasympathetic pathways. Thus, there appear to be afferent and efferent, as well as sympathetic and parasympathetic, components to the autonomic dysregulation associated with diabetes.

Glucose and blood pressure control may protect against neuropathic and microvascular complications and improve autonomic function. A recent study has evaluated the effects of prior intensive versus conventional insulin therapy on the prevalence of cardiac autonomic neuropathy in former subjects of the Diabetic Control and Complications Trial (DCCT).[17] DCCT autonomic measures (R-R variation with paced breathing, Valsalva ratio, postural blood pressure changes, and autonomic symptoms) were repeated in 1226 subjects,

studied 13 to 14 years after the end of the DCCT. Although the prevalence of cardiac autonomic neuropathy was higher in both groups after 13 to 14 years, the incidence was much lower (odds ratio [OR], 0.69; 95% confidence interval [CI], 0.51 to 0.96) in the former intensive group versus the conventional group, suggesting that the benefits of intensive insulin therapy in reducing risk of autonomic neuropathy may be sustained for many years.[17]

Amyloidosis can also result in secondary autonomic failure[18] (see Chap. 68). A recent retrospective study of 65 patients who had biopsy-proven amyloidosis and also had autonomic function testing suggested that patients with peripheral neuropathy of unknown origin should undergo autonomic testing, even in the absence of symptoms of autonomic failure.[19] Early recognition of autonomic failure in those patients may lead to earlier diagnosis of underlying amyloidosis, and hence earlier treatment.

Other common causes of secondary autonomic failure include renal failure[20] (see Chap. 93), paraneoplastic syndromes, and vitamin B$_{12}$ deficiency. If antibodies against components of the autonomic nervous system are present in the absence of clinically apparent neoplasm, further assessment for neoplasm should be made, given that clinical improvement can be achieved following treatment.[21] HIV infection can cause autonomic dysfunction independent of effects on cardiac function (see Chap. 72), as can heavy metal intoxication, particularly with copper, lead, mercury, or thallium.

AUTOIMMUNE AUTONOMIC FAILURE. Severe autonomic failure can result from autoimmune damage to neurons. Disease progression is variable and ranges from days to years. Because of the variable time of presentation, it may be difficult to separate autoimmune autonomic failure from other types of autonomic dysfunction. In addition to orthostatic hypotension, bowel and bladder dysfunction may occur. Plasma catecholamine levels are usually low and rise minimally with standing. Some reports have shown the beneficial effect of intravenous gamma globulin in treatment. One case report has also suggested a role for plasma exchange pheresis in treatment.[22]

In addition to autoimmune autonomic failure, autonomic dysfunction may be seen as a complication in severe cases of Guillain-Barré syndrome. In these patients, treatment is often supportive and orthostatic intolerance may be the only symptom. Furthermore, autonomic function may completely return with general motor function. Orthostatic intolerance may also occur as a sequela of prolonged bed rest in these patients.[1]

CONGENITAL AUTONOMIC FAILURE. The first autonomic disorder associated with a defined genetic abnormality was dopamine beta-hydroxylase deficiency. Dopamine beta-hydroxylase converts dopamine to norepinephrine in vesicles in noradrenergic neurons. Thus, this is a disorder of sympathetic noradrenergic function. As a result of the norepinephrine deficiency, patients cannot mount a vasoconstrictor response to upright posture and have marked orthostatic hypotension with a blunted rise in heart rate.[1] Also, they have excess quantities of dopamine, which is released in place of norepinephrine, resulting in increased urinary sodium excretion, ptosis, nasal stuffiness, joint hyperextensibility, and retrograde ejaculation in men. Dihydroxyphenylserine has been used with some benefit to restore norepinephrine levels because these patients have normal levels of dopa decarboxylase.[23]

Orthostatic Intolerance

Orthostatic intolerance (see Chap. 42) is an entity distinct from orthostatic hypotension and is only occasionally characterized by the rapid development of orthostatic hypotension. Generally, symptoms are seen in young women who report visual changes, poor concentration while standing, fatigue while standing, tremor, and often syncope. Several diseases are associated with orthostatic intolerance. These range from problems of localized excess noradrenergic stimulation to abnormalities of the baroreflex response. However, there is considerable overlap in terms of diagnosis, especially among postural

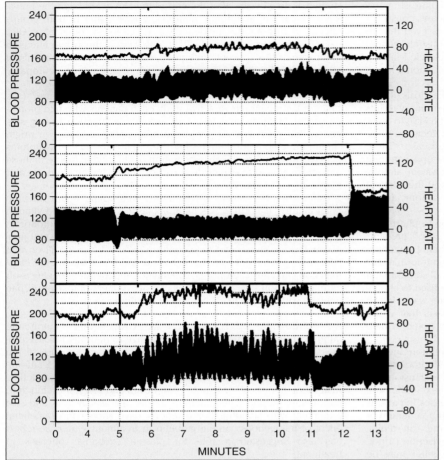

FIGURE 94-2 Examples of BP and heart rate recordings from a normal subject **(top panel),** a patient with neuropathic POTS **(middle panel),** and a patient with hyperadrenergic POTS **(bottom panel).** Note the modest reduction in BP in neuropathic POTS. Hyperadrenergic POTS is associated with prominent BP oscillations, an orthostatic increment in systolic BP, and a prominent norepinephrine response to head-up tilt. *(From Low PA, Sandroni P, Joyner M, Shen W-K: Postural tachycardia syndrome. J Cardiovasc Electrophysiol 20:352, 2009.)*

tachycardia syndrome, neurally mediated syncope, and chronic fatigue syndrome, which often coexist in patients presenting with orthostatic intolerance.

Postural Tachycardia Syndrome

Postural orthostatic tachycardia syndrome (POTS) presents primarily with orthostatic symptoms, tachycardia, and the absence of significant hypotension.[24] Symptoms of orthostatic intolerance include those elicited by brain hypoperfusion and by sympathetic excitation.[25] POTS affects females in a 5:1 ratio over males, and most patients are between 20 to 40 years of age. POTS is heterogenous in mechanisms, as well as in presentation. Major mechanisms are denervation (neuropathic POTS), deconditioning, and a hyperadrenergic state **(Fig. 94-2).** Each of these three major mechanisms is exacerbated by hypovolemia.

Diagnostic criteria for postural orthostatic tachycardia syndrome are controversial and may be based on several criteria, including the following:

- Orthostatic tachycardia greater than 30 beats/min, usually to 120 beats/min or higher
- Transient systolic blood pressure decrease of more than 20 mm Hg, with recovery within the first minute of tilt
- Standing plasma norepinephrine level higher than 600 pg/mL
- Severe orthostatic symptoms

Although patients with POTS often have increased anxiety and somatic hypervigilance, the excessive tachycardia during orthostatic stress is not secondary to anxiety, but is a physiologic response that helps maintain arterial pressure during venous pooling.[26] POTS patients also demonstrate excessive tachycardia during exercise. Recent data have suggested that the tachycardia during exercise in POTS is not secondary to abnormal baroreflex regulation of heart rate.[27] Treatment of POTS[25] includes increasing intravascular volume with high levels of salt and fluids, supplemented by compression garments. Pharmacologic interventions include low-dose beta blockers, and low dose vasoconstrictors such as midodrine and fludrocortisone. A recent, randomized, crossover acute drug trial has compared low-dose (20-mg) propranolol to placebo and found that propranolol reduces supine and standing heart rates and improves symptoms at 2 hours after dosing.[28] In a comparison between the low-dose and a higher (80-mg) dose propranolol, the higher dose had a great effect on attenuating standing heart rate and orthostatic tachycardia, but the lower dose elicited a greater improvement in symptoms at 2 hours after dosing. The therapeutic importance of exercise training and improved physical conditioning is becoming increasingly apparent as an important strategy for the deconditioned patient.

Neurally Mediated Syncope

Neurally mediated syncope, also known as *neurocardiogenic syncope,* is characterized by periodic syncopal episodes with normal autonomic function between episodes **(Fig. 94-3;** see Chap. 42). Patients frequently have vasovagal-like fainting and a reduction in vascular sympathetic activity during the syncopal episode. Several variants of neurally mediated syncope are discussed later in this chapter.

The mechanisms underlying neurally mediated syncope remain controversial but are presumed to be secondary to decreased venous return to the heart resulting from increased peripheral venous pooling of blood, which results in cardiac hypercontractility. One study has documented the complete disappearance of peroneal sympathetic nerve recordings during syncopal episodes in these patients. The hypercontractile response activates cardiac mechanoreceptors, resulting in a paradoxical reflex bradycardia and decreased systemic vascular resistance, despite the already decreased venous return, eliciting the characteristic presyncopal symptoms of weakness, light-headedness, feelings of warmth or cold, and ultimate brief loss of consciousness. This reflex bradycardia and hypotension are similar to those evoked by the Bezold-Jarisch reflex. In the absence of any underlying cardiovascular, neurologic, or other disease, isolated vasovagal syncope may represent a variation of normal; because spontaneous syncope may affect up to 50% of everyone, subjects are generally normotensive with otherwise normal blood pressure regulation,[29] and long-term prognosis is usually excellent,[30] aside from sequelae of any falls that may occur with a syncopal event.

Potential cardiac causes of syncope must be considered before this diagnosis of exclusion can be made. However, even then, diagnosis can be difficult. Situational syncope must be excluded, as well as phobia syndromes or other organic causes. Tilt-table testing has good specificity but uncertain sensitivity in diagnosis and is not always reproducible. Implantable loop recorders, which store 45 minutes of retrospective electrocardiographic data, may also be used and can be activated by patients after each syncopal event. However, the cost is high and the diagnostic benefit remains undefined.

Typically, treatment in these patients is conservative and involves education, particularly in determining potential predisposing factors and recognizing prodromal symptoms when they occur. Increasing fluid and salt intake may also help in avoiding the development of syncope. Pharmacologic therapy includes beta blockers, which presumably work via inhibition of mechanoreceptor activation; fludrocortisone, which expands central fluid volume via retention of sodium; and vasoconstrictors and selective serotonin reuptake inhibitors, which may have a role in regulating sympathetic nervous system activity. Although cardiac pacing addresses the bradycardia, it is incompletely effective because it does not compensate for the vasodepressor component.

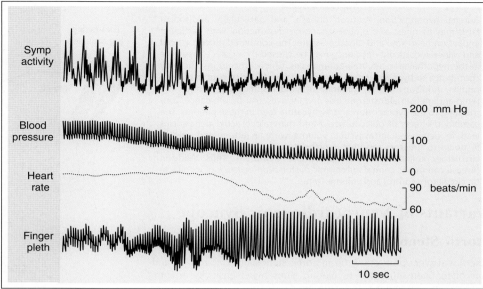

FIGURE 94-3 Recordings of sympathetic nerve activity and blood pressure before and during vasovagal syncope. Note the simultaneous reductions in sympathetic nerve activity, heart rate, and blood pressure associated with the episode of syncope (*). Pleth = plethysmography; symp = sympathetic. (*From Wallin BG, Sundlof G: Sympathetic outflow to muscles during vasovagal syncope. J Auton Nerv Syst 6:287, 1982.*)

Chronic Fatigue Syndrome

Chronic fatigue syndrome is characterized by new, unexplained fatigue that lasts for at least 6 months, is unrelieved by rest, and has no clear cause. The etiology of this syndrome is unclear. Some studies have suggested that dysautonomia may be common in patients with chronic fatigue syndrome. On the basis of tilt-table testing, more than 60% of patients with chronic fatigue show abnormal blood pressure or heart rate responses, with sudden hypotension or severe bradycardia or tachycardia, along with decreased consciousness. Syncopal episodes in these patients are usually associated with a decrease in sympathetic outflow in the absence of ventricular hypovolemia or hypercontractility.

Chronic fatigue patients have not been shown to benefit from treatment with fludrocortisone and high salt intake, unlike most patients suffering from orthostatic intolerance secondary to sympathetic neurocirculatory failure. Thus, the exact mechanism of orthostatic intolerance in these patients is unclear. Alternative treatments may include midorine or beta-adrenoreceptor blockers. Whether relief of any dysautonomic symptoms in these patients may relieve the symptoms of fatigue is unclear. Because these patients are often physically inactive, an exercise conditioning program implemented to improve well-being may help alleviate symptoms.

Baroreflex Failure

Causes of baroreflex failure most often include surgery, radiation therapy, and cerebrovascular accidents. Failure results from damage to afferent neuronal input (via the vagus and glossopharyngeal nerves) or from damage to brainstem nuclei or interneurons.[1] As a result, there is a loss of response to arterial baroreceptor stimulation.

These patients often present acutely with significant pheochromocytoma-like pressor crises associated with palpitations, diaphoresis, and severe headaches. Patients may present after surgical intervention, trauma, or stroke. Blood pressure is labile and may rise to extremely high levels. Some studies have shown that 9% to 30% of patients exhibit hypertension consistent with baroreflex failure after carotid endarterectomy.[1] Patients with unilateral involvement may show almost complete failure as well. The right carotid baroreflex may be more effective than the left carotid, suggesting a difference in clinical outcome depending on which carotid artery is affected.

The clinical presentation can vary over time, and acute episodes during waking hours may mimic a pheochromocytoma; severe hypotension and bradycardia may occur during sleep. Heart rate and blood pressure change together (concomitant rises or falls in both). Furthermore, there is little or no orthostatic hypotension initially, but it may appear later with prolonged standing. Apneic episodes may occur because of loss of neural afferents from carotid chemoreceptors.

Loss of the baroreflex buffering mechanism results in prolonged and exaggerated responses to a variety of tests, such as the cold pressor test. Plasma and urinary norepinephrine levels may be high, with plasma levels in the 1000- to 3000-pg/mL range. Minor stimuli can result in pressor crises, even after successful initial treatment in these patients, and long-term therapy may be necessary. Diagnostically, patients may show a depressor response to a small dose of clonidine but no heart rate response to depressor or pressor infusions, even though heart rate will change with sedation or cortical stimuli.[1]

Initial therapy over the first 72 hours can include nitroprusside and clonidine. Chronically, patients may continue to have labile hypertension and tachycardia alternating with hypotension and bradycardia. This may be effectively treated with clonidine and methyldopa. During periods of excess cortical stimulation (e.g., stress, anxiety), low-dose benzodiazepines and clonidine may help relieve symptoms.[1]

Carotid Sinus Hypersensitivity

Carotid sinus hypersensitivity is defined as a ventricular pause longer than 3 seconds and/or a fall in systolic BP of more than 50 mm Hg with carotid sinus massage.[30] Carotid sinus syndrome refers to the association of carotid sinus hypersensitivity with spontaneous syncope. Carotid sinus massage should be avoided in patients with prior transient ischemic attacks (TIAs), stroke within 3 months, or carotid bruits, unless Doppler studies exclude significant carotid artery disease. Cardiac pacing has been considered as a therapeutic option, although a recent randomized, double-blind, placebo-controlled crossover trial has shown no benefit of dual-chamber pacing[31] (see Chap. 38).

Norepinephrine Transporter Deficiency

In norepinephrine transporter deficiency, there is a deficiency of the membrane norepinephrine transporter. As a result, there is a more than 98% reduction in reuptake of norepinephrine at the sympathetic nerve ending. This results in elevated levels of norepinephrine at the synapse and resultant tachycardia, especially on standing, when norepinephrine delivery is increased, despite the already elevated synaptic concentration.

Addison Disease

Adrenal hypofunction, Addison disease, and particularly addisonian crisis may manifest as a global autonomic dysfunction, with particular impact on heart rate and blood pressure. The combined glucocorticoid and mineralocorticoid deficiency may be caused by a defect anywhere in the hypothalamic-pituitary-adrenal axis. Glucocorticoid insufficiency contributes to hypotension and may reduce myocardial contractility. In primary Addison disease, mineralocorticoid insufficiency disturbs the renin-angiotensin-aldosterone axis and intravascular fluid balance, contributing to the hypotension and tachycardia seen in these patients. The combined effects of glucocorticoid and mineralocorticoid deficiencies lead to decreased intravascular volume with an attenuated cardiac response to stressors, resulting in orthostatic hypotension and eventual circulatory collapse without appropriate treatment. Thus, Addison disease can mimic central autonomic dysfunction because of its effects on circulatory control and volume status.

Variants of Neurocardiogenic Syncope

Aortic Stenosis

Exertional syncope is common in aortic stenosis (see Chap. 66) and has often been attributed to carotid sinus hypersensitivity, arrhythmias, or left ventricular failure (**Fig. 94-4**). The normal compensatory response to exercise involves a rise in blood pressure and heart rate resulting from an increase in cardiac output, peripheral vasoconstriction in inactive muscles, and vasodilation in active muscles. The onset of near-syncope in patients with aortic stenosis has been associated with a large reduction in blood pressure and cardiac output to resting levels in the absence of appropriate reflex vasoconstriction. Patients with aortic stenosis and a history of exertional syncope develop paradoxical forearm vasodilation during leg exercise. This muscular vasodilation is presumed to be caused by activation of mechanosensitive vagal afferents in response to an outflow obstruction–associated increase in left ventricular end-diastolic pressure. The net effect of this process is a reflex vasodilation. However, the vasodilator response is not accompanied by bradycardia, suggesting that the syncopal response to exertion in aortic stenosis is primarily vasodepressor rather than cardioinhibitory in nature.

Renal Failure and Hemodialysis

Acute hypotension is a common complication of hemodialysis, although the precise cause is poorly defined (**Fig. 94-5**; see Chap. 93). Presumably, the mechanism may be similar to that in hypotension associated with acute hemorrhage, in which there is paradoxical sympathetic withdrawal, vasodilation, and bradycardia. This appears to result from activation of cardiac vagal afferents caused by tachycardia and decreased ventricular filling. Hypotension-prone hemodialysis patients have an initial tachycardia, sympathetic activation, and vasoconstriction, followed by profound hypotension caused by paradoxical bradycardia, vasodilation, and sympathetic inhibition. This is different from patients not prone to hypotension who exhibit progressive rises in heart rate and sympathetic activity during dialysis. Furthermore, there is a clear difference in cardiac adaptation to changes in fluid volume, with hypotension-prone patients exhibiting a progressive reduction to near-obliteration of left ventricular end-systolic dimensions, whereas there is little change in hypotension-resistant patients. This suggests that the mechanism whereby hypotension develops in hypotension-prone hemodialysis patients may be via excessive myocardial contraction around an empty chamber, resulting in activation of ventricular mechanoreceptors and consequent cardiac inhibition. The differential diagnosis of hypotension during dialysis should also include simple hypovolemia, pericardial effusion with development of tamponade as cardiac filling pressures decrease, and cardiac ischemia.

Right Coronary Thrombolysis

Patients with right coronary artery occlusion following intracoronary thrombolytic therapy and resultant reperfusion exhibit a greater inci-

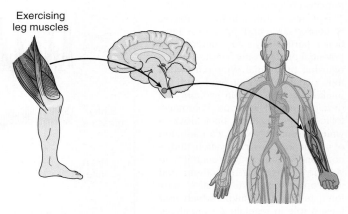

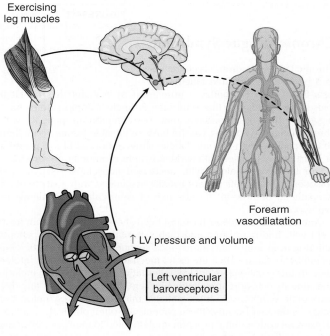

FIGURE 94-4 Syncope in severe aortic stenosis. The schematic shows how afferent impulses from exercising leg muscles relayed to the brainstem normally elicit reflex vasoconstriction in the nonexercising forearm. However, in patients with severe aortic stenosis, increased left ventricular pressure and volume during exercise inhibits and even reverses forearm vasoconstriction by inducing sympathetic withdrawal during exercise. This sympathetic withdrawal has the potential to result in exertional syncope. *(Modified from Mark AL: The Bezold-Jarisch reflex revisited: Clinical implications of inhibitory reflexes originating in the heart. J Am Coll Cardiol 1:90, 1983.)*

dence of bradycardia and hypotension (≈80%) than patients with left coronary occlusion (≈14%; see Chap. 58). This perceived difference may be caused in part by the preferential distribution of inhibitory cardiac receptors in the inferoposterior wall of the ventricle. Activation of the inhibitory reflex may be caused by sudden improvement in contractile force of the previously akinetic segment of myocardium, resulting in activation of mechanosensitive vagal afferents, or by the release of free radicals and other metabolic products, resulting in activation of chemosensitive vagal afferents.

Inferior Wall Myocardial Infarction

As noted, there is a preferential localization of inhibitory cardiac receptors in the inferoposterior wall of the left ventricle. With infarction, there would be an expected reflex tachycardia, and this is often the case in patients who suffer from an anterior wall infarction. However, patients suffering from an inferior wall infarction (see Chap. 55) may have a relatively increased incidence of bradycardia and hypotension. During Prinzmetal angina, spasm of vessels supplying the inferior wall more often results in bradycardia when compared with spasm of those vessels supplying the anterior wall, which more often results in tachycardia. This reflex activation of cardiac inhibitory signals also appears to result in inhibition of renal sympathetic activity, further potentiating neurogenic hypotension.

Reflex reduction in cardiac afterload and heart rate may be beneficial in the context of myocardial infarction caused by a decrease in myocardial oxygen demand. Thus, low-grade activation of the cardiac inhibitory reflex may conceivably contribute to the more favorable prognosis associated with inferior wall myocardial infarction.

Hypertrophic Obstructive Cardiomyopathy

Syncope in hypertrophic obstructive cardiomyopathy (HCM) is associated with a high risk of sudden death (see Chap. 69). In these patients, sudden death has generally been associated with a tendency to develop malignant arrhythmias. However, patients with HCM also demonstrate syncope during sinus rhythm and an abnormal blood pressure response to exercise, suggesting that activation of left ventricular baroreceptors may cause the associated hypotension and hemodynamic collapse. The predisposition to hypotension and bradycardia in these patients appears to result from activation of left ventricular mechanoreceptors. Studies with tilt-table testing in these patients resulted in hypotension in a significant number of patients with a prior history of syncope. Head-up tilt was paired with echocardiography, which revealed reduced cavity sizes and increased fractional shortening with head-up tilt, consistent with conditions that would be favorable to activation of left ventricular mechanoreceptors. This suggests that the cause of syncope in patients with HCM may not just be malignant arrhythmias but may also occur because of inappropriate activation of inhibitory left ventricular mechanoreceptors in response to vigorous ventricular contraction or reduced ventricular cavity size.

Blood Phobia

Many people suffer from blood or injury phobia and experience syncope or presyncope in response to these visual stimuli. Syncope in these patients has been thought to be largely neurogenic and anticipatory in origin because of the high correlation with situational stressors. It has been suggested that patients suffering from syncope secondary to blood or injury phobia actually have an underlying predisposition toward neurocardiogenic syncope. Patients with a history of blood phobia syncope have been shown to have a higher rate of tilt-induced syncope than controls. These findings suggest that fainting in response to blood or injury may be caused by dysfunction in neural circulatory control and has an associated organic origin. It has been proposed that this dysfunction may secondarily lead to the phobia because of repeated syncopal events.

Disorders of Increased Sympathetic Outflow

Increased sympathetic outflow may occur in a number of diseases, either as a primary event contributing to development of the disease or as secondary to the underlying disease. For example, many patients

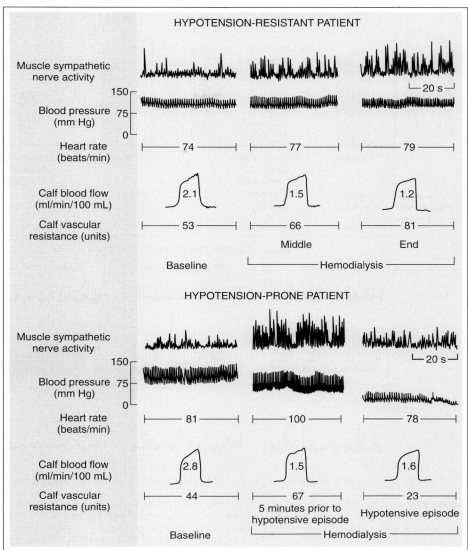

FIGURE 94-5 Mechanisms of hypotension during hemodialysis. **Top,** Measurements in a patient resistant to dialysis-induced hypotension. **Bottom,** Measurements in a patient prone to hypotension during dialysis. In a hypotension-resistant patient, hemodialysis induces a gradual increase in sympathetic activity and accompanying fall in calf blood flow and increased vascular resistance. This vasoconstriction works in concert with increased heart rate to maintain blood pressure. However, in a hypotension-prone patient, hemodialysis initially induces sympathetic activation that is qualitatively similar to that in the hypotension-resistant patient. However, further hemodialysis causes a marked fall in BP, with an associated reduction in sympathetic nerve activity, heart rate, and vascular resistance. This is likely caused by activation of ventricular mechanoreceptors because of volume depletion in the setting of tachycardia and increased contractility, resulting in a relative bradycardia and sympathetic inhibition with vasodilation and consequent profound hypotension. *(From Converse RL, Jacobsen TN, Jost CMT, et al: Paradoxical withdrawal of reflex vasoconstriction as a cause of hemodialysis-induced hypotension. J Clin Invest 90:1657, 1992.)*

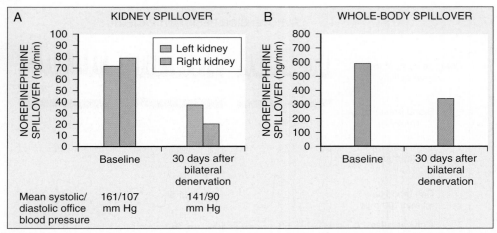

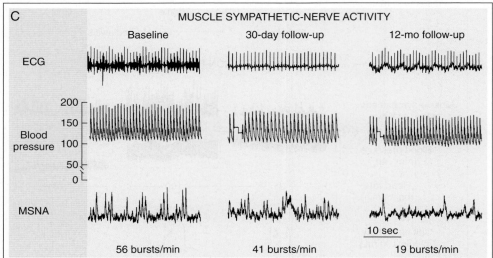

FIGURE 94-6 Norepinephrine renal and whole-body spillover and results of microneurography before and after renal nerve ablation. **A,** Results of bilateral renal denervation, as assessed by the radiotracer dilution method, at baseline and 30 days after the procedure. After ablation, decreases in renal norepinephrine spillover were observed in both kidneys (48% in the left kidney and 75% in the right kidney), indicating substantial modulation of renal sympathetic efferent-nerve activity after the procedure. Simultaneously, a marked reduction in whole-body sympathetic nerve activity was apparent, with a decrease in whole-body norepinephrine spillover of 42% **(B). C,** Reduction in muscle sympathetic nerve activity (MSNA), as assessed in the peroneal nerve on microneurography, after bilateral renal nerve ablation, which highlights the possibility that inhibition of afferent renal nerve activity may contribute to a reduction in central sympathetic drive. *(From Schlaich MP, Sobotka PA, Krum H, et al: Renal sympathetic-nerve ablation for uncontrolled hypertension. N Engl J Med 361:932, 2009.)*

nerve firing to skeletal muscle and elevated levels of norepinephrine in the heart and kidneys. High sympathetic outflow may be secondary to one or more of the following: impaired baroreflex gain, increased chemoreflex gain, insulin resistance, and/or genetic factors. Sympathetic activation stimulates the heart, elevating cardiac output, causing neurally mediated vasoconstriction, and augmenting renin secretion and tubular reabsorption of sodium, increasing total body fluid volume. In the long term, secondary end-organ and vascular changes may sustain established hypertension, even in the absence of overt sympathetic activation and tachycardia.

Recent studies have suggested that catheter-based radiofrequency ablation of renal nerves (efferent sympathetic and afferent sensory) bilaterally in patients with resistant hypertension may elicit significant and sustained (up to 12 months postprocedure) reductions in systolic and diastolic pressure.[34] In a recent case study, bilateral renal sympathetic nerve ablation was accompanied by marked falls in renal sympathetic activity, decrease of renin activity by 50%, reduced whole-body norepinephrine spillover, increased baroreflex gain, and decrease in BP.[35] At 12 months postprocedure, BP remained significantly lower, microneurography showed reduced sympathetic activity, and cardiac MRI showed a decrease in left ventricular mass (**Fig. 94-6**).

Panic Disorder

Cardiovascular events during a panic episode may be triggered by increased sympathetic outflow (see Chap. 91). Although the true risk is unknown, it seems that there may be some increased ischemic heart disease in patients with a history of panic disorder. During a panic attack, sympathetic nerve firing increases, as does adrenomedullary secretion of epinephrine. Patients who describe angina pectoris–like symptoms during a panic attack may or may not have electrocardiographic changes consistent with myocardial ischemia. It has been suggested that some patients may experience angina-like attacks secondary to coronary artery spasm.

Coronary Artery Disease

Sympathetic activity is increased in unstable angina and after a myocardial infarction[32] (see Chap. 54). The heightened sympathetic drive may persist for 6 to 9 months and may be implicated in subsequent cardiovascular morbidity and mortality.

Congestive Heart Failure

The failing heart becomes partly sympathetically denervated (**Fig. 94-7**; see Chap. 27). Thus, historically, adrenergic agonists were used to treat these patients, although this turned out to be more dangerous than helpful. In fact, beta blocker use in these patients contributed to long-term improvement rather than worsening of heart failure. The reason for this may be partially because although there is low myocardial tissue concentration of norepinephrine, cardiac norepinephrine spillover is increased to levels associated with near-maximal aerobic exercise. Heart failure patients may also exhibit baroreflex and chemoreflex dysfunction and disrupted heart rate variability and ventilatory control. In patients

with essential hypertension have chronic sympathetic activation, which may precede the development of sustained hypertension (see Chap. 40). Patients with panic disorder exhibit acute episodes that evoke sympathetic neuronal and adrenomedullary activation, with precipitation of coronary artery spasm. In heart failure patients, chronic elevation in sympathetic tone is noted, as is seen in patients with obstructive sleep apnea, in whom associated hypoxia and hypercapnia during nocturnal apneas may elicit further increases in sympathetic outflow.

Sympathetic activation increases with age, even in the absence of disease,[32] and can contribute to the age-related increased risk of hypertension.[33] Although women have lower muscle sympathetic activity than men, their age-related rise in sympathetic drive is greater, so the difference in sympathetic activation between men and women is attenuated by menopause.

Neurogenic Essential Hypertension

Patients with early essential hypertension (see Chap. 45) may have a hyperdynamic circulation driven by increased efferent sympathetic

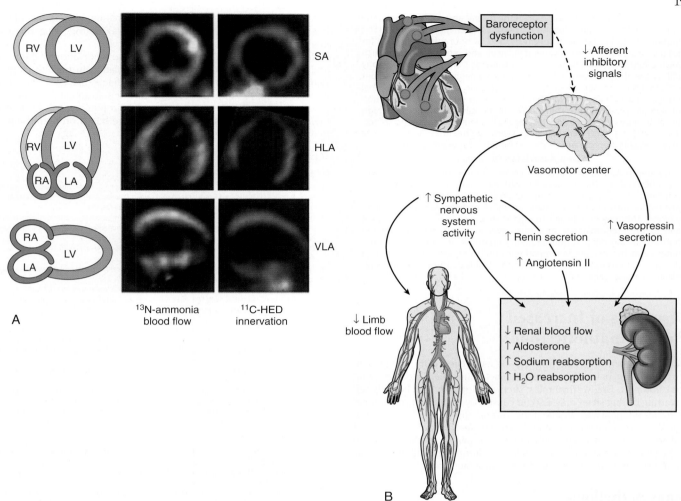

FIGURE 94-7 **A,** Autonomic denervation of the failing heart. Positron emission tomography images obtained from patients with congestive heart failure (CHF) demonstrate that there is partial denervation of the left ventricle in these patients. The images above demonstrate the short-axis (SA), horizontal long-axis (HLA), and vertical long-axis (VLA) views of the heart. Ammonia uptake is seen to be relatively homogeneous, which is consistent with intact myocardial perfusion. C-11 hydroxyephedrine (C-HED) uptake marks innervation of the heart and, in patients with heart failure, there is reduced retention that appears to be relatively heterogeneous, suggesting partial denervation of the left ventricle. A known association exists between the extent of denervation and clinical outcome, with higher degrees of denervation associated with increased mortality. Denervation of the heart may affect cardiac and vascular control secondary to defective afferent autonomic input from mechanoreceptors in the left ventricle. **B,** Increased sympathetic activity in CHF. Baroreceptor dysfunction may partly account for the increased sympathetic activity seen in patients with congestive heart failure. Baroreceptor function is impaired in heart failure, in part because of partial sympathetic denervation of the heart. Thus, inhibitory input from cardiac mechanoreceptors is decreased, despite increased intracardiac volumes. Typically, stimulation of these mechanoreceptors via increased stretch will result in vasodilation and depression of renal sympathetic nerve activity. However, because of partial denervation, there is a lack of appropriate inhibition of the sympathetic nervous system, leading to excess sympathetic activity to the kidney, worsening fluid retention, and to peripheral blood vessels, potentiating vasoconstriction. Therefore, partial denervation of cardiac mechanoreceptors may result in a neural circulatory profile mimicking that seen in hypovolemia and may, in part, explain the sympathetic activation and fluid retention seen in heart failure. (**A,** from Schwaiger M, Bengal F: Atlas of Heart Diseases: Nuclear Cardiology. In Dilsizian V, Narula J, Braunwald E [series eds]: Current Medicine LLC, Philadelphia, PA, 2006; **B,** modified from Nohria A, Cusco J, Creager M: Atlas of Heart Diseases: Heart Failure. In Colucci WS, Braunwald E [series eds]: Current Medicine LLC, Philadelphia, PA, 2004.)

with dilated cardiomyopathy, the presence of sleep apnea may further increase cardiac sympathetic activation,[36] perhaps because of heightened central chemosensitivity.[37] Increased cardiac sympathetic activation, altered baroreflex gain, chemoreflex dysfunction, blunted heart rate variability, and disordered breathing control have been associated with poorer long-term outcomes. It has been proposed that development of heart failure and increase in sympathetic outflow may occur in conjunction with and feed off one another to affect cardiac status further adversely. Although cardiac transplantation may improve some of the autonomic disturbances seen in heart failure, residual autonomic dysfunction may persist.

Obstructive Sleep Apnea

An increase in sympathetic outflow occurs during both sleep and waking hours in patients with obstructive sleep apnea (OSA; see Chap. 79). This is in part caused by the hypoxemia and hypercapnia during apneic episodes. During waking hours, the increased sympathetic outflow may be related to increased tonic chemoreflex sensitivity. Most OSA patients

are also obese, and the interaction between obesity and OSA in increasing sympathetic activity awaits further clarification. Continuous positive airway pressure treatment during sleep appears to attenuate sympathetic outflow, even during daytime wakefulness.

Pheochromocytoma

Pheochromocytoma is a rare catecholamine-secreting tumor derived from the chromaffin cells of the adrenal gland or the paraganglion chromaffin tissue of the sympathetic nervous system (see Chaps. 45 and 86). Most commonly, these tumors arise from the adrenal glands, but it is also possible to develop extra-adrenal pheochromocytomas in the sympathetic ganglia anywhere from the brain to the bladder. Because of the increased secretion of catecholamines, there is excess sympathetic drive, resulting in life-threatening hypertension or cardiac arrhythmias. The excess secretion is associated with lack of normal innervation to the adrenal medulla. The exact mechanism of secretion is not completely clear, although it may be caused by direct pressure or changes in tumor blood flow. Pheochromocytomas may also be sporadic or familial, with primarily norepinephrine secretion in the former and epinephrine in the latter. Diagnosis requires testing for plasma metanephrine, which has a higher sensitivity and lower specificity, and 24-hour urine collection for total catecholamines, vanillylmandelic acid, and metanephrines, which have a higher specificity and lower sensitivity. Computed tomography (CT) of the abdomen and pelvis is the typical imaging modality used but is neither the most sensitive nor the most specific, particularly for adrenal tumors smaller than 1 cm. MRI has almost 100% sensitivity for detection of adrenal pheochromocytomas. When the clinical suspicion is high because of positive laboratory test results but imaging reveals no source, a scan with ^{131}I-MIBG may be useful. Definitive treatment is via surgical resection with appropriate alpha and beta blockade preoperatively.

Sleep-Associated Disorders

In general, parasympathetic tone increases during non–rapid eye movement (REM) sleep. This is associated with a fall in heart rate during sleep. However, REM sleep, which is predominant in the later hours of sleep, just before waking, may be associated with significant sympathetic activation.[38] This may be relevant to nocturnal angina associated with REM and to the predominance of cardiac events during the early waking hours following sleep. Although parasympathetic activity largely dominates sleep, the increase in sympathetic outflow during REM sleep, when dreams are most likely to occur, may conceivably contribute to tachycardia and cardiac ischemia.

Disorders of Increased Parasympathetic Tone

Increased parasympathetic tone can be associated with a number of physiologic and pathologic conditions, including weight loss and spinal cord trauma.[39] Bradyarrhythmias, such as Mobitz type I heart block occurring during sleep, may also be caused by abrupt but physiologic increases in parasympathetic tone during REM sleep[38] (see Chap. 39). Also, the decrease in resting heart rate seen in well-conditioned athletes may be associated with an elevated parasympathetic outflow at rest. However, in general, pathologic disorders of sympathetic outflow are more common than those of parasympathetic tone.

Sinus Arrhythmia

Under normal circumstances, the heart is under parasympathetic dominance. Variations from the resting state occur with each breath because of the influence of breathing on the flow of sympathetic and vagal activity to the sinoatrial node.[40] With inhalation, vagus nerve activity is inhibited and heart rate begins to increase. With exhalation, this process reverses. This variation of heart rate with breathing is normal and is a sign of cardiac health. Absence of heart rate change with inspiration suggests cardiac disease and disturbed or diseased neural circulatory control (see Chap. 39).

Future Perspectives

Dysautonomias and other autonomic disorders can be debilitating and are often difficult to treat. Challenges in diagnosing and treating autonomic disorders include the ubiquitous nature of the autonomic nervous system, difficulties in differentiating autonomic symptoms from those caused by emotional or psychological disorders, relative paucity of quantitative measurements of autonomic dysfunction, and difficulties in accessing and modulating autonomic neural control. For example, evaluating cardiac sympathetic innervation requires expensive imaging techniques or invasive measures of cardiac norepinephrine spillover, and cardiac vagal activation is usually extrapolated from measures of heart rate control.

Technologies for inexpensive, noninvasive, and accurate measures of human autonomic tone are sorely needed to advance diagnosis and modulate therapeutic interventions. Improvements in information technology and rapid signal acquisition and processing are already forming the foundation for acutely responsive software and hardware, which can sense hemodynamic changes and respond in quick but measured fashion (e.g., could be enabled by an artificial baroreflex[41] or implanted cardiac[42] or vascular assist device). These could mimic autonomic function by modulating blood pressure via pharmacologic intervention (infusion of vasoactive agents) or triggering physical maneuvers, as needed.

Recent insights into the role of autonomic innervation of the heart and great vessels and the usefulness of ablation in treating tachyarrhythmias have also renewed interest in cardiac ganglia and their role in potentiating or inhibiting cardiac electrical instability. As methods develop for accessing these ganglia safely in humans, it is likely that therapeutic innovations will emerge that are based on perturbing or inhibiting their structure and function.

REFERENCES

Neural Circulatory Control

1. Robertson RH, Robertson D: Cardiovascular manifestations of autonomic disorders. In Zipes DP, Libby P, Bonow R, Braunwald E (eds): Braunwald's Heart Disease: A Textbook of Cardiovascular Disease, 7th edition. Philadelphia, WB Saunders, 2004, pp 2173-2184.
2. Ditting T, Hilgers KF, Scrogin KE, et al: Influence of short-term versus long-term cardiopulmonary receptor stimulation on renal and preganglionic adrenal sympathetic nerve activity in rats. Basic Res Cardiol 101:223, 2006.
3. DiBona GF: Physiology in perspective: The wisdom of the body: Neural control of the kidney. Am J Physiol Regul Integr Comp Physiol 289:R633, 2005.
4. Spicuzza L, Porta C, Bramanti A, et al: Interaction between central-peripheral chemoreflexes and cerebro-cardiovascular control. Clin Auton Res 15:373, 2005.
5. Caples SM, Gami A, Somers VK: Obstructive sleep apnea. Ann Intern Med 142:187, 2005.
6. Schrezenmaier C, Singer W, Swift NM, et al: Adrenergic and vagal baroreflex sensitivity in autonomic failure. Arch Neurol 64:381, 2007.

Autonomic Testing

7. Cooke WH, Convertino VA: Heart rate variability and spontaneous baroreflex sequences: Implications for autonomic monitoring during hemorrhage. J Trauma Inj Infect Crit Care 58:798, 2005.
8. Soriano F, Nogueira A, Cappi S, et al: Heart dysfunction and heart rate variability prognoses in sepsis. Crit Care 8:P75, 2005.
9. Cygankiewicz I, Wojciech Z, Vazquez R, et al: Heart rate turbulence predicts all-cause mortality and sudden death in congestive heart failure patients. Heart Rhythm 5:1095, 2008.
10. Tiukinhoy S: Heart rate profile during exercise as a predictor of sudden death. J Cardiopul Rehab 25:387, 2005.

Orthostatic Hypotension

11. Maule S, Papotti G, Naso D, et al: Orthostatic hypotension: Evaluation and treatment. Cardiovasc Hematol Disord Drug Targets 7:63, 2007.
12. Low PA, Singer W: Management of neurogenic orthostatic hypotension: An update. Lancet Neurol 7:451, 2008.
13. Mosnaim AD, Abiola R, Wolf ME, Perlmuter LC: Etiology and risk factors for developing orthostatic hypotension. Am J Ther 17:86, 2010.

Autonomic Dysregulation

14. Gilman S, Wenning GK, Low PA, et al: Second consensus statement on the diagnosis of multisystem atrophy. Neurology 71:670, 2008.
15. Lipp A, Sandroni P, Ahlskog E, et al: Prospective differentiation of multisystem atrophy from Parkinson disease, with and without autonomic failure. Arch Neurol 66:742, 2009.
16. Skrapari I, Tentolouris N, Katsilambros N: Baroreflex function: Determinants in health subjects and disturbances in diabetes, obesity and metabolic syndrome. Curr Diabetes Rev 2:329, 2006.
17. Pop-Busui R, Low PA, Waberski BH, et al: Effects of prior intensive insulin therapy on cardiac autonomic nervous system function in type 1 diabetes mellitus: The Diabetes Control and Complications Trial/Epidemiology of Diabetes Interventions and Complications Study. Circulation 119:2886, 2009.
18. Ito T, Sakakibara R, Yamamoto T, et al: Urinary dysfunction and autonomic control in amyloid neuropathy. Clin Auton Res 16:66, 2006.
19. Wang AK, Fealey RD, Gehrking TL, Low PA: Patterns of neuropathy and autonomic failure in patients with amyloidosis. Mayo Clin Proc 83:1226, 2008.
20. Koomans HA, Blankestijn PJ, Joles JA: Sympathetic hyperactivity in chronic renal failure: A wake-up call. J Am Soc Nephrol 15:524, 2004.
21. Low PA: Autonomic neuropathies. Curr Opin Neurol 15:605, 2002.
22. Schroeder C, Vernino S, Birkenfeld AL, et al: Plasma exchange for primary autoimmune autonomic failure. N Engl J Med 353:1585, 2005.
23. Vincent S, Robertson D: The broader view: Catecholamine abnormalities. Clin Auton Res 12(Suppl):I44, 2002.
24. Low PA, Sandroni P, Joyner MJ, Shen W-K: Postural tachycardia syndrome. In Low PA, Benarroch EE (eds): Clinical Autonomic Disorders. 3rd ed. Philadelphia, Lippincott Williams & Wilkins, 2008, pp 515-533.
25. Low PA, Sandroni P, Joyner M, Shen WK: Postural tachycardia syndrome (POTS). J Cardiovasc Electrophysiol 20:352, 2009.
26. Masuki S, Eisenach JH, Johnson CP, et al: Excessive heart rate response to orthostatic stress in postural tachycardia syndrome is not caused by anxiety. J Appl Physiol 102:896, 2007.
27. Masuki S, Eisenach JH, Schrage WG, et al: Arterial baroreflex control of heart rate during exercise in postural tachycardia syndrome. J Appl Physiol 103:1136, 2007.
28. Raj SR, Black BK, Biaggioni I, et al: Propranolol decreased tachycardia and improves symptoms in the postural tachycardia syndrome—less is more. Circulation 120:725, 2009.
29. Alboni P, Brignole M, Degli Uberti EC: Is vasovagal syncope a disease? Europace 9:83, 2007.
30. Moya A, Sutton R, Ammirati F, et al: Guidelines for the diagnosis and management of syncope (version 2009). The task force for the diagnosis and management of syncope of the European Society of Cardiology (ESC). Developed in collaboration with the European Heart Rhythm

Association (EHRA), Heart Failure Association (HFA), and Heart Rhythm Society (HRS). Eur Heart J 30:2631, 2009.

31. Parry SW, Steen N, Tynan M, et al: Pacing in elderly recurrent fallers with carotid sinus hypersensitivity: A randomised, double-blind, placebo controlled crossover trial. Heart 95:405, 2009.

Disorders of Increased Sympathetic Outflow

32. Charkoudian N, Rabbitts JA: Sympathetic neural mechanisms in human cardiovascular health and disease. Mayo Clin Proc 84:822, 2009.

33. Narkiewicz K, Phillips BG, Kato M, et al: Gender-selective interactions between aging, blood pressure, and sympathetic nerve activity. Hypertension 45:522, 2005.

34. Krum H, Schlaich M, Whitbourn R, et al: Catheter-based renal sympathetic denervation for resistant hypertension: A multi-centre safety and proof-of-principle cohort study. Lancet 373:1275, 2009.

35. Schlaich MP, Sobotka PA, Krum H, et al: Renal sympathetic-nerve ablation for uncontrolled hypertension. N Engl J Med 361:932, 2009.

36. Nanjo S, Yamashiro Y, Fujimoto S, et al: Evaluation of sympathetic activity by ^{123}I-metaiodobenzylguanidine myocardial scintigraphy in dilated cardiomyopathy patients with sleep breathing disorder. Circ J 73:686, 2009.

37. Mequro K, Toyama T, Adachi H, et al: Assessment of central chemosensitivity and cardiac sympathetic nerve activity using I-123 MIBG imaging in central sleep apnea syndrome in patients with dilated cardiomyopathy. Ann Nucl Med 21:73, 2007.

38. Verrier RL, Josephson ME: Impact of sleep on arrhythmogenesis. Circ Arrhythmia Electrophysiol 2:450, 2009.

Disorders of Increased Parasympathetic Tone

39. Gondim FAA, Lopes ACA, Oliveira GR, et al: Cardiovascular control after spinal cord injury. Curr Vasc Pharmacol 2:71, 2004.

40. Grossman P, Wilhelm, FH, Spoerle M: Respiratory sinus arrhythmia, cardiac vagal control, and daily activity. Am J Physiol Heart Circ Physiol 287:H728, 2004.

Future Perspectives

41. Yamasaki F, Ushida T, Yokoyama T, et al: Artificial baroreflex: Clinical application of a bionic baroreflex system. Circulation 113:634, 2006.

42. Birks EJ, Tansley PD, Hardy J, et al: Left ventricular assist device and drug therapy for the reversal of heart failure. New Engl J Med 355:1873, 2006.

DISCLOSURE INDEX

The following contributors have indicated that they have a relationship that, in the context of their participation in the writing of a chapter for the ninth edition of *Braunwald's Heart Disease*, could be perceived by some people as a real or apparent conflict of interest, but do not consider that it has influenced the writing of their chapter. Codes for the disclosure information (institution[s] and nature of relationship[s]) are provided below.

Relationship Codes

A—Stock options or bond holdings in a for-profit corporation or self-directed pension plan
B—Research grants
C—Employment (full or part-time)

D—Ownership or partnership
E—Consulting fees or other remuneration received by the contributor or immediate family

F—Nonremunerative positions, such as board member, trustee, or public spokesperson
G—Receipt of royalties
H—"Speaker's bureau"

Institution and Company Codes

001—Abbott Laboratories
002—Abiomed
003—ACC & ABIM
004—Accumetrics
005—Acorn Cardiovascular
006—Actelion Pharmaceuticals
007—Active Biotic
008—Adolor
009—AGA Medical
010—Alexion Pharmaceuticals
011—Alnylam
012—Alteon
013—American Board of Vascular Medicine
014—American College of Nutrition
015—American Heart Association
016—Amgen
017—Amorcyte Inc.
018—Anexon
019—Angiodynamics
020—Apnex
021—Apotex
022—Aptus Endosystems, Inc.
023—ARCA
024—Arena
025—Armgo Pharma
026—Arstasis
027—Astellas
028—AstraZeneca, Inc.
029—AtheroGenics, Inc.
030—Atlas Venture Advisors, Inc.
031—Automedics
032—Avanir
033—Aventis
034—Baker Brothers Advisors LLC
035—Barr-Teva Litigation
036—BASS Medical
037—Bayer Healthcare
038—Bayer Italy
039—Beckman-Coulter
040—Berkeley Heart Labs
041—BG Medicine
042—BGB-New York

043—Biomarin Pharmaceuticals
044—Bioscience Webster
045—Biosite, Inc.
046—Biotronik
047—Blackwell Publishing
048—Bluhm Cardiovascular Institute
049—BMS
050—BMS-Sanofi
051—Boeringer Ingelheim
052—Boston Scientific Corporation
053—Boston Scientific Inc.
054—Bracco
055—Brahms
056—Bristol Meyers Squibb, Co.
057—Bristol Meyers Squibb, Co. & BMS-Sanofi
058—Cardiac Concepts Inc.
059—Cardiac Dimensions
060—Cardio DX
061—CardioDynamics
062—Cardiokine Inc.
063—CardioMems Inc.
064—CDC
065—Centocor
066—Certification Board of Cardiovascular Computed Tomography
067—CHF Solutions
068—Circ HF
069—Circulation
070—Clinical Data Inc.
071—Cook Medical Inc.
072—Cordis Corporation
073—Corthera
074—Critical Diagnostics
075—Cryocor
076—Current Protocols in Human Genetics
077—CV Therapeutics, Inc.
078—Cytokinetics, Inc.
079—Dade Behring
080—Daiichi Sankyo
081—DebioPharm
082—Dime

083—Drugs for the Heart
084—Duke University
085—E Z EM
086—Edwards Lifesciences
087—Eisai
088—Eli Lilly and Company
089—Elsevier
090—Emisphere
091—Encysive
092—Endologix, Inc.
093—ErreKappa Terapeutici
094—European Union
095—F. Hoffmann–La Roche Ltd.
096—FoldRx
097—Forest Labs
098—GE Healthcare
099—Gene Ox
100—Genentech
101—Genzyme
102—Geron
103—Gilead Sciences
104—Glaxo SmithKline
105—Griffin & Schwartz Scientific Services
106—GSK
107—Guidant Corporation
108—Heart Ware
109—I3DNL
110—IBM
111—Intekrin Therapeutics
112—Interleukin Genetics
113—Int'l Life Sciences Health & Environmental Sciences Institue
114—Inverness Medical Inc.
115—ISIS
116—Johnson & Johnson
117—Kowa Research Institute
118—LabCorp
119—Laboratory of Molecular Medicine/ HPCGG
120—Lantheus Medical Imaging
121—Lippincott
122—LPath
123—Lung RX

124—Mallinckrodt
125—MAP Pharmaceuticals
126—Massachusetts Medical Society, Mayo Press
127—Mayo Health Solutions and Industry Partners
128—Medicines Company
129—Medicure
130—Medscape
131—Medtronic Vascular
132—Medtronic, Inc.
133—Merck & Co., Inc.
134—Merck-Schering Plough Corp.
135—Merck Cardiovascular Scientific
136—MG Medicine
137—Millennium Pharmaceuticals
138—Mitsubishi-Tanabe Pharma
139—Molecular Insight Pharmaceuticals
140—Myogen
141—Nanosphere
142—National Heart, Lung and Blood Institute
143—NCME
144—Nektar Therapeutics
145—Neurological Technologies
146—NIH
147—NIH/Agency for Healthcare Research and Quality
148—Nitromed
149—NormOxys
150—Northpoint Domain
151—NovaCardia
152—Novartis, Inc.
153—Ortho-Clinical Diagnostics
154—Otsuka Pharmaceuticals

155—PeriCor Therapeutics
156—Pfizer, Inc.
157—PGxHealth
158—Philips Medical
159—Physical logic
160—Pixel Velocity
161—Preventicum
162—Prime
163—Private companies
164—Proctor and Gamble
165—Protein Design Labs
166—Regado
167—Regeneron
168—Reliant Pharmaceuticals
169—Resmed Foundation
170—Respironics
171—Roche Diagnostics
172—SAB
173—Sanofi-Aventis
174—Sapphire Therapeutics, Inc.
175—Schering
176—Schering Plough Corp.
177—Sciele, Inc.
178—Scios, Inc.
179—Select research
180—Servier France
181—Shionogi
182—Siemens
183—Siemens Medical Solutions
184—Sigma Tau
185—Society of Cardiac Angiography and Interventions
186—Society of cardiovascular computed tomography
187—Society of Chest Pain Centers

188—Solvay Pharmaceuticals
189—Sorin Medical
190—Springer
191—St. Jude Medical
192—Stereotaxis
193—T2 BioSystems
194—T2cure
195—Takeda
196—Terumo Heart, Inc.
197—Tethys
198—Thoratec
199—Toshiba
200—Translational Research in Oncology
201—TriVascular Inc.,
202—United Health
203—United Therapeutics, Inc.
204—University of California
205—UpToDate (Wolters-Kluwer)
206—VA
207—Vanderbilt/Genaissance
208—Vascular Biogenics
209—Vascular Disease foundation
210—Vasculitis Foundation
211—Ventracor Inc.
212—Vertex
213—Viacor
214—Vifor
215—Visen Scientific
216—Vitae Pharamceutical
217—W.L. Gore & Associates, Inc.
218—Wyeth
219—Xceed Molecular Scientific Advisory Board
220—Xoma
221—Zoll

Contributors

Ackerman, Michael J. F-052, F-132, F-157, F-191, G-157
Ades, Philip A. B-146
Antman, Elliott M. B-080, B-088, B-173, F-015
Bhatt, Deepak L. B-028, B-056, B-087, B-128, B-173
Boden, William E. B-001, E-001, E-103, E-117, E-173, H-001, H-056, H-103, H-173
Bonow, Robert O. E-086
Bremner, James Douglas B-146, B-206
Cannon, Christopher A-031, B-004, B-028, B-104, B-111, B-133, B-195, E-011, E-057, E-152
Canty, John M. Jr. B-146, B-206, C-206
Chaitman, Bernard B-098
Creager, Marc B-146, E-101, E-134, E-149, F-013, F-209, G-089, G-190
Dilsizian, Vasken A-098, A-139, B-098, E-027, E-098, E-120, E-139
Douglas, Pamela S. B-002, B-016, B-086, B-125, B-142, B-147, B-213, C-084, E-060, E-200
Emanuel, Linda B-146, B-147, G-089
Felker, Michael B-016, B-041, B-078, B-116, B-142, B-171, E-016, E-041, E-078, E-102, E-171
Filippatos, Gerasimos B-073, B-094, B-114, B-141, B-171, B-184, B-214
Fisher, Stacy D. H-006

Force, Thomas H-133, H-134
Gaziano, Michael John B-016, E-037
Gheorghiade, Mihai E-001, E-027, E-028, E-037, E-073, E-078, E-081, E-093, E-104, E-116, E-132, E-133, E-152, E-154, E-155, E-165, E-173, E-184, E-188
Goldberger, Ary L. B-146, G-089
Goldhaber, Samuel Z. B-049, B-051, B-087, B-116, E-130, B-173, E-049, E-051, E-087, E-173
Gray, Andrew T. C-204
Greenberg, Barry A-122, B-146, E-045, E-077, E-103, E-132, H-103, H-133, H-152, H-173
Groh, William J. E-088
Hayes, David L. E-046, E-052, E-132, E-191, E-189, E-160, G-047
Jaffer, Farouc A-215, E-215
Jessup, Mariell B-108, F-015, E-053
Kaplan, Norman M. H-051, H-097, G-015, G-121
Krumholz, Harian M. B-147, E-202, F-003
Lange, Richard Allen B-146
Lipshultz B-142, B-146, B-152, B-156, B-171
Mann, Douglas L. A-062, B-142, E-005, E-104, E-132, F-025, G-089
Maron, Barry B-132, E-099
McGuire, Darren K. E-080, E-095, E-138, E-197
McManus, Bruce B-027, B-156

Mehra, Mandeep R. B-142, B-146, E-102, E-104, E-116, E-132, E-191
Miller, John M. E-052, E-132, E-191, E-192
Mirvis, David G-089, G-205
Morady, Fred E-107, E-132, E-191
Mueller, Paul S. E-053, E-126, G-126
Myerburg, Robert J. E-051, E-104, E-142, E-168, E-173, H-052, H-098, H-173, H-191
Newby, Kristin L. B-049, B-104, B-133, B-166, B-176, E-028, E-104, E-181, F-187
O'Gara, Patrick E-120, B-146
Oh, Jae K. B-146, B-199, G-121
Olgin, Jeffrey B-044, B-053, B-132, B-191, B-221
Opie, Lionel G-083, G-089
Otto, Catherine M. G-089, G-205
Redfield, Margaret M. B-130, B-146, B-218, E-068, E-152
Ridker, Paul M. B-016, B-028, B-146, E-101, E-208, G-028, G-079, G-182
Roden, Dan B-146, C-023, C-027, C-032, C-080, C-135, C-156, C-173, C-216, G-070
Rubart-von der Lohe, Michael B-146
Sabatine, Marc S. B-028, B-055, B-056, B-080, B-153, B-173, B-176, F-056, F-080, F-173, H-088
Sanchez, Luis A. E-022, E-071, E-092, E-201, E-217, E-131

A

Abciximab
  in myocardial infarction, with fibrinolytic, 1131
  in percutaneous coronary intervention, 1283
Abdomen
  in myocardial infarction, 1102
  physical examination of, 110
Abdominal aortic aneurysms, 1310-1313. *See also*
    Aortic aneurysm(s), abdominal.
Abetalipoproteinemia, 983
Ablation therapy, in arrhythmias, 730-731
  catheter, 730-731. *See also* Radiofrequency
    catheter ablation.
  chemical, 741-742
Abscess, splenic, in infective endocarditis, 1555
ACC. *See* American College of Cardiology (ACC).
Accelerated idioventricular rhythm, 798, 798f
  characteristics of, 772t-773t
  in myocardial infarction, 1152
Acceleration-dependent block, 148, 149f
Accessory pathways
  atriofascicular, 732-733, 787, 791f
  atrioventricular, 785
    in Wolff-Parkinson-White syndrome, 787
  clinical features of, 787
  concealed, 785-786
    electrocardiographic recognition of, 785-786,
      785f
  diagnosis of, 786-787
  location of, 731-732, 732f
  management of, 787
  radiofrequency catheter ablation of, 731-741,
    732f
  recognition of, 792
  schematic representation of, 790f
  septal, 731-732, 732f, 786
    electrophysiologic features of, 786-787
  variants of, 787-792, 790f-791f, 790t
Acupuncture, for coronary heart disease,
  1042-1043
ACE. *See* Angiotensin-converting enzyme (ACE).
Acebutolol, pharmacokinetics and pharmacology
  of, 1228t-1229t
Acetate, carbon-labeled, in oxidative metabolism
  and mitochondrial function imaging, 318-319
Acetylcholine test, in Prinzmetal variant angina,
  1196-1197
Acetylsalicylic acid. *See* Aspirin (acetylsalicylic
  acid).
Acidosis, in coronary resistance mediation, 1056
Acorn trial
  on cardiac support devices, 607-608
  on mitral surgery, 604-605, 605f
Acquired immunity, in myocarditis, 1601-1602
Acrocyanosis, significance of, 108-109
Acromegaly, cardiovascular manifestations of,
  1829-1830
Actin
  mutations of, causing hypertrophic
    cardiomyopathy, 71t, 72
  structure of, 460, 460f, 462f-463f
  troponin complex and, 461-462
Actin filaments, 57, 58f
Action potential(s)
  phase 0 (upstroke or rapid depolarization),
    665-668, 666f
    mechanism of, 665-666
    upstroke of, 666-668, 667t-668t
  phase 1 (early rapid repolarization), 668,
    669f-670f
  phase 2 (plateau), 668-669
  phase 3 (final rapid repolarization), 669
  phase 4 (diastolic depolarization), 669
  phase 4 (resting), 665
  fast response, 666

Action potential(s) *(Continued)*
  general considerations on, 664-665, 665t
  phases of, 664
  slow response, 666
Activity. *See* Exercise(s); Physical activity.
Acupressure, for obesity, 1044
Acupuncture
  description of, 1043t
  for hypertension, 1043
  for obesity, 1044
  for smoking cessation, 1044
  for stress, 1045
Acute coronary syndromes (ACSs), 1090, 1091f.
    See also Angina pectoris; Myocardial
    infarction (MI).
  cell therapy trials on, 630t
  in chronic kidney disease, 1941-1943. *See also*
    Chronic kidney disease (CKD), acute
    coronary syndromes in.
  clinical management of, 536, 536f
  in diabetes mellitus, 1401-1404. *See also*
    Diabetes mellitus (DM), acute coronary
    syndromes in.
  in elderly, 1740-1741. *See also* Elderly, acute
    coronary syndromes in.
  exercise testing in prognostic assessment of,
    181-182
  guideline algorithm for, 1202f
  history in diagnosis of, 107-108
  non–ST elevation, 1178. *See also* UA/NSTEMI.
  in pathology of myocardial infarction, 1090,
    1091f
  prevention of, statin therapy in, trials on,
    990-991
  prognosis for, renal dysfunction and, 1942, 1942f
  radionuclide imaging in, 327-330
    clinical questions answered by, 327-328
    in emergency room, 328, 328f
    research directions for, 329-330
  revascularization in, appropriateness criteria for,
    1297t
  risk stratification after, 1182
  secondary prevention trials on, 989
  secondary to coronary artery disease, signs and
    symptoms of, 1201t
  signs and symptoms representing, 1082t
Acute Decompensated Heart Failure National
  Registry Database (ADHERE), 517
Acute respiratory distress syndrome (ARDS),
  postoperative, 1804
Adaptive immunity, in atherogenesis, 904-905, 905f
Addison disease, 1832-1833, 1833f
  autonomic dysfunction and, 1956
Adeno-associated virus, as vectors, 69
Adenohypophysis, 1829
Adenosine
  adverse effects of, 727
  antagonists of, for acute heart failure, 538
  as antiarrhythmic, 727
  for atrioventricular nodal reentrant tachycardia,
    784
  in contraction-relaxation cycle, 474
  in coronary resistance mediation, 1055-1056
  dosage and administration of, 714t, 727
  electrophysiologic actions of, 713t, 715t, 727
  indications for, 727
  in myocardial infarction, 1140
  pharmacokinetics of, 727
  in stress myocardial perfusion imaging, 313-314,
    323f
    coronary hyperemia in, 314
    protocols for, 315, 315t
    reversal of, 314-315
    side effects of, 314
  vasodilation from, 1058

Adenosine diphosphate (ADP)
  antagonists of, in UA/NSTEMI, 1186-1189
  in coronary blood flow regulation, 1057
Adenosine monophosphate, cyclic (cAMP)
  compartmentalization of, 472
  protein kinase dependence on, 471-472
Adenosine triphosphate (ATP), diminished, in
  impaired ventricular relaxation, 482
Adenosine triphosphate (ATP) binding pocket, of
  myosin filament, 462
Adenoviruses
  infections from, myocarditis in, 1597
  as vectors, 68
Adenylyl cyclase
  in cAMP production, 471
  inhibition of, 471
Adolescents
  congenital heart disease in, 1415
  echocardiography in, transthoracic, in
    congenital heart disease, 1424
  permanent pacemaker indications for, 768t
Adrenal cortex, in myocardial infarction, 1099
Adrenal gland disorders
  Addison disease as, 1832-1833, 1833f
  hyperaldosteronism as, 1832
Adrenal medulla, in myocardial infarction,
  1099
Adrenergic agents, in stress myocardial perfusion
  imaging, 315-316
Adrenergic inhibitors
  alpha. *See* Alpha-adrenergic blocking agents.
  beta. *See* Beta blockers.
  in hypertension, 963-965, 963t
    alpha, 964
    beta, 964-965. *See also* Beta blockers.
    central, 964
    peripheral neuronal inhibitors as, 963-964
Adrenergic system
  in heart failure, pharmacogenetics and, 638t,
    639
  in pulmonary circulation, 1697
Adrenocorticotropic hormone (ACTH), 1830-1831
  excess, Cushing disease from, 1831-1832
Adrenomedullin, in heart failure, 493-494
Adriamycin (doxorubicin), cardiotoxicity of, 1896,
  1897f
Adrucil (fluorouracil), cardiotoxicity of, 1898
Advance care planning
  in end-stage heart disease, 646-647, 647t
  promoting, as ethical dilemma, 32
Advance directives, promoting, as ethical dilemma,
  32
Adventitia, of artery, 900, 901f
AEDs. *See* Automated external defibrillators
  (AEDs).
Aerobic exercise, definition of, 1037t
AF. *See* Atrial fibrillation (AF).
Affinity chromatography, in protein separation,
  66
African American Heart Failure Trial (A-HeFT), 27,
  27f
African American Study of Kidney Disease and
  Hypertension (AASK), 24-25
African Americans
  heart failure in, 26-27, 26f-27f, 27t
  hypertension in, 24-25
    therapy of
      drug, 969
      goals of, 956
After radiation therapy for cancer, 1902
Afterdepolarizations
  delayed, in arrhythmogenesis, 673
    intracellular calcium abnormalities and,
      673-675, 675f
  early, in arrhythmogenesis, 675